Essentials of Emergency Medicine

EDITOR IN CHIEF

Richard V. Aghababian, MD
University of Massachusetts Medical School

EDITORS

E. Jackson Allison, Jr., MD, MPH, FACEP
State University of New York Upstate Medical University

Edward W. Boyer, MD
University of Massachusetts Medical School

G. Richard Braen, MD, FACEP
State University of New York Buffalo

Mariann M. Manno, MD
University of Massachusetts Medical School

John C. Moorhead, MD, FACEP
Oregon Health Sciences University

Gregory A. Volturo, MD, FACEP
University of Massachusetts Medical School

JONES AND BARTLETT PUBLISHERS
Sudbury, Massachusetts
BOSTON   TORONTO   LONDON   SINGAPORE

D0209996
WIDENER UNIVERSITY

World Headquarters
Jones and Bartlett Publishers
40 Tall Pine Drive
Sudbury, MA 01776
978-443-5000
info@jbpub.com
www.jbpub.com

Jones and Bartlett Publishers Canada
6339 Ormindale Way
Mississauga, Ontario L5V 1J2
CANADA

Jones and Bartlett Publishers International
Barb House, Barb Mews
London W6 7PA
UK

Jones and Bartlett's books and products are available through most bookstores and online booksellers. To contact Jones and Bartlett Publishers directly, call 800-832-0034, fax 978-443-8000, or visit our website, www.jbpub.com.

Substantial discounts on bulk quantities of Jones and Bartlett's publications are available to corporations, professional associations, and other qualified organizations. For details and specific discount information, contact the special sales department at Jones and Bartlett via the above contact information or send an email to specialsales@jbpub.com.

Copyright © 2006 by Jones and Bartlett Publishers, Inc.

All rights reserved. No part of the material protected by this copyright may be reproduced or utilized in any form, electronic or mechanical, including photocopying, recording, or by any information storage and retrieval system, without written permission from the copyright owner.

Production Credits
Chief Executive Officer: Clayton Jones
Chief Operating Officer: Don W. Jones, Jr.
President, Higher Education and Professional Publishing: Robert W. Holland, Jr.
V.P., Sales and Marketing: William J. Kane
V.P., Design and Production: Anne Spencer
V.P., Manufacturing and Inventory Control: Therese Connell
Executive Publisher: Christopher Davis
Associate Editor: Kathy Richardson
Production Director: Amy Rose
Special Projects Editor: Elizabeth Platt
Director of Marketing: Alisha Weisman
Associate Marketing Manager: Laura Kavigian
Cover/Interior Design: Anne Spencer
Composition: Graphic World, Inc.
Cover Images (clockwise from top left): pills, © Shutterstock, Inc.; medical equipment, © Ablestock, Inc.; newborn infant, © E. Platt; ankle x-ray, © Jones and Bartlett, Inc.; injection, © Alamy Images.
Printing and Binding: Courier Stoughton
Cover Printing: Courier Stoughton

Library of Congress Cataloging-in-Publication Data

Essentials of emergency medicine/editor-in-chief, Richard V. Aghababian; editors E. Jackson Allison, Jr. . . . [et al.].
    p. ; cm.
  Includes bibliographical references and index.
    ISBN-10: 0-7637-3570-1 (hardcover: alk. paper)
  1. Emergency medicine—Handbooks, manuals, etc.   I. Aghababian, Richard.
  [DNLM: 1. Emergency Treatment—Handbooks. 2. Emergencies—Handbooks. 3. Emergency Medicine—Handbooks.   WB 39
E776
  2006]
  RC86.8.E77 2006
  616.02′5—dc22

2005030307

WIDENER UNIVERSITY
WOLFGRAM
LIBRARY
CHESTER, PA

The authors, editor, and publisher have made every effort to provide accurate information. However, they are not responsible for errors, omissions, or for any outcomes related to the use of the contents of this book and take no responsibility for the use of the products described. Treatments and side effects described in this book may not be applicable to all patients; likewise, some patients may require a dose or experience a side effect that is not described herein. The reader should confer with his or her own physician regarding specific treatments and side effects. Drugs and medical devices are discussed that may have limited availability controlled by the Food and Drug Administration (FDA) for use only in a research study or clinical trial. The drug information presented has been derived from reference sources, recently published data, and pharmaceutical research data. Research, clinical practice, and government regulations often change the accepted standard in this field. When consideration is being given to use of any drug in the clinical setting, the healthcare provider or reader is responsible for determining FDA status of the drug, reading the package insert, reviewing prescribing information for the most up-to-date recommendations on dose, precautions, and contraindications, and determining the appropriate usage for the product. This is especially important in the case of drugs that are new or seldom used.

Printed in the United States of America
09 08 07 06 05   10 9 8 7 6 5 4 3 2 1

CONTENTS

Eric Adar, MD
SUNY Downstate Medical Center/Kings County Hospital Center
Department of Emergency Medicine
Brooklyn, New York

Richard V. Aghababian, MD, FACEP
Associate Dean, Continuing Medical Education
University of Massachusetts Medical School
Chairman, Department of Emergency Medicine
University of Massachusetts Memorial Health Care
Worcester, Massachusetts

John L. Alexander, MD
EMS Director
Department of Emergency Medicine
Maine Medical Center
Portland, Maine
and
Clinical Instructor in Emergency Medicine
University of Vermont College of Medicine
Burlington, Vermont

E. Jackson Allison, Jr., MD, MPH, FACEP
Associate Dean & Professor of Emergency Medicine
College of Medicine, SUNY Upstate Medical University
and
Chief-of-Staff
Veterans Affairs Medical Center
Syracuse, New York

Harry L. Anderson III, MD, FACS, FCCM
Associate Professor of Surgery
Fellowship Director, Surgical Critical Care
Division of Trauma and Surgical Critical Care
Wright State University Department of Surgery
Miami Valley Hospital
Dayton, Ohio

Peter Angood, MD, FACS, FCCM
Professor of Surgery
Washington University School of Medicine
Director, Trauma Center
Washington University Medical Center/Barnes-Jewish Hospital
St. Louis, Missouri

Kavita Babu, MD
Fellow, Division of Medical Toxicology
Department of Emergency Medicine
University of Massachusetts Memorial Health Care
Worcester, Massachusetts

Richard Bachur, MD
Associate Chief/Fellowship Director
Children's Hospital, Boston
Boston, Massachusetts

Jerry R. Balentine, DO, FACOEP
Medical Director
St. Barnabas Hospital
Bronx, New York

Andrew R. Barnosky, DO, MPH, FACEP
Clinical Assistant Professor, Department of Emergency Medicine
Instructor, Program in Bioethics
Chairman, Medical Ethics Committee
Director, Bioethics Consultation Service
University of Michigan
Ann Arbor, Michigan

Christine Barron, MD
Clinical Director
Hasbro Children's Hospital
Providence, Rhode Island

Jeanne M. Basior, MD, FACEP
Associate Clinical Director, Emergency Department
Buffalo General Hospital
and
Assistant Program Director
Emergency Medicine Residency
SUNY Buffalo
Buffalo, New York

Marc Bayer, MD
Medical Director
Connecticut Poison Control Center
University of Connecticut School of Medicine
Farmington, Connecticut

Mary K. Bennett
Clinical Assistant Professor
Department of Emergency Medicine
School of Medicine and Biomedical Sciences
State University of New York at Buffalo General Hospital
Buffalo, New York

Genevieve Bensinger, MD
Resident Physician
The George Washington University
Department of Emergency Medicine
Washington, DC

Nicholas H. Benson, MD, MBA
Professor
Senior Assistant Dean for Operations
Department of Emergency Medicine
Brody School of Medicine at East Carolina University
Greenville, North Carolina

Anthony J. Billittier IV, MD, FACEP
Commissioner of Health
Erie County Department of Health
and
Assistant Professor of Clinical Emergency Medicine
University at Buffalo, SUNY
Buffalo, New York

Steven B. Bird, MD
Assistant Professor of Emergency Medicine
University of Massachusetts Memorial Medical Healthcare Center
Department of Emergency Medicine
Worcester, Massachusetts

Janice Blanchard, MD, MPH
Assistant Professor
Department of Emergency Medicine
George Washington University
Washington DC

Nicole C. Bouchard, MD
Fellow, Medical Toxicology
New York City Poison Control Center
Bellevue Hospital Center and New York University Medical Center
New York City Poison Control Center
New York, New York

Edward W. Boyer, MD
Associate Professor of Emergency Medicine
Chief, Division of Medical Toxicology
Director, Medical Toxicology Fellowship
University of Massachusetts Medical School
Department of Emergency Medicine
Worcester, Massachusetts

G. Richard Braen, MD, FACEP
Professor and Chair, Department of Emergency Medicine
Associate Dean for Graduate Medical Education
SUNY Buffalo
Buffalo General Hospital
Buffalo, New York

Alison Brent, MD
Medical Director
Pediatric Emergency Center
All Children's Hospital
St. Petersburg, Florida

Katherine Brinsfield, MD
Associate Medical Director, Boston EMS
Department of Emergency Medicine
Boston Medical Center
Boston, Massachusetts

Kerry B. Broderick, MD
Associate Professor of Emergency Medicine
University of Colorado Health Sciences Center
Denver, Colorado

James M. Brown, MD
Assistant Professor of Emergency Medicine
Texas Tech University Health Sciences Center
School of Medicine
El Paso, Texas

Jennifer L. Brown, MD
Department of Emergency Medicine
Erie County Medical Center
Buffalo, New York

Thomas A. Brunell, MD
Assistant Residency Director
Emergency Medicine Residency Program
Baystate Medical Center
Springfield, Massachusetts
and
Assistant Professor of Emergency Medicine
Tufts University School of Medicine
Boston, Massachusetts

John Burton, MD, FACEP
Medical Director, Maine EMS
Department of Emergency Medicine
Maine Medical Center
Portland, Maine

Beth Cadigan, MD
Ultrasound Fellow
Department of Emergency Medicine
Case Western Reserve University Hospital
Cleveland, Ohio

Gar Ming Chan, MD
Fellow, Medical Toxicology
New York City Poison Control Center
New York, New York

Kevin J. Corcoran, DO, FACEP
Clinical Assistant Professor
Medical Director
East Care Clinical Care Transport Service
Emergency Department
Brody School of Medicine
East Carolina University
Greenville, North Carolina

Jason E. Cross, PharmD
Assistant Professor of Pharmacy Practice
Massachusetts College of Pharmacy and Health Sciences-Worcester
Worcester, Massachusetts

Jeffrey M. Cukor, MD
Director of Emergency Medicine Residency Program
Assistant Professor
University of Massachusetts Medical School
Worcester, Massachusetts

Ronald J. DeBellis, PharmD, FCCP
Associate Professor of Pharmacy Practice
Massachusetts College of Pharmacy and Health Sciences-Worcester
Worcester, Massachusetts
and
Adjunct Assistant Professor of Medicine
Department of Pulmonary, Allergy and Critical Care Medicine
University of Massachusetts Medical School
Worcester, Massachusetts

Christopher J. DeFlitch, MD
Director and Vice-Chair
Department of Emergency Medicine
Hershey Medical Center
Hershey, Pennsylvania

Nicole DeIorio, MD
Assistant Professor of Emergency Medicine
Oregon Health Sciences University
Portland, Oregon

Michael David DiBella, MD
Director of Emergency Medicine
Associate Program Director of Internal Medicine Residency
Program
Clinical Assistant Professor Emergency Medicine and Internal
Medicine
State University of New York at Buffalo
Mercy Hospital of Buffalo
Buffalo, New York

Deborah B. Diercks, MD, FACEP
Assistant Professor of Emergency Medicine
University of California, Davis, School of Medicine
La Jolla, California

Djiby Diop, MD, MMS, MPH
Emergency Physician
Memorial Hospital
Belleville, Illinois

Kurt R. Dischner, MD
Resident Physician
Thomas Jefferson University
Department of Emergency Medicine
Philadelphia, Pennsylvania

Suzanne Dooley-Hash, MD
Resident
Department of Emergency Medicine
University of Michigan Health System
Ann Arbor, Michigan

James Ducharme, MD, CM, FRCP, DABEM
Professor, Emergency Medicine
Dalhousie University
Clinical Director, Department of Emergency Medicine
Atlantic Health Sciences Corporation
Saint John, New Brunswick
Canada

Michael D. Dunkerley, MD
Clinical Associate
Baystate Medical Center
Springfield, Massachusetts

Rob J. Edwards, MBBS
Consultant in Emergency Medicine
Emergency Department
Westmead Hospital
New South Wales, Australia

Tomer Feldman, MD
Emergency Department Attending Physician
Rockingham Memorial Hospital
Harrisonburg, Virginia

Eddie Fernandez, MD
Clinical Associate
Baystate Medical Center
Springfield, Massachusetts

James A. Fitch
Instructor, Emergency EMS Fellow
University of Massachusetts Medical School
Worcester, Massacusetts

Christopher J. Fullagar, MD, EMT-P
Clinical Assistant Professor & Flight Physician
Department of Emergency Medicine
SUNY Upstate Medical University
Syracuse, New York

Jessica Fulton, DO
Fellow, Medical Toxicology
New York City Poison Control Center
Bellevue Hospital Center and New York University Medical Center
New York City Poison Control Center
New York, New York

Gail Galletta, MD
Dept of Emergency Medicine
University of Massachusetts Memorial Medical Center
Worcester, Massachusetts

Michael Ganetsky, MD
Fellow, Division of Medical Toxicology
University of Massachusetts Medical School
Department of Emergency Medicine
Worcester, Massachusetts

Andrew L. Garrett, MD, FAAP, EMT
Instructor in Pediatrics and Emergency Medicine
University of Massachusetts Medical School
Department of Emergency Medicine
University of Massachusetts Memorial Health Care
Worcester, Massachusetts

Marc Gautreau, MD
Clinical Director, Emergency Medicine
Director of Tactical EMS
Associate Medical Director/EMS Life Flight
University of Massachusetts Memorial Health Care
Worcester, Massachusetts

Thomas Germano, MD
Attending Physician
Emergency Department
Kent County Memorial Hospital
Warwick, Rhode Island

Steven Go, MD
Assistant Dean for Medical Education
Director of Emergency Medicine Student Education
University of Missouri–Kansas City
School of Medicine
and
Department of Emergency Medicine
Truman Med CTR–Hospital Hill
Department of Emergency Medicine
Kansas City, Missouri

Rachel A. Goldstein, DO
New York Presbyterian Hospital
Westchester Division
White Plains, New York

Leonard G. Gomella, MD
The Bernard W. Godwin Professor of Prostate Cancer
Chairman, Department of Urology
Jefferson Medical College
Philadelphia, Pennsylvania

John E. Gough, MD, FACEP
Associate Professor
Department of Emergency Medicine
Brody School of Medicine
East Carolina University
Greenville, North Carolina

Louis G. Graff, MD
Associate Director Emergency Medicine
Director, Clinical Outcomes Management
New Britain General Hospital
New Britain, Connecticut
and
Professor, Emergency and Clinical Medicine,
University of Connecticut School of Medicine
New Britain, Connecticut

Susan Graham, MD
Mercy Medical Center–Durango/ER
Durango, Colorado

Howard A. Greller, MD
Assistant Professor of Emergency Medicine
New York University School of Medicine
Attending Physician
Department of Emergency Medicine
Bellevue Hospital
New York University Medical Center
New York, New York

Jill Griffin, MD
Assistant Clinical Professor
Department of Emergency Medicine
Tufts University
and
Baystate Medical Center
Emergency Medicine Department
Springfield, Massachusetts

Rosemary Guerguerian, MD
Best Practices
Potomac Hospital
Woodbridge, Virginia

Manisha Gupta, MD
Texas Tech University Health Sciences Center
School of Medicine
El Paso, Texas

Rania Habal, MD
Assistant Professor
New York Medical College
Valhalla, New York

Derek S. Halvorson, MD
Emergency Medicine Chief Resident
Oregon Health Sciences University
Portland, Oregon

Katie M. Hamblett, MD
Resident
Emergency Medicine
University of Massachusetts Medical Center
Worcester, Massachusetts

Kristin E. Harkin, MD
Assistant Professor of Emergency Medicine
Albert Einstein College of Medicine
Jack D. Weiler Hospital, Montefiore Medical Center
New York, New York

Katherine Harrison, MD
Department of Emergency Medicine
University Hospital
San Antonio, Texas

Daniel R. Hehir, MD
Department of Emergency Medicine
Michigan State University
Kalamazoo Center for Medical Studies
Kalamazoo, Michigan

Christina Hernon, MD
Fellow, Division of Medical Toxicoloy
Department of Emergency Medicine
University of Massachusetts Memorial Health Care
Worcester, Massachusetts

Michael Hirsh, MD, FACS, FAAP
Professor of Surgery and Pediatrics
University of Massachusetts Medical School
Chief, Division of Pediatric Surgery and Trauma
University of Massachusetts Memorial Children's Medical Center
Director, Trauma Services
University of Massachusetts Memorial Health Care System
Worcester, Massachusetts

Cherri Hobgood, MD
Director of Education
Department of Emergency Medicine
University of North Carolina School of Medicine
Chapel Hill, North Carolina

Robert J. Hoffman, MD
Research Director, Department of Emergency Medicine
Beth Israel Medical Center
New York, New York

Robert S. Hoffman, MD
Associate Professor of Emergency Medicine and Medicine
(Clinical Pharmacology)
New York University School of Medicine
New York, New York

Jon Hokanson, MD
Resident
Regions Hospital and University of Minnesota Medical School
St. Paul, Minnesota

Christopher P. Holstege, MD
Director, Division of Medical Toxicology
Medical Director, Blue Ridge Poison Center
Associate Professor, Departments of Emergency Medicine and Pediatrics
University of Virginia
Charlottesville, Virginia

Laura Roff Hopson, MD
Clinical Instructor
Department of Emergency Medicine
University of Michigan Health System
Ann Arbor, Michigan

Kurt R. Horst, MD
Clinical Instructor
Department of Emergency Medicine
University of Massachusetts Medical School
Worcester, Massachusetts

Gerald P. Igoe, MD
Clinical Assistant Professor of Emergency Medicine
Erie County Medical Center
Department of Emergency Medicine
Buffalo, New York

Dietrich V. K. Jehle, MD
Vice Chair and Associate Professor
Department of Emergency Medicine
School of Medicine and Biomedical Sciences
University of Buffalo
Erie County Medical Center
Buffalo, New York

Sandeep K. Johar, DO
Department of Emergency Medicine
SUNY Upstate Medical Univeristy
Syracuse, New York

Gary A. Johnson, MD, FACEP
Associate Professor
Department of Emergency Medicine
SUNY Upstate Medical University
Syracuse, New York

Nicholas J. Jouriles, MD, FACEP
Department of Emergency Medicine
Akron General Medical Center
Professor of Emergency Medicine
Northeastern Ohio Universities College of Medicine
and
Gems, Inc
Akron, Ohio

Daniel M. Joyce, MD
Attending Physician
Saint Vincent Hospital
Emergency Department
Green Bay, Wisconsin

Sig Karasch, MD
Director, Emergency Medicine
Boston Medical Center
One Boston Medical Center Place
Boston, Massachusetts

Eric M. Kardon, MD, FACEP
Emergency Physician
Athens, Georgia

Taryn Kennedy, MD
Assistant Professor
University of Massachusetts Memorial Medical Center
Worcester, Massachusetts

Arshad Khan, MD
Instructor in Medicine (Emergency Medicine)
Harvard Medical School
Cambridge, Massachusetts

Boris Khodorkovsky, MD
Resident, Emergency Medicine
SUNY Downstate Medical Center
Kings County Hospital Center
Brooklyn, New York

Samuel H. Kim, MD
Attending Physician
Tacoma General Hospital Emergency Department
Tacoma, Washington
and
Allenmore Hospital Emergency Department
Tacoma, Washington

J. Douglas Kirk, MD, FACEP
Associate Professor of Emergency Medicine
University of California, Davis, School of Medicine
and
Assistant Chief
Department of Emergency Medicine
Medical Director, Chest Pain Evaluation Unit
University of California, Davis, Medical Center
Sacramento, California

Robert Knopp, MD, MA, FACEP
Professor of Emergency Medicine
Regions Hospital and University of Minnesota Medical School
St. Paul, Minnesota

Richard S. Krause, MD
Program Director
Department of Emergency Medicine
SUNY Buffalo School of Medicine and Biomedical Sciences
Buffalo, New York

Baruch Krauss, MD, EdM, FAAP, FACEP
Division of Emergency Medicine
Children's Hospital Boston
and
Assistant Professor of Pediatrics
Harvard Medical School
Boston, Massachusetts

Ricky Kue, MD
Fellow, EMS Department of Emergency Medicine
University of Massachusetts Memorial Health Care
Worcester, Massachusetts

Melisa W. Lai, MD
Instructor in Medicine
Harvard Medical School
and
Fellow in Medical Toxicology
Massachusetts/Rhode Island Poison Control Center
Boston, Massachusetts

James M. Leaming, MD, FACEP
Assistant Professor
Tufts-New England Medical Center
Department of Emergency Medicine
Boston, Massachusetts

Chad W. LeBlanc, DO
Clinical Associate
Emergency Medicine
Baystate Medical Center
Springfield, Massachusetts

Lilly Lee
Attending Physician
Voluntary Assistant Professor
Jackson Memorial Hospital
Key Biscayne, Florida

Juraj Letko
Constantine the Philosopher University
Nitra, Slovak Republic

Robert L. Levine, MD
Associate Professor of Neurosurgery and Emergency Medicine
The University of Texas Medical School
Texas Memorial Hermann Hospital
Houston, Texas

Ivan Liang, MD
Attending Physician
Fellow, Division of Medical Toxicology
Department of Emergency Medicine
St. Elizabeth's Hospital
Brighton, Massachusetts

Rita Manfredi, MD, FACEP
Associate Professor of Emergency Medicine
Brody School of Medicine
East Carolina University
Greenville, North Carolina

Mariann M. Manno, MD
Associate Professor of Clinical Pediatrics and Emergency Medicine
University of Massachusetts Medical School
and
Division Chief, Pediatric Emergency Medicine
Children's Medical Center
University of Massachusetts Memorial Health Care
Worcester, Massachusetts

David E. Manthey, MD, FAAEM
Director, Undergraduate Medical Education
Assistant Professor
Department of Emergency Medicine
Wake Forest University School of Medicine
Medical Center Boulevard
Winston-Salem, North Carolina

Laura Matzkin
Clinical Associate
Bay State Medical Center
Springfield, Massachusetts

Douglas McAdoo, MD
University of Massachusetts Memorial Medical Center
Worcester, Massachusetts

Robert F. McCormack, MD
Clinical Chief, Emergency Medicine
Buffalo General Hospital–Kaleida Health
Assistant Professor of Clinical Emergency Medicine
University at Buffalo School of Medicine and Biomedical Sciences
Buffalo, New York

Jill McGovern
Clinical Associate
Baystate Medical Center
Springfield, Massachusetts

Charles McKay, MD, FACEP, ABIM
Director, Medical Toxicology
Medical Director, Department of Occupational Health Services
Department of Traumatology and Emergency Medicine

Hartford Hospital
and
Associate Medical Director
Connecticut Poison Control Center
Associate Professor of Emergency Medicine
University of Connecticut School of Medicine
Hartford, Connecticut

Darren Menditto, MD
Staff Physician
Department of Emergency Medicine
Beth Israel Medical Center
New York, New York

Chris J. Michalakes, DO, FAAEM
Chief, Emergency Medicine
Penobscot Bay Medical Center
Rockport, Maine

Anthony Montoya, MD
Resident
Department of Emergency Medicine
University of Massachusetts Memorial Medical Center
Worcester, Massachusetts

John C. Moorhead, MD, FACEP
Professor, Emergency Medicine
Oregon Health Sciences University
and
Attending Physician, OHSU Hospitals
Department of Emergency Medicine
Portland, Oregon

Ronald Moscati, MD
Emergency Room
Erie County Medical Center
Assistant Professor of Emergency Medicine
Buffalo, New York

Peter Murphy, MD
Assistant Professor of Pediatrics
University of Massachusetts Memorial Medical Center
Division of Pediatric Emergency Medicine
Worcester, Massachusetts

Bret P. Nelson, MD
Department of Emergency Medicine
Mount Sinai Hospital and Mount Sinai Medical School
New York, New York

Douglas Nelson, MD
Associate Professor of Pediatrics
Primary Children's Medical Center
Salt Lake City, Utah

Lewis S. Nelson, MD
Director, Medical Toxicology Fellowship Program
Assistant Professor of Emergency Medicine
New York University School of Medicine
New York, New York

Constance G. Nichols, MD, FACEP
Assistant Professor of Emergency Medicine
Department of Emergency Medicine
University of Massachusetts Medical School
Worcester, Massachusetts

Mary O'Neill, MD
Assistant Professor of Pediatrics
University of Massachusetts Memorial Medical Center
Division of Pediatric Emergency Medicine
Worcester, Massachusetts

Dr. David W. Osborne, MD
Resident
Division of Emergency Medicine
Harvard Medical School
Boston, Massachusetts

Michael Peikert, MD, FACEP
Clinical Faculty
Michigan State University
Kalamazoo Center for Medical Studies
Emergency Department
Kalamazoo, Michigan

Michael A. Pellegrino, MD
Attending Emergency Physician
Charlton Memorial Hospital
Southcoast Hospital System
Fall River, Massachusetts

Ruben Peralta, MD
Assistant Professor of Surgery/Anesthesia/Emergency Medicine
Department of Surgery
Division of Trauma and Surgical Care
University of Massachusetts Medical School
University of Massachusetts Memorial Medical Center
Worcester, Massachusetts

Tamas R. Peredy, MD, FACEP
Emergency Physician
Maine Medical Center
Portland, Maine

Alberto Perez, MD
Clinical Instructor of Emergency Medicine
University of Connecticut School of Medicine
Division of Medical Toxicology
Department of Traumatology and Emergency Medicine
Hartford Hospital
Hartford, Connecticut

Michael A. Peterson, MD, FAAEM
Assistant Professor of Medicine
The David Geffen School of Medicine at UCLA
Director of Emergency Ultrasound
Department of Emergency Medicine
Harbor–UCLA Medical Center
Torrance, California

David L. Pierce, MD
Vice Chairman, Department of Emergency Medicine
Associate Professor of Emergency Medicine
Clinical Director of Emergency Services, ECMC
Department of Emergency Medicine
School of Medicine and Biomedical Sciences
University of Buffalo
Buffalo, New York

Lauren Pipas, MD, FACEP
Department of Emergency Medicine
SUNY Upstate
Syracuse, New York

Laurel Plante, MD
Bay State Medical Center
Springfield, Massachusetts

Stephen J. Playe, MD
Assistant Professor of Emergency Medicine
Tufts University School of Medicine
Residency Program Director
Department of Emergency Medicine
Baystate Medical Center
Springfield, Massachusetts

N. Heramba Prasad, MD, FACEP
Associate Professor, Residency Director
Department of Emergency Medicine
SUNY Upstate Medical University
Syracuse, New York

Louise A. Prince, MD
Associate Professor of Emergency Medicine
SUNY Upstate Medical University
Syracuse, New York

Mark R. Pundt, MD, FACEP
Clinical Assistant Professor of Emergency Medicine
Millard Fillmore Emergency Room
SUNY at Buffalo School of Medicine
Buffalo, New York

Rama B. Rao, MD
Assistant Clinical Professor of Emergency Medicine
Bellevue Hospital Center and New York University Medical Center
New York, New York

Michael T. Rapp, MD, JD, FACEP
Clinical Professor
George Washington University
Department of Emergency Medicine
Washington DC

Timothy J. Reeder, MD, MPH
Assistant Professor
Vice Chair for Clinical Operations
Department of Emergency Medicine
Brody School of Medicine at East Carolina University
Greenville, North Carolina

Robert C. Reiser, MD, MS, FACEP
Associate Professor of Emergency Medicine
Medical Director, Emergency Department
University of Virginia
Charlottesville, Virginia

Marc C. Restuccia, MD, FACEP
Assistant Professor
University of Massachusetts Medical School
Department of Emergency Medicine
University of Massachusetts Memorial Health Care
Worcester, Massachusetts

Ralph J. Rivello, MD, FACEP, FAAEM
Assistant Professor
Director of Clinical Research
Department of Emergency Medicine
Thomas Jefferson University
Philadelphia, Pennsylvania

Walter C. Robey III, MD, FACEP
Clinical Associate Professor
Associate Residency Director
Department of Emergency Medicine
Brody School of Medicine at East Carolina University
Greenville, North Carolina

Colleen N. Roche, MD
Associate Residency Director
Assistant Professor
George Washington University
Department of Emergency Medicine
Washington DC

Luis E. Rodriguez, MD
Associate Clinical Professor
Department of Emergency Medicine
East Carolina University
and
Medical Director
Roanoke Chowan Hospital Emergency Department
Ahoskie, North Carolina

Brian Rose, MD
Staff Physician, Department of Emergency Medicine
Beth Israel Medical Center
New York, New York

Tina Rosenbaum, MD, MPH
Department of Emergency Medicine
George Washington University
Washington DC

Steven D. Salhanick, MD
Staff Toxicologist
Children's Hospital Boston
Boston, Massachusetts

Ramin R. Samadi, MD, FACEP, FACP
Assistant Clinical Professor
Emergency Medicine
University of Texas-Southwestern Medical School
Dallas, Texas
and
President and Chief Executive Officer
Tarrant Acute Care Physicians, P.A.
Forth Worth, Texas
and
Medical Director
Emergency Medicine
TrinityXpressMed Medical Center
Forth Worth, Texas

Joshua G. Schier, MD
Assistant Professor of Emergency Medicine
Emory University School of Medicine
Medical Toxicology Attending
Emory/CDC Medical Toxicology Fellowship
Chamblee, Georgia

Eric Schmidt, MD
Assistant Professor of Emergency Medicine
Department of Emergency Medicine
University of Massachusetts Medical School
Worcester, Massachusetts

Joseph C. Schmidt, MD
Assistant Professor
Tufts University School of Medicine
Department of Emergency Medicine
and
Bay State Medical Center
Belchertown, Massachusetts

Sandra M. Schneider, MD
Professor and Chair, Department of Emergency Medicine,
School of Medicine
University of Rochester
Rochester, New York

Gary Setnik, MD, FACEP
Assistant Professor
Division of Emergency Medicine
Harvard Medical School
Winchester, Massachusetts

Ralph J. Seymour, MD
Assistant Professor of Psychiatry
University of Massachusetts Medical School
University of Massachusetts Memorial Medical Center
Worcester, Massachusetts

Mark L. Shapiro, MD
Assistant Professor of Surgery
Associate Director of Trauma Services
University of Massachusetts Memorial Medical Center
Worcester, Massachusetts

Adhi N. Sharma, MD
Director, Division of Toxicology
Department of Emergency Medicine
Elmhurst Hospital Center
and
Assistant Professor
Department of Emergency Medicine
Mount Sinai School of Medicine
New York, New York

Jonathan E. Siff, MD, MBA, FACEP
Assistant Director, Medical Operations
Department of Emergency Medicine
MetroHealth Medical Center
and
Assistant Professor, Emergency Medicine
Case Western Reserve University
Department of Emergency Medicine
Cleveland, Ohio

Andrew Singer, MD
Emergency Department Attending
Sydney Adventist Hospital
Wahroonga, New South Wales, Australia

Ajeet Jai Singh, MD
Assistant Professor of Emergency Medicine
University of Massachusetts Medical School
Worcester, Massachusetts
and
Medical Director
Emergency Department
Clinton Hospital-UMMHC
Clinton, Massachusetts

Eunice M. Singletary, MD, FACEP
Clinical Associate Professor
Department of Emergency Medicine
University of Virginia
Charlottesville, Virginia

Brian Sloan, MD
Assistant Professor of Clinical Emergency Medicine
Indiana University School of Medicine
Indianapolis, Indiana

Patrick Smallwood, MD
Medical Director, Consultation
Liaison Psychiatry and Emergency Mental Health
University of Massachusetts Medical Center
Assistant Professor of Psychiatry
University of Massachusetts Medical School
Worcester, Massachusetts

Eustacia Su, MD
Associate Director of Emergency Medicine Residency Program
Director, Undergraduate and Pediatric Education
Associate Professor
Oregon Health and Science University
Portland, Oregon

Mark Su, MD
Assistant Professor of Emergency Medicine
Assistant Residency Director &
Director of Medical Toxicoloy
SUNY Downstate Medical Center
Kings County Hospital Center
Brooklyn, New York

Jeffrey R. Suchard, MD
Associate Clinical Professor of Emergency Medicine
Director of Medical Toxicology
Department of Emergency Medicine
University of California Irvine Medical Center
Orange, California

Jonathan M. Sullivan, MD, PHD
Assistant Professor
Department of Emergency Medicine
Wayne State University/Detroit Receiving Hospital
Detroit, Michigan

Lemeneh Tefera, MD, FAAEM
Attending Physician
Department of Emergency Medicine
Lincoln Medical and Mental Health
Bronx, New York

Stephen H. Thomas, MD
Director of Academic Affairs
Massachusetts General Hospital
Department of Emergency Services
and
Assistant Professor of Surgery
Harvard Medical School
Boston, Massachusetts

Jenna Timm, MD
Resident
Department of Emergency Medicine
Oregon Health and Science University
Portland, Oregon

Susan Torrey, MD
Assistant in Medicine
Children's Hospital, Boston
Division of Emergency Medicine
Boston, Massachusetts

Bradley J. Uren, MD
Resident Physician
Department of Emergency Medicine
University of Michigan Medical School
University of Michigan Medical Center
Ann Arbor, Michigan

Michele A. VanderHeyden, MD, MS
Medical Director, Pediatric Intensive Care Unit
Dartmouth-Hitchcock Medical Center
and
Assistant Professor of Pediatrics
Dartmouth Medical School
Lebanon, New Hampshire

Heidi S. Vermette, MD
Instructor in Psychiatry
University of Massachusetts Medical School
University of Massachusetts Memorial Medical Center
Worcester, Massachusetts

Carrie Vice, MD
Chief Resident, Emergency Medicine
University of North Carolina School of Medicine
Chapel Hill, North Carolina

Gregory A. Volturo, MD, FACEP
Professor of Emergency Medicine
Vice Chair, Department of Emergency Medicine
University of Massachusetts Memorial Health Care
Worcester, Massachusetts

Barbara M. Walsh, MD
Assistant Professor of Pediatrics
University of Massachusetts Memorial Medical Center
Division of Pediatric Emergency Medicine
Worcester, Massachusetts

Sheila Webb, MD
Emergency Medicine Resident
Michigan State University
Kalamazoo Center for Medical Studies
Kalamazoo, Michigan

Stacy N. Weisberg, MD
Clinical Assistant Professor
Department of Emergency Medicine
University of Massachusetts Memorial Health Care
Worcester, Massachusetts

Blaine C. White, MD
Professor of Emergency Medicine,
Wayne State University School of Medicine
Detroit Receiving Hospital
Detroit, Michigan

Sage W. Wiener, MD
Assistant Professor and
Assistant Director of Medical Toxicology
Department of Emergency Medicine
SUNY Downstate Medical Center
Kings County Hospital Center
Brooklyn, New York

James Winslow III, MD
Assistant Professor
Department of Emergency Medicine
Wake Forest University School of Medicine
Medical Center Boulevard
Winston-Salem, North Carolina

Richard V. Aghababian, MD, FACEP
Editor-in-Chief

DESPITE THREE DECADES of rapid growth and development, the specialty of Emergency Medicine (EM) continues to evolve more quickly than other medical specialties. The body of knowledge that an active emergency physician must command—and that a resident must learn—has increased dramatically in recent years. Examples of developments and events that have fueled this period of rapid growth in the EM knowledge base and patient demand include:

- Several published research trials have identified new interventions that improve outcome for patients presenting in the emergency department with acute cardiovascular, infectious disease, psychiatric and trauma-related illnesses or injuries. Recent technological advances in pharmacotherapy, medical imaging and laboratory measurement have contributed to making these improvements in patient care possible. Increasing emphasis on clinical practice guidelines for certain acute conditions assist emergency physicians who are managing several patients in a busy emergency department.
- Hospital closings, in the face of increasing demands for access to emergency care, have resulted in the overcrowding of many emergency departments. In addition, insufficient inpatient beds has resulted in delays in transferring the sickest patients to critical care settings. The increasing numbers of uninsured, the insufficient number of primary care providers in some areas, and the aging of the population as a whole suggest that the demand for emergency care will not soon abate. As hospitals are forced to expand their emergency departments, the departments are being redesigned to accommodate more and sicker patients for longer periods. Observation Units and Chest Pain Centers are being added to larger hospital emergency departments to improve efficiency and capacity. Emergency physicians are learning to adapt to the in-

creasing scope of care they must provide as a result of these environmental and demographic changes.
- Events such as the World Trade Center attack in New York City on September 11, 2001 have focused the attention of the media and the public on the critical role that emergency physicians and emergency departments play in disaster response. The EM subspecialty areas of disaster medicine, emergency medical services, and toxicology have experienced substantial increases in support for the development of rapid response capability and the performance of research in areas that will lead to improved management of terrorists threats.

The editors of this textbook have attempted to focus on the components of medical assessment and treatment that will assist the emergency physician functioning in a clinical setting by serving as a reliable source of clinical information. An attempt has been made to address significant recent advancements that are likely to alter the way the experienced emergency physician practices. This textbook is also intended to be helpful to residents and practicing emergency physicians who are assessing their need for further education, or who are preparing for an examination. Moreover, this book should also be of interest to medical students interested in emergency medicine, nurse practitioners, nurses practicing emergency medicine and to paramedics who are seeking to expand their body of knowledge in EM.

Finally, the editors are devoted emergency physicians committed to the practices of emergency medicine, the advancement of the specialty within organized medicine and to the support of research efforts that will improve the care provided to emergency patients.

The editors and authors wish to dedicate this textbook to their families and to the well being of the millions of patients being seen in the emergency departments across the globe.

Resuscitation

Richard V. Aghababian

No activities in medical care more dramatically typify the "life and death" nature of emergency practice than the efforts to resuscitate victims of cardiopulmonary arrest. Recognition of impending cardiorespiratory collapse, followed by rapid response; and appropriate intervention of educated laypersons are essential if the patient is to receive optimal care. Cardiopulmonary arrest patients must be rapidly turned over to EMS personnel, who further stabilize the patient before passing the patient to hospital-based medical professionals. One recent study of large city populations demonstrated survival rates for cardiac arrest to be as low as 3% to 4%, while another study cited a 71% survival rate of individuals who suffered a witnessed cardiac arrest in a casino, and who were then attended to within 3 minutes by a security guard trained to use an AED. Clearly, a huge opportunity to increase the number of survivors of cardiopulmonary arrest exists.

Consistent education and response capability at all levels—communities, laypersons, first responders, EMTs, RNs, and MDs—should be viewed as a public health imperative. In addition, research into improvement in our techniques—with regard to airway maintenance, effective ventilation, and restriction of an effective cardiac rhythm, while preserving of cerebral function—should be given high priority.

Adult Cardiopulmonary Resuscitation

Marc C. Restuccia

Introduction

The science of resuscitation, especially as it applies to victims of sudden cardiopulmonary collapse, has its roots in research conducted in the 1950s and 1960s. In 1966, a conference held under the auspices of the National Academy of Science recommended that cardiopulmonary resuscitation (CPR) be taught to all health care workers. The American Heart Association (AHA) actively took the lead in formulating curricula and training in reviving patients suffering cardiac emergencies. This has evolved over many years and conferences to include greater scientific evidence and international consensus to develop the current recommendations. During an international gathering of physicians and scientists in 2000, attendees looked at the latest scientific data to assess its relative merit for inclusion within a set of international standards for Advanced Cardiac Life Support (ACLS). The results of this conference were published in *Circulation* in 2000. This publication was remarkable for its attempt to place resuscitation into a rigorous scientific framework. The authors of this document characterized the available literature on resuscitation into levels of scientific validity. At the top were Level 1—randomized, double blind, controlled studies—progressing down to Level 3, 4, and 5, representing decreasing levels of evidence and finally anecdotal reports. Recommendations regarding appropriate intervention(s) were therefore based on the scientific evidence available, and on the quality of that evidence.

Recommendations were developed for all levels of providers, including typical pre-hospital personnel, first responders: police and fire personnel trained to do CPR and administer defibrillation via semi-automatic defibrillators (SAEDs) or automated external defibrillators (AEDs); basic emergency medical technicians (EMTs), who have some additional training; and EMT paramedics, who typically have a great deal more training. The scope of practice would encompass active airway management, defibrillation, cardioversion, and cardiac pacing, as well as a full range of cardiac medications. The hospital-based personnel (nurses and physicians) are likewise addressed in the guidelines. The theme is that the survival of any patient suffering from an acute cardiopulmonary arrest is dependent on the actions of many people, acting as a team, each trained and possessing unique and complementary skills, both in and out of the hospital.

This chapter outlines the interventions that are most scientifically valid for patients suffering from cardiac arrest and outlines general guidelines for all patients during the pre-, during, and post-arrest time frames.

Epidemiology of Cardiac Arrest

To understand the scope of the problem, it is necessary to recognize that roughly 1.25 million Americans will suffer myocardial infarctions this year. Of those, approximately 225,000 will suffer sudden cardiac death, dying before they reach the hospital.[1] Patients who experience acute cardiac or pulmonary insults that may or do lead to cardiopulmonary arrest are the focus of the current AHA Guidelines (**Table 1.1**).

The AHA Guidelines emphasize a few new and constantly changing concepts, as well as reinforcing some old ones (new guidelines are "in the works").

What can be seen at this time is that strict attention to the ABCs—airway, breathing, and circulation—must be of primary importance. Rapidly activating emergency medical services by calling 911; opening the airway and performing immediate CPR; early defibrillation; and rapid access to Advanced Life Support are appropriately stressed as the necessary links in the Chain of Survival. If all four links in this chain take place in a timely manner, survival from cardiac arrest is most likely to occur. By studying and ensuring the robustness of each link, every community can maximize the survivability of its citizens who suffer cardiac arrest. In this effort, the AHA has developed a program to recognize communities that have worked to assure each link in the Chain of Survival is optimized.

Next, antiarrhythmic medications are no longer considered *front line* therapy for such patients. Instead, early interventions with appropriate forms of electrical therapy (cardioversion, pacing, and defibrillation) are considered the cornerstones of intervention. It is only after such actions have failed that medication administration should be considered. Along these lines, emphasis has been placed on early defibrillation, via the positioning of SAED or AED devices where they can easily and quickly be used for patients suffering from sudden cardiac arrest. Options for

Table 1.1

Common Etiologies of Cardiac Arrest in Adults

I. Cardiovascular
Acute myocardial infarction (usually leading to one of the following):
a. Tachyarrhythmias/ventricular tachycardia
b. Ventricular fibrillation
c. High degree heart blocks
Pulseless electrical activity
Tension pneumothorax, pericardial tamponade, pulmonary embolism, hypoxia, hypovolemia, acidosis, electrolyte imbalance, cardiogenic shock, secondary to extensive left ventricular necrosis
Bradyarrhythmias
Asystole
II. Pulmonary
Hypoxia (multiple causes)
Pulmonary embolism, tension pneumothorax
Hypercarbia
Acidosis
III. Endocrine/Metabolic
Metabolic acidosis
Other electrolyte imbalance

this include training and equipping first responder agencies (police, fire, lifeguards, security officers and park rangers) with these machines, as well as the more controversial concept of placing public access defibrillations (PADs) in areas for public use.

Once the decision has been made to move to pharmacologic intervention, newer medications such as amiodarone should be considered over older, less well-proven medications, such as lidocaine (bretyllium has been entirely dropped from the resuscitation guidelines). Another medication, which may prove to be useful in resuscitating patients suffering cardiac arrest, is vasopressin, the effect of which, recent research suggests, is similar to epinephrine.

New guidelines are put forth for advanced airway management. Included are emphasis on the laryngeal mask airway (LMA) and the combi-tube as "rescue" airways when endotracheal intubation cannot be accomplished in the pre-hospital environment. In the hospital setting, additional adjuncts, which may facilitate endotracheal intubation are available, these include fiberoptic laryngoscopes, gum elastic (intubating) bougies, and use of paralytic medications.

Once endotracheal intubation has been performed successfully, new guidelines for confirming appropriate tube placement have been put forth. This would involve end tidal CO_2 measurement, either via color change in a colorimetric device or, preferably, via direct measurement of expired CO_2 via a capnometer. Additionally, other devices, such as the esophageal detector device (EDD) utilizing anatomical differences between the trachea and the esophagus, can be used to prevent the inadvertent cannulation of the esophagus rather than the trachea. This is later outlined in further detail.

The treatment of tachyarrhythmia's now emphasizes understanding the underlying rhythm and determining the functioning of the patient's heart, primarily the left ventricle. In patients with poorly functioning left ventricles, medications are likely to be pro-arrhythmic and early electrical intervention is encouraged. For those patients with intact left ventricular function, treatment with a single, most appropriate, medication is emphasized.

The acquisition of pre-hospital 12 lead ECGs is emphasized as a means to more rapidly triage and treat patients with an acute cardiac emergency.

Additionally, pre-hospital use of thrombolytic agents is considered to be beneficial in those patients with prolonged transport time to a hospital. This recommendation is controversial at this time and only those pre-hospital systems with prolonged transport times, and close medical oversight and quality assurance should be considering this intervention.

All patients with acute myocardial infarction (MI) should receive, if there are no contraindications, aspirin and β-blockers. Consideration of administration of angiotensin-converting enzyme inhibitor (ACE) medications in patients with large MIs, low ejection fractions, and left ventricular dysfunction (if not hypotensive), needs to occur in either the emergency department or the intensive care unit.

Finally, primary angioplasty is categorized as a Class 1 intervention in those locations where there is a large volume of angioplasties performed, the time to catheterization is short (<90 minutes), and/or there are contraindications to thrombolytic medications.

General Approach to Patients Who Are in Cardiopulmonary Arrest

The general approach to patients in arrest is similar no matter the etiology. The traditional "airway, breathing, and circulation" assessments are the first priorities.

Airway/Breathing

In patients who are in arrest, an adequate airway must be secured and the patient ventilated with 100% oxygen. This will usually mean placing an endotracheal tube and verifying its position. Multiple organizations have put forward guidelines for verification of endotracheal tube placement. In general, the paramedic or the emergency physician would be well advised to document the following in patients they intubate:

1. Visualization of the endotracheal tube passing through the vocal cords.
2. Some means of end tidal CO_2 measurement. This can be either quantitative via a capnometer or via color change with a colorimetric device.
3. Alternatively, an esophageal detector device (EDD) may be used. This device is designed to take advantage of the relative rigidity of the trachea with its cartilaginous rings and the contrasting characteristic of the esophagus, due to its muscular nature, to collapse when a negative pressure is applied. The EDD

can either be a collapsible bulb attached to an adaptor allowing it to be placed on the end of an endotracheal tube or can be a syringe type of device. By either compressing the bulb or applying negative pressure on the syringe, in either case attached to the endotracheal tube, a negative pressure is introduced into either the esophagus or trachea, whichever is intubated. If in the trachea, the bulb will rapidly inflate or the syringe will allow air to be drawn back due to the rigid nature of the wall. If in the esophagus, the walls will tend to collapse around the tube from the negative pressure and the bulb will either not inflate or very slowly inflate, while the syringe will not allow air to be drawn back.[2] Early studies showed the EDD to be very sensitive and specific.[3] This device may be useful in patients who are in arrest who are not generating enough CO_2 to be measured via capnometer.

4. Equal bilateral breath sounds.
5. Lack of sounds over the epigastrium.
6. Improving vital signs, including pulse oximetry (often not available in an arrest).

Of these, number 1 is the most important or "gold standard" to follow, with number 2 a close second. However, all of these, with the exception of direct visualization, have some potential for being incorrect and mislead the treating health care professional into which orifice is actually intubated. Therefore, it is probably wise to document as many of these as is possible and re-verify the placement of the endotracheal tube after each time the patient is moved (when it is most likely to become dislodged or moved). An additional benefit to measuring end-tidal CO_2 in patients in arrest is that a rising value is suggestive of adequacy of CPR and is always seen in patients who are successfully resuscitated. Conversely, in patients who have a properly placed endotracheal tube, who have been treated to the full extent of ACLS Guidelines for at least 20 minutes, who show end-tidal CO_2 readings of less than 10, survival is virtually 0%.[4]

Although endotracheal intubation is considered the gold standard for managing an airway, all emergency physicians must become skilled at managing an airway with a simple Bag-Valve-Mask (BVM) and with alternative/rescue airways. Such airways, like the laryngeal mask airway, the Combitube, and others will often allow ventilation in patients who cannot be intubated by one means or another. Likewise, familiarity with and competence in surgical airway management, either using a traditional cricothyrotomy set-up or (preferably) one of the commercially available kits (e.g., the Per-Trach, the Melkor/Cook Kit, and others) is mandatory. These kits are readily available and afford the emergency medical physician the opportunity to practice the technique in a number of models.

Recently, newer devices have been developed which may at some point in time replace the traditional BVM. One of these, the Oxylator, an oxygen powered pressure ventilator, has shown great promise. It has been used extensively in Europe and in a few systems in the United States. The advantages of this device are that it is very easy to use, far easier than the traditional BVM and when used appropriately leads to less gastric insufflation. Its disadvantage lies only in that it requires a compressed air or oxygen supply to function.

Circulation

Support of circulation in patients in arrest has, for many years, consisted of chest compressions. Although this has traditionally been done manually, there is at least one product being tested (which may supplant this writing) at least in some places and agencies. There has been some interest in chest-compression-only CPR, with a few studies, using it by otherwise untrained laypersons to allow the patient a potential bridge the first few minutes until first responders and EMS personnel arrive on scene. It is currently unclear if this will become more commonplace in the future. Finally, there have been studies suggesting that the patient suffering an unwitnessed cardiac arrest may do better if 60 to 90 seconds of CPR is performed prior to defibrillation.[5] Again, as mentioned above, it is unclear if this will become the standard of care for EMS and other health care providers.

Medications

For the patient who is in full cardiopulmonary arrest, the list of medications, which are used, is fairly brief. The vasopressor, positive inotropic and chronotropic medication, epinephrine, has long been a centerpiece of resuscitation. Recently the medication vasopressin has shown some promise either supplementing or supplanting epinephrine in arrest situations. However, data leading to improved outcomes is lacking at this time.[6] In addition to its hemodynamic effects, in the patient who is in arrest from angioedema or allergic reaction, leading to airway obstruction, administration of epinephrine may be life saving. The dose of epinephrine for patients in acute cardiac arrest is 1 mg (1:10,000), intravenous push, every 3 to 5 minutes. For patients with an anaphylactic reaction, either subcutaneous (1:1,000) or intravenous routes may be used. The dose sq is 0.3 to 0.5 mg, repeated every 15 to 20 minutes. If administered intravenously, typically when the patient is hypotensive, the usual dose is 0.1 mg slowly over 3 to 5 minutes. The usual dose of vasopressin for patients in cardiac arrest is 40 International Units via slow intravenous push.

Atropine, an anticholinergic medication, decreases the parasympathetic stimulation of the heart, leading to an increase in rate and blood pressure. It is used as well in symptomatic bradycardia, atrio-ventricular blocks, and in patients who are in full cardiac arrest. The usual dosage of atropine is 0.5 to 1 mg intravenously every 3 to 5 minutes to a total dose of 3 mg.

Dopamine is an excellent vasopressor for patients in shock especially after the patient has had adequate fluid resuscitation or adequate fluid resuscitation is contraindicated. It is also useful in the postresuscitaion period for patients in shock. The usual dose of dopamine is to begin an intravenous infusion at 2 to 5 $\mu m/kg/min$ and titrate to the desired blood pressure, typically a minimum systolic pressure of 100 mm Hg.

In the past few years, amiodarone has re-emerged as an excellent anti-arrhythmic. Its use is indicated in patients with ventricular fibrillation and pulseless ventricular tachycardia refractory to defibrillation. The usual dose of amiodarone is 300 mg via slow intravenous push.

Lidocaine, long the standard in anti-arrhythmic therapy, remains a useful medication. Like amiodarone, its use should be preceded by defibrillation. The standard dose of lidocaine is 1 to 1.5 mg/kg slow intravenous push, the dose being repeated in 3 to 5 minutes with a maximum dose of 3 mg/kg. In between the two "loading" doses, a continuous intravenous infusion of 1 to 4 mg/min should be started.

The choice of fluids used in resuscitation has likewise received much interest within the past 10 years. Traditionally, crystalloids, either normal saline or lactated ringers, have been used. They offer the advantages of being inexpensive, easy to store, and without having significant side effects. Downsides to their use are that they do not carry oxygen and remain in the central circulation for only a relatively brief period of time. This has spurred research into better volume resuscitation fluids.

Among these include colloids and hypertonic saline. Although each has shown promise, neither has shown improved outcomes, tend to be much more expensive and more difficult to store, and have not achieved widespread acceptance.

Blood, although an ideal resuscitation fluid, especially in hypovolemic and traumatic arrest, has significant drawbacks. It is difficult to store, is expensive and in short supply. Additionally, allergic reactions are a real concern. Despite this, there are pre-hospital agencies, primarily air medical services, which routinely carry blood products for resuscitation.

The search for an artificial blood product has gone on for many years. Ideally, such a product would be inexpensive, have a long shelf life, induce few reactions, and markedly improve hemodynamic parameters and oxygen carrying capacity. To date, no product has been found which fulfills all of the above criteria. Despite this, ongoing trials in new products continue.[7]

Electrical Therapy

As stated in the current AHA Guidelines, electrical therapy is considered the cornerstone of resuscitative efforts. Modern devices, such as the Life Pack-12, the Zoll M series, and machines by other manufacturers, offer unparalleled capabilities. Each has unique features recommending it for use. The determination of which device to use should be decided by each system and/or medical director.

Pacing

The ability to transcutaneous pace a patient has extended this ability to many patients both in the field and in the community ED. Classically, the use of pacing is seen in patients with symptomatic bradycardia, Type II second-degree AV blocks and complete (Type III) heart blocks. In addition, overdrive pacing may be used in patients suffering from prolonged QT interval tachycardias and/or torsades de pointes. Finally, transcutaneous pacing may be considered, although it is rarely successful in patients suffering asystolic arrest.

Defibrillation

Of the patients suffering sudden cardiac death, ventricular fibrillation and/or ventricular tachycardia are the predominant rhythms. Early defibrillation has long been, rightly, considered the "gold standard" of care. It has been argued, convincingly, that the earlier defibrillation is accomplished, the better the patient outcome in most circumstances. As stated above, in the unwitnessed cardiac arrest, a minute of CPR may be useful. The most modern defibrillation devices use a biphasic waveform, where the current switches polarity in mid-delivery. Long used for implantable defibrillators and for AEDs, the evidence is increasingly clear that biphasic defibrillation is superior to older monophasic defibrillators. An area of some controversy is the appropriate amount of energy to deliver to the patient. Traditional monophasic defibrillators had fairly routine energy delivery schedules, namely 200 to 300, then 360 joules. One of the potential advantages of biphasic defibrillation is the ability to defibrillate the patient with lower energy settings. This potentially could result in less myocardial damage during the shock and possibly better outcomes (citation). Despite this, different manufacturers of defibrillation equipment tout their different waveforms and energy settings for defibrillation with their device. Some manufacturers mirror the older defibrillation settings, while others limit their devices to lower energy levels. It is to be hoped that the science of resuscitation will resolve these conflicting claims in the next few years.

Cardioversion

Cardioversion, as opposed to defibrillation, assumes an organized cardiac rhythm that does not require total depolarization of the heart to achieve a more stable rhythm. In general, lower energy settings are required. Patients with a supraventricular tachycardia will usually require 50 to 100 joules of energy. Patients with atrial fibrillation require higher levels of energy, typically 100 to 200 joules. Finally, ventricular rhythms, such as stable ventricular tachycardia typically require greater energy settings, 100 to 200 or 300 joules. Just as in defibrillation, biphasic waveforms will, in all likelihood, require lower energy settings than traditional machines.

AED/SAED

Perhaps no other area of resuscitative science has generated as much interest and controversy as automatic defibrillators. Over the past 15 years these devices have become smaller, cheaper, easier to maintain, and incredibly easy to use. Their widespread deployment promises great hope for victims of sudden cardiac arrest. Today, they are to be found in many airports, most commercial aircraft, and are typical equipment of first responders (e.g., park rangers, police and fire departments, lifeguards and ski patrol personnel). Increasingly they are also to be found in physician's offices, clinics, and hospitals. There are even versions designed for home use. Although it would be hard to argue the use of these devices by trained personnel, the issue of public access defibrillation (PAD) is more controversial. The cost of placing such a device "on every street corner" would be prohibitive, yet the liability of not having such a device immediately available is not trivial.[8] It is to be hoped that each community, in conjunction with the local EMS, providers would develop a plan for the rational placement of such devices along with appropriate training of personnel and ongoing assessment of need.

Pre-Arrest Interventions

It is imperative that health care professionals be able to identify potentially life-threatening situations, such as acute myocardial infarction and allergic reaction and be able to intervene, preferably *before* the patient arrests. Examples of this would include:

1. Acute coronary syndromes
2. Acute pulmonary edema, and/or hypotension (cardiogenic shock)
3. Symptomatic bradycardia
4. Unstable tachycardias
5. Acute ischemic stroke

In addition, the following pre-arrest conditions must be recognized and treated in a pro-active fashion.

1. Hypovolemia, secondary to blood loss or dehydration
2. Anaphylactic shock
3. Trauma
4. Sepsis
5. Respiratory failure

In each of the above situations, rapid intervention, which is beyond the scope of this chapter, must be taken in a methodical, rational manner so as to prevent the patient from arresting.

Post-Resuscitation Management

The patient who has return of spontaneous circulation (ROSC) is particularly vulnerable to sustaining an arrest again. The reasons for this are multiple: such patients are susceptible to reperfusion injury, cerebral edema, coagulopathy, and the effect of toxic free radicals. In addition, the underlying cause for the patient arresting may still be present and need further treatment after resuscitation. Although the care of the resuscitated patient is beyond the scope of this chapter, meticulous attention should be paid to the following:

1. Appropriate fluid and/or blood for resuscitation and hemodynamic support.
2. Continued support and assessment of adequacy of airway interventions. Particular attention should be paid to the oxygenation and pH of the patient.
3. Continued assessment and intervention(s) directed at the cause of arrest.
4. Attention to the temperature of the patient. There is intriguing evidence that cooling patients who have suffered cardiac arrest may improve outcome.[9]
5. Exploration to determine if electrolyte or other lab abnormality may have contributed to the patient's arrest.

6. Early antibiotic therapy for patients who are considered potentially suffering from meningitis or encephalitis.
7. For patients suffering from cardiac arrest, early consideration of either fibrinolytic therapy or angioplasty.
8. In patients, particularly if unconscious, early consideration of neurosurgical intervention.

Thrombolytics versus Primary PTCA

The introduction of thrombolytics for use in patients suffering from acute myocardial infarction revolutionized cardiac care. Prior to then, the clinician treating such a patient could do little but support the patient during their infarct. With the introduction of streptokinase and then tPA, the ability to open occluded coronary arteries and salvage myocardial tissue and function meant markedly reduced morbidity and mortality from such infarcts. Later, in the early 1990s, the technique of percutaneous coronary angioplasty (PTCA) was demonstrated to also be quite effective in opening occluded arteries and salvaging heart muscle. Today, the controversy surrounding the use of these two modalities concerns their appropriate place in treatment algorithms. The advantages and disadvantages of each are listed below:

Thrombolysis

Advantages:
1. Readily available in almost any emergency department.
2. Able to be rapidly administered to most patients suffering from a myocardial infarct.
3. Requires little or no additional staff, training, or equipment.

Disadvantages:
1. Is not usable in patients who have had recent surgery, trauma or have uncontrollable hypertension.
2. Carries the risk of hemorrhage, including the requirement for transfusion and the possibility of intracranial hemorrhage, often fatal.

Percutaneous Coronary Angioplasty

Advantages:
1. May improve coronary flow in comparison to thrombolytics.
2. Carries a much reduced risk of hemorrhage.
3. Can be used in patients who have contraindications to thrombolysis.

Disadvantages:
1. Requires additional, expensive personnel and equipment.
2. May not be available in all institutions and to all patients.

Over the past few years, it has become standard practice for most emergency physicians, working in community departments, without immediate access to a cardiac catheterization lab to treat the patients they see with acute myocardial infarct, to treat them with thrombolytics and consider transferring them to cardiac catheterization capable hospitals. Those physicians typically practicing in larger teaching facilities, more commonly referred their patients with acute myocardial infarcts to the on-call interventional cardiologist for primary PTCA. Recently, this practice has been called into question, with publication of at least one article demonstrating that transferring such a patient, even if it delayed catheterization for several hours, was beneficial to the patient.[10] Such a strategy has not yet been proven to be cost effective and the cost to the health care system of such an increase in cardiac catheterization has not been determined, yet alone, whether it can be afforded. This remains a very active area of research and controversy.

Future Directions

The science of cardiopulmonary resuscitation is literally growing daily. Some areas of research, promise for the future include:

- Wider availability of SAEDs.
- Hypothermia for patients suffering cardiac arrest.
- New medications, perhaps, including vasopressin for resuscitation and free radical scavengers to minimize cellular injury and death following cardiac arrest.
- Improvements in CPR including early access to it via public education and possibly new technologies to improve the CPR delivery.
- Improvements in oxygen delivery including new devices such as the oxylator.

The past 20 years have seen an explosive growth in our ability to treat the adult in cardiopulmonary arrest. Advances in treatment have saved thousands of people who would have died or would have been severely disabled with the use of earlier interventions, medications, and knowledge. It is hoped that the next 20 years of research and treatment of this disease will be equally rewarding.

References

1. Eisenberg MS, Mengert TJ. Cardiac resuscitation, *N Engl J Med* 2001;344: 1304–1313.
2. Zaleski L, Abelo D, Gold MI. The esophageal detector device. Does it work? *Anesthesiology* 1993;79:244–247.
3. Takeda T, Tanigawa K, Tanake H, et al. The assessment of three methods to verify tracheal tube placement in emergency settings. *Resuscitation* 2003;56: 153–157.
4. Ahrens T, Schallom L, Bettorf K, et al. End tidal carbon dioxide measurements as a prognostic indication of outcome of cardiac arrest. *Am J Crit Care* 2001;10: 391–398.
5. Berg RA, Hilwig RW, Bern KB, Ewy GA. Precountershock cardiopulmonary resuscitation improves ventricular fibrillation median frequency and myocardial readiness for successful defibrillation from prolonged ventricular fibrillation: A randomized, controlled swine study. *Ann Emerg Med* 2002;40:563–570.
6. Wenzel V, Krismer AC, Arntz HR, et al. A comparison of vasopressin and epinephrine for out-of-hospital cardiopulmonary rescuscitation. *N Engl J Med* 2004;350:105–113.
7. Moore EE. Blood substitutes, the future is now. *J Am Coll Surg* 2003;196:1–17.
8. Sommers AL, Slaby JR, Aufderheide TP. Public access defibrillation. *Emerg Med Clin NA* 2002; 20:809–824.
9. The Hypothermia After Cardiac Arrest Study Group. Mild therapeutic hypothermia to improve the neurologic outcome after cardiac arrest. *N Engl J Med* 2002;8:549–556.
10. Dalby M, Bouzamondo A, Lechat P, et al. Transfer for primary angioplasty versus immediate thrombolysis in acute myocardial infarction. A meta-analysis. *Circulation* 2003;108:1809–1814.

Pediatric Resuscitation

Andrew L. Garrett

The resuscitation of infants and children is based upon the same fundamental principles as those used in adult patients. The "code" medications such as epinephrine, atropine, lidocaine, and normal saline are used, although they are dosed in a weight-based manner consistent with most pediatric drugs. The indications for interventions such as cardiopulmonary resuscitation and defibrillation are the same. The priorities of assessment—the "ABCs" of airway, breathing, and circulation—are identical.

It is essential, however, to appreciate the path that infants and children typically follow to cardiovascular decompensation and arrest, as it represents a departure from the "typical" cardiac arrest presentation in an adult patient. Adults commonly decompensate rapidly from a primary cardiac event such as acute myocardial infarction (AMI). In contrast, children typically follow an insidious and predictable path to cardiac arrest from origins of a primary respiratory (e.g., pneumonia, asthma), circulatory (e.g., dehydration, septic shock, or trauma), or at times metabolic instability (e.g., hypoglycemia). The assessment of the unstable child relies on an organized clinical evaluation of airway, breathing and circulation, looking for signs of inadequate oxygenation, ventilation, and perfusion. Using concrete physical exam findings such as capillary refill time and assessing mental status are essential. These qualitative assessments are as important as the quantitative data from vital signs, which can be falsely reassuring. Blood pressures in the pediatric patient can remain within the normal range in critically ill children until decompensated cardiopulmonary failure has occurred. Physical signs of hypoperfusion should always be considered an ominous sign of imminent arrest in infants and children. By aggressively identifying and treating signs and symptoms of compensated respiratory or circulatory impairment, it is frequently possible to prevent cardiac arrest.

Children and infants can remain in a compensated state with an evolving respiratory or circulatory disorder for prolonged periods of time. However, unrecognized and untreated respiratory distress or compensated shock can progress to a less stable decompensated state of respiratory failure or decompensated shock (**FIGURE 2.1**). This is the "golden window" when it is critical to identify and treat the sick or injured child in order to prevent subsequent decompensation, cardiopulmonary failure, and arrest.

A practical example of this model would be a child who develops severe wheezing from asthma and does not have access to treatment. Because of the decreased ability to ventilate, the child would move quickly into *compensated* respiratory distress. She would likely have tachypnea and a normal to high blood pressure. As the situation deteriorates, her tachypnea would become extreme, perioral cyanosis may develop, and her blood pressure would remain normal to high. She will pass into the *decompensated phase* of respiratory failure, as she becomes more acidotic, hypoxic, and hypercarbic. She is soon unable to maintain an adequate blood pressure, and becomes agitated and incoherent. After this she slows her respiratory rate, becomes somnolent, and then loses consciousness. Moments later she becomes apneic and bradycardic, and cardiac arrest occurs follows shortly.

This example illustrates the importance of early recognition of respiratory or circulatory distress (compensated states). With a treatable disease such as asthma, there are typically several opportunities for early intervention that can prevent an unfortunate outcome. The first would be the parent or patient's observation that the child needed treatment with her bronchodilator medication. The second is when she presents to the EMS provider or a clinician who recognizes that her worsening distress is a sign of impending trouble, even with a stable heart rate and blood pressure. The opportunity still exists to reverse her pathology with a bronchodilator and prevent further complications. If she worsens and presents to an emergency department in compensated respiratory distress, the ongoing tachypnea and respiratory distress should prompt rapid intervention with inhaled or parenteral bronchodilators, airway support, oxygen, fluid, and steroid medication. Once the patient progresses to cardiopulmonary failure (with global deficits in oxygenation, ventilation and perfusion; and presents with cyanosis, ineffective respiratory effort and bradycardia), aggressive and immediate resuscitation with assisted ventilation, oxygenation, vascular access, and resuscitation are needed to prevent cardiac arrest.

Young patients require a rapid yet organized and thorough assessment to detect the often subtle presentation

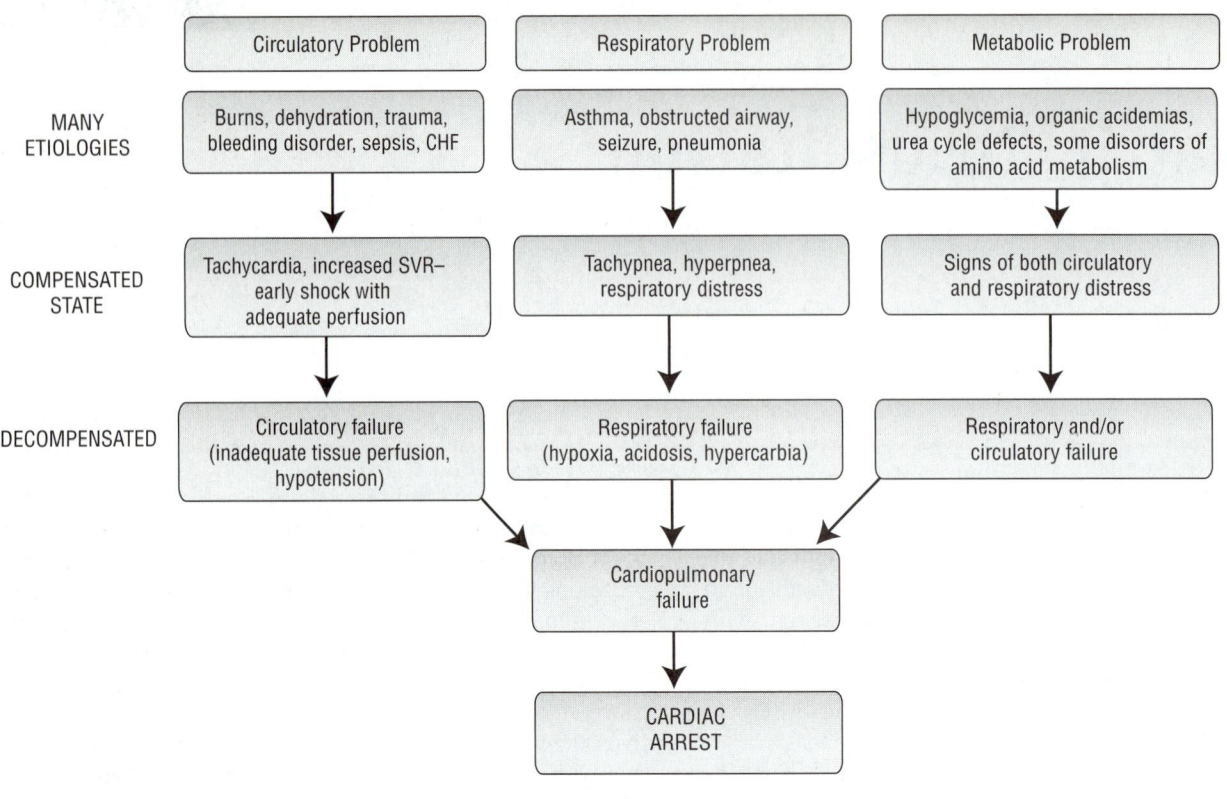

FIGURE 2.1 Cardiovascular decompensation can result from multiple problems and follows a common pathway.

of circulatory or respiratory distress and failure. Special training classes such as Pediatric Advanced Life Support (PALS), Advanced Pediatric Life Support (APLS), and the Neonatal Resuscitation Program (NRP) are useful for learning these specialized assessment skills and resuscitation strategies that are unique to infants and young children. There are also tools that can reduce some of the stress inherent in caring for a child who is sick or injured, such as a height-based weight estimation tape. An organized rapid cardiovascular assessment should help with the search for reversible disease, and it reflects the ubiquitous "ABC" (airway, breathing, circulation) approach of emergency medicine. Many courses will add the category of "first impression" or "appearance" to this first impression.

A rapid systemic cardiopulmonary assessment in a child at risk for decompensation begins with the airway. It is vital to rapidly identify and treat airway obstruction. In the setting of a functional obstruction from the tongue or secretions, this may be quickly done with positioning, suction and airway adjuncts. Remember that infants and young children have a large occiput and will typically benefit from a towel pad under the shoulders to help open the airway (**FIGURE 2.2**). When assessing the breathing, it is important to assess the respiratory rate over a minute as well as the qualitative aspects of the exam such as wheezing, stridor, chest expansion, symmetry of breath sounds, and the effort required to move air. Finally, assess the child's skin color for cyanosis or pallor. Imminent threats such as wheezing, pneumothorax or foreign body aspiration should be identified and treatment begun immediately. Administer oxygen (100% O_2 via nonrebreather mask) to any potentially unstable infant or child.

The cardiovascular assessment also has quantitative and qualitative components. Measurement of the heart rate (HR) and blood pressure (BP) (**Table 2.1**) can promptly identify the presence of instability, but reassuring numbers do not rule out serious pathology. Remember that the hemodynamic response to hypovolemia does not include a fall in BP until approximately half of the circulating vol-

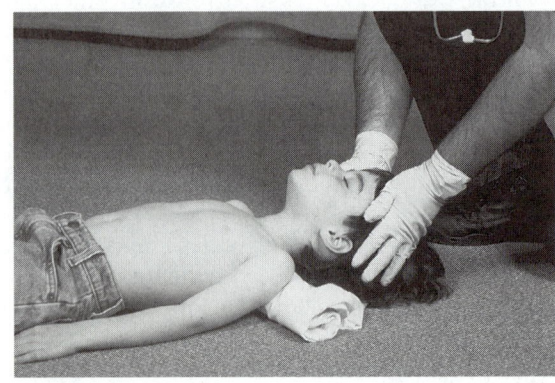

FIGURE 2.2 Use a shoulder roll or folded towel to position the airway of the infant and young child.

Table 2.1

Vital sign normal values in pediatric patients

Age	Mean Weight (kg)	Minimum Systolic BP	Normal Heart Rate	Normal Respiratory Rate
Premature	<2.5	40	120–170	40–60
Term	3.5	60	100–170	40–60
3 months	6	60	100–170	30–50
6 months	8	60	100–170	30–50
1 year	10	62	100–170	30–40
2 years	13	74	100–160	20–30
4 years	15	78	80–130	20
6 years	20	82	70–115	16
8 years	25	86	70–110	16
10 years	30	90	60–105	16
12 years	40	94	60–100	16

ume has been depleted. The same graph demonstrates the usefulness of assessing for signs of cardiac output and increased vascular resistance. These are much more useful indices of shock than BP alone. Assessment of the skin may show coolness, mottling, and a prolonged capillary refill time. Check these variables on the skin of the head or trunk for comparison with the extremities, especially if the child is in a cold environment where some vasoconstriction of the extremities is normal. Determining the peripheral pulse is another way of estimating cardiac output, as thready or absent distal pulses can be an indication of ongoing shock. Assessing end organ function is also useful. The central nervous system is susceptible to the effect of shock, so altered mental status—agitation or lethargy—is a serious sign. Monitoring urine output can be an important tool is useful in determining end organ perfusion in the setting of shock, as well as gauging the effectiveness of fluid resuscitation.

Metabolic instability can also contribute to or cause cardiovascular decompensation and arrest from processes such as hypoglycemia and acidosis. Euglycemia is essential for normal cardiac function, especially in the newborn and young infants. Glycogen storage capacity is normally lower in these very young patients, making them at a higher risk for hypoglycemia. This is especially true when a child is ill and may not have optimum oral intake. There are numerous inborn errors of metabolism, such as the organic acidemias, urea cycle defects, and amino acid metabolic disorders that can present with life-threatening acidosis or the accumulation of toxic metabolites. These can lead to cardiovascular instability through a cellular process.

Infants can present an especially difficult challenge for several reasons. Younger children have a higher metabolic rate and therefore a greater subsequent oxygen requirement. This lowers their ability to tolerate hypoxia, something seen clearly in premature infants, who may desaturate within moments and become bradycardic and asystolic very rapidly after airway obstruction. The cardiopulmonary assessment and the onset of interventions should occur via a team approach in a critically ill patient. It is not appropriate to delay interventions to wait for lab-

oratory results or radiography. Respiratory distress should be treated with oxygen, suction, and positioning, with airway interventions individualized based on the specific problem. This may require utilizing measures such as bronchodilators, obstructed airway maneuvers, or needle decompression of the chest. It is important to continually reassess the airway and breathing effort after any intervention, as rapid changes are common. If necessary, assistance through the use of the bag-valve mask (BVM) should be initiated. Most children and infants can be easily ventilated with the BVM, but it is a skill that must be frequently practiced to be effective. Intubation of children in actual or imminent respiratory failure should not be the first line treatment of respiratory distress or failure. BVM airway support is faster and very effective, allowing time to adequately prepare for a successful intubation. If the airway is difficult to secure with intubation or BVM, consider the use of the laryngeal airway mask (LMA), a device that has a high success rate for first time placement, but provides little protection of the airway from stomach contents.

A similar approach should be occurring with circulatory failure. The child with compensated shock will have tachycardia and possibly a diminished capillary refill time. Fluid resuscitation and hemorrhage control is the first line of therapy, using isotonic fluid (normal saline) (NS) or a Lactated Ringer's solution (LR). Hypotonic solutions such as 5% dextrose (D5W) for acute volume replacement are not indicated. Administration of rapidly infused NS or LR fluid boluses in increments of 20 mL/kg should occur with frequent reassessment until the vital signs and exam improve. Consider the possibility of congestive heart failure/congenital heart disease, third spacing, hidden bleeding or a surgical emergency if the patient worsens or does not improve after multiple fluid challenges have been administered. The use of broad-spectrum antibiotics or prostaglandins is indicated if sepsis or congenital cardiac disease is a possibility. Studies such as lumbar puncture should be deferred until first-line resuscitation is completed. Vasopressors are not first line treatment for patients in circulatory failure. They should be considered after adequate fluid resuscitation especially in the setting of distributive shock (sepsis, anaphylaxis) or congestive heart failure.

It has been described that primary cardiac disorders are a less likely cause for cardiovascular failure children outside of the neonatal age group. It is not uncommon, however, for arrhythmias such as ventricular fibrillation or ventricular tachycardia to present in an unstable child who has decompensated for other reasons. The indications for cardioversion and defibrillation are the same for infants and children as in adults. The use of the now ubiquitous automated external defibrillator (AED) is appropriate for children over 1 year of age, even if special energy modulating pads are not available.[1] It is expected that AED use in children under 1 year old may be indicated in the future.

Infants and children are efficient at maintaining a compensated state with most circulatory or respiratory insults. Conversely, once a child decompensates and develops cardiopulmonary failure, there is little time to reverse the process before cardiac arrest ensues. It is vital to have the skill to recognize the signs and symptoms of respiratory distress and circulatory failure and intervene as early as possible.

The child who ends up in or presents with cardiopulmonary arrest is treated in a similiar fashion to the adult. The ABC survey is performed, ventilation is secured (BVM followed by intubation), and prompt defibrillation at pediatric dosages is administered if it is indicated by ventricular tachycardia or fibrillation. The administration of ACLS medications is essentially the same as for adults, but it is necessary to know or estimate the patient's weight in kilograms for proper dosing. The American Heart Association 2000 guidelines contain some important updates in pediatric resuscitation:

1. Standard dose epinephrine has simplified the treatment of asystole.
2. The cause of PEA should be aggressively sought as resuscitation is ongoing (hypoxia, hypothermia, hyper/hypokalemia, hypovolemia, toxin, thromboembolus, tension pneumothorax, tamponade).
3. Amiodarone is an optional replacement for lidocaine as an antiarrhythmic for ventricular fibrillation or pulseless ventricular tachycardia.
4. Bretyllium is no longer recommended for pediatric use.

Because pediatric cardiac arrest may or may not be a primary cardiac event, it is important to search for reversible causes of airway and circulatory insult, such as pneumothorax, hemorrhage, seizure or head injury. Hypoglycemia and hypothermia are causes and complications of arrest in infants. They should be detected and treated during resuscitation. Once the infant has regained a perfusing rhythm, both of these parameters should be monitored closely. The larger surface-to-body ratio of children makes them especially vulnerable to hypothermia before and after they arrive at the hospital and needs to be addressed during and after resuscitation maneuvers are made. Lastly, consider a toxicologic insult (including alcohol) that could have caused the patient to decompensate, especially in the toddler or adolescent patient.

As in adult medicine, the science of pediatric resuscitation is constantly evolving. Some of it is specific to the pre-hospital environment, but much of it applies to both pre-hospital and in-house resuscitation. There are several topics that are being evaluated currently, many of which are extensions from adult resuscitation research, included here for informative purposes:

- Similar to adult patients, there is a growing support of the judicious use of IV crystalloid resuscitation in the pre-hospital environment rather than the aggressive use of IV boluses. This is especially true in patients injured traumatically. In contrast, there is a clear role for the use of prompt and repetitive fluid boluses in the resuscitation of pediatric patients with septic shock.
- During cardiopulmonary resuscitation (CPR), there is some controversy over the adequacy of coronary perfusion pressure that is achieved by a 5:1 ratio of compressions to ventilations. Alternatives being explored are the classic adult CPR radio of 15:2, which demonstrates an improved coronary perfusion pressure during compression for the latter $2/3$ of the compression phase. It is thought that it may take a series of approximately 5 compressions to generate forward coronary perfusion pressure with CPR. Other alternatives to traditional CPR are also being studied, such as interposed abdominal compressions to increase coronary and cerebral perfusion.
- Aufderheide, Sigurdsson et al published in 2004[2] that there are indications that the over-ventilation of patients by clinicians commonly seen in resuscitation may be contributing to the poor survival rates after cardiac arrest. This is likely due to an increase in intrathoracic pressure and a resultant drop in coronary perfusion pressure from a respiratory rate that is too high.
- Delaying defibrillation for several minutes of CPR was noted to result in a statistically increased survival rate in out-of-hospital ventricular fibrillation arrests according to Wik et al.[3] This is much more applicable to the adult population, where a primary cardiac arrhythmia is more likely to result in cardiovascular failure.
- In 2003, Gausche et al.[4] showed that in the Los Angeles and Orange County, California pre-hospital care system, the use of bag-valve mask resuscitation versus endotracheal intubation by paramedics on pediatric patients demonstrated no difference in outcome. At the same time, it was noted that patients who were intubated had longer scene times by 2 to 3 minutes and had an 8% rate of unrecognized tube displacement or misplacement. Based on this study, pediatric intubation protocols were modified in this service area. There are questions as to the generalizability of this extensive study to other pre-hospital systems or the emergency department, but it certainly emphasizes the role of excellent bag-valve mask skills in pediatric clinicians.
- The use of cuffed versus uncuffed endotracheal tubes in children under 8 years old is being considered. The PALS guidelines recommend uncuffed tubes in this age group for ease of placement, the presence of anatomic structure that obviates the need for a cuff,

risk of the cuff's damaging the airway, and the fact that the cuff reduces the inner diameter of the tube slightly. Proponents of cuffed tubes state that they can reduce air leak and prevent the need for tube changes as frequently. It is likely that end tidal carbon dioxide monitoring is more accurate with a cuffed tube.

- The use of vasopressin, as an alternative to epinephrine in pediatric cardiac arrest, is controversial. There is evidence that there may be a worse outcome in some animal models. The American Heart Association 2000 Guidelines state that "data is insufficient to allow a recommendation of vasopressin in children with cardiac arrest." Supporting the use of vasopressin, there have been several animal trials and a small case series, which indicate that its use may be beneficial. Studies in the adult realm have demonstrated improved outcomes for patients with asystole, but it was a subgroup analysis on a larger study that showed no difference between the use of epinephrine and vasopressin.[5]
- It is becoming evident that the use of high-dose (0.1 mg/kg) epinephrine in pediatric cardiac arrest may be detrimental. Perondi et al.[6] noted that in children with in-hospital cardiac arrest, there was a similar return of spontaneous circulation that was equivalent in the high- and low-dose groups. However, no patients receiving high-dose epinephrine survived to discharge versus 12% in the low-dose (0.01 mg/kg) group.

Skills and assessment classes such as PALS will help the new or experienced provider feel more confident with infant and pediatric assessment and resuscitation. The same can be said for frequent practice of these skills using full-context "mock code" scenarios in the workplace. This is especially important for trainees who need to feel comfortable with basic resuscitation skills prior to working without supervision.

References

1. Samson, RA et al. Use of automated external defibrillators for children: An update: An advisory statement from the pediatric advanced life support task force, international liaison committee on resuscitation. *Circulation* 2003;107:3250–3255.
2. Aufderheide TP, Sigurdsson G, Pirrallo RG, et al. Hyperventilation-induced hypotension during cardiopulmonary resuscitation. *Circulation* 2004;109:1960–1965.
3. Wik L, Hansen TB, Fylling F, et al. Delaying defibrillation to give basic cardiopulmonary resuscitation to patients with out-of-hospital ventricular fibrillation: A randomized trial. *JAMA* 2003;289:1389–1395.
4. Gausche-Hill M, Lewis RJ, Stratton SJ, et al. Effect of out-of-hospital pediatric endotracheal intubation on survival and neurological outcome: a controlled clinical trial. *JAMA* 2000;283:783–790.
5. Wenzel V, Krismer AC, Arntz HR, et al. A comparison of vasopressin and epinephrine for out-of-hospital cardiopulmonary resuscitation. *N Engl J Med* 2004;350:105–113.
6. Perondi MB, Reis AG, Paiva EF, et al. A comparison of high-dose and standard-dose epinephrine in children with cardiac arrest. *N Engl J Med* 2004;350:1722–1730.

Website References

PALS courses, www.americanheart.org.
American Academy of Pediatrics, www.aap.org.
The Center for Pediatric Emergency Medicine, www.cpem.org.
American College of Emergency Physicians, www.acep.org.
EMS For Children Organization, www.ems-c.org.

EMS Disaster

Richard V. Aghababian

Emergency Medical Services (EMS) is a critical component of the emergency care network. Often EMS is the patient's first encounter with a medical professional after experiencing an acute medical illness or injury. EMS has become an essential community resource in developed countries along with police and fire services. As public awareness of the importance of rapid access to emergency care increases and more and more citizens become first responders, EMS utilization should continue to grow.

The ability to provide medical direction to EMS personnel is an essential skill that must be mastered by emergency physicians. In addition, every emergency department should have at least one physician staff member actively involved in the supervision and training of EMS personnel. Emergency physicians must assure that they are adequately represented in the administration of EMS systems at the community, regional, and state level where they practice.

Emergency personnel must be prepared to respond to disasters involving medical casualties on a moment's notice. It is essential that advanced training and careful planning be in place to adequately respond to disasters that often occur with little or no warning. Effective response to disaster requires an immediate reassessment of existing emergency department patients and inventory of available patient care resources to prepare for the rapid triage and victim stabilization of a large number of patients. When the health care needs of the victims exceed human and material resources, emergency personnel may be confronted with "life and death" decisions that they are not accustomed to making. Therefore, preparation and experience are key to successful medical response in times of disaster.

A thorough review of all aspects of EMS operations and potential medical disaster scenarios (e.g., acts of terrorism) is beyond the scope of the book. This section is intended to cover the essential EMS and disaster operations issues that must be understood by physicians practicing in emergency settings. The authors have also provided references for readers wishing to explore additional aspects of EMS and disaster medical management.

Emergency Medical Services

Christopher J. Fullagar
N. Heramba Prasad

Introduction

Emergency Medical Services (EMS) is a broad term describing the many facets of out-of-hospital emergency care. Over the years, EMS has evolved from a simple means of rapidly transporting the sick and injured, to a complex system involving specialized health care professionals delivering high quality emergency medical care to the community. The term "out-of-hospital care" has replaced "pre-hospital care" to reflect the broadened scope of EMS.

EMS is much more than an extension of emergency department care to the field. Physicians involved in EMS have the responsibility to master the rapidly developing, unique body of knowledge that comprises out-of-hospital emergency care. Effective medical oversight by involved, knowledgeable EMS physicians is crucial to enable an EMS system to integrate into the continuum of medical care and to guide the system through the rapidly changing delivery of emergency care. EMS providers make house calls by delegation, and all members of the emergency department team should have a thorough knowledge of EMS, as well as an understanding of local protocols and guidelines that affect the delivery of care in the field. A thorough understanding can facilitate a seamless transfer of care from the scene through to hospital admission.

History

Prior to the 1960s, primarily volunteers staffed emergency services and many ambulances were based out of funeral homes. Emergency providers rarely had any medical education and as providers, their objective was simply to get the victim to the hospital as rapidly as possible. EMS, as understood today, was born of a 1966 white paper that helped to redefine "victims" as "patients" and "ambulance drivers" as "EMTs." The 1966 white paper was "Accidental Death and Disability: The Neglected Disease of Modern Society," published by the National Academy of Sciences' National Research Council, which identified the need for improving emergency care and specifically addressed out-of-hospital care. The Highway Safety Act of 1966, which established the National Highway Traffic Safety Administration (NHTSA) within the Department of Transportation (DOT), soon followed. The Highway Safety Act of 1966 also authorized the DOT to provide funding for ambulances, training programs, and communications for pre-hospital emergency services. By 1969 an eighty-one hour EMS training course was developed by the National Academy of Sciences (NAS) in cooperation with the American College of Orthopedic Surgeons.

In 1973 Congress passed Public Law 93-154, known as the EMS Systems Act. The goal of this legislation was to provide funding for the development of regional EMS systems in order to improve EMS on a national level. The Act defined fifteen elements to comprise an EMS system (**Table 3.1**). Interestingly, EMS medical oversight, now considered essential to the delivery of out-of-hospital care, was not included among the Act's original fifteen elements (Table 3.1).

Over the next decade, NHTSA and DOT developed national standard training curriculae for EMS providers. These curriculae became known as the EMT-Ambulance (EMT-A), the EMT-Intermediate (EMT-I), and the EMT-Paramedic (EMT-P). Later, the EMT-A became what is known today as the EMT-Basic (EMT-B) level. Since their inception, all of these curriculae have undergone continual adaptations and revisions. Many states have since developed varying levels of EMT certification, leading to a number of different certifications nationwide. In an attempt to redefine a national standard of expected knowledge base and skills, the National Emergency Medical Services Education and Practice Blueprint was published in 1993. While many states have moved toward implementing these national standards, there remains much variation among pre-hospital certification requirements from state-to-state.

Providers

The qualification levels of providers that comprise a particular EMS system are not uniform across the country. Although national curriculae for EMS provider levels do exist, the scope of practice for each level required of providers varies among states. Nationally recognized provider levels include basic, intermediate, and paramedic levels of the emergency medical technician (EMT). Some states do not recognize all of these provider levels, while other states recognize additional levels of training. In ad-

Table 3.1

The 15 Components of an EMS System According to the EMS Systems Act of 1973

1) Personnel
2) Training
3) Communications
4) Transportation
5) Facilities
6) Critical Care Units
7) Public Safety Agencies
8) Consumer Participation
9) Access to Care
10) Transfer of Care
11) Standardization of Patient Records
12) Public Education & Information
13) Independent Review & Evaluation
14) Disaster Linkage
15) Mutual Aid Agreements

dition, other providers, such as emergency medical dispatchers and first responders, are also integrated into many systems. The inclusion of EMS physician responders, especially medical directors, is becoming more common. In many areas, members of the general public are also included within the system. This is apparent in areas that have programs such as public access defibrillation (PAD) and community emergency medical education.

Emergency Medical Dispatcher

The emergency medical dispatcher (EMD) is an EMS provider who has been specially trained and certified in interrogation techniques, pre-arrival instructions, and call prioritization. They have been dubbed the "zero-minute responders" or the "first, first responders." EMDs provide medical instruction to the layperson over the telephone until EMS personnel arrive on scene. They often use a flip-card system to ensure that information is collected and provided in the most efficient manner. EMDs then use the information collected to prioritize calls and to determine the level of response using a verified method. The addition of EMDs to EMS systems has expedited the delivery of emergency medical care to the patient, improved the systems' liability posture, and has reduced the risk of EMS vehicle crashes on non-urgent calls. As part of the delivery of patient care, EMD constitutes part of the responsibility of the system medical director. Effective medical oversight and continuous quality improvement are important components of a successful EMD program.

First Responders

Many EMS systems utilize first responders to provide time-sensitive care until more advanced providers arrive on scene. The scope of practice of first responders varies and depends, in part, on state and local protocols. First responders are generally trained in professional level CPR and first-aid techniques. Police and fire personnel are of-

ten trained as first responders. Many first responders also have the capability to deliver automated external defibrillation (AED). First responders are of particular benefit in areas where there is a delay in the response of higher levels of care (e.g., EMTs and paramedics). In rural areas, many EMS agencies are staffed with volunteers. Response times may be delayed if the providers are responding from home or work versus centralized stations. Furthermore, some volunteer agencies may not always have a crew available to respond and, therefore, require mutual aid assistance from a neighboring unit, which may prolong the response. In urban settings, traffic delays are coupled with a relative paucity of EMS units, compared with the relatively high number of roving police units. Fire stations are often densely scattered throughout the urban community. In these areas, police and fire first responders may deliver prompt, basic emergency care while waiting for more advanced units to respond.

EMT-Basic

The EMT-Basic (EMT-B) undergoes approximately 110 to 160 hours of initial training. Examples of EMT-B skills include patient assessment, manual vital signs, oxygen administration, basic airway management including the use of the oropharyngeal and nasopharyngeal (nasal trumpet) airway, mass casualty incident management, spinal immobilization, traction splinting, extrication, and HAZMAT awareness. EMT-Bs may also assist the patient in the self-administration of certain medications such as the patient's own nitroglycerine, EpiPen, or albuterol inhaler. Otherwise, EMT-Bs do not administer medication or perform invasive procedures (e.g., intubation or venous cannulization). Although manual defibrillation is beyond the scope of practice of EMT-Bs, they are trained in the use of automatic and semi-automatic external defibrillators. In some areas, slightly more advanced airway management (e.g., the use of the laryngeal mask airway or LMA), has become an EMT-B skill.

EMT-Intermediate

In addition to EMT-B training, the EMT-Intermediate (EMT-I) undergoes an additional 120 to 400 hours of education. Skills generally include adult endotracheal intubation, use of Magill, forceps for clearing airway obstructions, initiation of intravenous access with or without administration of crystalloid solution, and manual defibrillation. The scope of practice for EMT-Is varies greatly from state to state. Some states do not recognize EMT-Is, whereas others may have more than one intermediate level of training between the EMT-B and paramedic levels.

EMT-Paramedic

The EMT-Paramedic (EMT-P) or paramedic is generally the highest level of out-of-hospital certification. Paramedic training programs may require from 600 to over 2,000 hours of didactic and clinical field learning. Most programs, however, average 1,000 to 1,500 hours of training. These professionals are trained to deliver full advanced life support care to the community. Despite the national curriculum, there is still a large variance in state and local practice.

Most paramedics provide advanced airway management, medication administration (including certain narcotics and intravenous drips), cardiac monitoring, defibrillation, external cardiac pacing, and synchronized cardioversion. In some areas, surgical airway management and rapid sequence intubation (RSI), including neuromuscular blockade, are performed.

Advanced paramedics, including critical care paramedics and flight paramedics, may undergo additional training and have a broader scope of practice than typical paramedics. These paramedics, especially in rural areas, are able to provide on-scene care for minor medical problems *instead of* monitoring transport to the hospital. In accordance, some paramedic programs have joined with local colleges and universities to offer 2- and 4-year degree programs.

Medical Director

The EMS medical director is a physician who is ultimately responsible for the medical care that is provided in their EMS district, and who may already serve as an EMS medical director at a state, regional or county, and local or organizational level. The medical director may delegate certain responsibilities of medical oversight to other physicians in the system to facilitate 24-hour physician availability. Delegation is the process by which emergency physicians are authorized by the system medical director to provide medical orders or consultation to field providers via a base station radio.

The term "medical oversight" has replaced the terms "medical command," "medical control," and "medical direction"; and is now the recognized term for the ultimate medical, legal, and moral responsibility for medical aspects of out-of-hospital care.

In the past the terms "on-line" and "off-line" were used to describe the functions of medical control. Today, the terms "direct medical oversight" and "indirect medical oversight" have replaced "on-line" and "off-line" medical control. Direct medical oversight refers to any concurrent provision or supervision of medical care. Indirect medical oversight includes activities (e.g., the implementation of standing orders and review of protocol adherence), which are removed by time or function from the immediate care of the patient.

There are now many areas of the country, especially in urban settings, where physician responders are integrated into the EMS system. As the field of EMS matures, many physicians are former past EMTs and paramedics have also maintained their involvement in out-of-hospital care. It is important to make the distinction between physician responders and the physician at-the-scene: physician responders are providers who are medical directors or other physicians who have a background in EMS and are approved by the medical director to provide patient care and direct, on-scene medical oversight. The physician at-the-scene refers to any physician who happens to arrive on the scene and offers assistance. The latter physician may not have the authority to provide medical oversight in most jurisdictions.

Communications

A reliable communication system is essential for successful operation of an EMS system. Providers should have a reliable way of communicating with dispatch or the public service answering point (PSAP); with other units both within and outside of their agency; other public service providers (e.g., police and fire personnel); medical oversight; and with the receiving hospital. Traditionally, radio systems have been the mainstay of EMS communication; however, cellular telephone, digital technology, microwave relays, radio telephone switching systems (RTSS), and land mobile satellite communications are also used. Although cellular technology is used in some regions, there may be certain emergency situations, such as disasters, in which cellular towers may be overloaded or otherwise not operational. Additionally, some agencies that use cellular technology have reported an inability to use cell phones during motor vehicular crashes that have required the closure of a major roadway due to overload of the system when other people made calls from their vehicles. For such instances, a reliable backup for cellular technology should be in place for EMS.

Communication between hospitals and from ambulances to hospitals can be utilized via the Hospital Emergency Administration Radio (HEAR), which operates on the designated frequency of 155.340 MHz. Having such universal emergency frequency is essential in a disaster situation when multiple agencies, normally operating on different frequencies, are responding to the same event.

Specialization

Emergency Medical Services for Children (EMS-C)

EMS-C is a federally established program that addresses all aspects of care pertaining to sick and injured children and which was created in response to the concern over the inadequacy of pediatric-specific training in EMS. The EMS-C program has enabled tremendous improvements in training and protocol algorhythm development for pediatric patients.

Air Medical Services

Air medical transport began on the battlefield as a means of evacuating injured soldiers from the field and transporting them rapidly to a safer area for medical treatment. Although some sources report the first use of an aircraft for medical evacuation in 1870, when injured soldiers were transported via balloon during the Prussian siege on Paris, this is now thought to be inaccurate. The first documented transport of an injured soldier by aircraft occurred in 1915, when a French pilot evacuated a Serb in an unmodified fighter airplane. The first reported use of helicopter medical transport was in Burma in 1944, just two years after the invention of the helicopter. Subsequently, large-scale medevac operations began in Korea and continued to develop throughout the Vietnam War.

In the late 1960s Helicopter Emergency Medical Services (HEMS) extended to civilian emergency functions for military, fire, and police operations. The first hospital-based HEMS began in 1972 at St. Anthony's Hospital in Denver, Colorado and has since continued to develop across the country, mostly within hospital-based programs.

Although civilian HEMS programs were initially designed around trauma, aircraft are being used today for a variety of applications, including critical care interfacility transfer, emergent cardiac transport to hospitals with coronary catheterization laboratories, and organ transplant missions. While there has been some controversy regarding the expense of HEMS programs, many have argued that HEMS is cost-effective, especially when compared with other medical therapies and interventions.

Crew configuration of HEMS varies significantly: most include two medical providers. Many are nurse-paramedic crews; however, nurse-nurse, nurse-physician, paramedic-physician, and paramedic-paramedic configurations also exist. Especially in rural areas, the air medical crew may be able to deliver a higher level of pre-hospital care that is otherwise not available locally. HEMS should be considered in any critical situation where the speed of the helicopter or the expertise of the crew (beyond that which is locally available) may be beneficial to the patient.

Fixed-wing air medical services are utilized primarily for long-distance interfacility transports. In contrast to helicopters, fixed-wing aircraft generally provide more cabin room, faster transport, and longer range. Fixed-wing services may also have the capacity to carry more crew members and specialized patient support equipment, beyond the capacity of a helicopter.

The effect of the cabin pressure while the aircraft is at altitude must be considered when selecting and treating patients during air medical transport. As altitude increases, pressure decreases, causing gas to expand and the partial pressure of oxygen to decrease. Oxygen delivery systems may need to be adjusted during flight to prevent hypoxia. Air-filled equipment (e.g., the cuff on an endotracheal tube) may need to be partially deflated at altitude. Sometimes the air in the cuff is replaced by water or saline to reduce volume fluctuations with changes in pressure. Because airplanes generally fly at higher altitudes than helicopters, cabin pressure is more of an issue during fixed-wing transports. Even airplanes with pressurized cabins are subject to changes in pressure with altitude. Most pressurized airplane cabins can create a cabin pressure equivalent of 8,000 feet when flying at an actual altitude of over 40,000 feet. At 8,000 feet the partial pressure of oxygen is almost 41 mm Hg less than at sea level (118.4 mm Hg versus 159.2 mm Hg).

Critical Care Ground Transport

There are many critical care ground transport services across the U.S. Many of these programs are operated by hospitals that also operate air medical services, which are often used when air medical transport is not available or not appropriate. Some of these programs operate specialty units with specially trained personnel, vehicles, and equipment designed for a specific mission (e.g., burn care or neonatal transport). Others may have providers (e.g., paramedics and nurses), who have special "critical care" training that covers the ongoing management and spectrum of critical patients.

Tactical Emergency Medical Support (TEMS)

TEMS is a relatively new area of out-of-hospital care developed from lessons learned during combat missions. TEMS providers are specially trained personnel who operate as part of a civilian special operations law enforcement unit, for example, within a special weapons and tactics (SWAT) team. TEMS providers deliver emergency medical care to officers, bystanders, and suspects injured during a tactical operation; and they are involved in all medically related aspects of the operation and are responsible for advising the tactical team leader on any medical aspects that can affect the mission. Preventative medicine and medical preplanning are a large part of TEMS. For example, during a mission occurring under conditions of high heat and humidity, the TEMS provider would advise the team leader on proper hydration, personnel rotation, and necessary periods of rest for team members. Medical preplanning responsibilities include maintaining timely information of the capabilities of local hospitals, mission-specific medical threat assessment, routes of evacuation, and coordination with local EMS and other emergency support resources. The term emergency medical *support* was chosen in place of emergency medical *services* to reflect the many facets of TEMS beyond the traditional scope of EMS.

During an incident, the TEMS provider must be prepared to deliver emergency medical care in an austere environment. There may be special hazards that pose mission-specific medical risks (e.g., booby traps or hazardous materials) encountered during a raid on a clandestine drug lab. The TEMS provider must have personal protective equipment, such as helmets, body armor, and gas masks, for protection in the event that they are required to deliver care in an area of higher risk. The decision whether or not to arm TEMS providers is generally left up to individual law enforcement agencies. TEMS providers may be civilian or law enforcement personnel, who may be trained to provide basic or advanced life support interventions.

Disaster Medicine

A disaster is a large-scale catastrophic event (e.g., tornado or earthquake) that affects hundreds or thousands of people. However, a disaster can be any situation in which the severity or number of patients exceeds the local resources available to provide immediate management. External resources are required in such instances. A plan must be in place to effectively triage and manage patients while waiting for further resources. The Incident Command System (ICS) is a universal emergency management tool for command and control in such an event. The ICS is a modular system that can be applied to any incident, regardless of scale, and is dynamic to expand or contract as the circumstances of an incident change. The five major components of the ICS are:

- Incident command
- Operations
- Planning
- Logistics
- Finance

On-scene medical care falls under the operations category of the ICS. In order to sort large numbers of patients quickly, Simple Triage and Rapid Transport (START) was developed. The system classifies patients based on respirations, presence or absence of a radial pulse, and mental status. Information can then be used to assign priority categories (e.g., immediate or delayed transport, minor or "walking wounded," deceased). Many systems use color-coded triage tags to classify patients respectively.

Disaster Medical Assistance Teams (DMATs) are federally supported local teams of health care providers (physicians, nurses, paramedics, EMTs, pharmacists, and support personnel), who can be activated in the event of a disaster. These teams are coordinated to respond based on the needs of the disaster-affected area.

Mass Gatherings

Preparation for organized emergency medical care is a critical part of planning for an event of mass gathering. Sporting events, parades, marathons, and concerts all must have dedicated medical support. Between 0.3 and 24 incidents requiring medical care per 1,000 people can be expected at any mass event, depending on its nature. In addition, weather, temperature, availability of adequate hydration, alcohol consumption, and illicit drug use are factors that significantly affect the number of people requiring medical care during mass gatherings. Preparations for disaster must also be in place for any mass gathering. Effective pre-planning for an event can effectively anticipate patient needs, and can help to minimize impact on the local EMS system.

HAZMAT

Traditionally, HAZMAT (hazardous materials) response teams have focused on dealing with the control of hazardous substance and to control threats of local effects. An area of EMS has recently developed that focuses on the effects of the hazardous substance on the *patient*. EMS training courses now include Advanced HAZMAT Life Support (AHLS) and ToxMedic that extend scope of practice to specifically include treatment of the HAZMAT patient.

While awareness of hazardous materials has always been an important component of EMS systems, the concern of terrorism has put HAZMAT preparedness in the forefront. The Occupational Safety and Health Administration (OSHA) and the National Fire Protection Association (NFPA) have developed levels of required education and standards for pre-hospital personnel. OSHA's Hazardous Waste Operations and Emergency Response (HAZWOPER) requirements include five levels of training:

1. First responder, awareness
2. First responder, operations
3. Hazardous materials technician
4. Hazardous materials specialist
5. Incident commander

Incident commander training requires 24 hours of training at the first responder operations level, plus additional scene management education regarding command and control of the HAZMAT incident. NFPA has also drafted guidelines to define the knowledge base for each of the five HAZWOPER levels.

The protection of the rescuers and maintaining overall scene safety is the top priority of a HAZMAT response team. When responding to a scene, EMS providers are encouraged to stay at a safe distance, uphill and upwind of the incident. This is imperative in order to protect rescue workers themselves and their equipment from any contamination.

To assist with the identification of hazardous materials, the U.S. Department of Transportation (DOT) has a system of labeling materials with diamond-shaped placards. Materials are identified on the placard by an identification number, which can be referenced in the DOT's *North American Emergency Response Handbook; A Guidebook for First Responders During the Initial Phase of a Hazardous Material/ Dangerous Goods Incident*. This book should be in every emergency vehicle to help HAZMAT teams determine evacuation areas, fire suppression methods, requisite protective equipment, and medical treatment. CHEMTREC, the Chemical Manufacturers Association, has a 24-hour national HAZMAT Emergency Communications Center (1-800-424-9300), which can provide information on the physical properties of the chemical. The Poison Control Center (1-800-222-1222) can also assist with clinical recommendations for patient treatment.

At a HAZMAT scene, there are three potential zones of operation, hot, warm, and cold. The hot zone is restricted to specially trained personnel wearing appropriate level personal protective equipment (PPE). The cold zone is an area determined to be free of hazards and is where most of the incident operations occur (e.g., command, triage, treatment, and staging). The warm zone is the location of the decontamination corridor and functions as the transition area between the hot and cold zones. Most emergency medical care is rendered in the cold zone after decontamination has occurred.

Decontamination is generally accomplished with copious irrigation. The use of household soap may also be of benefit. It is essential that all clothing and jewelry be removed prior to irrigation. While specialized decontamination may be required for certain chemicals, flushing the skin with water for 15 to 20 minutes is usually sufficient for dilution of most substances. It is important to remember, however, that certain substances, such as white phosphorous, may react with water. Brushing off the dry material may be an important initial step in decontamination of patients exposed to these materials.

Other Areas of EMS Specialization

There are many other areas of EMS specialization, too numerous to discuss in detail, but important to note.

Table 3.2

The 14 Aspects of the EMS System that Require Ongoing Attention According to the *EMS Agenda for the Future*

Integration of Health Services
Research
Legislation & Regulation
System Finance
Human Resources
Medical Direction
Education
Public Education
Prevention
Public Access
Communications
Clinical Care
Information Systems
Evaluation

Wilderness medicine, for example, has become an area of EMS with its own unique set of protocols and treatments. The FARMEDIC program covers special hazards and other situations that may be encountered on farms. The training of advanced scope paramedics to deliver specified treatment without patient hospital transportation has been implemented in certain rural areas. These specialized areas of EMS go above and beyond standard EMT or paramedic training. As EMS continues to evolve, so, too, will EMS specialization.

The Future of EMS

In 1996 the "EMS Agenda for the Future" was published by a multi-disciplined steering committee, a collaborative effort among NHTSA, the Health Resources and Services Administration (HRSA), and the Maternal and Child Health Bureau (MCHB). The document outlines a vision that includes fourteen aspects of the EMS system that require ongoing attention (**Table 3.2**).

For each of the fourteen aspects, the document cites present status and future goals, including suggestions for "how to get there." The committee also collaborated on two other significant documents, the "EMS Research Agenda for the Future" and "EMS Education Agenda" to assist in the realization of the visions outlined in the original agenda. NHTSA, HRSA, and MCHB have since collaborated to create an implementation guide.

Selected Readings

Air Medical Physician Handbook. Air Medical Physicians Association, 1999.

Arizona Emergency Medicine Research Center, University of Arizona Health Sciences Center, Advanced Hazmat Life Support Syllabus.

Bledsoe BE, Cherry RA, Porter RS. Paramedic Care: Principles and Practice. Saddle River, NJ: Prentice Hall, 2000.

Kuehl AE, NAEMSP. Prehospital Systems and Medical Oversight, 3rd Edition Dubuque, IA: Kendall/Hunt, 2002.

U.S. Department of Transportation, Pipeline and Hazardous Materials Safety Administration, Office of Hazardous Materials Safety. Emergency Response Guidebook 2004, Washington, DC: U.S. Government Printing Office, 2004.

Public Health Issues After a Disaster

Stacy N. Weisberg

Health Consequences of a Disaster

The health consequences of a disaster are variable and depend on many factors. First, the type of disaster may influence the health consequences. For example, a natural disaster, such as a hurricane, which damages electricity, hospitals, and power supplies, can have very different health consequences from a man-made disaster, such as a biological terrorism incident which may not damage any existing structures, but can overwhelm the health care system, which requires services such as quarantines and mass antibiotic prophylaxis.

Health consequences are also dependent on the duration of a disaster. A *simple disaster* is one which leaves the community's infrastructure (political, medical, EMS, fire, law enforcement) battered, but intact. Response to a simple disaster usually requires mutual aid. Examples of simple disasters include a 25 car pile-up on a major highway or a building collapse.

An *extended disaster* is one which cripples the community's infrastructure, is prolonged in nature, and covers a large geographical area. A federal response is required for an extended disaster. Examples of extended disasters are the 1993 floods in the Midwest and Hurricane Katrina in 2005. A *complex disaster* is defined as a disaster which involves an entire country and its population and overtakes all socio-economic and political priorities (for example, during the dissolution of Yugoslavia).[1] Both national and foreign government aid is required in this situation.

The initial health care response to a disaster usually emphasizes treating immediate needs, for example, illness and injury directly related to the disaster. These direct medical conditions usually predominate during simple and extended disasters. The injuries are usually traumatic in origin (e.g., crush injuries from a building collapse during an earthquake, respiratory emergencies from ash inhalation during a volcanic eruption, eye injuries from flying debris during a tornado).

However, there are also indirect medical consequences, most often seen during extended and complex disasters. People in affected areas with normally stable, chronic, medical conditions can become ill from the loss of the medical infrastructure. For example, a patient with diabetes may be unable to obtain insulin; or someone with emphysema may be unable to obtain aerosol therapy and may consequently suffer an exacerbation of his or her respiratory symptoms from a combination of lack of medication and decrease in air quality secondary to fires, or other environmental disasters.

Other indirect medical consequences include environmental emergencies from lack of intact shelter and clothing. Victims are susceptible to heat, cold, and sun exposure. They are also at increased risk of infection from decaying animals, insect bites and stings, and injuries from displaced animals wandering through the area. Persons residing in areas affected by an extended or complex disaster must be carefully monitored for infectious diseases and dietary deficiencies. Immunization programs may need to be implemented for these victims to prevent outbreaks of preventable illnesses.

It is also important to remember that there are psychological consequences to disasters. Not only can a disaster and its consequences cause new-onset psychological illnesses, such as depression and post-traumatic stress disorder, but such an event can exacerbate chronic conditions. People with pre-existing psychological illnesses may suffer from psychotic episodes, increased abusive behavior, or worsening depression.

The health consequences of a disaster can be varied and extensive and are both related to the immediate disaster and the recovery. It is important to remember that people will suffer from medical conditions beyond the immediate trauma from the disaster itself.[2]

One of the most recent examples of a devastating disaster, with an aftermath that may be worse than the disaster itself, is the tsunami in the Indian Ocean which struck in late December 2004. This was the world's worst earthquake in 40 years, measuring a 9.0 on the Richter scale. Per media reports, this disaster killed over 150,000 people from Malaysia to Somalia. However, this number will continue to rise, as those who initially survived the quake will die from the consequences.

Immediate needs for survivors have included trauma care, shelter, and safe water. Most survivable injuries are traumatic, including orthopedic injuries, lacerations, and contusions. Caring for these victims has constituted the majority of the immediate medical needs. As many people lost homes, leaving them susceptible to the elements, shelter also becomes an immediate need after such a disaster. The tsunami also caused the destruction of water purification systems, leaving a very large number of people without access to clean, safe water supplies. Safe water is critical to prevent morbidity and mortality from communicable water-borne diseases, such as cholera. The destruction of the transportation system, including railway, roads, and bridges has made delivery of water and supplies difficult, if not often impossible. Some alternative delivery methods used include elephants, which can traverse the rough and broken terrain, and aircraft, which can drop supplies down from above. After these immediate needs are met, public health interventions can then concentrate on longer term management plans. These include continuing to provide safe food and water to those in need and immunizations for highly communicable illnesses, such as measles for those living in close quarters, like shelters. Other public health needs include aid to reestablish medical facilities, long-term health care for those with chronic medical conditions, and mental health services.

As stated, not all disasters require the same public health services. Refugees and displaced persons resulting from civil wars and genocide demand a very different type of health care. The first issue in caring for such victims is patient access. These persons are often located in areas which are politically unstable and generally considered unsafe. Currently, one such area is Darfur, Sudan, where many African ethnic groups have attempted to escape to Chad to flee Arab Janjaweed attacks. Those that have relocated to the refugee camps in Chad have been able to receive medical care, while those still in Sudan cannot be accurately accounted for, let alone given medical care. The World Health Organization has been able to determine that mortality rates for those in West Darfur are above the emergency benchmark. Most people are dying from diarrhea due to clean water shortages. International organizations continue to have only limited access to some of these persons due to government restrictions.[3] In situations such as Darfur, the medical infrastructure has been completely disrupted, most especially for those in refugee camps. Besides suffering from illness and malnourishment, these persons are also often victims of torture and have, in addition, complex mental health needs.[4] Successful care requires practical knowledge of the culture and working with preexisting medical organizations, if available, and with the new government to reestablish health care capabilities for all persons.

Emergency Health Needs Assessment

An emergency health needs assessment following a disaster is an opportunity to uncover or predict deficiencies which can lead to further health consequences in a stricken community. The goal, early in the disaster response, is to identify urgent needs and to determine relief priorities for the affected population. These assessments are then used to match available resources to emergency needs. This assessment helps prevent decisions which could result in send-

ing useless medication and other unnecessary medical supplies to a disaster site. The emergency health needs assessment should evaluate the following areas:

1. Overall magnitude and effect of the disaster (e.g., geographical extent, number of affected persons, estimated duration of disaster).
2. Effect of the disaster on health (number of patients).
3. Integrity of the health services delivery systems.
4. Specific health care needs of survivors.
5. Disruption of other services relevant to public health (e.g., power, water, sanitation).
6. Available resources in the area.
7. Extent of the disaster response by local authorities.[5]

The health effects of a disaster can be determined by objective measurements, which include morbidity, mortality, number of damaged houses, number of homeless persons, number of nonfunctioning hospitals, and the status of community lifelines (e.g., water, electricity, gas, and sewage disposal).

Once collected, this information is used to plan the immediate responses. The goal of these immediate responses is to determine which early interventions will prevent the greatest loss of life or severe morbidity.

Disease Control and Prevention

A disaster-stricken area is more susceptible to infectious diseases. Large amounts of standing water in a flood-stricken region serve as a breeding ground for mosquitoes, which can transmit vector-born diseases (e.g., West Nile virus) to victims in the area. Breakdown in sanitation systems can also result in contaminated water supplies, and subsequent consumption of contaminated water can result in many bacterial and parasitic gastrointestinal illnesses.

Victims of a disaster-stricken area may leave their homes or lose their homes, then relocate to emergency shelter. Shelters house many people in very close quarters, which can lead to an increase in communicable diseases, especially those spread by respiratory droplets.

Although not all communicable diseases can be prevented after a disaster, incorporating some of the following steps into the disaster response can help limit the outbreaks and spread of disease. For example, although emergency shelters may be necessary, housing large numbers of people in close proximity or refugee camps should be discouraged. When possible, areas with standing water should be sprayed for mosquitoes. Potable water should be brought into a disaster-stricken area as soon as possible until the water and sanitation systems can be repaired. Residents should be discouraged from drinking water which cannot be clearly identified as safe.

Disease surveillance systems should also be implemented in the disaster area to track any illnesses. These are helpful for identifying diseases that can be controlled by immunization or quarantine. Monitoring the affected populations helps in early identification of the emergence or increased prevalence of an infectious disease.

Lastly, it should be noted that new diseases are unlikely to emerge in the disaster area. The most common illnesses are an increase in infections already seen in that geographical region. For example, a flood-stricken area of the Midwest is unlikely to experience an outbreak of cholera or malaria, whereas these diseases may be of serious concern in a refugee camp in Thailand.[6]

The best method of disease control is prevention. Knowledge of the region's common diseases, immunizations, where appropriate, and early intervention in a disaster region can greatly limit the spread of many highly contagious and disabling diseases.

References

1. Rega P, Bissell R. Disaster health: Health consequences and response. *NDMS Response Team Training Program Core Curriculum,* Section 141.
2. Noji EK. The public health consequences of disasters. *Prehospital Disaster Med* 2000;15:147–157.
3. Fowler J. Beyond human bandages—confronting genocide in Sudan. *N Engl J Med* 2004;351:2574–2576.
4. Shrestha NM, Sharma B, et al. Impact of torture on refugees displaced within the developing world. *JAMA* 1998;280:443–448.
5. Noji EK. Disaster epidemiology. *Emerg Med Clinics North Am* 1996;14:289–301.
6. Howard MJ, Brillman JC, Burkle Jr, FM. Infectious disease emergencies in disasters. *Emerg Med Clinics North Am* 1996;14:413–428.

5 Disaster Triage

Stacy N. Weisberg

Disaster Triage

Triage is defined as the medical screening of patients to determine relative priority for treatment. In the disaster situation, there are often large numbers of patients, limited medical resources, and prolonged scene times compared with triage in the general out-of-hospital setting. The overall goal of triage is to do the most good for the largest number of people using limited resources.

Disaster triage is divided into two phases: the immediate triage and the secondary triage. Immediate triage is usually carried out by local providers and follows the out-of-hospital model using the Simple Triage and Rapid Treatment method (START). Secondary triage is usually performed by disaster medical responders and follows Secondary Assessment of Victim Endpoint (SAVE) protocols.

START Triage

The START triage system was developed in California in the 1980s by Hoag Hospital and Newport Beach Fire and Marine. START was designed as the first triage or "start" of rapid approach to treating large numbers of casualties, where each patient is assessed in less than 60 seconds, allowing the opportunity to rapidly identify patients who require immediate interventions.

Each patient assessed is using a set of primary observations or RPM:

Respirations (>30), Perfusion (>2 seconds),
Mental Status ("can do").

According to assessment, patients are then immediately tagged by one of four categories by color and designation, indicating medical status:

1. Red, Immediate: altered RPM, designating immediate care
2. Yellow, Delayed: RPM normal, designating delayed care (majority of victims)
3. Green, Minor: designating minor care or "walking wounded" (may be later re-tagged)
4. Black, Dead: designating mortal wounds, including those who are dead or who will die despite medical attention

The method of START triage is shown in **FIGURE 5.1**.

In START triage, the first task of the triage officer is make the following announcement to the crowd (preferably with some type of public address system):

"If you can walk, please stand up and go over to the secondary assessment area." All victims who can follow this command are then tagged green as they proceed to the secondary triage area where their injuries can be evaluated. Patients can then be re-tagged as yellow or red depending on the severity of condition. At this stage, the only interventions performed by the triage officer include repositioning of the airway and control of bleeding (patients with uncontrolled bleeding are tagged red); and the triage officer should move on to the next patient in order to keep patient assessment within 60 seconds.

A patient who is not breathing upon initial assessment should be reassessed after repositioning of the airway. If respirations remain absent, patients are tagged black. Those who begin breathing and/or who have a respiratory rate greater than 30 breaths per minute should be tagged red. No further assessment of these patients is necessary. Patients breathing less than 30 times per minute who have absent or irregular pulse are also tagged red. Continued assessment of capillary refill should occur only in patients with a regular pulse. If capillary refill is more than 2 seconds, the patient is probably in shock and needs to be tagged red. Mental status should only be assessed in patients who are breathing less than 30 times per minute, with regular pulse and capillary refill of less than 2 seconds. Mental status is assessed by "can do": if the patient can follow a simple command (e.g., squeeze a hand upon request), then they can be tagged yellow. If the patient cannot follow this instruction, then it is assumed they have a head injury and are tagged red.

During the triage operation, a second group of rescuers follows behind the triage officer to bring patients to the different areas. Patients tagged red should be brought to where they can receive immediate medical care, or a medical crew should be brought to these patients. Those with yellow tags should be brought to an area where they can receive medical care after those requiring immediate inter-

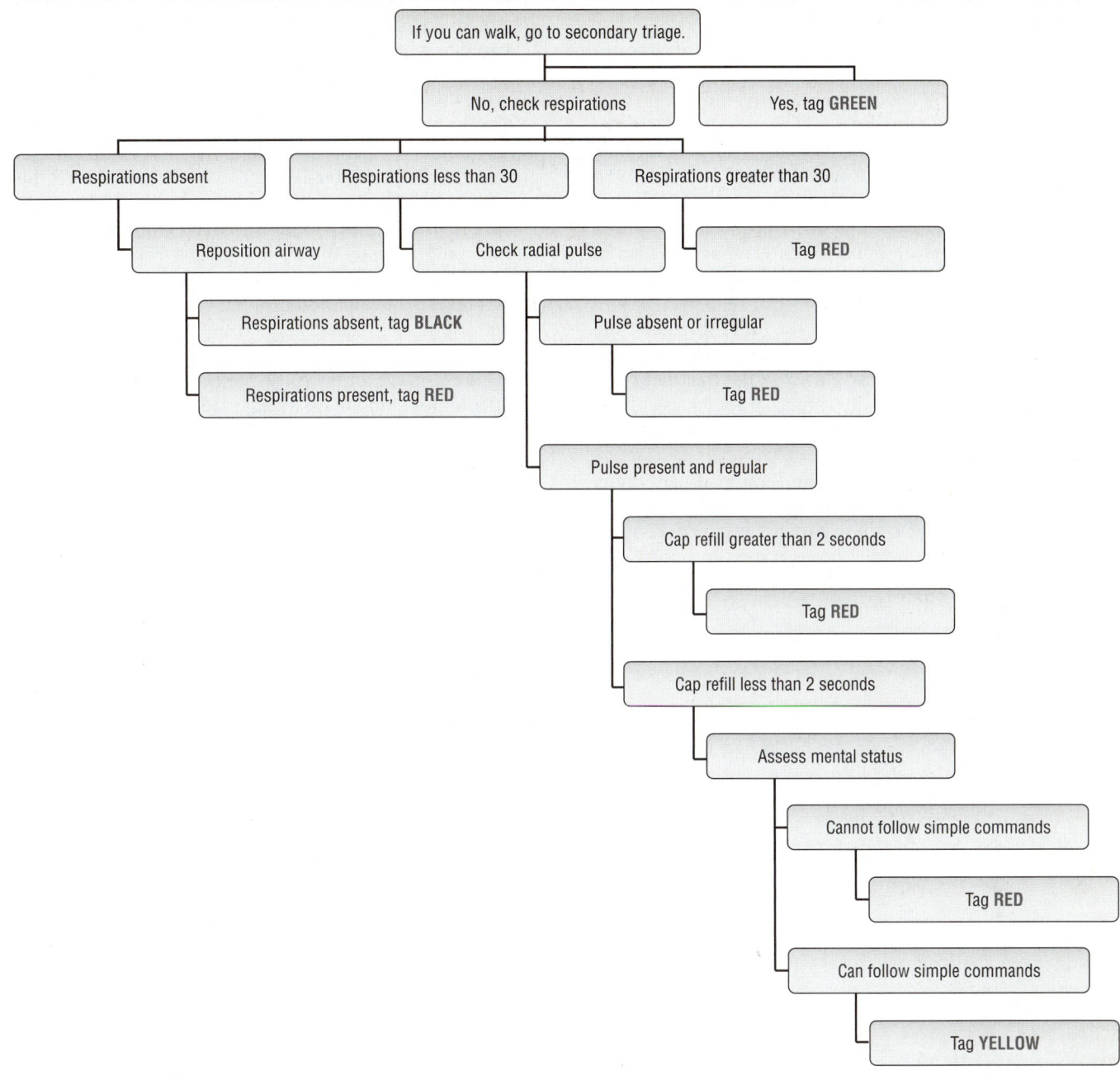

FIGURE 5.1 START triage algorithm.

ventions. Those tagged black should be brought away from the medical care area.

Victims can be identified by using tags with colored tear-off tabs that contain basic information or by using colored ribbons. Any triage system should use the same color system as noted above, so that all rescuers can understand which patients require immediate medical care.

Triage is a dynamic process: a patient's condition can quickly change, requiring re-classification. START triage is only intended for triaging adult patients (8 years of age or older). Triaging younger children requires use of a modified version of START (this is addressed in Chapter 7).

SAVE

The goal of SAVE is to direct limited resources to the subgroup of patients expected to benefit the most from their use. It is intended for catastrophic disasters where patients can receive immediate on-scene care, but transport from the disaster site to a hospital or other medical facility will be significantly delayed.

SAVE goes beyond START to assess survivability of patients with various injuries based on trauma statistics, using the following formula:

Benefit Expected $\times$ Probability of Survival $=$ Value of Resources Required

Patients are then placed into 3 categories:

1. Those who will die regardless of care.
2. Those who will survive whether or not they receive care.
3. Those who will benefit from limited immediate field intervention.

Based on these 3 categories, patients, who were initially assessed using START triage, are reassessed. Those who will die regardless of care are placed in an observation area where they can be reassessed for improvement. Those who will survive and do not need care are also placed in an observation area. Here, they can receive basic care and periodic reassessment.

Those patients who fall into the third category are brought to an area where they are treated in order of severity and resources. Patients are placed in the treatment category based on two critical questions:

1. What is the victim's prognosis if minimal treatment is provided?
2. What is the victim's prognosis with treatment using resources available at the treatment site?

The goal of treatment for these patients is to reduce morbidity and mortality, while not to use an inordinate amount of resources. Patients who do not respond to treatment are re-tagged and placed in the observation area.

Patients who would benefit most from early transport should be identified in the event that transportation and resources become available.

The purpose of triage is to do the most good for the most number of people through the use of the limited amount of resources available. This can be a difficult, but necessary task in the disaster setting. A simple, but rapid triage system like START, helps to make difficult decisions and to complete assessment of large numbers of victims in order to facilitate care to those with immediate need. SAVE and other evaluation programs help to ration and allocate resources in a disaster setting where there are large numbers of victims and limited resources. START and SAVE are not the only triage methods, but they are the most common and are easily adapted in most disaster and mass casualty incidents.

Selected Readings

Benson M, Koenig KL, Schultz CH. Disaster Triage: START then SAVE—a new method of dynamic triage for victims of a catastrophic earthquake. Prehospital Disaster Med 1996;11:117–124.

Disaster Triage. DMAT on-line training session. Basic Curriculum, Section 142.

Critical Incident Stress Debriefing

Stacy N. Weisberg

Critical Incident Stress Debriefing (CISD) is a single session, group crisis intervention process. The objective of CISD is for victims and responders of a stressful event to openly discuss their feelings with peers and mental health personnel.

The debriefing, usually lasting from one to three hours, is typically held within one week of the end of a disaster.

CISD was first introduced in 1974 by Jeffrey Mitchell, PhD, who had served as a volunteer firefighter in Maryland, after he had conducted debriefings of all emergency response personnel after unusually stressful response situations. Initially, the goal of Mitchell's research was to learn how to slow the attrition rate of first responders in his area. Mitchell published and formally introduced CISD into the fire and EMS community in 1982. At the time, several recent tragedies, including the 1978 Pacific Southwest Airlines Crash in San Diego, the fire at the MGM Grand hotel in Las Vegas in 1980, and the 1981 Hyatt Regency Skywalk Collapse in Kansas City had increased the country's awareness of the special needs of emergency services personnel.

The CISD process was designed to target emergency support services and personnel, including firefighters, police officers, soldiers, and emergency medical services (EMS) workers. CISD goals include prevention of chronic post traumatic stress disorder; screening of personnel for additional mental health treatment; facilitating verbalization of experiences; normalizing reactions to stressful events; and improving peer group support and cohesion.[1]

The Mitchell model, the original model for CISD, consists of seven phases to be covered during the single CISD session:

1. Introduction: The CISD team (mental health professionals and peer support personnel) introduces members, explains the process, sets expectations and ground rules.
2. Fact: Participants describe the trauma from their own perspective.
3. Thought: Participants describe their thoughts about the event.
4. Reaction: Participants can choose to speak about the most traumatic aspect of the crisis.
5. Symptom: The group can choose to share symptoms of distress and psychological discord.
6. Teaching: Participants are taught basic personal stress management techniques; participants' crisis reactions are normalized.
7. Re-entry. Closure of the CISD process, remembering the goal to provide psychological closure to the crisis event.[2]

The CISD process has been used by many emergency response agencies, including the Los Angeles County Fire Department (LACoFD) since 1986.[3] LACoFD members have participated in CISD after the Cerritos Air Crash, fire storms, earthquakes, and after any other smaller-scale incidents.

Professional responders were surveyed regarding incidents where they had participated in CISD and those where they had not. This was one of the largest studies to examine the effectiveness of CISD and found that those who participated were more likely to experience a reduction in stressful symptoms at a faster rate. A majority of the participants in the study would recommend the process to others, including those who did not find CISD personally helpful, underscoring the importance and perceived helpfulness of critical incident stress debriefing after a disaster situation.[4]

After the attacks of September 11, 2001, many rescue, pre-hospital, and health care workers participated in the CISD process. Recommendations from these events are that CISD should be incorporated into hospital and regional disaster plans. It is important that debriefing be conducted by experienced personnel who were not involved with the disaster. The debriefing should include all those involved, including dispatchers, who are a group frequently forgotten as part of emergency response efforts. Lastly, it must be recognized that all who have participated in the disaster response (including those who conduct the CISD) may require time beyond the briefing process before being able to return to regular duties.[5]

References

1. Bledsoe BE. Critical Incident Stress Management (CISM): Benefit or risk for emergency services? *Prehospital Emerg Care* 2003;7:272–279.
2. Mitchell JT. CISM at a glance. *J Emerg Med Services* 2002;57.
3. Hokanson M, Wirth B. The critical incident stress debriefing process for the Los Angeles County Fire Department: Automatic and effective. *Int J Emerg Mental Health* 2000;2:249–257.
4. Van Emmerik AAP, Kamphuis JH, Hulsbosch AM, et al. Single session debriefing after psychological trauma: A meta analysis. *Lancet* 2002;360:766–771.
5. Hammond J, Brook, J. The World Trade Center attack: Helping the helpers: The role of critical incident stress management. *Crit Care* 2001;5:315–317.

Pediatric Disaster Medicine

Andrew L. Garrett

The medical needs of infants and children in the disaster setting are an essential part of preparation for post-disaster care. After 2001, the paradigm of disaster medicine has expanded to include both natural- and human-caused disasters. Human-caused disasters may take the form of accidental incidents (e.g., a chemical spill) or a terrorism event (e.g., a nuclear or biological attack). Any disaster challenges even the most prepared providers when the victims include infants and children.

Children (including infants for the purposes of this discussion) are at a higher risk of injury during a disaster. In a chemical or biological exposure, children are more likely to be exposed due to hand-to-mouth behavior, proximity to the ground, and their higher respiratory rate. Due to their higher surface-to-body ratio, children are also much more susceptible to the effects of heat and cold (for example, when children have been decontaminated with cold water, even after arriving at the hospital). In a blast, the smaller mass of a child can become an airborne projectile, often head-first. The relatively large internal organs of a child are less protected by the skeleton, and more likely to receive an injury from projectiles, blast wave, or secondary impact. Additionally, a child is more likely to suffer the effects of malnutrition and/or dehydration as a disaster incident evolves.

The pediatric subpopulation is one that has traditionally been de-emphasized in disaster medicine, but this situation continues to improve as more attention has been given to disaster medicine in general. Children require a modified approach to routine disaster preparation.

Airway management is an excellent example. Contrary to adult physiology, cardiorespiratory decompensation in children is frequently due to a primary ventilatory disorder. This issue alone has led to the development of a modified triage protocol for children involved in a mass casualty situation. JumpSTART is a triage tool which has been objectively tested and which addresses the need to attempt airway maneuvers before black-tagging a child as unsalvageable, as one would with an adult in the same situation. Child-specific triage systems need to be in place in both the pre-hospital and in-hospital setting for any mass casualty incident (MCI) or disaster.

The area of pharmaceuticals for biological agent treatment and prophylaxis is another example. Many standard medications for disaster use are relatively contraindicated in children during day-to-day usage (e.g., ciprofloxacin and doxycycline). However, these drugs are commonly available and may be essential to use during a biological event when mass prophylaxis or treatment is required. Alternatives for children may exist, but clinicians must be familiar with them, have them available, and have a mechanism in place to guide their use. A failure to plan ahead could leave the pediatric segment of the population inadequately covered in planning and response capacities.

A third example is the need to maintain routine preventive care in children after a disaster. Children have many more routine immunization and health care needs than healthy adults; these should be maintained and emphasized after a disaster, especially vaccinations to prevent communicable disease.

There are special logistic circumstances to consider when planning to accommodate the handling and treatment of pediatric patients in the aftermath of a disaster. For example, a child may not be accompanied by a parent when a disaster occurs during school hours. Therefore, disaster response planning must include a mechanism to identify, track, supervise, and reunite unaccompanied minors with their families. Disaster planning must include consideration of emergency guardianship of children and the needs of medically complex children with special health care needs (CSHCN).

Disaster medical care for children can take place in a variety of situations, and each environment has its own special needs that must be addressed. The pediatric triage and treatment needs of a hospital require extensive pre-planning, especially as it pertains to decontamination, triage, emergency stabilization, and inpatient care. Medical clinics are not typically thought of as emergency rooms, but in times of disaster, clinics may become an important source of both urgent and routine medical care; therefore, clinics must also have emergency plans in place in order to remain functional during a crisis. The pre-hospital setting has its own needs, for example child-specific triage and the demand for specialized pediatric equipment that may be hard to come by in large quantities during an emergency.

Table 7.1

Pediatric Equipment and Skills Useful in a Disaster

- A child-based triage system (e.g., JumpSTART), previously practiced
- Child-friendly decontamination options (warm water, dry clothing)
- Emergency medication and antidotes (Atropine, 2-PAM, ACLS/PALS medications)
- Child-sized immobilization and restraint equipment (C-collar, backboard, car seats)
- Child-sized diagnostic equipment
- Child-sized airway equipment (laryngoscopes, O_2 masks, chest tubes, etc.)
- Child-sized vascular access equipment (18 to 24 gauge needles, butterflies, central line kits)
- Length-based weight estimation measuring tape (Broselow Tape)
- Toys or other distraction items (stuffed animal, pinwheel, etc.)
- Neonatal kits (clamps, suction, warmer, etc.)
- Routine childhood vaccinations (tetanus, pertussis, hepatitis, etc.)
- Plan for emergency guardianship of unaccompanied children
- Plan for communicating with parents who are searching for their children
- Plan for CSHCN children (coordinated with schools, specialists)
- Plan for emergency mental health care
- Plan for emergency social work response
- A site specific plan to respond to a disaster or MCI situation, one that is practiced and published for all appropriate staff members

Table 7.2

Antibiotic Therapy and Prophylaxis for Pediatric Patients

Disease	Therapy or Prophylaxis	Medication and Dosage
Inhalational Anthrax	Therapy—stable pts can switch to single oral agent after 2 weeks to treat for 2 mos total	ciprofloxacin 10-15 mg/kg IV q12h or doxycycline 2.2 mg/kg IV q12h (max 100mg) and clindamycin 10-15 mg/kg IV q8h and PCN G 400-600k U/kg/d div q4h
	Prophylaxis (60 days)	ciprofloxacin 10-15 mg/kg PO q12h (max 500 mg/dose) or doxycycline 2.2 mg/kg PO q12h (max 100 mg)
Cutaneous Anthrax, Endemic	Therapy	PCN V 40-80 mg/kg/d PO div q6h or amoxicillin 40-80 mg/kg/d PO div q8h or ciprofloxacin 10-15 mg/kg PO q12h (max 1 g/day) or doxycycline 2.2 mg/kg PO q12h (max 100 mg/dose)
Cutaneous Anthrax, Terrorism	Therapy	ciprofloxacin 10-15 mg/kg PO q12h (max 1 g/day) or doxycycline 2.2 mg/kg PO q12h (max 100 mg/dose)
Gastrointestinal Anthrax	Therapy	same as for inhalational
Smallpox	Therapy	supportive care
	Prophylaxis	?vaccination (early)
Plague	Therapy	gentamicin 2.5 mg/kg IV q8h or streptomycin 15 mg/kg IM q12h (max 2 g/day) or doxycycline 2.2 mg/kg IV q12h (max 200 mg/day) or ciprofloxacin 15 mg/kg IV q12h or chloramphenicol 25 mg/kg q6h (max 4 g/day)
	Prophylaxis	doxycycline 2.2 mg/kg PO q12h or ciprofloxacin 20 mg/kg PO q12h
Tularemia	Therapy	same as for plague
Botulism	Therapy	supportive, ?antitoxin (early)
Viral Hemorrhagic Fevers	Therapy	supportive care, ?ribavirin
Brucellosis	Therapy	TMP/SMX 30 mg/kg PO q12h plus rifampin 15 mg/kg PO q24h or gentamicin 7.5 mg/kg IM qd $\times$ 5

Finally, the field hospital operating during a disaster must also hold itself to a high standard with respect to its ability to triage and treat children appropriately.

In an emergency, unless the available facility routinely treats children, ensuring access to pediatric emergency supplies even on a day-to-day basis may be a challenge in its own right. Pediatric-sized gear typically comes in multiple sizes for different age groups, and it can be difficult to sort, store, and to use in a crisis if one is not familiar with its setup. The ability to promptly obtain a patient weight must also be planned for, especially if a parent is not present with the child. A length-based weight estimation tape or a scale is important to have available. Pediatric pharmaceuticals also frequently require refrigerated storage, which should be considered with regard to storage in the medical facility and at the child's home or shelter after leaving the hospital.

Pediatric Equipment and Supplies

Depending on the operational environment, the need for specialized pediatric emergency equipment may vary (**Table 7.1**).

Regardless of the equipment, triage system, or decontamination setup that is available to the provider, they are useless if their utilization is not practiced. It is essential to remember that disasters do not routinely occur during business hours and on a weekday—a disaster response system must include working with what you have during the initial phase of the incident while resources are assembled. In the preliminary stages of a public crisis, it is unlikely that you will be able to rely on an outside agency such as a fire department or state health department to provide services such as decontamination, pharmacy, or triage services.

Essential Pediatric Medications During a Disaster

Fortunately, most of the medications that we rely upon every day in Emergency Medicine are the same ones that will be utilized during a disaster, with a few exceptions. In the event of a chemical or biological attack, the ability to provide prompt administration of antidotes or antibiotic treatment may be paramount for patient survival.

The usual medications will be needed in larger quantities. A starting point is to stockpile a 2-day supply plus 100 doses. Much more may be needed depending on the situation. Examples in this category are the antibiotics amoxicillin, penicillin, trimethoprim/sulfate, ciprofloxacin, doxycycline, clindamycin, ceftriaxone, and gentamicin. **Table 7.2** illustrates some antibiotics that may be required for specific emergencies. Vaccinations such as tetanus, hepatitis B, pertussis, diphtheria, varicella, influenza, and measles/mumps/rubella are important to keep available. Standard emergency medications, antibiotics, and IV fluids must be available and the facility must have an established plan for restocking when demand is extreme.

Mass prophylaxis is an activity that can tax any medical system. The need for a pre-organized plan to screen patients and dispense antibiotic or antiradionuclide medication cannot be underemphasized. There are state and federal resources that may need to become involved if a large scale effort is undertaken. Extraordinary circumstances, for example, the 2001 U.S. Postal Service mass anthrax prophylaxis project, may require hundreds of providers and numerous federal resources to manage thousands of exposed patients.

It is the unusual medications that may be the most difficult to acquire and utilize during a disaster. After an exposure to nerve agent, the prompt administration of atropine and pralidoxime (2-PAM) may be lifesaving and is the primary treatment. Unfortunately, the ubiquitous Mark-I kit (one atropine autoinjector and one pralidoxime autoinjector) provides excessive dosing of both medications for an infant or child. Pediatric autoinjectors are available but not routinely deployed domestically. It has been described that the adult autoinjectors can be used to dispense agent into a sterile container such as a specimen cup, and then a pediatric dose can be obtained secondarily. Another agent that is not typically available in a pediatric dosage is potassium iodide (KI), which is indicated as prompt prophylaxis after a radiological release (**Table 7.3**). describes how to make an oral suspension of the

Table 7.3		
Potassium Iodide (KI) Oral Suspension Recipe for Pediatric Use After a Radiological Incident		
	130 mg Adult Tablet	**65 mg Adult Tablet**
grind with spoon in small bowl	↓	↓
add 4 tsp/ 20 ml water and mix to dissolve	↓	↓
add 4 tsp/ 20 mL of milk, soda, or flavored syrup	↓	↓
mixture concentration	16.25 mg/tsp (1 tsp=5 mL)	8.125 mg/tsp (1 tsp=5 mL)
dosing guideline for newborn-1 mo.	1 tsp	2 tsp
dosing guideline for 1 mo. to 3 yrs	2 tsp	4 tsp
dosing guideline for 4 yrs-17 yrs.	4 tsp or 1 130 mg tablet if > 70 kg	8 tsp or 1 65 mg tablet if < 70 kg. or 2 65 mg tablets if > 70 kg

medication for pediatric use. Other agents that may be useful after a radiation incident are the cell-line stimulators such as Epogen and Neupogen. Specific chelation drugs may also be utilized in certain types of radiation exposures.

Conclusion

The planning and preparation that is required to adequately care for children in the disaster setting are extensive and must be practiced to be effective. There are many unique needs that must be addressed, such as decontamination, triage, and emergency medication therapy. There are many resources that are available to the emergency medicine physician, including information that is on-line or that may be available by developing a relationship with the pediatricians in your area.

As the definition of disaster changes in our society, our commitment to providing equal disaster medical health care to children becomes even more important.

Resources

National Center for Disaster Preparedness, Pediatric Preparedness for Disasters and Terrorism: A National Consensus Conference, Executive Summary 2003.
Center for Disease Control Emergency Preparedness and Response Section, http://www.bt.cdc.gov.
Center for Pediatric Emergency Medicine, http://www.cpem.org/html/gf.html.
American Academy of Pediatrics, www.aap.org.
Jump START Pediatric Multiple Casualty Triage, www.jumpstarttriage.com.

Radiation Exposures, Blast Injury, and Bioterrorism

Kurt R. Horst
James A. Fitch

Blast Injury

The widespread availability and use of explosives has resulted in an ever-increasing number of casualties over the last several decades.[1] The terrorist bombings in Oklahoma City in 1995 as well as the attack on the World Trade Center in 2001 continue to highlight the growing number of events occurring within the United States.[2] An understanding of the mechanisms of blast injury is crucial for the emergency physician to properly triage, diagnose, and treat expected injuries.

Mechanism of Blast Injury

Injuries are typically divided into four categories: primary, secondary, tertiary, and miscellaneous.[1,3] Primary blast injury primarily effects gas containing organs and is caused directly by the blast wave as it spreads out from the initial explosion.[1,4,5] The wave passing through the body causes damage by four mechanisms. *Spalling* refers to the throwing of fluid particles from a more to less dense medium as the wave passes.[1,2] This occurs in tissues containing both liquid and gas, such as the lungs and gastrointestinal tract.[1] *Implosion* describes the initial compression of gas pockets that then reexpand with greater force after the blast wave passes.[1] This is the typical cause of tympanic membrane rupture.[1] A variety of injuries result from *inertia* whereby the victim is accelerated toward stationary objects.[1] At the moment the blast wave impacts the body, *pressure differentials* between liquid and air drives blood from the pulmonary capillaries into the alveolar spaces, contributing to pulmonary hemorrhage.[1,5]

Secondary injury is the result of surrounding debris being thrown into the air and impacting the body.[1-3] Objects deliberately attached to the bomb such as nails and bolts also cause damage by this mechanism.[1,3] Tertiary blast injuries are seen as the victim's body is thrown against stationary objects.[1-3] Miscellaneous injuries such as flash burns may result from the intense heat which is released from the explosion.[1,3] While this release of heat is brief, other combustibles in the room or the victim's clothing may ignite causing more significant thermal injury.[1,3]

General Management

As with any mass casualty incident, scene safety is paramount. With the risk of terrorist bombings, an awareness of the potential for a secondary device is essential to prevent further injuries amongst rescue personnel.[1] Appropriate and effective triage and decontamination when necessary will also hasten the care provided.[1,2] In general, mortality tends to be higher when the victim is closer to the blast, the blast occurs indoors or is associated with building collapse, and when there is a lack of medical resources available to provide care on-scene.[1-3] Some specific injury patterns and essential therapies are described below.

Specific Injury Patterns

Auditory

An array of hearing deficits arise after blast injury, and rupture of the tympanic membrane is common, and may be a marker of more severe injury.[1,3]

Nervous System

Head injury is common and the typical array of closed head and penetrating injuries will be seen.[1,2] Early diagnosis via CT scan and neurosurgical drainage and debridement when necessary are crucial.[1] Vertebral injuries, while commonly seen among fatalities, occur less frequently in survivors.[1]

Pulmonary

Primary blast lung injury (BLI) may be seen to varying degrees and may present with the classic triad of apnea, bradycardia, and hypotension.[1,4,5] Air embolism, bronchopleural fistula, pulmonary edema, and hemorrhage may occur and present with hypoxia and respiratory distress.[1,2,4,5] Infiltrates may appear early on chest radiograph in severe cases.[5] Supplemental oxygen should be provided.[1,2] Intubation and mechanical ventilation should be avoided if possible as this may increase the risk of air embolism and further barotrauma.[1,2] Unconventional therapies such as extracorporeal membrane oxygenation may have some benefit.[5] Fluids should be restricted when possible to avoid further exacerbation of pulmonary edema.[1,2] Additional injuries such as pneumothorax, penetrating wounds, and pulmonary contusion may be seen and treated as usual.[1,5]

Gastrointestinal

Primary blast injury may also be seen in the gastrointestinal tract, especially if the blast occurs while underwater.[1] Mesenteric injury, hemorrhage, and delayed perforation may arise as well as the typical array of penetrating and blunt abdominal trauma.[1,3] Intravenous fluids and nasogastric suction should be instituted early.[1]

Traumatic Amputation

Traumatic amputation deserves special note as it is a marker for severe injury, as less than 2% of such victims survive.[1,2,3] Reimplantation is generally impossible, and antibiotics and tetanus prophylaxis should be delivered.[1]

Miscellaneous

Penetrating wounds should be explored as foreign bodies are to be expected.[1] Excellent wound care, including debridement when needed, is imperative, and wounds should be reexamined frequently to identify secondary infection.[1] Tetanus prophylaxis should be given and prophylactic antibiotics may be of use.[1] Fractures are also commonly seen, and are often associated with lacerations that may require debridement and late amputations.[1]

Psychological

Victims as well as rescue workers are at increased risk of developing post traumatic disorders, and should be counseled accordingly.[1,2]

The majority of survivors will suffer common and often minor traumatic injuries.[2] However, an awareness of primary blast injury and other patterns of trauma will improve the recognition and treatment of these potentially life-threatening conditions.

Radiation Injury

The accidents at Three Mile Island in 1979 and at Chernobyl in 1986 have highlighted the potential and actual consequences of radiation exposure.[6,7] With the increased use of nuclear substances in research, in the generation of energy, and increased the risk of its use as a method of terrorism, radiation casualties present a new challenge to emergency workers around the world.[8,9] Exposure may occur through detonation of a nuclear weapon, release from a nuclear reactor, or more likely from detonation of explosives wrapped in radioactive material (a so-called dirty bomb).[6,8,9]

Ionizing radiation takes the form of alpha and beta particles, as well as gamma and x-rays.[6,10] Alpha particles are heavy, do not travel far and additionally do not penetrate intact skin.[9,10] They typically pose a threat when ingested, inhaled, or enter the body through wounds or breaks in the skin.[9,10] Beta particles can penetrate skin and travel a greater distance in air.[10] Both gamma rays and x-rays are forms of electromagnetic radiation which travel greater distances and have further penetration.[10] Radiation expo-

sure may be measured in rads (radiation absorbed dose) or Grays, with 1 Gray equivalent to 100 rads.[6,9] Exposure to 1 Gray produces nausea in vomiting in 10% of those exposed, while 6 Gray results in 100 percent mortality within 30 days without medical treatment.[9]

Localized radiation exposure produces an injury similar to a thermal burn.[9] Signs generally appear a few days and include erythema and blistering.[9] Ulceration and necrosis may appear months to years after the initial wound heals due to vascular insufficiency caused by the exposure.[7,9] Initial therapy includes treatment of infection and skin grafting when needed.[9] Acute radiation syndrome (ARS) occurs after whole body irradiation from a strong penetrating source usually over a short time period.[9,10] A prodromal phase consisting of nausea and vomiting generally occurs within 12 hours and may last up to 48 hours.[7,9] This is generally followed by an asymptomatic latent phase.[6,7,10] The symptoms of the illness phase depend on the specific syndrome and may include bone marrow suppression, infection, severe diarrhea, fever, convulsions, and coma.[6,7,9] This is followed by either recovery or death.[6,7,9]

Those who have sustained a radiation exposure, but who have not been contaminated, do not pose a risk to health care providers and should be treated as usual.[6,10] External decontamination should be performed at the scene when possible and levels of radioactivity should be monitored with a Geiger-Mueller instrument.[6] Rescuers should wear protective gloves, gown, mask, hat, and shoe covers.[6,9,10] Clothing should be removed and bagged.[6,9,10] Decontamination should begin with irrigation of wounds and areas of open skin with sterile saline.[6] Foreign bodies should be removed and the wound should be monitored for radioactivity.[6] The wound should be covered with plastic if contamination remains after multiple attempts of irrigation.[6] Intact skin should then be washed with soap and water, being careful not to abrade or irritate the skin.[6] Other agents such as surgical scrub soaps or bleach (diluted 1:10 with water) may also be utilized.[6] Internal contamination is suspected if radioactive material has entered the mouth, nose, eyes, or ears and sample swabs should be taken of these areas.[6,10] Gastric lavage may be used if material was swallowed.[10] Eyes should be irrigated with saline from inner to outer canthus, attempting to avoid flow into the nasolacrimal duct.[6] Decontamination should be stopped when measured levels fail to fall, levels are less than twice background, or when skin abrasion occurs.[6,10] Decontamination should begin or continue at the hospital as needed in the same fashion.[6] In the hospital, floors and surfaces should be covered with paper or waterproof disposable sheets to facilitate later decontamination.[10] An appointed radiation safety officer should continue to monitor radiation levels.[6,10]

A complete blood count should be collected initially and every 6 to 8 hours to identify any changes in lymphocyte count.[10] Lymphocytes are very radiosensitive and provide a marker for the level of radiation exposure.[6,10] Blood should also be sent for chromosomal analysis.[5] Samples of feces, urine, and secretions should also be examined if there is a possibility of internal contamination.[6] Supportive treatment should be provided, including antiemetics, wound care, antibiotics, and observation for other signs or symptoms of radiation exposure.[7,10] Consultation with a hematologist and administration of medications to stimulate hematopoiesis, as well as stem cell transplantation may be of benefit.[10] An array of therapies for internal contamination is available. Potassium iodide prophylaxis to prevent thyroid cancer should be given when exposure to radioactive iodines has occurred, such as after an accident at a nuclear power plant.[6] Prussian blue should be administered after internal contamination with radioactive cesium and thallium, while the chelating agent diethylenetriaminepentaacetate (DTPA) should be used to treat contamination with plutonium, americium, berkelium, curium, and californium.[10,12]

Bioterrorism

History

Biological warfare has been practiced for most of human history, and despite international treaties banning such activity, the development and testing of bioweapons has continued to present times. At its height the Soviet Biopreparat employed as many as 60,000 individuals in labs and production facilities across the Soviet Union, where they manufactured tons of weaponized anthrax, smallpox, tularemia, and plague.[13] Iraqi scientists pursued biological and chemical weapons technology and the Iraqi government admitted to weaponizing and deploying anthrax. Rogue states and terrorist groups have also sought biological weapons. Although conventional explosives remain the most commonly used weapon of terrorists, biological weapons have been used in terrorist attacks, and this threat is sure to continue.[14]

Characteristics of Biological Weapons

Biological weapons are traditionally grouped into one of three categories: bacteria, virus, or toxin. Certain characteristics are required for an organism or toxin to be an effective weapon. Because the most efficient way to expose large numbers of people is through inhalation, the agent must effectively aerosolized and able to induce disease in this form. The agent must be stable in storage and ideally will resist environmental degradation. Several diseases and toxins meet these criteria and are considered high risk for use as biological weapons. This chapter will discuss the agents currently thought to represent the greatest threat for use as biological weapons. The reader is encouraged to refer to the CDC website (http://www.bt.cdc.gov) and the references for more detailed information about individual agents.

Bacteria: Anthrax

Anthrax is caused by *Bacillus anthracis*, a Gram-positive spore-forming bacterium. Anthrax occurs naturally in sheep, cattle, and horses and in humans that work with these animals (hence the common name "wool sorters' disease"). In spore form, anthrax is hardy and can survive in the environment for decades. Human disease is produced when the spores enter the body through inhalation, inoculation into the skin, or ingestion, with the different routes of entry accounting for the three forms of human anthrax. Ingestion is rare and unlikely to be used in a bioterror attack, and therefore is not discussed here.[15,16]

Inhalational anthrax is the most deadly form of the disease and the form most likely to be seen in a terrorist attack. An accidental release of weaponized anthrax from a Soviet biological weapons plant in Sverdlovsk in 1979 killed at least 66 people downwind of the plant.[13,15,16] Once inhaled, the spores are ingested by macrophages and transported to tracheobronchial lymph nodes where they germinate, replicate and release toxins that cause edema, hemorrhage, and necrosis. Inhalational anthrax has a biphasic pattern. The initial phase is preceded by an incubation period lasting 1 to 6 days, and is characterized by a nonspecific, flu-like illness with malaise, fevers, myalgias, chest and abdominal pain, and a nonproductive cough. Initial chest radiography and laboratory studies will likely be nondiagnostic. Delays in onset of the initial phase of up to 60 days have been reported in experimental models.[15,16]

The second phase begins within 24 to 48 hours when the patient becomes acutely toxic with high fevers, sepsis, dyspnea, cyanosis, and shock. Chest radiograph will show a widened mediastinum and hilar lymphadenopathy, although these findings may be subtle. Bacteremia develops with as many as 10^8 organisms per milliliter of blood, and up to 50% of patients develop hemorrhagic meningitis with nuchal rigidity and altered mental status. Death occurs within 24 to 36 hours. There is no human-to-human transmission of anthrax.[15,16]

Cutaneous anthrax, the most common natural form of the disease, occurs when the spores enter the skin, usually through an abrasion or other wound. One to seven days later the primary lesion develops. It starts as a painless but pruritic papule that becomes vesicular over the next one to two days. The vesicle will enlarge and may have smaller satellite vesicles. A marked non-pitting edema develops surrounding the lesion and painful lymphadenopathy may occur. The patient may complain of low-grade fevers and malaise. The vesicle will then rupture, followed by necrosis and the formation of the characteristic black eschar. Over the next one to two weeks, the eschar will dry and slough off, usually without scarring. At this stage most patients will recover, but up to 20% will develop systemic disease that is fatal without treatment. Antibiotic treatment will not affect local disease but reduces progression to systemic disease to about 1%.

Diagnosis and Treatment

The early signs of anthrax are nonspecific; diagnosis requires a high index of suspicion. Presentation of cases of acute flu-like illness with a fulminant course and high fatality rate should raise suspicion. A chest radiograph showing a widened mediastinum in such a patient is virtually pathognomonic for inhalational anthrax. Blood cultures should show growth of Gram-positive rods within 24 hours. Gram stain of vesicular fluid will confirm the diagnosis of cutaneous anthrax. Gram stain and culture of sputum are nondiagnostic. Suspicion of anthrax should result in immediate notification of local and state public health departments. **Table 8.1** below describes treatment recommendations.

Table 8.1
Recommendations for Treatment of Selected Bioterror Agents*

Agent	Isolated/Contained Cases	Mass Casualty	Notes
Anthrax-Inhalational	Ciprofloxacin 400 mg IV q 12 hrs	Ciprofloxacin 500 mg PO bid	Treat for 60 days, transition to PO when possible
Anthrax-Prophylaxis	Ciprofloxacin 500 mg PO bid	Ciprofloxacin 500 mg PO bid	Treat for 60 days
Plague	Streptomycin 1 g IM q 12 hrs or Gentamicin 5 mg/kg IV/IM q 24 hrs	Doxycycline 100 mg PO bid or Ciprofloxacin 500 mg PO bid	Treat for 10 days for disease, 7 days for prophylaxis
Tularemia	Streptomycin 1 g IM bid or Gentamicin 5 mg/kg IV/ IM q 24 hrs	Ciprofloxacin 500 mg PO bid or Doxycycline 100 mg PO bid	Treat for 10 days (Doxycycline for 14–21 days)
Smallpox	Vaccinate	Vaccinate	Patients must be isolated. All contacts must be identified, vaccinated, and observed
Botulinum	Equine antitoxin, 1 10 mL vial	Equine antitoxin, 1 10 mL vial	Will prevent but not reverse paralysis

*Adapted from the Consensus Recommendations developed by the Working Group on Civilian Biodefense. The reader is referred to these sources for alternative regimens and recommendations for children, pregnancy, and immunosuppression.[9,12,15,16,19,22]

Plague

Plague is caused by the Gram-negative bacillus *Yersinia pestis* and has affected human populations since ancient times. Plague is endemic in much of the world; there have been several worldwide pandemics that killed millions of people. Smaller outbreaks continue to occur throughout the world, including the American Southwest. Both the United States and the Soviet Union developed weaponized plague.[13,17]

Plague is a zoonotic disease with rats and other rodents being the primary reservoir. Humans are infected through the bite of infected fleas or by inhalation of infectious rodent droppings. *Yersinia* is rapidly killed in the environment but persists for days in infected droppings, dried sputum, and human remains. Plague occurs in three forms: bubonic, pneumonic, and septicemic. In natural outbreaks, the bubonic form is the most common, but in a terrorist release of weaponized plague, the pneumonic form will predominate.[17]

Primary pneumonic plague develops when aerosolized *Yersinia* is inhaled into the lungs. Following a one- to six-day incubation, the patient will develop a flu-like illness with cough, dyspnea, fever and chills. Within 24 hours the patient will progress to a fulminant pneumonia with respiratory failure, hemoptysis, coagulopathy, sepsis, and shock. The patient may also complain of nausea, vomiting, diarrhea, and abdominal pain. Gangrene of the digits and nose may occur due to coagulopathy and is the origin of the term black death. The pneumonia ranges from lobar to diffuse bilateral infiltrates with ARDS. Without treatment death occurs within six days. Pneumonic plague is transmissible from person-to-person and requires strict respiratory and contact isolation.[17,18]

Diagnosis and Treatment

The primary diagnosis of plague is clinical and requires a high index of suspicion. Initial and isolated cases may be difficult to distinguish from more common bacterial pneumonias, but the presentation of unusual numbers of previously healthy patients complaining of fevers, respiratory distress and cough, chest pain and having a fulminant course must raise the suspicion of plague and inhalational anthrax. Hemoptysis is not present in anthrax and would be indicative of plague. Suspicion of plague must result in the isolation of the patient and notification of the local and state health departments.[17,18] **Table 8.1** below describes treatment recommendations.

Tularemia

Tularemia is a zoonotic disease caused by the Gram-negative coccobacillus *Francisella tularensis*. The bacterium is carried by wild and domestic animals including rabbits, squirrels, cats, and other small mammals. In nature it is transmitted to humans through arthropod bite or contact with a contaminated animal. Specific symptoms of tularemia differ depending on the route of exposure with six classical clinical syndromes described: ulceroglandular, glandular, oculoglandular, oropharyngeal and gastrointestinal, pneumonic, and typhoidal. Tularemia was weaponized by both the United States and the Soviet Union, although there is no record of its release.[13,19]

Tularemia infection begins with acute onset of fevers and chills, myalgias, arthralgias, sore throat, coryza, fatigue, and malaise after an incubation period ranging from 1 to 21 days. In an attack with aerosolized *F. tularensis*, the pneumonic form of the disease would be expected to predominate. Pneumonic tularemia may occur due to direct inhalation of organisms or hematogenous spread. It presents as pneumonia with non-productive cough, fever, dyspnea, and pleuritic chest pain. Typhoidal tularemia may develop with continuous high fevers and sepsis and may progress to septic shock.[19]

Diagnosis and Treatment

Diagnosis of tularemia is difficult and relies on clinical findings and suspicion. Non-specific lab abnormalities such as leukocytosis and mildly elevated transaminases may be seen. Chest radiograph will usually show multiple segmental or lobar infiltrates. Cavitary lesions, effusions, and mediastinal lymphadenopathy may be seen. Blood cultures are rarely positive. Direct fluorescent antibody staining is available but limited to reference laboratories. See Table 8.1 for treatment recommendations.

Viruses: Smallpox

Smallpox is caused by variola, a DNA virus from the genus *Orthopoxvirus*. Variola is transmitted easily from person-to-person as an aerosol and is highly infective, requiring only a few virions to cause disease. Prior to a successful international vaccination campaign smallpox was endemic worldwide. The virus was eliminated from human populations in 1977 and now officially exists only in two secure labs in the US and Russia. However, Soviet scientists are known to have produced tons of weaponized smallpox. These stocks of virus, as well as the scientists that produced them, are unaccounted for.[13,14] Vaccination against smallpox ceased in 1980, and immunity in vaccinated persons will have waned. This combination of high infectivity, easy transmissibility, lethality, and vulnerable population make smallpox an excellent biological weapon.

Smallpox begins when virus particles are inhaled and implant on the oropharyngeal or upper respiratory mucosa. The virus migrates to regional lymph nodes and begins to replicate. On day 3 to 4 an asymptomatic viremia develops and the virus spreads to bone marrow, liver, spleen, and other lymphatic tissue. Widespread replication begins, and a secondary viremia occurs about 8 to 10 days after the initial infection, causing fever, headache, and prostration. The virus then localizes to small blood vessels in the dermis. At the end of this incubation period (average 12 to 14 days but as long as 17 days) the patient becomes toxic with high fevers, headache, backache, and malaise. They may develop severe abdominal pain and mental status changes. At this point the exanthum develops, beginning as a maculopapular rash on the oropharyngeal mucosa, face, and forearms, and the patient becomes highly contagious. Over the next 1 to 2 days the rash spreads to the trunk and legs and becomes vesicular then pustular. Around the eighth or ninth day of rash, the pustules crust and form scabs, which slough off by day 14.

Variola infection presents in several clinical forms. The two most common, variola major and variola minor, make up about 90% of cases. Variola major, or classic smallpox has a mortality rate of about 30% and is the form described above. Variola minor is a milder disease with fewer pox and less systemic toxicity. The course of the disease tends to be shorter and mortality is only about 1%. The two other forms of the disease, malignant smallpox and hemorrhagic smallpox are much less common but have a mortality rate greater than 90%.[20,21]

Diagnosis and Treatment

The diagnosis of even a single case of smallpox constitutes an international public health emergency and requires immediate notification of public health authorities.[18,20] Diagnosis is based on clinical features. The rash of smallpox is distinguished from that of chickenpox by timing and distribution. The rash of smallpox begins on the face and extremities and is more scant on the trunk whereas chickenpox begins on the trunk and then spreads to the face and extremities. The smallpox rash is more deep-seated and lesions on any one part of the body will all be at the same stage. Chickenpox lesions are more superficial (dewdrop on a rose petal) and will be at various stages as lesions appear in crops. Lesions on the palms and soles are extremely rare in chickenpox. Diagnosis will be more difficult if the presenting case is malignant or hemorrhagic variant. Laboratory confirmation is possible from scabs and vesicular fluid, but requires a biosafety level 4 lab. Specimens should be collected and shipped according to instructions from the local or state health department.[20,21]

There is no specific treatment for smallpox once the infected individual develops symptoms, but vaccination early in the incubation period can attenuate or even prevent disease. The medical response to smallpox is aimed at containing the spread of the disease. Suspected patients must be isolated in a negative pressure room, and strict respiratory and contact precautions must be followed. Once the diagnosis of smallpox is confirmed, all other suspected cases should be isolated and vaccinated. All contacts of known or suspected patients should be vaccinated and put under surveillance. Those that develop symptoms of prodromal illness should be isolated. Because smallpox is spread via aerosol there is a high risk of widespread dissemination in a hospital, and care must be taken to avoid this.[18,22] Table 8.1 describes treatment recommendations.

Toxins: Botulinum

Botulinum toxin is produced by the anaerobic bacteria *Clostridium botulinum* and is one of the most toxic substances known to man. *Clostridia* species exist naturally in soil across much of the world and are easily isolated and cultured. The estimated lethal dose of the toxin for an adult is 0.09 to 0.15 μg IV or IM, 0.7 to 0.9 μg inhaled, and 70 μg ingested.[23] There are three naturally occurring forms of botulism—food-borne, wound, and intestinal—as well as man-made inhalational botulism. A bioterror attack would involve either an aerosol release or intentional contamination of food. Regardless of the route of toxin entry, disease is caused by the same mechanism and presents with the same signs and symptoms. The toxin binds and enters presynaptic cholinergic neurons where it inhibits acetylcholine release. Botulism is characterized by a symmetric, descending, flaccid paralysis. Paralysis always begins in the bulbar musculature and typical presenting complaints are diplopia, dysphagia, dysarthria, and dysphonia (the 4 Ds). Common signs include ptosis, dilated, sluggish pupils, and dry mucosa. Sensory nerves are not affected, and paresthesias are generally absent.

Diagnosis and Treatment

Botulism is often misdiagnosed as Guillain-Barré, Miller-Fisher syndrome, or myasthenia gravis. Botulism should be suspected in any cluster of acute, flaccid paralysis, and a common exposure should be sought. Botulism can be differentiated by its prominent bulbar symptoms with lesser peripheral weakness, symmetry, and lack of sensory nerve involvement. Treatment for botulism is with equine antitoxin, which is available from the CDC, or potentially with an experimental antitoxin held by the US Army. Antitoxin will bind circulating toxin but will not reverse existing paralysis and supportive treatment will be required.

References

1. Gens L, Kennedy T. Management of unique clinical entities in disaster medicine. *Emerg Med Clin North Am* 1996;14:301–326.
2. Frykberg E. Medical management of disasters and mass casualties from terrorist bombings: How can we cope? *J Trauma* 2002;53:201–212.
3. Leibovici D, Gofrit O, Stein M, et al. Blast injuries: Bus versus open-air bombings—a comparative study of injuries in survivors of open-air versus confined-space explosions. *J Trauma* 1996;41:1030–1035.
4. Guy R, Kirkman E, Watkins P, et al. Physiologic response to primary blast. *J Trauma* 1998;45:983–987.
5. Pizov R, Oppenheim-Eden A, Matot I, et al. Blast lung injury from an explosion on a civilian bus. *Chest* 1999;115:165–172.
6. Kilpatrick JJ. Nuclear attacks. *RN* 2002;65:46–52.
7. Centers for Disease Control and Prevention. *Acute Radiation Syndrome, Fact Sheet for Physicians.* 2003.
8. Helfand I, Forrow L, Tiwari J. Nuclear terrorism. *Br Med J* 2002;324:356–358.
9. Mettler F, Voelz G. Current concepts: Major radiation exposure—what to expect and how to respond. *N Engl J Med* 2002;346:1554–1561.
10. Oak Ridge Institute for Science and Education. Managing radiation emergencies: Guidance for hospital medical management. 2002, http://www.orau.gov/reacts.
11. Traynor K. FDA offers guidance on prophylaxis for exposure to radioiodines. *Am J Health System Pharmacy* 2002;59:324–326.
12. Centers for Disease Control and Prevention. Radiation emergencies: Facts about DTPA URL: www.bt.cdc.gov/radiation/dtpa.asp 2003, updated May 20, 2005.
13. Alibek K, Handelman S. *Biohazard: The Chilling True Story of the Largest Covert Biological Weapons Program in the World—Told from Inside by the Man Who Ran It.* New York: Random House, 1999.
14. Henderson DA. The looming threat of bioterrorism. *Science* 1999;283:12179–12182.
15. Inglesby TV, Henderson DA, Bartlett JG, et al. Anthrax as a biological weapon: medical and public health management. *JAMA* 1999;281:1735–1745.
16. Inglesby TV, O'Toole T, Henderson DA. Anthrax as a biological weapon, 2002: Updated recommendations for management. *JAMA* 2002;287:2236–2252.
17. Inglesby TV, Dennis DT, Henderson DA, et al. Plague as a biological weapon: medical and public health management. *JAMA* 2000;283:2281–2290.
18. CDC guidelines for state health departments on how to handle anthrax and other biological agent threats. Atlanta: Centers for Disease Control and Prevention. (Accessed June 2005 at http://www.bt.cdc.gov)
19. Cronquist SD. Tularemia: the disease and the weapon. *Dermatol Clin* 2004;22:313–320.
20. Henderson DA, Inglesby TV, Bartlett JG, et al. Smallpox as a biological weapon: medical and public health management. *JAMA* 1999;281:2127–2137.
21. Breman JG, Henderson DA. Diagnosis and management of smallpox. *N Engl J Med* 2002;346:1300–1308.
22. Chemical and Biological Defense Command. *Domestic Preparedness Training Program: Hospital Provider Manual.* Edgewood Arsenal, MD, 1999,
23. Arnon SS, Schecter R, Inglesby TV, et al. Botulinum toxin as a biological weapon: medical and public health management. *JAMA* 2001;285:1059–1070.

Abdominal and Gastrointestinal Disorders

John C. Moorhead

Patients complaining of abdominal pain present frequently to an emergency department and pose challenges for the emergency physician. Symptoms can represent acute, chronic, catastrophic, life-threatening, or simply benign conditions. Abdominal pain is frequently a manifestation of non-abdominal illnesses. Traditionally, about half of these patients leave the emergency department without a definitive diagnosis. Increasingly, however, a high level of suspicion for serious conditions in high risk patients and timely utilization of imaging in the ED have enhanced diagnostic specificity, patient outcomes, and both patient and physician satisfaction. Often patients require ongoing evaluation in hospital or ED observation units. Immediate intervention, appropriate, timely consultation, and follow-up are paramount to decreasing morbidity for many of these patients.

Approach to Abdominal and Gastrointestinal Disorders

Gary A. Johnson

Abdominal pain is one of the emergency physician's most challenging chief complaints. It is a common emergency department (ED) presentation that often does not result in a definitive diagnosis, but can represent a life-threatening disease that requires immediate intervention.

Epidemiology

After ED evaluation, various authors have found that nonspecific abdominal pain is the preliminary diagnosis in 41% to 50% of abdominal pain patients. These patients often have a benign prognosis. Many conditions that present as abdominal pain represent severe diseases that require immediate intervention. These diagnoses include appendicitis, acute cholecystitis, intestinal obstruction, intestinal ischemia, pelvic inflammatory disease, acute pancreatitis, AAA, perforated ulcer, and urolithiasis. Approximately 15% of patients seen for abdominal pain will require operation and 27% will require hospitalization.

The age of the patient greatly impacts on the differential diagnosis and incidence of severe disease and illness. One out of five children seeks medical help for abdominal pain by age 15. Approximately 5% of these require hospitalization. Presentations often vary by age. Infants commonly present with colic, gastroenteritis, and constipation. They also may have intussusception, malrotation, volvulus, renal neoplasm, necrotizing, or incarcerated hernia. Toddlers frequently have belly pain with pneumonia or pharyngitis, or other serious diagnoses including Meckel's diverticulum or appendicitis. Chronic illnesses may present acutely with belly pain. These illnesses include diabetes mellitus, sickle cell anemia, Mediterranean fever, porphyria, and cystic fibrosis. Adolescents may have other abdominal disorders such as pelvic inflammatory disease, urinary tract disease, and inflammatory bowel disease. Both school-age and adolescent children may have a psychosocial cause of abdominal pain.

Acute abdominal pain in the elderly is frequently a life-threatening illness. Nonspecific abdominal pain as a discharge diagnosis is relatively unusual (9% to 19%). Common diagnoses include malignant disease (13%), acute cholecystitis (26% to 41%), incarcerated hernia (5% to 10%), and pancreatitis (4% to 5%). Mortality in this patient population is significant (11% to 14%) and one-third of patients require operations.

Pathophysiology

Most abdominal pain is transmitted through visceral components. Possible neural mechanisms include stretch fibers, which are in the wall of all organs, as well as the capsules of solid organs. Input from these organs is conducted along afferent nerve fibers that return to the spinal cord at various levels. Visceral pain is often poorly localized and is characteristically vague. Somatic pain often originates in the peritoneum and is much better localized than visceral pain. Once the peritoneum is irritated, pain is well localized and more easily described.

Referred pain is frequently involved with evaluation of abdominal pain. Common referral patterns include pain originating in the chest (e.g., pneumonia, giving an upper quadrant tenderness, and pain near the diaphragm, giving a sensation in the neck or the back of the shoulder blade [C-3, -4, and -5 distribution]).

Emergency Department Evaluation

Historical Factors

For patients who present with abdominal pain, the history should include location of pain, movement of pain, time of onset, and duration of pain. Also, aggravating or palliative factors should be queried. Pain often moves and in many cases its final destination is more predictive of the final diagnosis than its original location (e.g., appendicitis). Episodic sharp pain that comes in increasing waves is often considered "colicky." Such pain may increase the suspicion of a hollow viscus as the origin (e.g., bowel or ureter). Pain that has been present for a long period of time is less likely to be emergent; however, many patients with acute appendicitis or cholecystitis present more than 12 to 24 hours after the onset of pain.

Associated symptoms provide important clues to the diagnosis. The presence of nausea or vomiting may help indicate the presence of hollow viscus disease. Appendicitis pain classically occurs before vomiting; however, this rule is violated in many appendicitis patients. Bowel symptoms including frequency and nature of stools, and presence or absence of bright red blood or melena must be queried. Dysuria, urinary frequency or discoloration of urine should be noted, as should menstrual history in female patients. Symptoms referable to organs in the chest or retroperitoneum must also be queried.

A past history that reveals prior abdominal pathology or prior surgical procedures may provide important clues as to the final diagnosis. Multiple medical diseases (cardiac or pulmonary disease, atherosclerotic risk factors, or diabetes) will impact and complicate the presentations of abdominal pain.

Physical Examination

Abnormal vital signs including tachycardia and elevation of temperature can be important clues to patients who have truly emergent or surgical presentation of disease. Often the general appearance of the patient can be helpful. Patients with peritonitis will lie very still to avoid any movement that may irritate their inflamed peritoneum. Patients with colic will frequently be very mobile and be difficult to examine because of their unwillingness to lie still.

Infrequently, simple inspection will reveal a localized mass or general distention of the abdomen. It is important to note location of prior surgical scars. The abdomen should be auscultated for presence or absence of bowel sounds. Very active bowel sounds may be a clue that the patient has increased gastrointestinal motility. The abdomen should be palpated for the point of maximal tenderness and total area of tenderness. It is wise to begin palpation away from the most tender area since the patient may provide more voluntary guarding after a tender area is elicited. Masses and organomegaly must specifically be searched for. Hepatic or sphenic enlargement should be noted.

Rebound tenderness may indicate peritonitis. A traditional method of testing for rebound tenderness is to palpate the abdomen somewhat deeply and then rapidly remove the hand. This withdrawal will move abdominal contents including the peritoneum and may indicate peritonitis. The test must be interpreted with care since abrupt movements startle patients and their response to the test may be difficult to interpret. Simply moving the stretcher, tapping the patient's heel in order to move the abdomen, or lightly percussing the abdomen are alternative tests for detecting peritonitis.

Many additional physical tests have been described. Murphy's sign tests for possible cholecystitis. While palpating the right upper quadrant the patient is asked to take a deep breath. If the patient suddenly halts inspiration in response to pain in the right upper quadrant, it is considered a positive Murphy sign. Rovsing's sign is positive when pain in the right lower quadrant occurs with palpation in the left lower quadrant. This may be indicative of appendicitis. The iliopsoas and obturator signs also look for possible appendicitis. A positive iliopsoas sign is pain that occurs when the patient has right lower quadrant pain when he tries to flex at the right hip against resistance. The obturator sign is elicited with the right leg flexed at the hip and the hip is rotated internally. The test is positive if pain is elicited with this motion. Rectal examination should be performed for presence or absence of mass, pain, and quality of stool. Testing for occult blood should be done.

Pelvic examination should be performed on all women with lower quadrant pain. Similarly, examination of male genitalia is mandatory in all patients with lower quadrant pain. Palpation of the back and percussion over costovertebral angles should always be performed. All patients should have pulmonary and cardiac examinations as well.

Laboratory Evaluation

Laboratory evaluations of patients with abdominal pain may be very specifically or very broadly undertaken. Certainly some patients may have a clear diagnosis based on history and examination alone and laboratory analysis is not required. Other patients may have a life-threatening presentation or a confusing presentation that requires multiple lab tests to be performed.

Complete blood count is often ordered to examine the patient's hematocrit and white blood cell count. Acute bleeding will have a normal hematocrit, but chronic blood loss with an insufficient compensatory mechanism will reveal a low hematocrit. Total white count and white count differential may imply presence of bacterial or surgical disease. The literature has addressed the place of leukocyte and neutrophil counts in the evaluation of appendicitis. Patients with appendicitis do tend to have higher white counts and higher percentage of neutrophilia. However, there is extensive crossover with other diagnoses including benign diagnoses.

Testing for hepatic enzymes may be very helpful in the setting of acute hepatitis, biliary tract disease, or pancreatitis. Hepatocellular enzymes (aspartate transaminase, alanine transaminase) will be elevated with hepatic inflammation or masses. This will also be more modestly elevated with biliary tract disease. Alkaline phosphatase will also be elevated in hepatic disease but more severely elevated in most cases of biliary tract disease. Bilirubin, both total and direct, should be measured to screen for hepatobiliary disease.

Amylase and/or lipase may be measured to look for pancreatic inflammation. These will also be elevated in other disease states. Amylase is present in nearly all hollow organs and therefore may be elevated with salivary gland or gastrointestinal disease. Lipase has been reported to have higher predictive value than serum amylase. However, it may be elevated in a large number of non–pancreatic disease states also.

Urinalysis should be performed on all patients with suspicion of urinary tract infection (UTI) or a suspected emergent cause of pain. Pyuria may occur with disease that is not intrinsically renal such as appendicitis. Hematuria may indicate renal disease (e.g., urolithiasis) or a more systemic insult (e.g., endocarditis).

A pregnancy test should be performed in all female patients of childbearing age who have not had a hysterectomy. It is clear that patients who have tubal ligation are still at risk for pregnancy-related diseases.

Abdominal radiography may be performed to look for evidence of bowel obstruction, calcifications, foreign bodies, or free intraperitoneal air. Special radiographic tests may be considered in patients after initial evaluation. These tests would include intravenous pyelogram, angiography, computed tomography, and ultrasonography.

Disposition

Since many patients have a potentially serious disease that is difficult to diagnose, a low threshold should be present for obtaining consultation and admitting patients with acute abdominal pain. Diseases that are notoriously difficult to diagnose include ischemic bowel disease, appendicitis, and pancreatic disease.

Treatment

Emergent treatment of these patients includes hemodynamic management, antibiotic therapy, and analgesia. A hemodynamically unstable patient should have two large-bore IV catheters placed and isotonic fluid administered. Control of emesis with antiemetics or nasogastric suction may aid in maintaining appropriate fluid hydration.

Administration of analgesics has always been controversial in the setting of acute abdominal pain. Despite traditional concerns, it is clear that judicious use of analgesics in closely observed patients can be safely performed.

Patients with suspected urinary tract infections or bowel perforations require antibiotic administration. Adequate Gram-negative coverage is required in either case. Anaerobic and enterococcal coverage should also be provided if bowel perforation is suspected.

Selected Readings

Gurleyik GA, Gurleyik EB. Age-related clinical features in older patients with acute appendicitis. *Eur J Emerg Med* 2003;10:200–203.

Jess P, Bjerregaard B, Brynitz S, et al. Prognosis of acute nonspecific abdominal pain: a prospective study. *Am J Surg* 1982;144:338–340.

Staniland JR, Ditchburn J, DeDombal FT. Clinical presentation of acute abdomen: study of 600 patients. *Br Med J* 1972;3:393–398.

Thomas SH, Silen W. Effect on diagnostic efficiency of analgesia for undifferentiated abdominal pain. *Br J Surg* 2003;90:5–9.

John C. Moorhead
Derek S. Halvorson

Anatomy and Pathophysiology

The stomach and esophagus arise from the foregut that extends from the oral cavity caudally to the descending portion of the duodenum. While each organ is subject to its own unique disease pathology, the presentation of stomach and esophageal disorders may be similar and thus are discussed together in this chapter. The pain from these organs is referred to a common mid-epigastric area. Inflammatory processes of both the esophagus and stomach can be described as burning, sharp or piercing and localize to the same region or, more common to esophageal pathology, in the substernal chest.

The esophagus is the proximal portion of the upper gastrointestinal tract and extends from the pharynx to the stomach. It is comprised of three distinct zones. The upper portion includes the cricopharyngeus muscle that initiates the contractions facilitating the transfer of a food bolus down the esophagus. The middle zone (body) is composed of an inner circular and outer longitudinal layer of muscle that continues the transfer of the food bolus with peristaltic action. Finally, the lower segment includes the lower esophageal sphincter (LES), which is a region of tonically contracted smooth muscle. The passage through the LES is modulated by inhibitory and excitatory parasympathetic nerves. The LES opens due to the activity of inhibitor nerve signals (mediated by vasoactive intestinal peptide and nitric oxide) and passes the food bolus into the stomach.

The esophagus travels along the curve of the vertebral column in the posterior mediastinum and pierces through the diaphragm at the level of T10 just left of the medial plane and empties in to the stomach. As it passes through the diaphragm, it is bound by the skeletal muscle forces of the crural diaphragm that provides further sphincter tone at the esophageal hiatus.

The stomach lies in the left upper quadrant of the abdomen and is fixed at the esophagocardiac junction. It is divided into four regions: the cardia, fundus, body, and antrum. Each region is characterized by different types of cells in the gastric mucosa that facilitate gastric secretions, digestions, and gastric emptying.

The arterial blood supply to the proximal and middle esophagus is through the inferior thyroid, bronchial and esophageal arteries. The stomach and distal esophagus are supplied by the branches of the celiac axis off the descending aorta. Parasympathetic innervation of the esophagus and stomach is provided by branches of the vagus nerve. Sympathetic innervation providing primarily inhibitory signaling travels through the celiac ganglia.

As a food bolus passes through the esophagus and passes the LES into the stomach it initiates a cascade of gastric secretions. Gastric acid secretion is stimulated by gastrin released by G-cells in the antrum, histamine release from mast cells in the mucosa and through parasympathetic release of acetylcholine. Pepsinogen is released by chief cells in the body of the stomach. The caudad region of the stomach contracts to mix the food bolus with gastric secretions and eventually propels the bolus into the duodenum. Gastric emptying is mediated by this process and can be slowed by fat and increased acid in the duodenum.

Disorders of the Esophagus

Motor Abnormalities

Esophageal Spasm

Esophageal spasm can be divided into two types of pathology. The first, diffuse esophageal spasm (DES) results from asynchronous contraction of esophageal smooth muscle. The result is dysfunctional propagation of a food bolus often accompanied by dysphagia and chest pain. Barium swallow can be used to aid in the diagnosis of DES. The study may show multiple simultaneous contractions often seen as a "corkscrew" appearance. Manometry is considered the gold standard for diagnostic tests.

The second type of esophageal spasm is a "nutcracker" esophagus. Manometry reveals high amplitude contractions, which are typically more synchronous than DES. These high amplitude spasms of the esophagus are less commonly associated with dysphagia however, chest discomfort is more likely. The chest pain in both entities can mimic more life-threatening pathology with substernal pain or pressure that may radiate to the arm, jaw or neck. Symptomatic relief may be gained from medications such as nitrates, calcium channel blockers and rarely anticholinergics and TCAs.[1]

Achalasia

As a food bolus passes into the oral cavity, the swallow center of the brainstem triggers the primary peristaltic wave that passes the bolus from the striated muscular portion of the upper esophagus to the smooth muscle body. The distention of the smooth muscle potentiates a secondary peristalsis coordinated by the vagus nerve, which propels the food bolus downward at a rate of 2 cm per second. Activation of inhibitory signals via vasoactive intestinal peptides and nitric oxide at the LES relaxes the smooth muscle sphincter allowing the food bolus to pass into the stomach.

Achalasia is a neuropathologic disorder of the esophageal smooth muscle which manifests as abnormal or absent esophageal motility. The problem often starts at the LES and progresses proximally. The loss of inhibitory nerves at the LES (marked by diminished levels of vasoactive intestinal peptides and nitric oxide) causes elevated LES pressures and failure of the LES to relax. Ganglion cell loss progresses throughout the esophageal mesenteric plexus causing aperistalsis and dilation of the esophagus. The dilated body of the esophagus leading to the tightly constricted LES appears as a classic "bird-beak" pattern on a barium swallow study. Manometry will show a diminished or absent peristalsis in the esophageal body.

Dysphagia, regurgitation, and chest pain are common complaints in patients with achalasia. Dysphagia is common early in its course and is typically associated with both solids and liquids. Chest pain is often substernal and may radiate to the neck, arm or jaw mimicking cardiac pathology. Chest pain may worsen with food. Patients with unrecognized achalasia often are diagnosed after an extensive cardiac workup.[1]

Scleroderma

The multisystem disorder, scleroderma or systemic sclerosis is due to overproduction and accumulation of collagen and fibrosis of various tissues including the esophagus. Esophageal involvement is manifest as impaired contractility of smooth muscle and subsequent decrease or loss of peristalsis. The lower two-thirds of the esophageal body is involved causing dysphagia more common with solid foods. Reflux is also a common complaint with chronic esophagitis which may lead to stricture formation, an increased incidence of Barrett esophagus and adenocarcinoma. Plain chest radiograph may show gas visualized in the middle and distal esophagus. Physical exam may reveal other manifestations of CREST syndrome including sclerodactyly, telangiectasias, calcinosis or Raynaud's phenomenon.[1]

Structural Disorders

Structural disorders of the esophagus may present with mechanical dysfunction, bleeding or pain. This group of disorders includes foreign body ingestion, traumatic disorders and anatomical disruption affecting the function of the esophagus.

GI bleeding accounts for up to 5% of all hospital admissions from the emergency department and carries significant morbidity and a mortality rate of 8% to 10%.[2] The vast majority of these patients have upper gastrointestinal (UGI) sources of bleeding commonly gastric, duodenal and esophageal sources.

Varices

Esophageal and gastric varices are dilated venous structures resulting from portal hypertension This causes a shunting hepatic blood flow from the high pressure portal system to low pressure systemic venous collateral channels. The lack of valves in the portal system allows a free passage of this collateral blood flow. Portal hypertension is most commonly associated with liver dysfunction due to cirrhosis or portal vein obstruction. As a result, patients may present with other stigmata of chronic liver disease. Mortality in the first year of a patients' first variceal bleeding episode is 25% to 50%.[3]

Patients with variceal bleeding typically present with hematemesis with or without melena. Patients often have clinical evidence of blood loss ranging from tachycardia and mild orthostatic hypotension to profound hypovolemic shock. While variceal bleeding accounts for approximately 20% of all UGI bleeds, patients with known varices present with UGI bleeding from other sources 50% of the time.[2] Therefore, the most definitive diagnostic and therapeutic procedure is endoscopy.

In the ED, management should include two large-bore IVs with rapid infusion of volume, type and crossmatch for blood, correction of any coagulopathy and metabolic derangement and a rapid gastroenterology consultation. NG tube placement is not contraindicated and should be performed in all patients with suspected upper GI bleeds as a diagnostic modality. Other therapeutic modalities include infusion of vasopressin or sandostatin, both of which act as splanchnic vasoconstrictors that decrease portal blood flow. In the event of continuous uncontrolled hemorrhage where endoscopy is unavailable, balloon tamponade may implemented with a Sengstaken-Blakemore or Minnesota tube. These interventions can halt bleeding in up to 80% of cases temporarily but have a significant complication rate.[2]

Tears (Mallory-Weiss Syndrome)

Mallory-Weiss tears are the second most common esophageal source of upper GI bleeding. They are longitudinal tears of the distal esophagus at the gastroesophageal junction that result from repeated regurgitation, retching or forceful coughing. Mallory-Weiss tears account for approximately 5% of all upper GI bleeds. They are more common in the third to fifth decade of life and have an association with significant alcohol and aspirin use and patients with hiatal hernias.[4] Classically they present with bright red hematemesis following several episodes of retching or regurgitation. Patients are generally hemodynamically stable and bleeding is self limited in 90% of cases. Rarely patients may have significant ongoing blood loss requiring endoscopy or vasopressin infusion. Admission and a GI consultation are indicated for all persistent or hemodynamically unstable GI bleeding patients.

Diverticula

Esophageal diverticular disease is relatively rare. The most common type is in the proximal esophagus, the Zenker's diverticulum, which is thought to erupt between the thyropharyngeal and cricopharyngeal muscle fibers in a posterior direction. These pouches occur most commonly in patients over 70 years old (>50%) and are rare in patients under 40.[5,6] The clinical presentation includes dysphagia, weight loss, chronic cough, regurgitation and aspiration. A barium swallow study is the diagnostic test of choice and definitive management includes surgical repair. There is a small risk of carcinoma within the pouch even after repair, thus long-term follow-up is indicated. Midesophageal and epiphrenic esophageal diverticula, which are outpouchings of the esophagus where the esophageal wall is weak, are much less common. These diverticuli are associated with abnormalities found on esophageal manometry such as "nutcracker" esophagus, diffuse esophageal spasm and achalasia. The clinical presentation is similar to Zenker's diverticulum as are diagnosis and management options.

Webs

Esophageal webs are outpouchings in the squamous epithelium of the esophageal mucosa that may be circumferential. When they occur in the distal esophagus they are also referred to as esophageal rings or Schatzkis rings. A hiatal hernia is often present with a ring. Plummer-Vinson syndrome is the combination of iron-deficiency anemia and symptomatic hypopharyngeal webs. As rings become less distensible with age, they commonly present with dysphagia after the onset of the fifth decade. If not discovered by endoscopy or contrast studies, webs may present with obstruction.[6]

Strictures

Esophageal stricture formation is a complication of prolonged esophageal inflammation or injury such as in reflux esophagitis or a single insult such as a caustic ingestion. Strictures are more likely to occur in patients with Barrett esophagus where the normal squamous epithelium of the esophagus is replaced with columnal epithelium. They may also arise from esophageal webs. Stricture from monilial esophagitis is also reported.

Both webs and strictures present with a history of dysphagia and often with a foreign body or food impaction. Diagnosis is made with endoscopy in the majority of cases, however, barium contrast radiography is also diagnostic. Treatment includes balloon dilation of the narrowing as well as treatment of the underlying disease process.[6]

Esophageal Tumor

Esophageal cancer is a significant disease process that carries a poor prognosis. In the western hemisphere, the incidence is around 5 per 100,000 people and rising.[1] The two main types of tumors include squamous cell carcinoma (SCC) and adenocarcinoma (AC), the latter accounting for the sharp rise in the overall incidence of esophageal cancers.

Risk factors for esophageal cancer include smoking, alcohol consumption, and dietary factors for both types.

Adenocarcinoma is often related to underlying mucosal changes in the setting of reflux esophagitis. Barrett's metaplasia due to chronic reflux esophagitis is thought to be one of the most significant factors associated with the rise in the incidence of AC. Obesity has also been linked to the increased risk of AC.[7]

Both types of esophageal cancers present with solid food dysphagia and weight loss. Often patient may have a history or GERD. Malignancy is often detected during screening for Barrett's metaplasia. Progressive cancer may present with other complications such as occult GI bleeding, tracheoesophageal fistula or voice changes due to recurrent laryngeal nerve involvement.

Diagnosis is made with endoscopy. Barium swallow studies are sensitive in evaluated for an underlying malignancy. Treatment includes primary resection of the tumor. Palliation with chemotherapy or radiation may be implemented if the tumor is advanced and thought to be unresectable. Esophageal cancer has a poor prognosis overall with a 5-year survival rate ranging from 10 to 30 percent.[7,8]

Foreign Body

Foreign body (FB) ingestion most commonly occurs in toddlers age 8 months to 3 years as a result of their natural instinct to explore their world with, among other means, their mouths. In adults, those at highest risk include alcoholics, denture wearers, patients with esophageal motility disorders or strictures, and prison inmates attempting to smuggle illicit materials past authorities. Although perforation is uncommon, children are at highest risk as the diagnosis may be delayed due to a lack of a history or the unwitting ingestion of erosive or sharp objects.

Small objects <2.5 cm are more likely to pass through the esophagus. Retained esophageal foreign bodies will predictably lodge at one of three esophageal narrowings: the cricopharyngeus muscle (thoracic inlet), the level of the aortic arch, and the lower esophageal sphincter (LES). In the airway, the carina and the right main stem bronchus are common sites for FB retention. Patients with esophageal cancer, webs and rings, strictures and motility disorders may lodge at any other level. A food bolus impaction in adults is related to an underlying physiologic abnormality in 95% of cases.

Asymptomatic children may present with a history of foreign body ingestion by a parent or sibling 35% of cases. In a review of 2,394 patients with foreign body ingestion, the most common symptoms were anorexia, salivation, pain, dysphagia and vomiting.[9] Other common symptoms include choking, foreign body sensation, dyspnea or respiratory symptoms, such as cough, wheezing, or recurrent pneumonia. Adults will present with a history of pain after eating or a FB sensation and dysphagia or odynophagia.

In light of a history or physical exam findings suggestive of FB ingestion, a PA and lateral chest and neck radiograph may be helpful in identifying and localizing a radio-opaque object. Coins are the most commonly ingested FB in children and will appear in the esophagus as a circular object ion the PA image and flat on the lateral view due to the flat coronal orientation of the esophagus.

Coins lodged in the airway are more commonly positioned in the sagittal plane appearing round on the later image. Contrast may aid in identifying a radiolucent FB, however, barium can obscure visualization with endoscopy and gastrograffin can cause pulmonary complications if aspirated. With a sensitivity of up to 100%, CT scan of the cervical esophagus may be helpful in identifying minimally calcified chicken or fish bones in cases not detected by conventional radiography.[10]

Retained FB may result in a wide range of complications. These include mucosal abrasions, esophageal strictures, retropharyngeal abscess, perforation leading to fistula formation, mediastinitis, pneumothorax or pneumomediastinum, vascular injuries and pericarditis or pericardial tampanade. Morbidity is often related to the size and duration of the FB entrapment. Small disk batteries pose a significant threat, leading to esophageal necrosis and perforation in as little as six hours.

Management is dependent on the location and type of object as well as clinical circumstances. Any evidence of airway compromise including stridor, wheezing, and dyspnea should be managed first by securing the airway if respiratory failure is imminent, then urgent consultation for endoscopic removal. If there is evidence for complete esophageal obstruction (i.e., persistent drooling), keep the patient in a sitting position with a suction catheter to aid with oral secretion.

Uncomplicated retained FB can be removed by other techniques. Single, smooth, blunt, radio-opaque item retained less than 72 hours can be removed using a Foley catheter. This procedure is most commonly done for objects retained high and the thoracic inlet and is often done under fluoroscopy. If the FB is at the distal esophagus, is smooth, not caustic and within 24 hours of ingestion, temporization with observation in the hospital or at home with a repeat x-ray in 24 hours is a good option. Lastly, a trial of medications that relax smooth muscle such as nifedipine, glucagons, or nitroglycerine can be attempted.

Retained button batteries in the esophagus are a serious threat and require urgent transfer and removal to prevent burns (within four hours) and perforation (within six hours). Batteries beyond the GE junction <15 mm can be observed with repeat x-rays in one week. If >15 mm, repeat x-ray within 48 hours is recommended. Endoscopic removal is indicated if battery is still found in the stomach at 48 hours.[11]

Clear guidelines for the removal of gastric foreign bodies do not exist. Most gastric FB can be safely removed with the use of an endoscope and should be considered for objects more than 2 cm in diameter or 5 cm in length, especially if the object has irregular edges. However, between 80% and 93% of FB that reach the stomach will pass spontaneously.[12] Sharp or pointed objects, such as sewing needles or razor blades, should be considered for emergent endoscopic removal since 15% to 35% will cause perforation, usually at the illeocecal valve.[13] Other points of obstruction for FB distal to the stomach include the pylorus, duodenum, ileocecal valve and anus. There is a great deal of controversy as to the timing of endoscopy to remove otherwise innocuous foreign bodies that do not pass through the stomach. These retained objects pose the risk of pressure necrosis, causing gastritis or ulceration. Generally, the patients are asked to follow up in one week for a repeat radiograph and subsequent endoscopic retrieval if the FB remains in the stomach.

Patients who are to have endoscopy for gastric FB should be placed in the left lateral decubitus position in an attempt to prevent the passage of the object through the pylorus. Outpatient management of benign FB should include close follow-up and a high-residue diet to promote passage through the gastrointestinal tract. Repeat radiographs weekly may be employed to follow the progression of the object through the gut. Patients should be advised to seek immediate medical attention for any abdominal pain, vomiting or fever.

Inflammatory Disorders

Reflux Esophagitis

Reflux esophagitis or gastroesophageal reflux disease (GERD) is a condition that involves retrograde flow of gastric acid or, rarely, alkaline bilious materials leading to erosive injury of the esophagus. The lower esophageal sphincter (LES) acts as a protective barrier separating the esophageal wall from the acidic environment of the stomach. Pathologic movement of gastric contents due to diminished LES tone or an anatomic abnormality affecting the LES, such as a hiatal hernia, is the hallmark of GERD. The level of esophagitis is more dependent on the frequency of refluxed gastric secretions than the quantity of secretion. Patients with esophageal motility disorders noted above, diabetes, or pregnancy are at higher risk for repeated esophageal erosion. Certain foods have a propensity for relaxing the LES including peppermint, alcohol, onions, tobacco products, chocolate, caffeine and fat. Other food items have a direct irritating effect on inflamed esophageal mucosa including tomato based foods, spicy foods, alcohol and tobacco products. Lastly, several drugs potentiate relaxation of the LES including calcium channel blockers, nitrates, progestins, estrogens, and anticholinergics.

Patients with GERD present most commonly with "heartburn" or a burning sensation in their epigastrium and lower substernal chest. The sensation may radiate into their back or upward into their throat leading to a sour taste in their mouth. Persistent airway irritation may cause persistent cough, wheezing, vocal changes or stridor. Patient often have more frequent nighttime symptoms when lying supine. Bending forward or eating large boluses of food may precipitate their symptoms. While symptoms occur equally in men and women, the incidence of endoscopically confirmed esophagitis and progression to Barrett metaplasia is higher in men.

A 24-hour esophageal monitor is considered the "gold standard" for the diagnosis of GERD. However, a two-week treatment trial with a proton-pump inhibitor (PPI) carries similar sensitivity and specificity compared with esophageal monitoring and is both diagnostic and therapeutic.[14] Lack of improvement strongly suggests that the patient needs further evaluation for a different etiology.

H2 receptor antagonists are less effective in clinical trials as compared to proton-pump inhibitors.[15]

Endoscopy is useful for evaluating complications of GERD. However, fewer than 50% of people with GERD have evidence of esophagitis on endoscopy. Complications of GERD include esophagitis, Barrett esophagus, and strictures.

Caustic Injury

Esophageal injuries from caustic agents are common with an annual incidence of 200,000 reported cases in 2000. The majority (80%) occurs in children as accidental ingestions. However, adult ingestions tend to be more serious as they are often in the setting of a suicidal attempt. Caustic ingestions include both acid and alkali material. They have both an acute phase with perforation, sepsis and/or death, and a chronic phase manifest by stricture formation and esophageal dysmotility.

Alkali Ingestions

Alkali ingestions account for the majority of caustic ingestions in the U.S. Alkalis are commonly found in household cleaning agents, drain openers and detergents. Bleach solutions often carry mild to moderate irritants, while drain cleaners carry more dangerous concentrations of alkali substances.

The severity of caustic alkali ingestions is dependent on several factors:
- The substance
- The concentration
- The amount
- The physical form
- The duration of contact[16]

Liquid caustic agents diffuse more rapidly and lead to more extensive field of injury, usually predominate in the esophagus and stomach. Solids and crystal particles however, are more likely to affect the mucous membranes and oral cavity. They tend to adhere to the mucosa and burn localized areas, and thus difficult to swallow and less likely to affect the esophagus and stomach. The duration of contact time until removal or dilution for both solids and liquid states correlates with the severity of injury. Solutions with a pH > 12 are highly corrosive. "A 22.5% solution of sodium hydroxide can produce a full thickness esophageal burn in 10 seconds while the same result can occur within 1 second if the concentration is 30%."[17] Anatomic and physiologic factors such as pyloric sphincter tone and laryngeal or esophageal spasm play a role in increasing the duration of contact. Lastly, stomach contents can affect the dilution rate.

The esophagus is the predominant site of injury for liquid alkali ingestions. Severe damage occurs rapidly prior to the patients presenting to the emergency department. Alkali produces suponification of tissues by liquefaction necrosis in the acute injury (phase 0) and is exacerbated by thrombosis of small blood vessels and heat production. This initial injury may last for minutes to several hours. Phase 1 injury occurs over the next four to seven days, marked by tissue sloughing, bacterial invasion, and a severe inflammatory response. Necrosis continues due to

vascular thrombosis and mediastinitis occurs with or without perforation due to translocation of bacteria into the mediastinal spaces. Perforation is more common during the first one to two weeks due to the low tensile strength of the early granulation tissue formation seen in phase 2 (days 5 to 15). During this phase, collagen deposition and mucosal reepithelialization begin and often last for several weeks. Endoscopy is avoided during this time due to the weak state of the esophagus and risk for perforation. Phase 3 is marked by retraction and stricture formation at week 3 and continues for many months. The contraction of collagen shortens both the length and circumference of the esophagus leading to stricture formation in up to 15% of patients. Anatomical derangement often leads to decreased LES pressure and persistent gastroesophageal reflux potentiating further stricture formation. Lastly, caustic injury affects esophageal motility resulting in abnormal or absent peristalsis.[17]

The clinical presentation is dependent on the timing of ingestion. Acute alkali ingestions are more likely to cause significant esophageal injury in the early stages and may progress rapidly to mediastinitis, perforation, sepsis and death. In all acute ingestions, the treating physician must first consider airway compromise. Hoarseness or stridor suggests laryngeal or epiglottis involvement where airway edema can progress rapidly. Definitive airway management with direct laryngoscopy and endotracheal intubation should be considered early in any patient with symptoms of airway involvement. Blind nasotracheal intubation is contraindicated. Patients may present with dysphagia or odynophagia indicating esophageal involvement, epigastric pain or hematemesis indicating gastric involvement or massive hematemesis in the setting of an aortoenteric fistula. The available literature is conflicted regarding the accuracy of clinical signs and symptoms in predicting esophageal injury. Anyone at risk for esophageal injury from caustic alkali ingestion should be evaluated thoroughly with a GI consultation before discharge from the emergency department.

Management of the patient with a caustic ingestion focuses on protecting the airway, and on preventing further damage by avoiding induced emesis or gastric lavage that allows the caustic agent to wick up to outside of the tube. Reexposure of the agent to the esophagus will cause further damage and may facilitate perforation. Milk and water have been used empirically as an antidote, but have no proven efficacy in this setting and may increase the risk of vomiting and are thus contraindicated.[17] Charcoal is contraindicated, as it obscures the endoscopic field and lacks any benefit in chemical absorption. Plain radiographs are helpful in determining mediastinal air or intra-abdominal free air suggesting perforation of the esophagus or stomach respectively. Prior to endoscopy, oral inspection and laryngoscopy should be employed to evaluate the airway. Any evidence of epiglottic or supraglottic erythema or edema is an indication to secure the airway with endotracheal intubation or tracheostomy. Endoscopy should be considered in most ingestions early within the first 12 to 24 hours. Household bleach ingestions or asymptomatic children may not need endoscopy. Patients should not undergo endoscopy between five and fifteen days due to a very high risk of perforation.

Esophageal rest in patients with severe burns is indicated for six to eight weeks following ingestion. Patients remain at high risk for perforation during the first two weeks following initial ingestion and should be evaluated should they present with severe chest or abdominal pain or sepsis. All patients are subject to lifelong endoscopic surveillance due to the increased risk of squamous cell esophageal carcinoma, especially in the setting of lye ingestions.[17] Also, close monitoring for GERD and other complications of stricture formation is necessary to prevent ongoing esophageal damage.

Acid Ingestions

Acids are much less common in the U.S. compared with alkali compounds and represent only 5% of all caustic ingestions. In the U.S., common acid compounds are found in household items such as toilet bowel cleaner, battery fluids or rust removal compounds. Solutions with a pH of <2 are highly caustic, although in general, acid ingestion are far less severe than alkali.

Acid ingestion produces a coagulation necrosis injury to the esophagus and stomach. They require a greater contact time, thus limiting the potential injury to the oropharynx. While it was generally accepted that the stomach assumes the majority of damage in acid ingestions, recent literature has implicated significant esophageal injury as well.[17] As tissue undergoes coagulation necrosis, an eschar is rapidly formed that can limit tissue penetration resulting in a decreased rate of perforation as compared to alkali ingestions. The location of injury in the stomach is somewhat dependent on the stomach contents. A solid-filled stomach will wick the caustic acid to the distal stomach while a liquid-filled stomach will have diffuse injury. Esophageal complications of acid ingestions are similar to those seen in alkali with stricture formation and motility disorders. Gastric complications are often more serious in acid ingestions and may result in gastric outlet obstruction.

Infectious Esophagitis

Infectious esophagitis is a common disorder of patients with an immunocompromised state. Patients at highest risk include HIV or AIDS patients, underlying malignancy, organ transplant patients or diabetes. The three main causes for infectious esophagitis include monilial infections, herpes simplex virus (HSV), and cytomegalovirus (CMV).

Monilial Esophagitis

Monilial or fungal esophagitis is most commonly due to *Candida* species and manifests as mild odynophagia, dysphagia, and retrosternal chest pain. It can represent an AIDS-defining opportunistic infection. An additional risk factor includes a disruption of mucosal integrity (e.g., following radiation, trauma, chemotherapy). Fluconazole has become the first-line drug of choice for *Candida* esophagitis due to its improved side-effect profile and its availability in both oral and IV dosing.[18]

Cytomegalovirus Esophagitis

CMV is the most common viral cause of infectious esophagitis. It is often associated with immunocompromised patients especially those who have undergone solid organ transplantation. Patients present with a similar history of dysphagia and odynophagia. Visualization of CMV lesions either directly or through endoscopy reveals deep, linear or longitudinal ulcerations. Treatment includes the antiviral medication gancyclovir or foscarnet.

Herpes Esophagitis

HSV esophagitis is another common cause of infectious esophagitis. The presentation is similar to those above with significant dysphagia and odynophagia. Patients may have oral or labial lesions present at the time of presentation as well, although not in all cases. HSV lesions can be distinguished from those of CMV or *Candida* as they appear to be erupting from the mucosa as a well circumscribed "volcano"-like appearance. Treatment includes topical anesthetics for all causes of infectious esophagitis as well as antiviral therapy such as acyclovir or valacyclovir.[19]

Disorders of the Stomach

Structural Lesions

Volvulus

Gastric volvulus is a potentially life-threatening surgical emergency that occurs when the stomach rotates upon itself. If not reversed, this abnormal rotation may lead to a closed loop obstruction with bowel ischemia, necrosis, perforation and ultimately death. Mortality in acute volvulus is up to 50%; however, with rapid diagnosis and treatment, current mortality rates are about 16%. Fifteen to 20% of cases occur in children less than 1 year of age due to congenital diaphragmatic defects.[20] The peak incidence in adults is in the fifth decade, with men and women being equally affected. While the majority of cases of gastric volvulus are chronic in nature, it is often under-diagnosed since it is frequently associated with transient, nonspecific symptoms such as heartburn, vomiting, or epigastric discomfort with meals.

The pathophysiology of gastric volvulus involves both a primary (subdiaphragmatic) and secondary (supradiaphragmatic) etiologies. Primary volvulus makes up one-third of all cases and is due to abnormal laxity of suspensory ligaments. Secondary volvulus is more common and is due to an underlying diaphragmatic defect. Predisposing factors of secondary volvulus includes (paraesophageal) hiatal hernia, elevation of the diaphragm, trauma to the diaphragm, gastric ulcer or neoplasm, diaphragm paralysis, intra-abdominal adhesions, and extrinsic pressure on the stomach. Rotation of the stomach can occur either on a longitudinal axis (organo-axial) or a horizontal axis (mesenteroaxial rotation).

Acute gastric volvulus presents with sudden onset of severe left upper quadrant pain or chest pain dependent on the location of the volvulus (above or below the diaphragm). The presenting pain is associated with vomiting progressing to nonproductive retching. Physical exam may reveal a distended upper abdomen with a normal soft lower abdomen and minimal abdominal tenderness. In 1904, Borchardt described a clinical triad associated with gastric volvulus that includes the following: severe epigastric pain with distention, violent non-productive retching and inability to pass a nasogastric tube.[20] In children, these symptoms are common and may also be associated with respiratory distress, dyspepsia, and dysphagia. Chronic volvulus is associated with recurrent vomiting, nausea, intermittent dysphagia, failure to thrive, irritability, and chronic, recurrent epigastric pain.

Patients with symptoms suggestive of gastric volvulus should get an upright chest and abdominal radiograph. In the acute presentation, gastric dilation is evident while the distal bowel has a paucity of gas. Barium swallow may aid in radiographic diagnosis. Acute gastric volvulus is a surgical emergency with complications that include perforation, hemorrhage, pancreatic and gastric necrosis, and omental avulsion. Emergency department interventions for patients suspected of gastric volvulus include IV hydration and gastric decompression with nasogastric tube. Immediate surgical consultation is warranted. Endoscopic decompression may be considered in some patients who are poor surgical candidates. Care should be taken as gastric perforation may occur with endoscopy or NGT placement.

Rupture

Gastric rupture refers to a tear in the stomach wall with release of gastric content into the peritoneum. The stomach is relatively resistant to rupture, with its muscular wall having the ability to greatly expand with increases in gastric content, a phenomenon known as receptive relaxation. Also, these muscular walls are mobile and can decompress through two valves, the gastroesophageal and the pyloric to decrease intragastric pressure. Gastric rupture is a rare condition with both traumatic and non-traumatic causes.

Non-traumatic or "spontaneous" gastric rupture appears to have preponderance among women and a mean age of occurrence of 43 years. Spontaneous gastric rupture occurs from an increase in intra-abdominal pressure and gastric distention combined with forceful emesis. It has also been described with overeating and overdrinking, sodium bicarbonate antacids, bag-valve-mask ventilation, esophageal intubation and oxygen therapy by nasal cannula. Predisposing factors include obstructing tumors of the esophagus, pylorus or duodenum that prohibit normal decompression.

The stomach's position in the abdomen is well protected by the rib cage and the liver with a high degree of mobility and thick muscular wall making it remarkably resistant to traumatic rupture. In fact, rupture due to blunt trauma has an overall incidence of 0.025 to 0.4% of all blunt trauma admissions in recent retrospective series.[21] Rupture is most commonly associated with motor vehicle accidents and has been seen with exertion with heavy lifting, forceful Heimlich maneuver or chest compressions

with CPR or with forceful coughing. A history of a recent meal prior to gastric rupture is common.

Patients with gastric rupture complain of an abrupt onset of pain associated with a bursting sensation. There is usually severe pain with signs of peritoneal irritation. Patients will have a distended and often rigid abdomen, and a small percentage will have subcutaneous emphysema with air passing through the mediastinum into the neck. Patients generally progress to shock rapidly.

Diagnostic studies to consider include an upright chest x-ray and/or lateral decubitus abdominal x-ray looking for free air. CT with oral and IV contrast is more sensitive than plain radiographs but takes more time and may compromise a patient in shock. Peritoneal lavage is one of the most sensitive indicators of gastric rupture after blunt trauma. Since most patients with gastric rupture present with impressive abdominal findings, there is little need for diagnostic workup prior to surgical exploration. The differential diagnosis includes all forms of abdominal catastrophe including aortic dissection and rupture, bowel infarction, rupture of the gallbladder and spleen and volvulus. Any perforated viscus, more commonly in the setting of peptic ulcer disease or appendicitis, may present with symptoms similar to stomach rupture.

ED management of gastric rupture should include aggressive fluid resuscitation and early administration of parenteral broad-spectrum antibiotics. Nasogastric suction may help reduce the amount of peritoneal soilage. Emergent surgical intervention is needed for peritoneal lavage and gastric repair.

Gastric Outlet Obstruction

Gastric outlet obstruction (GOO) is the result of a mechanical and/or pathophysiological abnormality that leads to restricted or blocked gastric emptying. The obstruction can be the result of either a benign or malignant underlying etiology. GOO was primarily a complication of peptic ulcer disease due to its prevalence and lack of definitive treatment. However, current studies have shown that it is now due to underlying malignancy the majority of the time. Currently, GOO is found in less than 5% of patients with peptic ulcer disease (PUD).[22] These patients typically have a long (>10 year) history of PUD, usually with a severe clinical course.

The predominant presenting symptoms associated with GOO include epigastric abdominal pain, vomiting, weight loss. Patients will also note early satiety and emesis after an evening meal with food from earlier in the day present in the emesis. Physical exam may reveal a palpable mass if the GOO is related to malignancy, a seccussion splash (splashing sound elicited by gently rocking the abdomen), and evidence of chronic malnutrition or dehydration.

In the ED, the workup should include an upright abdominal film, which often reveals a markedly dilated stomach shadow with a large air fluid level. Also, there may be a paucity of gas in the small and large intestine. Chemistries should be obtained to evaluate for hypokalemia, hypochloremic metabolic alkalosis due to chronic vomiting. Fluid and electrolyte replacement should be initiated as well as nasogastric tube insertion with wall suction to evacuate the distended abdomen.

Conditions that may mimic gastric outlet obstruction that more commonly present to the ED include gastroparesis and small bowel obstruction. Gastroparesis often occurs in the setting of predisposing illness, such as long-standing diabetes or scleroderma, and classically causes vomiting with little associated abdominal pain. Small bowel obstruction is often more acute onset than GOO and may have characteristic small bowel air-fluid level on x-ray. All patients with suspected GOO should be admitted to the hospital with a gastroenterology consultation. Endoscopy should be performed for definitive diagnosis and biopsy for malignant causes if indicated. Definitive management may include endoscopic balloon dilation or surgical pyloroplasty or gastric resection.

Tumors

Worldwide, gastric cancer has been a major cause of cancer death. It is the leading cause of cancer death in Japan. The incidence in the U.S. continues to decrease, however, gastric cancer remains the eighth leading cause of cancer death overall.

Gastric cancer has been linked to several factors. The relationship of diet and gastric cancer has been investigated extensively in the Japanese population. Foods high in nitrates such as smoked fish and meats, salty food and pickled foods prevalent in the Japanese culture have been implicated as a significant risk factor for developing gastric cancer. Genetic factors also appear to play a role. Families with a first-degree relative with gastric cancer have an eightfold increased risk of developing gastric cancer. Underlying gastric pathology such as atrophic gastritis (often related to *Helicobacter pylori* infection) as well as previous gastric ulcer surgery increases the risk for developing gastric cancer. Other risk factors include lower socioeconomic class, living in cold climates, age and male sex.

The majority of gastric cancers are adenocarcinomas (95%).[23] Other forms include, lymphoma, and leiomyosarcoma. In the United States, tumor staging is done using the standard TMN staging. Gastric cancer most commonly develops in the lower portion of the stomach (42%). It spreads locally and may invade the submucosal layer and directly invade surrounding structures such as the esophagus or duodenum, liver, pancreas, and colon. It can metastasize through the blood and lymphatics to these and other organs. It often presents with an initial left supraclavicular lymph node involvement (Virchow's node).

Clinical manifestation of gastric cancer is often vague. Patients will often have constitutional symptoms on review of systems such as weight loss, fatigue and night sweats. Patients often have a persistent abdominal pain that presents initially generalized and associated with early satiety. Abdominal distention and fullness are often noted after a bolus of food. Patients may present with gastric outlet obstruction with acute abdominal pain, nausea and vomiting as noted previously.

Diagnosis is made with endoscopy and biopsy of suspicious lesions. Workup can often be done in the outpatient setting. Those who present with failure to thrive or gastric outlet obstruction should be admitted for parenteral nutrition and more urgent endoscopy and diagnostic workup.

Five-year survival from gastric cancer in the U.S. is 15%.[23] Treatment is dependent of the grade and staging of each tumor. Tumor resection is widely curative for localized lesions without spread.

Inflammatory Disorders

Acute Gastritis

Injury to the gastric mucosa denoted by epithelial cell damage associated with local inflammation, seen histologically, is termed gastritis. The term gastritis, however, is often used broadly to describe all forms of epithelial cell damage with or without inflammation based on visualization by endoscopy. Gastric mucosal damage without inflammation is histologically distinct from gastritis and is properly referred to as gastropathy. Gastritis is most commonly due to infection, primarily *H. pylori*. Acute mucosal injury without inflammation is due to chemical irritants or drugs (NSAIDs), bile reflux, mucosal hypoxia (stress ulcers in trauma or burns) or chronic congestion. While the terms gastropathy and gastritis are often lumped into the broad category of acute or chronic gastritis, there are several classification systems that differentiate gastritis and gastropathy, acute and chronic disease, as well as variations in inflammatory cell infiltration.

Acute gastritis due to *H. pylori* infection has been demonstrated in studies where healthy volunteers were inoculated with *H. pylori* and developed a mild illness. While patients with acute infection may develop clinically relevant symptoms, they rarely undergo endoscopy or serologic *H. pylori* testing. These patients typically present later in the course with chronic inflammatory changes and peptic ulcer disease. The true incidence of acute gastritis is unknown due to the vast majority of cases going undiagnosed or diagnosed on clinical grounds leading to empiric treatment usually for dyspepsia.

Acute gastropathy however, is due to an irritant that can often be differentiated in the history. NSAIDs, corrosive agents, chemotherapeutic agents, radiation, bile reflux, physiologic stress, and alcohol have all been linked to destruction of epithelial gastric mucosa without local inflammation. Mucosal destruction is often transient and self-limited once the offending agent is removed. Chronic gastritis and gastropathy are on a clinical continuum with peptic ulcer disease (PUD). Acute ulceration can be seen in stress ulcer syndrome discussed later in this chapter.

Acute gastritis and gastropathy presents with vague upper abdominal complaints including dyspepsia or indigestion. Vomiting may be present. Acute gastritis/gastropathy can cause a significant amount of bleeding and patients may complain of hematemesis or have guaiac-positive stools. Patients with acute gastritis or gastropathy should not have signs of peritoneal inflammation.

Gastritis and gastropathy generally represents a diagnosis of exclusion for emergency physicians. Diagnostic workup in the ED should include a diligent search for other causes of upper abdominal pain and dyspepsia. A hematocrit or hemoglobin level, stool guaiac, transaminases, bilirubin, lipase or amylase should be performed with a consideration for an EKG and cardiac workup in the at risk patient population. Nasogastric suction should be performed in any patient with a history of hematemesis.

Treatment of acute gastritis should begin after a thorough evaluation of other possible causes has been done. The first-line therapy is to remove the offending agent. Antiemetics should be used to help control nausea and vomiting. Antisecretory medication such as H_2 blocker and proton-pump inhibitors have some clinical efficacy in treating acute gastritis/gastropathy as well as antacids, and the prostaglandin derivative misoprostol. Other recommendations should include cessation of smoking and alcohol use and the institution of a bland diet. Indications for admission include intractable vomiting, hematemesis with evidence of continued or massive hemorrhage, severe dehydration or further diagnostic workup for other possible diagnoses.

Drug-Induced Gastropathy

Several medications have been associated with gastric mucosal damage leading to gastric ulceration. Non-steroidal anti-inflammatory medications, including aspirin, are the most common offending agents in this category. The gastric mucosal injury is mediated by inhibition of mucosal cyclooxygenase activity and thus a decrease in prostaglandin production, leading to a breakdown in the mucosal barrier (mucin, bicarbonate and phospholipids secretion). The concomitant infection of *H. pylori* seems to increase the risk of ulceration and bleeding complications noted in a recent meta-analysis.[24] The risk of developing significant NSAID-induced gastropathy increases with duration of therapy. Other risk factors identified by the American College of Gastroenterology include:

- Age >60 (increases risk 5 to 6 times)
- Prior history of adverse gastrointestinal event (4 to 5 times)
- High dosage of NSAID (up to 10 times)
- Additional use of glucocorticoids (4 to 5 times)
- Additional use of anticoagulants (10 to 15 times)[25]

There is a strong correlation between dyspepsia and pathologic findings associated with drug-induced gastropathy. Treatment includes discontinuing the offending medication or changing from a nonselective NSAID to a selective COX-2 inhibitor, or the addition of an antisecretory agent such as an H_2 blocker or proton-pump inhibitor. Some authors advocate for primary prophylaxis against NSAID-induced gastropathy with synthetic prostaglandins such as misoprostol. Caution should be used by emergency physicians when prescribing NSAIDs, especially in elderly patients, or consider an alternative analgesic.

Corrosive Gastritis

The ingestion of caustic substances can cause severe gastropathy leading to both acute and chronic complications. The stomach is susceptible to damage from both highly acidic and alkali compounds. Alkaline compounds cause a liquefaction necrosis leading to saponification of tissues and a deeper penetration burn that more commonly affects the esophagus. Acid ingestion, less common in the U.S., leads to coagulation necrosis and an eschar formation, which is thought to be protective from deeper penetration. In general, acid ingestions are far less severe than alkali ingestions.

Swallowing a caustic substance and subsequent gastric injury causes severe epigastric pain that is often accompanied by retching and vomiting of blood and necrotic tissue. Airway compromise can occur early. Any patient with stridor, hoarseness or shortness of breath should be considered for immediate intubation. Blind nasotracheal intubation is contraindicated. Other early complications include hypovolemia, gastric or esophageal perforation and metabolic acidosis. Long-term complications include gastric outlet obstruction and stricture formation that can occur weeks to years post ingestion.

ED management of patients with corrosive gastritis should include IV hydration, chest and abdominal radiographs looking for evidence of perforation, and admission. Insertion of a nasogastric tube is contraindicated in caustic ingestions due to the risk of perforation and wicking of the caustic up the tubing leading to further esophageal injury and airway compromise. Likewise, emetic agents and administering "neutralizing" agents is also contraindicated. There is conflicting reports of benefit in preventing stricture formation with corticosteroids.

Stress-Related Gastropathy

In experimental models, stress predisposes to both gastric and duodenal injury. While it is well accepted that physical stressors lead to gastric mucosal injury, some debate exists as to whether psychological stress causes damage. Gastric damage is a significant problem in patients with large (>35% body surface area) burns (Curling's ulcers), sepsis, respiratory failure requiring prolonged mechanical ventilation, trauma, shock or prolonged hypotension, renal failure, and multi-organ failure. These physiologic stressors cause damage by mucosal hypoxia. Prolonged ICU stays or CNS injury (Cushing's ulcers) leads to inflammatory ulceration and are thought to be clinically distinct from stress ulcers. Of particular importance to the emergency medicine setting is the increased risk of patients at extended care facilities.

Stress-related gastropathy leads to acute hemorrhagic or erosive gastropathy. Therefore, the most common presentation is bleeding manifesting as hematemesis, guaiac-positive stools or frank melena.

Treatment involves primary prophylaxis in patients at risk. In the ICU setting, early enteral feeding can prevent ulcer formation. Antacids, H_2 blockers, proton-pump inhibitors, and sucralfate have been proven efficacious for prevention, as well. Initiation of therapeutic agents in the ED is warranted for clinically evident bleeding. [See section on peptic ulcer disease for specific guidelines regarding upper GI bleeding management.]

Peptic Ulcer Disease

Peptic ulcer disease (PUD) is the destruction of the gastric or duodenal wall beyond the submucosa and into the muscularis mucosa. PUD is caused by both the destructive forces of pepsin and acid secreted by the chief cells and parietal cells in conjunction with the breakdown or destruction of the gastroduodenal mucosal defenses. In general, PUD is a chronic disease process involving either the gastric or duodenal mucosal ulceration. There are approximately 500,000 new cases each year with a lifetime prevalence of 12% for men and 9% for women.[26] While there are some pathophysiologic differences between GU and DU, they are typically catalyzed by two main risk factors, *H. pylori* infection and NSAID use.

The gastric wall normally maintains a matrix of mucin and bicarbonate to protect the mucosal layer from the digestive juices ever present in the stomach. Breakdown of this layer is due to chronic infection with *H. pylori* that causes a chronic active gastritis leading to a disruption in mucosal integrity and a transient increase in acid secretion. *H. pylori* is the leading cause of PUD found in 80% of gastric ulcer cases and nearly 100% of duodenal ulcer cases.[27] The prevalence of *H. pylori* infection is around 5% to 15% in the U.S. in patients less than 18 years old and increases with age.[28] Aspirin and NSAID use accounts for 25% of all cases.[29] Their action decreases prostaglandin production which normally facilitates mucin layer building. The risk is highest in the first 3 months of NSAID use. Other risk factors for PUD include significant physiologic stress due to medical illness such as burns or trauma, renal failure, cirrhosis, pulmonary disease, smoking, genetics, Zollinger-Ellison syndrome, genetics, and radiation. Ethanol consumption, diet, corticosteroid use, and psychological stress all remain controversial risk factors for PUD.

Patients with PUD typically present with epigastric abdominal pain. It is often burning, cramping, sharp or gnawing. Pain is exacerbated with eating in 60% to 90% of cases and usually transiently improved with antacids or food. Patients may have variations of the pain syndrome often more localized with DU while GU are more vague and less localized. Both may present with radiation to the back, right or left upper quadrants. Up to 70% may experience more bloating, distention or belching. Nausea and vomiting often represent underlying gastric outlet obstruction. Physical exam may reveal epigastric or upper quadrant tenderness. Severe pain is more concerning as it may be a hallmark of more severe disease or complications of PUD. Abdominal distention, dizziness, lightheadedness or weakness may indicate bowel perforation or GI bleeding.

PUD cannot be diagnosed on clinical grounds alone. Definitive diagnosis includes endoscopy or barium swallow and should be arranged in consultation with the patient's primary care provider or a gastroenterologist. In the ED, focus is on evaluating for potential complications such as hemorrhage or perforation as well as pancreatitis, neoplasm, GERD or gastritis.

Treatment of presumed uncomplicated PUD in the ED is controversial. All potential ulcer causing medications and habits should be discontinued if possible. There is debate as to whether anti-ulcer medication should be started in the ED. Likewise, anti-*H. pylori* therapy should not be started without definitive diagnosis by biopsy or serum antibody test. Anti-ulcer treatment options include H_2 antagonists, proton pump inhibitors, prostaglandin analogue (Misoprostol), sucralfate, bismuth and antacids. H_2 antagonists, PPIs, and misoprostol have similar cure rates after six to eight weeks of treatment while misoprostol has better long-term prevention for patients who must remain on NSAIDs.[30] Outpatient treatment with one of these agents should be started only after consultation with gastroenterology or the primary care provider.

PUD Complications

Hemorrhage

Hemorrhage is the most common complication of PUD, occurring in approximately 15% of ulcer patients. Hemorrhage usually occurs in older, chronic ulcer patients with a peak incidence in the sixth decade. PUD accounts for 50 to 55% of all upper GI bleeding.[31] Complications due to PUD occur most commonly in chronic fibrosed ulcers that penetrate deep into the gastric wall. The ulcer erodes into vessels both venous and arterial leading to painless bleeding, hematemesis or melena in 95% of patients. If significant pain is present, perforation should be considered.

The differential diagnosis to consider in any patient with evidence of upper gastrointestinal bleeding includes gastritis, gastric or esophageal varices, Mallory-Weiss tears, esophagitis, and duodenitis. Endoscopy is needed to differentiate the source of the bleeding.

As a patient arrives in the ED, a rapid assessment of the hematocrit and coagulation studies as well as stool guaiac should be done. Blood for type and cross-match for packed red cells should be sent. Type O negative blood may be used if needed before cross-matched blood is available. Insertion of a nasogastric tube and aspiration is routinely performed despite its lack in sensitivity in ruling out active bleeding. Nevertheless, return of "coffee ground emesis" or frank blood helps to establish the bleeding as being upper GI in origin.

Pharmacologic interventions should be started early for those patients thought to have continuous active bleeding. Intravenous proton pump inhibitors have been proven to be effective in preventing rebleeding in patients with bleeding peptic ulcers. IV omeprazole was found to be both beneficial in preventing rebleeding and cost effective in these patients. At this time, omeprazole is not available in a parenteral form in the U.S. Pantoprazole is available in the U.S. and the suggested dose is an 80 mg bolus followed by 8 mg/hr infusion.

H_2 blockers have been shown to have only minimal benefit with parenteral administration and only in gastric ulcers. Without endoscopic diagnosis, H_2 blockers are not recommended as a first-line agent in this setting. There has been some proven benefit in the use of somatostatin and it analog octreotide. Their use is more common in the setting of variceal bleeding but have been proven to be of some benefit in reducing the risk of continued ulcer bleeding and should be considered especially with brisk bleeding or prolonged time to endoscopy.[32]

Endoscopy should be considered for all patients with upper GI bleeding (UGIB). In addition to locating the site of the bleed, several endoscopic modalities such as laser therapy, thermal probes and injection sclerotherapy are available. Endoscopic findings can also predict persistent or recurrent bleeding:

- Active bleeding during endoscopy has a 90% recurrence rate
- A visible vessel on endoscopy has a 50% recurrence rate
- An adherent clot has a 25% to 30% recurrence rate[33]

Any patient with evidence of significant UGI bleeding should be admitted to the hospital. Those patients with hemodynamic instability, repeated episodes of hematemesis or hematochezia, age over 60, a failure to clear with gastric lavage or significant cardiac, pulmonary or renal disease should be admitted to an ICU setting. Ten to 32% of patients admitted to the hospital because of UGIB caused by PUD will rebleed.[34]

Perforation

Perforation is the second most common complication of PUD occurring in 5% to 10% of patients with known PUD.[26] Perforation occurs when the ulcer extends through the muscle wall and serosa, establishing a communication between the lumen and the peritoneal cavity. PUD related perforation occurs most frequently in the duodenum (60%), followed by gastric (20%) and antral (20%),[35] and has classically been associated with chronic ulcerations. Males in their fourth and fifth decade with a history of smoking and frequent alcohol use fit the main profile for ulcer perforation. The demographics have shifted over the past ten to fifteen years with the advent of H_2 blockers with a fourfold rise in the number of women affected. Currently, women in their sixth decade on NSAIDs and corticosteroid therapy are at highest risk.[36] While most people with perforation have a history of dyspepsia, perforation is the first manifestation of their ulcer disease in 25% of patients.

Spillage of gastric or duodenal contents causes a chemical peritonitis that can quickly progress into bacterial peritonitis. In the initial phase, patients complain of sudden, severe epigastric or generalized abdominal pain. They are often tachycardic and have peripheral vasoconstriction. In the second phase, the pain improves except with movement and the abdominal wall is rigid. Lastly, the abdomen becomes increasingly distended and pain increases. By this time patients begin third spacing fluids causing intravascular collapse and shock. The time course is generally over 12 hours, but may last up to 24 hours.

Demonstration of free air on an upright chest x-ray or left decubitus abdominal film is diagnostic. However, this finding is present in only 60% to 70% of cases. Insufflation with 250 cc of air or instillation of a water-soluble contrast material through a nasogastric tube may be done to aid in the diagnosis.[37] An abdominal CT scan has a much greater sensitivity (>95%) however, and is arguably safer than insufflation or contrast.[38]

Treatment includes rapid fluid resuscitation, correction of electrolyte abnormalities, nasogastric suction and administration of broad-spectrum antibiotics. Timely surgical intervention is indicated in almost all cases. There is a statistically significant difference in time to definitive treatment at twelve hours showing fewer adverse events in patients with duodenal perforation. Therefore, rapid triage and surgical consultation is extremely important in improving outcome. Rarely, some perforations can be treated nonoperatively or with percutaneous drainage. The overall mortality for perforated PUD is 6% to 10%.

Penetration

Penetration describes the erosion of an ulcer through the entire thickness of the stomach or duodenal wall without leakage of digestive contents into the peritoneal cavity. The ulcerative process is contained by fibrous adhesions to adjacent structures, such as the pancreas (most common) and biliary tract. Penetration occurs most commonly with posterior wall ulcers.

Most patients with penetrating ulcers have had longstanding symptoms and present with a change in the pattern of their usual ulcer pain. They frequently describe a change in their pain from episodic to constant, with new referral of the pain to the midback. Ultrasound and CT may aid in the diagnosis.

References

1. Goyal RK. Diseases of the esophagus. In: Braunwald E, ed. *Harrison's Principles of Internal Medicine,* 15th ed. New York: McGraw-Hill 2001:1642.
2. Panacek A. Upper gastrointestinal bleeding. In: Harwood-Nuss A, ed. *The Clinical Practice of Emergency Medicine,* 3rd ed. Philadelphia: Lippincott, Williams & Wilkins, 2001:767–771.
3. Roerts LR, Kamath PS. Pathophysiology and treatment of variceal hemorrhage. *Mayo Clinic Proceedings* 1996;71:973–978.
4. Kortas DY, Haas LS, Simpson WG, et al. Mallory-Weiss tear: Predisposing factors and predictors of a complicated course. *Am J Gastroenterol* 2001;96:2863–2865.
5. Siddiq MA, Sood S, Strachan D. Pharyngeal pouch (Zenker's diverticulum). *Postgrad Med J* 2001;77:506–511.
6. Tobin R. Esophageal rings, webs, and diverticula. *J Clin Gastroenterol* 1998;27:285–295.
7. Shaheen N, Ransohoff DF. Gastroesophageal reflux, Barrett esophagus, and esophageal cancer: scientific review. *JAMA* 2002;287:1972–1981.
8. Fuchs CS, Mayer RJ. Gastric carcinoma. *N Engl J Med* 1995;333:32–41.
9. Nandi P, Ong GB. Foreign body in the oesophagus: review of 2394 cases. *Br J Surg* 1978;65:5–9.
10. Lue AJ, Fang WD, Manolidis S. Use of plain radiography and computed tomography to identify fish bone foreign bodies. *Otolaryngol Head & Neck Surg* 2000;123:435–438.
11. Litovitz T, Schmitz BF. Ingestion of cylindrical and button batteries: An analysis of 2382 cases. *Pediatrics* 1992;89:747–757.
12. Eisen GM, Baron TH, Dominitz JA, et al. Guideline for the management of ingested foreign bodies. *Gastrointest Endosc* 2002;55:802–806.
13. Webb WA. Management of foreign bodies of the upper gastrointestinal tract: update. *Gastrointest Endosc* 1995;419:39–51.
14. Schenk BE, Kuipers EJ, Klinkenberg-knol EC, et al. Omeprazole as a diagnostic tool in gastroesophageal reflux disease. *Am J Gastroenterol* 1997;92:1997–2000.
15. Chiba N, De Gara CJ, Wilkinson JM, Hunt RH. Speed of healing and symptom relief in grade II to IV gastroesophageal reflux disease: A meta-analysis. *Gastroenterology* 1997;112:1798–1810.
16. Goldman LP, Weigert JM. Corrosive substance ingestion: A review. *Am J Gastroenterol* 1984;79:85–90.
17. Ramasamy K, Gumaste VV. Corrosive Ingestion in Adults. *J Clin Gastroenterol* 2003;37:119–124.
18. Vazquez JA. Invasive oesophageal candidiasis: Current and developing treatment options. *Drugs* 2003;63:971–989.
19. McBane RD, Gross JB. Herpes esophagitis: Clinical syndrome, endoscopic appearance, and diagnosis in 23 patients. *Gastrointest Endosc* 1997;37:600.
20. Mayo A, Erez I, Ludwig L, et al. Volvulus of the stomach in childhood: The spectrum of disease. *Pediatr Emerg Care* 2001;17:344.
21. Nanji SA, Mock C. Gastric rupture resulting from blunt abdominal trauma and requiring gastric resection. *J Trauma* 1999;47:410.
22. Shone DN, Nikoomanesh P, Smith-Meek MM, Bender JS. Malignancy is the most common cause of gastric outlet obstruction in the era of H2 blockers. *Am J Gastroenterol* 1995;90:1769–1770.
23. Onishi K, Miaskowski C. Mechanisms and management of gastric cancer: A comparison between the Japanese and U.S. experiences. *Cancer Nursing* 1996;19:187–196.

24. Huang JQ, Sridhar S, Hunt, RH. Role of Helicobacter pylori infection and non-steroidal anti-inflammatory drugs in peptic-ulcer disease: A meta-analysis. *Lancet* 2002;359:14–22.
25. Lanza FL. A guideline for the treatment and prevention of NSAID-induced ulcers. Members of the Ad Hoc Committee on Practice Parameters of the American College of Gastroenterology. *Am J Gastroenterol* 1998;93:2037.
26. Yardley JH, Hendrix TR. Gastritis, duodentitis, and associated ulcerative lesions. *Textbook of Gastroenterology,* 3rd ed. Philadelphia: Lippincott, 1999.
27. NIH Consensus Conference. Helicobacter pylori in peptic ulcer disease. NIH Consensus Development Panel on Helicobacter pylori in Peptic Ulcer Disease. *JAMA* 1994;272:65.
28. Smoot DT, Go MF, Cryer B. Peptic ulcer disease. *Primary Care* 2001;28: 487–503.
29. Soll AH. Consensus conference. Medical treatment of peptic ulcer disease. Practice guidelines. Practice Parameters Committee of the American College of Gastroenterology. *JAMA* 1996;275:622–629.
30. Silverstein FE, Graham DY, Senior JR, et al. Misoprostol reduces serious gastrointestinal complications in patients with rheumatoid arthritis receiving nonsteroidal anti-inflammatory drugs. *Ann Intern Med* 1995;123:214.
31. Jutabha R, Jensen DM. Management of severe upper gastrointestinal bleeding in patients with liver disease. *Med Clin North Am* 1996;80:1035.
32. Barkun A, Bardou M, Marshall JK; Nonvariceal Upper G I *Bleeding Consensus Group.* Consensus recommendations for managing patients with nonvariceal upper gastrointestinal bleeding. *Ann Intern Med* 2003;139:843–857.
33. Bleau BL, Gostout CJ, Sherman KE, et al. Recurrent bleeding from peptic ulcer associated with adherent clot: A randomized study comparing endoscopic treatment with medical therapy. *Gastrointest Endosc* 2002;56:1.
34. Lau JY, et al. Effect of intravenous omeprazole on recurrent bleeding after endoscopic treatment of bleeding peptic ulcers. *N Engl J Med* 2000;343:310.
35. Gunshefsky L, Flancbaum L, Brolin RE, et al. Changing patterns in perforated peptic ulcer disease. *Am Surgeon* 1990;56:270.
36. Hudson N. Excess long-term mortality in patients with ulcer complications. *Lancet* 1997;349:968–969.
37. Upadhye AS, Dalvi AN, Nair HT. Nasogastric air insufflation in early diagnosis of perforated peptic ulcer. *J Postgraduate Med* 1986;32:82–84.
38. Chen CH, Huang HS, Yang CC, Yeh YH. The features of perforated peptic ulcers in conventional computed tomography. *Hepato-Gastroenterology* 2001;48: 1393–1396.

Liver

Kurt R. Dischner

Lemeneh Teferah

Ralph J. Riviello

Introduction

The liver is a dynamic organ that plays a central role in digestion, metabolism, and drug and toxin excretion. It is located in the right upper quadrant of the abdomen and is bordered by the right fifth rib superiorly and the right costal margin inferiorly. The liver is the largest intra-abdominal organ and weighs approximately 1,500 g. It has a smooth surface and is encapsulated by a fibrous connective tissue called Glisson's capsule. In addition, it has four anatomical lobes, the right lobe, left lobe, caudate lobe and quadrate lobe. However, the liver is divided into two functional lobes, the left lobe and the right lobe.

The liver has a dual blood supply. The portal vein, which accounts for 70% of its supply, carries nutrient rich venous blood from the digestive tract to the liver. The hepatic artery, which accounts for the remaining 30%, supplies oxygenated blood to the liver. Venous flow from the liver originates from drainage via central veins in the liver lobules, which form the hepatic vein, which then empties into the inferior vena cava. Histologically, the liver's basic anatomical unit is the lobule. Each lobule has a central vein, where blood empties into from tributaries of the portal vein and hepatic artery, both located on the periphery. Biliary canaliculi, which drain bile from the hepatocytes, are also located at the periphery of the lobule. The liver is innervated by both parasympathetic and sympathetic fibers.

The liver is multi-functional and is essential in homeostasis of the body. It is involved in the metabolism of proteins, lipids, and carbohydrates. It is one of the main sites for gluconeogenesis and it also produces and secretes bile. In addition, the liver transforms and excretes many drugs and toxins. It is a storage site for many vitamins (A, D, B_{12}) and iron. The liver also plays a role in the immunologic system. The liver's Kupffer cells are macrophages that secrete many cytokines and interleukins involved in the immunological response.

Liver Functions Test

The diagnostic approach to patients presenting with signs and symptoms consistent with hepatitis is easy once one understands the relevance of each test. Liver function tests (LFT) commonly include aspartate aminotransferase (AST), alanine aminotransferase (ALT), alkaline phosphatase (AP), total and direct bilirubin, prothrombin time, total protein, and albumin. These tests can be divided into markers associated with hepatocellular damage, obstruction of biliary flow, and measures of hepatic function.

AST and ALT are enzymes found in hepatocytes and become elevated when hepatocytes sustain injury. These are commonly elevated with viral hepatitis, alcoholic liver disease, Wilson's disease, hemochromatosis, toxins, medications, autoimmune hepatitis, and α_1-antitrypsin deficiency.[1] In acute viral hepatitis, ALT levels often are elevated from several hundred to several thousand units/L. This is in contrast to the higher levels seen in acute toxic hepatic injury (upper hundreds to 10,000 units/L) or to the lower AST levels (mid-hundreds of units/L) in alcoholic hepatitis.[2]

It should be noted that ALT levels only moderately correlate with hepatic inflammation in chronic liver diseases. This is especially true in cirrhosis, where patients may have normal to only slightly elevated ALT and AST levels. Therefore, ALT and AST are not as sensitive in identifying chronic liver injury.[2]

ALT and AST can also be elevated with skeletal muscle injury, myocardial infarction, and polymyositis. It is also interesting to note that elevations of AST and ALT within 1.5 times of normal may not be due to liver injury. Males, African-Americans, Hispanics, and obese individuals have been shown to have higher than normal ALT and AST levels.[2]

Obstruction of biliary flow results in cholestasis. In the presence of cholestasis, AP levels are elevated to several times normal in approximately 90% of patients.[2] Although, it can take AP several days to rise after biliary duct obstruction. As a result, AP may be normal early in the presentation of acute ductal obstruction, while the AST and ALT can be elevated into the 500 units/L range.[2]

AP is commonly found in both bone and liver. Therefore, one must account for the source of elevated AP levels. If γ-glutamyltranspeptidase (GGT) levels are also elevated, then a hepatic source is likely. A history of Paget's disease, fracture or bone pain would suggest a bone origin.[2]

The three labs that truly measure hepatic function are albumin, bilirubin, and prothrombin time. Albumin is synthesized by the liver. It is a serum protein that is used for transportation of certain ions and for maintaining serum oncotic pressure. Albumin levels are difficult to interpret with regard to liver capacity for several reasons.[2] First, the half-life of albumin is approximately three weeks, and levels change very slowly as a result of changes in synthesis.[2] In addition, the liver has the ability to double its basal albumin production rate and therefore compensate for albumin losses or changes in albumin production capacity.[2] Also, hypoalbuminemia may be due to non-hepatic etiologies. These include malnutrition, renal (i.e., nephrotic syndrome, proteinuria), and inflammatory states (i.e., trauma, burns, sepsis).[2]

In addition, the liver is responsible for the production of most of the body's blood clotting factors. Factors II, V, VII, IX, and X are synthesized by the liver. Prothrombin time does not become prolonged until the liver's synthetic capacity is decreased by 80%, and therefore is not a very sensitive test for diagnosing acute dysfunction.[2] It is, however, excellent for monitoring liver function in acute hepatic failure. This is due to factor VII having a half-life of approximately six hours.[2]

Another function of the liver is the excretion of bilirubin. Bilirubin is a degradation product of heme. A catabolic reaction turns heme into water insoluble unconjugated bilirubin. It is the liver's responsibility to conjugate the bilirubin with glucuronic acid to make it water soluble. Conjugated bilirubin is then excreted in bile by the liver.

In the evaluation of elevated bilirubin, one must analyze the different types of bilirubin. The total, direct (conjugated) and indirect (unconjugated) should be examined. The presence of elevated total and indirect bilirubin means that the problem is occurring prior to the conjugation step. The differential for this is hemolysis, drug-induced, Gilbert syndrome, or Crigler-Najjar syndrome.

The presence of elevated conjugated bilirubin is the result of the liver's inability to excrete bilirubin into the bile. This results in conjugated bilirubin being excreted by the kidneys into the urine. The presence of elevated serum direct bilirubin does not occur until the liver's excretory capacity has been reduced by 50%.[2] The differential diagnosis includes obstruction (gallstones, tumors, strictures), Dubin-Johnson syndrome, Rotor's syndrome, and hepatitis. An urinalysis positive for bilirubin is an easy test that is sensitive for presence of elevated direct bilirubin.[2] Jaundice is clinically apparent when the total bilirubin is greater than 2.5 mg/dL.

Hepatitis

Hepatitis is defined as inflammation of the liver. There are numerous etiologies that can cause hepatitis. Viral, autoimmune, drug or toxin-induced, and alcoholic are some of the causes that will be addressed in this chapter. Acute hepatitis is defined as symptoms lasting less than six months.

In acute viral hepatitis, patients can present with a viral prodrome that may include nausea, vomiting, malaise, myalgia, arthralgia, and a low-grade fever. This serum-sickness like prodrome is seen in about 10% of acute hepatitis B and about 5% to 10% of acute hepatitis C cases.[3] After the prodrome phase or in non-viral hepatitis, right upper quadrant pain, fever, nausea and/or vomiting may develop. If cholestatic disease is present, tea-colored urine, jaundice, and clay-colored stools may be seen. Patients with chronic hepatitis may present with symptoms consistent with complications of cirrhosis. These include fever, mental status change, increased abdominal girth, abdominal pain, and gastrointestinal (GI) bleed.

History is very important in helping to deduce the etiology of hepatitis. As a result, it is important during the medical interview to ascertain the following information: recent travel outside the U.S.; friends, family and/or acquaintances with similar symptoms; history of IV drug use or sharing needles; history of needle sticks; history of unprotected sex or sex with prostitutes; non-sterile body piercing or tattoos; history of blood transfusions; frequency and amount of ethanol use; raw seafood consumption; family history of certain diseases (Wilson's disease, hemochromatosis, α_1-antitrypsin deficiency, autoimmune disease); and use of medications or herbal remedies.

On physical exam, patients with acute hepatitis may have scleral icterus, right upper quadrant tenderness with or without liver enlargement, and jaundice. Jaundice is observed in less than 30% of patients with hepatitis C.[4] Patients with chronic hepatitis may have any of the following: fetor hepaticus, spider telangiectasia, palmar erythema, caput medusae, Dupuytren's contracture, pedal edema, gynecomastia, ascites, hemorrhoids, testicular atrophy, jaundice, asterixis, and splenomegaly. The liver itself varies in presentation. It can be enlarged or atrophied, as in cirrhosis.

The disposition of patients with hepatitis can vary from discharge to ICU admission. The indications for admission for patients presenting with acute hepatitis include the following signs of hepatic dysfunction: PT greater than three seconds above normal value, hypoglycemia, bilirubin greater than 20 mg/dL, or albumin less than 2.5 g/dL. In addition, the presence of dehydration, intractable vomiting or uncorrectable electrolyte abnormalities would be reasons for floor admission. If the patient has signs of fulminant liver failure, hepatic encephalopathy (HE), is pregnant, immunocompromised, or has toxic hepatitis, then ICU admission may be needed.[5]

However, most patients that present with acute hepatitis can be safely discharged home with appropriate follow-up. They should see their primary care physician or gastroenterologist within five to seven days. They should be advised to avoid hepatotoxins such as alcohol and acetaminophen. Also, they should avoid behaviors that might spread infection such as sexual contact, blood donation, food handling, etc. In many localities, viral hepatitis is reportable to the public health department.

Viral Hepatitis

Viral hepatitis can be caused by the following different strains of the hepatitis viruses; A (HAV), B (HBV), C (HCV), D (HDV), and E (HEV). In addition, Cytomegalovirus (CMV) and the Epstein-Barr virus (EBV) can cause hepati-

Table 11.1
Serological Patterns in Viral Hepatitis

Anti-HAV	HbsAg	Anti-HBs	Anti-HBc	HBeAg	Anti-HBe	HCV-Ag	HCV-Ab (IgG)	Interpretation
+	−	−	−	−	−	−	−	Acute hepatitis A
−	+	−	−	+	−	−	−	Early acute hepatitis B, highly infectious
−	+	−	IgM	+	−	−	−	Acute hepatitis B, highly infectious
−	+	−	IgG	+	−	−	−	Chronic hepatitis B, highly infectious
−	+	−	IgG	−	+	−	−	Chronic hepatitis B, low infectious
−	−	+	IgG	−	+/−	−	−	Recovery from hepatitis B
−	−	+	−	−	−	−	−	Hepatitis B vaccinated
−	−	−	−	−	−	+	+/−	Active hepatitis C infection
−	−	−	−	−	−	−	+	Past or recovered hepatitis C infection

Modified from Practical Guide to the Care of the Medical Patient.[8]

tis. **Table 11.1** illustrates the incidence and prevalence of viral hepatitis in the United States.[6]

Hepatitis A is a single-stranded RNA virus of the picornavirus family and hepatovirus genus. It represents the most common form of acute viral hepatitis. Hepatitis A is present in a worldwide distribution. It causes an acute infection only. The disease is mostly commonly seen in children and young adults. Transmission occurs mainly via a fecal-oral route, although parental and sexual transmission is possible. Incubation is approximately 15 to 45 days.[7]

Hepatitis B is a partially single-stranded, partially double-stranded DNA virus of the hepadnavirus family. It has both acute and chronic disease forms. Approximately 10% of patients will go on to develop chronic hepatitis. The disease affects mostly young adults, infants, and toddlers. It can be transmitted parentally, perinatally, and sexually. Saliva and semen are infectious, although to a lesser extent than serum. The incubation period can range from 30 to 180 days, with an average of 60 to 90 days.[7] Hepatitis B is also a risk factor for the development of hepatocellular carcinoma.

Hepatitis C is a single-stranded RNA virus in the Flaviviridae family. It has both acute and chronic forms. Approximately 50 to 70% of patients will develop chronic hepatitis.[7] In addition, there is an 8% to 20% risk of cirrhosis.[4] The disease can be seen in any age group and has an incubation period of 15 to 160 days, with an average of 60 days.[7] Transmission of the disease is mainly parenteral, through intravenous (IV) drug use, blood transfusions, occupational exposure, and non-sterile tattoo needles. There is a 5% chance of transmission via perinatal or sexual routes.[7] Patients with hepatitis C have an 8% chance of developing hepatocellular carcinoma.[4]

Presentation of viral hepatitis is consistent with the signs and symptoms of acute hepatitis mentioned earlier. Fulminant hepatic failure can be seen in viral hepatitis. There is a 0.1%, 0.1-1%, and 0.1% chance, of developing hepatic failure with hepatitis A, B, and C, respectively.[7] When children are infected with hepatitis A, approximately 80% are asymptomatic, or only have a minor illness.[3] Adults are more likely to have symptomatic hepatitis A infection. Interestingly, 50% of patients with acute hepatitis C infection are asymptomatic.[4]

Patients who present with signs and symptoms of hepatitis should have CBC with differential, chemistries, PT, acetaminophen level (if indicated by history) and LFT sent. Patients usually will have elevated AST, ALT, and total bilirubin may be elevated. Renal function should be normal, but may be elevated in cases of severe dehydration or in patients with hepatorenal syndrome. An ultrasound of the right upper quadrant may be indicated in the workup to rule out other etiologies including, biliary obstruction, hepatic vein thrombosis and cholecystitis.

In addition, a viral hepatitis serological panel should be sent. This commonly consists of IgM anti-HAV antibodies, hepatitis B surface antigen (HbsAg), IgM anticore antibody (IgM anti-HBc), and IgM anti-HCV antibodies. Table 11.1 shows the different possible serological findings and their clinical significance.[8] Serological testing for hepatitis C is often negative early in the acute hepatitis phase because of the time needed for IgM HCV antibodies to form. It takes an average of twelve weeks, but may take as long as six months, for these antibodies to form.[9] Therefore, in patients who HCV infection is suspected, enzyme-linked immunosorbent assay (ELISA) and recombinant immunoblot assay (RIBA) tests are useful to confirm the diagnosis. ELISA-2 and RIBA-2 test for specific antigens and have the respective sensitivities, 90 to 93% and 75 to 98% (4)[4] Third-generation tests are now available, but the sensitivity and specificity are only slightly increased.[4] Reverse transcriptase polymerase chain reaction (RT-PCR) is a superb diagnostic test because of its high sensitivity, specificity, and ability to detect virus within a few days.[4] However, its use is limited by cost and availability.

Management of acute hepatitis consists mainly of supportive care. The ABCs should be stabilized. Supportive care includes ensuring adequate hydration, pain control, anti-emetics, and correction of electrolyte abnormalities.

Hepatitis A usually resolves in a few weeks. If a patient presents within the incubation period, immuneglobulin

(Ig) has been shown to reduce the severity of illness. Emphasis is placed on preventing further disease spread and transmission. Daycare workers and food handlers should avoid work until symptoms are resolved.

In addition to supportive care, it is important to monitor hepatitis B patients for signs of fulminant hepatic failure due to its higher incidence. All patients should be referred to a specialist. They will need additional serial serological testing every three months to assess for ongoing viral replication and infection, until resolution of infection. Treatment for chronic hepatitis B consists of interferon-α (IFN-α) plus lamivudine. This treatment has been shown to improve survival and result in sustained clearance of HBV DNA. Patients being treated with interferon have a 40% chance of ceasing viral replication.[10]

Post-exposure prophylaxis (PEP) for hepatitis B has been shown to decrease disease transmission and is commonly administered in the ED to unvaccinated or incompletely vaccinated patients following needle-stick injury, sexual assault, unprotected sexual contact, and human bites. PEP treatment includes hepatitis B immunoglobulin (0.06 cc/kg IM) and the first hepatitis B vaccine. Patients need to be referred to their primary care physician or public health department to complete the vaccination series at one and six months.

The management of acute HCV also involves supportive care. In addition, early referral for these patients is crucial because clinical evidence has shown early treatment with IFN-α decreases the risk of chronic disease by 30% (10).[10] Treatment of chronic HCV consists of IFN-α plus ribavirin. This treatment results in 25 percent of patients having sustained remission.[4] Sustained viral clearance has been achieved in 30 to 40 percent of European patients with this regimen.[11] A positive response to interferon treatment is seen in patients with poor intrinsic interferon production, low viral RNA, less severe hepatic injury, and viral genotypes II and III.[4] Patients with end stage liver disease may need liver transplantation.

Autoimmune Hepatitis

Another type of hepatitis is autoimmune hepatitis. Autoimmune hepatitis is an idiopathic inflammation of the liver characterized by hypergammaglobulinemia, autoantibodies, and histologically has an interface hepatitis.

Autoimmune hepatitis has a prevalence of about 100,000 to 200,000 cases in the U.S.[12] The annual incidence is approximately 1.9/100,000.[12] Women typically have a higher prevalence of the disease as compared to men and it is found in all ages and races.

The diagnosis of autoimmune hepatitis is made by clinical suspicion. The presence of typical features of the disease and exclusion of other etiologies raises this suspicion. The typical features are hypergammaglobulinemia, female patient, presence of autoantibodies, and an interface hepatitis histologically (lymphoplasmacytic inflammatory infiltrate). In addition, other etiologies of hepatitis including viral, drug-mediated, and genetic must be excluded. The likelihood of the diagnosis is then evaluated by utilizing a complex system that analyzes different aspects of the disease devised by the International Autoimmune Hepatitis Group, based upon histological, biochemical, epidemiologic, and clinical criteria. This system is beyond the scope of emergency department (ED) treatment and management and is primarily used by the primary physician or hepatologist.

When treatment is indicated, corticosteroids are the cornerstone of treatment for autoimmune hepatitis. They result in laboratory, histological, and clinical remission in approximately 65% of patients by 18 months.[12] In addition, treatment also results in increased survival and decreased esophageal variceal bleeding.[12] Treatment may include monotherapy with prednisone or combination therapy with lower dose prednisone and azathioprine. Combination therapy is the preferred treatment secondary to fewer steroid induced side effects. The decision to initiate therapy should be left to the specialist.

Alcoholic Hepatitis

Alcoholic hepatitis is liver inflammation due to the hepatotoxic effects of ethanol. Consumption of ethanol results in fatty changes to the liver after a few consecutive days of consumption. These changes are reversible if consumption ceases. With continued ethanol use however, alcoholic hepatitis can occur. This is typically seen in patients who drink six to eight alcoholic drinks per day for several years.[13] Only 20 percent of chronic alcohol drinkers will develop alcoholic hepatitis and/or cirrhosis.[13] There are multiple factors including hepatitis C infection, female sex, genetic predisposition, and obesity that likely contribute to alcoholic hepatitis susceptibility.[13]

It is very important to ascertain a detailed alcohol consumption history from patients presenting to the ED. This is often difficult to do because patients frequently under report their alcohol use. It may be necessary to involve family members or use developed alcohol screens such as CAGE or AUDIT questions. Patients with alcohol hepatitis may present to the ED with signs of acute hepatitis following a drinking binge or with complications from cirrhosis.

The diagnostic workup for possible alcoholic hepatitis is the same as the general hepatitis workup mentioned above. Lab studies usually reveal an AST:ALT ratio of 1.5–2. A ratio higher than 2:1 is typically seen only with hepatic injury due to ethanol. ALT elevation more than fives times normal and AST elevation more than eight times normal are rarely seen in alcoholic hepatitis.[1] If the serum levels are higher than this, an alternative diagnosis or additional hepatitis etiologies may be present.

Emergency department management of these patients is similar to that of other hepatitis etiologies. The ABCs should be stabilized. Supportive treatment should be given. Fulminant hepatic failure should be ruled out. Furthermore, patients should be counseled on abstinence of ethanol and given the appropriate referrals for alcohol addiction and rehabilitation. Ethanol abstinence is the single most important factor for long- and short-term survival.[13] The seven-year survival rate for patients who continue to drink and for those who stop are 50 and 80 precent, respectively.[13]

Drug-Induced Hepatitis

Hepatitis secondary to drug toxicity is very common. There are numerous medications, and herbal entities that can cause hepatitis. Some of these medications are listed in **Table 11.2** Acetaminophen poisoning is one of the most common causes seen in the ED.

These patients typically present with an acute onset of hepatitis. There will be a history of acute ingestion or being on a specific medication. The diagnostic workup for these patients also includes a CBC with differential, chemistries, PT, LFT, and acetaminophen level (if indicated by history). The treatment for these patients is cessation of the hepatic-toxic drug, and supportive care. Patients should be monitored for the development of fulminant hepatic failure. If available, specific antidotes for the ingested drug should be administered. N-acetylcysteine (NAC) is commonly used to treat acetaminophen induced-hepatitis (see Chapter 134).

Cirrhosis

Cirrhosis is the diffuse fibrosis of the liver and its histological change to abnormal nodules. It is the endpoint of chronic liver disease where little or no hepatic function is left. Patients with cirrhosis present to the ED due to its complications. These include GI hemorrhage from esophageal varices, mental status changes from HE, ascites, and spontaneous bacterial peritonitis (SBP). In addition to the specific therapies discussed below, most patients require admission to the hospital and supportive care.

Ascites is the most commonly seen complication and develops in 50% of patients within ten years.[14] The formation of ascites is due to portal hypertension and the subsequent splanchnic arterial vasodilatation. This results in renal-mediated retention of salt and water that causes ex-

Table 11.2

Common Hepatotoxic Drugs*

acetaminophen	ibuprofen
amiodarone	isoniazid
amitriptyline	ketoconazole
anabolic steroids	methimazole
azathioprine	methotrexate
captopril	methyldopa
carbamazepine	nitrofurantoin
chlorothiazide	oxyphenisatin
dantrolene	phenothiazines
dapsone	phenytoin
daunorubicin	plicamycin
diltiazem	propylthiouracil
disulfiram	rifampin
divalproex	statins
erythromycin	sulfonamides
flutamide	valproic acid
halothane	zidovudine

*There are over 900 hepatotoxic drugs; this is not a complete list.

cess fluid to collect in the peritoneal cavity, thus forming ascites. History, physical exam and laboratory investigation are important in diagnosis. History may relieve increased abdominal girth and/or abdominal pain. Physical exam may show a fluid wave on percussion or shifting dullness.

Treatment is designed to reduce portal pressure and create a negative sodium and water balance.[14] This is achieved through sodium restrictions, bed rest, and diuretic therapy. Spironolactone and furosemide are commonly used diuretics. In patients with tense ascites, therapeutic paracentesis is recommended.[14] The procedure should be performed in the left lower quadrant to reduce the chance of injuring bowel.[14] It is also recommended that simultaneous plasma volume expansion with albumin be given during the procedure to reduce circulatory dysfunction from intravascular equilibration after paracentesis.[14] The suggested dose is 8 g/L of ascites removed. Transjugular intrahepatic portosystemic shunt (TIPS) and liver transplantation may be needed in refractory ascites.

SBP is a common occurrence in patients with ascites. It is a bacterial infection of the peritoneal fluid that results from gastrointestinal flora. SBP is a monomicrobial infection in 92% of patients.[14] Causative agents in order of most common to least common are *Escherichia coli, Klebsiella,* and other gram-negative organisms. Additionally, gram-positive organisms are present, and account for 25% of cases.[14] Anaerobic, polymicrobial, and fungal etiologies are rarely seen.

Patients typically have a history of ascites and develop abdominal pain and fever. The presence of fever, however, is variable. SBP should also be suspected in patients with ascites who have a change in their clinical condition. On physical exam, patients typically have diffuse tenderness and may have peritoneal signs. SBP is diagnosed by paracentesis. An ascites sample should be sent for Gram stain, protein, glucose, culture and sensitivity. A WBC greater than $1,000/mm^3$ or a neutrophil count greater than $250/mm^3$ (without evidence of an intra-abdominal source) is considered diagnostic for SBP. The presence of increased protein or decreased glucose is suspicious for SBP.

Examples of treatment for SBP include cefotaxime (2 g every eight hours) or alternatively, ampicillin plus tobramycin. However, a morality rate of 20 to 40% still exists for hospitalized patients.[14]

Esophageal varices are another complication of cirrhosis. Portal hypertension results in the dilation of the portosystemic collateral blood vessels in the esophagus, thus resulting in esophageal varices. The highest incidence of esophageal varices is in the distal esophagus. They represent 10% to 30% of upper gastrointestinal bleeds.[15] In addition, approximately one-third of patients with cirrhosis will experience a variceal hemorrhage and it is fatal in approximately 30% of initial episodes.[15]

Patients will present clinically with signs and symptoms consistent with blood loss. Patients may note hematemesis, coffee-ground emesis, melena or hematochiza. They may complain of dizziness or weakness. Physical exam may demonstrate abnormal vital signs (tachycardia and hypotension are common), heme-positive stools, bright red blood per rectum, or melena.

Diagnostic evaluation of these patients should include gastrointestinal lavage, CBC with differential, chemistries, PT, PTT, and type and screen (at minimum, may need type and cross). Nasogastric tube insertion is safe in patients with bleeding varices.

The emergency department management of these patients starts with the ABCs. Patients may need to be intubated to protect their airway if the bleeding is severe enough. Two large-bore IVs should be placed. The patient should be monitored hemodynamically. If variceal hemorrhage is suspected, pharmacologic therapy should be instituted with somatostatin or octreotide. They cease variceal hemorrhage in 80% of cases, similar to rates seen with vasopressin, and endoscopic therapy.[15] Somatostatin is given as an IV bolus of 250 μg initially, followed by a continuous infusion of 250 to 500 μg/hour. Octreotide is given as a 50 μg IV bolus, followed by a continuous infusion of 50 μg/hour. Emergent GI consultation for endoscopy should be placed. Endoscopic therapies include variceal band ligation or sclerotherapy, both of which have been shown to stop 80% to 90% of variceal hemorrhages.[15] Endoscopic therapy allows for confirmation of the diagnosis by direct visualization of the source and for direct control of the bleeding. When pharmacologic and endoscopic therapies fail to control hemorrhage, balloon tamponade and/or TIPS may be needed. In addition, intravenous antibiotics, such as third-generation cephalosporins have been shown to decrease mortality and infection rates.[15]

Hepatic Encephalopathy

Hepatic encephalopathy (HE) is a neuropsychiatric disorder that can develop in patients with cirrhosis. HE presentation can be quite variable depending on the severity. Patient presentations range from minor changes in personality to coma. The exact mechanism for HE is not completely understood. It is believed to involve elevated levels of neurotoxic substances in the brain. Some of these are ammonia and manganese.[16] Etiological reasons for the precipitation of HE include GI bleed, increased protein load, infection, hypotension, dehydration, TIPS, or sedatives.

The progression of neuropsychiatric signs and symptoms evolves from personality changes, altered sleep disturbances to asterixis, drowsiness to stupor to coma. In order to properly diagnosis a patient, other possible causes of mental status change must be excluded. These include subarachnoid hemorrhage, intracerebral hemorrhage, subdural hematoma, drug- or alcohol-induced, Wernicke's encephalopathy, hypoglycemia, and hyponatremia. Therefore, a workup should include a CBC with differential, chemistries, ammonia level, drug screen, a trial dose of thiamine, and possibly a CT of the head and/or lumbar puncture. Ammonia levels may be elevated in HE, but do not correlate with disease severity.

The main principle in the treatment of HE is the reduction of ammonia. Lactulose is the cornerstone of treatment. Lactulose's mechanism of action is through the reduction of intestinal microflora ammonia production and by the removal of dietary ammonia in the GI tract.[14] Lactulose can be given orally or as an enema. The oral dose is 20 to 30 g every six to eight hours until an endpoint of two to three soft stools per day is achieved. The rectal dose is 300 mL of a retention enema every four to six hours. Other possible treatments include antibiotics, ornithine aspartate, and flumazenil. Neomycin and metronidazole are two antibiotics that are commonly used. Ornithine aspartate has also been shown to be efficacious in clinical trials by enhancing the fixation of ammonia.[16] Flumazenil is another medication that has been shown to be useful, but only in patients with grade III or IV encephalopathy.[14]

Hepatocellular Carcinoma

Primary liver cancer is usually in the form of hepatocellular carcinoma (HCC). This is a malignant tumor that originates from hepatocytes. HCC has a very poor prognosis. The five-year relative survival rate for liver cancer is approximately 6.8%.[17] Untreated patients usually have three to six months to live following diagnosis. HCC is commonly seen in patients in their fifties and sixties. Risk factors for HCC include hepatitis B and C infections, cirrhosis, aflatoxin exposure, vinyl chloride exposure, hemochromatosis, and α_1-antitrypsin deficiency.

HCC is usually an asymptomatic cancer early in its course. Signs and symptoms do not become clinically apparent until the tumor is greater than 10 cm or greatly advanced.[18] Patients usually present with abdominal pain (91%), abdominal distention (43%), weight loss (35%), weakness (31%), vomiting (8%), and/or jaundice (7%).[18] On physical exam, patients are likely to have hepatomegaly (89%), splenomegaly (65%), ascites (52%), or/and jaundice (41%).[18] In addition, some patients may present with a paraneoplastic syndrome.[18] Some clinical findings that may suggest this are hypercalcemia, hypoglycemia, and erythrocytosis.

The work-up of patients with risk factors for HCC and the above signs or symptoms is extensive. However, while in the emergency department a CBC with differential, chemistries, PT, LFT, and a hepatitis panel should be sent. If ascites is found on exam, a paracentesis may be performed. Paracentesis may show bloody ascites in 20% of patients with HCC.[18] A sample of ascites fluid should be sent for cytology. Alpha-fetoprotein (AFP) is a cancer serum marker that is elevated in HCC, but is not routinely sent in the ED.

The next step in diagnostic evaluation is imaging. There are many different options available for imaging. Helical CT, MRI, angiography, and ultrasound can all be used. Ultrasound is usually used as a screening test in high-risk patients. Helical CT is commonly used and has a higher sensitivity.

Management of these patients also involves stabilization of the ABCs and screening for signs and symptoms of hepatic failure. A prompt outpatient follow-up or admission for inpatient work-up should be arranged depending on the severity of symptoms.

Fulminant Hepatic Failure

Fulminant hepatic failure (FHF) is the occurrence of hepatic encephalopathy in patients with an acute decline in their hepatic function with no history of prior hepatic disease. Hepatic encephalopathy usually develops within eight weeks of presentation of symptoms. This condition is rare, and there are approximately 2,000 cases per year in the U.S.[19] Etiologies for FHF are viral hepatitis, acetaminophen overdose, drug-induced (isoniazid, pyrazinamide, anti-depressants, NSAID, halothane), and some cardiovascular disorders (Budd-Chiari's syndrome, shock liver, veno-occlusive disease). Other possible causes include Wilson's disease, autoimmune hepatitis, fatty-liver of pregnancy, malignancies, and Reye's syndrome. Complications associated with FHF include ascites, hypoglycemia, SBP, sepsis, renal failure, hemorrhage, and cerebral edema.

Patients will present with signs and symptoms of acute hepatic failure. Mental status can range from normal to behavioral changes to coma. On physical exam, jaundice, right upper quadrant tenderness, ascites, and evidence of bleeding may be present.

The work up for FHF consists of a good history and laboratory tests. The clinician should attempt to deduce the etiology. It is important to ask about hepatitis risk-factors, medications, and ingestions. A CBC with differential, chemistries, PT, LFT, ammonia level, acetaminophen level (if indicated by history or history unknown) and a viral hepatitis serological panel should be sent. An ultrasound of the right upper quadrant may also be necessary to rule out anatomical etiologies.

The emergency department management of these patients is supportive and should be directed toward the correction of any complications that occur. The ABCs should be stabilized. Intubation may be required. If the INR is elevated and the patient is bleeding, the patient should receive fresh frozen plasma (FFP). Approximately 2 to 4 units of FFP should be given every six to twelve hours based upon the severity of the coagulopathy.[19] Hypoglycemia should be monitored for and corrected. Clinicians should be vigilante for the presence of infection and begin treatment early. Currently, there are no recommendations for prophylactic antibiotics. Also, there is a risk for cerebral edema in FHF and therefore patients should have the head of their bed at a 20-degree angle to increase jugular venous outflow.[19]

The precipitating etiology must be identified and treated. If acetaminophen toxicity is confirmed or suspected, then NAC should be given. If viral hepatitis is suspected as the cause, acyclovir or ganciclovir may be given.[19] Other specific treatments include delivery of the fetus in acute fatty liver of pregnancy, and TIPS or thrombolytic therapy for acute Budd-Chiari's syndrome.[19]

After stabilization of these patients, it is crucial to determine if a patient meets the criteria for needing a liver transplant. If the patient will likely die without a transplant, then initiating early referral to a transplant center is imperative. Liver transplantation can effectively save a patient's life; however, it is associated with a high financial cost, morbidity, and is limited secondary to organ availability.[19] In addition, 10% to 30% of patients will recover from FHF while awaiting their new liver.[19] Prior to transfer, these patients need to be admitted and monitored in an intensive care unit.

Liver Abscess

Hepatic abscesses can present with a variety of signs and symptoms but fever, right upper quadrant abdominal pain, leukocytosis, and abnormal LFTs are common.[20] Ultrasound and CAT scan will suggest a space-occupying lesion, and tissue densities might suggest that it is not solid. The chest x-ray will often reveal a pleural effusion. Percutaneous or open drainage will confirm the microbiology and is very important in the management. Smaller or multifocal abscesses may be treated with pharmacotherapy alone, but larger abscesses will require drainage. Pyogenic abscesses account for 90% of cases and often are caused by *E. coli, Streptococcus faecalis,* and *Proteus vulgaris.* Biliary tract infections, intra-abdominal infections (e.g., appendicitis), and hematogenous spread are common causes but nearly 20% do not have a clear etiology.[20] Amebic abscesses occur in approximately 10% of patients with liver abscesses. *Entamoeba histolytica* is transmitted by the fecal-oral route, proliferates in the colonic mucosa, migrates into the enterohepatic circulation, and finally lodges in the small portal venules of the liver. Single or multiple abscesses may form and there is a predeliction for the right lobe of the liver. Abscesses are more common in males. Abscesses are more common in areas where human feces is used as fertilizer or in institutions such as facilities for the mentally handicapped. Drainage of an amebic abscess should be undertaken if it appears large enough to rupture or when a pyogenic abscess is suspected. Anti-amebic therapy with metronidazole is effective against *E. histolytica* but, if a pyogenic abscess is suspected, treatment with broad spectrum antibiotics and drainage is recommended.[20]

Liver Transplantation

There are approximately 4,000 liver transplants per year in the U.S.[21] The rising frequency of liver transplantations will result in more ED visits and a challenge for the emergency practitioner. Liver transplant patients present with a constellation of symptoms including abdominal pain, jaundice, fever, shortness of breath, and lethargy.[22] In addition, the systemic immunosuppressants that these patients routinely take make them susceptible to potential life-threatening bacterial (e.g., *Pseudomonas aeruginosa*), viral (e.g., CMV, HSV, varicella), and fungal (e.g., *Candia albicans, Pneumocystis carinii*) systemic infections.[22] The physical exam in these patients can often be normal but many will have underlying active disease. The exclusion of possible organ rejection or occult infection involves extensive laboratory and radiographic studies and should include early consultation with the transplant team.[21,22] Considering the extensive wait time for organ donation, the immunocompromised host, and the high risk of sepsis, 70 percent of the patients are admitted for observation and/or treatment.[21] Any consideration of hospital discharge should be coordinated with the transplant service and patients should be evaluated in the ED by the transplant team before discharge.

References

1. Limdi JK, Hyde GM. Evaluation of abnormal liver function tests. *Postgraduate Med J* 2003;79:307–312.
2. Johnston DE. Special considerations in interpreting liver function tests. *Am Fam Physician* 1999;59:2223–2230.
3. Ryder SD, Beckingham IJ. Acute hepatitis. *Br Med J* 2001;322:151–153.
4. Morton TA, Kelen GD. Hepatitis C. *Ann Emerg Med* 1998;31:381–390.
5. Zagnoon A. Hepatitis. In: Rosen P, Barkin RM, Hayden SR, et al. *The 5 Minute Emergency Medicine Consult*. Philadelphia: Lippincott Williams & Wilkins 1999: 496–497.
6. Center for Disease Control and Prevention, Division of Viral Hepatitis; Viral Hepatitis Surveillance, http://www.cdc.gov/ncidod/diseases/hepatitis/resource/dz_burden02.htm.
7. Dienstag JL, Isselbacher KJ. Acute Viral Hepatitis. In: Braunwald E, Fauci AS, Kasper DL, et al. *Harrison's Principles of Internal Medicine, 15th ed.* New York: McGraw-Hill 2001:1721–1736.
8. Ferri FF. Gastroenterology. In: Ferri FF ed. *Practical Guide to the Care of the Medical Patient,. 4th ed.* St. Louis: Mosby 1998:429–430.
9. Walsh K, Alexander GJM. Update on Chronic Viral Hepatitis. *Postgraduate Med J* 2001;77:498–505.
10. Ryder SD, Beckingham IJ. Chronic viral hepatitis. *Br Med J* 2001;322: 219–221.
11. Gow PJ, Mutimer D. Treatment of chronic hepatitis. *Br Med J* 2001;323: 1164–1167.
12. Al-Khalidi JA, Czaja AJ. Current concepts in the diagnosis, pathogenesis, and treatment of autoimmune hepatitis. *Mayo Clinic Proceedings* 2001;76: 1237–1252.
13. Menon KVN, Gores GJ, Shah VH. Pathogenesis, diagnosis, and treatment of alcoholic liver disease. *Mayo Clinic Proceedings* 2001;76:1021–1029.
14. Menon KVN, Kamath PS. Managing the complications of cirrhosis. *Mayo Clinic Proc* 2000;75:501–509.
15. Sharara AI, Rockey DC. Medical progress: gastroesophageal variceal hemorrhage. *N Engl J Med* 2001;345:669–681.
16. Butterworth RF. Complications of cirrhosis III. Hepatic encephalopathy. *J Hepatology* 2000;32:171–180.
17. National Cancer Institute. Surveillance, Epidemiology, and End Results. http://www.seer.cancer.gov/csr/1975_2000/sections.html.
18. Ulmer SC. Hepatocellular carcinoma: A concise guide to its status and management. *Postgrad Med* 2000;107:117–124.
19. Vaquero J, Blei AT. Etiology and management of fulminant hepatic failure. *Curr Gastroenterol Rep* 2003;5:39–47.
20. Vukmir RB. Pyogenic liver abscesses. *Am Fam Physician* 1993;47:1435–1441.
21. Savitsky EA, Votey SR, Mebust, DP, et al. A descriptive analysis of 290 liver transplant patient visits to an emergency department. *Acad Emerg Med* 2000;7: 898–905.
22. Savitsky EA, Uner AB, Votey SR. Evaluation of orthotopic liver transplant recipients presenting to the emergency department. *Ann Emerg Med* 1998;31: 507–517.

12 Diseases of the Gallbladder and Biliary Tract

Laura Roff Hopson

Suzanne Dooley-Hash

Diseases of the gallbladder and biliary tract are significant causes of morbidity and mortality in the United States. It is estimated that up to 20% of women and half as many men will develop biliary problems over their lifetime. With the high incidence of these processes, a sizable number of patients will present for medical attention to the emergency department.

Cholelithiasis

Cholelithiasis is the presence of gallstones within the gallbladder. Gallstones are common, estimated to be present in more than 20 million Americans. The majority of gallstones remain asymptomatic; however, most symptomatic biliary disease is secondary to gallstones.

Pathophysiology

There are threes types of gallstones: cholesterol (70%), pigmented (20%), and mixed (10%). Cholesterol supersaturation of bile, delayed emptying of the gallbladder and resulting stasis cause the formation of cholesterol stones. Risk factors include female gender, age greater than 40 years, obesity, multiparity, and family history of cholelithiasis. Additional predisposing factors include cystic fibrosis, use of oral contraceptives, clofibrate therapy, and recent rapid weight loss or fasting.

Pigmented stones have two forms. Black stones, aggregates of hemoglobin breakdown products, are seen most often in the elderly and those with hemolytic disorders. Brown stones, composed of calcium bilirubinate, are most common in people of Asian descent and are increased in certain bacterial and parasitic infections.

Presentation

Biliary colic is the most common presentation of symptomatic gallstones. It is pain resulting from transient obstruction of the gallbladder outlet. This obstruction causes pain by increasing intraluminal pressure and distention of the gallbladder wall.

Right upper quadrant and/or epigastric pain often accompanied by nausea and vomiting are the most frequent symptoms of biliary colic. The pain may be intermittent, but is often a constant pain that may be described as burning, pressure-like, or heaviness. It may radiate to the back, flank, or right shoulder. Usually these symptoms are self-limited, lasting 4 to 6 hours and gradually resolving. The patient may relate a history of prior episodes or a temporal association of symptoms with a fatty meal.

Physical examination reveals only right upper quadrant or epigastric tenderness without signs of peritoneal irritation. Signs of dehydration such as tachycardia and dry mucous membranes may be present if the patient has had significant nausea and vomiting.

Differential Diagnosis

The differential diagnosis of biliary colic is broad and includes other disorders of the biliary tract such as cholecystitis or cholangitis. In addition, other gastrointestinal disorders with similar presentations include ulcer disease, gastritis or acid reflux, pancreatitis, and acute hepatitis. Gonococcal perihepatitis (Fitz-Hugh Curtis syndrome), pyelonephritis, and appendicitis may present similarly. Additional important considerations are atypical presentations of cardiac disease or pulmonary pathology such as a right basilar pneumonia or pulmonary embolus.

Diagnosis

The diagnosis of cholelithiasis is made based on clinical history, physical examination findings, and imaging studies. Laboratory studies are most useful to exclude the presence of other diseases. Typically they will reveal a normal white blood cell count, pancreatic enzymes and liver function tests. Ultrasound is the most commonly used modality to image the biliary system and has a greater than 95% sensitivity for detection of gallstones, and is noninvasive and readily available. Gallstones are seen infrequently on x-rays as only 10% to 20% contain the necessary 4% calcium to be radio-opaque. Therefore, plain radiographs are not useful diagnostically. CT has only about a 75% sensitivity for gallstones.

Treatment

Patients with an acute episode of biliary colic are treated symptomatically. This includes fluid resuscitation for volume losses, antiemetics, and analgesics. Non-narcotic pain medications, such as NSAIDs like ketorolac (Toradol), have been demonstrated to provide efficacious pain relief. Alternatively, opioids have traditionally been used for pain control with some research suggesting that meperidine (Demerol) may be preferred over other narcotic medications.

The definitive treatment of symptomatic cholelithiasis is surgical. Over 500,000 cholecystectomies are performed in the United States each year; however, the need for surgical intervention can often be delayed or even avoided with medical management. Dietary modification to eliminate fatty foods may significantly decrease the frequency of episodes of biliary colic. Less commonly, nonsurgical treatments including the use of oral bile acids or lithotripsy may be utilized to dissolve small stones.

Choledocholithiasis

Choledocholithiasis or the presence of a gallstone within the common bile duct system often presents with symptoms similar to biliary colic, but may have a more indolent course. Patients may be jaundiced with a conjugated hyperbilirubinemia and elevated alkaline phosphatase. Ultrasound may be able to demonstrate an obstructing calculus or proximal ductal dilatation. A minority (4% to 8%) of patients will develop acute pancreatitis as a consequence of pancreatic duct obstruction. Choledocholithiasis also predisposes to the development of cholangitis. Treatment involves removal of the calculus either surgically or via endoscopic retrograde pancreatography (ERCP).

Gallstone Ileus

Gallstone ileus is a rare cause of small bowel obstruction typically occurring in the elderly. It results when a gallstone erodes through a chronically inflamed gallbladder wall into an adjacent loop of intestine and subsequently obstructs the bowel, most commonly in the narrow distal ileum. Presentation is with abdominal distention and pain accompanied by nausea and vomiting. An acute abdominal series of radiographs will demonstrate air-fluid levels and distended bowel loops characteristic of an obstruction and, in up to 60% of patients, will also show pneumobilia. Treatment involves surgical removal of the obstructing calculus and cholecystectomy. Commonly, this diagnosis is only made intraoperatively.

Cholecystitis

Acute cholecystitis is inflammation of the gallbladder. Approximately 90% to 95% of cases of cholecyctitis are related to the presence of gallstones within the biliary tract.

Pathophysiology

Prolonged obstruction of the cystic duct or neck of the gallbladder by a gallstone leads to increased intraluminal pressure and distention of the gallbladder wall causing localized visceral hypoperfusion. The release of inflammatory mediators results in gallbladder inflammation and mucosal injury. In addition, bacterial infection develops in 50% to 75% of cases either through hematogenous spread or ascending from the duodenum. The most commonly isolated organisms are *Escherichia coli*, enterococci, bacteroides, and *Clostridium* species. Gas forming organisms such as *Clostridium perfringens* can cause an emphysematous cholecystitis, particularly in diabetics. This has a mortality rate of up to 15%.

Acalculous cholecystitis occurs in up to 10% of patients and is most common in the elderly, particularly those already critically ill or in the post-operative period. Patients present with a septic picture and tend to have a fulminant course with mortality rates of up to 40%. Cystic duct obstruction from stones or other processes such as compression from lymphadenopathy may contribute to this disease. Patients with advanced AIDS are also at risk for acalculous cholecystitis and cholangitis secondary to infection with atypical organisms such as cytomegalovirus, *Mycobacterium avium* complex, microsporida, and *Cryptosporidium*.

Presentation

Acute cholecystitis presents with right upper quadrant and/or epigastric pain sometimes radiating to the back, flank or right scapular tip. The pain is typically constant, and nausea and vomiting are common. In addition, the patient often complains of fever. A history of prior similar but less severe symptoms or known gallstones may also be elucidated.

Physical examination reveals an elevated temperature and tachycardia. Severe cases may present with signs of septic shock. Right upper quadrant or epigastric tenderness potentially with signs of peritonitis are the most consistent findings. Murphy's sign, which is pain and cessation of inspiration on deep palpation of the right upper quadrant, is classically associated with cholecystitis, but it is neither a particularly specific (87%) nor sensitive (65%) test. Evidence of dehydration secondary to significant vomiting may be present.

Differential Diagnosis

The differential diagnosis of cholecystitis is similar to cholelithiasis and includes cholangitis, hepatitis, hepatic abscess, ulcer disease, pancreatitis, appendicitis, gonococcal perihepatitis (Fitz-Hugh-Curtis syndrome) and pyelonephritis. Cardiopulmonary disorders may also present similarly.

Diagnosis

Laboratory studies may be normal or reveal an elevated white blood cell count with a neutrophilic predominance. Liver function tests vary from normal to mildly elevated and pancreatic enzymes are normal.

Ultrasound is considered the best initial test for diagnosis of cholecystitis. Findings of gallstones, gallbladder wall thickening, pericholecystic fluid, increased Doppler flow, and a positive sonographic Murphy's sign (presence of maximal tenderness with the ultrasound transducer directly over the gallbladder) are consistent with the diagnosis. While none of these signs alone are pathognomonic for the disease, the presence of 3 or more positive findings has a positive predictive value of 80% to 90% for acute cholecystitis.

Nuclear scintigraphy is the most sensitive and specific test for cholecystitis, but is often not as readily available as ultrasound and can be a time-consuming study. Technetium-99m labeled hepatic iminodiacetic acid (HIDA) is given intravenously and is secreted into bile. Cystic duct obstruction will prevent visualization of the gallbladder and common bile duct. Visualization of the gallbladder within one hour of injection has a 98% negative predictive value for cholecystitis. Overall, sensitivity of the HIDA scan for acute cholecystitis is 94% with a specificity of 65% to 85%. Opioid use and elevated total bilirubin above 5 mg/dL can cause falsely positive studies.

Treatment

Initial management of acute cholecystitis includes symptomatic therapy with intravenous fluids, antiemetics, and analgesics. In addition, nasogastric suction may help relieve nausea and vomiting and decrease biliary secretions. Parenteral administration of broad-spectrum antibiotics is indicated. A single agent such as ampicillin/sulbactam or a second or third generation cephalosporin is appropriate, unless there is evidence of sepsis in which case multi-drug coverage is warranted.

Cholecystectomy is generally required for cholecystitis. However, patients are often admitted for IV antibiotics for several days to decrease inflammation before surgery. Emergent cholecystectomy is indicated in complicated cases with evidence of gallbladder gangrene or perforation.

Complications

Gallbladder perforation occurs in up to 10% of patients with cholecystitis and is more common in acalculous and emphysematous cholecystitis. Other complications include cholangitis, pancreatitis, sepsis, gallstone ileus secondary to fistula formation, pericholecystic abscess or hepatitis.

Cholangitis

Cholangitis is infection of the biliary tree most commonly caused by a gallstone obstructing the common bile duct. The disease process and presentation show considerable overlap with that of acute cholecystitis. Although cholangitis is less common than acute cholecystitis, patients are generally sicker and the mortality rate is higher (up to 40%).

Pathophysiology

Cholangitis is caused by complete or, more commonly, partial obstruction of the common bile duct typically by a gallstone. However, bile duct strictures secondary to tumors, stenosis, sclerosis, parasitic infection or bile duct manipulation such as in cholecystectomy or ERCP can also be causative. Obstruction leads to bile stasis which predisposes to bacterial superinfection. The most common infecting organisms are the common enteric bacteria, particularly *E. coli*, *Klebsiella*, *Enterococcus*, and *Bacteroides* spp., as well as group D streptococci. Polymicrobial infection is common. Following infection of the common bile duct, the infection may ascend to the hepatic ducts, bile canaliculi and beyond, potentially causing bacteremia and sepsis.

Presentation

In 1877, Charcot first described cholangitis as a triad of right upper quadrant pain, fever and jaundice. These findings are present in up to 70% of patients. The addition of mental status changes and sepsis constitutes Reynold's pentad. Septic patients may present in extremis with hypotension, tachycardia, fever, and mental status changes. Other findings include nausea and vomiting, pruritus, and acholic stools. A history of known gallstones or biliary colic, prior episode of cholangitis, recent cholecystectomy or ERCP may also be found.

Differential Diagnosis

An important alternative diagnosis to consider is acute cholecystitis. The presence of jaundice is important in distinguishing the two processes. Bilirubin is frequently elevated in cholangitis (80%), but not in cholecystitis. Other considerations include hepatitic disorders such as cirrhosis, acute hepatitis or liver abscess, pancreatitis, perforated ulcer, appendicitis or diverticulitis.

Diagnosis

Common laboratory findings in cholangitis include an elevated white blood cell count (or potentially decreased in septic patients) and elevated liver function tests, including conjugated bilirubin. Pancreatic enzymes may also be elevated in a minority of patients. Additional laboratory evaluation should also include electrolytes, renal function, and blood cultures.

Ultrasound may demonstrate intra- or extrahepatic ductal dilatation and/or gallstones within the gallbladder or common bile duct. Sonography is, however, limited in its ability to demonstrate choledocholithiasis, and a HIDA scan may be better able to detect an early obstruction. Direct visualization and possible therapeutic benefit may be derived with ERCP or percutaneous transhepatic cholangiography (THC). These studies, however, are invasive and often difficult to obtain. CT scanning may not show gallstones, but may allow visualization of dilated ducts or other surrounding pathology that is either causative of cholangitis, such as extrinsic compression from a mass, or a complication, such as abscess formation. In addition, alternative diagnoses like appendicitis may be made.

Treatment

Along with initial stabilization and volume resuscitation particularly in patients showing signs of sepsis, all patients with cholangitis require broad-spectrum antibiotics. Mild cases may respond to medical therapy alone; however, immediate surgical, percutaneous, or endoscopic decompression is indicated for more seriously ill patients.

Tumors

Neoplasms involving the biliary tract are rare. Gallbladder carcinoma is the most common and is estimated to cause only 7,000 deaths in the United States annually. It occurs primarily in women over the age of 50 with a history of gallstones or porcelain gallbladder (calcification resulting from chronic gallbladder inflammation). Other risk factors include congenital biliary tract anomalies and Latin American ethnicity. The early course of the disease is indolent. Patients may be asymptomatic or have symptoms only of biliary colic such as intermittent nausea, vomiting and right upper quadrant pain. Invasive or metastatic disease is therefore the norm at the time of diagnosis. Right upper quadrant pain and jaundice are common presenting complaints and a palpable mass may be found in the right upper quadrant. Constitutional symptoms such as weight loss and fatigue may also be present.

Carcinoma of the extrahepatic bile ducts is less common, but occurs more frequently in men than does gallbladder carcinoma. Painless jaundice is the most common presenting complaint. Courvoisier's sign, which is a nontender, palpable gallbladder, is present in one-third of cases.

Diagnosis of biliary tract tumors is most often made by ERCP as ultrasound and CT will miss the majority of cases. Gallbladder and bile duct tumors both have an extremely poor prognosis. Surgical resection is the definitive treatment for all of these tumors. Patients with an emergency department diagnosis of such diseases merit prompt referral for a final diagnosis and definitive therapy.

Selected Readings

Aufderheide TP, Brady WJ, Tintinalli JE. Choloecystitis and biliary colic. In: Tintinalli JE, ed. *Emergency Medicine: A Comprehensive Study Guide,* 5th ed. New York: McGraw-Hill 1999;576–579.

Bartlett DL, Fong Y, Fortner JG, et al. Long-term results after resection for gallbladder cancer: Implications for staging and management. *Ann Surg* 1996;224:639–646.

Dula DJ, Anderson R, Wood GC. A prospective study comparing IM ketorolac with IM meperidine in the treatment of acute biliary colic. *J Emerg Med* 2001;20:121–124.

Gore RM, Yaghmai V, Newmark GM, et al. Imaging benign and malignant disease of the gallbladder. *Radiol Clin North Am* 2002;40:1307–1323.

Guss DA. Biliary tract disorders. In: Marx JA, ed. *Rosen's Emergency Medicine: Concepts and Clinical Practice,* 5th ed. St. Louis: Mosby, Inc. 2002;1265–1269.

Henderson SO, Swadron S, Newton E. Comparison of intravenous ketorolac and meperidine in the treatment of biliary colic. *J Emerg Med* 2002;23:237–241.

Henson DE, Albores-Saavedra J, Corle D. Carcinoma of the gallbladder. Histologic types, stage of disease, grade, and survival rates. *Cancer* 1992;70:1493–1497.

Kadakia SC. Biliary tract emergencies. Acute cholecystitis, acute cholangitis, and acute pancreatitis. *Med Clin* 1993;77:1015–1036.

Kalliafas S, Ziegler DW, Flancbaum L, Choban PS. Acute acalculous cholecystitis: incidence, risk factors, diagnosis, and outcome. *Am Surg* 1998;64:471–475.

Keaveny AP, Afdhal NH. Gallstone Ileus. In: Rose BD, ed. *UpToDate.* Wellesley, MA: UpToDate 2003.

Lipsett PA, Pitt HA. Acute cholangitis. *Front Biosci* 2003;8s:1229–1239.

Moscati RM. Cholelithiasis, cholecystitis, and pancreatitis. *Emerg Med Clin North Am* 1996;14:719–737.

Saini S. Imaging of the hepatobiliary tract. *N Engl J Med* 1997;336:1889–1894.

Singer AJ, McCracken G, Henry MC, et al. Correlation among clinical, laboratory, and hepatobiliary scanning findings in patients with suspected acute cholecystitis. *Ann Emerg Med* 1996;28:267–272.

Trowbridge RL, Rutkowski NK, Shojania KG. Does this patient have acute cholecystitis? *JAMA* 2003;289:80–86.

Wilson L. Diseases of the Gallbladder. In: Harwood-Nuss A, ed. *The Clinical Practice of Emergency Medicine,* 2nd ed. New York: Lippincott-Raven, 1996.

13 The Pancreas

Louise A. Prince
Daniel R. Hehir
Michael Peikert

The pancreas lies in the retroperitoneum and serves as both an exocrine and endocrine organ. It serves as an exocrine organ by secreting amylase, lipase, bicarbonate, trypsin, chymotrypsin, elastase, carboxypepditase, and phospholipase into the small intestine to facilitate digestion. As endocrine organ insulin, glucagon, and somatostatin are released into the bloodstream to maintain glucose homeostasis. The pancreas can be afflicted with many disease processes including pancreatitis, pancreatitic pseudocyst, pancreatic insufficiency, and pancreatic carcinoma to name the most common. An emergency physician must know the signs and symptoms of the presentations of pancreatic disease in order to provide timely intervention and treatment of these disease states.

Acute Pancreatitis

Pancreatitis can be of two types, acute and chronic. Acute pancreatitis is more common with prevalence being 0.5% in the United States. Incidence has increased tenfold from 1960 to 1980 possibly due to increased detection and increased alcohol abuse. Mortality rates are estimated between 2% to 9%.

Pathophysiology

There are many theories for the development of acute pancreatitis. Foremost among these is that a process develops by differing initiating factors that lead to the inappropriate activation of pancreatic enzymes. Proenzymes such as chymotrypsinogen, trypsinogen, proelastase and phospholipase are activated and this leads to the common final pathway of autodigestion of the organ. This autodigestion results in coagulation necrosis, fat necrosis, parenchymal cell necrosis and vascular injury causing hemorrhage, edema, and pain.

The list of known etiologies of acute pancreatitis is extensive (**Table 13.1**). However, in the United States 80% to 90% of adult cases can be attributed to alcohol ingestion and cholelithiasis. Etiology in children is somewhat different (**Table 13.2**) with the leading cause being trauma. It is important to consider occult child abuse in the child with

unexplained acute pancreatitis. Other common causes are complications of surgery and endoscopic retrograde cholangiopancreatography, hypercalcemia, hypertriglyceridemia and drugs (**Table 13.3**). Many drugs have been associated with pancreatitis but only those with a proven link are listed.

Presentation

Constant midepigastric pain accompanied by nausea and vomiting is the classic presentation of pancreatitis. The pain is variable from mild to incapacitating and can often be described as boring with radiation into the back. Abdominal tenderness in the epigastrium and periumbilical region is the norm, and guarding is often present. Loss of bowel sounds can represent an associated ileus. Grey Turner's sign, ecchymosis around the umbilicus, and Cullen's sign, ecchymosis in the flanks, are rare findings that indicate presence of severe necrotizing pancreatitis.

Diagnosis

The diagnosis of pancreatitis revolves around determining serum levels of amylase and lipase. It is important to note that levels of the two enzymes do not correlate with severity of disease.

Amylase

The presence of an elevated serum amylase often aids in the diagnosis of acute pancreatitis. However, it is only present in 75% to 90% of patients and elevation of amylase is somewhat non-specific for pancreatitis. Significant elevation of serum amylase often does not occur before 24 hours and then falls to within normal limits two to five days thereafter. Usually levels of two to three times the upper limit of normal are needed before the diagnosis is made. The specificity of this test is somewhat limited however by the myriad of conditions responsible for hyperamylasemia (**Table 13.4**).

Lipase

Lipase is found primarily in the pancreas and thus an elevated level has a higher specificity for pancreatitis than

Table 13.1
Etiologies of Acute Pancreatitis

Alcohol
Biliary tract disease (choledocholithiasis, carcinomas)
Hyperlipoproteinemias
Hyperlipidemia
Drugs
Posttraumatic
Postoperative
Post-ERCP
Pregnancy
Penetrating peptic ulcer
Carcinoma of the pancreas
Scorpion bites
Vasculitis
Infectious
    Mumps
    Coxsackie virus
    Mycloplasma
    Legionella
    Campylobacter
    Hepatitis B virus
    Ascariasis
    CMV
    Hepatitis B
    VZV
    HSV
    Salmonella

amylase. It is more sensitive than amylase, it rises sooner (within four to eight hours), and remains in the serum longer (eight to fourteen days), making it the most useful test for determining acute pancreatitis in the emergency setting.

Additional Studies

Ranson has outlined criteria for predicting the severity and mortality of acute pancreatitis (**Table 13.5**). These are useful for predicting outcome and are useful for managing supportive care. If 0 to 2 criteria are present on diagnosis mortality is 1%; 3 to 4 results in 15% mortality; 5 to 6, 40%; and greater than 6, 100% mortality. Additional studies may also identify the presence and severity of complications of the disease (**Table 13.6**).

Table 13.2
Additional Etiology of Pancreatitis in Children

Trauma (most common)
Familial
Cystic fibrosis
Vasculitides (Henoch-Schönlein purpura, Kawasaki
   disease)
Anatomic obstruction (i.e. pancreatic divisum, ductal
   abnormalities)

Table 13.3
Drugs Proven to Cause Pancreatitis

Azathioprine	Metronidazole
Cisplatin	Nitrofurantoin
Estrogens	Pentamidine
Furosemide	Methyldopa
Tetracycline	Cimetidine
Thiazides	Ranitidine
Corticosteroids	Didanosine
Sulfonamides	Acetaminophen
ACE inhibitors	Erythromycin
Pentamidine	Salicylates
Valproic acid	

Imaging

Plain abdominal x-ray may show calcifications in the epigastric region suggestive of chronic pancreatitis. Presence of a sentinel loop may be evidence of an associated ileus. Upright chest radiography may demonstrate free intraperitoneal air associated with perforated viscous. Ultrasonography may be useful for confirming diagnosis, etiology, or complications. Acute pancreatitis may be demonstrated by the presence of an enlarged hypoechoic gland or the presence of free intraperitoneal fluid. A stone impacted in the common biliary collecting system may signal an etiology for acute pancreatitis. Pseudocysts, abscesses, phlegmons, and hemorrhages may be identified as complications from the disease. Abdominal CT may demonstrate inflammation of the organ or surrounding tissues, phlegmons, abscesses, pseudocysts, and hemorrhage.

Management

The management of acute pancreatitis includes bowel rest, fluid resuscitation and management of complications. Oral intake is discontinued and insertion of a nasogastric tube may be necessary. This provides gastric and duodenal decompression and decreases stimulation of the pancreas by gastric contents. Use of nasogastric tubes have not been shown to increase patient comfort or decrease hospital times, but may be needed for those with severe vomiting. Pain control with narcotics is usually needed. Traditionally

Table 13.4
Nonpancreatic Causes of Hyperamylasemia

Salivary gland lesions
Pregnancy
Tumor
Burns
Renal disease
Diabetic ketoacidosis
Ruptured ectopic pregnancy
Peritonitis
Intestinal obstruction

Table 13.5

Ranson Criteria for Prognosis in Acute Pancreatitis

On Admission	In 48 Hours
Age > 55 years	Fluid sequestration > 6L
Serum glucose > 200 mg%	pO_2 < 60 mm Hg
WBC > 16,000/mm³	Hematocrit fall > 10%
LDH > 350 IU/L	Calcium < 8 mg%
SGOT > 250 SF units	Base deficit > 4 mEq/L
	BUN rise > 5 mg/dL

Adapted from Ranson JHC. Etiologic and prognostic factors in human acute pancreatitis: a review. *Am J Gastroenterol* 1982;77:663.

meperidine is used as the drug of choice. Meperidine is preferred over morphine, which may induce spasm of the sphincter of Oddi, worsening symptoms. Antiemetics may also be used as needed. Pancreatitis can result in large sequestration of fluid and often requires large amounts of fluid resuscitation. Insertion of a Foley catheter may be necessary to monitor results of IV fluid resuscitation.

Vigilance in the search for complications can help in decreasing mortality. Electrolytes and chemistry panels including glucose, calcium and magnesium should be monitored. PaO2 should be followed with arterial blood gases. Hypotension from fluid sequestration or hemorrhage needs to be aggressively managed. Falling hemoglobin or the presence of Grey Turner's or Cullen's signs may signal retroperitoneal hemorrhage. Transfusions may then be necessary. Antibiotics should be reserved for those who appear to be septic. Peritoneal lavage has not been proven to decrease morbidity or mortality. Surgical intervention may be necessary for those with complications of abscess, hemorrhage, pseudocyst, or necrotic tissue in need of debridement.

Table 13.6

Complications of Acute Pancreatitis

Hypovolemia
Pancreatic necrosis
Acute renal failure
Ileus
Sepsis
Shock
Acute respiratory distress syndrome
Pseudocyst
Abscess
Hemorrhage
Hydronephrosis
Coagulopathy
Hyperglycemia
Hypocalcemia
Retinopathy
Psychosis

Disposition

Most patients with acute pancreatitis require admission and if unstable admission to the intensive care unit is appropriate. A select few with mild disease and ability to tolerate oral intake may be discharged with close follow-up. These patients should initially be on clear liquids and return for worsening pain, fevers, or persistent vomiting.

Chronic Pancreatitis

Pathophysiology

In contrast to acute pancreatitis, the pancreas in chronic pancreatitis is abnormal both before and after the attack. Histological changes can be demonstrated such as the presence of necrosis, fibrosis, inflammation, loss of endocrine tissue, and duct obstruction and dilation. Acute episodes of pancreatitis result in the chronic form when complications such as ductal obstruction, irreversible parenchymal damage or pseudocyst formation occur. In the severe form of the disease, loss of acinar tissue and islet cells result in pancreatic insufficiency. The etiology of chronic pancreatitis is most often alcohol abuse, however other causes are known (**Table 13.7**).

Presentation

The classic presentation is that of an alcoholic patient with repeated attacks of upper abdominal pain. The pain is generally severe pain in the epigastrium often radiating into the back or scapula. Pain may improve with leaning forward. This presentation is variable though, and up to 20% of patients may have painless attacks, where symptoms may only be nausea, vomiting, diarrhea, weight loss, polyuria, diabetes, jaundice, or malabsorption.

Examination may reveal epigastric tenderness, often out of proportion to physical exam. The patient may appear chronically ill, malnourished and in varying amounts of distress.

Ancillary Tests

Laboratory testing may be unrevealing. Due to extensive paranchymal loss and fibrosis of the gland, lipase and amylase may be only slightly elevated, normal or even low. Due to strictures and ductal stenosis, sometimes bilirubin and alkaline phosphatase may be elevated. Glucose tolerance may be impaired with elevations in fast-

Table 13.7

Etiology of Chronic Pancreatitis

Alcohol abuse
Malnutrition
Hyperparathyroidism
Cystic fibrosis
Tropical pancreatitis
Pancreas divisum
Hereditary pancreatitis
Idiopathic

ing glucose. Exocrine insufficiency may be impaired resulting in steatorrhea. Sudan staining of feces and measurement of fecal fat content while on a fat controlled diet may be helpful in making the diagnosis in an outpatient or hospitalized setting.

Imaging by plain radiographs may demonstrate calcification in up to 30% of patients. Such calcifications are considered pathognomonic for chronic pancreatitis. CT may also reveal calcifications, cystic areas, abscess, or pseudocyst. ERCP may detect ductal changes and is considered the gold-standard for diagnosis.

Management

Treatment is generally symptomatic and supportive. Pain may be managed using narcotics such as meperidine; however, ketorolac may be used if there is no evidence of gastrointestinal hemorrhage or gastric ulcer. Nausea and vomiting should be managed with antiemetics. Fluid hydration with crystalloids may be necessary if the patient appears dehydrated or cannot tolerate oral hydration. Malabsorption can be treated with pancreatic enzymes and there is some evidence that these enzymes such as pancrelipase may reduce pain in these patients. Inciting factors such as alcohol must be removed; however, the disease may progress once alcohol use is halted or may not in patients who continue to abuse alcohol. The clinically stable, chronic patient who tolerates oral hydration and pain medication, and who has no complications of the illness, may be safely discharged with appropriate follow-up.

Pancreatic Pseudocyst

Pathophysiology

Pancreatic pseudocysts are collections of pancreatic tissue, debris, and secretory products surrounded by fibrous walls of granulation tissue. They are a complication of pancreatitis in 1% to 8% of cases. They are differentiated from true cysts by the lack of a true epithelial lining. Approximately 90% are located in the tail or body of the pancreas while the other 10% are in the head. They usually present in the fourth or fifth decade and are more common in men. Pseudocysts can present in about 10% of patients after both acute and chronic pancreatitis; 25% present after traumatic pancreatitis. They must be suspected in patients who have had a bout of pancreatitis and return with recurrent symptoms.

Presentation

The typical presentation is a patient who has pain, fever, and ileus 2 to 3 weeks after acute pancreatits or trauma, or in those known to have chronic pancreatits. This can be variable however, and up to 10% of patients may have no pain. Clinical suspicion must be raised when a patient known to have had pancreatitis presents with fever, nausea, vomiting, anorexia, or weight loss. Pain is mostly in the epigastrium, left upper quadrant or into the back. Physical examination may demonstrate variable degrees of tenderness. An abdominal mass may be palpated in up to 50% of patients.

Ancillary Tests

Elevation of amylase is present in up to 75% of patients and should be suspected in patients whose levels remain high two to three weeks after an episode of pancreatitis. Bilirubin may be slightly elevated due to duct compression, and hemoglobin may be decreased. Pseudocyst may be detected by ultrasound or CT. Generally ERCP is not required.

Management

A stable patient with the new diagnosis of pancreatic pseudocyst may be managed conservatively. Most pseudocysts resolve spontaneously over the course of four to six weeks. Complications include hemorrhage into the pseudocyst, rupture, and infection. If the mass enlarges or develops complications, immediate surgical intervention may be necessary. Catastrophic hemorrhage may be amenable to angiographic embolization. If the mass persists longer than six weeks, spontaneous resolution is unlikely and elective surgical decompression may be required.

Pancreatic Abscess

Pancreatic abscess is a feared complication of acute pancreatitis and occurs in 1% to 4% of patients after an acute episode. In lethal pancreatitis, autopsy reveals pancreatic abscess in 90% of patients. This occurs by infection of necrotic tissue during the acute episode or by secondary seeding of pancreatic pseudocyst weeks later. Pathogens are usually mixed, including *Escherichia coli*, Gram-negative anaerobes, and aerobic hemolytic streptococci.

Pancreatic abscess should be suspected in a patient with current or previous pancreatitis who destabilizes. Fever, abdominal pain, nausea, vomiting, and the development of an ileus are concerning symptoms. Physical examination reveals fever, abdominal tenderness, and eventually signs of septic shock.

Ancillary testing may reveal an elevated lipase, amylase, and increasing leukocytosis with left shift. Confirmation of clinical suspicion can be confirmed with ultrasound or CT scanning.

Pancreatic abscesses are not amenable to antibiotic therapy alone (mortality reaches 100%). In addition to broad-spectrum antibiotics, surgical debridement with removal of all necrotic material is necessary. Despite aggressive treatment, mortality for this condition remains high.

Pancreatic Insufficiency

Pancreatic insufficiency is the loss of endocrine and exocrine function of the gland resulting in diabetes and malabsorption. The common causes include chronic pancreatitis, cystic fibrosis (the most common pediatric cause), pancreatic carcinoma or surgical resection. In adults the history usually includes repeated attacks of pancreatitis, development of diabetes, and then chronic diarrhea and weight loss. Patients with cystic fibrosis may develop these symptoms in childhood often in conjunction with respiratory manifestations.

The loss of exocrine function leads to decreased ability to digest and absorb carbohydrates, lipids, and proteins.

This leads to steatorrhea, weight loss, and nutritional insufficiencies such as B_{12}, and fat-soluble vitamin (A, D, E, and K) deficiencies. Steatorrhea is most troubling as it leads to diarrhea and bloating. Diagnosis is dependent on quantitative fat excretion measurements.

Treatment is based on dietary counseling and enzyme replacement. A low-fat diet centered on medium-chain fatty triglycerides is helpful. Pancreatic enzyme replacement just before meals may be assisted with H_2 blockers or proton pump inhibitors that help decrease degradation of pancreatic enzymes in the acid-rich environment of the stomach. These preparations have varying degrees of effectiveness and are tailored to the patient's level of malabsorption. Pancreatic malabsorption is rarely an ED diagnosis; however, if suspected, appropriate referral for evaluation and treatment should be made.

Pancreatic Tumors and Carcinoma

Pathophysiology

Carcinoma of the pancreas is now the fourth leading cause of cancer-related deaths in the United States, and its incidence has increased over 300% in the past 30 years. Its presentation can be vague, and diagnosis may be difficult. Survival rates are poor, with an estimated five-year survival rate of less than 5%. The disease rarely presents before age 50 and is more common in males and blacks. Risk factors include cigarette smoking, diabetes, and the consumption of a diet high in fat and protein content. Chronic pancreatitis may also be a small risk factor. None of these factors greatly increase risk however, and this inability to identify strong risk factors makes screening for the disease very difficult.

Pancreatic carcinoma is classified as either endocrine or nonendocrine. Ductal carcinoma is the most common form of endocrine carcinoma and is responsible for 90% of cases. Exocrine tumors include insulinoma (most common), glucagonoma, VIPoma (secreting high levels of vasoactive intestinal peptide), somatostatinoma, and carcinoid tumor.

Presentation and Diagnosis

Pancreatic carcinoma is notoriously difficult to diagnose early in the disease process and a high level of suspicion must be maintained to make the diagnosis. Weight loss is present in 70% to 90% of patients with endocrine carcinomas. Pain is found in 50% to 80% of patients and is typically described as gnawing, with radiation to the back. Partial relief may be achieved by sitting forward. Diarrhea and malabsorption can signal a mass at the head of the pancreas, as can jaundice. Up to 40% of pancreatic cancer patients will have glucose intolerance up to 2 years prior to their carcinoma being discovered. For any patient over the age of 50 who presents with weight loss, vague abdominal pain, jaundice, irritable bowel-like symptoms, or carbohydrate intolerance, pancreatic carcinoma must be considered. Endocrine tumors are found by CT in over 80% of patients.

Nonendocrine tumors have variable presentations. Hypoglycemia with high insulin levels is characteristic of insulinomas. Glucagonamas present with insulin resistance and a necrotizing migratory erythematous rash. Glucagon levels will be elevated. Gastrinoma results in Zollinger-Ellison syndrome with the formation of multiple gastric ulcers. VIPomas present with diarrhea, which may be profuse, hypokalemia, and achlorhydria.

Treatment and Prognosis

For endocrine tumors the only cure is complete resection. For tumors less than 3 cm and without metastasis, a Whipple procedure may result in a cure rate of approximately 40% at two years. This is only possible in a minority of patients. Five-year survival rates are still only 10% after resection.

For patients in whom resection is not practical and obstruction is present, treatment is directed at improving symptomatology. Stenting bile ducts may result in some improvement of symptoms for these patients. Radiation and chemotherapy may improve survival for some select patients but for those with metastatic lesions, chemotherapy has shown little benefit.

Selected Readings

Baron T, Morgan D. Acute necrotizing pancreatitis. *N Engl J Med* 1999:340: 1412–1417.

Bruno MI, Haverkort EB, Tytgat G, et al. Maldigestion associated with exocrine pancreatic insufficiency: Implications of gastrointestinal physiology and properties of enzyme preparations for a cause-related and patient-tailored treatment. *Am J Gastroenterol* 1995;90:1383–1393.

Harwood-Nuss AL, Linden CH, Luten RC, et al. Pancreatitis. In: *The Clinical Practice of Emergency Medicine*. Philadelphia: Lippincott 1991:949–951.

Kadakia SC. Biliary tract emergencies. *Med Clin North Am* 1993;77:1015–1037.

May HL, Aghababian RV, Fleisher GR, et al. Acute pancreatitis. In: *Emergency Medicine, 2nd ed.* Boston: Little, Brown 1992:1480–1482.

Munoz A, Katerndahl DA. Diagnosis and management of acute pancreatitis. *Am Fam Physician* 2000;62:164–174.

Ranson JH. Etiologic and prognostic factors in human acute pancreatitis: A review. *Am J Gastroenterol* 1982;77:633–638.

Rosen P, Barkin R, Danzl DF, et al. Disorders of the liver, biliary tract, and pancreas. In: *Emergency Medicine: Concepts and Clinical Practice, 3rd ed.* St Louis: Mosby, 1992:1601–1626.

Schwartz S, et al. Pancreas. In: *Principles of Surgery, 5th ed.* New York: McGraw-Hill, 1989: 1413–1440.

Schwartz S, Shires G, Spencer F, et al. Peritonitis and intraabdominal abscesses. In: *Principles of Surgery, 5th ed.* New York: McGraw-Hill, 1989:1459-1490.

Steer M, Waxman I, Freedman S. Chronic pancreatitis. *N Engl J Med* 1995;332: 1482–1490.

Steinberg W, Tenner S. Acute pancreatitis. *N Engl J Med* 1994;330:1198–1210.

Tintinalli J, Ruiz E, Krome R, et al. Acute pancreatitis. In: *Emergency Medicine: A Comprehensive Study Guide, 4th ed.* New York: McGraw-Hill 1996:507–509.

Uretsky G, Golgschmiedt M, James K. Childhood pancreatitis. *Am Fam Physician* 1999.

Wilson J, et al. Acute and chronic pancreatitis. In Wilson J, Braunwald E: *Harrison's Principles of Internal Medicine, 12th ed.* New York: McGraw-Hill 1988: 1372–1382.

Wilson J, et al. Pancreatic cancer. In Petersdorf R, et al., eds: *Harrison's Principles of Internal Medicine, 12th ed.* New York: McGraw-Hill, 1988:1383–1387.

Small Bowel

Robert Knopp
Jon Hokanson

Small Bowel Obstruction

Assessment

Small bowel obstruction (SBO) is one of the most common abdominal emergencies that clinicians encounter. There are two broad categories of bowel obstruction: mechanical and functional (also known as adynamic ileus). Mechanical obstruction includes simple and closed-loop obstruction. In simple obstruction, there is a partial or complete obstruction of the bowel but no vascular compromise. Closed-loop obstruction involves an obstruction at two different sites in which vascular compromise may occur. Adynamic ileus is covered in a later section.

In the United States, adhesions (often secondary to prior surgery), Crohn's disease and neoplasm are the underlying etiologies for over 80% of cases of SBO.[1] Hernias, volvulus, intussusception, gallstones and foreign bodies are other less common causes.

Patients with SBO often present with a history of intermittent, crampy abdominal pain. If the obstruction is proximal, vomiting will frequently be present; in distal obstruction, vomiting may be absent. Distention is commonly present, but typically more pronounced with distal obstructions. If the obstruction is partial, the patient may continue to have stools and flatus. Although the pain is usually intermittent initially, with time it may become constant. The clinician should interpret this change in quality of pain as a cause for concern and consider the possibility of perforation or intestinal ischemia.

Initial evaluation should focus on the hemodynamic status of the patient. Volume depletion secondary to vomiting and/or redistribution of fluids from the vascular space may result in tachycardia and hypotension. Physical examination of the abdomen should include inspection to determine the presence of abdominal distention and surgical scars, auscultation of bowel sounds, and palpation for masses.

A recent European study has shown that hyperactive bowel sounds, abdominal distention, vomiting, patient age greater than 50, history of abdominal surgery and history of constipation are the most sensitive findings of the history and physical exam.[2] A history of Crohn's disease or previous obstruction is also important to elicit.

Hypovolemia, electrolyte abnormalities, bowel strangulation, bowel ischemia and sepsis are all potential complications of SBO.

The physician should suspect SBO in any patient who presents to the emergency department (ED) with acute abdominal pain and vomiting. If evaluation indicates a history of abdominal surgery, abdominal distention, crampy abdominal pain, and/or high-pitched bowel sounds, the level of suspicion should increase. Other diagnoses that must be considered: appendicitis, gastroenteritis, gallbladder disease, mesenteric ischemia, Crohn's disease, pancreatitis, hernia and pregnancy.

Management

The initial management of patients with suspected SBO is focused on rehydration with crystalloid fluids; aggressive resuscitation is required for those with overt signs of volume depletion. Pain relief, typically with intravenous morphine, is the second priority. In patients who are vomiting, electrolyte abnormalities may need correction.

Laboratory investigation is not usually helpful in diagnosing SBO. In volume depleted patients, electrolyte abnormalities, such as hypokalemia, may be present. Renal function requires assessment both for therapeutic and diagnostic purposes. If abdominal CT is considered, knowledge of the patient's renal function is essential in determining the ability to use IV contrast.

Imaging studies are essential once the patient is hemodynamically stable and pain relief is provided. In patients with severe continuous pain or peritonitis, surgical consultation should be obtained to determine whether the patient will go to the OR immediately or require an abdominal CT to confirm the diagnosis of SBO and determine the location and cause of the obstruction. Plain film radiography of the abdomen traditionally has been the initial imaging modality of choice. Multiple air-fluid levels, decreased colonic gas and stool, and distention of the small bowel are radiographic evidence of SBO. Thirty-three percent of plain films are non-diagnostic in cases of surgically proven SBO. When initial imaging is indeterminate, abdominal CT can provide a diagnosis and assist with delineating an underlying etiology. In patients with a history of abdominal malignancy, inflammatory bowel disease or an abdominal mass and an obstruction picture,

CT is essential. With more clinical experience and continued improvements in abdominal CT technology, CT may replace standard plain film radiography of the abdomen as the initial imaging modality; CT can more accurately diagnose SBO, detect the underlying etiology, and assist with the differential diagnosis in cases where no SBO is present. Helical CT has a sensitivity of 63% for all grades of SBO, ranging from 81% for high grade to 48% for low grade.[3] When detected, the underlying cause of the obstruction can be delineated in 93% to 95% of cases.[3] In patients with likely or definite SBO, oral contrast should be withheld, as it adds little to the imaging and can decrease the ability to assess bowel wall thickening. CT can assist with differentiating SBO from ileus and other causes of luminal dilatation with a sensitivity approaching 100%.[3]

Unless peritoneal findings are present or diagnostic imaging necessitates surgical intervention, the initial management is conservative. The initial therapy is hospitalization, nasogastric decompression, NPO status, and correction of fluid and electrolyte imbalances for the first 48 hours of treatment. If peritoneal findings are present or the obstruction does not resolve with conservative management, surgery is required.

Special Considerations

There are several conditions that warrant special consideration.

Gallstone Ileus

Accounting for 5% to 25% of obstructions in patients over 70 years old, this rare entity is caused by a large gallstone entering the intestine through a fistula and becoming impacted in the bowel.[4] Radiographic findings may include SBO, pneumobilia and an ectopic gallstone (Rigler's triad). If plain films are not diagnostic, CT is a more definitive imaging modality.

Intussusception

Intussusception is one of the most common causes of abdominal pain in infancy and the most common cause of intestinal obstruction in infants and young children. Sixty percent of cases occur in patients younger than 1 year; 80% in patients younger than 2 years old, with an overall 4:1 male predominance.

Intussusception occurs when the proximal bowel telescopes into distal bowel, pulling along mesentery. Constriction of the mesentery obstructs venous return, causing engorgement of the intussusceptum. "Current jelly stool," the classic late manifestation of intussusception present in 53% of cases, is secondary to the edema and bleeding caused by the engorgement.[5]

Clinically, a sudden onset of severe colicky pain, recurring at frequent intervals, accompanied by flexion of legs, is typical. These episodes can be followed by periods of normal playful behavior. Vomiting commonly occurs earlier in the course. Stools are normal in first few hours with the progression to current-jelly stool in a subset of patients. The classic triad of vomiting without diarrhea, intermittent abdominal pain and heme-positive stool, occurs in only 20 percent of infants (PPV 93%).[5]

On examination, palpation of the abdomen can reveal a sausage-shaped mass (63% of patients, PPV 94%), which may increase with size and firmness during a paroxysm of pain.[5] As the intestinal obstruction becomes more acute, abdominal distention and tenderness develop.

With a suggestive history and physical examination, radiographic studies are indicated. Early abdominal x-rays show a normal bowel gas pattern. As the intussusceptum progresses, a SBO pattern appears. A paucity of gas can be appreciated in RUQ. These signs, as well as the target sign and an absent liver edge are also radiographic evidence of intussusception.[5] A normal abdominal plain film does not exclude the diagnosis of intussusception. If the clinical suspicion is high, additional diagnostic interventions are required.

The air contrast enema has become the modality of choice for diagnosis and therapeutic intervention. If two attempts at reduction are unsuccessful, laparoscopic reduction becomes necessary. If that fails, intestinal resection may be required.

Other

Trauma and foreign bodies should be considered as the cause of SBO in patients with a suggestive history.

Adynamic Ileus

Functional obstruction, also referred to as *adynamic ileus,* has a variety of intra-abdominal etiologies. Adynamic ileus usually results from external trauma, severe electrolyte imbalances (especially hypokalemia), exposure of the peritoneum to irritants, intra-abdominal vascular accidents, pancreatitis, severe infections, uremia, renal colic or can occur in association with postoperative abdominal surgery. Anticholingeric medications altering the sympathetic tone also may cause an adynamic ileus.

In contrast to mechanical obstruction, the mild abdominal pain associated with functional obstruction is usually continuous rather than colicky. There may be associated vomiting and obstipation.

Physical examination of the abdomen reveals generalized distention and non-localized abdominal tenderness. Signs of peritoneal irritation are generally absent. Dehydration may develop secondary to vomiting or fluid shifts.

Similar to mechanical obstruction, patients with functional obstruction may show serum electrolyte imbalances and hemoconcentration on laboratory testing. Other laboratory abnormalities may reflect the underlying cause of the ileus, such as an increase in lipase with pancreatitis.

Abdominal x-rays may reveal gas-filled loops and air-fluid levels in the small bowel.

The treatment of functional obstruction is conservative medical management and treatment of the primary underlying condition. Supportive care includes nasogastric suction along with replacement of fluids and electrolytes as necessary. The patient should be restricted from any oral intake until normal intestinal function returns.

Appendicitis

Assessment

Acute appendicitis (AA) is the most common cause of surgery in patients with an acute abdomen.[6] Historically, AA was diagnosed on the basis of a suggestive history and physical examination, serial abdominal examinations, and a low threshold for surgical intervention. Since the mid-1990s, the evaluation of patients with acute abdominal pain and possible appendicitis has changed dramatically. The advent of the helical CT has resulted in more accurate assessments of patients with acute abdominal pain. CT is often the diagnostic test of choice for adolescent and adult patients without peritonitis or classical signs of AA.

AA is caused by an obstruction of the appendiceal opening to the intestines. This obstruction is most commonly secondary to lymphoid hyperplasia and fecaliths.[7] Classic symptoms include a history of pain that is initially periumbilical, later localizing to the right lower quadrant (RLQ), with associated anorexia, nausea, and vomiting. The onset of pain typically occurs before vomiting in AA.

Physical examination usually reveals some combination of the following signs: RLQ (McBurney's point) tenderness, fever, guarding, rebound, positive psoas sign, and Rovsing's sign. The most predictive signs and symptoms of AA are migration of the pain to the RLQ, RLQ pain, and abdominal rigidity.[8]

The differential diagnosis for these patients includes small bowel obstruction (SBO), Crohn's disease, pelvic inflammatory disease, ovarian torsion, ovarian cyst, intussusception, testicular torsion, gallbladder disease, kidney stone, mesenteric adenitis and urinary tract infection, among others.

Complications of AA include sepsis, peritonitis, perforation, and abscess formation.

Laboratory testing has limited utility. Tests can be suggestive of AA, but they usually are more helpful in considering other diagnoses. Leukocytosis, though frequently present, is very non-specific; in approximately 10% of patients with AA, the WBC will be less than 10,000. Urinalysis may show signs of pyuria or hematuria in patients with appendicitis. The clinician must determine whether these results represent urologic disease or are the indirect result of appendiceal inflammation. Any female of childbearing age should be screened with a urine pregnancy test.

Management

The initial management of patients with suspected AA is rehydration with IV fluids and judicious use of intravenous morphine to provide pain relief. Administration of morphine to patients with a non-traumatic acute abdomen has been advocated in consensus statements by the American College of Emergency Medicine and the Canadian Association of Emergency Physicians. Specific protocols for pain relief should be developed in collaboration with one's surgical colleagues. Early surgical consultation is essential when the diagnosis is strongly considered, peritoneal findings are present, or after the diagnosis has been made radiographically.

Radiographic investigation increasingly provides assistance with the diagnosis of AA. CT of the abdomen and pelvis has become the initial test of choice for the general population. There are certain subgroups where CT can be extremely helpful: non-pregnant women of childbearing age and the elderly. There is no consensus approach in the literature to the use of contrast in CT scanning of patients with potential AA. Intravenous (IV), oral and rectal contrast have all been administered solely or in some combination to evaluate the appendix. As technology continues to advance, use of the non-contrast abdominal CT also has become an acceptable option for evaluating specific patients with sufficient adipose tissue. The sensitivities, specificities, positive and negative predictive values for helical CT with all approaches (in appropriate patients) are similar (respectively: 92–96%, 89–99%, 90–97%, 95–98%); thus the most important determining factor should be the recommendation of the radiologist.

In general, unless the adult patient has sufficient adipose to allow a non-enhanced CT, IV and oral contrast should be used if the patient's creatinine allows. If this scan does not provide adequate visualization of the appendix, rectal contrast could then be considered. One option for reducing preparation time and contrast exposure in patients with sufficient adipose tissue would be to obtain a non-enhanced helical CT initially. If this test does not provide a definitive diagnosis, a second contrast-enhanced CT would be performed.[9] The exceptions to this approach would include young children and pregnant patients, in whom ultrasound is the initial investigation of choice, and adult males with classic symptoms; these patients should be evaluated by a surgeon before imaging is obtained to determine whether imaging is necessary or whether the surgeon is prepared to operate on the patient without a CT scan.

CT findings suggestive of appendicitis include an abnormally dilated appendix (>6 mm), appendiceal wall thickening, periappendiceal fat streaking, appendicolith, and a discrete fluid collection suggestive of a periappendiceal abscess.

The adjunctive use of abdominal CT has lowered negative laparotomy rates in patients with suspected AA from approximately 15% to 25% when the diagnosis is made clinically; to 4% to 8% with the addition of CT. CT can also assist with arriving at an alternative diagnosis in 23% to 46% of patients whose CT is negative for AA.

Antibiotics covering both Gram-negative aerobic and anaerobic bacteria should be considered before the patient is admitted to the hospital.

For patients with a negative CT, the disposition will depend on the patient's condition. Patients with moderate or severe abdominal pain on initial examination will likely need surgical consultation if the etiology of the pain remains unclear. Such patients should not be discharged from the ED until adequate time has elapsed to demonstrate that the patient's pain has improved sufficiently after analgesics have worn off. All patients discharged from the

ED with acute abdominal pain need explicit instructions describing under what circumstances the patient should return for evaluation and what additional follow-up is required.

Special Considerations

There are three subpopulations that present specific diagnostic challenges:

Infants/Children

Infants and young children are particularly difficult to diagnose as they cannot verbalize specific complaints and the physical exam can be complicated by age. Abdominal pain and tenderness are the most common presenting sign and symptom.[10] However, in small children who have pain, tenderness is not always easy to elicit. Vomiting and fever frequently occur. The rate of perforation is inversely proportional to the patient's age.[10] A first degree relative with a history of appendicitis confers a relative risk of 3.5 to 10 for developing appendicitis.[11] Leukocytosis and a left shift are common, but a normal leukocyte count and C-reactive protein do not exclude AA.[12] Gastroenteritis and upper respiratory tract infections are the most common initial misdiagnoses of childhood AA.[13] Ultrasound (US) and CT are the imaging modalities of choice. A relative lack of body fat and a smaller appendix makes identifying fat streaking and differentiating the appendix from lymph nodes on CT more difficult in younger patients. Thus, in these patients, the initial use of ultrasound followed by CT is appropriate if the US is non-diagnostic.

Pregnant

The diagnosis of AA should be strongly considered in any pregnant patient with new abdominal pain. An overall decrease in the incidence of appendicitis in pregnancy has been noted, especially in the third trimester.[14] A protective effect of female sex hormones has been suggested, but not proven. Right sided abdominal pain is the most common sign.[15] When present, appendicitis in the pregnant patient is associated with a significantly higher perforation rate. US is the initial imaging modality of choice. CT of the abdomen may be considered if the appendix was not appropriately visualized on US and the patient is not in the first trimester.[16]

Elderly

The perforation and overall complication rates in the elderly are 2.5 times that of younger patients; mortality is twelve times higher.[17] Classic symptoms are less common, frequently replaced by complaints of changes in bowel habits, primarily constipation, and generalized abdominal pain. Physical examination can reveal non-specific abdominal tenderness or suggest an acute abdomen with the presence of generalized tenderness, guarding and rebound secondary to later presentations.[17] Because of the significantly increased adverse outcomes in the elderly patient, physicians should have a high index of suspicion and a low threshold for imaging and surgical consultation.

Ischemic Disease: Mesenteric Ischemia

Assessment

Mesenteric ischemia is a potentially catastrophic emergency that must be considered when a middle-aged or elderly patient presents to the emergency department with severe abdominal pain. It is not a single disease, however, but a group of related conditions: acute mesenteric ischemia (AMI), mesenteric venous thrombosis (MVT) and chronic mesenteric ischemia (CMI). Patient presentation and underlying pathophysiology differentiate these entities.

AMI results from arterial occlusion (50%), non-occlusive mesenteric ischemia (NOMI) (20% to 30%), venous occlusion (MVT) (5% to 15%), and extravascular sources.[18,19] Arterial occlusion is the result of an embolus in >50% of cases (usually cardiac in origin) and thrombosis of pre-existing atherosclerotic lesions in 25%.[20] NOMI is caused either by a low-flow state (hypovolemia, shock, decreased cardiac output) or vasoconstriction. Extravascular pathology, such as intussusception, hernia and adhesions, also can impede mesenteric flow resulting in ischemia.

The classic presentation for AMI is the abrupt onset of severe abdominal pain out of proportion to the physical exam. Clinicians, however, cannot rely on this presentation. Many elderly patients will present with an altered level of consciousness that precludes obtaining an accurate history. The presentation also will vary depending on the length of time from the onset of ischemia until the patient is evaluated and whether infarction has occurred. Fever, vomiting and diarrhea also can be present.

The mortality rate of AMI approaches 70% even with advances in diagnostic testing. This high mortality rate is due to a combination of many factors: delayed recognition, delayed treatment, and associated medical problems in the elderly patient which adversely affect the outcome. In one study approximately 75% of patients had symptoms for more than 48 hours before they were evaluated.[21]

Mesenteric venous thrombosis accounts for 5% to 15% of mesenteric ischemia and is divided into primary and secondary MVT.[22] The "secondary" classification is based on delineating an underlying etiology, whereas "primary" is idiopathic. Secondary causes include the hypercoagulable states of protein C, protein S, Factor V Leiden, and antithrombin III deficiencies, oral-contraceptive use, postoperative state, cirrhosis, malignancy, and portal hypertension. The presentation can be acute, subacute or chronic, based on the underlying pathology. The clinical picture follows accordingly, mimicking either AMI or CMI. In acute or subacute conditions, patients usually will present with colicky, mid-abdominal pain. Hematemesis, hematochezia or melena occur in 15% of patients[23]; however, approximately 50% of patients have occult blood present in the stool.[24]

The characteristic presentation of CMI is diffuse abdominal pain, usually lasting for several hours after eating. Progression of stenosis or increasing obstruction of multiple vessels must occur to outstrip the diffuse collateral circulation and cause symptoms. Patients are typically over 50, have a history of atherosclerosis, and present with a history of vague mild postprandial pain that has worsened over the last several weeks. Symptoms of weight loss, decreased appetite and aversion to food are common.

The abdominal examination is normally not impressive initially in mesenteric ischemia. Diffuse, mild abdominal tenderness is common. Peritoneal findings and absent bowel sounds are late developments indicating bowel necrosis.

No laboratory investigation is diagnostic of mesenteric ischemia. Leukocytosis is commonly present. Late findings reflect the ischemic insult to the bowel and may include an elevated serum lactate and associated metabolic acidosis.

Management

The management of mesenteric ischemia depends on the presentation of the patient and the physician's clinical suspicion. The key to reducing the high mortality rate is early recognition and treatment. Initially, patients with acute severe abdominal pain and suspicion of AMI require assessment to determine hemodynamic stability. In cases where the patient is hypotensive or demonstrates signs of volume depletion, the physician should initiate fluid resuscitation. Oxygen should be administered in an effort to minimize potential intestinal ischemia. If the patient presents with signs of peritonitis, immediate surgical consultation is required to ensure rapid surgical exploration. A high suspicion of mesenteric ischemia, even without peritoneal findings, also necessitates early surgical consultation.

Hemodynamically stable patients without peritoneal findings should initially be investigated with plain abdominal radiographs and/or CT of the abdomen to assist with the differentiation of the patient's abdominal pain. This includes evaluation for conditions such as SBO, appendicitis, perforated viscous, and diverticulitis.

Abdominal CT with contrast has a sensitivity of 64 to 82% for diagnosing AMI.[25] The higher sensitivities are from studies requiring only one criterion for diagnosis. Technological advancements in CT scanners are continuing to increase the sensitivity for detecting AMI. Gas in the portal vein and pneumotosis intestinalis are highly suggestive for AMI, but are present after bowel gangrene has developed. The sensitivity of arterial occlusion on CT is 37% to 80%.[26] Other more non-specific findings on CT include abnormal bowel wall enhancement, luminal dilatation, and wall thickening. If the CT does not demonstrate the etiology of the pain and the clinician has a high index of suspicion for AMI, mesenteric angiography should be performed. Mesenteric angiography remains the gold standard evaluation of AMI with a specificity of 100% and a sensitivity >90%.[18,25,27] Treatment is specific to the recognized underlying etiology. Arterial embolus is usually treated surgically or, in patients who present <12 hours after onset of symptoms and have no clinical suggestion of infarction, with thrombolytic therapy. Patients identified with acute mesenteric arterial thrombus require

heparinization and surgical thrombectomy with resection of necrotic bowel and revascularization.

The imaging modality of choice in MVT is also abdominal CT. This should be obtained immediately in the patient with a suggestive clinical picture, specifically patients with acute abdominal pain and a history of a hypercoaguable state. Lack of venous opacification of the mesenteric veins is diagnostic. Sensitivity approaches 90%.[21,24] Heparinization is the standard treatment. Seven to 10 days of heparin therapy has been shown to improve survival and prevent clot propagation.[18] Surgery is required if peritoneal signs are present. The patient should be evaluated for an underlying hypercoagulable state if no etiology is obvious.

Angiography is the only imaging modality that can diagnose NOMI before infarction occurs. Immediate infusion of papaverine through the angiocatheter is required to reverse vasoconstriction. If no peritoneal signs are present, the patient should be admitted for serial exams, heparin, and repeat angiography in 24 hours.[18]

No test has been shown to be diagnostic of CMI. CMI is suggested by significant collateralization of mesenteric blood flow and vascular stenosis on CT. Angiography may show severely stenosed or obstructed 2 to 3 vessel (splanchnic) disease. CMI is treated with surgical revascularization or percutaneous transluminal mesenteric angioplasty with or without stenting.

In all patients, initial interventions include nasogastric decompression, broad spectrum antibiotics and fluid resuscitation to prevent worsening of ischemia and potential sepsis.

Special Considerations

A high index of suspicion is essential in the patient with abdominal pain that is inconsistent with the physical exam. Clinicians must be especially vigilant in elderly patients with altered mental status and abdominal pain. Early surgical consultation is required for expeditious management of these patients. Initial imaging modalities are similar; therapeutic options differ.

Crohn's Disease

Assessment

Crohn's disease (CD) is a chronic, recurring inflammatory disorder that may affect any part of the gastrointestinal tract. Although the exact etiology is unknown, it appears to involve the interaction of multiple factors, including environmental, immunologic and genetic. The result is an altered immune response. CD more commonly affects Caucasians and Jewish patients. The incidence of CD in North America is four to eight cases per 100,000. While a bimodal age distribution may occur with a peak incidence in the 20s and a smaller peak in the 60s, CD can present at any age; onset is most common between the ages of 18 to 40.[28]

The pathologic hallmark of CD is inflammation of all layers of the bowel wall. Although the terminal ileum is the most commonly affected region, these lesions are non-continuous and can occur anywhere along the alimentary tract. Advanced CD may lead to transmural ulcerations, strictures, and fistulas. Fistulas may develop between various segments of the GI tract, adjacent organs (bladder), or the skin. Perianal fistulas are common in CD and should always raise the index of suspicion. There is an increased risk of small bowel and large bowel cancer with CD. When CD is present in the mouth, it presents as aphthous ulcers of the lips, tongue, and buccal mucosa.

In patients presenting to the ED with crampy abdominal pain, diarrhea, weight loss and fever, CD must be considered. As these symptoms are not uncommon in ED patients, physicians must have a high level of clinical suspicion. Crampy abdominal pain is common in CD, regardless of the intestinal distribution of disease. Obstructive symptoms should also be investigated as the inflammatory nature of CD can cause fibrotic bands, scarring, and strictures, predisposing patients to bowel obstructions. It is important to elicit both a personal and family history of inflammatory bowel disease.

Patients with a known diagnosis of CD will also present to the ED, seeking intervention because of an exacerbation of their condition or a failure of their current drug regimen. In these patients it is important to review their medications and to determine the presence of a fever, ability to tolerate oral intake, weight loss, and abdominal tenderness. This allows for assessment of the severity of their exacerbation.

The physical examination can be normal in these patients. Examination of the abdomen may reveal tenderness, typically in the right lower quadrant, an abdominal mass or signs of obstruction. Rectal and perianal examination can provide suggestive clues including the presence of fissures or an enterocutaneous fistula. Suspicion should be increased in patients with aphthous ulcers in the oral cavity.

The differential diagnosis for these patients include appendicitis, infectious colitis, irritable bowel syndrome, ischemic bowel, diverticulitis, ulcerative colitis, gastroenteritis, bowel obstruction, peptic ulcer disease, urinary tract infection, renal calculi, and pelvic inflammatory disease in women.

Complications associated with CD include bowel obstruction (CD is the second leading cause of small bowel obstruction), abscess formation, fistula development, cancer, perianal disease (including fistulas and fissures), hemorrhage, malabsorption, renal calculi, and gallstones. Abscess formation occurs in 15% to 20% of patients with CD, originating most commonly in the terminal ileum.

Laboratory tests are not diagnostic. Mild anemia, leukocytosis and an elevated erythrocyte sedimentation rate and C-reactive protein are common, reflecting the inflammatory process. Depending on the patient's specific history, consideration should be given to testing the patient's stool for bacteria, ova, parasites, *Clostridium difficile* toxins, and other pathogens. There are serologic tests to assist with differentiating ulcerative colitis from Crohn's disease; this generally falls out of the realm of the emergency department physician. Urinalysis should also be obtained when the clinical situation dictates.

Plain films of the abdomen may demonstrate an obstructive picture, but more commonly the findings are non-specific or unremarkable. Although barium studies continue to be the main diagnostic modality of CD, with endoscopy and biopsy as confirmatory adjuncts, these studies are generally not performed in the ED. Patients will often present with non-specific abdominal pain or with a known diagnosis of CD and new abdominal pain (and fever): in the ED, CT of the abdomen and pelvis is the initial test of choice. CT can be suggestive of an inflammatory disorder; more importantly, it can show signs of complications including the presence of an abscess. The most common finding on CT is bowel wall thickening (target sign), often segmental with skip lesions; this is more common on the right side of the colon, whereas predominantly left-sided colonic involvement is characteristic of ulcerative colitis.[29,30] A normal CT does not rule out CD, although it suggests that a patient with Crohn's is not in an active phase of the disease. In patients with known CD, CT is a useful adjunct to evaluate for possible abscess or fistula. CT has been shown to affect disease management in 28% of cases.[30]

Management

ED management of CD depends upon the initial presentation of the patient to the emergency department, their current therapies, and the classification of the severity of their presentation.

In mild to moderate disease, the patient lacks a high fever, dehydration, abdominal tenderness, obstruction, or significant weight loss (<10%), while tolerating oral intake and ambulating. Although there remain questions about efficacy, mesalamine (5-aminosalicylic acid) is the initial drug of choice for mild to moderate disease.[31,32] It can be used safely in doses up to 4.8 g/day, with the incidence of side effects being dose dependent. Traditional corticosteroids such as prednisone and prednisolone, although effective for mild to moderate disease, should be limited to more severe disease because of their side effects. Budesonide, recently introduced in the United States, has the advantage of eliminating the majority of side effects seen with other corticosteroids because of its first-pass metabolism in the liver.[31]

Antibiotics, including metronidazole and ciprofloxacin, although used for luminal CD, have no proven efficacy; however, they are quite effective for perianal disease and may have a place in the management of such patients. Metronidazole does not induce remission, but at 20 mg/kg/d dosing, does decrease perianal manifestations. There is some evidence to support ciprofloxacin at 1 g/d as a remission induction agent. Combination therapy of metronidazole and ciprofloxacin is another option in this group; it has been shown to be superior to either therapy alone for perianal disease. Patients continuing to tolerate oral intake may be discharged home with close follow-up with the physician managing their CD.

Moderate to severe disease is defined by nausea, vomiting, significant anemia, weight loss (>10%), abdominal tenderness, and fever, or if the patient has failed therapy for mild to moderate disease. Oral systemic corticosteroids are the mainstay in treatment of these patients.[31,32] The equivalent of 40 mg of oral prednisone tapered over eight to twelve weeks has been shown to provide a clinical response in 50% to 70% of patients. Budesonide should be considered secondary to fewer side effects and less adrenal suppression than prednisone. The clinical picture determines disposition. If the patient is stable enough to be discharged, close follow-up is essential, otherwise hospital admission is necessary. Contacting the physician managing the patient's CD can help with this decision.

Severe exacerbations involve obstruction, rebound tenderness on abdominal examination, significant fever, intractable vomiting, evidence of wasting or abscess, or failure of outpatient steroid treatment. These patients require parenteral steroids, hospitalization and, if present, further investigation into any abdominal mass or rebound tenderness.[31,32] Surgical consultation should be obtained in the setting of the acute abdomen.

Special Considerations

The stratification of the Crohn's presentation is essential for managing these patients. Regardless of the patient's presentation, the emergency physician should consult gastroenterology regarding the specifics of management and the decision whether inpatient or outpatient management is appropriate.

Gastroenteritis

Assessment

Diarrhea, vomiting, and abdominal discomfort are exceedingly common complaints in patients presenting to the ED. Differentiating the underlying etiology can be difficult. Because so many conditions can present with one or more of these symptoms, the diagnosis of gastroenteritis should be made with great caution and usually as a diagnosis of exclusion in the ED.

Acute gastroenteritis is characterized by stomach and intestinal mucosal inflammation secondary to viral or bacterial infection, food poisoning, chemical irritants, or food allergies. Poor food preparation, a contaminated food source, fecal-oral transmission, person-to-person contact, and airborne transmission (viruses) can result in gastroenteritis.

Regardless of the source, patients often present complaining of some combination of anorexia, nausea, vomiting, cramping abdominal discomfort, and diarrhea. A history of other household members with similar symptoms is important to elicit. Recent travel can be associated with the underlying source of the diarrhea. Exposure to high-risk vectors, including day care and nursing homes, must be determined. Physicians should ask patients about the presence of blood or mucous in the stool; this is suggestive of a bacterial infection or inflammatory bowel disease. A review of the patient's medications also may provide clues to a causative agent. The state of the patient's immune system must be assessed, as susceptibilities change and the severity of reactions increase in the immunocompromised patient.

Gastroenteritis affects patients of all ages. Secondary to concomitant medical illnesses, the elderly are at risk for more severe outcomes. Patients older than 80 years have a 3% mortality rate associated with gastroenteritis, compared with 0.05% in patients less than 5 years old.[33] The incidence of an acute gastroenteritis episode is 1.2 to 1.5 per person-year.[34]

Viruses are the most common causes of acute gastroenteritis. The most frequent viral agents are rotavirus, Norwalk virus, caliciviruses, and adenoviruses. Illnesses induced by Norwalk and Norwalk-like viral agents account for up to 35 percent of all acute diarrheal outbreaks in the world. Their outbreaks are generally associated with contaminated food and water. Transmission is commonly via the fecal-oral route, although rotavirus can be spread by aerosolized means. Occurrences are more prevalent during the winter months. Viral gastroenteritis usually presents with diarrhea and vomiting over a 1-4 day course. Norwalk virus, however, may last for up to two to three weeks. In this clinical context, a viral cause is also supported by a lack of bloody diarrhea, severe abdominal pain, recent travel history or antibiotic use. Acute hepatitis A can present with acute diarrhea, frequently without jaundice, especially in children and adolescence.

Numerous bacterial agents can infect the small intestines. The highest incidence for hospitalizations caused by bacterial gastroenteritis occurs in August and September. Common bacterial species affecting the small intestine include *Escherichia coli*, *Staphylococcus aureus*, *Vibrio cholerae*, *Shigella*, *Salmonella enteritidis*, *Campylobacter jejuni*, *Yersinia enterocolitica*, and *Clostridium difficile*. The incubation period from infection to clinical symptoms for *Staphylococcus*, *E. coli*, and *Vibrio* is brief. The remaining organisms have a longer incubation period. Diarrhea in bacterial gastroenteritis is secondary to increased intestinal secretions resulting from decreased absorption.

E. coli species, commonly associated with travelers' diarrhea, cause diarrhea by both direct invasion and exotoxin release. The volume depletion associated with the diarrhea can be severe. The 0157:H7 strain of *E. coli* has been associated with contaminated meat products, causing hemorrhagic colitis and hemolytic uremic syndrome. Gram-positive *S. aureus* triggers diarrhea by exotoxin release and is the most common cause of food poisoning. *V. cholerae* also secretes an exotoxin. Cholera infection presents as severe rice watery stools with no pus. *Shigella* may cause large volumes of bloody diarrhea with mucus. *Shigella* has hundreds of serotypes that may cause diarrhea. The diarrhea is described as voluminous, watery with mucus, and frequently lasts less than a week. *Campylobacter* induced gastroenteritis often begins with malaise followed by abdominal pain and watery diarrhea that becomes bloody after three to five days. *Yersinia* is a common cause of acute diarrhea mediated by an enterotoxin.

Clostridium difficile–induced diarrhea frequently follows broad-spectrum antibiotic use that causes a pseudomembranous colitis. This allows *C. difficile*, which is also part of the normal intestinal flora, to proliferate and secrete an exotoxin. Only approximately 40% of antibiotic-induced diarrheas, however, are due to *C. difficile*. Risk factors include recent hospitalization or residence in a nursing home. Up to 25% of these patients will be colonized with *C. difficile* that, under the appropriate circumstances, can induce colitis. In contrast, up to 80% of infants harbor the bacteria, usually with no pathological consequences.

Physical examination in acute gastroenteritis is generally unremarkable. The primary goals of the examination are to evaluate for overt signs of dehydration and for findings suggestive of another cause of the patient's symptoms. Non-specific or mild LUQ abdominal tenderness may be present.

Depending upon the patient's presentation, the differential diagnosis may include parasitic infection, gastrointestinal bleeding, appendicitis, inflammatory bowel disease, small bowel obstruction, intestinal ischemia, or diverticulitis.

Major complications of gastroenteritis include bacteremia and dehydration. Electrolyte abnormalities and their sequela can develop with prolonged diarrhea and/or vomiting. Rotavirus has been associated with the development of necrotizing enterocolitis in neonates.

Laboratory investigation should include testing for electrolyte abnormalities. Examination of stool for fecal leukocytes is endorsed by the American Gastroenterology Association in the context of febrile patients with acute diarrhea. If this test is positive, empiric antibiotic treatment is recommended (the sensitivity of this test is 60% to 70%).[33] Stool culture should not be performed routinely but reserved for situations where the clinical presentation suggests an inflammatory diarrhea or fecal leukocytes are present in patients presenting with bloody diarrhea, high fever, and an elevated white count. Cultures can then be obtained to investigate for invasive bacteria.[33] Obtaining stool for ova and parasites should occur in the appropriate epidemiologic setting, such as recent travel, contact with day care centers, poor socio-economic status, the AIDS patient, an immunocompromised state, and homosexual males.[35] When a history of previous antibiotic use is elicited and *C. difficile* colitis is considered, assays for *C. difficile* toxins should be obtained. Commonly available enzyme immunoassays are available for rotavirus.

Management

Treatment is supportive for most patients with acute gastroenteritis, as the disease is almost always self-limited; diagnosis of a specific causative agent is usually not required. Rehydration and electrolyte replacement should occur as indicated. Antispasmodics and antidiarrheals are generally not advised, except for patients with presumed mild viral gastroenteritis. Unnecessary treatment with these drugs can prolong the carrier state of the individual.

In febrile patients with acute, severe, bloody diarrhea and positive fecal leukocytes or patients with a clinical picture suggestive of invasive bacteria, empiric antibiotic treatment for diarrhea of suspected bacterial etiology should be initiated. A fluoroquinolone (Cipro 500 mg PO bid × 3 days) or macrolide may be prescribed while awaiting stool cultures.[35] If *C. difficile* toxin presence is clinically suggested, treatment with metronidazole (Flagyl 500 mg PO tid × 10 days) should be initiated. Vancomycin (125 mg PO qid × 10 days) is equally effective as a first-tier therapy, but is substantially more expensive. It should be used in patients with contraindications to metronidazole or refractory patients.

Patients with severe disease, dehydration, or multiple comorbidities should be hospitalized for supportive care, monitoring, and if necessary, intravenous antibiotics; stool and blood cultures should be obtained. Most patients, however, can be managed as outpatients, provided they are able to maintain adequate hydration. Follow up with their primary physician is indicated within one week to ensure continued improvement and address other ongoing issues. If the source of the possible contamination is from a public facility, the physician should notify the local health authorities.

Special Considerations

Special consideration should be given to the immune-compromised patient as they may develop a more severe infection and more significant complications secondary to gastroenteritis. Common causes of immune deficiencies include diabetes, cirrhosis, AIDS, prolonged steroid use, chemotherapy, and immune suppression secondary to organ transplantation or autoimmune disorders. These patients are susceptible to the agents that cause gastroenteritis in the general population, but also to unusual organisms such as cytomegalovirus and aeromonas.

References

1. Miller G, Boman J, Shrier I, et al. Etiology of small bowel obstruction. *Am J Surg* 2000;180:33–36.
2. Bohner H, Yang Q, Franke C, et al. Simple data from history and physical examination help to exclude bowel obstruction and to avoid radiographic studies in patients with acute abdominal pain. *Eur J Surg* 1998;164:777–784.
3. Maglinte DDT, Heitkamp DE, Howard TJ, et al. Current concepts in imaging of small bowel obstruction. *Radiol Clin North Am* 2003;41:263–283.
4. Clavien PA, Richon J, Burgan S, et al. Gallstone ileus. *Br J Surg* 1990;77:737–742.
5. DiFiore JW. Intussusception. *Semin Ped Surg* 1999;8:214–220.
6. Owings MF, Kozak LJ. *Ambulatory and Inpatient Procedures in the United States, 1996. Vital and Health Statistics. Series 13. No. 139.* Hyattsville, MD: National Center for Health Statistics, November 1998:26. (DHHS Publication no. (PHS) 99–1710.)
7. Graffeo CS, Counselman FL. Appendicitis. *Emerg Med Clin North Am* 1996;14:653–671.
8. Wagner JM, McKinney WP, Carpenter JL. Does this patient have appendicitis? *JAMA* 1996;276:1589–1594.
9. Torbati SS, Guss DA. Impact of helical computed tomography on the outcomes of emergency department patients with suspected appendicitis. *Acad Emerg Med* 2003;10:823–829.
10. Nance ML, Adamson WT, Hedrick HL. Appendicitis in the young child: A continuing diagnostic challenge. *Pediatr Emerg Care* 2000;16:160–162.
11. Rothrock SG, Pagane J. Acute appendicitis in children: Emergency department diagnosis and management. *Ann Emerg Med* 2000;36:39–51.
12. Gronroos JM. Do normal leucocyte count and C-reactive protein value exclude acute appendicitis in children? *Acta Paediatr* 2001;90:649–651.
13. Rothrock SG, Skeoch G, Rush JJ, et al. Clinical features of misdiagnosed appendicitis in children. *Ann Emerg Med* 1991;20:45–50.
14. Andersson REB, Lambe M. Incidence of appendicitis during pregnancy. *Intl J Epidemiol* 2001;30:1281–1285.
15. Andersen B, Nielsen TF. Appendicitis in pregnancy: diagnosis, management and complications. *Acta Obstet Gynecol Scand* 1999;78:758–762.
16. Ames Castro M, Shipp TD, Castro EE, et al. The use of helical computed tomography in pregnancy for the diagnosis of acute appendicitis. *Am J Obstet Gynecol* 2001;184:954–957.
17. Kraemer M, Franke C, Ohmann C, et al. Acute appendicitis in late adulthood: incidence, presentation, and outcome. Results of a prospective multi-center acute abdominal pain study and review of the literature. *Langenbecks Arch Surg* 2000;385:470–481.

18. Tendler DA. Acute intestinal ischemia and infarction. *Semin Gastrointest Dis* 2003;14:66–76.
19. Sreenarasimhaiah J. Diagnosis and management of intestinal ischemic disorders. *Br Med J* 2003;326:1372–1376.
20. Stoney RJ, Cunningham CG. Acute mesenteric ischemia. *Surgery* 1993;114:489–490.
21. Rhee RY, Gloviczki P, Mendonca CT, et al. Mesenteric venous thrombosis: still a lethal disease in the 1990's. *J Vasc Surg* 1994;20:688–697.
22. Kumar S, Sarr MG, Kamath PS. Mesenteric venous thrombosis. *N Engl J Med* 2003;23:1683–1688.
23. Boley SJ, Kaleya RN, Brandt LJ. Mesenteric venous thrombosis. *Surg Clin North Am* 1992;72:183–201.
24. Harward TR, Green D, Bergan JJ, et al. Mesenteric venous thrombosis. *J Vasc Surg* 1989;9:328–333.
25. Kim AY, Ha HK. Evaluation of suspected mesenteric ischemia: efficacy of radiologic studies. *Rad Clin North Am* 2003;41:327–342.
26. Lee R, Tung HKS, Tung PHM, et al. CT in acute mesenteric ischemia. *Clin Rad* 2003;58:279–287.
27. Brandt LJ, Boley SJ. AGA technical review on intestinal ischemia. *Gastroenterology* 2000;118:954–968.
28. Loftus EV, Sandborn WJ. Epidemiology of inflammatory bowel disease. *Gastroenterol Clin North Am* 2002;31:1–20.
29. Rubesin SE, Scotiniotis I, Birnbaum BA, et al. Radiologic and endoscopic diagnosis of Crohn's disease. *Surg Clin North Am* 2001;81:39–70.
30. Carucci LR, Levine MS. Radiographic imaging of inflammatory bowel disease. *Gastroenterol Clin North Am* 2002;31:93–117.
31. Harrison J, Hanauer SB. Medical treatment of Crohn's disease. *Gastroenterol Clin North Am* 2002;31:167–184.
32. Hanauer SB, Present DH. State of the art in the management of inflammatory bowel disease. *Rev Gastroenterol Disord* 2003;3:81–92.
33. Ilnyckyj A. Clinical evaluation and management of acute infectious diarrhea in adults. *Gastroenterol Clin* 2001;30:599–609.
34. Garthright W, Archer D, Kvenberg J. Estimates of incidence and costs of intestinal infectious diseases in the United States. *Public Health Rep* 1998;103:107–115.
35. DuPont HL. Guidelines on acute infectious diarrhea in adults. The Practice Parameters Committee of the American College of Gastroenterology. *Am J Gastroenterol* 1997;92:1962–1975.

CHAPTER

15 Large Bowel

Nicole DeIorio

The colon, or large intestine, is the hollow tubular structure that constitutes the final portion of the alimentary canal. It begins at the ileocecal junction, extends to the anus, and averages 1.5 m in length. Approximately 12 cm of the distal colon is designated the rectum. The rectum has a separate arterial and venous system and is discussed in the next section. The colon absorbs up to 70% of the water from the fecal stream so that liquid stool becomes semi-solid. The distal colon and rectum also serve as a fecal reservoir, allowing convenient defecation. It is important to remember that the colon is not a vital organ: many individuals lead long and productive lives after colectomy. Newer surgical techniques allow for ileocanal anastomoses so that many patients who have undergone colectomies do not have ileostomies. Bleeding, colitis, diarrhea, constipation, irritable bowel syndrome, diverticulitis, obstruction, and neoplasia are commonly encountered (and often overlapping) colonic disorders. This section reviews common problems associated with the colon.

Bleeding

Bleeding is a common presentation of colonic pathology. It can manifest in a variety of ways from guaiac positive stools with or without anemia to massive acutely life-threatening hemorrhage. Visible bleeding routinely prompts patients to seek medical attention. Chronic low-grade blood loss may portend a worse outcome eventually, but evaluation and diagnosis are frequently delayed when bleeding is occult. The location of the bleeding site, the volume of blood lost, and the rapidity with which it is lost determines the form that the blood takes as it passes out through the rectum and anus. Melena (digested blood) often occurs as a result of upper gastrointestinal (UGI) bleeding, but can result from a proximal colonic bleed of lesser volume and slower transit time. Mahogany stools (partially digested blood) or bright red blood per rectum frequently denote a lower gastrointestinal (LGI) source of blood loss but can occur with a brisk and massive UGI bleed as well. Smaller amounts of bright red blood per rectum in a hemodynamically stable patient suggests a colorectal source. Hemorrhoidal bleeding is the most common form of lower gastrointestinal bleeding.

As in all gastrointestinal bleeding, the first step is to determine whether the patient is hemodynamically stable, and if not, to resuscitate the patient immediately. An attempt to quantitate the amount of blood lost should be made through questioning. If bleeding continues, direct observation is helpful. Vital signs, including orthostatic blood pressures, should be obtained immediately. Mental confusion, cool clammy skin, and hypotension suggest major blood loss. Clinicians should not be misled by "normal" hematocrit readings during any acute bleeding episode. The plasma volume can take 24 hours to equilibrate after large blood volume losses. A patient can exsanguinate acutely despite a "normal" hematocrit. Fluid resuscitation is indicated with any significant bleeding. Blood transfusions should be considered in the settings of significant anemia (significance may vary due to comorbid conditions), shock, and gross ongoing hemorrhage. If a patient is experiencing melena, mahogany stools or bright red blood per rectum with hypotension and an UGI bleed suspected, gastric lavage with room temperature water is recommended. Lavage water returned with bile staining, but without blood, argues against an active UGI bleed. The patient's coagulation status should be assessed and an effort to correct any coagulopathy detected should be considered.

Once resuscitative measures have been started, an effort can be made to diagnose the underlying problem, find the specific bleeding site, and control it directly if possible. Chronic bleeding in stable patients and small amounts of bright red blood per rectum associated with bowel movements can be handled definitively during follow-up after the ED visit. Anoscopy in the ED may confirm hemorrhoids, but follow-up should be arranged to make certain that they stop bleeding and that they represent the sole source of the blood loss. Significant, symptomatic anemia will generally require admission for transfusion. Ongoing larger volume bleeding requires an aggressive diagnostic approach beginning in the ED. Colonoscopy may be attempted in the setting of an active bleed. The unprepped colon with retained stool and blood can obstruct the endoscopist's view. If possible, the colon should be prepared using a standard oral lavage solution. In ongoing massive GI bleeds (both upper and lower) arteriography is used to localize the site of the bleeding, and when possible, to stop it via embolization of the culprit artery. Subsequent endoscopy may be required to determine the precise reason for the hemorrhage, but this can be arranged subsequently in a controlled setting. Luminal contrast studies, such as barium enemas, are not indicated in the evaluation of acute LGI bleeding. Even when they detect potential pathology they do not demonstrate that the lesions are actually bleeding. Furthermore, they obstruct the views of both the angiographer and the endoscopist. In the case of massive ongoing bleeding in an unstable patient, surgery may be indicated. Angiography and endoscopy have lessened the need for exploratory surgery in this setting. Surgery may be the definitive corrective action once the problem has been diagnosed.

Causes of colonic bleeding include diverticulosis, arteriovenous malformations (AVMs), neoplasia (benign and malignant), inflammatory bowel disease, infectious colitis, radiation colitis, and ischemic colitis. Anorectal bleeding is discussed elsewhere. Diverticulosis is common in Western societies with refined diets low in fiber. Diverticula are herniations of the mucosa and submucosa through the muscularis propria that result in outpouchings of variable size in continuity with the colonic lumen. Arterioles in the mucosa encounter sharp angles at the openings of these outpouchings. It is thought that bleeding occurs when sheer forces cause arteriolar rupture at the edges of a diverticulum. Bleeding is often brisk, bright red or mahogany in color, painless, and self-limited. Arteriovenous malformations are aberrant connections between arterioles and venules that largely bypass capillary beds. They may be congenital or acquired. Their pathogenesis remains a matter of speculation. They can present in a variety of ways including occult bleeding, massive bleeds with no warning, and at times as recurrent gastrointestinal bleeding of obscure etiology. Similar to diverticular bleeds, AVM bleeding is painless and usually self-limited. Both conditions may be suspected while definitive proof remains frustratingly out of reach. Arteriography may suggest AVMs, but without active bleeding during the study there is no proof they are actually responsible for the hemorrhage. Likewise, endoscopy may reveal that a patient with recent colonic bleeding has either diverticula or AVMs, or both, but if no visible bleeding site or adherent clot is detected, the diagnosis will remain "likely" while not actually confirmed. When the patient is hemodynamically stable and the bleeding is self-limited, it is generally advisable to prepare the colon properly for endoscopic evaluation rather than attempt emergent or urgent unprepared studies that ultimately prove to be suboptimal.

When colorectal neoplastic lesions bleed, they usually do so because they have outgrown their neovascular blood supply and tissue necrosis with sloughing results. Occasionally they serve as the lead point for intussusception wherein colonic mucosa is pulled into the more distal lumen, resulting in ischemia with tissue loss and bleeding. Bleeding is often occult but can become massive if a major vessel is disrupted. Weight loss, abdominal pain, and symptoms of anemia are common complaints heard from patients suffering from colon cancer. Such patients may never be aware that they have been bleeding.

A rare cause of gastrointestinal bleeding that should not be overlooked is that which results from aortoenteric or ilioenteric fistulae. These life-threatening conditions may present with smaller, temporarily self-limited "herald" bleeds before potential exsanguination. A patient with aortic or iliac artery aneurysms, or who has undergone repairs of such aneurysms, should be considered at risk for such an occurrence. The distal duodenum is the most frequent site for these fistulae, but other portions of the GI tract may be involved. Angiography is recommended.

Motor Abnormalities

Irritable Bowel Syndrome

The irritable bowel syndrome (IBS) may affect as much as a third of the population, although only about 5% of the population actually seeks medical care. Oversensitivity to bowel distention and disordered bowel motility are theorized to be the basis for the syndrome. Dyspepsia, bloating, abdominal cramping, diarrhea, constipation, and alternating diarrhea and constipation are common manifestations of IBS. Although IBS prompts many visits to health care providers, including ED usage, it is never fatal. It can occur concurrently with other conditions, for example, IBD. Unfortunately, it still remains largely a diagnosis of exclusion, although investigators have proposed diagnostic criteria. A single visit to the ED may prompt suspicion, but is not enough for a definitive diagnosis. Lack of bleeding, weight loss, and constitutional symptoms, as well as a chronic course, suggest the diagnosis. It is also common to see the symptoms (especially cramps and diarrhea) resolve when the patient sleeps. Patients presenting with changes in bowel habits of recent onset should not be given the diagnosis without a thorough evaluation for other causes. Although the ED can offer attempts at short-term symptomatic relief, it can probably do the most for patients with IBS by ensuring that they are referred for follow-up to physicians familiar with IBS who will provide the appropriate long-term care.

Constipation

Constipation refers to decreased frequency of bowel movements, increased stool firmness, or difficulty with stool passage. Soft but solid stools are generally passed painlessly and with minimal straining from once every three days to three times per day. The variability of patient perception as to what constitutes constipation is impressive. Some individuals become concerned with mild increases in stool solidity or after missing a single bowel movement. Others will not defecate for days or even weeks prior to seeking care. Two or three million U.S. medical visits per year result from constipation. Most such visits are not emergent. Short-term, self-limited constipation may result from changes in diet (usually decrease in dietary bulk), travel and immobility, intercurrent illness, certain medications, or even changes in daily schedules that disrupt stooling habits. Irritable bowel syndrome, which is often considered functional in nature, is a common cause of chronic or recurrent constipation. This will be discussed below. Medications, hypothyroidism, diabetes mellitus, colonic inertia, mechanical obstructions, anorectal disorders, and Hirschsprung's disease (a congenital disorder in which lack of colonic ganglion cells leads to lack of proper motor function) are organic causes for the syndrome of constipation. Anticholinergics, opiate narcotics, alumina-based antacids, and calcium channel blockers are common offenders. A careful history and physical examination should seek to elicit a medication profile, a family history of constipation, and the specific details of the problem per the patient, as well as looking for signs of systemic illness and localized disease. Painful defecation should prompt anoscopy and/or proctoscopy. Treatment of an anal fissure, for example, could lead to correction of resultant constipation. A barium enema or colonoscopy will rule out obstructing lesions. A barium enema would be more cost-effective unless there is concomitant bleeding. If the history, physical examination, blood glucose, thyroid function tests, proctoscopy, and barium enema are not revealing, the patient can usually be managed with increased dietary bulk and occasional laxatives. Cathartic laxative use on a regular basis may lead to neuromuscular degeneration in the colon, and is therefore not recommended. If simple measures do not work, referral to a gastroenterologist for more extensive evaluation is recommended. In the ED constipated patients must be distinguished from those who are obstructed. The history and physical examination as well as abdominal x-rays usually suffice.

Obstruction

Obstruction of the lumen of the colon can occur as the result of an intraluminal mass, kinking of the colon itself with a pinching off of the lumen, or external mass compression. The last is the rarest. Colony masses are most often tumors, although bezoars can occasionally obstruct the ileocecal valve area. Severe constipation, obstipation, results in generalized obstruction to forward flow of the fecal stream. Adhesions, hernias, intussusception, and volvulus (a twisting of the bowel with subsequent luminal compromise) are common causes of colonic obstruction. Rarely extracolonic tumor bulk will be great enough to obstruct the colon. Some tumors, such as adenocarcinomas of the prostrate, can grow into the colon and either bleed or obstruct. Colonic obstruction presents with abdominal pain, bloating, decreased or absent defecation and passage of flatus, and variable bowel sounds. Hyperactive bowel sounds are often noted earlier in the course with diminished or absent bowel sounds when ischemia or infarction ensues. Longer standing cases may be accompanied by nausea and the vomiting of feculent material. Urgent abdominal x-rays reveal dilated bowel loops, air-fluid levels, thumb-printing (with ischemia), and free intraperitoneal air if there has been a perforation. Intravenous fluid resuscitation should be started promptly and surgical consultation sought urgently. When there is

perforation broad-spectrum antibiotics are also necessary. Occasionally a volvulus, especially one involving the sigmoid colon, can be reduced endoscopically or by the administration of an enema. Most often complete bowel obstruction requires operative decompression. Partial bowel obstruction can present with paradoxical diarrhea as mentioned above.

Diverticulitis

Diverticulitis is a common inflammatory lesion of the colon originating from diverticula. Diverticula either bleed or become infected, but not both. In Western societies diverticula are more common in the left colon, hence so is diverticulitis. The precise reason for localized inflammatory lesions arising from diverticula is unknown. Abscesses can develop with luminal obstruction and/or perforation with generalized peritonitis. Muscular hypertrophy of the colonic wall adjacent to diverticula and diverticulitis can cause further luminal compromise. Abdominal pain (often in the left lower quadrant) with fever, nausea, and vomiting are common presenting symptoms. Laboratory analysis must include a complete blood count with differential. Mild diverticulitis can be evaluated with a water-based contrast enema. Sicker patients can be evaluated by CAT scan. Endoscopy is relatively contraindicated in suspected diverticulitis due to the risk of perforation. Bowel rest, hydration, and broad-spectrum antibiotics (including anaerobic coverage) are the mainstays of therapy for diverticulitis. The microbiology mirrors that of the gut flora. Some abscesses can be drained percutaneously if they do not respond to conservative measures. Perforations, strictures (especially with significant obstruction), and larger, refractory abscesses require surgical resection. Surgical management may require more than one step if there has been significant peritoneal contamination. Increasing dietary bulk is suggested as a means to forestall the development of diverticula and their complications.

Colitis

Colitis refers to inflammation of the colon. In general, the term implies that the lesion involves the mucosa or arises from it. Typhlitis is the much rarer condition in which the inflammation involves the serosa of the colon principally. The etiologies of colitis include infectious agents (including *Clostridium difficile*), radiation, ischemia, and idiopathic inflammatory bowel disease (IBD) (Crohn's colitis and ulcerative colitis). Symptoms of colitis include diarrhea, which may or may not be bloody secondary to frank mucosal disruption, abdominal pain and cramps, fever, nausea, and vomiting. Abdominal tenderness, fever, and guaiac positive stools are common signs. The amount of bleeding that results from colitis generally depends on the intensity of the mucosal disruption and the surface area involved. It can range from occult bleeding to massive life-threatening hemorrhage, although the latter is much less common. Unlike diverticular or AVM-related bleeding, prodromes are common with colitic bleeding. Infectious colitis may occur in outbreaks involving several people or more. Contaminated food and water may spread bacterial infections. Parasitic colitis in the United States generally means *Entamoeba histolytica,* and is seen most frequently among homosexually active men, those institutionalized due to developmental handicaps, and those who have traveled to areas where parasites are endemic. Antibiotic-related diarrhea may involve the overgrowth of bacteria that leads to diarrhea. *C. difficile* is a facultative anaerobe that can cause syndromes ranging from mild diarrhea to toxic megacolon and shock. *C. difficile* should be suspected in patients with colitis who have received antibiotics up to 8 weeks prior to presentation. Diarrhea, fever, malaise, nausea, and vomiting usually precede bleeding from colitis. Ischemic colitis occurs most often in individuals with significant atherosclerotic disease. On occasion, young patients with fibromuscular dysplasia of the major intestinal arteries will suffer ischemic events. The onset of severe abdominal pain followed by bloody diarrhea is the classic presentation. Radiation enterocolitis requires prior exposure to radiation, usually in therapeutic settings, but occasionally as the result of an industrial accident. It involves small vessel ischemia, although the resultant diarrhea may or may not be bloody.

IBD usually leads to recurrent episodes of active colitis with diarrhea with or without bleeding. Malaise, anorexia, weight loss, and extraintestinal manifestations including arthritis, cholangitis, skin lesions, and inflammation of ocular structures are seen in IBD patients as well. Ulcerative colitis presents as bloody diarrhea (unless an extraintestinal presentation occurs first). Crohn's disease may cause bloody or nonbloody diarrhea or manifest chiefly as abdominal pain or weight loss. Children may experience failure to thrive. Careful attention should be paid to searching for symptoms and signs of IBD that are extraintestinal. A rare complication of colitis is toxic megacolon. The colon dilates, becomes paralytic, and if untended, will often perforate. This surgical emergency is accompanied by serious constitutional symptoms that can include shock. Colectomy is usually required.

Gay bowel syndrome is a term, being used less often more recently, that refers to the sexually transmitted proctitis that occurs with anal intercourse. Gonorrhea, parasites, and other venereal proctidites are seen in greater numbers among sexually active homosexual males. They are not confined to this population, however, and all patients with proctocolitis should have their sexual practices reviewed while being evaluated.

Patients who present to the ED with symptoms and signs of colitis should have a thorough history and examination performed. Particular attention should be paid to food and water consumption, travel, sexual practices, the health of surrounding individuals, past similar histories, and comorbidities. Volume depletion should be corrected and hemorrhage managed as needed. Stool should be sent for white blood cell counts (WBCs), culture and sensitivity, *C. difficile* toxin titers, and (if the history is suggestive) ova and parasite examinations. Endoscopy may be required when ischemia is suspected but should be performed by a fully trained endoscopist. Flexible sig-

moidoscopy is often useful for the diagnosis of other types of colitis. Self-limited colitis (especially with a positive stool culture) does not require an invasive workup. Treatment is aimed at the underlying cause. Antibiotics are usually unnecessary in bacterial infectious diarrhea unless there is systemic illness. Metronidazole is used for *C. difficile* and *E. histolytica.* Ischemia requires supportive medical care and, often, surgical care. Radiation colitis is usually an insidious disease with a frustrating response to therapeutic attempts. Rarely, massive bleeding requires surgery. IBD is managed with 5-aminosalicylates and steroids. Patients with IBD are not immune to bacterial, parasitic, and clostridial infections. Increased disease activity in patients with IBD may represent such infections. Stool studies and endoscopy may be considered at such times. Significant volume depletion, serious hemorrhage, evidence of sepsis, metabolic derangement, and ischemic colitis warrant admission. Milder cases of colitis may be handled in the outpatient setting as long as medical care is readily available.

Although diarrhea is a prominent symptom of colitis, it has many causes. Diarrhea is technically defined as the passage of greater than 250 g of stool per day. Practically, it refers to more frequent stooling, greater stool volume, greater liquidity of the stools, or a combination of these symptoms. Colonic diarrhea is usually lower volume and higher frequency than that caused by small intestinal pathology. As above it may be bloody or "bland." In the ED it should be determined if volume or blood loss (or both) will require hospitalization. Stool studies should be sent as appropriate. Attention should be paid to any medications the patient might be taking that could cause diarrhea. Self-limited viral infections are a common cause of diarrheal illnesses in children and adults. Adequate fluids and antidiarrheal drugs maintain adequate volume status and minimize symptoms. Diarrhea may also occur paradoxically as a result of a partial obstruction with "overflow" incontinence. Relief of the obstruction restores normal bowel function. Obstipation may require manual disimpaction, enemas, and, in extreme cases, surgical decompression.

Tumors

Colonic neoplasia is very common in the United States and other developed nations of the world. Over 150,000 cases of colon cancer per year occur in the United States alone. Surgical removal affords the only true hope of cure, although adjuvant chemotherapy after surgery in stage C improves 5-year survival significantly. Most colon cancers form in previously benign adenomas. The type and size of the underlying adenoma determine subsequent malignant potential. Certain families are genetically prone to developing adenomas and adenocarcinomas of the colon. Screening regimens have been developed to prevent the development of frank colon cancer. These are not performed in the ED. However, guaiac positive stools, unexplained anemia, or a rectal adenoma found on proctoscopy should prompt a referral, as well as education of the patient as to the importance of follow-up. Most carcinomas occur in people over the age of 50, but familial syndromes occur at earlier ages. Juvenile polyps have little or no malignant potential, but may bleed and result in their disclosure. Hyperplastic polyps have no malignant potential and are usually found incidentally during endoscopy or contrast radiologic studies. Histologic review is required to determine the significance of colorectal neoplastic lesions. Elective endoscopy is the means by which the tissue is sampled, although surgery may be required for lesions unreachable or unresectable by endoscopic techniques.

Selected Readings

Blacklow NR, Greenberg HB. Viral gastroenteritis. *N Engl J Med* 1991;325:252–264.

Bleday R, Falchuk ZM. Diagnosis and Treatment of Constipation. *Comp Ther* 1994;20:44–49.

Ellis DJ, Reinus JF. Lower intestinal hemorrhage. *Crit Care Clin* 1995;11:369–389.

Freeman SR, McNally PR. Diverticulitis. *Med Clin North Am* 1993;77:1149–1167.

Guerrant RL, Bobak DA. Bacterial and protozoal gastroenteritis. *N Engl J Med* 1991;325:327–340.

Lynn RB, Friedman LS. Irritable bowel syndrome. *N Engl J Med* 1993;329:1940–1945.

Moriarty KJ. The Irritable bowel syndrome. *Br Med J* 1992;304:1166–1169.

Podolsky DK. Inflammatory bowel disease. Part One. *N Engl J Med* 1991;325:928–937.

Podolsky DK. Inflammatory bowel disease. Part Two. *N Engl J Med* 1991;325:1008–1016.

Rectum and Anus

Janice Blanchard
Tina Rosenbaum

There exist several disorders of the anorectum that prompt emergency department visits. After a brief review of the anatomy of the anorectum, the chapter will cover the conditions most commonly seen in the emergency department (ED).

Anatomy

The anorectum is the terminal end of the gastrointestinal (GI) tract. It begins at the rectosigmoid junction, follows the sacral curve for about 12 to 15 cm, and ends with the 4 cm anal canal which courses to the anal verge. Different types of epithelium line the anal canal at various levels; at its midpoint, approximately 2 cm from the anal verge, lay the anal valves at the thickened dentate line. The rectum has pink columnar epithelium that continues into the upper anal canal and then gradually transitions columnar to transitional (above dentate line) to squamous epithelium (below the dentate line). The rectum narrows into the anal canal forming the columns of Morgagni. At the base of the columns of Morgagni exist the anal crypts, which provide lubrication during defecation and create the possibility of infection if obstructed (**FIGURE 16.1**).

Proper function of the anorectum relies on the levator ani muscles and two sphincters (internal and external), which together control defecation. The large intestine down to the external anal sphincter receives innervation from the sympathetic and parasympathetic systems. The anal canal below the dentate line is innervated by somatic nerves. Sympathetic fibers from L1 to L3 and presacral nerves inhibit contraction of rectal smooth muscle and L5 fibers contract the internal sphincter. Defecation occurs as the rectum distends, parasympathetic fibers cause the rectal wall to contract and the internal sphincter relaxes (circular smooth muscle). The motor branches of the pudendal nerve (S2-S4) allow for the relaxation of the external anal sphincter (elliptical skeletal muscle). The anorectum receives blood supply from the superior, middle, and inferior hemorrhoidal arteries. The superior hemorrhoidal veins drain into the portal system and the inferior into the caval system.

Clinical Assessment

Examination of a patient with anorectal complaints should include retraction of the buttocks, observing the anus as the patient bears down, anal palpation with a well lubricated finger, circumferential exam, and anoscopy. History should include the duration of symptoms, onset of symptoms, association with defecation, bowel habits (frequency, color, melena, consistency, straining, incontinence), dietary changes, travel history, sexual history especially regarding anal intercourse, and medical history (leukemia, Crohn's, diabetes, etc.).

Structural Disorders

Anal Fissure

Fissure in ano or anal fissure is one of most common reasons for sudden, painful rectal bleeding. The classic symptoms include acute, shearing, knife-sharp pain associated directly with defecation and with usually small amounts of bright red blood on the toilet paper or on the outside of stool. Pruritus ani co-exists with anal fissures in half of the cases. Although anal fissures occur in patients of all ages and equally among men and women, they are most commonly present in young, healthy adults. Anal fissures are also the most common anorectal pathologic process in infants and children.

An anal fissure constitutes a longitudinal split in the squamous epithelium of the distal anal canal below the dentate line. The classic presentation (90% of women and 99% of men) is a linear tear occurring in the posterior midline; 10% of women and 1% men may have anterior midline fissures. Multiple fissures or fissures positioned other than in the midline should trigger a search for other etiologies including inflammatory bowel disease, syphilis, tuberculosis, herpes, HIV, occult abscesses, leukemia, and neoplasms.

Examination of a patient with fissure in ano includes retraction of the buttocks and observing the anus as the patient bears down. Lidocaine jelly is necessary to facilitate the digital part of the exam as the internal sphincter is

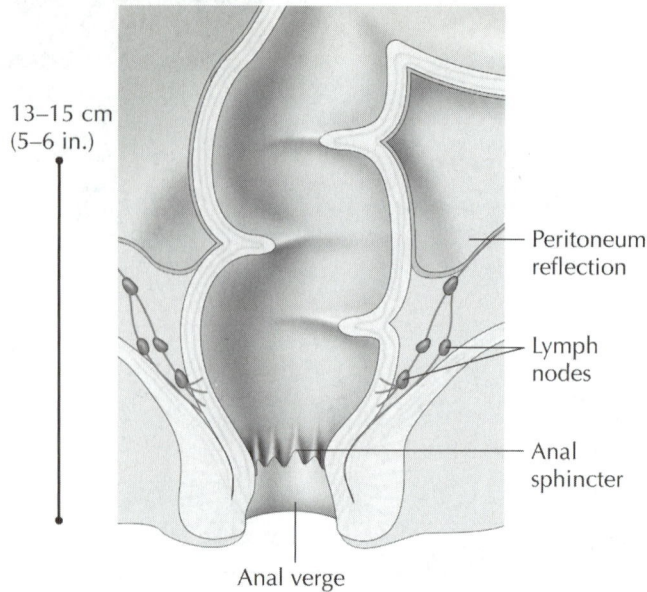

13–15 cm
(5–6 in.)

Peritoneum reflection

Lymph nodes

Anal sphincter

Anal verge

FIGURE 16.1 Structures of the anorectal area.

usually in spasm. Acute anal fissures appear as linear or elliptical mucosal tears with bleeding or granulation tissue at the base. Chronic fissures (usually non-healing after six weeks) have indurated edges: horizontal white fibers of the internal sphincter muscle may appear at the base, and often there will be hypertrophied anal papilla and a sentinel pile/skin tag surrounding the chronic fissure. As the anal papilla cephalad to the fissure hypertrophy, the area distal to the fissure enlarges and swells becoming the sentinel pile, which is, at times, confused with an external hemorrhoid.

The etiology of anal fissures has been attributed to the passing of hardened stool, particularly since most people feel the pain with defecation and most heal with high-fiber diets and stool softeners. However, the occurrence of anal fissures after episodes of diarrhea, as well as reports that only 25% of patients with anal fissures actually complain of constipation, have led to other theories of pathogenesis. Alternate explanations include trauma (e.g., pregnancy, foreign objects, etc.), internal sphincter hypertonia, and local ischemia with fibrosis.

Most acute anal fissures resolve completely with high-fiber diet, stool softeners, warm sitz baths, and analgesics as needed, preferably NSAIDS, as narcotics may cause constipation and aggravate the problem. Topical hydrocortisone and local anesthetics do not seem to accelerate healing, and may delay healing or lead to skin sensitization. For chronic fissures, in addition to the aforementioned treatments, there are a host of medications (see **Table 16.1**) which lower internal sphincter pressures and/or relax the smooth muscle to facilitate the healing process. The failures of medical treatment, deep fissures, infected fissures, and lateral fissures mandate surgical referral. There exist several surgical interventions for chronic anal fissures. Surgical interventions include anal dilation, lateral internal sphincterotomy, and anal advancement flaps.

Hemorrhoids

Common emergency department complaints associated with hemorrhoids include the sensation of a mass effect or rectal bleeding with or without pain and/or pruritus ani. Hemorrhoids result from swelling or deterioration of three discontinuous submucosal vascular cushions. External hemorrhoids, covered with squamous epithelium, begin below the dentate line and derive from the inferior hemorrhoidal plexus. Internal hemorrhoids, covered with mucosa, arise from the superior hemorrhoid plexus above the dentate line. Internal hemorrhoids are generally painless while external hemorrhoids can be painful if thrombosed. Internal hemorrhoids have a grading system from I to IV depending on the degree of prolapse from bulging with defecation without prolapse to permanent prolapse.

The precise etiology is unknown, but contributing factors including increasing age, pregnancy, pelvic tumors, chronic diarrhea, straining with stool, prolonged sitting, and diet. There have also been some proposed theories that hemorrhoids are varicose veins or result from vascular hyperplasia and deterioration of the supporting tissue around the vascular cushions producing venous dilation, erosion, bleeding, and thrombosis.

Patients with extremes of age, history of heavy bleeding or signs of anemia (such as pale skin or loss of color in palmar creases, gums, or conjunctiva) should have determination of their hemoglobin and hematocrit in the ED. The ED therapy of internal hemorrhoids consists of conservative measures, such as bulk laxatives. The definitive treatment is surgical. In the event of prolapse of an internal hemorrhoid, reduction in the ED is mandated to prevent strangulation and mucosal ulceration. Internal hemorrhoids should not have excisional or incisional

Table 16.1

Treatment of Chronic Anal Fissures

Medication	Pharmacology	Dose	Rate of Healing
GTN	Organic nitrate	0.2% topically BID for 8 wks	50–85%
Nifedipine	Calcium channel blocker	20 mg PO bid for 8 wks	60%
Botulinum toxin	Acetylcholine inhibitor	20 unit injection into internal sphincter	65–96%
Indoramin	Alpha-adrenoceptor agonist	20 mg PO	n/a
Salbutamol	Beta-adrenoceptor agonist	4 mg PO	n/a

GTN, glyceryl trinitrate; n/a, not applicable.

therapy even if thrombosed. Patients should also be taught to avoid defecation errors: not to wait too long after first feeling the urge to defecate, avoid straining, and spending too much time on the toilet (e.g., reading).

External hemorrhoids should be treated with conservative measures, unless they are thrombosed. Conservative measures in the treatment of nonthrombosed external hemorrhoids include high-fiber diet, stool softeners, and warm sitz baths. As with anal fissures, topical agents are of limited value. Thrombosed external hemorrhoids can be excised in the ED. Excision is felt to be of greatest benefit in the patient who presents in the first 48 hours following the onset of symptoms. Any elliptical incision over the thrombosed hemorrhoid allows for removal of the clot. The wound should then be packed and pressurized. Patients should remove the pack in six hours and start sitz baths.

The invasive treatment for both types of hemorrhoids, when conservative measures fail, include incisional therapy, excisional therapy, rubber band ligation, sclerosing injection, cryotherapy, infrared coagulation, or stapled hemorrhoidectomy. Of note, rectal bleeding may occur four to ten days after banding when the mucosa sloughs and the rubber band falls. Post-procedure severe anorectal pain, fever, or foul-smelling discharge may signal abscess or infection.

Rectal Prolapse

Patients with rectal prolapse commonly present with a painless mass, possibly with bleeding or mucoid discharge. Patients often complain of constipation and fecal incontinence in 20% to 100% of patients. There exists a predilection for women usually in the six and seventh decades. This is a diagnosis made simply by examining the perineum with or without straining, depending on the degree of prolapse.

Rectal prolapse or procidentia is the extrusion of all layers of the rectal wall through the verge of the anus. Rectal prolapse can include mucosal prolapse only or true, full-thickness prolapse. Mucosal prolapse is complete eversion of the anal mucosa and the anoderm. True rectal prolapse concentric folds are on the surface of the tissue, the anus is in normal anatomic position, and there is a sulcus between the anus the everted bowel. Mucosal prolapse occurs most commonly in children under 2 years of age and may indicate malnutrition, pinworms, paraplegia or cystic fibrosis.

In the absence of neuropathy (polio, stroke, etc.), true rectal prolapse occurs as a result of a weakening pelvic floor and anal sphincters. The most common etiology stems from childbirth or surgical trauma. Recurrent true rectal prolapse is associated with ulceration of the anterior anal mucosa, so this area should be examined closely.

Initial ED treatment starts with simple, gentle reduction if the tissue looks healthy and viable. After adequate sedation and analgesia, firm, slow, continuous pressure on the mass with moistened gauze for 5 to 15 minutes should reduce the prolapse. After reduction, patients can be discharged with surgical follow-up and clear instructions not to strain and lift. Stool softeners should be recommended.

Surgery is the definitive treatment. If the rectal tissue appears ischemic, necrotic, or, if reduction is unsuccessful, then immediate surgical consultation in the ED is required. The longer the rectum remains prolapsed, the higher the risk of incontinence because of sphincter tone loss, so surgical consultation should be immediate.

Foreign Body

The patient with anorectal foreign bodies presents complaining of a foreign body, fullness or pain, although patients can present with peritonitis secondary to perforation. It is imperative that the ED physician gain as much information in the most nonjudgmental manner. It is important to know what the object is, how long it has been retained, what attempts have been made to retrieve the object, and presence of fever, abdominal pain, and bleeding. In addition, the possibility of assault should be investigated. Rectal foreign bodies result from auto-eroticism, sexual play, ingestions, iatrogenic materials or assault. Iatrogenic foreign bodies usually involve enema equipment or rectal thermometers.

There exist a wide variety of approaches to removing rectal foreign bodies. Soft objects without sharp edges that lie below the rectosigmoid junction are easier to remove in the ED setting. Before attempting removal, bimanual examination, direct visualization, and radiographic evaluation should be completed. Successful removal of rectal objects demands adequate sedation and analgesia. A local perianal block can facilitate removal with or without conscious sedation. Options for removal include the use of a vaginal speculum, anoscope, proctoscope or sigmoidoscope to facilitate visualization. The item can be grasped with a number of items including polypectomy snares, ring forceps or suction devices. If there is a vacuum around the object preventing its release, passing a Foley proximal to the object and inflating it may break the seal and assist in passage. Agents that increase GI motility may result in obstruction or retrograde propulsion of the foreign object proximally in the GI tract. Very large, extremely fragile items, sharp objects or items that cannot be successfully removed in the ED should be removed surgically. Patient presenting with an acute abdomen, fever, abdominal pain or perforation should be admitted.

After object removal in the ED, all patients must be observed for bleeding. A careful proctosigmoidoscopy should be obtained to exclude the complications of perforation and laceration. Radiographs should be taken after removal of objects in order to detect perforation.

Inflammatory and Infectious Disorders

Proctitis

Proctitis is a general term relating to both inflammation and infection of the anal canal. Symptoms vary depending on the underlying etiology; however, the typical patient presents complaining of rectal discomfort, tenesmus, discharge, and constipation. Specific categories include infectious, traumatic, granulomatous, and radiation proctitis.

Infectious Proctitis

Infectious proctitis can have a number of etiologies. Pinworms (*Enterobius vermicularis*) is a common cause with the patient usually complaining of perianal itching that intensifies at night. *Candida albicans* proctitis can similarly present with itching and, as a frequent cause of perineal infection in infants, women, and diabetics, is a relatively rare cause of anal canal infection.

Sexually transmitted infections of anorectal region have a similar pathogenesis and treatment as those involving the genital region with the additional symptomatic benefit of adding a high-fiber diet, stool softeners, and warm sitz baths. The most common sexually transmitted organism is *Neisseria gonorrhea*. Examination may be normal or may reveal mucosal irritation and a purulent discharge. Anorectal syphilis presents with the chancre of primary syphilis or the condyloma lata of secondary syphilis, which are flat perianal warts. Herpes presents with painful vesicles often associated with adenopathy of the inguinal chain. *Chlamydia trachomati* can present as anorectal discomfort, inflammation, and discharge. HIV positive individuals may present to the ED with one or more of these anorectal disorders as their first manifestation of the disease. Potential opportunistic organisms include herpes simplex type I, *Mycobacterium avium intracellulare*, and cytomegalovirus (**Table 16.2**).

Cryptitis is the localized infection of one of the anal glands, or crypts. It can be identified as a bead of pus from the crypt while performing the anoscopic exam. Cryptitis may lead to anal fistulae and perianal abscesses, if left untreated. Treatment consists of normalization of stool consistency with fiber and stool softeners. Warm soaks, sitz baths, and rectal irrigation are thought to enhance healing. More advanced cases require surgical referral.

Traumatic Proctitis

Traumatic proctitis occurs from trauma including rectal prolapse, assault, enemas, manual disimpaction, or anal intercourse. It may also result from chemical irritants. This is usually discovered on anoscopy. As with anal ulcers from other etiologies, a biopsy to exclude malignancy must be obtained and treatment includes high-fiber diet, stool softeners, and warm sitz baths. Traumatic proctitis generally heals with discontinuation of the irritant.

Table 16.2

Treatment of Most Common Types of Infectious Proctitis

Infection	Presentation	Treatment
Candida albicans	Discomfort, rash	Cutaneous: topical antifungal 3-4 times a day for 7-14 days; ketoconazole 400 mg PO QD for 14 days. Additional treatment may be warranted depending on patient circumstances.[15]
Chlamydia trachomatis*	Discomfort, inflammation, discharge	Azithromycin 1 g PO × 1, or doxycycline 100 mg PO BID × 7 days. In pregnancy: erytho base 500 mg PO QID × 7 days; or, amoxicillin 500 mg PO TID × 7 days. Lymphogranuloma venereum: doxycycline 100 mg PO BID for 21 days
Enterobius vermicularis	Itching, especially at night	Albendazole 400 mg PO ×1 and repeat in 2 weeks; or, Mebendazole 100 mg PO × 1 and repeat in 2 weeks
Herpes	Painful vesicles, inguinal lymphadenopathy	Primary episode: acyclovir 400 mg PO TID for 7-10 days; valacyclovir 1,000 mg PO BID for 7-10 days; famciclovir 250 mg PO TID for 7-10 days. Recurrence: acyclovir 400 mg PO TID for 5 days; valacyclovir 500 mg PO BID for 3 days; famciclovir 125 mg PO BID for 5 days
Neisseria gonorrhoeae*	Mild discomfort, discharge	Ceftriaxone 125 mg IM, or Cefixime 400 mg PO × 1, or Cipro 500 mg PO × 1, or Oflox 400 mg PO × 1, or Levofloxacin 250 mg PO × 1, or Gatifloxacin 400 mg PO ×1
Syphilis	Primary chancre (can be painful)	Primary: Benzathine pen G 2.4 million units IM × 1; or, Doxycycline 100 mg PO BID × 14 days

*Always treat for both and screen for other sexually transmitted infections. Should be referred for HIV testing.

Granulomatous Proctitis

Granulomatous proctitis may occur with either ulcerative colitis or Crohn's disease, and, now less commonly, with tuberculosis. Most patients present to the ED with known disease.

Radiation Proctitis

Radiation proctitis usually presents 4 to 5 months following a course of pelvic ionizing radiation for cancers of testes, prostate, bladder, cervix, uterus, and anus. Patients present with bleeding, diarrhea, and tenesmus. Examination typically reveals a swollen, tender, brittle anal canal. Rectal strictures may be found.

Perirectal Abscess

A *perirectal abscess* presents as a painful mass. It starts as a polymicrobial anal gland infection composed of fecal flora that extends into the potential spaces around the anorectum. The different types, in order of frequency and classified by location, are perianal, ischiorectal, submucosal, and supralevator. Perianal abscesses may be drained in the ED, while all others should be referred to a surgeon. Patients who have incision and drainage require packing changes and surveillance for healing and the complication of fistula development. Even in cases where spontaneous draining occurs during the exam, formal incision and drainage is required to minimize the risk of recurrence. Other indications for surgical referral include perianal abcesses that are over 10 cm in size, necrotic, deep, undrainable or in an immunosuppressed host. Crohn's disease may present with this manifestation as their first indication of disease.

Antibiotics are indicated in patients who are at risk for endocarditis, who are immunosuppressed, have lymphangitis or systemic symptoms. Patients with constitutional complaints, fever, immunocompromise or cellulitis should be considered for admission and parenteral antibiotics.

Anorectal Fistula

The *anorectal fistula* or *fistula in ano* is an abnormal tract connecting the anal canal and the skin resulting from an infected anal gland. Patients typically complain of a discharge staining undergarments, unrelated to defecation. They may describe a cyclic history of discharge, quiescent period after cutaneous healing, progressive pain and tenderness during abscess formation, and back to purulent drainage with abscess rupture, thereby completing the cycle. The majority of cases are associated with Crohn's disease, anal fissures, anorectal trauma and/or surgery or infections (especially abscesses). Other predisposing etiologies include inflammatory bowel disease and tuberculosis. Infection of anorectal fistulae is common and they are particularly prone to abscess formation.

Examination during the fistulous phase reveals the draining ano-cutaneous tract, which may be palpable during digital rectal examination. A probe can be passed through the origin to assist in definition. Management is elective outpatient surgical repair when the traditional treatment does not work (which includes high-fiber diet, stool softeners, and warm sitz baths). In the ED any persistent local abscess should be incised and drained. Antibiotics are not felt to be of benefit in uncomplicated cases. However significant cellulitis, particularly in the immunocompromised patient, warrants antibiotics and admission.

Condyloma Acuminatum

Patients with *condyloma acuminatum* may complain of mass and some may experience anal pain or itching or bleeding. Raised perianal warts most likely represent condyloma acuminatum, a focal infection of human papillomavirus usually types 6 or 11. Usually this results from sexual contact. Although anal intercourse (homo- or heterosexual) increases the risk, any sexually active individual even without participating in anal intercourse may develop warts. The area should be soaked with 3% to 5% acetic acid to whiten the condylomata and thus better distinguish wart from normal tissue. Presence of condyloma should prompt further evaluation for other sexually transmitted infections including syphilis, which can present as condyloma lata (usually flat) and verrucous carcinoma.

Treatment for minor cases of perianal papillomata involves topical treatment with a variety of abrasive substances including 85% trichloroacetic acid, 25% podophyllin or cryotherapy, laser therapy, immune modifiers, or surgery. Refractory and more advanced cases require surgical care.

Condyloma lata are also sexually transmitted, but as a manifestation of secondary syphilis. On physical examination these may be differentiated from condyloma acuminata by their low horizontal plane, their more rigid texture, and that they are wetter lesions. Secondary syphilis is treated with 2.4 million units benzathine penicillin G by intramuscular injection. Penicillin-allergic patients may be given a ten-day course of either erythromycin or tetracycline.

Tumors

The most common presentation for anorectal tumors is that of inconsistent bleeding with, or more often, without pain. Any non-healing or suspicious lesions should be referred for excision and biopsy. There are several tumors of the anorectum, many of which are indistinguishable from more benign lesions and may be missed on exam. The majority of anorectal malignancies are squamous cell tumors (70%) and adenocarcinomas. Less frequent etiologies include basal cell carcinoma, melanoma, epidermoid carcinoma, Kaposi's sarcoma, Bowen's disease, extramammary Paget's disease, and others. Risk factors for anorectal tumor are family history of lower gastrointestinal cancer, personal history of breast or uterine carcinoma, pelvic irradiation, ureterosigmoidostomy, familial polyposis, and inflammatory bowel disease.

Anal cancers are staged and treated differently from rectal cancers. Most anal cancers respond well to chemotherapy and radiation. Colorectal cancer usually requires surgery. Tumors of the anorectum, when identified and referred early, are preventable causes of death, and it is imperative that the emergency physician do an appropriate visualization and evaluation for every anal and perianal complaint.

Selected Readings

Coates WC. Chapter 91: Anorectum. In: Marx JA, Hockberger RS, Walls RM et al, eds. *Rosen's Emergency Medicine Concepts and Clinical Practice,* 5th ed. St. Louis: Mosby 2002:1343–1359.

Farnsworth WJ. Rectum and anus. In: Aghababian RV et al., eds. *Emergency Medicine: Core Curriculum.* Philadelphia: Lippincott-Raven, 1998.

Felt-Bersma RJF, Cuesta MA. Disorders of the anorectum: Rectal prolapse, rectal intussusception, rectocele, and solitary rectal ulcer syndrome. *Gastro Clin* 2001;30:199–222.

Gilbert DN, Moellering RC, Sande MA. *The Sanford Guide to Antimicrobial Therapy 2003.* Hyde Park, VT: Antimicrobial Therapy, Inc., 2003.

Gopal DV. Disease of the rectum and anus: A clinical approach to common disorders. *Clin Cornerstone* 2002;4:34–48.

Gordon PH. Disorders of the anorectum: anorectal anatomy and physiology. *Gastroenterol Clin North Am* 2001;30:1–13.

Harrison BP, Cespedes RD. Genitourinary emergencies: Pelvic organ prolapse. *Emerg Med Clin North Am* 2001;19:781–797.

Hulme-Moir M, Bartolo DC. Disorders of the anorectum: Hemorrhoids. *Gastro Clin* 2001;30:183–197.

Jonas M, Scholefield JH. Disorders of the anorectum: Anal fissure. *Gastro Clin* 2001; 30:167–181.

Metcalf AM. Anal fissure. *Surg Clin North Am* 2002;82:1291–1297.

Moore HG, Guillem JC. Anal neoplasms. *Surg Clin North Am* 2002;82:1233–1251.

Nelson R. Anorectal abscess fistula: What do we know? *Surg Clin North Am* 2002; 82:1139–1151.

Pfenninger JL, Zainea GG. Common anorectal conditions: Part II. Lesions. *Am Fam Physician* 2001;64:77–88.

Sardinha TC, Croman ML. Hemorrhoids. *Surg Clin North Am* 2002; 82:1153–1167.

Vukasin P. Anal condyloma and HIV-associated anal disease. *Surg Clin North Am* 2002;82:1199–1211.

Cardiovascular Disorders

Louis G. Graff

Acute Coronary Syndrome: Rapid Assessment and Treatment Units

Scientific knowledge on diagnosing and treating cardiovascular disease is growing exponentially: The emergency physician has improved diagnostic capabilities with new technology, such as troponin cardiac biomarkers and sestimibi cardiac imaging; risk stratification tools help to identify high risk patients who are most appropriate for diagnostic evaluation; and more effective treatments are now available, such as anti-platelet drugs, ACE inhibitors, thrombolytics, and coronary angioplasty. The result has been improved outcomes with decreasing mortality from acute myocardial infarction.

Yet a major gap exists between our present knowledge of disease and the clinician's actual clinical practice. Acute myocardial infarction (MI) has been the number one killer in the United States. However, emergency department diagnosis is missed in 2% to 5% of patients, who are then discharged to home. These patients face a doubling of their risk of death. Thus, cardiovascular disease remains as emergency medicine's number one malpractice problem; it also remains one of emergency medicine's major therapeutic dilemmas. Aspirin and β-blockers have been shown to dramatically improve outcome, resulting in lower death rate, yet many acute MI patients do not receive these basic therapies.[8] The American College of Emergency Physicians and other specialty societies have established evidence-based guidelines on the care of patients with cardiovascular disease. Performance measures of interventions, such as aspirin and beta blocker treatment for acute MI, are now publicly reported due to initiatives from regulatory groups such as the Joint Commission and the Centers for Medicare and Medicaid Services. This has created an opportunity, but has also set an imperative for the clinician to meet the best practice standards.

Rapid assessment and treatment units or chest pain units (CPUs) are an important tool to aid clinicians in their difficult task. The emergency physician does not identify all acute MI patients during the emergency department (ED) evaluation because many acute MI patients have normal EKGs, and non-typical clinical findings. To help identify and stratify risk and probability of disease in such patients, multiple risk stratification models have been developed by different groups (Lee et al; Selker et al; Pozen et al; Goldman et al).[1-4] Risk stratification by the emergency physician with the initial clinical and EKG findings is a successful strategy to select patients: high to moderate risk patients are hospitalized for treatment of their acute coronary syndrome; low risk patients are evaluated in a CPU over a six- to twelve-hour time period; while very low risk patients are discharged.

Evaluation of the low risk patients in the CPU addresses both quality of patient care and cost-effectiveness. The "missed diagnosis" rate is inversely proportional to the "ruled out" rate. Evaluation of low risk patients in a CPU effectively identifies patients who can be discharged and, more importantly, identifies atypical presentation of acute MI patients.[5] Studies have also indicated that CPU evaluation reduces subsequent hospitalization numbers by one third and cuts overall costs in half. Gomez's randomized clinical trial shows a reduction in cost from $5,719 to $1,297 per patient.[6] Roberts's randomized clinical trial demonstrated cost reduction from $2,095 to $1,528 per patient.[7] Farkouh's randomized clinical trial evaluating costs over six-month follow-up periods indicated a 61 percent cost decrease.[8] Goodacre's randomized clinical trial in England found results similar to the American studies, where the hospitalization rate decreased from 54% to 37% and there was similar reduction in overall costs.[9]

Cardiovascular disease has continued to be the major killer in the United States since the birth of emergency medicine. Emergency physicians have long been in a holding pattern of care, but the advent of chest pain units and other technologic innovations will allow them to move forward.

References

1. Selker HP, et al. Use of the acute cardiac ischemia time-insensitive predictive instrument (ACI-TIPI) to assist with triage of patients with chest pain or other symptoms suggestive of acute cardiac ischemia: a multicenter, controlled trial, *Ann Intern Med* 1998;129:845–855.
2. Lee TH, Rouan GW, Weisberg WC, et al. Clinical characteristics and natural history of patients with acute myocardial infarction sent home from the emergency room. *Am J Cardiol* 1987:60;219–224.
3. Pozen MW, D'Agostino RB, Selker HP, et al. A predictive instrument to improve coronary-care-unit admission practices in acute ischemic heart disease. A prospective clinical trial. *N Engl J Med* 1984;310:1273–1278.

4. Goldman L, Cook EF, Brand DA, et al. A computer protocol to predict myocardial infarction in emergency department patients with chest pain. *N Engl J Med* 1988;318:797–803.
5. Tatum JL, Jesse RL, Kontos MC, et al. Comprehensive strategy for the evaluation and triage of the chest pain patient. *Ann Emerg Med* 1997;29:116–125.
6. Gomez MA, et al. An emergency department based protocol for rapidly ruling out myocardial ischemia reduces hospital time and expense: results of a randomized study (ROMIO). *J Am Coll Cardiol* 1996;28:25–33.
7. Roberts R, et al. Costs of an emergency department based accelerated diagnostic protocol vs hospitalization in patients with chest pain, *JAMA* 1997;278: 1671–1676.
8. Farkouh ME, et al. A clinical trial of a chest-pain observation unit for patients with unstable angina. *N Engl J Med* 1998;339:1882–1888.
9. Goodacre S, Nicholl J, Dixon S, et al. Randomised controlled trial and economic evaluation of a chest pain observation unit compared with routine care. *Br Med J* 2004;328:254.

Acute Coronary Syndrome (ACS)

Richard V. Aghababian
Djiby Diop

ACS Introduction

Acute Coronary Syndrome (ACS) represents a group of clinical entities that share impaired coronary blood artery flow as a common etiology. The human and economic burden of ACS is enormous. It is estimated that more than 12 million people carry the diagnosis of coronary artery disease (CAD) and that each year over 1 million patients in the United States have a new or recurrent acute coronary event.[1] Heart diseases of all types accounted for approximately 710,000 deaths in 2000 and has been the leading cause of death in the United States. The second most common cause of death in 2000 was malignant neoplasm at approximately 550,000 deaths and then cerebrovascular disease at approximately 168,000 deaths.[2] Deaths due to coronary artery disease, cerebrovascular disease, and peripheral vascular disease are combined together and reported as Cardiovascular Disease (CVD) deaths.

It is estimated that over 8 million patients present to Emergency Departments (ED) in the United States every year for the evaluation of chest pain and other symptoms that have been associated with ACS. Of these 5 million patients about 40% end up being discharged home after ED evaluation. Of those who are discharged home 2% to 5% are subsequently diagnosed as patients with acute myocardial infarction.[3] While in the past it was believed that "typical" ischemic symptoms including chest pain, shortening of breath and syncope were present in the majority of ACS patients, it is now recognized that symptoms such as weakness, back pain, dizziness, and indigestion previously referred to as "atypical" are also common. It is now understood that ACS symptoms can vary considerably based on sex, age and the presence of concomitant conditions such as diabetes mellitus or cerebrovascular disease.

Although (CVD) is the leading cause of death for adult women in industrialized nations, until recently CVD (and, therefore, ACS) was considered a disease that affected many more men than women. In 2001 in the United States CVD accounted for 499,000 deaths among women in contrast to the estimated number of deaths in 2001 from all cancers for women estimated at 272,810 of which 15% (or about 40,900) deaths are attributed to breast cancer.[4] Despite these figures women perceive the chance of dying from breast cancer to be far more likely than dying from ACS.[5] This misperception may in part be due to the belief that breast cancer generally occurs at an earlier age and causes more suffering. Many physicians share the perception that women's risk for ACS is lower than their male peers. Women are less often referred for cardiac catheterization than men following an acute myocardial infarction (AMI).[6] Recent reports have demonstrated that compared to men, women tend to have an AMI at an older age, are more likely to have unstable angina rather than AMI when presenting acutely. When women are determined to have an AMI they are more likely to also be suffering from conditions such as diabetes, hypertension, cerebrovascular disease, hyperlipidemia, and atrial arrhythmias. Studies have also shown that women with ST elevation have a worse prognosis than their male counterparts whereas women with unstable angina have a better prognosis than men.[7] Several explanations have been proposed to explain the gender difference with regard to onset of ACS symptoms, the nature of its symptoms, and subsequent various causes of mortality. The age at onset of symptoms is generally later in women than men and women live about 6 to 7 years longer than men, which may account for some of these differences. In addition it is postulated that estrogen/progesterone levels in pre-menopausal women afford some protection from the development of atherosclerosis, and subsequent ACS. This may be in part due to reduction in serum lipid levels.[8] While endogenous hormones appear to be beneficial to pre-menopausal women, estrogen/progestin therapy administered to post-menopausal women has not been demonstrated to provide any reduction in ACS events.[9]

Asking the patient about current and recent symptoms is an important part of ACS evaluation. When carefully interviewed many ACS patients will have had symptoms suggestive of ACS for several hours or days before seeking medical attention. Delays in seeking medical attention have been shown to increase morbidity and mortality associated with ACS. Public education efforts directed at aiding patients in recognizing the first signs and symptoms of acute coronary ischemia, and to appreciate the importance of early access to EMS assistance will help decrease the impact of ACS. Public education efforts should also emphasize the value of risk factor modification through adjustments in diet and exercise and the importance of regular visits to a primary care provider for patients with a strong family history for CAD, hypertension, hyperlipidemia, diabetes, mellitus, and those who are smokers.

Inadvertent discharge of a patient who is suffering from myocardial infarction is associated with a short-term mortality rate of 25%, twice that noted for AMI patients who are admitted. It is no surprise then given the incidence of ACS in the United States, that 21% of malpractice dollars paid on behalf of emergency physicians are assigned to claims for missed AMI.[10] The task of the ED physician caring for the patients with chest pain is therefore daunting. He or she must be vigilant enough to quickly recognize the varied signs and symptoms associated with the initial ACS presentation of a patient with ACS. Potentially lethal causes of chest pain other than ACS (for example, aortic dissection, pulmonary embolism, tension pneumothorax and pericardial tamponade) must be considered and ruled out during the initial patient assessment. Patients presenting with ACS, should be quickly stratified according to risk for acute coronary occlusion, and promptly provided the treatment most appropriate for the patients based on their risk stratification.

ACS Pathophysiology

ACS describes a spectrum of clinical presentations that includes Unstable Angina (UA), Non-ST Elevation Myocardial Infarction (NSTEMI), and ST Elevation Myocardial Infarction (STEMI). Cardiogenic shock and sudden death are the most severe consequences of ACS.[11] Stable angina or ischemic symptoms that occur during strenuous exercise and subside when the physical activity has ended, often precedes the development of ACS. For each of these presentations, a reduction in the blood supply to a portion of the myocardium causes the patient to experience one or more ACS symptoms, EKG abnormalities may or may not be detected, and if myocardial injury has occurred, characteristic patterns of cardiac biomarker release into the serum will be noted. Atherosclerosis is the most common cause of coronary artery narrowing and it typically develops over many years. Either sudden rupture erosion, or fissuring of the endothelial surface over pre-existing atheromatous plaque is frequently the catalyst for thrombus formation and further narrowing of the affected vessel. Signs and symptoms of ACS develop when there is critical narrowing or complete occlusion of the vessel lumen (**Table 17.1**).

Plaque fissuring, erosion and/or rupture, attracts platelets to the denuded vessel surface and begins the process of thrombus formation. Atherosclerotic plaque is more likely to fissure or rupture when it is characterized by a large lipid core, a thin fibrous cap, increased macrophage infiltration, high tissue factor levels and disorganized collagen formation.[12,13] A platelet rich thrombus forms after disruption of the endothelial surface of the plaque. Aggregating platelets from the developing thrombus release a prostaglandin thromboxane A_2. Thromboxane A_2 is a potent vasoconstrictor and therefore causes further narrowing of the vessel lumen. Serotonin and ADP are also released from activated platelets. These substances encourage further platelet aggregation and therefore thrombus enlargement. Circulatory macrophages, and activated T-lymphocytes converge on the site of plaque rupture. Activated T-lymphocyte release cytokines that activate macrophages. Activated macrophages encourage smooth muscle cell proliferation, which, over time, leads to further narrowing of the lumen of the coronary artery. They also release metalloproteases that digest components of the extracellular matrix, resulting in greater risk for erosion of the endothelial surface by atherosclerotic vessels.

The newly formed thrombus may present or undergo autolysis within minutes or hours. When this occurs, thrombus/platelet microemboli are released. These microemboli then travel in the coronary circulation to cause occlusion at a more distal site. If the microembolism causes persistent occlusion where it lodges, some myocardial necrosis may occur even though the patient's symptoms may have improved. Transient occlusion followed by thrombus autolysis may produce the fluctuating ACS symptoms associated with the diagnosis of UA or NSTEMI. Elevation of serum biomarkers may occur during transient periods of occlusion at the site of clot formation or the site where micro emboli eventually lodge. Positive serum markers without ST segment elevation define the NSTEMI patient. On the other hand, prolonged subtotal or total coronary artery occlusion that is commonly associated with persistent ischemic symptoms suggest a clinical diagnosis of STEMI.[11,14] Some patients who experience persistent ischemic symptoms are thought to have increased vasomotor tone resulting in vasoconstriction induced coronary artery narrowing. When vasoconstriction of coronary arteries is superimposed on vessels that have been narrowed by atherosclerosis, the extent of the myocardial ischemia may be considerable. Symptoms consistent with ACS have been shown to occur with the use of cocaine and may be a result of cocaine induced coronary vasoconstriction in cocaine using patients. Since repeated cocaine use may promote atherosclerosis, it is often difficult to determine whether the ACS symptoms experienced following cocaine use is a result of acute thrombus formation in a coronary vessel narrowed by chronic cocaine use or by coronary artery narrowing from cocaine-induced vasoconstriction.[15]

Regardless of the etiology, the sign and symptoms of ACS are indicative of an imbalance between oxygen supply and demand for myocardial cells and conduction system tissue. In the absence of oxygen, ischemia develops, and if unabated cell death follows. While coronary artery narrowing or occlusion is the most common etiology for

Table 17.1

Acute Coronary Syndrome and Related Conditions: Clinical Presentations

Stable Angina

Stable angina is characterized by transient symptoms of myocardial ischemia, that are induced by increased physical activity, stressful exercises. Exercise raises the need for glucose and oxygen delivery to exercising muscle and therefore increases demands for cardiac output. An increased demand for oxygen cannot be met by an increase in oxygen delivery to the myocardium in the setting of coronary artery atherosclerotic narrowing. Patients complain of chest pain, weakness, dizziness and/or shortness of breath during periods of increased activity that subsides with rest. Unlike unstable angina, the patient with stable angina can predict when the symptoms of angina will occur when the usual level of activity exceeds that which is usually tolerated. The pain in stable angina usually lasts for 1 to 5 minutes beginning during the period of exertion. Chest pain may be described as pressure like heaviness or tightness, radiating to the left arm, to the neck, jaw or back. The ECG at rest may suggest prior injury or may be within normal limits. ST-T changes suggesting ischemia may appear during vigorous activity, as for example during an exercise tolerance test.

Unstable Angina

Unstable angina (UA) is diagnosed when a patient with angina develops symptoms consistent with myocardial ischemia, that are more pronounced than the patient's usual pattern of symptoms in terms of the quality of pain, frequency and whether or not they occurred at rest or with minimal exertion. Unstable angina is diagnosed when ischemic symptoms occur at rest, and lasts longer than the patient has experienced with previous episodes or reaches 20 minutes, awakens the patient from sleep, and is increasing in severity and frequency with each successive episode. Patients with UA do not have elevated levels of serum biomarkers since no irreversible myocardial injury has occurred. The first occurrence of ischemic symptoms should be treated as UA regardless of the duration, if ST segment elevation is not present and serum biomarker levels are not elevated.

NSTEMI

Patients with NSTEMI present with ischemic symptoms similar to those described with unstable angina, however ST segment elevation is not present in the patient's ECG. Unlike UA, NSTEMI serum biomarker markers for myocardial necrosis are positive, indicating that some myocardial necrosis has occurred. Some NSTEMI patients will go on to develop ST segment elevation or Q waves in their ECG over time. Other NSTEMI patients will have ST segment depression or non-diagnostic ST segment and/or T-wave changes. Microembolization of platelet/thrombin debris in the coronary circulation may produce the fluctuating ischemic symptoms associated with elevated serum markers in the absence of ST segment elevation that defines NSTEMI.

STEMI

ST segment elevation myocardial infarction (STEMI) is diagnosed when a patient describes acute ischemic symptoms and ST segment elevation of more than 1 mm is noted in 2 or more EKG leads. The symptoms of acute ischemia associated with STEMI tend to be more persistent and more severe than those typically associated with UA or NSTEMI. Serum biomarkers should be elevated within 6 hours after the initial onset of acute symptoms. When a patient's ECG demonstrates left bundle branch block (LBBB) not known to be previously present in the presence of ischemic symptoms, the patient is managed in the same manner as those with STEMI. For some patients serial ECGs are needed to detect the presence of ST segment elevation.

Cardiogenic Shock

Soon after a severe myocardial infarction that results in ischemic/necrosis to a significant percentage of myocardium, the heart may not be able to propel blood through the ventricles into the pulmonary and systemic circulation adequately. Pressure with the arterial circulation begins to drop and plasma fluid is forced into lung alveoli as pressure within the pulmonary capillary bed rises. The patient may become pale and diaphoretic. As the blood pressure falls the patient's mental status will begin to deteriorate and mottling of the extremities may occur if the shock state is not reversed. When patients with AMI develop cardiogenic shock during hospitalization their risk of dying is 71.7%.[16]

Sudden Cardiac Death

Acute occlusion of the coronary vessels supplying the conduction system of the heart or ischemia to pre-existing unstable foci in the heart can stimuli electrical instability. Cardiac output ceases when electrical instability deteriorates to ventricular fibrillation or asystole. Death ensues in 4-8 minutes as major organs are irreversibly damaged. Properly performed CPR has been shown to maintain a fraction of normal coronary artery and cerebral artery flow, thereby extending the window of opportunity to restore electrical stability by defibrillation.

ACS, other conditions may produce ACS symptoms and myocardial injury if untreated. It is therefore important that all efforts be made to identify and treat conditions other than coronary artery disease that may have contributed to the patient's symptoms. Some such conditions have been listed in **Table 17.2**.

Initial Evaluation of Patients with ACS

Patients with symptoms and/or findings consistent with ACS should be triaged immediately to an area within the ED that is equipped and staffed to handle the life threatening complications that are associated with myocardial in-

Table 17.2

ACS Signs and Symptoms: Clinical Conditions to Consider in the Differential Diagnosis

- Acute coronary artery occlusion
- Pulmonary embolism
- Coronary artery dissection (often in association with thoracic aortic dissection)
- Uncontrolled hypertension
- Coronary artery spasm
- Coronary artery embolism (secondary to: atrial myxoma, platelet thrombi, valvular vegetation, etc.)
- Gastrointestinal diseases
  - acute gastritis
  - acute pancreatitis
  - acid reflux, esophagitis
  - peptic ulcer disease
  - Boehaave's syndrome
- Pneumonia, pleuritis
- Viral myocarditis/pericarditis
- Systemic vasculitis with coronary artery involvement
- Toxic exposure (cyanide or carbon monoxide, for example)
- Anemia or RBC dysfunction (sickle cell, for example)
- Shock (hypovolemic or septic)
- Cardiac arrhythmias
- Structural abnormalities of the heart (congenital or acquired)

jury. The initial evaluation must be focused on the history and the physical exam findings that, if present, would support a diagnosis of ACS. Administration of oxygen, cardiac monitoring and IV access should be established by members of the ED team while an emergency physician evaluates the patient. A chest x-ray should be obtained as well as blood tests to measure electrolytes, glucose, BUN, creatinine, cardiac biomarkers and the patient's coagulation status during the initial ED evaluation.

A team approach to possible ACS patient evaluation permits highly effective and time dependent therapy to be initiated promptly for patients who meet appropriate criteria. It is essential to consider potentially life-threatening conditions other than acute coronary ischemia during the initial evaluation, since some ACS treatment modalities, including fibrinolytic therapy, may increase the morbidity and mortality associated with other diagnoses (including thoracic aortic dissection).

ACS Diagnosis

The categories of information available to the emergency physician assessing a patient for possible ACS include: the patient's medical history, the physical exam, the ECG, and serum biomarkers. In some institutions stress tests or imaging studies can be arranged while the patient is in the emergency department when additional data is needed to establish a diagnosis. Such tests include stress testing, myo-

cardial perfusion imaging, echocardiography and coronary angiography.

The History

When evaluating ACS patients upon ED arrival, the history should be concise and targeted. It should focus on the quality of pain, the duration, location, radiation of pain (particularly the arm, neck or back), and if the pain is reproducible with pressure over the area identified by the patient. The examiner should inquire when the pain is associated with other symptoms such as nausea, vomiting, shortness of breath, diaphoresis, light headiness and/or dizziness. The history should also focus on any inciting factors such as exertion, emotional stress, cold exposure, fever, tachycardia, drug use or associated acute blood loss for any reason. The quality of the chest pain may be characterized by the patient as tightness, heaviness, squeezing, fullness, aching or indigestion. The duration of the pain is also important whether the patient has had a single or multiple episodes. As an example, pain that lasts only for a few seconds or is relieved by a change in position is less likely to be related to ACS than is persistent pain that cannot be relieved by a change in position. On the other hand, sharp pain that comes on suddenly and radiates through to the back is suggestive of thoracic aortic dissection. Comparing the patient's current symptoms to prior symptoms where the patient has had prior episodes of ACS can help to assess the patient's present risk for a catastrophic event. Patients who have had proven cerebrovascular accidents or who have been diagnosed as having peripheral vascular disease are at increased risk for ACS. Although many patients present with a combination of the described "typical" symptoms, some patients present with symptoms previously referred to as "atypical." This is especially true for patients who are 25 to 40 years old, patients with diabetes mellitus, and elderly women. Atypical symptoms include generalized weakness, nausea, dyspnea, difficulty sleeping or pain manifested only in the arms, epigastrium, shoulder, neck or jaw without being associated with any pain in the chest (**Table 17.3**).

Table 17.3

ACS-Associated Symptoms

- Chest pain
- Jaw pain
- Left shoulder and arm pain
- Back pain
- Epigastric pain, nausea
- Dyspnea (shortness of breath)
- General malaise or weakness (impending doom)
- Syncope or near syncope (dizziness)
- Diaphoresis
- Nausea
- Fear of death (impending doom), anxiety or restlessness

The examiner should determine if the patient has known hypertension, diabetes mellitus, hyperlipidemia, a smoking history, and whether a strong family history for CAD at an early age has been recorded.

The Physical Examination

Important clues for the presence and severity of ACS can be obtained from a careful physical exam; as with the history, patient examination provides an opportunity to narrow the list of possible causes for the patient's acute distress. Many patients with ACS will have a relatively normal physical exam. Findings may reflect concomitant conditions such as COPD, advanced diabetes mellitus prior cerebrovascular accident, peripheral vascular disease, congestive heart failure, chronic renal failure or a cardiac arrhythmia. The sudden appearance of new physical findings not previously described in the patient's medical record increase the likelihood that the patient is experiencing an episode of ACS. The most common of these findings are included in **Table 17.4**.

ECG

One of the most important tools that the ED physician has to aid in the diagnosis and management of ACS is the 12 lead ECG. It is therefore important that the ED physician be well versed in the interpretation of the ECG. Patients are candidates for fibrinolytic therapy or percutaneous coronary intervention (PCI) if there is more than 0.1 mV of ST segment elevation in 2 of the following leads: V_1, V_2, V_3, and V_4. ST segment elevation of at least 0.2mV in two or more of the following leads: aVL, I, II, III, aVf, V5 and V6 also identifies candidates for fibrinolytic therapy.

The presence of tall and slightly asymmetrical T waves without ST elevation, which may be the only ECG sign of ACS in the initial minutes of an acute event. However, marked hyperkalemia as may be seen in patients with chronic renal failure who miss dialysis may also cause tall (also called hyperacute) T waves. In the case of hyperkalemia the T waves are usually symmetrical as though picked up by tweezers. Repeating the ECG 10 to 15 minutes after the initial ECG in a patient with ongoing symptoms, may demonstrate progression from hyperacute T wave changes to commencement of ST segment elevation. The ECG can be used to monitor the impact of fibrinolytic treatment as manifested by reperfusion arrythmias and resolution of the ST elevation. The ECG and continuous monitoring are helpful in assessing patients with atypical presentations of ACS since ST-segment and T wave abnormalities may evolve over time. ECGs

Table 17.4		
Targeted ACS Physical Exam		
Critical Components of the Exam		**Important "Positive" Findings**
General appearance		• Diaphoresis
		• Cyanosis
		• Evidence of abnormal mental function
Vital signs:	Pulse	• Irregular: either too fast, or too slow
	Blood pressure	• Hypotension or hypertension (if aorta dissection is suspected) measure BP in upper and lower extremities
	Temperature	• Hypothermia or hyperthermia
	Oxygen saturation	• Hypoxemia
	Respiratory rate	• Labored respirations, either too fast or too slow
Breath sounds		• Rales, ronchi and/or wheezing are present
		• Distant or absent breath sounds in certain areas
Neck vein		• Jugular venous distention
		• Carotid pulse: irregular or diminished
Chest wall		• Surgical scars present
		• Paradoxical motion of the chest
		• Congenital deformity of the chest wall
Cardiovascular		• Irregular, rapid or slow rhythm
		• Murmurs, rubs, gallop rhythm, diminished heart sounds
Abdominal exam		• Hepatomegaly and or splenomegaly
		• Palpable midline mass and/or bruit on auscultation
Extremity exam		• Cyanosis, swelling, mottling or petechial rash
Appearance and arterial pulses		• Diminished or absent pulses
		• Pitting edema
Neurologic		• Evidence of impairment of motor function, sensation function, deep tendon reflexes and/or facial asymmetry coordination
		• Dysphasia or aphasia

also aid in the diagnosis of other conditions such as pericarditis, pulmonary embolism, transient arrhythmias and electrolyte abnormalities. Valuable data is collected when an ECG is performed while the patient is having chest pain. An old ECG for comparison becomes important if chest pain is atypical, or if the patient had a prior MI or left ventricle hypertrophy. The presence of ST segment depressions in leads opposite (180°) from those where ST segment elevation is present, are referred to as reciprocal changes. The presence of reciprocal changes implies that a proximal coronary artery occlusion has occurred.

STEMI: Common ECG Findings

ST segment elevation in leads V3 and V4 indicates anterior wall infarction. This type of infarction is usually associated with occlusion of the left anterior descending artery (LAD). ST segment elevation in leads V1 and V2 indicates injury to the interventricular septum, which is also supplied by the LAD in most patients. The distal LAD perfuses the lateral wall of the left ventricle in most patients and is associated with ST segment elevation in leads V5 and V6 in the pericardial leads.

Leads I and AVL may also exhibit ST segment elevation with LAD occlusion. Reciprocal changes (ST segment depression in leads opposite from the affected area) may be seen in limb leads II, II and AVF.

ST segment elevation in leads II, III, and AVF is indicative of an inferior wall infarction. Inferior wall infarction suggests a right coronary artery occlusion. Reciprocal changes (ST segment depression) may be seen in leads I and AVL. ST elevation may be detected if right precordial and posterior chest wall leads are recorded in patients with right-sided or posterior wall infarctions.

The presence of left bundle branch block (QRS complex > 0.12 seconds) may make interpretation of ST segment and T wave abnormalities difficult when a patient is being assessed for possible ACS.

In the setting of a left bundle branch block (LBBB), acute myocardial infarction is more likely recognized when the ST abnormalities are in the same direction as the QRS. This finding is referred to as "concordance." These concordant ST changes may also include ST depression in leads V1, V2, V3 or in leads II, III, AVF with ST elevation of at least 1 mm in V5. Sometimes one may note extreme ST elevation of greater than 5 mm.[17,18]

ECG Limitations

The ECG may be non-diagnostic in as high as 55% of patients suffering from AMI. This high rate of non-diagnostic ECG may be decreased by obtaining serial ECG every 10 to 15 minutes while the patient is symptomatic and also when the patient becomes pain free.

ECG interpretation may be difficult in the setting of a previous MI and an old ECG is not available for comparison. The presence of a LBBB may also make interpretation of the ECG in the setting of an MI difficult. The development of LBBB during an acute event or the presence of LBBB not noted at the time of the last EKG is believed to be consistent with a diagnosis of acute myocardial infarction.[19]

The ECG may be normal in two thirds of patients with unstable angina (**FIGURES 17.1–17.5**).

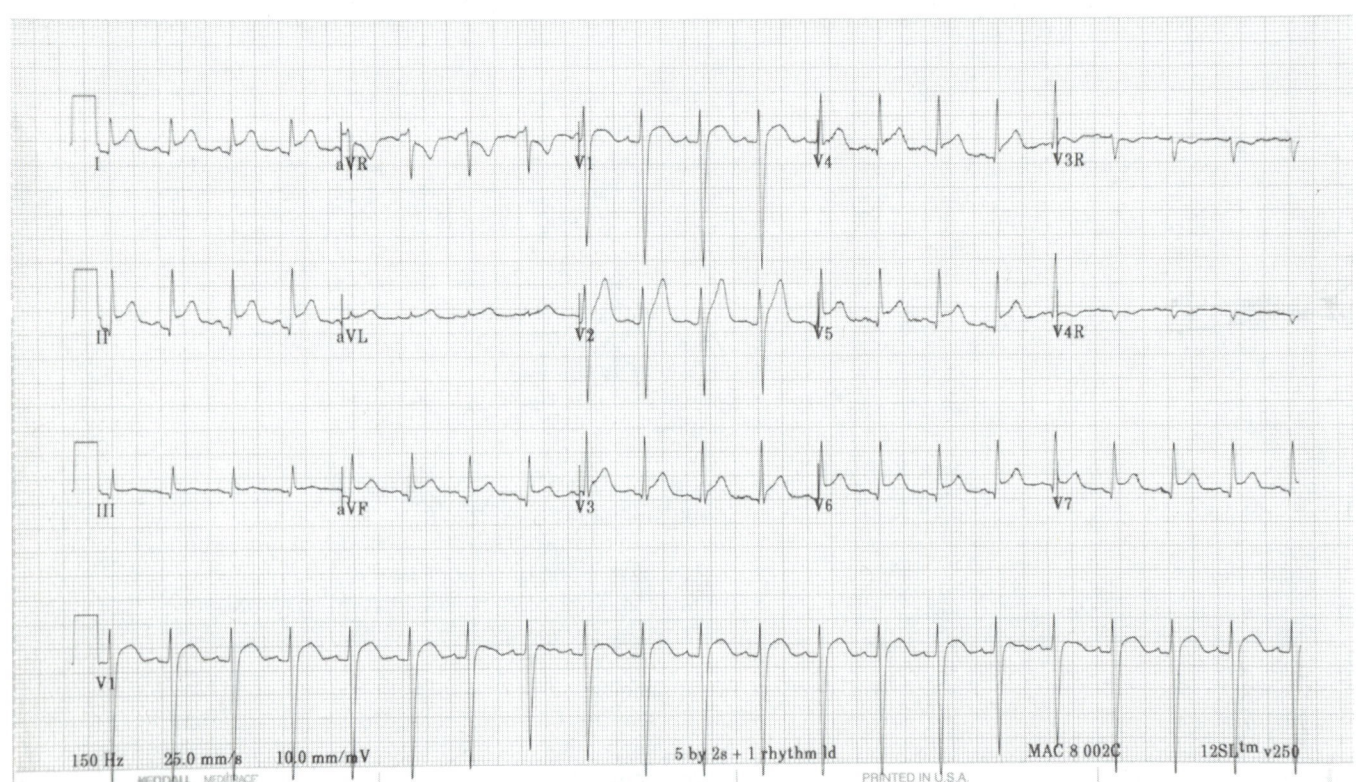

FIGURE 17.1 Diffuse ST-T segment changes and PR segment depression consistent with acute pericarditis.

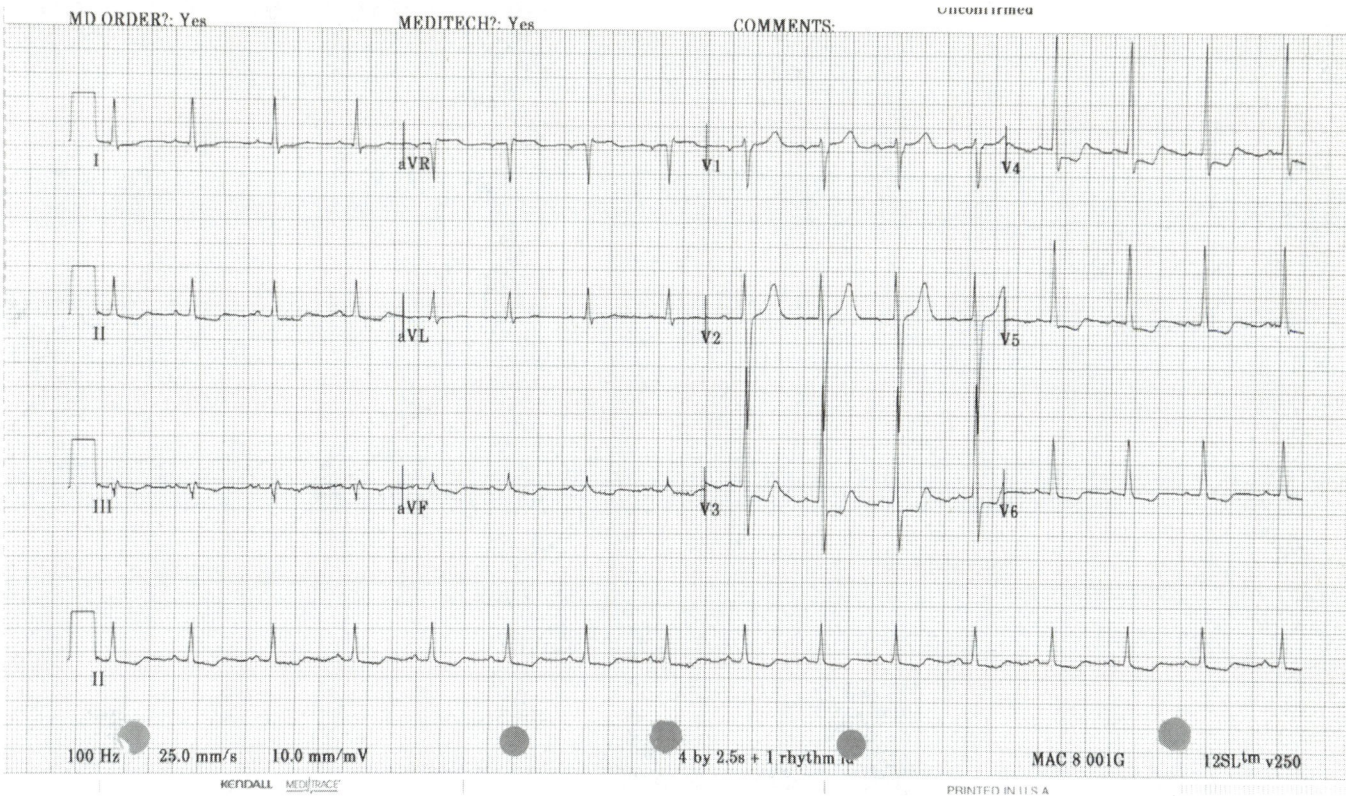

FIGURE 17.2 ST-T-segment depression consistent with myocardial ischemia.

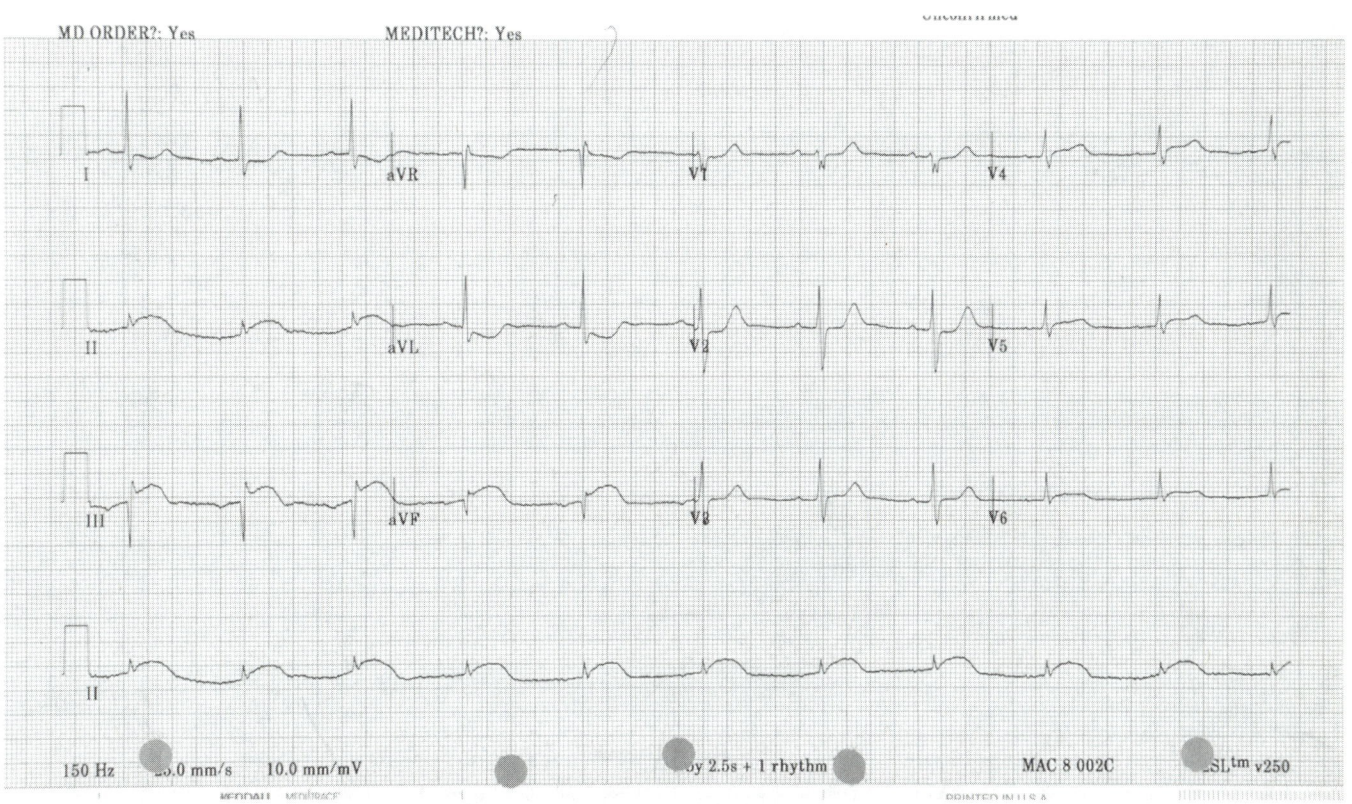

FIGURE 17.3 ST-T segment elevation of acute inferior myocardial infarction.

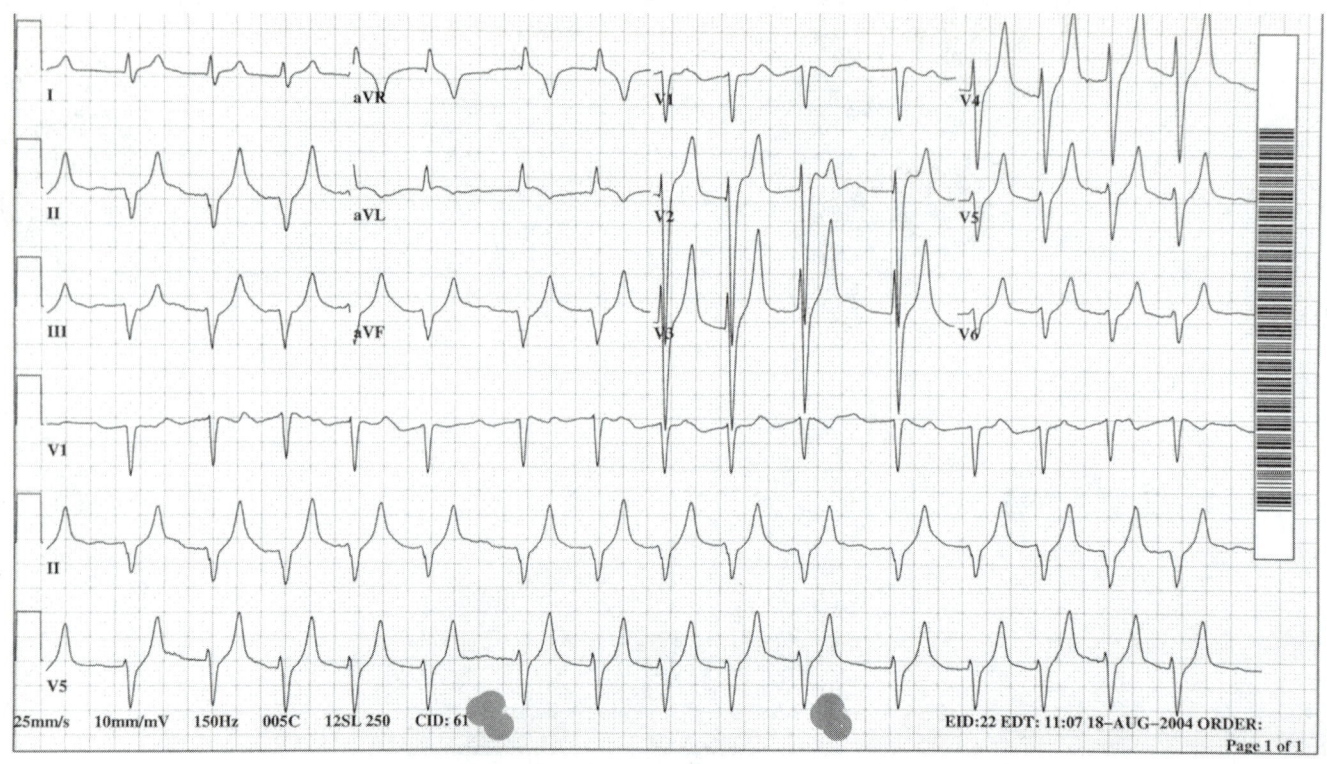

FIGURE 17.4 T wave abnormalities consistent with hyperkalemia.

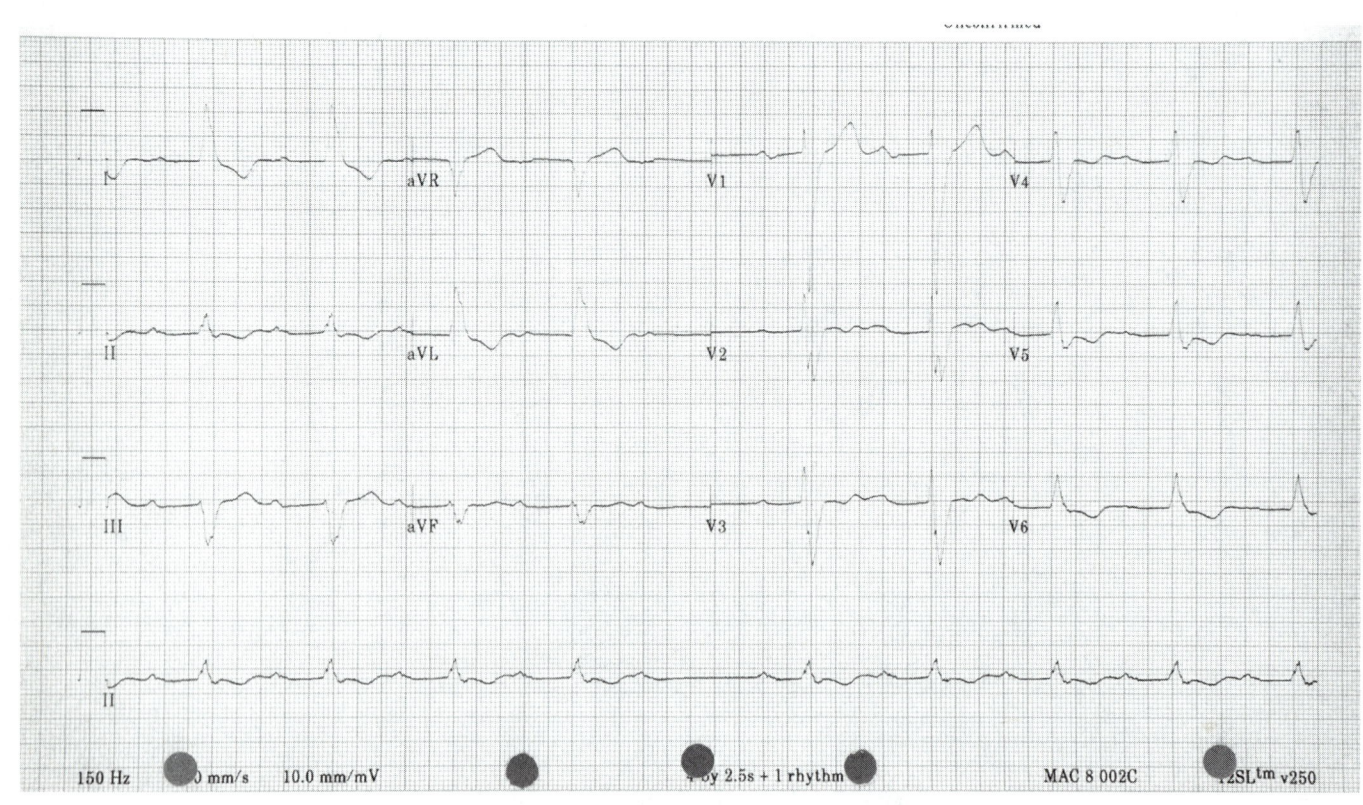

FIGURE 17.5 QRS widening of left bundle branch block.

Cardiac Serum Biomarkers

The diagnosis and management of ACS requires familiarity with the kinetics (appearance in, and clearance from the serum) of the biomarkers for myocardial necrosis. Most cardiac biomarkers are large molecules that are found in myocytes. In the setting of myocyte injury that leads to cell necrosis and cell death, these molecules are released in the bloodstream and are thus detected by sensitive immunoassays. Biomarkers found in the myocardial cell cytosol are released first, followed by biomarkers that are bound to other cellular elements. **FIGURE 17.6** demonstrates kinetic profile of release into, and clearance from the serum for the common biomarkers.

Biochemical markers should be measured in all patients who present to the ED with signs and symptoms consistent with ACS. The ED physician must, however, be careful not to attribute all rise in cardiac markers to myocardial ischemia, as mechanisms other than ischemic heart disease can cause cell injury and, thus, release of detectable levels of cardiac markers. For example, if the ED physician mistakenly interprets the rise in cardiac markers that can be seen in pericarditis, or myocarditis, and then treats the patient with an anticoagulant plus a fibrinolytic agent, the patient's condition may worsen.

If the patient presents within 6 hours of the start of the chest pain and the first set of cardiac enzymes is negative, but the clinical suspicion for NSTEMI or STEMI is high, then a second sample should be drawn in approximately 4 to 6 hours after the first draw and a third set after an additional 4-6 hours if the diagnosis remains unclear. Much has been written regarding the number of biomarker tests, that should be drawn, ECGs performed, and duration of ED observation needed before a suspected ACS patient can be safely discharged home. Strategies for biomarker utilization will continue to evolve as new biomarkers for cardiac necrosis are identified, assays for known biomarkers become more sensitive, and other means to rapidly detect acute cardiac ischemia are developed.

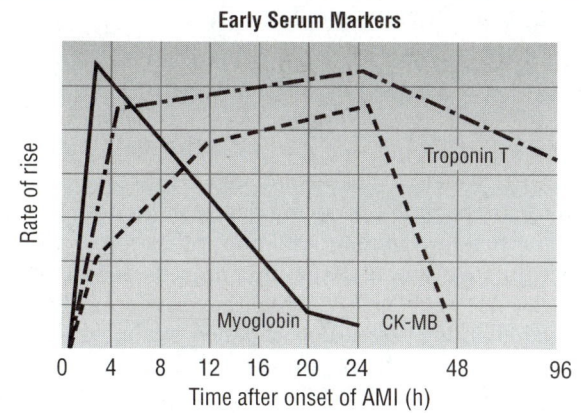

FIGURE 17.6 Release kinetics of early serum markers.

Myoglobin

Elevation of serum myoglobin leads can be detected within 1 to 2 hours following AMI. Elevated levels will persist for up to 24 hours after infarction. Myoglobin stored in cells is quickly released into the bloodstream following myocardial injury and therefore serum levels are detectable within a few hours. However myoglobin is also stored in the cytosol of cells from other organs besides myocardium, and therefore elevated levels of myoglobin does not distinguish ischemia injury to the myocardium from injury to other tissue. A normal level of myoglobin measured 4 to 6 hours after the onset of symptoms consistent with ACS can be helpful in ruling out AMI.[20]

Creatine Kinase

Creatinine kinase (CK) begins to rise within 3 to 6 hours of myocardial necrosis, and may remain elevated for as long as 48 hours. Creatinine kinase can be further divided into MM and MB fractions. The CK-MB fraction begins to rise within hours of the onset of acute symptoms and remains elevated for up to 48 hours. CK-MB is one of the cardiac markers that have enjoyed extensive use over recent years. CK-MB however is not totally specific for myocardial injury and it is important for the clinician to be aware of conditions other than myocardial ischemia that can cause an elevation in CK-MB. Other conditions known to cause a rise in the CK-MB include myocarditis, cardiac trauma, cardiac catheterization or recent coronary artery bypass surgery, disease of the uterus, renal failure, polymyositis and dermatomyositis.[21]

Troponin

The troponin complex is a molecule that is attached to the actin-myosin unit responsible for cardiac muscle contraction. And in conjunction with calcium, it has a role in regulating contractions. Troponin has 3 strict and distinct subunits, I, T, and C. Cardiac troponin I and T is structurally different from skeletal muscle troponin while Troponin C is not. Troponin I and troponin T can be detected in the blood as early as 3 to 4 hours following myocardial infarction. They remain detectable in the blood for as long as 10 days in the case of troponin I and up to 14 days in the case of troponin T.[21]

There are several reasons why troponins have become the preferred cardiac markers for myocardial cell necrosis: 1) both troponin I and troponin T are highly sensitive and specific for myocardial injury; 2) troponin I and T remain elevated for much longer than CK/CK-MB; 3) even in situations where there are only minor elevations of the troponins one can assume that an elevation is due to cardiac cell necrosis and not from leakage of the protein through reversible myocyte cell membrane permeability; or 4) the currently available assays of troponin I and T can reliably distinguish cardiac myocyte troponin from skeletal muscle myocyte troponin.

The downside of the longer duration of troponin in the blood when compared to CK is that it is not as reliable in detecting myocardial re-infarction. Since CK levels return to baseline within 48 to 72 hours of release, reinfarction will be noted as a secondary spike in measured levels. Due to their longer duration in the blood of 7 to 10 days in the case of troponin I and 7 to 14 days in the case of troponin T some episodes of reinfarction may go undetected. An advantage troponin has over other cardiac markers is that in the setting of AMI, it has the ability to predict patient outcomes such as death, based on the pack levels observed in the first 24 hours following AMI. Studies have shown that for both short- and long-term outcomes, the level of troponin elevation is directly correlated with the risk of death, whether the patient had ST elevation or non-ST elevation ACS.[22] Furthermore the risk of re-infarction, death and left ventricular dysfunction correlates with the degree of troponin elevation. The fact that troponin has a more accurate prognostic value than CK-MB was observed even among patients with renal failure, although troponin is largely cleared by the kidneys. Studies have now shown that cardiac troponin predicts outcome irrespective of the level of renal failure.[23] Interest in the white cell count (WBC) as a marker of coronary artery inflammation has recently been rekindled. It has been recommended that the WBC could play a role in early risk ST reinfarction of ACS since it is an independent predictor of in-hospital AMI mortality in a retrospective review of a large number of patients in an AMI registry.[24] B-type natriuretic peptide (BNP) is another serum marker that has been undergoing evaluation as a prognostic tool in ACS patients exhibiting left ventricular (LV) dysfunction.

Echocardiography

The use of two-dimensional echocardiography can be invaluable in the ED evaluation and management of patients with ACS. Echocardiography is helpful in situations where the patient presents with symptoms highly suggestive of ACS who do not have ST segment changes or elevated serum biomarkers. The presence of a ventricular wall motion abnormality suggests prior myocardial injury or ongoing ischemia. Echocardiography may also be very helpful in unstable angina by demonstrating (LV) wall motion akinesia or hypokinesia during ischemia that normalizes with resolution of the ischemia. Echocardiography can be helpful in: 1) in ruling in or out myocardial infarction when the ECG is normal; 2) identifying causes other than ischemia responsible for the patient's chest pain; 3) identifying and quantifying the mechanical complication of myocardial infarction such as mitral or aortic valve dysfunction; 4) providing information about left ventricular function. The echocardiogram can also be helpful for the purpose of patient risk assessment since a markedly reduced left ventricular ejection fraction indicates a poor prognosis, and may indicate the need for ACE inhibitor therapy.[25] Additional crucial information that the echocardiogram can provide includes the detection of right ventricular (RV) infarct, LV thrombus, pericardial effusion, mitral regurgitation, ventricular septal defect, and ventricular aneurysm. Transesophageal (TEE) echocardiography is helpful in assessing possible valvular abnormalities and in detecting aorta dissections involving the thoracic aorta.

Exercise Stress Testing (ETT)

Exercise stress testing (ETT) can very useful in further evaluating the cause of ACS symptoms in the ED when the ECG is non-diagnostic, cardiac markers are negative and the clinician cannot rule out ischemia as the cause of the patient's symptoms (see Table 17.3).

Although the risk of complication of undergoing ETT is low, estimated at a fatality rate of 1 per 10,000 tests, the ED physician should screen patients for contraindications prior to arranging for exercise stress testing (ETT).[26] Contraindications that have been traditionally listed for ETT include ischemic chest pain or angina within the past 48 hours, acute myocardial infarction within the last 4 to 5 days, acute myocarditis, uncontrolled congestive heart failure, infective endocarditis, unstable arrhythmia, severe aortic stenosis and suspected aortic dissection. Recent practice at many cardiac care centers has been to use ETT in low probability cases as a means to determine if discharge is warranted. A consultation from cardiology may be advisable before ETT in some patients.

A positive ETT test (ST-T changes during exercise) in a population with a pretest probability for ACS, makes it very likely that the patient has ACS. It is important to note that false positive occurs in patients taking digitalis or quinidine; those with ECG showing resting ST, T wave or conduction abnormalities; or with myocardial hypertrophy or abnormal serum potassium.

There are situations where the patient cannot adequately perform exercise testing on the treadmill due to age, arthritis, orthopedic impairment, peripheral vascular or neurological problems, and, therefore, cannot adequately increase their heart rate by exercising vigorously. Additionally, patients taking β-blockers may be unable to raise their heart rate sufficiently for an accurate ETT. Patients with a left bundle branch block and patients with ventricular pacemakers may not exhibit the ECG changes normally indicative of exercise-induced ischemia. Some patients, particulary women, may not have the muscle strength to attain the level of exercise required to test the cardiovascular system. The use of pharmacological vasodilatation drugs such as adenosine and dipyridamole can be used to simulate exercise-induced stress on the cardiovascular system in these patients.

Myocardial Perfusion Imaging

Myocardial perfusion imaging (MPI) is useful when a diagnosis of ACS is still suspected after serum markers; serial ECGs and stress testing have not confirmed the diagnosis. Single-photon emission computed tomography (SPECT) is widely available and can be used to measure coronary artery blood flow and cardiac function. Tc-99m based perfusion agents (sestamibi or tetrofosmin) are trapped in myocardial tissue after injection. Since these agents do not re-distribute over time, scanning that provides valuable images can be obtained for hours after injection. Decreased uptake of the labeled agent will be noted in the myocardial tissue of patients experiencing ischemic symptoms and the diagnosis of ACS is therefore highly likely. Normal imaging studies makes ACS much less likely. The ERASE demonstrated that the use of MPI as part of the ED education of suspected ACS patients reduced the number of unnecessary hospitalizations in a cost effective manner.[27]

Coronary Angiography

Coronary angiography is currently the "the gold standard" for confirmation that ACS is due to coronary artery narrowing. It provides a clear and definitive view of the culprit vessels and the degree of the lesion or lesions thus providing an assessment of whether or not the vessel or vessels is/are amenable to angioplasty with stent placement or require revascularization with coronary artery bypass surgery (CABG). Studies have found that when patients are determined to have multiple vessel disease, or left main disease, they have a higher risk of serious cardiac events. Coronary angiography is currently available on a continuous basis at approximately 20% of U.S. hospitals.

Hospitals without coronary angiography capability should maintain transfer agreements with cardiac care centers capable of receiving and managing complicated ACS patients 24 hours a day.

Coronary Magnetic Resonance Angiography

Coronary magnetic resonance angiography (CMRA) is a noninvasive diagnostic modality with high sensitivity that can assess the coronary artery lumen patency. CMRA is a promising innovation that may soon assist with the evaluation of patients with possible coronary artery disease and therefore ACS.

Recent data indicates that the overall accuracy of CMRA for diagnosing CAD was 72% (with a 95% confidence interval, 63% to 81%). The sensitivity, specificity and accuracy of diagnosing left main disease, or three vessel diseases were 100%, 85%, and 87% respectively. The negative predictive value for CAD and for left main or three vessel disease were 81% and 100% respectfully.[28] Studies that look at the correlation of CMRA findings with coronary angiographic studies in the presence of ACS symptoms will be helpful in defining the role for this new technology.

ACS Patient Risk Stratification

A useful step in the evaluation and management of patients with ACS involves "risk stratification." The use of risk stratifications strategy along with an ACS clinical pathway is very helpful in selecting the appropriate ED treatment, determining the most appropriate location within the hospital for the patient and deciding if the patient will require transfer to an institution with greater cardiac care capability (an operational catheterization lab). After the initial ED assessment, patients thought to have ACS should be provisionally diagnosed STEMI, NSTEMI or U/A. Patients in the UA/NSTEMI group should be further divided into low, intermediate and high risk. ACS patients with evidence of worsening heart failure, cardiogenic shock, arrhythmias refractory to manage-

Table 17.5
TIMI Score with High Risk Features

- TIMI Risk Score = 0-2 • Low Risk
- TIMI Risk Score = 3-4 • Intermediate Risk
- TIMI Risk Score = 5-7 • High Risk

High risk features:
- Persistent chest pain
- 20 min chest pain at rest
- Positive biomarker
- ST segment deviation > 0.5 mm
- Age > 75
- Hemodynamic instability
- Signs of heart failure
- Sustained VT

ment, or unremitting pain are high risk and should be considered for immediate transfer to a comprehensive cardiac care center.

An example of a risk stratification method is that developed by Antman et al. based on a 7 point risk score with one point assigned to each of the following category: age greater than 65 years; heart rate; more than 3 coronary risk factors; prior angiographic coronary obstruction; ST-segment changes; use of aspirin (ASA) within 7 days; more than 2 angina events within 24 hours; and elevated cardiac markers. These authors found that the risk of developing an adverse outcome defined as death, reinfarction, or recurrent severe ischemia requiring revascularization was 5% when the TIMI score was 0 to 1, and increased to 41% with a TIMI score of 6 to 7 (**Table 17.5**).[29]

Patients are stratified as "high risk" if at least two of the following features are present: acceleration of the symptoms in the preceding 48 hours; prolonged and ongoing pain at rest lasting longer than 20 minutes; pulmonary edema; new or worsening mitral regurgitation murmur; an S3 gallop; new or worsening rales; hypotension; tachycardia or bradycardia; age greater than 75; ST depression > 0.05 mV; new sustained ventricular tachycardia and bundle branch block; ST-segment or T-wave changes; or elevated cardiac markers. A patient should be considered to be high risk if he/she has one or more of the following features: a prior history of MI; CABG; cerebrovascular disease; claudication in association with peripheral vascular disease; prolonged angina at rest lasting more than 20 minutes and now resolved; age older than 75 years; T-wave inversions > 0.2 mV; and/or pathological Q-waves. Patients at low risk, on the other hand, lack high or intermediate-risk features and have none of the following features: new-onset worsening angina in the past 2 weeks; ischemic ECG changes; or biomarker changes.

Managing Patients with Presumed ACS

Evaluation and treatment of patients with presumed ACS begin together when the EMT first encounters the patient in the field, or on arrival in the ED. The man-

CHEST PAIN
Clinical Practice Guideline

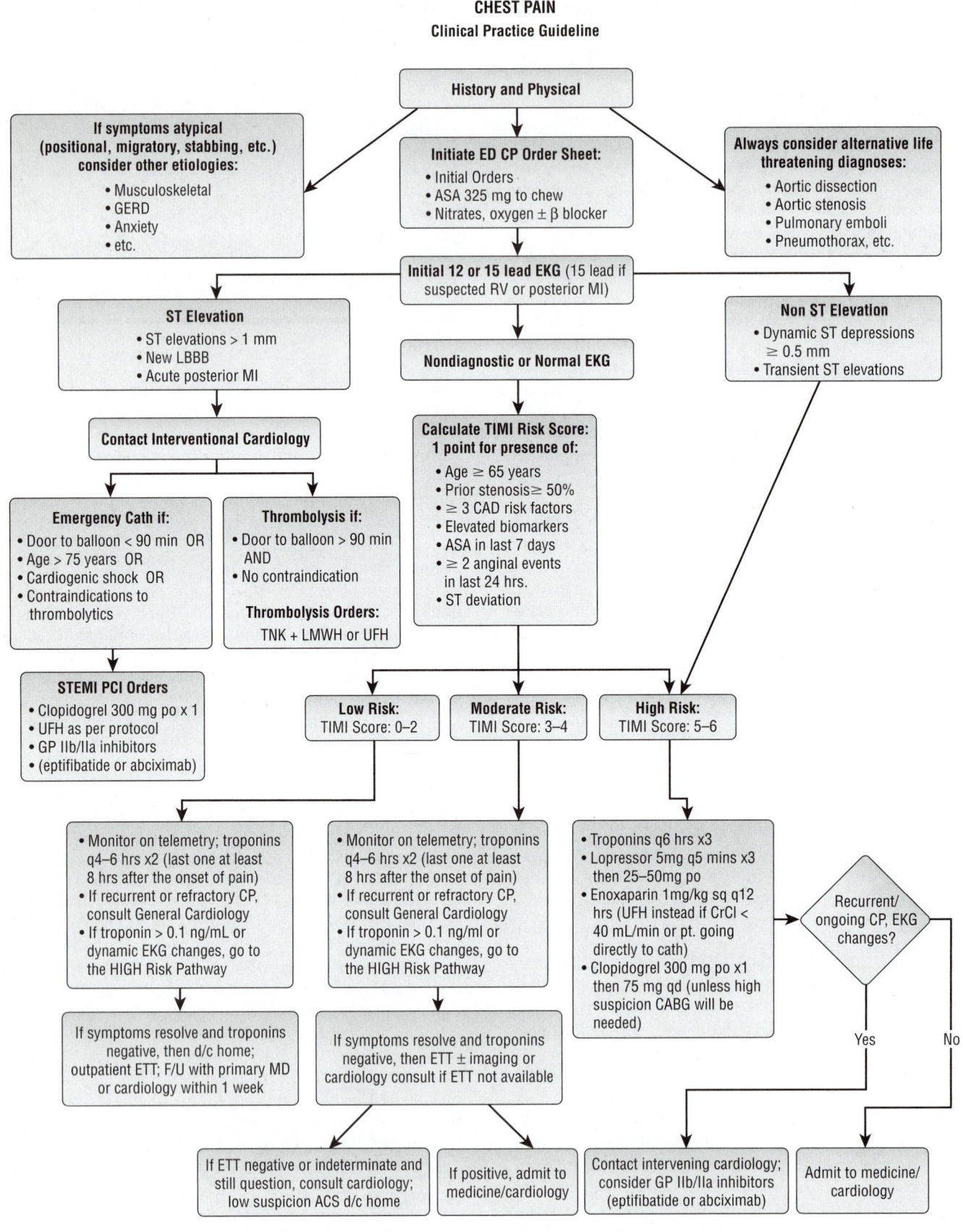

FIGURE 17.7 Chest Pain Clinical Practice Guideline.

Table 17.6

Initial Approach to a Patient with Presumed ACS

- Establish IV access
- Draw blood at the time of the IV placement and send for the following tests: CK, CKMB, Troponin, I or T, CBC, BUN, BS, Lytes—Also consider Myoglobin, PT/PTT/INR, BNP and D-Dimer tests
- Obtain and monitor vital signs including pulse oxymetry
- Obtain and interpret the 12-lead ECG
- Obtain a targeted but thorough history Focus on current symptoms, prior cardiovascular events, and current medications
- Perform a concise but thorough physical exam
- Order a portable chest x-ray and review for evidence of aortic dissection, pneumothorax, pneumonia or other conditions that could explain the patient's chest pain
- Ask for patient's medical records, including prior ECG tracings.

agement of ED patients with ACS proceeds in phases. In the initial phase, while the diagnosis is being confirmed, treatment is focused on improving oxygenation, relieving pain and making preparations to intervene if a life-threatening complication occurs (**Table 17.6**). In the second phase therapy is directed at reducing the ischemic insult to myocardium and to preventing further coronary occlusion is initiated. In the third phase specific therapy is instituted to re-establish flow in the affected coronary vessel and to present subsequent re-occlusion. The use of treatment pathways can improve efficiency particularly for patients presenting in the ED (**FIGURE 17.7**).

ACS Therapeutic Interventions

All ACS patients should receive the following interventions:
- Aspirin 162 to 325 mg chewed if possible (if no history of hypersensitivity).
- Oxygen at 2 to 4 liters by nasal canula or ventilatory assistance as needed to maintain SaO_2 at 90% or greater.
- Nitroglycerin SL, 1 tablet every 5 minutes, up to three doses, titrate to pain free; hold if SBP less or equal to 100 mm Hg. Nitroglycerin spray may also be used (patients with RV infarction can be very sensitive to the effects of nitroglycerine use). Use of medications for erectile dysfunction (Viagra, Cialis or Levitra) within 24 hours precludes the use of nitroglycerin.
- Morphine IV if pain persists after SL nitroglycerin.

After the above initial treatment is completed, the ED physician should then decide to tailor further therapy based on the ACS category that is suspect (STEMI, NSTEMI/UA) and on risk stratification (high, intermediate, low).

Stable Angina Treatment Considerations

While stable angina is not truly considered part of ACS, stable angina may be part of a constellation of symptoms noted by a patient who presents for care after because of a major accident, acute gastrointestinal bleeding or a serious systemic infection. These may include:

1. Anti-ischemic therapy: Add or increase nitroglycerine therapy or other nitrates; consider use of a β-blocker or increase the dose if the patient is taking a beta blocker (if no contraindications).
2. Suppression of platelet aggregation: Add clopidogrel if the patient has taking aspirin. Begin clopidogrel if the patient is unable to tolerate aspirin. Clopidogrel should be withheld if it is expected that the patient will require coronary artery bypass grafting within 5 days. Clopidogrel is given as 300 mg initial dose followed by 75 mg daily. This dose was shown to be effective in The Cure Trial, which included 12,562 patients.[30]
3. Additional treatment can be tailored to the patient's need after exercise stress testing, myocardial perfusion imaging or coronary angiography.

UA/NSTEMI: Treatment Considerations

1. Anti-ischemic therapy:
   a. Nitroglycerine (sublingual or IV)
   b. β-blockade (IV)
2. Suppression of platelet aggregation for moderate or high-risk patients:
   a. Add clopidogrel to aspirin unless it is reasonably certain that the patient will undergo CABG within 5 days.
   b. Consider platelet GP IIb/IIIa antagonists for high-risk patients with persistent symptoms. Eptifibatide or tirofiban may be started in the ED setting. Some angiographers may choose to start abciximab after the patient is in the catheterization lab for patients undergoing percutaneous intervention (PCI).
3. Antithrombin therapy:
   a. Consider either unfractionated heparin (UFH); or
   b. Low molecular weight heparin (LMWH) after screening the patient for possible heparin induced thrombocytompenia (HIT). If HIT is suspected, a direct thrombin should be started promptly.
4. Revascularization:
   a. Fibrinolytic therapy is **not** indicated for patients with UA/NSTEMI
   b. PCI
   c. CABG (if diffuse coronary disease is found during coronary angiography). Revascularization with PCI or CABG is indicated for patients whose symptoms persist despite conservative management.

For patients with worsening heart failure, cardiogenic shock or persistent ventricular, arrhythmias should be considered for immediate CABG surgery if "high grade" occlusion is found in more than a single, stentable coronary vessel.

STEMI: Treatment Considerations

1. **a.** Anti-ischemic therapy: Nitroglycerin if no contraindications. Administer nitroglycerin sublingual, by spray or via IV.
   b. Consider β-blockade of no contraindication.
2. Inhibition of platelet aggregation:
   a. Consider clopidogrel for patients who will undergo PCI. Since clopidogrel should be withheld if the patient is expected to undergo emergent CABG, some centers will administer clopidogrel in the Cath Lab and after the initial images confirm the presence of lesions that can be treated with a PCI procedure. Patients with diffuse coronary artery disease, who are likely to require immediate CABG should not be given clopidogrel.
   b. Consider a platelet GP IIb/IIIa Antagonist.
3. Anticoagulant therapy
   a. (UFH): After screening for HIT. If HIT is suspected a direct thrombin inhibitor should be used if PCI is planned. Argatroban is currently approved for HIT patients undergoing PCI.
   b. LMWH is an option if fibrinolysis with TNK is planned (and the patient has been screened for HIT).
4. Revascularization: Treatment strategy are influenced by the resources available at the receiving hospital and the ability to rapidly transfer a patient to a facility with ready catheterization lab and a cardiologist trained in invasive therapy.
   a. Early invasive therapy for PCI with stent placement. CABG if coronary angiography reveals diffuse atheromatous disease.
   b. Fibrinolytic therapy (TNK, Retevase, or Streptokinase), if an interventional center cannot provide PCI within 120 minutes for the time of the patient's symptom onset. LMWH may be substituted for UFH if TNK is the thrombolytic agent use.
   c. CABG surgery is indicted for patients who experience STEMI despite recent angioplasty.

ACS Therapeutic Interventions: Recommended Drugs and Initial Dose Recommendations

Anti-Ischemic Medications

Nitroglycerin

Sublingual or spray, 1/150 tablet sublingual or 2 sprays or IV nitroglycerin. Start IV nitroglycerin at 10 to 20 μg/min; increase by 5 μg/min every 1 to 2 minutes until symptoms are relieved or mean arterial blood pressure is decreased by 30% if patient is initially hypertensive. Hold if SBP is < 90 mm Hg. Start the oral dose 15 to 20 minutes after the last IV dose, starting with 25 to 50 mg PO q 6 hours for 48 hours, then 100 mg bid.

Patients who are having an inferior AMI with RV extension are extremely sensitive to nitroglycerin and in this set-

ting if nitroglycerin is to be used, the clinician should do so with extreme precaution in order to avoid profound hypotension with the potential of complication of further extending the infarction size. When indicated, Nitroglycerine produces favorable hemodynamic effects through venous as well as arterial dilatation, and by this mechanism reduces ischemic pain. Nitroglycerin should also be avoided in patients with severe bradycardia with pulse < 50 bpm. Nitroglycerin is contraindicated in patients who have taken medication for erectile dysfunction within the past 24 hours, since profound hypotension may occur. These agents inhibit phosphodiesterase resulting in the accumulation of the cGMP. cGMP stimulates vasodilatation via smooth muscle relaxation and adds to the vasodilatory effect already brought by the use of nitroglycerin.

β-Blockade Recommended Dose

Metoprolol, 5 mg slow IV q 5 min. Up to 3 doses or atenolol, 5 mg slow IV, repeat after 10 min, if needed. Check to be sure the SBP ≥ 100 mm Hg, pulse ≥ 60 bpm and no 2° or 3° AV block is present. Do not use if pulmonary edema is present.

β-blockers have been shown to reduce the progression of myocardial infarction by 13% and reduce mortality. β-blockers exert their effect in reducing risk of progression of MI and mortality by inhibiting the effect of circulating catecholamines on the myocardium thus preventing the occurrence of arrhythmias as well as decreasing oxygen consumption.

Suppression of Platelet Aggregation

Aspirin

Aspirin is a cyclooxygenase-1 inhibitor; the mechanism of its action is irreversible inhibition of the enzyme cyclooxygenase, thereby blocking the formation of thromboxane A2, a vasoconstricting agent and stimulus for platelet aggregation. Several studies have demonstrated that aspirin has been shown to reduce adverse outcomes in ACS patients when compared to placebo; aspirin should therefore be given to the patient as soon as possible after arrival in the emergency department.

Recommended Dose: Aspirin is given in a dose of 162 mg or 325 mg as an initial dose followed by a maintenance dose of 81–162 mg/d.

Thienopyridines

Clopidogrel and ticlopidine are classified as thienopyridines, and unlike aspirin, they block platelet aggregation induced by ADP. Of these two thienopyridines, ticlopidine has a shorter half live and is given at a dose of 250 mg twice a day. The use of ticlopidine has been severely limited for fear of causing severe neutropenia estimated at 2% to 3%. Clopidogrel has a better side effect profile than ticlopidine and was found to be better than aspirin in reducing ischemic complications such as AMI, stroke, and peripheral vascular disease during long-term use.[31,32] Clopidogrel is therefore recommended as a first-line adjunct therapy for patients with UA/NSTEMI in whom an early non-invasive therapy is planned or in situations in which catheterization has been deferred for an uncertain period of time, and patients who are not candidates for CABG surgery based on their coronary artery anatomy.[1] If a patient is to undergo elective CABG, clopidogrel should be discontinued 5 to 7 days before the surgery to reduce bleeding complications. Emergency CABG is not absolutely contraindicated in an unstable ACS patient who has received both aspirin and clopidogrel, however, the need for blood product transfusion will likely be increased. Recommended dosing of clopidogrel, based on the "CURE" Trial, has been covered. One study involving 40 patients suggested that a more rapid platelet inhibiting effect can be achieved in patients when a loading dose of 600 mg is given before coronary angiography. The implication is that ACS patients about to undergo PCI would benefit from earlier platelet aggregation from the larger loading dose of clopidogrel.[33]

Platelet GP IIb/IIIa Receptor Antagonists

Once activated, the GP IIb/IIIa receptors bind with fibrinogen to form bridges between the activated platelets thus leading to thrombus formation. The GP IIb/IIIa receptor inhibitors bind with the GP IIb/IIIa platelet receptor thus preventing attachment of the activated platelet to a fibrinogen molecule. There are currently three GP IIb/IIIa antagonists in use: eptifibatide, tirofiban and abciximab. The Gp IIb/IIIa antagonist abciximab has been shown to prevent AMI, abrupt vessel closure and death during angioplasty and is therefore used primarily in the catheterization lab. In the GUSTO–IV trial glucoprotein IIb/IIIa inhibition with abciximab demonstrated no benefit is ACS patients managed without PCI.[34]

Two trials involving tirofiban and eptifibatide have demonstrated reduction in subsequent AMI and refraction scheme or death in "high risk" ACS initially treated in the ED or during transport to a comprehensive cardiac center where PCI is available and a likely option. The combination of tirofiban, aspirin and intravenous heparin was studied in the Platelet Receptor Inhibition for Ischemia Syndrome Management (PRISM PLUS) study.[35] Major bleeding increased from 3% to 4% when tirofiban was added to heparin. In the Platelet IIb/IIIa antagonist Unstable Angina: Receptor Suppression Using Integrilin Trial (PURSUIT) study, eptifibatide was shown to reduce the risk of death or nonfatal AMI 31% at 30 days in patients undergoing percutaneous revascularization within 72 hours when compared to patients receiving placebo. The reduction was 7% for patients who did not undergo percutaneous revascularization. Bleeding requiring transfusion was increased in the patients receiving eptifibatide compared to placebo.[36]

Recommended dose of eptifibatide: 180 μg/kg IV bolus followed by 2.0 μg/kg/mm infusion for up to 48 hrs (if normal renal function). Recommended dose of tirofiban: 0.4 μg/kg loading dose over 30 min, followed by 0.1 μg/kg/min infusion for up to 48 hrs.

The Tactics-TIMI 18 trial added further support to recommendation that GP IIb/IIIa receptor antagonists were best used as part of an early invasive (PCI) strategy for UA/NSTEMI patients.[37]

Antithrombin Therapy

a. Unfractionated heparin recommended dose: 60 U/kg IV (maximum 4000 U) followed by 12 U/hr (maximum 1000 U/hr). Check patient in 4 to 6 hours and adjust infusion rate as needed to keep patient's INR at 2.5–3.0. Patients should be screened for HIT before administration.

b. Low molecular weight heparin (LMWH) Recommended Dose: enoxaparin 1 mg/kg SC q 12 hrs. Patients should be screened for HIT before administration. Enoxaparin is the most extensively studied LMH for use in ACS patients for patients with NSTEMI/ACS who are going to PCI, if the last dose of enoxaparin was given less than 8 hrs then no additional enoxaparin is needed. If the last dose was given more than 8 hours but less than 12 hours, then give enoxaparin 0.3 mg/kg IV bolus.

c. Direct thrombin inhibitors: Patients with suspected HIT should not receive unfractionated heparin or low molecular weight heparin. If anticoagulation is required a direct thrombin inhibitor (argatroban or lepirudin) should be used. For patients undergoing PCI argatroban is the only DTI approved.

Heparin

The heparins are a group of heterogenous molecules, ranging in size from 3000 to 30,000

Heparin is indicated in patients suffering AMI, who are receiving thrombolytics, undergoing PCI, and patients with unstable angina being treated with GP IIb/IIIa, and patients undergoing high-risk coronary angioplasty.

Heparin acts by binding to antithrombin III: this complex then inactivates factors thrombin (IIa), Xa, IXa, XIa and XIIa. UFH being an indirect thrombin inhibitor bind both factor Xa which blocks the step that converts prothrombin to thrombin and to thrombin (factor IIa) which inhibits thrombin activity namely platelet activation, fi_brin formation, activation of protein C, and the activation of factors V, VIII, and XIII. Most clinicians have extensive experience in using UFH in the treatment of patients with ACS. An additional benefit of heparin is its low cost. UFH, however, has the disadvantage of having an unpredictable bioavailability due to its binding to platelet factor-4, which readily inactivates it, as well as to other plasma proteins other than the intended antithrombin. For this reason, PTT must be monitored every time that the heparin dose is adjusted up or down.

Low Molecular Weight Heparins (LMWH) The LMWHs have a longer half-life than unfractionated heparin, a more predictable pharmacokinetic profile, a higher bioavailability and are easier to administer as they are given subcutaneously. As such they are administered to patients without the need to monitor the PTT and their usage is not limited to inpatients alone as patients, family member, or VNA can be trained to administer it in an outpatient setting.

Unlike unfractionated heparins (UFH), which are long chain polysaccharides with molecular weight ranging from 3,000 to 30,000, the LMWHs are short chain saccharides. They come in different preparations characterized by their molecular weight as well as their anti-factor Xa to anti-factor IIa ratio; the higher this ratio is, the more potent is their ability to inhibit the generation and biological activity of antithrombin.

Enoxaparin is the LMWH most widely studied in ACS patients. When enoxaparin was compared to unfractionated heparin in the SYNERGY trial, the incidence of death and non-fatal AMI for ACS patients was similar.[38] An overview of earlier trials has suggested enoxaparin was more effective then UH.[39] Some hospitals prefer enoxaparin because of ease of administration and monitoring.

Direct Thrombin Inhibitors

Heparin-induced thrombocytopenia (HIT) is a hypercoagulable state precipitated by increased thrombin production and micro particle release. Micro particles are released by activated platelets and are procoagulants. The result is an increased incidence of thrombosis. HIT occurs in most patients as a result of the development of an IgG antibody to heparin. HIT is less likely to occur when a LMWH is used rather than UFH, although the risk still exists.[40,41]

ACS patients suspected to have HIT based on history, a low platelet count or clinical presentation should not receive UFH heparin or LMWH. A direct thrombin inhibitor should be started in place of heparin or LMWH. Two direct thrombin inhibitors, argatroban and lepirudin, are indicated for use as anticoagulants for prophylaxis or treatment of thrombosis in patients with HIT. Argatroban alone is indicated as an anticoagulant in patients with or at risk for HIT who will be undergoing PCI. In the absence of an institutional protocol for the management of suspected HIT patients with ACS, the emergency physician may wish to consult with the call interventional cardiologist before administering a direct thrombin inhibitor.

Direct thrombin inhibitors approved for use in patients with HIT:

a. Argatroban, initial dose: 2 μg/kg/min as a continuous infusion in the absence of hepatic impairment.

The target is an aPTT of 1.5 to 3.0 times the initial baseline value. For patients undergoing PCI consult with the interventional cardiologist regarding the approved dosing.

b. Refludan: 0.4 mg/kg (up to 110 kg) over 15-20 seconds as a bolus, then 0.15 mg/kg/hr (up to 110 kg) as a continuous infusion. A target of an aPTT of 1.5 to 2.5 times the initial baseline is recommended. Refludan should be used with caution in patients with renal insufficiency.

Fibrinolytic Therapy

The "Danish Multicenter Randomized Trial on Thrombolytic Therapy versus Acute Coronary Angioplasty in Acute Myocardial Infarction" (DANAMI)-2 evaluated outcomes for STEMI patients following angioplasty at a specialized hospital when the patient did or did not receive fibrinolysis before transfer. This trial demonstrated that PCI at an Invasive Treatment Center is superior to on-site fibrinolytic treatment provided that the transfer to the Invasive Treatment Center is accomplished within 2 hours or less of symptom onset. Superiority was demonstrated by a reduction in the composite end point of death, reinfarction or disabling stroke at 30 days. The primary end point was reached in 8.5% of patients in the angiography group and 14.2% in the fibrinolysis group.[42] Other studies have also demonstrated superiority of primary angioplasty over on site fibrinolysis providing patients arrive in the catheterization lab within 2 hours of symptom onset.

Recommended Doses (Fibrinolytic Agents)

a. Tenecteplase (TNK) weight-based single bolus dosing (over 5 to 10 seconds)

< 60 kg:	30 mg IV bolus
< 60-69.9:	35 mg IV bolus
< 70-79.9 kg	40 mg IV bolus
< 80-89.9:	45 mg IV bolus
> 90 kg:	50 mg IV bolus

OR

b. Reteplase (rPA, Retavase): 10 U IV boluses (over 2 minutes), 30 minutes apart

OR

c. Streptokinase 1.5 MU over 30 to 60 minutes

Note: Do not use streptokinase if the patient has had a streptococcal infection within 2 years.

Contraindication and Relative Contraindications to Fibrinolytics

- **Absolute contraindications.** Confirmed or suspected aortic dissection, known intracranial neoplasm, any history of previous hemorrhagic stroke, head trauma within 6 months, brain surgery within 6 months, internal bleeding within 6 weeks, major bleeding within 6 weeks, active bleeding, known bleeding disorder, major surgery within 6 weeks, history of stroke within 1 year, history of central nervous system damage within 1 year, history of dementia within 1 year.
- **Relative contraindications.** Pregnancy, postpartum within 1 week, infective endocarditis, active peptic ulceration, oral anticoagulant therapy, transient ischemic attack within 6 months, active cavitating pulmonary tuberculosis, intracardiac thrombi, previous streptokinase therapy, dementia, uncontrolled hypertension defined as systolic blood pressure of >180 mm Hg, diastolic blood pressure of >110 mm Hg, puncture of a non-compressible blood vessels within 2 weeks.

Pain Management

Recommended Dosing:

a. Nitroglycerine (see anti-ischemic medications)

b. Morphine 4 to 6 mg IV initially, then an additional 2 to 4 mg IV q 10 minutes until pain is significantly reduced or eliminated. Observe the patient for evidence of hypoventilation.

c. Calcium channel antagonists: verapamil: 2.5 to 5.0 mg IV over 2 minutes or diltiazem: 10 to 20 mg IV over 2 minutes. Calcium channel antagonists may be used for pain control if pain persists despite nitroglycerin and β-blockers or if for some reason the patient cannot tolerate nitroglycerin or β-blockers. This should not be used in patients with severe LV dysfunction.

ACE Inhibitors

ACE inhibitors (ACE-Is) reduce mortality especially among patients with large or anterior AMI and who have evidence of heart failure. These agents appear to show the progressions of left ventricular dysfunction in patients without hypotension by preventing left ventricular remodeling. ACE also decreases the incidents of recurrent AMI and sudden death. Diabetic patients have also been shown to benefit from ACE-I use after AMI. ACE-Is should be started 6 to 12 hours after symptom onset of AMI symptoms. The ACE-I Ramipril was shown to be effective in the HOPE trial.[43]

Complications of ACS

There are several complications that are associated with ACS that are important to recognize and treat rapidly in order to decrease mortality and morbidity. These complications can be categorized into mechanical complications (such as cardiac rupture or cardiac valve incompetency), arrhythmias and conduction disturbances, pump failure or cardiogenic shock.

Rupture of the left ventricle is characterized by sudden cardiovascular collapse leading to pulseless electrical activity (PEA) that is fatal unless the patient can be taken to surgery immediately. If the ventricular wall rupture is subacute, blood can dissect into the pericardial cavity causing cardiac tamponade. Hypotension, distended neck vein muffle heart sound will follow. Echocardiography can assist with the diagnosis. Pericardiocentesis followed by surgery may be lifesaving.

Rupture of the intra-ventricular septum usually occurs early after myocardial infarction with an estimated incidence rate of 1% to 2 % of AMI. The diagnosis is clinically suspected by hemodynamic collapse associated with a loud systolic murmur and is confirmed by echocardiography with color Doppler that can locate the defect and the left to right shunt. If there is no cardiogenic shock, IV nitroglycerin or intra-aortic balloon counterpulsation while definitive surgery is being arranged.

In the past few years, the incidence of sudden cardiac deaths (SCD) in the United States has been between 400,000 and 500,000. In the 30 to 59 years of age group who participated in the Framingham Study, SCD accounted for 46% of the CAD deaths in men and 34% among women. While the actual number of SCDs increases with age for both sexes, CAD accounts for more SCDs in younger age groups when rapidly resuscitated patients in this younger age group can go on to lead highly productive lives. This observation further justifies current efforts in many cities and towns to achieve rapid deployment of first responders and EMTs with defibrillators to victims of SCD.[44]

The management of patients with sudden cardiac death who are bradycardic may involve the use of temporary transthoracic or transvenous pacemaker devices (**Table 17.7**). If sudden death was precipitated by a ventricular tachyarrhythmia and the patient is successfully resuscitated, then a search for a correctable cause is warranted and the use of an implantable cardioverter-defibrillator (ICD) should be considered. A recent trial suggests that while ICDs implanted in patients who have recently had an AMI reduces deaths due to arrhythmia, deaths from non-arrhythmia causes are increased.[45]

Mitral regurgitation is fairly common after myocardial infarction and can result from papillary muscle dysfunction, papillary muscle rupture or dilatation of the mitral valve annulus, due to the left ventricular dysfunction. The murmur in this setting is soft because of the elevated left atrial pressure. The diagnosis can be confirmed by Doppler echocardiography. For hemodynamically unstable patients, treatment is initiated with intra-aortic balloon counterpulsation while definitive valve replacement surgery is being arranged.

Left ventricular failure is manifested by shortness of breath, tachycardia a S3 heart sound and bilateral rales. Left ventricular failure is mostly the result of ischemic myocardial injury and the resulting of anatomical changes to the heart that occur. The diagnosis is confirmed with a chest x-ray consistent with congestive heart failure and an echocardiogram that demonstrates ventricular dysfunction. The treatment of the left ventricular failure depends on the severity of symptoms and the LV injury. If it is mild the patient should be given supplement oxygen as needed to maintain oxygen saturation of greater than 90%. If a $PaCO_2$ of at least 60 mm Hg cannot be maintained, despite 100% of supplemental oxygen and external ventilatory assistance, then the patient should be intubated and placed

Table 17.7
Indication for Pacemaker Placement
Class I
• Asystole
• Mobitz type II second-degree AV block
• Mobitz type I symptomatic, i.e., with hypotension
• Sinus bradycardia symptomatic, i.e., with hypotension
• Bilateral bundle branch block (alternating BBB, or right BBB with left anterior fascicular block or left posterior fascicular block
• Bifascicular block that is new or of indeterminate age (right BBB with LAFB of LPFB or left BBB) with a prolonged PR interval
Indication for Permanent Pacer
Class I
• Persistent 2° AV block in the His-Purkinje system, with bilateral BBB
• Persistent 3° AV block within or below the His-Purkinje
• Persistent and symptomatic 2° AV block and 3° AV block

on mechanical ventilatory support. In normotensive or hypertensive patients a loop diuretic and sublingual nitroglycerine (or spray) may improve patient's condition. In some patients nesiritide may help to stabilize the patient until the acute coronary event is definitely managed. Recommended dosing for nesiritide: 2 mg/kg initially, then 0.01 mg/kg per minute, IV.

Cardiogenic Shock

If hypotension develops in the face of an AMI and clinical findings of heart failure develop, the patient is in cardiogenic shock.

Cardiogenic shock still remains the leading cause of death in patients hospitalized for AMI. The overall mortality rate in patients determined to have cardiogenic remains high, estimated at 71.7%. Cardiogenic shock is said to be present if the patient's systolic blood pressure is < 90 mm Hg systolic with a wedge pressure of > 20 mm Hg or a cardiac index of > 1.8 L/min or if inotropic agents such as dobutamine or an intra-aortic balloon counterpulsation must be used in order to maintain a systolic blood pressure of > 90 mm Hg. Cardiogenic shock usually occurs in the setting of a large anterior myocardial infarction but it may also occur in the setting of a large right ventricular infarct. As in other situations where cardiac anatomy may be disrupted, a Doppler echocardiogram may help assess the left ventricular dysfunction. Cardiogenic shock patients should be considered as candidates for immediate PCI, and possibly CABG. If PCI is not available within 2 hours, then fibrinolysis should be considered while transfer to a hospital with available PCI is being arranged.

Right Ventricular Infarction

A right ventricular infarction (RVI) is suspected when, in the setting of an inferior myocardial infarction, the patient is profoundly hypotensive with distended neck veins, and clear lung fields. Right ventricular infarct is suggested by ST segment elevation in V_1 and the inferior leads. ST segment elevation, when the right chest lead V_{4r} is recorded is very helpful. A 15-lead ECG may be indicated when RVI is suspected. The diagnosing of RVI can be aided by Doppler echocardiogram which may show a dilated right ventricular which is hypokinetic, a dilated right atrium, and a significant mitral regurgitation. The treatment of the hypotension associated with right ventricular infarction is with an initial normal saline bolus of 250 mL, followed by additional bolus infusions of normal saline until the patient demonstrates normalization of their blood pressure or evidence of pulmonary congestion.

Pericarditis

The pain of pericarditis is worsened by recumbent position, inspiration, coughing, and relieved by sitting and leaning forwards. Another distinguishable feature is that pericarditis is manifested by consistent sharp pain. On auscultation the examiner may hear a pericardial rub that is present most often during expiration. The pain of pericarditis may radiate to the trapezius muscle, but it may also radiate to the left arm, right arm or to both arms. On the ECG pericarditis is recognized by diffuse ST, T wave changes, or a diffuse PR depression.

Cardiac tamponade is a serious complication of pericarditis and is recognized by a pulsus paradoxus defined as an exaggeration of the drop in arterial systolic arterial pressure of more than 10 mm Hg during inspiration.

Pericarditis may be secondary to an autoimmune or hypersensitivity reaction.

The treatment of pericarditis is with nonsteroid antiinflammatory drugs, aspirin, or steroids. Heparin and fibrinolytics are contraindicated in pericarditis as it may cause a hemopericardium leading to cardiac tamponade.

Arrhythmias Complicating Myocardial Infarction

Bradyarrhythmias occur often during an acute myocardial infarction.

Sinus bradycardia is defined as a rate of less than 60 bpm for patients on β-blocker medication. A lower rate may be accepted as the bradycardic threshold. Bradycardia occurs in one third of patients with AMI, and often occurs in the setting of inferior myocardial infarction, where it was thought to be secondary to the occlusion invading the right coronary artery (RCA). The RCA supplies perfusion to the sinus node and in most patients to the atrioventricular (AV) node. The correct treatment of sinus bradycardia is determined by the patient's symptoms and physical findings. Complaints of chest pain suggestive of ACS, and symptoms including premature ventricular complexes (PVCs), hypotension, diaphoresis, shortness of breath, lightheadedness, dizziness or change in mental status suggest immediate treatment is necessary.

Bradycardic Heart Block

First degree (1°) AV block: Defined as a constant prolongation of the PR interval greater than 0.20 seconds from cycle to cycle, with a normal P preceding every normal QRS on a one to one conduction.

Second degree (2°) AV block: Type 1 (also known as Wenckebach) is characterized by a series of cycles in which there is progressive prolongation of the PR interval until a P wave conduction is completely blocked, thus generating no QRS after the P wave. Immediately after the dropped QRS complex, the cycle starts again. The ratio of present QRS complexes to dropped complexes in a cycle is used to describe the ECG findings (2:1, 3:1, etc.). 2° AV block Type II (also known as Mobitz), occurs at the Purkinje fiber bundles of His or bundle branches and is characterized by a series of cycles in which the PR interval is constant until a P wave conduction is completely blocked, thus generating no QRS; immediately after the dropped beat, the cycle repeats again. The block can occur in a ratio of 2:1, 3:1, 4:1, and so on. Conduction block may occur below the AV node resulting in QRS widening that simulates a bundle branch block. This type of 2° heart block may progress to 3° heart block, particularly in the face of AMI and therefore treatment of 3° heart block should be ready.

Third degree (3°) AV block: Occurs when there is complete block of all atrial conduction to the ventricles giving rise to a situation in which there is no association between the atrial conduction and the ventricles activities. When the 3° AV block occurs above the AV junction then one sees normal QRS morphology with a ventricular rate generally between 40 to 60 bpm. However, when the 3° AV block occurs below the AV junction then one sees an abnormally widened QRS. Slow "ventricular escape" rhythm associated with 3° AV block are often accompanied by syncope due to cerebral hypoperfusion.

Treatment of 1° and type I 2° AV block is not required unless the patient is symptomatic as described above. When treatment is required, use atropine 0.5 to 1.0 mg IV every 3 to 5 minutes; a total of 0.03 mg/kg is usually effective. For the treatment of 2°, type II or 3° AV block, prepare to treat with transthoracic pacing as a bridge to transvenous pacing (Table 17.1) Transthoracic pacing may be preferred over transvenous pacing because it would avoid venipuncture in a non-compressible vessels in patients who have or will be getting fibrinolytics.

Avoid atropine in 3° AV block as it has no effect on infranodal AV block; by increasing the sinus rate, atropine may worsen the block or even precipitate 3° AV block. If the 3° AV block has been caused by an overdose of digoxin, β-blocker or a calcium channel blocker, the specific antidotes should be administered.

Ventricular fibrillation (VF) or pulseless ventricular tachycardia (PVT): Major cause of death within the first 24 hours in the setting of AMI; is noted to occur at a rate of 3% to 5% during the first 4 hours of AMI.

Recommended Treatment for VF or PVT

Amiodorone: 300 mg IV push, initial dose. 150 mg additional dose in 5 minutes, if the patient remains in VF or PVT.

Procaine amide may be used if the patient has recurrent episodes of VT or PVT; however, procaine amide cannot be given as an IV bolus.

Procainamide: 20 to 50 mg/min; IV infusion up to a total of 17 mg/kg.

Torsades de pointes is a form of ventricular tachycardia going at a rate of 250 to 350 bpm characterized by ventricular complexes that are twisting, giving the appearance of pointing up and then pointing down. Torsades de pointes may occur following AMI. It is also caused by conditions that prolong the QT interval, for example the use of certain medications in patients with congenital prolonged QT syndromes who are especially prone to torsades. Pharmacological treatment of Torsades consists of magnesium 1 to 2 g IV. Overdrive pacing may be beneficial in some instances.

Atrial fibrillation/atrial flutter are other common arrhythmias seen in the setting of AMI. Atrial fibrillation/atrial flutter arise from rapid, at 350 to 450 discharges per minute and numerous discharges from an irritable foci either from the atria giving rise to atrial fibrillation or from a foci in the ventricles, thus giving rise to ventricular fibrillation. The number of atrial impulses passing through the AV node will vary usually resulting in an irregular pulse.

Studies have shown that new onset atrial fibrillation in the setting of AMI occurs at a rate of 10% to 20% and is usually seen in the setting of large myocardial infarction, especially anterior myocardial infarction, CHF, LVH and occurs more frequently in the elderly.

Treatment of Atrial Fibrillation/Flutter

Beta blockers and calcium channel blockers are considered to be the "first line" agents to achieve slowing of the ventricular rate in patients with CAD unless WPW syndrome is suspected. If WPW is suspected then consider amiodarone or procaine amide. Cardioversion should be used if the patient is hemodynamically unstable. Anticoagulation therapy should be considered in order to decrease the risk of subsequent stroke or other embolic events.[46]

β-blocker Rx: Metoprolol: 5 mg IV every 5 min, up to 15 mg
Ca-blocker Rx: Diltiazem: 15 to 20 mg (or 0.25 mg/kg) IV over 2 min
Amiodarone: 150 mg over 10 min, then 1 mg/min
Procainamide: 20 to 30 mg/min, up to 17 mg/kg

Chest Pain Centers

Many comprehensive emergency departments have adopted the "Chest Pain Center" concept as a way to manage more efficiently patients with low or moderate risk of ACS who present for ED care. Some centers have designated space specifically for the management of such patients, given the number of diagnostic options currently available; the time needed to conduct a thorough evaluation; the need to carefully tailor treatment for each ACS patient during evaluation; and the fact that inpatient beds are often unavailable. These "Chest Pain Centers" have been shown to improve patient care while allowing more efficient use of ED and hospital resources.[46]

Conclusion

Proper management of ED patients who present with symptoms of ACS is one of the most challenging aspects of emergency medicine practice. Such patients may have one of several life-threatening conditions. The emergency physician may have little information about the patient's medical history or treatment at the level of symptom onset. As the portion of population of older age group continues to grow over the next three decades and as greater numbers of people survive illnesses such as cancer and serious infection, the incidence of ACS will grow. Close attention to research developments that will result in improved clinical care is, therefore, warranted in this area.

References

1. American Heart Association. *Heart Disease and Stroke Statistics—2005 Update.* Dallas, TX: American Heart Association 2004.
2. Mokdad AH, Marks JS, Stroup DF, Gerberding JL. Actual causes of death in the United States, 2000. *JAMA* 2004;291:1238–1246.
3. Pope JH, Aufderheide TP, Ruthazer R, et al. Missed diagnosis of acute cardiac ischemia in the emergency department. *N Engl J Med* 2000;342:1163–1170.
4. Jemal A, Tiwari RC, Murray T, et al. Cancer statistics, 2004. *CA Cancer J Clin* 2004;54:8–29.

5. Mosca L, Jones WK, King KB, et al. Awareness, perception and knowledge of heart disease risk and prevention among women in the United States. *Arch Fam Med* 2000;9:506–515.

6. Rathore SS, Chen J, Wang Y, et al. Sex differences in cardiac catheterization. *JAMA* 2001;286:2849–2856.

7. Malacrida R, Genoni M, Maggioni AP, et al. A comparison of the early outcome of acute myocardial infarction in women and men. The Third International Study of Infarct Survival Collaborative Group. *N Engl J Med* 1998;338:8–14.

8. Mendelsohn ME, Karas RH. The protective effects of estrogen on the cardiovascular system. *N Engl J Med* 1999;340:1801–1811.

9. Mason JE. Estrogen plus progestin and the risk of coronary heart disease. *N Engl J Med* 2003;349:523–534.

10. Karcz A, Holbrook J, Burke MC, et al. Massachusetts emergency medicine closed malpractice claims: 1988-1990. *Ann Emerg Med* 1993;22:553–559.

11. Braunweld E, Antman EM, Beasley JW, et al. ACS/AHS 2002 guideline update for the management of patients with unstable angina and non-ST segment elevation myocardial infarction: summary article: a report of the American College of Cardiology/American Heart Association task force on practice guidelines (committee on the management of patients with unstable angina). *J Am Coll Cardiol* 2002;40:1366–1374.

12. Libby P. Current concepts of the pathogenesis of the acute coronary syndrome circulation. *Circ J Am Heart Assoc* 2001;104:365–372.

13. Topol EJ. A guide to therapeutic decision-making with non-ST segment elevation acute coronary syndrome. *J Am Coll Cardiol* 2003;41:123s–129s.

14. Antman EM, Anbe DT, Armstrong PW, et al. ACC/AHA guidelines for the management of patients with ST-elevation myocardial infarction: executive summary. A report of the ACC/AHA task force on practice guidelines (Writing Committee to revise the 1999 guidelines on the management of patients with acute myocardial infarction). *J Am Coll Cardiol* 2004;44:671–719.

15. Weber JE. Validation of a brief observation period for patients with cocaine-associated chest pain. *N Engl J Med* 2003;348:510–517.

16. Goldberg RJ, Samad NA, Yarzebski J, et al. Temporal trends in cardiogenic shock complicating acute myocardial infarction. *N Engl J Med* 1999:340:1162–1168.

17. Sgarbossa EB, Pinski SL, Barbagelata A, et al. Electrocardiographic diagnosis of evolving acute myocardial infarction in the presence of left bundle-branch block. *N Engl J Med* 1996;334:481–487.

18. Chan TC, Brady W, Harrigan R, et al. *ECG in Emergency Medicine and Acute Care.* St. Louis, MO: Mosby, Inc., 2005.

19. Clinical policy: critical issues in the evaluation and management of adult patients presenting with suspected acute myocardial infarction or unstable angina. *Ann Emerg Med* 2000;35:521–544.

20. McCord J, Nowak RM, Hudson MP, et al. The prognostic significance of serial myoglobin, troponin I, and creatine kinase-MB measurements in the emergency department for acute coronary syndrome. *Ann Emerg Med* 2003;42:343–350.

21. Braunwald E, Zipes DP, Libby P, eds. *Heart Disease: A Textbook of Cardiovascular Medicine,* 6th ed. Philadelphia: W.B. Saunders Co., 2001.

22. Antman EM, Tanasijevic MJ, Thompson B, et al. Cardiac-specific troponin I levels to predict the risk and mortality in patients with acute coronary syndromes. *N Engl J Med* 1996;335:1342–1349.

23. Aviles RJ, Askari AT, Lindahl B, et al. Troponin T levels in patients with acute coronary syndromes, with or without renal dysfunction. *N Engl J Med* 2002;346:2047–2052.

24. Grzybowski M, Welch RD, Parsons L, et al. The association between white blood cell count and acute myocardial infarction in-hospital mortality: findings from the natural report of myocardial infarction. *Acad Emerg Med* 2004;11:1049–1060.

25. Khalid MA, Bhatia A, Gal R. Echocardiographic assessment of complications related to left ventricular function in acute myocardial infarction. *Echocardiography* 1999;16:281–288.

26. Isselbacher KJ, Braunwald E, et al. *Harrison's Principles of Internal Medicine,* 13th ed. New York: McGraw-Hill, 1994:1079.

27. Udelson JE, Beshansky JR, Ballin DS, et al. Myocardial perfusion imaging for evaluation and triage of patients with suspected acute coronary ischemia. *JAMA* 2002;288:2693–2700.

28. Kim WY, Danias PG, Stuber M, et al. Coronary magnetic resonance angiography for the detection of coronary stenoses. *N Engl J Med* 2001;345:1863–1869.

29. Antman EM, Cohen M, Bernink PJ, et al. The TIMI risk score for unstable angina/non-ST elevation MI: A method for prognostication and therapeutic decision making. *JAMA* 2000;284:835–842.

30. CAPRIE Steering Committee. A randomized, blinded, trial of clopidogrel versus aspirin in patients at risk of ischemic events (CAPRIE). *Lancet* 1996;349:1329–1339.

31. Bertrand ME, Rupprecht HJ, et al. Double-blind study of the safety clopidogrel with and without a loading dose in combination with aspirin compared with ticlopidine in combination with aspirin after coronary stenting. *Circ J Am Heart Assoc* 2000;102:624.

32. Yusuf S, Zhao F, Mehta SR, et al. Effects of clopidogrel in addition to aspirin in patients with acute coronary syndromes without ST-segment elevation. *N Engl J Med* 2001;345:494–502.

33. Kastrati A, von Beckerath N, Joost A, et al. Loading with 600 mg clopidogrel in patients with coronary artery disease with and without chronic clopidogrel therapy. *Circulation* 2004;110:1916–1919.

34. Simoons ML, GUSTO IV-ACS Investigators. Effect of glycoprotein IIb/IIIa receptor blocker abciximab on outcome in patients with acute coronary syndromes without early coronary revascularisation: the GUSTO IV-ACS randomised trial. *Lancet* 2001;357:1915–1924.

35. PRISM-PLUS Study Investigators. Inhibition of the platelet glycoprotein IIb/IIIa receptor with tirofiban in unstable angina and non-Q-wave myocardial infarction. *N Engl J Med* 1998;338:1488–1497.

36. The PURSUIT Investigators. Inhibition of platelet glycoprotein IIb/IIIa with eptifibatide in patients with acute coronary syndromes. *N Engl J Med* 1998;339:436–443.

37. Synergy Trial Investigators. Enoxaparin vs. unfractionated heparin in high-risk patients with non-ST-segment elevation acute coronary syndromes managed with an intended early invasive strategy. *JAMA* 2004;292:45–54.

38. Peterson JL, Mahaffey KW, Hasselblad V, et al. Efficiency and bleeding complications among patients randomized to enoxaparin or unfractionated heparin for antithrombin therapy in non-ST-segment elevation acute coronary syndromes. *JAMA* 2004;292:89–96.

39. Hirsh J, Heddle N, Kelton JG. Treatment of heparin-induced thrombocytopenia. *Arch Intern Med* 2004;164:361–369.

40. Levine R, Hursting MJ, Drexler A, et al. Heparin-induced thrombocytopenia in the emergency department. *Ann Emerg Med* 2004;44:511–515.

41. Anderson HR, Nielsen TT, Rasmussen K, et al. A comparison of coronary angioplasty with fibrinolytic therapy in acute myocardial infarction. *N Engl J Med* 2003;349:733–742.

42. Pitt B. ACE inhibitors for patients with vascular disease without left ventricular dysfunction—may they rest in peace? *N Engl J Med* 2004;351:2115–2117.

43. Myerburg RJ, Interian A Jr, Mitrani RM, et al. Frequency of sudden cardiac death and profiles of risk. *Am J Cardiol* 1997;80:10F–19F.

44. Hohnloser SH, Kuck KH, Dorian P, et al. Prophylactic use of an implantable cardioverter-defibrillator after acute myocardial infarction. *N Engl J Med* 2004;351:2481–2488.

45. Page RL. Newly diagnosed atrial fibrillation. *N Engl J Med* 2004;351:2408–2416.

46. Kugelmass AD, Anderson AL, et al. Does having a chest pain center impact the treatment and survival of acute myocardial infarction patients? *Circulation* 2004;110:111–409.

Acute Decompensated Heart Failure

J. Douglas Kirk
Deborah B. Diercks

Introduction

Heart failure is frequently seen in the emergency department (ED) and is a clinical syndrome rather than a specific disease entity. It is not characterized by a single finding or diagnostic test, but rather by a constellation of symptoms, signs, and diagnostic test findings. It results from a structural or functional disorder that impairs the ventricle's ability to fill with blood (diastolic dysfunction) or pump blood (systolic dysfunction). It is important to identify the correct type of heart failure to manage these patients accurately and effectively. Appropriate recognition of patients with heart failure and differentiation from other causes of dyspnea, a very common chief complaint in the ED, are difficult.

The diagnosis of heart failure is on the rise, with a prevalence of more that 5 million patients and more than 500,000 new cases per year.[1] This is a disease primarily of the elderly and its recent increase is likely due to the general aging of the population, as well as improved survival of patients after myocardial infarction or other index events that lead to impaired ventricular function and subsequent heart failure. The most common causes of heart failure are listed in **Table 18.1**.

Pathophysiology

Heart failure occurs when the ventricles are unable to generate sufficient pressure during systole, or when high pressures are required to fill the ventricles during diastole. The understanding of heart failure pathophysiology has progressed considerably over the past two decades, from a relatively simple hypothesis of impaired contractility and pump failure, to one of complex neurohumoral activation. Although pump failure is a key component of heart failure, the progression of the disease and exacerbations of ADHF are manifestations of maladaptive processes of neurohumoral activation that result in vasoconstriction, pulmonary congestion, ventricular remodeling, and myocardial toxicity.

The neurohumoral compensatory mechanisms resulting from low cardiac output are initially beneficial, as they contribute to maintaining perfusion of vital organs. This is mediated primarily by the sympathetic nervous system, the renin-angiotensin-aldosterone system (RAAS) and antidiuretic hormone (ADH). One of the first responses to a fall in cardiac output is the release of norepinephrine, which results in increases in myocardial contractility and heart rate, both of which improve cardiac output. In addition, norepinephrine is a potent vasoconstrictor that helps maintain systemic pressure and end-organ perfusion.

Similar to the sympathetic nervous system, activation of the RAAS promotes vasocontriction via angiotensin II. This is particularly true of renal vasoconstriction, primarily at the efferent arteriole, to maintain glomerular filtration rate despite an overall reduction in renal blood flow due to poor cardiac output. Renin release is further stimulated by a reduction in sodium delivery to the distal tubule. As a result, angiotensin II and norepinephrine stimulate proximal tubular sodium reabsorption, which contributes to retention of fluid and an increase in extracellular volume. The latter is valuable, as an increase in preload results in an improvement in cardiac output via the Frank-Starling equation. In addition, low cardiac output stimulates the release of ADH, promoting water reabsorption in the collecting tubules. This also contributes to an increase in fluid volume and results in hyponatremia, an important prognostic indicator of heart failure.

While it is true these neurohumoral responses are beneficial in the short term, their deleterious effects predominate over the long term. Persistent elevated filling pressures lead to pulmonary congestion and peripheral edema. Ongoing increases in afterload due to these potent vasoconstrictors lead to myocardial toxicity and a further reduction in ventricular performance, as well as renal injury secondary to relative hypoperfusion. Finally, both norepinephrine and angiotensin II promote myocardial cell death, hypertrophy, and remodeling, which lead to progressive cardiac dysfunction.

Contrary to the aformentioned vasoconstrictors, natriuretic peptides are counterregulatory hormones released in response to an increase in atrial or ventricular volume or stretch. They are potent vasodilators that reduce both preload and afterload, both of which serve to improve myocardial performance and reduce pulmonary congestion. They cause renal efferent arteriolar constriction and afferent dilatation to promote both natriuresis and diuresis. They also antagonize the RAAS.[2] Unfortunately, the release of these agents is insufficient to balance the effects of the sympa-

Table 18.1

Causes of Heart Failure

- Ischemia
- Hypertension
- Valvular disease
- Myocarditis
- Restrictive
- Cardiomyopathy
  - Idiopathic
  - Hypertrophic
  - Peripartum
  - Drug induced (ethanol, methamphetamine, cocaine)
  - Other (infiltrative, HIV, connective tissue disorder)

thetic nervous system and the RAAS. However, it does provide insight into a new hypothesis of heart failure as not only a disease of pump failure, but also as a neuroendocrine disorder. This provides rationale not only for developing assays to measure these markers of elevated left ventricular filling pressures, but may also explain the benefits of neurohumoral antagonists, including angiotensin converting enzyme inhibitors (ACEI), β-blockers, aldosterone inhibitors, and natriuretic peptides in the management of heart failure.

Diagnosis

The majority of symptoms and signs of heart failure are secondary to compensatory mechanisms responding to a fall in cardiac output, regardless of the cause. An initial index event such as myocardial infarction may result in a first-time presentation of heart failure, but the majority of ED visits are in patients with known heart failure. Frequently a secondary event or condition, such as atrial fibrillation, myocardial ischemia, progressive renal insufficiency or just disease progression, precipitates an acute exacerbation of heart failure. Patient behavior, especially noncompliance with diet or medications, also plays a major role. The clinical assessment of patients with suspected heart failure typically incorporates the history, physical examination, electrocardiogram (ECG) and chest radiograph (CXR). This is usually followed by an array of diagnostic tests to secure the diagnosis, determine the etiology, and assess the severity.

Clinical Assessment

The value of the history and physical examination, although critical components to any disease assessment are less than ideal in heart failure recognition. The predominant symptom is dyspnea, followed by edema and fatigue. Dyspnea is present in essentially all cases, but obviously is a common presenting complaint for numerous diseases in the differential diagnosis of patients with suspected heart failure, including chronic obstructive pulmonary disease, asthma, and pneumonia. The most valuable piece of information may come from the past medical history, not the

history of present illness. A history of myocardial infarction or previous diagnosis of heart failure, especially if earmarked by prior presentations to the ED, may be the best clue to a heart failure etiology of dyspnea.

The physical examination is important to establish the presence and degree of volume overload, the predominant finding in ADHF. The most common physical findings mirror this: pulmonary congestion, leg edema, ascites, and hepatomegaly. Surprisingly, the typical physical findings we associate with an elevated filling pressure (S3 gallop, jugular venous distention, hepatojugular reflux, and rales) are very specific for heart failure, yet not very sensitive. The absence of rales in as many as half the cases is probably most surprising, owing to an increase in venous capacitance and lymphatic drainage in chronic heart failure. Although the majority of ADHF patients are warm (perfused) and wet (congested), a significant number present with evidence of low cardiac output; therefore, assessment of the adequacy of tissue perfusion is necessary. Typical findings include tachycardia, hypotension, narrowed pulse pressure, and vasoconstriction. The latter is typically manifested by cool, pale extremities or lethargy.

Diagnostic Tests

The CXR is a mainstay in the evaluation of heart failure, but its value is limited in securing a definitive diagnosis. It is helpful in identifying other pulmonary diseases as a cause of dyspnea. Findings suggestive of heart failure include Kerley B lines, pleural effusion, cardiomegaly, and evidence of vascular redistribution or cephalization, with the latter two being the key findings. Overt pulmonary edema is often absent despite markedly elevated filling pressures, likely due to the aforementioned increase in venous capacitance and lymphatic drainage.

Performing an ECG is routine in patients with undifferentiated dyspnea and rarely is it normal in patients with heart failure. Unfortunately, it seldom establishes the specific diagnosis or etiology of heart failure. Potentially helpful findings include evidence of myocardial infarction (acute or old), left ventricular hypertrophy, low voltage, or arrhythmias such as atrial fibrillation. Other laboratory tests, such as the complete blood count or chemistry panel, may uncover comorbid disease or provide some prognostic data, but they typically afford little discriminating information as to the presence or absence of heart failure.

The clinical evaluation of heart failure, including the use of commonly available tests in the ED such as the ECG and CXR, are inexact at best. The most definitive diagnosis would come from placing a right heart catheter and measuring hemodynamics or by performing an echocardiogram in the ED in all patients with unexplained dyspnea, but obviously neither of these is practical. However, it is critical that the correct diagnosis be arrived at as soon as possible, as earlier recognition carries important prognostic and cost implications.

Natriuretic Peptide Assays

The pathophysiology of the counterregulatory hormones found in ADHF provided impetus to investigate their role as diagnostic tests in patients with dyspnea in whom heart failure is suspected. The FDA approved the β-type natriuretic peptide (BNP) assay (Biosite) in 2000 and the majority of the subsequent literature reflects this assay. Other natriuretic peptide assays, such as atrial natriuretic peptide, which is available in Asia, and the recently approved N-terminal pro-BNP (Roche will not be discussed in detail here due to their limited availability or recent release).

Since an elevated filling pressure is the hallmark of ADHF, regardless of type (systolic versus diastolic) or etiology, a marker that identifies its presence is invaluable in distinguishing heart failure from other pulmonary causes of dyspnea. Natriuretic peptides are elevated in response to increases in ventricular volume or stretch, regardless of the etiology. The value of BNP as a diagnostic test was best demonstrated in the Breathing Not Properly trial.[3] In this study of 1,586 patients, heart failure was confirmed in half of the patients and other pulmonary causes were found in the rest. Using a cut-off value of 100 pg/mL, the sensitivity and specificity was 90% and 76% respectively. Reducing the cut-off value improved specificity at the expense of sensitivity. Predictably, raising it had the opposite effect, neither of which led to an appreciable effect on overall accuracy. BNP levels were markedly higher in patients with a final diagnosis of heart failure compared to those without heart failure (675 pg/mL versus 110 pg/mL). The predictive accuracy of an abnormal BNP (83%) was superior to Framingham criteria (73%) and the National Health and Nutrition Survey criteria (67%). Compared to historical or physical examination findings, BNP was the best at distinguishing heart failure from other pulmonary causes of dyspnea (**Table 18.2**).[2]

Arguably, the most valuable finding from clinical trials of BNP is the excellent negative predictive value of a low BNP (50 to 100 pg/mL). This has been the most consistent and useful datum to date. It is important to recognize that mild elevations of BNP (100 to 500 pg/mL) can be found in diseases other than heart failure, typically those with elevated right-sided filling pressures (pulmonary embolism with right ventricular strain, cor pulmonale, pulmonary hypertension) or general volume overload states (renal failure, liver cirrhosis).[4] Interpretation of these results requires clinical correlation. However, in the appropriate context, especially with BNP levels greater than 500 pg/mL, heart failure remains the most likely etiology of dyspnea.

BNP assays are also valuable tools in correcting initial misdiagnosis based upon clinical data alone. Dao et al. showed that in 250 patients with unexplained dyspnea, 15 were overdiagnosed with heart failure and 15 were underdiagnosed with heart failure. Adding BNP results to the clinical information correctly identified 29 of the 30 cases that were initially misdiagnosed.[5]

BNP also provides significant prognostic information in patients with ADHF. In a study of 325 ED patients with unexplained dyspnea, the BNP level was predicative of subsequent adverse events (death, recurrent heart failure) during 6 month follow up.[6] Patients with BNP levels greater than 480 pg/mL had event rates of 51%, while those with levels less than 230 pg/mL had only a 2.5% probability of adverse events.

Therapeutic Management

Although there are guidelines from various sources about the management of patients with heart failure, most pertain to chronic management. There is little consensus regarding the management of patients with acute decompensation in the ED. Furthermore, there are limited data from randomized controlled trials to help guide the management of these patients in the ED, adding to the inconsistent care of heart failure patients.

General Support

The majority of patients who present to the ED with ADHF have a chief complaint of dyspnea. Supplemental oxygen should be administered in essentially all patients, at least initially. Pulse oximetery should be used to measure the effectiveness, with a target to maintain an oxygen saturation greater or equal to 95%. This may require high flow oxygen by face mask in some patients, while others may only need oxygen by nasal cannulae.

Patients with severe dyspnea or hypoxia, as typically seen with acute pulmonary edema or in cases of "flash pulmonary edema" from severe hypertension and diastolic dysfunction may require more aggressive airway maneuvers. In such cases, endotracheal intubation may be warranted or inevitable, but every attempt should be made to avoid this because of the associated increased morbidity in these patients. The use of aggressive airway adjuncts, such as non-invasive ventilation (NIV), may assist in avoiding the need for intubation while maintaining adequate oxygenation and ventilation. NIV should not be considered a substitute for intubation or, more importantly, other pharmacologic management, but rather as a bridge to therapies directed at reducing filling pressures and pulmonary congestion. NIV typically includes either continuous positive airway pressure (CPAP) or bi-level positive airway pressure (BiPAP), both of which are beneficial in reducing the work of breathing and improving alveolar ventilation. In

Table 18.2

Predictors of Heart Failure

Predictor	P Value	Odds Ratio
Age	0.04	1.02 (1.00-1.03)
JVD	0.04	1.87 (1.04-3.36)
Rales	<0.001	2.24 (1.41-3.58)
History of MI	<0.001	2.72 (1.63-4.54)
Edema	<0.001	2.88 (1.81-4.57)
Cephalization	<0.001	10.69 (5.3-21.5)
History of HF	<0.001	11.08 (6.6-18.8)
BNP ≥ 100 pg/mL	<0.001	29.60 (17.8-49.4)

BNP, B-type natriuretic peptide; HF, heart failure; JVD, jugular venous distention; MI, myocardial infarction.
Adapted from Maisel AS, Krishnaswamy P, Nowak RM, et al. Rapid measurement of B-type natriuretic peptide in the emergency diagnosis of heart failure. *N Engl J Med* 2002;347:161-167.

addition, the increase in intrathoracic pressure provided by positive pressure ventilation reduces venous return (preload) and increases the pressure gradient between the left ventricle and arterial circulation, thereby reducing afterload.

Both CPAP and BiPAP have been successfully used to treat the hypoxia and hypercapnea associated with ADHF. However, there is some concern, or at least controversy, with the safety of BiPAP. Early trials of BiPAP in ADHF suggested an increased risk of acute myocardial infarction, but the trials were small and inconsistently designed. Subsequent larger trials, albeit still with few patients, provided support for this modality. In a randomized controlled trial of 130 patients with ADHF, Nava et al. demonstrated physiologic improvement was faster in the NIV group with no increased risk of acute myocardial infarction.[7] Furthermore, there were trends toward a lower rate of intubation and death in the non-invasive group, which with respect to intubation rates became significant (6% versus 29%) in patients with hypercapnea ($pCO_2 > 45$ mm Hg). Therefore, the best evidence available suggests BiPAP is safe and effective in reducing the need for intubation in patients with severe respiratory distress and should be considered as a useful adjunct to the pharmacologic management of patients with ADHF.

Pharmacological Therapy

Although general supportive measures such as maintaining adequate oxygenation are critical, the mainstay of therapy is pharmacological. The primary goal is to decrease filling pressures. Additional important goals include improving cardiac output through a reduction in afterload or improvement in contractility. In patients with diastolic dysfunction, improving the ventricle's ability to fill with blood is key through efforts that improve myocardial relaxation.

Initial Management of Acute Pulmonary Edema

In patients with severe respiratory or hemodynamic instability, time is critical and the emergency physician may only have a few minutes to significantly reduce filling pressures to avoid respiratory collapse, or even worse, cardiac arrest. Concurrent with the aforementioned airway maneuvers, all efforts should be directed at reducing pulmonary congestion. Although diuretics are important, their net effects are not fast enough to be of initial benefit. The most rapid improvement is achieved with potent vasodilators such as nitroglycerin, nesiritide, or nitroprusside. Although each are quite effective, their immediate intravenous use often requires too much time to set up, a luxury these patients do not have. Initiation of sublingual nitroglycerin therapy in doses larger than those typically used for chest pain (2 to 6 0.4-mg tablets or sprays) can be quite effective.[8] This medication's availability and onset of action are quite rapid. Significant reductions in pulmonary capillary wedge pressure and blood pressure (afterload) with an improvement in respiratory symptoms, can be achieved often within minutes. Patients can then be transitioned to one of the aforementioned intravenous

vasodilators. In settings where the availability of rapid intravenous vasodilators is possible, this is an attractive alternative. The addition of an intravenous diuretic to this strategy only makes sense as it will result in significant diuresis, which, in turn, leads to a drop in preload, although not immediately. There is some evidence that the initial improvement in symptoms with intravenous diuretics prior to significant diuresis is related to a transient venodilation, resulting in decreased pulmonary congestion.

The use of sublingual ACEI in this setting has been advocated based on a small trial of 21 patients who showed symptomatic improvement after treatment with sublingual captopril.[9] Although data are limited in the use of these agents in the setting of acute pulmonary edema and imminent respiratory failure, there appears, however, to be a benefit in the rapid administration of sublingual nitroglycerin with or without an intravenous loop diuretic. Further recommendations on the combination of these agents cannot be made until further research elucidates the utility and safety of such an approach.

Diuretics

Diuretics are often first-line therapy in the ED management of patients with ADHF. The rationale is that patients are "volume overloaded" and although this may be true, more important than a total increase in volume is the acute elevation in filling pressures. Nonetheless, diuretics are effective at reducing preload and removing excess fluid. The loop diuretic furosemide is most commonly used although other loop diuretics are equally effective. Suggested starting doses are 40 mg of intravenous furosemide in "diuretic virgins" or an amount equivalent to the patient's total usual daily dose given intravenously. Peak diuresis should occur within 30 to 60 minutes. Repeated doses, usually double the initial dose, can be used in patients who fail to respond. Doses greater than 160 to 320 mg of furosemide are likely to produce as many side effects as results and should, therefore, be discouraged. In patients with diuretic resistance, use of an additional diuretic that works on the proximal tubule, e.g., metolozone, may produce an effective diuresis. Caution should be exercised with excessive diuretic use. In addition to well described electrolyte depletion (K^+, Mg^+, Ca^{++}), recent literature demonstrates that diuretics result in decreased renal perfusion and neurohormonal activation by increasing RAAS and norepinephrine.[10] The short-term gains with diuretic therapy may be offset by the decrease in renal perfusion and resultant deleterious long-term effects (**Table 18.3**).

Vasodilators

In the majority of patients with ADHF in the ED, initial therapy with oxygen and loop diuretics will not be sufficient to reduce preload and improve symptoms. The addition of vasodilators is frequently necessary. This is particularly true in patients with severe hypertension and/or diastolic dysfunction. A majority of patients are well-perfused, despite having an increase in filling pressures, and are best treated with vasodilators such as nitroglycerin, nesiritide, or nitroprusside. Some patients with

Table 18.3

Untoward Effects of Therapeutic Agents for ADHF

Diuretics	Vasodilators	Inotropes

• Decreased renal perfusion
• Volume depletion
• Electrolyte abnormalities
  (K^+, Ca^{++}, Mg^+)
• Neurohormonal activation
  ↑ renin-angiotensin aldosterone
    system
  ↑ sympathetic nervous system
	• Tachycardia (NTG, NTP)
	• Tachyphylaxis (NTG)
	• Neurohormonal activation
	  (NTG, NTP)
	• Thiocyanate toxicity (NTP)
	• Need for titration (NTG, NTP)
	• Need for invasive monitoring
	  (NTP, ± NTG)
		• Increased mortality
		• Proarrhythmic
		• Tachycardia
		• Neurohormonal activation

ADHF, Acute decompensated heart failure; NTG, nitroglycerin; NTP, nitroprusside.

mild exacerbations of heart failure may respond to sublingual or topical nitrates, but a significant number will require intravenous therapy. Data from ADHERE, a multicenter heart failure registry, suggest that patients treated with any intravenous vasodilator, initiated in the ED versus later in the hospital or not at all, had lower mortality (4.3% versus 10.9%, unadjusted, $P < 0.0001$) and shorter hospital lengths of stay (3 versus 7 days, $P < 0.001$).[11] These agents decrease both systemic and pulmonary pressures and result in fairly rapid reductions in filling pressures and congestive symptoms. Surprisingly little trial data on clinical outcomes exist for nitroglycerin or nitroprusside to support their use in ADHF. Nitroprusside can be particularly useful in patients with acute pulmonary edema associated with hypertensive emergencies and extreme elevations of systolic and diastolic blood pressures. However, there are numerous limitations to these therapies, including the need for titration, hemodynamic monitoring, and the deleterious effects of neurohormonal activation (Table 18.3).

Nesiritide

Approved by the FDA in 2001, nesiritide is the first commercially available natriuretic peptide used for the treatment of ADHF. It is identical to human endogenous BNP. Although plasma levels of endogenous BNP are elevated in ADHF, the administration of additional exogenous BNP has beneficial effects. Several mechanisms have been suggested to explain this paradox, including BNP receptor down regulation, increased BNP degradation, and postreceptor uncoupling at the tissue level. Probably the most important is the general counter-balancing of vasoconstrictive neurohormones in patients with poor cardiac output. BNP serves as an antagonist to pathologic neurohormonal activation that occurs in heart failure. This is a necessary characteristic of all heart failure pharmacologic agents with a proven mortality benefit, including ACEI and β-blockers.

Nesiritide produces significant reductions in pulmonary capillary wedge pressure, right atrial pressure, and systemic venous resistance within minutes and concomitant increases in stroke volume and cardiac output.[12] It has significant advantages over other agents, including balanced vasodilation, diuresis, and naturesis, as well as beneficial effects in myocardial cells (**Table 18.4**). In addition, it does not possess many of the deleterious properties associated with diuretics, inotropes, or other vasodilators (Table 18.3).

In the VMAC trial, nesiritide decreased pulmonary capillary wedge pressure more than either nitroglycerin or placebo at three hours and more than nitroglycerine at 24 hours (**FIGURE 18.1**). Dyspnea and global clinical status were improved compared to placebo, similar to nitroglycerin.[13] Nesiritide is typically administered as a bolus of 2 µg/kg, followed by an infusion of 0.01 mg/kg/min. There is no occurrence of tachyphylaxis and typically no need for titration as there is with nitroglycerin or nitroprusside. In patients with relatively low systolic blood pressure (90 to 110 mm Hg), the bolus can be reduced or eliminated. If hypotension occurs, the infusion can be discontinued and then restarted at a lower dose when the blood pressure has stabilized. Diuretics may be continued but often at lower doses due to the potentiation of effects from nesiritide. ACEI may also be used but not at the expense of curtailing the dose of nesiritide. The use of β-blockers is not con-

Table 18.4

Pharmacologic Actions of Nesiritide

- Hemodynamic (balanced vasodilation)
  - Venous
  - Arterial
  - Coronary vasodilation
- Neurohormonal
  - Decreased renin-angiotensin-aldosterone
  - Decreased norepinepherine
  - Decreased endothelin
- Renal
  - Increased diuresis
  - Increased natriuresis
- Myocardial
  - Lusitropy (diastolic relaxation)
  - Antifibrotic
  - Reverse remodeling

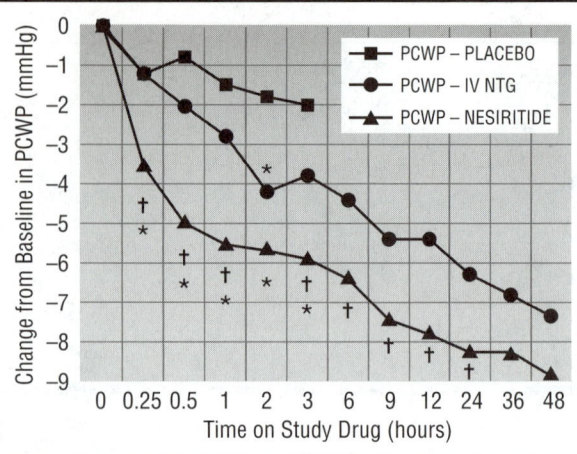

FIGURE 18.1 Change in pulmonary capillary wedge pressure (PCWP) from baseline.

*Comparison of nesiritide vs. placebo, P , 0.05.
†Comparison of nesiritide vs. nitroglycerin, $P < 0.05$.
Adapted from VMAC Investigators. Intravenous nesiritide versus nitroglycerin for treatment of decompensated congestive heart failure: a randomized controlled trial. *JAMA* 2002;287:1531-1540.

traindicated although their use in patients with ADHF is typically discontinued until patients are hemodynamically stable. The concurrent use of inotropes may be indicated in patients with poor cardiac output and evidence of hypoperfusion, although this may necessitate employing invasive monitoring with a right heart catheter to guide this complex therapy. After therapeutic targets have been achieved, typically in one to three days, nesiritide may be discontinued (**Table 18.5**). Patients should be started back on previous outpatient regimens (ACEI, β-blockers, diuretics) with appropriate adjustments in dosing based on clinical status.

Recent data suggest that nesiritide is associated with reduced need for readmission and an overall reduction in hospital length of stay. In the PROACTION trial, 237 patients were randomized to either standard care or at least 12 hours of nesiritide therapy in an observation unit.[14] Mortality rates and complications were similar in the two groups. However, nesiritide use was associated with a 21%

decrease in heart failure readmissions and a substantial decrease in the sum length of stay over the ensuing months after the index visit (2.5 versus 6.5 days, $P < 0.032$).

Nesiritide is not only effective in the management of ADHF, it possesses several characteristics that provide convenience and ease of use, making it quite suitable for ED or observation unit patients (**Table 18.6**). Recent meta-analyses have raised concerns about the safety of nesiritide with respect to renal insufficiency and mortality. However, the data are limited, the findings were only trends, and some questions have been raised regarding the research methodology of these reports. Further outcome studies are planned or ongoing to address these important issues.[15,16]

Inotropes

The use of inotropes in patients with ADHF is frequently employed to improve hemodynamics and symptoms in patients' refractory to management with diuretics and vasodilators. The β-agonist, dobutamine, and phosphodiesterase inhibitor, milrinone, are effective at improving cardiac output and tissue perfusion. However, recent literature suggests that these hemodynamic improvements come with a price (Table 18.3): both cause neurohormonal activation, an increase in ventricular ectopy, and appear to be associated with an increase in long-term mortality.[17,18] Unless patients exhibit clear signs of decreased perfusion or have overt cardiogenic shock, these agents should be used with caution as their long-term deleterious effects may outweigh any short-terms gains.

Hemodynamic Monitoring

Although not typically employed in most EDs, invasive monitoring with placement of a right heart catheter can be quite useful in certain patients. Indications would include critically ill patients not responsive to initial therapies or those with cardiogenic shock. In addition, patients with unclear etiologies of pulmonary edema or those in which the history and physical examination cannot determine

---

Table 18.5

Therapeutic Targets in ADHF Management

- Improvement in dyspnea, resolution of orthopnea
- Ambulatory without dizziness or dyspnea on exertion
- Stable vital signs (heart rate < 100 bpm, systolic blood pressure > 90 and < 200 mm Hg
- Urine output > 1 liter
- Normal electrolytes
- Normal cardiac injury markers
- Stable renal function

ADHF, Acute decompensated heart failure.

Table 18.6

Salient Features of Nesiritide

- Onset of action is very fast
- No need for complex monitoring
- Safety comparable to nitroglycerin
- Useful in patients with renal insufficiency or failure
- Enhances the effects of conventional diuretics
- Efficacious in both systolic and diastolic dysfunction
- Simultaneously lowers preload and afterload in patients with severe hypertension
- Vasodilates coronary arteries and lowers myocardial oxygen demand
- Not proarrhythmic
- Triage from emergency department to a non-intensive care unit bed
- No need for titration
- No tachyphylaxis

the perfusion status or amount of pulmonary congestion may be good candidates for invasive hemodynamic monitoring. Such patients are often so complex that multiple therapeutic agents are required and having hemodynamic, goal-directed therapy is essential. Other options include assessment with bioimpedance monitoring, which allows rapid determination of cardiac output and volume status. In addition to being noninvasive, bioimpedance monitoring is low risk and is relatively inexpensive.

Disposition

Patient disposition is one of the most challenging tasks an emergency physician faces in heart failure management. Poor decisions may have profound effects on mortality, morbidly, repeat visits, readmissions, and overall cost. Unfortunately, few patients have an obvious disposition after initial management in the ED. Critically ill patients require hospital admission (**Table 18.7**), while those with

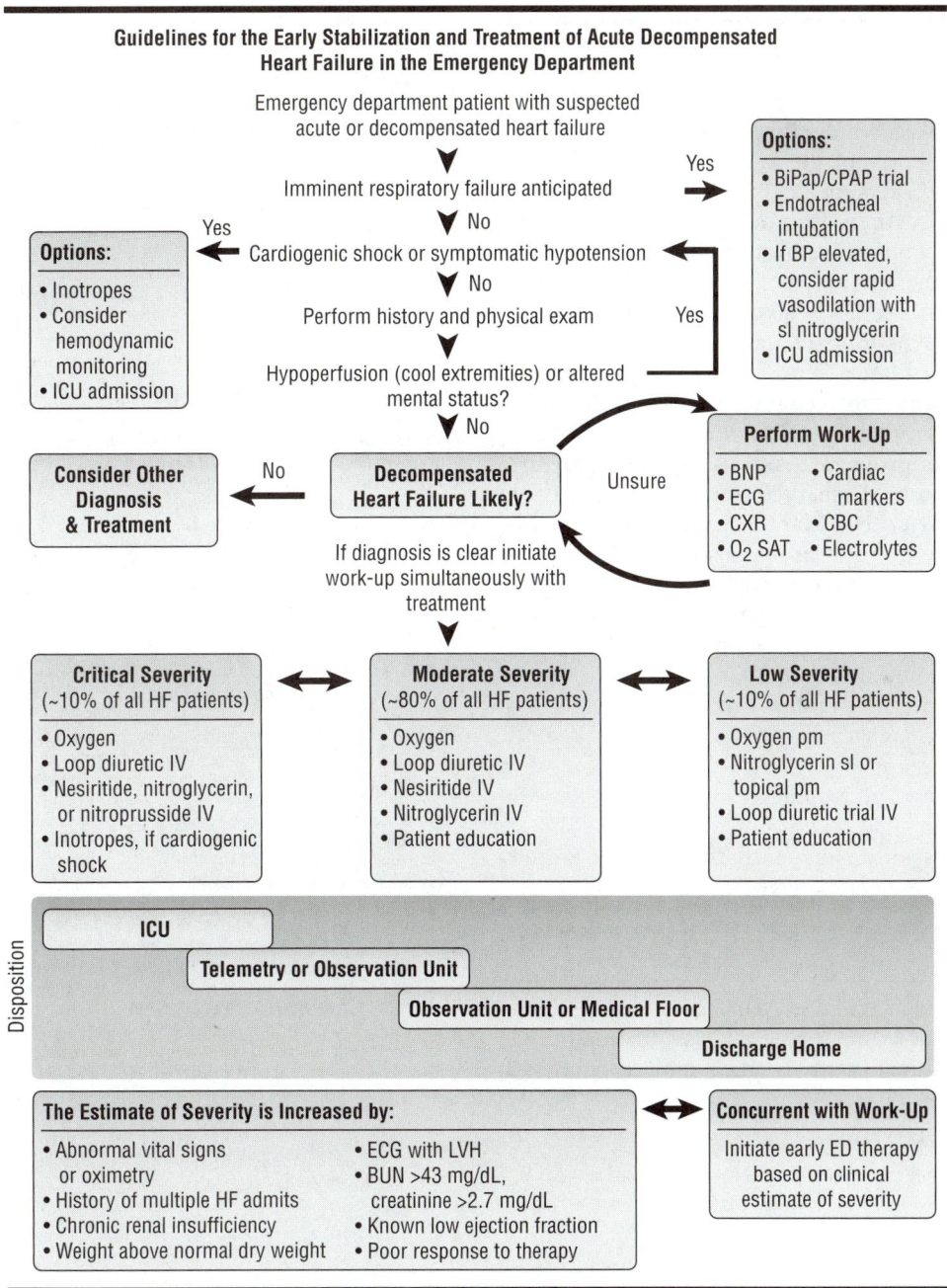

FIGURE 18.2 BiPAP, bi-level positive airway pressure; BNP, B-type natriuretic peptide; BUN, blood urea nitrogen; CBC, complete blood count; CPAP, continuous positive airway pressure; CXR, chest radiograph; ECG, electrocardiogram; ICU, intensive care unit; LVH, left ventricular hypertrophy; O₂SAT, oxygen saturation; sl, sublingual; prn, as needed.

Adapted from Peacock WF, Allegra J, Ander D, et al. Management of acutely decompensated heart failure in the emergency department. CHF 2003; 9(suppl 1):3-18.

Table 18.7

Criteria for Hospital Admission

- Unstable vital signs
  - Systolic blood pressure < 90 or > 200 mm Hg after therapy
  - Heart rate > 130 bpm
  - Temperature > 38.5°C
- Persistent hypoxemia (O^2 saturation < 90%)
- Evidence of myocardial ischemia/infarction
- Severe comorbidity (COPD, pneumonia)
- Requirement of ventilatory support

COPD, Chronic obstructive pulmonary disease.

mild symptoms may be discharged relatively quickly. These two groups represent the minority, as the majority will require complex decision making. The recent development of ED management or observation unit protocols has given the emergency physician an additional option for patient disposition. Therapy for patients managed in the ED or observation unit should be goal oriented and protocol driven, including supplemental oxygen, intravenous diuretics and vasodilators, the mainstays of therapy. Responses to therapy and recognition of complications are keys to successful disposition. Identifying *a priori* targets of clinical improvement and using them to determine if patients can be discharged home from the ED or observation unit are crucial (Table 18.5). Critical to successful ED or observation unit management and appropriate disposition is appropriate aftercare. The initial improvements gained in the ED can be quickly negated if the outpatient disease management plan is inadequate. Important components include:

1. Appropriate physician follow-up
2. Nursing case management
3. Patient education
4. Optimizing medical regimens
5. Social support

Hospital readmission is frequently the result of failure of one or more of these components.

Conclusion

Recognition and management of ADHF in the ED entail a complex process that requires systematic evaluation of the undifferentiated patient with dyspnea and/or hemody-namic derangement. Therapy for patients with imminent respiratory failure or cardiogenic shock must accompany the concurrent investigation of the etiology of presenting symptoms. Selection of diagnostic tests, prognostic assessment, and appropriate therapeutic maneuvers are paramount. An algorithm shown in **FIGURE 18.2** for the early stabilization and treatment of ADHF provides guidelines to assist the emergency physician in the management of these patients.

References

1. American Heart Association. *2002 Heart and Stroke Statistical Update*. Dallas TX: American Heart Association, 2001.
2. Schrier RW, Abraham WT. Hormones and hemodynamics in heart failure. *N Engl J Med* 1999;341:577–585.
3. Maisel AS, Krishnaswamy P, Nowak RM, et al. Rapid measurement of B-type natriuretic peptide in the emergency diagnosis of heart failure. *N Engl J Med* 2002;347:161–167.
4. Peacock WF, IV. The B-type natriuretic peptide assay: a rapid test for heart failure. *Cleve Clin J Med* 2002;69:243–251.
5. Dao Q, Krishnaswamy P, Kazanegra R, et al. Utility of B-type natriuretic peptide in the diagnosis of congestive heart failure in an urgent-care setting. *J Am Coll Cardiol* 2001;37:379–385.
6. Harrison A, Morrison LK, Krishnaswamy P, et al. The B-type natriuretic peptide predicts future cardiac events in patients presenting to the emergency department with dyspnea. *Ann Emerg Med* 2002;39:131–138.
7. Nava S, Carbone G, DiBattista N, et al. Noninvasive ventilation in cardiogenic pulmonary edema: a multicenter randomized trial. *Am J Respir Crit Care Med* 2003;168:1432.
8. Bussmann W, Schupp D. Effect of sublingual nitroglycerin in emergency treatment of severe pulmonary edema. *Am J Cardiol* 1978;41:931–936.
9. Hamilton RJ, Carter WA, Gallagher EJ. Rapid improvement of acute pulmonary edema with sublingual captopril. *Acad Emerg Med* 1996;3:205–212.
10. Kaplan NM. Treatment of hypertension: drug therapy in clinical hypertension. In: Kaplan NM, Lieberman E, Neal WW, eds. *Clinical Hypertension*, 1994:203
11. Peacock WF, Emerman CL, Costanzo MR, et al. Early initiation of intravenous vasoactive therapy improves heart failure outcomes: an analysis from the AD-HERE registry database. *Ann Emerg Med* 2003;42:S26.
12. Mills RM, LeJemtel TH, Horton DP, et al. Sustained hemodynamic effects of an infusion of nesiritide (human b-type natriuretic peptide) in heart failure: a randomized, double-blind, placebo-controlled clinical trial. Natrecor Study Group. *J Am Coll Cardiol* 1999;34:155–162.
13. VMAC Investigators. Intravenous nesiritide versus nitroglycerin for treatment of decompensated congestive heart failure: a randomized controlled trial. *JAMA* 2002;287:1531–1540.
14. Peacock WF, Emerman CL, Young J. On behalf of the PROACTION study group. Safety and efficacy of nesiritide for treatment of decompensated heart failure in emergency department observation unit patients. *J Am Coll Cardiol* 2003;4(suppl a):336A.
15. Sackner-Bernstein JD, Skopicki HA, Aaronson KD. Risk of worsening renal function with nesiritide in patients with acutely decompensated heart failure. *Circulation* 2005;111:1487–1491.
16. Sackner-Bernstein JD, Kowalski M, Fox M, Aaronson K. Short-term risk of death after treatment with nesiritide for decompensated heart failure. A pooled analysis of randomized controlled trials. *JAMA* 2005;293:1900–1905.
17. O'Connor CM, Gattis WA, Uretsky BF, et al. Continuous intravenous dobutamine is associated with an increase risk of death in patients with advanced heart failure: insights from the Floan International Randomized Survival Trial (FIRST). *Am Heart J* 1999;138:78–86
18. Cuffe MS, Califf RM, Adams KF Jr, et al for the OPTIME-CHF Investigators. Short-term intravenous milrinone for acute exacerbation of chronic heart failure: a randomized controlled trial. *JAMA* 2002;287:1541–1547.

Pericarditis

Luis E. Rodriguez
John E. Gough

Etiology/Pathophysiology

The heart is surrounded by connective tissue called the pericardium. It is made up of visceral pericardium, which is adherent to the myocardium, and the parietal pericardium which is the outer layer. When this tissue becomes inflamed, it is called pericarditis. Acutely, when this tissue is inflamed it may produce a pericardial effusion. As time progresses this inflammation may pass to a chronic phase leading to a constrictive disorder. Pericarditis may further be classified as idiopathic, constrictive or restrictive, with the most common being idiopathic. There are numerous etiologies of pericarditis, and the physician should always maintain a wide differential such as viral, malignancy, uremia, and tuberculosis (**Table 19.1**).

Clinical Findings

The most common symptom produced by pericarditis is chest pain. This pain is usually pleuritic, sharp, and may radiate to the back or shoulder. Pericarditis should be in the differential for any patient presenting with chest pain. The pain is most often described as worsening with recumbency and improving with leaning forward. Often with idiopathic pericarditis the patient may complain of dyspnea as well as a mild fever.

The physical examination may be normal; however, a pericardial friction rub may be present. This is not a murmur although it may be confused with one. It is a high-pitched sound heard best over the left sternal border and is heard both through systole and diastole. The friction rub may be accentuated by having the patient lean forward. Other pericardial etiologies such as tamponade may cause muffled heart sounds, jugular venous distention, and hypotension (Beck's triad). Jugular venous distention upon inspiration (Kussmaul's sign) may also be seen in constrictive disorders.

Evaluation

All patients suspected of having pericarditis should have an electrocardiogram, chest x-ray, and an echocardiogram. Laboratory analysis may consist of rheumatological factors and ppd testing, although this is often not practical in the ED because of time constraints. Cardiac markers such as troponin I may be elevated.[1]

The classic teaching of EKG findings in pericarditis are diffuse ST elevation with no evidence of reciprocal changes, and PR segment depression (best seen in the inferior leads) in the acute phase. After the ST segments normalize, T wave inversion may occur. Not all patients will manifest these findings, and some may have a normal

Table 19.1

Etiologies of Pericarditis

Bacterial	Viral	Systemic Diseases	Neoplastic	Direct Cardiac Insult
Mycobacterium sp.	Coxsackie A & B	Lupus erythematosus	Lupus erythematosus	Trauma
Staphylococcus	Adenovirus	Rheumatoid arthritis	Rheumatoid arthritis	Acute MI
Streptococcus	Echovirus type 4	Sarcoidosis	Sarcoidosis	Surgery
Borrelia burgdorferi	Influenza	Myxedema	Myxedema	Radiation
Legionella	Cytomegalovirus	Uremia	Uremia	
Rickettsia sp.	Epstein-Barr	Inflammatory disease	Inflammatory disease	
Gram-negative rods	Mumps	Connective tissue disease	Connective tissue disease	
	Varicella			
	Herpes simplex			
	Hepatitis B			

electrocardiogram. It may also be difficult to distinguish these findings from J point elevation, which may represent a normal variant or acute coronary ischemia.[2] If an effusion is present, low voltage may occur as well as electrical alternans. Arrhythmias are unusual.

The CXR is frequently normal; however small pleural effusions nay occur. An echocardiogram is recommended by most authorities and may help exclude other pericardial diseases such as effusions, tamponade or restrictive phenomena.

Treatment

Treatment is etiology-based. For idiopathic acute pericarditis, the treatment is based on non-steroidal anti-inflammatory agents such as ketorolac, ibuprofen or indomethacin. Rheumatological causes may respond to prednisone. For uremic pericarditis, dialysis is the mainstay of therapy. Most patients with acute pericarditis may be safely discharged from the ED, with appropriate treatment and close follow up with their primary care physician. Those with arrhythmias, tamponade, high fevers, intractable pain, or uncertain diagnosis should be admitted for further evaluation and treatment.

References

1. Imazio M, Demichelis B, Cecchi E, et al. Cardiac troponin I in acute pericarditis. *J Am Coll Cardiol* 2003;42:2144–2148.
2. Jaume-Boscio FH, Jaume-Anselmi F, Ramirez-Rivera J. ST segment elevation: is it a possible infarct? *Bol Asoc Med P R* 2001;93:28–31.

Endocarditis and Myocarditis

John E. Gough
Luis E. Rodriguez

Endocarditis

Etiology/Pathophysiology

Endocarditis is an infection of endothelial surface of the heart, and may have acute and subacute presentations. The infection may affect either normal or damaged native heart valves as well as prosthetic valves. Rarely the infection may also involve a septal defect, chordae tendinae, or mural endocardium. Although the incidence of endocarditis is low (1.5 to 6 cases per 100,000 per year and up to 15 cases per 100,000 per year in patients older than 50 years), it is associated with high morbidity and mortality.[1] There is a high incidence of complications (greater than 50%) seen with endocarditis, most commonly CHF, paravalvular abscess, and embolism (stroke). Also seen are septic arthritis, vertebral osteomylitis, pericarditis, metastatic abscesses, glomerulonephritis, and renal abscesses.[2] Furthermore, there are potential complications associated with the medical treatment, such as ototoxicity, nephrotoxicity, skin rashes, and serum sickness.

Clinical Findings

The patient frequently presents with fever, malaise, and systemic toxicity. Chest pain and shortness of breath are also common findings. Congestive heart failure (CHF) may be present and is the leading cause of death in patients with endocarditis. CHF is most often caused by valvular insufficiency secondary to valvular dysfunction (aortic more frequently than mitral) from infectious endocarditis.[2] Valvular vegetations can embolize to coronary arteries resulting in an acute MI and subsequent CHF. Paravalvular abscesses are associated with a 75% death rate if surgery is not performed. Embolic events may result in an acute stroke. Hemorrhagic strokes are particularly associated with bacterial endocarditis. Endocarditis should be considered in a patient with stroke symptoms who has a fever and history of valvular disease.[2] Mycotic aneurysms in the middle cerebral arteries can present like subarachnoid hemorrhages and stroke. Other physical findings may include petechiae, Janeway lesions (small non-tender erythematous, hemorrhages, or pustular lesions on the palms and soles), splinter hemorrhages (subungual dark red–brown streaks), Osler's nodes (small, tender nodules on the finger or toe pads), and Roth spots (retinal lesions). Janeway lesions, Osler's nodes, and especially Roth spots are rare findings, but are very specific (however, not diagnostic) for endocarditis.

Evaluation

Laboratory findings generally include a leukocytosis, a normochromic normocytic anemia, increased ESR, and increased C-reactive protein. Blood cultures should be obtained, however, cultures are negative in 2% to 5% of patients. Common infectious agents are *Viridans strep*, enterococci, and *Staphylococcus aureus* (high mortality).[2] The EKG is rarely diagnostic, but may show an infranodal heart block (associated with greater mortality than when present without endocarditis). Other EKG findings may include changes consistent with ischemia or infarction. As with the EKG, the CXR is not diagnostic, but may demonstrate CHF and valvular calcifications. Echocardiography, specifically TEE should be performed, as transthoracic echocardiography is insensitive to paravalvular abscesses.[2] Cerebral angiography may be used to evaluate intracranial abscesses.

Treatment

The patient should be admitted and started on antibiotics. A cardiac surgery consult should be obtained especially if the patient presents with CHF or aortic regurgitation. Patients with *S. aureus* infections, paravalvular abscesses, and fungal endocarditis should also receive surgical consultations.

Myocarditis

Etiology/Pathophysiology

Myocarditis affects 1 to 10 per 100,000 in United States every year. Myocarditis may affect any or all chambers of the heart. Causes of myocarditis include viral and bacterial infectious agents; immunologic (e.g., rheumatic fever), toxins (EtOH, doxorubicin, ementine); pseudohypertrophic muscular dystrophy; metabolic causes (hyper/hypothyroidism, beriberi, glycogen storage diseases); infiltrative diseases (amyloidosis, hemochromatosis); neoplastic causes; physical stresses (hyperthermia); and peripartum.

More recently myocarditis has been associated with the smallpox vaccine.[3] In developing countries, viral causes such as coxsackievirus B-related virus, hepatitis C, and CMV are frequently implicated. Myocarditis often presents with an associated pericarditis.

Clinical Findings

The clinical presentation is dependent upon the severity of disease and the amount of myocardial involvement/depression. Cases of myocarditis may be subclinical. Often there is a viral prodrome. The patient frequently presents with fever and sinus tachycardia (out of proportion of extent of fever). Myalgias, headache, rigors, fatigue, and decreased exercise tolerance are common. Other findings include dyspnea, orthopnea, and rales. The patient may complain of retrosternal or precordial chest pain especially if there is a concurrent pericarditis. On auscultation there may be a S3 or S4 gallop, murmurs of mitral/tricuspid insufficiencies or a pericardial friction rub with myopericarditis. Physical findings consistent with right ventricular failure (e.g., JVD, hepatomegaly, peripheral edema) can be seen. In rare cases sudden death may occur.

Evaluation

The CXR is usually normal, however, it may show cardiomegaly and pulmonary vascular congestion. EKG findings include non-specific ST-T changes, ST elevation (which may mimic acute MI), AV block, BBB, ventricular extrasystoles, flat or inverted T waves, and low voltage QRS complexes.[4] Cardiac enzymes may be elevated. Echocardiography often demonstrates decreased ventricular function. Radionucleotide studies have been utilized in the past but do not offer much information over echocardiography. Endomyocardial biopsies may be used, but are only 35% sensitive.

Treatment

The mainstay of treatment is supportive. The patient should be instructed to rest. Antibiotics, immunotherapy, anti-viral agents, and steroids may be used. NSAIDs are not effective, and may actually worsen the condition and should be avoided. Medications such as antiarrhythmics, anticoagulants, and those used to treat CHF may be indicated on an individual basis. In rare cases, such as with giant cell myocarditis, heart transplantation may be necessary. Hospital admission may be needed, especially if CHF is present.

References

1. Sexton DJ, Spelman D. Current best practices and guidelines. Assessment and management of complications in infective endocarditis. *Cardiol Clin* 2003;21: 273–282.
2. Mylonakis E, Calderwood SB. Infective endocarditis in adults. *N Engl J Med* 2001;345:1318–1330.
3. Halsell JS, Riddle JR, Atwood JE, et al. Myopericarditis following smallpox vaccination among vaccina-naïve US military personnel. *JAMA* 2003;289: 3283–3289.
4. Wang K, Asinger RW, Marriott HJL. ST-segment elevation in conditions other than acute myocardial infarction. *N Engl J Med* 2003;349:2128–2135.

Cardiomyopathies

John E. Gough
Luis E. Rodriguez

Dilated Cardiomyopathy

Etiology/Pathophysiology

The etiology of dilated cardiomyopathy is often unknown. It is thought that approximately 30% of cases result from infectious causes and greater than 50% are idiopathic. In many cases dilated cardiomyopathy is a diagnosis of exclusion. It is estimated to occur in 7.5 per 100,000 population; however, this is probably an underestimation as many cases go undiagnosed. Seventy-five percent of patients die within 5 years of diagnosis. Dilated cardiomyopathy is more common in males and most commonly occurs between the ages of 40 to 65 years old. Common risk factors include infections, tobacco and alcohol abuse, hypertension, and pregnancy.[1]

Clinical Findings

Frequently the patient presents with dyspnea, orthopnea, and exertional chest pain. Left heart failure is common and is present in 75% to 85% of patients. Right heart failure presents late and is a poor prognostic sign. The patient may also present with embolic events (e.g., stroke).

Evaluation

The CXR will generally demonstrate cardiomegaly and changes consistent with CHF. The EKG is nonspecific and frequently demonstrates non-diagnostic findings of ventricular ectopy, LBBB, and poor R wave progression. Sudden death is a rare presentation. Central venous pressures, pulmonary capillary wedge pressures, and end diastolic volumes are all increased. Echocardiography is the diagnostic test of choice and typically shows LV dilatation, reduced systolic function, wall motion abnormalities, and reduced ejection fractions (less than 45%).

Treatment

The mainstay of treatment is supportive, including rest, weight control, and avoidance of tobacco and alcohol. ACE inhibitors are the drugs of choice for long-term therapy. If CHF is present, administration of oxygen, nitrates, diuretics, and possibly vasodilators may be utilized. Thromboembolism is a rare complication; therefore, anticoagulation should be considered in individual cases.

Antiarrhythmics are of questionable value. Medical treatment is not always efficacious, and dilated cardiomyopathy remains a leading cause of heart transplants.[1]

Peripartum Cardiomyopathy

Etiology/Pathophysiology

Peripartum cardiomyopathy is a specific type of dilated cardiomyopathy. The occurrence of peripartum cardiomyopathy is uncommon (28 per 100,000 pregnancies); accounting for less than 1% of pregnancy related heart problems. The specific cause is unknown. The onset is most common in the last 3 months of pregnancy to the first 6 months postpartum. Risk factors include age greater than 30, twin gestations, and multiparous patients.[2]

Clinical Findings

Common presenting complaints include tachypnea, tachycardia, an S3 gallop, palpitations, and CHF. Thromboembolic events are not common, but do occasionally occur.

Evaluation

The EKG findings are nondiagnostic and typically include changes consistent with LVH, and nonspecific ST abnormalities. The CXR frequently has findings of CHF and cardiomegaly. Echocardiography will demonstrate enlargement of all four chambers, decreased LV systolic function, and may also show a pericardial effusion. Endomyocardial biopsy may be performed to rule out myocarditis.

Treatment

The patient should be instructed to rest. Diuretics are utilized to decrease preload and treat CHF. Afterload reduction may be accomplished with the use of hydralizine during pregnancy and ACE inhibitors in the postpartum period. Digoxin may be used to increase ventricular contractility. Anticoagulation should be considered to reduce the risk of embolic events. Despite treatment, approximately 25% of the cases may result in death within three months. Of the survivors approximately one half will return to normal in 6 months.[2]

Hypertrophic Cardiomyopathy

Etiology/Pathophysiology

Hypertrophic cardiomyopathy commonly presents between 30 to 40 years of age: however, it may occur at all ages (7% occur in patients younger than 10 years old). The etiology is thought to be mutations in genes that code for sarcomere contractile proteins.[3] The patient will have a hypertrophic, nondilated LV without an identifiable cause such as hypertension or aortic stenosis. The LV and RV cavities are typically small or normal. In approximately one-fourth of cases there is an associated obstruction of LV outflow, known as hypertrophic obstructive cardiomyopathy.[3]

Clinical Findings

Common presenting complaints include chest pain, syncope and palpitations. Patients may present with sudden death, especially associated with exertion. On auscultation there will be an S4 gallop, reversed splitting of second heart sound, and a crescendo/decrescendo midsystolic murmur. The intensity of the murmur is enhanced by valsalva or standing and decreased with squatting, lying down, and isometric hand grips. There may be a bifid arterial pulse, and multiple dysrhythmias are possible.

Evaluation

The EKG may show LVH, non-specific ST abnormalities, atrial enlargement, T-wave inversions, Q waves, and decreased or absent R waves in the lateral leads. The CXR may be normal, or may have LV or LA enlargement. Echocardiography remains the most important diagnostic tool and may demonstrate LVH, LV outflow tract narrowing, a small LV cavity, and decreased septal motion. Nucleotide studies may be used to evaluate systolic and diastolic function. EP studies may be performed to evaluate arrhythmias. Patients should be referred for genetic screening.

Treatment

Beta blockers and calcium channel blockers may be used to decrease heart rate and myocardial oxygen demand.[3] Nitrates are contraindicated as they may decrease LV volume. Amiodarone is frequently indicated for treatment of dysrhythmias. Prophylactic antibiotics should be instituted to prevent endocarditis. The presence of atrial fibrillation may represent a medical emergency and anticoagulation and cardioversion should be performed. If the patient fails medical management a surgical consultation should be obtained for possible septal myomectomy.[3]

Restrictive Cardiomyopathy

Etiology/Pathophysiology

Restrictive cardiomyopathy is the least common type of cardiomyopathy in developed countries. There is progressive limitation of ventricular filling due to endocardial and myocardial lesions.[4] As the disease progresses the ventricular cavities fill with fibrous tissue, scarring, and thrombus. It is unknown whether the cause is infectious or immunologic. The most common proposed cause in developed counties is amyloidosis.[4] Also seen as causal are sarcoidosis, hemochromatosis, scleroderma, neoplastic infiltration, radiation, glycogen storage disease, Fabry's disease, and Gaucher's disease.

Worldwide the most common cause is endomyocardial fibrosis, especially in India, Africa, and Latin America.

Clinical Findings

The patient often presents with dyspnea and exercise intolerance. Peripheral edema is common. The CVP will be elevated. On auscultation S3 or S4 gallops are frequently present.

Evaluation

Steps should be undertaken to differentiate restrictive cardiomyopathy from constrictive pericarditis. The CXR and EKG findings will be nonspecific. Early on the CXR is often normal, as the disease progresses, cardiomegaly and vascular congestion is a common finding. The EKG often demonstrates AF, ectopy, and conduction delays. On echocardiography there will be a thickened LV, and the atrial cavities will be enlarged.

Biopsy remains the gold standard of diagnosis.[4]

Treatment

There is no specific treatment beyond supportive measures. Despite supportive measures 70% to 90% of patients will die within 10 years of diagnosis.[4]

References

1. Felker GM, Hu W, Hare JM, et al. The spectrum of dilated cardiomyopathy. The John Hopkins experience with 1,278 patients. *Medicine* 1999;78:270–283.
2. Avila WS, Carneiro de Carvalho ME, Tschoen CK, et al. Pregnancy and peripartum cardiomyopathy. A comparative and prospective study. *Arq Bras Cardiol* 2002;79:489–493.
3. Yoerger DM, Weyman AE. Hypertrophic obstructive cardiomyopathy: Mechanism of obstruction and response to therapy. *Rev Cardiovasc Med* 2003;4:199–215.
4. Ammash NM, Seward JB, Bailey KR, et al. Clinical profile and outcome of idiopathic restrictive cardiomyopathy. *Circulation* 2000;101:2490–2496.

Valvular Disease

John E. Gough
Luis E. Rodriguez

Mitral Valve Stenosis

Etiology/Pathophysiology

Although the incidence has been declining, rheumatic heart disease remains the leading cause of mitral valve stenosis and incompetence.[1] Scarring from rheumatic endocarditis results in fusion of the commissures and matting of the chordae tendonae: this along with calcifications on the valve prevents proper closure of the valve. The disease process is progressive: commonly there is 20 years between the onset of rheumatic fever and the symptoms of mitral stenosis.[1] Approximately 40% to 65% of elderly patients with mitral valve stenosis relate a history of rheumatic heart disease during childhood.[2] Less common causes include congenital abnormalities, atrial myxoma, thrombus, and calcification of annulus and leaflets (almost always present in older patients).[2] Interference of blood flow between left atrium (LA) and left ventricle (LV) leads to LA hypertension, pulmonary hypertension, pulmonary and tricuspid valve dysfunction, LV failure, atrial fibrillation (AF), and pulmonary edema. After onset of symptoms there is an 85% mortality rate if surgery is not performed.[1]

Clinical Findings

Onset of symptoms typically occurs between 30 and 50 years of age. The most common finding is dyspnea on exertion (~80% of patients).[1] Paroxysmal nocturnal dyspnea (PND) and orthopnea may be present, and is thought to be due to an elevation of LA pressure secondary to increased central blood flow during recumbency. Additionally, hemoptysis may be seen and may be secondary to pulmonary infarction, rupture of bronchial veins, and pulmonary edema. Other symptoms include fatigue, cool extremities, abdominal swelling and discomfort, and recurrent bronchitis.

Obstruction of blood flow through the mitral valve (MV) may lead to LA enlargement, pulmonary hypertension, congestive heart failure (CHF), and right heart failure. The patient may note palpitations, particularly if premature atrial contractions (PACs) or AF are present. If AF is present, there is a risk of systemic embolization, most commonly to the cerebral circulation followed by the renal, splenic, and other vessels.

Auscultation of the lungs frequently reveals rales. The cardiac examination often demonstrates a loud S1 with high pitched opening snap heard best just to right of apex, and a rumbling mid-diastolic murmur crescendo toward S2 heard best at apex. One may appreciate an apical diastolic thrill. If right heart failure is present ascites and jugular venous distention may be present. The systolic blood pressure is usually low to normal. The extremities are cool and peripheral edema is not uncommon. Elderly patients may have pink or purple patches on the face.[2]

Evaluation

The EKG will typically show evidence of LA enlargement; notched or biphasic P wave in lead II ("P mitrale"), negative terminal deflection of P wave in V1, and a right axis deviation. As mentioned above, AF and PACs are common. The chest x-ray (CXR) may be normal or may show straightening of left heart border, left atrial enlargement, and/or calcifications of mitral orifice. Eventually pulmonary congestion, Kerley B lines, and increased vascular markings will be present. The diagnostic test of choice is transesophageal echocardiography (TEE); however, a bedside transthoracic echo is frequently performed as an initial test.

Treatment

Medical management includes treatment of CHF (e.g., oxygen, diuretics, nitrates) if present. Avoidance of physical exertion is recommended. Prophylactic antibiotics should be administered if endocarditis is suspected. If AF occurs, medications to control the ventricular rate and anticoagulation to prevent embolic events may be necessary. In rare instances, severe hemoptysis may require blood replacement. If the degree of stenosis is mild, balloon valvuloplasty may be attempted. The patient should have a surgical evaluation for valve replacement.

Mitral Valve Incompetence

Etiology/Pathophysiology

Common etiologies of mitral valve incompetence include infective endocarditis, myxomatous leaflet degenerative changes in MV, CAD, acute myocardial infarction (MI) [usually right coronary occlusion leading to inferior MI with ischemia and rupture of papillary muscles], rheumatic heart disease, collagen vascular disease, and trauma. Recently associations with diet medications (fenfluramine/phenteramine, dexfenfluramine) have been noted.[3] In the acute setting mitral incompetence can be rapidly fatal. If chronic, LA enlargement and LV dilatation occurs, and the LV stroke volume will increase in an attempt to compensate.

Clinical Findings

Acutely, dyspnea is the most common finding. This may rapidly progress to pulmonary edema, circulatory collapse, and shock. If infective endocarditis is present, fever and septicemia may be seen. There is typically an apical systolic murmur, loud S3, and also an S4.

If chronic, findings include DOE, palpitations (especially if AF is present), and easy fatigability. Typically a holosystolic murmur, S3, and diastolic rumble are heard on auscultation.

Evaluation

The EKG commonly demonstrates changes consistent with LVH and LA abnormality. AF, PACs, atrial flutter, and findings of an acute inferior MI may be seen. The CXR will show LA enlargement, and pulmonary congestion/edema. Diagnosis is best made with echocardiography (TEE preferred).

Treatment

Treatment of pulmonary edema should occur, including oxygen, endotracheal intubation, nitrates, and diuretics. Treatment of concomitant arrhythmias (including anticoagulation, if AF is present) may be necessary. Prophylactic antibiotics to treat endocarditis are indicated. A combination of sodium nitroprusside and dobutamine may be used, although if the patient is hypotensive, dopamine may be necessary. In unstable patients, an aortic balloon pump and referral for emergency surgery may be indicated.

Mitral Valve Prolapse

Etiology/Pathophysiology

Mitral valve prolapse (MVP) or "click murmur syndrome" is the most common of valvular abnormality in industrialized civilization.[4] One or both leaflets prolapse into atrium during systole, and there may be mild regurgitant flow. The onset of MVP may occur at any time of life. The cause is generally unknown; however, MVP may be associated with congenital valve abnormalities, myxomatous degeneration of the mitral valve, Marfan's syndrome, collagen vascular disease, and/or coronary artery disease. Unlike other mitral problems, mitral valve prolapse is not associated with rheumatic heart disease. There is no increased risk of AF, stroke, syncope or sudden death.

Clinical Findings

Most patients are asymptomatic. The most common symptoms are atypical chest pain, fatigue, palpitations,

lightheadedness, and dyspnea unrelated to exertion. Symptoms are more common if the patient is aware of diagnosis. Patients may have asthenic build, skeletal abnormalities such as pectus excavatum, a straight thoracic spine, or scoliosis. On auscultation there is a midsystolic click, as redundant valve tissue bulges back into LA, and a late systolic murmur. Maneuvers that make heart larger (when lying down or squatting) and make the heart click occur later; while maneuvers that decrease heart size (standing up), may bring click closer to S1 and increase the intensity of the murmur.

Evaluation

The EKG is commonly normal. There may be nonspecific ST-T changes. The CXR is usually normal with a normal heart size. Cardiology referral for echocardiogram is indicated if a murmur is present.

Treatment

Often there is no treatment necessary, especially in the emergency department setting. Antibiotic prophylaxis is indicated if endocarditis is suspected. Often these patients may be prescribed aspirin and a β-blocker or calcium channel blocker.

Aortic Valve Stenosis

Etiology/Pathophysiology

Aortic stenosis is the most common of primary valvular heart diseases. In younger patients aortic stenosis is commonly congenital, often associated with bicuspid valve. In adults the most common cause is usually degenerative (calcifications on valve).[2] The cause of calcifications is not clear; however, risks include smoking, hypertension, hypercholesterolemia, diabetes mellitus, renal disease, and hypercalcemia. Aortic valve thickening and a systolic murmur are seen in approximately half of patients greater than 65 years old.[2] Rheumatic heart disease is an uncommon etiology in industrialized countries. The stenosis of the aortic valve interferes with blood flow across the valve creating a gradient. The degree of the murmur heard is associated with the degree of gradient. Over time there is a decrease in LV compliance and LVH develops. Diastolic dysfunction will lead to pulmonary congestion.

Clinical Findings

Typical presenting complaints include chest pain, dyspnea, syncope, presyncope (associated with exertion), dyspnea on exertion, angina, PND, MI, AF (although less common than with mitral disease), and sudden death. The 5-year survival rate is poor if CHF, syncope, and angina are present in unoperated patients.[1] There is a low intensity medium pitch systolic ejection murmur that is harsh and radiates to the carotids. Secondary to decreased stroke volume the pulse may be of small amplitude (pulsus parvus). There is also a slow carotid upstroke (pulsus tardus), and brachio/radial delay; however, decreased vascular compliance may interfere with perception of slow rise.[4] The blood pressure is usually low or normal, often with a narrow pulse pressure, although the presence of hypertension does not rule out aortic stenosis. On auscultation, a split S2, as well as an S3 and S4, are commonly present.

Evaluation

Suspicion of aortic stenosis should occur in any patient who presents with syncope and a new systolic murmur. The EKG may be normal; however, criteria for LVH may be present, as well as BBB and AF (especially in the elderly patient). The CXR also may be normal in the early stages, later LVH (boot-shaped heart) and CHF are common findings. Echocardiography is the main diagnostic test. Cardiac catheterization my be preformed; this is not as common as in the past, as color doppler can give a good estimate as to the degree of gradient present,[5] although, cardiac catheterization may be used to determine the extent of underlying CAD. In stable patients, MRI is now being utilized in the evaluation of aortic stenosis.[6]

Treatment

The patient should be admitted, placed on bed rest, and a cardiology consultation should be obtained. If present, treatment of CHF is indicated; however, nitrates should be used with caution as the decreased preload may lead to significant hypotension. If AF is present, it should be treated as it may decrease cardiac output. AF may also necessitate need for anticoagulation. Surgical referral for aortic valve replacement should be obtained.

Aortic Valve Incompetence

Etiology/Pathophysiology

In 20% of cases of aortic valve incompetence, there is an acute onset when the cusp perforates or tears. This is most commonly a result of infective endocarditis.[5] The majority of cases are chronic (80%), with calcific degeneration and prolapse of aortic leaflets.[4] Risk factors include hypertension; volume overload; LV congenital disease (bicuspid valve); myxomatous proliferation; rheumatic heart disease; patients who are debilitated; immunosuppressed; aortic dissection; and/or intravenous drug use. Less common predisposing factors include Marfan's syndrome; syphilis; anklyosing spondylitis; Erlos-Danler's syndrome; Reiter's syndrome; and use of diet medications (fenfluramine/phenteramine, dexfenfluramine).[3] Aortic valve incompetence may also be secondary to blunt or penetrating trauma.

Clinical Findings

In the acute setting, common presentations include dyspnea, acute pulmonary edema, tachycardia, and tachypnea. If there is an associated endocarditis the patient will appear ill and septicemic, often with fever and chills. If the incompetence is due to an aortic dissection, the patient will frequently note a "tearing" chest pain, anxiety, confusion, and shock. Typically, there will be a high-pitched blowing early diastolic murmur immediately after S2. The pitch and loudness will depend upon the amount of regurgitant blood and the diastolic pressure gradient. An S3 and systolic flow murmur best heard at the left sternal border is usually present. In chronic presentations the patient may be asymptomatic for years. Often the patient will state that they are aware of their heartbeat. This may be secondary to palpitations, PVCs, and increased stroke volume. Other complaints include chest pain, fatigue, and dyspnea. Physical exam findings may include: a wide pulse pressure; Musset's sign (bobbing head movement with pulse); Hill's sign (femoral systolic blood pressure [SBP] 30 mm Hg or more, greater than brachial SBP); Quincke's sign (capillary pulsations in extremities—best seen with pressure on nail beds); Duroziez's sign (systolic and diastolic bruit over femoral artery); Corrigans or "water hammer" pulse; LV impulse heaving; and/or a hyperdynamic carotid pulse (brisk quality with a "double hump" on palpation or "bisferiens pattern").

Evaluation

The CXR typically demonstrates pulmonary edema with not as much cardiomegaly as would otherwise be suspected (especially if acute), LV dilatation, and aortic dilatation. The EKG will have changes of LVH and left axis deviation. Less commonly seen are BBB. Diagnosis is best confirmed by echocardiography (TEE is preferred). Cardiac catheterization may be utilized to determine extent of underlying CAD.

Treatment

In the acute presentation, treatment is aimed at alleviating pulmonary edema. Providing supplementary oxygen, often via endotracheal intubation, will be necessary. Diuretics and nitrates may not be effective. A combination of sodium nitroprusside and dobutamine or dopamine may be used. Antibiotics should be started if endocarditis is suspected. In chronic patients, ACE inhibitors may be utilized. A patient should receive a surgical referral for evaluation for possible valve replacement.

References

1. Petty GW, Khandheria BK, Whisnant JP, et al. Predictors of cerebrovasular disease and death among patients with valvular heart disease. *Stroke* 2000;31: 2628–2635.
2. Segal BL. Mitral valve disease in older adults. *Geriatrics* 2003;58:26–31.
3. Loke YK, Derry S, Pritchard-Copley A. Appetite suppressants and valvular heart disease—a systematic review. *BMC Clin Pharm* 2002;2:6–16.
4. Segal BL. Diagnosis and surgical management of aortic valve disease in older adults. *Geriatrics* 2003;58:31–35.
5. Borer JS, Bonow RO. Contemporary approach to aortic and mitral regurgitation. *Circulation* 2003;108:2432–2438.
6. Caruthers SD, Lin SJ, Brown P, et al. Practical value of cardiac magnetic resonance imaging for clinical quantification of aortic valve stenosis: Comparison with echocardiography. *Circulation* 2003;108:2236–2243.

Dysrhythmias

John E. Gough
E. Jackson Allison, Jr.

In this discussion of specific dysrhythmias and their recognition and treatment, it is assumed that the basic tenets of emergency care such as stabilization (the ABCs), supplemental oxygen, intravenous access, continuous cardiac monitoring, assessment/monitoring of the vital signs, and obtaining an ECG will be applied to all patients.

Sinus Bradycardia

Sinus bradycardia is characterized by a decrease in the rate of atrial depolarization secondary to a slowing of discharges from the sinus node. The ECG findings of sinus bradycardia include an atrial rate less than 60 beats per minute (bpm), normal P waves and PR intervals, and one-to-one AV conduction (**FIGURE 23.1**).

There are many etiologies of sinus bradycardia. Some are representative of pathologic causes such as acute inferior myocardial infarction, hypothyroidism, and increased intracranial pressure. Other etiologies may be the result of certain medications, for example digoxin, β-blockers, calcium channel blockers, sedatives, or narcotics. Furthermore, sinus bradycardia may occur in settings unrelated to pathologic processes such as during sleep, vagal maneuvers or in conditioned athletes.

Clinical manifestations vary based on the etiology. The need for treatment, if any, is based on the patient's condition. If the patient is asymptomatic, addressing possible pathologic causes and continued monitoring are indicated. In the rare instance where sinus bradycardia causes hemodynamic compromise, treatment should begin with transcutaneous pacing. If a pacemaker is not immediately available, agents such as atropine, epinephrine, dopamine, and isoproterenol may be utilized (**Table 23.1**).

Sinus Tachycardia

Sinus tachycardia occurs when there is an increase in atrial depolarization secondary to an acceleration of discharges from the sinus node. The characteristics of sinus tachycardia seen on ECG are an increased atrial rate (usually between 100 and 160 bpm), one-to-one AV conduction, and usually normal P waves and PR intervals (**FIGURE 23.2**).

Like sinus bradycardia, sinus tachycardia may represent pathologic conditions or drug effects or be physiologic.

Pathologic conditions associated with sinus tachycardia include hyperpyrexia, pulmonary embolus, hypovolemia, hypoxia, hyperthyroidism, and congestive heart failure (both high- and low-output states). Medications that can cause sinus tachycardia include cocaine, atropine, epinephrine, β-agonists, xanthenes, and sympathomimetics. Physiologic etiologies of sinus tachycardia are exercise, emotional stress, and fear. Sinus tachycardia is a normal finding in resting heart rates of infants and small children.

Sinus tachycardia rarely requires treatment. Initial measures should be aimed at eliminating the underlying cause(s). In the setting of suspected ongoing myocardial ischemia or infarction, treatment may be required with administration of β-blockers. (**Table 23.2**)

Atrial Flutter

Atrial flutter is a dysrhythmia that usually originates in the right atria. Although thought by some to be the result of a reentry circuit, the exact mechanism is unknown. ECG characteristics of atrial flutter include a regular atrial rate ranging from 220 to 350 bpm (usually around 300 bpm), and absence of normal P waves (the "saw-tooth" flutter waves are best seen in leads II, III, and aVF). The PR interval and QRS complexes are usually normal, but may be variable. The ventricular response depends on the degree of

---

Table 23.1

Treatment of Sinus Bradycardia

Rarely requires treatment
Search for underlying causes (e.g., drug effects, hypothyroidism, acute MI) and institute appropriate treatment
If hemodynamically unstable:
Transcutaneous pacemaker
Atropine 0.5 to 1.0 mg IV (may repeat q 5 min to total dose of 0.4 mg/kg)
Epinephrine drip 2 to 10 μg/min
Isoproterenol drip 2 to 10 μg/min (drug of choice in patients status post-heart transplant)
Dopamine drip 2 to 20 μg/kg/min

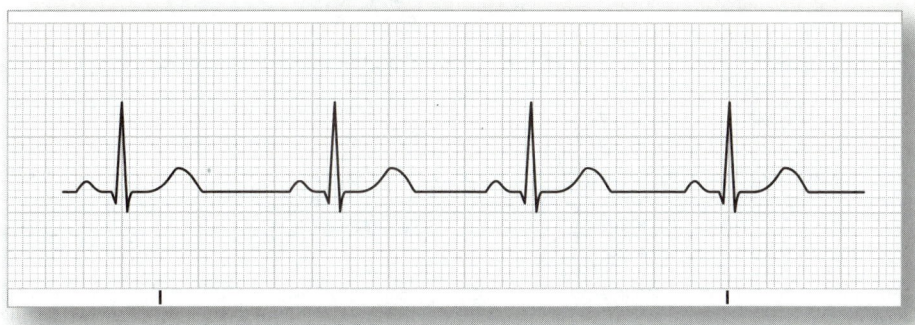

FIGURE 23.1 Sinus bradycardia.

(Reprinted from Garcia TB, Miller GT, *Arrhythmia Recognition: The Art of Interpretation*. Sudbury, MA: Jones and Bartlett Publishers, Inc., 2004.)

block at the AV node. The block may be constant (usually 2:1) or variable. When 2:1, the patient frequently presents with a ventricular rate of 150 bpm, and the rhythm may initially be mistaken for a sinus tachycardia or SVT. Vagal maneuvers or an intravenous dose of adenosine may be helpful in making the diagnosis by decreasing the ventricular response and exposing the flutter waves (**FIGURE 23.3**).

The possible etiologies for atrial flutter are many; however, it seldom presents in patients without underlying heart disease. Causes of atrial flutter include ischemic heart disease, acute myocardial infarction (AMI), hypoxia, hypokalemia, pulmonary embolism, thyrotoxicosis, myocarditis, congestive cardiomyopathy, valvular disease, and drug toxicity (digoxin).

Clinical manifestations of atrial flutter are dependent on the etiology, the patient's existing medical condition, and the ventricular response. The patient may complain of minimal symptoms such as palpitations or mild shortness of breath or may present with severe respiratory distress, hypotension, and ischemic pain.

Treatment of the patient with atrial flutter is based on the clinical presentation. If an etiology listed above is identified, measures to correct that condition should be instituted. If the patient is tachycardic and hemodynamically unstable, immediate synchronized cardioversion is indicated. The majority of cases of atrial flutter respond to low-energy cardioversion (50 to 100 J). If unsuccessful, repeated cardioversion at progressively higher energy levels may be necessary. Recently, biphasic defibrillators have shown

equal or greater effectiveness of successfully converting dysrhyhtmias compared to monophasic defibrillators, while utilizing lower energy levels. If time and patient's condition permits, sedation and/or analgesia with appropriate short-acting and reversible agents (i.e., fentanyl, midazolam) should be administered prior to cardioversion.

In the stable patient, control of the ventricular response is the immediate goal. Many agents such as diltiazem, amiodarone, verapamil, digoxin, and β-blockers may be utilized. Verapamil and β-blockers should be used with caution in patients presenting with congestive heart failure (CHF) as they may exacerbate this condition. If the patient is presently taking digoxin, blood levels should be obtained prior to administering additional digoxin as atrial flutter is a rare consequence of digitalis toxicity. The above agents are used primarily for rate control; however, they do exhibit a low incidence (20% to 30%) of conversion of atrial flutter to a sinus rhythm. Once rate control has been achieved, a type I antiarrhythmic such as procainamide or quinidine can be administered to help convert the dysrhythmia and prevent recurrence (**Table 23.3**).

Atrial Fibrillation

Atrial fibrillation results from multiple areas within the atria continuously discharging. This may be caused by many ectopic foci or multiple areas of reentry. The result is a lack of orderly depolarization and effective contraction of the atria. While the rate of atrial electrical discharges

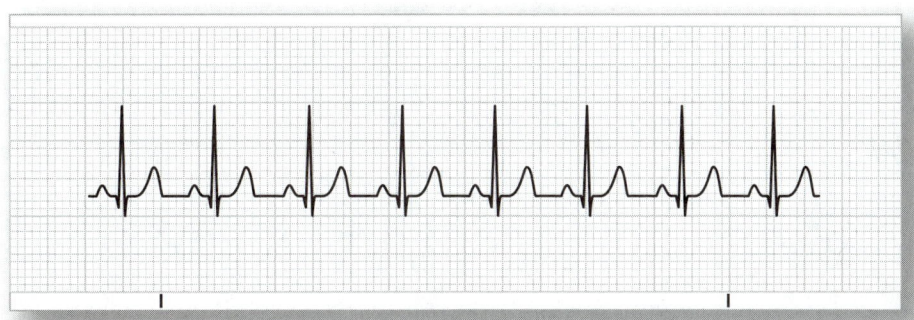

FIGURE 23.2 Sinus tachycardia.

(Reprinted from Garcia TB, Miller GT, *Arrhythmia Recognition: The Art of Interpretation*. Sudbury, MA: Jones and Bartlett Publishers, Inc., 2004.)

Table 23.2
Treatment of Sinus Tachycardia

Rarely requires treatment
Search for underling cause (e.g., pulmonary emboli, drug effects, fever) and institute appropriate treatment
If unstable or suspect ongoing cardiac ischemia:
β-blockers: propranoloI 1.0 to 3.0 mg IV, atenolol 5.0 mg IV (may repeat up to 15.0 mg total dose)
Benzodiazepines: diazepam 2.0 to 5.0 mg IV, lorazepam 1.0 to 2.0 mg IV (especially useful in setting of cocaine toxicity)

Table 23.3
Treatment of Atrial Flutter

If hemodynamically unstable:
Synchronized cardioversion 25 to 50 (if unsuccessful, reattempt at progressively higher energy levels) with appropriate sedation/analgesia
If stable, initial goal is rate control:
If diagnosis is unclear, vagal maneuvers or adenosine 6.0 mg rapid IV push may slow ventricular response enough to establish dysrhythmia identification
Amiodarone 150 mg IV over 15 minutes (drug of choice in patient with impaired ejection fraction)
Diltiazem 0.25 mg/kg IV (may repeat at 0.35 mg/kg if no response); if successful, may begin continuous IV infusion at 10 mg/hr
Verapamil 2.0 to 5.0 mg IV
Digoxin 0.4 to 0.6 mg IV (if patient presently on digoxin, consider digitalis toxicity as potential cause of dysrhythmia)
β-blockers-propranolol 1.0 to 3.0 mg IV, atenolol 5.0 mg IV (may repeat to total dose of 15.0 mg IV). Use with caution in the setting of CHF.
When rate control is achieved:
Procainamide 50 mg/kg/day po
Quinidine 1-2 tabs q po 8-12 hr

typically ranges from 400 to 700 per minute, decreased conduction by the AV node results in an average ventricular response of 160 to 180 bpm. Characteristics of atrial fibrillation seen on the ECG include no discernible P waves, a chaotic baseline of fibrillatory waves best seen in leads VI, V 2, V 3, and a VF, and an "irregularly irregular" ventricular response usually at 160 to 180 bpm (**FIGURE 23.4**). The ventricular rate may be faster or slower based on preexisting cardiovascular status and the presence of certain drugs, especially digoxin. The QRS width is usually unaffected unless aberrant conduction exists. Atrial fibrillation may be constant or intermittent; therefore, continuous monitoring is indicated.

The most common conditions associated with atrial fibrillation are rheumatic heart disease, ischemic heart disease, hypertension, and thyrotoxicosis. It may also be seen with pericarditis, atrial septal defects, acute myocardial infarction, and acute alcohol intoxication (holiday heart).

As with atrial flutter, the clinical manifestations seen with atrial fibrillation are variable. In patients with compromised cardiac output, the loss of effective atrial contractions may precipitate congestive heart failure. Angina, respiratory distress, and hypotension are also common presentations with acute atrial fibrillation, particularly with a rapid ventricular response. Patients with long-standing atrial fibrillation may remain relatively asymptomatic, if the ventricular rate is controlled. Chronic atrial fibrillation predisposes the patient to arterial embolic events (up to 15% of patients per year). If the onset of the atrial fibrillation is not clear, it is not recommended to convert the patient to a sinus rhythm without first instituting anticoagulants. Administration of heparin, warfarin or more recently enoxaparin, for a period of 1 to 3 weeks prior to cardioversion will help prevent the sequelae of arterial embolism of an intraatrial thrombus.

While it is ideal to first anticoagulate patients in atrial fibrillation of chronic or uncertain duration prior to attempting conversion of the rhythm to sinus, if the patient's condition warrants, the treatment of choice is synchronized cardioversion. Atrial fibrillation usually requires higher energy levels for conversion to a sinus rhythm than does atrial flutter, and some authors recommend beginning doses of 200 to 300 J (lower energies, if

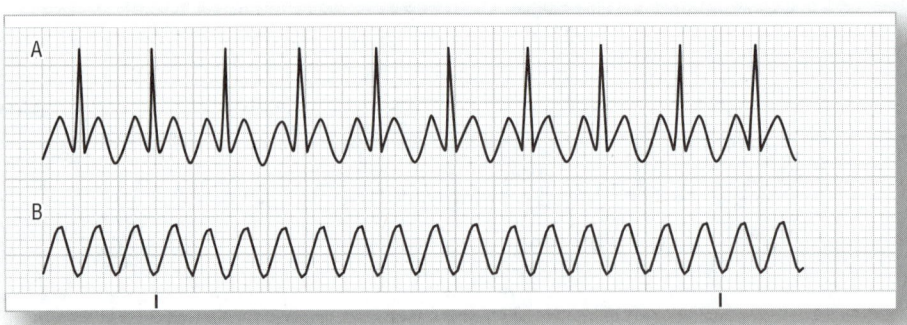

FIGURE 23.3 Atrial flutter.

(Reprinted from Garcia TB, Miller GT, *Arrhythmia Recognition: The Art of Interpretation*. Sudbury, MA: Jones and Bartlett Publishers, Inc., 2004.)

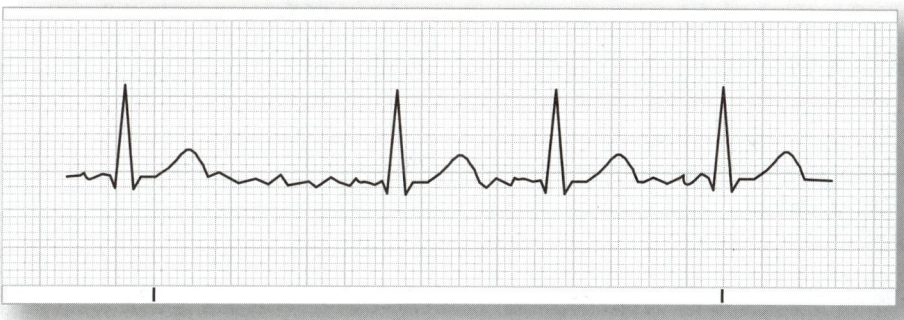

FIGURE 23.4 Atrial fibrillation.

(Reprinted from Garcia TB, Miller GT, *Arrhythmia Recognition: The Art of Interpretation*. Sudbury, MA: Jones and Bartlett Publishers, Inc., 2004.)

using a biphasic defibrillator). However, the American Heart Association's ACLS guidelines recommend starting at 100 J and escalating the dose, as needed. If the first attempts at cardioversion are unsuccessful, administration of intravenous procainamide may enhance success. Appropriate analgesia/sedation is suggested. If the patient is hemodynamically stable, control of the ventricular response is desirable. Many agents may be used. Digoxin has long been used and is effective; however, the onset of action may be slow (mean time to conversion of approximately 11 hours). Diltiazem is very effective in slowing the ventricular response, often in less than 10 minutes. Amiodarone may be used; however, if duration of atrial fibrillation is greater than 48 hours there may be a risk of conversion to sinus rhythm and therefore the risk of embolization is increased. Once rate control has been established, attempts to pharmacologically convert the atrial fibrillation to a sinus rhythm may be attempted with the use of procainamide, amiodarone, quinidine, or verapamil (**Table 23.4**). In atrial fibrillation associated with an acces-

sory pathway, most commonly Wolff-Parkinson-White syndrome, it is recommended to avoid medications which increase refractoriness of the AV node. A mnemonic to remember which drugs to avoid is **ABCD**: adenosine, beta-blockers, calcium channel blockers, and digitalis. The concern is that if the AV nodal pathway is blocked, the impulse may preferentially opt for the accessory pathway, leading to uncontrolled arrhythmias and even sudden cardiac death. Medications that may increase the refractoriness of the accessory pathway are preferred (e.g., procanamide, quinidine, amiodarone, dofetilide, ibutilide, sotalol).

Supraventricular Tachycardia

Supraventricular tachycardias (SVTs) are the result of a reentry circuit or an ectopic foci occurring above the bundle of His. A reentry mechanism accounts for approximately 80% of SVTs, with three-fourths of those occurring in the AV node. The other 20% involve the presence of bypass tracts. Bypass tracts, as seen in Wolff-Parkinson-White (WPW) syndrome, are accessory pathways located outside the AV node (e.g., Kent's bundle) that can conduct impulses into the ventricle.

The ECG typically demonstrates a regular rate of 160 to 200 bpm; however, ranges between 100 and 250 bpm have been reported. The P wave is often obscured by the QRS complex and difficult to identify. Patients with WPW may exhibit a shortened PR interval (<0.12 seconds) and a slurring of the upstroke of the QRS complex (delta wave). The AV conduction in SVTs is usually 1:1. The QRS complexes are usually narrow, even in the setting of bypass tracts. Wide QRS complexes may be rate-related, resulting from abnormal conduction through a bypass tract or seen with preexisting bundle branch blocks. Aberrantly conducted SVTs are often mistaken for ventricular tachycardia.

Reentry SVTs can be seen in patients with normal hearts or may be associated with rheumatic heart disease, pericarditis, myocardial infarction, mitral valve disease, stimulant use, or in the presence of an accessory pathway. Acute paroxysmal episodes (PSVTs) are more commonly associated with a reentrant phenomenon than with ectopic foci. Ectopic SVTs are commonly associated with digitalis toxicity, myocardial infarction, hypoxemia, COPD, and alcohol

---

Table 23.4

Treatment of Atrial Fibrillation

If hemodynamically unstable:
Synchronized cardioversion, 100 (if unsuccessful, reattempt at progressively higher energy levels) with appropriate analgesia/sedation

If stable, but tachycardic, attempt to control ventricular response:
Amiodarone 150 mg IV over 15 minutes
Diltiazem 0.25 mg/kg IV (may repeat at 0.35 mg/kg if no response); if successful, may begin continuous IV infusion at 10 mg/hr
Digoxin 0.4 to 0.6 mg IV (if patient presently on digoxin, consider digitalis toxicity as potential cause of dysrhythmia)

When rate control is established:
Procainamide 50 mg/kg/day po
Quinidine 1 to 2 tabs po q 8-12 hr
Verapamil 240 to 320 mg/day (divided tid or qid). Use with caution in the setting of CHF.

Table 23.5

Treatment of Supraventricular Tachycardia

If hemodynamically unstable:
Synchronized cardioversion 50 J (if unsuccessful, reattempt at progressively higher energy levels)

Reentrant SVT in a stable patient:
Vagal maneuvers (e.g., Valsalva, carotid sinus massage)

Adenosine 6.0 mg rapid push (if unsuccessful, may repeat at 12.0 mg for 2 doses)

Diltiazem 0.25 mg/kg IV (may repeat at 0.35 mg/kg if no response); if successful, may begin continuous IV infusion at 10 mg/hr

Amiodarone 150 mg IV over 15 minutes

Verapamil 2.0 to 5.0 mg IV

Digoxin 0.4 to 0.6 mg IV (if patient presently on digoxin, consider digitalis toxicity as potential cause of dysrhythmia)

β-blockers: propranolol 1.0 to 3.0 mg IV, atenolol 5.0 mg IV (may repeat to total dose of 15.0 mg)

Overdrive pacing (rarely necessary)

If ectopic SVT:
Digoxin 0.4 to 0.6 mg IV (if patient presently on digoxin, consider digitalis toxicity as potential cause of dysrhythmia)

Amiodarone 150 mg IV over 15 minutes

Diltiazem 0.25 mg/kg IV (may repeat at 0.35 mg/kg if no response); if successful, may begin continuous IV infusion at 10 mg/hr

Verapamil 2.0 to 5.0 mg IV

β-blockers-propranolol 1.0 to 3.0 mg IV, Atenolol 5.0 mg IV (may repeat to total dose of 15.0 mg)

If SVT thought to be secondary to digitalis toxicity:
Digitalis specific antibodies (Fab)

Phenytoin 15.0 mg/kg (infuse no greater than 25 to 50 mg/min); cardioversion ineffective

---

intoxication. Symptoms range from mild palpitations to severe respiratory distress, hypotension, and anginal-like chest discomfort.

Treatment is based on suspected etiology and patient condition. Regardless of suspected cause, if the patient presents with severe distress and hemodynamic instability, synchronized cardioversion is the treatment of choice. Like atrial flutter, PSVT usually responds to low energy levels and it is recommended to begin at 50 J.

Vagal maneuvers are sometimes helpful to both diagnose and treat SVTs. As vagal maneuvers are generally safe and noninvasive, they should be attempted first in the stable patient. By slowing the ventricular response, the underlying rhythm is much easier identified in cases when the diagnosis is unclear. With reentry SVT, vagal maneuvers can terminate the circuit by increasing the refractory period in the AV node.

If vagal maneuvers are unsuccessful, adenosine should be administered as the drug of choice. Adenosine will produce a transient AV block that is successful in terminating approximately 90% of reentrant SVTs. Diltiazem is as effective as adenosine, but due to its mechanism of action as a calcium channel blocker, it may be associated with more adverse effects, particularly hypotension. However, if adenosine is ineffective, diltiazem is the next agent of choice. Other medications such as amiodarone, verapamil, β-blockers, and digoxin may also be utilized, if necessary. In rare cases, overdrive pacing may be used. Once the acute event has been terminated, referral to an internist, cardiologist, or electrophysiologist may be indicated. Patients with WPW have been successfully treated with radiofrequency catheter ablation of their bypass tracts.

If the SVT is thought to be of an ectopic nature (excluding digitalis toxicity), medications that may be helpful for rate control include digoxin, verapamil, diltiazem, amiodarone, and β-blockers. Long-term antidysrhythmic therapy with either procainamide or quinidine may be necessary. Ectopic SVT in the presence of digitalis toxicity warrants the use of digoxin-specific antibody fragments (Fab). Phenytoin was traditionally utilized as the antiarrhythmic of choice with varying success. Lidocaine and magnesium may also be used. Cardioversion in the presence of digitalis toxicity is generally ineffective and may precipitate more serious dysrhythmias; therefore, it is not recommended (see **Table 23.5**).

Multifocal Atrial Tachycardia

Multifocal atrial tachycardia (MAT), otherwise known as "wandering atrial pacemaker," is an irregular dysrhythmia caused by multiple atrial ectopic foci. ECG characteristics include P waves with three or more different morphologies, variable PR and RR intervals, and a ventricular rate usually between 100 and 180 bpm. As the initiation of the impulse is in the atria, the QRS complex is usually of normal width unless a bundle branch block exists. Due to the abnormal P wave morphologies and the irregular ventricular rate, it is often mistaken for atrial fibrillation (**FIGURE 23.5**).

MAT occurs primarily in patients with chronic lung disease. Hypoxemia associated with the chronic lung disease appears to be the major initiating factor. Theophylline and rarely digitalis toxicity are also possible etiologies. Clinical response is variable; however, the tachycardia may exacerbate associated congestive heart failure. Treatment is directed toward correcting hypoxemia with oxygen and bronchodilators. Rate control has also been accomplished with magnesium, verapamil, and β-blockers. Cardioversion is ineffective and should not be used (**Table 23.6**).

Atrial Ectopy

Premature atrial contractions (PACs) arise from ectopic foci within the atria. PACs are very common and are seen in patients of all ages in the absence of heart disease. ECG features include an abnormal P wave (P') that occurs earlier than the next expected sinus P wave. The P' has a different morphology than the preceding sinus P waves, and the interval to the next sinus P wave following a PAC is longer but less than fully compensatory when compared to normal. The P' may be difficult to identify if it occurs early enough to be obscured by the preceding T wave. If the PAC occurs too early during the absolute refractory

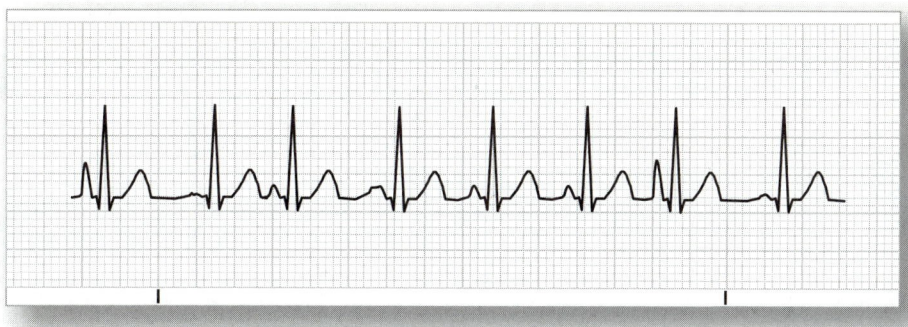

FIGURE 23.5 Multifocal atrial tachycardia (MAT).

(Reprinted from Garcia TB, Miller GT, *Arrhythmia Recognition: The Art of Interpretation*. Sudbury, MA: Jones and Bartlett Publishers, Inc., 2004.)

period of the AV node, it will not be conducted or "blocked," exhibiting a P′ with a QRS. The majority of PACs are conducted normally through the AV node, resulting in a normal-appearing QRS complex. Multiple etiologies include fatigue, alcohol, tobacco, caffeine, COPD, and emotional stress. Digitalis toxicity is a potential cause and if seen in this setting, the PACs may be a precursor to SVT. Myocardial ischemia/infarction and distention of the atria as seen with CHF are also potential causes.

Clinical effects are usually minimal. Some patients may note the sensation of a "skipped beat" as a result of increased ventricular filling after the PAC. PACs have been shown to precipitate SVT, atrial flutter, and atrial fibrillation.

Treatment of PACs is directed toward eliminating any underlying etiology (discontinuing drugs, avoiding stimulants). If the PACs trigger sustained tachycardias, anti-dysrhythmics such as quinidine, procainamide, and β-blockers are sometimes used (**Table 23.7**).

Junctional Rhythms

While the conducting tissues surrounding the AV node and bundle of His above the bifurcation can serve a pacemaker for myocardial contraction, the sinus node normally serves this function. In situations when no impulse from the sinus node reaches the AV node for 1.0 to 1.5 seconds, this specialized tissue can fire, initiating a junc-

tional escape beat. If the sinus node continues to fail to generate an impulse, or if the sinus initiated impulse is blocked from reaching the AV node, repeated impulses from the tissue surrounding the AV can establish a junctional rhythm. Junctional rhythms are usually regular and between 40 and 60 bpm; however, accelerated junctional rhythms (60 to 100 bpm), and junctional tachycardias (>100 bpm) can occur. P waves may be inverted (retrograde) in leads II, III, and aVF, and may precede, follow, or be obscured by the QRS complex. The PR interval is often shorter than the normal preceding PR interval. The QRS complexes are usually normal (**FIGURE 23.6**).

Junctional rhythms may occur with severe bradycardias, AV blocks, CHF, myocarditis, hypokalemia, and digitalis toxicity. Accelerated junctional rhythms are seen with myocardial ischemia/infarction, rheumatic heart disease, and digitalis toxicity.

Clinical manifestations may include CHF and worsening of ischemic symptoms, particularly if the ventricular response is slow. Treatment may not be necessary in the stable patient. If digitalis toxicity is suspected, it should be treated with Fab antibodies. Atropine may be useful to increase the discharges from the sinus node in an effort to initiate a sinus rhythm. Transcutaneous pacing should be standing by in the rare event of severe decomposition (**Table 23.8**).

Premature Junctional Contractions

Premature junctional contractions (PJCs) occur when an ectopic pacemaker around the AV node initiates the impulse for ventricular depolarization. ECG findings include a P′ wave of differing morphology than the sinus P wave (as with junctional rhythms, the P′ may be retrograde and

---

Table 23.6

Treatment of Multifocal Atrial Tachycardia

Treat underlying hypoxia (oxygen, bronchodilators)
Control ventricular rate
Amiodarone 150 mg IV over 15 minutes
Diltiazem 0.25 mg/kg IV (may repeat at 0.35 mg/kg if no response); if successful, may begin continuous IV infusion at 10 mg/hr
Verapamil 2.0 to 5.0 mg IV.
β-blockers: propranolol 1.0-3.0 mg IV, atenolol 5.0 mg IV (may repeat to total dose of 15.0 mg). Use with care in the setting of CHF.
Magnesium sulfate 1.0 to 2.0 g IV

Table 23.7

Treatment of Premature Atrial Contractions

Treat underlying cause
Discontinue medications (digitalis)
Avoid stimulants (caffeine. tobacco)
Decrease fatigue and stress

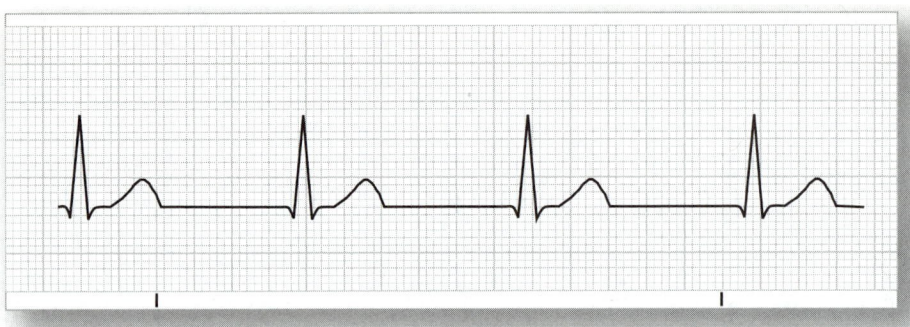

FIGURE 23.6 Junctional Rhythm.

(Reprinted from Garcia TB, Miller GT, *Arrhythmia Recognition: The Art of Interpretation*. Sudbury, MA: Jones and Bartlett Publishers, Inc., 2004.)

occur anytime in relation to the QRS complex); a QRS complex that is earlier than expected and usually of normal configuration; a shortened P'R interval; and a fully compensatory pause before the next sinus beat.

PJCs are rare in an undiseased heart. Etiologies include myocardial ischemia/infarction, CHF, and digitalis toxicity. PJCs are generally asymptomatic. Treatment is directed at correcting any underlying causes and continued observation for the appearance of other dysrhythmias (**Table 23.9**).

Ventricular Fibrillation

Ventricular fibrillation (VF) results from multiple areas within the ventricles spontaneously depolarizing and contracting. There is no organized ventricular depolarization; hence no effective contraction occurs. The ventricle appears to quiver and produces no cardiac output. The ECG displays an erratic baseline without defined P waves, QRS complexes, or T waves. The amplitude of the baseline may vary from very coarse deflections to an almost flat line that can be mistaken for asystole (**FIGURE 23.7**).

VF may occur without warning (sudden death) with or without associated acute myocardial infarction. VF may also be the result of trauma, hypothermia, drug toxicity (digitalis, quinidine), electric shocks, or electrolyte abnormalities. Iatrogenic causes include direct myocardial stimulation during transvenous pacemaker or central line placement. Furthermore, unsynchronized cardioversion of a tachydysrhythmia is also a potential iatrogenic cause.

Clinically, since there is no cardiac output, the patient will be without pulse or blood pressure. The patient will be apneic; however, early in the course of the dysrhythmia, ineffective agonal respirations may be present. If a defibrillator is not immediately available, airway control and support (ideally through endotracheal intubation and bag-valve-mask), cardiopulmonary resuscitation (CPR), and intravenous access should be initiated. While there are ongoing investigations as to the optimal timing of defibrillation, the American Heart Association's Advanced Cardiac Life Support (AHA ACLS) guidelines state that treatment of choice for VF is immediate defibrillation. The initial three defibrillations should be delivered at 200 J, 200 to 300 J, and 360 J. As stated earlier, trials with biphasic defibrillators have shown comparable or better results than monophasic defibrillators at lower energy levels. Some manufacturers recommend the initial three defibrillations occur at 150 J, 150 J, and 200 J with a biphasic machine. If an automated external defibrillator (AED) is utilized, the pre-set energy levels will be programmed into the machine, typically 200 J, 200 J, or 360 J. If the patient does not respond to the initial three defibrillations, the above resuscitative measures should be started and medications given, keeping in mind that some of the major resuscitative medications can be administered both intravenously and endotracheally. Endotracheal administration of epinephrine, atropine and lidocaine are approved; however, it should be noted that the doses should be increased 2.0 to 2.5 times the IV dose. After each medication administration, an attempt to circulate the drug should be made through continued CPR for 30 to 60 seconds. At this point, the patient should be reassessed, and if VF is persistent, repeated defibrillations at 360 J (200 J biphasic) should be delivered.

Table 23.8
Treatment of Junctional Rhythm

May not be necessary in stable patient
If bradycardic and symptomatic:
  Pacemaker
  Atropine 0.5-1.0 mg IV (may repeat q 5 min to
    total dose of 0.4 mg/kg)
  Epinephrine drip 2 to 10 µg/min
  Isoproterenol drip 2 to 10 µg/min (drug of choice
    in patients status post-heart transplant)
  Dopamine drip 2 to 20 µg/kg/min
If digitalis toxicity is suspected:
  Digitalis specific (Fab) antibodies

Table 23.9
Treatment of Premature Junctional Complexes

Generally asymptomatic
Treatment is directed at alleviating precipitating
  causes (CHF, MI, digitalis toxicity)

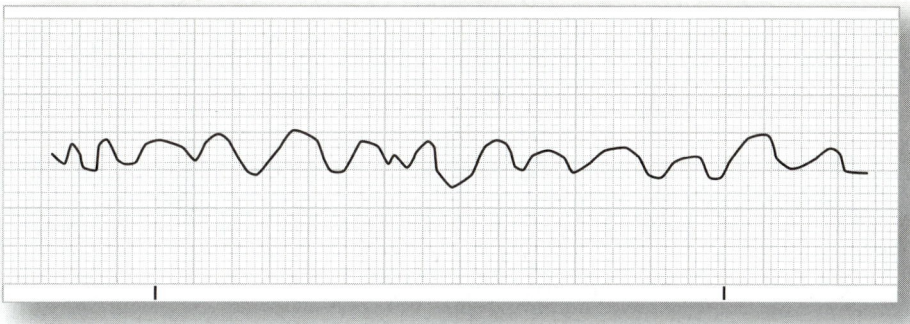

FIGURE 23.7 Ventricular fibrillation.

(Reprinted from Garcia TB, Miller GT, *Arrhythmia Recognition: The Art of Interpretation*. Sudbury, MA: Jones and Bartlett Publishers, Inc., 2004.)

There now exists choice over the first drug that should be administered: epinephrine 1.0 mg repeated q 3 to 5 minutes, which makes VF more susceptible to defibrillation; or a one-time dose of 40 U vasopressin. Following delivery of epinephrine or vasopressin, antidysrhythmic agents (e.g., lidocaine, amiodarone, procainamide, and magnesium) may all be utilized as per the AHA ACLS guidelines (**Table 23.10**). It should be noted that it is recommended to administer the maximum dose of the antiarrhythmic medication before moving on to the next choice. This will decrease the risk of adverse effects of mixing medications, and help eliminate any confusion over which medication was successful in helping to terminate the dysrhythmia. Sodium bicarbonate may be used to alleviate the acidosis that inevitably occurs with VF. However, since the acidosis is a result of metabolic by-products of hypoxic lactic acidosis, it is recommended that acidosis first be treated by hyperventilation and that sodium bicarbonate be utilized with caution. While defibrillation is effective in some cases of VF, particularly if delivered early, VF is often a preterminal rhythm, and the decision concerning when to terminate resuscitative measures will need to be addressed on an individual basis.

Ventricular Tachycardia

Ventricular tachycardia (VT) occurs when there are three or more consecutive beats from an ectopic ventricular focus firing at a rate greater than 100 bpm. The ECG will typically display wide QRS complexes; a usually regular ventricular rate between 100 and 220 bpm; ST segments and T waves of opposite polarity to the QRS; and a usually constant QRS axis. Because there is often AV dissociation, the sinus node may still be firing and depolarizing the atria. Therefore, a P wave can sometimes be seen between the QRS complexes; however, there will not be a fixed relationship between the P wave and the QRS complex (**FIGURE 23.8**).

VT is rarely seen in the setting of a normal heart. VT most commonly occurs in the presence of myocardial ischemia and/or infarction. Other causes include mitral valve prolapse, drugs (quinidine, procainamide), hypoxia, alkalosis, electrolyte abnormalities, and cardiomyopathy.

VT is often difficult to distinguish from an SVT with aberrant conduction, and clinical presentation is of little help since both can present with similar symptomatology. A QRS width of greater than 0.14 seconds suggests VT; however, it is not absolute. It is generally thought best to assume that all wide complex tachycardias are VT. It would be uncommon for VT treatment to cause harm to the patient with SVT. In the stable patient, vagal maneuvers or adenosine administration are considered to be safe and may occasionally demonstrate an underlying SVT.

The clinical manifestations of VT are varied and the treatment is dependent on the clinical presentation. Polymorphic VT or VT presenting without a pulse is treated as VF. If a pulse is present but the patient exhibits significant symptoms or hemodynamic compromise, synchronized cardioversion is the treatment of choice. An energy level of 100 J is generally effective. As with all cardioversion attempts, administration of sedation and/or analgesia is de-

---

Table 23.10

Treatment of Ventricular Fibrillation

If defibrillator immediately available:

Immediate defibrillations (200 J, 200-300 J, 360 J or 150 J, 150 J, 200 J, if biphasic defibrillator used)

Airway control-endotracheal intubation

Support ventilations with bag-valve-mask

Cardiopulmonary resuscitation

Initiate intravenous access (if access not immediately available, several resuscitative drugs [epinephrine, atropine and lidocaine] can be delivered via the endotracheal tube)

Either: Epinephrine 1.0 mg IV (may repeat q 3 to 5 min as long as the dysrhythmia persists); or a one-time dose of vasopressin 40 U IV

After every medication administration, circulate drug via CPR and repeat defibrillations at 360 J (200 J biphasic)

Amiodarone, 300 mg IV (may repeat second dose of 150 mg in 5 to 10 minutes) or

Lidocaine, 1.0 to 1.5 mg/kg bolus (may repeat q 5 min to total dose of 3.0 mg/kg)

Magnesium sulfate, 1.0 to 2.0 g IV

Procainamide, 20 to 50 mg/min (to total dose of 17 mg/kg). Consider termination of resuscitative efforts.

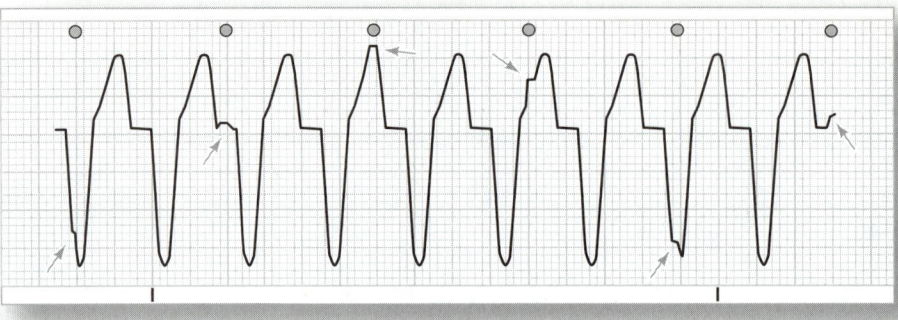

FIGURE 23.8 Ventricular tachycardia (VT).

(Reprinted from Garcia TB, Miller GT, *Arrhythmia Recognition: The Art of Interpretation*. Sudbury, MA: Jones and Bartlett Publishers, Inc., 2004.)

sirable if the patient's condition permits. If the patient is hemodynamically stable, then medication administration is indicated. Lidocaine is the first agent of choice followed by procainamide (**Table 23.11**). Patients who survive episodes of VT or VF should be evaluated as to the potential need for automatic implantable cardiodefibrillators (AICDs).

Ventricular Ectopy

Premature ventricular contractions (PVCs) may arise from ectopic foci located in either ventricle, which cause depolarization of the ventricle prior to the next expected sinus beat. Since the depolarization does not occur through normal pathways, the resulting QRS complex is often bizarre in appearance and abnormally widened (>0.12 seconds). Another ECG characteristic is a missing or abnormal P wave. The next sinus P wave is usually hidden within the PVC's QRS complex; however, occasionally the PVC causes retrograde depolarization of the atria resulting in an abnormal P wave. Most PVCs are associated with a fully compensatory pause before the next sinus beat; however, PVCs may occur between sinus beats without associated pauses (interpolated

PVC). Since PVCs may arise from separate foci, the resulting QRS complexes are of differing morphologies (multifocal PVCs). Due to the prematurity of the PVC, the ventricular rhythm is usually irregular. PVCs may occur alone, in pairs (couplets), or in groups of three or more (VT). Certain nomenclature has been developed for PVCs occurring in regular patterns after every sinus beat (bigeminy), after every two sinus beats (trigeminy), and after every three sinus beats (quadrageminy, i.e., every fourth beat is a PVC) (**FIGURE 23.9**).

PVCs are common and often occur in the absence of heart disease. Common causes of PVCs include myocardial ischemia/infarction, hypoxemia, CHF, drugs (stimulants, digoxin), and electrolyte abnormalities. Patients experiencing PVCs may be asymptomatic or may complain of palpitations.

The need to treat PVCs is based on multiple factors such as their frequency, timing, number of ectopic foci, and the clinical condition of the patient. In the setting of acute myocardial ischemia or infarction, the goal should be to treat the underlying ischemia and not simply to suppress the PVCs.

PVCs seen with ischemia may represent potential instability and be a precursor of VT or VF. If the PVCs do not resolve with measures to restore myocardial perfusion, treatment may be indicated. PVCs that occur during or immediately after the T wave (ventricular repolarization) carry a risk of precipitating VT or VF (R on T phenomena). If treatment is indicated, amiodarone or lidocaine are the first drugs of choice; if unsuccessful, procainamide may be utilized (**Table 23.12**).

Pulseless Electrical Activity

Pulseless electrical activity (PEA), otherwise known as electromechanical dissociation (EMD), occurs in settings other than VT or VF where there is electrical activity noted on the cardiac monitor or ECG without an associated palpable pulse. The appearance on the ECG may range from normal appearing complexes to chaotic, bizarre complexes with no uniformity.

In the setting of cardiac arrest associated with acute myocardial infarction, PEA often represents profound dysfunction of the myocardium ("pump failure") and is gen-

---

Table 23.11

Treatment of Ventricular Tachycardia

If pulseless, treat as VF (Table 23.11)

If a pulse is present, but the patient is hemodynamically unstable:

Synchronized cardioversion 100 J (if unsuccessful, reattempt at progressively higher energy levels); lower energies with biphasic defibrillator.

If a pulse is present and the patient is hemodynamically stable:

Amiodarone 150 mg IV over 15 minutes, if successful may begin continuous drip of 1.0 to 2.0 mg/min

Lidocaine 1.0 to 1.5 mg/kg bolus (may repeat q 5 min to total dose of 3.0 mg/kg); if successful, may begin continuous infusion of 1.0 to 4.0 mg/min

Procainamide 20 to 30 mg/min (to total dose of 17 mg/kg); if successful, may begin continuous infusion of 1.0 to 4.0 mg/min (drug of choice in recurrent VT)

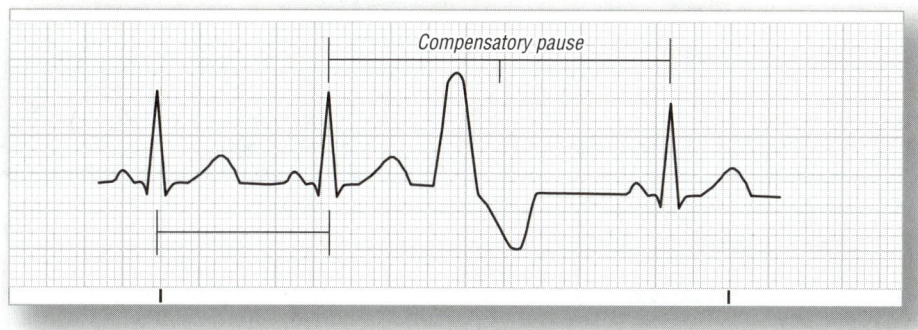

FIGURE 23.9 Ventricular rhythms: premature ventricular contraction (PVC).

(Reprinted from Garcia TB, Miller GT, *Arrhythmia Recognition: The Art of Interpretation.* Sudbury, MA: Jones and Bartlett Publishers, Inc., 2004.)

erally resistant to treatment. Potentially treatable causes of PEA include tension pneumothorax, hypovolemia, hypoxemia, severe acidosis, cardiac tamponade, ventricular rupture, drug overdoses (tricyclic antidepressants or TCAs, digoxin, calcium channel blockers), pulmonary emboli, hypothermia, and hypo- or hyperkalemia.

Treatment is directed at the identification and alleviation of the underlying causes. Epinephrine and atropine (if the rate is less than 60 bpm) are also utilized to total dose of 0.4 mg/kg (**Table 23.13**).

Asystole

Ventricular asystole occurs when there is an absence of ventricular electrical activity. Since no electrical activity is present, ventricular depolarization cannot occur, and thus there is no ventricular contraction or cardiac output. The ECG generally demonstrates a "flat line," though occasionally P waves or wide, irregular complexes (agonal beats) may occur. Asystole should be documented in at least two different leads because fine VF may be mistakenly identified as asystole. Asystole is the most common dysrhythmia seen in pa-

tients sustaining cardiac arrest of greater than 10 minutes. Etiologies of asystole include hypothermia, hypoxemia, severe acidosis, hypo/hyperkalemia, electrical shocks, and drug overdoses. The patient is unresponsive and pulseless.

Treatment of asystole consists of addressing potential treatable causes. Additionally, transcutaneous pacing, epinephrine, and atropine are utilized. However, it should be noted that asystole is a preterminal rhythm that rarely responds to treatment. Cessation of resuscitative measures should be considered (**Table 23.14**).

Torsades de Pointes

Torsades de pointes is an atypical form of VT in which the QRS axis appears to be constantly changing. The ECG generally demonstrates a rate of 200 to 240 bpm with the QRS axis alternating between positive and negative in the same lead. Torsades de pointes usually occurs in short bursts (<15 seconds). The QT interval of the beats preceding torsades de pointes is usually prolonged.

Torsades de pointes is felt to be secondary to a triggered automaticity mechanism. Drugs that may precipitate torsades de pointes are type IA antidysrhythmics (e.g., quinidine, procainamide, disopyramide), TCAs, phenothiazines, and organophosphates. Electrolyte imbalances such as hypomagnesemia, hypokalemia, and hypocalcemia may also contribute to the onset of torsades de pointes. Other etiologic factors are myocardial ischemia/infarction, hypothyroidism, myocarditis, mitral valve prolapse, left ventricular failure, and severe bradycardias.

Table 23.12

Treatment of Premature Ventricular Contractions

Often do not require treatment
If treatment is indicated, first priority is to restore adequate oxygenation and perfusion
Supplemental oxygen
Support blood pressure
If significantly bradycardic, increase heart rate (pacemaker, atropine)
Amiodarone 150 mg over 15 minutes (if successful may begin continuous drip of 1.0 to 2.0 mg/min)
Lidocaine 1.0 to 1.5 mg/kg bolus (may repeat q 5 min to total dose of 3.0 mg/kg); if successful, may begin continuous infusion of 1.0-4.0 mg/min
Procainamide 20 to 30 mg/min (to total dose of 17 mg/kg); if successful, may begin continuous infusion of 1.0 to 4.0 mg/min

---

Table 23.13

Treatment of Pulseless Electrical Activity

Search for and correct underlying causes
Epinephrine 1.0 mg IV (may repeat q 5 min if dysrhythmia persists)
If rate is < 60/min:
Atropine 0.5 to 1.0 mg IV (may repeat at 5 min intervals if heart remains below 60 bpm, not to exceed a total dose of 3 mg.)

Table 23.14

Treatment of Asystole

Identify and treat potential correctable causes
Transcutaneous pacemaker (if considered, use early)
Epinephrine 1.0 mg IV (may repeat q 5 min if
 dysrhythmia persists)
Atropine 0.5 to 1.0 mg IV (may repeat to total dose of
 0.4 mg/kg)
Consider termination of resuscitative measures

Initial treatment consists of removing or alleviating underlying causes. Accelerating the heart rate to a rate greater than the torsades de pointes (overdrive pacing) is the most effective treatment. Magnesium sulfate has also been demonstrated to be effective (**Table 23.15**).

Conduction Blocks

Sick Sinus Syndrome

Sick sinus syndrome (SSS), also known as tachy-brady syndrome, is a clinical entity that involves both intermittent tachydysrhythmias and bradydysrhythmias. Common tachydysrhythmias include atrial fibrillation, atrial flutter, re-entrant SVTs, and junctional tachycardias. The bradydysrhythmias commonly seen include severe sinus bradycardias and sinus and AV blocks.

The etiology of SSS includes rheumatologic diseases (e.g., sarcoidosis), rheumatic heart disease, ischemia, myocarditis, pericarditis, cardiomyopathy, and cardiac surgery. A variety of medications (digoxin, quinidine) and medical conditions (hyperthyroidism, electrolyte imbalances) can potentiate the tachy- or bradydysrhythmias.

Symptoms such as palpitations, syncope, dyspnea, and chest discomfort may be precipitated by the dysrhythmias. As the dysrhythmias are intermittent, continuous cardiac monitoring either in the inpatient or outpatient setting may be necessary to make the diagnosis. Treatment is directed at rhythm control. Patients often require pacemaker placement to prevent untoward sequelae from the bradydysrhythmias. It is recommended that pacemaker placement be considered prior to treatment of tachydysrhythmias as the treatment may exacerbate the bradycardias.

Atrioventricular Blocks

Atrioventricular (AV) blocks are divided into first, second, and third degree. The block may occur in the AV node it-

Table 23.15

Treatment of Torsades de Pointes

Alleviate underlying causes
Overdrive pacing
Magnesium 1.0 to 2.0 g IV

Table 23.16

Treatment of First-Degree AV Block

No treatment needed, except identification and
 correction of precipitating factors

self or may be infranodal. A first-degree AV block represents a delay in AV conduction; however, all impulses are conducted. A second-degree AV block is characterized by an intermittent lack of conduction through the AV node and is further divided into Mobitz I and II AV blocks. A third-degree AV block represents complete interruption of AV conduction (AV dissociation).

First-Degree AV Block

With a first-degree AV block, there is a delay in normal AV conduction. ECG characteristics of first-degree AV block include a prolonged PR interval (>0.20 seconds); one-to-one conduction of P waves to QRS complexes; usually a regular rhythm; and normal-appearing QRS complexes. The PR interval is usually constant but may be variable (**FIGURE 23.10**).

First-degree AV blocks may be the result of myocardial infarction, myocarditis, or drug effects (digitalis). They may occur in normal individuals and are not associated with increased mortality. The patient is typically asymptomatic. There is usually no need to initiate treatment other than correcting underlying causes (**Table 23.16**).

Second-Degree AV Block, Mobitz I

Second-degree AV block, Mobitz I, also known as Wenckebach's disease, is a condition where there is progressive delay in AV conduction until there is complete block of the sinus impulse. The ECG demonstrates a progressively lengthening PR interval until a P wave is seen without a corresponding QRS complex. The P waves and QRS complexes are usually of normal morphology. The R-R intervals shorten prior to the dropped beat. Once the complete block occurs, the PR interval lessens and the pattern is repeated. Wenckebach's may occur in patterns such as 4:3, 3:2, or 2:1. The pulse will be irregular unless

Table 23.17

Treatment of Second-Degree AV Block, Mobitz I (Wenckebach)

Generally no treatment needed
Consider discontinuing drugs that may have initiated
 the block
If bradycardic and symptomatic
 Pacemaker
 Atropine 0.5 to 1.0 mg IV (may repeat q 5 min to
  total dose of 0.4 mg/kg)
 Epinephrine drip 2 to 10 μg/min
 Isoproterenol drip 2 to 10 μg/min (drug of choice
  in patients status post-heart transplant)
 Dopamine drip 2 to 20 μg/kg/min

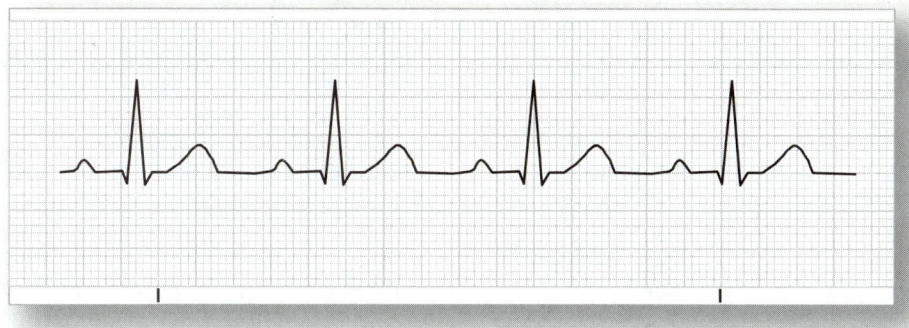

FIGURE 23.10 Heart blocks: First degree heart block.

(Reprinted from Garcia TB, Miller GT, *Arrhythmia Recognition: The Art of Interpretation*. Sudbury, MA: Jones and Bartlett Publishers, Inc., 2004.)

the pattern is 2:1. It is often difficult to initially differentiate a 2:1 Wenckebach from a second-degree AV block, Mobitz II. However, Wenckebach's is more commonly associated with a normal QRS length than is a Mobitz II block (**FIGURE 23.11**).

Wenckebach's disease is often transient and intermittent. Common causes include acute myocardial infarction, cardiac surgery, and myocarditis. Drugs such as digitalis, verapamil, and propranolol can also produce a second-degree Mobitz I AV block. Patients are usually asymptomatic and do not require treatment. If there is associated symptomatic bradycardia, atropine or pacing may be utilized (**Table 23.17**).

Second-Degree AV Block, Mobitz II

Mobitz II AV blocks occur infranodally, usually at the bundle branches and, less commonly, at the bundle of His. ECG characteristics include a normal P wave with more P waves than QRS complexes; a PR interval that may be prolonged from normal but remains constant; and an irregular ventricular rate associated with a regular atrial rate. Mobitz II AV blocks are usually seen in association with bundle branch or fascicular blocks; therefore, the QRS complexes are usually wide (**FIGURE 23.12**).

Mobitz II AV block generally represents structural damage to the conducting system below the AV node. There is a potential for the block to progress to complete heart block, particularly in the setting of myocardial ischemia/infarction.

Treatment involves increasing the ventricular rate with either atropine of pacing. Since patients with Mobitz II AV blocks can precipitously decompensate, it is advisable to have transcutaneous pacing pads in place even with the stable patient (**Table 23.18**).

Third-Degree AV Block

In third-degree AV block there is no AV conduction. The block may occur at the AV node, the bundle of His, or the bundle branches. Since no atrial impulses reach the ventricles, the ventricular response is controlled by a ventricular ectopic focus. ECG findings include a ventricular response that is slower than the atrial rate and usually regular; an atrial rate that is typically normal with normal P waves; and since the atria and ventricles are being depolarized at different rates from different foci, the PR interval is variable. If the ventricular pacemaker is located near the junction, the rhythm is typically between 40 and 60 bpm and may have a normal QRS configuration. If the ectopic pacemaker is located lower in the ventricles, the intrinsic rate will more likely be slower (<40 bpm) and be associated with widened QRS complexes.

Third-degree AV blocks occurring at the AV node may result from acute inferior myocardial infarction, structural damage to the AV node, and drug toxicities

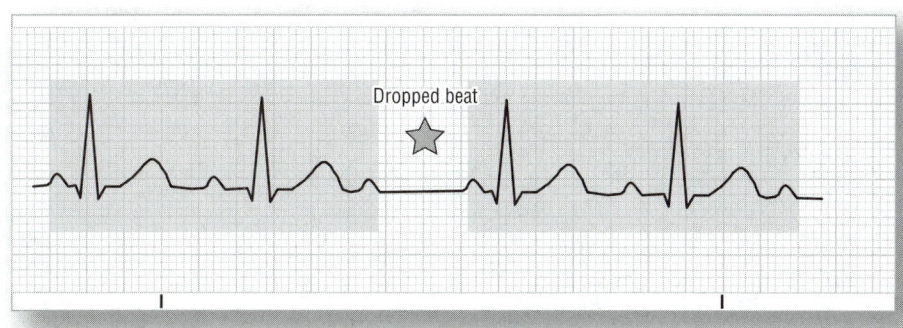

FIGURE 23.11 Second-degree heart block, Mobitz I (Wenckebach).

(Reprinted from Garcia TB, Miller GT, *Arrhythmia Recognition: The Art of Interpretation*. Sudbury, MA: Jones and Bartlett Publishers, Inc., 2004.)

Table 23.18
Treatment of Second-Degree AV Block, Mobitz II

Increase ventricular rate
  Pacemaker
  Atropine 0.5 to 1.0 mg IV (may repeat q 5 min to
    total dose of 0.4 mg/kg)
  Epinephrine drip 2 to 10 µg/min
  Isoproterenol drip 2 to 10 µg/min (drug of choice
    in patients status post-heart transplant)
  Dopamine drip 2 to 20 µg/kg/min

Table 23.19
Treatment of Third-Degree AV Block

If hemodynamically unstable
Transcutaneous pacemaker
Atropine 0.5 to 1.0 mg IV (may repeat to total dose of
  0.4 mg/kg) may not be effective since the
  mechanism of action of atropine is increasing SA
  node discharges through vagolytic action. Atropine
  may be potentially dangerous as it may cause
  increased refractoriness around AV node, therefore
  paradoxically slowing ventricular rate.
Epinephrine continuous infusion 2 to 10 µg/min
Isoproterenol drip 2 to 10 µg/min (drug of choice in
  patients status post-heart transplant)
Dopamine drip 2 to 20 µg/kg/min

(e.g., digitalis, propranolol). Infranodal blocks are most commonly associated with acute anterior myocardial infarction.

Clinical manifestations depend on the level of the block and the resulting bradycardia. Patients with blocks occurring at the AV node may initially present with stable vital signs secondary to the junctional escape rhythm, which may maintain perfusion. These patients should have transcutaneous pacemakers at the bedside as they may decompensate, particularly in the setting of ongoing ischemia/infarction. Patients presenting with infranodal blocks generally necessitate emergent pacing as the intrinsic rate of their ectopic pacemaker is generally too slow to maintain perfusion. Atropine and catecholamines may be utilized as needed; however, pacing is preferred in the unstable patient. All patients with third-degree AV blocks should receive an evaluation by a cardiologist to determine the need for a permanent pacemaker (**Table 23.19**).

Bundle Branch Blocks

Bundle branch blocks can occur in any of the three major ventricular conduction pathways: the right bundle branch (RBB), the left anterior superior fascicle (LASF), or the left posterior inferior fascicle (LPIF). The block may involve one (unifascicular), two (bifascicular), or all three (trifascicular) pathways.

ECG characteristics of right bundle branch blocks include increased QRS width (>0.12 seconds), RSR′ in lead V1, and wide S waves in leads I, V5, and V6. Blocks

involving the LASF demonstrate QRS axis of <−45 degrees, R wave in lead I greater than that in leads II or III; a normal QRS width; deep S waves in the inferior leads; and a qR complex in lead aVL. LPIF blocks present with a normal QRS duration; QRS axis > 110 degrees; deep S and small R in lead I; R wave in lead III greater than that in lead II; and a qR complex in lead III. Left bundle branch blocks (LBBB) have the following ECG findings: a wide QRS (>0.12 seconds); large R waves in leads I, aVL, V5, and V6; small r and deep S waves in leads II, III, aVF, VI, and V3; and no q waves in leads I, aVF, V5, and V6.

Bundle branch blocks may be the result of ischemia, myocarditis, surgery, cardiomyopathy, valvular disease, and congenital conditions. Bifascicular and trifascicular blocks are associated with severe heart disease. In the presence of ongoing ischemia/infarction, patients with these blocks are at increased risk of developing third-degree heart block and should be treated with pacemakers.

Summary

Diseases of the cardiac conduction system, manifested as cardiac dysrhythmias, are commonly encountered clinical

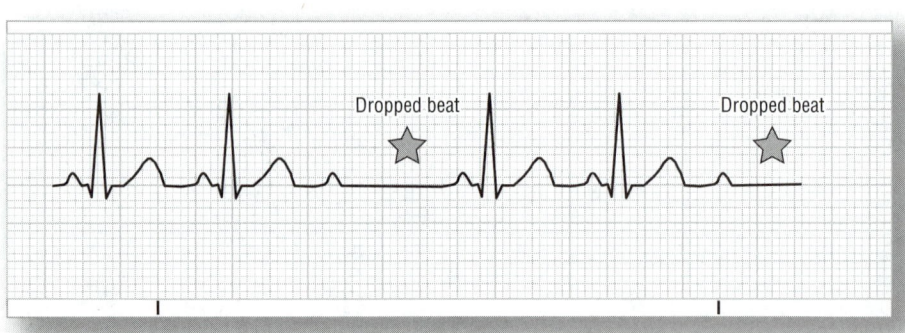

FIGURE 23.12 Second-degree heart block, Mobitz II.

(Reprinted from Garcia TB, Miller GT, *Arrhythmia Recognition: The Art of Interpretation*. Sudbury, MA: Jones and Bartlett Publishers, Inc., 2004.)

entities in the emergency department. Patients presenting with cardiac dysrhythmias may demonstrate little to no clinical effects or may present with life-threatening symptoms. Understanding of potential causes and having the ability to properly identify and treat cardiac dysrhythmias are essential skills for all emergency physicians.

Selected Readings

American Heart Association. *ACLS Provider Manual*. Dallas, TX: American Heart Association 2001.

Capucci A, Aschieri D, Piepoli MF, et al. Tripling survival from sudden cardiac arrest via early defibrillation without traditional education in cardiopulmonary resuscitation. *Circulation* 2002;106:1065–1070.

Dorian P, Cass D, Schwartz B, et al. Amiodarone as compared with lidocaine for shock-resistant ventricular fibrillation. *N Engl J Med* 2002;346:884–890.

Faddy SC, Powell J, Craig JC. Biphasic and monophasic shocks for transthoracic defibrillation: Meta-analyis of randomized controlled trials. *Resuscitation* 2003; 58:9–16.

Hoffmann T. Clinical application of enoxaparin. *Expert Rev Cardiovasc Ther* 2004; 2:321–337.

Joglar JA, Kowal RC. Electrical cardioversion of atrial fibrillation. *Cardiol Clin* 2004;22:101–111.

Krismer AC, Wenzel V, Stadlbauer KH, et al. Vasopressin during cardiopulmonary resuscitation: A progress report. *Crit Care Med* 2004;32:432–435.

Lobel RM, Lustgarten DL. Treatment of arrhythmias in patients with congestive heart failure. *Curr Treat Options Cardiovasc Med* 2004;6:519–529.

Somberg JC, Bailin SJ, Haffajee CI, et al. Intravenous lidocaine versus intravenous amiodarone (in a new aqueous formulation) for incessant ventricular tachycardia. *Am J Cardiol* 2002;90:853–859.

24 Hypertension

Gary Setnik
Arshad Khan

Introduction

Hypertension is one of the most common illnesses in the Western world. It is a major cause of office visits and prescription drug use. Due to a lack of symptoms and the requirement of sometimes painful or difficult lifestyle changes, most patients are unwilling to either seek care or to exercise due diligence. Hypertension is, therefore, a frequent problem encountered in the emergency department (ED). Since rapid identification and treatment of hypertension is associated with a critical difference in patient outcome, it is incumbent upon the emergency physician to be thoroughly familiar with the evaluation and treatment of all aspects of this condition.

Blood pressure should be checked in a standardized manner, with several readings over a period of time, before diagnosing hypertension. The use of blood pressure measurements using inexpensive semi-automatic or automatic machines should be encouraged to provide an improved baseline. Indeed, the rationale for obtaining blood pressure in normal healthy people presenting to the ED for reasons unrelated to hypertension has been questioned.

The following conditions should be met for obtaining blood pressure: patient relaxation (to prevent "white coat hypertension"); no alcohol, tobacco, caffeine, or food for a half hour prior to examination; an empty bladder; a sitting patient with arm resting on a table and the cuff at heart level. Of course, the circumstances of practice emergency medicine may well prevent any or all of these conditions to be met.

Definitions and Overview

The traditional classification of hypertension into mild, moderate, and severe categories, arbitrarily based on blood pressure recordings, is no longer used. Traditional classification has been replaced by a new standard based on the risk of developing cardiovascular disease (**Table 24.1**). Men and blacks overall have a higher prevalence of hypertension as compared to women and whites, although the incidence of hypertension in women accelerates in young adulthood and middle age. Blacks and whites in the southeastern U.S. have a higher risk for hypertensive stroke than do similar populations elsewhere. Blacks have more severe disease, with greater mortality, across all income strata. These demographic differences apply to both primary and malignant forms of the disease. Severe disease is generally more common in the middle aged with peak incidence occurring between 40 to 50 years. Improvements in the early recognition and treatment of hypertensive patients have led to a much lower incidence of severe complicated disease, but it still occurs quite frequently, especially in the underserved or those who are non-compliant with their treatment regimen. Over the last two decades, there has been a steady increase in the number of patients aware of their condition, those taking medication, and those with controlled hypertension. This has resulted in dramatic decreases in the cardiovascular mortality (50%) and stroke (75%) over the same time span.

The ED management of hypertension can be broadly divided into three categories, depending upon the level of treatment required: 1) emergencies, 2) urgencies (severe hypertension), and 3) uncomplicated and transient hypertension.

Hypertensive Emergencies

The presence of "target" or end organ damage, or dysfunction, with elevated blood pressure is a hypertensive emergency. The brain, heart, kidneys and large arteries constitute end organs. The treatment goal is to reduce blood pressure within an hour. Diastolic blood pressure, in these cases, will generally exceed 120 mm Hg. There are, however, circumstances where end organ damage can occur with seemingly mild to moderate elevations of blood pressure. Less than 1% of all hypertensive patients ever experience a hypertensive crisis. However, given the large number of patients with the disease, this still represents a significant segment of the population.

Untreated severe or malignant hypertension has a dismal prognosis. Mortality rates approaching 90% within one year have been reported. Uremia, stroke, congestive heart failure, and myocardial infarction account for the vast majority of deaths, while severe complications, such as aortic dissection, are less common. The degree of renal involvement is a good prognostic indicator of the severity of hypertension. While it is true that hypertension affects every organ system, in a critical situation, signs and symp-

Table 24.1		
Classification of Blood Pressure for Adults (JNC7)		
BP Classification	**SBP mm Hg**	**DBP mm Hg**
Normal	<120	and <80
Prehypertension	120–139	or 80–89
Stage 1 hypertension	140–159	or 90–99
Stage 2 hypertension	≥160	or ≥100

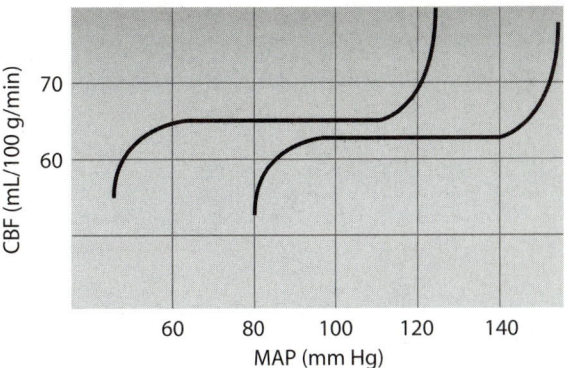

FIGURE 24.1 Cerebral blood flow and mean arterial blood pressure in normal (left curve) and hypertensive (right curve) patients.

toms of failure of one organ system may predominate, hence the classification. The clinical syndromes that will be discussed generally coexist, in the same patient, to varying degrees.

Hemodynamics and Pathophysiology

Blood pressure is a function of a complex interplay between cardiac output and resistance of the systemic vascular bed. Cardiac is dependent upon heart rate and stroke volume. Stroke volume is affected by pre-load, after-load, and the inotropic state of the heart. Systemic vascular resistance is a function of peripheral vascular resistance, which, in turn, is determined by complex neurohumoral control and renal vascular resistance. Under resting conditions, arteriolar tone is the major determinant of arterial pressure, while cardiac output plays a major role during muscular exercise. A useful concept is the determination of mean arterial pressure (MAP), which is the average pressure during a cardiac cycle. It is a geometric mean that takes into consideration both magnitude and duration of the pressure pulse and can be roughly represented by the equation: MAP = diastolic pressure + $\frac{1}{3}$ pulse pressure.

The degree of end organ damage is not entirely dependent on the absolute degree of BP elevation, but is also related to control of baseline blood pressure, the rapidity of rise of blood pressure from that baseline, as well as age and gender. Chronically hypertensive patients may not exhibit end organ dysfunction until diastolic pressure is over 140 mm. In a previously normotensive patient, however, even modest blood pressure elevation may precipitate complications. Patients at risk for neurological, renal, and cardiac complications are children with acute glomerulonephritis, young women with eclampsia, and patients who discontinue their normal regimen of anti-hypertensive medication. Diastolic pressures as low as 100 mm Hg have been known to precipitate complications in these circumstances.

In an effort to render effective treatment, concepts of autoregulation and perfusion (especially cerebral) should be well understood. Cerebral blood flow (CBF) is maintained within specific limits in normal patients. The same is true for hypertensive patients, although the limits are reset at a higher level of MAP, the so-called "shift to right" (**FIGURE 24.1**). Normal CBF is in the range of 50–60 mL/min/100 gm of brain. If MAP falls below the lower limits of autoregulation, normal vasodilatory compensation fails, leading to diminished CBF. Similarly, a MAP exceeding the upper limit of autoregulation overcomes the compensating vasoconstrictor response, resulting in a forced pressure vasodilatation. In a normotensive individual, this autoregulatory mechanism is primarily controlled by blood carbon dioxide concentrations. At extremes of blood pressure fluctuations, neurohormonal mechanisms usurp control of autoregulation. Normal aging impairs this compensatory mechanism, and patients with prior cerebral vascular disease (e.g., hypertensive encephalopathy, stroke, TIA, etc.) are at even greater risk. Minor reductions in BP can lead to profound CNS hypoperfusion, causing syncope, stroke, and cerebral infarction.

Management Principles

A systematic but rapid evaluation is required in the ED for a severely hypertensive patient. End organ dysfunction should be ascertained rapidly by detailed history, physical examination, laboratory data and imaging studies. Attempts at uncovering secondary causes of hypertension should be made after end organ damage has been excluded. Simple rest and relief of anxiety may suffice to reduce blood pressure.

History

The duration of hypertension, compliance with treatment plans and past history of emergency or urgency are elicited (**Table 24.2**). History of cigarette smoking, genetic predisposition, and use of oral contraceptives should be sought in the initial encounter with the patient. History of current or recent use of medications known to cause hypertension is sought as well as discontinuance of anti-hypertensive drugs. Nonspecific symptoms, such as dizziness, blurred vision, headache and anorexia, should be correlated with funduscopic examination. Concurrent chronic illness may also cause a predisposition for hypertension. Symptoms of cardiovascular decompensation such as chest pain or dyspnea may indicate end organ damage. A history of seizures, stroke, focal neurological deficits, or acutely altered mental state are indicative of CNS dysfunction.

Table 24.2

Conditions Predisposing to Hypertensive Crises

Acute elevation of blood pressure in a previously well controlled hypertensive
Renovascular disease
History of pregnancy and toxemia
Acute nephritis or history of parenchymal renal disease
Pheochromocytoma
Head injury
Withdrawal from antihypertensive
Burns
Autoimmune disorders
Concurrent drug use known to cause hypertension (MAO inhibitors, sympathomimetics, cocaine, antihistamines/decongestants and other anticholinergics, tricyclic antidepressants, oral contraceptives, NSAIDs, non-selective β-blockers in hypoglycemic patients and ergots

Examination

A detailed examination of the CNS, renal, cardiovascular, and pulmonary systems should be performed, searching for clues of end organ damage. Funduscopic examination is often useful, as well as documentation of the patients mental state. A finding of abdominal or flank bruits may be indicative of renal stenosis as the cause of hypertension. Rales, murmurs, and jugular venous engorgement are signs of ventricular failure. A brief neurological examination may reveal a focal process.

Laboratory

A complete blood count, chemistry profile, renal function tests and urinalysis should be performed on all patients if a hypertensive emergency is suspected. Proteinuria and microangiopathic hematuria are clues to renal damage and complications. Urine should be sampled for the presence of cocaine and amphetamine by-products, if indicated. Renin and aldosterone levels, while probably neither immediately helpful nor available, should be obtained prior to commencing treatment. An EKG may determine the presence of myocardial ischemia or strain and a chest x-ray may show pulmonary edema or aortic dissection. If dissection is a significant consideration, more advanced imaging (i.e., CT, MRI, TEE) may be appropriate. CT scan of the head is mandatory if signs of CNS dysunction are present.

Therapy

Treatment should be guided by the principle of reducing blood pressure to safe levels, in a timely fashion, and preventing ongoing end organ damage, while not provoking further ischemia by too rapid a reduction in blood pressure. Each patient has to be evaluated individually and treatment focused on the organ involved, for example, in a patient with aortic dissection the pressure needs to be reduced immediately while a patient with stroke may need gradual reduction.

The criteria for selection of antihypertensive drugs should be based not only on the pathophysiology of the underlying condition, but should also include consideration of the route of administration (intravenous versus oral), availability of monitoring systems, onset and duration of action, effects on cardiac rate and output, renal blood flow, systemic vascular resistance and side effects. Older drugs, such as diazoxide and trimethaphan, are no longer used routinely, and have been replaced by drugs from all the major classes of antihypertensive medications. These drugs are generally shorter acting, easily titratable, and less toxic.

Patients with CNS involvement ideally need an agent that decreases systemic vascular resistance without affecting cardiac output or cerebral blood flow. These include nitroprusside, fenoldopam, selective β-blockers (labetalol) and calcium channel antagonists. Fenoldopam is a recently approved dopamine-receptor agonist that is administered intravenously. Its advantages are that it doesn't require extremely close intra-arterial monitoring or the need to maintain the solution in darkness as it doesn't cause thiocyanate toxicity.

Situations where immediate relief from hypertension is required in minutes include aortic dissection, acute pulmonary edema, and unstable angina, anti-coagulated patients, crisis from pheochromocytoma and tyramine-MAO inhibitor reaction. Nitroprusside, fenoldopam, nitrates, labetalol and phentolamine are all appropriate in this group of patients. Hypertension complicating pregnancy (eclampsia) will require use of drugs (e.g., magnesium sulphate, hydralazine and methyldopa) not normally used for other hypertensive crises, as the safety issues of the newer drugs regarding the fetus have not been resolved.

Hypertensive CNS Disorders

Malignant and Accelerated Hypertension

This is defined as hypertension with diastolic blood pressure exceeding 120 mm Hg with retinopathy and papilledema. A host of factors are held responsible for converting stable and controlled blood pressure to the malignant type (**Table 24.3**).

A deadly combination of increased vascular tone, high levels of vasoactive substances (angiotensin II, norepinephrine, ADH), diminished vasodilating hormones, and substances leading to increased urinary water and sodium loss, is responsible for malignant transformation of benign hypertension. In fact, onset of malignant transformation may be heralded by a natriuresis.

A vicious cycle of increased vascular hyper-reactivity, most pronounced in renal efferent vessels, leads to higher glomerular filtration and forced diuresis. Timely replenishment of these losses may interrupt the cycle, and sodium and water restriction are, therefore, contraindicated in patients with malignant hypertension.

The pathological lesion in malignant hypertension is a fibrinoid necrosis with proliferative endarteritis. There is a loss of structural integrity, due to necrosis, of the vessel with focal areas of dilatation, alternating with constric-

Table 24.3

Associated Factors for Development of Malignant Hypertension

Severe hypertension—high baseline levels, rapidity of rise, target organ damage

Genetic predisposition

Smoking

High circulating levels of renin, angiotensin II, ADH and catecholamines

Immunologic abnormalities

Diminished natural vasodilators—kininogens, kinins, and prostacyclins

tion. Deposition of fibroblasts on the damaged intima and generalized edema causes a marked thickening of the vessel wall. There is a loss of normal compensatory mechanisms, and a sudden surge in blood pressure may lead to malignant hypertension.

These changes are usually apparent on fundoscopy arteriovenous (AV) "nicking." This is a result of dilatation and hypertrophy of retinal arterioles compressing normal venules with distal dilatation of venule at "crossing points." Eventually, high arteriolar pressure will cause flame-shaped hemorrhages around the optic disc as blood escapes from the vessels. Retinal exudates are seen, signifying cellular death with protein leakage. With intracranial pressure exceeding venous pressure, papilledema ensues, manifested as loss of venous pulsations, generalized hyperemia, obscured disc margins and increased cup-to-disc ratio.

Patients with malignant hypertension present most commonly with headache (85%), which is often worst in the morning, and usually occipital or frontal. Blurred vision, loss of acuity, and blindness may also occur. Confusion, neurological deficits, excessive sleepiness, depressed sensorium, convulsions, and ultimately coma, may be present.

Hypertensive Encephalopathy

This condition is caused by ischemia of the brain, secondary to failure of protective auto-regulatory mechanisms. The collapse of normal compensatory mechanisms responsible for arteriolar constriction and dilation to maintain a constant flow of blood to the brain, when MAP fluctuates over a wide range, leads to ischemia and encephalopathy. This mechanism may become impaired with aging, chronic hypertension, and cerebral vascular disease. Elevation of the blood pressure, past a certain threshold, causes failure of protective arteriolar constriction with resulting dilatation and flooding of the brain with transudate leading to cerebral edema. Postmortem examinations reveal petechial hemorrhages, microinfarcts, edema, and mural thrombi of the brain. Microscopic damage to the intima leads to fibrinoid necrosis, and a loss of the ability of vessels to respond to the pressure surge. Retinal examination reveals this as segmental spasm and "sausage linking" of arterioles, loss of flow, and hemor-

rhages. Since carbon dioxide tension regulates CBF, hypercapnea and acidosis will accelerate cerebral edema, hence, the nocturnal development of symptoms of encephalopathy. Use of opiates, sedatives, and respiratory depressants should be avoided in patients at risk.

The onset of hypertensive encephalopathy may be insidious, and often progresses over several days. These patients will typically have headache, dizziness, nausea, vomiting, aphasia, transient hemiparesis, nystagmus, confusion, somnolence, apprehension and anxiety, visual disturbance, loss of acuity, and even blindness. Retinal examination will show papilledema, arteriolar spasm and hemorrhages. If not treated promptly, the patient may have seizures, increasing CNS metabolic demands, and eventually deteriorate into coma. The blood pressure in these cases can be extremely high (greater than 250/150 mm Hg). Children frequently have abdominal symptoms and vomiting, occasionally projectile, and unless the blood pressure is checked (frequently overlooked) the diagnosis may be missed entirely. It has been shown that blood pressure, over a 24-hour period, in patients with benign hypertension may not be very different than in malignant hypertension, and indeed may be higher. As always, the total clinical picture should be considered and the dictum, "treat the patient, not the disease" should be followed. Hypertensive encephalopathy is a diagnosis of exclusion. Stroke syndromes, such as intracranial hemorrhage, thrombosis, and embolism, must be ruled out by CT or MR imaging prior to instituting treatment.

The treatment of hypertensive encephalopathy is based on the principle of decreasing blood pressure to allow the patient's inherent autoregulatory mechanisms to resume functioning. A precipitous fall, past the lower limits of autoregulation, may provoke worsening ischemia, and has been known to cause stroke, blindness, paraplegia, and may precipitate myocardial infarction. A 25% reduction in the MAP is a reasonable goal.

The ideal drug for this condition should maintain cerebral blood flow, have rapid onset of action, last a short time, and not adversely affect the heart or other organs. Nitroprusside is the drug of choice for hypertensive encephalopathy. Optimally this will require admission to intensive care and insertion of arterial catheters for continuous blood pressure readings. Fenoldopam is an attractive alternative, as it does not require cumbersome monitoring and special tubing, is titratable, and does not cause thiocyanate toxicity. The second-line alternatives are labetalol, nicardipine, and esmolol, administered intravenously, as an infusion, or in boluses. The majority of patients with hypertensive crises are volume depleted and do not require diuretics, unless volume overload can be specifically documented. There may be reflex volume retention after several days of non-diuretic anti-hypertensive therapy, at which time diuretics can be administered.

Stroke

Hypertension is the major risk factor for stroke. It has been well documented that long term control of hypertension will reduce the incidence and severity of stroke. Treatment of hypertension in the post-stroke period is,

Table 24.4

Parenteral Drugs for Treatment of Hypertensive Emergencies*

Drug	Dose	Onset of Action	Duration of Action	Adverse Effects†	Special Indications
VASODILATORS					
Sodium nitroprus-side	0.25–10 µg/kg/min as IV infusion‡	Immediate 1–2 min	Nausea, vomiting, muscle twitching, sweating, thiocy-anate and cyanide intoxication	Most hypertensive emergencies; caution with	High intracranial pressure or azotemia
Nicardipine hydrochlo-ride	5–15 mg/h IV	5–10 min	15–30 min, may exceed 4 h	Tachycardia, headache, flushing, local phlebitis	Most hypertensive emergencies except acute heart failure; caution with coronary ischemia
Fenoldopam mesylate	0.1–0.3 µg/kg per min IV infusion	5 min	30 min	Tachycardia, headache, nausea, flushing	Most hypertensive emergencies; caution with glaucoma
Nitroglycerin	5–100 µg/min as IV infu-sion§	2–5 min	5–10 min	Headache, vomiting methemo-globinemia, tolerance with prolonged use	Coronary ischemia
Enalaprilat	1.25–5 mg every 6 h IV	15–30 min	6–12 h	Precipitous fall in pressure in high-renin states; variable response	Acute left ventricular failure; avoid in acute myocardial infarction
Hydralazine hydrochlo-ride	10–20 mg IV, 10–20 mg IM	10–20 min IV, 20–30 min IM	1–4 h IV, 4–6 h IM	Tachycardia, flushing, headache, vomiting, aggravation of angina	Eclampsia
ADRENERGIC INHIBITORS					
Labetalol hydrochlo-ride	20–80 mg IV bolus every 10 min, 0.5–2.0 mg/min IV infusion	5–10 min	3–6 h	Vomiting, scalp tingling, broncho-constriction, dizziness, nausea, heart block, orthostatic hypo-tension	Most hypertensive emergencies except acute heart failure
Esmolol hydrochlo-ride	250–500 µg/kg/min IV bolus, then 50–100 µg/kg/min by in-fusion; may repeat bolus after 5 min or increase infusion to 300 µg/min	1–2 min	10–30 min	Hypotension, nausea, asthma, first-degree heart block, HF	Aortic dissection, perioperative
Phentolamine	5–15 mg IV bolus	1–2 min	10–30 min	Tachycardia, flushing, headache	Catecholamine excess

*These doses may vary from those in the Physicians' Desk Reference (51st edition).
†Hypotension may occur with all agents.
‡Requires special delivery system.

however, controversial. While the cause and effect relationship is not clear, blood pressure is frequently elevated in acute stroke, with higher incidence of death. This hypertension usually declines over several days in the post-stroke period, and whether it is the cause of increased mortality is not known.

It has been shown that ischemic stroke will result in an area of severe ischemia immediately surrounding a blocked artery. Areas of brain farther away from this central area, the penumbra, may then be subject to relative ischemia, where there is a temporary cessation of function, with potential return to viability. This is dependent on persisting high cerebral perfusion pressures, and any decrease in this pressure may put this area at risk.

An argument for acutely decreasing arterial pressure in syndromes of intracerebral and subarachnoid hemorrhage can be made; however, the same general principles still hold true: High blood pressure levels may be necessary to maintain brain viability and therapy should be guided by these principles.

Very high blood pressure can be lowered by judicious use of agents that optimally have very few CNS effects and that are short acting. Blood pressure should be reduced gingerly (approximately 20% of MAP) and if there is any worsening of neurological deficit, this treatment should be suspended immediately. This will necessitate use of drugs such as sodium nitroprusside, fenoldopam, or labetalol. These drugs need to be administered intravenously and require an intensive care setting with arterial blood pressure monitoring (**Table 24.4**).

Hypertensive Cardiovascular Complications

Acute Aortic Dissection

About 2,000 new cases (5 to 10 per million) of aortic dissection occur annually in the U.S. It is a catastrophic event that kills 25% of victims within 24 hours and 90% within a year. Hypertension is responsible for more than 50% of the cases, but Marfan's syndrome, Ehlers Danlos syndrome, bicuspid aortic valve, coarctation, luetic aortitis, and pregnancy are other causative factors. Cystic medial degeneration with loss of cohesiveness between layers of aortic wall can initiate dissection. There is a sudden tear of aortic intima with extravasation of blood into the media of the aorta. Anatomical (rigid sternum and vertebral column) and hydrodynamic (dP/dTmax) factors subject the proximal aorta to maximal flexion and shearing stress. With each heartbeat, blood dissects for varying distances in either direction, occluding various ostia in the affected segment and stretching the aortic root. Depending upon the area(s) involved, any number of injuries may occur: acute hemopericardium, acute aortic incompetence, myocardial infarction, stroke, paraplegia, intestinal infarction, and ischemic extremities.

Aortic dissection is classified into three types, depending upon the location of intimal injury: Type I (proximal) is most common with the intimal tear just distal to coronary take-off and extends distally to involve the arch and descending aorta to a varying distance; Type II (proximal)

is similar to Type I, but spares the arch; and Type III (distal) where the intimal tear is located distal to left subclavian artery and dissects distally.

Patients with aortic dissection usually complain of acute and severe pain that is maximal at onset and often described as "tearing" or "ripping." It may be present in the anterior chest or in the interscapular area and is often not controlled with opiates. Depending upon the degree of distal aortic involvement there may be acute neurological deficits, back pain, abdominal pain or extremity pain. There may be a significant difference in blood pressure between the two upper extremities, indicating partial compression of a subclavian artery. New aortic valvular murmurs may be heard and a chest x-ray may show mediastinal widening, hemothorax/effusion, or extension of the aortic shadow beyond atherosclerotic calcium deposition. If dissection is suspected then diagnosis should be made rapidly utilizing any one of the available modalities. These include CT and MRI scanning, aortography, and echocardiography.

It is vital to immediately lower blood pressure to prevent further dissection. Systolic blood pressure should be reduced to less than 110 mm Hg with nitroprusside, and the shearing stress (dP/dTmax) on the aorta should be relieved by administering β-blocking agents such as propranolol, labetalol or esmolol. Dissection of Types I, II, and complicated Type III will require surgical repair, while treatment of uncomplicated Type III is controversial and is often treated medically.

Acute Coronory Syndrome and Acute Pulmonary Edema

Chronic hypertension commonly results in left ventricular hypertrophy and strain. These patients frequently have coronary artery disease, increased oxygen demands, and depressed ejection fraction. Any disruptions caused by a sudden increase in blood pressure may cause unstable angina, myocardial infarction, and pulmonary edema.

Therapeutic interventions are governed by the need to reduce cardiac work or oxygen demand, and to preserve myocardial tissue by enhancing coronary perfusion. Decreasing heart rate, after-load, pre-load, and wall tension accomplish these. Intravenous nitroglycerin and nitroprusside are first-line drugs for the critically ill. Oral ACE inhibitors like captopril or enalaprilat can also be used. Captopril can be used orally or sublingually. Intravenous nesiritide, a natriuretic peptide that is also a vasodilator and a diuretic has recently been approved for use in refractory hypertension with acute pulmonary edema. The early use of high-dose furosemide has been questioned and has been implicated in worsening hypertension. It should be avoided as a first-line drug unless volume overload is suspected. Drugs inducing tachycardia are contraindicated. While β-blocking agents are of benefit in chronic congestive heart failure patients, they should generally not be used in acute pulmonary edema.

Hypertensive Renal Crises

Underlying renal dysfunction is a major cause of hypertension in African Americans and the young. While progression of uncontrolled chronic hypertension is the most common cause, acute glomerulonephritis, IgA nephropathy, vasculitides, and renal artery stenosis may accelerate the process.

The presence of fibrinoid necrosis and proliferative endarteritis in the afferent arteriole may result in its total occlusion. Higher perfusion pressure is required, eventually leading to endothelial damage, manifested by marked proteinuria and microscopic hematuria.

ACE inhibitors should be used with caution as acute renal failure may have resulted in elevated potassium levels. If signs of encephalopathy predominate, parenterally administered rapidly acting agents such as nitroprusside, are indicated. Renal artery lesions may require angioplasty and stenting.

Pre-Eclampsia and Eclampsia

Normal pregnancy is characterized by a gradual reduction in blood pressure. Beginning around the 20th week of gestation it gradually returns to normal levels at term. Diastolic readings of 75 mm Hg and 85 mm Hg in the second and third trimester, respectively, are the upper limits of normal. As is evident, these values are lower than those considered normal for the non-pregnant adult. An increase in systolic pressure of more than 30 mm Hg and a similar increase of 15 mm Hg in the diastolic reading, over normal baseline blood pressure, indicates the presence of hypertension. The patient may also develop edema and proteinuria, in which case the definition of pre-eclampsia is met. However, the sudden rise in blood pressure in itself justifies the use of aggressive monitoring and treatment.

Women at risk for developing pre-eclampsia are those with chronic hypertension, molar pregnancy, diabetes mellitus, nulliparity, renal insufficiency, and prior gestational hypertension.

Pre-eclamptic patients who develop seizures, with or without coma, indicate that the patient has eclampsia. The pre-term phase of pregnancy is when most eclamptic fits occur, however they can occur well into the first three weeks of the postpartum period.

The definitive treatment for pre-eclampsia and eclampsia is delivery of the fetus. The preferred method is vaginally, to avoid the stress of surgery and anaesthesia. Intravenous magnesium sulphate is used for control of seizures. Benzodiazepines and phenytoin are second line drugs. Hydralazine, used parenterally, is the drug of choice for control of hypertension. Labetalol can also be used safely, although nitroprusside use past four hours can cause fetal cyanide toxicity, and should be avoided generically. A more extended discussion of pre-eclampsia and eclampsia may be found in Chapter 84.

Pediatric Hypertension

A diagnosis of hypertension is made when the BP remains elevated on repeated measurement at the 95th percentile or greater for age, height, and gender, in the pediatric and adolescent population (**Table 24.5**).

Younger children will tend to have secondary causes of hypertension while adolescents are prone to essential hypertension. Children will present with nonspecific symptoms, such as poor feeding and growth, and behavioral problems. Acute elevations may result in vomiting, abdominal crises. It is essential that blood pressure be checked as a routine in all children. Substance abuse as a cause of severe hypertension should be considered in the adolescent.

The approach to treatment is the same as for adults. Nitroprusside, labetalol, and phentolamine are the first line drugs, preferably in an intensive care setting.

Drugs Used to Treat Hypertensive Emergency

Sodium Nitroprusside (SNP)

SNP is a potent direct-acting vasodilator, reducing preload by venodilatation of capacitance vessels and afterload by general arteriolar dilatation. Its effects are manifest within a minute of starting the infusion; blood pressure response can be closely titrated, which makes it an ideal drug for acute hypertensive emergencies. SNP decreases vascular resistance and pulmonary wedge pressure, has no appreciable effect of cardiac output or rate and increases cerebral and renal blood flow. It is metabolized to cyanide and

Table 24.5

95th Percentile of Blood Pressure by Selected Ages, by the 50th and 75th Height Percentiles, and by Gender in Children and Adolescents

Age	50th Percentile for Height, Girls	75th Percentile for Height, Girls	50th Percentile for Height, Boys	75th Percentile for Height, Boys
1	104/58	105/59	102/57	104/58
6	111/73	112/73	114/74	115/75
12	123/80	124/81	123/81	125/82
17	129/84	130/85	136/87	138/88

Source: Adapted from Update on the 1987 task force report on high blood pressure in children and adolescents: a working group report from the national high blood pressure education program. *Pediatrics* 1996;98:649-658.

then to thiocyanate in the liver. Thiocyanate is excreted in the urine. Liver disease will therefore exacerbate cyanide toxicity while impaired kidney function will lead to elevated thiocyanate levels and toxicity. Prolonged administration of SNP in high doses, generally beyond 72 hours, increases the risk of toxicity, and levels of cyanide and thiocyanate should be monitored. Treatment should be augmented by the addition of antihypertensive agents from other classes of drugs (e.g., SNP reacts adversely with clonidine and methyldopa), and intravascular volume should be maintained. Potential side effects are hypotension, nausea, vomiting, apprehension, delirium, psychoses, convulsions, muscle spasms and tinnitus.

Fenoldopam

This is a dopamine receptor agonist, recently approved for parenteral use in acute hypertensive emergencies. Unlike SNP, it does not require BP monitoring with arterial catheters and the solution is stable in light. Its effect is manifest within 5 minutes and lasts for 30 minutes. It may cause reflex tachycardia, which may require β-blockade to control. Intraocular pressure tends to rise with its use. It is also expensive, although its cost may be offset by diminished monitoring requirements.

Labetalol

It is an alpha 1, β1 and β2-antagonist. It not only reduces blood pressure but also the shearing forces on the proximal aorta, which makes it particularly useful in the treatment of aortic dissection and hypertension due to high catecholamine levels (e.g., pheochromocytoma, antihypertensive drug withdrawal). It can be administered as a continuous infusion or in intravenous boluses. It may precipitate severe hypotension so close monitoring of patients is essential. It is relatively contraindicated in patients with reactive airway disease, CHF, diabetes or atrioventricular block.

Phentolamine

This is a pure alpha antagonist, with more affinity for alpha 1 receptors, and is the drug of choice for "hypercatecholamine" states. While its use has declined in recent years, it is the drug of choice for crises due to pheochromocytoma, MAO inhibitor reactions, clonidine withdrawal, cocaine and amphetamine intoxication and overdose of epinephrine preparations. It can be administered as bolus or as an infusion, and may cause profound hypotension in volume-depleted patients. Other side effects are tachycardia, nausea, vomiting, diarrhea and headache.

Hypertensive Urgency

Hypertensive urgency is a condition of markedly elevated blood pressure with no evidence of end-organ damage.

Table 24.6

Recommendations for Follow-Up Based on Initial Blood Pressure Measurements for Adults Without Acute End Organ Damage (JNC7)

Initial Blood Pressure, mm Hg*	Follow-Up Recommended†
Normal	Recheck in 2 years
Prehypertension	Recheck in 1 year‡
Stage 1 hypertension	Confirm within 2 months‡
Stage 2 hypertension	Evaluate or refer to source of care within 1 month. For those with higher pressures (e.g., 180/110 mm Hg),evaluate and treat immediately or within 1 week depending on clinical situation and complications.

*If systolic and diastolic categories are different, follow recommendations for shorter time follow-up (e.g., 160/86 mm Hg should be evaluated or referred to source of care within 1 month).
†Modify the scheduling of follow-up according to reliable information about past BP measurements.

The degree of blood pressure elevation necessary is variably defined although diastolic levels in the range of 115 to 140 have been suggested. This may be too simplistic a characterization.

The ED visit may have been prompted by an entirely unrelated problem. Frequently, the same individual may have a nearly normal BP if checked a short time later. These patients may or may not have chronic hypertension. They may have discontinued their normal antihypertensive regimen or have used substances leading to severe, but transient, BP elevation. After determining the absence of end-organ damage, the patient's prior therapy should be restarted and follow up should be arranged. If the patient has not been on antihypertensives previously, he may be started on an appropriate medication in consultation with the primary care physician with whom he will have to follow up. **Table 24.6** summarizes JNC7 recommendations for the approach to management of hypertension.

Selected Readings

The Seventh Report of The Joint National Committee on Prevention, Detection, Evaluation, and Treatment of High Blood Pressure. Washington, DC: US Department of Health and Human Services. PDF file prepared by the National Heart, Lung, and Blood Institute. December, 2003.

Shayne PH. Severely increased blood pressure in the emergency department. *Ann Emerg Med* 2003;41:513–529.

Kaplan NM. Management of hypertensive emergencies. *Lancet* 1994;344:1335–1338.

Khan IA. Clinical, diagnostic, and management perspectives of aortic dissection. *Chest* 2002;122

Peripheral Vascular Disease

John E. Gough

Luis E. Rodriguez

Peripheral Arterial Disease

Etiology/Pathophysiology

Peripheral arterial disease (PAD) is usually a manifestation of systemic atherosclerosis, where there is stenosis or occlusion of the arteries especially those of the lower legs. This ischemia prevents blood supply from meeting tissue oxygen and nutrient demands and can lead to limb loss. PAD is a widespread problem, affecting an estimated 8 to 12 million people in the U.S., and possibly just as many in Europe. The risk factors are similar to those of coronary artery disease (CAD), with potentially modifiable factors (e.g., tobacco abuse, hypertension, DM, hypercholesterolemia) and non-modifiable factors (e.g., age, sex, family history). Recently elevated homocysteine levels have been demonstrated to be a significant risk factor for CAD and PAD.[2] Not surprisingly, patients with PAD are at higher risk for angina, MI, stroke, CHF and vascular death. Patients with PAD have a sixfold risk of death from cardiovascular events. There is a similar incidence of PAD in both men and women, and the risk increases with age: PAD is present in approximately 20% to 30% of patients greater than 70 years old.[1]

Clinical Findings

Approximately 25% to 50% of patients experience claudication, which can significantly impact their quality of life. Claudication may be described as aching, fatigue, and/or discomfort in the legs associated with walking, and is generally relieved within 10 minutes of rest.[1] However, as the disease progresses the patient may also experience pain at rest. About 5% to 8% of patients will encounter severe ischemia at rest and this can lead to non-healing wounds, gangrene, amputation, and decreased survival. The feet may exhibit signs of ischemia such as discoloration, cool skin, chronic changes, skin breakdown, and decreased pulses; however, these findings are not specific for PAD.

Evaluation

The most important initial screening test is the ankle-brachial index (ABI). A standard blood pressure cuff and doppler are all that is needed to perform this test. The systolic pressure is obtained at both brachial arteries and the higher of the two is used as the denominator. Then the systolic pressure is obtained in both legs utilizing either the posterior tibial or dorsalis pedis pulse. This number is used as the numerator to determine the ABI for each leg. Values greater than 0.9 are considered normal; while those less than 0.9 suggest PAD. To improve accuracy, the ABI may be evaluated both pre- and post-exercise. Other tests that may be utilized are pulse volume recordings, exercise doppler, duplex doppler, and transcutaneous oximetry. More recently, CT angiography,[3] and MR angiography[4] are noninvasive tests that are being used to determine the degree of PAD. The above tests are usually sufficient to make the diagnosis and contrast angiography is reserved for those failing medical management, and to plan for surgical intervention.

Treatment

The initial plan of treatment is to correct modifiable risk factors, with smoking cessation being the most important. A supervised exercise program should be initiated to treat claudication. Additionally the physician should aggressively treat hypertension and diabetes. Lowering lipid has shown to be helpful with a 12% reduction in mortality in one study.[5] Antiplatelet agents such as long-term aspirin or clopidogrel are also recommended.[1] Pentoxifylline is an agent that improves red cell deformability, lowers fibrinogen, and decreases platelet aggregation. Use of this medication has been shown to increase treadmill walking; however, overall clinical benefits are questionable.[1] Cilostazol, a phosphodiesterase III inhibitor, promotes arterial vasodilatation, and has shown a positive impact on improved walking and quality of life; however, it is contraindicated if CHF is present.[1] Percutaneous angioplasty and stents may be used.[6] Surgical revascularization may be necessary if the patient fails the above methods.

Thromboembolism

Arterial Thrombosis

Etiology/Pathophysiology

Acute arterial occlusion remains a significant health problem in the U.S. It is estimated that there are at least

60,000 major limb amputations that occur in the United States every year.[1] Arterial thrombosis, thromboembolism, and PAD are the major predisposing factors to acute limb ischemia and limb loss. Other factors may include vasospasm, arterio-venous fistulas, and trauma. Additionally, some arterial thromboembolism may actually be venous in origin and cross through a patent foramen ovale.[7] Patients who present in the first six hours after the onset of symptoms are considered to have an acute occlusion.

Clinical Findings

The major symptoms of patients with an acute occlusion are pain, diminished or absent distal sensation and motor function, and loss of a peripheral pulse. On the physical exam, attention should be given to temperature demarcation, sensory and motor function, and quality or absence of pulses. An assessment of tissue perfusion (appearance, discoloration, lesions and/or ulcerations, capillary refill) should be performed.

Evaluation

If the clinical presentation is consistent with an acute occlusion, a vascular surgery should be obtained immediately. Contrast angiography, or MR or CT angiography[3,4] may be employed. So as not to delay definitive treatment, the decision on which modality utilized should cooperatively be decided upon based on a discussion with the vascular surgeon.

Treatment

Initial treatment should be supportive including adequate hydration and pain management. Heparinization may be considered, again in consultation with a vascular surgeon. Many possible treatments may be utilized, including thrombolytic (fibrinolytic) medications, catheter thrombectomy, rheolytic thrombectomy catheters, laser-assisted angioplasty, balloon angioplasty, endarterectomy, and surgical bypass.

Venous Thromboembolism

Etiology/Pathophysiology

Venous thromboembolism (VTE) remains a major health problem in the U.S. The estimated incidence of VTE in the general population is 1 to 2 per 1,000 persons per year, with a 90-day survival after onset of VTE being 69%.[8] Common disorders with VTE are deep vein thrombosis (DVT) and pulmonary embolism (PE). VTE significantly contributes to patient morbidity and mortality, with an estimated 60,000 deaths annually attributed to PE.[7] Many acquired and inherited risk factors have been identified (**Table 25.1**).[8,9]

Clinical Findings

DVT: The incidence of DVT is 2 to 3 times more frequent than that of PE. Often the initial presentation may be of discomfort in the lower calf muscles and may be misinterpreted as a simple muscle strain. As

Table 25.1	
Risk Factors for VTE	
Inherited	**Acquired**
Factor V gene mutation (G1691A) *Factor V Leiden*	Age
	Recent surgery/trauma
Prothrombin gene mutation (G20210A)	Hospitalization/immobilization
Methylenetetrahydrofolate reductase gene mutation homozygous (c677T)	Thrombophilia *Hyperhomocysteinemia*
Antithombin deficiency	*Antiphospholipid syndrome*
Protein C deficiency	*Myeloproliferative disorders*
Protein S deficiency	Antipsychotic medication use
Dysfibrinogenemia	Oral contraceptive use
Homozygous homocystinuria	Personal hx VTE
Increased levels of Factors VIII, IX, XI or fibrinogen	Obesity
	Secondary antiphospholipid syndrome
	Family hx VTE
	Smoking
	Hormone replacement therapy
	Malignancy
	Prolonged travel
	Venous catheters
	Venous insufficiency
	Pregnancy/peripartum
	CHF
	Acute MI
	Ischemic stroke

the course progresses, there is more pain in the area with associated swelling, warmth, and erythema. Commonly there is swelling and tenderness of the associated veins and a palpable cord may be present. The "Homan's sign" (increased pain and resistance to dorsiflexion of the foot) is not a reliable indicator of the presence or absence of a DVT. Other conditions to consider include cellulitis, ruptured Baker's cyst, venous insufficiency, hematoma, and trauma.

PE: There are many potential presentations of an acute PE, which can make diagnosis difficult. It is estimated that less than half of those who die from an acute PE were correctly diagnosed antemortem. The most common presenting complaints are dyspnea and tachypnea. Frequently, the patient will appear anxious and complain of pleuritic chest pain. There may be an associated cough, hemoptysis, tachycardia, and low-grade fever. Massive PE may present with right heart failure, severe dyspnea, cyanosis, syncope or sudden death. Other diagnoses to consider include acute MI, pneumonia, cardiomyopathy, myocarditis, pericarditis, costochondritis, and CHF.

Evaluation

DVT: D-dimer assays are increasingly being utilized in the evaluation of suspected DVT. There are several conditions that can falsely elevate D-dimer levels such as pregnancy, malignancies, renal failure, acute MI, and sepsis. However, a normal D-dimer level has a high negative predictive value and may be useful, particularly when the clinical suspicion of DVT is low. Duplex venous ultrasonography is commonly the initial test utilized to diagnose DVT. Ultrasonography may miss isolated calf DVTs; however, most emboli are caused by leg or pelvic thrombi. If the ultrasound is negative and clinical suspicion remains high other modalities such as pelvic CT scanning, MRI, or contrast venograms may be used.

PE: Arterial blood gases were traditionally used in the diagnosis of PE; however, neither the pO_2 nor the alveolar-arterial gradient can reliably be used to rule out a PE. As with DVT, the D-dimer assay may be useful in the setting of low clinical suspicion. An EKG should be obtained, particularly to evaluate for the presence of an acute MI. The "classic" EKG findings of PE are an S-wave in lead I, a Q-wave in lead III, and a T-wave inversion in lead III. Other possible EKG manifestations of an acute PE include right ventricular strain, right BBB, and right axis deviation. The CXR may be useful in identifying conditions that mimic PE. In approximately 25% of cases the CXR will be completely normal, and a normal CXR in the setting of significant dyspnea should increase the physician's suspicion for the possibility of PE. The "classic" findings of an enlarged descending right pulmonary artery, Westermark's sign (focal oligemia), and Hampton's hump (pleural based wedge density above the diaphragm) are not commonly present. Recently, the most common definitive test for the evaluation of a potential PE is the CT scan. Current scanners are very fast and accurate and, in most institutions, these have replaced more traditional modalities, such as ventilation-perfusion lung scans and angiography. Lung scanning may still be utilized in special cases, such as dye allergies, pregnancy, and renal insufficiency.

Treatment

Traditionally, patients with an acute DVT or PE were admitted to the hospital and started on unfractionated heparin. Once anti-coagulation was obtained the patient would be switched to oral warfarin for long-term therapy. Recently, several studies have demonstrated the safety and efficacy of low molecular weight heparin (LMWH) in the treatment of DVT. Additionally, while not as extensively studied as DVT, LMWH is now also being proposed as an initial treatment of patients with an acute PE. Patients to be treated as outpatients with LMWH should be chosen based on the patients' clinical presentations, the severity of the thrombus, and patient comorbidities. LMWH is given subcutaneously and does not require intravenous administration or laboratory monitoring, which also allows patients to return home and to avoid the cost and inconvenience of hospital admission. LMWH may be used as a bridge to warfarin therapy; however, it has also been proposed that long-term anticoagulation with LMWH has advantages over warfarin, including improved safety and no need to follow laboratory measurements.[7] If there are contraindications for anticoagulation (GI/intracerebral bleeding, trauma), inferior vena cava (IVC) filters may be utilized. IVC filters have been shown to decrease the short-term risk of PE; however, IVC filers are associated with an increased long-term risk of recurrent thrombus.[7] To help avoid this potential sequelae, newer IVC filters are being designed to be used on a short-term basis (2 weeks to 2 months).[1] After the acute treatment has been initiated, consideration should be given to a referral for a work-up of potential causes of hypercoagulablity.

References

1. Alving BM, Francis CW, et al. Consultations on patients with venous or arterial disease. *Hematology* 2003;2003:540–558.
2. Ciccarone E, DiCastelnuovo A, Assanelli D, et al. Homocysteine levels are associated with the severity of peripheral arterial disease in type 2 diabetic patients. *J Thromb Haemost* 2003;1:2540–2547.
3. Lookstein RA. Impact of CT angiography on endovascular therapy. *Mt Sinai J Med* 2003;70:367–374.
4. Goldman JP. New techniques and applications for magnetic resonance imaging. *Mt Sinai J Med* 2003;70:375–385.
5. MRC/BHF heart protection study of cholesterol lowering with simvastatin in 20,536 high-risk individuals: A randomized placebo-controlled trial. *Lancet* 2002;360:7–22.
6. Ellozy SH, Carroccio A. Drug-eluting stents in peripheral vascular disease: Eliminating restenosis. *Mt Sinai J Med* 2003;70:417–419.
7. Shafer AI, Levine MN, et al. Thrombotic disorders: Diagnosis and management. *Hematology* 2003;2003:520–539.
8. Samama MM, Dahl OE, Quinlan DJ, et al. Quantification of risk factors for venous thromboembolism: A preliminary study for the development of a risk assessment tool. *Haematologica* 2003;88:1410–1421.
9. Seligsohn U, Lubetsky A. Genetic susceptibility to venous thrombosis. *N Engl J Med* 2001;344:1222–1231.

Cutaneous Disorders

Constance G. Nichols
Eric Schmidt

Skin diseases and cutaneous manifestations of systemic disease make up a large part of emergency practice. Few dermatologic complaints are life-threatening emergencies, yet many conditions cause significant distress. Emergency physicians should approach cutaneous disorders as all other complaints: identify and initiate treatment of emergent conditions, and provide relief from less serious entities.

Anatomy

The skin is the largest organ system of the body. It is a protective shield, as well as the primary guard against dehydration and infection.

The skin is divided into three layers: from external to internal they are the epidermis, the dermis, and the subcutaneous fat. The epidermis is further subdivided into four histologically distinct layers. Separated from the dermis by an epithelial basement membrane, the basal cell layer (stratum germinativum) is the deepest germinal layer. Cells mature, producing more and more keratin through the prickle cell layer (stratum spinosum) and granular layer (stratum granulosum). The final horny layer (stratum corneum) is composed of flattened nonviable cells. It takes roughly 2 to 3 weeks from the time a cell is generated in the basal layer until it is exposed and sloughed to the environment. Pigment-producing melanocytes are found in the basal layer and immunologically active Langerhans cells are found in the prickle cell layer.

The dermis is divided into two layers, the more pliable papillary dermis and the deeper more resilient reticular dermis. The dermis is composed of several cell types including fibroblasts and mast cells and has a base material of collagen, ground substance, and elastin forming the structural integrity of skin, allowing for significant distortion prior to loss of integrity. Many nerves course through the dermis terminating in various endings. An elaborate network of capillaries supplies sustenance to the dermis as well as the epidermis. Thermoregulation is achieved under central and humoral regulation of deep and superficial capillary networks.

The skin appendages, sweat glands, nails, and hair follicles are specialized invaginations of the epidermis into the dermis. The sweat glands are an integral part of thermoregulation as well as fluid balance, especially in hot environments. Sebum is a protective oily emollient secreted from the sebaceous gland part of each follicle. The subcutaneous fat layer serves for protection and insulation, and is minimally metabolically active.

Age greatly affects all the functions of the skin. Decreased metabolic rate results in thinner, far less elastic dermis that is much more subject to injury, even from minor trauma. Venous stasis, atherosclerosis, and diabetes further limit the dermal and subsequent epidermal blood supply. This decreased perfusion limits regenerative capabilities as well as infection response and the ability to dissipate a heat load. Cumulative solar radiation injury, as well as medications, especially cardiac and anticholinergic agents, decrease the skin's protective capabilities.

History and Physical Examination

The evaluation of the patient with a dermatologic complaint should begin with a detailed history and physical examination. The examiner should ask questions common to all historical examinations, such as significant past medical history, current medications, including over-the-counter preparations, allergies, travel history, and possible animal, home or workplace exposure. Ascertaining whether the patient has been treating himself prior to presentation and whether there were any past occurrences is important, as is obtaining a history of familial complaints or potentially inherited conditions.

The history should include particular attention to onset, change, and progression of the condition, as well as the nature and extent of pain or pruritus, if present. The history should also cite any general or systemic complaints. The dermatologic examination should be preceded by a general examination, including a review of the vital signs, the patient's general appearance, and signs of systemic disease. Lighting and the ability to completely expose the patient are important to determine the color and pattern of distribution of the dermatologic condition. Palpation of the lesions may elicit tenderness, induration or fluctuance, which are helpful in making a determination.

Dermatitis

Constance G. Nichols
Eric Schmidt

Dermatitis

Dermatitis is a catchall dermatologic category of multiple entities predominantly of unknown or complex etiology. Each condition has a suspected immunologic, constitutional or mechanical irritant. Pruritus is the universal complaint, resulting in a cycle of scratching, inflammation, and more pruritus.

Acne

Acne is a multi-factorial inflammatory condition of the pilosebaceous complex. It is the most common complaint seen by dermatologists. Half the population shows some degree of acne by the age of puberty, and 80% to 90% by their high school years.

The lesions may include papules (white heads), comedones (black heads), pustules, or cysts. Any or all of these lesions may be present with the distribution usually involving the face, neck, back, and chest.

Similar lesions may be seen in the older patient involving the nose and alar areas. This condition is called acne rosacea and is treated similarly.

Differential Diagnosis

Emergency physicians should seek signs of secondary infection of the lesions predominantly by staphylococcus or streptococcus. Impetigo, cellulitis, furuncles, or carbuncles may be found.

Treatment

Secondary infections should be treated with topical antibiotics such as bacitracin or mupirocin. Systemic antibiotics primarily active against gram-positive species may be required for extensive involvement or signs of toxicity. Cautious incision and drainage may be required for larger cystic lesions.

Topical benzoyl peroxide application may be recommended. Many other excellent therapies exist including retinoids and systemic antibiotics. The patient, however, should be referred for these therapies as they require monitoring for toxicity and contraceptive considerations.

Atopic

Atopic dermatitis is the most common form of eczema. Five percent of the population exhibits the condition early in childhood. There is frequently a strong family history and an association with allergic rhinitis and reactive airway disease. It is suspected that these patients have relatively inactive suppressor T-cell function.

Atopia usually presents in the first few years of life and generally, but not always subsides by adulthood. The rash begins on the face, diaper area, and extensor surfaces. If the condition continues, one is more likely to find the lesions on the flexor surfaces of adults, especially the popliteal and antecubital fossae.

Differential

Chronic itching, lichenification of the skin, and dryness are the *sine qua non* of atopia. No other skin disease fits these criteria.

Treatment

Diphenhydramine is helpful when initiating therapy. After topical steroids in the lowest possible potency or immunomodulators such as tacrolimus and pimecrolimus have been used for about two weeks, the diphenhydramine may be stopped.

Contact

Contact dermatitis is a delayed hypersensitivity reaction to an environmental exposure. The reaction may appear as soon as 12 hours post-exposure, but usually occurs in 1 to 2 days. The reaction usually begins with pruritus and erythema. Urticaria, edema vesicles, and crusting may follow. Chronic exposure may lead to an eczematous lesion. Identifying the offending agent and the pattern of the exanthem is the key to diagnosis.

Rhus dermatitis (**FIGURE 26.1**) is the most common form of contact dermatitis. It is estimated that three-fourths of the population will eventually become sensitized to the volatile oils found in poison ivy, oak, and sumac. Exposure to any part of the plants usually leads to linear

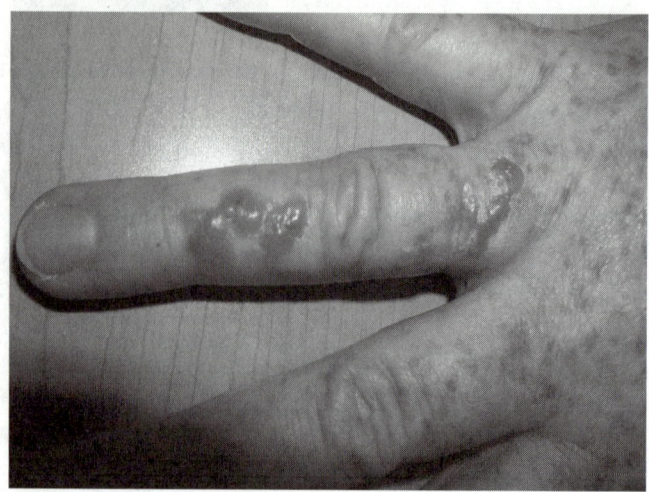

FIGURE 26.1 Rhus dermatitis.

streaks of erythema that may progress to weeping vesicles subject to secondary infection. Generally the agents have oxidized by the time symptoms appear and cannot be spread by scratching. The lesions may continue to appear for up to 8 days after the initial symptoms depending on the amount of oleoresin and the thickness of the epidermis. The epidermis of the soles and palms are thick enough to prevent exposure and symptoms. Oxidation of the resin results in dark black lines on exposed clothing. A patient sensitive to the resins may minimize the reaction by washing with detergents or alcohol after noting these lines. Rhus dermatitis generally takes 10 to 14 days to run its course, though the initial course may be more prolonged.

Nickel dermatitis from jewelry is common in areas of direct contact. Topical medications or cosmetic preparations may also precipitate contact eruptions.

Differential Diagnosis

Eczema should be considered in a patient with a history or signs of atopia such as reactive airway disease. Pruritus should be the predominant complaint, with pain suggesting a primary or secondary infection. Signs of acute hypersensitivity, such as wheezing and urticaria, although rare, should be carefully excluded. Urticaria, edema, or excoriation as the primary finding suggests an ingested agent or photodermatitis reaction.

Treatment

Identification of the irritant aids the clinician in tailoring the therapeutic regimen. The patient may not be aware of any new irritant, and a review of any over-the-counter exposure may be fruitful. Avoidance of further exposure is critical.

Topical steroids are appropriate for small areas, whereas severe or widespread eruptions require systemic therapy.

Short courses of prednisone starting with 40 to 60 mg per day may be sufficient. Longer courses of 10 to 14 days with taper will be necessary for rhus dermatitis, as well as other entities if exposure continues. Pruritus may be controlled with antihistamines.

Frequent sunscreen use, effective against UVA and UVB, should be recommended in photodermatitis reactions, along with sun avoidance.

Dyshydrotic Eczema

Dyshydrotic eczema is limited to the hands and feet. Tiny, pearly cysts may be seen in the hypertrophic epidermis. The possibility of chronic contact dermatitis should be considered especially in this entity.

Psoriasis

Psoriasis is a chronic inflammatory rash, which has multifactorial causalities. There are genetic and environmental factors as well as evidence that T cells are involved in the development of psoriasis. The onset usually occurs in the fourth decade of life, and a strong family history is common. The condition results from rapid acceleration of epidermal proliferation, resulting in well-demarcated erythematous plaques with a characteristic silvery scale. The lesions are most commonly found on the elbows, scalp, back, gluteal fold, and popliteal area. The initial presentation may begin suddenly, involving the trunk. Half of the patients have nail involvement, demonstrating the characteristic pits. Pruritus is the predominant complaint.

Nonsteroidal anti-inflammatory agents, lithium, and β-blockers, as well as recent streptococcal infection, have been associated with exacerbations.

Differential Diagnosis

Nummular eczema and pityriasis are frequently mistaken for psoriasis, as well as many of the fungal infections. Early presentation, especially in the absence of a family history, may suggest underlying HIV infection.

Treatment

Moisturizing agents and moderate to strong topical steroids are the treatment of choice. Systemic steroids should be avoided due to a strong rebound of symptoms after therapy.

Many other therapies, including tar, anthralin, psoralen, Eucerin, phototherapy, methotrexate, retinoids, and cyclosporine, are effective, but require referral for appropriate long-term management.

Selected Readings

Cottam JA, Shenefelt PD, Sinnott JT, et al. Common skin infections in the elderly. *Infect Med* 1999;16:280–290.

Fitzpatrick TB, Johnson RA, Wolff K, et al. *Color Atlas and Synopsis of Clinical Dermatology*, 4th ed. New York: McGraw Hill 2001:18–27, 39–41, 826–833.

Gordon KB, McCormick TS. Evolution of biologic therapies for the treatment of psoriasis. *SKINmed* 2003;2:286–294.

Hansen RC. Atopic dermatitis: Taming the itch that rashes. *Contemp Pediatr* 2003; 20:79–87, 97.

Bacterial Infections

Constance G. Nichols
Eric Schmidt

Bacterial Infections

The skin is one of the most important barriers to infection. Emergency physicians are frequently presented with a variety of lesions with differing skin elements involved. Gram-positive organisms predominate, primarily *Staphylococcus* and *Streptococcus* species.

Abscesses and Furuncles

Abscesses and furuncles are collections of purulent material from *Staphylococcus aureus* infections. Furuncles are expansions from folliculitis, whereas abscesses are deeper, often from trauma. Intra-epidermal inclusion cysts may become secondarily infected and mimic an abscess. The presence of a central pore or the finding of caseous or purulent material during incision and drainage indicates an area subject to recurrence.

Cellulitis/Lymphangitis

Cellulitis is an infection of the deeper dermis. The painful erythematous infection causes an orange peel–like induration and may be associated with regional adenopathy, lymphangitis or systemic signs of infection. Erysipelas is a distinction given to cellulitis of rapidly spreading cellulitis involving the face. Trauma is postulated as the causative event in this Gram-positive infection. Facial cellulitis in the pediatric patient without a history of trauma and commonly a recent upper respiratory infection may suggest *Haemophilus influenzae* infection.

Lymphangitis is erythematous local streaking from any infection and indicates involvement of lymphatics. Regional adenopathy and systemic signs of infection are not uncommon.

Treatment

Topical mupirocin may be sufficient for small areas of impetigo. Oral penicillinase–resistant agents or macrolides may be prescribed for cellulitis, impetigo, and mild lymphangitis in the immunocompetent patient. Parenteral therapy with elevation of the involved area may be necessary for septic or immunocompromised patients or for those not improving on oral therapy.

In pediatric patients, especially with facial cellulitis, expanding the coverage to include *Haemophilus* should be considered. Incision and drainage is the only therapy required for abscesses and furuncles in the absence of significant associated cellulitis, lymphangitis, or systemic signs of infection.

Folliculitis

Folliculitis is a pustular, most commonly staphylococcal infection of the hair follicle apparatus. The pustular follicles may be seen in areas of impetigo or cellulitis. Gram-negative organisms may be involved in patients on antimicrobial therapy or hot tub exposure. The most common "hot tub" folliculitis organism is *Pseudomonas aeruginosa*. This requires treatment with either topical gentamicin ointment applied three to four times daily and 0.25% acetic acid solution applied three to four times daily or a course of oral ciprofloxacin 500 mg taken twice daily for seven to ten days.

Differential Diagnosis

Candida infections may cause pustules and should be considered in intertriginous areas or if antibacterial therapy is ineffective. Cellulites and impetigo must also be considered.

Treatment

Local care with careful shampooing and washing may be all that is required. More widespread outbreaks may require topical or systemic antibiotic therapy. Empiric therapy may include topical ointments, such as clindamycin or erythromycin, both of which are used twice daily; gentamycin ointment three times daily; or benzoyl peroxide ointment applied once or twice daily. Oral therapy choices include minocycline 100 mg bid, erythromycin 250 to 500 mg qid or amoxicillin/cavulanate 875/125 mg twice daily. All oral therapies should be taken for seven to ten days or longer, if infection persists.

Impetigo

Impetigo is a superficial infection of the dermis with epidermal or intraepidermal elevation and characteristic amber- or honey-colored crust formation over an erythematous bed. Historically, erythema and crusting without any pustules or folliculitis was caused by *Streptococcus* or *Staphylococcus* only and termed erythema, although both organisms may be present. Most commonly seen in the peri-oral area or as a complication of dermatophyte diaper dermatitis, the infection has been associated with poststreptococcal glomerulonephritis and scalded skin syndrome. In bullous impetigo, less traumatized areas allow for larger discrete bullae to form as on the extremities or in the diaper area.

Differential Diagnosis

Contact dermatitis or eczematous lesions are frequently mistaken for impetigo. In both pruritus is the primary complaint, and there is usually more hemorrhagic crust than impetigo. Herpes simplex may initially resemble impetigo, especially in the perioral area. Vesicles and recurrent episodes should suggest herpes in both these painful exanthems.

Treatment

Topical mupirocin ointment applied three times daily for five to ten days may be effective for small areas of impetigo. If a more widespread area of skin is involved oral antibiotics such as dicloxacillin 250–500 mg every 4 to 6 hours; cloxacillin 500–1,000 mg every 6 hours days; clindamycin 150–300 mg every 6 hours; or erythromycin 250–500 mg every 6 hours for 5 to 10 days may be used.

Selected Readings

Fitzpatrick TB, Johnson RA, Wolff K, et al. *Color Atlas and Synopsis of Clinical Dermatology*, 4th ed. New York: McGraw Hill 2001:18–27, 39–41, 826–833.
Goldblum OM. Acne vulgaris. *SKINmed* 2003;2:309–311.
Koay J, Hsu S. *Folliculitis. Best Practice of Medicine*. www.merckmedicus.com 2002.
Stevens DL. 20 clinical pearls: skin and soft tissue infections. *Infect Med* 2003; 20:483–493.

Fungal Infections

Constance G. Nichols
Eric Schmidt

Candida

Candida albicans may cause an infection of any moist area. The beefy red areas cause burning and may be surrounded by small pustules from local follicular infection. These pustules may be confused with folliculitis or miliaria rubra (prickly heat). The perineal area is commonly involved.

"Prickly heat" is an uncomfortable condition due to a new exposure to a hot moist environment. Skin maceration, from profuse sweating in intertriginous areas or tight-fitting clothing, causes gland plugging with secondary rupture and inflammation. Desquamating agents and antipruritic therapy along with antibiotics if infection is present is the treatment of choice.

The diagnosis of *Candida* is best made with KOH preparation demonstrating hyphae and pseudohyphae. Recurrent *Candida* infections of the skin, vulvovaginal area or mouth (thrush) may be caused by antibiotic therapy, diabetes, pregnancy, or immune suppression.

Treatment

Candida infections may be controlled with zinc or selenium solutions or shampoos, although the use of imidazole agents is more convenient and effective. Topical miconazole 2% cream applied twice daily; clotrimazole 1% cream or solution twice daily; econazole 1% cream applied daily; or ketoconazole 2% cream applied once or twice daily may be used for localized infections. Oral ketoconazole 200 to 400 mg daily, fluconazole 100 mg daily; or itraconazole 200 mg once or twice daily may be used in short courses for widespread or severe outbreaks. Prolonged therapy, especially with ketoconazole, requires liver function and CBC monitoring. Recurrent vulvovaginitis, seborrhea, or onychomycosis may be treated with a five- to seven-day daily dose, followed by a weekly dose as the skin acts as a reservoir for some of the agents.

The intense burning of *Candida* infections may require mild topical steroids, but caution must be taken to avoid secondary infections.

Tinea

Tinea is a collection of epidermal keratin layer fungal infections by *Trichophyton, Microsporum,* or *Epidermophyton* species. The fungae produce keratolytic enzymes causing stratum corneum loosening and scaling. These scaly mildly pruritic lesions are usually oval in shape, developing a well-demarcated, serpiginous border when large. As the organisms are limited to the keratin layer, the patient complaint is usually the presence of the lesion, unless it is located in an area subject to maceration and secondary bacterial or yeast infection. The finding of hyphae on a KOH preparation is diagnostic.

Tinea capitis may be one of the causes of alopecia. Head dermatophyte infections may be confused with seborrheic dermatitis, which has a thicker oily scale.

Tinea faciale may mimic photosensitivity reactions, although the presence of uninvolved sun-exposed skin should suggest tinea, systemic lupus or seborrheic dermatitis. Seborrhea is mostly associated with facial fold involvement. A negative KOH preparation and systemic complaints suggest lupus.

Tinea corporis may easily be confused with pityriasis. Impetigo should demonstrate a honey-colored crust. Pityriasis does not show hyphae on KOH preparation and may exhibit the larger herald patch.

Tinea cruris is a dermatophyte infection of the intertriginous areas. The fine scales, a serpiginous border, and a positive KOH preparation distinguish these fungal infections from the noninfectious skin maceration, as seen especially in obese patients. Intense burning or a beefy-red base suggest *Candida* involvement.

Onychomycosis is a fungal infection of the nails causing thickening and separation. Psoriatic nail changes may mimic early fungal infections. Contact dermatitis or prolonged dyshydrotic eczema may also be confused with fungal infection.

Tinea pedis is an interdigital fungal infection causing maceration (**FIGURE 28.1**) and cracking (**FIGURE 28.2**). Contact dermatitis or hyperhidrosis may mimic the condition.

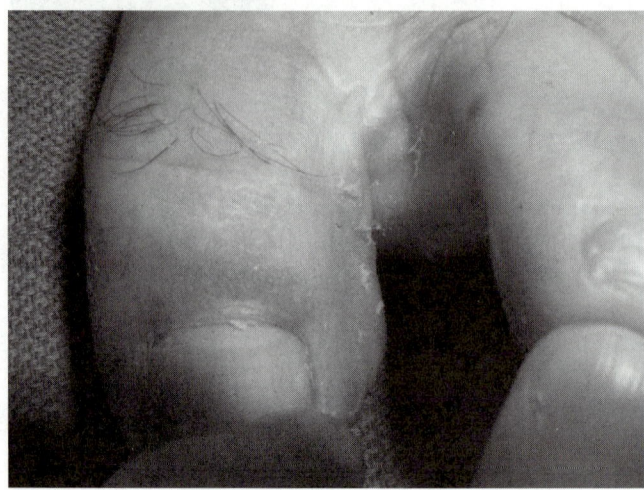

FIGURE 28.1 Tinea pedis maceration.

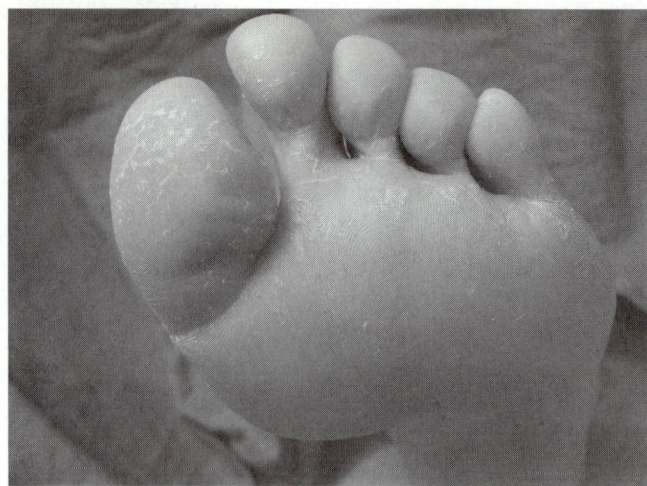

FIGURE 28.2 Tinea pedis cracking.

Seborrheic dermatitis is a pruritic superficial inflammation of areas with high concentrations of sebaceous glands. The condition is currently felt to be secondary to *Pityrosporum* yeast. The condition causes scaling and dandruff in mild outbreaks, to moist pruritic plaques with greasy brown to white scales. The scalp, facial folds, central chest, back, and intergluteal area are most commonly involved. The tinea has a finer scale, while psoriasis also involves areas without sebaceous glands and has a less greasy scale.

Differential

Tinea may be confused with other noninfectious cutaneous conditions such as eczema and psoriasis. The observation of fungus in KOH preparation is diagnostic.

Treatment

Topical or systemic antifungal agents such as topical terbinafine 250 mg daily for 2 to 8 weeks; ketoconazole 200 mg daily for 4 weeks; itraconazole 200 to 400 mg daily for 30 days; or griseofulvin 500 mg daily for 4 to 6 weeks are effective in treatment of tinea capitis. Recommendations for tinea cruris, corporis, and pedis include creams, sprays, and powder forms of the common antifungals. These include miconazole 2% cream powder or spray used twice daily for 2 to 3 weeks; clotrimazole 1% topical cream solution or lotion applied twice daily for 2 to 3 weeks; econazole 1% topical cream twice daily for 2 to 3 weeks; naftifine 1% topical cream twice daily for 2 to 3 weeks; or ciclopiroxolamine 1% cream, gel, or lotion applied twice daily for 2 to 3 weeks.

Selected Readings

Fitzpatrick TB, Johnson RA, Wolff K, et al. *Color Atlas and Synopsis of Clinical Dermatology,* 4th ed. New York: McGraw Hill 2001:18–27, 39–41, 826–833.

Stevens DL. 20 clinical pearls: skin and soft tissue infections. *Infect Med* 2003; 20:483–493.

Parasitic Infections

Constance G. Nichols
Eric Schmidt

Pediculosis

Pediculosis is caused by one of three types of sucking lice. Crab lice (*Phthirus pubis*) most commonly involve the genital area and are spread by sexual contact. Head and body lice (*Pediculosis humanus capitis* and *corporis*) may also infest the genital area, but are more commonly found in the other hairy areas of the body. They are spread among institutional patients and among people in close contact. With all lice infestations the chief complaint is pruritus with frequent biting or stinging sensations.

Nits, louse eggs, are droplet-shaped opalescent bodies found on hair, clothing, and bedding of patients. They may be the only physical finding, especially with head and body lice, which are only on the patient during feeding and survive up to 24 hours.

Differential Diagnosis

Localized pruritus of the head, axillae, or genital area suggests pediculosis and should instigate a search for nits. Other arthropod infestations are more common on the extremities and waistband area. Folliculitis and contact dermatitis are frequently confused with lice infestation.

Treatment

Pyrethrins, permethrin or lindane may be used. The nits should be removed by combing. Bedding and clothing should be hot washed and dried or ironed. The pruritus may last for 1 to 2 weeks and should signal reexamination at one week for more nits and treatment, if any are found.

Scabies

Scabies is an intradermal infestation of the *Sarcoptes scabiei* mite. The mite produces intensely pruritic papules and characteristic linear burrows involving the web spaces, extremities, and trunk, sparing the head. Infestations are cyclic with close contact infection common. Diagnosis is best made with skin scraping of the burrow or papule demonstrating the mite or eggs.

Differential Diagnosis

Scabies infestations are frequently confused with folliculitis, which is rarely as widespread or pruritic as scabies. The finding of nits on any hair-bearing area is diagnostic of pediculosis. Flea or other arthropod bites may produce similarly pruritic papules without web space involvement or burrow formation.

Treatment

Lindane lotion or cream applied for 8 hours to all areas other than the face or head, with careful application to the hands, is effective. Repeat therapy at one week may be necessary. Sexual contacts should be treated. Lindane is not recommended for pediatric and pregnant or lactating patients due to the risk of absorption with subsequent vomiting, blood dyscrasias, and seizures. Permethrin is recommended in these situations or in recurrent cases.

The pruritus may last longer than two weeks after therapy, as the irritant mite material remains until epidermal turnover has occurred. Antihistamines are helpful with short courses of steroids postulated, but are not proven for severe infestations.

Selected Readings

Fitzpatrick TB, Johnson RA, Wolff K, et al. *Color Atlas and Synopsis of Clinical Dermatology*, 4th ed. New York: McGraw Hill 2001:18–27, 39–41, 826–833.
Stevens DL. 20 clinical pearls: skin and soft tissue infections. *Infect Med* 2003; 20:483–493.

30 Viral Infections

Constance G. Nichols
Eric Schmidt

Herpes Simplex

Herpes simplex is a painful, contagious, and recurrent vesicular eruption. Both HSV-I and HSV-II are the causative viruses presumably lying dormant in the dorsal root ganglion between eruptions. Classically, HSV-I has been associated with oral infections and HSV-II with genital outbreaks. Either virus may cause outbreaks in any distribution.

The eruption usually begins approximately one week after exposure with up to 80% transmission for genital herpes. The initial symptom is intense local burning with vesicular eruption 1 to 2 days later. There may be a viral prodrome. Lesions are small intraepidermal vesicles on a common erythematous region. The vesicles are filled with clear fluid with a central dark spot or umbilication. Over the 10- to 14-day course of the eruption, the vesicles break and crust over, leaving the area subject to secondary bacterial infection and only rarely scarring. The initial eruption is usually the most severe.

Herpes neonatorum may occur after vaginal delivery from asymptomatic mothers, with two-thirds of the outbreaks more than a month postpartum. Neonatal herpes carries a high mortality of roughly 50% from secondary infection.

Differential Diagnosis

Impetigo may mimic HSV infection if all the vesicles have crusted. The history of recurrent outbreaks in the same area should suggest a herpes infection. A Tzanck smear of the crust or fluid looking for the diagnostic multinucleated giant cells or viral cultures may be helpful. Multiple areas or chronic outbreaks should suggest immunosuppression. HIV patients commonly have chronic painful outbreaks.

Treatment

Acyclovir is a well-tolerated agent specific for herpes virus that shortens the course and decreases the intensity of the outbreak. Topical 5% acyclovir may be adequate for small outbreaks.

Oral acyclovir 200 mg five times daily or 5 mg/kg every 8 hours for 5 to 10 days is recommended for immunocompetent patients and, for immunocompromised patients, twice the dose for 1 to 14 days with additional topical dosing. Recurrent episodes may be treated for 5 to 7 days with chronic suppression doses of 400 mg three times daily, effective in preventing symptomatic recurrences. Treatment with famciclovir (500 mg every 8 hours for 7 days) and valacyclovir (1,000 mg 2 to 3 times daily) is a more recent treatment and offers more convenient dosing regimens. Acyclovir resistance is emerging, especially in the HIV population and may require foscarnet therapy.

The pain of herpes is neuropathic in origin and responds poorly to usual analgesic therapy, although tricylic antidepressants have been used with some success.

Varicella

Varicella (chickenpox) is a common herpes virus infection. The vast majority of the population demonstrates the infection in childhood, 90% prior to the age of 10.

Infection occurs 8 to 20 days later after exposure via the nasopharynx. There is an initial prodrome of fever, headache, and anorexia. The lesions are 2 mm to 3 mm in diameter, appear in crops, and rapidly progress from macules to papules and vesicles demonstrating umbilication. The lesions may become pustular prior to crusting. Rarely, encephalitis, hepatitis, and pneumonitis are complications. Fetal infection in titer-negative mothers has potentially devastating results and requires isolating pregnant females from infected patients. Patients will defervesce 3 to 4 days into the course, with persistent fever suggestive of secondary skin or lung infection. Viral shedding and possible contagious contact risk last for roughly 1 week, from 1 to 2 days prior to eruption until after all the lesions have crusted.

Differential Diagnosis

Coxsackievirus, echovirus, and disseminated herpes simplex infections may mimic varicella. Viral cultures are not useful with varicella, although a Tzanck prep will show the characteristic multinucleated cells.

Treatment

Antipyretics and antihistamines remain the cornerstone of therapy. Acyclovir lessens the symptoms and shortens the course, although its general use is still debated. Use in immunocompromised patients or cases of severe stomatitis is indicated. Of course, use of aspirin as an anti-pyretic is not considered safe in children, due to the possibility of Reyes syndrome.

Herpes Zoster

Herpes zoster is caused by reactivation of latent varicella. Up to one-fourth of the population may suffer the condition, with two-thirds of the cases occurring over the age of 50. Immunocompromised patients have a higher incidence of multidermatomal outbreak. Without other known immunocompromising conditions, this is highly suggestive of HIV.

The outbreak is usually preceded by intense burning pain over a single dermatomal distribution with vesicles appearing over an erythematous bed 1 to 2 days later and lasting 10 to 14 days. Patients shed virus over the course of symptoms until crusting has occurred.

Molluscum Contagiosum

Infection of the epidermal cells with a common unclassified DNA poxvirus produces a smooth, umbilicated, painless papule known as molluscum contagiosum. These lesions are very common, especially in children. They are spread by direct contact. They are usually pearly, skincolored, small (2 mm to 5 mm) nodules, occurring singularly or in groups on the trunk, face, and extremities, sparing the palms and soles. They can also occur on the genitals of sexually active individuals. The lesions are of little clinical significance, but are often removed by simple curettage for cosmetic reasons.

Treatment

Without treatment, most resolve spontaneously within 6 to 9 months. Sudden appearance of many molluscum lesions that do not spontaneously regress should raise the suspicion of an immunocompromising illness. Molluscum contagiosum is seen in approximately 9% of individuals with AIDS.

Warts

Warts are among the most common benign tumors of the skin. Common warts can be seen in up to 25% of the general population. Approximately 1% of sexually active adults have genital warts with 10% to 20% harboring latent or asymptomatic infection. Warts are caused by infection of the keratinocytes by one of several strains of the human papillomavirus. It is felt that different strains are responsible for different types of warts.

The common wart (verruca vulgaris) is found on the hands and fingers. It appears as an isolated, firm, skincolored papule with a rough, scaling surface. Its presence interrupts the normal architecture of the skin. It can vary in size, from barely visible to greater than 1 cm. The plantar wart is similar in appearance to the common wart but as its name suggests is found on the plantar aspect of the foot. It is often painful due to its location on the weight-bearing areas of the foot. A central black dot or "seed" can frequently be seen that represents thrombosed blood vessels. Genital warts (condyloma acuminatum) affect the rectum, external genitalia, and surrounding skin as well as the urethra and vagina. Warts found in these areas appear soft, moist, and skin-colored to pink. They may be singular or multiple and can be sessile or pedunculated with a cauliflower-like appearance. Soaking the affected area with 5% acetic acid for 5 minutes turns the questionable lesions white (acetowhitening), allowing improved visualization.

Treatment

Patients usually seek treatment due to the unsightly nature of these lesions or due to pain caused by excessive pressure on plantar warts. Without treatment, 35% to 65% resolve spontaneously within 2 years. Treatment with keratinolytic agents, such as salicylic acid plaster, is effective for common and plantar warts. After soaking the wart in water for 5 minutes, the surface tissue should be removed. The plaster is painted on the wart and left in place under an occlusive dressing. This procedure is repeated daily. Other commonly utilized therapies include cryotherapy with liquid nitrogen, trichloroacetic acid, and cantharidin (a blistering agent from the blister beetle) treatment. Genital warts should be treated aggressively as human papilloma virus (HPV) infection has been found to be associated with cervical cancer. Treatment includes podophyllin resin and cryotherapy. Infected women should be screened periodically for cervical changes with pelvic examination and Pap smears. Infected patients and their partners should be screened for other sexually transmitted diseases. Treatment of viral warts results in a cure in up to 80% of cases.

Selected Readings

Fitzpatrick TB, Johnson RA, Wolff K, et al. *Color Atlas and Synopsis of Clinical Dermatology*, 4th ed. New York: McGraw Hill 2001:18–27, 39–41, 826–833.
Stevens DL. 20 clinical pearls: skin and soft tissue infections. *Infect Med* 2003;20:483–493.

Maculopapular Lesions

Constance G. Nichols
Eric Schmidt

Pityriasis Rosea

Pityriasis rosea is a mildly pruritic self-limited rash of un-known etiology. Small (1 cm to 2 cm) oval, salmon-colored lesions are characteristic with a fine, frequently centrally-oriented scale. The lesions are truncal and may exhibit a Christmas tree pattern. A larger, up to 10 cm, herald patch may be present or described as preceding the other lesions.

Differential Diagnosis

Pityriasis may be confused with fungal infections, which are usually more erythematous and pruritic. These may also be distinguished by a KOH preparation. Lesions that greatly involve the extremities or involve the palms and soles should raise the possibility of secondary syphilis.

Treatment

Reassurance is the cornerstone of therapy as most cases resolve spontaneously over several weeks. Antihistamines may be used to control the pruritis.

Selected Readings

Fitzpatrick TB, Johnson RA, Wolff K, et al. *Color Atlas and Synopsis of Clinical Dermatology,* 4th ed. New York: McGraw Hill 2001:18–27, 39–41, 826–833.
Hansen RC. Atopic dermatitis: taming the itch that rashes. *Contemp Pediatr* 2003;20:79–87, 97.

Purpura and Petechiae

Constance G. Nichols
Eric Schmidt

Description

Purpura is a collection of entities in which blood has extravasated from the vasculature. Since the blood is in the tissues, the lesions do not blanch when pressure is applied. The word purpura derives from the word purple, although these lesions may range from erythematous through purple to necrotic in color.

The entities are generally divided into palpable and nonpalpable purpura. The nonpalpable purpuras are most commonly from thrombocytopenia and generally involve the superficial vasculature. Palpable purpura involves the deeper vasculature and should suggest a true vasculitis.

If the lesions are 3 mm or less, they are referred to as petechiae: larger ones are macules.

Thrombocytopenia with platelets of less than 50,000/mm^3 may produce petechiae. Platelet counts of 10,000/mm^3 put the patient at risk of severe hemorrhage.

Drugs including sulfonamides, heparin, quinine, Dilantin, and chemotherapeutic agents may cause thrombocytopenia. Malignancy or viral infections, such as HIV, may cause decreased platelets. Autoimmune or suspected postviral autoimmune reactions may cause low platelet counts.

Vasculitis (FIGURE 32.1) from autoimmune, infectious or idiopathic processes may produce purpura in the face of normal platelet function. Severe presentations may produce a consumptive thrombocytopenia.

Schönlein-Henoch purpura is an idiopathic, probably immunoglobulin A (IgA) vasculitis seen most commonly in children and is frequently self-limited, although renal involvement should be considered.

Cryoglobulinemia and collagen vascular diseases, such as rheumatoid arthritis and systemic lupus erythematosus, may also present as vasculitic purpura.

Infectious vasculitis from disseminated gonorrhea, meningococcal, staphylococcal, streptococcal, rickettsial, or pseudomonal infections produce the most acute presentations. An unstable septic shock presentation requires aggressive fluid resuscitation, pressors, and empiric broad-spectrum antibiotic therapy.

Differential Diagnosis

The history of a preceding viral syndrome or the presence of a potentially offending drug aids the clinician.

Treatment

Early initiation of broad-spectrum antibiotics is key in treating patients subject to a fulminant course. Antistaphylococcal and a third-generation cephalosporin along with tetracycline or chloramphenicol may be considered until the etiologic agent or underlying process is identified.

Severe thrombocytopenia may require steroids, gammaglobulin infusions, and/or plasmaphoresis.

Selected Readings

Cottam JA, Shenefelt PD, Sinnott JT, et al. Common skin infections in the elderly. *Infect Med* 1999;16:280–290.
Fitzpatrick TB, Johnson RA, Wolff K, et al. *Color Atlas and Synopsis of Clinical Dermatology*, 4th ed. New York: McGraw Hill 2001:18–27, 39–41, 826–833.

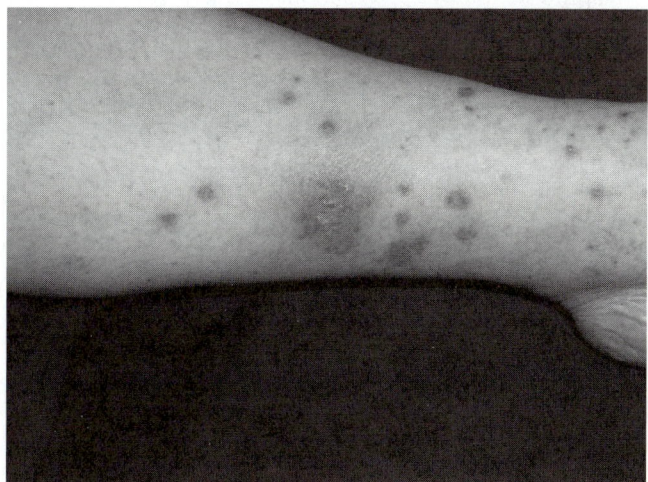

FIGURE 32.1 Leukoclastic vasculitis.

Urticaria/Angioedema

Constance G. Nichols
Eric Schmidt

Description

Urticaria (**FIGURE 33.1**) is a common complaint involving up to 25% of the population, most commonly young adults. The condition presents with diffuse pruritus and evanescent wheals lasting not more than 24 hours. Urticaria may be immunologically precipitated from medications, food allergies or even over-the-counter preparations. Aspirin and nonsteroidal anti-inflammatory agents have been associated with urticaria. Other suspected non-immunologic precipitants are cold, sunlight, and emotional stress. A serum sickness like picture of arthralgias or a history of a viral syndrome may be present.

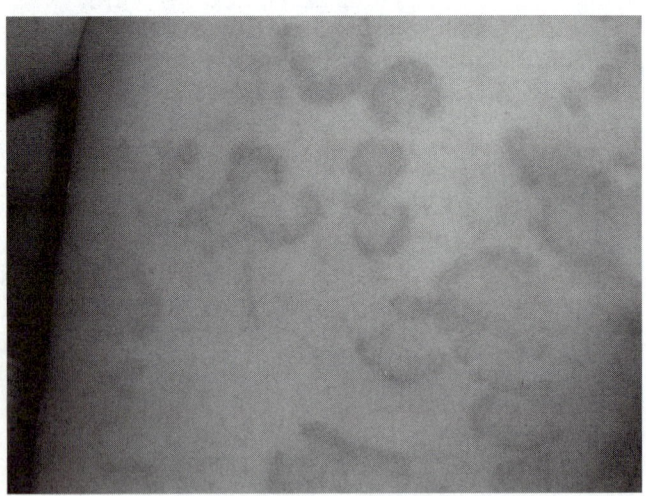

FIGURE 33.1 Urticaria.

Angioedema is edema of the deeper dermis with less pruritus. A strong association with angiotensin-converting enzyme (ACE) inhibitors has been made. Familial angioedema is associated with C1q esterase deficiency and may present after trauma.

Differential Diagnosis

Erythema multiforme more often involves the palms and soles and demonstrates the classic target lesion. Erythema migrans is most commonly a solitary lesion. Signs of systemic hypersensitivity reactions should be sought.

Treatment

A new environmental factor or medication exposure should be sought, although the search is frequently unfruitful. Urticaria is usually self-limited to 7 days, with short courses of oral steroids significantly decreasing the duration of symptoms. Avoidance of any suspected precipitant as well as aspirin and non-steroidal anti-inflammatory agents should be encouraged. The pruritus may be controlled with antihistamines.

Familial angioedema responds to fresh frozen plasma infusion.

Urticaria lasting longer than 6 weeks could suggest a missed precipitant or connective tissue disorder.

Selected Readings

Fitzpatrick TB, Johnson RA, Wolff K, et al. *Color Atlas and Synopsis of Clinical Dermatology,* 4th ed. New York: McGraw Hill 2001:18–27, 39–41, 826–833.
Hansen RC. Atopic dermatitis: taming the itch that rashes. *Contemp Pediatr* 2003;20:79–87, 97.

Papular/Nodular Lesions

Constance G. Nichols
Eric Schmidt

Epidermoid Inclusion Cyst

The epidermoid cyst is a keratin-containing cyst, lined by epidermal cells. Commonly, but incorrectly, known as a sebaceous cyst, the epidermoid does not contain sebum. These lesions are very common in adults. They appear as a firm, freely mobile, dome-shaped, skin-colored nodules and are most commonly seen on the face, neck, chest, and back. They are slow-growing and asymptomatic unless they become irritated or infected. When infected, cultures reveal a polymicrobial environment, with *Staphylococcus aureus* being the most frequently isolated organism.

Treatment

Lesions that are cosmetically unappealing can be easily removed by incision with a number 11 scalpel blade or a needle, followed by gentle pressure to express the contents of the cyst.

Millium

A millium is a lesion that is histologically identical to the epidermoid cyst, differing only in size. A millium is a su-

perficial, epidermis-lined cyst that contains keratin. It is found commonly on the face, cheeks, and eyelids. When found on the palate it is known as Epstein's pearl. It appears as a 1 mm to 2 mm, superficial, pearly white papule.

Treatment

Treatment with incision and drainage is usually required when these cysts become inflamed or infected. Antibiotic therapy should be aimed at the most common pathogen, *S. aureus*. Removal of the entire cyst and lining is required to prevent recurrence. This should be performed after any infection has been adequately treated and the inflammation resolved.

Selected Readings

Cottam JA, Shenefelt PD, Sinnott JT, et al. Common skin infections in the elderly. *Infect Med* 1999;16:280–290.
Fitzpatrick TB, Johnson RA, Wolff K, et al. *Color Atlas and Synopsis of Clinical Dermatology*, 4th ed. New York: McGraw Hill 2001:18–27, 39–41, 826–833.

Erythemas

Constance G. Nichols
Eric Schmidt

Erythema Multiforme

Erythema multiforme is an immune complex–mediated exanthem. The lesion may demonstrate erythematous macules and blisters, but needs to show the classic target lesion for diagnosis. The target lesion demonstrates central blistering erythema surrounded by a clear edematous area and another erythematous ring. The lesions are usually found on the soles and palms, with mucous membrane involvement occurring in the most severe form referred to as Stevens-Johnson syndrome.

Drugs, especially penicillins, sulfas, and hydantoin, have been associated with erythema multiforme. Viral, mycoplasmal or recurrent herpetic infections have been etiologic precipitants.

Differential Diagnosis

Urticaria may be confused with erythema multiforme, but is usually more pruritic and less likely to involve the soles and palms. Pemphigus or pemphigoid may be confused early on but do not demonstrate target lesions, and the blistering of erythema multiforme is usually more discrete.

Treatment

Erythema multiforme is usually self-limited and clears in 2 to 3 weeks. Cessation of suspected drugs should be encouraged. Treatment of suspected underlying mycoplasma infection with erythromycin may be considered in the patient with an atypical pneumonia presentation. Acyclovir may be used to suppress recurrent herpes, although the exanthem usually occurs after the herpetic flair.

There is little evidence for the role of steroids except in severe cases involving mucous membranes (e.g., Stevens-Johnson syndrome). It is hoped that the corticosteroid may prevent coalescence of the lesions resulting in toxic epidermal necrolysis in which the entire epidermis and mucous membranes can slough, resulting in severe secondary infection and dehydration and associated with high mortality.

Erythema Nodosum

Erythema nodosum presents as deep, painful, well-demarcated lesions, mostly in the pre-tibial area. The condition is a localized inflammation of the subcutaneous fat. This inflammation is secondary to immune complexes from some other inflammatory process. Fever and arthralgias may also be present.

Tuberculosis, sarcoidosis, and inflammatory bowel disease have been associated with the lesions.

Differential Diagnosis

The lesions may resemble bruises with a history of repeated trauma.

Treatment

Mild analgesics are appropriate as well as initiating evaluation for the causative underlying process.

Selected Reading

Fitzpatrick TB, Johnson RA, Wolff K, et al. *Color Atlas and Synopsis of Clinical Dermatology*, 4th ed. New York: McGraw Hill 2001:18–27, 39–41, 826–833.
Requena L, Requena C. Erythema nodosum. *Dermatol Online J* 2002:8.

Vesicular/Bullous Lesions

Constance G. Nichols
Eric Schmidt

Pemphigus/Pemphigoid

Pemphigus is an uncommon autoimmune blistering disorder. IgG-mediated intraepidermal lysis causes clear blisters that readily spread laterally with pressure (Nikolsky's sign).

Pemphigoid is an immunoglobulin, compliment mediated, subepidermal necrolysis with clear fluid-filled bullae that do not spread with pressure.

Both rare conditions present in the fifth to seventh decade, and although the prognosis of pemphigoid resolving in several months is good, pemphigus historically has a high mortality. Both conditions respond well to immunosuppressant therapy, including initially systemic steroids.

Scalded Skin Syndrome

Scalded skin syndrome, also known as toxic shock syndrome, was initially described in menstruating women. Toxins from phage group II *Staphylococcus aureus* were initially implicated from infected tampons. Subsequently, similar toxins have been associated with Group A streptococcal infections of the conjunctiva or nasal pharynx.

Patients present in septic shock with a diffuse erythroderma resembling sunburn. The erythroderma includes non–sun-exposed areas. The condition produces an intraepidermal lysis and sloughing during convalescence.

Differential Diagnosis

Viral exanthems show a less toxic presentation, as well as a more diffuse exanthem. Kawasaki's syndrome (mucocutaneous lymph node syndrome) demonstrates a sandpapery erythema, strawberry tongue, prominently red lips, mucous membrane conjunctivitis, and adenopathy.

Treatment

Vigorous support with broad-spectrum antibiotics with consideration of gammaglobulin and aggressive fluid and vasopressor therapy may be necessary. Any foreign body in contact with mucous membranes should be sought and removed. While tampons are the most likely offenders, stents from nasal procedures have also been the culprit.

Selected Readings

Fitzpatrick TB, Johnson RA, Wolff K, et al. *Color Atlas and Synopsis of Clinical Dermatology*, 4th ed. New York: McGraw Hill 2001:18–27, 39–41, 826–833.
Stevens DL. 20 clinical pearls: skin and soft tissue infections. *Infect Med* 2003; 20:483–493.

37 Cancers

Constance G. Nichols
Eric Schmidt

There are approximately 500,000 new cases of skin cancer yearly in the United States. The incidence of these tumors has been steadily increasing throughout the past decade. The majority of these cases can be directly related to one of several risk factors. The skin type of an individual, exposure to ultraviolet radiation, common skin viruses, x-ray exposure, chemicals, infrared radiation, and chronic wounds and scars all can contribute to the development of neoplasms of the skin.

Light-complexioned, fair-haired, blue-eyed individuals have been shown to be at increased risk for development of certain malignancies of the skin. Common viruses such as HPV have also been shown to produce abnormal cell division and have been linked to cervical cancer. Chronic low level x-ray exposure can produce damage at the DNA level and result in abnormal cell growth and replication.

Occupational, environmental, and medicinal exposure to certain chemicals can be carcinogenic. Skin cancer has been induced experimentally by exposure to hydrocarbon derivatives of tar and oil. Carcinogenesis seems to be augmented by ultraviolet radiation exposure. Arsenic found in contaminated well water, kelp and shellfish, pesticides, and several medicinal preparations (Fowler's and Donovan's solutions) has been linked to skin cancers that can appear several decades after exposure.

Frequent and prolonged exposure to infrared radiation in the form of heat can result in skin cancer. Chronic scar formation has been associated with the delayed development of skin cancer. Rarely, the site of a scar, nonhealing ulcer, sinus tract, and chronic dermatoses may develop skin cancer. Chronic immunosuppression, seen in transplant patients, as well as those with AIDS, predisposes to the development of certain skin cancers. In these patients, the disease often has a more aggressive course.

Basal Cell Carcinoma

Basal cell carcinoma is a malignant epithelial tumor that arises from the basal cells of the epidermis. Some texts refer to this lesion as basal cell epithelioma because it rarely metastasizes. Still others prefer the term basal cell carcinoma to reflect the malignant, locally invasive, destructive

nature of this tumor. Basal cell carcinoma affects more than 400,000 individuals each year in the United States. It is the most common malignancy of humans, and its incidence is increasing. Basal cell carcinoma occurs more commonly in light-skinned individuals on sun-exposed areas, particularly on the head, face, and neck. It is relatively uncommon in dark-skinned individuals. This lesion is rarely seen before the age of 40, and is more common in men than women.

Chronic sun exposure is the cause of most basal cell carcinomas. Individuals with genetic defects in DNA repair mechanisms (xeroderma pigmentosum) or lack of melanin pigments (albinism) are at increased risk for development of basal cell tumors. Exposure to arsenic found in insecticides, contaminated well water, and medicinal preparations used in the past to treat asthma and psoriasis (Fowler's and Donovan's solutions) have been linked to basal cell carcinoma that can appear several decades after exposure.

A typical lesion is a small, smooth, pearly nodule found on sun-damaged skin of the face. The surface may reveal many fine telangiectasias. As the lesion enlarges, the delicate surface often ulcerates and bleeds, leading to the characteristic rodent ulcer, a ragged, relentless, destructive ulcerating tumor.

The diagnosis of basal cell carcinoma is based on history, appearance, clinical course, and biopsy results.

Treatment

The goal of treatment should be to cure with the best possible cosmetic result. The best cosmetic result is most often achieved with surgical excision. This tumor is often slow growing, and is frequently ignored by individuals. There is often significant damage to the surrounding tissue requiring skin grafting and reconstructive surgery. Basal cell carcinoma rarely metastasizes (incidence between 0.003% and 0.1%) to the regional lymph nodes, lung, and bone. Close follow-up is recommended as up to 35% develop additional lesions within 5 years. All individuals with basal cell carcinoma should be counseled to avoid sun exposure and to use sunscreens on sun-exposed areas.

Melanoma

Malignant melanoma is a cancerous neoplasm of the pigment-forming cells of the skin. Greater than 30,000 new cases of malignant melanoma are diagnosed each year in the United States. The incidence of this cancer has been rapidly increasing over the past several decades for reasons that are not clear, although increase in sun exposure has been implicated. Malignant melanoma can be divided into four types: lentigo maligna, superficial spreading, nodular, and acral lentiginous.

Lentigo maligna melanoma is the least common form of melanoma. Seen in approximately 5% of cases, it is almost exclusively found on the sun-exposed areas of the head and neck. It presents as a flat, often large (3 cm to 6 cm) macule with variable coloration. It can be tan, brown, black, or occasionally blue or white. The lesion often contains scattered black nodules on its surface. This lesion is characterized by a radial growth phase of 3 to 15 years before vertical growth and invasion of the deep tissues is seen. Lentigo maligna melanoma is most commonly diagnosed in the seventh decade.

The most common form of melanoma is superficial spreading melanoma. Seen in approximately 70% of cases, it can be found anywhere on the skin surface. It is most commonly found on the back and trunk of men and the legs of women. It presents as a slightly raised, palpable, asymmetric, less than 2.5 cm, unevenly pigmented lesion. The color varies from brown to black with scattered areas of gray or white. The radial growth phase is somewhat shorter than that seen with lentigo maligna melanoma, usually evolving over 1 to 5 years. Superficial spreading melanoma is usually diagnosed in the fourth or fifth decade.

The second most common type of melanoma, seen in 10% to 15% of cases, is nodular melanoma. The most common sites affected are the trunk in men and the legs in women. The lesion presents as a small, 1 cm to 2 cm, elevated, dark, uniformly pigmented nodule or plaque with frequent central ulceration. Nodular melanoma is characterized by a very short radial growth phase and a rapid vertical growth phase and is, therefore, less likely to be diagnosed in a pre-metastatic stage. Nodular melanoma is usually diagnosed in the fifth decade.

Acral lentiginous melanoma represents less than 10% of melanomas in Caucasians, but is the most common form of melanoma seen in dark-skinned individuals. The lesions are found on the palms, soles, and nail beds and appear as irregular, small, 2 cm to 3 cm, brown to black macules. Papules and nodules are often seen. When found under the nails, the lesions appear as linear streaks. Acral lentiginous melanoma evolves over 2 to 3 years and metastasizes early. It is most often diagnosed in the sixth decade.

Treatment

All patients with suspicious lesions should be referred promptly to a dermatologist for evaluation, biopsy, and follow-up care. Diagnosis, treatment, and prognosis of malignant melanoma is based on history, clinical appearance, and biopsy results. Treatment involves surgical excision with or without regional lymph node dissection. Those individuals with stage I disease (thin tumors without nodal metastases) have a greater than 85% 8-year survival. Long-term survival with Stage II (nodal metastases) and Stage III (systemic metastases) disease drops off sharply. Radiation therapy is used for palliative treatment of brain, bone, and skin metastases. Chemotherapy has been used with little success.

Squamous Cell Carcinoma

The development of squamous cell carcinoma is related to the amount of sun exposure and degree of pigmentation of the skin. Other factors such as common skin viruses, x-ray exposure, chemicals, infrared radiation, and chronic wounds and scars all can contribute, to a lesser degree, to the development of neoplasms of the skin.

Squamous cell carcinoma is a malignancy of the keratinocytes of the epidermis. There are 80,000 to 100,000 new cases of squamous cell carcinoma each year in the United States. The incidence of skin cancer in general has been increasing during the past decade. The development of squamous cell carcinoma is primarily related to the amount of sun exposure and degree of pigmentation of the skin. Squamous cell carcinoma usually appears as a small, distinct, skin-colored, slightly erythematous, firm nodule. The surface may be smooth, rough, or scaling. As it grows it increases in elevation as well as area. Ulceration may occur earlier in fast-growing tumors. As the tumor invades the deeper tissues it may become fixed to the structures below. Metastasis occurs in up to 50% of cases of invasive squamous cell carcinoma, and is most likely to occur with larger, fast growing tumors, as well as in association with tumors of the dorsa of the hands, lips, mucous membranes, and temples.

Treatment

Treatment options include excision, cryotherapy, and topical chemotherapy. Only surgical excision allows pathologic examination to detect occult squamous cell carcinoma. Patients with suspicious lesions should be referred to a dermatologist for evaluation and treatment.

Primary prevention is probably the most important intervention that can be offered. Routine use of topical sunscreens with SPF ratings of 15 to 30 should be encouraged. High-risk (i.e., fair-skinned) individuals should avoid sun exposure during the hours of peak sun intensity. Contact with environmental and occupational carcinogens should be avoided. Smoking and chewing of tobacco should be discouraged. Finally, routine skin examination should be performed by the patient, as well as by the physician to increase opportunity for early detection and treatment of suspicious lesions.

Selected Readings

Cottam JA, Shenefelt PD, Sinnott JT, et al. Common skin infections in the elderly. Infect Med 1999;16:280–290.

Fitzpatrick TB, Johnson RA, Wolff K, et al. Color Atlas and Synopsis of Clinical Dermatology, 4th ed. New York: McGraw Hill 2001:18–27, 39–41, 826–833.

Humphreys TR. Skin cancer: Recognition and management. Clin Cornerstone 2001;4:23–32.

Endocrine and Metabolic Disorders

G. Richard Braen

Emergency physicians evaluate patients with potential endocrine and metabolic problems on a daily basis. Acid-base abnormalities, along with fluid and electrolyte disturbances, are frequent among patients who suffer a cardiac arrest; have a diabetic crisis; develop an episode of an alcohol-related illness; have an acute overdose; or who become septic, to name a few of the related conditions. Each emergency physician should know the basics of acid-base, fluid, and electrolyte disorders and should understand at which times these disorders demand immediate attention and correction.

The patient with diabetes can present an extremely broad spectrum of problems and presentations. In the Emergency Department we not only deal with patients whose glucose levels are either life-threateningly high or life-threateningly low, but also with diabetics who present with increased coronary artery occlusion rates; decreased ability to fight infections, if not well controlled; kidney diseases; and a number of other end organ pathologies. The chapter on glucose metabolism in this section addresses a number of these issues.

Adrenal diseases, parathyroid diseases, pheochromocytoma, and thyroid disorders can present with manifestations that bring patients to the Emergency Department; though these are relatively uncommon events, when compared to occurrence of diabetic problems and acid-base, fluid and electrolyte problems. These areas and related conditions and diseases are each described in corresponding chapters within this section.

Acid-Base Disturbances

Andrew Singer

Classification

Acid-base disorders are classified as follows:

Acidosis or Alkalosis

An acidosis should be considered if the pH is below 7.35; while an alkalosis should be considered when the pH is above 7.45.

Metabolic or Respiratory

In metabolic disorders the primary change is in $[HCO_3^-]$ with compensatory changes in PCO_2, while in respiratory disorders, the primary change is in PCO_2 (i.e., carbonic acid) with compensatory changes in $[HCO_3^-]$. Respiratory disorders are further classified into acute or chronic, based on the amount of renal adaptation. These changes are summarized in **Table 38.1**.

Simple or Mixed

In simple disorders, the changes in $[HCO_3^-]$ and PCO_2 are in the same direction (increase or decrease), and occur in the expected range shown in Table 38.1. If the changes in $[HCO_3^-]$ or PCO_2 are outside of these patterns, or the $[HCO_3^-]$ or PCO_2 is abnormal in the presence of a relatively normal pH, a mixed disorder is usually present.

The anion gap is used to further categorize metabolic disorders. The anion gap (AG) is the difference between the unmeasured cations and unmeasured anions, and can be estimated in the following way:

$$\text{Anion Gap} = Na^+ (Cl^- - HCO_3^-)$$

The normal anion gap is approximately 12 mmol/L, due to a greater concentration of unmeasured anions than unmeasured cations. Where there is excess organic acid leading to a metabolic acidosis, bicarbonate is consumed, replaced by the organic acid in maintaining electroneutrality. This increases the proportion of unmeasured anions, leading to a larger anion gap (typically > 30 mmol/L, but a gap over 18 is considered abnormal).

Buffer Base and Base Excess

Buffer base refers to the body's chemical buffering capacity (approximately 15 mmol/kg). Many blood gas analyzers calculate various measures of buffer base to allow quantification of changes in buffer base independent of the influence of PCO_2.

One of these is the standard bicarbonate, which is the $[HCO_3^-]$ corrected for a PCO_2 of 40 mm Hg. The deviation from 24 indicates the severity of the metabolic disorder.

The base excess is the deviation of the extracellular fluid buffer base concentration from normal. The figure calculated represents the amount of HCO_3^- (in mmol/L)

Table 38.1

Simple Acid-Base Disorders

Disorder	pH	PaCO$_2$	HCO$_3^-$	Expected change
Metabolic acidosis	↓	↓	↓	PaCO$_2$ drops 1-1.5 mm Hg for each 1 mmol/L drop in HCO$_3^-$
Metabolic alkalosis	↑	↑	↑	PaCO$_2$ rise is 0.5-1.0 mm Hg for each 1 mmol/L HCO$_3^-$ rise
Acute respiratory acidosis	↓	↑	↑	HCO$_3^-$ rises 1 mmol/L for each 10 mm Hg PaCO$_2$ rise (±3 mmol/L) up to 30 mmol/L
Chronic respiratory acidosis	↓	↑	↑	HCO$_3^-$ rises 4 mmol/L for each 10 mm Hg PaCO$_2$ rise (±4 mmol/L) up to 36 mmol/L
Acute respiratory alkalosis	↑	↓	↓	HCO$_3^-$ falls 1-3 mmol/L for each 10 mm Hg fall in PaCO$_2$ to a minimum of 18 mmol/L
Chronic respiratory alkalosis	↑	↓	↓	HCO$_3^-$ falls 2-5 mmol/L for each 10 mm Hg fall in PaCO$_2$ to a minimum of 14 mmol/L

that theoretically would need to be added to or subtracted from the extracellular fluid (ECF).

In a metabolic acidosis, HCO_3^- needs to be added, and so the base excess is negative, or a base deficit. In a metabolic alkalosis, there is excess HCO_3^-, so the base excess is positive. In acute respiratory disorders, the base excess is ±2 mmol/L from 0, as the HCO_3^- is usually close to normal.

Differential Diagnosis

Acid-base disorders are the metabolic effect of an underlying disease process. The possible causes of the disorder are often apparent from the history and examination, as well as from calculating the anion gap as demonstrated above, or, in the case of a metabolic alkalosis, measuring the urinary $[Cl^-]$.

Metabolic Acidosis

Etiology

The etiology of metabolic acidosis is usually divided into two groups: those associated with an increased anion gap, and those without (**Table 38.2**).

High-Anion Gap Metabolic Acidosis

Diabetic ketoacidosis. The lack of insulin leads to gluconeogenesis by the liver, with the production of the ketoacids acetoacetate (33%) and β-hydroxybutyrate (66%) from short chain fatty acids. These produce a high-anion gap metabolic acidosis with $[HCO_3^-]$ typically 5 to 10 mmol/L. The situation is made worse by the osmotic diuresis from the hyperglycemia.

Diagnosis is usually made with the combination of a high-anion gap, a metabolic acidosis (pH < 7.30), ketonuria and glycosuria. Tests measuring ketones measure acetoacetate but not β-hydroxybutyrate, and so may underestimate the extent of ketosis.

Starvation. Gluconeogenesis from fatty acids induced by starvation will also create a ketosis. It is usually only mild.

Alcoholic ketoacidosis. Chronic alcoholics often have a combination of both a ketoacidosis induced by starvation and a lactic acidosis. The picture may be further complicated by vomiting, which adds a metabolic alkalosis. This will show a relatively normal or alkalotic pH with a high-anion gap.

Lactic acidosis. Lactate is the end product of the anaerobic metabolism of glucose. It is normally converted by lactate dehydrogenase and nicotinamide adenine dinucleotide (NAD) to pyruvate for aerobic metabolism. Excess production (usually due to tissue hypoxia) or underutilization will lead to a high-anion gap acidosis. Lactic acidosis is usually categorized into two types, based on the presence or absence of tissue hypoxia.

Nonketotic hyperosmolar coma. Occasionally some diabetics may have a high AG acidosis without a significant ketosis, but due presumably to other organic acids.

Salicylate poisoning. Salicylate poisoning, either through aspirin or methyl salicylate (in muscle ointments), has two effects that lead to acid-base abnormalities. Salicylate is a direct central stimulator of ventilation, which in adults often leads to an initial respiratory alkalosis with hypocapnia. Eventually, the second effect of salicylate intervenes, namely the direct acid load of salicylate itself, as well as organic acids formed by metabolic pathways affected by salicylate. This may initially be a mixed picture, but in time the metabolic acidosis predominates. The acidosis enhances the salicylate toxicity, which has a direct toxic effect on the brain.

Methanol poisoning. Methanol is an alcohol used in solvents, lacquers, and windscreen-washer fluid (methylated spirits used to be 5% methanol, but this is no longer the case). It is metabolized by alcohol dehydrogenase to

---

Table 38.2

Etiology of Metabolic Acidosis

1. High anion gap metabolic acidosis
   A. Increased acid production
      i. Ketoacidosis
         a. Diabetic
         b. Starvation
         c. Alcoholic
      ii. Lactic acidosis (types A and B)
      iii. Nonketotic hyperosmolar coma
      iv. Inborn errors of metabolism
      v. Ingestion of toxic substances
         a. Salicylates
         b. Methanol
         c. Ethylene glycol
         d. Solvent inhalation
         e. Other drugs: strychnine, iron, isoniazid, papaverine, expired tetracycline, H_2S, CO, paraldehyde
   B. Failure of acid excretion
      i. Renal failure
2. Normal anion gap metabolic acidosis
   A. HCO_3^- loss
      i. Gastrointestinal
         a. Diarrhea
         b. Drainage or fistulas involving small intestine or pancreas
         c. Urinary diversion via ureterosigmoidostomy, or a long or obstructed ileal loop conduit
         d. Anion exchange resins
         e. Ingestion of $CaCl_2$, $MgCl_2$
      ii. Renal
         a. Carbonic anhydrase inhibitors
         b. Renal tubular acidosis (RTA)
         c. Hyperparathyroidism
         d. Hypoaldosteronism
   B. Acid gain
      i. Recovery from ketoacidosis
      ii. Dilutional acidosis
      iii. Addition of HCl or its congeners
      iv. Parenteral alimentation acidosis
      v. Sulfur ingestion

formic acid and formaldehyde, with a resultant severe metabolic acidosis.

Another diagnostic clue can be made from the calculation of the osmolar gap. This is the difference between the measured osmolality (by freezing point depression) and a calculated osmolality (from serum electrolytes). The calculated osmolality is derived as follows:

Calculated osmolality = $1.86[Na^+]–[glucose]–[urea]$ (all measured in mmol/L)[1]

If using non-SI units the equation is as follows:

$1.86[Na^-]–[glucose]/18–[BUN]/2.8$

If one is also measuring ethanol, this can also be added to the formula as:

$[ethanol]/4.6.$

Ethylene glycol poisoning. Ethylene glycol is an alcohol found in radiator antifreeze fluid, brake fluid, and solvents. It is metabolized by alcohol dehydrogenase into the toxic metabolites glycolic, glyoxylic, and oxalic acids. These lead to severe metabolic acidosis.

Diagnosis can be made in the same way as methanol, based on symptoms such as intoxication without a raised ethanol concentration, and the presence of a high anion and osmolar gap acidosis.

Other drugs, such as strychnine, iron, isoniazid, papaverine, expired tetracycline, hydrogen sulfide, and carbon monoxide can cause a metabolic acidosis, mainly by the production of lactate. Toluene and paraldehyde also cause a metabolic acidosis by direct effects.

Acute renal failure. In acute renal failure, the acute fall in renal function prevents the kidney from handling the body's normal daily nonvolatile acid load. This usually leads to a fall in $[HCO_3^-]$ by 2 mmol/L/day, but there are often other processes such as infection, trauma or corticosteroids that lead to increased catabolism and, thus, to an increased acid load.

Chronic renal failure. With the more gradual loss of functioning nephrons in chronic renal failure, those nephrons still functioning maximize NH_4^+ excretion to maintain the acid-base balance, as well as enhancing phosphate excretion of titratable acidity. The secondary hyperparathyroidism that occurs is believed to depress proximal tubular reclamation of HCO_3^-, leading to a bicarbonate wasting state.

Normal Anion Gap Metabolic Acidosis.

Diarrhea. This is the commonest cause of a normal AG acidosis. Diarrheal fluid has a $[HCO_3^-]$ of 30 to 50 mmol/L, and a $[K^+]$ of 20 to 40 mmol/L, and so leads to significant losses of both ions.

Small bowel or pancreatic drainage or fistula. Surgery involving drainage of the small bowel, biliary system, or pancreas drains fluid rich in HCO_3^-, and low in Cl^-.

Carbonic anhydrase inhibitors. Acetazolamide and methazolamide are drugs used as diuretics and in the treatment of glaucoma. They function by inhibiting carbonic anhydrase. This results in a marked slowing of the conversion of H_2CO_3 to H_2O and CO_2, and so HCO_3^- is not regenerated to replace that filtered or lost. Na^+ and Cl^- resorption is af-

fected (though less so), and H^+ secretion is reduced (due to a urinary acidosis), so a net loss of HCO_3^- occurs, along with a diuresis of HCO_3^-, Na^+, and K^+.

Renal tubular acidosis. Renal tubular acidosis (RTA) is a group of disorders involving either primary or secondary renal disease, where there is a reduction of renal H^+ secretion, but normal GFR. They are normally divided based on the likely site of the defect. In distal disorders, H^+ secretion and NH_4^+ production in the collecting duct are insufficient to match net acid production. There are a number of possible causes, including hypercalcemia, multiple myeloma, hepatic cirrhosis, systemic lupus erythematosus (SLE), and renal transplant rejection. Distal RTA may be further divided according to the effect on serum $[K^+]$.

In proximal RTA, the defect affects reclamation of HCO_3^- in the proximal tubule. As 85% of filtered HCO_3^- is reclaimed here, large amounts of HCO_3^- are lost. The plasma $[HCO_3^-]$ falls and eventually reaches a new steady state, where the reduced plasma $[HCO_3^-]$ means a reduced filtered load of bicarbonate, which can then be regenerated by mechanisms in the distal nephron. Thus urinary acidification is maintained.

The main causes are inborn errors such as cystinosis and Wilson's disease; heavy metal toxicity from lead, mercury, or cadmium; amyloidosis; multiple myeloma; medullary cystic disease; nephrotic syndrome; or early transplant rejection.

Treatment

In an acute metabolic acidosis, the main focus of treatment must be the correction of the underlying disease process. Treatment of a severe acidosis (pH < 7.1) is controversial. The theoretical advantage is an avoidance of the adverse effects of a severe acidosis. The disadvantages are:

1. An increased Na^+ load: 50 ml of 8.4% $NaHCO_3$ contains 50 mmol of sodium (equivalent to 333 ml of 0.9% NaCl);
2. A paradoxical intracellular acidosis, due to an inability to excrete the extra CO_2 load produced by the buffering effect of the added bicarbonate, with reduced cardiac and respiratory function, and its diffusion across cell membranes;
3. A paradoxical decrease in cerebrospinal pH.

The trend now is to avoid giving bicarbonate, even if the pH is < 7.1. If it is felt bicarbonate has to be given, the dose to restore $[HCO_3^-]$ to a given level is:

$$NaHCO_3 = (desired\ [HCO_3^-] – measured\ [HCO_3^-]) \times .5\,BW$$

where the amount of sodium bicarbonate is in millimoles and the body weight (BW) is in kilograms.

Alkalosis

Etiology

A metabolic alkalosis occurs when a disease process raises the pH via a primary increase in plasma $[HCO_3^-]$. There are three main causes of a primary increase in plasma $[HCO_3^-]$:

1. Net loss of $[H^+]$ from ECF. This can occur through the gut (via loss of gastric HCl), or through the kid-

neys (via accelerated acid excretion from diuretics, excess mineralocorticoid effect, or increased anion excretion). There may also be induced deficits of potassium, which leads to the shift of H^+ into cells in exchange for K^+ with a further rise in pH.

2. Net addition of HCO_3^- or precursors to extracellular fluid. Administration of HCO_3^- or its precursors lactate, citrate or acetate in excess of acid production leads to an alkalosis. If renal function is normal, most of this load is excreted, so the rise in pH is usually only modest.

3. Loss of fluid with a higher $[Cl^-]$ and lower $[HCO_3^-]$ than ECF. This occurs in specific situations such as an intestinal villous adenoma or diuretic-induced Cl^- losses, or following a hypercapnic state (e.g., severe respiratory failure or cardiac arrest).

There are two ways to categorize the etiology of metabolic alkalosis: either according to the mechanism of generation (**Table 38.3**) or according to the response to ECF replacement with NaCl.

Pathophysiology

Maintenance of Metabolic Alkalosis

Normally, the body is able to rapidly reverse any increase in HCO_3^- by increasing HCO_3^- excretion. There are some mechanisms, though, that will interfere with HCO_3^- excretion by the kidney, and work to maintain a metabolic alkalosis:

1. ECF volume depletion. This reduces HCO_3^- excretion in three ways: by reducing GFR and thus filtering of HCO_3^-, by stimulating increased reabsorption of Na^+ and HCO_3^- in the proximal tubule (with enhanced Na^+-H^+ exchange), and through mineralocorticoid-stimulated Na^+ reabsorption (with K^+ and H^+ secretion and HCO_3^- generation) in the distal tubule.

2. Mineralocorticoid excess. The distal tubule mechanism described above can occur in the absence of ECF volume depletion if there is excess mineralocorticoid activity present. H^+ excretion is enhanced if there is K^+ depletion present as well.

3. Chloride depletion. Because of the importance of Cl^- as an extracellular anion, and in the reabsorption of Na^+ in the kidney, any significant Cl^- depletion will have to be replaced by HCO_3^- until the Cl^- loss is corrected. There is also low Cl^- stimulated secretion of renin, which encourages aldosterone effects.

4. Potassium depletion. This can effect H^+ secretion as described above, though it would appear to be a small contribution, as K^+ replacement is not necessary to reverse a metabolic alkalosis.

5. Hypoventilation and hypercapnia. It appears that hypercapnia itself may increase HCO_3^- reclamation by the kidney.

Assessment and Diagnosis

Metabolic alkalosis should be suspected in situations where conditions generating and maintaining it are present, e.g., vomiting, gastric drainage, diuretic therapy, muscle cramps/weakness, or hypertension (due to mineralocorticoid effect).

Serum electrolytes show an increased bicarbonate or total CO_2 with hypochloremia and hypokalemia. Arterial blood gases show a pH > 7.35 with hypercapnia and an increased $[HCO_3^-]$.

Treatment

In treating a metabolic alkalosis, the mechanism that is both generating and maintaining the condition needs to be addressed.

NaCl responsive situations respond to volume replacement with 0.9% NaCl (normal saline), and with the addition of KCl to help replenish potassium stores.

Mineralocorticoid excess needs the source of the mineralocorticoid to be removed, or spironolactone should be used to block the mineralocorticoid effect on the kidney.

Severe potassium depletion with NaCl resistance requires large doses of KCl before any NaCl will be effective.

Mixed Acid-Base Disorders

Diagnosis

The expected changes for each of the simple acid-base disorders are given in Table 38.1

Changes outside these predicted patterns, either in the direction of change or the level of change, are usually due to mixed acid-base disorders. They may be of three types:

1. Those where the effects are opposite, leading to excessive adaptation and a relatively normal pH (so-

---

Table 38.3

Etiology of Metabolic Alkalosis Categorized by Mechanism of Generation

1. Loss of H^+
   A. Renal
      i. Mineralocorticoid effect
         a. Conn's syndrome (primary hyperaldosteronism)
         b. -Secondary hyperaldosteronism with K^+ depletion
         c. Cushing's syndrome (glucocorticoid excess)
         d. Bartter's syndrome
         e. ACTH secreting tumors
         f. Exogenous steroids
      ii. Drugs—carbenoxolone, diuretics, liquorice
      iii. Posthypercapnic alkalosis
   B. Gastrointestinal
      i. Vomiting or gastric drainage
      ii. Villous adenoma
      iii. Congenital alkalosis with diarrhea
2. Gain of HCO_3^-
   A. $NaHCO_3$ administration
   B. Metabolic conversion of citrate, acetate, lactate
   C. Milk-alkali syndrome

called benign disorders). These include a mixed metabolic acidosis and respiratory alkalosis or mixed metabolic alkalosis and respiratory acidosis.

2. Those where the effects on the pH are additive, and, thereby, lead to a failure of adaptation and a worsening of the pH changes. These include a combined respiratory and metabolic acidosis or alkalosis.

3. So-called triple disorders, where a metabolic acidosis and alkalosis is combined with a respiratory acidosis or alkalosis as well.

Classification

Respiratory Acidosis and Metabolic Alkalosis

Chronic lung disease produces a chronic respiratory acidosis. The patient then develops cardiac failure and is given diuretics, which adds a metabolic alkalosis. This leads to a $[HCO_3^-]$ much higher than predicted on the basis of either primary disorder alone. Treatment should be directed at improving excretion of HCO_3^- by using NaCl and KCl, though one must be wary of the risk of worsening cardiac failure. This treatment will lower the pH and will maintain a better respiratory drive.

Respiratory Acidosis and Metabolic Acidosis

The combination of respiratory acidosis and metabolic acidosis may occur in cardiac arrests, in the combination of chronic obstructive airway disease (COAD) and shock, or in respiratory failure in a patient who already has a metabolic acidosis. The pH falls markedly, as buffering and kidney are unable to compensate. The $PaCO_2$ and $[HCO_3^-]$ depend on which disorder is dominant. Treatment needs to be directed at both the metabolic and respiratory components of the acidosis, with attention to both ventilation and bicarbonate.

Respiratory Alkalosis and Metabolic Acidosis

The combination of respiratory alkalosis and metabolic acidosis can have various causes. Examples include hepatic or renal failure combined with sepsis, and salicylate intoxication, which initially produces a respiratory alkalosis that is then replaced by a metabolic acidosis. The pH is usually close to normal, but the $PaCO_2$ and $[HCO_3^-]$ are lower than can be explained by either simple disorder.

Respiratory Alkalosis and Metabolic Alkalosis

This combination is probably the most common mixed disorder. The causes include a combination of hepatic failure with hyperventilation and diuretic use or vomiting, or it can occur in someone with a compensated respiratory acidosis who is placed on a ventilator, resulting in a rapid fall in $PaCO_2$. It is characterized by a marked rise in pH, with $PaCO_2$ and $[HCO_3^-]$ out of proportion to what is expected.

Respiratory Acidosis

Etiology

The etiology of a respiratory acidosis is essentially that of hypercapnia. There are two main mechanisms: hypoventilation or ventilation-perfusion mismatching. The difference between acute (**Table 38.4**) and chronic respiratory acidosis relates to whether renal compensation has had time to come into play, usually requiring about 1 to 5 days to take effect.

Pathophysiology

Renal compensation for the acidosis caused by hypercapnia occurs by the increased $PaCO_2$ inducing increased secretion of H^+ (excreted as NH_4Cl), with regeneration of HCO_3^-. This adds an HCO_3^- ion to the body, and so moves the pH toward normal, but has no effect on the $PaCO_2$. Eventually a new steady state is reached, with acid excretion matching production, but with a persistently raised $PaCO_2$.

Assessment and Diagnosis

In an acute respiratory acidosis, arterial blood gases (ABGs) demonstrate a low pH, raised CO_2, and a bicarbonate concentration less than 30 mmol/L. A low O_2 may also be present, especially if the sample is taken while the patient is breathing room air.

In chronic respiratory acidosis, the patient exhibits few symptoms and signs related to the hypercapnia (unless there has been an acute decompensation). ABGs show a lowered pH (but usually > 7.25), a raised $PaCO_2$, and a

---

Table 38.4

Etiology of Acute Respiratory Acidosis

1. Hypoventilation
   A. Central
      i. Brain stem injury
      ii. Cardiopulmonary arrest
      iii. High spinal cord injury
      iv. Opiate or sedative overdose
      v. Coma
   B. Peripheral
      i. Guillain-Barré syndrome
      ii. Myasthenia gravis
      iii. Botulism
   C. Mechanical
      i. Laryngeal edema
      ii. Flail chest
      iii. Multiple rib fractures
      iv. Inadequate mechanical ventilation
          a low breath rate or tidal volume
          b. excessive dead space
2. Ventilation-perfusion mismatching
   A. Airway obstruction
      i. Foreign body
      ii. Aspiration
      iii. Severe bronchospasm
   B. Chest disorders
      i. Pneumothorax
      ii. Severe lung infection
      iii. Smoke inhalation
      iv. Severe pulmonary edema
   C. Vascular disease
      i. Massive pulmonary embolism

raised $[HCO_3^-]$ (rising 4 mmol/L $\pm$ 4 mmol/L per 10 mm Hg rise in $PaCO_2$). $[Cl^-]$ is reciprocally decreased.

Alkalosis

Etiology

The etiology of a respiratory alkalosis (**Table 38.5**) is hyperventilation, whether mechanical, neurochemical or psychological in origin.

Pathophysiology

Adverse Effects. Adverse effects mainly relate to the effects of the acute alkalosis on the concentrations of K^+ and ionized Ca^{2+}, which are both reduced. Neuromuscular irritability is increased, with paresthesias, increased reflexes, tetany (spasms), and possibly even seizures. Hypocapnia is also a potent cerebral vasoconstrictor, which may cause problems in patients with compromised cerebral blood flow.

Buffering and Compensation. Buffering occurs by cells releasing H^+ from body buffers, which leads to a reduction in $[HCO_3^-]$ by converting to CO_2 to correct the low level; 99% of the H^+ comes from intracellular sources, with the remainder from plasma proteins. Cells also are able to respond by increasing lactate production.

Renal compensation usually occurs rapidly and takes place over 24 to 48 hours. Bicarbonate is reduced either by decreasing the reclamation of filtered HCO_3^- or by reducing the production of HCO_3^- used to replace that lost to buffering normal acid loads.

Assessment and Diagnosis

Patients with an acute respiratory alkalosis hyperventilate. They may develop symptoms of neuromuscular irritability secondary to the reduction in ionized Ca^{2+}, such as perioral and extremity paresthesia, muscular cramps, tetany (such as carpopedal spasms), or in extreme cases seizures. There may be ECG and cardiovascular effects secondary to effects on both Ca^{2+} and K^+.

The typical ABG changes are a raised pH, with a reduced $PaCO_2$ and a mildly reduced $[HCO_3^-]$, in the range of 1 to 3 mmol/L for each 10 mm Hg drop in $PaCO_2$. Serum electrolytes may show a reduced $[K^+]$ and ionized $[Ca^{2+}]$.

Selected Readings

1. Bidani A. Electrolyte and acid-base disorders. *Med Clin North Am* 1986; 70:1013–1036.
2. Gennari FJ. Serum osmolality. Uses and limitations. *N Engl J Med* 1984;310: 102–105.
3. Goodkin DA, Krishna GG, Nairns RG. Role of the anion gap in detecting and managing mixed metabolic acid-base disorders. *Clin Endocrinol Metab* 1984;13: 333–349.
4. Kassirer JP. Serious acid base disorders. *N Engl J Med* 1974;291:773–776.
5. Nairns RG, Emmer M. Simple and mixed acid base disorders: a practical approach. *Medicine* 1980;59:161–187.
6. Oh MS, Carroll HJ. The anion gap. *N Engl J Med* 1977;297:814–817.
7. Ventriglia WJ. Arterial blood gases. *Emerg Med Clin North Am* 1986;4:235–251.

Table 38.5

Etiology of Respiratory Alkalosis

1. Central stimulation of respiration
   A. Anxiety
   B. Head trauma
   C. Cerebral tumors or CVA affecting the brain stem
   D. Salicylates
   E. Fever
   F. Pain
   G. Pregnancy
2. Hypoxemia
   A. Pulmonary embolism
   B. Congestive cardiac failure
   C. Interstitial lung disease
   D. Pneumonia
   E. Altitude
   F. Asthma
3. Multiple mechanisms
   A. Hepatic failure
   B. Gram-negative sepsis
   C. Mechanical or voluntary hyperventilation

Adrenal Disease

G. Richard Braen

Adrenal crisis is a clinical syndrome caused by the lack of cortisol, the primary product of the adrenal cortex. Adrenal insufficiency is the lack of cortisol production by the adrenal gland. This may be due to a lesion in the adrenal gland or the anterior pituitary gland, which is primarily responsible for control of the adrenal gland. Primary adrenal insufficiency is a functional or structural lesion in the adrenal gland itself, where a lesion disrupting control of the gland by the pituitary or hypothalamus is known as secondary adrenal insufficiency. Adrenal crisis is a clinical syndrome reflecting an acute loss of adrenal function, usually involving a chronic deficiency of cortisol that is exacerbated by an acute medical, surgical, or traumatic event.

Hyperadrenalism, or Cushing's syndrome, is a state where continuing high levels of steroid hormones (adrenal or exogenous) cause structural and physiologic changes.

Adrenal Insufficiency

The adrenal glands, located at the superior border of each kidney, weigh approximately 4 to 6 g each. The outer cortex is of mesodermal origin; the medulla is of neural crest (ectodermal) origin, and is responsible for the release of epinephrine and norepinephrine. Control of the cortex is hormonal, while control of the medulla is through direct sympathetic stimulation.

The adrenal cortex is divided into three levels structurally and functionally. The zona glomerulosa (outer) layer produces aldosterone, stimulating the kidney in response to potassium and angiotensin. The zona reticulata (inner) produces androgens, and small amounts of other sex steroids. The zona fasciculata (middle) produces cortisol, contributing to control of blood pressure, inflammatory response, and fat and carbohydrate metabolism.

Pathophysiology

Control over secretion of cortisol from the zona fasciculata is exerted by the hypothalamic-pituitary axis in the form of adrenocorticotropin (ACTH). Cortisol-releasing factor (CRF) from the hypothalamus causes release of ACTH, which directly stimulates cortisol release from the adrenal gland tissue. Negative feedback by cortisol on the pituitary suppresses the release of ACTH. Chronic hyperstimulation of the pituitary by exogenous steroids or a cortisol-secreting tumor suppresses the pituitary, an effect that may last several weeks to months before recovery.

Aldosterone is secreted from the zona glomerulosa and is controlled via the renin-angiotensin system and potassium ion concentration. Angiotensin II, converted from angiotensin I by angiotensin converting enzyme, directly stimulates aldosterone, which acts at the renal tubules to retain potassium, sodium, and water.

Primary Adrenal Insufficiency

Primary adrenal insufficiency involves a lesion in the adrenal gland, which affects secretion of both aldosterone and cortisol. There are numerous causes, most of which are insidious in onset. Decreased secretion of cortisol leads to chronic release of corticotropin-releasing hormone (CRH) and ACTH, important factors in the diagnosis of primary adrenal insufficiency. In a manner similar to the melanocyte-stimulating hormone (MSH), ACTH often causes a darkening of the skin in patients with primary adrenal insufficiency. This process develops over a course of weeks to months, and reflects a chronic elevation in ACTH levels.

Idiopathic autoimmune causes of immune deficiency are the most common. Polyglandular autoimmune syndromes (PGA) constitute the majority of autoimmune adrenalitis. Other causes of primary adrenal insufficiency include surgical adrenalectomy, metastatic cancer, granulomatous disease (TB, blastomycosis), infiltrative disease (sarcoid or amyloid), and bilateral adrenal hemorrhage caused by Waterhouse-Friderichsen syndrome, trauma, or disseminated intravascular coagulation (DIC). Addison's disease occurs when the production of cortisol is reduced, requiring a destruction of 90% of the glandular tissue. Onset in most of these conditions is gradual, but an acute crisis can be precipitated in times of stress, causing a state of persistent, vasopressor-resistant shock. Common stressors precipitating cardiovascular collapse in adrenal insufficiency include trauma, infection, surgery, myocardial infarction, and alcohol withdrawal.

Secondary Adrenal Insufficiency

Secondary adrenal insufficiency results from a loss of stimulation of the adrenal cortex by ACTH. Destruction of the pituitary, hypothalamus or a loss of ACTH secretion causes a loss of cortisol production, resulting in the clinical syndrome.

Chronic suppression of ACTH by exogenous steroids is the most common cause of secondary adrenal insufficiency. The effect of steroids on the ACTH axis may persist for up to a year after therapy is withdrawn. Patients on long-term steroid therapy may develop the clinical syndrome of adrenal crisis when steroids are abruptly withdrawn or when the dose of steroids is not increased under times of stress.

Other causes of secondary adrenal insufficiency include pituitary tumors, infarction, hemorrhage, trauma, autoimmune destruction of the pituitary, and infiltration (sarcoid). Sheehan's syndrome is acute pituitary necrosis in the postpartum period due to hemorrhage and shock. The loss of ACTH stimulation causes the adrenal to stop producing cortisol, and an adrenal crisis results. Aldosterone secretion (controlled by renin-angiotensin) remains unaffected, with a preservation of sodium and potassium balance.

Clinical Presentation

Initial presentation of adrenal dysfunction is often characterized by vague systemic symptoms, including weakness, malaise, lethargy, vomiting, abdominal pain, and weight loss. Due to the vague nature of these complaints, the diagnosis is often delayed. Eventually, the more severe symptoms of adrenal crisis, such as shock, will develop, leading to the diagnosis.

Laboratory Assessment

Laboratory findings in acute adrenal insufficiency classically include hypoglycemia, hyponatremia, and hyperkalemia. Hypercalcemia, azotemia, and acidosis may also be present. Hyponatremia is due to a syndrome similar to the syndrome of inappropriate secretion of antidiuretic hormone (SIADH), one that is caused by the loss of cortisol and the resulting increased antidiuretic hormone (ADH) secretion. Sodium is usually >120 mEq/L. Hyperkalemia is due to loss of aldosterone's effect on the kidney, with a net retention in potassium. This rarely becomes high enough to require treatment beyond fluids. Hematocrit and BUN are increased due to dehydration, and hypercalcemia is due to volume depletion. These usually require no treatment besides fluids and reversal of the adrenal crisis.

Emergency Management

Two areas of therapy are important in adrenal insufficiency: volume resuscitation and steroid replacement. Aggressive volume replacement with D5 normal saline should begin immediately: in symptomatic adults at least 1 or 2 L of deficit is present. If necessary the patient may be started on vasopressor agents to maintain blood pressure. Immediate steroid replacement is lifesaving. Hydrocortisone 100 mg IV is an excellent choice, although steroids with minimal mineralocorticoid activity may be chosen, as aldosterone's replacement in the acute phase of therapy is not critical. Dexamethasone 4 mg IV immediately, repeated as needed, provides adequate activity in most situations. Dexamethasone may have an advantage over hydrocortisone in that it does not interfere with further serum cortisol measurements.

Patients who present in shock with suspected adrenal crisis should be admitted to an intensive care unit for further therapy. Patients who are hemodynamically stable may be admitted for further workup. Blood drawn for analysis during the initial IV placement can be sent for a cortisol level, considerably shortening the time period necessary for diagnosis of the type and etiology of the patient's adrenal insufficiency.

Author's Note

This chapter contains information originally written by Dr. Mark D. Crockett in *Emergency Medicine, The Core Curriculum*, R.V. Aghababian et al., eds. Philadelphia: Lippencott-Raven 1998.

Fluid and Electrolyte Disturbances

Daniel M. Joyce

Calcium

The adult body contains approximately 25 mg/kg of calcium: more than 99% is found in the skeleton. The remainder, the miscible pool, is divided into three fractions. Approximately 40% is protein bound (predominantly albumin), 10% is complexed to polyvalent anions (phosphate, citrate, sulfate, and others), and 50% is found ionized. The ionized component is the most important physiologically.

Various conditions affect calcium levels. Most frequently, hypoalbuminemia decreases the protein-bound portion, and, thus, the total serum calcium level, without affecting the ionized portion. A convenient formula to correct this apparent decrease in total serum calcium is as follows: increase the total serum calcium by 0.8 mg/dl for each decrease of 1 g/dl (below 4) in the serum concentration of albumin. Alterations in acid-base status also alter the protein binding of calcium, with alkalosis decreasing the ionized component, roughly a 0.1 mg/dl decrease for every 0.2 unit increase in pH. Additionally, increases in serum anions or free fatty acids decrease the ionized concentration of calcium. Measurement of the ionized fraction of calcium is recommended.

Parathyroid hormone (PTH) is secreted by the parathyroid gland in response to a decrease in the serum ionized calcium. This hormone stimulates osteoclastic bone resorption, increases renal tubular reabsorption of calcium, promotes renal production of calcitriol [$1.25(OH)_2D_3$, the most active metabolite of vitamin D], and, in concert with calcitriol, promotes intestinal absorption of calcium. These cumulative actions of PTH all result in a return to normal calcium levels and reduced PTH secretion via negative feedback.

Hypocalcemia

Symptoms

Commonly, calcium's effect on neuromuscular function predominates the signs and symptoms of hypocalcemia. Circumoral and distal extremity (acral) paresthesias may be the initial complaint. Patients may complain of weakness, fatigue, muscular cramps, and/or difficulty breathing secondary to laryngeal spasm and stridor. Frank tetany may be evident in severe cases. In other patients, the neuropsychiatric manifestations of hypocalcemia may be more prominent, as exhibited by emotional lability, depressive affect or psychosis.

Signs/Findings

Chvostek's and Trousseau's signs denote latent tetany. The cardiac effects of hypocalcemia include decreased myocardial contractility and prolongation of the QT interval. Unfortunately, QT interval prolongation lacks sensitivity and should not be used to screen for hypocalcemia. Hypocalcemia may lower the cerebral excitation threshold, and seizures, usually of the Jacksonian type, may result, especially in a patient with a preexisting seizure disorder. Long-standing hypocalcemia results in calcification of the basal ganglia, cerebellum, and cerebral cortex. As a result, extrapyramidal syndromes, such as choreoathetosis and parkinsonism, may result. Other symptoms result from smooth muscle spasm, including wheezing, dysphagia, and abdominal pain.

Differential Diagnosis

Hypoalbuminemia is the most common cause of hypocalcemia, but as previously discussed, only the total calcium and not the ionized calcium is affected. It is encountered in a variety of conditions, most notably advanced cirrhosis, nephrotic syndrome, and chronic illness. Many of the conditions that result in hypoalbuminemia—nephrotic syndrome and acute pancreatitis, to name two—also concomitantly cause a decrease in ionized calcium.

Treatment

Intravenous calcium is the treatment for symptomatic hypocalcemia. The recommendation is to give 10 ml of a 10% calcium gluconate solution (4.65 mEq, 2.2 mmol, 93 mg) over 10 minutes. This is repeated until patient is asymptomatic. An infusion containing 15 mg/kg of calcium given over 4 to 6 hours may be necessary. Cardiac monitoring and caution are in order for the patient on digoxin. Magnesium levels should be checked and replaced accordingly. Asymptomatic patients may be managed with oral replacement; daily doses of 1 g are usually initiated. Serum phosphorus, PTH, and calcitriol levels should be done in the initial workup if a specific etiology is not readily apparent.

Hypercalcemia

Most patients with hypercalcemia are ultimately diagnosed with primary hyperparathyroidism (PHPT) and are unlikely to develop hypercalcemic crisis. In the emergency department (ED), most of the patients who present with hypercalcemic crisis develop this as a complication of malignancy.

Symptoms, Signs and Findings

Frequently the symptoms of hypercalcemia may masquerade as those of the underlying disease (malignancy) and its treatment. Weight loss, anorexia, weakness, constipation, and changes in mental status are attributed to advancing cancer. Lethargy and disorientation are ascribed to analgesics. The severity of the symptoms relate to the rate at which the calcium level rises. If rapid, lower levels in the 12 to 14 mg/dl range may be sufficient to be symptomatic. Other complaints relate to the obligatory osmotic diuresis that ensues: dehydration, polydipsia, and polyuria. Gastrointestinal symptoms may predominate, such as nausea, vomiting, and constipation.

Patients exhibit evidence of dehydration, at times profound, with weakness, confusion, hyporeflexia, obtundation, and, rarely, seizure activity. The dehydration should result in hypotension, but relative hypertension to the state of volume status may be present due to calcium's effect on vascular tone. Renal insufficiency may be evident on the initial labs. Cardiac effects include bradycardia, bundle-branch blocks, heart block, prolonged PR interval, shortened QT interval, wide T waves, and atrial and ventricular dysrhythmias. Hypercalcemia potentiates the effect of digoxin, and the cardiac side effects may be clinically more apparent.

Differential Diagnosis

Emergency treatment of the patient's profound dehydration should start before the cause of the hypercalcemia is confirmed. In general, the higher the serum calcium level, the more likely that malignancy is the underlying cause of the hypercalcemia.

Malignancy. Hypercalcemia is the most common metabolic complication of malignancy. It occurs in 10% to 20% of patients with cancer at some point during their disease. Roughly 80% of hypercalcemic episodes associated with malignancy are from solid tumors. Hematologic malignancies such as multiple myeloma, lymphoma, and leukemia compose the remaining 20%. There are several mechanisms whereby malignant tumors can result in life-threatening hypercalcemic crisis. Humoral hypercalcemia of malignancy (HHM) results from elaboration by the tumor of a bone-resorbing substance, most often PTH-related polypeptide (PTHrP). This is secreted by solid tumors and their metastases in a manner not subject to a feedback mechanism. The hematologic malignancies, most notably multiple myeloma, secrete a number of cytokines that act locally in the bone marrow to stimulate osteoclastic bone resorption.

Primary Hyperparathyroidism. Parathyroid adenomas cause more than 80% of cases of primary hyperparathyroidism (PHPT). In the outpatient setting, this is the most prevalent cause of hypercalcemia, which results from a primary increase in PTH secretion. The elevation in calcium levels is usually mild and only infrequently results in hypercalcemic crisis.

Other Causes. Less common causes of hypercalcemia are granulomatous disease (sarcoid, tuberculosis) in which calcitriol is elaborated. Infrequently, vitamin D intoxication, milk-alkali syndrome, and adrenal insufficiency may be associated with severe hypercalcemia; the hypercalcemia seen with hyperthyroidism and lithium administration is usually of a milder degree.

Treatment

The kidney can accommodate a significant calcium load. The osmotic diuresis that occurs with hypercalcemia leads to volume depletion and decreasing GFR and a secondary decrease in calcium excretion. Vomiting further advances volume depletion. Encephalopathic changes resulting from increasing calcium levels interfere with thirst mechanisms, further decreasing GFR; thus, calcium levels rise even further, and a true hypercalcemic crisis develops. Initial treatment is aimed at restoring intravascular volume aggressively and enhancing renal excretion of calcium. The solution of choice is normal saline. Patients may require 2 to 3 L of saline over the first few hours. After volume status is adequately restored, then furosemide (40 mg to 80 mg) is administered to augment renal sodium and calcium excretion. Fluid and electrolyte status must be carefully followed to avoid problems with volume depletion and hypokalemia and hypomagnesemia. Thiazide diuretics should be discontinued, as they may aggravate calcium excretion. If renal failure is present, dialysis is indicated.

Steroids have been shown to be beneficial for patients with lymphoma, multiple myeloma, vitamin D intoxication, and granulomatous disease. In severe life-threatening hypercalcemia, calcitonin, which has a quick onset but is hindered by tachyphylaxis, is administered at a dosage of 4 to 8 units/kg every 6 to 12 hours. Currently, pamidronate, a biphosphonate that directly inhibits osteoclast function, is first-line antiresorptive therapy. Plicamycin (formerly mithramycin) and gallium nitrate, although effective, have fallen out of favor due to their toxicities.

Magnesium

Alterations in serum magnesium (Mg^{2+}) represent the single most underdiagnosed electrolyte abnormality in current clinical practice. The normal adult total body magnesium content is approximately 25 g, 60% of which resides in bone. Extracellular Mg^{2+} accounts for 1% of total body Mg^{2+}. The normal serum magnesium concentration is 0.71 to 0.91 mmol/L (1.4 to 1.8 mEq/L, 1.7 to 2.2

mg/dl). The kidney is the principal organ involved in Mg^{2+} homeostasis.

Magnesium Deficiency

Magnesium is principally an intracellular cation, and the serum Mg^{2+} concentration may not reflect the intracellular Mg^{2+} content. Many intracellular Mg^{2+} assays have been utilized experimentally, but currently serum Mg^{2+} analysis appears to be clinically the most practical method of identifying alterations in Mg^{2+} homeostasis.

Symptoms and Signs

Frequently a coexisting and precipitating disease process may mask the signs and symptoms of hypomagnesemia. Commonly found symptoms include central nervous system manifestations, such as tremulousness, twitching, and weakness. Patients may complain of dysphagia.

Signs consistent with neuromuscular hyperexcitability and possibly coexistent hypocalcemia (latent tetany, carpal-pedal spasm, seizures) may be evident. Hyperactive tendon reflexes, ataxia, mental obtundation, and nystagmus can occur in association with hypomagnesemia. Electrocardiographic abnormalities of Mg^{2+} deficiency include prolonged PR and QT intervals. Mg^{2+} deficiency may result in supraventricular and ventricular dysrhythmias (torsades de pointes being a classic example).

A common associated laboratory feature of Mg^{2+} deficiency is hypokalemia. With magnesium deficiency there is renal potassium wasting, and attempts to replete the potassium deficit without simultaneous Mg^{2+} therapy are unsuccessful.

Precipitating Conditions

Hypomagnesemia usually results from losses of Mg^{2+} through the gastrointestinal tract or the kidney. Diabetes mellitus is the most common condition associated with magnesium deficiency. **Table 40.1** lists the causes of hypomagnesemia.

Treatment

Patients who have signs and symptoms of Mg^{2+} deficiency should be treated with Mg^{2+}, usually parenterally. In the ED setting 2 to 4 g of magnesium sulfate given intravenously over 4 hours can start the repletion process. In critically ill patients with ventricular tachycardia and or fibrillation, 2 g intravenously as a bolus over 1 minute is advocated. This may be followed by 10 g of $MgSO_4$ in 500 cc saline over the next 5 hours. Parenteral Mg^{2+} therapy should be interrupted whenever hypotension or bradycardia occurs, or when deep tendon reflexes disappear.

Special Therapeutic Circumstances

Myocardial Infarction. There has been much debate regarding the usefulness of magnesium administration in the setting of acute MI. There is presently no consensus for treating MI patients with magnesium.

Asthma. Magnesium's role in asthma treatment began with anecdotal reports more than 50 years ago, but more

Table 40.1
Causes of Magnesium Deficiency

Gastrointestinal disorders
  Nasogastric suctioning, malabsorption, intestinal fistula, malnutrition, acute hemorrhagic pancreatitis
Renal loss
  TPN therapy, osmotic diuresis (glucose, mannitol, urea)
Renal disease
  Chronic pyelonephritis, interstitial nephritis, glomerulonephritis, non-oliguric ATN, RTA, postrenal transplant
Drugs
  Loop diuretics, alcohol, aminoglycosides, cisplatin, amphotericin B, pentamidine, cyclosporine
Endocrine and metabolic disorders
  Diabetes mellitus, primary hyperparathyroidism, hyperthyroidism, hungry bone syndrome, primary aldosteronism, Bartter's syndrome, metabolic acidosis

ATN, acute tubular necrosis; TPN, total parenteral nutrition.
Adapted from Nadler JL, Rude RK. Disorders of magnesium metabolism. *Endocrinol Metab Clin North Am* 1995;24(3):623-641; and Whang R, Hampton EM, Whang DD. Magnesium homeostasis and clinical disorders of magnesium deficiency. *Ann Pharmacother* 1994;28:220-226.

recently has begun to be demonstrated in clinical trials. There are several conflicting studies regarding efficacy. Despite this, many clinicians administer magnesium to patients with severe asthma not adequately responding to routine treatment.

Alcoholic Patients. Alcohol use is a well-recognized precipitant of magnesium depletion due to both poor intake and renal magnesium wasting. Although thiamine replacement is widely accepted empiric treatment in alcoholic patients, the importance of empiric treatment with Mg^{2+} is probably underestimated. Adding 2 g of $MgSO_4$ to IV fluids in these patients is likely warranted.

Phosphorus

The storage and liberation of cellular energy (adenosine triphosphate, ATP), the delivery of oxygen to peripheral tissues (2,3-diphosphoglycerate, 2,3-DPG), the contraction of muscles, and the structural integrity of the skeleton all depend on the presence of phosphorus and may fail when phosphate stores are depleted.

Hypophosphatemia

Phosphate deficiency most commonly occurs in hospitalized patients. The symptoms of anorexia, muscle weakness, and bone pain rarely become evident until the phosphorus concentration is less than 1 mg/dl. Patients with severe burns experience transient, at times severe, hypophosphatemia. Alcoholic patients are also predisposed to low levels of phosphorus. The severe catabolic events that occur with diabetic ketoacidosis (DKA) deplete phosphate stores, only becoming apparent once hydration and insulin therapy begin. Treatment entails replacing some of the obligatory potassium deficit as potassium phosphate.

Hyperphosphatemia

Hyperphosphatemia may be caused by a decrease in urinary phosphate excretion (renal failure), increased tubular reabsorption (hypo- and pseudohypoparathyroidism), or sudden release of intracellular stores into the extracellular space (rhabdomyolysis and tumor lysis syndrome).

Mild hyperphosphatemia has no apparent harmful effects. There are two major consequences of more severe degrees of hyperphosphatemia: hypocalcemia and metastatic calcifications. Extreme phosphate elevations as a result of cell lysis can be treated with saline bolus and mannitol if renal function is normal, and dialysis if not.

Potassium

Potassium is the principal intracellular cation with a concentration of 140 to 160 mEq/L. In the extracellular fluid (ECF), the concentration of K^+ varies from 3.5 to 5.0 mEq/L. Potassium excretion occurs mainly in the urine, although formed stools contain 5 to 10 mEq/L. Potassium is filtered at the glomerulus and reabsorbed passively along the proximal tubule. It is then secreted by the distal nephron in association with Na^+ reabsorption and H^+ secretion. Aldosterone is released in response to increased plasma potassium levels and to hypovolemic stimulation of the renin-angiotensin-aldosterone axis. It is necessary for normal and augmented K^+ elimination.

Hypokalemia

Symptoms and Signs

Although usually nonspecific, patients complain of weakness, easy fatigability, muscle cramps, paresthesias, and nausea and constipation from an ileus. The most worrisome of presentations result from the cardiac effects on conduction, rhabdomyolysis, and severe weakness progressing to paralysis.

Signs. Generalized weakness and hyporeflexia may be evident. Electrocardiographic findings include diffuse ST and T wave changes, PR prolongation, T wave flattening, and U waves. The action potential and refractory period are prolonged, predisposing the patient to reentrant and atrial and ventricular tachycardias, atrioventricular (AV) dissociation, and ultimately ventricular fibrillation.

Differential Diagnosis

Diuretic use and malnutrition, especially in association with chronic alcohol use, are the most frequent etiologies in the ED setting. **Table 40.2** outlines a rather complete listing of the causes of hypokalemia.

Treatment

The treatment of hypokalemia is simple for the most part. Rough estimates of requirements in replacement are 200

Table 40.2
Causes of Hypokalemia

Gastrointestinal losses
  Diarrhea, laxative abuse, ureterosigmoidostomy, fistulas, vomiting
Transcellular shifts
  Metabolic or respiratory alkalosis, insulin therapy, β-adrenergic agonist therapy, B_{12} therapy, periodic paralysis, hypothermia
Renal losses
  Polyuria (DKA, diuretics, hypercalcemia); RTA, mineralocorticoid excess; Conn's, Bartter's, Cushing's, Liddle's syndromes; renal tubular damage (nephrotoxins, chronic pyelonephritis, or interstitial nephritis); magnesium depletion
Toxicologic
  Clay ingestion, theophylline, insulin overdose, β-agonist overdone, barium (Pa Ping disease), chloroquine, licorice
Miscellaneous
  Hypocalcemia, antibiotics (penicillin, gentamicin, carbenicillin, amphotericin B)
DKA, diabetic ketoacidosis

mEq for a K^+ equal to 3.0, and 400 to 600 mEq for a K^+ equal to 2.0. These are conservative estimates. Treatment varies with severity. With mild or asymptomatic hypokalemia, foods rich in K^+ should be given, especially to patients on laxatives or diuretics. Many of these patients need added oral replacement, occasionally as much as 3 to 5 mEq/kg/day of KCL. In patients with severe symptoms, significant ECG findings or marked hypokalemia, potassium must be given rapidly. However, rapid administration may precipitate arrhythmias even in severely depleted patients. The first goal is to get the patient out of danger rather than complete restoration of body stores. The maximum rate of repletion is generally 0.3 mEq/kg/hour or 40 mEq/hour, whichever is less. Cardiac monitoring is essential at these high rates. Solutions containing greater than 60 mEq/L should be delivered through a central vein, with the distant femoral vein preferred over a more central location.

Hyperkalemia

Hyperkalemia is the most dangerous acute electrolyte abnormality. Potassium homeostasis is dependent on intake and output, and potassium shifts between extracellular and intracellular compartments. As with most electrolyte abnormalities, the severity of the hyperkalemia depends on the rapidity of rise of the potassium level and the absolute level achieved. It may be classified as follows: mild, where level is 5.5 to 6.5 mEq/L, without ECG changes; moderate, where level is 6.5 to 8.0 mEq/L; and severe, where level is greater than 8.0 mEq/L.

Symptoms and Signs

Although exceptions exist, clinical symptoms are rare unless the hyperkalemia is severe, and when present, they are primarily muscular and cardiac in origin. Patients may complain of weakness or dyspnea. Paradoxically, patients may complain of tetany-like symptoms of muscle twitching and tingling, during the early stages of rapidly rising levels of K^+. If hyperkalemia is severe, flaccid paralysis may be present. Most frequently, though, no outward clinical symptoms occur, and cardiac dysrhythmias are the initial manifestation.

Cardiac Signs. Although the following progressive levels of hyperkalemia may be roughly correlated with ECG changes, the rate of rise is more important than absolute levels:

- Tall, narrow, peaked T waves in precordial leads (5.5 to 6.0 mEq/L).
- Prolongation of PR interval and QRS duration, shortened QT interval (>6 to 7 mEq/L).
- Progressive flattening of P wave (>7 to 8 mEq/L).
- Merging of QRS and T wave to produce sine wave (>8 to 10 mEq/L).
- Ventricular fibrillation and asystole (>10 to 12 mEq/L).

A normal or nonspecific ECG does not rule out hyperkalemia. The sensitivity for predicting moderate hyperkalemia in one series was only ~60%: the specificity, though, was >85%. The cardiac effects may be exacerbated by hypocalcemia, hyponatremia, hypermagnesemia, and acidemia.

Neuromuscular. Hyperkalemia produces an ascending flaccid paralysis of proximal limb muscles with hypoactive reflexes. Cranial nerve function is usually spared and sensory changes are minimal. Respiratory muscles may be involved. Paralysis has been reported with levels as low as 6.8 mEq/L, but levels greater than 8.5 mEq/L are more common.

Predisposing Factors and Associated Conditions

There are multiple causes of increased potassium levels and, frequently, more than one condition coexists. Aside from spurious or pseudohyperkalemia, the most common cause is renal failure (40%), either acute or chronic. See **Table 40.3** for a detailed listing of the multiple causes.

Treatment Strategies

Patients with respiratory insufficiency, either secondary to paralysis or rhythm disturbances with hypotension, should be monitored and intubated. Avoid succinylcholine during rapid sequence intubation in patients suspected of having hyperkalemia.

In the asymptomatic patient, if an unsuspected elevated potassium level is encountered, the test of the level should be repeated to confirm or rule out. An ECG should be performed prior to receiving the results from the repeat test. Once true hyperkalemia is documented, there are three goals to treatment: (1) reverse cell membrane abnormalities; (2) restore transcellular gradient by moving potassium into the cells; and (3) remove potassium from the body. The treatment varies depending on the severity

---

Table 40.3

Causes of Hyperkalemia

Pseudohyperkalemia
- Hemolysis from aggressive aspiration, polycythemia, leukemia (>50 100,000 /mm^3), thrombocytosis (>800,000 /mm^3), familial leaky RBC membrane

Decreased renal excretion
- Renal failure (acute, oliguric most severe), Addison's, hypoaldosteronism, medications (ACE inhibitors, potassium sparing diuretics), distal RTA-type IV

Increased release from cells
- Metabolic acidosis and to lesser extent respiratory acidosis, familial hyperkalemic periodic paralysis, tissue catabolism (trauma, hemolysis, chemotherapy, tumor lysis, burns, rhabdomyolysis), medications (succinylcholine, β-adrenergic blockers, NSAIDs), toxicologic (digoxin, fluoride), hypersmolality

Increased intake
- Iatrogenic, salt substitutes, transfusions, potassium penicillin
- NSAID, nonsteroidal anti-inflammatory drug.

---

of effects from the hyperkalemia. Agents available for use to achieve the goals of treatment include calcium, glucose/insulin, bicarbonate, cation exchange resins, dialysis, b-agonists, and hydration/diuretics to a lesser degree (**Table 40.4**).

Treatment Algorithm

Severe Hyperkalemia. If there is evidence of ECG abnormalities (loss of P waves and QRS widening), severe neuromuscular manifestations, or serum potassium level above 8 mEq/L:

- Calcium chloride 10%, 5 to 10 cc IV over 5 minutes; may repeat in 5 minutes PRN.
- Glucose 50 g (100 cc of D50W) intravenous push (IVP).
- Insulin 10 units regular IVP.
- Bicarbonate 1 mEq/kg over 10 minutes, IVP if sine wave or pulseless electrical activity (PEA).
- Kayexalate 30 to 60 g in 100 to 200 cc sorbitol PO or 50 g in sorbitol as retention enema.

Moderate Hyperkalemia (K^+ 6.5–8.0 mEq/L). If chronic in nature and without ECG findings, treatment is Kayexalate alone. Patients with acute onset of hyperkalemia should receive more aggressive treatment (glucose/insulin, bicarbonate, Kayexalate).

Mild Hyperkalemia (K^+ < 6.5 mEq/L, No ECG findings). Mild Hyperkalemia may be managed with restriction of dietary potassium and stopping any potassium-sparing drugs. Patients with a serum potassium level less than 6.0 mEq/L and without ECG changes may be dis-

Table 40.4

Medications for Hyperkalemia

	Mode of Action	Onset/Duration
Calcium	Increases threshold potential	2 to 3 min/20 min
Insulin/glucose	Uptake of potassium into cells	20 to 30 min/several hours
Bicarbonate	Intracellular shift of potassium	<20 min/several hours
Cation exchange resins	Increase colonic potassium excretion	1-2 hours/4-6 hours
Dialysis	Elimination; useful if fluid overload	Immediate/variable
β-Agonists	Intracellular shift	Variable
Volume/diuretics	Kaliuresis	Variable

charged if diagnosis is clear and further increases in potassium concentration are not expected.

Sodium

Sodium is the major extrcellular fluid (ECF) cation and accounts for the majority of the intravascular osmotic pressure. Changes in serum sodium concentration produces a similar change in plasma osmolality. The balance of sodium, water and osmolality is maintained and regulated by the kidney, the neurohypophysis of the posterior pituitary, and the hypothalamic thirst center. Under normal circumstances, ECF osmolality is tightly controlled within a narrow range (275 to 295 mOsm/kg). Increased plasma osmolality stimulates thirst and secretion of ADH or vasopressin from the neurohypophysis; a decrease in plasma osmolality suppresses both.

Hyponatremia

Hyponatremia is the most common electrolyte disturbance. Hyponatremia does not indicate a patient's total body water or total body sodium status, but rather reflects an abnormal sodium-to-water ratio. Hyponatremia may result from sodium loss, water excess, or both.

Pseudohyponatremia

Sodium is confined to the aqueous phase of the serum. Excessive quantities of lipids and proteins decrease the proportion of serum that is water, increasing the solid phase of the plasma above the normal 6% to 8%. The most common method for determining sodium concentration (flame emission spectrophotometry) includes the whole sample when determining the sodium concentration. The sodium concentration of the total sample may be artifactually low because the aqueous proportion of the sample containing the electrolytes is decreased as a result of hyperlipidemia or hyperproteinemia. The true serum sodium concentration may be normal or elevated. A direct ion select electrode, in greater use today, measures only the liquid phase and alleviates this problem. A normal serum osmolality would be expected in this situation.

Hyponatremia with Hyperosmolality

Excess serum concentrations of osmotically active substances, such as glucose, mannitol, and glycerol, cause water to move from the intracellular space to the extracellular space, thus causing a dilutional lowering of the serum sodium concentration. The presence of these osmotically active substances causes a true increased measured serum osmolality, although the calculated osmolality will be lower using Na^+, glucose, and BUN in the following equation:

2Na minus (glucose/18) minus (BUN/2.8)

If the difference between the measured and calculated osmolality is greater than 10 mOsm/kg water, an osmolal gap is present. In addition to the agents above, sorbitol and other organic alcohols (ethanol, methanol, ethylene glycol) typically produce an osmolal gap. This occurs most commonly in the setting of hyperglycemia.

Hyponatremia with Hypo-Osmolality

Acute hyponatremia develops within 72 hours, and results in a serum sodium concentration of less than 120 mEq/L. It is rare for these patients to be asymptomatic.

Symptoms and Signs

If symptomatic, patients present with complaints of headache, nausea, vomiting, and weakness. Symptoms vary from subtle changes in mentation or level of energy to severe alterations, such as coma or seizures. Symptoms generally correlate with the rate of development and the degree of hyponatremia (**Table 40.5**). These features are caused by cerebral edema resulting from cellular overhydration.

Patients are typically without clinical signs except for mild weakness. Advanced encephalopathy is heralded by impaired response to verbal and painful stimulus, hypoventilation progressing to respiratory arrest, seizure activity, coma, and ultimately death.

Differential Diagnosis

The differential diagnosis is best approached by categorizing affected individuals into one of three extracellular volume categories: dehydrated, euvolemic or edematous. During the initial evaluation, the volume status should be assessed clinically and a urinary sodium concentration test should be done.

Central Pontine Myelinolysis (CPM). Mention should be made of a devastating consequence of too ag-

Table 40.5

Clinical Symptoms of Hyponatremia

Early Signs/Symptoms	Moderate Signs/Symptoms	Advanced Signs/Symptoms (Increased ICP)
Nausea	Impaired response to verbal/painful stimuli	Unresponsive/coma
Vomiting	Hallucinations	Hypothermia/hyperthermia
Headache	Obtundation	Seizures
Weakness	Incontinence	Bradycardia/hypertension
Muscle Cramps		Respiratory arrest

gressive correction of the serum sodium. Demyelination is a response of white matter to injury not noxious enough to cause cell death. The classic presentation is that of a hyponatremic patient (most commonly chronic hyponatremia) whose serum sodium is rapidly normalized with resolution of symptoms, but who 3 to 5 days later, develops severe disturbances of the corticobulbar, corticospinal, and cerebral function. The result is mutism, dysphagia, quadriparesis, pseudobulbar palsy, delirium, and even death. Confirmatory findings on CT or MRI may lag behind the clinical findings by several days.

Treatment Strategies

Basic laboratory tests should be obtained: serum electrolytes, BUN, creatinine, glucose, and serum osmolality along with urinary sodium and osmolality.

Asymptomatic Hyponatremia. The emphasis should be on correcting the underlying disturbance. In the hypovolemic patient, restoration of the circulating volume with normal saline solution is indicated. The sodium level should be reassessed every 2 hours at the start of treatment, avoiding a greater than 2 mEq/L/hour rise in the serum sodium concentration. The edematous patient benefits from water restriction, diuretics, inotropic or afterload reducing agents, dialysis, or organ transplantation. For the asymptomatic euvolemic patient with sodium values above 115 to 120 mEq/L, water restriction is all that is usually necessary.

Symptomatic Hyponatremia. Patients developing symptomatic hyponatremia out of the hospital generally have chronic hyponatremia, unless thiazide diuretics or excessive water drinking are etiologic. These patients are unlikely to have the severe complications of hyponatremia (seizures, respiratory arrest, herniation, neurologic damage) but are at risk for the development of central pontine myelinolysis (osmotic demyelination syndrome) during cor-

rection. Initial treatment consists of water restriction, removal of offending drugs, and treatment of the underlying condition. Stabilize the blood pressure and perfusion with normal saline solution before beginning tailored therapy (**Table 40.6**). In moderately symptomatic acute cases (Na^+ 115–120 mEq/L), normal saline infusion supplemented with furosemide to counteract the ADH released in response to sodium infusion may be all that is necessary. It is important to monitor urinary output and to repeat the sodium level in 2 hours. In severe acute cases (Na^+ usually less than 115 mEq/L) in which altered mental status, seizures, or coma are present, hypertonic saline is indicated. Start 3% (not 5%) hypertonic saline solution (HSS) at 100 cc/hr or 1 cc/kg/hr. Maximum initial infusion duration should be 2 to 3 hours. Check the serum sodium every 1 to 2 hours. The serum sodium concentration may rise 1 mEq for every 1.2 cc/kg HSS. Add Lasix 20 mg intravenous to counteract the ADH released; maintain a negative water balance. Correct the serum sodium concentration by a maximum of 8 to 12 mEq during the first 24 hours or an average of 0.5 mEq/hr. If the patient clinically improves (stops seizing) and the sodium is only 113 mEq/L, slow the correction.

Water

Water homeostasis is indirectly maintained by regulation of osmolality and intravascular pressure. The human body is composed of approximately 60% water (range 50% to 70%, obese to lean). Total body water is divided into three compartments: intracellular 67%, interstitial 25%, and intravascular 8%.

Syndrome of Inappropriate Secretion of Antidiuretic Hormone

The syndrome of inappropriate secretion of antidiuretic hormone (SIADH) is a disorder characterized by impaired water excretion and secondary hyponatremia in the ab-

Table 40.6

Treatment of Hyponatremia

Dehydrated	Euvolemic	Edematous
Volume expansion with 0.9% NcCI or 3.0% NcCI solution in severe cases	Fluid restriction Dietary salt	Fluid restriction (treat specific condition)

sence of hypovolemia, hypotension, and cardiac, renal, thyroid or adrenal dysfunction.

Antidiuretic hormone (vasopressin) is synthesized and secreted by the neurohypophysis. Its physiologic role is to reduce the urinary excretion of water. Thirst is equally as important as vasopressin for body water homeostasis. It is regulated by osmoreceptors in the hypothalamus near those for vasopressin release. Studies have found that both impaired urine dilution from inappropriate ADH secretion and excessive fluid intake, frequently iatrogenic, are necessary for the clinical signs and symptoms of SIADH to become manifest.

Clinical Forms

For the most part, the inappropriate antidiuresis in patients with SIADH results from endogenous secretion rather than administration of vasopressin or deamino-8-D-arginine vasopressin (DDAVP). Patients with von Willebrand's disease taking vasopressin are rarely seen with hyponatremia owing to the compensation from their thirst mechanism.

Endogenous secretions can be ectopic from a malignant tumor or eutopic from the neurohypophysis as a result of damage to the gland or inappropriate stimulus. Most frequently hyponatremia develops after or during admission to the hospital when intravenous fluids are injudiciously prescribed to a patient with a condition that causes inappropriate secretion of vasopressin. **Table 40.7** details the many conditions associated with SIADH.

Table 40.7

Conditions Associated with Syndrome of Inappropriate Antidiuretic Hormone

Malignant tumors (ADH-producing)
- Carcinoma (bronchogenic, pancreas, duodenum, ureter, prostate), thymoma, ALL, lymphoma, mesothelioma, Ewing's sarcoma

CNS disorders
- Infection (meningitis, encephalitis, abscess), CVA, trauma, hypoxia, tumors, psychosis

Pulmonary disorders
- Infection (tuberculosis, bacterial, viral, fungal, mycoplasma), respiratory failure (RDS, ventilation, asthma, pneumothorax)

Drugs
- Exogenous ADH (vascopressin, desmopressin, oxytocin), promote ADH release (TCAs, vinca alkaloids, carbamazepine, colchicine), potentiates ADH action (chlorpropamide, cyclophosphamide)

General surgery
- 3-days of increased ADH release postoperatively

ADH, antidiuretic hormone; ALL, acute lymphatic leukemia; CNS, central nervous system; CVA, cardiovascular accident; RDS, respiratory distress syndrome; SIADH, syndrome of inappropriate secretion of antidiuretic hormone; TCA, tricyclic antidepressants.

Clinical Manifestations

The signs and symptoms elaborated above in the section on hyponatremia are seen in SIADH. The severity of the signs and symptoms is related to the rapidity, as well as the absolute level of hyponatremia. Acute hyponatremia occurring over less than 24 hours to a concentration less than 120 mEq/L usually causes significant disability and mortality.

Diagnosis

The clinical and laboratory criteria for diagnosis of SIADH are shown in **Table 40.8**.

The first step is to check serum osmolality and to confirm that the hyponatremia is associated with hypo-osmolality. Measure urine osmolality and confirm that the urine is not maximally dilute. This is a key point: in the setting of low sodium and osmolality, the urine should be maximally diluted, that is, less than 100 mOsm/kg.

Therapy

Since much of the morbidity associated with SIADH results from iatrogenic administration of hypotonic fluids, this practice should be avoided in the ED setting. If euvolemic hyponatremia is confirmed, water restriction is all that is necessary in the vast majority of patients. Severely symptomatic patients (seizing, coma) can be treated with small amounts of 3% hypertonic saline as detailed above.

Hypernatremia

Hypernatremia, and its attendant hyperosmolality, is seen most commonly in patients with no access to fluids or with an impaired thirst mechanism. Contributors include febrile illnesses, vomiting, diarrhea, and burns. The normal compensatory response is an increase in thirst and renal water conservation through ADH secretion. Hypernatremia is rarely seen in an alert patient with an intact thirst mechanism and access to water.

Symptoms and Signs

The clinical features result from loss of intracellular water from brain cells; like hyponatremia, they are primarily central nervous sytem (CNS) related. Anorexia, nausea, and vomiting are the early features, with lethargy, increased reflexes, confusion, seizures, and coma occurring as the serum sodium level rises (**Table 40.9**).

Table 40.8

Diagnostic Criteria for SIADH

Plasma [Na] < 135 mEq/L and plasma osmolality < 280 mOsm/kg
Urine osmolality > 100 mOsm/kg (not maximally dilute); contains sodium
No dehydration, edema, hypotension
Renal, adrenal, thyroid, and cardiac function normal

Table 40.9		
Clinical Symptoms of Hypernatremia		
Muscle weakness		
Mental confusion		
Irritability		
Seizures/coma		
Hyper reflexia		
Treatment of Hypernatremia		
Dehydrated	**Euvolemic**	**Edematous**
Volume Expansion	Water replacement	Diuretics and water replacement
0.9% NcCI Solution until stable, then switch to hypotonic solution	Consider a vasopressin trial	

If the clinical status of the patient is such that volume contraction is present, signs of dehydration predominate. Otherwise, weakness, increased reflexes, and seizure activity are found, as noted above. The physical decrease in brain volume caused by cellular dehydration can put unusual stress on the cerebral vasculature, leading to subcortical and subarachnoid hemorrhage in the rare patient.

Differential Diagnosis

Again, as with hyponatremia, it is relevant to divide the etiologies of hyponatremia based on clinical volume status: dehydrated, euvolemic, and hypervolemic. The reported causative factors of diabetes insipidus are listed in **Table 40.10**.

Treatment Strategies

Initially one should obtain an accurate history, including water and salt intake, daily urine output, investigation of extrarenal fluid losses, a review of medications, and prior history of CNS, renal, or endocrine disease. Routine laboratory analysis, including serum osmolality and urinary electrolytes and osmolality, should be performed. Potas-

sium replacement should be aggressive, if hypokalemia is present in the absence of significant acidosis.

Most important when determining treatment is an understanding of how the brain adapts to dehydration. In hypertonic states, brain cell dehydration is prevented by an accumulation of intracellular idiogenic osmoles (thought to be electrolytes and amino acids). These idiogenic osmoles are not dissipated rapidly and aggressive correction with hypotonic fluids can lead to rapid uptake of water by the brain cells, resulting in cerebral edema and CNS dysfunction.

The treatment of hypernatremia is guided by the patient's volume status. The formula—water deficit = 0.6 kg $[(Na^+ - 140)/140]$—may be helpful: however, only frequently repeated sodium measurements define therapy. If the patient is volume depleted, restore intravascular volume with normal saline solution, then switch to half-normal saline (or D5W) at a rate equal to their daily losses or 100 cc/hr, once the patient is stable. The goal of sodium correction should be no greater than a 0.5 mEq/L/hour: if faster, reduce fluid infusion by 50. The very rare patient who is volume expanded may require diuretic therapy. Patients with central diabetes insipidus (DI) require fluids and hormone replacement. Aqueous Pitressin is a short-acting preparation for the treatment of acute DI. Give 5 units SQ/IM/IV every 3 to 4 hours, as guided by urine volume and specific gravity.

Selected Readings

1. Avner ED. Clinical disorders of water metabolism: hyponatremia and hypernatremia. *Pediatr Ann* 1995;24:23–30.
2. Bilezikian JP. Management of acute hypercalcemia [see comments]. *N Engl J Med* 1992;326:1196–203.
3. Bourke E, Delaney V. Assessment of hypocalcemia and hypercalcemia. *Clin Lab Med* 1993;13:157–172.
4. Bourke E, Yanagawa N. Assessment of hyperphosphatemia and hypophosphatemia. *Clin Lab Med* 1993;13:183–207.
5. Bradberry SM, Vale JA. Disturbances of potassium homeostasis in poisoning. *J Toxicol Clin Toxicol* 1995;33:295–310.
6. DeVita MV, Michelis MF. Perturbations in sodium balance. Hyponatremia and hypernatremia. *Clin Lab Med* 1993;13:135–148.
7. Edelson GW, Kleerekoper M. Hypercalcemic crisis. *Med Clin North Am* 1995;79:79–92.
8. Haycock GB. The syndrome of inappropriate secretion of antidiuretic hormone [Review]. *Pediatr Nephrol* 1995;9:375–381.
9. Hodgson SF, Hurley DL. Acquired hypophosphatemia. *Endocrinol Metab Clin North Am* 1993;22:397–409.
10. Kinirons MT. Newer agents for the treatment of malignant hypercalcemia. *Am J Med Sci* 1993;305:403–406.

Table 40.10	
Causes of Diabetes Insipidus	
Central	
• Primary (congenital and familial, nonfamilial)	
• Secondary (head trauma or surgery, supra- and intrasellar tumors, granulomas, infection, vascular lesions, hemorrhage, thrombosis)	
Nephrogenic	
• Primary (genetic)	
• Secondary (renal disease, electrolyte imbalance)	
Drugs	
• Inhibit ADH release (ethanol, diphenylhydantoin, CO, clonidine)	
• Inhibit ADH action (lithium, amphotericin B, cisplatin, propoxyphene, osmotics)	

ADH, antidiuretic hormone.

11. Kovacs L, Robertson GL. Syndrome of inappropriate antidiuresis [Review]. *Endocrinol Metabol Clin North Am* 1992;21:859–875.
12. McDonald RA. Disorders of potassium balance. *Pediatr Ann* 1995;24:31–37.
13. McLean RM. Magnesium and its therapeutic uses: a review. *Am J Med* 1994;96:63–76.
14. Mulloy AL, Caruana RJ. Hyponatremic emergencies. *Med Clin North Am* 1995;79:155–168.
15. Nadler JL, Rude RK. Disorders of magnesium metabolism. *Endocrinol Metab Clin North Am* 1995;24:623–641.
16. Nussbaum SR. Pathophysiology and management of severe hypercalcemia. *Endocrinol Metab Clin North Am* 1993;22:343–362.
17. Reber PM, Heath H 3rd. Hypocalcemic emergencies. *Med Clin North Am* 1995;79:93–106.
18. Stedwell RE, Allen KM, Binder LS. Hypokalemic paralyses: a review of the etiologies, pathophysiology, presentation, and therapy. *Am J Emerg Med* 1992;10:143–148.
19. Whang R, Hampton EM, Whang DD. Magnesium homeostasis and clinical disorders of magnesium deficiency. *Ann Pharmacother* 1994;28:220–226.

Disorders of Glucose Metabolism

Sandra M. Schneider

Diabetes Mellitus

Elevation in glucose triggers release of insulin by the beta cells of the pancreas. Insulin transports glucose, amino acids, phosphorus, and potassium across the cell membrane in target tissues. Insulin is required for the transport of glucose into the cells of all tissues except red blood cells and brain. Very small levels of insulin inhibit ketogenesis, glycogenolysis, lipolysis, and gluconeogenesis.

In absence of insulin, fat metabolism and release of glycogen is controlled by the counterregulatory enzymes glucagon, epinephrine, cortisol, and growth hormone.

Diabetes is the most common endocrine abnormality in humans; 1% to 3% of the population has some form of diabetes. Nearly 6% of health care costs in the United States arise from diabetes or its complications.

Type 1 diabetics are insulin dependent and predisposed for diabetic ketoacidosis. Type 1 diabetics make no insulin. It is an autoimmune disease affecting primarily Caucasian children with peak incidence at puberty. Type 2 diabetes is likely hereditary. It is prevalent in Native Americans, Blacks, and Mexican Americans. The prevalence of type 2 diabetes increases through life and is related to obesity. All patients with type 2 diabetes have low but detectable levels of insulin. Some type 2 diabetics progress to type 1 diabetes.

Rarely, diabetes mellitus has a secondary cause, such as severe pancreatitis, pheochromocytoma, acromegaly, Cushing's disease, and the exogenous use of corticosteroids. Drugs and chemical exposures, such as salicylate overdose, thiazide diuretics, and propranolol, may result in reversible glucose intolerance. Genetic diseases, such as lipodystrophy, myotonic dystrophy, and ataxia telangiectasia, are associated with insulin deficiency.

Hypoglycemic Syndromes

Hypoglycemia causes two types of symptoms, those secondary to a loss of glucose and those secondary to counterregulatory hormone release, specifically the action of glucagon. Hypoglycemia below a critical level results in CNS dysfunction, seen as confusion, abnormal behavior, and/or deceased level of consciousness. As the glucose falls, there is a mobilization of counterregulatory hor-

mones. Glucagon is the most critical of these hormones as it results in immediate release of glucose from liver, fat, and muscle storage. In the absence of glucagon, epinephrine mobilizes glucose. Epinephrine release causes side effects of sweating, tachycardia, restlessness, hunger, and tremor, often alerting the individual to the onset of hypoglycemia, allowing for self-treatment. While CNS symptoms begin when glucose falls <70 mg/dL, catecholamines are not released until glucose levels are <50 to 55 mg/dL. Symptoms are related to the degree of hypoglycemia and the rate of fall. Type 1 diabetics quickly lose the capacity to release glucagon, and catecholamines are often depleted or ineffectively released. Without these symptoms, Type 1 diabetics are at high risk for severe hypoglycemia and coma. Hypoglycemia at night can cause night sweats, nightmares, and headaches.

Up to 7% of deaths among insulin-dependent diabetics are secondary to hypoglycemia. Nearly 8% to 15% of insulin-dependent diabetics have one or more severe hypoglycemic episodes each year. Repeated hypoglycemia may produce cognitive deficiencies. The common causes of hypoglycemia are shown in **Table 41.1**.

Diagnosis

Hypoglycemia is easily diagnosed. Bedside glucose levels are accurate if done correctly; however, they require meticulous attention to detail. If the symptoms appear to be classic but the bedside test does not demonstrate hypoglycemia, it is best to treat the patient. Hyperlipidemia causes displacement of glucose and falsely low glucose levels. Some women and neonates tolerate glucose levels as low as 35 mg/dL without symptoms. Patients may develop symptoms of counterregulatory hormone release without the presence of hypoglycemia. These patients may respond to food intake, aborting the catecholamine-type symptoms.

Treatment

The goal of treatment of hypoglycemia is to resupply the body with glucose. In patients who are alert and have no risk of aspiration, oral replacement is preferred. This is done with sugar and orange juice. Regular granulated sugar contains only 4 g of glucose per teaspoon. Glucola,

Table 41.1

Common Causes of Hypoglycemia

Fasting
1. Endocrine disorders—hypopituitarism, adrenal insufficiency
2. Enzyme defects—G6PD
3. Decreased glucose intake deficiency
   - Starvation, malnutrition
   - Infancy
   - Late pregnancy
4. Liver disease
5. Hepatic congestion
6. Hepatic failure—hepatitis, cirrhosis
7. Hypothermia
8. Uremia
9. Toxins—alcohol, insulin, sulfaureas, quinine, pentamidine, disopyramide
10. Endotoxic shock
11. Pancreatic tumors—insulinoma
12. Carnitine deficiency

Reactive (postprandial)
1. Reactive hypoglycemia—alimentary hyperinsulinism
2. Hereditary fructose intolerance
3. Idiopathic

used primarily for glucose tolerance tests, contains 75 g of glucose. Glutose and instant glucose are gel-like substances that can be absorbed from the oral mucus membranes.

For patients who have a decreased level of consciousness, are at risk of aspiration or are unable to take oral medication, intravenous dextrose (25 g of 50% dextrose) rapidly reverses hypoglycemia, raising the blood glucose level by 35 to 350 mg/dL (mean 50 mg/dL). In children, a 25% dextrose solution is given, and in neonates, a 10% dextrose should be used. The majority of adults respond to a single ampule of 50% dextrose (D50); however, in some patients a second dose is necessary. Adrenal insufficiency should be considered in patients who fail to respond appropriately after two ampules of IV 50% dextrose. Such patients should have a plasma cortisol drawn, and should receive hydrocortisone 100 to 200 mg IV. The plasma cortisol drawn prior to cortisone replacement is used to confirm adrenal insufficiency. Another important cause of treatment failure in hypoglycemia is the presence of large amounts of exogenous insulin or sulfonylureas, such as with intentional overdose.

Treatment should resolve both CNS symptoms and catecholamine-induced effects within 5 to 10 minutes. The time for resolution of the symptoms is dependent on the duration and severity of the symptoms. While catecholamine-related symptoms such as restlessness, tremor, and hunger may be relieved within minutes, CNS symptoms may take longer, because the blood-brain barrier has a slower diffusion of glucose.

Intramuscular glucagon may be used to reverse hypoglycemia. Glucagon increases gluconeogenesis and glycogenolysis, thereby raising serum glucose. Glucagon can be given intravenously, intramuscularly, or subcutaneously in doses of 1 to 2 mg (0.5 mg for children younger than 1 year). Glucagon takes two to six times longer than intravenous dextrose to achieve a normal glucose level and reversal of CNS effects. Plasma glucose rises an average of 100 mg/dL after glucagon 1.0 mg IM. Glucagon can also be administered intranasally. This may eventually prove to be effective for home use.

Intravenous dextrose and glucagon effects last for only 60 minutes. Oral feeding with complex carbohydrates will maintain a steady supply of glucose. Patients who cannot tolerate oral feeding because of nausea, vomiting or decreased level of consciousness should receive intravenous 5% dextrose solution. In general, 8 g to 10 g of glucose per hour is sufficient to prevent hypoglycemia. Treatment of insulin overdose requires special consideration. Administration of D50 is the appropriate initial treatment. In most patients, 10% dextrose solution via central line maintains euglycemia. Overdose patients with ongoing severe hypoglycemia should be started on either diazoxide (a direct insulin inhibitor) or octreotide (a somatostatin analogue). Overdose with oral hypoglycemics may require higher concentrations of glucose, but more importantly may require prolonged glucose support.

Patients should be admitted if they display hemodynamic instability, particularly after the return of glucose to normal or with signs of concomitant illness. Patients on long-acting oral hypoglycemics often require hospitalization with frequent serum glucose estimation. Prior to discharge, attention should be paid to prevention of further recurrences. The cause of the incident is usually obvious— skipped meals, excessive exercise, insulin adjustment. In some cases, the cause may not be identified and close home monitoring or at times inpatient observation may be necessary. Family members should be available to monitor the patient for the next several hours and instructed in the use of supplemental glucose.

Differential Diagnosis

Although most cases of hypoglycemia are related to over-use of insulin, patients who are not diabetic and who deny use of insulin or sulfaurea products can pose a diagnostic dilemma (**Table 41.2**). Insulinoma is a β-cell tumor of the pancreas that secretes insulin, causing recurrent hypoglycemia. Sepsis is another important cause of hypoglycemia.

Hypoglycemia is seen in patients with alcohol use, primarily in those patients with glycogen deficiency due to prolonged malnutrition. Treatment of patients with alcohol-induced hypoglycemia is identical to that of other patients with hypoglycemia. Small children may have ethanol-induced hypoglycemia from drinking either alcohol or perfumes or colognes.

Hyperglycemia

Two syndromes are seen with hyperglycemia: diabetic ketoacidosis and hyperglycemic hyperosmolar coma.

Diabetic Ketoacidosis

Diabetic ketoacidosis (DKA) occurs in Type 1 diabetics, where insulin levels are absent. Its incidence is approximately 12.5 episodes of DKA per 1,000 individuals with Type 1 diabetes. DKA is the initial sign of diabetes in approximately 10% of patients. Diagnostic criteria include glucose greater than 250 mg/dL, pH less than 7.35, low bicarbonate, high anion gap, and positive serum ketones.

Pathophysiology

Diabetic ketoacidosis is a two-hormone disorder: too little insulin and too much glucagon (and other counterregulatory hormones). Lack of insulin causes muscle, adipose tissue, and cells to starve. The liver increases glycogenolysis and gluconeogenesis. Adipose tissue releases free fatty acids that, when delivered to the liver, result in ketogenesis and hyperketonemia. Proteolysis yields a catabolic transfer of amino acids, potassium, phosphate, and magnesium from the intracellular fluid to the extracellular fluid and loss of nitrogen and electrolytes in the urine.

While the cells are starving, there is increasing hyperglycemia. The renal threshold for glucose is rapidly reached. Marked increase in urine output creates extracellular fluid, and sodium and potassium loss. Overall, there is a shift of water due to the hyperosmolality; this leads to hyponatremia, ketosis, and acidemia, resulting in nausea and vomiting, further increasing dehydration.

The brain is unaffected by the lack of insulin. Glucose easily diffuses across the blood-brain barrier and across brain cells and is easily utilized by the brain. Mental status deteriorates with increasing hyperosmolality and acidosis.

Approximately 80% of DKA episodes have an identifiable precipitating factor: infection in 37%; insulin administration error in 21%; drugs or alcohol use in 10%; other endocrine abnormalities in 8%; pancreatitis and abdominal disease in 5%; and acute myocardial infarction in 5%. Infection causes an increase in plasma cortisol levels, secondary to stress, leading to insulin resistance.

Clinical Presentation

Diabetic ketoacidosis should be suspected in any patient with known Type 1 diabetes who presents with decreased level of consciousness, abdominal pain or who has concomitant illness that would lead to DKA (e.g., sepsis). Many will have a fruity odor of acetone detected on their breath, although a significant percentage of normal individuals lack the ability to smell acetone. Careful physical examination of the patient should be performed, looking for sites of infection. Any skin ulcers need to be examined fully. The nasal turbinates and palate should be examined for necrotic lesions indicating mucormycosis, aspergillosis or candidiasis. Bedside glucose determinations, if done correctly, confirm the presence of hyperglycemia. A spot check of serum on a nitroprusside tablet confirms ketosis. Typical values obtained from the laboratory include glucose of approximately 600 mg/dL (range 200 to 2000 mg/dL), β-hydroxybutyric acid and acetoacetate 12 mmol/L (range 6 to 20), pH 7.15 (range 6.8 to 7.3), bicarbonate 10 mEq/L (range 4 to 15 mEq/L), PCO_2 20 mm Hg (range 14 to 26 mm Hg), and anion gap $[Na^-(CL + HCO_3)]$ greater than 18.

Hyponatremia may be reported by the laboratory; however, true sodium levels are normal to elevated:

True sodium = measured sodium + [(serum glucose – 100)/100] × 1.6 or
Na = [1.6 × glucose (mmol/L)–5.5]/5.5.

In the formula above, sodium is measured in mEg/L and serum glucose is measured in mg/dL.

Potassium is reported by the lab as normal to elevated, but there is often severe total body depletion of potassium. Potassium is driven out of the cells by acidosis.

Hypotension indicates a severe dehydration; aggressive fluid replacement is mandatory. Leukocytosis is caused by demargination by catecholamines, and does not by itself

Table 41.2
Differential Diagnosis of Hypoglycemia Unrelated to Diabetes

	Insulin	Insuli:glucose ratio	Insulin antibodies	C peptide	Drug screen for sulfaureas
Insulinoma	↑	>0.4	↑	−	−
Surreptitious insulin	↑	>0.4	↓	+	−
Surreptitious sulfaureas	↑	>0.4	↑	−	+

indicate the presence of infection. Elevations in amylase and lipase do not indicate pancreatitis.

Variations on Presentation

Patients with hypoperfusion may have an increased anion gap with low ketones because of high lactate and b-hydroxybutyric acid levels. As the patient recovers, ketones may appear to rise as b-hydroxybutyrate is metabolized to acetone.

Occasionally, patients present with normal to slightly elevated glucose levels. These patients have excellent hydration or an elevation in glomerular filtration rates, such as pregnant patients. DKA occurs at a lower glucose level (150 to 300 mg/dL) and more rapidly in pregnant patients. Metabolic changes associated with pregnancy lower buffer capacity. There is increased bicarbonate excretion by the kidney. Hormones, which act as insulin antagonists, including placental lactogen, cortisol, and prolactin, are produced in higher amounts during pregnancy.

Some patients present with a normal or elevated pH due to the presence of vomiting (contraction alkalosis), alkali ingestion (antacids), diuretic use, and/or Cushing's disease.

Differential Diagnosis

Starvation can cause urinary ketones; however, glucose is normal and serum ketosis is not present. Uremia, lactic acidosis, and some toxic ingestions may have a metabolic acidosis and elevated glucose, and no serum ketone bodies. Patients with hyperosmolar nonketotic syndrome may present with an elevated glucose, but they do not form ketone bodies because of the presence of low insulin levels. Patients with prolonged alcohol ingestion, particularly accompanied by nausea and vomiting, present with starvation ketosis that can become a systemic ketosis because of the presence of dehydration. In this case, b-hydroxybutyric acid is classically elevated while other ketone bodies are low, causing a false-negative nitroprusside test. Ketone bodies clear with hydration and the patient recovers quickly. Hyperglycemia with an elevated anion gap may be seen with ingestion of methanol, ethylene glycol, and salicylates; however, systemic ketosis is rare. Isopropyl alcohol ingestion causes a significant ketonemia; however, glucose levels and the anion gap are normal.

Treatment

The goal of treatment of DKA is to decrease the action of counterregulatory hormone and restore normal glucose transport. Care can be divided into three phases: acute stabilization, elimination of ketosis, and reinstitution of normal diabetic regimen.

Phase I—Acute Stabilization

Acute stabilization of the patient often takes place before there is a definitive diagnosis of diabetic ketoacidosis. Treatment is initiated on the basis of history, physical examination, and bedside screens showing elevation in glucose and urinary ketosis. Particular attention should be placed on early restoration of the blood volume with the immediate replacement of 1 to 2 L of normal saline (10 to 20 cc/kg in children). All patients should receive supplemental oxygen, ECG monitoring, and close monitoring of urine output. A Foley catheter should be avoided when feasible.

Fluid Therapy

After assuring the ABCs, 1 L of intravenous normal saline is infused over 30 minutes and a second liter over 60 to 90 minutes to rapidly restore extracellular fluid (in children 20 cc/kg over 2 hours). Restoration of the intracellular fluid should then take place using half normal saline 150 to 200 cc/hour for 8 to 12 hours. In children, half normal saline is given at a maximum rate at 5 cc/kg per hour. As an alternative to intravenous therapy, oral rehydration salt therapy can be given at 1 L/hour orally or via nasogastric (NG) tube.

Insulin

Lipolysis is inhibited by insulin levels of 5 mU/mL. Proteolysis is inhibited by insulin levels of by 10 mU/mL and hepatic glucagon production by 20 mU/mL. Insulin clearance rates are approximately 12 cc/kg per minute. Peripheral glucose utilization is maximum at levels of 100 mU/mL. To allow for some presence of insulin resistance, it is appropriate to maintain a concentration of 200 mU/mL. Insulin administration of approximately 0.1 U/kg per hour achieves this level and saturates most insulin receptors.

An optional insulin bolus of 10 units regular insulin IV is followed by insulin infusions of 4 to 8 units/hour (0.1 U/kg/hr) of regular insulin. The same results can be achieved by an intravenous bolus of insulin followed by 10 units (0.1 U/kg) of regular insulin IM every hour. The onset of action of intravenous insulin occurs within minutes, and has a half-life of 30 to 45 minutes. Serum glucose levels should be expected to fall 75 mg/dL per hour. If there has not been a decrease in 4 hours, then insulin rates should be increased. Insulin infusion should be continued until the glucose becomes < 250 mg/dL and all ketones are cleared.

Bicarbonate

As ketone bodies are metabolized, bicarbonate is generated. The use of exogenous bicarbonate has been associated with severe side effects including a paradoxical lowering of intracellular pH, a shift in the oxygen dissociation curve (which negatively affects tissue oxygenation), hypernatremia, hypertonicity, and hypokalemia (bicarbonate shifts potassium to reenter the cell). Other effects include cerebral dysfunction caused by a pH gradient across the CNS (bicarbonate cannot readily enter the brain) and late alkalemia secondary to bicarbonate regeneration. Even in the presence of severe acidosis (pH ranges 7.1 to 6.9), there appears to be no significant benefit for patients treated with bicarbonate. Bicarbonate therapy should be reserved for patients with pH < 6.9, severe hyperkalemia (ECG presence of peak T-waves and a widened QRS), or hypotension refractory to aggressive fluid therapy. Patients in deep coma with very low pH may benefit by bicarbonate replacement.

Even within these indications, there is no place for large boluses of bicarbonate in the treatment of DKA.

Patients should receive 50 to 100 mEq IV over 1 to 2 hours. Patients who have severe hyperkalemia with ECG changes may receive 50 to 100 mEq of IV bicarbonate over 15 minutes.

Potassium

The most common serious error made in DKA therapy is the failure to replace potassium. Acidosis drives potassium from the cells into the intravascular fluid, leading to hyperkalemia and potassium loss in the urine. With hydration and correction of acidosis, potassium returns to the cell and serum levels decrease rapidly. The goal is to maintain the serum potassium level in excess of 3.5 mEq/L. If the initial potassium is less than 3.5, immediate potassium replacement is necessary. In all patients, potassium replacement should begin once urine output is established.

Phosphate and Magnesium

Phosphate falls with the development of DKA; levels <1.5 mg/dL are not unusual. Hypophosphatemia decreases red blood cell 2,3-bisphosphoglycerate, which shifts the oxygen dissociation to the left and causes left ventricular dysfunction. Severe hypophosphatemia contributes to rhabdomyolysis and confusion. Phosphate replacement with potassium phosphate 60 mmol (in children approximately 1 mmol/kg) over a 6-hour period generally replaces phosphate loss. Replacement can cause hypocalcemia and tetany. Phosphate replacement is not necessary unless the patient shows clear symptoms of hypophosphatemia.

Hypomagnesemia may cause ventricular irritability; however, treatment is rarely needed. In the face of severe symptomatic hypomagnesemia, magnesium 10 to 20 mEq can be given intravenously as 5% magnesium sulfate (25 to 50 cc) over 30 to 60 minutes. ECG monitoring is essential during the replacement of magnesium salt.

Variations In Treatment

Patients with congestive heart failure and DKA present a difficult therapeutic challenge. These patients require central pressure monitoring, preferably using a Swan-Ganz catheter. Patients with serious fluid overload may be managed with insulin alone. Likewise, patients in acute or chronic renal failure may be fluid overloaded and unable to excrete excessive water and potassium. Such patients may require dialysis.

Phase II: Eliminating Ketosis

Once the initial therapy is established, the patient's blood sugar, electrolytes, ketone bodies, and urine output should be measured on an hourly basis. Blood glucose should be expected to fall at 75 to 125 mg/dL per hour. Insulin infusion levels can be adjusted on an hourly basis to assure that this fall rate is achieved. The initial fall may be greater due to rehydration.

Once the patient's glucose has fallen to 250 mg/dL, it is imperative that the patient's ketones be reassessed. Despite the correction of glucose, continued insulin therapy is required to clear ketosis. Fluids are changed to D5 with the

insulin infusion and adjusted to maintain a serum glucose of 200 mg/dL, and continued until ketosis has cleared.

Phase III: Reestablishing Insulin Regimen

The patient may eat when there is no further nausea or vomiting. Additional insulin may be required to cover the ingested glucose bolus. Once the acidosis and ketone bodies have cleared, the patient can be switched to his or her regular dose of insulin. The patient can be discharged once the ketone bodies have cleared and regular insulin regimen has been reestablished, provided that all other symptoms, such as nausea, vomiting, abdominal pain, and central nervous system depression, have cleared. Insulin dosages may need to be adjusted, and factors contributing to the patient's diabetic ketoacidosis state need to be eliminated.

Complications

The mortality rate for DKA is less than 5%. Many of the deaths due to DKA are seen in "brittle diabetics" with recurrent DKA. These patients are generally adolescent females with a myriad of psychosocial problems. In one study there was a 19% mortality rate among this subset of diabetic patients in a 10-year period.

Fetal mortality from maternal DKA is 35% and is due to decreased uterine blood flow. Perhaps the most common maternal complication is due to thromboembolic disease. Thromboembolism and disseminated intravascular coagulation accounts for 20% to 50% of the total mortality rate. Patients at risk are at prolonged bed rest in a hypercoagulable state due to immobility and fluid depletion. In addition, hyperosmolality causes hyperactivation of platelets and hyperfibrinogenemia. There is also a decrease in fibrinolysis and an increase in plasminogen activator inhibitor.

Children are at risk for cerebral edema, which may occur anywhere from 2 to 24 hours after the onset of therapy for DKA. Patients appear to be doing well and their electrolytes and fluid status are normalizing. Patients then develop a headache and experience a gradual decrease in level of consciousness. In many cases, herniation of the brain stem occurs despite aggressive therapy. Cerebral edema may be far more common than the few patients who develop clinically obvious cerebral edema. Subclinical edema is noted to be present by CT scan in many asymptomatic children and adults. In addition there is evidence of some edema existing before therapy is started.

Cerebral edema is seen 0.7% to 1% of patients with DKA below the age of 28 and carries a mortality rate of 70%. Surviving patients have permanent neurologic impairment and recovery without impairment is present in only 7% to 14% of the patients. It is more likely in young individuals with new-onset DKA who have had a longer duration of symptoms. There is some evidence that aggressive fluid replacement may be associated with the presence of cerebral edema. Centers reporting the lowest incidence of cerebral edema use less fluid of lower tonicity.

Nonketotic Hyperosmolar State (NKHS)

This syndrome is known by a variety of names including hyperosmolar nonketotic coma, nonketotic hyperosmolar state (NKHS), hyperglycemic hyperosmolar coma, and others. "Coma" is a misnomer as it occurs in less than 10% of patients. Hyperosmolar state was first described in 1881, but the syndrome of nonketotic hyperosmolar syndrome was not recognized until 1957. This syndrome is generally seen in elderly individuals with chronic medical conditions, and Type 2 diabetics. However, 50% of NKHS occurs in patients who have no known diagnosis of diabetes. Patients gradually develop progressive hyperglycemia, complicated by dehydration. Characteristically, no ketone bodies are formed; therefore, the classic signs of tachypnea, abdominal pain, and CNS confusion seen with acidosis are not present or form very late. Because of the patient's underlying debilitated conditions, progressive dehydration can extend over many days until the patient is quite moribund. Progressive dehydration is often inapparent to caregivers.

Pathophysiology

The cause of NKHS is the underutilization of glucose because of decreased insulin supply or insulin resistance. Only very small amounts of insulin are required to suppress lipolysis. Many non–insulin-dependent diabetics are resistant to glucagon, a key contributor to the generation of ketone bodies. Without the presence of ketone bodies and acidosis, hyperglycemia increases to dramatic amounts. Osmotic diuresis causes loss of sodium, calcium, phosphorus, magnesium, urea, and uric acid. There is a severe total body dehydration seen chemically in increased serum sodium and BUN. Marked dehydration continues because of obtunded state, limited fluid ingestion, and the aggressive osmotic diuresis.

Focal and diffuse CNS symptoms occur because of cerebral dehydration and changes in neurotransmitter levels. In addition, many patients have underlying microvascular disease that causes focal ischemia. Hallucinations, lethargy, and focal findings, particularly in areas in old ischemia, are common and often correct with the lowering of the serum osmolality. Seizures may occur in up to 25% of the patients, many of which are unusual seizures such as occipital seizures and epilepsia partialis continua, seen in up to 6% of patients with NKHS.

Many diseases cause an increase cortisol or stress, thereby making the patient insulin resistant and predisposing them to NKHS. These states are listed in **Table 41.3**. In addition, many drugs are associated with NKHS (the most frequent of these are listed in **Table 41.4**). Of particular note are diuretics that cause increased serum glucose, as well as decreased body fluid. β-blockers, diazoxide, and phenytoin inhibit insulin release.

Clinical Presentation

Patients present with a decreased level of consciousness and classic signs of severe dehydration (dry mucus membranes, poor skin turgor, etc.). Osmolality is generally greater than 350 mosm/L, glucose greater than 600 mg/dL, and ketones classically absent. Patients may show the presence of acidosis due to lactate formation. Sodium is extremely high, particularly in patients who have a decreased level of consciousness. Potassium is usually nor-

mal, but may be elevated due to impaired entry into the cell. Hypokalemia may be seen because of renal losses. Osmolality correlates with cerebral function and level of consciousness, and the lowering of the osmolality toward normal should cause the patient to regain consciousness.

Treatment

Therapy is directed at the replacement of fluid and, to a lesser extent, the reestablishment of normal insulin levels. Initially, the patient is given normal saline 1 to 2 L over 1 to 2 hours. The average fluid loss is approximately 24% of total body water or 10% to 15% of total body weight. Fluid therapy alone should be able to decrease glucose 36 to 70 mg/dL per hour. Approximately 50% of the estimated fluid loss should be replaced in the first 24 hours. The initial normal saline reestablishes intravascular volume. After the initial 1 to 2 L, one-half normal saline is substituted and continued at 200 cc/hour, until the patient is rehydrated. Treating patients with NKHS who have poor left ventricular function, yet who require aggressive fluid management, is often difficult. These patients require central pressure monitoring. In many cases, invasive monitoring is necessary to assure that the patient is not overhydrated. Colloid fluids are not recommended unless the patient is resistant to initial fluid challenge.

Total insulin requirements are less than those for the patients with DKA. In general 10 units of insulin IV are given initially, followed by 0.1 to 0.15 units/kg IV per

Table 41.3
Conditions Predisposing to Nonketotic Hyperosmolar State
Burns
Cerebral vascular accident/bleed
Diabetes mellitus
Dialysis
Drug ingestion
GI hemorrhage
Gram-negative infection
Hyperthermia
Myocardial infarction/cardiac surgery
Pancreatitis
Pulmonary embolism
Trauma

Table 41.4
Drugs Predisposing to Nonketotic Hyperosmolar State
Diuretics—thiazide, furosemide
Diazoxide
Steroids
Phenytoin
Propranolol
Cimetidine

hour. Fluid resuscitation and insulin infusion are continued until the patient develops a normal glucose level and fluid losses are replaced, which often takes 48 to 72 hours. Therefore, all or nearly all patients are admitted.

It is important that underlying causes are diagnosed and treated. Once the acute event is over, many patients require continuous insulin supplementation.

Complications

Mortality rates of 14% to 18% have been reported. Mortality increases with age and initial osmolality, and is highest in patients who reside in long term care residences.

The most common complication is vascular thrombosis secondary to the hyperglycemia, hypercoagulable state, and stasis. Heparin should be avoided due to increased incidence of hemorrhage. Cerebral edema is uncommon, but the mortality associated with it is 50% to 70%. The etiology of cerebral edema is unknown, but idiogenic osmoles are thought to form in the brain.

Seizures are common, occurring in 10% to 15% of patients. Seizures are generally focal and quite resistant to standard anticonvulsants. Lowering the glucose level and osmolality resolves the seizures. Phenytoin is not used as it further inhibits insulin release.

Other complications are due to the low flow state: acute renal failure, rhabdomyolysis, cardiac failure, and respiratory failure. Deaths are due to adult respiratory distress syndrome, cardiac events, and underlying sepsis.

All complications are best prevented by aggressive and rapid fluid replacement.

Selected Readings

1. Basu A, Close CF, Jenkins D, et al. Persisting mortality in diabetic ketoacidosis. *Diabetic Med* 1993;10:282–284.
2. Cruz-Caudillo JC, Sabatini S. Diabetic hyperosmolar syndrome. *Nephron* 1995;69:201–210.
3. Fleckman AM. Diabetic ketoacidosis. *Endocrinol Metab Clin North Am* 1993;22:181–207.
4. Hagay ZJ. Diabetic ketoacidosis in pregnancy: etiology, pathophysiology, and management. *Clin Obstet Gynecol* 1994;37:39–49.
5. Kent LA, Gill GV, Williams G. Mortality and outcome of patients with brittle diabetes and recurrent ketoacidosis. *Lancet* 1994;344:778–781.
6. Kitabshi AE, Wall BM. Diabetic ketoacidosis. *Med Clin North Am* 1995;79:9–37.
7. Lebovitz HE. Diabetic ketoacidosis. *Lancet* 1995;345:767–772.
8. Lorber D. Nonketotic hypertonicity in diabetes mellitus. *Med Clin North Am* 1995;79:39–52.
9. Mel JM, Werther GA. Incidence and outcome of diabetic cerebral oedema in childhood: are there predictors? *J Paediatr Child Health* 1995;31:17–20.
10. Seltzer HS. Drug-induced hypoglycemia. *Endocrinol Metab Clin North Am* 1989;18:163–183.

CHAPTER

42 Nutritional Disorders

Rob J. Edwards

This chapter is not an exhaustive review of nutritional deficiency syndromes, but rather concentrates on the more important and more common nutritional emergencies that may be seen in the emergency department (ED).

Wernicke-Korsakoff Syndrome

Thiamine (Vitamin B$_1$)

Thiamine is important for the metabolism of carbohydrates, especially glucose, and amino acids. It is a water-soluble vitamin found in meat, especially liver, and unrefined cereals and grains.

Thiamine is absorbed readily in the upper small bowel. Increased requirements are seen in pregnancy, lactation, thyrotoxicosis, and fever. Increased losses are seen with diuretic therapy and peritoneal dialysis.

Thiamine deficiency causes syndromes affecting the cardiovascular and neurologic systems. They are better known by the names beriberi and Wernicke-Korsakoff syndrome. There are two forms of beriberi, wet and dry.

In developed countries, thiamine deficiency is seen mostly in chronic alcoholics. However, it has been reported to occur in others, such as pregnant women with hyperemesis gravidarum on prolonged intravenous fluid therapy, patients on parenteral nutrition, and elderly patients. In alcoholics, thiamine deficiency is due to decreased intake consequent upon a poor diet and also decreased absorption from the intestine. Neurologic and cardiovascular manifestations are the common presenting symptoms of thiamine deficiency. Sensorimotor neuropathy, or dry beriberi, is a condition of slow onset. It is usually symmetrical and characterized by loss of ankle jerks and eventually foot drop and wrist drop if the upper limbs are affected. Wernicke's encephalopathy is a characterized by increasing confusion, mental dullness, decreasing level of consciousness, ataxia, insomnia, nystagmus, and diploma arising from disturbances of extraocular movement. MRI scanning demonstrates focal lesions in patients with Wernicke's encephalopathy. Korsakoff's syndrome is typified by a disproportionate impairment in memory relative to other aspects of cognitive functioning. Short-term memory is usually affected more than long-term memory.

Anterograde amnesia often leads to the phenomenon of confabulation. Cardiac failure, or wet beriberi, is a high-output cardiac failure, as evidenced by tachycardia, vasodilatation, cardiomegaly, and peripheral edema.

A diagnosis of thiamine deficiency can be confirmed by a rapid response to thiamine replacement therapy. Recovery is not always complete and there may be residual neurologic impairment that may be severe. The best laboratory investigation to confirm thiamine deficiency is the measurement of erythrocyte transketolase activity. Transketolase is an enzyme that depends on the thiamine ester thiamine pyrophosphate (TPP). Transketolase activity is measured with and without added TPP. An increase in enzyme activity is called TPP effect. TPP effect of 15% to 25% is borderline deficient and over 25% indicates definite deficiency.

Thiamine replacement therapy in the first instance is obviously important, followed by attention to the underlying cause, such as alcoholism and/or poor diet. The route of thiamine replacement depends on the acuity and severity of the clinical manifestations. Parenteral therapy (100 mg IM or IV) should be used in acute presentations such as Wernicke-Korsakoff syndrome. Oral replacement therapy can be used (200 mg/day).

Vitamin B$_{12}$ (Cyanocobalamin) Deficiency

The most common cause of vitamin B$_{12}$ deficiency is pernicious anemia, where antibodies to intrinsic factor prevent absorption of vitamin B$_{12}$. Other causes include gastric or ileal resection, tropical sprue, and dietary cobalamin malabsorption. In a recent study on patients infected with HIV, vitamin B$_{12}$ deficiency was found in 7% of HIV-infected patients and in 15% of those with AIDS. The etiology is thought to be in part due to malabsorption. Up to 75% of patients with low cyanocobalamin levels have neurologic manifestations. These include peripheral neuropathy and a myelopathy (subacute combined degeneration of spinal cord). Typically the myelopathy of vitamin B$_{12}$ deficiency affects the posterior columns of the thoracic cord initially. This syndrome is characterized by loss of vibration and proprioception, spastic weakness of the legs with brisk reflexes, and ataxia. Patients may have a combination of neuropathy and myelopathy. Dementia with either a global reduction in cognitive functioning or recent memory loss are also manifestations of vitamin B_{12} deficiency. Rarely, deficiency may manifest as a psychosis.

The anemia of vitamin B_{12} deficiency is typically a macrocytic anemia, although in up to 23% of cases the mean corpuscular volume (MCV) may be normal. When the MCV is raised, it is frequently markedly raised (>110).

Investigations

Measurement of serum vitamin B_{12} level establishes a diagnosis of a deficiency state. To determine the etiology, a Schilling test establishes malabsorption of vitamin B_{12}, and detection of antibodies to intrinsic factor establishes a diagnosis of pernicious anemia. MRI has recently been described as demonstrating spinal cord lesions in subacute combined degeneration of the spinal cord. Electromyographic studies may be useful in assessing cases of peripheral neuropathy.

Vitamin B_{12} replacement therapy is usually the only treatment required. Some patients with neurologic manifestations may deteriorate initially, however. Generally, there is a good response to treatment; however, patients are often left with residual neurologic manifestations. If anemia is severe enough to warrant blood transfusion, care should be taken not to precipitate fluid overload.

Hypervitaminosis A

Hypervitaminosis A presents in many different ways. Neurologic symptoms of headaches, dizziness, ataxia visual disturbances, irritability, and psychosis may occur with acute toxicity. Pseudotumor cerebri (benign intracranial hypertension) can occur in chronic toxicity. Vitamin A has been shown to induce osteolysis and enhances the osteolytic effect of parathyroid hormone (PTH). This may manifest as bone pain as well as the usual features of hypercalcemia. Ingestion of excessively large amounts of provitamin carotenoids in fad diets has been documented as a cause of yellow skin. Alopecia, brittle nails, and desquamation of the skin usually beginning at the mucocutaneous junction of the lips can be seen, especially in chronic toxicity. In addition to bone pain, there are some typical radiologic features of chronic hypervitaminosis A that have been described. These include hyperostosis (especially in the ulnar and metatarsals) associated with overlying soft tissue swelling. The high incidence of localization in the ulnars and metatarsals has been described as the most diagnostic feature of these skeletal lesions. There have been reports of vitamin A–induced cirrhosis.

Apart from stopping intake from vitamin A and managing hypercalcemia, hypervitaminosis A requires no other active treatment.

Vitamin D Deficiency and Excess

Because vitamin D is produced endogenously in the skin, deficiency states are often due to factors such as lack of sunlight; however, inadequate dietary levels or problems with absorption are often also involved. Nutritional dietary deficiency is seen in patients with malabsorption due to bowel disease, such as Crohn's disease, and poor dietary intake in developing countries; in breast-fed children of deficient mothers; and in homebound elderly patients, who remain indoors and have an inadequate vitamin D intake. Developed countries, however, are not free of vitamin D deficiency, even despite fortification of foods with vitamin D. This condition and its effects on bone are underdiagnosed. In children, vitamin D deficiency leads to rickets and in adults, it leads to osteomalacia.

Rickets is essentially caused by failure of calcium deposition in growing bone. Infants may present with hypocalcemic seizures. Skeletal deformities are the hallmark of this disease. These include prominence of the costochondral junctions ("rachitic rosary"), bossing of the frontal bone, cartilaginous softening of the skull (craniotabes), and bowing of the tibias. These patients are prone to fractures. Short stature may also be noted.

Typical radiologic findings include widening of the epiphyseal space, and disappearance of the normally sharp metaphyseal line with a cupped appearance of the end. In the skull the fontanelles may remain open, and the overall appearance of the bony trabeculae is coarsened with demineralization. There may be bulbous enlargement of the costochondral junctions. Subperiosteal calcification also occurs. Pseudofractures are pathognomonic.

Patients with osteomalacia may complain of bony pain and tenderness or suffer fractures. Radiologically, there is a loss of the normal bony trabeculae and a decrease in bone density. This is often difficult to distinguish from osteoporosis.

Vitamin D excess is usually caused by ingestion of vitamin D preparations. Heavy ingestion of vitamin-fortified milk is another cause. Other causes include ectopic production of vitamin D_3. This may occur in sarcoidosis, tuberculosis, and lymphoproliferative disorders. Hypercalcemia persists for months when vitamin D_1 and vitamin D_2 are involved. When vitamin D_3 is involved, it persists for days to weeks. The major manifestation of vitamin D excess is hypercalcemia.

Selected Readings

1. Dordain G, Deffond D. Pyridoxine neuropathies. *Review of the Literature Therapy* 1994;49:333–337.
2. Gloth FM, Grungberg CM, Hollis BW. Vitamin D deficiency in homebound elderly persons. *JAMA* 1995;274:1183–1186.
3. Hathcock JN, Haltan DG, Jenkins MY, et al. Evaluation of vitamin A toxicity. *Am J Clin Nutr* 1990;52:183–202.
4. Healton EB, Savage DG, Brust JC, et al. Neurological aspects of cobalamin deficiency. *Medicine* 1991;70:229–245.
5. Kopelman MD. The Korsakoff syndrome. *Br J Psychiatry* 1995;166:154–173.
6. Naidoo DP, Singh B, Malfeyee A. Cardiovascular complications of parenteral nutrition. *Postgrad Med J* 1992;68:629–630.
7. O'Keefe ST, Tormey WP, Glasgow R. Thiamine deficiency in hospitalized elderly patients. *Gerontology* 1994;40:18–24.

Parathyroid Disorders

Tomer Feldman

Parathyroid Disease

In 85% of the population there are four parathyroid glands. When there is failure during a parathyroidectomy, it is commonly due to ectopic glands or extra glands not seen by the surgeon. The average size of a gland is $2 \times 3 \times 7$ mm, with a total weight of the four glands of only 150 mg. The arterial supply to the glands typically comes from the inferior thyroid artery, and occasionally from the superior thyroid artery.

Epidemiology

The annual incidence of primary hyperparathyroidism continues to rise as more cases are detected by regular screening tests. The annual incidence is reported as 25 to 50 per 100,000. This increases with age, with figures climbing to 100 per 100,000 for men older than 60 years of age. Among women in this age group, the number is 200 per 100,000.

Parathyroidism is the foremost cause of hypercalcemia in the outpatient population. It is the second most prevalent cause of hypercalcemia in the inpatient population, after malignancies (**Table 43.1**).

Physiology

The parathyroid glands, with the aid of calcitonin (from the thyroid glands) and vitamin D, are responsible for calcium balance. In the average 70-kg man there is 1,000 g of calcium, most of which is stored in bones. Only 1% is located in bodily fluids (plasma, extracellular, etc.) and soft tissue.

Many life-sustaining enzyme systems (ATPase, lipase, amylase, etc.) use calcium as a metal cofactor. Calcium is indispensable for bone formation, blood clotting, muscle function, nerve conduction, cellular structure, and many secretory mechanisms. Calcium balance is linked to phosphorus balance secondary to the fact that calcium-phosphorus salt is required for bone mineral formation.

Parathyroid hormone (PTH) is produced by the chief cells of the parathyroid gland. It is a protein hormone with a half-life of only 15 to 20 minutes in blood. The chief function of PTH is to increase serum calcium levels. This is achieved by three pathways: (1) increasing the amount of calcium (and phosphate) removed from bone; (2) decreasing the amount of calcium excreted by the kidneys, and increasing the amount of phosphorous excreted into the urine; (3) increasing the levels of $1,25\text{-}(OH)_2$–vitamin D in the intestines.

The primary regulatory mechanism to keep PTH in check is a negative feedback system. As calcium levels in the blood rise, there is suppression on the chief cells to produce less PTH. When the levels of calcium are lowered there is a rise in adenosine 38,58-cyclic monophosphate (cAMP), prostaglandin E, and b-adrenergic agonist—all PTH promoters.

Calcitonin, produced by the thyroid gland's clear cells, has an antagonistic relationship with PTH. Its function is to reduce the amount of calcium in extracel-

Table 43.1
Most Common Causes of Hypercalcemia
Hyperparathyroidism
Primary
Secondary
Ectopics
Malignancies
Breast cancer
Metastatic tumor
PTH secreting tumor
Multiple myeloma
Leukemias
Lab error
Vitamin D overdose
Thiazide diuretic use
Hyperthyroidism
Milk-alkali syndrome (calcium carbonate ingestion)
Sarcoidosis
Benign familial hypocalciuric hypercalcemia
Immobilization
Paget's disease
Acute renal failure with rhabdomyolysis

Table 43.2

Table 43.2

Regulators of Calcium-Phosphate

	PTH	Calcitonin	1,25 (OH)$_2$-Vitamin D$_{3C}$
Calcium (serum)	Increases (at bone, kidney)	Decreases	Increases (at intestine, kidney)
Phosphate (serum)	Increases (at bone), decreases (at kidney)	Decreases	Increases (at intestine, kidney)

lular spaces. Its half-life is also very short, at approximately 20 minutes. 1,25-(OH)$_2$–vitamin D is the third factor in determining calcium levels. It assists PTH in raising calcium serum levels. A deficiency in vitamin D$_3$ leads to bone disease (rickets in children and osteomalacia in adults), while an excess causes fragile bones. PTH assists vitamin D$_3$ by promoting it in one of its synthesis steps (**Table 43.2**).

Hyperparathyroidism

The most common cause of hypercalcemia is hyperparathyroidism, and the most common type is primary hyperparathyroidism. Primary hyperparathyroidism is due to an excess of PTH secretion from the parathyroid, usually due to a single adenoma, multiple adenomas, hyperplasia, or carcinoma. Peak incidence is from ages 20 to 49, with women at two to three times greater risk. For other causes of hypercalcemia see Table 43.1.

The common clinical findings are suggested in the following rhyme, "Stones, bones, abdominal groans, psychic moans, and fatigue overtones." In other words, patients present with a wide range of findings, such as renal stones, peptic ulcers, pancreatitis, and depression. The signs and symptoms include muscle fatigue, nausea and vomiting, constipation, polydipsia, polyuria, arthralgias, and psychiatric difficulties. On physical examination patients may have hypertension, gout, pancreatitis, osteitis fibrosa cystica, peptic ulcer disease, kyphosis, band keratopathy, clubbing, renal stones, weakened muscles, or psychiatric behavior. Lab findings include increased serum calcium, PTH, chloride, uric acid, and urine phosphate, and decreased serum phosphate and urine calcium. X-rays might show bone cysts, subperiosteal resorption of phalanges, skeletal demineralization, and renal stones.

The role of the emergency physician is primarily to treat the underlying complications. Many patients who are asymptomatic are diagnosed with hyperparathyroidism after routine lab tests pick up high levels of calcium. After a careful search, these patients are often found not to be asymptomatic, with many having subclinical depression, fatigue, and constipation.

The patient who presents in hypercalcemic crisis needs to be treated to lower the calcium level as quickly as possible. Fluid rehydration is the first step. Calcitonin (4 IU/kg subcutaneous or IM q 12 hours) is another option, although it has a short time of action with a risk of rebound hypercalcemia. Fluid therapy is outlined in the section above on hypercalcemia.

Hypoparathyroidism

Hypoparathyroidism, clinically defined as a low serum calcium, high serum phosphate, and low PTH, is a rare medical entity. The most common cause, in 80% to 90%, is as a complication of surgery of the parathyroids or the thyroid. The next most common cause is idiopathic, believed to be an autoimmune disorder. Less common causes include congenital (DiGeorge syndrome), and infiltrative (Wilson's disease, hemochromatosis, radioactive iodine). Another unusual presentation is secondary to hypomagnesemia.

Whatever the underlying etiology, the presentation is usually secondary to hypocalcemia. While a rare entity, the clinician must recognize severe cases. Patients can present with symptoms as varied as depression and laryngeal stridor. The severity of presentation is dependent not only on the overall level of serum calcium, but also on the rate at which the calcium is falling. The causes of hypocalcemia are many (**Table 43.3**).

The classic acute presentation includes tetany (positive Chvostek's or Trousseau's sign), paresthesias, muscle cramps, carpopedal spasm, convulsion, or neuropsychosis. One should always look for a history of thyroidectomy, since it is the most common cause.

Table 43.3

The Most Common Causes of Hypocalcemia

Hypoparathyroidism
  Surgical 80% to 90%
  Idiopathic (? autoimmune)
  Infiltrative (Wilson's, hemochromatosis, radioactive iodine)
Functional
  Hypomagnesemia
Pseudohypoparathyroidism
  X-linked autosomal syndrome
Pseudopseudohypoparathyroidism
Miscellaneous
  Anxiety—secondary to hyperventilation causing alkalosis
  Intestinal malabsorption
  Renal failure
  Pancreatitis
  Vitamin D deficiency
  Osteoblastic metastasis

The signs, symptoms, and therapy for hypocalcemia are discussed in an earlier part of this section.

Selected Readings

1. Akerstrom G, Rastad J, Juhlin C, Ljunghall S. Primary hyperparathyroidism—aspects of pathophysiology, symptoms, and treatment. *Surg Ann* 1991;23:133–151.
2. Akerstrom G, Malmaeus J, Berstrom R. Surgical anatomy of human parathyroid glands. *Surgery* 1984;95:14.
3. Dufour W. The normal parathyroid revisited. *Hum Pathol* 1982;13:717.
4. Kaplan EL, Yashiro T, Salti G. Primary hyperparathyroidism in the 1990's. *Ann Surg* 1992;215:300–318.
5. Moore KL. *Before We Are Born—Basic Embryology and Birth Defects,* 3rd ed. Philadelphia: Saunders 1989:139–157.
6. Packman KS, Demeure MJ. Indications for parathyroidectomy and extent of treatment for patients with secondary hyperparathyroidism. *Surg Clin North Am* 1995;75-3:465–481.
7. Way LW. *Current Surgical Diagnosis and Treatment,* 9th ed. Stamford, CT: Appleton and Lange 1990:275–285.

Pheochromocytoma

Michael A. Pellegrino

Clinical Presentation

Pheochromocytomas are tumors that release catecholamines, usually norepinephrine. The clinical presentation of patients with such tumors may vary greatly but the hallmark is markedly elevated blood pressure, either sustained or paroxysmal. The hypertensive crisis associated with catecholamine secreting tumors is usually sudden, and most commonly associated with headaches (80%), sweating (70%), and palpitations and/or arrhythmias (65%). Many patients have severe anxiety, nausea or vomiting, and even chest pains or shortness of breath. Some clinicians feel that the presence of sinus tachycardia with severe hypertension is an important clinical factor suggesting the diagnosis. Although the paroxysms of hypertension are often of short duration (less than 1 hour), severe uncontrollable systolic and diastolic pressures can rapidly result in myocardial infarction, encephalopathy, renal failure, and, ultimately, shock and death. Some patients clearly have an inciting stimulus that precipitates the attack, such as lifting, twisting, or any activity that shifts the abdominal contents resulting in a large catecholamine release. There are reported cases of a crisis being brought on by physical examination of the abdomen. Half of the patients who ultimately are diagnosed with a pheochromocytoma are clearly able to give a history consistent with paroxysmal crisis.

Paroxysms may also be induced by administration of tricyclic antidepressants, opiates, glucagon, radiocontrast dyes, droperidol, naloxone, phenothiazines, pancuronium, and other drugs. This occurs as a result of either a direct stimulus for release of catecholamines from tumor cells or by blocking the reuptake of epinephrine or norepinephrine.

The cardiovascular complications associated with pheochromocytoma range from ventricular or supraventricular arrhythmias to myocardial infarction, even in the absence of coronary artery disease. Cardiogenic and noncardiogenic pulmonary edema have been noted as well as myocarditis and catecholamine-induced cardiomyopathy. Severe lactic acidosis in a seemingly well-perfused patient should make the emergency physician consider the diagnosis. This occurs in the absence of other identifiable etiologies for the acidosis.

Another distinctive clinical feature of pheochromocytoma is orthostatic hypotension. This is usually noted in an otherwise hypertensive patient. Orthostatic hypotension is thought to be due to a reduction of intravascular volume from prolonged vasoconstriction and down regulation of peripheral receptors to circulating catecholamines.

Incidence and Pathophysiology

The incidence of pheochromocytomas in the hypertensive population ranges from 0.1% to 1.9%. Pheochromocytoma occurs at about the same frequency in men and women and most commonly presents between 40 and 50 years of age.

Pheochromocytomas arise from neural crest cells anywhere along the sympathetic or paraganglionic nervous tissue. Approximately 90% are found in the adrenal medulla and are specifically termed pheochromocytoma. The remaining tumors found outside the adrenal glands are called paragangliomas. Most of these are found in the sympathetic ganglia of the abdomen, i.e., upper abdomen (40%), para-aortic organ of Zuckerkandl (30%), or bladder (10%). Sometimes, however, tumors are located in the posterior mediastinum (10% to 20%) or are associated with ganglia of the neck (2%).

Pheochromocytomas may be associated with inherited conditions. These include multiple endocrine neoplasia (MEN)-1, -2A, and -2B; neurofibromatosis; von Hippel–Lindau disease; or simple familial pheochromocytoma. Ten percent of all tumors are malignant with metastatic lesions to bone (44%), liver (37%), lymph nodes (37%), lungs (27%), CNS (10%), pleura (10%), kidney (5%), omentum (2%), and pancreas (2%).

Diagnosis

The diagnosis is made by detection of elevated levels of catecholamines and their metabolites in a 24-hour urine sample. Biochemical serum tests for free catecholamines, metanephrines, and vanillylmandelic acid are also employed in the diagnosis. CT, MRI, and iodobenzylguanidine scanning are all used in the localization of such tumors. Laboratory data in the ED is typically of little value but may help exclude other causes of hypertension. Elevation of hematocrit, hypoglycemia, and hypercalcemia are sometimes seen, but are not diagnostic. Evaluation of the ECG, electrolytes, urinalysis, blood gas, chest x-ray, and, if indicated, specific toxins (e.g., amphetamines and cocaine) should be performed. The differential diagnosis of paroxysmal hypertension should also include thyroid storm, monoamine oxidase inhibitor (MAOI) overdose or in combination with tyramine-containing foods, alcohol, or medication withdrawal (e.g., clonidine, β-blockers), carcinoid, and other endocrine-secreting tumors.

Management

The medical management of emergencies associated with pheochromocytomas generally centers around the management of associated hypertension. If pheochromocytoma is highly suspected, the α-blocker phentolamine is the drug of choice. This may be administered in doses of 2 to 5 mg every 5 minutes until blood pressure is controlled and then a continuous infusion is usually needed. Nitroprusside also acts quickly and is easily titrated to effect at doses of 0.5 to 10 mg/kg/min. Beta blockade can be applied if severe tachycardia is present, but should not be undertaken until adequate alpha blockade has been achieved to avoid paradoxical hypertension from unopposed alpha effects. Esmolol, propranolol, or labetalol are agents of choice for tachycardia, and, along with lidocaine, are also used for arrhythmias.

Disposition

Most often, symptomatic patients require admission. Those who are suspected to have a catecholamine-secreting tumor and are asymptomatic should have urgent referral to a primary care physician or to an endocrinologist.

Selected Readings

1. Bergland BE. Pheochromocytoma presenting as shock. *Am J Emerg Med* 1989;7:4448.
2. Bravo EL, Gifford RW. Pheochromocytoma: diagnosis, localization and management. *N Engl J Med* 1984;311:12981303.
3. Bravo EL, Gifford RW. Pheochromocytoma: endocrine crisis, endocrinology, and metabolism. *Endocrinol Metab Clin North Am* 1993;22:329341.
4. Cohen CD, Dent DM. Pheochromocytoma and cardiovascular death (with special reference to myocardial infarction). *Postgrad Med J* 1984;60:111115.
5. Sheps SG, Nai-Siang J, Klee GG, et al. Recent developments in the diagnosis and treatment of pheochromocytoma. *Mayo Clin Proc* 1990;65:8895.
6. Werbel SS, Ober KP. Pheochromocytoma: update on diagnosis, localization and management. *Med Clin North Am* 1995;79:131153.

Pituitary Disorders

Jerry R. Balentine

CHAPTER

45

Patients presenting to the ED with pituitary-related emergencies can present as an acute and devastating event (pituitary apoplexy, Sheehan's syndrome) or as vague complaints with long-standing symptoms (acromegaly, chronic hypopituitarism). Pituitary disorders are relatively rare presentations in the emergency department (ED) and evaluation of the hormones produced by the pituitary are usually not available in the ED. A careful history and physical, as well as a high level of suspicion, are required to make the correct diagnosis or at least to start the workup, which will ultimately lead to the correct diagnosis.

Anatomy and Physiology

The pituitary is under the control of the hypothalamus and produces six hormones (**Table 45.1**). The feedback loop between the anterior pituitary and its three target glands (thyroid, adrenal cortex, and gonads) can be destroyed at the pituitary level, giving rise to secondary hypothyroidism, adrenal insufficiency or hypogonadism. If the thyroid gland, adrenal cortex or gonads are removed or fail to produce hormones, primary hypothyroidism, primary adrenal insufficiency or primary hypogonadism result. Symptoms of isolated hormone loss are not discussed in this section (with the exception growth hormone disturbances).

The pituitary gland sits within the sella turcica of the sphenoid bone at the base of the skull. The adult pituitary measures approximately $12 \times 9 \times 6$ mm, but enlarges during pregnancy or if a tumor is present. Adjacent structures (optic chiasm, cavernous sinus with cranial nerves III, IV, V, and VI) can be invaded or impinged upon by pituitary tumors, leading to visual field defects and cranial nerve palsies as presenting signs.

Pituitary Apoplexy

Pituitary apoplexy describes a clinical syndrome of sudden headache, visual impairment, and ophthalmoplegia caused by the enlargement of a pituitary adenoma due to either hemorrhage or infarction.

Pituitary tumors have a significantly higher incident of spontaneous bleeding than other primary CNS tu-

mors, and the incidence of apoplexy has been reported from as low as 1% up to 10% in patients with pituitary adenomas.

Emergency Department Presentation

The presentation depends on the size of the original tumor and the amount of bleeding. The majority of patients presenting to the ED have no prior knowledge of having a pituitary tumor. The typical case is described as a middle-aged man who develops sudden frontal headache, followed within hours or days by extraocular ophthalmoplegia, impaired visual acuity, visual field defects, signs of meningeal irritation, and progressive deterioration of level of consciousness. To distinguish this entity in the ED from other intracranial events, the ophthalmologic findings have to be detected.

The majority of patients who retain consciousness complain of diplopia occurring with their headache. This diplopia is due to direct pressure of the expanding tumor on cranial nerves III, IV, or VI in the cavernous sinus, whose medial wall forms the lateral boundary of the pituitary fossa.

Pituitary apoplexy has been linked to head trauma and a sudden increase in intracranial pressure (ICP). Case reports and series have also described pituitary apoplexy with anticoagulant treatment, DKA, bromocriptine, and estrogen therapy, as well as following CNS radiation therapy.

Differential Diagnosis

The most commonly considered diagnoses in patients presenting with pituitary apoplexy are aneurysmal subarachnoid hemorrhage and meningitis. This distinction is made even more difficult, as patients with pituitary apoplexy frequently have blood leaking into the subarachnoid space.

Diagnosis and ED Management

The primary responsibility of the ED physician is protecting the patient's airway should altered level of consciousness be part of the presenting symptoms. Steroid therapy should be started as soon as the diagnosis is suspected

Table 45.1

Pituitary Hormones

Pituitary Hormone	Function
Thyrotropin (TSH)	Regulates thyroid function
Adrenocorticotropin (ACTH)	Controls glucocorticoid function of adrenal cortex
Prolactin	Lactation
Growth hormone	Regulates growth; metabolic effects
Follicle-stimulating hormone (FSH) and luteinizing hormone (LH)	Controls gonads in men and women

even if no apparent endocrinopathy is present (hydrocortisone 100 mg IV stat, followed by 100 mg IV every 8 hours). Electrolytes and fluid status have to be monitored closely to avoiding drastic changes in intracranial pressure. CT scan or MRI is essential in helping with the diagnosis of pituitary apoplexy. The radiologist needs to be alerted to the possible diagnosis to allow especially thin cuts and possible use of contrast material.

Neurosurgical consultation should be obtained to evaluate the patient for possible neurosurgical decompression. Decreasing mortality from pituitary apoplexy over the last 40 years seems to be due to aggressive neurosurgical intervention and endocrinologic management.

Sheehan's Syndrome

The typical emergency department presentation of Sheehan's syndrome is a patient who, after postpartum shock, fails to lactate and has amenorrhea. This is followed by loss of scalp, axillary, and pubic hair, and atrophy of the breasts and genitals. Signs and symptoms of hypothyroidism and adrenal insufficiency follow, as well as sterility. These symptoms usually start while the patient is still in the hospital and presentation to the ED should therefore be rare, although with shorter hospital stays for obstetrical patients, the emergency physician has to be prepared to make this diagnosis.

ED Treatment and Diagnosis

The ED care should be based on a thorough obstetric and gynecologic history, evaluation for signs of hypopituitarism, and admission if the patient shows acute signs or symptoms.

This diagnosis can be excluded in women who have no history of complications during childbirth (especially hypovolemic shock).

The IV administration of 200 mg of thyrotropin-releasing hormone followed by prolactin measurements may be used as a simple test to distinguish patients with Sheehan's syndrome from patients with no endocrine abnormality. If no acute reason for admission is found, the patient can be discharged with an appropriate follow-up.

Selected Readings

1. Abboud CF. Laboratory diagnosis of hypopituitarism. *Mayo Clin Proc* 1986; 61:35–48.
2. Cardosa ER, Peterson EW. Pituitary apoplexy: a review. *Neurosurgery* 1984; 14:363–373.
3. DiZerega G, Kletzky OA. Diagnosis of Sheehan's syndrome using a sequential pituitary stimulation test. *Am J Obstet Gynecol* 1978;132:348–353.
4. Edwards OM. Post-traumatic hypopituitarism: six cases and a review of the literature. *Medicine* 1986;65:281–290.
5. Findling JW, Tyrell JB, Aron DC, et al. Silent pituitary apoplexy: subclinical infarction of an adrenocorticotropin-producing pituitary adenoma. *J Clin Endocrinol Metab* 1981;52:95–97.
6. Sheehan HL. Postpartum necrosis of the anterior pituitary. *J Pathol Bacteriol* 1937;45:189–214.

Thyroid Disease

Gary A. Johnson

Thyroid disease is rarely diagnosed or treated in the emergency department (ED). However, hyperthyroidism and hypothyroidism combined represent the second most common endocrine emergency after complications of diabetes.

Thyroid Physiology

Release of thyroid hormone is influenced by the hypothalamus, the pituitary gland, and the thyroid gland itself. The hypothalamus produces thyrotropin-releasing hormone, which stimulates the release of thyrotropin (TSH). The hypothalamus also produces somatostatin, which inhibits TSH release. Within the thyroid gland, thyroid globulin is united with iodine to produce mono- and diiodotyrosine, which is combined to form thyroxine (T_4), and then may be deiodinated to triiodothyronine (T_3) (or reverse T_3). T_3 and T_4, which are circulated in plasma, are almost entirely bound by proteins including thyroxine-binding globulin (TBG) and albumin. Most activation of T_4 to T_3 occurs in the liver and the kidney.

Hyperthyroidism/Thyroid Storm

Hyperthyroidism is caused by excess thyroxine and leads to a clinical spectrum of metabolic hyperactivity without elevated serum catecholamines. Various terms—hyperthyroidism, thyrotoxicosis, thyrotoxicrisis, and thyroid storm—have been used for hyperthyroid states of different severities, but they are not universally well defined. Signs and symptoms of hyperthyroidism include fever, tachycardia, weight loss, agitation, tremor, and thyromegaly. Graves' disease is a triad of hypermetabolism, thyromegaly, and ophthalmopathy. Eye findings include exophthalmos, lid lag, upper lid retraction, and extraocular muscle weakness. Gastrointestinal symptoms are common with hyperthyroidism and include nausea, vomiting, diarrhea, and intermittent abdominal discomfort.

Thyrotoxicosis or thyroid storm usually presents with fever, tachycardia, and severe manifestation of hyperthyroidism. Central nervous system findings, tachydysrhythmias, or congestive heart failure may complicate thyrotoxicosis. Thyrotoxic patients may also have pretibial myxedema, hyperpigmentation, and fine, straight hair.

Older patients may present with apathetic hyperthyroidism. Rather than having prominent symptoms of hypermetabolism, they may present with depression or weight loss and symptoms of congestive failure as predominant findings. Dysrhythmias such as atrial fibrillation and other supraventricular tachycardias may also be present.

Laboratory Evaluation

Nearly all patients with hyperthyroidism have elevation of free T_4 (the metabolically active form of T_4). Assays for total T_4, free T_4, total T_3, and free T_3 are all available. Patients may have an abnormally high total T_4 or total T_3 level despite normal free T_4 levels because of abnormalities of thyroid-binding globulin. TSH levels may differentiate between primary and secondary hyperthyroidism. TSH levels are low in primary hyperthyroidism (the gland is overproducing T_4 despite a lack of TSH). If a patient has a normal free T_4 or total T_4 test and symptoms of hyperthyroidism, a free T_3 assay should be performed to look for T_3 toxicosis. T_3 toxicosis occurs primarily in areas of iodine deficiency and may occur disproportionately in patients with Graves' disease or multinodular goiter.

The screening test of choice for hyperthyroidism is controversial. Sensitive thyrotropin (TSH) assays can adequately screen for both hyper- and hypothyroid disease. These tests are more costly than other thyroid assays and there is a lack of consensus as to whether they are a cost-effective screen. The choice of a screen for laboratory evaluation of hyperthyroidism needs to be based on the sensitivity and specificity of tests available, as well as the cost.

Management and Disposition

Management of hyperthyroidism patients with mild illness may not require emergent therapy. However, patients with tachycardia, fever, congestive heart failure or other manifestations of severe disease require immediate therapy. Beta blockade is the treatment of choice for thyroid storm. Propranolol IV may be used. It can be given in 1 mg aliquots and titrated to a reasonable heart rate. Ten milligrams is frequently considered the maximum initial dose. It acts by blocking the peripheral effect of excess thyroid hormone. Other treatments include propylthiouracil (PTU), which blocks synthesis of thyroid hormone; potassium iodine solution, which blocks release of hormone; and glucocorticoids (e.g., dexamethasone 2 mg or hydrocortisone 100 mg), which help block peripheral T_4 conversion.

It is important to diagnose and treat possible precipitating factors, such as infections, traumatic injuries or metabolic diseases. Congestive heart failure may require diuretic therapy.

Patients with congestive heart failure or neuromuscular manifestations should be admitted. Patients whose primary symptoms are tachycardia or tremor may be safely discharged once therapy is initiated successfully in the ED.

Hypothyroidism/Myxedema

Hypothyroidism is the end result of an insufficient amount of thyroid hormone production. It may be primary (the thyroid gland does not produce adequate thyroid hormone) or secondary (the thyroid gland is not stimulated by the pituitary or hypothalamus).

Signs and Symptoms

Hypothyroidism may be very subtle and diagnosed only by a screening lab test or result in myxedema coma. Symptoms of hypothyroidism include lassitude, cold intolerance, paresthesias, generalized weakness, and constipation. Cold intolerance occurs from the body not being able to generate calories in the face of a cold stressor. Therefore, most cases of hypothyroidism are recognized in winter months.

Hypothyroidism in its extreme can cause coma based on lack of thyroxine or complications from lack of thyroxine. Such complications would include sepsis, drug interactions, hypothermia, hypotension, and hypoglycemia. Signs and symptoms of sepsis may be difficult to illicit, since fever and tachycardia may be absent in hypothyroidism.

Symptoms of hypothyroidism present in a very subacute manner and years of delay between onset of symptoms and diagnosis may occur.

Physical examination findings in hypothyroidism include delay in muscular contraction when testing deep tendon reflexes, hypothermia, hair loss, weight gain, and non–pitting-dependent edema. Some patients with hypothyroidism have a goiter. Cerebellar symptoms and progressive hearing loss are also common signs.

Laboratory Evaluation

Patients who are suspected of being hypothyroid have low free T_4 levels and high TSH levels (in primary hypothy-

roidism). Alterations in thyroxine-binding globulin will alter T_4 levels. T_3 levels are usually not diagnostically helpful. However, low T_3 levels may occur in the "sick euthyroid" state. Patients with systemic illness may have decreased peripheral conversion of T_4 to T_3, and therefore manifest low T_3 levels despite the physiologically euthyroid state. ED patients who may be hypothyroid can be effectively worked up by simply doing a thyrotropin (TSH) level test.

Therapy

Patients with mild hypothyroid states may be treated with oral thyroid replacement with a low initial dose that is adjusted over several weeks time. Obtunded patients must be treated more aggressively and often need therapy to be given before laboratory confirmation occurs.

Myxedema coma should be treated by intravenous thyroxine. Appropriate dose and indication is somewhat controversial because of the possibility of intravenous thyroid replacement causing dysrhythmias or ischemic cardiac disease. Initial dose of 300 mg of T_4 intravenously may be given and followed by dosages of 50 mg each day. Such patients should have continuous cardiac monitoring.

Supportive care is necessary in myxedema coma for metabolic, respiratory, and cardiac complications of the disease. Possible precipitating factors must be diagnosed and treated. Glucocorticoid therapy is frequently given (for possible adrenal failure). Hypothermia does not require active rewarming, and passive measures with hormone replacement are sufficient.

Selected Readings

1. de los Santos ET, Starich GH, Mazzaferri EL. Sensitivity, specificity, and cost-effectiveness of the sensitive thyrotropin assay in the diagnosis of thyroid disease in ambulatory patients. *Arch Intern Med* 1989;149:526.
2. Franklyn JA. The management of hyperthyroidism. *N Engl J Med* 1994;330:1731–1738.
3. Hellman R. The evaluation and management of hyperthyroid crisis. *Crit Care Q* 1980;77.
4. Klein I, Becker DV, Levey GS. Treatment of hyperthyroid disease. *Ann Intern Med* 1994;121:281–288.
5. Menendez CE, Rivlin RS. Thyrotoxic crisis and myxedema coma. *Med Clin North Am* 1973;57:1463.
6. Mokshagundam S, Barzel US. Thyroid disease in the elderly. *J Am Geriatr Soc* 1993;41:1361–1369.
7. Senior RM, Birge SJ, Wessler S, et al. The recognition and management of myxedema coma. *JAMA* 1971;217:61.
8. Smith SA. Commonly asked questions about thyroid function. *Mayo Clin Proc* 1995;70:573–577.

Endocrine Manifestations of Neoplasia

Jerry R. Balentine

In addition to direct effects due to their mass or tissue invasion, cancers can also cause symptoms secondary to hormonal effects. These paraneoplastic syndromes are related to ectopic hormone secretion. As survival increases and hormone assays and imaging techniques further improve, more of these hormonal manifestations become apparent. The hormonal active substances that are produced may reflect the normal function of the tissue (pituitary adenomas secreting growth hormone) or may be a hormonal action usually not performed by this tissue (small cell lung cancer; vasopressin). These hormones are usually not under the direct control of hormonal feedback systems that balance the normal hormone production. Many of these ectopic hormones are inactive precursors or fragments and a wide variety of hormones have been produced by neoplasms (**Table 47.1**). Although most of the ectopic paraneoplastic syndromes do not present with significant symptoms, some hormonal effects (SIADH, hypercalcemia, hypoglycemia) can bring the patient to the emergency department with life-threatening signs and symptoms.

Syndrome of Inappropriate Antidiuretic Hormone

The syndrome of inappropriate antidiuretic hormone (SIADH) or the syndrome of inappropriate AVP (arginine vasopressin = ADH) secretion is a failure of the normal feedback mechanism on ADH secretion. This condition is described in another section.

Hypercalcemia

Hypercalcemia occurs in up to 20% of cancer patients and is the most frequent metabolic emergency in oncology. Hypercalcemia generally implies progression of the tumor, with the exception of patients with metastatic breast cancer, who can develop hypercalcemia when a new hormonal therapy is initiated. Hypercalcemia rarely presents as the first sign of malignancy.

Four mechanisms can cause hypercalcemia in patients with neoplasms: (1) Solid tumors can secrete proteins that bind to the parathyroid hormone receptors. (2) Hemato-logic malignancies can produce substances (cytokines and prostaglandins) that act locally to activate bone calcium. (3) Solid tumors may secrete parathyroid hormone (rare). (4) Neoplasms with widespread bone metastasis can cause hypercalcemia by osteolysis.

Emergency Department Presentation

Symptoms of hypercalcemia are nonspecific and are summarized in **Table 47.2**. The GI symptoms tend to be the earliest findings with anorexia, vomiting, constipation, and nonspecific abdominal pain. Patients with hypercalcemia due to hyperparathyroidism have increased incidence of pancreatitis and peptic ulcer disease (PUD), but this correlation is not seen in patients with increased calcium secondary to malignancy.

Renal manifestations can lead to polyuria and polydipsia due to renal tubular defects. ECG changes are a shortened QT interval, although at very high calcium levels (> 16 mg/dl) bradyarrhythmias, bundle branch block, and complete heart block can occur. In general, calcium levels above 14 mg/dl cause symptoms and should be considered a medical emergency, although calcium levels as high as 15 mg/dl may only cause mild symptoms in patients chronically hypercalcemic.

Hypoglycemia

Hypoglycemia has been described in conjunction with most common neoplasms. There are four mechanisms by which patients present with hypoglycemia due to a neoplasm: (1) secretion of insulin by a tumor (insulinoma;

Table 47.1
Hormones Produced by Neoplasms
ACTH
Chorionic gonadotropin
Calcitonin
Vasopressin (AVP or ADH)
Growth hormone
Erythropoietin

Table 47.2

Signs and Symptoms of Hypercalcemia

Gastrointestinal
   Nausea, vomiting, constipation, abdominal pain
Renal
   Polyuria, polydipsea
Cardiovascular
   Increased cardiac contractility and irritability
   Shortening of QT

islet cell tumors); (2) increased glucose utilization by a tumor; (3) secretion of an insulin-like substance; and (4) alterations in glucose homeostasis. Cancer patients seem to have decreased rates of hepatic gluconeogenesis, reduced glycogen breakdown in response to stress, and decreased glycogen stores in the liver. At the time hypoglycemia is noted, the underlying neoplasms are usually quite large, averaging 2400 g. Two-thirds are retroperitoneal or peritoneal and the remainder arise in the thorax.

Selected Readings

1. Bajorunas DR. Clinical manifestations of cancer related hypercalcemia. *Semin Oncol* 1990;17:16.
2. Besarab A, Caro JF. Mechanisms of hypercalcemia in malignancy. *Cancer* 1978;41:2276.
3. Markman M. Common complications and emergencies associated with cancer and its therapy. *Cleve Clin J Med* 1994;61:105–114.
4. Pimentel L. Medical complications of oncologic disease. *Emerg Med Clin North Am* 1993;11:407–419.
5. Schiller JH, Jones JC. Paraneoplastic syndromes associated with lung cancer. *Curr Opin Oncol* 1993;5:335–342.
6. Sorensen JB, Andersen MK, Hansen HH. SIADH in malignant disease. *J Intern Med* 1995;238:97–110.

Head, Ears, Eyes, Nose, and Throat Disorders

Lilly Lee

In 1995 there were approximately 700 million office and clinic visits for complaints related to the ears, nose, and throat (ENT). A vast majority of these visits did not require emergency department intervention or consultation with specialists: One study has shown that only approximately 10% of these visits represented real medical emergencies, while only 0.5% were life-threatening. Given the proximity of these structures to the central nervous system (CNS), however, the great vessels, the airway, and the mediastinum through facial planes, failure to recognize life-threatening ENT emergencies or potential complications of more common ENT problems can lead to significant morbidity and mortality with catastrophic outcomes. This section will focus on acute evaluation and emergency department (ED) management and indications for specialist referral of ENT emergencies.

Clinical evaluation of patients in the ED with ENT disorders requires specialized physical examination skills and a clear understanding of the function and anatomy of the head and neck. Adequate illumination and exposure with the appropriate equipment is imperative. A focused and carefully elicited history and thorough physical examination of adjacent areas ensure a correct diagnosis and avoids potential pitfalls.

Examination of the nose in the ED involves external inspection to check for deformities and interior inspection with anterior rhinoscopy. The latter is achieved with a nasal speculum and ideally a headlight that follows the line of sight and leaves both hands free. The nasal speculum should be opened in the vertical direction so as to avoid pressure on the septum. This technique should allow for visualization of the anterior ends of the turbinate and the septum. Possible abnormalities include swollen turbinates, masses and polyps, bleeding sites, septal perforation, and septal hematoma.

Examination of the Oral Cavity and Throat

Complete examination of the mouth includes inspection of the recesses inferior and posterior to the tongue, inspection of the gingivobuccal sulci, and bimanual palpation of the tongue and the floor of the mouth. This can be achieved with a good light source and tongue blades. Dentures should be removed to ensure exposure of the alveolar surface.

The posterior wall of the oropharynx can be visualized easily via the mouth by depressing the tongue. Inspection of the hypopharynx, larynx, and nasopharynx requires the use of either indirect mirror examination or endoscopy. The mirror technique is a skill that requires practice and often not well tolerated by the patients. Visualization with a fiberoptic nasopharyngoscope has become more common in the ED. For patient comfort and easier introduction, the nose should be treated with Neo-Synephrine or oxymetazoline prior to insertion of the scope. Topical lidocaine (4%) can also be used. The scope is passed into the nose under direct visualization, and then advanced by viewing through the scope. The best route is along the floor of the nose; and when the scope is at the back of the nasal cavity, the scope should be flexed downward in order to enter the nasopharynx. The patient should be instructed to breathe through the nose so that the palate will relax and open the nasopharyngeal inlet. The tip of the scope can then be advanced to the hypopharynx.

Life-Threatening Emergencies

Lilly Lee

Life-threatening emergencies in the ear, nose, throat, head, and neck are rare. The initial management of these patients should be based on evaluation of the patient's airway, breathing, circulation, and neurological status. Immediate specialist consultation is indicated, as well as prompt initiation of antibiotic therapy.

Penetrating Wounds of the Neck

Trauma to the neck is either immediately life-threatening or not immediately life-threatening. The patient with severe injuries, who presents in shock and with airway and neurological compromise, requires immediate, skilled evaluation, and management. Airway control is the first priority, as approximately 10% of patients with penetrating neck trauma experience significant airway compromise. Intubation via nasotrachael, orotrachael or cricothyrotomy is often indicated and in-line cervical stabilization must be maintained while the airway is secured. Vascular injuries occur in more than 20% of these patients. Hemorrhage needs to be controlled by direct pressure. Large bore intravenous catheters should be placed and volume resuscitation started with colloid or crystalloid as deemed appropriate. Wound exploration or removal of penetrating objects from the neck wound is not indicated in the emergency department (ED). Patients with massive hemorrhage should be taken directly to the operating room. Stable patients with penetrating trauma to the neck are managed based on whether the platysma is penetrated or not and by the anatomic location of the neck wound. The evaluation and management of these patients is discussed elsewhere.

Major Infections of the Head and Neck

Despite significant advances in antibiotic therapy, major infection in the head and neck remains a potentially life-threatening emergency. As in all life-threatening emergencies, the first priority is airway management. Ludwig's angina is a rapidly spreading gangrenous cellulitis of the submandibular and sublingual spaces. The airway is compromised by the edema of the floor of the mouth, which displaces the tongue upward and backward, and significant trismus. The airway can also be directly compressed by a large abscess collection or by abscess rupture into the airway. Nasotrachael fiberoptic intubation is generally the preferred technique secondary to trismus and edema. In severe respiratory distress, emergency tracheotomy or cricothyrotomy may become necessary.

After stabilization of the airway, treatment of this infection dictates prompt initiation of the appropriate intravenous antibiotics in the ED and surgical drainage by the specialist consultants. This condition most often results from dental infection, but it may also be caused by mandible fracture or a submandibular gland infection. This infection is polymicrobial with a mixture of anaerobic and aerobic oral flora. Traditionally, penicillin or clindamycin has been the drug of choice, but with the emergence of resistance, treatment should include the addition of a β-lactamase inhibitor, such as clavulanic acid or metronidazole (clindamycin 600 mg to 900 mg IV every 8 hours or penicillin G 24 million units every 4 to 6 hours, plus metronidazole 1 g load, then 0.5 g every 6 hours). Untreated or inadequately treated infections in the neck can lead to septic thrombosis of the internal jugular vein (Lemierre's syndrome) and potentially metastatic embolic abscesses to the brain and the lungs. Carotid artery erosion can also occur, with a fatality in 20% to 40% of the cases. Other life-threatening complications include inferior extension of the infection, resulting in mediastinitis, and bacteremia, leading to sepsis.

Craniocervical necrotizing fasciitis, though rare, is a rapidly progressive necrotizing process of the superficial layer of the cervical fascia. It is most commonly odontogenic in origin, and approximately 50% of the patients affected have co-morbid conditions, such as diabetes mellitus, alcoholism or cirrhosis. The process extends rapidly from the superficial fascia to the deep cervical fascia into the anterior chest wall and the mediastinum. The classic radiographic appearance of craniocervical necrotizing fasciitis on plain films or CT imaging reveals extensive subcutaneous emphysema. As in all life-threatening emergencies, the first priority is to secure the airway, which often necessitates a tracheotomy given the distortion of normal anatomic landmarks. The definitive treatment is aggressive and radical debridement of the necrotic tissue in the operating room and, hence, immediate ENT consultation is indicated. Broad-spectrum intravenous antibiotic therapy should be initiated in the ED when this diagnosis is suspected. Initial coverage should include a penicillinase-resistant penicillin, such as imipenem 500 mg every 6 hours or clindamycin, and often an aminoglycoside. Craniocervical necrotizing fasciitis has a mortality ranging from 20% to 70% in patients with predisposing co-morbidities.

Epiglottitis in the pediatric population is a rapidly progressing, life-threatening bacterial infection of the supraglottic larynx. Symptoms usually progress within 4 to 8 hours from fever to respiratory distress requiring rapid airway management. The incidence in the pediatric population continues to fall with the widespread use of the newer conjugate *Haemophilus influenzae* type B (HIB) vaccine. Examination or intravenous line placement is usually deferred until the airway is stabilized, as agitation of the patient may precipitate complete airway obstruction. Airway management in these patients requires a multi-disciplinary team comprising of otolaryngologists, anesthesiologists, intensivists, and emergency physicians experienced in the care of children with airway compromise. This should ideally be performed in the surgical suite under controlled conditions and with specialists prepared for a tracheotomy, should oral intubation prove difficult.

Facial trauma and sinusitis can lead to orbital infections. The orbital veins drain posterior to the cavernous sinus and serve as access of orbital infection to the CNS. Untreated orbital cellulitis has mortality rates of 17% with blindness in 25% of survivors. These patients should have immediate treatment with intravenous antibiotics covering polymicrobial infections and anaerobic infections. Prompt ophthalmologic and ENT consultation should be obtained.

Bleeding

Vascular emergencies of the head and neck most often occur in the operating room or in the postoperative period. Less common are life-threatening hemorrhages in patients with cancer or severe infections in which high flow vascular structures such as the carotid arteries or the jugular veins are eroded by these lesions. Similarly, penetrating trauma of the neck involves vascular injuries in 20% to 40% of cases.

Tonsillectomy with or without adenoidectomy is one of the most commonly performed surgical procedure in children. Beyond those associated with anesthesia, its most serious complication is hemorrhage. Primary hemorrhage, defined as within the first 24 hours of surgery, is less common, whereas rates of secondary hemorrhage have been reported to range from 0.5% to 9.3%. Postoperative hemorrhage after adenotonsillectomy creates two major issues:

airway management to avoid aspiration of blood and the management of hypovolemia secondary to blood loss. In cooperative patients, hemorrhage can be temporarily controlled by packing the area with tonsil sponges. In most cases of brisk bleeding, definitive control of hemorrhage is obtained in the operating room.

The prevalence of acute epistaxis is estimated at 10% to 15% of the adult population. Life-threatening nasal hemorrhage is rare and is usually associated with trauma. Treatment of intractable bleeding (i.e., bleeding resistant to topical vasoconstriction, compression, local cautery, anterior and posterior packing,) is surgical ligation or angiographic embolization of the involved arteries. In addition to control of active bleeding, major priorities in the management of epistaxis are airway management to avoid aspiration of blood and the evaluation and treatment of blood loss.

Examination of the Ear

The ear can be divided into three parts: external, middle, and inner. The external ear is that portion lateral to the tympanic membrane and includes the auricle and the external auditory canal. The auricle consists of elastic cartilage covered with skin. In the adult, the external ear canal (EAC) consists of the medial bony segment that curves anteriorly and the lateral cartilaginous segment, which points inferiorly. The skin of the lateral canal is thicker and contains all the skin appendages, such as cerumen glands and hair follicles. By contrast, the bony aspect of the canal is covered by a thin layer of skin devoid of appendages and easily abraded by instrumentation.

Examination of the ear should include inspection and palpation of the auricle, mastoid areas, and the external meatus and otoscopic examination of the EAC and the tympanic membrane. The largest speculum that would fit in the external auditory meatus should be used to provide maximal visualization and illumination. It will lodge itself in the narrower lateral segment and not extend into the sensitive and easily traumatized bony canal. Given the curved shape of the ear canal, to allow proper visualization of the tympanic membrane in the adult, the auricle should be pulled superiorly and posteriorly. In the young pediatric patients, the auricle should be pulled inferiorly. The tympanic membrane is inspected completely to look for perforation and to locate the important landmarks: the annulus and the malleus. The tympanic membrane is usually pearly gray, shiny, translucent, and concave. White patches, retraction or a dull membrane suggest chronic infectious processes. Pneumatic otoscopy assesses the motion of the drum as the air pressure changes in the auditory canal. It is useful for detecting occult perforation and the presence of fluid in the middle ear.

Disorders of the External Ear

Lilly Lee

Cellulitis

Cellulitis of the auricle and subsequent infection of the underlying cartilage may occur as a complication of otitis externa or from a traumatic injury to the auricle. Patients characteristically present with warmth, erythema, and induration of the auricle, and systemic signs of infection. The most common causative organisms are *Staphylococcus aureus* and *Pseudomonas aeruginosa*. Empiric treatment should provide coverage for both organisms. Follow-up visit to the emergency department (ED) or an ear, nose, and throat (ENT) consultant is imperative, as failure to respond to antibiotic may necessitate surgical debridement of sequestered cartilage. Erysipelas of the auricle is a result of hemolytic streptococci entering abraded skin near the external auditory meatus. A well-defined, painful, raised erythema can spread to involve the face. Treatment is with a synthetic penicillin or first generation cephalosporin, such as cephalexin 1 g IV every 6 hours or oxacillin 2 g IV every 6 hours.

Furuncles

Furuncles represent a *S. aureus* infection involving the hair follicles in the lateral cartilaginous segment of the external auditory canal (EAC). It is characterized by severe localized pain, redness, and swelling. Preauricular and mastoids nodes may be enlarged. Treatment consists of excision and drainage, anti-staphylococcal antibiotics, and pain medication. A nasal swab to test for colonized *S. aureus* may be indicated in recurrent furunculosis, as patient may be transferring the organism with his finger from the nasal vestibule to the ear. Patients with recurrent infections should be evaluated for diabetes mellitus and referred to ENT follow-up.

Otitis Externa

Otitis externa is an inflammation of the skin of the EAC. The EAC is normally protected by a mildly acidic pH of 4 to 5 and the lipid film from the skin. Its squamous epithelium is susceptible to similar dermatological conditions as those affecting other parts of the body. Otitis externa causes drainage, swelling, and intense pain. This condition is usually precipitated by trauma to the EAC (often caused by attempt to clean ear) and increased moisture either from swimming or from showering. Irrigation of the EAC to remove cerumen is a well-recognized risk factor for otitis externa.

Otitis externa causes intense tenderness over the tragus and pain when the auricle is displaced. The canal may be too swollen to allow for visualization of the tympanic membrane. This disease entity needs to be differentiated from otitis media and, in fact, both may co-exist and the patient may require treatment both topically and systemically. The usual causative organisms are *S. aureus* and *P. aeruginosa,* but otitis externa may also be caused by fungus, either *Candida albicans* or *Aspergillus niger.* Careful inspection of the auricle, pre- and postauricular areas, and upper cervical lymph node chain is necessary to evaluate for extension of disease. Herpes zoster involving the geniculate ganglion may present as grouped vesicles in the EAC. In addition to ear pain, patients present with facial nerve palsy, hearing loss, and other cranial nerve impairment.

Treatment consists of gentle cleansing if possible followed by administration of antibacterial/acidic-corticosteroid otic or ophthalmic drops (**Table 49.1**).

If the canal is extremely swollen, a wick may be placed in the canal to facilitate administration of drops. Treatment with oral antibiotics may be needed if there is extension of the inflammatory process beyond the EAC. Fungal otitis externa should be treated with lotrimin or tolnaftate solution and the patient should have prompt referral to an otolaryngologist. Patient with Ramsey Hunt syndrome (reactivation of the varicella-zoster virus dormant since appearing as childhood chickenpox) should be treated with an antiviral agent. Corticosteroids should not be administered in cases of known fungal otitis externa or Ramsey Hunt syndrome. In immunocompromised patients, a cautious approach is to add systemic antibiotics to provide added *Pseudomonas aeruginosa* coverage and to ensure close follow-up.

Pain management is important in the first 24 to 48 hours of treatment. Anti-inflammatory drugs or oral narcotics should be prescribed as needed. Patient should be instructed to avoid precipitating factors, i.e. humidifica-

Table 49.1
Medication for Otitis Externa

Name	Comments
For Bacterial Infections	
Neomycin + polymyxin B +/− hydrocortisone	Covers Gram + and − bacteria; neomycin potentially ototoxic if tympanic membrane perforation; neomycin has potential for skin sensitization. Solution causes discomfort if contacts middle ear mucosa.
2% acetic acid +/− hydrocortisone	Broad coverage; depends on antibacterial effects of low pH solution; middle ear irritant
Ofloxacin 0.3%	Approved for OM and OE with tympanic membrane perforation
Ciprofloxacin 0.2% with hydrocortisone	Able to use for patient one year or older
For Fungal Infections	
Tolnaftate	Off-label use
Clotrimazole 1% solution	Off-label use

tion of EAC or trauma. Follow-up visit is unnecessary in uncomplicated otitis externa, but patient should be instructed to return if symptoms persist or recur.

Malignant Otitis Externa

Simple otitis externa in the diabetic or immunocompromised host (e.g., those with carcinoma, human immunodeficiency virus or those on chronic immunosuppressive therapy) may progress to a life-threatening disorder known as malignant otitis externa. This represents a necrotizing osteomyelitis of the skull base with mortality rate as high as 53%. The causative organism is most often *P. aeruginosa*. Once the epithelial barrier in the EAC is breached in a susceptible host, the infection becomes invasive, spreading rapidly anteriorly into the parotid space and inferiorly into the retromandibular fossa. Classically, granulation tissue replacing the lost epithelium is present on the floor of the EAC at the bony/cartilaginous junction, and the patient complains of pain disproportionate to the physical findings. The disease progresses rapidly to deep tissue necrosis, osteomyelitis, intracranial extension, and systemic toxicity. Late in the course of the disease, these patients present with severe trismus and progressive cranial nerve palsies, with the facial nerve being the most common nerve involved. In cases of suspected malignant otitis external, immediate ENT consultation is needed to evaluate the need for surgical debridement. Intravenous antibiotics with anti-pseudomonal coverage should be administered in the ED.

Foreign Bodies

Foreign bodies in the EAC are a relatively common problem faced by emergency physicians. The adult patient usually presents shortly after accidental entry of a foreign body. Children are often brought in when an otitis externa has developed secondary to the presence of a foreign body. Sudden pain, ear fullness, and altered hearing are all common symptoms of a retained EAC foreign body. Unusual presentation may include symptoms such as dizziness,

chronic cough, hiccup, and persistent noise. Patients with tympanic membrane perforation may present with severe bleeding, marked hearing loss, vertigo, and facial paralysis. A judicious and limited attempt to extract the foreign body should be carried out in the ED provided that the patient is cooperative and the tympanic membrane is not perforated. It is of vital importance not to convert a relatively benign condition to an emergency by pushing the foreign body further into the canal and possibly damaging the tympanic membrane and middle ear structures.

The clinician should be familiar with various techniques of foreign body removal, as the approach taken differs, depending on the type and location of the foreign body and the patient's clinical presentation. Irrigation is the least invasive method, although it is contraindicated in a perforated tympanic membrane and may cause swelling of vegetative matters. Adding isopropyl alcohol to the irrigant will prevent swelling of organic material. Irrigation will not work either when the foreign body obstructs the entire ear canal, as water cannot pass beyond it to provide the back pressure needed for removal. Living insect should be drowned by mineral oil or sedated by 2% lidocaine solution prior to extraction with either alligator forceps or suction. Alligator forceps should not be used to extract round foreign bodies; these can be best removed by using a curet or wire loop, which is passed just beyond the foreign body, then dragged laterally. Whenever possible, instrumentation should be confined to the lateral cartilaginous portion of the canal, as the medial bony canal is extremely sensitive to pain and susceptible to hemorrhage.

No routine follow-up is necessary after atraumatic extraction. Minor laceration or excoriation in the ear canal will heal with or without antibiotic solution, as long as the canal is kept clean and dry. The lack of specialized instrumentation in most ED makes atraumatic removal difficult at times and most patients can be referred to the ENT consultant for next day follow-up, if attempts in the ED prove unsuccessful. Patients with suspected tympanic perforations from the foreign body, those in severe discomfort or those with a caustic foreign body (e.g., button battery) require prompt ENT consultation.

Disorders of the Internal Ear

Lilly Lee

Otitis Media

Otitis media is the most common cause of pediatric visits to the physician and generates the largest number of antibiotic prescriptions in the United States; yet a clear, descriptive classification system does not exist for this entity. It is not clear that all cases of otitis media are infectious processes that require treatment with antimicrobial therapy. Review of the literature suggests considerable controversy regarding the medical and surgical management of otitis media. Studies have shown that 28% of the case have no bacteria or have nonpathogenic bacteria; and that approximately 30% to 40% of patients have respiratory viruses that may be present in combination with bacterial pathogens. *Streptococcus pneumoniae* remains the primary bacterial cause of otitis media (40%), followed by *Haemophilus influenzae* (25%), and *Moraxella catarrhalis* (12%). Some European studies have advocated nontreatment of otitis media given that approximately 60% of cases may resolve spontaneously. However, approximately 20% of *Streptococcus pneumoniae* infection may persist if left untreated, and may result in extension and development of intratemporal and intracranial complications. Antibiotic treatment also results in a slight decrease in the duration of symptoms, which may be important for children in daycare or school.

Acute otitis media can be defined as a purulent middle ear effusion with associated otalgia, fever, acute onset of irritability, and slight loss of hearing. Otoscopic findings should include the presence of a purulent middle ear effusion and a bulging erythematous tympanic membrane with loss of tympanic landmarks, decreased drum mobility with pneumoscopy; and possibly the presence of an acute draining perforation. The first line of treatment for acute otitis media remains amoxicillin (40 mg/kg per day in three divided doses per day) unless local resistance pattern suggests need for higher dosing of amoxicillin (60 mg to 90 mg/kg per day in two doses) or use of amoxicillin or clavulanate or one of the newer expanded spectrum macrolides. The length of treatment has been reassessed and most authorities advocate a 5-day course of antibiotics for treatment of simple acute otitis media in children over two years, and 10 days for those under two years. Single dose treatment with ceftriaxone has also demonstrated efficacy and may be useful in certain social settings.

Pediatric patients should have follow-up with their primary pediatrician in approximately 2 to 4 weeks. Patients with persistent or worsening pain and fever after 48 hours of antibiotics are considered treatment failure and should be evaluated for mastoiditis. They should return to the emergency department (ED) for further evaluation and ENT consultation.

Mastoiditis

The mastoid air cells are contiguous with the middle ear cavity; hence, fluid in the middle ear will involve the mastoid cells. Fluid may be an incidental finding on imaging. This stage of mastoiditis represents an extension of an otitis media and not strictly a complication. Acute mastoiditis with periosteitis involves the periosteum in the post auricular area. Patients may present with signs and symptoms of acute otitis media. They also have postauricular erythema, tenderness, and auricular protrusion secondary to periosteal elevation over the mastoid cortex. Bezold's abscess (abscess in the lateral aspect of the neck inferior to the mastoid tip) may also be present. CT of the mastoid will show loss of the normal bony trabecular pattern of the mastoid cells, in addition to fluid density. Mixed bacterial flora, including aerobic and anaerobic organisms is common. The treatment of acute mastoiditis includes prompt administration of intravenous antibiotics such as Imipenem 500 mg IV every 6 hours in the emergency department. Urgent ENT consultation is needed to perform a simple mastoidectomy, if a collection is present, and insertion of a tympanostomy tube is required.

Tympanic Membrane Perforation

Tympanic membrane perforation can result from direct trauma due to an attempt to clean the ear or from debris falling into the EAC. Indirect trauma, such as a slap to the auricle or barotrauma from scuba diving, may also result in perforation of the drum. In traumatic perforation, it is important to assess for injury to the ossicular chain or inner ear. The presence of sensorineural hearing loss, nystagmus, and significant vestibular symptoms suggest the possibility of a perilymph leak, and the case should be referred to an ENT specialist for urgent consultation. Most otherwise uncomplicated perforations heal spontaneously. Clean perforations do not require antibiotics. However, the patient must prevent water from entering the ear canal. If the perforation occurred under contaminated situation, cleaning of the canal is imperative and antibiotics are often prescribed. The tympanic membrane should be re-examined within 10 days by an ENT specialist, or sooner if drainage occurs after the first two days. Injury by hot slag during welding accidents should be referred promptly to ENT, as these seldom heal and may be complicated by bacterial superinfection.

Tympanic membrane perforation can also result from acute otitis media. Streptococcal infections can result in rapid rupture; or an organism not sensitive to the prescribed antibiotic, often *Staphylococcus aureus*, can also lead to tympanic membrane rupture. With infection, the drainage should be cultured, and a topical antibiotic suspension as well as oral antibiotic should be prescribed. These usually heal spontaneously within a few weeks after the drainage has subsided.

Labyrinthitis (Vestibular Neuronitis)

This syndrome is characterized by acute onset of intense true vertigo associated with nausea and vomiting. Associated aural symptoms (decreased hearing, aural pressure, and tinnitus) are usually not present and there is an absence of other neurological symptoms and findings. This represents one of the most common forms of vertigo to present to the ED. The patient may have had a viral illness prior to onset of vertiginous symptoms. Patients are usually in their 30s and 40s and without a history of prior medical problems. Other factors associated with vestibular neuronitis are recent large ingestion of alcohol, allergic reactions, extreme fatigue or administration of ototoxic antibiotics.

These patients should have a thorough ENT and neurological exam and if normal, no additional testing is needed. Clinical examination will reveal normal tympanic membranes, symmetrical hearing, spontaneous nystagmus in the acute phase, unilateral reduced or absent caloric response and otherwise normal neurological testing. Treatment is supportive and consists of tapering doses of vestibular suppressants. Meclizine, 12.5 mg to 25 mg every 8 hours or diazepam, 2 mg to 5 mg every 8 hours, are effective for managing symptoms of vestibular neuronitis. These medications can be increased from twice daily to three times a day, if no response in 24 hours, and then to four times a day, if no response in 48 hours. Once vertigo is controlled, the frequency can be reduced by one dose every five days. Continued vestibular suppressant therapy can delay central nervous system compensation mechanisms and prolong vestibular symptoms. Reso-

lution is expected within a six to eight week time frame. Resistant and recurrent symptoms should be referred to an ENT specialist for further evaluation to assess for CNS disease, atypical Meniere's or migraine related vestibulopathy. Rarely patients may need to be hospitalized for intravenous hydration and medication secondary to intractable vomiting or severe vertigo.

Suppurative Labyrnthitis

Suppurative labyrinthitis represents the most serious form of labyrinthine disease. Extension of acute otitis media or chronic otitis is the usual cause of this process. The perilymph becomes infected and this results in permanent loss of hearing and vestibular function secondary to the destruction of sensory elements in the labyrinth and cochlea. The patient presents with severe vertigo with associated nausea and vomiting on minimal movement. On examination, the patient has a purulent otitis media, usually with drainage out the external canal; is deaf on the affected side; and shows a horizontorotary nystagmus with the fast component to the affected side. Treatment with intravenous antibiotics to cover aerobic and anaerobic pathogens, and ENT consultation should be initiated immediately.

Meniere's Disease

Review of the ENT literature suggests that the diagnosis and management of patient's with Meniere's disease represent one of the most controversial subjects in neurotology. It is a chronic condition characterized by a progressive dysfunction of the inner ear or the cochleovestibular nerve, or both. The precise pathophysiology of this problem remains poorly elucidated, but is classically thought to be secondary to excess fluid in the perilymph system. The cause is presumed to be idiopathic. The official definition proposed by the American Academy of Otolaryngology requires that the following symptoms be present for a diagnosis of Meniere's disease: recurrent spells of vertigo, lasting at least 20 minutes, with associated sensorineural hearing loss, and aural fullness or tinnitus, particularly in the low tone type. Some patients will have these symptoms (Meniere's syndrome), which are secondary to other causes such as food allergies, immune disease, syphilis, and CNS lesions and these should be treated as such. The typical course of Meniere's disease is clusters of vertiginous episodes separated by remission. When patients present to the ED with an acute exacerbation, the treatment is supportive with vestibular suppressants and anti-emetics. Occasionally, patients may need to be admitted for intravenous hydration and medication. Long-term management of this disease (including medication, diet, and surgery) should be handled by the ENT consultant.

Selected Readings

Alper CM, Myers EN, Eibling DE. *Decision Making in Ear, Nose, and Throat Disorders*. Philadelphia: W.B. Saunders, 2001.

Bull TR. *Color Atlas of ENT Diagnosis.* Stuttgart, Germany: Georg Thieme Verlag, 2003.

Eisele WE, McQuone SJ, eds. *Emergencies of the Head and Neck.* St. Louis: Mosby, 2000.

Pensak ML. *Controversies in Otolaryngology.* New York: Thieme Medical Publishers, 2001.

Stair T, ed. *Emergency Medicine Clinics of North America: ENT Emergencies.* Philadelphia: W.B. Saunders, 1987.

Wilson WR, Nadol JB, Randolph GW. *The Clinical Handbook of Ear, Nose and Throat Disorders.* New York: Parthenon, 2002.

Woodson Gayle E. *Ear, Nose and Throat Disorders in Primary Care.* Philadelphia: W.B. Saunders, 2001.

John L. Alexander
Ramin R. Samadi
John Burton

Anterior Epistaxis

Epistaxis is one of the most common nasal emergencies. Although usually self-limited, nasal hemorrhage may be profuse and life-threatening. Proper management of patients with epistaxis requires an understanding of the underlying anatomy and pathophysiology associated with significant nasal bleeding. The goal of treatment of epistaxis is to maximize patient comfort, diagnose underlying pathology, and prevent life-threatening hemorrhage.

Anterior epistaxis is the most common etiology for all nasal hemorrhages, with more than 90% of bleeds originating in the anterior-inferior part of the nasal septum. Most episodes of simple anterior epistaxis are controlled by the patient outside the emergency setting. However, up to 10% of patients with anterior epistaxis will present to the emergency department (ED).

The nasal mucosa is supplied with a dense network of submucosal blood vessels. The most common site of anterior epistaxis is Little's area in the anterior-inferior septal plexus, known as Kiesselbach's plexus. This complex is supplied by branches of the anterior ethmoidal artery and the nasopalatine artery.

In most cases, anterior epistaxis is caused by direct trauma. This may include digital manipulation, nasal foreign bodies, or nasal bone and other facial bone fractures. Other local causes of anterior epistaxis include mucosal inflammation due to infection or allergy, neoplastic disease, or anatomic deformities, such as septal deviation. Systemic causes of epistaxis include blood dyscrasias, such as hemophilia or von Willebrand's disease, anticoagulant therapy, arterio-venous malformations, and arteriosclerosis. Although hypertension is associated with prolonged, active bleeding, it is not considered to be a primary cause of epistaxis. The causes of epistaxis are listed in **Table 51.1**.

The management of epistaxis should follow three simple guidelines: (1) identify patients in need of resuscitation and initiate resuscitative efforts, (2) determine the location and cause of the bleeding, and (3) establish hemorrhage control.

Patients with anterior epistaxis rarely present with life-threatening hemorrhage. In most cases, the patient cannot accurately determine the amount and duration of bleeding. However, a full set of vital signs and cardio-respiratory monitoring, when appropriate, should be obtained in every patient to verify the patient's hemodynamic stability.

A focused history should be obtained from the patient to assist in narrowing the differential diagnosis for anterior epistaxis. Important elements of the history include the duration and severity of bleeding, list of current medications, history of medical conditions predisposing the patient to excessive bleeding, recent history of trauma or surgery, and history of prior episodes of epistaxis and the means by which the bleeding was controlled.

The examination of the patient with anterior epistaxis is best achieved with the patient seated and the patient's head in the upright position. Use of a nasal speculum, opened in the superior-inferior direction, is recommended for proper visualization of the entire nasal cavity. Adequate lighting, as provided by the head mirror, headlamp, or fiberoptic lighting source, is essential to illuminate the area completely. In anterior epistaxis, sites of common bleeding include anterior septum, sphenopalatine artery distribution to superior and middle turbinates, and turbinates of lateral walls of the nasal cavity. Sites of bleeding should be properly identified prior to administration of any medications. Examination of the mucosa of the anterior nose should be done to document mucosal hypertrophy, mucosal disruption, or irritation, and presence or absence of septal perforation. Posterior sources of epistaxis should be suspected if the patient has continued bleeding even after pressure is applied, has drainage to the posterior oropharynx with occlusion of the nostrils, or sites of active bleeding are not visualized on anterior examination.

A stepwise algorithm for the treatment of anterior epistaxis in the ED is presented in **Table 51.2**.

Initial therapy for anterior epistaxis is digital pressure applied anterior to the nasal bone occluding both of the nostrils. Pressure should be applied for 10 to 15 minutes to providing adequate tamponade of the bleeding. If hemostasis has been achieved after digital pressure alone, the emer-

Table 51.1

Causes of Epistaxis

Local	Systemic
Traumatic	Hematologic
• Digital manipulation	• Anticoagulant therapy (e.g., warfarin)
• Foreign body	• Anti-inflammatory therapy (e.g., ibuprofen)
• Facial bone fractures	• Platelet dysfunction (e.g., thrombocytopenia)
• Blunt facial trauma	• Inherited disorders (e.g., hemophilia A)
Inflammatory	• Disseminated intravascular coagulation
• Rhinitis/sinusitis	Vascular
• Nasal polyps	• Atherosclerosis
Anatomic	• Connective tissue disorders
• Septal deviation	• Hereditary hemorrhagic telangiectasia
• Septal perforation	Endocrine
Neoplastic	• Endometriosis
• Benign	Idiopathic
• Malignant	
Iatrogenic	
• Nasotracheal intubation	
• Nasal packing	

gency provider should consider further intervention to ensure that the patient will not re-bleed after discharge.

If a complete examination of the nasal cavity is not possible due to excessive bleeding, topical anesthesia and vasoconstrictors may be necessary. A variety of agents can be used including 4% cocaine hydrochloride, 0.5% to 1.0% phenylephrine (Neo-Synephrine) with 2% to 4% lidocaine mixture, 0.05% oxymetozaline (Afrin) with 2% to

Table 51.2

Stepwise Approach to the Treatment of Epistaxis

Technique	Examples
Digital pressure	
Chemical cauterization	Topical vasoconstrictors
	Silver nitrate
Electrical cauterization	
Placement of hemostatic material	Gel foam
Nasal packing	Antibiotic-impregnated vaseline gauze
	Nasal sponge (e.g., Merocel)
	Nasal tampon (e.g., Rhino Rocket)
Balloon tamponade	
Surgical intervention	Ligation of the maxillary artery
Radiologic intervention	Angiographic embolization

4% lidocaine mixture, 0.25 mL of 1:1,000 epinephrine in combination with 2% to 4% lidocaine. Agents of choice should be applied directly to the bleeding area using soaked cotton applicators or cotton pledgets on a bayonet forceps. Multiple pledgets may be required to completely anesthetize the entire nasal cavity and should be left in place for 10 to 15 minutes. After anesthetic/vasoconstrictors have been removed, further examination of the bleeding site should be undertaken.

When bleeding is minimal or has ceased and no coagulopathy is present, attempts at cautery with either electrocautery or silver nitrate can be made. Contact with the cautery device should occur concentrically in a circle around the vessel from the outside in. This technique decreases collateral flow and creates a drier field for contact. Excessive attempts at cautery risk destruction of the underlying cartilage of the nose and possible septal perforation and should be avoided.

If bleeding continues or non-localizable bleeding is present, or if the patient has a coagulopathy, the use of a hemostatic material, such as gel-foam, may be effective. Placement of the material should occur with the use of bayonet forceps, and direct pressure should be re-applied to ensure adherence to the mucosal surface.

In the patient with a coagulopathy, a significant area of involved mucosa, repeated episodes of anterior epistaxis, or continued anterior epistaxis, anterior nasal packing is a good means of hemostasis. Several alternative methods for anterior nasal packing exist.

Antibiotic-impregnated petrolatum jelly gauze is an effective tool for hemostasis in the patient with severe hemorrhage, complex or distorted anatomy, or in whom the site of bleeding is located beneath the middle or inferior turbinate. The gauze should be placed with a bayonet forceps in a pleated manner, beginning inferiorly along the floor of the nasal cavity and progressing superiorly.

Placement of one of the commercially available nasal sponges or tampons may be preferred for uncontrolled anterior epistaxis. The benefits of use of these nasal packs include rapid placement, ease of placement, and procoagulant materials. The technique for insertion of these devices is similar to the introduction of nasal pledgets. The pack should be coated with a lubricant jelly or antibiotic cream. Insertion should be directed posteriorly through the nares with a bayonet forceps only after adequate anesthesia of the nasal mucosa. Once in place, the sponge should be expanded using normal saline or an antibiotic solution, either via direct injection with an 18-, 20-, or 22-guage needle or via droplets.

Patients without hemodynamic compromise, coagulopathy, and who have achieved control of simple, anterior epistaxis are good candidates for outpatient management. The patient should be advised of the need to avoid manipulation of the packing material, and avoid the use of salicylates and other non-steroidal anti-inflammatory drugs for several days. The patient should be instructed of the need to seek the attention of a physician for removal of the nasal packing within 48 hours. The patient should receive antibiotic prophylaxis for bacterial sinusitis and toxic shock syndrome. Commonly used antibiotics include cephalexin, 500 mg orally three times daily, and amoxicillin-clavulanic acid, 500 mg orally three times daily or 875 mg orally twice daily. If re-bleeding occurs with the anterior nasal packing in place, the patient should be instructed on how to apply pressure to the nose to tamponade bleeding and when to return to the ED. Admission should be considered for hemodynamic instability, coagulopathy, inadequate hemostasis, frail, elderly patients, and patients with respiratory or cardiac diseases compromised by the presence of the anterior nasal packing.

Posterior Epistaxis

Posterior epistaxis occurs in approximately 10% of patients presenting with nasal hemorrhage. It is more common in persons older than 50 years, and it is more likely to present with signs of hemodynamic instability. A posterior source of bleeding should be suspected when bleeding continues despite external compression, in the presence of bilateral anterior nasal bloody discharge or when bleeding persists despite adequate anterior nasal packing.

Posterior epistaxis can be defined as bleeding from sites in the nasal cavity not visualized from the anterior approach. The most common site of posterior bleeding in the nose is Woodruff's plexus, which is supplied by the lateral nasal branch of the sphenopalatine artery. Sources of posterior epistaxis may also occur in areas supplied by the posterior ethmoidal artery. Posterior epistaxis can result from the multiple causes of epistaxis listed in Table 51.1, but systemic causes, such as anticoagulant therapy and atherosclerosis, are most common.

Management of posterior epistaxis is similar to that of anterior epistaxis. The recognition and treatment of hemodynamic instability is of paramount importance. Any patients with vigorous posterior epistaxis, coagulopathy, recent surgery to the nose, or recurrent posterior epistaxis represent situations requiring special attention and possible immediate otolaryngologist consultation. In the presence of severe hypertension, efforts to reduce anxiety and improve patient comfort should be made. Uncontrolled hypertension should be treated aggressively with medications, if necessary.

In patients with multiple co-morbid conditions, elderly patients, or unstable patients, several ancillary tests should be considered. Coagulation studies (i.e., prothrombin time and partial thromboplastin time) should be obtained from the patient on anticoagulation therapy or having any bleeding abnormalities due to hepatic dysfunction or other underlying medical problems. A complete blood count should be considered in patients with any hemodynamic instability, platelet abnormalities, prolonged and excessive blood loss, or a history of carcinoma or recent chemotherapy. Patients in whom there is hemodynamic compromise or likely coagulopathy should have cross-matched blood products available.

If other attempts at hemorrhage control have been unsuccessful, the patient with posterior epistaxis may require the use of a posterior nasal packing to obtain hemostasis. The traditional method of posterior nasal packing involved the placement of a rolled, 4×4 gauze against the posterior nasopharynx, held in place by silk ties exiting the nares. This method can be cumbersome to employ, difficult to tolerate by the patient, and ineffective at hemostasis.

An easier method of controlling posterior epistaxis is to insert a 12F to 16F Foley catheter with a 30 cc balloon into the nose along the floor of the nasopharynx until the tip of the catheter is visible in the posterior oropharynx. The balloon is then inflated with 15 cc of saline or sterile water, and eased anteriorly until coming in firm contact with the posterior choana. The Foley catheter is then secured with a 0-0 sink tie or umbilical tape to a dental roll or gauze roll to prevent pressure necrosis of the ala or columella.

The most commonly used device for posterior packing is the triple-lumen, double-balloon intranasal catheters. The nasal balloon may provide anterior and/or posterior hemostasis via a single efficient procedure. A further advantage of this system is the design of the device as a nasal airway in combination with the low-pressure, dual-balloon combination.

Insertion of the nasal balloon is similar to that of a nasal sponge or tampon. The device should be lubricated with bacteriostatic or anesthetic jelly and introduced through the nares, directed posteriorly until the tip can be seen in the posterior pharynx. The distal balloon should be filled with 10 cc to 15 cc of normal saline, and the device pulled anteriorly until gentle resistance is met. The proximal balloon should then be filled with 20 cc to 30 cc of normal saline. The packing is left in place for between 3 and 5 days, depending on the extent of bleeding and underlying medical conditions that may retard hemostasis.

Any patient receiving posterior packing should have consultation with an otolaryngologist. These patients require strict cardiac and respiratory monitoring after placement, supplemental, humidified oxygen via facemask, and prophylactic antibiotic therapy. Patients with a nasal balloon in place should be admitted to a monitored unit due to the risk of hypoxia secondary to intrapulmonary shunting as a result of the nasopulmonary reflex. Complications associated with posterior nasal packing are listed in **Table 51.3**.

Table 51.3	
Complications Associated with Posterior Nasal Packing	
Organ System	**Complication**
Respiratory	Hypoxia
	Hypoventilation
	Hypercapnia
	Exacerbation of obstructive sleep apnea
	Aspiration
Cardiovascular	Hypertension
	Bradycardia
	Dysrhythmias
	Myocardial infarction
Mechanical	Pressure necrosis of mucosa and cartilage
Infectious	Sinusitis
	Otitis media
	Toxic shock syndrome

Finally, bleeding refractory to the methods described above requires intervention by an otolaryngologist. The techniques for surgical intervention include ligation of the external carotid artery, maxillary artery or ethmoidal artery. Other means for controlling severe epistaxis include angiographic embolization by an interventional radiologist.

Nasal Foreign Body

Nasal foreign bodies represent a common nasal emergency, especially among pediatric patients. Although most patients present soon after insertion of the foreign body, a small number of children will present with unilateral, mucopurulent nasal discharge in which the possibility of nasal foreign body should be considered. The majority of nasal foreign bodies can be appropriately removed without complication by a trained emergency provider.

There are endless possibilities to the type of objects, which may present as a nasal foreign body. These include most small items found in the household, such as raisins, beads, crayons, seeds, nuts, paper, and erasers. Although benign, these objects can provide a nidus for infection. Other items that deserve particular mention include button batteries and small insects or worms. Button batteries are composed of various heavy metals and produce a severe local tissue reaction and liquefaction necrosis, resulting in septal perforation, synechiae, and stenosis of the nasal cavity. Small insects or larvae may produce a range of responses, from a mild inflammatory reaction to destruction of the nasal bones and cartilaginous spaces.

Location of the nasal foreign body may occur anywhere in the nasal cavity. The most common locations include the floor of the nasal cavity below the inferior turbinate and directly anterior to the middle turbinate. Nasal foreign bodies are typically painless, unless they have been present long enough to promote an inflammatory response or localized infection. A classical set of symptoms related to a retained foreign body in the nasal cavity is unilateral purulent rhinorrhea, foul odor, and unilateral epistaxis; however, incidental diagnosis has been reported after routine dental examination, routine medical examination, or on radiographs done for other reasons. Other signs or symptoms that may lead to diagnosis of a foreign body are a sensation of unilateral nasal obstruction, nasal or facial cellulitis, nasal pain, episodic sneezing and failure of antibiotic therapy for presumed sinusitis.

The examination of the patient is best achieved with the patient seated in the upright position, with the nose extended in the sniffing position. In the pediatric patient, the child should be placed in a position of comfort to provide a more optimal examination setting. Examination of the involved side requires the use of a nasal speculum, inserted in a superior-inferior fashion, and adequate lighting, as provided by the head mirror, head lamp or fiberoptic lighting source. If the foreign body is not located on initial examination despite adequate visualization of the entire nasal cavity, topical anesthesia and vasoconstrictors may be used to provide patient comfort and improve the visual field. Cotton pledgets soaked with anesthetic solutions may be used, or droplets of anesthetic solutions may also be effective. After examination of the nose and verification of the foreign body, further examination should be undertaken to include transillumination and percussion of the sinuses, a complete ear examination, and pertinent further physical examination.

Multiple techniques for nasal foreign body removal have been developed by emergency physicians. Initial attempts should involve the patient forcefully attempting to expel the object while compressing the uninvolved nares. For children not old enough to cooperate, the unaffected side may be held closed by the physician while air is blown into the open mouth by the parent using the mouth-to-mouth technique. An additional positive pressure technique described in the literature involves placement of a male-to-male adapter attached to oxygen tubing with 10 L to 15 L/min of flow rate into the unaffected nostril. In a small case series, this technique was found to be 100% effective and well tolerated by patients.

Various extraction devices may be employed for foreign body removal, depending on the size, shape, and consistency of the object. For objects that have a smooth surface or are rounded, a suction catheter with a flange-tip may be used. For irregularly shaped and soft or compressible objects, bayonet forceps, Noyes forceps, long right-angle alligator forceps, or a right-angle probe may provide the greatest chance at removal of the material. A further means of extraction of foreign bodies from the nose involves the use of a No. 4 Fogarty vascular catheter. The catheter is inserted from an anterior approach, passing the balloon past the foreign body into the posterior nasal cavity. The balloon is then inflated and slowly eased forward to provide a solid base for removal of the object with retraction.

After removal of any foreign material, the nose should further be inspected to examine for the presence of further foreign bodies, infection, trauma, or pressure necrosis. Unlike other areas of the body, removal of foreign bodies from the nasal cavity should not involve irrigation or pushing the object into the posterior oropharynx, as the risk of aspiration is significant. Routine antibiotic prophylaxis is not indicated for simple foreign bodies removed within 24 hours of insertion. Tetanus prophylaxis should be performed, if indicated.

Urgent follow-up with an otolaryngologist is indicated for the patient with symptoms indicating foreign body but no evidence of an object on examination. Should attempts at removing a visualized nasal foreign body be unsuccessful, the simple foreign body is amenable to an outpatient visit to an otolaryngologist within the next 24 hours. Immediate consultation of an otolaryngologist and possible hospitalization are reasonable in the patient who has systemic symptoms (such as fever, malaise, hypoxia, or lethargy), a button battery that is not rapidly removed from the nose, facial cellulitis, or evidence of tissue destruction by parasitic infection, or where there is a significant possibility of aspiration by the patient.

Cavernous Sinus Thrombosis

Cavernous sinus thrombosis (CST) is the generation of a thrombus in the cavernous sinus(es). In the post-antibiotic era, CST is uncommon, but is still a very fulminant and rapidly progressing disease. It is usually a late complication of a sinus, facial, or ear infection. Even with the proper therapy, CST is associated with a 30% mortality and an extremely high neurological and ophthalmologic morbidity rate. Complete recovery is extremely rare. In the United States, approximately 5% of all the ophthalmoplegias are secondary to the involvement of the cranial nerves in the cavernous sinuses. Fortunately, with the advent of antibiotic therapy, both the incidence of CST and its mortality has decreased significantly. Without antibiotic therapy the mortality of CST may exceed 80% to 100%.

Etiology and Pathophysiology

CST may be secondary to either infectious or aseptic causes. The majority of the CSTs are as a result of an infectious process involving middle of the face, also known as "triangle of death." This space, which is centered around the nose, involves the area between the glabella and the two lateral corners of the upper lips. Infections of the paranasal sinuses (specifically sphenoid or ethmoid sinuses), facial skin and soft tissue, middle ear, eye, or eyelids are considered the primary culprits. In as many as 25% of cases, a "manipulated" nostril furuncle is the precipitant etiology. On rare occasions, the infectious CST may occur following "minor" oral or maxillofacial surgeries, such as dental extraction or rhinoplasty. Most patients are previously healthy; however patients with diabetes mellitus or a compromised immune system may be at a higher risk of acquiring CST.

The majority of infections are caused by *Staphylococcus aureus* and *Streptococcus pneumoniae*. Other less commonly involved pathogens include *Haemophilus influenzae* and anaerobic bacteria. Exotic organisms, such as *Fusibacterium, Aspergillus, Mucor,* and *Rhizopus* have also been rarely implicated in infectious CST.

Aseptic CST may occur as a result of a space occupying lesion involving the cavernous sinuses. These parasellar lesions may include a variety of benign or malignant tumors, carotid-cavernous fistula, cavernous sinus aneurysm, and internal carotid artery aneurysm. Primary tumors are most commonly meningiomas, pituitary tumors and neurofibromas. Malignant tumors are usually nasopharyngeal, pulmonary, prostatic or breast metastatic neoplasms. Less commonly, various hypercoagulable or hyperproliferative states, and diseases such as polycythemia, hematological malignancies, or vasculitis may be the underlying etiology of a non-infectious CST.

Anatomy

The knowledge of the anatomy of the cavernous sinuses and their relationship to various other structures are paramount to the understanding of the clinical presentation of CST.

The irregularly shaped, trabecular paired cavernous sinuses are basically two large veins. They are located at the base of the skull, immediately posterior to the orbits. They lie lateral and superior to the sphenoid sinus, posterior to the optic chiasm, and on the sides of the sella turcica. These sinuses are formed from layers of dura and are connected to each other via the intercavernous sinus. These venous reservoirs do not possess any valves and the direction of the blood flow is decided by the existing pressure gradients. The cavernous sinuses receive facial venous blood, from the superior and inferior ophthalmic, middle cerebral, and sphenoidal veins. Subsequently, utilizing the inferior and superior petrosal veins, cavernous sinuses drain into the internal jugular veins and superior petrosal sinuses. The infected thrombosis of the cavernous sinus results in upstream venous stasis. In addition to the venous blood, cavernous sinuses contain the internal carotid arteries and their adjacent autonomic plexus, and the cranial nerves III, IV, VI, and the ophthalmic and maxillary divisions of VI. The carotid arteries are centrally located and the cranial nerves are lined up on the lateral wall of the sinuses. The disruption of the delicate proximity of these vital structures can explain the clinical presentation of CST.

Clinical Presentation

CST has a characteristic presentation. Acute and rapidly progressing systemic symptoms may include fever, chills, malaise, retro-orbital pain and headache. Venous stasis will result in unilateral periorbital edema, the swelling of the eyelids and chemosis. These signs will proceed to ptosis and proptosis of the involved eye. With the progression of the disease, ophthalmologic signs become prominent. Lateral gaze palsy is the most common and the earliest ophthalmologic sign. This can be followed by a generalized ophthalmoplegia. The intraocular pressure is usually elevated. At this stage of the disease, the presence of a very sluggish or a fixed and dilated pupil is very common. Visual acuity will also be significantly decreased. These signs are secondary to the increased intraocular pressures and the traction on the optic nerve. The corneal reflex will be abnormal. Patient may complain of painful diplopia. The involvement of the sensory branches of cranial nerve V is omnipresent. Papilledema and retinal hemorrhages may also be present. Patient may complain of stiff neck and manifest signs of meningismus. Generalized seizures and hemiparesis will commonly develop. Although not occurring universally, one of the characteristics of infectious CST is progression of the infection through the intercavernous sinus and the involvement of the contralateral cavernous sinus and the subsequent manifestation of bilateral disease. Sepsis, delirium, and shock will follow shortly thereafter.

In aseptic CST, the disease usually presents as a subacute or even chronic illness. Systemic symptoms and signs are usually absent and painful diplopia or another isolated ophthalmoplegia may be the only initial complaint.

Diagnosis

CST is a clinical diagnosis and laboratory tests are rarely specific. Manifestation of ophthalmoplegia in a patient with either sinusitis or a mid-facial infection must be considered as an indication for the pursuit of the diagnosis of CST. The involvement of the contralateral eye is considered pathognomonic for CST.

Patients will present with an elevated white blood cell count and a left shift. Lumbar puncture, if performed, will suggest bacterial meningitis. Cerebro-spinal fluid (CSF) will reveal an elevation of opening pressure, elevated white blood cell count and protein, and a decreased glucose. Blood culture must be obtained and may reveal the causative pathogen.

Although nonspecific, diagnostic imaging may include plain radiographs of the orbit and the paranasal sinuses. Computed axial tomography (CT) of the brain and the orbit can visualize the bony structures. Magnetic resonance imaging (MRI) and magnetic resonance angiography (MRA) provide a better detail of the soft tissue and a higher diagnostic resolution. The signal void of the carotid artery and the visualization of the superior and inferior orbital veins are highly suggestive of CST. The gold standard for diagnosis of CST is the seldom-performed orbital venography. Carotid angiography can be obtained as an alternative modality and as a surrogate substitute.

Differential Diagnosis

Early on, CST maybe confused with and must be differentiated from diseases, such as periorbital and orbital cellulitis, exophthalmic goiter, epidural hematoma, epidural and subdural infections, acute angle-closure glaucoma, subarachnoid hemorrhage, and subdural hematoma.

Treatment

CST must be considered a medical emergency. Therapeutic modalities include antibiotics, anticoagulation, and surgery. Once the diagnosis is considered, intravenous broad spectrum antibiotic therapy must be initiated promptly. Antimicrobial agents should provide coverage for Gram-positive, Gram-negative, and anaerobic organisms. Commonly used antibiotic regiments include semisynthetic penicillinase resistant penicillins, third generation cephalosporins, and metronidazole. Appropriate choices of intravenous antimicrobial agents are: oxicillin or nafcillin 2 g every 4 hours (adults) or 150 to 200 mg/kg per day (pediatrics) every 6 hours, not to exceed 12 g per day; ceftriaxone 2 g every 12 hours (adults) or 75 mg/kg every 12 hours (pediatrics); metronidazole (in combination with either one of the above-mentioned agents) 500 mg every 6 hours (adults). Despite its rare but potentially lethal side effects, cloramphenicol 1.5 g every 6 hours (adults) or 50 to 75 mg/kg per day every 6 hours (pediatrics) is an acceptable alternative intravenous antibiotic. In diabetic or immunocompromised patients, use of antifungal medications should also be seriously considered.

Although still considered controversial, anticoagulation therapy, with either unfractionated heparin or a low molecular weight heparin, is generally supported by the available data and should be considered as a therapeutic modality. This therapy will prevent the recurrence of thrombosis and new infarctions, and reduce the incidence of septic embolization. However, it may increase the incidence of hemorrhagic events. Anticoagulation therapy may also be beneficial in aseptic CST.

Surgical drainage of an identifiable septic focus, e.g., sinusitis or facial abscess, should be attempted and may be lifesaving. Surgery on the cavernous sinus is technically difficult and has not been proven efficacious in reduction of mortality or morbidity.

Use of steroids, as an adjunct therapy has been debated and may reduce the secondary inflammatory processes and edema. The related published data has been fairly disappointing. Use of thrombolytic agents, e.g., urokinase, in treatment of isolated CST has not been fully studied.

Prognosis

In surviving patients neurological sequelae are fairly common. Major long-term complications include significantly diminished vision or total blindness and persistent ophthalmoplegia. Around 17% of patients will suffer from some degree of visual impairment and 50% from cranial nerve deficits.

Rhinosinusitis

Definition

Recent reviews have suggested the advantage of the term "rhinosinusitis" as preferable to the terms rhinitis and sinusitis. While there are patients who suffer from chronic, isolated rhinitis complaints, the majority of emergency physician encounters will involve patients with acute or chronic inflammation and/or infection of both the paranasal sinuses and nasal mucosa. Hence, consideration should be directed toward rhinosinusitis symptoms with an understanding and approach consistent with accepted treatment principles for the paranasal sinuses and contiguous nasal mucosa.

Background

Rhinosinusitis has a substantial impact on health with estimates of between one and two of every ten Americans suffering rhinosinusitis at some time in their lives. Approximately 10 million work and school days are lost each year with annual physician visits exceeding 25 million. Infection of the paranasal sinuses and complaints that result from these infections are frequent causes for ED visits. Rhinosinusitis is frequently cited as the fifth most common cause for physician-prescribed antibiotic therapy in acute care.

The paranasal sinuses are a group of pneumatized cavities with a mucociliary lining. Proper function of the mucociliary lining and mucous membranes allows for host defense against the normal nasopharynx flora. Mucus production, ciliary mucosa, ciliary movement, and drainage of the sinuses through ostial openings provide cleansing of the sinuses and a sterile environment. If any part of this apparatus is defective, the flora from the nasopharynx in proximity to the sinus may be transported into the sinus and result in bacterial overgrowth and infection. The most common cause of abnormal sinus function is due to obstruction; however, nasopharyngeal anatomic abnormalities, ciliary dysfunction, and others may also contribute to this problem (**Table 51.4**).

Acute Versus Chronic Rhinosinusitis

The approach to the rhinosinusitis patient should initially be directed toward the distinction between acute and chronic rhinosinusitis. Rhinosinusitis can be considered chronic when symptoms are present beyond 12 weeks in duration and recalcitrant to initial acute rhinosinusitis management. The causes of chronic rhinitis can be further subdivided into allergic and nonallergic causes. Acute rhinosinusitis is considered recurrent when patients suffer greater than three episodes per year with each episode lasting in excess of seven days.

Acute Rhinosinusitis

Investigations describing patients with common cold or viral rhinosinusitis have described the symptoms associated with these illnesses as typically lasting less than seven days in duration. Therefore, many guidelines for the approach to the acute rhinosinusitis patient have cited patients with symptoms exceeding seven days to be at higher relative risk (increased specificity) of bacterial infection.

Clinical Assessment

Acute rhinosinusitis patients typically present with complaints including rhinorrhea—clear or purulent, paranasal congestion/drip, cough, headache, sneezing, sore throat, fever, facial fullness, facial pain, and tooth pain. These symptoms are not exclusive to acute rhinosinusitis, and a complete history and physical examination should be done to exclude other causes of similar symptoms (**Table 51.5**).

Physical examination of the rhinosinusitis patient may reveal fever and rhinorrhea. Inspection of the nasopharynx may demonstrate clear or purulent drainage from the middle or superior meatus of the nasal turbinates. Tenderness to percussion of the tissues overlying the frontal sinus or maxillary sinus region may be present. Percussion of the maxillary teeth may also elicit pain.

Table 51.4

Common Causes of Malfunction of the Sinuses

Viral infection
Allergic rhinitis
Chemical irritants
Mechanical obstruction
Vasomotor abnormalities
Nasal instrumentation
Nasal surgery
Tumor
Fungal infection
Barometric pressure changes
General anesthesia

Table 51.5

Etiologies to Include in Differential Diagnosis of Rhinosinusitis

Intranasal abscess
Dental abscess
Intracranial abscess
Facial cellulitis
Orbital cellulitis/abscess
Fungal infection
Allergic rhinitis
Viral upper respiratory infection
Tension headache
Migraine headache
Intranasal foreign body
Nasal polyp
Chemical irritant
Dental disease
Rhinitis medicamentosa

Transillumination of the sinuses may show differential opacification of the affected sinuses.

In the immunocompetent patient, acute rhinosinusitis is a diagnosis that should be made on a clinical basis, without the need for further ancillary tests. Over a 20-year period in medical literature (1976 to 1996), at least eight studies with sample sizes exceeding 100 patients were published assessing the relative strength of clinical and historical findings for the diagnosis of acute bacterial rhinosinusitis. These studies found a history or finding of purulent nasal discharge, unilateral maxillary tooth pain or tenderness, and unilateral facial pain or tenderness to be most predictive of the presence of a bacterial infection.

Radiographic Assessment

Should radiographic evaluation be deemed necessary, a standard sinus series, including Waters, Caldwell, and lateral views should be included. Findings most consistent with a diagnosis of rhinosinusitis include a sinus air and/or fluid level, periosteal thickening in excess of 5 mm, and sinus opacification. In the acute setting, the presence of orbital swelling or periorbital erythema should prompt consideration of evaluation by computed tomography (CT) scan to rule out extension of the infection into the orbit or periorbital tissues.

In the acute rhinosinusitis patient, the routine use of radiographs or CT should be discouraged. Although studies have cited an approximate 90% sensitivity of radiographic findings for bacterial rhinosinusitis, the same radiographic findings are also prevalent in viral rhinosinusitis patients rendering a very poor specificity. Additionally, given the cost and inconvenience of radiographic screening to the large population of acutely symptomatic patients, a routine approach incorporating sinus imaging is rendered impractical. Radiographic evaluation, however, should be considered routine in the complicated or chronic rhinosinusitis patient.

ED Management

Treatment of the patient with acute rhinosinusitis should be focused toward symptom improvement and prevention of further exacerbation. The mainstay of treatment employs the strategy of reducing inflammation and edema in the nasal mucosa, thinning sinus secretions, promoting sinus decongestion and analgesia. During the period 1967 to 1994, as many as eight trials have evaluated the effect of various non-antibiotic medications, prescribed as well as over-the-counter, with varying results.

Alpha-adrenergic, topical spray vasoconstrictors (e.g., phenylephrine, oxymetazoline) are believed to be efficacious in reducing edema and inflammation within the nasopharynx. These agents are limited by the potential for vasomotor dependency and rebound congestion if utilized for continuous periods in excess of 72 hours. Oral decongestants (e.g., pseudophedrine) offer the possibility of congestion reduction to deeper tissues and should be employed routinely. Antihistamines, given their drying effect on the mucous membranes, may impede mucous clearance and decongestion and should not be routinely utilized. Topical and systemic steroids are known to reduce inflammation; however, their use is likely more efficacious in prevention and reduction of chronic symptoms rather than the acutely symptomatic patient.

Analgesia is best achieved via non-steroidal agents (e.g., ibuprofen) and/or acetaminophen (many oral decongestants are available in combined preparations and can be convenient). Selected patients may require short-term analgesia with oral narcotics (e.g., hydrocodone, oxycodone).

In uncomplicated acute rhinosinusitis, no follow-up medical care is required if symptoms improve. However, if symptoms persist for greater than three weeks or despite initial treatment, outpatient referral is warranted with an allergist or otolaryngologist.

Antimicrobial Therapy

The most common offending organisms in acute bacterial rhinosinusitis are *Streptococcus pneumonia* and *Haemophilus influenzae*, although *Streptococcus pyogenes*, *Staphylococcus aureus*, *Moraxella catarrhalis*, and anaerobic organisms have also been implicated.

The gold standard for diagnosis of the acute bacterial infection remains sinus puncture, aspiration and culture. Given the complexity of the intervention, this standard cannot be applied to patients routinely. Further, many published series of patients with acute bacterial rhinosinusitis do not achieve this standard and opt for more convenient and noninvasive radiographic imaging as the diagnostic standard.

The clinical approach to determination for the appropriateness for antibiotic therapy should incorporate length and severity of symptoms, previous history of sinus infections, and findings of history and physical examination. The decision to use antibiotics will typically be prompted by a history of symptoms in excess of 5 to 7 days, fever, mucopurulent nasal discharge, and unilateral face or dental pain.

It is estimated that approximately 1% to 2% of patients with acute rhinosinusitis will have accompanying bacterial infection. However, the percentage of patients seeking medical care may lend a bias toward those with more prolonged and/or severe symptoms. If this is the case, the percentage of patients presenting for medical treatment may represent an increased prevalence of bacterial infections allowing for estimates of as many as 10% to 15% of patients as being appropriate for antibiotic therapy.

Two meta-analyses of the effects of antibiotics on the course and cure of suspected acute bacterial rhinosinusitis patients have demonstrated a small benefit to those patients prescribed antibiotics. However, no investigation has demonstrated a benefit derived from the routine use of broad-spectrum antibiotics in preference to less costly narrow-spectrum agents. Therefore, the prescribing physician should emphasize cost, convenience and a narrow spectrum agent in the selection of a first-line antibiotic (**Table 51.6**).

The primary, first-line antibiotic for suspected acute bacterial rhinosinusitis should be amoxicillin, with doxycycline, trimethoprim-sulfamethoxazole, and macrolides (specifically, azithromycin and clarithromycin) alternate choices and/or considerations in the penicillin-allergic patient. Antibiotic resistance patterns within one's community may affect antibiotic selection. High dose amoxicillin (80 mg/kg per day divided bid) has been suggested in many communities due to increasing *Streptococcus pneumonia* resistance. Additionally, trimethoprim-sulfamethoxazole has demonstrated high *Streptococcus pneumonia* resistance thereby affecting its utility as a first-line agent. In those patients with a more complicated history, suspected high prevalence of drug-resistant *Streptococcus pneumonia* or failure of initial therapy, amoxicillin-clavulanate is often recommended as a primary agent with second generation cephalosporins, azithromycin, clarithromycin, telithromycin, and fluoroquinolones representing alternatives.

The treatment duration of systemic antibiotics should include approximately ten days of therapy and antibiotic

Table 51.6

Indicated Antibiotics for Suspected Acute Bacterial Rhinosinusitis

FIRST-LINE AGENT(S)
Amoxicillin: 250 mg tid or 500 mg bid (40 mg/kg/day)
Doxycycline: 100 mg bid
Trimethoprim/Sulfa: 1 double-strength tablet bid
Azithromycin: 500 mg q day × 3 days

ALTERNATIVE AGENT(S)
Amoxicillin: 500 mg tid or 875 mg bid (80 mg/kg/day)
Amoxicillin/Clavulanate: 250–500 mg tid or 500–875 mg bid
2nd Generation cephalosporins (e.g., cefuroxime axetil 250–500 mg bid)
Fluoroquinolones* (e.g., moxifloxacin 400 mg q day)
Clarithromycin: 250–500 mg bid
Telithromycin: 800 mg qd

* Avoid with patients younger than 18 years of age.

tissue penetration to be effective. Longer courses may be necessary in refractory cases. Selected antibiotics, specifically azithromycin, may offer the benefit of 3- or 5-day dosing for 10 days of sustained antibiotic tissue levels.

Chronic Rhinosinusitis

Rhinosinusitis symptoms that have been present for greater than three months are considered chronic rhinosinusitis. The two major classifications of chronic rhinosinusitis: allergic and nonallergic, have vastly different pathophysiologic causes involved.

Allergic rhinitis is an immunologic-mediated entity that is prompted by repetitive exposure to allergens. After initial sensitization to the allergen, the patient produces IgE antibodies specific against the allergen. These antibodies attach to the mast cells and basophils in the nasal mucosa. When the patient is presented with the allergen again, the allergen attaches to the IgE antibody on the mast cell and causes the cell to "degranulate," releasing histamines, leukotrienes, and other allergic inflammatory chemicals. These substances cause rhinitis, ocular itching, congestion of the nasal passages, and sneezing.

Often chronic sinusitis develops in patients with recurrent allergic rhinitis or in people who, earlier in life, had recurrent episodes of acute rhinosinusitis. These patients appear to be at higher risk of chronic disease due to irreversible damage to the paranasal mucociliary clearance mechanism. In these patients, the ostia of the sinuses are often nonfunctional due to similar damage at their mucosal boundaries. This recurrent cycle of bacterial inflammation, followed by ciliary dysfunction, creates an environment for development of chronic infection.

Patients with chronic rhinosinusitis most often present with symptoms similar to those of patients with acute rhinosinusitis: facial pain, purulent postnasal or anterior rhinorrhea, headache, malaise, and facial fullness. Physical examination findings are also similar to those found in acute rhinosinusitis.

The most common bacterial organisms in chronic rhinosinusitis include anaerobic bacteria such as *Corynebacterium, Bacteroides,* and *Veillonella* species. Aerobic bacteria, including *S. pyogenes, S. aureus,* and *M. catarrhalis,* have also been isolated in chronic sinusitis. In immunocompromised patients, fungal infection and other chronic granulomatous disorders should be included as possible etiologies of chronic or recurrent rhinosinusitis.

Relevant history to the diagnosis of chronic sinusitis is aided by a history of recurrent sinus infections or recurrent allergies. The findings on examination of the patient should be noted as described for acute rhinosinusitis. If clinical symptomatology is vague and the patient has recurrent or chronic sinus infections, sinus imaging via radiographs or CT should be strongly considered. High-resolution CT scan technology has enabled imaging of the anterior ethmoid region and the ostio-meatal complex. Likewise, coronal CT scan provides excellent imaging of the soft tissues of the region and adequately illustrates anatomic abnormalities. Radiographic imaging of the chronic rhinosinusitis patient should prompt consideration of consultation and/or referral for acute and follow-up management.

Chronic rhinosinusitis presents difficult treatment options. Chronic rhinosinusitis in an otherwise healthy patient will usually be managed on an outpatient basis. As with acute sinusitis, therapeutic efforts should be directed to relief of sinus obstruction and promotion of sinus drainage. Systemic antibiotic therapy is often prescribed in chronic sinusitis, requiring as much as four weeks of therapy to be effective (Table 51.6).

Selected Readings

Anonymous. Antimicrobial treatment guidelines for acute bacterial rhinosinusitis. Sinus and Allergy Health Partnership. *Otolaryngol Head Neck Surg* 2000; 123:5–31.

Campbell RJ, Okazaki H. Painful ophthalmoplegia (Tolosa-Hunt variant): autopsy findings in a patient with necrotizing intracavernous carotid vasculitis and inflammatory disease of the orbit. *Mayo Clin Proc* 1987;62:520–526.

de Bock GH, Dekker FW, Stolk J, et al. Antimicrobial treatment in acute maxillary sinusitis: a meta-analysis. *J Clin Epidem* 1997;50:881–890.

Dinubile MJ. Septic thrombosis of the cavernous sinuses. *Arch Neurol* 1988; 45:567–572.

Ellie E, Houang B, Louail C, et al. CT and high field MRI in septic thrombosis of the cavernous sinuses. *Neuroradiology* 1992;34:22–24.

Goodwin WJ. Orbital complications of ethmoiditis. *Otolaryngol Clin North Am* 1985;18:139–147.

Heckmann JG, Tomandl B. Cavernous sinus thrombosis. *Lancet* 2003;362: 1958.

Henry DC, Riffer E, Sokol WN, et al. Randomized double-blind study comparing 3- and 6-day regimens of azithromycin with a 10-day amoxicillin-clavulanate regimen for treatment of acute bacterial sinusitis. *Antimicrob Agents Chemother* 2003; 47:2770–2774.

Hickner JM, Bartlett JG, Besser RE, et al. Centers for Disease Control and Prevention. Principles of appropriate antibiotic use for acute rhinosinusitis in adults: background. *Ann Emerg Med* 2001;37:703–710.

Horowitz M, Purdy P, Unwin H, et al. Treatment of dural sinus thrombosis using selective catheterization and urokinase. *Ann Neurol* 1995;38:58–67.

Kalan A, Tariq M. Foreign bodies in the nasal cavities: a comprehensive review of the aetiology, diagnostic pointers and therapeutic measures. *Postgrad Med* 2000;76:484–487.

Karlin RJ, Robinson WA. Septic cavernous sinus thrombosis. *Ann Emerg Med* 1984;13:449–455.

Lessner A, Stern GA. Preseptal and orbital cellulites. *Infect Dis Clin North Am* 1992;6:933–952.

Mahmood S, Lowe T. Management of epistaxis in the oral and maxillofacial surgery setting: an update on current practice. *Oral Surg Oral Med Oral Pathol Oral Radiol Endod* 2003;95:23–29.

Manthey DE, Harrison BP. Otolaryngologic procedures. In: Roberts JR, Hedges JR, eds. *Clinical Procedures in Emergency Medicine,* 3d ed. St. Louis, MO: Mosby 1998:1120–1149.

Piccirillo JF, Mager DE, Frisse ME, et al. A. Impact of first-line vs second-line antibiotics for the treatment of acute uncomplicated sinusitis. *JAMA* 2001;286: 1849–1856.

Poole MD. A focus on acute sinusitis in adults: changes in disease management. *Amer J Med* 1999;106:38S–47S.

Saah D, Schwartz AJ. Diagnosis of cavernous sinus thrombosis by magnetic resonance imaging using flow parameters. *Ann Otol Rhino Laryngol* 1994;103: 487–489.

Sparacino LL. Epistaxis management: what's new and what's noteworthy. *Lippincott's Primary Care Practice* 2000;4:498–507.

Stam J, de Brujin SFTM, DeVeber G. Anticoagulation for cerebral sinus thrombosis. *Cochrane Rev* 2003;4.

Tan L, Calhoun KH. Epistaxis. *Medical Clinics of North America.* 1999;83:43–56.

Williams JW Jr, Aguilar C, Makela M, et al. Antibiotic therapy for acute sinusitis: a systematic literature review (Cochrane Review). In: The Cochrane Library. Oxford, UK: Update Software 2002.

Williams JW, Simel DL. Does this patient have sinusitis? Diagnosing acute sinusitis by history and physical examination. *JAMA* 1993;270:1242–1246.

Yanofsky NN. The acute painful eye. *Emerg Med Clin North Am* 1988;6:21–42.

Throat and Oropharynx

Christopher J. DeFlitch

The third most common reason patients present for medical care are related to complaints of the throat and oropharynx. These disorders can be as innocuous as the common cold or as life threatening as epiglottitis. The expert emergency physician must have knowledge of anatomy, physiology, microbiology, and pathophysiology in the fields of otorhinolaryngology, dental medicine, and gastroenterology to diagnose and treat this common complaint. This chapter reviews the diagnosis, evaluation, and treatment of many of these disorders.

Foreign Body

Airway foreign bodies (FBs) are a major source of morbidity and mortality in the pediatric population, especially in children under age 4, accounting for nearly 2,000 deaths per year in the United States. Critical occlusive foreign bodies in adults are frequently seen with food boluses, often described as the "café coronary." Other patients can present with a foreign body sensation, but have the ability to talk. These non-obstructed foreign body presentations are still marked with significant morbidity, especially in the setting of perforation, and must be managed aggressively.

The location in which a FB lodges is age- and foreign body-type specific. Sharper objects, such as fish bones, are frequently lodged in the oropharynx. With the anatomical changes of age, the pediatric population will more commonly have upper esophagus obstructions, whereas the adults more commonly present with distal esophageal obstructions. By far, the most common location to identify a foreign body is just below the cricopharyngeus.

The evaluation of patients with a potential foreign body always begins with the ABCs (airway, breathing, circulation). It is critical for the emergency physician to determine if a life-threatening or potentially life-threatening obstruction exists. If there are no immediate risks to airway occlusion, a clear and complete history is essential, as this may be the only suggestion of a possible foreign body. It is important to determine patient information, including history of difficulty with obstruction or foreign bodies, persistent cough, sore throat, stridor, or drooling. Adults may complain of a foreign body sensation, where children

may not admit to any complaints. If the FB is above the cricopharyngeal muscle, dysphagia with odynophagia radiating to the suprasternal notch may be the presenting symptoms. The patient's ability to tolerate liquids, including saliva, and/or solids is important, but does not eliminate the diagnosis of a foreign body. Patients with esophageal abrasions present with foreign body sensations, however, most have symptom resolution within 24 hours. Persistent foreign body sensation and/or recurrent foreign bodies should raise the suspicion of underlying pathology or anatomic abnormalities. Physical exam should include inspection of the patient's general appearance (respiratory distress, handling secretions, etc.) as initial presentation can be varied. Specific attention should be paid to visual inspection to the hypopharynx, determining if the foreign body can be visualized directly, or other signs such as erythema, edema, or abrasion. A complete neck and chest exam are necessary to identify subcutaneous air if perforation is present or external compression from a mass (adenopathy, goiters, etc.).

The diagnosis of foreign body is definitively made with direct visualization. Soft tissue radiography is occasionally helpful and may identify subcutaneous air but is limited to foreign bodies that are radio-opaque. Fiberoptic nasopharyngoscopy or traditional direct or indirect laryngoscopy is needed to completely evaluate the hypopharynx. Once identified, occasionally the foreign body can be manually removed by the emergency physician using McGill or foreign body forceps. This should not be attempted by individuals who lack sufficient experience in performing this procedure or by those who are not skilled in advanced airway management. These procedures are frequently referred to an otolaryngologist.

Esophageal foreign body is best identified by esophagoscopy. This procedure is frequently therapeutic as well and requires consultation with an experienced endoscopist. Gastrographin swallow study may be helpful in diagnosing non-obstructive foreign bodies. Occasionally, these cases may require referral to another facility, especially in the case of pediatric patients. A patient unable to tolerate secretions requires immediate referral and esophagoscopy. Stable patients able to tolerate secretions or if the clinician has a low index of suspicion for a foreign body, may be referred on an urgent basis (within 24 hours). Patients with a "button battery" lodged in the esophagus must be referred for immediate FB removal, due to the corrosive nature of the battery.

There are a number of non-invasive treatments for esophageal foreign body available, with variable results. Glucagon, a smooth muscle relaxant, may dislodge the foreign body. In addition, the side effect of vomiting induction frequently caused by this agent may also relieve the foreign body. Glucagon is given 1 mg IV slow push, and may be repeated at 2 mg IV after allowing 20 minutes to determine results. Many emergency physicians attempt this maneuver prior to emergently involving the endoscopist. Calcium channels blocker, such as nifedipine, and sublingual nitroglycerin, are alternatives with variable results. In the distant past, proteolytic enzymes, such as meat tenderizer, had been used. These agents are contraindicated, as there is an increased risk of esophageal perforation. With any removal of an FB, caution must be used to prevent compromise of the airway or aspiration of the foreign body. Independent of the mechanism of resolution, all patients with esophageal foreign bodies should be referred for definitive diagnosis of possible underlying esophageal pathology.

Gingivitis

Gingivitis, in general, is an inflammatory response to an irritant, frequently bacterial plaque that may present with foul-smelling breath and does not involve bacterial invasion of the oral mucosa. Acute necrotizing ulcerative gingivitis (ANUG) or trench mouth is distinguished by bacterial invasion of the soft tissue and is frequently accompanied by periodontal infection and/or disease. Unlike gingivitis, ANUG is associated with painful, bleeding gingiva, a metallic taste, and systemic symptoms, such as fever, malaise, and lymphadenopathy. Caused by invasive fusiform bacillus and spirochetes, ANUG can extend to the tonsils, producing sore throat, as well. ANUG involving the tonsils and fauces is termed Vincent's angina. Risk factors for this disease include immunocompromised state, poor oral hygiene, smoking, local trauma, and emotional stress.

Patients with ANUG have edematous, bright red gingiva covered in a gray pseudomembrane. This tissue is very friable and is frequently bleeding. The diagnosis is made on visual inspection and history. No cultures or invasive tests are needed unless the patient is toxic appearing. Treatment of this disease consists of warm saline rinses and systemic analgesics for pain. Antibiotics are indicated (penicillin, 250 mg PO every 6 hours, or, for patients over age 8, tetracycline, 250 mg PO every 6 hours for 10 days). Patients can be discharged with follow-up to a dentist or oral surgeon for continued care and dental hygiene education.

Periodontal Abscess

Periodontal disease represents a spectrum of disease: from gingivitis progressing to periodontitis that forms a pocket, which can then develop periodontal abscess. A true periodontal abscess frequently is caused by food being caught in these periodontal pockets. This should not to be confused with a periapical abscess, which is generally caused by dental caries, eventually invading and infecting the dental pulp and/or root, and which is entirely surrounded by alveolar bone. Both periapical and periodontal abscesses can present similarly with dental pain, swelling, tooth sensitivity, and fever. If the abscess has previously spontaneously drained, the patient may complain of a foul taste. There is rarely associated systemic symptomatology, but depending on the tooth location, regional pain such as dental, jaw, ear or sinus pain may be an accompanying complaint. Both periodontal and periapical abscesses may appear similar, especially if the alveolar bone surrounding the periapical abscess has been eroded. The surrounding tooth is tender, and sensitive to hot or cold. A discrete area of fluctuance and pus is frequently identified.

Treatment includes local and/or regional dental block with a long acting local anesthetic, such as bupivicaine. After adequate anesthesia, the abscess is incised and drained with a puncture incision using an 11 blade and irrigated with normal saline. Antibiotics such as penicillin, or tetracycline (for patients over age 8) and systemic analgesics should be prescribed. Follow-up with a dentist and/or oral surgeon is needed.

Epiglottitis

Epiglottitis is a critical, life-threatening diagnosis that is caused by bacterial infection of the epiglottis and surrounding tissue and traditionally described as having a bimodal distribution of age range of infection in children (ages 1 to 4) and in adults (ages 20 to 40 years). Immunizations are changing the distribution this disease to adults and the unimmunized. *Haemophilus influenzae* type B (HIB) is the etiology in more than 90% of the epiglottitis cases, while the HIB vaccine has significantly decreased the presentation of this disease in the pediatric population in recent years. The presentation of epiglottitis is sporadic and can occur throughout the year.

The clinical presentation can be as a benign as an upper respiratory tract infection, with fever and adenopathy, especially in adults. However, it can rapidly progress within 6 to 24 hours to airway obstruction. The common sign of fever may be absent in 30% to 50% of the cases. Sore throat, tachycardia, dysphasia, dysphagia, muffled "hot potato" voice, and drooling may occur. Stridor is frequent. Patient often assumes a "sniffing" position with the jaw jutted forward in an attempt to protect and to keep an open airway. If the patient has stridor or is drooling, it is essential that there is minimal manipulation of the oropharynx. Maintenance of the patient's airway is first and foremost. Soft-tissue radiographs are 79% to 90% sensitive in diagnosing epiglottitis, but the absence on plain x-rays does not exclude the diagnosis. The films should be completed in an area where the patient's airway can be effectively managed in an emergency. This frequently means portable radiographs. The classic finding on plain radiographs is the "thumb" sign and thickened aryepiglottic folds. If the diagnosis is remotely entertained and there is no respiratory distress or concern with airway compromise, direct fiberoptic pharyngoscopy or indirect pharyngoscopy are diagnostic options. At all times in the diagnostic work-up, consideration for the ability of obtaining a definitive airway should be maintained.

Patients with dramatic presentations should have immediate airway stabilization including endotracheal intubation and, if unsuccessful, tracheostomy. Less dramatic presentations should have the diagnostic work-up in a rapid fashion. Once the diagnosis is made, airway management maneuvers in a controlled setting should be considered, frequently in consultation with ENT and anesthesiology specialists. All patients should be admitted to the intensive care unit and receive broad-spectrum IV antibiotics, such as ceftriaxone 100 to 200 mg per kg per day divided every 6 hours or cefuroxime 100 to 150 mg per kg per day every 8 hours. Some consider adjuvant IV steroid therapy, but there is no documented prospective benefit.

Laryngitis

Common in the winter months, this viral upper respiratory infection (URI) typically presents with hoarseness and dysphonia secondary to swelling of the larynx and vocal cords. Bacteria such as diphtheria and streptococci are found to be the etiology in fewer than 10% of cases. Typical physical findings include low-grade temperature elevation, with a mildly edematous and erythematous pharynx. If the larynx and vocal cords are visualized, they are also edematous. With these constellations of physical finding, the diagnosis is made and no further invasive tests are required. Treatment includes antipyretics, fluids, rest, and limited phonation. Some suggest humidified air or steroids. Antibiotics are not indicated.

Ludwig's Angina

A potentially lethal disease first described in 1836, Ludwig's angina is an infection of the sublingual and submandibular space that frequently extends from an existing dental infection and is caused by oral flora, including anaerobes. The edema from the infection, though not frequently abscessed, causes such significant soft tissue swelling so that the tongue is pushed upward and forward, causing concern for airway occlusion. Young adult males with peridontal disease are most frequently affected. Polymicrobial infection has been reported in diabetics and other immunodeficiency syndromes.

Clinical symptoms usually present as dental pain and infection, then progress to neck pain, swelling and fever. Dysphagia, odynophagia, and trismus may also be present. On examination, these patients appear ill with fever and tachycardia. Palpation of the sublingual space with the thumb and the submandibular space with the index finger, externally, reveals a tender, tense mass with a wood-like consistency. In addition to these distinct clinical findings, the leukocyte count may be elevated and air may be detected in the sublingual or submandibular space.

Airway management is of immediate concern. The presence of stridor is significant for impending airway obstruction. Options include awake oral or nasotracheal intubation or assistance with fiberoptic laryngoscopy. One should always be prepared for emergent cricothyroidotomy or tracheostomy. Broad-spectrum antibiotics, such as high-dose penicillin or clindamycin, are suggested. Admission to the ICU with ENT consultation is indicated, with tracheostomy kit at the bedside.

Oral Candidiasis

Oral candidiasis is an opportunistic infection that consists of overgrowth of the normal flora, *Candida albicans*. Immunocompromised states such as diabetes, hypopituitarism, steroid therapy, leukemia, lymphoma, and advanced HIV disease facilitate candidiasis. In addition, pregnancy, some antibiotic therapy, radiation therapy, and wearing of dentures may also precipitate oral candidal infection. Patients may present with oropharygneal pain and bleeding. Infection extending into the esophagus may cause significant odynophagia.

The diagnosis is frequently made by history and the identification of the easily removed white plaques in the oropharynx. When removed, the uncovered areas may bleed. For laboratory confirmation, the emergency physician can observe hyphae on a slide prepared with a smear of the plaque and 20% KOH.

Treatment consists of antifungal mouthwash, oral nystatin solution or anti-fungal lozenges. Non-AIDS patients may be treated with fluconazole (200 mg orally as a single dose). Additional work-up or referral may be indicated if the reason for the flora overgrowth is not obvious.

Pharyngitis

Sore throat is one of the most common complaints of any emergency department or outpatient clinic. Pharyngitis, a common component of an URI, can be caused by bacteria, virus, or fungi, all of which can be spread by direct and respiratory contact. Most common in young adults, teenagers, and children, β-hemolytic streptococcus receives the most attention, due to its association with rheumatic fever. In addition, *H. influenzae*, *Corynebacterium diphtheriae*, *Staphylococcus aureus* and other strep groups have been shown to also cause pharyngitis. The overwhelming cause of pharyngitis, however, is viral. Adenovirus, enterovirus, influenza, parainfluenza viruses are among the most common.

Patients are febrile with varying degrees of toxicity, headache, dehydration, and difficulty swallowing. Tonsils may be involved with the pharynx or alone and could be associated with trismus. It is very difficult to distinguish between bacterial and non-bacterial pharyngitis based on clinical exam alone. Frequently, the first step in physical exam is to determine the presence of exudates. Whitish exudates on the tonsils or grayish membranes are somewhat more likely to be bacterial (*Streptococcus*). Non-exudative pharyngitis or the presence of tonsil ulcerations is more consistent with viral etiology.

The common distinction between pharyngitis and tonsillitis is arbitrary with tonsillar enlargement as the distinguishing difference, though etiology is similar. Complications, however, can be more pronounced with tonsillitis. Both are complicated by persistent fever, dehydration, and poor feeding.

Evaluation to determine etiology frequently consists of a rapid strep screen, a test that is very specific but less sensitive. All negative strep screens should be routinely confirmed with a formal culture. Monospot and a CBC differential with lymphocyte or monocyte predominance may be helpful in viral diagnoses. Simple pharyngitis or tonsillitis does not require imaging, unless deeper space infection or abscess is suspected.

Treatment of most patients is supportive with antipyretics, fluids, and rest. Confirmation of bacterial pharyngitis warrants treatment with penicillin or erythromycin for 10 days. High dose IM benzathine penicillin G (1.2 million units) is a viable option for patients in whom compliance is questionable.

Peritonsillar Abscess

Peritonsillar abscess is a complication of suppurative bacterial tonsillitis. Pus collects between the tonsillar capsule and the superior constrictor muscles. Similar to pharyngitis, this disease frequently affects teenagers and young adults, but can occur at any age. Immunocompromised states and previous mononucleosis may be a predisposing factor. Patients frequently present with a few days of fever and sore throat, progressing to unilateral throat pain and dysphagia. As the abscess grows, the voice may be muffled, with difficulty swallowing and trismus. As suggested, this disease is the end of a spectrum that progresses from simple tonsillitis to peritonsillar cellulitis to a phlegmon to a frank abscess cavity. Complications may extend beyond the local area resulting in deeper space infection, erosion of the neck vessels, mediastinitis, and sepsis. The physical finding of uvular deviation away from the mass and unilateral tonsillar enlargement is very concerning for this diagnosis.

Definitive management as with any abscess is incision and drainage. The emergency physician should insure adequacy of the airway, obtain IV access, and frequently fluid resuscitation is required. High-dose penicillin or clindamycin 600 mg IV every 8 hours should be started. When abscess drainage is attempted, caution should be used to avoid injury to the underlying vasculature. After use of an initial local anesthetic, such as Cetacaine, it is recommended that an initial aspiration be performed. The needle should be directed toward the midline as much as possible, to identify the cavity. Then an incision using an 11 blade can be made, usually superior and lateral to the tonsil, but at the area identified by the aspirate. ENT consultation should be obtained for assistance with the aspiration or follow-up. Patients who are toxic appearing, have evidence of infection beyond the local area, or in whom there is concern for airway compromise should be admitted to the ENT service.

Retropharyngeal Abscess

Suppurative bacterial infection in the retropharyngeal space is most common in children under age 3, but is also frequently caused by local trauma from foreign body, intubation, endoscopic procedures, or cervical injury. This potential space between the posterior pharyngeal mucosa and the fascia overlying the paraspinal cervical muscles is connected directly to the mediastinum, hence these infections may be potentially life-threatening. Presentation is similar in course and symptoms to the peritonsillar abscess, with fever progressing to difficulty swallowing and potential airway compromise. These patients are frequently toxic appearing. The presence of chest pain strongly suggests the feared complication of mediastinitis. Evaluation should include a lateral soft tissue radiograph of the neck. Typical soft tissue measurements should be <7 mm at C2. At C6, in children, the soft tissue should be <14 mm, where adults should remain <22 mm. CT can be helpful in distinguishing cellulitis from abscess. CXR is indicated for any patient with associated chest complaints.

Because of concerns with airway compromise, it is not recommended that the emergency physician attempt surgical drainage. Initial management includes obtaining IV access, fluid resuscitation as indicated, obtaining diagnostic studies to confirm the diagnosis and referral of all patients to an ENT specialist for admission and consideration of abscess drainage in the OR. IV antibiotics, with similar spectrum as the treatment of peritonsillar abscess, should be started. Most patients will require admission to the acute care hospital.

Sialadenitis

Acute suppurative sialadenitis is an infection of the parotid or submandibular glands. With predisposing factors such as salivary stones, dehydration, and poor oral hygiene, these infections are more common in post-operative patients and in patients ages 60 to 70. Both aerobic and anaerobic bacteria are causative. Patients present with fever, pain, and unilateral glandular/face swelling. On physical exam, pus may be expressed from Stenson's or Warton's duct.

These patients can frequently be managed as an outpatient with antibiotics, such as amoxicillin-clavulanate and analgesia. Patients should be encouraged to massage the gland externally and to use tart candy to induce salivation. Follow-up with ENT specialists is indicated to monitor progress and, if complications arise, to surgically intervene.

Sialolithiasis

As with sialadenitis, the patient with sialolithiasis will present with a tender, swollen face/gland, but fever may not be present. Patient may describe increasing pain with eating (salivation). On exam, the gland is tender and there may be no flow of saliva from the ducts. Stones occur most frequently in the salivary duct, where they can cause intermittent or continuous occlusion, and stones can be painful, indicating a predisposing factor to sialadenitis. The majority of these stones are calcium-based. The stones can be identified by plain film or ultrasonography, but is frequently missed. Sialography, reportedly 100% effective in determining diagnosis, is rarely available to the emergency physician; therefore diagnosis of sialolithiasis is typically clinical.

Treatment is similar to sialadenitis (analgesia, tart candy, and massage of the gland and ducts). In patients with persistent symptoms, surgical removal of the stone is recommended. Antibiotics are indicated when sialadentis is present.

Selected Readings

Fleisher GR, Ludwig S. *Textbook of Pediatric Emergency Medicine.* 3rd ed. Baltimore: Williams & Williams 1993.

Rice BR, Spiegel PK, Dombrowski PJ. Acute esophageal food impaction treated by gas-forming agents. *Radiology* 1983;146:299–301.

Roberts JR, Hedges JR. *Clinical procedures in Emergency Medicine.* 2nd ed. Philadelphia: WB Saunders 1991.

Rosen P, Barkin R. *Emergency Medicine Concepts and Clinical Practice.* 4th ed. St. Louis, MO: Mosby 1998.

Spires J, Owens JJ, Woodson GE, Miller RH. Treatment of peritonsillar abscess. *Arch Otolaryngol Head Neck Surg* 1987;113:984–986.

Wurtule P. Acute epiglottitis in children and adults: a large scale incidence study. *Otolaryngol Head Neck Surg* 1990;103:902–908.

CHAPTER

53 External Eye

James M. Leaming

The structures of the external eye include the eyelid, lacrimal ducts and glands, and conjunctiva ending at the cornea. These structures have in common the function of protection of the eye from dehydration and mechanical injury. Patients with disorders involving these structures often have complaints that include swelling, redness, and often, dull pain of the eye.

Blepharitis

Blepharitis is irritation and inflammation of the lid margins. This disorder occurs due to bacterial infection. Blepharitis caused by bacterial etiologies results in an ulcerative appearance to the lids and most commonly results from staphylococcal infection. Nonulcerative blepharitis (seborrheic blepharitis) is associated with the presence of *Pityrosporum ovale*; however, often a mixed picture of ulcerative and non-ulcerative blepharitis is present.

Blepharitis is commonly a chronic infection, often affecting the lids bilaterally for a period of months to years. The patient often presents with irritation, burning, and itching of the lid margins. The eyes appear "red-rimmed" and obviously inflamed. Poor hygiene and the use of eyeliner cosmetics have been shown to be possible etiologies for initiation of the staphylococcal infection. In staphylococcal blepharitis, scaling appears as dry, small ulcerations that can be seen along the lid margins, and the eyelashes tend to easily fall out of the eyelids. Poor hygiene causes seborrheic blepharitis, with scaling and build-up of sebaceous secretions leading to inflammation.

Examination of the patient with blepharitis should begin with visual acuity testing of the affected and the unaffected eye. Next, the lid margins should be examined for erythema, scaling, crusting, ulceration, lash loss, and irregularity. The upper eyelid should be everted to examine the eye for evidence of retained foreign material as a source of irritation. The external aspect of the face should also be examined for evidence of scaling, inflammation, or trauma. Conjunctival inflammation or ulceration should be noted, and any purulent discharge should be examined as to the source. In the absence of other findings, blepharitis can be diagnosed and treated by the emergency department (ED) physician without the need for further ancillary studies.

As a result of chronic staphylococcal blepharitis, many patients will develop conjunctivitis or keratitis of the lower third of the cornea. If ulcerative blepharitis is present, appropriate antimicrobial therapy should be started to cover staphylococcal organisms. Sulfonamide eye ointment or other antistaphylococcal ointment should be applied to the lid margins twice daily. Seborrheic blepharitis does not require antibiotic treatment if isolated and if it responds well to improved hygiene. The scalp, eyebrows, and lid margins should be kept clean by means of soap and water. Scaling should be removed from the lid margins daily with a damp cotton applicator. Contact lens wearers should avoid use of the contact lens until therapy is completed. Patients should receive outpatient follow-up with their primary physician in 3 to 5 days to insure improvement while on antibiotic therapy.

Chalazion/Hordeolum

Another common ocular complaint is related to the development of swelling and pain secondary to a chalazion or hordeolum. A chalazion is a sterile granulomatous inflammation of a meibomian gland. The chalazion is often seen in patients with chronic eye inflammation; however, no specific etiology has been determined. The chalazion most often affects the tarsal aspect of the lid, but can be seen on the lower lid as well. The hordeolum is an infection of the follicle or sweat gland (Zeis' gland) along the lid margin. When it involves the meibomian gland, it is referred to as an internal hordeolum and may "point" or drain to the conjunctival side of the lid or to the skin side. The smaller more superficial lid margin infection is known as the external hordeolum (sty) and will "point" or drain to the skin side of the lid margin. The hordeolum is most commonly caused by staphylococcal infection of the lid glands, and may result from poor hygiene and use of eye cosmetics.

Patients with a chalazion present with localized swelling in the upper or lower eyelid that may be in multiple locations and recurrent. The swelling may begin with inflammation and tenderness that develops over a period of weeks; commonly, however, the eye reveals no acute inflammatory signs. The hordeolum differs from the chalazion in presentation in that pain is the primary symptom. The affected lid margin is erythematous, with swelling and localized tenderness and inflammation of the eyelid margin. The patient may describe spontaneous drainage from the lid.

The duration of swelling, age of the patient, visual deficit, fever, and purulent discharge from the affected eye are significant historical elements. Also important is assessment for systemic illnesses, trauma, occupational exposures, uses of contact lenses or corrective lenses, prior ocular surgery, and similar presentations. Examination of the patient with complaints of eye swelling should begin with visual acuity testing. The lid margins should be examined for erythema, pustular eruptions, discharge, and localized swelling or irregularity. The upper eyelid should be everted to examine the eye for evidence of retained foreign material as a source of irritation. The external aspect of the face should also be examined for evidence of inflammation and trauma. The diagnosis of the chalazion or hordeolum should be able to be made on physical examination, without the need for any further testing by the ED physician.

The treatment of the patient with localized swelling due to a chalazion or hordeolum depends greatly on the severity of the lesion. In the chalazion, if the swelling is minimal, the patient should be instructed to apply warm compresses to the eye and, optionally, the patient can be treated with topical erythromycin to prevent infection of the meibomian gland. Often the small, uncomplicated chalazion will spontaneously resolve. However, if the chalazion is large, vision can be distorted due to compression of the globe, detracting from cosmesis, or is refractory to treatment by the patient, where incision and curettage of the gland may be required. The hordeolum often will respond well to conservative treatment with warm compresses, topical erythromycin ointment, and consistent hygiene with avoidance of cosmetics around the eyes. Surgical intervention is rarely required since most hordeolum spontaneously drain; however, a very painful or enlarging abscess may require drainage. Most patients with uncomplicated chalazions or hordeola respond well to conservative therapy and require no further consultation or referral.

Conjunctivitis

Inflammation of the conjunctiva (conjunctivitis) is the most common eye disease in the Western hemisphere, varying from mild hyperemia with tearing to a severe necrotic process. The etiology of conjunctivitis can be exogenous or endogenous, and many of the most common causes of conjunctivitis are listed in **Table 53.1**. In the otherwise healthy patient, bacterial and viral conjunctivitis are by far the most common causes of "red eye"; other etiologies, however, cannot be discounted. Conjunctivitis is considered common in the United States, representing nearly 30% of all eye complaints in the ED.

Bacterial conjunctivitis often results from inoculation of the eye with skin pathogens and generally affects all ages. Three categories of bacterial conjunctivitis include suppurative, acute, and chronic bacterial infection. Suppurative bacterial conjunctivitis is most often caused by infection with *Neisseria gonorrhoeae* and has predominance in the neonate, the sexually active adult, and in health-care workers. The patient often presents with complaints of diffuse erythema of the eye, chemosis (edema of the conjunctiva), itching foreign body sensation, purulent discharge from the affected eye, and crusting of the eyelids with the lids which are stuck together upon awakening. Typically, the symptoms have begun less than 5 days after inoculation with *N. gonorrhoeae*, with worsening redness and chemosis, increasing purulence, and probable spread to both eyes. Care should be taken in triage and in the ED to use universal precautions with these patients to avoid further spread of the infection. The history of the patient may reveal the source of the infection based on sexual contacts, occupational exposure, or self-inoculation due to gonococcal urethritis. Pain should not be prominent, but the eye involved is severely irritated and inflamed. Examination of the eye may show diffuse conjunctival injection, profuse tearing, exudate, chemosis, and swelling of the eyelids. The pupil is symmetrical and reactive; visual acuity may be diminished due to tearing and purulence, but it improves after repeated testing and clearing of the visual fields. In the patient with suspected *N. gonorrhoeae* conjunctivitis, Gram's stain of the exudate should be obtained and culture obtained to confirm the diagnosis. Since this infection can rapidly penetrate the intact cornea and cause severe visual complications, these patients should receive rapid ophthalmologic consultation and intravenous antibiotic therapy, frequent irrigation of the eye, and topical erythromycin or tetracycline. Trials of single-dose intramuscular ceftriaxone have made possible outpatient treatment in certain groups of patients. All patients with *N. gonorrhoeae* conjunctivitis should advise their sexual partners to seek treatment to prevent public health outbreaks of the disease.

Acute bacterial conjunctivitis is most commonly a result of infection due to *Staphylococcus aureus* and *pneumococcus,* the latter occurring in epidemics in cooler climates. Another common cause of acute bacterial conjunctivitis is *Haemophilus influenzae*, occurring in up to 25% of cases and also causes epidemics of conjunctivitis. Symptoms include generalized conjunctival injection, chemosis, itching, crusting of the eyelids, and profuse tearing. *H influenzae* infection usually begins unilaterally, then spreads to both eyes. Care should again be taken to use universal precautions to avoid direct contact with the patient's mucous membranes. Examination shows conjunctival erythema, profuse tearing, and little to no purulent discharge. The pupil is symmetrical and reactive; visual acuity may be diminished due to tearing, but it improves after repeated testing and clearing of the visual fields. All age groups are equally affected, and response to antimicrobial therapy is usually excellent. No culture or other testing needs to be done, with diagnosis by the ED physician being accomplished based on history and physical examination. Treatment with sulfacetamide, erythromycin, or gentamicin ophthalmic preparations (aminoglycosides have some epithelial toxicity and may slow healing) for 7 days is the

Table 53.1

Types of Conjunctivitis and Common Causes

Viral
  Acute follicular
  Adenovirus
    Herpes simplex
    Enterovirus
    Coxsackie virus
    Newcastle disease

  Chronic follicular
    Molluscum contagiosum
  Others
    Vaccinia
    Varicella zoster
    Measles
Bacterial
  Acute catarrhal
    Pneumococcus
  Subacute catarrhal
    Haemophilus influenzae
  Chronic
    Staphylococcus aureus
  Suppurative
    Neisseria gonorrhoeae
    Pseudomonas
    Proteus
  Rare types
    Catscratch fever
    Tuberculosis

Rickettsial
  Typhus
  Murine typhus
  Rocky Mountain spotted fever
  Q fever

Systemic disease-related
  Thyroid disease
  Gouty conjunctivitis
  Carcinoid conjunctivitis
  Erythema multiforme (Stevens-Johnson Syndrome)

Chlamydial
  Chlamydia trachomatis
  Chlamydia oculgenitalia
  Lymphogranuloma venereum
  Psittacosis

Fungal
  Candida
  Actinomyces
  Aspergillus
  Blastomyces
  Mucor
  Sporotrichum schenckii
  Coccidioides immitis (San Joaquin Valley fever)

Parasitic
  Acantamoeba
  Phthirus pubis
  Ascaris lubricoides
  Trichinella spiralis
  Schistosoma haematobium
  Toxoplasma

Atopic
  Hay fever conjunctivitis
  Vernal keratoconjunctivitis

Autoimmune
  Sjogren's syndrome
  Psoriasis
  Mucous membrane pemphigoid
  Wegener's granulomatosis

Irritative
  Iatrogenic
  Occupational

Idiopathic
  Reiter's syndrome
  Ocular rosacea
  Folliculosis

standard for uncomplicated acute bacterial conjunctivitis. Artificial tears help the discomfort of keratitis and photophobia. Cold compresses improve the swelling and discomfort of the lids. Antibiotic drops help prevent a secondary bacterial infection. Polytrim (trimethoprim/sulfamethoxazole) is a reasonable choice particularly in children. If the patient does not have improved symptoms within 2 to 3 days of antibiotic therapy, ophthalmologic consultation, Gram's stain, and culture should be obtained. Reserve topical corticosteroids for use by an ophthalmologist when substantial inflammation is present and herpes simplex is excluded.

In chronic bacterial conjunctivitis, the patient often presents with symptoms similar to that seen in acute bacterial conjunctivitis, but with symptoms persisting for more than 2 weeks. In addition to these symptoms, the patient may also have scant discharge from the eyes, worse upon awakening in the morning. Most commonly, chronic bacterial conjunctivitis results from *S. aureus* infection, but *Moraxella lacunata* also presents with chronic symptoms. As with uncomplicated acute bacterial conjunctivitis, sulfacetamide, erythromycin, and gentamicin topical ophthalmic preparations are effective within 3 days of initiation of therapy. Broad-spectrum antibiotics, such as Ciloxan (ciprofloxacin) or Ocuflox (ofloxacin), are good choices.

Viral infection is also a very common cause of conjunctivitis, often confused with bacterial etiologies. As with bacterial conjunctivitis, erythema, profuse tearing, chemosis, and itching of the eyes predominate. Patients with viral conjunctivitis have an increased incidence of fever, myalgias, generalized malaise, and preauricular lymphadenopathy associated with the viral infection causing the conjunctivitis. Viral conjunctivitis often produces a follicular response in the palpebral conjunctivae, giving the patient a foreign body sensation. Viral pathogens of greatest concern include herpes simplex and herpes zoster; however, adenovirus is perhaps the most common etiology. The conjunctiva is injected, papillary reaction may be noted in the conjunctiva, and clear discharge occurs from the affected eye. The pupils are symmetrical and reactive, and no photophobia is present. Slit-lamp examination should be accomplished with fluorescein stain instilled into the eyes. If herpes simplex virus is the etiology, ulcerations and vesicles may be seen on the eyelids. Corneal ulceration in the form of dendritic lesions is a serious finding, resulting from rapid corneal spread of the virus.

Treatment of viral conjunctivitis varies depending on the etiology. Simple viral conjunctivitis will often improve spontaneously; however, due to confusion with bacterial causes for conjunctival inflammation, ocular preparations of sulfacetamide, erythromycin, or gentamicin should be used for 7 days. If findings of herpetic infection are evident on examination, ophthalmologic consultation should be obtained.

Chlamydial conjunctivitis is characterized by follicular hypertrophy, usually bilateral; redness, itching, chemosis, and concomitant urethritis may be found. This etiology can be seen in the neonate after passing through the birth canal and also should be considered highly in the young sexually active adult presenting with complaints of conjunctival irritation. A high suspicion for this disease in the given population and physical findings should be enough for the ED physician to begin therapy with systemic doxycycline, tetracycline, or erythromycin. Concurrent gonococcal infection rate is high, and, therefore, any patient with chlamydial infection should also be treated for *N. gonorrhoeae*. Partners of treated patients need to be examined and given appropriate therapy also to prevent public health risks.

Fungal pathogens are an etiology of conjunctivitis that should be considered in any patient with immunocompromised, diabetes, or those patients taking systemic corticosteroids. Fungal infections should also be suspected in any patient relating a history of trauma to the eye that resulted from contact with vegetation. Fungal conjunctivitis does not usually present with significant disease; instead, it often appears as chronic inflammation and discharge from the eyes. Consultation should be obtained, and treatment based on the fungal etiology and symptomatology can range from topical antifungal medications to intravenous antifungal therapy.

Corneal Abrasions

The cornea is an avascular protective layer of the external eye that often is subjected to mechanical trauma that results in abrasion of the cornea. The patient may describe moderate photophobia secondary to iritis, redness of the eye, and possibly decreased vision from the affected eye. Tearing may be present, but no other discharge is present. Initial assessment should include evaluation for the presence of foreign body, determination of visual acuity, and examination for evidence of trauma to the eye. By history, the patient should be able to relate the immediate time at which pain began and the probable etiology for the abra-

Table 53.2
Diffential Diagnosis of Acute Eye Pain and Redness
Conjunctivitis
Bacterial
Viral
Fungal
Other
Keratitis
Acute angle-closure glaucoma
Trauma
Foreign bodies
Optic neuritis
Chemical or thermal injury
Conjunctivitis medicamentosus
Uveitis
Stevens-Johnson syndrome

sion. It is important to assess, however, the timing of the onset of symptoms, nausea or vomiting associated with symptoms, flashing lights or floaters, other medical problems or new medications. Finally, the patient's current level of immunization against tetanus should be documented.

Topical anesthetic may be used to facilitate examination. The upper eyelid should be everted to examine the eye for evidence of retained foreign material as a source of irritation. Conjunctival inflammation or ulceration should be noted, and any purulent discharge should be examined as to the source. After thorough external examination, slit-lamp examination of the eye should be performed with fluorescein staining, followed by examination under cobalt-blue light or a Wood's lamp. Any evidence for corneal ulceration, abrasion, or laceration should be noted. The differential diagnosis for eye pain and redness can be found in **Table 53.2**. No ancillary tests are required for further evaluation if the diagnosis of corneal abrasion can be made.

After diagnosis of corneal abrasion is made, treatment in the ED consists of ophthalmic antibiotic suspensions of gentamicin, sulfacetamide, or erythromycin to prevent secondary infection of the denuded cornea. Prolonged use of topical anesthetics should be avoided due to delay in healing and secondary development of keratitis. Repair of the cornea occurs rapidly, especially if the abrasion is small. Cycloplegic agents may also be supplied to prevent ciliary spasm and diminish pain. Follow-up with an ophthalmologist is recommended for patients with persistent symptoms for more than 72 hours and for patients with large corneal abrasions. Delayed healing and recurrent corneal erosions due to imperfect healing after the initial insult are the main dangers to consider in corneal abrasions, and both are indications for further outpatient follow-up.

Dacryocystitis/Dacryoadenitis

Dacryocystitis is a common acute or chronic disease that usually occurs in infants or in persons over the age of 40. Dacryocystitis can be seen in all age groups after trauma or as a result of a fungal infection. It is most often unilateral and results from obstruction of the naso-lacrimal duct. Acute episodes are usually exacerbations of chronic dacryocystitis or severe conjunctivitis. The usual infectious etiologies include *S. aureus, S. pneumococcus,* and *Haemophilus influenzae,* but *Candida albicans* and mixed infections are also seen. Infantile dacryocystitis results from incomplete canalization of the lacrimal duct in the first month of life, leading to a secondary *H. influenzae* dacryocystitis. The chief symptoms are profuse tearing and purulent discharge from the lacrimal duct. In acute cases, inflammation, pain, swelling, and localized tenderness is present in the area of the lacrimal gland. In chronic cases, however, the only symptoms may be those of tearing and mucus discharge from the lacrimal duct.

On physical examination, the patient will have swelling in the area of the lacrimal gland, and if pressure is applied to this region, purulent material may be expressed. Patients can be treated with oral preparations of ampicillin, with acute dacryocystitis responding well to treatment. Chronic cases may be recurrences of acute dacryocystitis or may result from latent infection. These cases may be treated with antibiotic eye drops, but relief of the obstruction is the definitive cure. In infantile dacryocystitis, sulfacetamide, gentamicin, or erythromycin eye drops should be used, and the gland should be massaged to attempt to promote opening of the lacrimal duct. If conservative treatment is unsuccessful, referral to an ophthalmologist is necessary for probing of the duct and further therapy.

Dacryoadenitis is an acute inflammation of the lacrimal gland and has a similar presentation to dacrocystitis. This is a rare unilateral condition seen in children as a complication of mumps, measles or influenza. This disorder can be seen in the adult population and is exclusively associated with gonorrhea. Dacryoadenitis may also develop following a penetrating injury to the lacrimal gland or secondary to bacterial conjunctivitis. In the acute case, swelling, pain, and injection over the upper temporal aspect of the eye occurs, deforming the upper lid into a serpentine deformity. Chronic dacryoadenitis may result as a manifestation of systemic sarcoidosis, tuberculosis, leukemia, and lymphosarcoma. History of systemic diseases, trauma, and surgery is important to the diagnosis. Systemic antibiotic therapy is effective in bacterial dacryoadenitis, but if the gland is extremely enlarged, consultation for incision and drainage may be indicated.

Foreign Body

Complaint of foreign body sensation in the eye is a common presentation to the ED and can range from the uncomplicated corneal foreign body to globe penetration and intraocular foreign bodies. The patient with the corneal foreign body will most often present with complaint of pain, profuse tearing, sensation of the foreign body, and conjunctival injection. Depending on the size of the foreign body, the patient may have secondary keratitis and resulting photophobia.

Important aspects of the history include onset of pain, velocity of the object upon impact, the nature of object suspected to have been involved, decrease in vision, occupational exposure, and presence of pain; special concern should be given to injuries resulting from explosions, metal working, or other high-velocity projectiles. Physical examination should begin with visual acuity testing, followed by examination of the external eye with eversion of the upper lid and, if needed, double eversion of the lid to inspect the ocular cul-de-sac for foreign bodies. Slit-lamp examination can be done to aid in visualization of the surface of the eye and aid in magnification of small objects. If there is not an obvious corneal foreign body seen, fluorescein should be applied, and repeated slit-lamp examination should be done with cobalt-blue light or Wood's lamp. Small corneal foreign bodies may be able to be flushed from the eye with saline, but more often will have to be removed with a moistened cotton swab, commercially developed eye spud, or 25-gauge needle. Adequate local anesthesia and patient cooperation are required to remove the object and to prevent perforation of the globe in attempts to remove the foreign body. After removal of the object, the site should further be inspected for other foreign material and evidence for any "rust ring" that developed secondary to iron-containing metallic foreign bodies. Rust rings in the cornea are important to diagnose and remove as photophobia, visual impairment, and visual field glare can result. The presence of corneal abrasions prior to removal and after removal of the foreign body should be noted. Tetanus immunization status should also be established at the time of ED visit and given, if appropriate. The patient should be given ophthalmic preparations of topical sulfacetamide, gentamicin, or erythromycin to prevent secondary infection. An eye patch may be used to provide patient comfort, but this severely limits patient activity due to loss of binocular vision and peripheral vision.

Any patient with multiple corneal foreign bodies, especially in the visual field, large corneal foreign bodies, possible intraocular foreign material, or foreign bodies not easily removed with the above techniques should be consulted with an ophthalmologist for evaluation. Patients successfully treated should return in 24 hours for re-evaluation or should have ophthalmologic evaluation within 24 hours.

Intraocular foreign bodies are a much more severe injury and can be less obvious in presentation. Small foreign bodies, especially those at high speed, may penetrate the globe of the eye without significant signs of penetration. Commonly, work-related eye injuries result in intraocular foreign bodies, and a high suspicion for this should be raised. Any large intraocular foreign body should be left in place prior to ED presentation. The ED physician should also leave the foreign body in place and seek immediate ophthalmologic consultation. Depending on the velocity and nature of the intraocular foreign body, penetration of the cranium and involvement of the nervous system may be present. Substances poorly visualized on initial examination may be evident on plain film x-rays or CT scan. Immediate consultation for any intraocular foreign body is required, as treatment may vary.

Hyphema/Hypopyon

Hyphema and hypopyon represent abnormal collections of fluids in the anterior chamber that result from trauma or infection. Hyphema is a layering or clotting of blood inferiorly in the anterior chamber, and hypopyon is a similar layering, composed, however, of white blood cells. Patients with these disorders often complain of eye pain, progressive blurring of the vision, and photophobia. They may relate a history of trauma or irritation in the affected eye. Historical items of importance in the presence of trauma include the type of injury, time of the injury, and time of visual compromise if present. If a history of trauma is not elicited, sources of ocular infection, systemic causes for bleeding disorders, recent surgery, and contact lens use may provide important historical information to the presenting problem (**Table 53.3**). Physical examination of these patients in the upright position will reveal layering of cells inferiorly forming a discrete meniscus. The size of the collection can vary from very minor to complete occlusion of the anterior chamber. It is important to note that in traumatic causes for hyphema, often damage can be found in the other eye; therefore a complete ophthalmologic examination as described above should be performed, first ruling out a ruptured globe. The quantity of the effusion at examination should be noted as a percentage of the anterior chamber size, and the intraocular pressure of the patient should also be determined.

Management consists of immediate consultation, and hospitalization for any significant hyphema especially in the presence of increased intraocular pressure and for patients with sickle-cell disease or sickle-cell trait-positive. The patient should be kept at rest with the head elevated at >30 degrees. An eye shield should be applied to the involved eye, and mild analgesics can be given. Due to risks of development of glaucoma, especially in the patient with sickle-cell

Table 53.3
Causes of Hyphema and Hypopyon
Hyphema
Bleeding from the iris
Corneal wound neovascularization
Herpes simplex iritis
Herpes zoster iritis
Blood dyscrasias
Clotting disorders
Intraocular tumor
Trauma
Intraocular surgery
Hypopyon
Infectious corneal ulcer
Endophthalmitis
Severe iritis
Reaction to intraocular foreign body
Intraocular tumor necrosis
Tightly adherent contact lens

Table 53.4
Risk Factors Predisposing to Glaucoma
Elevated intraocular pressure
Systemic hypertension
Genetic predisposition
African ancestry
Diabetes mellitus
Myopia
Age of >40 years
Vasospastic vascular disease

homozygous or heterozygous disease, these patients need careful observation and follow-up to ensure resolution of the collection and decrease the risk of re-bleeding.

Glaucoma

Glaucoma is best described as a group of ocular disorders characterized by pressure-related damage to the optic nerve. Although glaucoma damage is associated with multiple risk factors, its major determinant is an intraocular pressure that is too high for the normal functioning of the optic nerve. **Table 53.4** lists several associated risk factors for the development of glaucoma. If not treated, glaucoma results in progressive and irreversible contraction of the visual field that may ultimately lead to blindness. Glaucoma is usually insidious and asymptomatic, affecting the central vision only in late stages (**Table 53.5**). In its acute, overtly symptomatic form, however, glaucoma can cause rapid visual loss within hours to days. Although several theories exist for the mechanisms of optic nerve damage, lowering the intraocular pressure is the only treatment for glaucoma.

Glaucoma develops as a result of an increase in the resistance to aqueous outflow due to malfunction or obstruction of the trabecular meshwork of the eye. Increasing age, trauma, inflammation, ischemia, and many other factors may alter production and outflow of aqueous humor. As a result, intraocular pressure rises, further decreasing outflow by impairing the function of the trabecular meshwork. Eventually, a new steady state is reached as aqueous humor production decreases and the intraocular pressure plateaus. The location of the obstruction to aqueous outflow is the main determinant of the type of glaucoma and its treatment. The three main categories are developmental, open angle, and closed angle glaucoma. Developmental glaucoma is characterized by an anterior chamber angle defect caused by abnormal differentiation of embryonic tissue. Infants afflicted with this disorder may present as irritable, photophobic, profusely tearing, rubbing the eyes, and preferring to keep the eyes closed. Penlight examination reveals haziness and bluish appearance to the cornea, corneal diameter of greater than 10.5 mm, and conjunctival inflammation. The cornea may also appear edematous with epithelial blistering and breakdown. Examination of the child with suspected glaucoma requires a comprehensive examination of all eye struc-

Table 53.5

Causes of Painless Loss of Vision

Acute
- Retinal hemorrhage
- Vitreous hemorrhage
- Retinal detachment
- Maculopathy
- Central retinal artery occlusion (CRAO)
- Central retinal vein occlusion (CRVO)
- Ischemic neuropathy
- Occipital infarction
- Cytomegalovirus retinitis

Chronic
- Chronic corticosteroids
- Ocular trauma
- Toxic exposure
- Congenital cataract
- Cataracts secondary to intraocular disease
  - Uveitis
  - Glaucoma
  - Retinitis pigmentosa
  - Retinal detachment
- Cataracts secondary to systemic disease
  - Diabetes mellitus
  - Hypoparathyroidism
  - Myotonic dystrophy
  - Atopic dermatitis
  - Galactosemia
  - Lowe's syndrome
  - Werner's syndrome
  - Down's syndrome

tures and is best performed with the child sedated and with consultation of an ophthalmologist.

Open angle glaucoma (OAG) can be divided into primary and secondary classifications, with primary OAG occurring in over 60% of adults with glaucoma. Secondary causes of OAG include inflammation, drug-related or mechanical obstruction, and dysfunction of the trabecular meshwork. OAG is usually bilateral, with one eye more greatly involved than the other, insidious in onset, and slowly progressive. Symptoms are usually minimal in the initial phase, with the patient in the late phases of the disease complaining of decreased vision, aching of the eyes, cloudy vision, or impaired peripheral vision. Patients may also give a family history of glaucoma. Examination of the patient presenting in the late phases of the disease can be variable. Visual acuity testing may show decrease in vision bilaterally, the external eye appears unremarkable, and examination of the anterior chamber angle appears normal. Visual field testing may show loss of peripheral vision early and central visual field defects late in the disease. Funduscopic examination may show important early findings in the optic disk, including thinning of the disk margins in the temporal region and widening and cupping of the optic disk. The large vessels become nasally displaced, and the affected area of the disk becomes atrophic. The intraocular pressure is usually increased, but can be normal

(10 to 20 mm Hg). The ED treatment of primary OAG is medically oriented and consists of ophthalmic drops of various medications, including pilocarpine, acetazolamide, timolol, and other topical treatments. The goal of these medications is to reduce intraocular pressure by improving aqueous flow through the trabecular meshwork and decreasing the rate of aqueous humor formation. Side effects of these medications include miosis and loss of accommodation. Any patient with suspected primary OAG should have consultation with an ophthalmologist for referral and further treatment as an outpatient.

More common and more urgent in presentation is acute closed angle glaucoma or acute ACG. This disease results when there is a sudden increase in the intraocular pressure due to a block of the anterior chamber angle by the root of the iris. This results in complete cessation of aqueous flow, severe pain, and sudden visual loss. ACG is much less common than OAG, occurring in only 10% of cases, but is the most common presentation for glaucoma in the ED. The patient classically has sudden onset of severe localized pain in the eye or orbit, or generalized in the head that develops after entering a darkened area or after going to sleep, after emotional upset, or after beginning sympathomimetic or anticholinergic medications. The patient may also complain of blurred vision or halo vision, nausea, vomiting, and photophobia. The patient with suspected acute ACG should be urgently triaged to the ED to prevent further ischemic damage to the optic nerve. The patient with acute ACG reveals decreased visual acuity, conjunctival hyperemia, corneal edema, hazing, and a fixed, mid-dilated pupil. The uninvolved eye continues to have a consensual response to light and has no visual deficit or inflammation present. The anterior chamber angle is decreased, and intraocular pressures are usually high (>50 mm Hg); however, in prolonged attacks, the ciliary body becomes ischemic and intraocular pressure decreases to normal or low levels. Suspected acute ACG should be differentiated from other diseases with similar presentations such as acute iritis and conjunctivitis, as well as the other etiologies listed in Table 53.2. ED treatment of acute ACG consists of lowering the intraocular pressure, followed by pupillary-constricting agents to disrupt the lens-iris apposition and open the area of aqueous blockage. Topical pilocarpine produces miosis, decreasing blockage of the trabecular meshwork. Topical timolol can be used to decrease the intraocular pressure and augment the effect of miotic agents. The use of carbonic anhydrase inhibitors and hyperosmolar agents such as glycerol and mannitol decrease the intraocular pressure by removing fluid from the eyes into the plasma and by decreasing production of the aqueous humor. Immediate consultation of an ophthalmologist is imperative to prevent serious visual complications, ensure continuation of treatment, and prevent recurrence of the acute attack.

Complications of untreated acute ACG include formation of peripheral anterior synechias as a result of apposition of the lens and iris, cataract formation, ischemic atrophy of the retina and optic nerve, and absolute glaucoma with constant pain and blindness. An acute attack occurs in the second eye in at least 50% of cases, even when the patient has conscientiously carried out miotic prophylactic treatment.

Iritis

In any patient with complaint of eye redness and pain, acute iritis (or uveitis) should be considered as an etiology. Acute iritis can develop as a result of many systemic inflammatory diseases, systemic infectious diseases, or trauma (**Table 53.6**). Patients present with complaints of moderate to severe pain, photophobia, eye redness, blurred vision, and copious tearing. Often the onset of symptoms is gradual. History of trauma to the eye should be elicited, as well as a history of other systemic diseases or symptoms. Classic physical examination findings of uveitis are conjunctival injection with inclusion of the perilimbal region of the conjunctiva, corneal edema, ocular pain when light is shined into the eye, and a miotic pupil in the involved eye. Other signs of iritis on physical examination may include decreased intraocular pressure, hypopyon, keratitic precipitates in the anterior chamber, and normal anterior chamber depth. If the iritis is chronic or recurrent, macular edema and cataract may also be evident on examination.

The differential diagnosis in patients with these symptoms should include conjunctivitis, keratitis, acute ACG, posterior pole tumors, and possible intraocular foreign body. If history and complete ocular examination, including determination of intraocular pressure, are unremarkable, and the iritis is bilateral or recurrent, consultation should be obtained and ancillary studies appropriate to suspect systemic causes of iritis obtained by the ED physician.

Corneal Keratitis

A further cause of eye redness that can often be confused with iritis is corneal keratitis. Keratitis involves inflammation of the cornea due to trauma or infection. Patients present with complaints of moderate to severe sharp pain, profuse tearing, purulent discharge (if infectious), foreign body sensation, blurred vision, and eye redness. Patients may give a history of trauma to the involved eye. Onset is usually subacute as compared to other etiologies of eye redness. On physical examination, the patient will exhibit conjunctival injection with involvement of the limbal region of the conjunctiva, the pupil is reactive and normal in size, and intraocular pressure is normal. Visual acuity is normal to slightly decreased in the affected eye. When fluorescein stain is instilled into the eye, the affected cornea will have increased uptake and staining in characteristic patterns depending on the etiology of the keratitis. Possible etiologies of keratitis are listed in **Table 53.7**. Specific treatment in the ED depends on the pat-

---

Table 53.6

Causes of Iritis

Trauma
Inflammatory
  Ankylosing spondylitis
  Inflammatory bowel disease
  Reiter's syndrome
  Psoriatic arthritis
  Lens-induced uveitis
  Behçet's disease
Infectious
  Herpes simplex, herpes zoster, varicella
  Lyme disease
  Mumps
  Influenza
  Adenovirus
  Measles
  Chlamydia
  Rickettsial disease
  Leptospirosis
Other
  Kawasaki's disease
  Postoperative iritis
  Uveitis-glaucoma-hyphema syndrome
  Glaucomatocyclitic crisis
  Tight contact lens

Table 53.7

Etiologies of Keratitis and Fluorescein Uptake Patterns

Fungal keratitis
  History of trauma (especially vegetable matter) or chronic eye disease
  Fluorescein uptake in area of infection with satellite lesions surrounding primary lesion
Bacterial keratitis
  History of trauma or chronic eye disease
  Fluorescein uptake in area of infection
Ultraviolet keratitis
  History of welding or sunlamp use without protective eyewear
  Fluorescein uptake in a confluent superficial punctate lesion in the distribution of the interpalpebral region
Exposure keratitis
  History of inadequate blinking or closure of the eye
  Fluorescein uptake in a horizontal band in the region of the palpebral fissure or on the lower one-third of the cornea
Acanthamoeba keratitis
  Poor contact lens hygiene, hot tub use, or swimming with contact lenses in place
  Fluorescein uptake in ring shape or pseudododendrite pattern
Herpes simplex keratitis
  Prior attacks in the same eye, vesicles on erythematous base on eyelids
  Fluorescein uptake as branching dendritic lesions, superficial punctate lesions, or stellate lesions
Herpes zoster keratitis
  Prior attacks in the same eye, vesicular skin rash in dermatomal pattern
  Fluorescein uptake in pseudodendritic pattern or superficial punctate lesions

tern of uptake and findings on physical examination. Consultation should be obtained when iritis results from trauma or infection, and follow-up is crucial in most types of keratitis.

Choroiditis

Choroiditis is inflammation of the vascular layer between the retina and the sclera that can be seen in patients with herpes zoster infection, posterior uveitis or other inflammatory diseases. Patients often present with complaints of unilateral blurred vision, floaters, eye redness, mild pain, and photophobia that is insidious in onset. Physical examination is remarkable for possible vitreous or anterior chamber inflammatory cells. Funduscopic examination may show inflammatory lesions on the retina, mild disc edema, and neovascularization of the choroid plexus. If herpes zoster is the suspected etiology, the patient should be admitted for intravenous acyclovir and steroid therapy. If choroiditis results from an inflammatory etiology, consultation and oral steroid therapy often can improve symptoms. In severe choroiditis with significant neovascularization, laser photocoagulation may be required.

Optic Neuritis

Optic neuritis is a serious cause of subacute visual loss. Etiologies for optic neuritis include multiple sclerosis, viral infections, childhood infections, and inflammatory diseases of the eye and surrounding structures (**Table 53.8**). Patients present with loss of visual acuity that worsens over a period of hours to days that is usually unilateral, but can present with bilateral visual involvement. Often, the patient also complains of eye pain with movement of

the eye and decreased color vision. Patients may give a history of antecedent viral syndromes or systemic diseases. Other elements of historical significance include toxic or metabolic causes such as alcohol, malnutrition, heavy metal exposure, anemia, and multiple other toxins. Complete physical, ophthalmologic, and neurologic examinations should be performed, including pupillary response, visual field testing, and funduscopic examination for papilledema. Further causes often confused with optic neuritis include acute papilledema from increased intracranial pressure, ischemic optic neuropathy, orbital tumor compression of the optic nerve, and toxic or metabolic optic neuropathy. Ancillary tests to consider include a CBC, erythrocyte sedimentation rate (ESR), rapid plasma reagin RPR, and CT or magnetic resonance imaging (MRI) of the orbits and brain. All patients with optic neuritis respond to some degree to intravenous steroids, and therefore consultation and admission for observation and treatment are warranted.

Papilledema

Patients can also develop visual loss due to optic disc swelling produced by increased intracranial pressure. Increased intracranial pressure results from swelling or mass effect in the confined space of the cranium. Specific etiologies for increased intracranial pressure are listed in **Table 53.9**. Patients with papilledema, present with episodic, transient, visual loss that can be precipitated by changes in posture. Visual loss is often bilateral, lasting seconds, and is recurrent. Patients may also complain of headaches, diplopia, nausea, vomiting, and, in chronic papilledema, loss of central visual acuity. Complete physical examination (blood pressure evaluation, ophthalmologic examination, and neurologic examination) should be performed. The patient with acute papilledema will have bilaterally swollen, hyperemic disks with indistinct

---

Table 53.8

Causes of Optic Neuritis

Multiple sclerosis
Viral infection
  Mononucleosis
  Viral encephalitis
  Herpes zoster
Childhood diseases
  Chickenpox
  Measles
  Mumps
Inflammatory diseases
  Meningitis
  Orbital inflammation
  Sinusitis
  Tuberculosis
  Syphilis
  Sarcoidosis
  Cryptococcus
  Intraocular inflammatory processes
Idiopathic

Table 53.9

Causes of Increased Intracranial Pressure

Tumor
  Primary
  Metastatic
Hemorrhage
  Subdural hematoma
  Epidural hematoma
  Subarachnoid
  Arteriovenous malformation
Infection
  Meningitis
  Abscess
  Encephalitis
  Sagittal sinus thrombosis
Other
  Pseudotumor cerebri
  Hydrocephalus

disk margins, papillary retinal hemorrhages (flame hemorrhages), obscuring of the blood vessels, and enlarged physiologic blind spot to visual field testing. In chronic papilledema, optic atrophy is present, and hemorrhages resolve, with other findings being consistent with acute papilledema. Determination of the pathology causing papilledema is a priority, and patients should receive emergent CT or MRI of the brain. If no intracranial pathology is noted in these studies, lumbar puncture recording of opening pressure should be performed. Specific therapy for the causes of increased intracranial pressure varies for each and should be directed at the specific underlying disease.

Retinal Detachment

Retinal detachments constitute a separation of the retinal layers resulting from accumulation of fluid in the potential space that lies between the sensory layer and the underlying retinal pigmented epithelial layer. Most retinal detachments result from one or more retinal holes that allow for passage of fluid. Specific causes of retinal detachments can be found in **Table 53.10**.

Patients with retinal detachment may present with light flashes, dark floating specks, a curtain-like visual field defect, and peripheral or central vision loss. Symptoms may be minimal or may result in significant loss of vision unilaterally, but can be bilateral. A history of antecedent trauma, prior retinal detachment or retinal surgery, and systemic disease may be important to the diagnosis of retinal detachment. Complete physical, ophthalmic, and neurologic examinations should be performed, including visual acuity, visual field testing, and fundoscopic examination. Funduscopic examination may readily show retinal detachment or tears. Immediate consultation should be obtained to prevent further progression of the retinal detachment, especially if encroaching on the macula of the retina.

Table 53.10
Etiologies of Retinal Detachment

Trauma
Retinopathy
  Diabetic retinopathy
  Sickle-cell retinopathy
  Retinopathy of prematurity
Neoplasia
  Choroidal malignant melanoma
  Hemangioma
  Multiple myeloma
  Metastasis
Inflammatory disease
  Scleritis
  Chronic inflammatory processes
Congenital disease
Idiopathic

Central Retinal Artery Occlusion

Vascular diseases of the retina often result in acute visual loss that is not associated with pain. Central retinal artery occlusion (CRAO) presents with unilateral, painless, acute loss of vision that occurs over a matter of seconds to the extent of mere light-dark perception. The central retinal artery develops arterial narrowing as a result of atherosclerosis similar to any other artery. Acute occlusion results from decreased blood flow or embolic phenomena that arise from the carotid arteries or cardiac sources (**Table 53.11**). Patients may give a history of significant atherosclerotic disease, prior intracranial vascular insufficiency, or prior episodes of amaurosis fugax. Physical ex-

Table 53.11
Etiologies of Central Retinal Artery Occlusion and Central Retinal Vein Occlusion

Central retinal artery occlusion
  Embolic
    Carotid plaques
    Cardiac valvular disease or endocarditis
  Thrombosis
    Sickle-cell disease
    Polycythemia
    Oral contraceptives
    Antiphospholipid syndrome
  Collagen vascular diseases
    Giant cell arteritis
    Other
  Trauma
  Other
    Migraine
    Behçet's disease
    Syphilis
    Sickle-cell disease
    Hypotension
    Homocystinuria
Central retinal vein occlusion
  Atherosclerosis
  Hypertension
  Papilledema
  Glaucoma
  Hypercoagulability
    Polycythemia
    Lymphoma
    Leukemia
    Sickle-cell disease
    Multiple myeloma
    Others
  Vasculitis
    Sarcoidosis
    Syphilis
    Systemic lupus erythematosus
  Others
    Migraine
    Drugs

amination may reveal evidence of atherosclerotic disease with the presence of carotid bruits, and complete ophthalmologic examination and neurologic examination should be done. Often, a relative afferent pupillary defect will be noted in the affected eye, and funduscopic examination shows narrowed retinal arterioles, and superficial opacification or whitening of the retina in the posterior aspect with a cherry-red spot in the center of the fovea.

The differential diagnosis for CRAO includes acute ophthalmic artery occlusion, which presents with similar symptoms, but without a cherry-red spot in the fovea. ED treatment consists of attempts to lower intraocular pressure. Massage of the globe of the eye, and use of medications such as carbonic anhydrase inhibitors or beta-adrenergic blockers are preferred methods of reduction of intraocular pressure. Patients should have blood drawn for ESR, CBC, and coagulation profile, and immediate consultation of an ophthalmologist should be obtained. Delay of more than 12 hours after onset of symptoms is associated with poor restoration of vision. If the ESR is greatly increased, giant cell arteritis should be suspected and the patient should be started on high-dose systemic steroids in the ED.

Central Retinal Vein Occlusion

Central retinal vein occlusion (CRVO) also presents with painless loss of vision that is acute in nature and usually unilateral. Specific etiologies for CRVO can be found in Table 53.11.

Complete physical, ophthalmologic, and neurologic examinations should be done. A relative pupillary defect may or may not be present, depending on the type of venous obstruction, and intraocular pressure may be elevated. Funduscopic examination shows diffuse retinal flame hemorrhages in all quadrants of the retina, dilated and tortuous retinal veins, cotton-wool spots, optic disk edema, and retinal edema. The differential included in CRVO includes ocular ischemic syndrome, diabetic retinopathy, papilledema, and radiation retinopathy. Patients should have blood work as mentioned above, and ophthalmologic consultation should be obtained as patients need close follow-up. Treatment in the ED consists of correction of underlying medical disorders and lowering intraocular pressure if elevated.

Vitreous Hemorrhage

A final cause of painless loss of vision is vitreous hemorrhage. Patients present with sudden onset of painless, unilateral loss of vision or sudden appearance of black spots with flashing lights. Symptoms result from physical obstruction of light reaching the retina due to the presence of blood in the vitreous body. Patients prone to vitreous hemorrhage include diabetics and patients with prior retinal detachment, CRVO, trauma, sickle-cell disease, or subarachnoid or subdural hemorrhage. Physical examination reveals mild afferent pupillary defect, absent red reflex in severe vitreous hemorrhage, or blood in the posterior pole of the eye partially or completely obstruct-

ing the view of the fundus. The major differential diagnosis is retinal detachment as symptoms can be very similar. Patients should be admitted, with ophthalmologic consultation, for bed rest, with the head of the bed elevated, NSAID avoidance, and treatment of the underlying etiology of hemorrhage.

Panophthalmitis/Periobital Cellulitis

Trauma that results from vegetable matter can result in a rapidly progressive and fulminant panophthalmitis. Periorbital and orbital cellulitis are infections that involve the structures around the eye. Periorbital cellulitis involves infection in the region anterior to the orbital septum, not extending into the tissues within the orbit. Orbital cellulitis is infection that is anatomically posterior to the orbital septum and involves any of the structures in the orbit. More than half of these infections result from sinusitis, URIs, and otitis media. Children are most commonly affected, but adults may develop periorbital and orbital cellulitis. Common bacterial causes of these diseases are *H. influenzae, S. aureus,* and *S. pneumococcus.* Patients with orbital cellulitis often present with ocular pain, decreased visual acuity, diplopia, ophthalmoplegia, swelling, redness, and proptosis of the affected eye. Periorbital cellulitis presents with erythema and swelling, but lacks ocular pain, ophthalmoplegia, and proptosis. Physical examination will reveal erythema, warmth, and tenderness to palpation. Conjunctival chemosis, injection, proptosis, and restricted ocular motility with pain on movement of the eye are more often seen with orbital cellulitis. The differential diagnosis for orbital and periorbital cellulitis includes subperiosteal abscess, orbital abscess, and cavernous sinus thrombosis (CST). Any patient with suspected periorbital or orbital cellulitis should receive appropriate intravenous antibiotic therapy as soon as diagnosis is made (cefuroxime or nafcillin are excellent choices), but pediatric patients should receive blood culture prior to beginning antibiotic therapy. If question remains as to the extent of the infection beyond the orbital septum, CT scan of the orbits should be obtained. Immediate ophthalmologic consultation should be obtained, and the patient should be admitted for continued intravenous antibiotic therapy.

Preseptal Orbital Cellulitis

Orbital cellulitis can be a rapid cause of death if not treated adequately, as it can easily extend into the cranium if not rapidly controlled. A common site for extension is the cavernous sinus, resulting in thrombosis of the sinus and significant morbidity and mortality. CST develops as a result of thrombophlebitis or septic emboli spread from facial veins draining from sites of infection. Patients present with complaints of bilateral eye pain, headache, bilateral eye swelling, blurred vision, diplopia, and ophthalmoplegia. Findings on physical examination are dramatic and include those symptoms listed above, as well as proptosis, paresis of the third, fourth, and sixth cranial nerves, and decreased sensation of the first and second divisions of the trigeminal nerve. CT scan or MRI should be obtained to confirm diagnosis, but intravenous antimicrobial therapy should not be delayed if infection is suspected (cefuroxime or nafcillin). Neurosurgical evaluation should also be obtained, and the patient should be admitted for further intravenous medications and observation.

Selected Readings

Bergin DJ, Wright JE. Orbital cellulitis. *Br J Ophthalmol* 1986;70:174–178.

Chandler PA, Grant WM. *Glaucoma*, 2d ed. Philadelphia: Lea & Febiger, 1979:132.

Colenbrander A. Principles of ophthalmology. In: Tasman W, Jaeger E, eds. *Duane's Clinical Ophthalmology*. Vol. 1. Philadelphia: Lippincott, 1992.

Cullom D, Chang B. *The Wills Eye Manual: Office and Emergency Room Diagnosis and Treatment of Eye Disease*, 2d ed. Philadelphia: Lippincott, 1994.

Lowe RF. Aetiology of the anatomical basis for primary angle-closure glaucoma. *Br J Ophthalmol* 1970;54:161–169.

Miller MR. Optic neuritis. In: Miller N, ed. *Walsh and Hoyt's Clinical Neuro-Ophthalmology*. Baltimore: Williams and Wilkins, 1982:227–248.

Newell FW. *Ophthalmology: Principles and Concepts*, 6th ed. St. Louis, MO: CV Mosby 1986.

Scott J, Ghezzi K, eds. Emergency treatment of the eye. *Emerg Med Clin North Am* 1995;13(3):521–701 [issue devoted to eye emergencies].

Towbin R, Han BK, Kaufman RA, et al. Postseptal cellulitis: CT in diagnosis and management. *Radiology* 1986;158:735–737.

Vargas E, Drance SM. Anterior chamber depth in angle-closure glaucoma. Clinical methods of depth determination in people with and without the disease. *Arch Ophthalmol Visual Sci* 1973;90:438.

Vaughn D, Asbury T. *General Ophthalmology*, 11th ed. Los Altos, CA: Lange Medical Publications, 1986.

Yanofsky N. The acute painful eye. *Emerg Med Clin North Am* 1988;6:21–42.

Hematologic Disorders

G. Richard Braen

Bleeding and anemia from multiple causes frequently need to be evaluated in emergency departments. This section covers hemostatic disorders and red blood cell disorders which lead to the need for evaluation and, in more severe cases, transfusions.

Also included in this section are considerations of lymphomas, white blood cell disorders, and heparin-induced thrombocytopenia (HIT). Of these, HIT is the most recently described condition, and emergency physicians should be familiar with the principals of diagnosis and treatment.

Hemostatic Disorders

Jeffrey R. Suchard

Hemostasis involves a complex interaction of physiologic processes that result in the arrest of blood flow from or within a blood vessel. A brief description of normal hemostasis is necessary before discussion of its disease states. When a blood vessel is damaged, tissue factor, collagen, and other components of the subendothelial matrix are exposed. Platelets then aggregate at the site of injury by direct adhesion and by the mediation of von Willebrand's factor (vWF). Platelets and fibrinogen form a soluble occlusive plug that provides phospholipid surfaces for the reactions of the coagulation cascade. Tissue factor also activates the extrinsic coagulation pathway. Intrinsic pathway proteins become activated by factor VII, thrombin, or by surface contact factors. Both the intrinsic and extrinsic pathways activate factor X, which converts prothrombin to thrombin. Thrombin in turn cleaves fibrinogen to fibrin, which forms an insoluble clot. Fibrin is then crosslinked, and the hemostatic plug gets anchored into place via clot retraction. Modulating proteins limit extension of the clot by thrombin inhibition and inactivation of clotting factors. Eventually, the clot is lysed by plasmin once the vessel is sufficiently healed.

Uncontrolled bleeding is a common presenting complaint to the emergency department (ED). Most cases are traumatic and treatment is directed toward anatomic repair. When bleeding is a result of impaired hemostatic mechanisms, however, specific therapy directed against the pathophysiology is often needed. Most problems are caused by deficiencies or abnormalities in clotting factors or platelets. Although specific therapy is intellectually gratifying, no patient should suffer for lack of general supportive measures. All patients with significant bleeding require immediate stabilization with airway management (if necessary), direct pressure, venous access, and infusion of crystalloid solution. Packed red blood cell (PRBC) transfusion is directed by clinical status, presence and rate of continued hemorrhage, and the hematocrit.

Laboratory tests frequently used to evaluate hemostatic disorders are the hematocrit, platelet count, prothrombin time (PT), and partial thromboplastin time (PTT). The PT is a measure of the extrinsic and common pathways, while the PTT reflects the intrinsic and common pathways.

Clotting Factor Disorders

Hereditary

The Hemophilias

Hemophilia A Classic hemophilia (hemophilia A) is an X-linked recessive bleeding disorder occurring in approximately 1 in 10,000 live male births. Hemophilia A results from abnormal production of factor VIII, a coenzyme in the intrinsic pathway of the clotting cascade. One-third of cases are due to spontaneous mutations. Clinically apparent disease occurs when factor VIII activity is severely reduced, usually at less than 1% of normal. Milder forms may only be recognized after significant trauma or surgery.

The hallmarks of hemophilia are easy bruising, joint and muscle hemorrhages, and profuse posttraumatic/postsurgical bleeding. Minor cuts and abrasions are not typically associated with excessive bleeding. The platelet count and prothrombin time (PT) are normal, but the partial thromboplastin time (PTT) is prolonged. Specific clotting factor assays show decreased factor VIII activity.

About 90% of all bleeding in hemophilia is into joints or muscle. Hemarthrosis is the most common acute presentation, with the knee affected in over 50% of cases. Some hemophiliacs develop "target joints" that undergo a vicious cycle of rebleeding. Early treatment of hemarthrosis is crucial to relieve pain and to reduce complications. Factor replacement is indicated for all joint bleeding, even if objective findings are absent but the patient reports typical symptoms of their bleeding. If treatment is initiated later, ice packs, compressive elastic dressings, or splinting may be necessary. Hematology consultation should be considered, since repeat doses of factor replacement may be needed. Septic arthritis should also be considered, and joint aspiration is indicated if the patient is febrile, exhibits systemic toxicity or has joint pain that is unresponsive to factor replacement.

Intramuscular (IM) hemorrhage is next most common presentation. IM bleeding into fascial compartments puts the patient at risk for neurologic and vascular compromise, while bleeding in the tongue, pharynx, and neck can obstruct the airway. Most IM bleeds are recognized by the patient's complaint of pain, localized tenderness, and swelling. Hemorrhage into the iliopsoas muscles is more difficult to detect. Typical symptoms include groin pain, flexion of the hip, passive resistance to extension, and paresthesias from femoral nerve compression. Diagnosis is confirmed by ultrasound or computed tomography (CT) scan. Treatment of intramuscular hemorrhage is factor replacement, splint immobilization, and hematology consultation to evaluate for admission.

Intracranial hemorrhage (ICH) used to be the leading cause of death in hemophiliacs in the pre-AIDS era. Death occurs in roughly one-third of patients, while half suffer from long-term neurologic sequelae. In children, ICH is almost always posttraumatic. In adults, half of cases occur without any known antecedent trauma. Treatment must be initiated prior to confirmatory head CT in any hemophiliac with history of head trauma (even in the absence of lacerations, external contusions, or neurologic signs) or severe headache lasting longer than 4 hours. Intraspinal hemorrhage may also occur and is characterized by backache with or without immediate neurologic deficits. Treatment is the same: factor replacement to 100% of normal activity, neurosurgical consultation, and confirmatory radiologic studies if the patient's condition permits.

Oral bleeding from the gingiva or after dental extraction is common. Most patients are pretreated with factor replacement and prophylactic oral antifibrinolytics (e.g., ∈-aminocaproic acid and tranexamic acid). Intraoral lacerations generally need factor replacement and antifibrinolytics.

Subcutaneous hemorrhages and minor cuts rarely need specific therapy; however, any wound requiring sutures also requires factor replacement, both acutely and for suture removal. Epistaxis often responds to direct pressure. Packing with porcine fat or microfibrillar collagen can be useful, although factor replacement is necessary in serious epistaxis. Other presentations in hemophiliacs that require factor replacement include fractures, gastrointestinal bleeding, and severe abdominal pain where bleeding is not, or cannot be, ruled out.

Patients with mild hemophilia A and non–life-threatening bleeding can be treated with DDAVP (1-desamino-8-D-arginine vasopressin, desmopressin). DDAVP releases factor VIII and von Willebrand's factor from endothelial and other storage sites, increasing plasma levels three to five times. Ideal candidates for DDAVP have a baseline factor VIII activity level of more than 8%, so a threefold increase reaches a hemostatic level of about 30% normal. DDAVP is ineffective in moderate or severe hemophilia. Dosage is 0.3 mg/kg IV in 50 mL NS, given over 10 to 15 minutes. Patients requiring serial dosing of DDAVP need admission for periodic electrolyte monitoring and assessment of clinical effect, since tachyphylaxis occurs.

Many blood-derived products are available for factor VIII replacement therapy. Fresh frozen plasma (FFP) contains all clotting factors, but requires too much volume to be clinically useful. Cryoprecipitate contains about 100 units, factor VIII per bag, but contains many other un-

needed proteins and carries the risk of viral disease transmission. Concentrates pooled from several thousand donors contain about 15 units, factor VIII per milligram of total protein. Although widely used in the past, these concentrates have fallen out of favor due to the frighteningly high rate of transmission of hepatitis B and C, and HIV seroconversion. Recombinant factor VIII products are currently the preferred agents for factor replacement. These products carry virtually no risk (except for hypersensitivity reactions) but may be prohibitively expensive.

The amount of factor VIII to administer is determined by the severity of the patient's bleeding and the risk for complications. Guidelines vary, but generally the more severe the presentation, the higher the dose. For minor bleeding episodes (atraumatic joint/muscle hemorrhage, epistaxis, oral bleeding [greater than oozing]) painless hematuria lasting longer than 2 to 3 days, and minor procedures such as lumbar puncture and thoracentesis) raising the factor activity level to 40% should be sufficient. For major bleeding episodes (advanced or traumatic joint or muscle hemorrhage, significant trauma [even without apparent bleeding], and severe, atraumatic headache without focal neurologic signs) the goal should be 60% of normal activity. We further recommend raising the level to 100% in potentially fatal situations, such as intracranial hemorrhage, hematomas threatening the airway, and the need for emergent surgery.

Factor VIII is reconstituted from its lyophilized form and administered intravenously. One unit per kg body weight raises factor VIII activity levels by 2% of normal. Dosing by the above guidelines, therefore, would be 20, 30, or 50 U/kg, depending on the indication. The half-life of factor VIII is 8 hours, so repeated doses are required. Once the patient is initially evaluated, stabilized, and treated, a hematologist should be contacted, whether to admit the patient, act as consultant while the patient is hospitalized or to arrange for timely follow-up and outpatient therapy.

Hemophilia B Hemophilia B is another X-linked recessive hemorrhagic disorder that is clinically indistinguishable from hemophilia A. First described in the December 25, 1952 issue of the British Medical Journal, hemophilia B is also known as Christmas disease, and factor IX is called the Christmas factor. Factor IX deficiency occurs in 1 in 30,000 to 40,000 live male births. Clinical presentation and laboratory tests are identical to hemophilia A, except for specific clotting factor assays.

Treatment of bleeding episodes is similar to hemophilia A with a few exceptions. DDAVP is ineffective, since it does not cause release of factor IX. Also, the dose of factor IX administered to achieve a given level of activity is twice the amount of factor VIII that is given in hemophilia A. One unit of factor IX per kilogram body weight raises the activity level by 1% (versus 2% for factor VIII).

Historically, hemophilia B was treated with FFP and prothrombin-complex concentrates (PCCs). Purified factor IX concentrates are currently recommended for hemophilia B, both in acute and chronic management. There are several preparations available that are variably treated with heat, solvents, and chromatographic separation depending on the specific product. Genetically engineered factor IX products are also available, which eliminate the possibility of viral transmission but are very expensive. The half-life of factor IX is 18 to 30 hours, so daily dosing is appropriate.

Other Clotting Factor Disorders   Congenital deficiencies of several other coagulation factors (II, V, VII, X, XI) have been described, but are quite rare. Diagnosis of these conditions will probably never be made in the ED. If a bleeding patient has no known history of congenital hemostatic disease and has an abnormal PT and/or PTT, treat with FFP transfusion. Further workup is deferred to the primary physician or hematologist.

Acquired

Warfarin Therapy and Overdose

Warfarin interferes with vitamin K metabolism, resulting in less γ-carboxylation of factors II, VII, IX, and X, impairing formation of activation complexes in the coagulation cascade. Peak plasma concentrations occur within a few hours, and absorption is essentially complete. Warfarin is roughly 97% protein bound. The anticoagulant effect is seen within 24 hours, and half-life is about 60 hours. Warfarin is metabolized in the liver, excreted into the bile, reabsorbed, and ultimately excreted in the urine. Warfarin dosage ranges from 2 to 10 mg orally per day, with a typical dose of 5 to 7.5 mg. Given warfarin's relatively narrow therapeutic window and variability of patient response, frequent monitoring is necessary.

The prothrombin time is the first laboratory measurement to change, and is the traditional marker of antithrombotic effect. Interlaboratory differences in PT control values and materials used has led to the general adoption of monitoring the International Normalized Ratio (INR) as the test of choice, because it corrects for these confounding factors. Low-intensity anticoagulation, with an INR in the 2 to 3 range, is effective for most indications. High-intensity anticoagulation (INR = 3–4.5) is sometimes necessary with mechanical heart valves or recurrent thrombosis.

Patients taking warfarin can develop either thrombotic or hemorrhagic complications through several mechanisms. Lack of compliance is always a potential problem. Fluctuations in dietary vitamin K intake may confound warfarin therapy. Green leafy vegetables are especially rich in vitamin K. Many illnesses, such as acute viral infections or progression of chronic heart or liver failure, reduce requirements for therapeutic anticoagulation. Concurrent treatment with other drugs may affect warfarin metabolism by competition for protein binding sites (dilantin), inhibition or acceleration of drug clearance (trimethoprim-sulfamethoxazole, barbiturates) or may effect in reduced absorption (cholestyramine). Aspirin or NSAIDs potentiate any bleeding complications through their antiplatelet effect.

Treatment of warfarin-associated bleeding depends on the severity of hemorrhage. Studies of the annual incidence of hemorrhage in patients taking warfarin put mi-

nor episodes at 9.6%, major episodes at 3%, and fatal bleeding at 0.6%. Minor bleeding episodes (e.g., epistaxis with a therapeutic INR) can often be managed with local measures, brief discontinuance of warfarin, and close follow-up for coagulation profile monitoring. Vitamin K is indicated for more serious bleeding, since the result of toxicity is a functional vitamin K deficiency. The ideal dose and route of administration is undergoing constant reevaluation in the medical literature, with the current trend toward conservative "watch and wait" management. For asymptomatic patients with an elevation in the INR, many authorities recommend simple discontinuation of warfarin or low-dose oral vitamin K (1 to 2 mg) with follow-up evaluation and labs the next day. If rapid reversal of warfarin-induced coagulopathy is necessary, FFP transfusion is indicated, starting with at least 4 to 6 units. Prothrombin-complex concentrate infusion may be used in life-threatening situations, such as intracranial hemorrhage with deteriorating neurologic status, but this carries significant risk of thrombosis in other sites. General resuscitative measures, including IV access and PRBC transfusion as needed, should be performed in all patients with significant bleeding from warfarin overdose.

Vitamin K Insufficiency

Vitamin K insufficiency may arise by malabsorption, malnutrition, or drug therapy, particularly antibiotics and oral anticoagulants. Because it is a fat-soluble vitamin and requires bile salts for absorption, biliary obstruction or fistulae can lead to vitamin K deficiency. Ulcerative colitis, regional enteritis, extensive bowel resection, celiac disease and other malabsorption syndromes may also be implicated. Malnutrition, prolonged fasting, and even inadequate hyperalimentation may also cause vitamin K deficiency. While a healthy liver contains a 30-day store, deficiency can occur in 7 to 10 days in acutely ill patients. Even with adequate intake, hepatocellular disease causes a functional vitamin K deficiency from impaired synthetic ability. In addition to oral intake, vitamin K is also produced by normal colonic bacteria, so prolonged antibiotic therapy can impair hemostasis by altering the intestinal flora. Warfarin, cephalosporins with a N-methyl-thiotetrazole side chains (cefamandole, moxalactam, cefoperazone, cefazolin, cefazedone), and salicylates inhibit vitamin K epoxide reductase, the enzyme that regenerates the active form of the cofactor, disrupting the vitamin K salvage pathway. Maternal anticonvulsant therapy is associated with increased incidence of hemorrhagic disease of the newborn; routine neonatal prophylaxis with parenteral vitamin K is performed in most hospitals.

With a half-life of only 5 hours, factor VII is the first protein in the coagulation cascade to decrease in vitamin K insufficiency. The earliest laboratory abnormality, then, is an increased PT. Later, the PTT also increases as factors II, IX, and X become depleted. Isolated vitamin K deficiency should not cause abnormalities in the thrombin time, platelet count, or fibrinogen levels.

Nonemergent treatment for vitamin K deficiency, by PO or IM replenishment, is both effective and relatively rapid; therefore, ED treatment is reserved for significant hemorrhage. At least 4 to 6 units of FFP, which contains all necessary clotting factors, is given to adults, and proportionately less to children. Parenteral vitamin K is also given, either IM or by slow IV infusion. Dosage is 1 to 5 mg in infants/small children, 5 to 10 mg in older children, and 10 to 20 mg in adults. Cessation of bleeding and correction of laboratory abnormalities usually occurs within 8 hours.

Liver Disease

Bleeding due to liver disease is multifactorial in origin. The most common sites are localized lesions, such as esophageal varices and peptic ulcers; however, control of bleeding is complicated by defects in the coagulation cascade, platelet number and function, consumption of coagulation factors, and systemic fibrinolysis, which are all associated with liver disease.

Because nearly all components of the clotting cascade are synthesized in the liver, some of the earliest signs of hepatic dysfunction are reflected in coagulation abnormalities. Most patients with a bleeding tendency from liver disease have a chronic, progressive hepatitis from ethanol, persistent viral infection, or primary biliary cirrhosis. Vitamin K deficiency is a frequent confounding factor. Nonemergent correction of coagulation defects in liver disease is by a trial of vitamin K repletion, either by PO or IV routes. IM injections are avoided due to risk of hematoma formation. Serious bleeding is treated with transfusions of FFP, and possibly cryoprecipitate if associated with hypofibrinogenemia.

Liver disease also causes abnormalities in platelet number and function. Thrombocytopenia is due to ethanol-induced inhibition of thrombopoiesis and sequestration of platelets from hypersplenism. Concomitant folate deficiency also impairs platelet production. Platelet function defects are due to decreased hepatic clearance of circulating platelet inhibitors. DDAVP infusion (0.3 mg/kg IV) produces a significant, if transient, improvement in platelet function in over half of patients with liver disease. Platelet transfusions are indicated for active bleeding associated with thrombocytopenia, platelet count less than 50,000/mL.

Hypofibrinogenemia

Fibrinogen is a glycoprotein essential for normal hemostasis. In the common coagulation pathway, thrombin converts fibrinogen to fibrin, which forms a soluble clot. Factor XIII then stabilizes the clot by fibrin polymerization. Normal serum levels range from 200 to 400 mg/dL. Primary hypofibrinogenemia is caused by a number of uncommon genetic diseases; secondary hypofibrinogenemia may occur due to liver disease, ascites, DIC or drugs (L-asparaginase, ticlopidine, ethanol, pentoxifylline, valproate). Isolated hypofibrinogenemia rarely requires treatment; when associated with significant hemorrhage, cryoprecipitate transfusion is indicated.

Cryoprecipitate (cryo) is produced by slow thawing of FFP at 4° C and recovering the cold-insoluble fraction of plasma proteins by centrifugation. Cryo contains 100 to 250 mg fibrinogen in 5 to 30 mL volume. In addition, cryo contains greater than 80 U factor VIII activity per bag (average 100 U), 40% to 70% of original vWF, and several other clotting factors. Usual dosing is one bag per 6 kg body weight, which will increase fibrinogen by 75 to 100 mg/dL, the minimal level for hemostasis. Initial doses as high as one bag per 2 kg body weight are recommended for patients with hypofibrinogenemia-associated hemorrhagic shock.

Disseminated Intravascular Coagulation

Disseminated intravascular coagulation (DIC) is characterized by simultaneous unregulated activation of the coagulation and fibrinolytic pathways. DIC has been called a "consumptive coagulopathy," in that clotting factor and platelet levels fall as microthrombi are produced, but the most prominent clinical feature is bleeding. DIC is not a primary disease entity; it is always secondary to an underlying, usually severe, and most often systemic illness.

Pathophysiology

DIC is initiated by the entrance of procoagulant substances into the circulation. Tissue factor is released from damaged tissue, activating the extrinsic coagulation pathway. Exposure of subendothelial tissue activates the intrinsic pathway and induces platelet aggregation. Plasminogen is converted to plasmin by tPA released from damaged endothelial cells and/or by activated intrinsic pathway factors. Fibrinolysis then produces FDPs that are nonclottable, and inhibit fibrin polymerization and platelet aggregation.

DIC may be initiated by many primary illnesses. The most common causes are sepsis, malignancy, obstetrical complications, trauma, and liver disease. Overwhelming infection causes DIC due to the procoagulant nature of endotoxin, bacterial cell wall components, and WBC-released factors. Malignant cells can release tissue factor and other procoagulants. Late pregnancy and childbirth is a particularly DIC-prone period for both the mother and infant, because amniotic fluid and the placenta are rich in tissue factor. Burns, crush injuries, and other trauma are obvious sources of tissue factor. Chronic liver disease is a common cause of low-grade, compensated DIC, which rarely needs treatment.

Diagnosis

The diagnosis of DIC is suggested in patients with unexplained and often widespread bleeding manifestations in the appropriate clinical setting. The average patient bleeds from three or more unrelated sites. DIC also causes microvascular thrombosis that is present even if clinically inapparent. Such microthrombi may present as end-organ damage to the lung (hypoxemia, adult respiratory distress syndrome), kidney (oliguria, renal failure) or central nervous system (stroke). A thrombotic manifestation of the skin called purpura fulminans can also occur, appearing initially as ecchymotic lesions that subsequently demarcate and necrose. Large vessel thrombosis can cause acral cyanosis, necrosis or even gangrene of the extremities.

DIC causes a number of laboratory abnormalities. The most useful diagnostic test is measurement of FDPs. Elevation of FDPs is found in more than 95% of patients with DIC, representing the effects of fibrinolytic activation. FDPs impair coagulation and therefore act as an acquired anticoagulant. The D-dimer assay is more specific for DIC than FDPs, but less sensitive. This test measures the degradation product of cross-linked fibrin, reflecting concurrent coagulation and fibrinolysis. PT and PTT are elevated in fulminant DIC, but may occasionally be normal in early or mild disease. Thrombocytopenia is prominent, and may be the presenting finding in low-grade, compensated disease, as found in chronic liver failure. Hypofibrinogenemia with levels less than 100 mg/dL is expected, given the pathophysiology of the disease. In early DIC, levels may be normal, because fibrinogen is an acute-phase reactant; however, serial fibrinogen levels show a decline. Microangiopathic hemolytic anemia (decreased hematocrit, fragmented red cells on peripheral smear) is present in over half of cases.

Treatment

The paramount issue in DIC is treatment of the underlying disease process. Treating thrombocytopenia, clotting factor depletion, thrombosis, and hemorrhage is futile until the inciting event is reversed. The vast majority of cases of DIC seen in the ED are secondary to trauma, sepsis, and malignancy. Although complete resolution of DIC is dependent on subsequent management, emergency physicians can impact patient outcome by addressing the ABCs of resuscitation, correcting metabolic abnormalities, and rapidly initiating antibiotic treatment in sepsis.

Specific treatment of DIC remains controversial. Some authorities insist on heparin as initial therapy. Despite the apparent paradox in anticoagulating a bleeding patient, there is a sound theoretic basis to this course of action. First, although bleeding is the most obvious clinical problem in DIC, the thrombotic component has the greatest impact on morbidity and mortality. Second, there is some evidence that repletion of clotting factors may "feed the fire," by providing substrate for generating more thrombosis and more FDPs, impairing hemostasis further. Third, the patient is already bleeding, and heparin is unlikely to make it significantly worse. The other option for DIC therapy is transfusion of depleted coagulation factors: platelets, clotting proteins, and fibrinogen. The effect may be temporary as the transfused factors are consumed; however, the goal is to have the patient admitted for definitive therapy by the time repeat laboratory values would return.

Platelet Disorders

Immune Thrombocytopenic Purpura

Immune thrombocytopenic purpura (ITP) is a bleeding disorder caused by increased clearance of circulating platelets by the reticuloendothelial system. ITP was formerly known as idiopathic thrombocytopenic purpura, until the 1950s, when autoantibodies against platelets were identified as the etiologic agent. There are two distinct clinical forms of ITP, acute and chronic. The acute form is found most often in children and has an excellent

prognosis. Adults more commonly develop chronic ITP, a lifelong recurrent disease.

The typical clinical picture of acute ITP is the sudden onset of a "rash"—petechiae, purpura, and ecchymoses—in an otherwise healthy child. The incidence is equal for males and females, peaks between 2 and 5 years of age, and has a seasonal predominance in winter and fall. Childhood ITP often follows an acute viral illness or immunization. Chronic ITP accounts for 75% to 85% of all adult cases. There is a 3:1 male to female predominance, and, frequently, an associated family or personal history of autoimmune and lymphoproliferative disorders. Common manifestations of both acute and chronic ITP are epistaxis, gingival bleeding, easy bruising, and petechiae on the lower arms and legs without trauma; 10% to 20% of patients have hematuria, hematochezia, or menorrhagia. Life-threatening GI or CNS bleeds are rare, occurring in less than 1% of ITP patients.

Other than bleeding manifestations, the physical examination should be normal in ITP. Hepatosplenomegaly, adenopathy, history of weight loss, and fever all suggest alternate diagnoses, such as acute infections with Epstein-Barr virus (EBV) or cytomegalovirus (CMV), malignancy, collagen vascular disease, or AIDS. Between 5% to 10% of children with ITP have splenomegaly—the same percentage as for normal children.

Isolated thrombocytopenia should be the most significant laboratory abnormality in ITP. Anemia may result from hemorrhage or an associated autoimmune hemolysis (Evan's syndrome). Pancytopenia suggests bone marrow failure or infiltration rather than ITP.

Most cases of ITP do not require emergent treatment. Oral prednisone (1 to 2 mg/kg/day) or intravenous immune globulin (IVIG, 0.4 to 1.0 mg/kg per day) is usually effective. The proposed mechanism is by downregulating or binding of Fc receptors on monocytes and macrophages, thereby decreasing platelet clearance. Refractory cases are managed by splenectomy, antineoplastics or hormone therapy.

Transfused platelets are generally ineffective because of rapid destruction and removal from circulation. In cases of uncontrollable bleeding, however, transfusion may provide needed, if transient, hemostasis. Life-threatening CNS or GI bleeding (or intraocular bleeding) from ITP are clear indications for emergent treatment. IV methylprednisolone and IVIG are administered. Plasmapheresis may also be used, and if so, IVIG is initially withheld. If splenectomy, craniotomy, or other surgery is necessary, platelet transfusion is absolutely indicated prior to and during the procedure.

Thrombotic Thrombocytopenic Purpura and Hemolytic Uremic Syndrome

Thrombotic thrombocytopenic purpura (TTP) and hemolytic uremic syndrome (HUS) are two closely related disorders of microvascular occlusion by platelet microthrombi. Both disorders tend to occur abruptly in previously healthy individuals, and have significant risk for morbidity and mortality if not promptly recognized and treated.

HUS occurs mostly in young children, with greater than 90% of cases following a prodromal illness, frequently acute bloody diarrhea. *Escherichia coli* 0157:H7 is the most commonly associated infectious agent; however, *Shigella* gastroenteritis and many other infections (*Mycoplasma, Pneumococcus,* viral) may precede the onset of HUS.

The hemolytic uremic syndrome is heralded by the acute onset of a triad of symptoms: acute renal failure (oliguria); thrombocytopenia (petechiae, purpura, and ecchymoses); and microangiopathic hemolytic anemia (weakness/fatigue). CNS involvement and fever may be present but are unusual, in distinction from TTP. Anemia, with fragmented red cells on peripheral smear, thrombocytopenia, leukocytosis, and elevations in BUN, creatinine, and lactate dehydrogenase (LDH) are expected. Coagulation tests should show a normal PT/PTT, elevated FDPs, and raised fibrinogen levels; however, DIC may occur in complicated cases.

Patients diagnosed with HUS require admission for close supportive care and monitoring for development of complications. About 75% of cases need dialysis before return of adequate renal function, but most patients need no other specific therapy. Potential complications include CNS involvement (hyponatremic seizures, cerebral infarction), pancreatic islet cell necrosis leading to diabetes mellitus, bowel infarction, arterial thrombosis, and congestive heart failure. Heparinization, plasmapheresis, or plasma exchange with FFP may become necessary. Fortunately, the vast majority of patients survive with mild renal impairment as the only sequela. Recurrence of HUS is uncommon.

TTP is found most often in young adults with a 2:1 female predominance. Symptoms are variable, with vague, nonspecific complaints such as fatigue, malaise, abdominal pain, and weakness. Onset is usually acute, over hours to days, without a distinct prodromal illness. The classic pentad of neurologic signs and symptoms, hemolytic anemia, thrombocytopenia, renal disease, and fever is seen in 40% to 50% of patients. Kidney failure is significantly less common than in HUS. Diagnosis of TTP can be difficult, requiring exclusion of diseases with similar presentations, such as autoimmune hemolytic anemia, systemic lupus erythematosus (SLE), preeclampsia/eclampsia, postpartum renal failure, sepsis/endocarditis, vasculitis, and drug reactions. Laboratory abnormalities are similar to those in HUS, but also include hyperbilirubinemia.

Diagnosis or suspicion of TTP mandates admission. Treatment consists of PO or IV glucocorticoids depending on the severity of illness. Lack of response, deterioration, and prominent CNS involvement are indications for plasmapheresis and plasma exchange with FFP. Splenectomy may help in refractory cases. Unlike HUS, recurrences of TTP are common. Treatment reduces mortality from approximately 80% to less than 10%.

Drug Inactivation of Platelets

A variety of vascular diseases are treated with drugs that block platelet deposition on the surface of disrupted atherosclerotic plaques, preventing thrombotic and embolic complications. Typical indications for antiplatelet therapy include myocardial infarction, stable and unstable angina, stroke, transient ischemic attacks, atrial fibrillation, and chronic lower extremity ischemia.

Acetylsalicylic acid (ASA or aspirin) is the most commonly used antiplatelet drug due to its low cost, wide availability, relative safety, and demonstrated efficacy. Aspirin permanently acetylates the prostaglandin-producing enzyme cyclooxygenase, preventing production of thromboxane (TXA_2). Prolongation of bleeding time and decreased platelet aggregation are seen within 2 hours after ingestion, and since this inhibition is permanent, the effect lasts 2 to 4 days. Aspirin simultaneously inhibits endothelial cyclooxygenase, blocking production of prostacyclin (PGI_2), a platelet function inhibitor. However, this latter effect is mitigated by renewal of endothelial cyclooxygenase in 24 to 48 hours and lower sensitivity of the endothelial enzyme to ASA. With the generally recommended administration of aspirin (60 to 325 mg QD or QOD), the net effect is antithrombotic.

Complications of aspirin therapy are well known and potentially serious. Gastrointestinal symptoms are related to dose and especially common with more than 975 mg (three regular tablets) daily. Bruising, GI bleeding, postoperative hemorrhage, and epistaxis are more common in patients taking aspirin.

NSAIDs are reversible cyclooxygenase inhibitors. The antiplatelet effect of NSAIDs lasts only 6 to 24 hours, depending on the drug's half-life. β-Lactam antibiotics in sustained, high doses can impair platelet function by membrane binding, and lasting up to 7 to 10 days after withdrawal of therapy.

Discontinuation of the offending agent is the first line of therapy in bleeding associated with antiplatelet drugs. Severe hemorrhage is managed with DDAVP (0.3 mg/kg IV), and platelet transfusions if necessary.

von Willebrand's Disease

von Willebrand's disease (vWD) is a collection of quantitative and qualitative deficiencies of von Willebrand factor (vWF). vWD is the most common genetic bleeding disorder, with a prevalence of roughly 1% in the general population, although many cases are mild or clinically asymptomatic. The majority of identified patients are heterozygotes, for these autosomal dominant traits and have mild bleeding manifestations. Homozygotes or mixed heterozygotes have severe disease.

vWF is a glycoprotein synthesized by endothelial cells and megakaryocytes, and stored in the endothelium and in platelet granules. vWF acts as a bridge between platelets and exposed subendothelium, serving as the basis for formation of a hemostatic plug. In addition, vWF complexes with and stabilizes factor VIII, protecting it from rapid clearance. vWF is found in multimers of varying sizes; large multimers are the active form.

vWD is classified according to the type of vWF deficiency. Roughly 80% of patients have type I-vWD, a quantitative deficiency where all multimers are affected. Type II-vWD occurs in 15% to 20% of cases and results from a relative paucity of large multimers. Type IIB-vWD is a subclass characterized by platelet hyperaggregability. DDAVP is contraindicated in this type due to risk of inducing thrombocytopenia. Type III-vWD is a severe, usually homozygous form of the disease where all multimers are absent or nearly so. Acquired vWD can occur with or without autoantibodies, usually in association with myelo- or lymphoproliferative disorders, gammopathies or tumors.

Bleeding tendencies from vWD are typical of the kind found in platelet disorders: cutaneous manifestations (petechiae, purpura, ecchymoses), postoperative oozing (surgical wounds, dental extraction), and mucosal bleeding (epistaxis, gastrointestinal, menorrhagia). Routine coagulation studies are usually normal; however, the PTT is variable. Although bleeding time is prolonged, it does not distinguish among quantitative and qualitative platelet disorders. The platelet count is normal, except in type IIB-vWD where significant thrombocytopenia can occur. Often the most useful diagnostic aid is a positive family history or the patient's prior diagnosis of vWD.

Theoretically, treatment of bleeding in vWD depends on which type of the disease the patient has. However, clinically when a new diagnosis of vWD is suspected, a trial of DDAVP (0.3 mg/kg IV in 50 mL NS, over 10 to 15 minutes) is generally recommended as initial therapy (in the absence of known contraindications) for the following reasons:

1. Type I-vWD is most often encountered and should respond to this therapy, as well as most type II subclasses.
2. Some authorities report that type IIB-vWD is not an absolute contraindication to DDAVP, and that a drop in platelet count represents a pseudothrombocytopenia.
3. DDAVP does not affect type III-vWD, and is neither indicated nor contraindicated.

The next line of therapy is replacement of normal vWF through blood product infusions. Purified factor VIII concentrates also contain vWF. Of the commercially available preparations, Humate-P (Armour) is most recommended because it has the highest relative concentration of vWF. Dosage is by factor VIII activity, 50 to 60 U/kg given over 5 to 10 minutes. FFP could potentially be used, but the volume necessary would be prohibitive. Cryoprecipitate primarily contains factor VIII/vWF complexes and fibrinogen, but in a much smaller volume. Dosage is one to two bags per 10 kg body weight depending on severity of bleeding.

Selected Readings

Bell WR, ed. *Hematologic and Oncologic Emergencies*. New York: Churchill Livingstone, 1993.

Gilbert JA, Scalzi RP. Disseminated intravascular coagulation. *Emerg Med Clin North Am* 1993;11:465–480.

Hathaway WE, Goodnight SH. *Disorders of Hemostasis and Thrombosis: A Clinical Guide*. New York: McGraw-Hill, 1993.

Hoyer LW. Hemophilia A. *N Engl J Med* 1994;330:38–47.

Logan LJ. Treatment of von Willebrand's disease. *Hematol Oncol Clin North Am* 1992; 6:1079–1094.

Mammen EF. Coagulation defects in liver disease. *Med Clin North Am* 1994;78: 545–554.

Pfaff JA, Geninatti M. Hemophilia. *Emerg Med Clin North Am* 1993;11:337–363.

Tardio DJ, McFarland JA, Gonzalez MF. Immune thrombocytopenic purpura. *J Gen Intern Med* 1993;8:160–163.

Thorp JA, Gaston L, et al. Current concepts and controversies in the use of vitamin K. *Drugs* 1995;49:376–387.

55 Lymphomas

Robert F. McCormack

Lymphomas are a diverse group of solid tumors of the immune system. Primary categorization is between Hodgkin's disease and non-Hodgkin's lymphoma. Both Hodgkin's and non-Hodgkin's lymphoma have a variety of pathologic and clinical subtypes with unique clinical manifestations and prognoses. While Hodgkin's disease spreads locally to contiguous lymphoidal tissue, non-Hodgkin's lymphoma disseminates via a hematogenous route. The prognosis of treated Hodgkin's disease is excellent with a cure rate of 85% whereas treatment of non-Hodgkin's lymphoma results in a 30% to 40% cure rate. Emergency physicians need to recognize the primary presentations and recurrences of lymphoma as well as the complications of disease progression and treatment. Sophisticated staging protocols and evolving treatment options are beyond the necessary expertise of the field of emergency medicine (**Table 55.1**).

Initial presentation of Hodgkin's disease (HD) and non-Hodgkin's lymphoma (NHL) may be very subtle. Diagnosis is typically made on an outpatient basis but certain findings should prompt the emergency physician to assure adequate follow up. A single isolated lymph node of greater than 1 cm size which persists longer than 4 weeks, in the absence of infection, should prompt an investigation for lymphoma. Unexplained mediastinal adenopathy on a CXR may also be due to lymphoma. Patients with advanced undiagnosed disease or recurrence may present with a multitude of complaints which may require in-depth evaluation in the emergency department.

Hodgkin's Disease

Clinical Features and Differential Diagnosis

Hodgkin's disease (HD) in 70% of cases presents as a solitary or group of persistent lymph nodes that are nontender, mobile, and firm. The adenopathy tends to be axial with the majority in the neck or supraclavicular region. Most patients (60%) will have hilar adenopathy. Growth of these nodes may be very slow and occasionally may show temporary regression. A minority of HD patients will have symptoms related to their disease. Thirty percent will have constitutional symptoms (night sweats, low grade fever, or unexplained weight loss). Occasionally, a pruritic generalized skin rash may be present.

Advanced disease may present with cough, chest pain, shortness of breath, obstruction of the superior vena cava, bone pain, spinal cord compression, abdominal pain, bowel disturbances, ascites or, rarely, with headache or visual disturbances.

Differential diagnosis of cervical adenopathy includes bacterial or viral pharyngitis, infectious mononucleosis, toxoplasmosis, non-Hodgkin's lymphoma and nasopharyngeal or thyroid cancers. Mediastinal adenopathy can be related to pulmonary infections, sarcoid, tuberculosis, histoplasmosis, or lung cancer.

Epidemiology and Classification

There are 7,500 new cases of Hodgkin's disease diagnosed each year in the United States. There is a bimodal age peak between ages 15 to 35 and over 50 years. It is more prevalent in males. Epstein Barr virus genome is found in a subset of cases suggesting a causative role. Identical twin studies indicate a genetic contribution. An increased risk of both HD and NHL is seen in patients with immunodeficiencies (including AIDS) and autoimmune disorders.

Diagnosis is made by tissue biopsy demonstrating Reed Steinberg cells in the appropriate cytoarchitectural milieu. Four different subtypes have been identified: lymphocyte predominant, nodular sclerosis, mixed cellularity, and lymphocyte depleted. Treatment and prognosis is dependent upon the stage of disease. Staging is determined by the Ann Arbor Classification (**Table 55.2**). Constitutional symptoms of fever, weight loss, and sweats are designated by suffix B, and their absence by suffix A. Extralymphatic disease is designated by a suffix E. Solitary involvement of the lung or bone may be classified as E, whereas multifocal involvement, bone marrow, or liver involvement is always disseminated disease.

Lab Abnormalities

Moderate normochromic normocytic anemia and a moderate to marked leukocytosis may be present before treatment.

Table 55.1

Lymphomas

	Hodgkin's	Non-Hodgkin's
Localized	Common	Uncommon
Nodal spread	Contiguous	Discontiguous
Extranodal	Uncommon	Common
Mediastinal	Common	Uncommon
Abdominal	Uncommon	Common
Bone marrow	Uncommon	Common
Systemic Symptoms	Common	Uncommon
Curability	>85%	30–40%

Treatment

Stage IA or IIA is treated with radiation therapy. Stage IB or IIB is treated with radiation therapy with or without the addition of chemotherapy because of a greater risk (20%) of recurrence. Stage II with bulky mediastinal disease is treated with combined chemotherapy and radiation therapy. Stage III and IV is treated with combination chemotherapy. Salvage therapy with high dose chemotherapy and bone marrow transplant may be necessary for recurrent disease.

When radiotherapy is considered, a staging laparotomy may be indicated. Patients who undergo staging laparotomy will undergo splenectomy as well.

Hodgkin's disease impairs cellular immunity (anergy). Humoral immunity is usually preserved (except postsplenectomy). HD patients experience a higher than normal incidence of herpes zoster and warts, but are not typically plagued by opportunistic infections.

Table 55.2

The Ann Arbor Staging System for Hodgkin's Disease

Stage I: Involvement of a single lymph node region or single extralymphatic site

Stage II: Involvement of two or more lymph node regions on the same side of the diaphragm

Stage III: Involvement of lymph node regions or extralymphatic sites on both sides of the diaphragm, and may include the spleen

Stage IV: Disseminated involvement of one or more extralymphatic organs with or without lymph node involvement

  A: Absence of systemic symptoms (fever > 38°, sweats, weight loss > 10%, TBW < 6 months)

  B: Presence of systemic symptoms

  E: Localized extranodal contiguous extension

Prognosis

Eighty-five percent of patients with Hodgkin's disease are curable. Fifty percent of patients with recurrent disease are cured with salvage therapy.

Non-Hodgkin's Lymphoma (NHL)

Clinical Features and Differential Diagnosis

More than two-thirds of patients diagnosed with NHL present with persistent, painless, peripheral adenopathy. The adenopathy may be generalized and may wax and wane with time. Waldeyer's ring (tonsils, base of tongue, nasopharynx) and epitrochlear adenopathy is more common with NHL. Systemic symptoms of weight loss, night sweats and fever, as well as mediastinal adenopathy occur in 20% of cases, and are less common than in HD. Retroperitoneal, mesenteric, and pelvic nodes are not uncommon but rarely cause symptoms. Aggressive forms of NHL can present as abdominal obstruction or distention, spinal cord compression or rarely as meningitis. Bone pain with lytic lesions may indicate primary bone lymphomas.

Generalized adenopathy must be distinguished from infectious mononucleosis, CMV or HIV infection.

Epidemiology and Classification

The Ann Arbor staging system (Table 55.2) is used for both HD and NHL. Since NHL typically disseminates hematogenously, this staging system is not as useful as with HD. In contrast to HD, only a small number of NHL patients have localized disease on staging and are appropriate for radiation therapy.

The histologic classification of NHL is based upon assessment of the overall pattern of lymph node architecture, as well as on the cytologic classification of the neoplastic cell. A number of different classification systems are in use for NHL. Most helpful to the clinician is the Revised European American Lymphoma (REAL) classification, which divides lymphomas into indolent, aggressive and highly aggressive. Indolent lymphomas (survival of untreated disease measured in years) account for 35% to 40% of all NHL. In 1999, 24,000 cases were diagnosed in the United States. Aggressive lymphomas (survival of untreated disease measured in months) accounted for 50% NHL with 30,000 cases in United States in 1999. Highly aggressive lymphomas (survival of untreated disease measured in weeks) represent 5% of all NHL, with 3,000 cases diagnosed in the United States in 1999 (**Table 55.3**).

Lab Abnormalities

Anemia, thrombocytopenia, and less commonly leukopenia may be seen on diagnosis. Hypercalcemia or hyperuricemia are more common after treatment has been initiated.

Table 55.3

WHO/REAL Classification of the Non-Hodgkin's Lymphomas, According to Clinical Aggressiveness

The indolent lymphomas
  B-cell neoplasms
    Small lymphocytic lymphoma/B-cell chronic lymphocytic leukemia
    Lymphoplasmacytic lymphoma (+ Waldenström's macroglobulinemia)
    Plasma cell myeloma/plasmacytoma
    Hairy cell leukemia
    Follicular lymphoma (grade I and II)
    Marginal zone B-cell lymphoma
    Mantle cell lymphoma
  T-cell neoplasms
    T-cell large granular lymphocyte leukemia
    Mycosis fungoides
    T-cell prolymphocytic leukemia
  Natural killer cell neoplasms
    Natural killer cell large granular lymphocyte leukemia
The aggressive lymphomas
  Follicular lymphoma (grade III)
  Diffuse large B-cell lymphoma
  Peripheral T-cell lymphoma
  Anaplastic large cell lymphoma, T/null cell
The highly aggressive lymphomas
  Burkitt's lymphoma
  Precursor B lymphoblastic leukemia/lymphoma
  Adult T-cell lymphoma/leukemia
  Precursor T lymphoblastic leukemia/lymphoma

Treatment

Indolent lymphomas may be observed for years with minimal clinical symptoms. Single or combination chemotherapy may be necessary, but complete cures are uncommon. Aggressive lymphomas are commonly cured with combination chemotherapy but are rapidly fatal if not treated or unresponsive to therapy. Treatment failures may require a more aggressive chemotherapy and bone marrow transplant.

Hodgkin's Disease and Non-Hodgkin's Lymphoma Treatment Complications

Transient xerostomia, pharyngitis, fatigue, and weight loss are common with local radiation therapy. Fifteen percent of patients experience Lhermitte's syndrome (paresthesias in the lower extremities upon flexion of neck or thighs), which resolves spontaneously and has no correlation to irreversible spinal injury. Pulmonary fibrosis, pneumonitis, cardiac effusion, accelerated coronary artery disease (threefold increase in risk of fatal myocardial infarction), and hypothyroidism are less common, but known side effects. There is a 0.5% to 1% risk per year of second malignancies. Pelvic radiation may cause diarrhea, bladder irritation, and infertility.

Chemotherapy complications include nausea, vomiting, and bone marrow suppression. Neutropenic patients are susceptible to infection and require aggressive evaluation and antibiotic coverage when they present with fever. Two percent of patients who receive chemotherapy develop myelodysplasia or acute leukemia within 4 to 6 years. Fatal pulmonary toxicity and infertility are possible, depending upon the chemotherapy agents administered.

Acute tumor lysis syndrome following initial treatment can produce hyperuricemia, renal failure, and hyperkalemia requiring emergent treatment.

Selected Readings

Armitage JO, Longo DL. Malignacies of lymphoid cells. In: *Harrison's Textbook of Medicine,* 15th ed. New York: McGraw-Hill, 2001:715–727

Urba WJ, Longo DL. Hodgkin's disease. *N Engl J Med* 1992;326:678–687.

Canellos GP, Lister TA, Sklar JL. *The Lymphomas.* Philadelphia: W.B. Saunders Company, 1998.

Red Blood Cell Disorders

Jeanne M. Basior

Anemia

The primary function of erythrocytes is the transport of hemoglobin, which transfers oxygen and carbon dioxide at the cellular level. Anemia results from hemorrhage, dilution, insufficient production of red blood cells (RBCs), production of abnormal erythrocytes, or increased peripheral destruction (hemolysis) (**Table 56.1**).

Insufficient Production

Hypochromic/Microcytic

This group of anemias occurs as a result of marrow hypoproliferation. The most common is iron deficiency anemia. Causes of iron deficiency include physiologic changes (pregnancy, menstruation), bleeding, chronic hemolytic disease, or decreased iron intake (dietary deficiency, malabsorption). Erythrocyte precursors require iron to synthesize heme from porphyrin. Insufficient iron results in erythrocytes that are smaller in size. Lab abnormalities include decreased serum iron levels and decreased transferrin saturation. Transferrin is a protein that binds and delivers iron to tissues. The total of all binding sites of circulating transferrin make up the total iron binding capacity (TIBC) of plasma. In the normal state, 20% to 45% of the transferrin binding sites are filled with iron. Thus the TIBC is higher than normal. The reticulocyte count is usually normal, because there is insufficient substrate for erythroid precursors to proliferate. Serum ferritin levels, which reflect iron stores in the body, are decreased.

Patients with suspected iron deficiency anemia should be evaluated for hemodynamic compromise. Possible extravascular blood loss should be determined, and menstrual or pregnancy status verified. Treatment of severe anemia may require packed red cell transfusion, but more commonly is accomplished with iron replacement therapy. Oral ferrous sulfate 325 mg (65 mg elemental iron) three times daily for 6 months restores total body stores.

Microcytic iron-deficiency anemia is an important manifestation of chronic lead toxicity, especially in the pediatric population. Free erythrocyte protoporphyrin (FEP) and serum lead assays confirm the diagnosis.

Hereditary or acquired sideroblastic anemias involve the inhibition of heme synthesis. Ineffective utilization of iron results in accumulation of iron around the nuclei of erythroid precursors resulting in a morphologically peculiar cell within the marrow, termed the ringed sideroblast. The acquired forms may be associated with inflammatory or neoplastic processes or due to specific agents including isoniazid, alcohol, lead, and chemotherapy agents. Most commonly, acquired sideroblastic anemia is idiopathic and occurs in older patients. Treatment is supportive and includes marrow stimulators, such as erythropoietin.

Normochromic Normocytic

Anemias with normal RBC indices include a wide variety of disorders of diverse etiology, but generally fall into two groupings: marrow hypoproliferation and hemorrhage. Acute extravascular blood loss, whether apparent or occult, must be ruled out in any patient presenting with a low hematocrit and normal indices. Mild iron deficiency anemia presents with a normal mean corpuscular volume (MCV). Aplastic anemia is also characterized by normal indices. Pure red cell aplasia is manifest by a normochromic, normocytic anemia with normal leukocyte and platelet counts. Chronic renal failure results in a deficiency of erythropoietin, a glycoprotein hematopoietic growth factor synthesized by kidney cells in response to alterations in tissue oxygen tension in the renal microcirculation. Erythropoietin replacement is the treatment.

A wide variety of miscellaneous disorders are associated with a chronic normocytic, normochromic anemia. These include chronic inflammatory conditions, such a rheumatoid arthritis, systemic lupus erythematosus, the vasculitides, and sarcoidosis. Chronic infectious processes such as tuberculosis, subacute bacterial endocarditis, osteomyelitis, and lung abscesses demonstrate a similar type of anemia. A group of hormone deficiency states (hypothyroidism, panhypopituitarism, and Addison's disease) include anemia as a manifestation. These are correctable by adequate hormone replacement. The diagnosis of these disorders is usually one of exclusion after a trial of iron replacement fails to improve the hematocrit. Treatment is aimed at correction of underlying pathology.

Table 56.1
Types of Anemia

Hemorrhage: acute, chronic
Dilutional
Insufficient RBC production
  Microcytic: iron deficiency, lead toxicity, sideroblastic
  Normocytic: chronic disease, aplastic anemia
  Megaloblastic: folate, B12 deficiencies
Abnormal RBC production
  Cell defects: G6PD deficiency
  Hemoglobinopathies: SCD, thalassemia
Increased RBC Destruction/Hemolysis
  Immune-mediated: drugs, transfusions, toxins, venoms, cold agglutinins
  Microangiopathic: HUS, abnormal heart valves, eclampsia, intravascular trauma
  Membrane defects: spherocytosis

Megaloblastic

Megaloblastic anemia is due to impaired DNA synthesis with continued precursor cell growth, resulting in a macrocytosis. Megaloblastic cells are destroyed within the marrow, resulting in ineffective erythropoiesis. Abnormal cell morphology is evident on the peripheral smear, including macrocytosis with an MCV over 100, hypersegmented neutrophils, and giant platelets. The reticulocyte index is characteristically normal.

Folate deficiency results in a megaloblastic anemia. Dietary deficiencies of fruits and vegetables, malabsorption disorders, increased physiologic demands (e.g., pregnancy), and toxins can cause folate deficiencies. Ethanol depletes hepatic stores of folate. Methotrexate acts as a folate antagonist by inhibiting dihydrofolate reductase, the enzyme that converts folate to its active state. Other toxins such as triamterene and trimethoprim act as folate antagonists. Diagnosis is confirmed by serum folate assay. Treatment consists of oral folate replacement, 1 mg daily, with dietary correction.

Vitamin B_{12} (cyanocobalamin) deficiency results in a megaloblastic anemia. Dietary deficiency of animal products, malabsorption or competition for vitamin B_{12} are the principal causes. A spectrum of neurologic symptoms, including peripheral and central manifestations, as well as organic psychoses, is associated with B_{12} deficiency. Absorption of vitamin B_{12} depends on a glycoprotein (intrinsic factor), produced by parietal cells of the gastric mucosa. Ingested B_{12} joins with intrinsic factor, allowing absorption of B_{12} in the terminal ileum. Pernicious anemia is the most common cause of B_{12} deficiency. This involves an autoimmune destruction of parietal cells with gastric mucosal atrophy, reducing the production of intrinsic factor. This condition occurs most frequently in patients over age 60.

Other causes of vitamin B_{12} deficiency include partial and total gastrectomy, congenital abnormalities of the gastric mucosa, and competitive absorption of B_{12} due to ex-

cessive bacterial colonization of the small intestine within strictures, diverticula, or blind loops. Antineoplastic drugs may result in megaloblastic anemia due to inhibition of DNA synthesis. Macrocytosis may also be cause by hemolysis, alcoholism, hypothyroidism, and hepatic disease.

B_{12} deficiency is confirmed by serum assay. The Schilling test can define etiology. Oral radiolabeled cobalamin is administered, and a 24-hour urine collection reflects the absorption of cobalamin. In the second part of the Schilling test, a radiolabeled cobalamin–intrinsic factor complex is administered, and absorption is again measured. Low absorption in the first stage, with normalized absorption in the second, suggests pernicious anemia. Low absorption in both stages suggests bacterial overgrowth. Treatment consists of replacement with vitamin B_{12}.

Abnormal RBC Production

Glucose-6-Phosphate Dehydrogenase Deficiency

Enzymatic defects in erythrocyte ability to metabolize cellular toxins result in premature RBC death. The most common of these is glucose-6-phosphate dehydrogenase (G6PD) deficiency, frequently seen in descendants of populations from central African and eastern Mediterranean areas. Clinically significant hemolysis develops only when the cellular environment is stressed beyond capacity. Common precipitating factors include infections, drugs such as sulfa compounds and antimalarials, metabolic acidosis, and exposure to fava beans. Mediterranean-type G6PD deficiency may present with a chronic hemolytic anemia due to a more severe enzymatic deficiency.

Hemoglobinopathies

Sickle Cell Disease/Trait

Adult hemoglobin (Hg A) consists of four globin chains, two α and two β, linked to a heme moiety. Many hemoglobin variants exist, but the most clinically significant is due to HgS. HgS differs from HgA by the substitution of valine for glutamic acid at the sixth position of the β chain. This substitution results in an alteration of the physical molecular structure, providing the basis for the pathophysiology of sickle cell disease (SCD). When HgS is deoxygenated, the strands elongate, causing the characteristic sickle-shaped erythrocytes. Such RBC deformities obstruct the microcirculation, producing microinfarcts within organs. The chronic hemolytic anemia associated with SCD is a result of mechanical fragility.

SCD occurs in populations descended from areas where malaria is endemic, and is thought to provide a protective mechanism in this disease, which resulted in genetic selection. In the United States, 8% of the African-American population carries the HgS gene. The homozygous state, HgSS, occurs in 0.15% of this population and results in SCD. The heterozygous population, HgSA, is termed sickle trait. With trait, there is no sickling unless patients are subject to significant hypoxia, e.g., high altitude.

There is an increased incidence of spontaneous hematuria, splenic infarcts, hyphema, and leg ulcers in these individuals. Hemoglobin electrophoresis is diagnostic.

Multiple heterozygous variants occur. HgSC results in a variable phenotypic expression, from asymptomatic to full disease. Retinopathy, avascular osteonecrosis, and acute chest syndrome are common. HgSbthal is prone to symptomatic disease and splenomegaly.

Diagnosis is usually made at 6 to 12 months of age, as fetal hemoglobin (HgF) declines. Infants often present with acute dactylitis, a symmetric painful swelling of the hands and feet due to bony infarcts.

Vascular occlusion and susceptibility to infection account for the manifestations of SCD. Infections due to encapsulated microorganisms (*Streptococcus pneumoniae, Haemophilus influenzae,* and *Salmonella*) are particularly severe because these patients are functionally asplenic. The lungs, urinary tract, and bones are frequently affected. Pediatric patients are susceptible to meningitis and sepsis. Chronic penicillin prophylaxis may alter the clinical and culture data. Sickle cell patients younger than 5 years should be admitted for intravenous antibiotic therapy when infection is clinically suspected or proven.

Acute painful crises are the most common emergency presentation in adult sicklers. The long bones are more frequently affected than the axial skeleton. There is local tenderness on examination in the absence of a history of trauma. Repeated episodes result in avascular necrosis, especially in the hip and digits. There is no objective method to confirm this diagnosis, either clinically or in the laboratory. Precipitating factors that elicit or worsen sickling should be sought. These include infection, emotional stress, hypoxia, acidosis, dehydration, hemorrhage, and exposure to cold ambient temperatures.

Acute painful crises may also involve the chest, presenting with severe pain usually of a pleuritic nature, accompanied by dyspnea and hyperventilation. This is most frequently seen in the pediatric population. This is a diagnosis of exclusion and other causes of chest pain such as pneumonia, pulmonary infarcts, and myocardial ischemia must be eliminated.

An acute painful crisis involving the abdomen may occur. The examination is generally benign. This is also a diagnosis of exclusion, and a coordinated emergency evaluation, (including lab tests, x-rays, ultrasound examination, and CT scan) is usually required to rule out other causes of abdominal pain. Intraabdominal processes unique to SCD, such as splenic and hepatic infarcts and splenic sequestration syndrome, should be sought during the evaluation.

Moderate leukocytosis of 12,000 to 17,000 cells/mm is common in sickle cell crisis, and at baseline. Low-grade fever may be present with pain crises. Lab evaluation should be tailored to the presenting complaint and findings on physical examination, and specifically focused to exclude infection. This should include a CBC, and comparison with baseline values. The reticulocyte count is elevated in acute crises, unless there is an aplastic crisis. Hematuria may occur independent of urinary tract infections or nephrolithiasis. Laboratory evaluation should generally be more inclusive in the pediatric population.

Treatment of painful crisis includes aggressive oral or intravenous hydration. Although there is tissue hypoxia, supplemental oxygen has not been demonstrated to be of any benefit in limiting or relieving painful crises in the absence of hypoxemia. Sufficient analgesia must be provided in a timely manner. Patients can often guide their own therapy: They may be familiar with analgesics and doses that have been successful in the past. Patients may be maintained at home for chronic pain with daily analgesic therapy and an additional agent for breakthrough pain symptoms. Potent oral narcotics are available (e.g., morphine elixir) with a relatively rapid onset (usually within 30 minutes), and can be titrated with additional doses every 30 minutes. If IV access is initiated for other indications, titration of intravenous narcotics (morphine or hydromorphone) is effective. Patients who require admission may benefit from continuous infusion devices involving patient-controlled analgesia regimens (PCA pumps). Other parenteral routes of administration, such as intramuscular and subcutaneous, should be avoided since absorption is erratic, doses are more difficult to titrate, and areas of repeated injections develop scarring. Antiemetics may be provided parenterally or by suppository. NSAIDs can be used for additive analgesia. Infections should be treated with appropriate antibiotic coverage.

Pain crises usually resolve within 4 to 6 days, and may require admission if not adequately controlled in the ED. Patients who can be discharged from the ED should be provided with adequate oral analgesia and close follow-up.

Patients with SCD are subject to several processes affecting the cardiopulmonary system. Pulmonary infarcts from vaso-occlusion may occur and accumulate over time. Chronic tissue hypoxia may lead to the development of pulmonary hypertension and cor pulmonale. Cardiomegaly develops as a response to a high-output type of congestive heart failure and may progress to cardiomyopathy. Adult sicklers may have atypical chest pain, baseline hypoxia or a widened arterial to alveolar oxygen gradient. The typical chest radiograph shows bibasilar congestion due to a low-level congestive heart failure. Patients are also at risk for chronic pulmonary emboli from peripheral venous thrombosis or fat emboli from marrow.

A pediatric complication is the aplastic crisis with acute marrow failure due to infection or folate deficiency. A reduced reticulocyte count is pathognomonic.

Acute splenic sequestration of sickle cells occurs spontaneously and may result in a sudden precarious drop in hemoglobin to levels as low as 1 to 2. Presentation may be dramatic, with hypotension, syncope, and painful splenomegaly. Vigorous fluid resuscitation and transfusion, as well as a search for underlying infection, are indicated. Acute splenic sequestration of sickle cells occurs in children under age 6; after this age, the spleen autoinfarcts and is no longer functional. Acute sequestration may occur into adulthood in patients with HgSC or HgSbthal disease in whom splenomegaly persists.

Neurologic complications in SCD include transient ischemic attacks and stroke, with a high incidence in the pediatric population. Ischemic cerebral infarction results from sickle occlusion of large vessels. Treatment and diagnosis should parallel that of non-SCD patients. In addition, exchange transfusion may be indicated to improve blood flow to the infarcted area. Sicklers also have an increased risk of cerebral and subarachnoid hemorrhage.

Genitourinary complications of SCD may include gross painless hematuria secondary to renal parenchymal vaso-occlusion. Renal colic with gross hematuria results from renal papillary necrosis. Management is the same as that for non-SCD patients, with generous hydration prior to the administration of hyperosmolar contrast, or the use of nonionic contrast. Sickle sludging in the corpora cavernosa of the penis may cause priapism, which may persist for days if untreated. Management includes hydration, analgesia, and sedation as needed. Urgent urologic consultation for needle aspiration of the corpora, α-blockers or an operative shunting procedure may be indicated.

Other complications of SCD include leg ulcers; pathogenesis and treatment is the same as that for the microvasculopathy of diabetes. Ophthalmologic complications include proliferative retinopathy, retinal infarctions, and retinal detachment. Avascular necrosis, particularly of the digits in children and of the femoral head in young adults, is a complication that must be differentiated from osteomyelitis. The chronic hemolysis associated with SCD results in accumulation of pigment cholelithiasis. Acute cholecystitis is treated surgically.

The psychosocial aspects of SCD cannot be underestimated. Most SCD patients suffer complications less than yearly. A minority of SCD patients has frequent clinical deteriorations resulting in frequent hospitalization and ongoing debility. Patients with chronic pain syndrome and insufficient coping mechanisms have organic depression and dependent-type personality traits. Because there is no objective evidence for painful sickle crisis, some caregivers may tend to underestimate the behavior of SCD patients. There are no data that demonstrate an increase in drug-seeking behavior or drug addiction in this population. Many SCD patients are from disadvantaged backgrounds and use the emergency department (ED) as a primary source for acute care. Nonjudgmental compassion and appropriate medical care should guide the evaluation of each SCD patient.

Thalassemia

The thalassemias are a group of hereditary anemias resulting from defects in globin chain synthesis. They are found among patients descending from the Mediterranean and African countries, the Middle East, and Southeast Asia. The anemia is more profound than that found in iron deficiency.

There are a variety of genotypes and subsequent complications. Diagnosis is made by hemoglobin electrophoresis. Treatment includes genetic counseling and transfusions if necessary. Iron therapy is contraindicated. Life expectancy is decreased. Definitive therapy is bone marrow transplantation.

Hemolytic Anemia

This group of disorders is characterized by an increased destruction of erythrocytes. RBC destruction occurs most commonly through extravascular hemolysis within the spleen and liver. RBCs with abnormal structures or surfaces (e.g., bound immunoglobulins) are trapped within the microcirculation where they are removed by the reticuloendothelial system. Intravascular hemolysis is the other mechanism of RBC destruction. Erythrocyte trauma, complement fixation or exogenous toxins cause RBC lysis within the circulatory system.

Hemolytic anemia may be either acute or chronic. Acute crises produce marked anemia, and are the result of intravascular hemolysis. The anemia of chronic hemolysis is usually less severe. Findings include icterus, pallor, bony tenderness, splenomegaly, pigment cholelithiasis and signs of cholecystitis.

Laboratory findings include reticulocytosis (unless there is concomitant marrow failure), hemoglobinuria and hemoglobinemia. Unconjugated (indirect) bilirubin is elevated. Unconjugated bilirubin is bound to albumin and is not filtered by the kidney; thus, no bilirubin is excreted in the urine. In contrast, the hyperbilirubinemia of primary liver disease results in bilirubinuria. Haptoglobin is a plasma protein that binds free hemoglobin within the circulation and is subsequently rapidly removed from the circulation by phagocytosis. Thus, serum haptoglobin levels are decreased in hemolytic anemia. Free hemoglobin is bound by albumen to form methemalbumin; methemalbumin levels are increased with intravascular hemolysis.

The peripheral blood smear may demonstrate a number of abnormalities, depending on the etiology of the hemolytic anemia. Fragmented RBCs suggest traumatic injury, such as that due to cardiac valvular disease or to a microangiopathic process. Spherocytes, sickle cells, spiculated erythrocytes (acanthocytes), and target cells each suggest specific disease processes.

Extracorpuscular defects include a group of disorders that result in microangiopathic hemolysis. Mechanical trauma may occur when RBCs in the microcirculation are impacted by physical activities. Prolonged jogging or marching may result in hemolysis of normal RBCs. Mechanical trauma from shear stresses may fragment RBCs as they flow across pressure gradients created by diseased or prosthetic cardiac valves. Intrinsic vessel disease leading to fibrin deposition and hemolytic anemia occurs in eclampsia, malignant hypertension, renal graft rejection, and hemangiomas.

Congenital hemolytic anemia due to red cell defects includes three membrane abnormalities: spherocytosis, elliptocytosis, and stomatocytosis, which render cells more susceptible to lysis because of osmotic fragility of the cell membrane.

Hemolytic uremic syndrome, a disorder of unclear etiology with a mortality rate that approaches 20%, occurs primarily in children. It consists of a constellation of findings, including acute hemolysis, thrombocytopenic purpura, and acute oliguric renal failure. Often there is a viral prodrome. Treatment consists of transfusion and dialysis.

A similar clinical picture occurs with thrombotic thrombocytopenic purpura (TTP), which most commonly affects young women and is of unknown etiology. Acute hemolysis and thrombocytopenia occur in the face of normal coagulation tests. Fever, hemorrhage, constitutional symptoms, hepatosplenomegaly, and progressive renal failure occur. The clinical hallmark of TTP is neurologic involvement including altered mental status, focal findings, seizure, and coma. Treatment consists of high-dose corticosteroids and plasmapheresis.

Immune hemolysis occurs when antibodies coat RBCs and induce lysis. There is a spectrum of clinical presentations, from laboratory abnormalities with normal hemoglobin levels to fulminant hemolysis. This process may complicate lymphomas or systemic lupus erythematosus; it may occur as an idiosyncratic reaction to drugs (α-methyldopa, penicillin, quinidine) or it may be idiopathic. Treatment consists of steroids, splenectomy or immunosuppressive drugs. Complement fixation causes hemolysis in a group of disorders in which antibodies become reactive in colder ambient temperatures. So-called cold agglutinin disease is associated with infectious mononucleosis, mycoplasma pneumonia, and lymphoproliferative diseases. Transfusions may accelerate the hemolytic process and are contraindicated. Immunosuppressive therapy may be palliative. A similar immunohemolytic process occurs with transfused RBCs via previously acquired antibodies or pregnancy.

The Coombs test is diagnostic of immune hemolysis. A direct Coombs test is positive if specific animal antisera cause agglutination of a patient's RBCs. An indirect Coombs test distinguishes whether there is an antibody in a patient's serum that may react against other human RBCs.

Polycythemia

Polycythemia is a condition of increased hemoglobin (>18 g/dL) and hematocrit (>56%). It may be due to an absolute increase in red cell mass, or to a relative decrease in plasma volume. This relative erythrocytosis may be caused by any source of dehydration, and treatment is aimed at correction of the underlying disorder. Absolute erythrocytosis may be a physiologic response to any condition resulting in chronic hypoxia, such as chronic lung disease or high altitude. Tobacco smoking causes a polycythemia due to the relative tissue hypoxia caused by chronically elevated carboxyhemoglobin levels. Polycythemia causes increased blood viscosity and sludging in the microcirculation.

Polycythemia rubra vera is a disease process where there is absolute erythrocytosis in the absence of hypoxemia and splenomegaly. The minor associated criteria for this diagnosis are thrombocytosis, leukocytosis, increased leukocyte alkaline phosphatase, and increased vitamin B_{12} levels. The common presentations are ischemic cerebral infarcts and acute Budd-Chiari syndrome, an acute thrombosis of the hepatic veins or the infrahepatic vena cava resulting in the acute onset of massive ascites. Treatment is surgical thrombectomy. Maintenance treatment of polycythemia vera is chronic phlebotomy.

Selected Readings

Babior BH, Bunn HF. Megaloblastic anemias. In: Isselbacher KJ, Braunwald E, Wilson JD, et al, eds. *Harrison's Principles of Internal Medicine,* 13th ed. New York: McGraw-Hill, 1994:1726–1732.

Bayless PA. Selected red cell disorders. In: Moore GP, Jorden RC, eds. *Emergency Medical Clinics of North America: Hematologic Oncologic Emergencies.* Philadelphia: W.B. Saunders, 1993:481–493.

Bridges KR, Bunn HF. Anemias with disturbed iron metabolism. In: Isselbacher KJ, Braunwald E, Wilson JD, et al. *Harrison's Principles of Internal Medicine,* 13th ed. New York: McGraw-Hill, 1994:1721–1726.

Bunn HF. Disorders of hemoglobin. In: Isselbacher KJ, Braunwald E, Wilson JD, et al, eds. *Harrison's Principles of Internal Medicine,* 13th ed. New York: McGraw-Hill, 1994:1734–1743.

Bunn HF. Anemia associated with chronic disorders. In: Isselbacher KJ, Braunwald E, Wilson JD, et al, eds. *Harrison's Principles of Internal Medicine,* 13th ed. New York: McGraw-Hill, 1994:1732–1734.

Pollack CV. Emergencies in sickle cell disease. In: Moore GP, Jorden RC. *Emergency Medical Clinics of North America: Hematologic Oncologic Emergencies.* Philadelphia: WB Saunders, 1993:365–378.

Rappeport JM, Bunn HF. Bone marrow failure: aplastic anemia and other primary bone marrow disorders. In: Isselbacher KJ, Braunwald E, Wilson JD, et al. *Harrison's Principles of Internal Medicine,* 13th ed. New York: McGraw-Hill, 1994:1754–1757.

Rosse W, Bunn HF. Hemolytic anemias. In: Isselbacher KJ, Braunwald E, Wilson JD, et al, eds. *Harrison's Principles of Internal Medicine,* 13th ed. New York: McGraw-Hill, 1994:1743–1754.

Transfusions

Anthony J. Billittier IV

Component Therapy

Techniques for crossmatching, anticoagulation, preservation, and storage of blood have allowed for the practical use of blood since World War II. Type O universal donor blood was used successfully during the Vietnam War, and in the 1970s, transfusion of blood components, rather than whole blood, became standard. Advances in blood banking and transfusion technology continue to improve the safety and efficacy of blood component therapy; and nearly 29 million units of blood components were transfused in 2001.

Blood Banking and Compatibility Testing

Each unit of donor blood is typed for ABO and Rh red cell antigens, is screened for unusual antibodies to other red cell antigens, and is tested for infectious disease markers. If a unit of donor blood has no evidence of infectious disease it may be used as whole blood, or separated into up to four components such as packed red blood cells (PRBC), fresh frozen plasma (FFP), platelets, albumin, cryoprecipitate, or leukocytes. To produce these components, whole blood is centrifuged at low speed to separate the red cells from plasma and platelets. The platelet-rich plasma is then centrifuged at high speed to separate plasma from the platelet pellet. Albumin can be isolated from plasma by ethanol fractionation, and cryoprecipitate can be produced by freezing plasma and then collecting the insoluble proteins that separate out as the plasma is slowly thawed. Alternatively, greater quantities of platelets, plasma, red blood cells (RBC) or leukocytes can be collected from a single donor by apheresis. This technique involves collecting and centrifuging donor blood. Unneeded components are then returned to the donor.

Storage of separate blood components is superior to storage of whole blood since each component can be stored under different conditions to optimally preserve its function. PRBC can be stored up to 42 days when refrigerated between 1° and 6° C. Red cells can also be frozen with glycerol and stored up to 21 years. Platelets are stored at room temperature since their function is impaired by freezing and refrigeration; and platelets must be used within 5 days of collection because of the risk of bacterial contamination. FFP is plasma that has been frozen within 8 hours of collection to prevent plasma proteins from degenerating. Cryoprecipitate is also frozen and, like FFP, can be stored up to one year.

When the potential need for blood arises, a type and screen should be ordered. It takes 5 to 10 minutes to type a sample of the recipient's blood for ABO and Rh antigens. Type specific blood could then be made available to the patient. The recipient's blood is also screened for preexisting antibodies to other red cell antigens. This screen usually requires at least 30 minutes to complete. A type and crossmatch can then be completed within another 5 to 10 minutes. Units of blood that have been typed and crossmatched are typically not made available to other patients for 72 hours.

A and B antigens or agglutinogens are genetically determined molecules found on red cell membranes. Individuals with red cells that do not contain A and/or B antigen instead produce anti-A and/or anti-B immunoglobulin M (IgM) isohemagglutinin antibody, respectively. For example, type A individuals produce anti-B and type AB individuals produce neither anti-A nor anti-B. Identification of ABO blood type is important since transfusion of as little as 30 mL of ABO incompatible blood could result in agglutination, or an intravascular acute hemolytic transfusion reaction (AHTR), that can be life threatening. Individuals with type O blood (45% of Caucasians and 49% of African-Americans) are referred to as universal donors since their red cells can be given to patients with any ABO blood type; and those with type AB blood (4% of Caucasians and African Americans) are referred to as universal recipients since they have no anti-A or anti-B antibodies and can receive red cells of any ABO type. Forty percent of Caucasians and 27% of African Americans have type A blood, and 11% and 20% have type B blood, respectively.

The Rh antigen (most commonly the D antigen) is present on the red cell surface of approximately 85% of individuals. Unlike the ABO system, those who are Rh negative have no naturally occurring antibodies to the Rh antigen. However, they may become sensitized and produce antibodies (usually IgG), with a 30% to 50% incidence following fetal/maternal blood mixing or transfusion of Rh positive blood. Sensitized individuals are at risk of transfusion reactions in the future. Rh positive fetuses of sensitized Rh negative mothers are at risk of erythroblastosis fetalis or isoimmune hemolytic disease of the newborn. Therefore, when transfusing an Rh negative woman of childbearing potential, only Rh negative blood products should be used. If Rh negative blood products are not available, anti-D immunoglobulin (RhoGAM), 300 mg intramuscularly should be given with the transfusion. It should also be administered whenever fetal/maternal blood mixing is suspected in a mother who is Rh negative. RhoGAM contains human anti-Rh IgG and produces passive immunity. Circulating Rh positive antigen is thereby neutralized, and the development of active immunity in an Rh negative patient is suppressed.

Over 350 other potential red cell antigens are known to exist to which blood recipients may either have naturally occurring antibodies or produce antibodies following an exposure to these foreign antigens. These latter alloantibodies may cause clinical sequelae during subsequent transfusions; however, naturally occurring antibodies rarely cause hemolysis or other transfusion problems. Rather than complete testing of donor and recipient blood for all possible red cell antigen/antibody incompatibilities, a screen for the most common (yet rarely found) alloantibodies (e.g., Duffy, Kell, Kidd, Lutheran, MNS, P) is performed during a type and screen.

Crossmatching, or compatibility testing, refers to mixing recipient and donor blood and observing for macroscopic or microscopic agglutination (antigen–antibody reaction). Mixing recipient plasma with donor red cells is called the major crossmatch. The minor crossmatch is performed by mixing recipient red cells with donor plasma, but is no longer routinely performed. The crossmatch contributes little additional safety to a transfusion, but may reveal an error made during the donor or recipient type and screen.

Administration of Blood Products

Transfusion of blood and blood products (blood component therapy) can be used to correct hypovolemia, anemia, thrombocytopenia, and coagulopathy. Specific component therapy should be determined by the clinical needs of the patient.

Red Cells

Transfusion of red cells may be indicated whenever tissue oxygen delivery is inadequate secondary to an insufficient amount of hemoglobin, and the delay necessary for correction of the anemia (e.g., iron, vitamin B_{12}, folic acid, and erythropoietin) cannot be tolerated. Hematocrit and hemoglobin values may not be reliable, especially in cases of acute blood loss; and the decision to transfuse should be based on clinical status rather than an automatic numerical threshold (e.g., hemoglobin less than 8 or 10 g/dL). Physiologic compensation for chronic anemia may allow patients to remain relatively asymptomatic even with hemoglobins of 7 g/dL or less. However, patients with more rapidly developing anemia (e.g., secondary to

acute blood loss) and those with advanced age or co-morbidities such as pulmonary, peripheral vascular, or cardiac disease may not tolerate low hemoglobin states as well, although this has not been clearly defined.

Red blood cells undergo significant biochemical changes over time during storage. This storage lesion includes a decrease in red cell pliability; diminished red cell concentrations of 2,3-diphosphoglycerate (2,3-DPG) and adenosine triphosphate (ATP); a left-shift of the hemoglobin-oxygen dissociation curve; hemolysis resulting in elevation of plasma potassium, lactate dehydrogenase (LDH), and free hemoglobin; and production of waste products, including ammonia and lactate, resulting in a decreased plasma pH. The benefits from transfusion may diminish with the age of the PRBC.

A unit of whole blood contains about 450 mL of blood with a hematocrit between 35 and 40% and 50 mL of anticoagulant/preservative. Whole blood provides red cells, volume expansion, and some coagulation factors, and remains the ideal resuscitation fluid for patients with significant acute blood loss. However, the banking of fresh whole blood is not practical or efficient, so it is rarely available in the emergency department (ED) setting. Stored whole blood is devoid of functional platelets and contains decreased amounts of labile clotting factors (i.e., factors V and VIII).

PRBC have become the component of choice for correction of reduced oxygen carrying capacity. A unit of PRBC has a hematocrit between 65% and 80% and contains about 300 mL of volume. Unlike whole blood, a unit of PRBC has only about 50 mL of plasma that may contain ABO alloantibodies. Therefore, compatible, but not necessarily ABO identical, PRBC can be given if necessary since the risk of graft-versus-host reaction is minimal. Type specific or type O universal donor blood can be given safely to patients presenting with hemorrhagic shock resistant to crystalloid therapy who cannot wait the minimum of 45 minutes necessary to complete a type and crossmatch. PRBC are also devoid of functioning platelets and clotting factors, and administration of FFP and/or platelets may be necessary.

Each unit of whole blood or PRBC ideally should be infused within 2 to 4 hours. However, there is no limit to the rate of red cell transfusion or to the number of units that can be simultaneously infused in the unstable patient. A diuretic (e.g., furosemide) may be given for patients who are at risk of fluid overload. Standard blood infusion sets containing an in-line 170-mm filter to remove large particles allow for rapid infusion of 2 to 3 units before becoming obstructed. Filters with 40-mm pores may be used for newborns, patients needing multiple units, or patients with significant pulmonary dysfunction. Addition of 60 to 100 mL of 0.9% sodium chloride to each unit of PRBC reduces viscosity and allows for more rapid infusion.

A rise in the hemoglobin of 1 g/dL (hematocrit rise of 3%) can be expected after transfusion of one unit of whole blood or PRBC in an adult. In a child, a hematocrit rise of 1% can be expected after transfusion of 1 mL/kg of PRBC.

Leukocytes can be removed (leukoreduction) from PRBC by apheresis collection or filtration shortly after collection (prestorage) or during administration (bedside). Leukoreduction may be necessary for patients with a history of nonhemolytic febrile transfusion reactions or to minimize the risk of cytomegalovirus (CMV) infection. There are also conflicting reports that leukocytes may be responsible for posttransfusion immunosuppression. Although leukoreduction is the largest incremental blood production expense to date (about $30 per unit) and the cost-benefit ratio remains controversial, routine prestorage leukoreduction is becoming commonplace. Washed PRBC may be needed for patients who cannot tolerate leukocytes, plasma, platelet debris, or the extra potassium normally contained in PRBC.

Plasma

A unit of FFP contains between 180 and 300 mL of anticoagulated plasma, including most of the coagulation factors, albumin, and other proteins present in a unit of fresh whole blood. FFP contains no cells, platelets, or cellular debris, but may have red cell antibodies. Therefore, FFP must be ABO compatible but does not need to be Rh compatible or crossmatched. FFP should be ordered as soon as the need is recognized since thawing time is approximately 1 hour.

FFP is indicated for correction of coagulopathies of unknown etiology and coagulopathies caused by deficiencies of multiple coagulation factors including those vitamin K–dependent factors affected by Coumadin therapy. FFP may also be given for known factor deficiencies, such as hemophilia A or B, if specific factor concentrates or cryoprecipitate are not available. FFP is not indicated for nutritional purposes or for volume expansion since it has no proven benefit over crystalloid therapy.

Each unit of FFP contains about 200 units of each coagulation factor, and should raise these levels to 30% of normal in an average adult. Infusion of 5 to 10 mL/kg of FFP rapidly corrects most coagulopathies and bleeding caused by Coumadin. The usual initial dose of FFP is one or two units, but larger volumes may be required depending on the extent of the coagulopathy. Laboratory assays of coagulation function (e.g., PT, aPTT, INR) along with the patient's clinical status should be monitored to evaluate the response to FFP administration.

Each unit of FFP may be given over 15 to 20 minutes to patients with healthy cardiovascular systems. Patients prone to fluid overload should be given FFP more slowly, and administration of furosemide should also be considered. FFP can be infused through a filter with pores as small as 5 mm, but standard filters are probably adequate.

Platelets

A single unit of platelets contains most of the platelets separated from a single unit of donor whole blood. These are resuspended in 20 to 70 mL of plasma. Platelet concentrates may contain red cells, red cell fragments, lymphocytes, platelets with some A and/or B antigens, as well as anti-A and/or anti-B antibody depending on preparation technique. Therefore, platelets should be type specific, but do not need to be crossmatched. ABO typing is not an absolute requirement in an emergency; however, an Rh negative patient can become sensitized by platelets from an Rh positive donor.

Typically 6 or 10 single units of platelets are pooled and administered as a six-pack or a ten-pack as quickly as possible. Alternatively, a similar quantity of platelets may be harvested from a single donor by apheresis or plateletpheresis to minimize the risk of bacterial contamination and infectious disease, and/or to provide HLA-matched platelets. Platelet concentrates may be infused through a standard 170 mm filter. Microaggregate filters (20 to 40 mm) can trap platelets and slow infusion, and their use is controversial.

Platelet administration may be indicated for patients with platelet dysfunction and/or platelet counts less than $50,000/\mu L$ who have either evidence of microvascular bleeding or a planned invasive procedure (e.g., surgery). Surgery involving the eye or central nervous system should raise this "trigger" to $100,000/\mu L$. Prophylactic platelet administration should be considered for patients with platelet counts less than $10,000/\mu L$. However, in the presence of complicating conditions such as fever, other coagulopathy, or sepsis, this threshold should be increased to $20,000/\mu L$. Platelet counts between 20,000 and $50,000/\mu L$ are usually adequate for patients undergoing lumbar puncture and central venous catheter insertion. Bleeding time may have little predictive value in patients with thrombocytopenia.

Ten minutes to 1 hour after infusion of a single unit of platelets, an increase of 5,000 to $10,000/\mu L$ in the platelet count can be expected. A poor response to platelet transfusion may be secondary to a consumptive process such as disseminated intravascular coagulation (DIC), sequestration from splenomegaly, or destruction due to fever, sepsis or idiopathic thrombocytopenic purpura (ITP). Some patients may be refractory to random donor platelet administration because of antiplatelet alloantibodies that have developed as a result of prior exposure to foreign platelets. These patients may benefit from administration of platelets that are HLA-specific, crossmatched, donated by family members, or especially leuko-reduced.

Platelet administration may have a limited and temporary role in patients with conditions such as ITP and DIC, and whose underlying pathology also consumes, sequestrates, destroys, or otherwise inactivates the transfused platelets. Both uremia and recent aspirin ingestion can result in poorly functioning platelets. An individual with aspirin-induced thrombocytopathy may benefit from platelet transfusion; however, uremia must be corrected to improve platelet function. Platelet administration is relatively contraindicated in patients with heparin-induced thrombocytopenia, and may actually aggravate the thrombotic process in patients with thrombotic thrombocytopenic purpura (TTP) and HELLP syndrome (hemolysis, elevated liver enzymes, and low platelets).

Cryoprecipitate and Clotting Factor Concentrates

Cryoprecipitate is rich in some clotting factors such as fibrinogen, von Willebrand factor, and Factors VIII and XIII. It can be administered to patients with hemophilia and von Willebrand's disease bleeding, when more specific clotting factor concentrates are not available. Plasma concentrates including Factors VIII and IX, albumin, immune globulins (such as Rh immune globulin, or anti-thrombin III concentrate) are produced from pooled plasma. Despite the significantly increased risk of infectious disease from the pooling process, the enveloped viruses including HIV, hepatitis B and C viruses, HTLV-I and II, and West Nile Virus are able to be routinely heat or solvent-inactivated.

Complications

Increased awareness of infectious complications resulting from blood and blood component administration by both the public and medical community has changed the practice of transfusion therapy more than any other factor in the last few decades. Although careful donor screening and testing of donated blood have made the current blood supply safer than ever (i.e., blood safety), recipients of red cells, platelets, plasma, and cryoprecipitate are still at slight risk of transfusion-related infections. Albumin and other coagulation factor concentrates currently available are free from risk of infection because of improved purification and washing techniques. Unfortunately, these strides have not been matched by improvement in the non-infectious reactions and complications resulting from the actual process of transfusion (i.e., transfusion safety); and these risks (1 in 12,000 to 1 in 19,000 transfusions) are now much greater than the threat from infections (1 in 34,000 transfusions). Use of information technology (e.g., bar coding patients and units of blood products) does offer opportunity to reduce some of these ongoing risks.

Infections

Blood is not accepted from donors who participate in high-risk behaviors, such as intravenous drug use, homosexual activity, and encounters with multiple sex partners or those who have other risk factors, such as potential exposure to Creutzfeldt-Jakob disease (CJD) or variant CJD (vCJD), history of babesiosis or Chagas' disease or other recent illness. Blood that is collected is tested for evidence donor infection with HIV-1 and 2, hepatitis B and C, human T-cell leukemia viruses (HTLV-I and II), and syphilis. The Alanine aminotransferase testing (a surrogate marker for occult hepatitis infection) may also be performed, but is no longer routinely required by the FDA. Donor blood is discarded if any of these infectious disease markers are abnormal.

Although transfusion-related hepatitis infection has been more prevalent, greater public awareness, and almost certain mortality have made HIV the most feared pathogen. Only about 2.7% of all AIDS cases were thought to have resulted from administration of infected blood products; and pooled clotting factors were responsible for nearly one-third. Most transfusion-related HIV transmission occurred between 1982 and 1985 before widespread HIV antibody screening with a protein-based enzyme-linked immunosorbent assay (ELISA) resulted in a significant improvement in the safety of the US blood supply.

Since 1999, implementation of nucleic acid amplification testing (NAT) for the actual HIV-1 virus has further reduced the number of HIV infected units to less than 1 in 1,900,000.

Transmission of hepatitis B has become extremely rare because of testing for hepatitis B surface antigen (HBsAg) and core antibody (anti-HBc); and the frequency is not distinguishable from the background rate of the general population. However, documented cases of transfusion related hepatitis B infections still occur because of the "window period" between positive HBsAg and anti-HBc tests. It is estimated that the risk of hepatitis B transmission is 1 case per 137,000 to 200,000 units transfused; however, routine NAT for hepatitis B is currently under consideration.

Hepatitis C is now recognized as the agent formerly known as non-A, non-B hepatitis. Risk of hepatitis C transmission prior to the initiation of donor unit testing was 1 per 200 units transfused. In 1990, an ELISA test for hepatitis C protein became available. Since 1999, NAT for the hepatitis C virus has been routinely performed; and today, it is estimated that the transmission rate is less than 1 case per 1,000,000 to 3,000,000 units screened by NAT.

While normally transmitted by the bite of a mosquito during summer and fall months, West Nile Virus (WNV) was first documented to have been transmitted through transfusion in 2002. Blood centers have since begun stock piling frozen blood products collected during WNV-free months, as well as deferring donors who report recent fever and headache during WNV months. Routine nucleic acid technology (NAT) screening for WNV is also under development.

Human T-cell leukemia (HTLV) viruses have been causally associated with adult T-cell leukemia, spastic paraparesis, polymyositis, and progressive myelopathy. HTLV-I and HTLV-II have been identified, and screening of all blood products in the United States for anti–HTLV-I antibody began in 1989. This assay also has some cross-reactivity so that some HTLV-II antibodies may also be detected. Risk of transfusion-related infection with HTLV-I or -II is estimated at 1 per 641,000 units transfused. However, only approximately 5% of those infected will develop serious clinical disease.

Neonates and immunodeficient individuals including bone marrow and organ transplant patients are at risk of transfusion-related CMV infection. Risk for CMV infection is estimated to be less than 1 case per 1 million units transfused although roughly 50% of donors will be CMV-positive. Blood products can be tested for anti-CMV antibody. Alternatively, leukocyte-depleted blood can be used for these patients since CMV is associated with leukocytes.

Parvovirus B19, the cause of fifth disease or erythema infectosium, can also cause fetal death or serious disease following maternal infection. It may rarely induce aplastic crises in immunocompromised patients. Risk of transfusion-related infection is estimated at 1 per 10,000 units transfused.

Bacteria and/or bacterial toxins are 50 to 250 more likely to cause transfusion-related infection than viruses.

Serious bacterial infection, including septic shock, may result from transfusion of contaminated blood products. Because they are stored at room temperature, platelets are the most commonly contaminated component and must be used within 5 days to minimize this risk. Although underdetection and underreporting are likely, it is estimated that 1 in 100,000 platelet transfusions are clinically significantly contaminated. Some cold-growing bacteria, especially *Yersinia enterocolitica*, may infect PRBC stored between 1° and 6° C. Patients developing high fever and hypotension during a transfusion should be cultured and started on broad-spectrum antibiotics. The nontransfused portion of the offending blood product should also be sent for Gram stain and culture.

Transmission of syphilis, Lyme disease, malaria, Chagas' disease, leishmaniasis, toxoplasmosis, Babesiosis, hepatitis A, SEN virus, transfusion-transmitted virus (TTV), Epstein-Barr virus (EBV), exanthum subitum (roseola infantum), hepatitis GB virus (GBV-C), hepatitis G virus (HGV), and filariasis are theoretically possible, but exceedingly rare in the United States. While there are currently no screening tests for CJD or vCJD, there has never been a documented case of transmission through blood or blood component transfusion.

Transfusion Reactions

Non-infectious transfusion reactions are either hemolytic or non-hemolytic. Acute hemolytic transfusion reactions (AHTR) secondary to complement-mediated lysis of transfused red cells result from ABO incompatibility and occur within minutes of the start of transfusion. Complement-fixing antigen/antibody systems cause mast cell degranulation. Pulmonary dysfunction may result from granulocyte migration to the pulmonary capillary beds. Antibody-coated red cells may induce renal vasoconstriction and result in renal tubular acidosis and renal failure. DIC may also result from activation of the coagulation system.

Patients with AHTR may develop fever, chills, headache, dizziness, flushing, nausea, vomiting, joint or low back pain, bronchospasm, shortness of breath, chest pain, tachycardia, hypotension, shock, and sense of impending doom. Abnormal bleeding may be seen if DIC occurs. Hemoglobinuria and hemoglobinemia also acutely develop and are suggested by red urine or pink plasma. A decrease in the haptoglobin level and an elevation of the bilirubin and LDH levels may be seen within hours.

Treatment of a suspected AHTR should be initiated immediately since a mild, treatable reaction may become life-threatening. Transfusion should be stopped immediately, and any remaining blood product should be returned to the blood bank for testing. Copious intravenous fluids should be administered to maintain urine output of at least 100 mL per hour for 24 hours. Diuretics may be helpful, but the use of mannitol has become controversial. Pressors and bronchodilators may also be required. Administration of FFP and/or heparin may be indicated if DIC occurs. Close monitoring of urine output, renal function, electrolytes, and coagulation status is prudent. Hemodialysis may become necessary.

Extravascular AHTR develop secondary to ABO incompatibility when complement activation, but not fixation, of C3a and C5a occurs. Red cells with IgG antibodies on their surfaces are cleared by the liver and the spleen. These reactions result in a low-grade fever and mildly decreasing hemoglobin. They rarely cause hemoglobinuria and hemoglobinemia but do produce a positive antibody test.

Delayed hemolytic transfusion reactions (DHTR) result from gradual development of red cell antibodies following a transfusion. This condition usually does not present as an emergency, but rather is manifested as slowly decreasing hemoglobin 4 to 14 days posttransfusion. Gradual generation of C3a and C5a results in mild, sustained hemoglobinuria and hemoglobinemia. These reactions are often secondary to Rh incompatibility and acute development of Rh sensitivity, or anamnestic antibody production to the non-ABO system (e.g., Kidd). DHTR are not likely to require acute intervention, and patients are usually asymptomatic.

The most common causes of incompatible transfusion (called biological product deviations by the FDA) include clerical, laboratory, sample or patient misidentification or other human error. However, reactions can also be the result of preexisting alloantibodies missed on antibody screening of the recipient's blood.

A febrile nonhemolytic transfusion reaction should be suspected if the recipient's temperature rises more than 1° C during or after transfusion and no other etiology can be found. Fever and shaking chills, without hemoglobinuria and hemoglobinemia, are the hallmark of these reactions. These reactions are caused by agglutinating antibodies in the patient's plasma against antigens present on leukocytes or platelets in transfused products. The mediators of febrile transfusion reactions are interleukins, cytokines, and tumor necrosis factor. Symptoms usually begin shortly after the start of the transfusion, but may occur hours later. Symptoms worsen as the rate and volume of transfusion increase and may include true rigors, nausea, and vomiting. These reactions are self-limiting with defervescence occurring within 8 hours after transfusion, although elderly and compromised patients may experience respiratory failure or shock. Treatment consists of acetaminophen and patient reassurance. The transfusion should be interrupted temporarily while a sample of the donor blood is rechecked to assure that ABO incompatibility has not occurred. Patients with a history of febrile transfusion reactions should be premedicated and/or receive leukocyte-depleted blood products.

Allergic reactions to transfused products are characterized by the attachment of preformed antibodies to foreign plasma proteins (as opposed to cellular elements) leading to mast cell degranulation and histamine release. The majority of life-threatening anaphylactic reactions occur in recipients who have an IgA deficiency and therefore make antibodies to IgA. The incidence is higher in patients who have a history of prior blood transfusion. Blood recipients may also develop an allergic reaction to donor ingested food or medications. Less severe allergic reactions are termed anaphylactoid-type.

Symptoms of allergic reaction may include flushing of the skin, hives, increased respiratory tract secretions, increased vascular permeability, smooth muscle contraction causing bronchospasm, a sense of impending doom, and shock. Fever is not part of the symptomatology. Most allergic reactions occur within the first hour after the start of the transfusion. Treatment of a mild, urticarial reaction consists of temporarily stopping the transfusion and administering antihistamines until symptoms improve. If more significant sequelae do not develop, the transfusion may be slowly restarted. Therapy for anaphylactic-type reactions includes halting the transfusion; administering parenteral epinephrine, antihistamines, and steroids; and providing supportive care.

Other non-infectious complications of blood and blood component transfusion include volume overload, hypothermia, air embolism, and transfusion-related acute lung injury (TRALI), which resembles adult respiratory distress syndrome. TRALI, which is believed to be immune-mediated, begins within a few hours of administration, and is thought to occur in 1 in 5,000 transfusions. It usually resolves within 86 hours without sequelae but is fatal in 5% to 10% of cases. Treatment includes stopping the transfusion and supportive care.

Massive Blood Transfusion

Although many definitions have been suggested, transfusion of more than 10 units of PRBC acutely may be considered a massive transfusion. Complications of massive transfusion may be overshadowed by the danger of persistent shock and continued tissue hypoxia. In fact, many of the metabolic derangements often ascribed to massive transfusion such as acidosis, coagulopathy, and pulmonary injury may actually be due to persistent shock.

Hypothermia may be caused by the infusion of cold blood products and other fluids. Complications of this condition include decreased metabolism of lactate and citrate, increased hemoglobin-oxygen affinity, platelet dysfunction, coagulopathy, and cardiac arrhythmias. Devices may be used to warm blood to 40° C, but these may not be readily available. Infusion of warm crystalloid with red cells may be a practical alternative.

Red cell solutions contain significant amounts of citrate and lactate. Citrate is the anticoagulant used to keep blood products from clotting and lactate is produced by stored red cells. Metabolism of citrate and lactate in the liver usually occurs shortly after transfusion. However, if the transfusion rate exceeds one unit per 5 minutes or if liver function is impaired secondary to hypothermia, shock or chronic disease, citrate and lactate will not be cleared adequately. The excess citrate and lactate may cause metabolic acidosis.

Citrate also binds to ionized calcium in the circulation and may produce hypocalcemia. Severe hypocalcemia can cause ventricular fibrillation, decreased myocardial function, and hypotension. Routine calcium replacement is not recommended in such patients and should only be given if persistent hypotension or documented hypocalcemia are present. Calcium administration through the same intra-venous line used for transfusion may cause clotting in that line. Similarly, citrate has an affinity for magnesium; and administration of magnesium should be considered when conditions remain refractory to calcium administration.

Hyperkalemia may result from massive transfusion and can cause cardiac arrhythmias, especially with coexistent hypocalcemia. Potassium moves out of red blood cells during storage, resulting in high concentrations in the supernatant plasma. Excess potassium is usually drawn into cells or excreted shortly after transfusion. However, transient hyperkalemia may develop if transfusion occurs rapidly. Treatment of hyperkalemia is usually not indicated, but all patients receiving large-volume transfusion should be on a cardiac monitor. Patients with renal compromise are also at increased risk of significant hyperkalemia. Conversely, significant amounts of potassium may actually be taken back up by the depleted red blood cells and result in hypokalemia. This is more likely to occur with less rapidly administered massive transfusions.

A coagulopathy may be associated with massive transfusion. Thrombocytopenia and coagulation factor deficiencies may result from the delusional effects of blood products not containing platelets or adequate amounts of coagulation factors. Platelet counts, however, are usually not as low as would be predicted based on simple dilution. This is probably due to the release of platelets from the spleen and bone marrow. Further, even low concentrations of coagulation factors are usually adequate to prevent microvascular bleeding. Therefore, significant bleeding due to clotting dysfunction does not usually occur until 15 to 20 units of PRBC have been transfused. Shock, DIC, and platelet dysfunction can also contribute significantly to abnormal bleeding. Platelet dysfunction can be caused by hypothermia. DIC may occur in up to 30% of massively transfused patients probably secondary to diffuse hypoxic tissue damage from shock.

Although PT and aPTT levels greater than 1.5 times mean control suggest a significant coagulopathy warranting FFP administration, correction of coagulopathy often must be a clinical decision since platelet counts and clotting times are not immediately available and may not correlate well to a patient's actual coagulation status. Platelets and coagulation factors should not be administered prophylactically, but should be based on the presence of shock and the degree of microvascular bleeding. Transfusion of platelet concentrates may be considered for first-line therapy since thrombocytopenia may be the major factor and 6 units of platelets include about 300 mL of plasma that contains significant amounts of active coagulation factors. If bleeding continues, large volumes of FFP may be required. Cryoprecipitate may be helpful in patients with DIC since it contains significant amounts of fibrinogen.

Adult respiratory distress syndrome (ARDS) may result from sequestration of microaggregates in the lungs of patients receiving massive transfusions. Microaggregates are composed of fibrin, platelets, and white cells that accumulate in stored blood. It is difficult, however, to separate the effects of microaggregates from the effects of shock on the lung; and even the use of specialized filters to eliminate microaggregates (20 to 40 μ) does not completely prevent this pathology.

Anti-A and anti-B antibodies contained in the small amount of plasma of type O PRBC can become problematic for non-type O recipients following transfusion of large quantities of type O PRBC, as can future type and crossmatching. Of course, the risk from infectious disease transmission increases proportionately to the number of units transfused. The same is true for non-infectious transfusion complications.

Again, it is difficult to delineate complications of massive transfusion from those caused by the underlying condition that necessitated the massive transfusion. Aggressive and adequate treatment of hemorrhagic shock should be the first priority in these patients, especially since studies have failed to delineate a specific number of units beyond which transfusion efforts become medically futile.

Alternatives to Transfusion of Blood Products

Salvage of lost blood for the purpose of autotransfusion is done routinely in operating rooms via a cell saver apparatus. Blood from a sterile operating field is collected by suction and then separated, washed, and stored by the cell saver. This blood can then be reinfused, decreasing the need for homologous blood products. The use of a cell saver in the ED may not be as practical, since expensive equipment and setup time for collection of noncontaminated blood are necessary. Blood from a hemothorax is probably the only sterile blood that can be practically salvaged in the ED. Special chest tube suction reservoirs are available that can be attached to a standard chest tube collection system. The reservoirs can then be hung for immediate reinfusion of chest tube output. DIC is a complication and may be secondary to reinfusion of activated coagulation products especially if more than 1,500 mL are autotransfused.

The perfection of an oxygen-carrying blood substitute would be a significant breakthrough in resuscitation medicine. A practical substitute for red cell transfusion should effectively deliver oxygen to tissues, remove carbon dioxide from tissues, and maintain acid-base balance in the circulation. The product should be nontoxic and non-immunogenic, free from infectious disease, as well as have a reasonable storage profile and long half-life in the circulation. Hemoglobin is the ultimate oxygen transport molecule, and a useful blood substitute will most likely be a derivative of the hemoglobin molecule.

The infusion of non-modified cell-free hemoglobin is not an option since this has been shown to increase pulmonary vascular resistance and decrease cardiac output. Also, free hemoglobin is unstable, raises oncotic pressure, and is excreted by the kidneys. To circumvent these shortcomings, either free hemoglobin (collected from outdated human blood or genetically engineered or blood from animal species) may be attached to large molecules, crosslinked or polymerized. Phase II and III trials of a number of such compounds are now in progress. A more recent approach involves encapsulating hemoglobin using biodegradable polymers without surface antigens into synthetic RBC. Inclusion of antioxidants and other elements naturally found in RBC may result in a more physiologic product and reduce side effects.

The development of perfluorocarbons (e.g., Fluosol-DA) is a different approach to a practical blood substitute. Perfluorocarbon emulsions are inert halogenated liquids in which oxygen and carbon dioxide are extremely soluble, but are not yet routinely available.

Jehovah's Witnesses and Blood Transfusion

Jehovah's Witnesses are members of a Christian denomination that forbids the acceptance of blood transfusions. Whole blood, packed red blood cells, white blood cells, platelets, fresh-frozen plasma, and autologous stored blood are clearly prohibited. Other blood components and related therapy are accepted by some but not all Witnesses. Many Witnesses accept hemodialysis and heart-lung bypass, as long as the necessary equipment is used as an essentially uninterrupted extension of the circulatory system and blood is not used as a primer. The same principle is applicable to chest-tube reservoir autotransfusion systems. Albumin, hemophiliac factor preparations, serum-based immunizations, organ transplants, and epidural blood patches are also accepted by many but not all Witnesses. If the Witness believes the particular blood component therapy is not given to feed the body, but rather to fight against disease, it is more likely to be allowed.

When treating an adult Witness who is conscious and has decision-making capacity and who emergently needs blood component therapy, the emergency physician should consider the following:

- Discuss the need for transfusion with the patient when no family members, friends, or religious advisors are present.
- Inform the patient of the risks of refusing and of accepting the recommended blood component therapy. Specifically address whether the risk of HIV and hepatitis infection is a significant concern and put such risks in perspective. Alternatives to blood should also be discussed if they are reasonable options.
- Tell the patient that any decision he or she makes in regard to refusing or accepting blood products will be respected and, if desired, will remain absolutely confidential. If the patient accepts blood products, reducing the risk of death as a result of anemia or a coagulopathy, the appropriate blood product should be administered. However, transfusing with strict confidentiality in the ED setting is potentially difficult. Extra staff and resources should be devoted to this task, and resuscitation in the privacy of the operating room could be considered for trauma patients. If the patient refuses blood, make appropriate modifications in monitoring and treatment (e.g., admit to the ICU instead of a regular ward, surgery instead of observation for splenic trauma).
- Consider asking the patient whether blood will be allowed if it is ordered by a court. Some Witnesses have accepted a transfusion, as long as they did not

personally consent to it. A judge might order a transfusion under these circumstances.

A Witness who presents to the ED unconscious and in need of blood with a signed "No Blood" advance medical directive creates a dilemma encompassing potentially conflicting medical, ethical, and legal concepts. There are no rigid standards for blood to be withheld or given in such circumstances. Courts have both supported and ruled against physicians who have transfused unconscious patients in the presence of a "No Blood" advance directive. If an advance directive does not exist or is not available in a timely manner and the patient needs blood emergently, consider beginning transfusion—even if family or friends object. If an advance directive does exist, assess its authenticity. However, the presence of a "No Blood" advance directive, particularly a wallet card, does not necessarily ensure that informed refusal requirements are satisfied. Withhold blood if you believe that a "No Blood" advance directive satisfies informed refusal requirements, but transfuse if you do not believe informed refusal requirements are satisfied.

Contact a hospital administrator and/or attorney as soon as possible if an unconscious Witness in need of blood presents to the ED. However, do not assume they will have answers. Consult with a second physician, as well. Whether you withhold blood or transfuse, carefully provide and meticulously document evidenced-based care, as these cases are likely to be scrutinized extensively.

If time permits, an emergency court order can be obtained authorizing transfusion for a minor who needs blood emergently and whose Jehovah's Witness parent refuses to consent. However, blood should be given immediately if a legal proceeding will result in an unacceptable delay in treatment. A hospital policy should delineate the procedure for obtaining a court order to transfuse minors.

Selected Readings

America's Blood Centers. Detection of bacterial contamination in platelet components. In: Menitove JE, ed. *Blood Bulletin* 2003;6. http://www.americasblood.org/download/bulletin_v6_n4.pdf.

America's Blood Centers. Hemolytic transfusion reactions; part 1: biological product deviations (errors and accidents). In: Strong M, ed. *Blood Bulletin* 2002;3. http://www.americasblood.org/index.cfm?fuseaction=display.showPage&pageID=125.

America's Blood Centers. Infectious risks of blood transfusions. In: Strong M, ed. *Blood Bull* 2001;4. http://www.americasblood.org/index.cfm?fuseaction=display.showPage&pageID=123.

America's Blood Centers. Indications for platelet transfusion therapy. In: Strong M, ed. *Bulletin* 1999;2. http://www.americasblood.org/index.cfm?fuseaction=display.showPage&pageID=130.

America's Blood Centers. Leukocyte reduction of blood components. In: Strong M, ed. *Blood Bull* 1998;1. http://www.americasblood.org/index.cfm?fuseaction=display.showPage&pageID=134.

America's Blood Centers. The transfusion trigger updated: current indications for red cell therapy. In: Menitove JE, ed. *Blood Bull* 2003;6. http://www.americasblood.org/download/bulletin_v6_n2.pdf.

America's Blood Centers. West Nile Virus and the blood supply. 2003. In: Menitove JE, ed. *Blood Bull* 2003;6. http://www.americasblood.org/download/bulletin_v6_n1.pdf.

American Association of Blood Banks. *All About Blood.* www.aabb.org/All_About_Blood.

Beutler E, et al., eds. *Williams' Hematology,* 5th ed. New York: McGraw-Hill 1995.

Choudhry VP. Platelet therapy. *Indian J Pediatr* 2002;69:779–783.

Corazza ML, Hranchook AM. Massive blood transfusion therapy. *AANA J* 2000;68:311–314.

Dale DC, Federman DD, et al., eds. *Scientific American Medicine.* New York: Scientific American, 1995.

Dodd RY. Transfusion transmitted hepatitis virus infection. *Hematol Oncol Clin North Am* 1995;1:137.

Dodd RY. Viral contamination of blood components and approaches for reduction of infectivity. *Immunol Invest* 1995;24:25.

Donaldson MDJ, Seaman MJ, Park GR. Massive blood transfusion. *Br J Anaesthesiol* 1992;69:621.

Downes K, Sarode R. Massive blood transfusion. *Indian J Pediatr* 2001;68:145–149.

Draker RA. The development and use of oxygen-carrying blood substitutes. *Immunol Invest* 1995;24:403.

Drews RE. Critical issues in hematology: anemia, thrombocytopenia, coagulopathy, and blood product transfusions in critically ill patients. *Clin Chest Med* 2003;24:607–622.

Dzik S. Non-infectious serious hazards of transfusion. *Blood Bulletin.* America's Blood Centers. May 2002;5. http://www.americasblood.org/download/bulletin_v5_n1.pdf.

Dzik WH. Leukoreduction of blood components. *Curr Opin Hematol.* 2002;9:521–526.

Fakhry SM, Sheldon GF. Blood administration, risks, and substitutes. *Adv Surg* 1995;28:71.

Hellstern P, Haubelt H. Indications for plasma in massive transfusion. *Thromb Research* 2002;107:S19–S22.

Janatpour K, Holland PV. Noninfectious serious hazards of transfusion. *Curr Hematol Rep* 2002;1:149–155.

Jeter EK, Spivey MA. Noninfectious complications of blood transfusion. *Hematol Oncol Clin N Amer* 1995;1:187.

Kleimann I. Written advance directives refusing blood transfusion: ethical and legal considerations. *Am J Med* 1994;96:563–567.

Krombach J, Kampe S, Gathof BS, et al. Human error: the persisting risk of blood transfusion: a report of five cases. *Anesth Analg* 2002;94:154–156.

Labadie LL. Transfusion therapy in the emergency department. *Emerg Med Clin N Amer* 1993;2:379.

Lackritz EM, et al. Estimated risk of transmission of the human immunodeficiency virus by screened blood in the United States. *N Engl J Med* 1995;333:1721.

Lo B. *Resolving Ethical Dilemmas: A Guide For Clinicians.* Baltimore: Williams & Wilkins, 1995.

Lowe KC, Ferguson E. Benefit and risk perceptions in transfusion medicine: blood and blood substitutes. *J Intern Med* 2003;253:498–507.

Lozano M, Cid J. The clinical implications of platelet transfusions associated with ABO or Rh(D) incompatibility. *Transfus Med Rev* 2003;17:57–68.

Menitove JE. Transfusion medicine-2003: a comprehensive review, part 1. *Missouri Med* 2003;100:256–261.

Nacht A. The use of blood products in shock. *Crit Care Clin* 1992;2:255.

Prati D. Transmission of viral hepatitis by blood and blood derivatives: current risks, past heritage. *Digest Liver Dis* 2002;34:812–817.

Radhakrishnan KM, Chakravarthi S, Pushkala S, et al. Component therapy. *Indian J Pediatr* 2003;70:661–666.

Regan F, Taylor C. Blood transfusion medicine. *Brit Med J* 2002;325:143–147.

Roberts JR, Hedges JR, eds. *Clinical Procedures in Emergency Medicine.* 2nd ed. Philadelphia: WB Saunders 1991.

Rosen P, Barkin RM, et al., eds. *Emergency Medicine Concepts and Clinical Practice.* St. Louis, MO: CV Mosby 1992.

Tremblay LN, Rizoli SB, Brenneman FD. Advances in fluid resuscitation of hemorrhagic shock. *Cana J Surg* 2001;44:172–179.

Vaslef SN, Knudsen NW, Neligan PJ, et al. Massive transfusion exceeding 50 units of blood products in trauma patients. *J Trauma* 2002;53:291–296.

Viele MK, Weiskopf RB. What can we learn about the need for transfusion from patients who refuse blood? The experience with Jehovah's Witnesses. *Transfusion* 1994;34:396–401.

Walker J, Criddle LM. Massive transfusion: don't stop. *J Emerg Nurs* 2002;28:176–178.

Weil MH. Blood transfusions. *Crit Care Med* 2003;31:2397–2398.

Wright-Kanuth M, Smith LA. Transfusion-transmitted viruses. *Clin Lab Sci* 2003;16:221–229.

58 White Blood Cell Disorders

Robert F. McCormack

The complete blood count is one of the most frequently ordered laboratory tests in the emergency department (ED). The white blood cell count (WBC) is often incorporated in clinical decision making and many physicians would find it difficult to work without it. However, WBC is often over-utilized as a screening test and incorrectly relied upon to exclude significant disease. It is imperative that the emergency physician (EP) has an awareness of both the usefulness and limitations of the WBC in clinical practice.

A review of leukopoiesis (WBC development), normal age-related WBC counts and differentials, and physiologic leukocyte responses are covered in this chapter. Leukopenia and the clinical consequences are discussed. The significance of leukocytosis and bandemia are reviewed. Leukemia and multiple myeloma are discussed in detail.

Leukopoiesis

All WBCs are derived from multipotential stem cells in the bone marrow (**Table 58.1**). Stem cells develop into blast cells, promyelocytes, myelocytes, and metamyelocytes. Metamyelocytes then differentiate into neutrophils, basophils, and eosinophils. Blast cells also develop into monocytes, lymphocytes, and platelets. Maturation occurs within 2 to 9 days and primary disease processes may occur at any stage. Immature neutrophils may appear in the peripheral blood and are referred to as band cells.

Physiologic WBC Responses

An equal number of mature neutrophils adhere to the walls of blood vessels as are present in the peripheral circulation. These cells are undetected in the CBC as they are not circulating in the peripheral blood. Any stressors (i.e., trauma, seizure, intoxication) can move these cells into the peripheral blood elevating the WBC count, specifically the neutrophil count. This is referred to as demargination and may double the WBC (20,000 cells/mm^3). The differential should remain in the normal range and immature cells should not be seen in the peripheral blood (i.e., no

band cells). Steroid administration may also increase the neutrophil count to a similar degree but should peak within 4 to 6 hours and return to baseline in 24 hours.

A large number of developing cells exist in the bone marrow. WBCs may be released from the marrow into the circulation in response to infection or inflammation. Immature WBC forms may be seen in the peripheral blood elevating the band count. This is referred to as a left shift (toward more immature cells). This may increase the neutrophil count by 15-fold.

Leukopenia

Leukopenia (4,000 cells/mm^3) describes a decreased number of white blood cells. Accurate diagnosis requires a WBC differential and is usually due to a decrease in neutrophils. Neutropenia is an absolute neutrophil count [total WBC count × % (neutrophils + bands)] less than 1,500 cells/mm^3. Neutropenia may be caused by a multitude of processes (**Table 58.2**) including immunosuppressive therapy, sepsis, and drug reactions.

Neutropenic states below 500 cells/mm^3 are particularly worrisome for infectious complications. The EP should always consider neutropenia with a fever (>100.4° F) a true medical emergency. Neutropenia often masks what would otherwise be an obvious infection. The lack of neutrophils results in a diminished or absent inflammatory response, thereby dampening the usual signs and symptoms associated with infection. The production of purulent material is minimal, also are redness and swelling at the site of infection. Fever, however, is usually preserved in the neutropenic patient as a result of endogenous pyogens released from fixed macrophages in the liver, spleen, and lungs, and should be taken seriously when present.

Neutropenia with a fever requires a complete evaluation for the cause of the fever and prompt antibiotic therapy (**Table 58.3**). A complete history should be obtained to determine source of the infection. Headache, neck stiffness, cough, abdominal pain, diarrhea, pain on defection or ill contacts are particularly important. A through physical exam should be done with particular attention to the skin (rashes or cellulitis), meningeal signs (may be sub-

Table 58.1

Normal WBC Counts (with differential counts in absolute numbers)

Age	WBC ($\times 1000$/ mm^3)	Segmented Neutrophils ($\times 1000$/ mm^3)	Bands ($\times 1000$/ mm^3)	Lymphocytes ($\times 1000$/ mm^3)	Monocytes ($\times 1000$/ mm^3)	Eosinophils ($\times 1000$/ mm^3)	Basophils ($\times 1000$/ mm^3)
Newborn	9.1–34.0	6.0–20.0	<3.5	2.5–10.5	<3.5	<2.0	<0.4
1–23 mo	6.0–14.0	1.0–6.0	<1.0	1.8–9.0	<1.0	<0.7	<0.1
2–9 yrs	4.0–12.0	1.2–6.0	<1.0	1.0–5.5	<1.0	<0.7	<0.1
10–17 yrs	4.0–10.5	1.3–6.0	<1.0	1.0–3.5	<1.0	<0.7	<0.1
>18 yrs	4.0–10.5	1.3–6.0	<1.0	1.5–3.5	<1.0	<0.7	<0.1

Modified from *Interpretation of Diagnostic Tests,* 7th ed. Wallach J, ed. Boston: Little, Brown 2000.

tle), rectal exam (to exclude an abscess), and close inspection of any indwelling catheters including central lines, shunts, intrathecal catheters or urinary catheters. It may be judicious to initiate antibiotics prior to gentle rectal exam in the neutropenic patient to avoid bacteremia in the setting of a perirectal abscess. Laboratory investigation is listed in Table 58.3.

The majority of infections are caused by endogenous flora particularly from the skin and gastrointestinal tract. Gram-negative bacteria have previously accounted for up to 50% of infections. However, there has been a rise in gram-positive bacteria due to the increasing use of indwelling catheters and invasive critical care.

If the history, physical exam, and available test results reveal a source, antibiotic therapy should be directed at the cause of infection. Those patients with neutropenia and fever without a clear etiology of infection should receive broad-spectrum antibiotics and potentially broad-spectrum antifungal therapy (**Table 58.4**). Standard antibiotic regimens include broad coverage of synergistic and bactericidal combinations such as an aminoglycoside and extended-spectrum penicillin or third-generation cephalosporin. Treatment should begin as soon as possible and should not be delayed awaiting a lumbar puncture or lab results.

Patients should be continued on broad-spectrum antibiotics until the fever resolves, the neutrophil count increases and cultures are definitively negative. Most of these patients will require hospitalization, as the risks for sepsis and shock are significant.

Leukocytosis

An elevated WBC is a common finding with limited diagnostic value. The causes of leukocytosis are extensive and include infection, inflammation or any stressor that may cause demargination. Leukocytosis may also represent a primary blood disorder, such as leukemia.

A number of studies have looked at the reliability of an elevated WBC as an indicator of specific diseases and have demonstrated less than desirable results. Appendicitis may be present with a normal WBC, as may other infectious processes. Use of a normal WBC as exclusionary evidence of a significant infection is not supported by the literature. Differential counts, although helpful in theory, have been shown to rarely influence the clinical treatment and the EP should critically evaluate the benefit before reflexively ordering differential counts on all CBCs.

Leukemias

The leukemias are a heterogeneous group of neoplastic disorders derived from a hematopoietic cell line which in-

Table 58.2

Causes of Neutropenia and Neutrophilia

Causes of Neutropenia	Causes of Neutrophilia
Infections: Bacterial, Parasitic, Viral, Rickettsial	Infections: Bacterial, Parasitic, Viral, Fungal
Drugs: Sulfonamides, Antibiotics, Analgesics, Chemotherapeutic Agents	Inflammation
Ionizing Radiation	Drugs: Lithium, Glucocorticoids
Hematopoietic Diseases: Leukemias, Aplastic Anemia	Hemorrhage, Myocardial Infarction, Burns, Gangrene
Autoimmune disorders: SLE	Myeloproliferative Disorders: Leukemia, P. Vera
Hypersplenism, hemodialysis	Physiologic: Exercise, Stress, Menstruation, Labor
Nutritional: Alcoholism, B$_{12}$/Folate Deficiency	Metabolic: DKA, Acute Renal Failure

Table 58.3

Suggested Diagnostic Testing for Neutropenia with a Fever

- CBC, basic metabolic panel, LFTs, coagulation profile, two sets of blood cultures
- Urinalysis and urine culture (consider obtaining by catheter)
- Sputum Gram stain and culture
- Chest x-ray (consider sinus films)
- Consider lumbar puncture (symptoms of meninigitis may be minimal)
- Consider computed tomography of abdomen & pelvis (to exclude an intraabdominal process)
- Consider stool culture, ova and parasites, *Clostridium difficile* toxin

filtrates the blood, bone marrow, and other tissues. Leukemias may proliferate rapidly and invade the bone marrow, leading to suppression of the normal marrow function. Over time, these malignant cells spread to the peripheral blood, spleen, lymph nodes, and other tissues, ultimately causing death in the untreated patient.

Although difficult, classification of the leukemias is of major importance in determining both prognosis and treatment. In this regard, it has been useful to determine whether the cell line of origin is lymphoid or myeloid (derived from bone marrow) and whether the patient's clinical presentation is acute or chronic. Although the etiology of leukemia is largely unknown, there have been associations made to both environmental and genetic factors.

Classification

The leukemias are categorized by their cell of origin and rapidity of clinical course into four major classes: acute lymphocytic leukemia (ALL), acute myeloid leukemia (AML), chronic lymphoid leukemia (CLL), and chronic myeloid leukemia (CML). The acute leukemias demonstrate younger and less differentiated cells than those seen in the chronic leukemias. In addition, they are characterized by a rapid progression of illness. Modern biological, antigenic, and molecular techniques have allowed for greater detail in classifying and subdividing the leuke-

Table 58.4

Recommended Therapy for Neutropenia with a Fever

- Cefepime (Maxipime) 2 g IV + aminoglycoside (gentamicin 1.5 mg/kg IV)
- Imipenem/cilastatin (Primaxin) 500 mg IV + aminoglycoside (gentamicin 1.5 mg/kg IV)
- Consider vancomycin for MRSA, skin or catheter site infection, hypotension, mucositis, recent quinolone prophylaxis
- Consider antifungal therapy with fluconazole or amphotericin B

mias; however, these general categories remain useful and continue to facilitate our understanding of the disease.

During the early stages of leukemia there may be no morphologically distinguishable cells in the peripheral blood. More invasive testing, such as bone marrow biopsy, may be required to achieve a correct diagnosis and classification. Despite advances in this field, it is not always possible to verify the diagnosis of leukemia or to accurately classify the disease. Lymphomas that originate in the lymph nodes and spread to the bone marrow can be quite difficult to distinguish from leukemia because both diseases have phenotypically identical cells.

Incidence and Epidemiology

The overall incidence of leukemia in the United States is approximately 13 cases per 100,000 people each year. The overall incidence of both acute and chronic leukemia is higher in men than in women. There are age differences in the incidence of leukemia according to specific class.

ALL is a disease primarily occurring in children and young adults with a peak incidence at 2 to 4 years of age. ALL is the most common form of pediatric cancer. The incidence of CLL increases with age. AML is primarily a disease of older adults. The median age at diagnosis is 60 to 65 years. The incidence of CML increases slowly with age until 40 then rapidly rises.

Etiology

Both environmental and genetic elements have been demonstrated to increase the incidence of this disease. Ionizing radiation, chemicals, and viruses have been implicated in the development of leukemia.

Clinical Manifestations, Diagnosis, and Treatment

Chronic Myelogenous Leukemia

The onset of CML is usually insidious. Diagnosis may be made during an evaluation for a complaint unrelated to the leukemia or a general health screening. Symptoms consistent with anemia such as fatigue, weight loss, and malaise may be the presenting complaint. Left upper quadrant pain is common in patients with CML due to the infiltration of leukemic cells into the spleen, and splenomegaly is the most consistent physical finding in CML.

CML is characterized by a marked increase in myelopoiesis, splenomegaly, and the presence of the Philadelphia chromosome. Bone marrow aspirate/biopsy is confirmatory. The WBC is typically in the range of 100,000 to 300,000 cells/mm^3 at the time of diagnosis and can reach levels of 800,000 cells/mm^3 or more. A normochromic normocytic anemia is common as the bone marrow becomes infiltrated with white blood cells. Anemia is rarely observed until the peripheral white blood cell count has exceeded 100,000 cells/mm^3. Often there is an associated thrombocytosis in the range of 300,000 to 600,000/mm^3 with a majority of patients having a level of greater than 450,000/mm^3. Hyperuricemia is quite common due to high cell turnover.

CML has classically been separated into three phases: chronic phase, accelerated phase, and blast phase. The most common course of disease is a stepwise progression from chronic to accelerated to blast phase. The majority of patients are first diagnosed while in chronic phase. Chronic phase is designated when blast cells make up no more than 15% of cells on bone marrow biopsy or peripheral smear. The chronic phase is characterized by mild symptomatology including left upper quadrant discomfort and complaints from an anemic state. Bone pain and splenic infarction are rare this early in the disease. The duration of this phase can be quite variable with a median time of 3 to 4 years. Usual survival is 4 to 5 years from the time of diagnosis.

The accelerated phase is defined by the presence of between 15% to 30% blast cells in the peripheral blood or marrow. In this phase, there is worsening of symptoms such as left upper quadrant discomfort resulting from hepatosplenomegaly, anorexia, and weight loss. A chronic low-grade fever is associated with this phase and may require a careful evaluation to rule out an underlying infection or sepsis. White blood cell counts increase during this phase and can be associated with either severe thrombocytosis or thrombocytopenia.

Progression to the blast phase is the most ominous stage of this disease and is characterized by greater than 30% of the peripheral blood or marrow cells consisting of blast forms. Occasionally, patients will undergo direct transformation from the chronic stage to blast crisis. Blast crisis may involve any cell line: myeloid, lymphoid or erythroid. Treatment of all forms of blast crisis is generally ineffective. Patients develop diffuse lymphadenopathy and begin to experience bone pain. During the blast phase, central nervous system (CNS) involvement may produce a variety of neurologic manifestations. Survival in this phase is measured in weeks to months with a median of 2 to 4 months. Death from infection, hemorrhage, or thrombosis occurs rapidly in 85% of patients once the blast phase has begun.

Currently the only possible curative treatment for CML is bone marrow or stem cell transplant (BM/SCT). Long-term disease-free survival is achievable in 50% to 70% of chronic phase patients after receiving an allogenic transplant from an HLA-matched sibling. BM/SCT is much less successful in the accelerated phase or blast phase, with 30% and 10% long-term survival, respectively.

When BM/SCT is not feasible, interferon-α is the treatment of choice. Interferon therapy produces flu like symptoms early in the course of treatment followed by fatigue, lethargy, weight loss, myalgias, and arthralgias. Several chemotherapeutic drugs have been used in the treatment of CML but remissions have been short lived. Hydroxyurea may be used to control the blood cell counts in those patients who are not BM/SCT candidates.

Treatment of the blast crisis is usually determined by the cell type that predominates in the crisis. Myelogenous blast crisis follows the same treatment recommendations for AML induction therapy. Lymphogenous blast crisis follows the same treatment pathway recommended for ALL. Emergency treatment of CML is usually not required unless the patient presents with acute symptoms that are produced by a leukostasis-related complication or hyperuricemia.

Leukostasis may occur when the myeloblast count increases to levels over 100,000 cells/mm^3. There is an increased risk for microinfarction and hemorrhage in small blood vessels as a result of sludging and thrombus formation. The pulmonary vasculature is frequently affected, resulting in radiologic infiltrates and hypoxemia. Involvement of the CNS vasculature leads to changes in mental status, cerebral infarction, and death. Treatment is aimed at vigorous hydration and reducing the WBC count with hydroxyurea. Leukapheresis and whole-brain irradiation may be indicated in more extreme cases.

Acute Myelogenous Leukemia

Patients with AML often present with nonspecific symptoms that are a consequence of anemia, leukocyte dysfunction, or thrombocytopenia. Fatigue, anorexia, weight loss, pallor, and dyspnea on exertion are common initial complaints. Infections of the pharynx, lung, perirectal area, blood, skin, and gingiva may cause the patient to seek medical evaluation. Petechiae, easy bruising, and gingival hemorrhage secondary to thrombocytopenia are noted in about 5% of patients at diagnosis. Physical findings may include fever, splenomegaly, hepatomegaly, lymphadenopathy or other evidence of infection.

Laboratory analysis usually reveals a moderate to severe anemia. The median leukocyte count is about 15,000 cells/mm^3. Approximately 30% of patients will have counts lower than 5,000 cells/mm^3 and 20% will have counts greater than 100,000 cells/mm^3. A majority (75%) of patients will have a platelet count of under 100,000 cells/mm^3. Twenty-five percent will have a count of less than 25,000 cells/mm^3. By definition, AML patients have more than 30% of the bone marrow occupied by myeloblasts.

AML therapy is divided into two phases: induction and postremission management. The goal of induction chemotherapy is a complete remission which is attained in 70% to 80% patients under 60 and about half of older patients. Post remission management may include intensive chemotherapy or BM/SCT. Survival in these patients is inversely proportional to age. Long-term survival in those over 60 years remains poor, despite intensive chemotherapy.

Symptomatic treatment often includes filtered platelet transfusions for bleeding secondary to thrombocytopenia. Platelet counts should be maintained between 10,000 and 20,000 and may need to be greater in febrile patients because of an increased risk of bleeding. Leukocyte depleted, irradiated transfusions should be used to maintain a hemoglobin level more than 8 g/L. Fever is of major concern in these patients especially when the absolute neutrophil count is less than 500/mm^3. Infectious complications remain the major cause of death and morbidity during the induction and post remission phase. Fever or symptoms suggestive of infection should be aggressively investigated. Patients should be pan-cultured and broad-spectrum antibacterial and antifungal antibiotics should be initiated as early as possible.

Electrolyte abnormalities are also common. Hypokalemia may be present secondary to renal tubular damage. A complication of leukemia treatment is tumor lysis syndrome which is caused by the turnover of rapidly proliferating neo-plastic cells. Tumor lysis syndrome can produce hypocalcemia (due to precipitation of calcium phosphate), hyperphosphatemia, hyperkalemia, and hyperuricemia. Hyperuricemia and hyperphosphatemia can lead to nephropathy and often requires treatment with hydration, allopurinol to block conversion of xanthine to uric acid, and potentially temporary hemodialysis. Tumor lysis syndrome is typically a complication of therapy but the incidence has decreased with the use of prophylactic allopurinol and aggressive oral hydration. Occasionally, tumor lysis syndrome occurs before treatment as a result of the rapid cell turnover of the malignancy.

Acute Lymphogenous Leukemia

ALL is the proliferation of immature lymphoid cells in the bone marrow. It is most common in children younger than 10. Patients present with signs of marrow failure: fatigue, pallor, weakness, tachycardia, bleeding, bruising, or fever. Diagnosis of ALL is determined by greater than 30% lymphoblasts in the peripheral blood or bone marrow. Patients with classic childhood ALL may have low, normal, or high leukocyte counts but rarely have counts over 25,000 cells/mm^3. Anemia and thrombocytopenia are common. Neutropenia and fever should be immediately addressed with a septic workup and broad-spectrum antibiotics. Thrombocytopenia with bleeding may require platelet transfusions. CNS involvement, often without clinically apparent neurologic changes, may occur in 2% to 10% of patients. Leukemia meningitis may present with headache, nausea, and cranial nerve palsies. Tumor lysis syndrome may be a prominent feature. Leukostasis complications become a concern with the blast counts above 50,000 cells/mm^3.

Treatment is dependent upon various prognostic factors and includes induction chemotherapy as well as maintenance chemotherapy to prevent relapse. Aggressive therapy has improved childhood overall cure rate to more than 85%, but only 50% of adults have a long-term disease-free period. BM/SCT remains an option, but long-term leukemia-free survival remains low.

Chronic Lymphogenous Leukemia

The most common form of adult leukemia in western countries, CLL is more prevalent in males than females and has no known risk factors. It should be suspected when a sustained increase in small mature-appearing lymphocytes is encountered on a peripheral smear. The white cell count usually ranges between 10,000 to 200,000 cells/mm^3, including 70% to 95% small lymphocytes. The absolute neutrophil count is usually normal. Red cell and platelet counts are mildly decreased. Although many lymphocytes may appear morphologically mature, extensive immune dysfunction is associated with CLL. The B cells produce decreased amounts of immunoglobulin in response to antigenic presentation. The number and function of T cells and natural killer cells are also decreased.

Staging of CLL involves the degree of lymphocytosis and the presence or absence of adenopathy, splenomegaly, anemia and thrombocytopenia. Secondary malignancy,

particularly lung cancer and melanoma, occurs with increased frequency in patients with CLL. A small proportion of CLL patients can progress to a more aggressive disease. Richter syndrome is the most common form of advanced and aggressive CLL, characterized by worsening adenopathy, fevers, abdominal pain, and anemia. There is a rapid rise in peripheral lymphocyte count and a decreased response to treatment. Median survival once CLL has progressed to this stage is 4 to 5 months. Several other transformations are possible from the chronic course of CLL, including the development of ALL, multiple myeloma (MM), and even Hodgkin's lymphoma.

Since most patients are asymptomatic at presentation, with a very long natural history without treatment, observation is the common recommendation. Indications for beginning treatment include lymphadenopathy, cytopenia, systemic symptoms or autoimmune phenomena (hemolytic anemia, thrombocytopenia). Single agent chemotherapy is the initial treatment. BM/SCT and radiotherapy are not routinely recommended in the treatment of CLL but may be used as salvage therapy. An increased frequency of opportunistic infections is seen during advanced stages of disease due to diminished opsonization and the adverse effects of chemotherapy.

Leukemoid Reaction

A leukemoid reaction is typically defined as a persistent neutrophilia of 30,000 to 50,000 cells/mm^3 or greater. Anemia, young WBC forms, thrombocytopenia, splenomegaly, and fever can be present in both leukemia and leukemoid reaction, making the clinical presentations nearly indistinguishable. There are many causes of a leukemoid reaction, including infection, intoxication, and malignancy. Adding to the complexity of this entity is the fact that there are numerous grades of leukemoid reaction ranging from simple leukocytosis without immature forms to a complex picture indistinguishable from AML. Differentiation between leukemia and a leukemoid reaction may require thorough testing of the bone marrow and/or lymph node biopsy, including cultures and specialized stains. A logical approach to the patient with suspected infection and an otherwise unknown source of leukocytosis is to obtain cultures and treat with broad-spectrum antibiotics. Antileukemic therapy should only be instituted once it is clear that the patient is presenting with a true leukemia and not simply a leukemoid reaction.

Multiple Myeloma

Multiple myeloma (MM) is a disorder in which there is a malignant proliferation of plasma cells stemming from a single clone. In MM, the maturation of B lymphocytes into antibody-secreting plasma cells is no longer controlled. The normal process in which conversion into mature plasma cells requires exposure to a particular antigen is lost in these cells.

About 95% of patients with MM possess an increased concentration of hypersecreted immunoglobulin referred to as the monoclonal or "M-component." Immunoglobulins are constructed of both heavy and light chains.

Approximately 20% of MM patients have only the light chain detectable, referred to as Bence Jones protein.

Incidence and Epidemiology

MM accounts for 10% to 15% of hematologic neoplasms in Caucasians and up to one-third of hematologic neoplasms in African-Americans. The incidence is approximately 4 cases per 100,000 per year and is currently rising. The median age at onset is 68 years with more than 90% of patients over the age of 50.

Diagnosis and Clinical Manifestations

Bone marrow plasmacytosis, lytic bone lesions and the finding of an M-component make up the classic triad of MM. The most common presentation of MM is that of bone pain affecting nearly 70% of patients. Typically, this manifests as unexplained back pain. The bone pain of MM is worsened by movement; in contrast to the bone pain of metastatic cancer, which is often worse at night and while resting. Lytic bone lesions can lead to pathologic fractures. Spinal cord compression syndromes may occur. A high index of suspicion should be utilized when encountering prolonged or unexplained back pain in the older individual.

The finding of a normochromic, normocytic anemia in an older individual is another common presentation of MM. This is caused by bone marrow myelophthisis, resulting in decreased erythropoiesis in addition to increased destruction of red blood cells. Platelet dysfunction as a result of the M-component predisposes to bleeding, which contributes to the anemic state. Anemia complicates up to 80% of myeloma patients.

Approximately 25% of patients present with recurrent bacterial infection. Pneumonia and pyelonephritis are common, and frequent pathogens include *Staphylococcus*, *Streptococcus*, and Gram-negative organisms. These infections are due to hypogammaglobinemia and diminished neutrophil migration. Hypogammaglobinemia results from increased destruction of both monoclonal and normal antibodies. Regulatory mechanisms lead to decreased production of normal antibodies due to the high concentration of total immunoglobulin.

Several other abnormalities are often encountered in MM. Renal failure eventually complicates approximately one-fourth of myeloma patients and results from Bence Jones proteinuria and hypercalcemia. Neurologic symptoms occur in the setting of hyperviscosity and hypercalcemia. Hypercalcemia results from the osteoclastic activating factors released by the increased number of plasma cells. Symptoms of hypercalcemia include weakness, anorexia, abdominal cramping, constipation, and mental status changes.

Hyperviscosity commonly leads to blurred vision, headache, fatigue, and mental status changes.

CBC can demonstrate the anemia commonly associated with myeloma. Rouleaux formation is another useful finding on CBC that is seen as the M-component concentration increases. Pseudohyponatremia may be observed also, due to the high concentration of M-component. X-ray investigation of the skull, pelvis, lumbar, and any tender areas is often useful in locating lytic lesions.

Treatment and Disposition

Symptomatic treatment is usually the first priority in MM and should be directed by the individual presentation. Treatment of bone pain, dehydration, and hypercalcemia is the main focus of the EP. Dehydration can worsen renal failure and intensify symptoms due to hyperviscosity. Severe hypercalcemia may require high-dose steroid treatment or dialysis when hydration and diuresis are not sufficient.

Chemotherapeutic treatment of MM provides only modest prolongation of survival. Due to the toxic nature of treatment, it is generally delayed until the patient is sufficiently symptomatic to warrant such medications. Occasionally treatment is initiated to control severe hypercalcemia. The most common medications are alkylating agents combined with oral steroids. Treatment leads to a mild neutropenia and a gradual decline in the concentration of M-component. Complete remission is only achieved in approximately 10% to 15% of patients as defined by disappearance of the M-component. Approximately 50% of myeloma patients achieve control of their disease once treatment is initiated. The asymptomatic patient should be followed with laboratory testing every 3 to 6 months and periodic x-ray evaluation. Median survival period is approximately 3 years from the time of presentation.

Acknowledgment

Dr. Thomas Nowicki and Dr. Marc Borestein contributed this chapter to *Emergency Medicine: The Core Content,* and some elements of that chapter have been retained in this edition.

Selected Readings

Appelbaum FR. Bone marrow and stem cell transplantation. In: Fauci A, et al., eds. *Harrison's Textbook of Medicine.* 15th ed. New York: McGraw-Hill 2001:739–744.

Armitage JO, Longo DL. Malignacies of lymphoid cells. In: Fauci A, et al., eds. *Harrison's Textbook of Medicine,* 15th ed. New York: McGraw-Hill, 2001:715–727.

Longo DL. Plasma cell disorders. In: Fauci A, et al., eds. *Harrison's Textbook of Medicine,* 15th ed. New York: McGraw-Hill, 2001:727–733.

Lowenberg B, Downing JR, Burnett A. Acute myeloid leukemia. *N Engl J Med* 1999;341:1051–1062.

Pui CH. Childhood leukemias. *N Engl J Med* 1995;332:1618–1630.

Sawyers CL. Chronic myeloid leukemia. *N Engl J Med* 1999;340:1330–1340.

Wetzler M, Byrd JC, Bloomfield CD. Acute and chronic leukemia. In: Fauci A, et al., eds. *Harrison's Textbook of Medicine,* 15th ed. New York: McGraw-Hill, 2001: 706–714.

59 Heparin-Induced Thrombocytopenia

Robert L. Levine

Frequency and Pathophysiology

Heparin-induced thrombocytopenia (HIT) is a serious, immune-mediated prothrombotic condition that occurs in approximately 1% to 5% of patients who receive heparin. The frequency of HIT is greater with bovine versus porcine heparin usage, with unfractionated versus low-molecular-weight heparin usage, and in post-surgical versus medical or obstetrical patients.

HIT is caused by antibodies against a complex of heparin and platelet factor 4 (PF4). The antibody-antigen complex activates platelets, leading to the release of procoagulant platelet microparticles, excessive thrombin generation, thrombocytopenia, and often thrombosis. Depending on the patient population and the type of heparin used, 7% to 50% of patients develop heparin-PF4 antibodies following heparin exposure. These antibodies circulate for at least 4 months in approximately 40% of patients, although their longevity thereafter remains unclear. No distinguishing clinical or laboratory feature has yet been identified to predict the individual with heparin-PF4 antibodies who will progress to HIT. Among patients with the antibodies, orthopedic surgery patients are more likely to develop HIT than cardiac surgery patients.

Clinical Presentation

Clinically, HIT manifests as platelet count drop of at least 30% to 50% from the pre-heparin value, often under 150×10^9/L, typically beginning 5 to 14 days after starting heparin. The thrombocytopenia may occur earlier, even within hours if a patient has circulating heparin-PF4 antibodies from a recent heparin exposure. Conversely, the onset of HIT may be delayed up to approximately 20 days in some patients. The thrombocytopenia is typically moderate in its severity (median platelet count of approximately 50 to 70×10^9/L). However platelet counts of under 15×10^9/L occur in about 5% of patients with HIT, and platelet count drops of greater than 50% may occur.

Complications include deep venous thrombosis, pulmonary embolism, myocardial infarction, stroke, limb artery occlusion leading to amputation, and other thromboembolic events. These events more frequently manifest in the venous than arterial circulation (approximate 4 : 1 ratio). Thrombosis often leads to the initial recognition of HIT. Bleeding is rare, despite the thrombocytopenia.

Thrombosis will occur within a month in 38% to 52% of HIT patients treated by heparin cessation alone, and 22% to 28% of these patients will die. Because patients administered heparin during hospitalization may be discharged before their HIT is manifested or recognized, patients may develop HIT-related thrombosis as an outpatient. Approximately 10% of recently (under 6 months) hospitalized patients coming to the emergency department with chest pain or symptoms of thrombosis have circulating heparin-PF4 antibodies. Patients often, but not always, have thrombocytopenia when returning to the hospital with HIT-related thrombosis. It should be recognized however that patients may have a relative, yet not absolute, thrombocytopenia and that platelet counts may normalize within days of discontinuing heparin despite an increased risk of thrombosis persisting for several weeks.

Diagnosis

The diagnosis of HIT is based on its typical clinical picture, most often isolated thrombocytopenia in a patient treated with a heparin product or an acute thrombotic event associated with thrombocytopenia and a similar history, and the exclusion of other causes of thrombocytopenia. In contrast with most thrombocytopenic conditions, bleeding is rare in HIT.

Furthermore, thrombocytopenia associated with quinine or other drug-induced immune thrombocytopenic purpura, as well as abciximab-induced thrombocytopenia, is typically more severe than found in HIT.

The differential diagnosis of thrombocytopenia with thrombosis includes disseminated intravascular coagulation (DIC), thrombotic thrombocytopenic purpura (TTP), and hemolytic uremic syndrome (HUS). DIC is a consumptive coagulopathy in which patients characteristically have prolonged global clotting tests, decreased fibrinogen, and increased fibrin degradation products. TTP is characterized by the classic pentad of neurologic symptoms, microangiopathic hemolytic anemia, thrombocytopenia, renal impairment, and fever. HUS presents with a triad of symptoms including severe renal impairment, variable thrombocytopenia, and thrombotic microangiopathic hemolytic anemia, usually after a prodromal illness with acute, bloody diarrhea.

Patients presenting with thrombosis-related symptoms after a recent hospitalization should be considered to be at increased risk of HIT. Due to the ubiquitous use of heparin in most institutions, it is reasonable to assume that a patient, if hospitalized, was exposed to heparin. A careful history concerning any recent hospitalization or procedure, heparin exposure, "heparin allergy" or "platelet problem" is important. Review of platelet counts from the recent hospitalization, if available, may be useful. Assessment of the current platelet count is essential, particularly before initiating heparin therapy.

The College of American Pathologists recommends heparin-PF4 antibody testing for patients in whom there is suspicion of HIT based on the temporal features of the thrombocytopenia or based on the occurrence of new thrombosis during, or soon after heparin treatment. Such tests typically take several hours to perform. Because of the increased thrombotic risk early in the progression of HIT, appropriate therapy should be delayed pending laboratory confirmation.

Treatment

The initiation of heparin therapy for thrombosis in a patient with HIT or reactive heparin-PF4 antibodies could be catastrophic. When HIT is suspected, all heparin must be avoided, including low-molecular-weight heparins, heparin flushes, heparin-coated catheters, and any other sources. In addition, alternative non-heparin anticoagulation must be initiated immediately.

Two alternative anticoagulants—the direct thrombin inhibitors argatroban and lepirudin—are approved in the United States for use in patients with HIT. Argatroban is also approved as an anticoagulant for patients with or at risk for HIT undergoing percutaneous coronary intervention. Argatroban and lepirudin have been shown in prospective, historical controlled studies to improve the outcomes of HIT, including reducing new thrombosis. Associated major bleeding rates were 6% to 7% with arga-

troban (7% in control) and 13% to 17% with lepirudin (9% in control). For argatroban therapy, the recommended dose is 2 μg/kg/min adjusted to achieve an activated partial thromboplastin time or 1.5 to 3 times the baseline value. Because argatroban is primarily hepatically metabolized, reduced doses are used in patients with hepatic impairment. For lepirudin therapy, the recommended dose is a 0.4 mg/kg initial bolus followed by a 0.15 mg/kg/hour infusion, adjusted to achieve activated partial thromboplastin time ratios of 1.5 to 2.5. Lepirudin, which is renally cleared, requires reduced doses in renal impairment and should be avoided in acute renal failure. Anticoagulation with argatroban or lepirudin should be continued until the platelet cout has recovered, or until HIT is no longer suspected and/or the lack of circulating heparin-PF4 antibodies has been confirmed.

Warfarin should not be used as the sole acute therapy in HIT because it can paradoxically worsen the thrombosis and cause venous limb gangrene. Initiation or warfarin for the long-term treatment of HIT must be delayed until adequate alternative parenteral anticoagulation has been provided and platelet counts have recovered substantially. Warfarin therapy is appropriate for a minimum of 3 to 6 months after an episode of HIT-associated thrombosis and is adjusted to maintain an international normalized ratio of 2:3. Platelet transfusions should not be used for prophylaxis of bleeding because they may exacerbate the hypercoagulable state, leading to additional thrombosis. Surgical thromboembolectomy or systemic or local thrombolysis, as adjunctive therapy to alternative parenteral anticoagulation, may be appropriate for selected patients with large vessel arterial thromboembolism or severe pulmonary embolism, respectively.

Selected Readings

Hirsh J, Heddle N, Kelton JG. Treatment of heparin-induced thrombocytopenia: a critical review. *Arch Intern Med* 2004;164:361–369.

Levine RL, Hursting MJ, Drexler A, et al. Heparin-induced thrombocytopenia in the emergency department. *Ann Emerg Med* 2004;44:511–515.

Rice L, Attisha WK, Drexler A, et al. Delayed-onset heparin-induced thrombocytopenia. *Ann Intern Med* 2002;136:210–215.

Warkentin TE, Greinacher A, eds. *Heparin-Induced Thrombocytopenia,* 3rd ed. New York: Marcel Dekker, 2004.

Warkentin TE, Kelton JG. Delayed-onset heparin-induced thrombocytopenia and thrombosis. *Ann Intern Med* 2001;135:502–506.

Introduction to Immune System Disorders

G. Richard Braen

During the past three decades, the science of immunology has made great advances in the understanding of the complex humoral and cellular components, which interact when our bodies are challenged with a multitude of antigenic stimuli, and with the diagnostic approach and treatment of the disorders caused by immunologic dysfunction. At times, these complex interactions "overreact," creating hypersensitivity responses, or "under-react," leaving the body vulnerable to infections and other diseases.

This section deals with hypersensitivity reactions, transplant-related problems (particularly as they affect the heart), autoimmune diseases, and immune deficiency syndromes. Emergency physicians are commonly presented with hypersensitivity reactions. Less often, emergency physicians are presented with problems related to immune deficiency syndromes, autoimmune diseases, and transplant-related problems. Each of these presents unique diagnostic and therapeutic challenges, and each emergency physician should have a general knowledge of these immune system disorders.

Autoimmune Diseases

David L. Pierce
Dietrich V. K. Jehle

Immune responses occur constantly in normal individuals and are a part of normal homeostasis. They involve multiple interactions eventually resulting in a response characterized by a particular type of cellular activity and requiring assistance from other cells and systems for the response to be effective. This is particularly true of the interactions between B and T lymphocytes.

Lymphocytes arise from progenitor cells that have migrated to the primary lymphoid organs and have undergone a process of development and maturation. In the thymus these progenitor cells develop into T lymphocytes, and in the fetal liver and in bone marrow they develop into B lymphocytes. With help from activated T-helper cells the B lymphocytes will proliferate and secrete antibody that can specifically recognize and bind to the antigen that initiated the process.

Antibody binding to antigen can lead to opsonization, neutralization of free antigen, and further stimulation of immunocytes, platelets, and other cells (such as mast cells), in addition to stimulation of vascular smooth muscle and increased vascular permeability.

Inappropriate reactivity of components of the immune system with aberrant responses to self antigens are features of those diseases that are described as autoimmune. The mechanisms by which these processes occur are incompletely understood but include cross-reactivity of epitopes (e.g., hepatitis B and polyarteritis nodosa), loss of active suppression, release of hidden antigens (e.g., Dressler's syndrome), generation of modified self antigens, T-cell bypass, and superantigen stimulation of T-cell populations (e.g., by streptococcal antigens in rheumatic fever).

Acute Rheumatic Fever

Rheumatic fever is most often a disease of children between the ages of 5 and 15 years. The disease has a degree of familial predominance, and affected individuals are prone to recurrent attacks.

While the exact pathophysiologic mechanisms remain unproven, rheumatic fever is thought to be due to an uncommon dysfunctional immune response following pharyngeal infection with some strains of group A β-hemolytic streptococcus resulting in inflammatory changes in the heart, skin, joints, and other tissues. While the history of antecedent pharyngitis is often lacking, patients with acute rheumatic fever usually have increased titers of antibodies to streptococcal antigens, indicating infection within the preceding month.

The clinical presentation is most commonly as an acute febrile illness with fever greater than 38° C and migratory polyarthritis of the larger limb joints. Cardiac symptoms and signs are less common, although the murmurs of mitral or, less often, aortic incompetence usually appear if carditis is present.

Marked tachycardia, pericarditis, and in severe cases, cardiac enlargement and failure may occur. First- or second-degree heart block may also be seen.

Sydenham's chorea, when present, occurs late in the illness and may develop insidiously. It is characterized by sudden erratic jerking movements that are most marked on effort, anxiety, or excitement, and that are not present during sleep. Muscle weakness may be quite severe and emotional lability may also be present.

Erythema marginatum is an evanescent, macular, pink rash that is nonpruritic and has irregular borders with central clearing. It occurs most often on the trunk and proximal limbs and appears in only a small percentage of patients during the acute phase of rheumatic fever. Subcutaneous nodules tend to be pea-sized, painless, and positioned over prominences of bone.

Other symptoms that may occur include fatigue, weight loss, and abdominal pain.

Rheumatic fever is a clinical diagnosis using the revised Jones criteria. The major criteria are carditis, polyarthritis, chorea, erythema marginatum, and subcutaneous nodules. The minor criteria are fever, arthralgia (in the absence of arthritis), previous rheumatic fever or rheumatic heart disease, acute phase reaction such as leukocytosis, elevated erythrocyte sedimentation rate (ESR) or abnormal C-reactive protein (CRP), and ECG changes such as prolonged PR interval. Evidence of recent streptococcal throat infection (e.g., positive throat swab culture or raised antistreptolysin antibodies) and either two major or one major and two minor criteria are required to make the diagnosis.

History, physical examination, ECG, and chest x-ray are all of importance in establishing the diagnosis. Laboratory tests may determine the presence of recent group A streptococcal pharyngeal infection by throat swab culture or by serologic testing and may demonstrate nonspecific markers of inflammation such as raised ESR, CRP, leukocytosis, and anemia. Further investigations such as echocardiography should be undertaken in conjunction with specialist consultation.

Having established the diagnosis, bed rest and supportive therapy are instituted as clinically indicated. Parenteral penicillin or an acceptable alternative antibiotic should be administered. The nature and duration of long-term antibiotic prophylaxis to prevent rheumatic fever recurrence must be determined on an individual basis. Patients with subsequent rheumatic heart disease require prophylaxis to prevent bacterial endocarditis.

Salicylates are usually adequate to relieve the symptoms of arthritis. Corticosteroids are prescribed for several weeks in patients with carditis who have not responded to salicylate therapy. Sedatives, tranquilizers, reassurance, and appropriate nursing care are indicated in the management of chorea. Rheumatic fever typically is self-limiting and can be expected to last for several months. The ESR and CRP are useful laboratory markers of disease activity.

Prevention of recurrent attacks and subsequent cumulative cardiac damage is important. In some patients emergency management of significant cardiac failure, arrhythmias, or other complications may be urgently required.

Collagen Vascular Diseases

Collagen vascular diseases are a group of disorders characterized by abnormalities of the immune system, vasculitis, and varying multisystem involvement. They may be difficult to diagnose and may themselves mimic infections, malignancies, thromboses or a number of other diseases. Some collagen vascular diseases such as thyroiditis are relatively organ specific, others such as systemic lupus erythematosis are less so. The types and sites of vessels involved also vary and this largely determines the clinical manifestations. As the clinical presentations of this group of disorders are legion, they must be considered as a part of the differential diagnosis in a wide variety of clinical settings.

Despite a number of attempts to standardize classification, the incomplete understanding of the underlying processes has meant that all systems have their limitations and that many patients will not fit easily into one category. Such patients may display features of several diseases and may continue to evolve for quite some time before conforming to a recognizable pattern.

Dermatomyositis and Polymyositis

Polymyositis is an uncommon inflammatory disease of muscle characterized by lymphocytic infiltration without suppuration; when it is associated with skin involvement, it is called dermatomyositis. A significant propor-

tion of patients also have connective tissue disease such as rheumatoid arthritis or systemic lupus erythematosus, and up to 10% are ultimately found to have an underlying malignancy, most commonly in patients over 60 years of age. There is some familial predominance, and the disease is more common in patients with some particular HLA epitypes. The role of viral infection in pathogenesis is as yet unclear. Polymyositis can occur in patients with AIDS and less commonly as a side effect of zidovudine therapy.

The clinical symptoms usually appear gradually. Proximal muscle weakness sometimes with pain and tenderness may precede or be preceded by a rash. The rash may appear lilac colored (heliotrope) and present in a butterfly facial distribution or it may present in a variety of ways, including erythema or even as an itchy dermatitis. Rarely the onset may be as dramatic weakness, sometimes with rhabdomyolysis.

Reflexes may be normal or brisk. Involvement of striated esophageal muscle leads to dysphagia, and cardiac involvement may manifest as arrhythmias or as heart failure. Typically ESR and creatine kinase (CK) elevation can be expected.

The electromyogram often demonstrates muscle irritability as well as changes typical of myopathy. Muscle biopsy may provide confirmation.

Reiter's Syndrome

Reiter's syndrome is a relatively common form of reactive arthritis, triggered by urogenital chlamydial infection. It is most common in HLA-B27–positive young men and is part of the spectrum of reactive arthritis that also includes arthritis following gastrointestinal infection with salmonella, shigella, or other enterobes.

Reiter's syndrome is characterized by arthritis, urethritis, conjunctivitis, and mucocutaneous lesions. The initial symptoms are typically of intermittent, sometimes painless, urethral discharge, followed by constitutional symptoms such as fever, fatigue, and malaise. Prostatitis may also be present. The arthritis is acute, painful, and asymmetrical, involving few joints at first, with others being affected over days to weeks. The lower limbs, feet, and low back are common sites, although upper limb joints including fingers (dactylitis) may also be involved. Fasciitis and tendonitis are also common. Mild conjunctivitis and less frequently uveitis is seen. Superficial, relatively painless oral and penile ulcers may be present. Typical skin lesions (keratoderma blenorrhagica) consist of vesicles on the palms, soles, and elsewhere, which later become hyperkeratotic and encrusted.

Initial laboratory investigations demonstrate nonspecific markers of acute inflammation. Rheumatoid factor and antinuclear antibody (ANA) are usually negative and most patients are HLA-B27 positive.

Treatment with tetracyclines should be initiated when chlamydial infection is present. Nonsteroidal antiinflammatory drugs (NSAIDs) are effective in treating arthritis. In some situations local steroid injection may be helpful.

Rheumatoid Arthritis

Rheumatoid arthritis is a relatively common disease that can be seen in all age groups but is most common in women between the ages of 35 and 50 years. Its pathogenesis is incompletely understood, but it is highly likely that an element of genetic predisposition is present.

The predominant pathologic changes initially seen in joints consist of synovial hyperplasia, T cell infiltration, and microvascular injury, resulting in damage to cartilage and bone. Rheumatoid nodules are thought to be a result of vasculitis in periarticular structures. Vasculitis may also involve skin, nerves or other organs, although renal disease is rare.

Low-grade fever and constitutional symptoms such as fatigue and lethargy are in part due to cytokine release. Joint disease often begins as the slow onset of a symmetrical, peripheral polyarthritis, with morning stiffness. The wrists, metacarpophalangeal and proximal interphalangeal joints, elbows, knees, and feet are commonly involved. Spinal disease usually involves the upper cervical region. Long-standing disease leads to deformities, especially in the wrists, fingers, and feet. Synovial inflammation spreading beyond the knee into the popliteal space is a cause of Baker's cyst.

Extraarticular manifestations are relatively common. Rheumatoid nodules occur around joints and occasionally on serous membranes such as pleura. Pulmonary nodules may cause respiratory impairment and may sometimes cavitate. Vasculitis may present as necrotic areas of skin, digital ischemia or following infarction of gut or other organs. Neurologic manifestations may be related to compression entrapment or vasculitis. Dry eyes (Sjögren's syndrome) are relatively common; however, other ophthalmic complications such as scleritis are much rarer. A number of syndromes such as Caplan's syndrome (pulmonary rheumatoid nodules in patients with pneumoconiosis and pulmonary fibrosis) and Felty's syndrome (rheumatoid arthritis, splenomegaly, neutropenia, and thrombocytopenia) have been described.

Immune Deficiency Syndromes

Immunodeficiency syndromes are characterized by a remarkable susceptibility to infections, autoimmune disease, and lymphoreticular malignancies. The most common infectious cause is acquired immunodeficiency syndrome (AIDS) caused by the human immunodeficiency virus (HIV).

HIV Disease/AIDS

HIV disease is an infection of the immune system that results in progressive premature destruction of the T-helper (CD4) lymphocytes. There is a broad range of disease seen in HIV-infected individuals, from asymptomatic to AIDS; with a myriad of associated infections and disorders.

The current definition of AIDS includes all patients with HIV infection and a CD4 count less than $200/\mu L$ or

Table 60.1
AIDS-Defining Disorders

Laboratory evidence of HIV with any of the following:
- Candidiasis: pulmonary or esophageal
- Cervical cancer
- Coccidioidomycosis
- Cryptococcosis, extrapulmonary
- Cryptosporidiosis
- Cytomegalovirus: chronic (more than 1 month) or esophageal
- Histoplasmosis
- Kaposi's sarcoma
- Lymphoma
- *Mycobacterium avium*
- *Mycobacterium kansasil*
- *Mycobacterium tuberculosis*
- Pneumocystis
- Pneumonia, recurrent
- Progressive multifocal leukoencephalopathy
- Salmonellosis

patients with an AIDS-indicator condition (i.e., unusual secondary infections, specific neoplasms or neurologic disease). (**Table 60.1**).

There are two types of HIV viruses that have been identified in humans; HIV-1 (responsible for AIDS) and HIV-2 (most frequently identified in West Africa).

Epidemiology

Incidence   It is estimated that there are more than 42 million people worldwide infected with the HIV virus, with over 950,000 individuals living in the United States. In 1999 there were approximately 44,000 new cases of HIV reported in North America.

Transmission   HIV infection is most frequently transmitted via sexual intercourse, parenteral routes, or maternal-fetal transmission (horizontal or vertical). The HIV virus is concentrated in cells; therefore, cellular fluids are potentially more infectious than acellular secretions. Other documented sources of HIV transmission include semen, cervical/vaginal secretions, breast milk, cerebrospinal fluid, and pleural/peritoneal fluids. There is no evidence to date that HIV infection can be spread by routine casual contact. Of note, although antiretroviral therapy can potentially decrease HIV viral load and reduce the risk of infection, it does not prevent an HIV-infected individual from transmitting the virus.

Sexual behaviors that are associated with the highest rates of transmission of HIV are anal intercourse and sex during menses, while parenteral transmission occurs most frequently from sharing needles among IV drug abusers. In addition, donation of blood products prior to 1985 (before antibody screening) by HIV-infected individuals was associated with many documented cases of HIV. Healthcare workers who receive an HIV-contaminated needle-stick have a 0.3% to 0.4% risk of viral transfer. Maternal-fetal transmission occurs in 13% to 39% or infants born to HIV-infected mothers, with additional risk of viral transmission from breast milk.

Testing The interval between HIV infection and antibody response is from 1 to 3 months. Antibodies to HIV usually appear within 2 weeks of onset of the acute retroviral syndrome (when present) and are usually present within 8 weeks. Enzyme-linked immunosorbent assay (ELISA) for HIV antibody is currently the best screening test with sensitivities and specificities of over 99.5% and 99%, respectively. The Western blot assay, with sensitivities and specificities that approach 100%, is most frequently utilized as a confirmatory test for positive ELISA test results. In addition, a single use diagnostic system (SUDS) assay can be prepared in less than one hour. This is a useful test in the health care setting to help determine the need for post-exposure prophylaxis.

Natural History

Acute Retroviral Infection The primary infection with the HIV virus is estimated to be symptomatic in only 30% to 70% of cases, and generally occurs 3 to 6 weeks after the primary exposure to HIV. It usually presents as a mononucleosis-type illness with fever, pharyngitis, lymphadenopathy, headache, nausea, myalgias, arthralgias, and malaise. An erythematous maculopapular rash, hepatosplenomegaly, meningismus, and an encephalitic picture have also been described. Symptoms are usually self-limiting and resolve in 7 to 10 days. Most HIV specialists recommend treatment in this setting.

Clinical Staging The addition of viral load measurements has significantly improved HIV disease management. It is interpreted in the context of CD4 count to help determine the need to initiate antiretroviral therapy and monitor the effectiveness of such therapy. The viral load correlates with the decline of CD4 count and disease progression. However, the probability of developing an opportunistic infection appears to be rare with viral loads below 5,000 copies/μL (regardless of CD4 count). Viral load is considered the better indicator of rapid progression in early stage disease.

Most experts of HIV disease consider the CD4 count to be the most important indicator of prognosis in the later stages of the disease. Patients are often stratified based on their CD4 count; Early disease (>500/μL), Intermediate disease (200 to 500/μL), Late symptomatic disease (50 to 200/μL),and Advanced disease (<50/μL).

Clinical Manifestations and Management of Associated Disease

The symptomatic phase of HIV infection is characterized by infections encompassing a wide variety of bacteria, viruses, parasites, and fungi. The following section will focus on some of the most common HIV-related diseases.

HIV-Related Malignancies Patients with HIV disease are at greater risk of developing malignancies. The cancers most commonly associated with HIV disease include Kaposi's sarcoma, non-Hodgkin's lymphoma, and anogenital malignancies.

Kaposi's sarcoma (KS) is the most common cancer associated with HIV disease and may present at any stage of HIV; however, most of the reported cases (96%) have occurred in homosexual or bisexual men. Typically, these sarcomas appear as raised, reddish to purple macules measuring from a few millimeters to several centimeters. The lesions may involve skin, mucous membranes, lymph nodes, GI tract, or lungs; but are most commonly found on the face, genitalia, and feet. The diagnosis is confirmed by the pathologic appearance on tissue biopsy. Treatment with interferon-alpha decreases tumor bulk and improves survival in patients with CD4 counts greater that 200/μL.

Non-Hodgkin's lymphoma (NHL) is usually a late manifestation of AIDS (CD4 < 200/μL). The majority of HIV-related lymphomas are high-grade B-cell tumors, with a higher prevalence seen in hemophiliacs. Epstein-Barr virus (EBV) genetic material is often identified in HIV-related lymphomas. Characteristically, patients note a rapidly growing mass; however, nonspecific symptoms may prevail (fever, night sweats or weight loss). Extranodal disease is found on presentation in 98% of AIDS patients. Standard intensive chemotherapy regimens have been rejected due to poor response rates and complicating opportunistic infections.

HIV-related primary CNS lymphoma can present with focal neurologic findings, headache, altered mental status or seizures. Computed tomography (CT) scanning (with contrast) classically demonstrates a ring-enhancing nodule that is greater than 3 cm at the time of presentation. CNS toxoplasmosis, which classically shows two or more ring enhancing lesions, may be mistaken for lymphoma (as 43% have solitary lesions). In addition, cerebral cryptococcal granulomas appear as low or isodense lesions, with or without ring-enhancement, and metastases to the brain may demonstrate contrast enhancement on brain imaging as well.

Anogenital malignancies (cervical and anal squamous cell carcinomas) have a higher incidence in HIV patients, most likely secondary to coincidental infection with human papilloma virus (HPV).

Pulmonary Involvement In the patient with early or intermediate disease, there is an increased incidence of bacterial pneumonia and tuberculosis. As the HIV disease progresses to the late stages (CD4 < 200/μL), a variety of opportunistic pulmonary infections are encountered. The most common of these is *Pneumocystis carinii* pneumonia (PCP).

Bacterial pneumonia and sinusitis are found in all stages of HIV infection. There may be a slightly increased incidence of infections with encapsulated bacteria (*Streptococcus pneumoniae* and *Haemophilus influenzae*) in AIDS. Bacterial pneumonia typically presents with a relatively sudden onset of symptoms: fever, productive cough, and pleuritic chest pain. Radiographically, bacterial pneumonia tends to display focal consolidation or cavitary disease; however, diffuse bilateral infiltrates are occasionally reported. Sinusitis, which generally involves the maxillary sinuses, should be treated with broad-spectrum antibiotics and decongestants.

Prophylaxis against PCP in patients with CD4 counts less than 200/μL (or higher CD4 counts with prominent constitutional symptoms) has markedly reduced the incidence of this infection. Patients often describe prodromal symptoms of fever, fatigue, and weight loss for several weeks prior to onset of dyspnea and nonproductive cough. The chest radiograph most often demonstrates bilateral interstitial or alveolar infiltrates, yet focal infiltrates; cavitary lesions, pleural effusions, nodular densities, and pneumothorax have been reported. Upper lobe infiltrates may be seen in patients receiving aerosolized pentamidine prophylaxis. Diagnosis is usually clinical, but induced sputum or bronchoalveolar lavage (BAL) with fluorescein staining provides good sensitivity for detection. Some experts recommend a 21 day course of tapering prednisone (40 mg BID × 5 days, 40 mg QD × 5 days, followed by 20 mg QD × 11 days), if the PaO_2 is less than 70 and A-a gradient greater than 35 on room air. The steroids act by decreasing inflammatory cytokines in the lung, stabilizing capillary permeability, and thus improving oxygenation.

Fungal disease of the lung in the AIDS patient may also be secondary to *Cryptococcus, Coccidiomycosis,* or *Histoplasmosis.* Although *Aspergillus* is an important cause of pneumonia in immunocompromised hosts, it is an infrequent pathogen in the AIDS patient.

The incidence of tuberculosis (TB) has increased significantly due to the spread of HIV disease. The risk of reactivation and primary infection with *Mycobacterium tuberculosis* is strikingly higher in the HIV-infected patient. Reactivation tuberculosis frequently occurs with only mild to moderate decreases in CD4 counts. The radiologic appearance of pulmonary tuberculosis in these patients is usually classic, with apical and cavitary infiltrates. When tuberculosis occurs, the x-ray findings in patients with advanced HIV disease (CD4 < 50/μL) may be more atypical (lower lobe or military patterns). A positive purified protein derivative (PPD) may support the diagnosis of TB; however, a negative test is less useful, since anergy is common in patients with HIV disease. Multiple drug-resistant TB (MDR-TB) has emerged as a problem, particularly among HIV-infected patients in institutional settings. Treatment response is usually poor with MDR-TB.

Neurologic Manifestations Central nervous system disorders associated with HIV disease include primary and secondary CNS infections, peripheral neuropathies, myopathies, vascular complications, and neoplasms. Neurologic involvement occurs in 75% to 90% of patients with CD4 counts less than 100/μL.

Toxoplasma gondii is a protozoon that typically infects humans early in life through the ingestion of substances contaminated by cat feces or consumption of undercooked meat. Toxoplasmosis in patients with AIDS usually occurs secondary to reactivation of *T. gondii* cysts and generally presents as encephalitis; however, it may manifest as transverse myelitis, retinochoroiditis, pulmonary disease, peritonitis or orchitis.

Patients with CNS toxoplasmosis typically present with altered mental status, focal neurologic deficits, or seizures. In addition, fever and headache are commonly present. *T. gondii* is the most frequently encountered secondary CNS infection in HIV disease and the leading cause of intracranial mass lesions in patients with AIDS. Lumbar puncture may show mononuclear pleocytosis and an elevated protein level; however, this is contraindicated in patients with significant mass lesions. CT or MRI is the preferred technique to confirm presence of brain lesions. As discussed earlier, the differential diagnosis for ring-enhancing lesions includes lymphoma, metastasis, and CNS cryptococcus. The definitive diagnosis of CNS toxoplasmosis can only be made with a brain biopsy. Chemoprophylaxis to prevent toxoplasmosis reactivation is indicated in toxo-seropositive patients with CD4 counts less than 200/μL.

Cryptococcus neoformans is the most common cause of meningitis in individuals with CD4 counts less than 100/μL. Headache, fever, meningismus, and photophobia are the most commonly reported symptoms. India ink stains and CSF cryptococcal antigen are more helpful than other CSF studies; however, neither test is as sensitive as the serum cryptococcal antigen (98%). The definitive diagnosis is based on culturing *C. neoformans* from the CSF.

AIDS dementia complex (also called HIV encephalopathy and HIV dementia) usually occurs late in the course of HIV. Deficits in attention, forgetfulness, and decreased cognitive function are the initial symptoms. Apathy, withdrawal, ataxia, and deterioration of fine motor skills follow as the disease advances. During the later stages of this disorder, patients may develop severe motor dysfunction with incontinence of the bowel and bladder. Neuroimaging (CT/MRI) typically shows cerebral atrophy, ventricular enlargement, subcortical gray matter lesion, and parenchymal changes in the white matter. CSF may demonstrate elevated protein and mild pleocytosis.

Peripheral neuropathies are common in HIV disease. Painful and painless sensory neuropathies, pure motor, mixed, and autonomic dysfunction have been described. An inflammatory demyelinating neuropathy similar to Guillain-Barré syndrome has been reported in early HIV disease. In addition, many of the antiretroviral medications can cause peripheral neuropathies.

Myopathy associated with HIV disease is characterized by slowly progressive proximal muscle weakness, wasting of the upper/lower extremities, elevated CPK, and a myopathic picture on electromyography. Prolonged treatment with ZVD (AZT) may also result in myopathy that presents in a similar fashion. The diagnosis is confirmed with muscle biopsy.

Gastrointestinal Complications Diarrhea is the most common gastrointestinal disturbance in AIDS patients. HIV enteropathy, Kaposi's sarcoma, *Cryptosporidium, Mycobacterium avium* complex (MAC), and *Microsporidia* can all cause chronic diarrhea. In addition, patients with HIV disease are at risk for other causes of diarrhea; including *Isospora, Giardia, Entamoeba histolytica,*

Campylobacter, Salmonella, and *Shigella. Cryptosporidium parvum* is the most frequent cause of diarrheal illness in AIDS. It is characterized by copious watery diarrhea and cramping abdominal pain. In addition, it may involve the biliary tract, resulting in acalculous cholecystitis or cholangitis (also seen with CMV). Therapy is symptomatic with anti-motility agents and nutritional supplements.

The most common pathogen of esophagitis in HIV patients is *Candida,* which usually presents once the CD4 count is less than 200/μL. The differential diagnosis of esophageal symptoms in HIV disease includes herpes simplex virus (HSV), CMV, lymphoma, and Kaposi's sarcoma. If clinical suspicion of esophagitis is high, empiric treatment with fluconazole is initiated. If there is no response in 7 to 14 days, an upper endoscopy with biopsy is indicated. In fluconazole-refractory cases, voriconazole, itraconazole, caspofungin, amphotericin B, and higher-dose fluconazole are acceptable alternatives.

Cutaneous Manifestations
Dermatologic conditions are described in over 90% of AIDS patients. The cutaneous manifestations of HIV disease may be secondary to infection, malignancies, drug therapies, nutritional deficiencies, or autoimmune phenomenon.

Oropharyngeal candidiasis typically presents as "pseudomembranous" candidiasis this is characterized by an easily removable white plaque. Less commonly, patients present with candidal leukoplakia, with white patches that cannot be removed. Treatment with topical or oral antifungal agents is usually effective for both oral and vaginal candidiasis. *Candida albicans* is the etiologic agent in most cases; however, prolonged use of systemic antifungal agents has led to resistant yeast infections which may require treatment with high dose "azoles" or amphotericin B.

Oral hairy leukoplakia (an Epstein-Barr virus associated condition) presents with painless thick white lesions on the lateral surface of the tongue that cannot be removed when scraped. No specific treatment is indicated; however, there have been reports of improvement with oral acyclovir, ZVD, and topical tretinoin.

Herpes simplex virus (HSV) infection is similar to that in an immunocompetent host; however, it usually presents in a more aggressive manner when CD4 counts fall below 200/μL. Treatment is initiated with either acyclovir or famciclovir, with intravenous foscarnet reserved for resistant strains of HSV.

Herpes zoster (shingles), which represents reactivation of latent varicella zoster virus (VZV), develops more commonly in HIV patients. Young, otherwise healthy patients who present with VZV infection should be tested for HIV disease. Dermatomal VZV can be treated with oral agents, while disseminated, ophthalmic or visceral disease should receive IV antiviral medication (acyclovir).

Treponema pallidium, the etiologic agent of syphilis, is a spirochete that enters the body through mucous membranes or broken skin. The course of primary and secondary syphilis in the patient with HIV disease is basically unaltered; however, treatment failure after standard therapy may occur more frequently in AIDS. There are several unusual manifestations of late syphilis that develop in the AIDS patient, including lues maligna (necrotizing vasculitis) and atypical early neurosyphilis (meningitis, stroke, blindness, or deafness)

Ophthalmologic Manifestations
Cytomegalovirus (CMV) retinitis is the leading ocular complication of advanced HIV disease (CD4 < 50/μL). Approximately 90% of patients with invasive disease develop eye involvement. Patients generally describe floaters, decreased visual acuity, or field deficits. The diagnosis is based on retinal findings (hemorrhage, exudates, dense opaque lesions, and vasculitis) from indirect ophthalmoscopy. If untreated, CMV retinitis is rapidly destructive, leading to blindness. The role of oral valganciclovir or ganciclovir for CMV prophylaxis of patients with CD4 counts less than 50/μL appears promising.

Other less frequent causes of retinitis in the AIDS patient include herpes zoster, *Pneumocystis carinii, T. gondii,* and ischemic retinitis.

Renal Manifestations
HIV nephropathy is characterized by striking proteinuria, hypoalbuminemia, anasarca, and rapidly progressive azotemia. This condition occurs more frequently in young black males. The course of HIV nephropathy is rapidly progressive with the development of end-stage renal disease within 4 months. A urinalysis, BUN, and creatinine should be obtained as part of the work-up in the emergency department. Diagnosis is confirmed with renal biopsy; however, there is currently no effective therapy for HIV nephropathy.

Treatment
Prescribing, monitoring, and adjusting antiretroviral regimens is outside the purview of the emergency medicine physician; however, it is important to recognize the indications for initiating treatment, the potential for opportunistic pathogens, and the inherent side effects of the medications.

During the past decade, there has been a dramatic decrease in the mortality and morbidity associated with HIV disease. Highly active antiretroviral therapy (HAART) is largely responsible for this change. Although the potential benefits derived from the newer regimens are considerable, they are not without their risks. The medications are costly, have significant side effects, and not all patients respond equally. The United States Department of Health and Human Services (DHHS) and the International AIDS Society-USA publish guidelines for initiating antiretroviral therapy on the basis of demonstrated benefit in clinical trials, clinical experience, and minimization of serious side effects.

HIV Vaccination
Unfortunately, no effective vaccine against the HIV virus has been produced to date despite many prototypes. However, there are several trials using a proposed vaccine (AIDSVAX) under way. Despite enthusiasm for the vaccine there are concerns about its effectiveness against current strains of HIV in the population.

Antiretroviral Therapy

The typical treatment regimens consist of combinations of the available antiretrovirals: NNRTIs (non-nucleoside reverse-transcriptase inhibitors), PIs (protease inhibitors), NRTIs (nucleoside analog reverse-transcriptase inhibitors), and NtRTIs (nucleotide analog reverse transcriptase inhibitor). The recommended treatment options are:

Two NRTIs + PI, Two NRTIs + NNRTI, Triple Nucleoside therapy,

or

One or two NRTIs + an NNRTI + PI.

Side Effects of Antiretroviral Medications Lipodystrophy is commonly seen in all patients taking PIs (Agenerase, Crixivan, Kaletra, Viracept, Norvir, Fortovase). This usually manifests as central obesity, gynecomastia, or a "buffalo hump" fatty distribution. Nausea, vomiting, bloating, hyperglycemia, hyperlipidemia, and osteopenia are also common.

Many NRTIs (Ziagen, Epivir, Zerit, Hivid, Retrovir, Combivir, Trizivir) have been associated with macrocytic anemia, peripheral neuropathy, lactic acidosis, steatosis, nausea, vomiting, diarrhea, and headache. There is also the potential for mitochondrial toxicity and lipodystrophy, as well.

Currently, the only approved NtRTI medication is Tenofovir (Viread). The most common side effects are nausea and diarrhea, with reports of lactic acidosis and hepatic steatosis as well.

NNRTIs (Sustiva, Rescriptor, Viramune) commonly cause nausea, diarrhea, vomiting, and headaches. There have been reports of rashes, including Stevens-Johnson syndrome and erythema multiforme.

Prevention

Sexual Transmission Prevention of sexual transmission of HIV includes avoidance of behaviors associated with increased likelihood of transmission (e.g., anal intercourse and sex during menses) and limiting the number of sexual partners, coupled with the use of latex condoms.

Postexposure Prophylaxis The optimal duration of post-exposure prophylaxis for health care workers is unknown. However, based on the current available occupational and animal studies, therapy should be administered as soon after exposure as possible (within 1 to 2 hours, up to 36 hours) and continued for 4 weeks, if tolerated. Therapy typically consists of a dual-drug regimen (Retrovir and Epivir). The National Clinician's Post Exposure Hotline can be accessed by phone (1-888-448-4911) or via internet (www.ucsf.edu/hivcntrl).

Maternal-Fetal Transmission

Antiretroviral therapy significantly reduces the incidence of maternal-fetal HIV transmission. Treatment of the mother with Zidovudine (Retrovir) should start in the second half of pregnancy, followed by a maternal loading dose during labor, then treatment of the infant for an additional 6 weeks. HIV-infected mothers should also be discouraged from breastfeeding, as this has been associated with significant viral transmission.

Selected Readings

Ammassari A, Scoppettuolo G, Murri R, et al. Changing disease patterns in focal brain lesion-causing disorders in AIDS. *J Acquir Immune Defic Syndr Hum Retrovirol* 1998;18:365–367.

Cardo DM, Culver DH, Ciesielski CA, et al. A case-control study of HIV seroconversion in health care workers after percutaneous exposure. *N Engl J Med* 1997;337:1485–1490.

Carr A. HIV Protease Inhibitor-Related Lipodystrophy Syndrome. *Clin Infect Dis* 2000;30(Suppl 2):S135–S142.

Colson AE, Sax PE. Primary HIV-1 infection: Diagnosis and treatment. UpToDate; 2004.

Cooper ER, Charurat M, Mofenson L, et al. Combination antiretroviral strategies for the treatment of pregnant HIV-1-infected women and prevention of perinatal HIV-1 transmission. *J Acquir Immune Defic Syndr Hum Retrovirol* 2002;29: 484–494.

Dworkin MS, Hanson DL, Kaplan JE, et al. Risk for preventable opportunistic infections in persons with AIDS after antiretroviral therapy increases CD4+ T lymphocyte counts above prophylaxis thresholds. *J Infect Dis* 2000;182:611–615.

Fortgang IS, Belitsos PC, Chaisson RE, Moore RD. Hepatomegaly and steatosis in HIV-infected patients receiving nucleoside analog antiretroviral therapy. *Am J Gastroenterol* 1995;90:1433–1436.

Friedland GH. Early treatment for HIV: the time has come. *N Engl J Med* 1990;322: 1000–1002.

Gerberding JL. Management of occupational exposures to blood-borne viruses. *N Engl J Med* 1995;16:444–451.

Grant RM, Dahn J, Warmerdam M, Liu L, et al. Transmission and transmissibility of drug-resistant HIV-1. 9th Conference of Retroviruses and Opportunistic Infections. Seattle, 2002.

Guidelines for the use of antiretroviral agents in HIV-infected adults and adolescents; 2003. http://aidsinfo.nih.gov/guidelines.

Hirschtick RE, Glassroth J, Jordan MC, et al. Bacterial pneumonia in persons infected with the human immunodeficiency virus. Pulmonary Complications of HIV Infection Study Group. *N Engl J Med* 1995;333:845–851.

Kaplan JE, Hanson D, Dworkin MS, et al. Epidemiology of human immunodeficiency virus-associated opportunistic infections in the United States in the era of highly active antiretroviral therapy. *Clin Infect Dis* 2000;30(Suppl 1):S5–S14.

Kovacs JA, Gill VJ, Meshnick S, Masur H. New insights into transmission, diagnosis, and treatment of Pneumocystis carinii pneumonia. *Ann Int Med* 1990;112: 750–757.

Mellors JW, Munoz A, Giorgi JV, et al. Plasma viral load and CD4+ lymphocytes as prognostic markers of HIV-1 infection. *Ann Int Med* 1997;126:946–954.

MinKoff H. Prevention of mother-to-child transmission of HIV. *Clin OB-GYN* 2001;44:210–225.

Palella FJ, Delaney KM, Moorman AC, et al. Declining morbidity and mortality among patients with advanced human immunodeficiency virus infection. *N Engl J Med* 1998;338:853.

Reef SE, Mayer KH. Opportunistic candidal infections in patients infected with HIV: prevention issues and priorities. *Clin Infect Dis* 1995;21(S1):S99–S102.

Sun XW, Kuhn L, Ellerbrock TV, et al. Human papillomavirus infection in women infected with the human immunodeficiency virus. *N Engl J Med* 1997;337: 1343–1349.

Weverling G, Lange J, Jurriaans S, et al. Alternative multidrug regimen provides improved suppression of HIV-1 replication over triple therapy. *AIDS* 1998;12: 117–122.

Cardiac Transplantation

Susan Graham

Complications

Within the past twenty years, cardiac transplantation has evolved from an experimental procedure to an accepted treatment for end-stage heart failure. Each year approximately 1,600 transplants are performed in the United States, and nearly 3,000 worldwide. One-, five-, and ten-year survival rates are approximately greater than 90%, 70%, and 50%, respectively. As the number of transplant operations performed each year increases and survival rates improve, emergency physicians must become increasingly skilled in the evaluation of the cardiac transplant patient in the emergency department (ED).

The most common reason for cardiac transplantation is end-stage heart failure from ischemia or non-ischemic etiology. Occasionally, transplantation will be performed for benign cardiac tumors, for coronary occlusive disease in previously transplanted patients, and for congenital heart defects in pediatric patients.

The transplanted heart functions differently from the normal heart in several ways. The transplanted heart remains denervated, and, therefore, lacks efferent and afferent fibers. Reinnervation may occur in some patients a few years after transplant. The resting heart rate is usually higher (e.g., 90 to 100 beats per minute) due to the lack of parasympathetic control on the sinoatrial node. Similarly, cardiac transplant patients depend on circulating catecholamines to increase their heart rate and contractility in order to increase cardiac output in response to stress or exercise; therefore, transplant patients are instructed to shift gradually from the supine to a standing position, and to perform warm-up and cool down exercises for 5 to 10 minutes prior to and after strenuous physical activity. Cardiovascular drugs should be used with caution in these patients since these medications may have an altered effect due to denervation. **Table 61.1** lists the effect of commonly used cardiac drugs in transplant patients. In general, cardiac function of the transplanted heart is excellent, with a nearly normal left ventricular ejection fraction. However, levels of brain natriuretic peptide (BNP) may remain elevated even after successful transplantation of a heart.

Advances in immunosuppressive therapy account for much of the improved survival rate in cardiac transplant pa-

tients. Most immunosuppressive protocols are divided into two periods. The first period is the induction phase, and involves the administration of high doses of immunosuppressive drugs for the first few weeks following surgery to prevent rejection. The second period is the maintenance phase, during which immunosuppressive medications are given at lower doses and steroid withdrawal is attempted. The most common regimens are a combination of cyclosporin or tacrolimus, azathioprine or mycophenolate mofetil, and low dose prednisone. Other immunosuppressive medications may be used for induction to treat episodes of rejection or for rescue therapy. Successful long-term immunosuppressive therapy requires depressing the patient's immune response enough to prevent rejection, but not so much as to invite infection. Similarly, there are a number of drugs that interact with the immunosuppressives, resulting in increased or decreased levels, or in increased organ toxicity. Common drugs which interact in such a way are: diltiazem, verapamil, ketoconazole, fluconazole, bromocriptine, methylprednisone, metoclopramide, erythromycin, phenobarbital, phenytoin, carbamazepine, rifampin, and St. John's Wort. Emergency physicians should alter the doses or add or withdraw immunosuppressive medications only after discussion with the patient's transplant physician or with a pharmacist.

The leading causes of morbidity and death following cardiac transplantation are rejection and infection. Other serious complications include allograft coronary artery disease, malignancy, and complications associated with the use of immunosuppressive medications, such as progressive renal failure.

Rejection

Allograft rejection remains one of the leading causes of morbidity and mortality in transplant recipients. Cell-mediated rejection is responsible for the vast majority of such episodes. Rejection may occur at any time, but 90% occur within the first 6 months: rejection is less common after 1 year without significant alterations in immunosuppression. The most important risk factors for rejection include female recipient (particularly multiparous females), having a human leukocyte antigen (HLA) mismatch, and receiving a fe-

Table 61.1

Cardiovascular Drugs after Cardiac Transplantation

Drug	Effect in Recipient	Mechanism
Digitalis	Normal increase in contractility, minimal AV nodal effect	Denervation
Atropine	None	Denervation
Epinephrine, norepinephrine	Increased contractility and chronotropy	Denervation Hypersensitivity
Isoproterenol	Normal increase in inotropy, chronotropy	No neuronal uptake
Adenosine	Normal AV block	Direct effect
Verapamil	Normal AV block	Direct effect
Nifedipine, hydralazine	No reflex tachycardia	Denervation
Beta-blockers	Increased antagonist effect during exercise	Denervation

male or younger donor heart, or having a hepatitis C mismatch (particularly if the donor has had hepatitis C).

The majority of patients with acute rejection are asymptomatic. Patients may present with complaints of fatigue, malaise, or palpitations. Less than 10% of patients with rejection present with hemodynamic compromise. Arrhythmias have been shown to be associated with rejection, although not all arrhythmias are caused by rejection.

The gold standard for the diagnosis of acute rejection in adults is endomyocardial biopsy. Echocardiography may prove useful as a screening tool but clinical suspicion confirmed by tissue biopsy is required for definitive diagnosis. Therapy for acute rejection involves a pulse of high-dose corticosteroids and reevaluation of other drug therapy.

Infection

The use of immunosuppressive medications to prevent allograft rejection results in an increased risk of infection. Infectious complications are categorized by the time since transplant. The majority of life-threatening infections occur in the first 3 months following surgery (i.e., occurring early), when immunosuppression is maximal. During this period, many infections are nosocomial, often catheter-related, and usually involve *Staphylococcus* species and Gram-negative organisms. Late infections (following 3 months post-transplant) occur in approximately 20% of patients per year of follow-up. The lungs remain the most common site of infection in cardiac transplant patients, followed by blood, urine, the gastrointestinal tract, and the sternal wound. Cytomegalovirus in a common infection may affect numerous organs and can occur early or late after transplant.

All cardiac transplant patients with signs or symptoms of infection require a thorough evaluation. Fever may not always be present in these patients; similarly, fever does not always indicate infection (i.e., a sign of rejection). Blood, urine, and sputum should be sent for analysis and culture. All patients require a chest x-ray. Prophylactic antibiotics should be initiated in the ED, after culture; and the specific drug regiment to be used is best determined in consultation with the patient's transplant physician.

The total artificial heart and implanted ventricular assist devices are available at transplant centers. Currently, these devices serve as a bridge to cardiac transplantation. Complications such as thromboembolism and infection remain a challenge.

Allograft Coronary Artery Disease

Allograft coronary artery disease (also known as graft atherosclerosis or transplant coronary artery disease) is the leading cause of death occurring in these patients one year posttransplantation. The disease is detectable by intracoronary ultrasound in at least 50% of recipients within three years after surgery. Unlike normal atherosclerosis, the disease is concentric and tubular, and is a diffuse process that affects both the proximal and distal coronary vessels. Risk factors for allograft coronary artery disease include hyperlipidemia, obesity, donor age, donor ischemic time, rejection, or hepatitis C mismatch.

Because the heart is denervated, cardiac transplant patients do not experience angina. Rather, they may present with new-onset or worsening shortness of breath, chest fullness, or signs and symptoms of congestive heart failure. Graft failure, myocardial infarction, and sudden death, alone or in combination, may be the presenting symptoms of allograft coronary artery disease. The baseline ECG is usually a right bundle branch pattern. Abnormal cardiac enzymes are helpful in discerning the correct diagnosis, although systemic viral infections can also cause global left ventricular function.

Because of the disease's diffuse nature, percutaneous transluminal coronary angioplasty (PTCA) and coronary artery bypass grafting (CABG) are not usually effective in the treatment of allograft coronary artery disease.

Malignancy

The development of malignant neoplasms is a potential consequence of immunosuppressive therapy. The current estimate of the risk of malignancy after cardiac transplantation is 1% to 2% per year. The frequency depends primarily on the specific immunosuppressive drugs utilized. Cutaneous malignancies (usually squamous cell) are the most common tumors. The next most common tumor is a unique form of lymphoma, referred to as posttransplant lymphoproliferative disease. The clinical presentation of posttransplant lymphoproliferative disease ranges from a mild lymphadenopathy and fever to widely disseminated disease. Other malignancies may occur, which may be rapidly progressive due to the chronic immunosuppression.

Complications of Immunosuppressive Medications

A number of side effects are associated with the use of immunosuppressive medications. The two most common are hypertension and nephrotoxicity. Hypertension occurs in 50% to 100% of cardiac transplant patients on cyclosporine. The hypertension develops within days after surgery, includes diastolic hypertension, and usually requires multiple drug therapy to control. Calcium channel blockers and angiotensin-converting enzyme (ACE) inhibitors are the drugs most frequently used to treat this complication. β-blockers are withheld early after transplantation due to denervation hypersensitivity.

Declining renal function is a major short- and long-term concern in transplant patients. Hypertension, transplant drug toxicity, and pre-existing medical conditions act synergistically to accelerate the decline in kidney function. The ED physician must be aware of the potential for drug interaction when prescribing medicine and, further, of the potential for worsening renal function from dye studies.

Selected Readings

Chin C, Naftel D, Singh T, et al. Risk factors for recurrent rejection in pediatric heart transplantation: a multicenter experience *J Heart Lung Transplant* 2004;23:178–185.

Grauhan O, Patzurek J, Hummel M, et al. Donor-transmitted coronary atherosclerosis. *J Heart Lung Transplant* 2003;22:568–573.

Hollenber S, Klein L, Parrillo J, et al. Changes in coronary endothelial function predict progression of allograft vasculopathy after heart transplantation. *J Heart Lung Transplant* 2004;23:1265–1271.

Hosenpud JD, Morton MJ. Physiology and hemodynamic assessment of the transplanted heart. In: Hosenpud JD, Cobanoglu A, et al, eds. *Cardiac Transplantation.* New York: Springer-Verlag 1991:169–189.

Kirchhoff W, Gradaus R, Stypmann J, et al. Vasoactive peptides during long-term follow-up of patients after cardiac transplantation. *J Heart Lung Transplant* 2004;23:284–288.

Miller LW. Long-term complications of cardiac transplantation. *Prog Cardiovasc Dis* 1991;33:229–282.

Oaks TE, Wallwork J. Cardiac transplantation: a review. *Br J Biomed Sci* 1993;50:200–211.

Petri WA. Infections in heart transplant recipients. *Clin Infect Dis* 1994;18:141–148.

Rosenthal D, Chin C, Nishimura K, et al. Identifying cardiac transplant rejection in children: diagnostic utility of echocardiography, right heart catheterization and endomyocardial biopsy data. *J Heart Lung Transplant* 2004;23:323–329.

Rubel JR, Milford EL, McKay DB, et al. Renal insufficiency at end-stage renal disease in heart transplant population. *J Heart Lung Transplant* 2004;23:289–300.

Senechal M, LePrince P, Tezenas du Montcel S, et al. Bacterial mediastinitis after heart transplantation: clinical presentation, risk factors and treatment. *J Heart Lung Transplant* 2004;23:165–170.

Shao-Zhou G, Chaparro S, Perlroth M, et al. Post-transplantation lymphoproliferative disease in heart and heart-lung transplant recipients: 30-year experience at Stanford University. *J Heart Lung Transplant* 2003;22:505–514.

Shiba N, Chan M, Kwok B, et al. Analysis of survivors more than 10 years after heart transplantation in the cyclosporine era: Stanford Experience. *J Heart Lung Transplant* 2004;23:155–164.

Showkat H, Starling R, Avery R, et al. Donor hepatitis-C seropositivity is an independent risk factor for the development of accelerated coronary vasculopathy and predicts outcome after cardiac transplantation. *J Heart Lung Transplant* 2004;23:277–283.

Yamani M, Youssufuddin M, Starling R, et al. Does acute cellular rejection correlate with cardiac allograft vasculopathy? *J Heart Lung Transplant* 2004;23:272–276.

Hypersensitivity

Richard S. Krause

Anaphylactic/Anaphylactoid Reactions

The term *anaphylaxis* was first used in 1902 to describe a paradoxical reaction to an immunization protocol in which dogs repeatedly injected with an allergen developed increased sensitivity rather than immunity. Later, it became clear that the phenomenon required an initial exposure to an allergen followed by a delay of days to weeks before the reaction could be elicited by re-exposure. Subsequently, it has been demonstrated that the clinical features of anaphylaxis are mediated by activation of antigen-specific IgE attached to mast cells and basophils. When re-exposed to the allergen, IgE causes the release of mediators from mast cells and basophils. These mediators are responsible for the observed clinical manifestations. The classic anaphylactic reaction is thus an immune-mediated phenomenon. A nearly identical clinical syndrome known as an anaphylactoid reaction does not require previous exposure. It immediately follows an exposure to an inciting substance. Anaphylactoid reactions involve the same mediators implicated in anaphylaxis, but are not IgE-mediated. In the clinical setting, the term anaphylaxis is often used to describe both types of phenomenon. In this chapter anaphylaxis will be used to represent both conditions unless otherwise specified.

A variety of substances including foreign proteins and drugs can elicit anaphylaxis. In the classic mechanism, exposure to a foreign substance, either in isolation or bound as a hapten to a carrier protein, elicits the generation of an IgE antibody. The antibody binds to receptors on mast cells and basophils. The receptors are activated on re-exposure and mediators are released, causing the clinical manifestations of anaphylaxis. Certain other agents, such as radiocontrast, can directly trigger mediator release. A third mechanism that may produce anaphylaxis involves complement activation after exposure, with subsequent generation of mediators known as anaphylatoxins. For some substances, exposure leads to anaphylaxis with no clearly identified mechanism (NSAIDs are one example). In addition, in the entity known as idiopathic anaphylaxis, no inciting agent can be identified.

The most commonly implicated medical agents that cause anaphylaxis are antibiotics. Penicillins and cephalo-sporins are the most often cited. Reactions are much more common after parenteral administration and are more severe than those that follow oral exposures. Approximately 1 in 5,000 exposures leads to anaphylaxis. More than 100 deaths per year are reported. Approximately 10% of patients sensitive to penicillin may have cross-sensitivity to cephalosporins, even with no history of previous cephalosporin exposure. Aspirin and NSAIDs are common causes of medication-induced anaphylaxis. Radiocontrast media administered intravenously may cause an anaphylactoid reaction that is clinically very similar to true anaphylaxis, although it is not IgE mediated and does not require previous exposure. One to two percent of patients experience reactions, but fatalities are rare. The use of low molecular weight contrast media or pretreatment with antihistamines and steroids leads to lower rates of anaphylaxis. Gastrointestinal administration of contrast is an unlikely cause of anaphylaxis.

Hymenoptera stings are the most common environmental cause of anaphylaxis. The rate of reactions is not well established. The fatality rate is low, with fewer than 100 deaths occurring per year, in spite of the large numbers of exposures. Less serious allergic reactions (e.g., urticaria, local reactions) are also very common with stings. Foods are another common cause of anaphylaxis. Most cases are mild, but fatal anaphylaxis due to foods has been reported. Nuts and seeds, legumes, shellfish, and chocolate are common offending agents.

The major physiologic events in anaphylaxis include increased mucous secretion, bronchospasm, decreased vascular smooth muscle tone, and increased capillary permeability. Mucous secretion and bronchospasm are responsible for the signs and symptoms of shortness of breath, chest tightness, tachypnea, wheezing, and hypoxia. Airway mucosal edema also contributes to respiratory difficulty. Decreased vascular smooth muscle tone and increased capillary permeability can cause cardiovascular collapse. Many of the clinical and physiologic manifestations of anaphylaxis can be explained by the actions of histamine released from mast cells. Elevated plasma histamine has been measured in patients experiencing anaphylaxis. Additional mediators have also been implicated and include leukotriene C_4, prostaglandin D_2, and tryptase.

The degree of sensitivity and the dose, route, and rate of administration of the offending agent determine the timing of onset of an anaphylactic reaction. Large intravenous doses are most likely to produce immediate, severe reactions. Most reactions occur within minutes to hours, but symptoms may be delayed up to 3 days after an oral exposure. It is a generally accepted clinical maxim that the more rapidly the symptoms develop, the more severe the reaction is likely to be. A biphasic reaction in which recurrent symptoms develop hours after initial improvement has been described. The incidence is not precisely known, but has been reported in up to 20% of cases of severe anaphylaxis. Biphasic reactions are associated with a delayed onset of symptoms after initial exposure.

Airway obstruction from upper airway edema is the most common cause of death in anaphylaxis. Bronchospasm with wheezing, shortness of breath, and chest tightness are lower airway manifestations of anaphylaxis. Respiratory failure can occur. Cardiovascular abnormalities are responsible for the remaining major clinical manifestations of anaphylaxis. Hypotension is common and thought to result from increased vascular permeability with intravascular volume depletion and vasodilation. Frank cardiovascular collapse may occur with profound hypotension leading to confusion, syncope, or seizures. While ECG changes of ischemia may be seen, there is no evidence that mediators have direct cardiotoxicity. The cardiac effects are probably secondary to ischemia, resulting from volume depletion, loss of vascular tone, hypotension, and decreased oxygen delivery.

The clinical picture of anaphylaxis almost always involves the skin. One or more manifestations of pruritus, erythema, urticaria, or angioedema are noted in more than 90% of patients. Mucosal edema and erythema of the nose, eyes, or mouth may also be seen with resultant tearing, itching, nasal congestion, and sneezing. The GI tract is also affected. Symptoms of abdominal pain, nausea, vomiting, and diarrhea are often observed. Visceral congestion is a common finding at autopsy.

The diagnosis of anaphylaxis is clinical and based on the observation of the typical features. When these are associated with a history of exposure to a foreign substance, the diagnosis is virtually certain. Cutaneous reactions, airway obstruction, bronchospasm, cardiovascular effects or GI symptoms may occur singly or in any combination. Diagnostic confusion may occur when cutaneous manifestations are lacking. Anaphylaxis should be considered when a patient presents in shock or syncope without an obvious cause.

The differential diagnosis of acute airway obstruction includes infections of the upper airway and foreign body aspiration. The history and physical examination usually allow these to be differentiated. Angiotensin-converting enzyme (ACE) inhibitors may cause angioedema of the upper airway, and this diagnosis should be considered in patients taking these medications who develop facial or airway swelling. Treatment for this condition is similar to that for anaphylaxis. Status asthmaticus may mimic the lower airway manifestations of anaphylaxis, but a history of asthma is almost always present and a history of exposure less likely. Myocardial infarction can cause hypotension, pulmonary congestion, and changes in mental status, but is usually accompanied by typical chest discomfort and ECG changes. Pulmonary embolism can cause respiratory distress and shock, but symptoms are usually limited to the respiratory system and the lungs are usually clear. Chest pain is often present and there are often risk factors for deep venous thrombosis. Hereditary angioedema is due to a deficiency of the enzyme C_1 esterase inhibitor. It can cause airway obstruction, angioedema, and GI symptoms. The GI symptoms are often prominent and there may be a family history. Urticaria does not occur and cardiovascular effects are not noted.

The symptoms of scombroid fish poisoning are very similar to those of anaphylaxis. They occur when spoiled fish with a high histadine content are ingested. The histidine is broken down to histamine and this is responsible for the symptoms. Exposure to monosodium glutamate (MSG) can cause flushing, chest discomfort, and nausea in individuals susceptible to the "Chinese restaurant" syndrome. Headache is common and urticaria does not occur. Patients may present with respiratory distress, stridor, and inability to swallow due to globus hystericus. In this condition there is no identified pathology on indirect or fiberoptic laryngoscopy. Globus hystericus is a diagnosis of exclusion, and may be a form of Munchausen's syndrome.

Prehospital assessment and stabilization of patients with signs and symptoms of anaphylaxis begin with standard interventions provided to all patients with potentially serious conditions. After airway patency is assured, high-flow oxygen and cardiac monitoring should be applied. Intubation, if needed, may be difficult due to airway edema. Bag–mask ventilation may be effective as a temporizing measure while drugs are administered. Surgical airway intervention may be needed in rare cases. A large bore intravenous line with isotonic crystalloid solution is advisable, even for a normotensive patient. Hypotensive patients should receive vigorous fluid resuscitation. An initial bolus of 1 L for adults or 20 mg/kg for children is often appropriate. In patients with known or suspected cardiac or renal disease, fluid resuscitation should be cautious. A systolic blood pressure of 80 to 100 mm Hg is acceptable in adults. The mainstay of management is pharmacologic. Epinephrine is the primary agent and should be available on all advanced life support ambulances. Many patients with a history of hymenoptera sting or food-induced anaphylaxis have an epinephrine autoinjector. If epinephrine is not available on the ambulance, the patient's autoinjector should be sought and used.

Epinephrine increases intracellular production of adenosine 38, 58-cyclic monophosphate (cAMP) in mast cells and basophils with resultant inhibition of mediator release. In addition, epinephrine is a physiologic antagonist to the vasodilatory, bronchoconstricting, and cutaneous effects of histamine and other mediators. It counteracts bronchospasm, hypotension, urticaria, and angioedema. Subcutaneous administration is recommended except for patients in profound shock, in which case epinephrine may be given intravenously. Sublingual injection is an alternative for patients in severe distress who lack IV access. The adverse effects of epinephrine are predominantly cardiovascular. Hypertension and dysrhythmias occur, predominantly when the intravenous route is used in patients with preexisting cardiac disease or hypertension. Malignant dysrhythmias, myocardial infarction, and death have been reported, especially after intravenous use in patients older than 50 years. Dosages for epinephrine and other drugs are noted in **Table 62.1**.

Patients taking β-receptor blocking agents may be resistant to the pressor effects of epinephrine. Glucagon may be effective as a treatment of refractory hypotension in these patients, due to positive inotropic and chronotropic effects that are not mediated by β-receptors. Inhaled β-agonists are useful as secondary therapy for bronchospasm. Upper airway edema may respond to nebulized racemic epinephrine. Antihistamines and corticosteroids are not primary agents in serious anaphylactic or anaphylactoid reactions. While some authors have theorized that corticosteroids decrease the incidence or severity of biphasic or protracted reactions, this has not been verified. Antihistamines seem to affect predominantly the cutaneous manifestations of anaphylaxis, although in theory histamine-induced vasodilatation should also respond. While both the H_1 and H_2 effects of histamine may play a role in anaphylaxis, H_1 blocking agents have a more logical role and should be used first. Some authors have suggested a role for H_2 blockers in prevention of biphasic or protracted reactions, but this has not been verified.

Corticosteroids are useful in treatment of bronchospasm and urticaria. The slow onset of action of corticosteroids and their lack of effect on the cardiovascular manifestations of anaphylaxis make them second-line agents.

Pretreatment with antihistamines and corticosteroids prevents or ameliorates reactions to intravenous contrast agents. Prior to administration of contrast to patients at high risk of an anaphylactoid reaction, pharmacologic prophylaxis should be administered with antihistamines and corticosteroids. There are also short-term desensitization regimens effective in preventing reactions to penicillin antibiotics. These should be considered when a patient with a history of a serious anaphylactic reaction requires penicillin as a first-line agent for a life-threatening infection.

Most patients treated in the emergency department (ED) for anaphylaxis respond rapidly to treatment, but patients with persistent manifestations involving the cardiovascular or respiratory systems require admission for further treatment and observation. Published materials regarding the majority of patients who respond to treatment also recommend a period of observation up to 24 hours. These recommendations are based on the occurrence of a second phase of the anaphylactic response occurring 4 to 8 hours after the initial stimulus. Anaphylaxis with a delayed second phase is known as biphasic anaphylaxis and is reported in up to 20% of cases. Prevention of biphasic anaphylaxis with corticosteroids is theoretically attractive, but the true incidence of biphasic anaphylaxis and the ef-

Table 62.1
Pharmacologic Treatment of Anaphylaxis

Drug	Dosage	Indications
β-Agonists		
Epinephrine	Adults: 0.3 mL 1:1,000 dilution SQ q 15 min or 1.0 mL 1:10,000 dilution slow IV Children: 0.01 mL/kg 1:10,000 dilution SQ q 15 min or 0.01 mL/kg 1:10,000 dilution slow IV	Shock, angioedema, airway obstruction, brochospasm, urticaria
Albuterol	Adults: 0.5 mL of 0.5% soln in 2.5 mL NS nebulized q 15 min Children: 0.03 mL/kg of 0.5% soin via nebulized q 15 min	Brochospasm
Antihistamines		
H_1-Blocker	Adults: diphenhydramine, 25–50 mg IV, IM, or po q 6-8h Children: diphenhydramine, 2 mg/kg IV, IM or po q 6–8h	Hypotension, urticaria
H_2-Blocker	Adults: cimetidine, 300 mg IV or po q 6h Children: cimetidine, 5 to 10 mg/kg IV or po q 6h	Hypotension, urticaria
Corticosteroids		
Hydrocortisone	Adults: 250 to 500 mg IV q 6h Children: 5 mg/kg IV q 6h	Bronchospasm, urticaria, possible modification biphasic reactions
Methylprednisolone	Adults: 40 to 125 mg IV q 6h Children: 1 to 2 mg/kg IV q 6h	
Other agents		
Glucagon	Adults: 1 to 2 mg slow IV or IM Children: dosage not established, adult dose is equivalent to 150 μg/kg	Shock, for patients with beta-blockade

ficacy of corticosteroids is not well established. Given the lack of definitive data, hospital admission for patients with airway compromise or hypotension represents the most conservative approach and is therefore advised. Other patients may be considered for discharge after a period of observation.

Angioedema and Urticaria

Urticaria is a common cutaneous condition, also known as hives. Three major mechanisms of pathogenesis have been described. Most commonly, urticaria is a manifestation of acute IgE-mediated hypersensitivity. As with the classic anaphylaxis, IgE-mediated urticaria occurs when a sensitized host is re-exposed to an antigen. Preformed mediators are then released from mast cells and basophils. Histamine is the primary mediator. As with anaphylaxis, urticaria also may be caused by complement-mediated reactions or specific drug reactions, or may be idiopathic. Physical agents such as cold, sun exposure, and pressure also cause urticaria. Urticaria is characterized by superficial dermal edema and vascular dilation with capillary leakage of plasma. Angioedema can be regarded as a more severe form of urticaria. It is characterized by vasodilation and exudation of plasma into the deeper layers of the dermis and may also occur on the mucosal surfaces of the respiratory or gastrointestinal tract. Causes of angioedema include those listed for urticaria. In addition, there is an inherited form of angioedema known as hereditary angioneurotic edema (HAE). HAE is inherited as an autosomal dominant, but may also occur sporadically. It is caused by a deficiency of the enzyme C_1 esterase inhibitor. This deficiency results in an inappropriate activation of the complement pathway with the resultant clinical manifestations of angioedema.

Urticarial lesions are also known as hives. The lesions are red and raised and vary in size from very small (papular urticaria) up to many centimeters (giant urticaria). There may be only a few, small lesions or they may be numerous and become large and confluent. Urticarial lesions are pruritic. The individual lesions are evanescent and tend to first enlarge and then resolve over several hours with new lesions occurring at other locations. When lesions are fixed in one location and persist for more than 24 hours, the diagnosis of vasculitis should be considered. Urticarial lesions may occur on any part of the body. The deeper lesions of angioedema are nonpitting and are often nonpruritic. Angioedema may involve the face, oral cavity, palms, soles, and genitalia. Airway compromise can result from edema of the tongue or pharynx. In HAE, symptoms of abdominal pain, nausea, and vomiting are common and result from localized edema of the gastrointestinal mucosa. The diagnosis of urticaria is based on the history and observation of the characteristic skin lesions. Angioedema is diagnosed by observing the typical pattern of asymmetric, nonpitting edema. Patients with HAE and abdominal pain usually carry the previous diagnosis of HAE. Other causes of abdominal pain must be ruled out.

Most cases of urticaria are idiopathic. Specific causes include many drugs and foods. Commonly implicated drugs include the penicillins and sulfonamide antibiotics, salicylates, other NSAIDs, insulin, codeine, and other narcotics. Food substances associated with urticaria include shellfish, chocolate, aged cheeses, peanuts, and many others. Viral infections including hepatitis, varicella, and infectious mononucleosis are frequently associated with urticaria. Occult infections such as sinusitis and prostatitis may also precipitate urticaria. Physical urticaria may also occur due to a variety of physical stimuli including cold, heat, pressure or sun exposure. Urticaria may occur as a local allergic phenomenon at the site of exposure to an allergen. Acquired (i.e., nonhereditary) angioedema is most often idiopathic. The ACE inhibitors used for treatment of hypertension and congestive heart failure may cause angioedema by an unknown mechanism.

After the diagnosis is established, the ED evaluation of urticaria or angioedema is aimed at differentiating among common possible causes by the history and physical examination. Laboratory testing is not usually part of this evaluation unless the history or physical points to an underlying systemic illness. Important historical factors include exposure to commonly implicated agents and other inciting factors. Patients should be questioned about the signs and symptoms of either systemic or local infections. The past history should include questions about previous episodes and any previous evaluation. A family history of similar episodes suggests HAE. The physical should seek signs suggesting that the urticaria is a manifestation of a more severe episode of systemic anaphylaxis. Airway patency should be assured and hypotension or tachycardia regarded as possible indications of anaphylaxis. The symptoms of faintness, dizziness, or syncope are also indications of a possible anaphylactic reaction.

The treatment of urticaria and angioedema is empiric and symptomatic. If potential inciting agents are identified, further exposure should be avoided. Mild cases of urticaria or angioedema may be treated with an oral antihistamine alone. Parenteral routes may be utilized for a more rapid effect. Typical regimens are diphenhydramine (Benadryl), 25 to 50 mg, or hydroxyzine (Vistaril, Atarax) 25 mg every 6 hours until the symptoms are resolved. Severe cases of urticaria with generalized hives and severe itching or angioedema involving the upper airway should be treated with both subcutaneous epinephrine and a parenteral antihistamine. Epinephrine often produces dramatic relief. Doses are outlined in Table 62.1. Corticosteroids are often used in the treatment of acute urticaria and angioedema but should be considered second-line agents. H_2 blockers have also been used, but their efficacy is unproven. Insect stings may cause reactions that are purely local (swelling and itching adjacent to the sting) or progress to generalized urticaria or anaphylaxis. Urticaria and anaphylaxis are treated in the usual manner. Local reactions may be treated with ice and antihistamines.

Most patients with urticaria or angioedema may be discharged for outpatient follow-up. Patients with airway involvement or possible anaphylaxis should be considered for observation. When a patient experiences generalized urticaria or anaphylaxis as a result of an envenomation, they are at risk of anaphylaxis on subsequent exposure. They should be instructed to avoid situations likely to lead to an exposure, and consideration should be given to prescribing an epinephrine autoinjector. When angioedema is associated with ACE inhibitor use, the drug should be discontinued and an agent from another class of antihypertensives selected.

Allergic Rhinitis

Allergic rhinitis is an antibody-mediated reaction localized to the nasal mucous membranes. It is very common in adolescents with a reported prevalence of up to 25%. The clinical manifestations include nasal congestion, drainage, and sneezing. Conjunctivitis is a commonly associated symptom. The pathophysiology involves sensitization and re-exposure of mucosal mast cells to an environmental allergen. Allergic rhinitis may occur in a seasonal or perennial pattern. In the seasonal form pollen is the inciting allergen and the condition tends to recur at the same time each year. In perennial allergic rhinitis, dust, dander, or chemical exposure may elicit symptoms at any time.

The diagnosis of allergic rhinitis is based on the history and the presence of characteristic symptoms. Typical findings on physical examination include swollen, pale, boggy nasal mucosa. There may be associated conjunctivitis, but systemic signs and symptoms are lacking. The main differential diagnosis is upper respiratory tract infection, which is not seasonal and is unrelated to environmental factors. Upper respiratory infections are usually associated with systemic symptoms of fever, malaise, and myalgias.

Symptomatic treatment of allergic rhinitis consists mainly of antihistamines. The newer nonsedating agents are effective, but are more expensive than older H_1 blockers. Nasal corticosteroids are also expensive but are effective and have few adverse effects. Topical nasal decongestants are effective, but tachyphylaxis and rebound nasal congestion limit their utility. Perennial rhinitis also responds to antihistamines but is best treated by avoiding inciting agents. If allergens cannot be avoided, immunotherapy may be effective.

Drug and Food Allergies

Allergic reactions to foods and food additives are common. Nuts, eggs, legumes, chocolate, peanuts, and dairy products are often implicated. Most reactions are mediated by IgE-coated mast cells, which line the mucosa of the GI tract. After prior sensitization, ingestion of the allergen causes release of histamine and other mediators. Non–IgE-mediated reactions may also occur.

The diagnosis of food allergies depends on the history. Prior reactions are usual. Many patients give a history of multiple allergic symptoms. The most common symptoms of food allergy are limited to the GI tract. Crampy abdominal pain, nausea with or without vomiting, and local

swelling of the lips, tongue, and pharynx are observed. Occasionally, generalized urticaria or anaphylaxis is seen. Treatment is symptomatic, with antihistamines used for mild symptoms and epinephrine for severe urticaria or anaphylaxis. If the offending agent can be identified, avoidance should be advised as a preventative measure.

Drugs are commonly implicated in allergic reactions. Most drugs are not true allergens, but function as haptens. When the drug molecules are bound to plasma proteins, they may become immunogenic. Many adverse allergic effects are not immunologically mediated, but mimic true allergic reactions. ACE inhibitor associated angioedema and reactions to IV contrast are prominent examples. Penicillin is the most commonly implicated drug in severe allergic reactions, but allergy to almost any drug can occur. The clinical manifestations and treatment of acute drug allergy does not differ from other acute allergic reactions. Topical reactions may be treated by avoidance and topical corticosteroids or by oral antihistamines. Generalized urticaria or angioedema is treated using antihistamines with epinephrine added in more severe cases. When an allergic reaction occurs in the setting of exposure to a likely offending agent, patients should be counseled regarding avoidance.

Serum Sickness

Serum sickness provides the classic model of an immune-complex disease and is most often caused by drug hypersensitivity. When an allergen is introduced into a sensitized individual, it binds to specific antibody and immune complexes are formed. Usually, these immune complexes are cleared by the reticuloendothelial system without complications. When the immune complexes exceed a certain size and are present in large amounts, they may be deposited in tissues with resultant inflammation and tissue damage. The kidney, joints, skin, and blood vessels walls are the tissues usually affected.

In drug-induced serum sickness, drug molecules act as haptens, with resulting sensitization and formation of specific antibody. Upon re-exposure, immune complexes form and serum sickness may result. Implicated agents include sulfonamides, penicillins, diphenylhydantoin, and thiazides. Blood products may also cause serum sickness. Serum sickness and late-onset anaphylaxis has also been reported to occur after insect stings. Clinical manifestations of serum sickness typically begin 1 to 3 weeks after the initial exposure to an agent and may occur much sooner (12 to 36 hours), if there has been prior sensitization. Typical signs and symptoms include fever, malaise, arthralgias, and cutaneous rashes. Gastrointestinal symptoms, lymphadenopathy, and proteinuria also occur, but are less common. The skin eruption may be morbiliform or urticarial and is often confined to the trunk, though it may be generalized. Less often, frank arthritis or vasculitis may occur. Vasculitis may affect the kidney, central nervous system, and the coronary arteries.

The diagnosis of drug-induced serum sickness is based on the clinical presentation and a history of exposure to a likely offending agent. Laboratory tests to detect circulating immune complexes are available, but are not helpful during the initial patient encounter in the ED. Drug-induced serum sickness typically resolves within days of withdrawal of the offending drug, so no specific treatment is usually needed. Antihistamines may provide relief from the cutaneous manifestations. Corticosteroids are recommended for severe cutaneous manifestations or if there is significant vasculitis. Acetaminophen may be used for arthralgias and fever.

Selected Readings

Atkinson TP, Kaliner MA. Anaphylaxis. *Med Clin North Am* 1992;76:841.

Austen KF. Diseases of immediate type hypersensitivity. In: Wilson JD, et al, eds. *Harrison's Principles of Internal Medicine,* 12th ed. New York: McGraw-Hill 1991.

Bochner BS. Anaphylaxis. *N Engl J Med* 1991;324:1785.

Cochrane CB, Koffler D. Immune complex disease in experimental animals and man. *Adv Immunol* 1963;16:185.

Greenberger PA. Contrast media reactions. *J Allergy Clin Immunol* 1984;74:600.

Lawley TJ, Frank MM. Immune-complex diseases. In: Wilson JD, et al, eds. *Harrison's Principles of Internal Medicine,* 12th ed. New York: McGraw-Hill 1991.

Stark BJ, Sullivan TJ. Biphasic and protracted anaphylaxis. *J Allergy Clin Immunol* 1986;78:76.

Systemic Infectious Diseases

Gregory A. Volturo

Management of infectious disease is vitally important to the practice of emergency medicine. Illness from infection precipitates a large number of emergency department (ED) visits. Illness may range from benign self-limiting conditions to more severe life-threatening infections. Some infections are routine and common, while others are elusive, rare or are completely foreign to a specific geographic area; therefore all emergency care providers should have a broad breadth of knowledge about infectious disease.

Infectious disease management issues facing emergency physicians are often different from those confronted by physicians in other practice settings. The ability to differentiate between serious and minor illness based on the data that is immediately available determines the initial management, as well as subsequent patient outcome. Admission and discharge decisions are routinely made in the ED. Culture and sensitivity results are usually not available, and, as a result, presumptive diagnoses are made based on clinical presentation. Treatment with antibiotics is frequently empiric. Many ED patients do not have continuing care physicians, fail to comply with medical follow-up, and/or tend to be non-compliant with treatment; therefore, the emergency physicians must consider these tendencies when make decisions regarding antibiotic selection, dosage, and route of delivery.

As they have relatively high exposure to communicable disease, emergency care providers must have solid knowledge regarding both treatment and prevention of disease. Human immunodeficiency virus (HIV)-related infections, emerging antibiotic resistance, and the increasing incidence of tuberculosis have further burdened the ED, requiring emergency physicians to have much more in-depth knowledge regarding infectious diseases.

Lastly, with an overburdened health care system, the ED is pivotal in developing and implementing new strategies to manage more severe infections in the outpatient setting. Many infectious diseases are discussed in detail throughout this text; however, this section focuses on systemic infectious diseases not elsewhere discussed in this book.

Bacterial Infections

Gregory A. Volturo
Jill Griffin
Thomas Germano
Thomas A. Brunell
Joseph C. Schmidt

Ajeet Jai Singh
Chad W. Le Blanc
Ramin R. Samadi
Stephen J. Playe

Botulism

Botulism is a rare, descending paralytic disease caused by neurotoxins produced by the Gram-positive spore-forming obligate anaerobic bacilli *Clostridium botulinum*. Derived from the Latin botulus, for sausage, the disease was first described as "sausage-poisoning" in 18th century Europe. On a molecular weight basis, botulinum toxin is the most lethal human toxin. Targeting the neuromuscular junction in a non-reversible manner causing a classic descending paralysis.

C. botulinum belongs to a group of antigenic toxin producing organisms (*C. botulinum* Types A, B, C1, C2, D, E, F, and G). Human disease is primarily attributed to types A, B, E, and F. Cases of botulism are rare in the United States (fewer than 200 cases reported annually). Ubiquitous in soil, it has a worldwide distribution. The spores of *C. botulinum* are resistant to radiation, heat and desiccation. The toxin is heat labile and easily destroyed by boiling but spores persist to 120° C and require pressurized sterilization to insure complete destruction. Botulism can be classified by mode of acquisition into six distinct entities: (1) food-borne, (2) wound-borne, (3) intestinally absorbed (infant and adult), (4) iatrogenic, (5) bioterrorism associated, and (6) idiopathic.

Food-Borne Botulism

The most common cause of food-borne outbreaks is home canned products with a low acid content (e.g., green beans, corn, beets, etc.). More unusual sources include chopped garlic in oil; potatoes wrapped in foil from a fast food establishment, beached whale blubber, fermented fish, stews, and frozen food products. In 2001 there were 33 cases of food-borne botulism reported in the United States. The age of those affected ranged from three to 78 years old. The majority of cases were caused by Type A and Type E toxins. Four clustered outbreaks occurred. In Texas sixteen patients were infected by contaminated chili and nine people in Alaska developed disease in three different outbreaks (involving beaver products, white fish, and stink egg ingestion).

Wound Botulism

Prior to 1980, less that one case per year of wound botulism was reported in the United States. Since that time, nearly forty cases have occurred annually, with the vast majority being attributed to the subcutaneous or intramuscular injection of black tar heroin. Although the mechanism of contamination of the heroin is not known, it is thought to be a result of soil spores being introduced into the heroin during the cutting process. Heating does not destroy the spores, and the use of sterile injection equipment does not protect against disease. Of the 23 cases of wound botulism reported in 2001, all but one was secondary to injection drug use. The remaining case was from a wound that occurred in a motor vehicle crash.

Intestinally Absorbed (Infant and Adult) Botulism

In 2001 there were 112 reported cases of infant botulism and one adult case due to intestinally absorbed toxin. Type B toxin was isolated from 60% of patients and Type A from 40%. Distribution of cases was nationwide. One death occurred. Although consumption of honey is a risk factor for development of botulism, in most cases the source of contamination is never determined. Incubation time for infants is three to 30 days and peak incidence is two to four months.

Iatrogenic Botulism

Botulinum toxin Type A has been used to treat various spasticities and dystonias since the 1980s. In 1989 Botox (botulinum toxin type A) became FDA approved for treatment of blepharospasm and strabismus. In 2000 Botox and Myoblock (type B toxin) were approved for the treatment of cervical dystonia. Off-label use of the drugs is common, with 1.6 million people having received injections for cosmetic purposes in 2001, one year prior to

FDA approval for injections for the cosmetic treatment of frown lines. Although no cases of full-blown iatrogenic botulism have been reported, symptoms consistent with mild disease have been seen and include headaches, muscle weakness, fatigue, ptosis, and flu-like symptoms.

Bioterrorism

Botulinum toxin has been used as a biological weapon in the past. In the 1930s the Japanese fed the toxin to prisoners of war during the occupation of Manchuria. During the Second World War the United States produced botulinum toxin for biological warfare but did not use it. In 1990, a Japanese cult (Aum Shinrikyo) unsuccessfully released *C. botulinum* over two U.S. military installations. Although no large-scale attacks have been carried out, the use of botulinum toxin is a potential threat to national security. Botulinum toxin is 100,000 times more toxic than Sarin, and one gram of botulinum toxin could kill 1.5 million people. It is believed that aerosolized spread would represent the most likely form of deliberate release. Hospitals would rapidly become overwhelmed with patients presenting with respiratory failure. Food-borne and water-borne outbreaks are also possible.

Idiopathic Botulism

Several cases of idiopathic botulism have been reported. In addition to *C. botulinum*, *C. baratti*, and *C. butyricum* have also been implicated in disease.

Over the past 50 years, the death rate from botulism in the United States has decreased from about 60% to the current estimate of 5%. Respiratory failure is the primary cause of death, and improved critical care support measures are largely responsible for the dramatic decrease in mortality.

Pathophysiology

All forms of *C. botulinum* that cause disease act through a common pathway. After *C. botulinum* toxin is ingested or produced in vivo it is systemically absorbed and binds irreversibly to the presynaptic cleft of cholinergic nerve terminals blocking release of acetylcholine. Its effects are exerted at the neuromuscular junction, postganglionic parasympathetic nerve endings, and peripheral ganglia.

Food-borne botulism is caused by toxin ingestion. Wound botulism and intestinally absorbed botulism both result from exposure to spores which enter the gut or a wound, proliferate and produce toxin which is then absorbed. Intestinal acquisition is more likely when normal gut defenses are compromised. Lack of bacterial competition (infants and patients on broad spectrum antibiotics), non-acidic gut pH (post-gastrectomy or patients on H_2 blockers or proton pump inhibitors) and inflammation of the gastrointestinal mucosa (inflammatory bowel disease) all increase the risk of botulism. Injection drug users are at highest risk for developing wound botulism.

Clinical Presentation

Food-borne Botulism

Symptoms of food-borne botulism can appear as early as 6 hours and as late as ten days after exposure to *C. botulinum*

depending on the amount of toxin ingested. In most patients, however, symptoms will begin appearing within about twelve hours. Some patients will initially present with GI symptoms (nausea, vomiting, diarrhea, abdominal cramping), however, the dominant clinical picture is one of neurological impairment. Cranial muscles are affected first with dysphagia, dyplopia, dysarthria, and ptosis mimicking an initial presentation of myasthenia gravis. Blurring of vision occurs due to loss of pupillary accommodation. In severe cases weakness and paralysis progress in a descending, symmetric fashion; upper extremities are affected first, followed by respiratory muscles and finally lower extremity paralysis occurs. Weakness is usually symmetric, and deep tendon reflexes tend to be preserved until the involved muscle group is completely paralyzed. Autonomic dysfunction causes dry mouth, constipation, urinary retention, and postural hypotension mimicking an anticholinergic overdose.

Wound Botulism

Although botulism is primarily considered a food-borne disease, *C. botulinum* can also be transmitted through wounds. While food-borne disease severity depends directly on the amount of toxin ingested, wound botulism is dependent upon toxin production following spore proliferation in the wound, which continues until the bacillus is debrided from the wound. As toxin enters systemic circulation, the classic symptoms of botulism appear.

Intestinally Absorbed Infant Botulism

The clinical presentation of infant botulism is a constipated child less than one year of age that is afebrile, but appears septic. Average age of onset is 13 weeks, with only 10% of cases occurring in children greater than six months of age. Symptoms of floppiness, poor feeding, weak cry or suck, as well as the musculoskeletal features of botulism are common. Approximately three fourths of children will require ventilatory support. CNS penetration with seizures and EEG abnormalities is reported rarely.

Intestinally Absorbed Adult Botulism

Adults suffering from achlorhydria, inflammatory bowel disease, or other conditions that may disrupt intestinal flora are at risk for developing botulism in the same manner that infants develop it (ingestion of spores). Clinically the symptoms mimic food-born botulism without the clustering of cases.

Iatrogenic Botulism

Patients affected by injection of Botox (type A) or Myoblock (type B) toxin may present with headaches, ptosis, flu-like symptoms, and weakness.

Diagnosis

The diagnosis of botulism is clinical, and is frequently underdiagnosed. Botulism should be considered in any adult presenting with descending paralysis and any afebrile infant who appears septic. The differential diagnosis includes Guillaine-Barre (ascending paralysis with loss of reflexes), myasthenia gravis (dysarthria, dysphagia, ptosis, diplopia), tick paralysis (resolves within 12 hours of tick removal), polio (typically asymmetric), organophosphate toxicity (anticholinergic toxidrome without paralysis), and hypermagnesemia (loss of reflexes, muscle weakness, hypotension, arrhythmias). The tensilon test cannot be used to differentiate myasthenia gravis from botulism, as the test is positive in up to one fourth of botulism patients.

Routine labs drawn in the emergency department (ED) are of no value in diagnosing botulism, however samples of serum, gastric aspirate, stool, and food should be collected for analysis before treating with antitoxin. Analysis of CSF may help narrow the differential, as patients with botulism have normal CSF. Electromyography findings of low-amplitude compound muscle action potential (CMAP) are suggestive of botulism, however these studies are very painful and are impractical in the ED setting.

Treatment

The mainstay of treatment for botulism is supportive care with special attention paid to the respiratory status of the patient. The decision to intubate is based on bedside assessment of upper airway competency and monitoring of vital capacity. Intubation is frequently necessary and should be accomplished before hypoxia or hypercapnea develop. Ventilatory support is generally needed for two to eight weeks. Whole bowel irrigation should be considered if contaminated food may still be in the GI tract and ileus has not yet developed.

Adults with either wound or food-borne botulism should be treated with trivalent (types A, B, and E) equine botulinum antitoxin, one vial IV and one vial IM, which can be obtained from state health departments or the CDC (telephone 404-639-2206 daytime Monday through Friday or 404-639-288 evenings and weekends). Prior to IV administration, a skin test should be performed since as many as 2% of patients will have an anaphylactic reaction. Desensitization can be accomplished before treatment if necessary. All treated patients should be watched closely for anaphylaxis. Since antitoxin blocks only toxin that is still circulating, it should be administered as early as possible. It is safe to give in pregnancy but is not recommended for infant botulism.

Infant botulism is treated with human botulinum immunoglobulin (BIG). Antibiotics should not be given, as they may lyse bacteria in the gut and, thus, spur release of more toxin. Extracorporeal adsorption is being evaluated as an adjunct therapy to the above treatment regimens.

Wound botulism caused by injection drug use is treated locally, with debridement, and systemically, in the same manner as food-borne disease. While antimicrobial use has not been studied in botulism, penicillin G, or alternatively, metronidazole, are often recommended.

Antibiotics are often indicated to treat the bacterial complications of prolonged intensive supportive care (i.e., pneumonia and UTI). Antimicrobials associated with neuromuscular blockade (i.e., aminoglycosides and tetracycline) should be avoided in botulism patients.

Botulism caused by bioterrorism requires large-scale decontamination procedures. In an aerosolized attack, the toxin will not be absorbed through intact skin. People should be advised to cover the mouth and nose with a cloth, wash exposed skin with soap and water, disinfect contaminated objects with hypochlorite bleach (0.1%) and seek medical attention immediately. The military has a heptavalent antitoxin-containing antibody to all *C. botulinum* toxins. It is not currently available for civilian use.

Prevention

Many cases of botulism are preventable. Home canned food should be processed following strict hygiene procedures: cans with bulging lids should be discarded, unopened. Home made oils infused with garlic or herbs require refrigeration and home canned products should be boiled for ten minutes prior to ingestion to destroy the toxin. Spores are difficult to destroy, therefore, infants less than 12 months old should not be fed honey and injection drug users should seek medical care immediately if skin wounds become infected.

Gonococcal Disease

There are nearly one million gonococcal infections that occur in the United States annually, making gonorrhea second only to *Chlamydia trachomatis* as the most common bacterial sexually transmitted disease. Clinical infection occurs as the result of mucosal colonization by *Neisseria gonorrhoeae*, a Gram-negative bacteria. Untreated Gonococcal infection may lead to locally invasive disease with serious sequelae, including pelvic inflammatory disease (PID) with resultant infertility, ectopic pregnancy, septic abortion, or blindness. Disseminated disease can result in septic arthritis, endocarditis, or meningitis. The clinical presentation of infected patients may range from classic urethritis or cervicitis to sepsis of uncertain etiology. The infection may also be asymptomatic or sub-clinical in a significant percentage of both male and female patients. In recent years, the bacteria have developed resistance to several commonly recommended antibiotics. Emergency practitioners must be well-acquainted with the myriad of presentations of gonococcal infections, as well as with current modalities of diagnosis and treatment, as the ED will continue to be the point of entry to the health care system for a vast number of these patients.

Epidemiology

Gonorrheal disease may affect individuals of any age; however, approximately three quarters of cases occur in individuals aged 15 to 30, with the highest risk in sexually active adolescents. Risk factors for gonorrheal disease include being single, indigence, prostitution, and an early age at the onset of sexual activity. Transmission of the disease between individuals may occur without knowledge of either party since in both males and females the infection is frequently either asymptomatic or produces minimal non-specific symptoms. The disease appears to be more easily transmitted from male to female during vaginal intercourse rather than vice versa.

Pathophysiology

Neisseria gonorrhoeae is a Gram-negative cocci that is round or ovoid shaped, and characteristically grows in pairs, although it may occur singly. They are fastidiously aerobic. The organism is frequently covered by fimbrae that assist in adherence to host mucosal epithelial cells. Humans are the only reservoir. Several protein mediators of host inflammation are present in the bacterial cell wall. An IgA protease secreted by the organism appears to be important in overcoming secreted human immunoglobulin.

Nearly any mucosal surface may become infected with the bacteria. Most commonly involved are the male urethra and the female urogenital tract. The pharynx may be involved during oral sex. The rectum may be colonized following anal intercourse or via infectious vaginal secretions in the female. The conjunctiva in the adult may be inoculated by contact with infected vaginal or seminal fluids during or following sex or in the neonate via vertical transmission.

In the heterosexual male, the usual manifestation of the disease is acute urethritis. The typical period of incubation is 2 to 5 days, but may occur within several weeks. Complications of this initial urethral infection include epididymitis and prostatitis. The degree of symptoms that an individual will experience is likely related to the particular infecting gonococcal strain, as well as host factors.

In women the clinical manifestations of gonorrhea usually occur as a result of an initial infection of the cervix. It is estimated that about 15% of patients with cervicitis will develop upper genital tract disease involving the uterus, fallopian tubes, ovaries, or the peritoneal cavity resulting in clinical PID. Salpingitis in addition to placing the patient at risk for peritoneal infection is also responsible for the serious sequelae of PID, pelvic adhesions, chronic pain, infertility, and ectopic pregnancy. The risk of infertility has been estimated to be as high as 25% for each episode of gonococcal salpingitis with a concomitant six-fold increase in the risk for ectopic pregnancy. It should be remembered that PID may be caused by organisms other than *N. gonorrhoeae,* such as *C. trachomatis,* and is also frequently polymicrobial.

Other acute complications of PID include Fitz-Hugh-Curtis syndrome (perihepatitis) and the formation of tubo-ovarian abscesses. In addition to the ascending genital infection localized infection may occur in the female urethra, as well as the Skene's or Bartholin's glands, resulting in labial edema or abscess. Obstetrical complications of gonococcal infection include septic abortion, premature rupture of membranes, preterm delivery, and intrauterine growth retardation.

Neisseria gonorrhoeae is an infrequent but important cause of conjunctivitis in both adults and neonates, and may be blinding. When responsible for conjunctivitis in the neonatal period, the illness is usually acquired at birth from passage through the vaginal canal and usually presents within the first five days of life.

Disseminated gonococcal infection (DGI) occurs in approximately 0.5% to 3% of cases and is more common in females. It results from the bacteremic spread of the organism from the original site of mucosal infection. Pharyngeal infection is associated with a higher risk of dissemination. Pathologic manifestations typically include a migratory polyarthritis, tenosynovitis, and dermatitis.

Patients may present with all or only one of these entities. Rare but devastating sites of dissemination include the heart, with resultant endocarditis, and the meninges.

Clinical Evaluation

Gonorrheal disease should be considered in the differential diagnosis of any patient who presents with complaints regarding the urogential tract (most common), as well as the pharynx, rectum, and conjunctiva. The symptoms of a male with urethritis include dysuria and urethral discharge. The discharge is usually characterized as purulent, but may also be described as white, mucoid, or cloudy. Complaints in females with genital tract infection include vaginal discharge or bleeding, pelvic or abdominal pain, dyspareunia, labial pain or swelling, and dysuria. Additionally, the diagnosis should be carefully considered in patients presenting with rash or arthralgias, as well as in those with clinical tenosynovitis, endocarditis or meningitis. The arthralgias typically involve several joints (oligoarthralgia or polyarthralgia) and are often migratory. When gonococcal disease is considered in the differential diagnosis a thorough sexual history should be sought for.

Pharyngeal infection is usually sub-clinical, but a minority of patients may complain of sore throat. Likewise, a high percentage of rectal infection occurs without overt symptoms although rectal pain, discharge, bleeding, and tenesmus may occur.

Clinicians should bear in mind that the disease in both sexes frequently remains either asymptomatic, or only minimally so, resulting in failure of patients to seek medical attention or alter their sexual behavior resulting in spread of the organism to other individuals. In one study of females aged 12 to 21 presenting to an adolescent inner city clinic, both with and without gynecologic complaints, the prevalence of gonorrhea was 6.3%. Of these approximately one third reported no symptoms. In another inner city population the prevalence of untreated gonorrheal infection in a probability sample of individuals aged 18 to 35 was 5.3%. It was also determined that the number undiagnosed infections in the community vastly outnumbered those that were diagnosed and treated. These investigations strongly suggest that emergency physicians should never minimize a seemingly minor genitourinary complaint in either sex.

Upon examination, males with symptomatic urethritis frequently have a penile discharge. In some cases, it may be helpful to have the patient "milk" the penis to elicit the discharge. Patients who have voided just prior to examination may reveal no discharge at all. Therefore, urine specimens in males with chief complaints of dysuria or penile discharge should be collected after physician examination and specimen acquisition if at all possible. Inspection of the patient's undergarments or trousers may provide a clue to the nature and quantity of the discharge. Scrotal tenderness suggests epididymitis. Prostate tenderness or swelling may be noted on digital rectal exam.

In the female pelvic examination may reveal cervical injection and friability, a mucopurulent cervical or vaginal discharge as well as labial swelling or mass suggestive of abscess involving Bartholin's or Skenne's glands. Low abdominal tenderness, cervical motion tenderness and adnexal tenderness suggest a diagnosis of PID. Additional findings supporting PID include fever greater than 38° C, an elevated WBC count or sedimentation rate, a mucopurulent cervical discharge, a positive Gram stain for Gram-negative intracellular diplococci, and the presence of a mass on examination or ultrasound. PID may present with a wide range of clinical severities: from the well-appearing patient with uncomplicated cervicitis, to the toxic-appearing patient with tubo-ovarian abscess or peritonitis, presenting with severe abdominal pain, rebound tenderness, and fever.

The differential diagnosis of the reproductive age female with low abdominal pain is complex. Conditions such as appendicitis, ruptured ovarian cyst, and ectopic pregnancy may be difficult to distinguish from PID. In these instances, judicious use of laboratory testing and radiology studies can be especially helpful. Qualitative HCG testing should never be overlooked. Other ancillary studies, including quantitative HCG, CBC, sedimentation rate, liver profile and urinalysis, should be considered when appropriate. Abdominal or vaginal probe, ultrasound or CT scanning may all prove valuable to elucidate the correct diagnosis. Rarely the true nature of a patient's problem will be diagnosed only with laparoscopy or surgical exploration.

While PID can and does occur in the pregnant patient, a diagnosis of PID should be made with caution beyond about twelve weeks gestation, since, by this time, the attachment of the chorion to the uterine decidua makes ascending genital tract disease less likely. If previous documentation that the pregnancy is intrauterine has not been established, a confirmatory ultrasound would seem prudent.

Disseminated gonococcal infection presents a particular diagnostic challenge, since at the time of dissemination the initial site of mucosal infection is often asymptomatic. Women have higher incidences of asymptomatic infection and, thus, are at higher risk for dissemination than their male counterparts. Dissemination is more likely to occur during the beginning of the menstrual cycle or in the pregnant patient. While a toxic appearance, elevated WBC count and fever may be present, these findings may be notoriously absent in the patient with disseminated disease. Blood cultures are positive in less than 50% of DGI cases.

The typical pattern of joint involvement is that of an oligoarthralgia or polyarthralgia, which is migratory or less commonly additive and may be associated with constitutional symptoms, such as fever and chills. While any joint may be a potential site of involvement, the knees, elbows, wrists, hands, and ankle joints are the most frequently affected sites. Of these, the knee is the most common. Less than half of the patients with arthralgia will have a proven septic arthritis. Only approximately one third will develop a synovial effusion. Permanent joint destruction may occur. The differential diagnosis of the patient with arthralgias due to DGI includes Reiter's syndrome, septic arthritis, gout and pseudogout, rheumatic fever, secondary syphilis, hepatitis, other rheumatologic associated arthritides, and Lyme disease. An associated tenosynovitis frequently occurs and

usually involves the dorsum of the hands and wrists, fingers, ankles, or toes.

The skin lesions of DGI are pustular on an erythematous base, are usually relatively few in number (less than twenty), and generally occur on the extremities. They frequently will become hemorrhagic, necrotic, or ulcerative. In general, the rash is painful and may infrequently be macular or petechial. Approximately 1% of patients with DGI develop meningitis or endocarditis. Cardiac involvement usually involves the aortic valve and may be rapidly progressive.

The diagnosis of disseminated disease is confirmed by the identification of the diplococci from the blood, synovial fluid or from a mucosal surface, such as the urethra, cervix, rectum, or oropharynx, along with clinical signs of disseminated disease. The highest yield for a definitive diagnosis is via the identification of the organism from a mucosal surface of a patient with the appropriate clinical scenario. It is important that all potential sites of infection be swabbed. Cultures of the mucosal site of involvement may have a sensitivity of 60% to 80%, with cultures of the cervix and urethra having the highest yields. The newer nucleic acid amplification tests such as polymerase chain reaction (PCR) and ligase chain reaction (LCR) have demonstrated excellent sensitivity.

The Gram stain should not be overlooked especially in the presence of a male with a symptomatic urethral discharge as it has sensitivity of greater than 90%. The sensitivity for a cervical Gram stain is considerably less, possibly in the 60% range. The sensitivity is also poor for men with asymptomatic urethral infection, as well as those with rectal disease. The specificity of a Gram stain which shows Gram-negative intracellular diplococci is about 95% if taken from the urethra, cervix, rectum or joint fluid, but is less reliable from the mouth due to native flora. In addition to being highly sensitive, some of the newer non-culture modalities can be performed on voided urine instead of by genital swabs, making them convenient screening tools.

When a joint effusion is present arthrocentesis should be performed and the fluid analyzed for white blood cell count, glucose, crystal analysis, Gram stain and culture. The leukocyte count will usually range from 30,000 to 100,000 WBC/mm^3 with a predominance of polymorphonuclear cells. Gram staining and culture of synovial fluid have sensitivities less than 50%.

If the diagnosis of gonorrhea is considered likely in a prepubertal patient beyond the neonatal stage, there must be a prompt evaluation for sexual abuse. The identification of *N. gonorrhoeae* from such a patient is strongly suggestive of sexual abuse. Furthermore, there may be no other physical clues on examination. The most frequent clinical manifestation of gonorrhea in girls is vulvovaginitis, with clinical PID being uncommon. For medicolegal considerations, the presence of the organism must be documented by culture, and reports to the local health department and child protective services are mandated.

Treatment and Disposition

Guidelines for the evaluation and treatment of sexually transmitted diseases were updated by the CDC in 2002 (online at www.cdc.gov/std/treatment). Co-infection with *C. trachomatis* is common. One study determined that the prevalence of co-infection with *C. trachomatis* in patients treated for proven gonococcal infection at STD clinics was 20% in men and 41% in women. Since the sequelae of this infection is similar to that of *N. gonorrhoeae*, its presence should be assumed and empiric treatment instituted in the ED setting. In other clinical venues, treatment based on testing may be more cost-effective if the prevalence of co-infection in the community is low.

When choosing a treatment regimen it should be remembered that quinolone antibiotics are contraindicated in pregnancy, lactating females, and in patients below 18 years due to the potential risk of arthropathy. Additionally, in recent years there has been an emergence of quinolone-resistant *N. gonorrhoeae* primarily involving the nations of the Pacific Ocean, Asia, and the state of Hawaii. As such, a travel history from both the patient and any available sex partner is important. Quinolone therapy is no longer advised if infection is believed to have been acquired in a Pacific basin nation, Asia or Hawaii and is considered "inadvisable" in California. Local outbreaks of quinolone-resistant *N. gonorrhoeae* have also occurred sporadically in the rest of the continental United States, as well. Physicians are encouraged to remain abreast of recommendations from local health departments regarding this point.

Women with upper genital tract disease should be treated with an effective regimen for anaerobic bacteria given that anaerobic isolates have been cultured from patients with PID. The use of metronidazole or ampicillin/sulbactam should strongly be considered. Finally, uncomplicated pharyngeal infection has proven more difficult to treat and, thus, fewer regimens are recommended.

For reasons of public health, as well as the wellness and reproductive health of at risk individuals, the sexual partners of individuals treated for gonorrhea and other sexually transmitted diseases should be referred for evaluation and treatment. Limitation of the number of sexual partners and the use of condoms are effective means of controlling the transmission of the disease, and physicians should advise patients of these preventive means whenever possible.

Finally, patients with disseminated disease or with locally invasive disease (e.g., complicated PID), as well as patients, who for social reasons are unable to comply with outpatient treatment and follow up, cannot be treated with a one-time regimen. In these patients hospitalization is advisable. **Table 63.1** summarizes the CDC 2002 treatment recommendations.

Table 63.1

Treatment of Gonococcal Infections

Uncomplicated infections of the cervix, urethra or rectum[a,b]
1. Ceftriaxone 125 mg IM single dose
2. Ciprofloxacin 500 mg PO single dose
3. Ofloxacin 400 mg PO single dose
4. Cefixime 400 mg PO single dose
5. Levofloxacin 250 mg PO single dose
6. Spectinomycin 2 g IM single dose may be useful for those who are not candidates for either cephalosporin or quinolone therapy.

Uncomplicated Pharyngeal Infection[b]
1. Ceftriaxone 125 mg IM single dose
2. Ciproflaxacin 500 mg PO single dose
3. Spectinomycin 2 g IM single dose[c]

PID—Outpatient treatment[a,d]
1. Ceftriaxone 250 mg IM single dose[e,f]
2. Cefoxitin 2 g IM single dose concomitant with Probenicid 1 g PO[e,f]
3. Ofloxacin 400 mg PO bid × 14 days[f]
4. Levofloxacin 500 mg PO once daily × 14 days[f]

[a]Other treatments using alternative quinolones and/or cephalosporins are available and reviewed in the CDC 2002 guidelines.
[b]The presumptive treatment of concomitant infection with *Chlamydia trachomatis* is suggested in clinical settings of uncertain patient follow up such as the emergency department. Chlamydial infection may be treated using Doxycycline 100 mg PO bid × 7 days or azithromycin 1g PO single dose.
[c]Spectinomycin has limited efficacy for infection of the pharynx and patients require a pharyngeal culture 3 to 5 days post treatment to verify eradication of the organism.
[d]Admission criteria for inpatient treatment with parenteral antibiotics include possible emergent surgical diagnosis, pregnancy, the patient who fails to respond to outpatient treatment, toxic appearance, nausea and vomiting, tubo-ovarian abscess, and unusual social circumstances making outpatient management difficult.
[e]Chlamydial infection should be treated using doxycycline 100 mg PO × 14 days. In inpatients not tolerating oral medication doxycycline 100 mg IV bid may be used.
[f]Metronidazole 500 mg PO bid × 14 days may be added to any of these regimens.
[g]Parenteral antibiotics should be continued for 24 to 48 hours after improvement begins. Oral therapy should be continued for 14 days.
[h]Metronidazole 500 mg IV Q 8 hours may be added.
[i]Parenteral antibiotics should be continued for 24 to 48 hours after improvement begins. Oral therapy should be continued for 7 days.
[j]Treatment for meningitis should continue for 10 to 14 days. Treatment for endocarditis should continue for 4 weeks.
[k]Testing for concomitant *C. trachomatis* is recommended. Irrigate purulent material from eye. Admission to hospital is warranted. The mother of the patient and her sexual partners warrant treatment.

Table 63.1

Treatment of Gonococcal Infections—continued

PID—Inpatient treatment[d,g]
  1. Cefotetan 2 g IV q 12 hours[e]
  2. Cefoxitin 2 g IV q 6 hours[e]
  3. Clindamycin 900 mg IV q 8 hours with Gentamicin 2 mg/kg IV or IM loading dose followed by 1.5 mg/kg q 8 hours. Single daily dosing may be used.
  4. Ofloxacin 400 mg IV q 12 hours.[h]
  5. Levofloxacin 500 mg IV q 24 hours.[h]
  6. Ampicillin/Sulbactam 3 g IV q 6 hours.[e]
Disseminated Gonococcal Disease[i]
  1. Ceftriaxone 1 g IV or IM q 24 hours[b]
  2. Cefotaxime 1g IV q 8 hours[b]
  3. Ceftizoxime 1 g IV q 8 hours[b]
  4. Ciprofloxacin 400 mg IV q 12 hours
  5. Ofloxacin 400 mg IV q 12 hours
  6. Levofloxacin 250 mg IV q 24 hours
  7. Spectinomycin 2 g IM q 12 hours
Gonococcal Meningitis or Endocarditis
  1. Ceftriaxone 1 to 2 g IV q 12 hours.[j]
Gonoccocal Conjunctivitis—Neonate
  1. Ceftriaxone 25 to 50 mg/kg IV or IM (not to exceed 125 mg), single dose.[k]
Gonoccocal Conjunctivitis—Adults 2
  1. Ceftriaxone 1 g IM single dose.

Meningococcemia

Meningococcemia is bacteremia from *N. meningitidis*, an aerobic, Gram-negative diplococcus responsible for causing bacterial meningococcal meningitis. There are at least thirteen known serotypes of *N. meningitidis*, but only three of these serotypes; serogroups A, B and C, are responsible for about 90% of human disease. Bacteremia from *N. meningitidis* is frequently found in the absence of central nervous system infection (30% to 50% of cases of meningococcemia occur without meningitis).

Meningococcemia is significant for its predilection for rapid clinical progression from a mild, non-specific presentation to severe illness, with significant sequela and death. Mortality from meningococcal disease ranges from 5% to 15%. Mortality from fulminant meningococcemia is higher (and death within two days of diagnosis is not uncommon). Early recognition of meningococcemia appears to be the key to preventing more serious sequelae. The usual route of entry for the bacterium is via the nasopharynx. Humans are the sole reservoir for *N. meningitidis*. The organism can enter and colonize the nasopharynx, causing mild symptoms or no symptoms at all. A general estimate is that between 5% to 20% of the population may be asymptomatic carriers. For certain subgroups living in crowded, close quarters, the carrier state may be much higher. It has been estimated that over 90% of military recruits may be asymptomatic carriers of *N. meningiditis*. For bacteremia to occur, the organism must gain entry to the bloodstream through some breakdown in the host's defenses. Meningococcemia can be rapidly progressive and severe. In most industrialized nations, meningococcal diseases occur annually with a bimodal peak, occurring

during the spring and fall. The populations which are especially at risk for meningococcal diseases are children younger than five years of age, military recruits, persons having close contacts with patients affected with the disease, and the immunocompromised. Recent studies suggest that the incidence of meningococcal infections within the first five years of life may not vary as much as once believed. It is currently thought that the highest incidence of infection occurs in children from 5 to 24 months, but recent data points to a more uniform infectivity rate for children under age 2. In industrialized countries, there is a secondary peak in occurrence in late adolescence and early adulthood. Dormitory living style may be a contributing factor to this secondary peak. Other factors which appear to put patients at higher risk are alcohol abuse, cigarette smoking (or a high exposure to cigarette smoke), low socioeconomic status, and crowded living conditions. Meningococcal diseases occur in outbreaks. Epidemics occur sporadically throughout the world. The highest incidence of meningococcal diseases is in sub-Saharan Africa, with over 250,000 cases reported and over 25,000 deaths. There have been recent outbreaks in the United States, Canada, Spain, and New Zealand.

N. meningitidis is spread via respiratory droplets from either an infected host or a colonized individual. The organism comes in contact with the new host's oropharyngeal mucosa. The conditions necessary for the bacterium to enter the bloodstream are multiple and complex. Co-transmission with viral entities (e.g., influenza A), as well as specific compliment deficiencies may play a role in the bacterium's ability to circumnavigate a host's defenses. The incubation period from exposure to the onset symptoms is usually between two and ten days. There is an increased risk of infection for individuals following close exposure to an affected host for as long as sixty days.

Clinical Presentation

The most frequently considered presentations of meningococcal disease are of meningitis and meningococcemia. There is however, an extremely wide range of clinical presentations. Meningococcemia may be indolent and chronic, acute and severe, and may also be self-limited. The initial presenting complaints may be vague and non-specific, and may also be limited to a single organ or system. N. meningitidis has been found in conjunctivitis, proctitis, urinary infections, as well as in primary pneumonias.

It is most common for acute meningococcemia to be preceded by a respiratory infection. Initial signs and symptoms are non-specific and "flu-like." It is at this stage that the entity is extremely difficult to differentiate from any of a number of benign disorders. Duration of mild symptoms varies from as short as twelve hours to as long as two weeks. But rapid progression to severe sepsis and shock is the hallmark of meningococcemia. The most common presenting complaint is fever. Other common complaints include: sore throat, rigors or chills, myalgias, nausea, vomiting, and diarrhea. Some form of rash is common on initial presentation and may be present in 75% to 80% of cases on initial exam. The classic petechial rash is found only about half of the time. Other forms of dermatitis may include a macular or maculopapular rash, diffuse erythema, nodules, or pustules. On occasion, the diagnosis has been made retrospectively by positive blood cultures in an individual whose condition improved spontaneously. In children, especially infants, the presentation may be with high fever and behavioral or feeding changes alone.

Fulminant meningococcemia, also known as purpura fulminans or Waterhouse-Friderichsen Syndrome, presents with an abrupt onset of fever and, usually, a rapidly progressing course to sepsis and shock. Common presenting complaints are high fever, rigors, profound malaise or change in mental status, severe arthralgias, and headache. Acute delirium is not uncommon. Usually the history is replete with a short duration of symptoms, which worsened over a matter of hours. Petechiae and purpura are common findings. They may initially have appeared as small petechiae on the distal extremities: wrists, ankles, and axilla being common sites. Petechiae can also be found early on the conjunctiva, the oral mucosa, and on areas of the body where gentle pressure has been applied (e.g., the belt line or in a sock distribution). The palms of the hands and the soles of the feet are often spared. Purpura appears later. Most likely the purpura occur not as a result of a confluence of the initial petechiae, but as a result of progressive disseminated intravascular coagulation. Purpura fulminans is also a term used to describe the skin lesions—the confluent areas of purpura, with tissue necrosis and skin sloughing. Shock typically occurs with purpura. Respiratory, gastrointestinal, and cutaneous sloughing may occur and may be associated with significant bleeding and hypotension. The findings of fever, purpura, and shock are characteristic of fulminant meningococcemia.

Chronic or indolent meningococcemia is an unusual form of the disease. It may present with fevers lasting from days to weeks. Typical presenting complaints (other than fever) include rigors or chills, headaches, arthralgias and myalgias, and rash. In the case of chronic meningococcemia, the rash is rarely petechial, and is much more likely to be represented by a number of small patches of macular or maculopapular eruptions. These patients rarely appear acutely ill. In these cases the diagnosis is usually made by blood culture. The entity is easily confused with other clinical entities like influenza, Lyme disease, Rocky Mountain spotted fever, Kawasaki syndrome or Henoch-Schönlein purpura. Overall, patients with chronic meningococcemia experience fewer long-term complications, but a failure to make the diagnosis can lead to meningitis in as many as 20% of these patients.

Meningitis is probably the most familiar form of meningococcal disease. But meningitis implies central nervous system involvement. Meningitis is present in approximately 55% of patients presenting with meningococcal septicemia. Mortality and morbidity are much higher in the set of patients that have both entities (meningitis and meningococcemia). Of the subset of patients that have meningococcal infections, outcomes are best in patients presenting with meningitis alone. Patients with meningococcemia, alone or in association with meningitis, have much poorer outcomes than those diagnosed with meningitis alone. The classic presentation for meningitis is a high fever (plus or minus rigors), headache, stiff neck, and mental status change. This constellation often occurs two to ten days after an upper respiratory infection. If the patient also presents with skin findings, especially petechiae, a presumptive diagnosis of meningococcal infection should be made.

Meningococcal pneumonia can occur as a primary entity. It may be diagnosed less frequently because it is not usually associated with hematogenous spread. The clinical entity may be indistinguishable from pneumonia caused by other organisms. Classically, meningococcal pneumonia is thought of as a lower lobe pneumonia. They become clinically significant when they are the source for bacteremia and meningococcemia. Fortunately, most of the guidelines that are utilized to treat community-acquired pneumonia will also be effective at treating primary N. meningitidis pneumonia. Secondary N. meningitidis pneumonia occurs as a result of hematogenous spread to the lung. In these instances, the overall clinical picture of meningococcemia, and its associated damage to other organ systems, usually overshadows the pulmonary findings of the disease.

Virtually any organ system can be secondarily affected by N. meningitidis. Rarely, primary organ systems are affected without causing meningococcemia. Although cases of primary N. meningitidis monoarthritis have been reported, the most common arthritides occur after a documented meningococcal disease. Arthritis can complicate up to 15% of all cases of meningococcemia. Most frequently, post-meningococcal arthritis is polyarticular and without effusion. However, the arthritis may be septic and may require aspiration to differentiate a reactive (or sterile) arthritis from a septic arthritis. Similarly, pericarditis may complicate the course of meningococcal diseases. Early pericarditis is usually a result of direct hematogenous spread of bacteria. Late pericarditis is usually reactive and sterile.

Diagnosis

Meningococcemia is diagnosed by growing *N. meningitidis* by blood culture. Other forms of meningococcal disease may be diagnosed by similar cultures of the affected systems; e.g., meningitis by cerebrospinal fluid culture, arthritis by synovial fluid culture. The organism can be cultured from the pharynx (but this is useful only as an adjunctive test as there is a high rate of colonization of *N. meningitidis* in the oropharynx of healthy individuals. The organism can be isolated in CSF by Gram stain, where it appears as a gram-negative diplococcus. It may also be isolated approximately 70% of the time in skin scrapings from purpuric lesions. There are a variety of rapid antigen tests available which can be performed on CSF, blood, urine, and other body tissues/fluids. These tests lack specificity, but may be useful in cases where a patient was pretreated with antibiotics and culture methods may be unreliable. PCR can also be performed on CSF to confirm a specific serogroup. Specific antibody titers to *N. meningitidis* are also available but are of limited utility to the emergency physician. Because early recognition and treatment are essential in cases of meningococcemia, when clinical suspicion is high, treatment should not be withheld pending a confirmative test. The most useful measures (cultures) will often take one to two days to be confirmative.

Treatment

Once the diagnosis of meningococcemia is entertained, treatment should be rapidly instituted. In cases where other diagnoses may also be considered (e.g., Rocky Mountain spotted fever or pneumococcal sepsis), initial broad-spectrum therapy and consultation with an infectious disease specialist is the preferred treatment. Initiation of early antibiotic therapy is crucial and it is appropriate to begin antibiotic therapy before confirmative studies (e.g., lumbar puncture) are performed. It is preferable; however, to obtain blood cultures prior to instituting antibiotics, but this should not delay antimicrobial pharmacotherapy. Accepted antibiotic regimens include penicillin G, amoxicillin, ceftriaxone, cefotaxime, and chloramphenicol. Broader spectrum antimicrobial therapy at higher doses is generally instituted in the ED. Inpatient therapy can be narrowed pending later test results. Dexamethasone is currently recommended for cases of meningococcal meningitis, but is not indicated for meningococcemia in the absence of neurological involvement. Fluid resuscitation is required in all cases of suspected meningococcemia. Often, blood pressure support with inotropic agents is also required. Meningococcemia often produces a low central venous pressure in conjunction with high peripheral vascular resistance and hypotension. End organ damage and peripheral ischemia may be complicated by the use of inotropes in this setting. Management of the coagulopathies inherent in fulminant meningococcemia is a complex task. The institution of heparin should be done in consultation with a critical care physician or a hematologist.

Respiratory support and adequate tissue oxygenation is imperative. Supplemental oxygen should be given to all suspected patients. Intubation and ventilatory support should be initiated if needed. Patients with fulminant meningococcemia are more likely to rapidly decompensate into respiratory distress for many reasons including hypotension, bleeding, acidosis, and ARDS.

Prophylaxis

Prophylaxis should be considered for all close contacts of a patient with confirmed meningococcal disease. This includes family members, roommates, day-care center members, and medical personal who had intimate contact with the patient (e.g., the intubating physician, the ICU taking care of the patient or any other health care personnel who had prolonged, close contact with the patient or who were exposed to high concentrations of respiratory secretions). When the diagnosis is in question, it is appropriate and safe to wait one or two days until confirmatory tests return prior to instituting prophylactic therapy for those who would require it. Appropriate prophylactic regimens include oral Rifampin (for 2 days), a single dose of oral ciprofloxacin, or a single IM/IV dose of ceftriaxone.

Commercial vaccinations against *N. meningitidis* are available but they are not currently recommended for all individuals. The vaccine offers protection from the predominant serogroups. Overall, the vaccine appears to be well tolerated and safe, but is not proven to be effective at providing protection for children less than two years of age. It is available as a single injection and is relatively inexpensive. Once given lifelong protection can be maintained with a booster dose every three to five years. The vaccine is utilized if there is an outbreak of meningitis or can be given to a person who is traveling to an area where the disease is prevalent (e.g., "The Meningitis Belt" in Africa). Within the last few years, many colleges have begun to offer incoming students information regarding the vaccine and vaccination upon informed consent.

Summary

Meningococcemia is a serious clinical entity which can present with subtle and non-specific symptoms. It is associated with significant mortality and morbidity and requires a high degree of suspicion to diagnose in its early stages. Prognosis and outcome is highly dependent on early recognition and initiation of appropriate antibiotic therapy. The disease can progress rapidly to shock, multi-system organ failure, and death. When the diagnosis is considered, confirmatory tests should not delay antibiotic administration. Aggressive supportive measures are often necessary in serious cases. Consultation with infectious disease, critical care and hematology may be needed. Prophylaxis should be given to close contacts of the patient and to health care personnel who were intimately involved with the patient's care (or were exposed to respiratory secretions).

Plague

Plague is a bacterial infection of humans and animals, caused by the aerobic, Gram-negative, nonmotile, coccobacillus *Yersinia pestis*. The disease may vary from a local reaction at regional lymph nodes proximal to the site of inoculation—acute regional lymphadenitis called bubonic plague, to a fulminant disseminated infection without adenopathy—septicemic plague. Pneumonic plague, the most serious epidemic form of plague, may be transmitted from person to person via aerosols. Plague may be rapidly fatal, if left untreated. Plague is usually transmitted to humans by the bites of fleas that parasitize wild rodents. Plague borne by rat fleas devastated Europe during the Middle Ages, and has been recognized in North America since the early part of this century. Significant foci of plague also exist in Africa and Asia.

Since 1925 all known cases of plague reported in the United States have been associated with exposures to wild rodents and their fleas in the western half of the country. American Indians are disproportionately represented among plague cases in the United States, possibly because many reside in rural areas in the western part of the country. Plague in the United States is most frequently transmitted to humans from flea bites from infested rock squirrels, California ground squirrels, prairie dogs, chipmunks, and wood rats. Occasional cases of human plague have been reported in hunters exposed to the incidentally infected carcasses of deer, antelope, gray fox, badger, bobcat, and coyote. These animals rarely develop overt illness and are not thought to be part of the usual endemic transmission cycle. Only rarely, during epidemics of human pneumonic plague, is the infection passed directly from person to person.

The occurrence of human plague is always linked to the transmission of plague among the natural animal reservoirs, and the incidence of human plague is a function of both the frequency of infection in the local rodent population and the rate of exposure to the infected rodents and their fleas. Typically plague occurs in very focal areas, involving one town or a city street, with adjacent areas being plague free. This has been attributed to the parochial behavior of rats, which tend to stay near one food supply for extended periods of time. Rapid suburbanization of endemic states has increased the number of persons living in or near active plague foci. Plague predominantly occurs in warm tropical climates, and outbreaks tend to occur during humid warm seasons. In the United States, the majority of cases tend to occur during the months of May through September, with the peak incidence during the month of July. Due to the mild winter months in some of the southwestern states, however, cases can occur during any month of the year.

The most common clinical form of human plague is bubonic plague. Bubonic plague usually presents as a febrile illness beginning 2 to 7 days following a bite from an infected flea. During the incubation period, bacteria proliferate in regional lymph nodes. Patients typically present with the sudden onset of fever, chills, weakness, and headache, followed by painful lymphadenopathy (buboes) proximal to the infected bite, usually at the same time or within 12 to 24 hours. Pain and tenderness often precede palpable and visible adenitis. The most common sites are the groin and the axillae, resulting from the inoc-

ulation of the extremities by flea bites. Pain may be so intense so as to restrict any movement of the affected areas. Buboes are oval swellings that may vary from 1 to 10 cm in length. The overlying skin may be elevated, or appear stretched or erythematous. The buboe may appear smooth and egg shaped or may feel like an irregular cluster, with surrounding edema, which may be pitting or gelatinous in nature. Palpation typically elicits tenderness and warmth.

In uncomplicated bubonic plague, patients are usually prostrate and lethargic. They often exhibit restlessness and agitation; seizures are common in children. The temperature is usually in the 38.5° to 40° C range. Pulse is elevated and the blood pressure is usually in the range of 100/60 mm Hg due to vasodilatation. The liver and spleen may be palpable and tender. There is no characteristic skin rash; however, pustules may develop at the sites of flea bites. With fulminant systemic disease, patients may develop purpura that may become necrotic resulting in gangrene—the probable basis for the term black death. A fulminant clinical course can produce death within 2 to 4 days of the onset of symptoms. Nearly all fatal cases of plague in the United States are a result of delays in seeking treatment or in making the diagnosis.

Primary pneumonic plague is caused by the inhalation of an infectious respiratory droplet, which may have originated from another human pneumonic plague case. While this distinction is of little therapeutic importance, the public health implications are significant. Plague pneumonia is highly contagious by airborne transmission, it has a short incubation period, and it can spread rapidly in close person-to-person contact. While primary pneumonic plague is now rare, it is a potential threat to any person who is exposed to a patient with plague who has a cough. It may be so rapidly fatal that individuals have been reported to have been exposed, become ill, and die in the same day. Pneumonic plague is invariably fatal if antibiotic therapy is delayed more than 20 hours after the onset of symptoms. Gram-negative septicemia and endotoxic shock account for many of the early deaths from pneumonic plague. In patients with septicemic plague, hematogenous spread of bacteria from the bubo to the lung may result in pneumonia. Plague pneumonia is characterized by fever, lymphadenopathy with cough productive of purulent sputum, chest pain, and often hemoptysis. Chest radiography may reveal a patchy bronchopneumonia or consolidation. When septicemic plague results in pneumonia, it is classified as secondary plague pneumonia.

Primary pneumonic plague has also been reportedly transmitted to humans by animals—most often domestic cats, in which plague produces a severe, often fatal infection. These animals probably develop secondary pneumonic plague after ingesting infected wild rodents, and may transmit the infection via infectious aerosols from the animal's cough to their owners or veterinary professionals caring for them.

Plague meningitis, a rare complication of bubonic plague, occurs usually as a result of inadequately treated plague. It is characterized by fever, headache, meningismus, and CSF pleocytosis. As in secondary pneumonic plague, it is a result of hematogenous spread of bacteria from a bubo. When compared to uncomplicated bubonic plague, the mortality rate is very high. There may be an association between buboes located in the axilla and the development of meningitis. Occasionally, plague meningitis may appear as a primary infection, without any antecedent lymphadenitis.

Plague pharyngitis, a rare clinical form of plague, is thought to result from the inhalation or ingestion of the plague bacilli. It may resemble acute tonsillitis with inflamed anterior cervical lymph nodes. *Y. pestis* may be recovered by throat culture.

World events of recent years have raised public awareness of the potentially deadly use of biological agents as weapons of mass destruction. The Centers for Disease Control and Prevention has created a classification system for Critical Biological Agents that pose substantial risk to the public. Pneumonic plague from the intentional release of *Y. pestis* into a populated area has been classified as a category A risk, the most dangerous of the identified potentially infectious agents. Other agents in this category include anthrax, smallpox, tularemia, and the viral hemorrhagic fevers. These agents are noted for their ease of dissemination, potential for person-to-person transmission, high mortality rate, potential for major impact on public health, ability to incite public and social disruption, and the need for major public health preparation and resources. Investigations into the preparation and modes dissemination of these agents, as well as the surveillance, treatment and prevention of the infections they cause are currently underway.

Diagnosis

The diagnosis of plague should be suspected in febrile patients, who have been exposed to rodents or other mammals in known endemic areas of the world. Eliciting a history of recent travel in plague endemic areas of the United States, South America, Africa, or Southeast Asia is of obvious value. Because of the similarities between plague and the hantavirus pulmonary syndrome, the diagnosis of plague may be further complicated. A bacteriologic diagnosis may be made in many patients by smear and culture of bubo aspirate. This may be obtained by inserting a 20-gauge needle on a 10-cc syringe containing 1 mL of sterile saline solution into a bubo. The solution is then injected and aspirated several times until it is blood tinged. Drops of the aspirate should then be placed onto slides and air dried for both Gram and Wayson's or Giemsa stain. These will readily demonstrate the bipolar ("safety-pin") morphology that is characteristic, but not diagnostic, of *Y. pestis*. Pus from a fluctuant bubo or sputum also may be smeared and treated in the same fashion. Rapid presumptive identification of the organism can also be made using a fluorescent antibody test. Aspirate as well as blood should be sent for culture, which will confirm the diagnosis. Recognizing the patient with plague requires a heightened suspicion for rare causes of infectious illness with prominent, severe respiratory symptoms. A clinician who suspects pneumonic plague must not only provide appropriate treatment for their patient, and close contacts, but must also alert the public health authorities to the possibility of a mass exposure of a potentially deadly biological agent.

Treatment

Untreated plague may evolve into a fulminant illness complicated by septic shock, with an estimated mortality of greater than 50%. Hospitalization, fluid hydration, and early treatment with effective antibiotics can be lifesaving. Streptomycin is the drug of choice for the treatment of plague. It can reduce the case fatality rate to less than 5%. No other drug has been demonstrated to be more efficacious or less toxic. Streptomycin should be administered intramuscularly, in two divided doses daily, totaling 30 mg per kilogram of body weight per day for 10 days. Most patients improve rapidly, and they defervesce in approximately 3 days. A 10-day course of therapy is recommended because viable bacteria have been isolated from buboes of patients with plague during convalescence. During a 10-day course of streptomycin, the risk of vestibular damage and hearing loss is minimal. The antibiotic, however, should be used cautiously during pregnancy, in the elderly, and in patients with previously impaired hearing. In such patients, the course of therapy may be shortened to 3 days after the patient becomes afebrile. Renal failure with this regimen is rare; however, the serum creatinine should be monitored, and the dose of streptomycin reduced if the creatinine concentration rises significantly. In patients who present with renal impairment, the dosage of streptomycin should be adjusted accordingly. Other aminoglycosides known to be effective for treatment of plague are gentamicin and kanamycin.

Doxycycline 100 mg twice daily is an alternative therapy for plague in patients who are allergic to streptomycin or who prefer oral treatment. Doxycycline is contraindicated in children and in pregnant women to avoid staining developing teeth.

Intravenous chloramphenicol is the drug of choice for patients who may have profound hypotension resulting in poor absorption of an intramuscular injection, and in patients who have meningitis and require a drug with good cerebrospinal fluid penetration. Chloramphenicol should be administered intravenously with a loading dose of 25 mg per kilogram of body weight followed by 60 mg per kilogram per day in four divided doses. After clinical improvement, oral chloramphenicol should be continued to complete a total course of 10 days. The dosage may be reduced to 30 mg per kilogram per day to reduce the magnitude of bone marrow suppression.

Plasmid mediated resistance to aminoglycosides has been reported with plague in some parts of the world. Buboes usually resolve spontaneously. Occasionally they may become fluctuant and require incision and drainage. Despite the development of disseminated intravascular coagulation and purpura in severely ill patients, neither heparin nor steroids have had any proven benefit in the treatment of plague. Many patients who present with plague are dehydrated due to fever, nausea, and vomiting, or they may be hypotensive. In either case they may require vigorous fluid resuscitation with a balanced saline solution.

In treating individual patients, careful consideration of the indications and contraindications of the various antimicrobial agents that are effective against plague is warranted. Parenteral therapy with streptomycin or gentamicin would be the most efficacious. However, in the event of a mass exposure the standard health care system would be quickly overwhelmed, and choice of therapy would be limited to the oral agents, doxycycline, and ciprofloxacin. These would also be the agents of choice for post-exposure prophylaxis to any contacts of those with pneumonic plague.

Prevention

As soon as a diagnosis of plague is suspected, public health officials should be notified. Patients with uncomplicated infections who are promptly treated are not a health hazard to other persons. If pulmonary symptoms were prominent from the beginning of the illness, a human or animal source and other contacts of that source must be rapidly identified. Those patients with cough or other signs of pneumonic plague must be placed in respiratory isolation for at least a period of 48 hours after the start of antibiotic therapy, or until sputum cultures are negative. The close (within 2 m) contacts of an index case of plague must be identified and evaluated for prophylaxis. Reliable contacts can be instructed to take their temperatures and to seek medical attention immediately should they develop a fever or any respiratory symptoms, including a sore throat. Antibiotic prophylaxis may be given to heavy contacts. Doxycycline is an excellent drug for the prophylaxis of plague in patients for whom it is not contraindicated.

The production of the US-licensed formaldehyde-killed whole bacilli vaccine was discontinued in 1999 and is not currently available. This vaccine did not appear to provide protection against the pneumonic form of plague. Research continues on a recombinant vaccine effective against pneumonic plague.

The control of plague by local health departments requires the knowledge of the epidemiology of the infected animals, the vectors of transmission, and the potential sources of human contact. Control measures usually involve the use of insecticides to control fleas, trapping of animals, and the education of people to avoid contact with certain animals. Persons living in endemic areas should provide themselves with personal protection, such as living in rat-proof houses, wearing shoes and garments that cover the legs, and by applying insecticides. Sick animals, especially cats, should not be handled.

Tetanus

Introduction

Tetanus is a toxin-mediated disease first described by the ancient Egyptians. In the early 19th century, the use of curare, coupled with artificial ventilation, was suggested as a treatment for tetanus. However, only in the 1950s, with the development of hand-held manual ventilators for polio, did this mode of therapy become available.

There are fewer than 100 cases of tetanus yearly in the United States, the majority in the elderly. Worldwide, over a million cases per year are recorded; 50% of these occur in neonates, a reflection of inadequate maternal immunization and unsterile obstetrical practices, with an estimated mortality rate of 90%.

When introduced into a wound under appropriate anaerobic conditions, *Clostridium tetani*, a ubiquitous, Gram-positive, anaerobic bacillus, forms a highly stable spore. The spores germinate and elaborate two toxins: tetanolysin, of unclear significance, and tetanospasmin, the prime etiologic agent of tetanus.

Tetanospasmin is a 151-kd polypeptide that requires cleavage for activation. The heavy chain facilitates attachment and neurocellular internalization, whereas the light chain inhibits neurotransmitter release. Initially, alpha motor neurons are involved. The toxin is then transferred to the neurons and the extracellular space of the central nervous system via retrograde transport and diffusion. Once in the CNS, the toxin affects presynaptic g-aminobutyric acid (GABA)ergic and postsynaptic glycinergic neurons, preventing the release of their inhibitory neurotransmitters. The resulting disinhibition permits uncontrolled agonist and antagonist muscular contraction and spasm characteristic of generalized tetanus. In addition to its local neuromuscular actions and CNS disturbance, tetanospasmin also affects the autonomic nervous system, clinically manifested as a labile, sympathetic overflow, not unlike a pheochromocytoma. An important consideration during management is that once internalized in a neuron, the toxin is no longer accessible to antitoxin, resulting in prolonged recovery until new presynaptic receptors are formed.

Diagnosis

Tetanus is a clinical diagnosis; cultures are of minimal value. Up to 21% of patients have no obvious demonstrable wound. There are essentially four variants of tetanus, a reflection of the groups of neurons involved:
- Generalized
- Cephalic
- Neonatal
- Localized tetanus

Trismus, "lock jaw," is the most common presenting symptom of generalized tetanus. Also common is risus sardonicus or "sneering grin." The most dramatic presentation, however, is generalized muscular contractions with opisthotonos and maintenance of consciousness. The diffuse spasms result in severe pain. Diaphragmatic and vocal cord involvement may result in respiratory compromise. Progression of the disease for up to 2 weeks followed by a prolonged recovery period may occur.

Cephalic tetanus usually involves the lower cranial nerves. A Bell's palsy is often the first presenting complaint. Cephalic tetanus has been linked to otitis media/externa and has occurred in fully immunized individuals.

Neonatal tetanus generally results from an infected umbilical stump. Nonimmunized mothers cannot confer passive immunity to their neonates. Newborns present 1 to 2 weeks after birth with a weak sucking reflex rapidly progressing to generalized spasms. A high mortality is associated with severe autonomic dysfunction.

Localized tetanus is characterized by rigidity within the vicinity of the initial wound. Additionally, there is muscular weakness and often enhanced deep tendon reflexes (DTRs). Symptoms usually resolve with appropriate treatment, but progression to generalized tetanus may occur.

Treatment

- Early airway maintenance. Patients may require orotracheal intubation or tracheostomy in the event of vocal cord and/or diaphragmatic spasms.
- Benzodiazepines for control of unregulated muscular contractions with the use of paralytics, if needed.
- Pain medication.
- Human tetanus immunoglobulin (HTIG) (500 U IM) and tetanus-diphtheria toxoid (Td), diphtheria-pertussis-tetanus (DPT) or tetanus toxoid (TT) at a separate site (deltoid muscle), should be given.
- Control of autonomic dysfunction with the use of labetolol, clonidine, morphine, $MgSO_4$ or epidural blockade.

Key prognostic indicators include the incubation period and onset of symptoms; the shorter the period of incubation and onset of symptoms, the worse the prognosis. The portal of entry is also an important prognostic sign; burns, umbilical stumps, surgical procedures, open fractures, IM injections, and septic abortions all potentiate the likelihood of severe disease.

Strychnine poisoning is the only close mimicker of generalized tetanus and involves postsynaptic glycinergic neurons. Dystonic reactions, meningitis, peritonsillar and retropharyngeal abscesses, seizures, hypocalcemia and "stiff-man syndrome," a consequence of antibodies toward GABAergic neurons, should be considered in the differential diagnosis.

Complications associated with tetanus include hypoxic organ injury, pneumonias, autonomic lability, rhabdomyolysis, spine and long bone fractures, gastrointestinal stress ulcerations, deep venous thrombosis (DVT) and pulmonary emboli, and decubitus ulcers.

There is no natural immunity to tetanus and infection does not confer immunity.

Immunization

- DPT (3 initial doses) 1 to 2 months apart during infancy followed by a booster at age 1 and just prior to entering grammar school. Children younger than 7 receive DPT unless allergic to the pertussis component.
- Td (0.5 mL IM) every 10 years following the initial immunization series.
- Patients with non-tetanus prone wounds but with unclear immunization history should receive a Td and two subsequent boosters, the first 1 to 2 months and the second 6 to 12 months following the primary Td.
- Td (0.5 mL IM) if the wound is tetanus prone (penetration wounds, those with dirt or saliva, burns, frostbite injuries, wounds with devitalized tissue) and the

last booster was greater than 5 years but less than 10 years. If Td was given greater than 10 years ago, both HTIG (250 U IM) and Td should be administered but at separate sites.
- Patients with tetanus-prone wounds and incomplete immunization or those with uncertain immunization should receive a Td and HTIG followed by complete immunization.
- TT should be considered for patients with sensitivity to the diptheria component of Td.

In general, reactions to tetanus immunization are mild and include localized swelling, erythema, and pain. Rarely, a hypersensitivity reaction may occur.

Wound Management

Proper wound management to reduce the risk of tetanus includes thorough wound irrigation and the debridement of devitalized tissue.

Toxic Shock Syndrome

Introduction

In the late 1970s, Todd et al. first described toxic shock syndrome (TSS) as a distinct clinical entity characterized by profound hypotension, fever, multi-organ involvement, and a diffuse erythroderma that subsequently desquamates. TSS gained public notoriety in the early 1980s due to an unsettling number of cases noted in menstruating women, epidemiologically related to the use of highly absorbent tampons. With the withdrawal from the market of these tampons and heightened awareness of the occurrence of TSS, and most likely other concomitant factors, the number of catamenial-related cases of TSS has been greatly reduced, with non-menses-related cases now constituting the greater fraction.

The development of TSS requires colonization or infection by a toxigenic strain of *Staphylococcus aureus* (approximately 20%) elaborating the exotoxin toxic shock syndrome toxin-1 (TSST-1), a 22- to 24-kd protein. Greater than 90% of the *S. aureus* isolates from patients with menstrual-related TSS produce TSST-1, whereas approximately 60% of isolates from non-menstrual-derived cases elaborate TSST-1. The effects of TSST-1 are protean and it is likely that the manifestation of TSS is related both to the direct activity of the toxin as well as induction of other mediators such as interleukin-1 and tumor necrosis factor. In addition, host susceptibility is related to a deficiency in protective antibodies directed toward TSST-1. An anaerobic, neutral pH, magnesium-deficient microenvironment is the ideal condition for the elaboration of TSST-1 by toxigenic *S. aureus*.

Diagnosis

Staphylococcal toxic shock syndrome is characterized by:
- Hyperpyrexia.
- Erythroderma that is fine, diffuse, spreads centrifugally, and desquamates in 1 to 2 weeks (especially palms and soles).
- Nausea, vomiting, and diarrhea.

- Headache and sore throat.
- Myalgias.
- Hypotension.

TSS is a clinical diagnosis that must meet the CDC's strict case definition criteria (**Table 63.2**). Renal involvement is common and may be secondary to prerenal failure, acute tubular necrosis, or rhabdomyolysis, resulting in elevated BUN, creatinine, metabolic acidosis, and diminished urine output. Diarrhea, preceded by vomiting, is often seen as is elevation in hepatic transaminases, most often the γ-glutamyl transpeptidase (GGTP). Adult respiratory distress syndrome (ARDS) may occur, and pleural effusions are commonly present in severe cases. Muscle breakdown may result in gross elevation of creatine kinase with resultant myoglobinuria.

Central nervous system encephalopathy may range from a mild headache to severe disorientation and seizures. Dermatologically, the classical rash associated with TSS is a scarlatiniform exanthem that is nonpruritic, blanching, and generally begins on the lower torso, eventually spreading and involving the extremities. Conjunctival and tympanic membrane hyperemia is often noted along with erythematous mucous membranes and a "strawberry tongue." Hematologic abnormalities may include mild anemia, microangiopathic hemolysis, leukocytosis, eosinophilia, thrombocytopenia, and disseminated intravascular coagulation. A pelvic examination is essential in any woman with TSS for the removal of a tampon or other foreign object. The vaginal walls are usually erythematous and a "strawberry cervix" may be appreciated. Menstrual blood and a malodorous discharge may be present, with Gram stain of the discharge revealing Gram-positive cocci in clusters.

Treatment

- Infusion of intravenous crystalloid solution (normal saline or lactated Ringer's). In the presence of refractory hypotension, peripheral pressors are employed.
- Identifying and removing the source of the infection (e.g., tampon, nasal packs, surgical wound infection, soft tissue abscess) is essential.
- Antistaphylococcal antibiotics may serve to eradicate toxin-producing staphylococci, thereby lowering the overall toxic burden.
- Immunoglobin therapy may benefit patients with TSS who have a low anti-TSST-1 antibody titer.
- Corticosteroids use is controversial and not well established.
- Estrogens may improve catamenial-related TSS by the cessation of menses.

The differential diagnosis of TSS includes staphylococcal-scalded skin syndrome, Kawasaki disease, scarlet fever, Rocky Mountain spotted fever, leptospirosis, erythema multiforme major, typhus, Lyme disease, menigococcemia, staphylococcal food poisoning, Gram-negative urosepsis, necrotizing fasciitis, and toxic streptococcal syndrome. Toxic streptococcal syndrome warrants special mention as it is a toxin-related condition that closely mimics staphylococcal TSS. Streptococcal pyrogenic exotoxin A, synthesized by *Streptococcus pyogenes,* a group A *Streptococcus* species, is thought to be the etiologic agent responsible for the hypotension, multi-system failure, hypocalcemia, and thrombocytopenia observed in toxic streptococcal syndrome, similar to staphylococcal TSS. Skin and soft tissue portals of entry, as well as respiratory and genitourinary sources have been identified as potential sites of infection by toxigenic strains of *S. pyogenes.*

Lyme Disease

Lyme disease, originally termed Lyme arthritis, was first described in 1975 after an unusual epidemic of arthritis occurring in a group of children in the town of Lyme, Connecticut. The arthritis was often preceded by a distinctive skin rash, erythema migrans (EM). The correlation between the bite of a tick and EM was already known in Europe. Lyme disease is a complex immune-mediated multi-system disorder that may affect patients of any age or either sex. The disease is caused by the spirochete *Borrelia burgdorferi,* which is transmitted to humans via a tick bite from either *Ixodes scapularis* (Northeast or North Central United States) or *Ixodes pacificus* (California). The entire genome of *B. burgdorferi* has been sequenced, demonstrating that the likely virulence factor is a surface

---

Table 63.2

Centers for Disease Control Case Definition of Toxic Shock Syndrome

Fever: temperature ≥ 38.9° C (102° F)

Rash: diffuse macular erythroderma

Desquamation: 1 to 2 weeks after onset of illness, particularly of palms and soles

Hypotension: systolic blood pressure ≤ 90 mm Hg, orthostatic drop in diastolic ≥ 15 mm Hg; orthostatic syncope or dizziness

Involvement of three or more of the following organ systems:
- Gastrointestinal: Vomiting or diarrhea at onset of illness
- Muscular: Severe myalgia or twice-normal creatine phosphokinase
- Mucous membranes: Vaginal, oropharyngeal, or conjunctival hyperemia
- Renal: Twice-normal BUN or creatinine or pyuria (>5 WBC/hpf)
- Hepatic: Twice-normal bilirubin or transaminases
- Hematologic: Platelets < 100,000/mm^3

Central nervous system: disorientation or alterations in consciousness without focal neurologic signs when fever and hypotension are absent.

Negative results on following tests, if obtained:
- Blood, throat, or cerebrospinal fluid cultures (blood culture may be positive for *S. aureus*)
- Serologic tests for Rocky Mountain spotted fever, leptospirosis, or measles
- BUN, serum urea nitrogen; WBC, white blood cells; hpf, high-power field.

protein that allows the spirochete to attach to mammalian cells leading to Lyme disease.

Epidemiology

B. burgdorferi infection is particularly prevalent in North America and Europe, and has also been reported in South America, Asia, and Africa. Lyme disease is now the most common vector-borne disease in the United States with over 23,000 cases reported in 2002. The peak incidence of Lyme disease correlates with the density of the tick and white-tailed deer populations and is contracted by humans at the end of spring and early summer; however, late manifestations may occur throughout the year. Humans may be exposed when frequenting woodlands where Lyme disease is endemic. Endemic areas include three primary foci: the Northeast (from Maine to Maryland), the North Central region (Wisconsin and Minnesota), and the Pacific Northwest (northern California and Oregon).

Clinical Findings

Lyme disease cases can be divided into three groups based on the timing and type of symptoms: (1) early localized disease, (2) early disseminated disease, and (3) late Lyme disease. Early localized disease occurs from three to 30 days after the tick bite and is characterized by the classic bull's-eye rash, erythema migrans (EM), without any other manifestations. The lesion can be primary (at the site of the tick bite) or secondary (other locations on the skin). It starts as an erythematous maculopapular lesion that concentrically expands, has a well-demarcated border, and is usually larger than 5 cm in size. Only one third of cases have the classic central clearing to the rash. EM appears after an incubation period of seven to 14 days and is noted in only about half of the cases of Lyme disease. If left untreated, the rash resolves without scarring, several days to several weeks after onset.

Early disseminated disease occurs days to weeks after the appearance of EM and is characterized by EM and systemic manifestations primarily affecting the nervous system, musculoskeletal system, and heart. Symptoms range from minor complaints in well appearing patients to debilitating symptoms in toxic-appearing patients. Symptoms to look for include headache with or without meningismus, fever, dry cough, myalgias/arthralgias, joint effusions, focal neurologic deficits or paresthesias, and prostration.

Lyme carditis occurs in 10% to 15% of patients with early, disseminated Lyme disease. Lyme carditis is characterized by a mild myocarditis with minor left ventricular dysfunction and is usually associated with atrioventricular node conduction abnormalities. Approximately half of patients with Lyme carditis develop complete heart block, which is always reversible, but may require temporary cardiac pacing. Lyme carditis has not been shown to affect the distal conduction system of the heart or the heart valves. Five percent of untreated individuals will develop myopericarditis and, more rarely, pancarditis or cardiomegaly.

Late Lyme disease occurs weeks to months after the initial rash. Symptoms and signs are generally either neurologic or arthritic.

Neurologic manifestations occur in 10% to 40% of patients with early or late disseminated disease and can affect both the central and peripheral nervous systems. The central nervous system involvement often leads to cranial neuropathies. The facial nerve is most commonly involved (70% of all cranial neuropathies), presenting as unilateral Bell's palsy; however 33% may be bilateral. Other cranial neuropathies include ophthalmoplegia with diplopia, and abnormalities of lacrimation, the stapedius reflex, and taste sensation. The spirochete also causes meningitis with typical symptoms of headache, fever, and stiff neck. Lyme encephalitis usually occurs as a late process characterized by confusion, cognitive difficulties and emotional lability.

Peripheral manifestations of Lyme disease present as upper motor neuron signs with radicular pain and paresthesias. If not treated, the neurologic manifestations of Lyme disease may last for months, but will usually resolve even without antibiotic therapy. However, 5% of untreated patients have symptoms that persist into late Lyme disease and now carry the diagnosis of "chronic Lyme disease" or "post Lyme disease syndrome."

Lyme arthritis usually occurs in late, disseminated disease, but many patients develop arthralgias early in the illness. Overall, sixty percent of patients will develop arthritis. Lyme arthritis is an asymmetric, oligoarticular arthritis occurring in large, weight-bearing joints with or without effusion, with the knee being the most commonly affected site. The joint is often painful and warm. Symptoms are migratory and intermittent. Attacks last from days to weeks. Although most patients' symptoms resolve as the disease is treated, 10% of cases develop a chronic arthritis that may last two to three years after a period of remission. Some of these patients require a repeat course of antibiotics or long-term antibiotic therapy.

Diagnosis

Lyme disease diagnosis is based primarily on the history and physical exam as well as seasonal and geographic consideration. Characteristic symptoms and clinical signs classic for Lyme disease are sufficient to make the diagnosis and begin treatment.

The timing of the onset of symptoms determines the appropriateness of supportive laboratory data. In early localized disease, EM biopsy cultures grow *B. burgdorferi* more than 80% of the time. Culture is thought to be more sensitive than serology this early in the disease course. The required medium (Barbour-Stoenner-Kelly), however, is not available in most laboratories and lengthy observation times are needed. Serologic testing in early localized disease has a sensitivity of only 20% to 30%, due to the physiologic delay in antibody response.

Early disseminated disease occurs weeks to months after the tick bite. By this time an immunologic response may have developed making serologic or CSF testing more useful. The best initial test is a second or third generation ELISA or immunofluorescence assay (IFA). If positive, a confirmatory Western immunoblot should be ordered. ELISA tests have a sensitivity of 40% to 60% in early Lyme disease. This increases to 95% in late Lyme disease.

The immunologic response to *B. burgdorferi* is unusual and makes interpreting serologic results difficult. The following facts may be helpful in deciding when to perform supporting laboratory tests and how to interpret them. Prior antibiotic use does not significantly change serological reactivity. Seroreactivity alone cannot be used as a marker of active disease as antibodies will persist for years following infection, whether or not it is treated. Antibodies do not confer complete immunity in previously infected patients, as there are documented reports of repeat infections. Background seropositive rates of 5% to 20% in endemic areas result in many false-positive results.

CSF should be tested in patients with possible Lyme disease and who have neurologic symptoms (meningitis, encephalitis, radicular signs, and cranial neuropathies). CSF abnormalities usually appear within three to four weeks after inoculation and may persist for months. Microscopic analysis in Lyme disease with CNS involvement shows a lymphocytic and monocytic pleocytosis, with elevated protein and normal glucose. Antibodies to *B. burgdorferi* are found in the CSF of infected individuals more often in acute disease than in chronic Lyme disease. Overall, PCR is more sensitive than culture in CSF studies.

Arthrocentesis can confirm the diagnosis of Lyme disease with either culture or PCR. If the patient has late disseminated or chronic disease, PCR is more sensitive than culture.

Treatment

Treatment of Lyme disease is based primarily on clinical signs and symptoms. Patients with early, localized disease, and most patients with early disseminated disease can be treated with oral doxycycline. An added benefit of doxycycline is its coverage of other tick-borne infections such as ehrlichiosis. If neurologic or cardiac symptoms are present, ceftriaxone IV is the preferred agent (**Table 63.3**).

The treatment of Lyme disease in pregnancy is an area of special concern. Transplacental transmission of *B. burgdorferi* has been reported in the first trimester. There have been several documented cases of neonatal death as a result of untreated or inadequately treated Lyme disease during pregnancy. In general, pregnant women are treated as non-pregnant adults, except that tetracyclines, including doxycycline, should be avoided. Also, a lower threshold for post-tick bite antibiotic prophylaxis has been recommended for pregnant patients.

In most instances Lyme disease can easily be managed in the outpatient setting. Coordination with primary care providers and home nursing providers can even allow for the administration of intravenous antibiotics without admission to the hospital. Patients with Lyme carditis and meningitis should be admitted to the hospital and monitored.

Prevention

Avoidance of the tick habitat is difficult since most infections likely occur in residential areas during routine activities. Effective landscaping that reduces leaf litter and creates desiccating barriers between forest vegetation and the land owner's property with stone walls or wood chips will reduce tick density and possibly rates of infection. Spraying an acaricide (carbaryl, cyfluthrin, deltamethrin) on residential properties also reduces tick density by 68% to 83%.

A vaccine was available until February 2002, but was removed from the market due to lack of efficacy as a multi-dose regimen and lack of sales.

Wardrobe considerations will also aid in prevention. Wearing light-colored clothing to make ticks visible, tucking pant cuffs into socks to prevent ticks from gaining access to exposed skin, and applying skin repellents con-

---

Table 63.3

Clinical Setting	Treatment†
Endemic area and partially engorged deer tick	Doxycycline 200 mg PO single dose
Early localized/disseminated disease† • 1O AV block and • Absence of neurologic symptoms* • Absence of 2O/3O heart block	Doxycycline 100 mg PO bid 14 to 21 days or Amoxicillin 500 mg PO tid 14 to 21 days or Cefuroxime axetil 500 mg PO bid 14 to 21 days or Erythromycin 250 mg PO qid 14 to 21 days
Early/late disseminated disease • CNS involvement (meningitis) or • Radicular symptoms or • 2O/3O heart block	Ceftriaxone 2 g IV qd 14 to 28 days or Cefotaxime 2 g IV q4h 14 to 28 days or Penicillin 24 million units IV qd 14 to 28 days
Lyme arthritis • Absence of neurologic symptoms	Doxycycline 100 mg po bid 30 to 60 days or Amoxicillin 500 mg PO tid 30 to 60 days

Pregnancy	Amoxicillin 500 mg PO tid 21 days
	 If penicillin allergic:
	  Azithromycin 500 mg qd 7 to 10 days or
	  Erythromycin 500 mg qid PO 14 to 21 days

Recommendations based on *Sanford Guide to Antimicrobial Therapy 2003*.
* An isolated facial palsy, with normal CSF testing though a CNS finding, may be treated with the oral 14- to 21-day regimen listed for early disseminated disease.
† All oral regimens are dosed for 14 to 21 days. Note that there is a high incidence of failure with both erythromycin and azithromycin.

taining DEET (N,N-diethyl-m-toluamide) are all helpful. Daily inspections for attached ticks should be routine in endemic areas. Attached ticks should be removed immediately with fine forceps, as transmission of *B. burgdorferi* increases with time. The maximum efficiency of transmission by the infected tick does not occur until after attachment for 24 to 48 hours.

Routine antibiotic prophylaxis after all tick bites is not recommended. Recent evidence shows that patients that live in or traveled to endemic areas and present within 72 hours after discovery of an engorged deer tick or a tick that was attached for more than 36 hours, have a lower risk of developing erythema migrans if treated with a single 200 mg dose of doxycycline. This new treatment recommendation is based on the simplicity, low cost, safety, and high efficacy of single dose doxycycline among adults who live in areas where Lyme disease is endemic.

Chlamydia

Chlamydia species are unique microorganisms that are classified as bacteria. However their specific properties differentiate them from both the viruses and bacteria. *Chlamydia* species are obligate intracellular organisms and grow in the eukaryocyte cells, which closely resemble the viruses. However the possession of deoxyribonucleic acid (DNA) and ribonucleic acid (RNA), their division by binary fission, and the presence of a distinct cell wall very similar to the Gram-negative microorganism, has a close semblance to the bacteria. Due to their lack of electron transport chain enzymes, *Chlamydia* species utilize the host's adenosine triphosphate (ADP) and nutrients for their growth and are considered energy parasites. These organisms cause a wide range of diseases in humans.

Etiology and Epidemiology

In the last two decades multiple *Chlamydia* species have been identified. These species include *C. trachomatis*, *C. pneumoniae*, *C. psittaci*, and *C. pecorum*. The incubation period for chlamydial infections is between 1 to 3 weeks.

C. trachomatis

C. trochomatis is the most common cause of sexually transmitted bacterial infections (STD) in the United States, and probably the rest of the world. Furthermore, this organism is one of the main causes of mucopurulent cervicitis (MPC), pelvic inflammatory disease (PID), and subsequent infertility and ectopic pregnancies. It is estimated that 25% to 50% of the PIDs are due to this infection. The precise incidence and prevalence of this infection is unknown. However the prevalence of chlamydial genital infections in women has been reported from 8% to 40%. It is estimated that the incidence of chlamydial STD is 2.5 times that of gonococcal disease. Close to 50% of all non-gonococcal urethritis and acute epididymitis in men are secondary to a chlamydial infection. Compared to heterosexual men, the prevalence of urethritis is reduced by two thirds in homosexual men, however 4% to 8% of these patients have rectal chlamydial infection. *C. trochomatis* is also responsible for procto-colitis in women. This organism can also cause orchitis in men. A large number of infected patients, specifically women, are asymptomatic. The reported rate for asymptomatic women and men exceeds 70% and 30%, respectively. This phenomenon is a major contributor in the transmission of the infection to new patients. In the United States annually 4 million new cases of the disease is the cause of more than 50,000 cases of involuntary infertility. It is estimated that at least 5% of all the pregnant patients are infected with genital chlamydia. Furthermore, annually more than 155,000 infants are born to chlamydia-infected mothers. Contact with the mother's infected cervico-vaginal secretions, predispose these newborns to neonatal inclusion conjunctivitis (ophthlamia neonatorum) and afebrile inclusive pneumonia. Conjunctivitis will develop between one to three weeks after birth in 15% to 80% of the infants born to infected mothers. The symptoms are often mild and can be missed. It is usually self-limiting and does not cause any long lasting sequelae. This infection is usually associated with peri-auricular adenopathy. Pneumonia or bronchitis occurs in 3% to 18% of this subset of newborns. The onset of the subacute and afebrile pneumonia is usually from the 1 to 3 months of age. It presents with repetitive staccato cough, tachypnea, hyperventilation, and diffuse infiltrates on chest radiographs. Although the infection is generally mild, need for hospitalization in severe cases has also been reported. Infected children are also at a slightly higher risk for otitis media and bronchiolitis. Maternal infection during pregnancy is also associated with postpartum endometritis and possibly with an increase in perinatal mortality. Additionally, this pathogen is closely linked with Reiter's syndrome and Fitz-Hugh-Curtis syndrome (perihepatitis).

Risk factors for chlamydial genital infections include young age, marital status, number of sexual partners, low socioeconomic status, sexual preference and use of oral birth control. Co-infection with *Neisseria gonorrhoeae* occurs in 15% to 30% and 25% to 50% of afflicted men and women, respectively. Women suffering from trichomoniasis and bacterial vaginosis are at higher risk for chlamydial genital infections.

C. trochomatis serotypes A, B, and C are also the causative pathogens for trachoma. Although rare in the United States, worldwide this chronic conjunctivitis is the leading cause of preventable blindness. Worldwide, there are an estimated 500 million cases of active trachoma. Persistent infections or frequent re-infections result in 20 million cases of blindness secondary to conjunctival scarring and eyelid deformities.

Several serotypes of *C. trochomatis*, e.g., L1, L2, and L3, are also the causative agents for lymphogranuloma venereum (LGV). This disease is rare in the United States, but is relatively prevalent in Asia, Africa, and South America.

C. pneumoniae

C. pneumoniae was first identified in 1989 and is a common cause of acute respiratory infections accounting for 6% to 10% of all the community acquired pneumonias. The majority of infections with *C. pneumoniae* are either asymptomatic or mild in nature. These infections include pharyngitis, sinusitis, bronchitis, and pneumonia. In elderly patients, specifically those with co-morbidities, the disease may present as a severe infection. This pathogen is unique to humans and spread from person to person. Most primary infections occur in childhood or young age. This pathogen's seroprevalence in adults is 40% to 70% suggesting an extraordinary high prevalence rate. Antibodies are not protective and re-infections are common. Reported outbreaks or epidemics have been are documented. Co-infections with viruses, e.g., influenza and respiratory syncytial virus, and other bacteria are a common occurrence. Recurrent infections are relatively common.

Clinical manifestations associated with *C. pneumoniae* infections continue to emerge beyond respiratory illnesses. Recent published data is suggestive of an association of chronic *C. penumoniae* infections with atherosclerosis, coronary artery disease, acute myocardial infarction, and acute exacerbation of bronchial asthma.

C. psittaci

C. psittaci is found in more than 130 species of birds, and has also been isolated in kittens. The related infections are considered a zoonosis. The spread of the infection is through respiratory droplets and by means of contact with the nasal secretions or fecal material of the infected animal. Birds can be healthy carriers. Human infections can result in severe pneumonia, with mortality rates exceeding 40%. Despite the use of antibiotics in feeds and the screening of poultry, sporadic outbreaks of psittacosis continue to be reported. Other infections caused by *C. psittaci* include conjunctivitis, endocarditis, hepatitis, glomerulonephritis, and disseminated intravascular coagulation (DIC). This pathogen may cause placentitis and resultant spontaneous abortion in infected pregnant patients. In spite of proper therapy, protracted recovery and high relapse rates have been reported.

Presentation

Non-Gonococcal Urethritis and Cervicitis

In infected men, symptoms and signs include dysuria, frequency, penile discharge, meatal itching, meatal erythema, tenderness and inflammation. In infected women, the disease predominantly presents as purulent vaginal discharge or leucorrhea.

Lymphogranuloma Venereum (LGV)

Manifestations of the disease is initiated with a painless skin lesion in the genital area. This lesion will develop into a shallow ulcer or become vesicular or papular. Subsequently, e tender unilateral inguinal lymphadenopathy will develop in two thirds of cases. The excessive growth of these nodes will produce the characteristic "groove sign." Systemic signs, such as fever, chills, malaise, and headaches are common. Patients involved in anal intercourse may develop procto-colitis, anal fissures, and strictures. LGV may be complicated with late manifestations of fistula formation, chronic ulcerative lesions, inguinal sinus tract formation, lymphatic obstruction and secondary elephantiasis. Rare complications include arthritis and meningitis.

C. pneumoniae Pneumonia

Symptoms and signs of this form of pneumonia include nonproductive cough, upper respiratory symptoms, fever, and a small infiltrate on the chest radiograph.

C. psittaci Pneumonia

The incubation period for this infection is 7 to 14 days. Manifestations of this infection include fever, chills, headache, malaise, nonproductive cough, myalgia, arthralgia, rash, and gastrointestinal symptoms. Chest radiographs will reveal diffuse patchy infiltrates.

Diagnosis

The gold standard for diagnosis of chlamydial infection is isolation of the pathogen in cell culture. However, this procedure is very difficult and expensive, and has a 2- to 3-day turn around time. Recent advancements in molecular amplification tests have drastically simplified the task of diagnosis of chlamydial infections. In addition to urethral and cervical specimens, this test can be performed on the patient's urine. Polymerase chain reaction (PCR) assays on urethral or cervical swabs in symptomatic patients have a sensitivity of 89% to 100% and specificity of 99% to 100%. Sensitivity of PCR assays for urine specimens are 87% to 100% and 96% to 100%, and a corresponding specificity of 96% to 100% and 95% in men and women, respectively.

Patients with genital chlamydial infection are also at increased risk for infections with treponema pallidum and HIV. In patients who are suspected of having a chlamydial STD, obtaining a serological test for syphilis is highly recommended. Counseling for HIV testing is also recommended in all patients who are being treated for a STD.

Treatment

Uncomplicated Genital and Ocular Chlamydial Infection

Azithromycin prescribed as a single oral one gram dose is the treatment of choice. There is limited data for the use of this regimen in pregnancy, PID, and cervicitis. Other alternative therapeutic modalities include 7-day oral regimens of doxycycline, 100 mg twice a day, or erythromycin, 500 mg every 6 hours. In pregnancy, erythromycin must be prescribed either in its base or ethyl succinate forms, and use of doxycycline should be avoided. The therapeutic regimen must include therapy for possible concomitant gonococcal infection.

Neonatal Conjunctivitis or Pneumonia

Oral erythromycin 50 mg/kg per day, divided in 4 doses for 14 days. Topical antibiotics are not indicated in treatment of conjunctivitis.

C. pneumoniae Infections

Treatment of choice includes use of the standard doses of either azithromycin or clarithromycin for 2 to 3 weeks. Other alternative therapies include standard doses of doxycycline or erythromycin for 2 to 3 weeks. With the occurrence of a relapse, a second course of antimicrobial therapy may be required.

C. psittaci Infections

Treatment of choice for this infection is either oral tetracycline or erythromycin 500 mg, every 6 hours for 21 days.

Prevention

Genital Chlamydial Infections

All individuals exposed through sexual contact with a symptomatic patient, within 30 days of the onset of symptoms or clinical evaluation must be assessed for the presence of the disease and should be treated for presumptive infection. Furthermore, all female patients afflicted by bacterial vaginosis or trichomonas vaginitis should also be screened for STD.

Neonatal Conjunctivitis

Prophylactic therapy with ophthalmic silver nitrate drops or topical antibiotic ointments are ineffective for chlamydial infections. Prevention of this infection, as well as neonatal pneumonia, is fulfilled through screening of all the pregnant patients. Infected patients should be promptly treated prior to the initiation of labor. Considering its efficacy in prevention of neonatal ophthalmic gonococcal infections, the utilization of ophthalmic silver nitrate drops or topical antibiotic ointments should be continued.

Selected Readings

Al-Suleiman S, Grimes E, Jonas H. Disseminated gonococcal infections. *Obstet Gynecol* 1983;61:48–51.

American Academy of Pediatrics Committee on Child Abuse and Neglect. Gonorrhea in prepubertal children. *Pediatrics* 1998;101:134–135.

Angulo F, Getz J, Getz J, et al. A large outbreak of botulism: the hazardous baked potato. *J Infect Dis* 1998;178:172–177.

Balmelli C, Gunthard H. Gonococcal tonsillar infection—a case report and literature review. *Infection* 2003;31:362–365.

Bardin T. Gonococcal arthritis. *Ballieres Best Pract Res Clin Rheumatol* 2003;17: 201–208.

Bauwens JE, Clark AM, Stamm WE. Diagnosis of Chlamydia trachomatis endocervical infections by a commercial polymerase chain reaction assay. *J Clin Microbiol* 1993;31:3023.

Biro F, Rosenthatl S. Gonococcal and chlamydial infections on symptomatic and asymptomatic adolescent women. *Clin Pediatr* 2003;34:419–424.

Bleck TP. Tetanus: pathophysiology, management, and prophylaxis. *Dis Mon* 1991; 37:547–603.

Bonacorsi SP, Scavizzi MR, Guiyoule A, et al. Assessment of a fluoroquinolone, three beta lactams, two aminoglycosides and a cycline in the treatment of murine Yersinia pestis infection. *Antimicrob Agents Chemother* 1994;38: 481–486.

Brady WJ, DeBehnke D, Crosby DL. Dermatological emergencies. *Am J Emerg Med* 1994;12:217–237.

Butler T. Yersinia infections: centennial of the discovery of the plague bacillus. *Clin Infect Dis* 1994;19:655–663.

Cartwright KAV, Jones DM, Smith AJ, et al. Influenza A and meningococcal disease. *Lancet* 1991;338:554.

Caugant DA, Hoiby EA, Magnus P, et al. Asymptomatic carriage of Neisseria meningitidis in a randomly sampled population. *J Clin Microbiol* 1994;32:323.

Centers for Disease Control and Prevention. Prevention and control of meningococcal disease: recommendations of the advisory committee on immunization practice (ACIP). *Morb Mort Wkly Rep* 2000;49:1–10.

Center for Disease Control and Prevention. Sexually transmitted disease treatment guidelines. *Morb Mort Wkly Rep* 2002;51:180.

Coleman EA, Yergler ME. Botulism. *Am J Nurs* 2002;102:44–47.

Craven RB, Barnes AM. Plague and tularemia. *Infect Dis Clin North Am* 1991; 5:165–175.

Craven RB, Maupin GO, Beard ML, et al. Reported cases of human plague in the United States, 1970–1991. *J Med Entomol* 1993;30:758–761.

Darling RG, Catlett CL, Huebner KD, et al. Threats in bioterrorism I: CDC category A agents. *Emerg Med Clin N Am* 2002;20:273–309.

Doll J, Fink TM, et al. Plague. *Morb Mort Wkly Rep* 1992;41:787–790.

Food and Drug Administration. *Product Approval Information-Licensing Action-Botulism Immune Globulin, United States Food and Drug Administration, 2004.* Washington, DC: US Government Printing Office 2003.

Freedman JD, Beer DJ. Expanding perspectives on the toxic shock syndrome. *Adv Intern Med* 1991;36:363–397.

Giangrasso J, Smith RK. Misuse of tetanus immunoprophylaxis in wound care. *Ann Emerg Med* 1985;14:573–579.

Gordon S, Carlyn C, Doyle L, et al. The emergence of Neisseria gonorrhoeae with decreased susceptibility to ciprofloxacin in Cleveland, Ohio. *Ann Intern Med* 1996;125:465–470.

Granier S, Owen P, Stott NCH. Recognizing meningococcal disease: The case for further research in primary care. *Br J Gen Pract* 1998;48:1167–1171.

Hakakha MM, Davis J, et al. Leukorrhea and bacterial vaginosis as in office predictors of cervical infection in high risk women. *Obstet Gynecol* 2002;100: 8080–8012.

Hayes E, Piesman J. Current concepts: how can we prevent Lyme disease? *N Engl J Med* 2003;348:2424–2430.

Hedberg K, White KE, et al. An outbreak of psittacosis in Minnesota turkey industry workers: implications for modes of transmission and control. *Am J Epidemiol* 1989;130:569–577.

Hook E, Hansfield H. Gonococcal infections in the adult. In: Holmes K, et al, eds. *Sexually Transmitted Diseases.* 3rd ed. New York: McGraw Hill 1999: 451–466.

Hook EK, Holmes K. Gonococcal infections. *Ann Intern Med* 1985;102:229–243.

Hussey J, Edirisinghe DN, Pattman RS, et al. Does bacterial vaginosis alter the sensitivity of screening tests of Chlamydia trachomatis? An analysis of patient characteristics. *Int J STD AIDS* 2003;14:448–450.

Ilowite NT. Muscle, reticuloendothelial, and late skin manifestations of Lyme disease. *Am J Med* 1995;98:s63–s69.

Increases in fluoroquinolone resistant Neisseria gonorrhoeae—Hawaii and California—2001. *Morb Mort Wkly Rep* 2002;51:1041–1044.

Inglesby TV, Dennis DT, Henerson DA, et al. Plague as a biological weapon. *JAMA* 2000;283:2281–2290.

Jackson LA, Shuchat A, Reeves MW, et al. Serogroup C meningococcal outbreaks in the United States: an emerging threat. *JAMA* 1995;273:383.

Jafari H, McCracken GH. Dexamethasone therapy in bacterial meningitis. *Pediatr Ann* 1994;23:82–88.

Judson, F. Gonorrhea. *Med Clinics North Am* 1990;74:1353–1366.

Kefer MP. Tetanus. *Am J Emerg Med* 1992;100:445–448.

Kerle, K, Mascola J, Miller T. Disseminated gonococcal infection. *Am Fam Phys* 1992;45:209–214.

Klempner MS, Hu LT, Evans J, et al. Two controlled trials of antibiotic treatment in patients with persistent symptoms and a history of Lyme disease. *N Engl J Med* 2001; 345:85–92.

Klempner MS. Prolonged antibiotic treatment did not relieve chronic symptoms in Lyme disease. *ACP J Club* 2002;136:57.

La Force M, et al. Tetanus in the United States: epidemiologic and clinical features. *N Engl J Med* 1969;280:569–574.

Larkin M. Meningitis risks multiply. *Lancet Infect Dis* 2002;2:772.

Lastavica CC, Wilson ML, Bernardi VP, et al. Rapid emergence of a focal epidemic of Lyme disease in coastal Massachusetts. *N Engl J Med* 1989;320:133–137.

Lyss SB, Kamb ML, Peterman TA, et al. Chlamydia trachomitis among patients infected with and treated for Neisseria gonorrhoeae in sexually transmitted disease clinics in the United States. *Ann Intern Med* 2003;139:178–185.

Magid D, Douglas JM, Schwartz JS. Doxycycline compared with azithromycin for treating women with genital Chlamydia trachomatis infections: an incremental cost effective analysis. *Ann Intern Med* 1996;124:389–399.

Mandell GL, Douglas R, et al. *Mandell, Douglas, and Bennett's Principles and Practice of Infectious Diseases.* Philadelphia: Churchill Livingstone 2002.

McNeely G. Gonococcal infections in women. *Obstet Gynecol Clin North Am* 1989;166:467–477.

Merrison AF, Chidley KE, et al. Wound botulism associated with subcutaneous drug use. *Br Med J* 2002;325:1020–1021.

Meyers SA, Sexton DJ. Dermatologic manifestations of arthropod-borne diseases. *Infect Dis Clin N Am* 1994;8:689–712.

Nadelman RB, et al. Prophylaxis with single-dose doxycycline for the prevention of Lyme disease after an Ixodes scapularis tick bite. *N Engl J Med* 2001;345:79–84.

Nafissi S. Current concepts in botulism: clinical and electrophysiological aspects. *J Clin Neuromusc Dis* 2003;4:139–149.

O'Brien KK, Higdon MJ, Halverson JJ. Recognition and treatment of bioterrorism infections. *Amer Fam Phys* 2003;67:1927–1934.

Opulski A, MacNeil E, et al. Pneumonic plague—Arizona, 1992. *Morb Mort Weekly Rep* 1992;41:737–739.

Outbreak of botulism type E associated with eating a beached whale—Western Alaska, July 2002. *Morb Mortal Wkly Rep* 2003;52:24–26.

Pachner AR. Early disseminated Lyme disease: Lyme meningitis. *Am J Med* 1995; 98:s30–s42.

Peebles TC, Levine L, Eldred MC, Edsall G. Tetanus-toxoid emergency boosters. *N Engl J Med* 1969;280:575–581.

Peeling RW. Chlamydia trachomatis and Neisseria gonorrhoeae: Pathogen in retreat? *Curr Opin Infect Dis* 1995;8:26–34

Peterson H, Galaid E, Cates W. Pelvic inflammatory disease. *Med Clin North Am* 1990;74:1603–1613.

Poland G. Prevention of Lyme disease: a review of the evidence. *Mayo Clinic Proceedings* 2001;76:713–724.

Reingold AL. Toxic shock syndrome: an update. *Am J Obstet Gynecol* 1991; 165:1236–1239.

Resnick SD. Staphylococcal toxic-mediated syndromes in children. *Semin Dermatol* 1992;11:11–18.

Rice P, Hansfield H. Arthritis associated with sexually transmitted disease. In: Holmes KK, et al, eds. *Sexually Transmitted Diseases.* 3rd ed. New York: McGraw Hill 1999:921–935.

Rosenstein NE. Meningococcal vaccines. *Infect Dis Clin North Am* 2001;15: 155–169.

Sato Y, Kimata N, et al. Extracorporeal adsorption as a new approach to treatment of botulism. *ASAIO J* 2000;46:783–785.

Schoen RT. Identification of Lyme disease. *Rheum Dis Clin North Am* 1994;20: 361–369.

Scopelitis EP, Martinez O. Gonococcal arthritis. *Rheum Dis Clin North Am* 2003; 19:363–377.

Seligson R, Pollack C. Update on emerging infections: news from the Centers for Disease Control and Prevention. *Ann Emerg Med* 1998;32:748–750.

Sigal LH. Management of Lyme disease refractory to antibiotic therapy. *Rheum Dis Clin North Am* 1995;21:217–230.

Stanwell-Smith RE, Stuart JM, Hughes AO, et al. Smoking, the environment and meningococcal disease: a case-control study. *Epidemiol Infect* 1994;112:315.

Steere AC. Medical progress: Lyme disease. *N Engl J Med* 2001;345:115–125.

Strausbaugh LJ. Toxic shock syndrome: Are you recognizing its changing presentations? *Postgrad Med* 1993;94:107–118.

Sutton DN, Tremlett MR, Woodcock TE, Nielsen MS. Management of autonomic dysfunction in severe tetanus: the use of magnesium sulphate and clonodine. *Intensive Care Med* 1990;16:75–80.

Taylor S. Infant botulism in a 10-week-old male: a wolf in sheep's clothing. *J Emerg Nurs* 2002;28:581–583.

Teoh D, Reynols S. Diagnosis and management of pediatric conjunctivitis. *Pediatr Emerg Care* 2003;19:48–55.

Thaisetthawatkul P, et al. Peripheral nervous system manifestations of Lyme borreliosis. *J Clin Neuromusc Dis* 2002;3:165–171.

Toye B, Peeling RW, Jessamine P, et al. Diagnosis of Chlamydia trachomatis infections in asymptomatic men and women by PCR assay. *J Clin Microbiol* 1996; 34:1396–1400.

Turner C, Rogers S, Miller H, et al. Untreated gonococcal and chlamydial infection in a probability sample of adults. *JAMA* 2002;287:726–733.

Werner, SB, Murry R, et al. Human plague. *Morb Mort Weekly Rep* 1994;43:242–246

Wiesenfeld HC, Uhrin M, et al. Diagnosis of male Chlamydia trachomatis urethritis by polymerase chain reaction. *Sex Transm Dis* 1994;21:268–271.

Wiesenfeld HC, Hillier SL, Krohn MA, et al. Bacterial vaginosis is a strong predictor of Neisseria gonorrhoeae and Chlamydia trachomatis infection. *Clin Infect Dis* 2003;36:663B.

Wilske B. Microbiological diagnosis in Lyme borreliosis. *Internat J Med Microbiol* 2002;291:114–119.

World Health Organization. Meningococcal meningitits. *WHO Fact Sheet* 2003;451.

World Health Organization. Sexually transmitted diseases. *WHO Press Release* 1995;64.

Wormser GP, et al. Practice guidelines for the treatment of Lyme disease. *Infect Dis Soc Amer* 2000;31:1–14.

Parasites

Stephen J. Playe
Michael D. Dunkerley

Thomas A. Brunell
Eddie A. Fernandez

Malaria

Malaria kills over 2.5 million persons throughout the world each year. Due to increasing international travel and immigration, there were over 1,300 cases diagnosed in the United States in 2001. Many of these cases are first seen in emergency departments. Despite global eradication efforts, malarial infection plagues humankind in increasing numbers due to mosquito resistance to pesticides and parasite resistance to antimalarial drugs. Malaria, especially due to *Plasmodium falciparum* is a medical emergency and must be considered in anyone returning from the tropics with unexplained fever.

Epidemiology

Malaria is found in tropical areas including Central and South America, the Caribbean, sub-Saharan Africa, the Indian subcontinent, Southeast Asia, the Middle East, and the South Pacific. The vast majority of domestic cases are found in travelers, with the risk of malaria dependent on destination. Sub-Saharan Africa dominates the risk profile with more than 50% of reported cases originating there (compared to much lower rates in Asia and Latin America, 15% to 20% each), despite at least a 10:1 ratio of travelers to Asia and Latin America versus Africa. The risk of malarial infection is greatest immediately after return to the United States (with less than 2% of all cases presenting one year after return) and in those who did not follow chemoprophylaxes guidelines.

Pathophysiology

Malaria is transmitted by the bite of a female Anopheles mosquito (only the female takes blood meals) infected with the plasmodial parasite. There are four species of plasmodia that can cause malaria in humans: *Plasmodium falciparum*, *P. vivax*, *P. ovale*, and *P. malariae*. They share a basic life cycle—relevant to understanding of the disease, its prevention, its clinical presentations, and treatment—with some important differences between species. Sporozoites of the mosquito salivary gland are injected into the human blood stream, where they migrate to the liver.

There, the exoerythrocytic reproductive cycle begins in infected hepatocytes, maturing into tissue schizonts, which in turn rupture and release 10,000 to 30,000 merozoites into the blood. These then invade erythrocytes, where further reproduction, differentiation and maturation take place from ring forms to trophozoites and finally the schizont stage. Schizont-parasitized erythrocytes then rupture releasing merozoites, which re-infect a new subpopulation of erythrocytes, and the cycle then continues in the host. The schizont may also differentiate into erythrocytic sexual forms (gametocytes), which are subsequently taken up by the mosquito vector in which they fertilize and differentiate finally into sporozoites to infect another host.

Each of the four species is endemic to different, overlapping geographic areas. Each has different reproductive cycles in the host, a preference for different age red blood cells, and different prevalence and virulence in various host populations; however, all can produce the cyclic "malarial paroxysm" related to erythrocyte rupture. Symptomatology corresponds with the lysis of infected erythrocytes, the release of antigenic products, the activation of macrocytes and the production of proinflammatory cytokines. Acutely ill patients have either *P. falciparum* or *P. vivax* infections, with approximately a 1% incidence of co-infection with an additional species in domestic cases. Identification is important clinically because of the severity of disease and drug resistance seen with *P. falciparum*.

P. vivax and *P. ovale* do not cause the microvascular and end-organ damage seen with *P. falciparum* infections. These species only infect reticulocytes. While anemia may stimulate hematopoiesis and reticulocytosis, the subsequent parasitemia is markedly less than that seen in *P. falciparum*. *P. malariae* also has intrinsically low levels of parasitemia with a tropism for older erythrocytes. The infection, though, may exist subclinically for up to 30 years.

P. falciparum causes the most virulent form of malaria. Its ability to infect erythrocytes of all ages results in high levels of parasitemia and marked anemia. Erythrocytes infected with *P. falciparum* are prone to deformation and cytoadherence in microvasculature, leading to obstruction of capillaries and post-capillary venules, which damages the brain, kidney, lung and heart. Furthermore, *P. falciparum* is the most resistant to various antimalarial therapies.

Prevention

Chemoprophylaxis is started two weeks before travel to permit a change in regimen, should significant side-effects occur. Therapy should be continued for four weeks after return. Chloroquine, which is safe for pregnant women and young children, should be used for travel to areas free of chloroquine-resistant (CR) malaria. For areas with CR *P. falciparum*, mefloquine is preferred, but doxycycline, malarone or primaquine can also be used.

Chemoprophylaxis is not 100% effective in preventing disease, so contact with mosquitoes must still be avoided. Bed nets impregnated with permethrin or deltamethrin should be used and DEET containing repellant should be applied to the skin.

Clinical Presentation

The hallmark of malarial infection is the "malarial paroxysm," with cyclic fever and influenza-like symptoms. Symptoms may develop as early as one week after exposure. There is generally a prodrome of nonspecific malaise within one to several days prior to the paroxysms. The malarial paroxysm (**Table 64.1**) is defined by a "cold stage" that lasts 15 minutes to several hours during which the patient feels cold and has rigors. The "hot stage" is characterized by 2 to 8 hours of high spiking fevers up to 41° C (105° F), typically with extreme weakness, tachycardia, nausea and mild diaphoresis. Other signs and symptoms can include orthostatic hypotension, dizziness, cough, headache, myalgias, nausea, vomiting, abdominal pain, diarrhea, and altered mental status. Finally, there is a "wet stage," marked by diaphoresis with decreased temperature, exhaustion, and sleep. The cycles tend to become increasingly regular, as lysis becomes synchronous. However, patients with *P. falciparum* infection and those who received chemoprophylaxis may have a constant low-grade temperature with irregular fever spikes.

Patients with *P. falciparum* often appear acutely ill, with jaundice, pallor, altered level of consciousness, delirium, fever, tachycardia, and tachypnea. Splenomegaly, hepatomegaly, and a tender abdomen can be found in cases of advanced disease. Findings of maculopapular skin rash and lymphadenopathy are atypical and suggest alternative diagnoses.

The "benign" malarial infections (*P. vivax*, *P. ovale*, and *P. malariae*) are limited in their clinical course to fever, mild anemia, and hypersplenism. Acute mortality rates from these infections are very low. Anemia is due, acutely, to hemolysis of parasitized erythrocytes and, more chronically, from the anti-hematopoietic effects of TNF-α, as well as sequestration due to splenomegaly, which can cause pancytopenia.

Table 64.1

Stages of Malaria

Stage	Duration	Presenting Symptoms	Presenting Signs
"Cold Stage"	15 minutes to several hours	Chills or rigors (84%)	Afebrile (20–50%) Febrile (50–80%)
"Hot Stage"	Several hours (2–8)	Fever (99%) as few as $\frac{1}{2}$ febrile at exam Headache (74%) Arthralgia/myalgia/backache (47%) Nausea/vomiting (40%) Abdominal pain (23%) Diarrhea (19%) Altered mental status (12%) cough	Splenomegaly (34%) Hepatomegaly (25%) Jaundice (16%) Tachycardia Orthostatic hypotension Cough Vomiting Diarrhea Altered mental status Diaphoresis
"Wet Stage"	Variable	Malaise/fatigue/anorexia (53%)	

Stage	Duration	Signs and Symptoms
"Cold Stage"	15 minutes to several hours	Feels cold, rigors
"Hot Stage"	Several hours (2–8)	High spiking fever, extreme weakness, tachycardia, nausea. Can include orthostatic hypotension, dizziness, cough, headache, myalgias, nausea, vomiting, abdominal pain, diarrhea, altered mental status.
"Wet Stage"	Variable	Diaphoresis, decreased temperature, exhaustion and sleep

More severe clinical disease is due to *P. falciparum* infection. Sequestration of parasitized erythrocytes in vascular endothelium leads to stagnant anoxia of vital organs. Common metabolic derangements include both hypoglycemia and lactic acidosis due to microvascular obstruction and tissue hypoxia. End organ damage—most importantly cerebral malaria, renal failure and pulmonary edema—may also complicate the clinical course. Patients at greatest risk are the very young, elderly, pregnant, immunocompromised, asplenic, those without chemoprophylaxis, and those who delay seeking medical care.

Cerebral malaria is due to intracerebral small vessel occlusion and cellular damage. It can lead to seizures, altered level of consciousness, coma or delirium, and is lethal in approximately 20% of cases. Reversible encephalopathy of alternate etiologies must be excluded. One third of all *P. falciparum* patients have some degree of renal insufficiency, usually reversible (with renal tubular acidosis due to microvasculature susceptibility to cytoadherence, occlusion and tissue hypoxia, in the setting of increased Hb pigments from erythrocyte lysis). Pulmonary edema can result from TNF-α mediated capillary leak, often with overzealous fluid resuscitation. Splanchnic vessel involvement may lead to symptoms of gastroenteritis, hepatic necrosis, or hepatomegaly. Splenic involvement may lead to splenomegaly with pancytopenia and risk of splenic rupture. Coronary vessel obstruction can occur. More chronically, malarial infection may lead to a number of immunologic disorders, notably immune mediated glomerulonephritis.

Diagnosis

Early symptoms are nonspecific, with symptomatology consistent with viral syndromes, including influenza and hepatitis. Malaria should be considered in any febrile patient who has traveled to a malaria-prone region within the past year.

Diagnosis is confirmed by the presence of parasites on Giemsa-stained peripheral blood smears. Both thick and thin smears are necessary. Thick smears ensure adequate concentration for parasite detection, and thin smears provide better visualization for species identification. Blood smears need to be obtained at the time the diagnosis is first considered (generally their highest yield is during the transition from cold to hot stage). The first smear is 90% sensitive. Smears should be repeated two to three times per day for 48 to 72 hours, if there is persistent clinical suspicion. If no parasites are seen on smears collected over 48 to 72 hours, the diagnosis of malaria is very unlikely.

Hemolysis can lead to anemia, hyperbilirubinemia, and elevated lactate dehydrogenase. Splenic sequestration can lead to thrombocytopenia; renal involvement results in elevated serum creatinine, as well as proteinuria and hemoglobinuria.

Disposition and Treatment

Patients with suspected or confirmed acute malaria should be admitted to the hospital. Patients with cerebral malaria, renal failure or ARDS should be admitted to the ICU. Treatment should include supportive care (hemodynamic monitoring, fluid repletion, electrolyte monitoring, and correction) and therapy for end-organ dysfunction (seizure control, mechanical ventilation, hemodialysis, etc.), as well as anti-malarial chemotherapy. Neither exchange transfusions nor steroids have been shown to decrease morbidity or mortality.

The most important factors in selecting chemotherapy are to determine the severity of disease and to predict drug sensitivity. Severe disease (high burden of parasitemia, inability to tolerate oral fluids, evidence of end organ damage) requires aggressive parentral treatment. The CDC maintains an up-to-date Web site with global drug resistance patterns and also operates a 24-hour hotline; if treatment options are uncertain, empirical treatment for chloroquine-resistant *P. falciparum* should be given.

Anti-malarial therapies include quinoline derivatives (chloroquine, quinidine, quinine, mefloquine, halofantrine), antifolates (pyrimethamine and sulfonamides), ribosomal inhibitors (aminoglycosides, clindamycin), and artemisinin. Should treatment be required, the regimen should not include continued chemoprophylactic medications (**Table 64.2 and Table 64.3**).

Anti-malarial medication choice will depend upon the age and possibility of pregnancy, as well as the plasmodium susceptibilities in the area where the disease was contracted. Up-to-date treatment recommendations can be obtained from the CDC's Malaria Hotline (770) 488-7788, Monday through Friday, 8 am–4:30 pm EST; (404) 639-2888 at other times and ask the operator to page the person on call for the Malaria Epidemiology Branch.

Toxoplasmosis

Toxoplasmosis is caused by the obligate intracellular protozoan *Toxoplasma gondii*, and toxoplasma infection refers to the presence of parasite in the infected person. Toxoplasma infection is one of the most common latent parasitic infections in the world. In humans it can be congenital or acquired, and the infection can be acute or chronic. Acute toxoplasmosis in the immunocompetent host results in a self-limited illness of short duration, and after its resolution is considered chronic toxoplasmosis. Congenital toxoplasmosis is usually asymptomatic, but later manifests in a wide array of clinical signs and symptoms, including, chorioretinitis, strabismus, epilepsy, and psychomotor retardation. Immunocompromised hosts, i.e., patients with HIV infection, lymphomas, and cardiac or bone marrow transplants are at greatest risk for severe infections and complications from acute or reactivation of chronic infection. Cases in the immunocompromised tend to be long term and devastating, with costs, in addition to human suffering, of millions of dollars per year in treatment and therapy.

Epidemiology

Toxoplasma gondii is ubiquitous in nature, infecting all mammals, some birds, and some reptiles. The domestic

Table 64.2

Treatment of Malaria

Clinical Setting	Drug	Adult Dosage	Child Dosage
Uncomplicated infection with *P. vivax, P. ovale, P. malariae* and chloroquine sensitive *P. falciparum*	Chloroquine phosphate	1 g (600 mg base) PO initially, followed by 500 mg (300 mg base) 6 hrs later, and again on days 2 and 3	10 mg/kg of base (maximum 600 mg base load), then 5 mg/kg base after 6 hrs and again on days 2 and 3.
	(Primaquine—for *P. vivax* and *P. ovale* only)	15 mg PO qd × 14 d after completion of chloroquine	0.3 mg/kg × 14 d after completion of chloroquine
Uncomplicated infection with chloroquine resistant *(CR) P. falciparum*	(a) Quinine sulfate	650 mg PO tid for 3-7 d	25 mg/kg/d (max 200 mg) divided tid × 3-7 d
	+ Doxycycline[a]	100 mg PO bid for 7 d	3 mg/kg/d PO qd (max 200 mg/d) × 7 d
	± Fansidar (pyrimethamine-sulfadoxime[b])	3 tablets (75/1500) PO × 1 dose	15 mg/kg (max 1250 mg) followed by 10 mg/kg 8-24 hrs later.
	(b) Mefloquine (+ doxycycline[c])	750 mg PO initially followed by 500 mg in 6-8 hrs	>40 kg adult dose 31-40 kg 3 adult tabs × 3 d 21-30 kg 2 adult tabs × 3 d
	(c) Atovaquone-proguanil (Malarone)	4 adult strength (250/100) tabs qd × 3 d	11-20 kg 1 adult tabs × 3 d
Complicated infection with chloroquine resistant *P. falciparum*	Quinidine gluconate plus	10 mg/kg load IV over 2 hrs (max 600 mg) then 0.02 mg/kg/min IV until stable or able to tolerate PO or × 7 d	10 mg/kg load IV over 2 hrs (max 600 mg) then 0.02 mg/kg/min IV until stable or able to tolerate PO or × 7 d
	Doxycycline[1]	100 mg IV q12 h until tolerating PO	3 mg/kg/d PO qd (max 200 mg/d) × 7 d

[a]Clindamycin may be used as an alternative to doxycycline at dose of 10 mg/kg (max 900 mg) every 8 h for 3-7 d.
[b]Optional; unlikely benefit if infection acquired with Fansidar prophylaxis.
[c]Optional.
[d]Not for use in children under 8 years old. Alternatively may add pyrimethamine-sulfadoxime (Fansidar) as single PO dose after quinine: 4-9 kg: $1/4$ tab; 10-14kg: $1/2$ tab; 15-29 kg: 1 tab; 30-50 kg: 2 tabs; >50 kg: 3 tabs) or clindamycin (30 mg/kg/day PO divided TID, max 900 mg/dose, × 7 d)
[e]Emergent consultation with Pediatric Infectious Disease specialist recommended.

cat is the only definitive host for *T. gondii,* and functions as a reservoir of disease. Humans can be infected by one of four ways: ingestion of undercooked meat from an infected animal (25% of pork and 10% of lamb and beef in the United States); through ingestion of oocytes from exposure to soil contaminated with cat feces; vertical transmission from infected mother to fetus; or via blood transfusion and organ transplant. Congenital transmission is the most common form of human infestation, with an estimated 400 to 4,000 cases of congenital transmission annually in the United States.

Pathophysiology

Once absorbed through the digestive tract, the trophozoite form invades all types of mammalian cells via an un-

known mechanism, and proliferates. This leads to cell rupture and subsequent necrotic tissue foci surrounded by an intense inflammatory response. In the immunocompetent host, this area is walled off and becomes a localized tissue cyst, provoking little or no further inflammatory response and persisting in a latent, viable form for the life of the host. If host immunity, particularly cell-mediated, is impaired, cell invasion can lead to persistent lesions like necrotizing encephalitis, pneumonitis, or myocarditis.

Congenital transmission of toxoplasma occurs from placental infection, with transmission of parasites following a primary maternal infection accompanied by parasitemia. Infection of the mother prior to conception rarely translates into transmission of infection to the fetus, the rare exception being the immunocompromised mother. The risk

Table 64.3

Antimalarial Agents

Drug	Minor Side Effects	Major Side Effects/Toxicity	Comments
Chloroquine	Pruritus esp. in dark skinned individuals, n/v, dysphoria, HA, blurry vision, dizziness	Rare: hypotension/shock after parenteral therapy. Transient neuropsychiatric syndrome, cerebellar dysfunction.	May cause decreased response to rabies vaccine. Drug of choice in pregnancy.
Quinine and Quinidine	GI upset/v (if vomiting occurs < 1 hr and repeat full dose; pretreatment with antipyretics may decrease incidence of v). Cinchonism (n/v/dysphoria/tinnitus/high tone deafness/HA/visual disturbances) that resolves after treatment.	QT prolongation and arrhythmias at high doses. Never bolus, always IV infusion; decrease rate of QT interval increases by >25%. May cause hyperinsulinemia and hypoglycemia. May cause myasthenia.	PO quinine is drug of choice in uncomplicated malaria. Drugs of choice in children. Parenteral quinine is available only from the CDC. Contraindicated in cardiac disease; cautiously in pregnancy and myasthenia gravis.
Mefloquine	n/v, HA, blurry vision, dizziness, diarrhea, nightmares	Rare: acute confusional states, seizures. Rare: cardiotoxicity with underlying heart disease or medications	Precaution in pregnancy, children <10 kg, heart disease, seizure disorder or major neuropsychiatric disorder.
Fansidar (pyrimethamine/sulfadoxime)	GI disturbances, phototoxicity, HA, dizziness	Hypersensitivity reaction-Stevens-Johnson Syndrome; agranulocytosis.	Contraindicated in pregnancy and in children.
Malarone (atovaquone-proguanil)	Infrequent AP, n/v, HA, oral ulcers.	Rare: serious allergic reactions.	Contraindicated in pregnancy and in children <11 kg.
Doxycycline	GI disturbances, phototoxicity, vaginal candidiasis	Rare, esophageal ulcerations if not taken with fluids.	Photosensitivity drug reaction. Contraindicated in pregnancy and in children < 8 yo. Women at risk for yeast infection.
Primaquine	n/v/diarrhea, methemoglobinemia.	Severe in hemolysis in those with G6PDH deficiency.	Required only for infections with *P. vivax* and *P. ovale*. All persons must be tested for G6PDH before administration. Contraindicated in pregnancy.

AP, abdominal pain; n, nausea; v, vomiting; HA, headache; G6PDH, glucose-6-phosphate-dehydrogenase.

of infection increases with the duration of pregnancy, but severity of infection in the fetus depends on its age at the time of transmission, with earlier transmission being most significant. In the untreated, infected mother, transmission to the fetus occurs 25% of the time in first trimester pregnancies with severe impairment to the fetus (miscarriage, stillbirth or severe sequelae in the newborn), while the transmission rate is 54% and 65%, respectively, in the second and third trimesters, with milder consequences.

Clinical Findings

In the immunocompetent individual acute toxoplasmosis infection is most frequently asymptomatic and may go unrecognized up to 90% of cases. The other 10% of the clinical manifestations can be so diverse and resolution so spontaneous that making a diagnosis is a challenging process. The serious morbidity associated with the congenital infection makes the disease critical to recognize and diagnose in expectant mothers.

The most common manifestation of symptomatic toxoplasmosis in the immunocompetent hosts (80% to 90% of acute infections are asymptomatic) is benign mild lymphadenopathy. The lymphadenopathy can be localized or diffused and is characterized by nodes that are single or multiple, and, frequently, non-tender cervical lymphadenopathy is most common. The presentation of toxoplasmosis can mimic mononucleosis or CMV infection, and it may be the ultimate cause of "fever of unknown origin." Lymphadenopathy is often benign and self-limited, usually resolving within months and rarely lasting beyond 12 months. Generalized lymphadenopathy occurs in 20% to 30% of symptomatic individuals, and of those 20% to 40% will have associated headache, malaise, fatigue, and fever. The elusive presentation of toxoplasmosis necessitates an extensive differential that includes Hodgkin's disease and other lymphomas, to establish a definitive diagnosis often requires biopsy and serologic testing.

Congenital toxoplasmosis, is frequently asymptomatic and without apparent abnormalities in as many as 75% of infected infants at birth. Any clinical signs in the neonate indicate a high likelihood of severe sequelae. Signs of infection at birth represent a wide range from fever, maculopapular rash, hepatosplenomegaly, microcephaly, seizures, jaundice, thrombocytopenia, and, rarely, generalized lymphadenopathy. The overall incidence of sequelae exceeds 85%, usually by age 8. Later effects include sensorineural hearing loss, chorioretinitis, hydrocephalus, and delayed psychomotor development. Markedly elevated CSF protein is the hallmark of congenital toxoplasmosis, and differentiates it from the other diseases included in the TORCH syndrome (rubella, cytomegalovirus, herpes simplex), as well as congenital syphilis and sepsis.

Ophthalmologic toxoplasma infections account for 35% of all cases of chorioretinitis in the United States and Europe, most cases being congenital transmission. However ocular toxoplasmosis occurs only in 1% of all cases of acquired disease, but is more common in the immunocompromised host. Usually unilateral when acquired, and bilateral when congenital, most cases occur in the second and third decades of life; it is rare after age 40. Symptoms include blurred vision, scotomata, pain, photophobia, and epiphoria. Resolution of the inflammation brings restoration of vision, but flares are common with eventual development of glaucoma and destruction of the retinal tissue. Fundoscopic examination reveals retinal lesions caused by focal necrosis. Initially appearing as a yellow-white "cotton patch," it becomes an atrophic white-gray plaque with black pigment and distinct borders. The differential diagnosis includes the posterior uveitis of syphilis, leprosy, and tuberculosis.

In the immunocompromised host, toxoplasmosis is the most common opportunistic infection and can be either acquired or reactivated from a latent infection that was acquired when the host was healthy; the latter is more common. In patients with AIDS, toxoplasmosis usually occurs when the CD4 count drops below 100. AIDS patients have an approximately 30% probability of developing reactivated toxoplasmosis if they are not receiving effective prophylaxis, with 95% of toxoplasma encephalitis believed to be due to recrudescent infection. The CNS is the most common site of reactivation, with more than 50% of patients having findings referable to the CNS. Toxoplasmosis is the most common cause of intracerebral mass lesions in patients with AIDS (in the United States, the rate is currently 5% to 10%). Patients usually present with symptoms compatible with a mass lesion; hemiparesis, focal seizures, visual disturbances, confusion, and lethargy are the most common. Computed tomography (CT) scanning usually reveals multiple lesions, 90% of which will be ring-enhancing. This finding is nonspecific, also being seen in association with bacterial, fungal, or tubercular lesions. Routine analysis of the CSF may be normal or it may reveal low WBCs, low to normal glucose or high-normal protein. Serologic testing rarely confirms the diagnosis, but a negative serum IgG diminishes the likelihood of the diagnosis. The rare severe illnesses in the immunocompetent host are associated with pneumonitis, acute respiratory distress syndrome, myocarditis, pericarditis, polymyositis, hepatitis, or encephalitis.

Diagnosis

The diagnosis of toxoplasmosis cannot be made on clinical findings alone. In the symptomatic infant, the diagnosis of congenital toxoplasmosis may be strongly suggested by history and physical examination. Ophthalmologic, auditory, and neurological examinations, including lumbar puncture and CT of the head, should be performed. In the AIDS patients, the diagnosis is frequently inferred based on the response to empiric therapy. Isolation of *T. gondii* in tissue sections, smears or body fluids, characteristic lymph node histology, placenta, umbilical cord, infant blood or serology may prove only the presence of latent cysts, not active infection. Currently, the most useful serologic tests for *T. gondii* are immunofluorescence (IFA), IgM-ELISA, and immunosorbent agglutination assay (ISAGA, which is used mainly in Europe). Of these IgM-ELISA and ISAGA are more sensitive than IFA, but most experts currently recommend a combination of serologies.

Due to the considerable morbidity and mortality, as well as the great difficulty of accurately diagnosing *T. gondii,* considerable attention should be emphasized on prevention and early prenatal diagnosis of toxoplasmosis in the fetus. Women planning pregnancy should be tested serologically for evidence of previous toxoplasmosis infection. If they test positive for antibodies, they have little or no risk of transmitting the disease to a fetus, unless immunocompromised for some other reasons. If they test negative, they should be followed for possible seroconversion during pregnancy. Detecting the parasite in fetal blood or amniotic fluid or documenting the presence of *T. gondii* IgM or IgA antibodies in fetal blood has been used to make a prenatal diagnosis of congenital toxoplasmosis.

Treatment

Acquired toxoplasmosis infections in the immunocompetent host do not require treatment. Acutely infected pregnant women should be treated immediately with spiramycin (1 g taken orally every 8 hours, without food). Spiramycin, a macrolide antibiotic similar to erythromycin, is concentrated in the placenta, where it is thought to treat placental infection and, thereby, help to prevent transmission to the fetus. However, spiromycin does not cross the placenta well; thus, it is not effective for treatment of an infected fetus. If fetal infection is confirmed then additional therapy of sulfadiazine (75 mg/kg per day in two divided doses for 2 days, followed by 100 mg/kg per day in 2 divided doses [maximum dose for each of 4 g per day]) and pyrimethamine (100 mg/day in two divided doses for 2 days followed by 50 mg per day) to the mother is recommended. Folinic acid (5 to 20 mg/d) must be taken with pyrimethamine to rescue human cells; *T. gondii* cannot use exogenous folinic acid.

Studies have shown that the treatment of asymptomatic newborns with evidence of congenital toxoplasmosis appears to improve outcome. One study found improved neurologic and developmental outcomes for patients treated with pyrimethamine and sulfadiazine compared to untreated children or those treated for only one month.

Ocular toxoplasmosis should be treated with pyrimethamine and sulfadiazine or clindamycin for one month, with repeat courses, as clinically indicated. Systemic corticosteroids are required for lesions involving the macula, optic nerve head or papillomacular bundle.

Combination therapy with pyrimethamine and sulfadiazine or clindamycin has traditionally been the treatment of choice for immunocompromised patients with toxoplasmosis. Trimethoprim-sulfamethoxazole has also been used as chemoprophylaxis. Because treatment is only effective against trophozoites and not the cysts, therapy must be continued until the host cell-mediated response can prevent recrudescence. In some patients 6 to 8 weeks may suffice; in AIDS patients the treatment is frequently lifelong. All patients treated with pyrimethamine combination therapy must be followed for the development of blood dyscrasias.

Currently, azithromycin has also been successfully used to treat *T. gondii* in humans with AIDS, and clarithromycin is still being tested as treatment for toxoplasmosis and for prevention of in utero infection.

Prevention

Acquired toxoplasmosis can be prevented through the adequate cooking of meat (to 60° C) or freezing meat to less than −20° C for 24 hours (U.S. freezers typically do not reach this temperature). People should be instructed to wash their hands after any contact with raw meat: to wash fruits and vegetables; to clean areas of food preparation well before and after cooking; and to avoid consumption of raw eggs or unpasteurized milk. Pregnant women in particular should avoid areas likely to be contaminated with cat feces.

Research is being conducted into the feasibility of a vaccine for non-immune women of childbearing age, and/ or for the prevention of cysts in household cats.

Selected Readings

Centers for Disease Control, National Center for Infectious Disease, Travelers' Health. www.CDC.gov/travel.

Centers for Disease Control and Prevention. Surveillance summaries. *Morb Mort Wkly Rep* 2003:52.

Chandy J. Drug treatment of malaria in children. *Ped Infect Dis J* 2003;22:649–652.

Cook AJ, Gilbert RE, Dunn DT. Sources of toxoplasma infection in pregnant women: European multicentre case-control study. European Research network on congenital toxoplasmosis. *Br Med J* 2000;321:142–147.

Dorsey G, Ghandi M, Oxygi JH, et al. Difficulties in prevention, diagnosis and treatment of imported malaria. *Arch Intern Med* 2000;160:2505.

Hänscheid T, Grobusch MP, et al. Avoiding misdiagnosis of imported malaria: screening of emergency department samples with thrombocytopenia detects clinically unsuspected cases. *J Travel Med* 2003;10:155–159.

Humar A, Keystone J. Evaluating fever in travelers returning from tropical countries. *Br Med J* 1996;312:953–956.

Foulon W, Pinon JM. Prenatal diagnosis of congenital toxoplasmosis: a multicenter evaluation of different diagnostic parameters. *Am J Obstet Gynecol* 1999;181: 843–847.

Jones JL, Lopez A. Congenital toxoplasmosis: a review. *Obstet Gynecol Surv* 2001; 56:296–305.

Krogstad, DJ. Plasmodium species (malaria). In: Mandell GL, Bennett JE, Dolin R, eds. *Mandell, Douglas and Bennett's Principles and Practice of Infectious Diseases,* 5th ed. New York: Churchill Livingstone 2000:2817–2831.

Moore DAJ, et al. Assessing the severity of malaria. *Br Med J* 2003;326:808–809.

New LC, Holliman RE. Toxoplasmosis and human immunodeficiency virus (HIV) disease. *J Antimicrob Chemother* 1994;33:1079–1082.

Perlmann P, Björkman A. Malaria research: host-parasite interactions and new developments in chemotherapy, immunology and vaccinology [Review Article]. *Curr Opin Infect Dis* 2000;13:431–443.

Roizen N, Swisher CN. Neurologic and developmental outcome in treated congenital toxoplasmosis. *Pediatrics* 1995;95:11–20.

Riddle MS, Jackson SL, Sanders JW, et al. Exchange transfusion as an adjunct therapy in severe Plasmodium falciparum malaria: A meta-analysis. *Clin Infect Dis* 2002;34:1192.

White NJ. The treatment of malaria. *N Engl J Med* 1996;335:800.

Wong SY, Remington JS. Toxoplasmosis in pregnancy. *Clin Infect Dis* 1994;18: 853–861.

World Health Organization. Expert committee on malaria, 20th report. *WHO Technical Report Service* 2000;892:1.

Rickettsial Infections

Thomas A. Brunell
Jill McGovern
Laurel Plante

Rocky Mountain Spotted Fever

Rocky Mountain spotted fever (RMSF) is the most virulent rickettsial disease of the spotted fever group. First identified in Idaho and Montana in the late 1800s, most cases of RMSF today are concentrated in the south central and southeastern United States. RMSF is caused by the obligate, intracellular coccobacillus *Rickettsia rickettsii*. *R. rickettsii* elicits moderate to severe systemic illness by causing a generalized vasculitis that may involve any organ system. RMSF presents with a broad range of symptoms, depending on the stage of infection. The classic presentation includes fever, headache, rash, myalgias, and history of tick exposure. The disease is transmitted by the American dog tick (*Dermacentor variabilis*) in the eastern United States, and by the wood tick (*Dermacentor andersoni*) in the Rocky Mountain states. Although highly sensitive tests are available for confirmation (including indirect fluorescent antibody and indirect hemagglutination), they are not positive early enough for help in establishing the diagnosis. Prognosis depends heavily on prompt recognition of the disease and appropriate initiation of antibiotic therapy.

Epidemiology/Pathophysiology

Ticks infected with *R. rickettsii* will remain infected for their life, and can pass the infection to their offspring. The ticks harbor *R. rickettsii* in their gut and transmit it to humans during feeding. *Rickettsia* organisms invade and multiply in the vascular endothelium of their host. This induces a generalized vasculitis that leads to activation of the clotting cascade, capillary leakage, and microinfarctions in various organs. These pathophysiologic mechanisms are responsible for the rash, headache, myalgias, and gastrointestinal symptoms that commonly occur with RMSF infection.

The seasonal distribution of cases of RMSF is a distinct feature of the illness. Most cases occur during spring and summer. This time period parallels peak occurrences of *Dermacentor* tick bites. Cases have infrequently been reported during fall and winter months.

Although first identified in Idaho and Montana in the late 1800s, the name Rocky Mountain spotted fever is something of a misnomer, as relatively few reports of RMSF have originated from the Rocky Mountain states in the last several decades. Most cases of RMSF today are concentrated in the southeastern and mid-western states. The disease has been reported in all the contiguous United States except for Maine and Vermont; among the top 10 states in national surveillance summaries of RMSF are North Carolina, Oklahoma, Tennessee, Arkansas, South Carolina, Maryland, and Virginia.

Rocky Mountain spotted fever remains the most lethal tick-borne infection. Persons aged less than 10 years have the highest age-specific incidence. Untreated, the mortality for RMSF is high, with a case-fatality ratio (CFR) of untreated RMSF approaching 25% across all age groups. The annual CFR for RMSF declined during the 1980s and into the 1990s. There are many factors which likely have contributed to the decline in CFRs for RMSF: increased public awareness of the disease, recognition of the early indicators of infection, and the increased use of tetracycline-class antibiotics for treatment. Studies evaluating fatal and non-fatal cases of RMSF have identified older patient age, black race, delay or lack of treatment, and failure to treat with a tetracycline antibiotic as risk factors for death from infection.

Clinical Findings

Rocky Mountain spotted fever is an acute febrile, multisystemic disease. Fever, malaise, myalgia, and severe headache are the most common initial features of RMSF. The rash classically begins on day 4 of illness (range 1 to 15 days) on the ankles and wrists; it then spreads to the palms and soles. Later, the rash spreads centrally to the proximal extremities and trunk. This classic centripetal spread is the hallmark of RMSF, though it is not always seen. The absence of rash does not exclude the diagnosis, as 10% of patients never develop rash, thereby manifesting "spotless" fever. Additionally, the rash may develop late during the course of the disease. When present, the dermatologic findings consist of small pink or red macules that blanch with pressure. Over time, the rash becomes petechial and purpuric. Dermatologic complications include gangrene of the fingers, toes, nose, ears, scrotum, and vulva. Patients with darker skin tones are less likely than Caucasian patients to present with a reported tick attachment, rash, headache or myalgia, which makes the diagnosis in these subgroups more elusive.

In its early stages, RMSF may resemble other infectious and noninfectious conditions and can be difficult to diagnose. Nonspecific signs and symptoms are often prominent early in the course and include nausea, vomiting, diarrhea, and abdominal pain. These symptoms may suggest gastroenteritis or an acute surgical abdomen. Focal neurologic deficits, transient deafness, meningismus, and photophobia may suggest meningitis or meningoencephalitis. Between 3% to 18% of patients with RMSF present with the classic triad of rash, fever, and history of tick exposure, thus absence of tick exposure should not dissuade the clinician from suspecting RMSF, as this feature may be absent in up to 40% of patients.

Devastating complications of RMSF include gangrene, pulmonary hemorrhage and edema, acute respiratory distress syndrome, myocarditis, acute renal failure, meningoencephalitis, and cerebral edema. Presenting symptoms of these complications include cough, dyspnea, hypoxemia, confusion, stupor, delirium, ataxia, coma, seizures, and sensory neuropathy. In patients with delayed diagnosis, these complications may result in significant morbidity, if not mortality.

Diagnosis

The clinical diagnosis of RMSF can be difficult, particularly in the early stages of illness, since serologic evidence of infection occurs no earlier than the second week of illness in any of the rickettsial diseases. Early clinical manifestations and laboratory data are nonspecific and pose a challenge in diagnosis. A classification of "confirmed" RMSF requires signs and symptoms compatible with disease and at least 1 confirmatory laboratory finding. Criteria for laboratory confirmation include a ≥4-fold change in titer of antibody to *R. rickettsii* antigen between acute- and convalescent-phase serum specimens, measured by latex agglutination, microagglutination, indirect hemagglutination assay, indirect immunofluorescence assay or complement fixation. Additional criteria for laboratory confirmation include PCR assays with specific primers for *R. rickettsii,* isolation of *R. rickettsii* from clinical specimens, or identification of rickettsial antigens by immunostaining of biopsy or autopsy specimens. Unfortunately, these clinical laboratory findings seldom offer effective assistance in diagnosing RMSF in its acute stages. Detectable antibodies are often absent by available assays early in the course of illness and diagnostic skin biopsy immunochemistry requires the presence of rash lesions that are often not present.

Potentially corroborating, yet nonspecific laboratory data that may occur in patients with RMSF include leukopenia, thrombocytopenia, anemia, hyponatremia and elevated liver enzyme function tests. Though the majority of patients have a normal white blood cell count, increased quantities of immature myeloid cells may also occur. The cerebrospinal fluid of patients with RMSF is typically normal, yet one third of patients demonstrate an increased leukocyte count. The CSF protein is elevated in one third of patients, as well.

Treatment

Treatment of RMSF should never be delayed pending a laboratory diagnosis: it should be initiated immediately when clinical and epidemiologic clues suggest RMSF. Most broad-spectrum antibiotics are ineffective treatments for RMSF. Use of tetracycline-class antibiotics for treatment of RMSF significantly increased in the 1990s, whereas chloramphenicol-only treatment decreased. Doxycycline (intravenous or oral) is now the mainstay of treatment for RMSF in both adults and children. Given the potential for fatal illness secondary to RMSF, the American Academy of Pediatrics and the Centers for Disease Control and Prevention recommend doxycycline as the treatment of choice in all children, regardless of age. The risk of tooth staining in children is not significant with short-term therapy. For adults, the recommended dosage of doxycycline is 200 mg/d or 3 mg/kg of body weight, whichever is greater. In children less than 45 kg, the recommended dosage is 4.4 mg/kg. Typical length of treatment is for a minimum of 7 days. Chloramphenicol may be used in pregnant women or in patients with known hypersensitivity to tetracyclines. Those at risk for CFR include patients in whom treatment is delayed more than 5 days after the onset of symptoms, older patients, and patients in whom tetracycline-class antibiotics were not the primary therapy.

Management should also include close monitoring of fluid and electrolyte balance, secondary to the fluid losses associated with increased vascular permeability. Most patients with RMSF should be considered for hospitalization. Supportive care may be needed for the severely ill patient. In mild cases, patients can be closely followed as an outpatient, assuming they are able to tolerate oral antibiotics and compliance is not an issue.

Prevention

Individuals in endemic areas who spend time outdoors should take measures to protect themselves from tick bites. Such measures include wearing light-colored clothing, tucking pant cuffs into socks, and using repellents. These measures make ticks more easily visible and prevent access to exposed skin. Permethrin repellents can be applied to the clothes and repellents containing DEET (*N,N*-diethyl-m toluamide) can be applied to exposed skin areas. Thorough inspections of head, body, and clothes for ticks should be routine in endemic areas after time spent in wooded or grassy areas. Attached ticks should be immediately removed with tweezers or forceps by grasping the tick close to the skin and pulling gently with steady pressure. Although the use of antibiotics during the incubation period may delay the onset of the illness, it does not prevent the development of the disease.

Ehrlichiosis

Human Monocytic Ehrlichiosis (HME) was first recognized in the United States in 1986 as a nonspecific febrile disease, caused by the small, Gram-negative obligate intracellular bacteria, *Ehrlichia chaffeensis*. Later, in the early 1990s, a second similar disease termed human granulocytic ehrlichiosis (HGE) was identified. The bacterium causing this disease was not identified until approximately a decade later, and was subsequently found to be caused by two separate but related bacteria: *Anaplasma (Ehrlichia) phagocytophilia* and *Ehrlichia ewingii*. In total, five species have been shown to cause human ehrlichial disease; however, the most common agents are those above.

The vector of HME is the Lone Star tick, *Amblyomma americanum*; thus, HME occurs in areas in which this tick is endemic, namely the southeastern and midwestern parts of the United States. HGE, in contrast, is transmitted principally by *Ixodes scapularis* in the northeastern and upper midwestern United States, and by *Ixodes pacificus* in the western coastal United States. The diagnosis of human ehrlichiosis can be difficult because its nonspecific initial clinical presentation is easily confused with less significant viral illnesses, as well as with other tick-borne zoonoses such as Lyme disease and RMSF. Furthermore, as the vectors for ehrlichial bacteria are also the main vectors for other tick-borne illnesses, it is imperative to consider all diseases, as treatment can differ considerably.

Epidemiology/Pathophysiology

As of 1997, HME had been reported in 47 states, with a total of 742 probable or confirmed cases. The actual number of cases is believed to be much higher. The main natural reservoir of *E. chaffeensis* is the white-tailed deer. HGE has been described in Europe, as well as in North America, where 449 cases had been documented as of 1997. The main identified reservoir is the white-footed mouse, but it is also carried by other animals, such as the white-tail deer and the coyote.

Both forms of ehrlichiosis are strongly related to tick bites, although this can be difficult to document, especially when nymphs attach to the body. The nymph bite tends to be painless. Nymphs, being especially small, are easily overlooked by the human host. The bite must be sufficiently long for transmission to occur (24 to 48 hours). The main target cell of HGE and HME are the neutrophil and mononuclear phagocytes, respectively.

The illness is seasonal, following the life cycle of the vector: in HGE, the incidence of disease peaks during the summer, when the nymphs and adults are feeding on mammalian hosts, and again in mid-autumn. In HME, most cases occur between April and September. The incubation period is 1 to 2 weeks, and there is a male predominance of disease, with HGE showing a 3:1 male-to-female ratio, and HME showing an even larger 4:1 ratio. Age-dependent severity has been shown in most series of cases. There has also been documented risk of transfusion-related disease.

Clinical Presentation

The clinical presentation of ehrlichiosis is almost identical to that of RMSF. The clinical spectrum of HME ranges from moderately ill to fatal disease. The onset of symptoms is usually abrupt, occurring 7 to 10 days after the tick bite. There have been reported cases of low-grade fever and malaise for 24 to 48 hours before the onset of symptoms. Symptoms are non-specific and include fever, severe headache, malaise, chills, myalgias, arthralgias, lymphadenopathy, anorexia which may be profound enough to lead to weight loss, abdominal pain, diarrhea, nausea, vomiting, confusion (especially in the elderly), vertigo, ataxia, cough, shortness of breath, delirium, and coma. More severe symptoms tend to occur in the elderly. A rash has been reported in 20% to 80% of HME cases however, rash is present at onset in only 6% of cases. The rash typically appears on days 3 to 8, ranging from day 0 to day 13 of illness. In children, in whom 10% of HME cases occur, rash is more common, occurring in up to 67% of patients. It is most often described as petechial or maculopapular, but can be variable and is thus an unreliable sign of disease. The usual distribution is on the trunk and extremities.

Complications from HME include ARDS, acute respiratory insufficiency, renal failure, hypotensive shock, gastrointestinal hemorrhage, coagulopathy, severe central nervous system disease, cardiomyopathy and opportunistic infections. The disease is fatal in 2% to 3% of cases.

The clinical picture of HGE is very similar to that of HME, with a few differences. The incidence of rash in HGE is lower than that of HME (2% to 5%), and central nervous system manifestations are rarely seen in HGE. It is believed that HGE tends to be a milder illness than HME, but some studies have shown severe illness to be present in up to 16% of patients, particularly in the Midwest. The case-fatality rate has been shown to be 0.5% to 1%, as opposed to 2% to 3% in HME. Complications, which appear to be less frequent than in HME, include acute respiratory insufficiency due to diffuse alveolar damage, opportunistic infections, rhabdomyolysis, myocarditis, plexopathy, and a demyelinating polyneuropathy The duration of illness of both diseases is about 2 to 4 weeks, with a median duration of 23 days. Chronicity generally does not appear to occur. Asplenic patients may develop some atypical features in the course of HGE. Due to the common vectors, co-infection with RMSF, Lyme disease or babesiosis is being seen more often and a high index of suspicion should be maintained.

Diagnosis

The diagnosis of ehrlichiosis depends mainly on clinical findings. Early clinical diagnosis based on a high degree of suspicion and early administration of antibiotics is necessary to ensure a good clinical outcome. Characteristic laboratory abnormalities that suggest the diagnosis include the progressive development of leukopenia (often with a left shift), thrombocytopenia, and, less frequently, anemia. These findings are usually present during the first week of illness and the values then return to normal. During the second week of illness, one will often see a lymphocytosis, with an excess of T lymphocytes. Mild to moderate elevations (2 to 8 times the normal upper limit) in the serum hepatic transaminase concentration and elevation of C-reactive protein are also typically present. Elevations of bilirubin and alterations in coagulation time are not commonly seen. Infiltrates may be seen on chest x-ray. Indirect fluorescent antibody (IFA) is the primary diagnostic tool, and is considered the gold standard for diagnosis of both HME and HGE. These tests are in the process of being standardized. For HME, titers of 1:64 to 1:128 are considered probable cases of HME, while single titers of 1:256 or greater are considered confirmed cases. For HGE, titers of 1:80 or greater are considered positive. Due to the lack of standardization, this may vary between labs.

Ehrlichial infections may also be recognized by the presence of morulae (microcolonies consisting of 3 to 50 bacteria) in circulating peripheral blood leukocytes. This method, however, is insensitive in diagnosing ehrlichiosis, and the characteristic intracytoplasmic inclusions are seen in only 50% of patients with HGE and in only 7% to 17% of patients with HME. Patients in an immunocompromised state tend to show a higher incidence of morulae in HME. Culture requires incubation of cell cultures for 2 months and is thus of little help in diagnosis.

Treatment

Because of the similarities between RMSF and human ehrlichiosis, human ehrlichiosis was initially treated with doxycycline, tetracycline, and chloramphenicol with reported success. Chloramphenicol treatment is now controversial, as both bacteria show significant resistance to this antibiotic.

Due to the potentially fatal nature of ehrlichiosis, the initiation of treatment in any patient suspected of having the disease should not be delayed until diagnosis is confirmed. The specimens used for confirmatory tests should be obtained before starting antibiotic therapy.

Both forms of ehrlichiosis respond to the tetracyclines, although doxycycline is better tolerated and has a longer half-life than tetracycline. The recommended therapy for adults is doxycycline, oral or intravenous, 100 mg twice a day, and for children, doxycycline 3 mg per kilogram per day in two divided doses for children weighing less than 45 kg. Children weighing greater than 45 kg should be given the adult dose. Although there is no well-designed, randomized, double-blind study with these drugs as the treatment for ehrlichiosis, there is general agreement on these doses. In younger children, the total dose of doxycycline should be minimized to avoid staining of the teeth. Most patients defervesce within the first 24 to 48 hours after initiation of therapy. If no improvement is seen after 48 hours, other diagnoses should be entertained. Doxycycline should be continued for at least 3 days after defervescence, and is often continued for a total of 14 days. In pregnant women or tetracycline-allergic patients, rifampin may be used for 7 to 10 days for suspected HGE, but there is no clear choice for similar HME patients, as rifampin does not appear to treat this as well. In these patients, chloramphenicol or rifampin may be used in an attempt to lessen the severity of the disease, but the effect is not clear. Elderly patients, patients with underlying illness, and patients in whom therapy has been delayed should all be admitted to the hospital for intravenous therapy, as morbidity and mortality is high in these groups. In these patients, HME appears to carry a worse prognosis than HGE.

Chronic ehrlichiosis and relapsing infection in humans has thus far been reported only once. Close follow-up should be established for recrudescence. Recovery is usually complete in those in which the disease is not fatal. However, there have been anecdotal reports that easy fatigability, irritability, and difficulty concentrating may persist for months after the organism is cleared from the body. Due to the potentially severe nature of ehrlichiosis and its common vector with other tick-borne illnesses, one must have a high degree of suspicion for co-infection. Given the fact that some antibiotics cover one infection, but not the other (i.e., amoxicillin for treatment of Lyme disease in children), care must be taken to consider all possible tick-borne illnesses. Caution must be used with prescribing trimethoprim-sulfamethoxazole for nonspecific febrile illnesses, as this has been suspected in a few case studies to worsen the clinical course of ehrlichiosis, causing a fulminant disease.

Prevention

Prevention of ehrlichiosis is the same as for other tick-borne illnesses: individuals who are outdoors in endemic areas should take measures to protect themselves from tick bites. These measures include wearing light-colored clothing to make crawling ticks visible, tucking pant cuffs into socks to prevent ticks from gaining access to exposed skin, and using repellents. Permethrin repellents can be applied to the clothes, which will enhance their protection, and repellents containing DEET (N,N-diethyl-m-tolumide) can be applied to exposed skin areas. Daily inspections for attached ticks should be routine in endemic areas. Attached ticks should be removed immediately with a fine forceps. The use of antibiotics during the incubation period delays the onset of the illness, but is not believed to prevent the eventual development of the disease. A vaccine is in the early stages of development.

Selected Readings

Bakken JS, Krueth J, Wilson-Nordskog C, et al. Clinical and laboratory characteristics of human granulocytic ehrlichiosis. *JAMA* 1996;275:199–205.

Centers for Disease Control and Prevention. Consequences of delayed diagnosis of Rocky Mountain spotted fever in children—West Virginia, Michigan, Tennessee, and Oklahoma, May-July 2000. *Morb Mortal Wkly Rep* 2000;49: 885–888.

Childs JE, Paddock CD. Passive surveillance as an instrument to identify risk factors for fatal Rocky Mountain spotted fever: is there more to learn? *Am J Trop Med Hyg* 2002;66:450–457.

Drage LA. Life-threatening rashes: dermatologic signs of four infectious diseases. *Mayo Clinic Proc* 1999;74:68–72.

Dumler JS, Bakken JS. Ehrlichial disease of humans: emerging tick borne infections. *Clin Infect Dis* 1995;20:1102–1110.

Dumler JS, Dawson JE, Walker DH. Hematopathology and immunohistologic detection of Ehrlichia chaffeensis. *Hum Pathol* 1993;24:391–396.

Dumler JS, Walker DH. Diagnostic tests for Rocky Mountain spotted fever and other rickettsial diseases. *Dermatol Clin* 1994;12:25–36.

Goodman JL, Nelson C, Vitale B, et al. Direct cultivation of the causative agent of human granulocytic ehrlichiosis. *N Engl J Med* 1996;334:209–215.

Herron, MJ et al. Intracellular parasitism by the human granulocytic ehrlichiosis bacterium through the P-selectin ligand, PSGL-1. *Science* 2000;288:1653–1656.

Holman RC, Paddock CD, et al. Analysis of risk factors for fatal Rocky Mountain spotted fever: evidence for superiority of tetracyclines. *J Infect Dis* 2001;184: 1437–1444.

Jantausch BA. Lyme disease, Rocky Mountain spotted fever, ehrlichiosis: emerging and established challenges for the clinician. *Ann Allergy* 1994;73:4–11.

Javed, MZ et al. Concurrent babesiosis and ehrlichiosis in an elderly host. *Mayo Clin Proc* 2001;76:563–565.

Krause, PJ. Successful treatment of human granulocytic ehrlichiosis in children using rifampin. *Pediatrics* 2003;112:252–253.

Masters EJ, Olson GS, et al. Rocky Mountain spotted fever: a clinician's dilemma. *Arch Intern Med* 2003;163:769–774.

McGinley-Smith, DE. Dermatoses from ticks. *J Am Acad Dermatol* 2003;49:363–392.

Moss WJ, Dumler JS. Simultaneous infection with Borrelia burgdorferi and human granulocytic ehrlichiosis. *Pediatr Infect Dis J* 2003;22:91–92.

Olano JP, Walker DH. Human ehrlichiosis. *Med Clin North Am* 2002;86:375–392.

Sexton, DJ. Rocky Mountain spotted fever. *Med Clin North Am* 2002;86:351–360.

Pancholi P, Kolbert CP, Mitchell PD, et al. Ixodes dammini as a potential vector of human granulocytic ehrlichiosis. *J Infect Dis* 1995;172:1007–1012.

Singh BD, et al. Tick-borne infections. *Dermatol Clin* 2003;21:237–244.

Tan HP, et al. Human monocytic ehrlichiosis: an emerging pathogen in transplantation. *Transplantation* 2001;71:1678–1680.

Wormser G, McKenna P, Aguero-Rosenfield M, et al. Human granulocytic ehrlichiosis—New York 1995. *MMWR* 1995;44(32):593–595.

Yawetz S, Mark EL. Weekly clinicopathological exercises: case 37-2001: a 76-year-old man with fever, dyspnea, pulmonary infiltrates, pleural effusions and confusion. *N Engl J Med* 2001;345:1627–1634.

Viral Infections

Rosemary Guerguerian
Ajeet Jai Singh
Thomas A. Brunell

Laura Matzkin
Stephen J. Playe
Ramin R. Samadi

Human Immunodeficiency

Acquired immunodeficiency syndrome (AIDS) was first described in 1981, when a cluster of otherwise healthy young homosexual men in Los Angeles inexplicably developed *Pneumocystis carinii* pneumonia. By 1984, human immunodeficiency virus (HIV) was identified as the cause of AIDS. The United Nations estimated that over 40 million people were living with HIV/AIDS worldwide by the end of 2001. Since the start of widespread use of highly active antiretroviral therapy (HAART) in 1996, the number of AIDS deaths has declined. However, the total number of people living with HIV-AIDS continues to increase steadily over time. The current surveillance case definition of AIDS in adults includes any HIV-infected individual who has either: 1) a CD4 T-lymphocyte count of less than 200 cells/mm^3; 2) a CD4 T-lymphocyte percentage of less than 14%; or 3) an AIDS-defining illness. In patients without known HIV infection, an AIDS-defining illness, in the absence of other causes of immune deficiency, also defines AIDS (**Table 66.1**).

Emergency physicians should be alert as to the possibility of HIV infection when any patient with risk factors for HIV presents with fever of unknown cause or with a clinical presentation consistent with an opportunistic infection. HIV testing is rarely indicated in the emergency department (ED); however, if suspicious of diagnosis, proper referral for counseling is indicated.

Pathophysiology

HIV is a cytopathic retrovirus that carries its genetic material in the form of RNA and, with the enzyme reverse transcriptase, can convert the viral RNA to DNA. This DNA is then incorporated into the host cell's genetic material. At least two types of this virus have been identified: HIV-1 and HIV-2. HIV-1 is the primary cause of infection in the United States, while HIV-2 is more prevalent in West Africa. HIV affects modulation of the immune system by cytokines and impairs the function of monocytes, macrophages, neutrophils, B lymphocytes, and T lymphocytes, in particular CD4 T helper cells. This results in a defect in cellular immunity. Once viral exposure occurs, seropositivity develops in as little as 4 weeks to as long as 6 to 8 months. The mean time between exposure and diagnosis of AIDS, if untreated, is 8.23 years for adults and 1.97 years for children under 5 years of age. The virus has been isolated in blood, semen, vaginal secretions, urine, CSF, tears, breast milk, synovial fluid, saliva, and other bodily fluids. However, only a few proven modes of transmission have been identified, including sexual contact with both homosexual and heterosexual exposure, intravenous drug abuse (IVDA), blood transfusion (especially prior to 1985), maternal-neonatal transmission, and occupational exposures.

Diagnosis

A presumptive diagnosis of AIDS can be made by the clinical criteria outlined by the CDC in 1993. The definitive diagnosis is most often made using serologic tests for HIV-1 antibodies or antigen. Screening is achieved using antibody assays, starting with the ELISA test, which is then confirmed by Western blot. IgG antibodies are first detectable at 6 to 12 weeks. By 6 months, HIV IgG antibodies are present in greater than 95% of patients. False-negative tests can occur if patients are tested after exposure but prior to seroconversion or in patients infected with HIV-1 subtype O or HIV-2 (predominantly African strains). HIV RNA and HIV core protein p24 antigen levels are detectable prior to the presence of antibodies. Polymerase chain reaction (PCR) detection of the p24 HIV-1 antigen can be employed to determine the presence of HIV if exposure is too recent for antibody testing to be accurate. Alternative choices have also become available, such as home kits, rapid screening tests, salivary tests, and urine tests. Early identification of HIV infection is important as initiation of HAART can slow the decline of immune system function and the development of opportunistic infections. Also, diagnosis of HIV can alert the health care provider to the possibility of opportunistic infections such as tuberculosis, *Pneumocystis carinii* pneumonia (PCP), and bacterial pneumonias, for which preventative regimens are available. Finally, HIV affects the diagnosis, evaluation, and

Table 66.1

AIDS Defining Illnesses

CDC 1993 Revised Classification System for HIV Infection and Expanded Surveillance Case Definition for AIDS among Adolescents and Adults:

- Candidiasis of bronchi, trachea, or lungs
- Candidiasis, esophageal
- Cervical cancer, invasive
- Coccidioidomycosis, disseminated or extrapulmonary
- Cryptococcosis, extrapulmonary
- Cryptosporidiosis, chronic intestinal (greater than 1 month's duration)
- Cytomegalovirus disease (other than liver, spleen, or nodes)
- Cytomegalovirus retinitis (with loss of vision)
- Encephalopathy, HIV-related
- Herpes simplex: chronic ulcer(s) (greater than 1 month's duration); or bronchitis, pneumonitis, or esophagitis
- Histoplasmosis, disseminated, or extrapulmonary
- Isosporiasis, chronic intestinal (greater than 1 month's duration)
- Kaposi's sarcoma
- Lymphoma, Burkitt's (or equivalent term)
- Lymphoma, immunoblastic (or equivalent term)
- Lymphoma, primary, of brain
- *Mycobacterium avium* complex or *M. kansasii*, disseminated or extrapulmonary
- *Mycobacterium tuberculosis,* any site (pulmonary or extrapulmonary)
- *Mycobacterium* spp., other species or unidentified species, disseminated or extrapulmonary
- *Pneumocystis carinii* pneumonia
- *Pneumonia* spp., recurrent
- Progressive multifocal leukoencephalopathy
- *Salmonella septicemia,* recurrent
- Toxoplasmosis of the brain
- Wasting syndrome due to HIV

treatment of many diseases. HIV counseling is recommended, and informed consent is required prior to testing.

The CD4 T-lymphocyte count is the best laboratory test indicating severity of clinical progression. Patients with counts > 500 cells/mm^3 usually do not show manifestations of clinical immunosuppression. Patients with CD4 counts < 200 cells/mm^3 are at a high risk for developing complicated AIDS presentations.

Clinical Presentation

Acute HIV Infection Syndrome

Within the first 2 to 6 weeks after infection with HIV, an acute viral illness may develop consisting of fever, weight loss, myalgias, headache, and fatigue (seen in 81% patients). The previously described mononucleosis-like syndrome of fever, lymphadenopathy and pharyngitis is not as common. Initial infection is easily missed given the non-specific nature of the symptoms. In addition to constitutional symptoms, patients with acute infection may also complain of symptoms involving nearly every organ system, including rash, oral and esophageal ulcerations, abdominal pain, nausea, vomiting and diarrhea, genital ulceration, encephalopathy, and neuropathy. In some cases, acute infection may present with opportunistic infections.

Mucous Membrane and Cutaneous Manifestations

Xerosis and Pruritus

Xerosis (dry skin) and pruritus (itching) are common among HIV-infected patients. Treatment with emollients or topical steroids is the mainstay. Patients should also be encouraged to avoid long, hot showers, harsh soaps, and fragrances.

Kaposi's Sarcoma

Kaposi's sarcoma (KS) is the most common neoplasm in patients with AIDS. An otherwise rare tumor, KS is a mesenchymal tumor involving blood and lymphatic vessels. KS lesions are firm, painless, nonpruritic, purple-reddish-brown plaques or nodules of the squamous epithelial and mucous membranes. In AIDS, they may arise within few days, beginning with macules that can evolve into erythematous papules and then tumors. The disease can progress to extensive skin and visceral involvement. Lymph nodes, the gastrointestinal tract, and the lungs are affected the most, although any organ can be involved.

Kaposi's sarcoma is now thought to be caused by human herpesvirus 8 (HHV8) or by Kaposi's sarcoma herpes virus (KSHV). Viral oncogenesis and cytokine-induced growth, combined with some states of immunocompromise, appear to be primary factors in tumor development. KS seems to have a male predominance, though that may be due to low rates of HHV8 infection in women in the western world. In Africa, KS occurs with a more equal distribution. There is some suggestion that HHV8 may be sexually transmitted.

With the advent of antiretroviral therapy, there has been a significant decline in the incidence of AIDS related KS, likely due to immune reconstitution and anti-HHV8 immune response. Current therapy for KS is palliative and is recommended in cases of cosmetically disfiguring lesions, problematic oral lesions, severe pain and edema associated with lymphadenopathy or extensive cutaneous disease. Current techniques include local therapies such as excision, cryotherapy, laser, and radiation that induce an inflammatory response, and chemotherapies, such as interferon and liposomal doxorubicin. Recurrence and drug-induced toxicity limit the use of these current treatments. Studies for the role of antiviral agents such as ganciclovir, cidofovir, adefovir, and foscarnet have been encouraging.

Varicella Zoster

Varicella zoster eruptions are common in HIV, though it is rarely a life-threatening complication. Recent data has suggested an increased rate of eruptions in patients newly started on combination antiretroviral therapy. This is actually thought to represent improving immune function, particularly of CD8 T-lymphocytes. With advanced HIV disease, lesions can involve one or several dermatomes or may become widely disseminated or ulcerative. The possibility of systemic involvement should be considered. Herpes ophthalmicus, involvement of the trigeminal nerve branch V_1, can lead to ocular complications if treatment is not initiated early. Treatment of focal varicella zoster consists of oral acyclovir and pain management. Admission and IV acyclovir (5 to 10 mg/kg IV every 8 hours) until clinical resolution is recommended for debilitating disseminated cutaneous lesions or systemic infection. Varicella zoster immune globulin (VZIG) is recommended for HIV patients with primary varicella zoster infection and for those with visceral involvement.

Herpes Simplex Infections (HSV-1 and HSV-2)

Most individuals with HIV are also infected with HSV. These patients may have prolonged episodes of genital, oral, or anal herpes. Lesions in HIV can be atypical, more frequent, recurrent (more than 6 per year) medication resistant, and unusually located. In some, they may become chronic, large and ulcerative, or necrotic. Ulcerative lesions may also become secondarily infected. Patients may benefit from oral antiviral medications, such as acyclovir, famciclovir, and valacyclovir, for episodic infections or for daily suppressive therapy. In a nonimmunocompromised patients with local infection, oral acyclovir 400 mg three times daily or 200 mg five times daily for 5 to 10 days can be used. IV acyclovir at 5 to 10 mg/kg every 8 hours is used for immunocompromised patients or patients with severe, disseminated cases. Patients with acyclovir-resistant HSV can be prescribed foscarnet at a dose of 40 mg/kg intravenously every 8 hours until clinical resolution. These patients should be admitted.

Direct viral culture from suspected lesions is the diagnostic procedure of choice. Tzanck smear showing inclusions or multinucleated giant cells, direct immunofluorescent staining of infected cells for virus antigen, and antibody detection methods are also used. HSV serology is rarely useful and does not change the management.

The severity of the illness depends on whether HSV infection is primary or recurrent, on the site of infection, and on the degree of HIV-induced immunosuppression. Other HSV infections include herpes proctitis, herpes gingivostomatitis, herpes esophagitis, and herpes encephalitis.

Molluscum Contagiosum

Molluscum contagiosum is a superficial cutaneous viral infection occurring in up to 20% of HIV-infected patients. The lesions appear as multiple, small, flesh-colored umbilicated papules with a whitish core in the center of each papule. They occur most frequently on the head, neck, and intertriginous areas. The lesions can be sexually transmitted with papules forming in the pubic area. Once the CD4 count falls below 200 cells/mm^3, lesions tend to proliferate. Because the lesions rarely cause medical complications, treatment is primarily for cosmetic reasons.

Cryosurgery or topical agents are used, yet lesions often recur.

Intertriginous Infections

Intertriginous infections are common among HIV-infected patients and are usually caused by fungi such as *Candida* or *Tricophyton*. Diagnosis is made by examining microscopic potassium hydroxide (KOH) slides of lesion scrapings. Topical antifungal creams are the mainstay of treatment.

Human Papillomavirus Infection

Human papillomavirus (HPV) infection, which causes genital warts, occurs in HIV patients with increased frequency and severity. The lesions may be extensive and resistant to therapy. The genital and perianal areas are usually involved.

Treatment consists of cryotherapy, topical therapy containing salicylic and lactic acids, and in extreme cases laser surgery. Cervical dysplasia and carcinoma are clearly associated with HPV infection. Careful evaluation and close follow-up are necessary once premalignant lesions have been diagnosed.

Other Cutaneous Manifestations

Other cutaneous manifestations of disease that occur with increased frequency and severity in HIV patients include Epstein-Barr virus, scabies, Reiter's syndrome, seborrheic dermatitis, eczema, psoriasis, and onychomycosis. Common bacterial infections in HIV include *Staphylococcus aureus* (folliculitis, impetigo, and furuncles), group A β-hemolytic *Streptococcus* (impetigo and lymphangitis), and *Pseudomonas aeruginosa* (folliculitis and ecthyma). Folliculitis may be present in up to 25% of HIV-infected patients and presents with intense pruritus. Disseminated cryptococcosis, coccidioidomycosis, and histoplasmosis may also present with cutaneous lesions.

Neoplasms

There is a higher incidence of certain malignancies among HIV patients including Kaposi's sarcoma (as discussed above); lymphoma; Hodgkin's disease, multiple myeloma, squamous cell carcinoma of the cervix, anus, and mouth; CNS lymphoma and basal cell carcinoma. Pediatric HIV patients have a higher incidence of embryonic carcinomas. The incidence of KS and CNS lymphomas has decreased since the advent of HAART.

The risk of non-Hodgkin's lymphoma (NHL) in untreated AIDS patients is 113 times that of the normal population. The advent of HAART has not had as dramatic an effect with NHL. Occurrence is related to severe immunosuppression with CD4 counts of less than 150 cells/mm^3. These lymphoma tumors are mostly B-cell type and high to intermediate grade. Extra-lymphatic disease is common with involvement of the bone marrow, CNS, skin and GI tract. CD4 counts greater than 50 cells/mm^3 increase the risk of CNS lymphoma. Computed tomography (CT) imaging will reveal single or multiple ring enhancing lesions with areas of low attenuation that can cross the midline. Oncologic consultation is recommended.

Cervical dysplasia, a precursor lesion that may progress to cervical cancer, is common among HIV-infected women and increases in severity as immunosuppression worsens.

Neurologic Complications

HIV Encephalopathy

HIV encephalopathy, or AIDS dementia, is caused by infiltration by circulating macrophages. Infected peripheral monocytes have been shown to invade the CNS and serve as a reservoir. Astrocytes, microglia, multinucleated giant cells, and myelin are affected. Neurotoxins released from the infected macrophages may also be a culprit. HIV encephalopathy presents with impairment of recent memory, cognitive impairment, inattention, behavioral changes, and motor dysfunction. This syndrome occurs in over one third of HIV patients and is progressive, leading to severe mental deterioration. CT or MRI scans show cerebral atrophy and widening of the sulci. HAART has had little effect on the prevalence of HIV encephalopathy.

Progressive Multifocal Leukoencephalopathy (PML)

Progressive multifocal leukoencephalopathy is caused by the Jakob-Creutzfeldt (JC) virus, a polyoma virus that affects approximately 4% of patients with advanced HIV disease. This rapidly progressive demyelinating disease is characterized by focal neurologic findings such as hemiparesis, gait disturbances, visual field defects, and personality changes. With severe disease one can see dementia, encephalopathy, and coma. CT or MRI scans show focal or diffuse lesions in the white matter, particularly in the periventricular areas. Most cases of PML progress to death within 4 to 5 months. No specific therapy is available for PML, though HAART has reduced the incidence.

Toxoplasmosis

Toxoplasmosis is the most common cause of focal encephalitis in patients with AIDS and the most common cause of intracranial mass lesion in AIDS. Patients with a CD4 count less than 100 cells/mm^3 have a 30% chance of reactivation of a latent toxoplasmosis infection if they are not on prophylaxis. The CNS is the most common site. Patients may present with a severe, incapacitating headache and fever. Patients may also have focal neurological deficits, altered mental status, and seizures. Frank meningismus is uncommon. Involvement of other organs, especially the lungs and eyes, are common.

Diagnosis of CNS involvement is made with contrast-enhanced CT scan showing multiple ring-enhancing lesions (abscesses). Lesions in the basal ganglia are highly suggestive. MRI or delayed CT scanning or brain biopsy may be needed to make the diagnosis. Lumbar puncture results are nonspecific, but can rule out other opportunistic infections. The presence of serum anti-toxoplasma IgG or IgM antibodies may determine infection, though the absence of these antibodies does not exclude infection.

First-line treatment include pyrimethamine (200 mg loading dose PO, followed by 75 mg per day) plus sulfadiazine (6 to 8 g per day PO in 4 divided doses) or pyrimethamine plus clindamycin (600 to 1,200 mg IV or 450 mg PO QID).

Folinic acid therapy should be given since these medications block folic acid metabolism. Corticosteroids are suggested in patients with noted midline shift. Chronic suppressive therapy is needed after the initial episode is treated.

Cryptococcal Meningoencephalitis

Cryptococcus neoformans is the most common cause of meningitis in HIV patients and is by far the most common life-threatening fungal pathogen in patients with HIV infection. The most common source is soil contaminated by bird droppings. Altered host immune defenses allow local proliferation of fungus and dissemination. The two most common sites of involvement include the central nervous system (CNS) and pulmonary system. Cryptococcal CNS infection occurs in patients with CD4 count of less than 100 cells/mm^3, causing meningitis, encephalitis, and a focal granulomatous disease. Patients with CNS involvement present with the indolent onset fever, headache, malaise, mental status changes, and cranial nerve palsies. These symptoms may be subtle and unimpressive, and are commonly missed. Seizures are rare. Respiratory involvement leads to symptoms such as cough and fever. Chest radiograph may reveal multiple subpleural nodules or infiltrates. Both the CNS and respiratory involvement can lead to disseminated infection with painless skin lesions (macules, pustules, or ulcers) and can involve other organs such as the heart, kidneys, adrenals, bones, lymph nodes, and eyes.

Diagnosis of cryptococcal infection is by CSF India ink preparation, culture, or by detection of cryptococcal antigen in the CSF via a latex agglutination test. The latter is positive in more than 90% of HIV-infected patients with culture-proven cryptococcal meningitis. Other CSF findings include an elevated opening pressure and protein, low glucose, and a lymphopleocytosis, though 25% of AIDS patients have normal initial CSF values. Cryptococcal meningoencephalitis is uniformly fatal if untreated. It may be treated with either IV amphotericin B plus oral flucytosine or with fluconazole. Infectious disease specialists should be consulted immediately. Sixty percent of patients respond to therapy. Chronic suppressive therapy is also required after recovery.

Herpes Simplex Virus (HSV) Encephalitis

HSV encephalitis usually occurs in the setting of reactivated HSV infection. The majority of cases are secondary to HSV-1. Symptoms include headache, seizures, altered mental status, and coma.

Diagnosis of HSV encephalitis in HIV patients with advanced disease by clinical presentation alone is difficult. Some patients present with subtle abnormalities, while others present with frank mental status changes, seizures, and coma. In general, with the presence of headache, fever, and seizure in the absence of other clear etiologies in an HIV patient, empirical treatment for HSV encephalitis should be started. CT scan may reveal enhanced cortical uptake in the temporal area. Lumbar puncture findings in HSV encephalitis are nonspecific with elevated protein, normal glucose, and a lymphocytic pleocytosis. Detection HSV DNA in CSF by PCR approaches 100% specificity and 75% to 98% sensitivity, though brain biopsy is the only mode of definitive diagnosis,

Intravenous acyclovir 10 mg/kg every 8 hours is the treatment of choice for 14 to 21 days or until clinical resolution. Early diagnosis and treatment is imperative. All of these patients require hospitalization.

HIV Neuropathy

HIV neuropathy usually presents with a painful peripheral neuropathy. Toxic neuropathies associated with didanosine (ddI) or calcitabine (ddC) always present initially with symptoms in the feet or the hands. Some patients receive symptomatic relief from amitriptyline.

Pulmonary Complications

Pneumocystis carinii Pneumonia (PCP)

Pneumocystis carinii pneumonia (PCP) is the most common opportunistic infection in patients infected with HIV. *P. carinii*, once considered to be a protozoan, has recently been shown through studies of RNA to show a similarity with fungi. *P. carinii* is ubiquitous in nature and commonly exists in a latent phase in many asymptomatic individuals. The mode of transmission is unknown but is presumed to be by the airborne route. The opportunistic pathogen can cause severe disease when the host's immune system becomes depressed. This infection is most likely to occur when the CD4 count is less than 200 cells/mm^3.

Symptoms usually have an insidious onset including fever, chills, sweats, nonproductive cough, and dyspnea, particularly on exertion. Physical findings include tachypnea, tachycardia, and cyanosis, lung auscultation however, usually reveals minimal abnormality. In patients with HIV disease, extrapulmonary infection is common and can include the eyes, skin, thyroid, pituitary, bone marrow, kidneys, heart, liver, and lymph nodes.

Serum lactate dehydrogenase (LDH) is elevated in 90% of infected patients. Arterial blood gas measurements usually show an increased P(A-a)O$_2$ gradient and a low PaO$_2$. A P(A-a)O$_2$ gradient greater than 29 mm Hg and a PaO$_2$ less than 70 mm Hg are associated with a poor outcome. Diffuse interstitial infiltrates with peripheral sparing is the most common chest radiograph finding. Other findings include abscesses, cavitations, lobar consolidation, nodular lesions, pneumothoraces, and normal chest radiographs. Pleural effusions are rare. High resolution computed tomography has a high sensitivity for PCP in HIV patients and usually shows patchy or nodular ground-glass attenuation.

Sputum stains are not very sensitive. Fluorescent antibody stain has been shown to be as high as 90% sensitive. Sputum induction with hypertonic saline solution has a sensitivity of approximately 75%. If negative, the diagnosis should be confirmed with the combination of bronchoalveolar lavage (BAL), bronchial brushings, and washings with a transbronchial biopsy, which has become the gold standard with a diagnostic yield of near 100%. BAL alone has a sensitivity of approximately 80% to 90%.

Serologic testing for PCP is not helpful. Gallium scanning of the lung is very sensitive for PCP but specificity is low at 20%. Diagnosis by PCR is under investigation.

Treatment of PCP is with trimethoprim (TMP), 15 mg/kg per day, and sulfamethoxazole (SMX), 100 mg/kg per day. Adverse reactions occur in 50% to 100% of HIV patients and include rash, increased liver function tests, vomiting, and neutropenia. Steroids have been shown to be beneficial for patients with PO$_2$ less than 70 mm Hg or P(A-a)O$_2$ gradient greater than 35. It should be started within 72 hours of antimicrobial treatment. In patients who have adverse reactions or fail to respond to the above regimen, pentamidine at 4 mg/kg/day intravenously can be given. About 50% of patients on pentamidine develop adverse reactions, including hypotension, renal toxicity, hypoglycemia, neutropenia, thrombocytopenia, rash, elevated liver enzymes, and pancreatitis. The usual length of treatment is 21 days. Oral dapsone/TMP in combination has been used for outpatient treatment of PCP. Dapsone is contraindicated in patients with glucose-6-phosphate dehydrogenase deficiency and pretreatment screening is recommended. Other drug regimens used to treat PCP are clindamycin plus primaquine.

Prophylaxis is recommended in anyone with a CD4 count less than 200 cells/mm^3. Prophylaxis consists of oral TMP (5 mg/kg per day) and SMX (25 mg/kg per day), or oral dapsone (50 to 100 mg per day). Aerosolized pentamidine (300 mg for 4 weeks) is also used for pulmonary prophylaxis but is not effective for systemic prophylaxis secondary to poor systemic absorption. In patients with HIV disease, the mortality rate for the first episode is now 10% to 15%, which is reduced from earlier rates of 60% to 70%. This is thought to be secondary to better drug regimens and earlier diagnoses. Since HIV patients with PCP can decompensate quickly, they should be admitted for initial treatment of pneumocystis infection.

Tuberculosis

Tuberculosis (TB) is a frequent and treatable cause of morbidity and mortality in HIV-infected patients. The majority of these cases are due to the reactivation of dormant infection secondary to immunodeficiency. Racial and ethnic minorities, immigrants, and residents of overcrowded institutions, such as shelters and prisons, account for the majority of cases. *Mycobacterium tuberculosis* is an obligate aerobic organism that is spread mainly by the respiratory route. The clinical presentation of tuberculosis in HIV-infected patients may be atypical, and diagnosis may be more difficult, requiring more invasive diagnostic procedures. Pulmonary involvement of tuberculosis is the major manifestation in immunocompetent patients, as well as in HIV-infected patients with a CD4 count greater than 300 cells/mm^3. Patients usually present with fever, weight loss, malaise, cough, and night sweats. These patients usually have focal pulmonic infiltrates and cavitations. In HIV-infected patients with CD4 counts less than 200 cells/mm^3, the presentation is more atypical with a much greater frequency of extrapulmonary involvement and diffuse pulmonary disease without cavitations. These patients more often have miliary tuberculosis and involvement of lymph nodes, central nervous system, soft tissues, bone marrow, and liver.

Physical examination findings include tachypnea due to lung involvement, hepatosplenomegaly, and lymphadenopathy. Bacteremia caused by *M. tuberculosis* has been recently described. Chest radiographs show diffuse interstitial lower lobe infiltrates with hilar enlargement as opposed to typical radiograph findings of upper lobe infiltrates seen in immunocompetent patients. Pleural effusions and intra-thoracic lymphadenopathy are also common and may be the only finding.

Diagnosis is difficult in patients with HIV disease. Approximately 30% to 40% of these patients react to the tuberculin skin test. Infected patients with a CD4 count greater than 300 cells/mm^3 are the most likely to have a positive skin test. Sputum should be sent for acid-fast bacillus smear and culture. Diagnosis may require smear and culture of tissue specimens from involved sites or by bronchoscopy with biopsy. The role of PCR in the diagnosis of TB in AIDS is under investigation.

Treatment recommendation for HIV patients with tuberculosis is 2 months of isoniazid, rifampin (or rifabutin), pyrazinamide, and ethambutol, followed by 4 to 7 months of isoniazid and rifampin. Adverse reactions are more frequent with rifampin than with other tuberculosis antimicrobial agents, and include rash, hepatitis, thrombocytopenia, and renal failure.

The emergence and transmission of multi-drug resistant *Mycobacterium tuberculosis* (MDRTB), defined as strains resistant to two or more first-line drugs, is an alarming trend. Treatment regimens involving five or six drugs are necessary. Other choices of therapy include ciprofloxacin, amikacin, and imipenem. Initial drugs should be chosen depending on drug susceptibilities from tuberculosis organisms in the patient's geographic location followed by susceptibility testing of the organism isolated from the patient. Recommended treatment duration is 18 to 24 months.

All patients with HIV and tuberculin skin test reaction greater than or equal to 5 mm who don't have active TB should receive isoniazid prophylaxis (300 mg per day for 9 months). HIV patients with possible TB exposure should be evaluated with an anergy panel including control antigens such as mumps, *Candida*, or tetanus toxoid. Even if the PPD skin response is negative, those patients with anergic panels should receive isoniazid prophylaxis for 1 year.

Coccidioidomycosis

Prior to the widespread use of HAART, coccidioidomycosis was a major cause of opportunistic infection in HIV patients living in endemic areas. *Coccidioides immitus* is a dimorphic fungus that is endemic in the southern United States, including southern Arizona, central California, southwest New Mexico, and west Texas. In normal hosts, it is typically a self-limited pulmonary infection. HIV patients with CD4 counts less than 250 cells/mm^3 may develop a diffuse pulmonary process clinically indistinguishable from PCP. They can also present with focal pulmonary disease, meningitis, and disseminated disease. Chest x-ray may reveal bilateral diffuse reticulonodular pulmonary infiltrates. Diagnosis is best made by isolation of the fungus on bronchoalveolar lavage.

Serologic tests are less useful in HIV-infected patients that in immunocompetent hosts. Treatment is with ketoconazole, itraconazole, or fluconazole.

Other Pulmonary Manifestations

Patients with HIV are also susceptible to bacterial, viral, and fungal pulmonary infections common in immunocompetent patients. They also have an increase susceptibility to the more uncommon fungal pulmonary and disseminated infections in certain endemic areas, such as histoplasmosis and blastomycosis.

Nonspecific interstitial pneumonitis (NIP) may also develop in HIV-infected patients. NIP is similar to PCP in presentation, but may affect immunocompetent HIV patients. Histologic examination reveals patchy lymphocytic infiltrates, predominantly composed of B cells. Pediatric patients may present with lymphocytic interstitial pneumonitis (LIP).

Ophthalmologic Manifestations

Cytomegalovirus Retinitis

Cytomegalovirus retinitis infection affects up to 40% of patients with HIV infection. The virus can be spread by sexual contact, blood transfusion, organ transplantation, or breast milk. In patients with a CD4 count less than 100 cells/mm^3, the virus may reactivate, causing colitis, pneumonia, esophagitis, and neurologic complications. The most common involvement in HIV patients is ocular disease. There has been a dramatic decline in the incidence of CMV retinitis since the development of HAART. However, initiation of HAART in patients with CMV retinitis can result in intraocular inflammation, called immune recovery uveitis and vitreitis. This can be counteracted with the administration of corticosteroids. Symptoms of CMV include painless loss of vision, visual field defects, and a complaint of floaters. Fundoscopic examination reveals large, yellow-white granular areas with perivascular exudates and hemorrhage. Treatment is with ganciclovir 5 mg/kg intravenously every 12 hours for 14 to 21 days. Foscarnet 90 mg/kg intravenously every 12 hours can also be used. Maintenance treatment is necessary.

Other Ophthalmologic Complications

Other ocular infectious manifestations of HIV include varicella zoster virus, KS, molluscum contagiosum, HSV, toxoplasma, and syphilis. Microvascular changes of the conjunctiva and retinal microvasculopathy (AIDS retinopathy) is also found in AIDS patients. AIDS retinopathy is characterized by cotton wool spots, intraretinal hemorrhage, and retinal microaneurysms. Patients are usually asymptomatic. The lesions may regress spontaneously and patients usually have an excellent prognosis. No specific treatment is necessary. Follow-up examinations are recommended.

Gastrointestinal Complications

Esophageal and Oral Candidiasis

Candida species are the most common fungal pathogens in HIV-infected patients. Clinical presentations include mucocutaneous infections and rarely systemic involvement. The majority of cases are caused by *Candida albicans*. Oral involvement demonstrates curd like patches on the tongue and buccal mucosa. The underlying mucous membranes are usually inflamed. Esophageal involvement includes symptoms of odynophagia, dysphagia, and retrosternal pain. Esophageal candidiasis is included as one of the AIDS-defining criteria. Rare extensive involvement with pseudomembrane formation has been known to cause partial obstruction. Oral thrush is nearly always present in patients with HIV and candidal esophagitis. Other mucocutaneous findings include balanitis, folliculitis, intertrigo, and onychomycosis. Systemic *Candida* is rare in HIV-infected patients, yet should be considered in patients with severe neutropenia, indwelling catheters or in those treated with prolonged broad-spectrum antibiotics. Dissemination of *Candida* to sites such as the lung, central nervous system, heart, and kidney has been documented.

The diagnosis of oral thrush is made by microscopic evaluation of oral scrapings treated with 10% potassium hydroxide solution identifying yeast and pseudohyphae. Cultures of oral lesions are not useful.

Diagnosis of esophageal involvement by barium swallow is not as sensitive as esophagoscopy with biopsy for definitive diagnosis. A presumptive diagnosis of candidal esophagitis in a patient with esophageal complaints and oral candidiasis should be made and the patient should be started on empiric therapy with an antifungal agent for 2 weeks. If no oral thrush is evident, esophagoscopy should be attempted to rule out other causes of esophagitis such as CMV or HSV. In systemic involvement, blood cultures are often negative. Diagnosis is usually made postmortem.

Standard treatment of oral and esophageal candiasis in AIDS patients involves fluconazole (200 mg PO on day one, then 100 mg PO qd for 7 to 14 days) or itraconazole or caspofungin. There is an increased incidence of fluconazole resistant strains, particularly in patients with CD4 counts less than 50 cells/mm^3, for which higher doses of the above medications or parenteral amphotericin B may be required. Oral topical agents such as clotrimazole troches (10 mg, 5 times a day) or nystatin may be tried for oral candidiasis without esophageal involvement in patients with CD4 counts greater than 50 cells/mm^3 or those on HAART. Systemic infection requires intravenous amphotericin B (0.6 to 0.8 mg/kg per day) for 6 to 8 weeks.

HSV Gingivostomatitis and Esophagitis

HSV gingivostomatitis in HIV-infected patients, which is usually secondary to HSV-1, may be more protracted than in the normal host with extensive tissue destruction, poor healing of ulcerative lesions, and occasional virus dissemination. Herpes esophagitis affecting patients with HIV disease presents with similar complaints as esophageal candidiasis with dysphagia and retrosternal discomfort, yet visible oral lesions are often not present. The diagnosis of HSV esophagitis often requires endoscopic evaluation with Tzanck smear and biopsy obtained for viral culture. Treatment is with acyclovir 200 to 400 mg orally five times per day for mild or moderate HSV infection. Intravenous acyclovir at 5 mg/kg every 8 hours is used to treat more severe HSV esophagitis. Treatment is usually for 7 days or until all external lesions have crusted.

Other Oral Manifestations

Oral hairy leukoplakia, believed to be related to Epstein-Barr virus reactivation, can sometimes be confused with oral candidiasis. However, unlike candidal thrush, these lesions cannot be scraped off. They are usually seen on the lateral borders of the tongue.

Causes of ulcerative oral lesions not related to HSV include CMV, aphthous ulcers, occurring predominantly on nonkeratinized mucosal surfaces, and VZV, which affect the oral mucosa along with trigeminal nerve branches and tend to be unilateral. Periodontal disease, such as linear gingival erythema, necrotizing gingivitis, necrotizing periodontitis, and necrotizing stomatitis, are also more commonly seen. AIDS-related neoplasms, such as Kaposi's sarcoma or lymphoma, may have oral manifestations, as well.

Hepatomegaly and Splenomegaly

Tender hepatomegaly and splenomegaly occur frequently with acute HIV infection. Acute hepatitis has also occurred with hepatic enzymes, returning to normal within 6 weeks. Hepatomegaly occurs in more than 50% of patients with advanced HIV disease. *Mycobacterium avium-intracellulare* (MAC) is the most frequent hepatic pathogen in advanced HIV disease. CMV is also noted to be a frequent infectious pathogen of the liver in patients with HIV. *M. tuberculosis*, KS, cryptococcus, *P. carinii*, and non-Hodgkin's lymphoma have also been cited. Drug-induced hepatitis, mainly with sulfonamides, has been implicated. Hepatitis B and C are common among HIV patients with a history of intravenous drug use. Treatment depends on underlying cause and includes antimicrobial agents for specific infection or chemotherapy for neoplasms, such as KS.

Biliary Tract and Pancreatic Disorders

Acalculous cholecystitis and AIDS cholangiopathy as specific AIDS-related illnesses are frequently related to opportunistic infection. Acalculous cholecystitis has a similar presentation to calculus cholecystitis and is frequently attributable to CMV or *Cryptosporidium* species. It requires surgical intervention. AIDS cholangiopathy includes a number of illnesses including papillary stenosis, sclerosing cholangitis, and long extrahepatic bile duct strictures. Patients present with fever, right upper quadrant pain, diarrhea, and weight loss. Jaundice is rare. The etiology may be infectious, caused by CMV, *Cryptosporidium* species, *Microsporidia* species, MAC, or due to chronic inflammation. Pancreatitis in HIV is similar in presentation to non-HIV-infected patients. Causes include infection (CMV, MAC, *Cryptosporidium*, *Cryptococcus*, and *Toxoplasma* species), malignancy, hypertriglyceridemia, and medications (pentamidine, dideoxyinosine, dideoxycytidine, lamivudine, and TMP-SMX).

Mycobacterium Avium-Intracellular Complex

Mycobacterium avium-intracellulare complex (MAC) refers to infection by one of two non-tuberculous mycobacteria species (*M. avium* or *M. intracellurare*). *M. avium-*

intracellulare is found in soil, dust, and water. Patients may either have disseminated or local disease. Local disease presents primarily with focal adenopathy. Patients with disseminated disease may present with fever, anorexia, malaise; and weight loss, diarrhea, and abdominal pain are secondary to involvement of the gastrointestinal tract. Pulmonary symptoms are less common. Disseminated MAC infections seem to occur later in course of HIV infection, most often when the CD4 count is less than 50 cells/mm. Use of HAART has decreased the incidence of disseminated MAC.

Diagnosis is made by obtaining positive blood cultures. Bacteremia is common with disseminated disease. Soft tissue biopsy and culture of involved sites also aids in diagnosis. Rapid diagnosis by acid-fast bacilli smear is helpful for initiating empiric therapy for *M. tuberculosis* until the culture results become available. Treatment for active infection is clarithromycin (500 mg PO BID) or azithromycin (600 mg PO qd) plus ethambutol (15 to 25 mg/kg per day) plus rifabutin (300 mg PO qd). Prophylaxis is recommended with azithromycin (1,200 mg PO weekly) or clarithromycin (500 mg PO bid) for patients with CD4 count of less than 100 cells/mm^3.

Diarrhea

Diarrhea is the most common gastrointestinal complaint in HIV patients. It occurs in 50% to 90% of patients with advanced HIV disease. There are a wide variety of protozoan, viral, and bacterial pathogens known to cause diarrhea in HIV patients, and should be suspected in any HIV patient with diarrhea for greater than ten days. Protozoan organisms include *Isospora belli, Giardia, Microsporidium,* and *Cryptosporidium.* The bacterial pathogens, primarily *Salmonella, Shigella,* and *Campylobacter,* have higher rates of bacteremia and antibiotic resistance in HIV patients. Infections are also more frequent and more severe. Viruses such as CMV and HSV as well as fungi including *Candida,* histoplasmosis, and coccidiomycosis have also been known to cause diarrhea in these patients. Malignancies with KS or lymphoma are other diagnostic possibilities. MAC should always be ruled out in immunocompromised HIV patients who present with gastrointestinal symptoms.

An idiopathic AIDS enteropathy has been proposed to account for the diarrhea in HIV-infected patients who lack an identifiable pathogen. The pathogenesis is unknown. It is thought that enteric HIV infection leads to mucosal atrophy, causing diarrhea and weight loss. HIV medications may also be culprits.

Diagnostic measures include microscopic evaluation of stool for leukocytes, ova and parasites, acid-fast organisms, and occult blood. Cultures also should be done. Treatment involves hydration and correcting electrolyte disturbances. Some bacterial dysenteries may require antibiotics.

Herpes Proctitis

Herpes proctitis is a frequent cause of nongonococcal proctitis in sexually active homosexual men. Symptoms include anorectal pain, perianal ulceration, difficulty with urination, obstipation, and sacral neurologic findings. Sacral paresthesias occur more frequently with HSV proctitis than with other causes of proctitis. Diagnosis is by direct inspection of rectal mucosa and virologic testing such as direct antigen detection or viral culture.

Cardiovascular Complications

Cardiac manifestations can be seen in up to 70% of HIV-infected individuals. They are seen most commonly in late stages of the disease and in patients not on HAART. The most common cardiac disturbances include pericarditis, endocarditis, myocarditis, pericardial effusion, dilated cardiomyopathy, dilation of the right ventricle secondary to pulmonary hypertension, and malignancy. Endocarditis is frequently involved with IV drug use and, hence, right-sided heart valves are more commonly involved. *Staphylococcus aureus* and *Streptococcus viridians* are the most common pathogens. Myocarditis is frequently due to lymphocytic involvement secondary to the HIV infection itself, though other causes include CMV, *Cryptococcus neoformans, Candida* species, *Toxoplasmosis gondii, Histoplasma capsulatum,* tuberculosis, *Aspergillus* species, *Sarcosporidium,* and Coxsackie virus. Myocardial infection may lead to dilated cardiomyopathy, which is a significant cause of morbidity in late HIV infection.

Renal Complications

Acute renal failure most commonly includes acute tubular necrosis, acute interstitial nephritis secondary to drug toxicity, tubular obstruction secondary to tumor lysis syndrome, and hemolytic uremic syndrome or thrombotic thrombocytopenic purpura. Parenchymal renal disease may be from opportunistic infections, such as CMV, *Cryptococcus, Candida, Mycobacterium, Aspergillus,* and tumors, such as KS and lymphoma that invade renal parenchyma. HIV nephropathy occurs in 5% to 10% of patients with HIV infection. It is more common in black patients than white (12:1) and is more common in IV drug users. This usually progresses to end-stage renal disease requiring dialysis. The clinical presentation includes heavy proteinuria, azotemia, normal blood pressure, and enlarged kidneys on ultrasound.

Psychiatric Disorders

The most common psychiatric disease presentations seen in patients with HIV infection include delirium, dementia, depression, and psychosis. Depression is common among AIDS patients and is exacerbated especially in those with a history of depression before their HIV illness. Treatment consists of hospitalization and psychosocial intervention. Antidepressants may be used in those patients with symptoms of depression that last longer than 6 weeks.

Delirium and dementia may be a manifestation of a primary physiologic disease that should be thoroughly investigated since treatment can be offered.

Psychosis in AIDS patients can present with a variety of symptoms including hallucinations, abnormal behavior, and delusions. The etiology is unclear. Treatment is similar to other psychosis. A full workup is recommended for the initial presentation.

Other Miscellaneous Conditions

Arthritis

HIV-associated arthritis has been described in some patients. Arthritis tends to be oligoarticular, self-limited, and affect primarily the lower extremities. The cause is unclear.

Polymyositis

Polymyositis associated with HIV presents with proximal muscle wasting and an elevated CPK from breakdown of affected muscles. It is not associated with level of immunosuppression and the cause is unknown. Myositis associated with zidovudine has also been described with myalgias, proximal muscle weakness, tenderness, and elevated CK. Symptoms improve with discontinuation of the drug.

Metabolic Disturbances

The most common metabolic disturbance in HIV is hyperlipidemia. This is in part due to increased lipid synthesis in the liver. In addition, use of protease inhibitors is also implicated as they may reduce hepatic uptake of lipids. High levels of lipids result in fat redistribution, insulin resistance, and hyperglycemia. Another metabolic abnormality commonly seen, lactic acidosis, is due to the use of nucleoside analogue reverse transcriptase inhibitors, and can be fatal.

Anemia

Anemia is a common complicating factor in HIV infection. It is typically caused by anemia of chronic disease infections, such as MAC and parvovirus B19, or drug therapy, such as with zidovudine.

Thrombocytopenia

Idiopathic thrombocytopenia (ITP) is more common in HIV-infected patients and presents with complications associated with low platelets. The primary causes are decreased platelet production and immune mediated destruction of platelets. Other causes include hypersplenism in liver disease, bone marrow infiltration by opportunistic infection or neoplasm, the myelosuppressive effects of therapy, and thrombotic thrombocytopenic purpura. Hematologic consult should be obtained in cases of severe thrombocytopenia.

Antiviral Drugs in Clinical Practice

While antiretroviral therapy is rarely initiated in the emergency department, except in cases of occupational exposure and sexual assault, the emergency physician should be familiar with the commonly used drugs and potential side effects. A few commonly seen side effects will be covered below excluding minor side effects.

Nucleoside Reverse Transcriptase Inhibitors (NRTI)

These medications include abacavir (Ziagen), didanosine (Videx), lamivudine (Epivir), stavudine (Zerit), zalcitabine (Hivid), and zidovudine (Retrovir). All of these medications have been associated with lactic acidosis, severe steatosis, and lipodystrophy. Didanosine is associated in particular with pancreatitis. Zidovudine is known for causing anemia and granulocytopenia in some patients. Many of these medications also cause peripheral neuropathy.

Nucleotide Reverse Transcriptase Inhibitors (NtRTI)

Tenofovir (Viread) is in this group and is commonly associated with lactic acidosis and hepatic steatosis. This drug interacts with didanosine.

Non-Nucleoside Reverse Transcriptase Inhibitors (NNRTI)

These medications include delavirdine (Rescriptor) and nevirapine (Viramune), and efavirenz (Sustiva), which can all have associated rash. Efavirenz is also associated with teratogenicity and CNS effects, such as insomnia, dizziness, somnolence, and abnormal dreams.

Protease Inhibitors (PI)

These medications include amprenavir (Agenerase), indinavir (Crixivan), nelfinavir (Viracept), ritonavir (Norvir), saquinavir (Invirase or Fortovase) and lopinavir/ritonavir (Kaletra). All the PIs have been associated with lipodystrophy, hyperlipidemia and hyperglycemia. Some patients develop diabetes mellitus and glucose intolerance. These patients may also be at higher risk of developing osteopenia and osteoporosis. Spontaneous bleeding has been noted in hemophiliacs with HIV on PIs. Many are also associated with diarrhea. Indinavir has been associated with indinavir kidney stones. Amprenavir has been associated with skin rashes that may become severe and life threatening, including Stevens-Johnson syndrome.

Prevention and Post-Exposure Prophylaxis

There has been a great deal of progress in the prevention of transmission of AIDS today. Blood products are now much safer due to screening and heat treatment. Hospitals need to continue encouraging medical personnel to follow universal precautions when dealing with blood products. Prevention of sexual transmission has been a challenge. The use of condoms has markedly reduced transmission in major segments of the population but continued education is still needed. Trials for HIV vaccine are underway.

In the event of high risk HIV exposure, postexposure prophylaxis (PEP) is recommended. In an occupational setting, initiation of PEP within 72 hours should be considered for exposure to blood, bloody fluid, semen, or vaginal fluid. Contact of fluids with intact skin is not an indication, nor is exposure to fluids from a non-HIV-infected person (although hepatitis B and C prophylaxis and counseling may still be required). For a source of unknown HIV status, the basic regimen is zidovudine and lamivudine (or didanosine and stavudine, or stavudine and lamivudine). It is recommended for fluid contact with mucous membranes or un-intact skin, particularly if exposure is to a large amount of fluid, and for percutaneous exposures (needle stick or scratch). An expanded regimen with the addition of indinavir, nelfinavir, abacavir, or efavirenz is recommended for high-risk exposures (puncture with a large bore hollow needle, deep puncture, visible blood, and needle used in vein of source patient) with a source that is known HIV-positive. Baseline complete blood count, renal panel, hepatic panel, and pregnancy test should be drawn, as well as baseline HIV, hepatitis B and C serology. Prophylaxis is given for four weeks with careful monitoring for adverse effects. Repeat HIV testing should occur at three to four weeks, at three and at six months. Most patients will seroconvert by three months. Delayed seroconversion beyond six months is rare. The initial dose of PEP may be given in the emergency department and close follow up should be arranged with an infectious disease specialist. PEP should also be considered in persons who have had a sexual encounter with an HIV+ individual if seen within 72 hours. Prophylaxis for *Neisseria gonorrhoeae, Chlamydia trachomatis,* and syphilis should also be considered. It has been estimated that transmission of HIV following a single exposure to an HIV-infected individual is 0.1% to 0.2% for receptive vaginal exposure and 0.1% to 0.3% in receptive penile-anal exposure.

Infectious Mononucleosis

Infectious mononucleosis (IM) is a virally mediated, generally benign, lymphoproliferative disease characterized by tonsillitis, pharyngitis, lymphadenopathy, hepatosplenomegaly, fever, fatigue, and malaise. Usually children and young adults are affected, with the vast majority of the population exposed and immune to re-infection by age 25. In countries with poorer hygiene, IM is a disease of early childhood and is rarely encountered in adults.

In 1967, the Epstein-Barr virus (EBV), a double-stranded DNA, herpes virus, strongly trophic toward B lymphocytes and epithelial cells of the oropharynx and cervix, was identified as the etiologic agent of IM. Infection of B lymphocytes by EBV permits unrestricted, indefinite, cellular proliferation in the absence of adequate immune control, as witnessed in immunodeficiency syndromes and transplant recipients. The oncogenetic potential of EBV-infected cells is demonstrated through the association of EBV with malignancies such as Burkitt's lymphoma, nasopharyngeal carcinoma, T cell lymphoma, Hodgkin's and CNS lymphomas, and some thymomas. Additionally, oral hairy leukoplakia, an overgrowth of epithelial cells on the tongue and buccal mucosa, often noted in AIDS patients, is caused by EBV. Unlike other herpes viruses, however, reactivation of EBV disease rarely occurs in immune-competent hosts.

The differential diagnosis for patients presenting with symptoms compatible with IM includes streptococcal pharyngitis, *Corynebacterium diphtheriae,* CMV, rubella, HIV, adenovirus, hepatitis A and B, *Toxoplasma gondii,* and other lymphoproliferative disorders.

Diagnosis

Three to seven weeks following the exposure to respiratory droplets or oropharyngeal secretions, patients with IM frequently present with the following triad:

- Pharyngitis
- Adenopathy
- Fever

The pharyngitis of IM is often exudative. Three to thirty percent of patients with IM will throat culture positive for a concomitant group A β-hemolytic streptococcal infection. Occasionally, the tonsillo-pharyngitis of IM is severe enough to threaten the patency of the airway. The adenopathy associated with IM can be prominent and persistent. Posterior cervical adenopathy, in association with pharyngitis and fever, can be quite suggestive of IM. Up to 50% of patients with IM also develop *splenomegaly,* making them vulnerable to splenic rupture from seemingly even minor trauma. Blood analysis reveals a predominant lymphocytosis, with greater than 10% atypical lymphocytes and, frequently, a mild thrombocytosis. The presence of heterophile antibodies capable of agglutinating sheep erythrocytes with a titer of 1:56 or greater, as measured by the Paul-Bunnell-Davidsohn assay, along with the above clinical and hematologic parameters, is generally adequate for the diagnosis of IM. The Paul-Bunnell-Davidsohn assay has subsequently been refined into the rapid latex agglutination test, the *Monospot.* It is essential to note that up to 20% of adults and an even greater percentage of children under 4 years of age fail to produce heterophile antibodies resulting in a false-negative Monospot. Additionally, anywhere from 5% to 15% of patients demonstrate a false-positive Monospot in response to heterophile antibodies produced to other infections, such as cytomegalovirus, adenovirus, and toxoplasmosis. In the few instances where it is imperative to definitively identify the presence of EBV, specific assays are available to detect various EBV components.

Treatment

The vast majority of patients with IM require only supportive care: rest, fluids, analgesics, and antipyretics. It is important to advise patients to refrain from contact sports until splenomegaly has resolved, usually within a month. Splenic ultrasound may be used to verify resolution of splenomegaly if this determination is necessary (e.g., a pressing desire to return to contact sports. Spontaneous splenic rupture, though rare, is also known to occur. Splenic rupture is the most common cause of death due to IM. Patients who culture positive for a concomitant group A β-hemolytic strep infection of the throat should receive an appropriate antibiotic. Ampicillin or amoxicillin must not be used due to their frequent association with rash in patients with IM. Special attention should be paid to the patency of the airway with the use of corticosteroids to reduce tonsillar and pharyngeal edema and obviate airway obstruction. Additionally, steroids may be beneficial for the treatment of other complications of IM such as severe hemolytic anemia, thrombocytopenia, or neurologic manifestations such as Guillain-Barré syndrome, encephalitis, meningitis, transverse myelitis, neuropathies, optic neuritis, cranial nerve palsies, and cerebellar ataxia.

Influenza

Influenza is a virally mediated disease, characterized by frequent epidemics and episodic global pandemics. It has a seasonal predilection and occurs in the winter months in the northern hemisphere and summer months in the southern hemisphere and year round in the tropics. Thousands of deaths are attributed yearly either directly to influenza or to its related complications. Additionally, the four pandemics this century have resulted in millions of lost lives. The pandemic of 1918 to 1919 alone resulted in 20 million deaths, more than those due to the First World War. Further, absenteeism from work, and school due to influenza has significant economic consequences.

The influenza viruses are single-stranded RNA viruses belonging to the orthomyxovirus family. Influenza types A, B, and C are distinguished by their nuclear material. Types A and B are clinically relevant to human disease. Influenza virus has two protein surface antigens, hemagglutinin and neuraminidase, that allow for the formation of unique subtypes through antigenic shift. There is minimal to no immune cross-reactivity of the new subtype relative to prior strains, thus exposing large masses of the global population to disease and subsequent worldwide pandemics. *Antigenic drift* permits minor alterations of the surface antigens of both influenza A and B and accounts for the observed yearly variations in viral strains. Vaccines for influenza A and B are generated based on predicting which strains will be prevalent during the infectious season.

Diagnosis

One to two days following respiratory or contact exposure to the influenza virus, symptoms of influenza appear abruptly and include high fever, myalgias, headache, nonproductive cough frequently associated with chest discomfort, rhinorrhea, malaise, and photophobia.

Systemic symptoms usually resolve within 5 days with conservative therapy alone, although the fatigue of influenza may persist for several weeks. The diagnosis of influenza is most often clinical and based on the presence of known influenza in the community and the above symptomatology. Rapid tests for influenza A and B are available and may be helpful, if positive. However, their limited sensitivity frequently makes definitive viral culture or serologic evaluation necessary, though these studies are not adequately rapid to be clinically relevant but may serve epidemiologic needs. The differential diagnosis of influenza includes mycoplasma, early measles, Q fever, and other viral upper respiratory tract infections.

Infection rates during epidemics is highest among young children and adolescents; however, complications due to influenza most commonly occur in the very young, in the elderly with superimposed medical conditions or in immune-compromised individuals. Influenza pneumonitis is a rare, but aggressive and potentially devastating complication of influenza that most often affects patients with underlying cardiopulmonary disease. Secondary bacterial pneumonias due to *Staphylococcus aureus, Streptococcus pneumonia* or *Haemophilus influenzae* may occur 1 to 2 weeks following the initial viral disease. Other complications include encephalitis, pericarditis, myocarditis, and myositis. Reye's syndrome has been associated with the use of salicylates in young children with influenza B and varicella zoster.

Immunization

Prevention of influenza through effective immunization of the high-risk population remains the cornerstone of influenza control. The elderly and those with pre-existing cardiac or pulmonary disease or immune compromise are primary targets for vaccination. Additionally, those living in close quarters who desire to limit exposure and reduce out of work/school time should receive vaccine prophylaxis. Pregnant women who are at moderate risk of influenza complications should be vaccinated during the second or third trimester; however, vaccination should not be withheld at any time should the patient be at high risk for complications. Despite the recent FDA approval of Flumist, an attenuated, intranasally administered vaccine cleared for immunocompetent recipients aged 5 to 50 years, inactivated, trivalent (antigens of influenza B strain and two strains of influenza A), intramuscular vaccine continues to be the cornerstone of large scale vaccination in the United States. The effectiveness of the vaccine is in part related to the antigenic proximity of the influenza vaccine to wild strains of the season in addition to host response factors. The vaccine is most efficacious when given intramuscularly within 2 to 4 months but at least 2 weeks prior to exposure. Children less than 9 years of age should receive two doses of vaccine 4 weeks apart to ensure an adequate immune response. Children less than 12 years of age should receive the "split-virus" (disrupted virus) vaccine since this is less reactogenic. Those older than 12 years of age receive the "whole-virus" vaccine. The vaccine is produced in fertilized hens' eggs; consequently, hypersensitivity to egg proteins is a contraindication to the administration of the vaccine. Reactions to the vaccine include localized erythema and discomfort, fever, chills, and myalgias. Anaphylaxis is rare and most likely related to egg protein, neomycin or polymyxin allergy. Children under 6 months should not receive the vaccine due to the frequent occurrence of febrile reactions. Immunization should be postponed in any person acutely febrile until the fever has subsided.

Treatment

Chemotherapy utilizing amantadine, oseltamivir, oral antiviral agents, and zanamivir, an inhaled drug, provides effective influenza prophylaxis, as well as attenuates the severity of the disease if given within 48 hours of the onset of symptoms. Amantadine has minimal if any activity against influenza B because the virus lacks the target M2 protein of the drug. Oseltamivir and zanamivir are effective against both influenza A and B as they block the activity of neuraminidase, a viral enzyme present on both viruses that is necessary for viral dispersion after replication. Amantadine is administered for five days at a dose of 200 mg daily, 100 mg daily in the elderly and those with renal impairment. Up to one third of patients treated with amantadine may shed resistant virus at the end of their five-day course, making this medication a poor choice for hospitalized patients living in close proximity. Amantadine has few serious side effects. Intolerance is manifested by central nervous system symptoms of insomnia, headache, light-headedness, vertigo, and difficulty concentrating. These symptoms usually resolve with discontinuation of the drug. Oseltamivir is available in pill and liquid form and given at a dose of 75 mg twice daily for 5 days. It is well tolerated, but mild nausea and vomiting occurs in approximately 7% of cases. Similarly, zanamivir is generally well tolerated, but may exacerbate asthma or COPD due to bronchospasm. Ten milligrams (10 mg) are inhaled twice daily for five days.

Mumps

Mumps is generally a benign and self-limited disease caused by a paramyxovirus. It predominantly afflicts young children and peaks during the late winter and early spring months. Despite a radical reduction in the number of yearly cases since the introduction of the mumps vaccine in 1967, the case-fatality ratio remains relatively unchanged at approximately 1.8 deaths per 10,000 cases.

Diagnosis

The transmission of the mumps virus is via respiratory secretions. Following replication in the respiratory epithelium and local lymph nodes, a blood-borne viremia leads to seeding of other organs. Unilateral or bilateral parotitis is nearly always present and occurs within 3 weeks of exposure. Additionally, fever and malaise are often noted. Meningoencephalitis associated with mumps occurs at a rate of about 2.6 per 1,000 cases with a fatality rate of 1.4%. In one study, orchitis occurred in nearly 10% of males over 12 years of age. Of significance is the rare case of sterility due to mumps orchitis. Other complications of mumps include arthritis, pancreatitis, thyroiditis, myocarditis, nephritis, cerebellar dysfunction, and hearing loss. The vast majority of these complications are self-limited.

Immunization

Vaccination is the primary mode of mumps control. A live, attenuated virus vaccine was approved for use in 1967 and is currently administered in association with measles and rubella vaccine as the "MMR." Seroconversion to the mumps vaccine is on the order of 95%. Adverse reactions to mumps vaccination are infrequent, but include parotitis, fever, rash, pruritus, purpura, and rare cases of CNS dysfunction.

Rabies

Annually, thousands of people die from rabies throughout the world. The majority of these cases occur in developing nations, a reflection of widespread disease in the animal population and inadequate rabies immunization.

Over half a million people are bitten by animals in the United States yearly. Between 20,000 and 30,000 receive post-exposure rabies prophylaxis (PEP). Although most cases of rabies in the United States have been secondary to *wild* animal bites, the administration of PEP has been overwhelmingly skewed toward dog and cat bites. The overall economic burden, inclusive of animal vaccination, is estimated at approximately $300 million yearly.

In the 1940s, dogs and cats were the primary reservoir for rabies. Now the vast majority of rabid animals in the United States are wild. Aggressive rabies vaccination of domesticated animals has resulted in a radical reduction of human rabies occurrences.

The skunk is the most commonly reported rabid animal, followed by raccoons, foxes, and bats. Bats are the most ubiquitous source of rabies. Rodents are very rare carriers of rabies. Only about 15% of all rabid animals isolated are domestic. Since their introduction to the hunting clubs of West Virginia in the late 1970s, raccoons have established themselves as a major source of rabies in the mid-Atlantic states. Their subsequent northeasterly migration has resulted in the spread of rabies into New York and New England. Cats are particularly at risk for acquiring rabies from raccoons, owing to their natural nocturnal behavioral tendencies and inadequate vaccination status.

Rabies virus is from the viral family Rhabdoviridae. When introduced into a wound, the virus remains at the site of inoculation from 1 to 4 days, then presumably migrates into the CNS via nerve pathways. Involvement of the salivary glands is most likely secondary to hematologic spread. Once symptoms begin, the disease is nearly always fatal, with death occurring within 3 to 10 days.

The presence of Negri bodies, cytoplasmic inclusion particles in neurons, is diagnostic of rabies, although a newer method, immunofluorescent labeling, is often the test of choice.

Transmission

Bite wounds, with virally contaminated saliva, are the most common mode of rabies transmission. Bite wounds cause almost all cases of rabies, with bites to the face considered most serious due to rapid involvement of cranial nerves. Nonbite exposures rarely result in rabies infection. Corneal transplants have resulted in the only cases of human-to-human transmission. A few isolated cases of rabies via viral inhalation have also been reported (i.e., in bat caves and laboratory exposure). Bat exposure requires special attention. Because of their thin, needle-like teeth, bat bites may go unnoticed. Rabies treatment should be strongly recommended to anyone who awakens to find a bat in their room, or when a child, mentally handicapped individual or impaired person is similarly exposed.

Diagnosis

Symptoms of rabies infection are often nonspecific, and include fever, malaise, headache, upper respiratory infection (URI), GI symptomatology, and, at times, subtle alterations in mentation. Sialorrhea, agitation, weakness, or paralysis may also be present. The incubation period is variable and can often be long.

The most characteristic symptoms are hydrophobia due to dysphagia, a result of bulbar palsy, and paresthesias around the wound site. However, no single finding is diagnostic of rabies. Once established, the disease nearly always progresses to fatal encephalitis. Antiviral agents appear of little value in altering the course of the infection.

Treatment

Rabies is the only disease where post-exposure immunotherapy results in a cure. Ideally, treatment should be initiated within 24 hours of exposure, but should not be withheld whenever the risk of rabies is suspected, owing to the virus's often extended incubation period. Treatment includes:

- Wound cleaning (soap and water).
- Human rabies immunoglobulin (HRIG)-passive immunization:

  HRIG is given (20 IU/kg), as much as possible is infiltrated around the wound site and the remainder IM in the gluteal region. HRIG suppresses the body's response to rabies vaccine so no more than the recommended dose should be given. HRIG may be administered up to 8 days after rabies vaccine.
- Human diploid cell vaccine (HDCV), rabies vaccine adsorbed (RVA), purified chick embryo cell culture (PCEC) vaccine-active immunization:

  HDCV, RVA, or PCEC vaccine is given IM in the deltoid (1 mL on days 0, 3, 7, 14, and 28) for maximal immune response. HRIG and rabies vaccine should never be injected at the same site since HRIG will inactivate rabies vaccine.

Pre-exposure prophylaxis rabies vaccine should be considered for individuals with a higher likelihood of encountering rabid animals. The recommended vaccination sequence is HDCV, RVA, PCEC vaccine 1 mL IM in the deltoid on days 0, 7, and 21, or 28. A booster of rabies vaccine 1 mL IM in the deltoid is given on days 0 and 3 following exposure. HRIG is not administered. Rabies vaccination does not confer lifelong immunity to rabies.

Rabies exposure is reportable to public health departments. Animals should be evaluated and appropriately observed, quarantined, or sacrificed for pathology inspection, depending on the circumstances of the attack as well as their immunization and health status.

Rubella

Rubella, also known as German measles, is generally a benign acute exanthematous viral infection of children and adults. Clinical manifestations of the virus will vary with age. Many rubella infections are subclinical, but if acquired early in pregnancy rubella can cause multiple fetal abnormalities, collectively known as the congenital rubella syndrome (CRS).

Epidemiology

Rubella, from the *Rubivirus* genus, is transmitted without a vector and humans are the only known natural host. The virus is spread via droplets emanating from the respiratory secretions of an infected person. Close and prolonged contact with the carrier seems to be required for transmission; a single brief encounter does not appear to lead to infection. Patients are most contagious when the virus is erupting. However, the virus may shed from the throat from 10 days before the rash to 15 days after the onset. Re-infection with rubella virus can occur but most are asymptomatic. Re-infections are more common in patients who have received vaccine, rather than in persons who had natural rubella.

With the licensure of a live attenuated rubella vaccine in 1969, there have been no large epidemics of the virus since 1964 in the United States. The incidence of clinical cases of rubella tends to be higher in the spring. Rubella was once thought to be most common in children age 5 to 9 years; however, it is increasing in frequency in older age groups secondary to widespread use of the vaccine. Persons older than 20 years now comprise 62% of cases of rubella reported in the United States. Limited outbreaks still occur among non-immunized young adults in prisons, colleges, and the military, where susceptible individuals are in close contact with one another.

The widespread use of the vaccine in the United States has drastically reduced the overall incidence of rubella, and virtually eliminated congenital rubella syndrome. However, 10% to 20% of women of childbearing age in the United States are still susceptible to rubella. During the first two months of gestation the fetus has a 65% to 85% chance of being infected with the rubella virus. The risk of development of CRS decreases to virtually nil by 20 weeks' gestation. In addition, infants born with CRS are contagious for the virus for many months after birth.

Pathophysiology

The incubation period for rubella ranges from 12 to 23 days, with viremia present 7 days before the presence of the exanthem. Within 24 to 48 hours of the development of the rash immunity develops and the virus disappears from the blood. Virus can be recovered during the viremic phase of infection from all bodily fluids. After it disappears from the blood, it continues to be shed from the nasal passages for up to 2 weeks.

When a woman in early pregnancy contracts rubella, the virus can be transmitted to the fetus through the placenta and thus entering the fetal circulation. There are four mechanisms that are thought to be responsible for the development of congenital rubella syndrome:

1. a persistent infection that causes reduced cellular mitotic activity and retardation of organ growth;
2. a vasculitis that interferes with the blood supply to developing organs;
3. direct tissue necrosis without inflammation;
4. an increased incidence of chromosomal breakage and damage.

All of these can result in fetal death, premature delivery, and/or an array of congenital defects. The severity of the outcome to a large extent is dependent on the time of infection.

Clinical Findings

A few days before the appearance of the classic rubella rash, there is usually a mild prodrome, especially in young adults. This consists of conjunctivitis, headache, low-grade fever, malaise, and tender lymphadenopathy, particularly in the posterior auricular, posterior cervical, and suboccipital chains. The adenopathy peaks during the rash and can persist for weeks to, occasionally, months afterward. These symptoms are not specific for rubella and can resemble measles, roseola, scarlet fever, toxoplasmosis, and parvovirus.

The classic rubella exanthem is a discrete pink maculopapular eruption starting on the face and spreading rapidly downward, and fading in the same order in which it appeared lasting 3 to 5 days in total. In adults, the rash can be very pruritic, which can lead to a misdiagnosis of contact dermatitis if the associated adenopathy is missed. Forscheimer's spots, which are petechial lesions of the soft palate, have also been described for rubella but unlike Koplik's spots for measles they are not diagnostic.

The prodrome, lymphadenopathy, and rash are all a part of classic rubella, but any one or all of these manifestations may not be apparent in every case. The frequency of "occult rubella" ranges from 1 in 9 in the general population to 6 in 7 in military recruits. In general, it is considered that 30% of rubella cases are subclinical and are, therefore, not detected.

Complications of acquired rubella are rare. Cases of arthritis or arthralgias have been reported in one third of women with rubella, but are rare in children and adult males. It can range from a mild arthralgia to overt arthritis, usually involving the fingers, wrists, and knees. It is generally self-limited and clears without residua in 2 to 30 days. In addition, skin and mucous membrane hemorrhage, myocarditis, pericarditis, hepatitis, hemolytic-uremic syndrome, and testicular pain have all been rarely described as associated with rubella. Encephalitis is an extremely rare complication (1 in 5,000 cases), and more likely to occur in adults. Mortality is high ranging from 20% to 50%, but survivors have a low incidence of permanent sequelae.

Congenital rubella syndrome involves every fetal organ system. The classic triad of CRS consists of sensorineural hearing loss occurring in 58% of patients, ocular abnormalities including cataracts, glaucoma and pigmentary retinopathy, and congenital heart disease, particularly patent ductus arteriosus and pulmonary artery stenosis.

Diagnosis

Rubella is typically a mild disease with nonspecific symptoms, making clinical diagnosis difficult. Acquired rubella can be clinically diagnosed with assurance only in the presence of all the classic findings, or in an epidemic. Sporadic cases are almost impossible to diagnose clinically. Specific diagnosis is usually made by serologic testing. Several tests are available for detection of the rubella antibody. A four-fold or greater rise in titers in samples obtained 1 to 2 weeks apart indicates a recent infection. The presence of antibody is a reliable indicator of past infection and therefore a presumptive indicator of immunity.

The diagnosis of congenital rubella syndrome is made by identification of a series of malformations, with serologic testing confirming rubella (in the neonate, this is usually both active IgM and passive maternal IgG). It may be necessary to perform several antibody assays on infant serum to determine whether the titer of rubella antibody is falling indicating passively acquired maternal antibody or rising indicating congenital rubella infection.

Treatment

The treatment of acquired rubella is symptomatic in the vast majority of cases with an excellent prognosis for full recovery. Supportive therapy is indicated in the event of complications. NSAIDs and rest are recommended for severe arthritis and for patients with rubella encephalitis adequate fluid and electrolyte maintenance are necessary. Bacterial complications are rare and there is no evidence that antimicrobials alter the course of uncomplicated disease.

Treatment for congenital rubella syndrome is supportive. Some manifestations, such as glaucoma and hearing loss, require early detection and intervention to ensure optimal future development. Thus vision screening and hearing screening should be provided to all asymptomatic newborns.

Prevention

The United States Public Health Advisory Committee on Immunization Practices recommends that the current live attenuated rubella vaccine be given (usually in combination with measles and mumps vaccines) to all children between the ages of 12 months and puberty; to adolescent and adult males; and to adolescent and adult females who are not pregnant (and who will not get pregnant within 3 months) and are shown to be seronegative. The first dose of MMR is given at 15 months and the second dose between 4 to 6 years. The immunization programs in the United States have decreased the transmission of rubella and have prevented major epidemics.

Vaccination during early pregnancy carries a small theoretical risk of 2% for congenital rubella syndrome. However as of 1987, a CDC study of 812 women inadvertently immunized against rubella in early pregnancy did not result in one of CRS. The vaccine is also contraindicated in patients with acute febrile illnesses or the immunocompromised. Complications of the vaccine are related to the transient viremia causing fever, adenopathy, and arthralgias. The complications are more common in adults, are mild, and are self-limited.

Human immune serum globulin has been used prophylactically to prevent rubella infection in seronegative women exposed to the virus early in pregnancy. Although IG might suppress symptoms, it wouldn't necessarily prevent the viremia; thus, its efficacy has not been established. It should not be given routinely in these situations, but it may be considered in cases where a therapeutic abortion would not be an acceptable alternative. If serologic testing confirms the presence of rubella during the first trimester of pregnancy, therapeutic abortion should be considered due to the high risk to the fetus. During the period of communicability, patients with suspected rubella should be advised to avoid contact with women of childbearing age.

Roseola

Roseola is a common pediatric exanthem. The causative agent of this disease has recently been attributed to human herpesvirus 6. It is a disease of many names; "roseola infantum," "exanthema subitum," and "sixth disease." The latter name predates its association with its herpesvirus 6. It is considered the sixth pediatric exanthem (the other five being measles, scarlet fever, rubella, atypical scarlet fever, and erythema infectiosum).

Epidemiology

HHV-6 is a very common infectious agent. It has a worldwide distribution. Estimates range that between 90% to 95% of the adult population globally is seropositive for HHV-6. The disease has been recognized for almost a century as a distinct clinical entity. It is seen almost exclusively in children less than two years of age, and it is extremely rare for it to be seen in immunocompetent children over 3 years of age. The disease has a bimodal distribution, with most cases occurring in the spring and fall. Although only about 50% of children will exhibit the symptoms of roseola infantum, greater than 85% will be seropositive for antibodies to the HHV-6 virus by their third birthday. It is well established that viral shedding occurs in saliva, but the precise mechanism by which the agent achieves its high rate of infectivity is unclear.

Clinical Findings

Roseola is a generally benign infection, which follows a characteristic course. The bulk of cases occur between 6 and 15 months of age. The first symptom of roseola is fever. Diarrhea may occur. Children may be less active, especially when febrile. Fevers with roseola tend to be high (average 103° F, 39° C). Classically, the fever lasts for 3 to 5 days (3 days is most common). With defervescence appears a fine, "rose-colored" rash. The rash is usually most prominent on the neck, trunk, back and upper arms. It may be slightly raised, but it is blanching, does not form pustules or petechiae, and is non-pruritic. The rash lasts for approximately 24 to 48 hours before resolving. Clinical symptoms may appear more from the loss of maternal antibodies than from the infecting agent alone. This might explain why there are many cases in which children seroconvert without demonstrating the classic rash. Generally, roseola is self-limited, without any significant sequelae.

Disease Associations

There have been a number of diseases that have been recently attributed to HHV-6. But the most common associations are with febrile seizures and dehydration. Rarely, liver dysfunction and encephalitis can occur. Other diseases linked to HHV-6 are chronic fatigue syndrome, "gloves-and-socks" syndrome, hypersensitivity drug reactions, Gianotti-Crosti syndrome, lymphomas, leukemia,

and multiple sclerosis. In immunocompromised patients the complications may include demyelinating diseases (especially in AIDS patients) and graft-versus-host disease in transplant patients.

Diagnosis

For almost all cases, the diagnosis of roseola is made clinically. There are a number of methods to directly and indirectly detect HHV-6. It can be cultured in lymphocytes. There exist ELISA assays but they may not differentiate well between different strains of herpesvirus. Serologically, HHV-6 IgG and IgM can be measured. Plasma PCR testing also exists to detect acute HHV-6 infections. Usually none of these tests are necessary.

Treatment

Treatment for HHV-6 infections is predominantly supportive. Fever control is utilized to keep the child comfortable and to help prevent dehydration. Although there is mounting evidence that there are antiviral agents with some activity against HHV-6 (ganciclovir and acyclovir included), the generally benign course of the disease in immunocompetent patients makes these agents not indicated in almost all cases.

Summary

Roseola is a benign, self-limited disease of infancy. It occurs almost exclusively in children less than two years of age. The disease is ubiquitous throughout human populations globally. The causative agent is human herpesvirus-6. Roseola is characterized by a three to five day febrile illness. The appearance of a fine, blanching rash on the neck and trunk after defervescence is its hallmark. There is no specific treatment for roseola.

Varicella-Zoster

Varicella-zoster virus (VZV) is a herpesvirus that causes two distinct clinical diseases. The primary infection is varicella (chickenpox), the reactivation of infection is herpes zoster (shingles). While childhood VZV remains endemic worldwide, widespread vaccination, which began in the United States in the mid-1990s, has already resulted in a marked reduction of childhood cases. It is anticipated that decreased rates of primary infection will ultimately also result in a decrease in the rate of herpes zoster and the frequently associated post-herpetic neuralgia. The severity of VZV infection in immunocompromised patients has been a major impetus for the development of preventive and treatment measures.

Epidemiology

Varicella-zoster virus has been recognized as a highly communicable disease for centuries. It occurs worldwide, and it is most prevalent in large urban centers and in temperate climates where it is most frequent in late winter and early spring. Humans are the only known species naturally infected. Most are in children ages 5 to 9. Infants under the age of 1 and adults over the age of 19 (the populations with the highest risk of complications), account for less than 3% of all cases. VZV remains an important pathogen in this country, leading to approximately 100 deaths annually.

The virus is transmitted via aerosolized respiratory secretions from a person in the early stages of varicella. Virus is also shed in the vesicle exudate, although not in the vesicle scab. Therefore, patients are generally considered to be contagious for a period extending from 4 days before the appearance of the rash to 4 to 5 days after, or until all the vesicles are crusted. Transmission from a person with herpes zoster requires direct contact with vesicle exudate.

Reactivation of VZV, which is presumed to establish latency in the dorsal root ganglia, leads to herpes zoster which occurs at a rate of 300,000 cases per year and accounts for 1.5 million physician visits per year. The incidence increases steadily with age. It is estimated that half the people who live to age 85 will have at least one episode of zoster. Approximately four percent of herpes zoster patients experience a second reactivation.

Clinical Findings

Varicella

After an incubation period of about two weeks (range 10 to 21 days) there is often a mild prodromal stage of fever and malaise 24 hours before the onset of the rash. The fever may persist for several days but rarely exceeds 39° C. Patients do not appear acutely ill, although they may be uncomfortable due to pruritus. The initial lesions are on the face and trunk with centrifugal spread as the disease progresses. The classic rash consists of a clear superficial vesicle surrounded by a halo of erythema ("dewdrop on a rose petal"), the fluid then becomes purulent, the lesion umbilicates and finally crusts over. The hallmark of this disease is the coexistence of lesions in varying stages of maturation in the same area of the body. This helps distinguish varicella from other vesicular exanthems, including smallpox.

Previously healthy children have varicella-associated mortality in less than two cases per 100,000. The risk is increased 15-fold in adults. Immunocompromised children have more severe and protracted disease and develop visceral complications in 30% to 50% of cases, with a fatality rate as high as 15%.

The most common complications of childhood varicella are due to secondary bacterial infections and CNS involvement. Bacterial infections range from relatively benign impetigo to varicella gangrenosa and necrotizing fasciitis, caused by group A streptococci, and toxigenic *S. aureus*. One must search carefully for bacterial infection in any child who presents with worsening fever, increasing rash or with any respiratory symptoms.

CNS complications occur in 1 in 5,000 children. Cerebellar ataxia is a benign, self-limited condition that presents with vomiting, ataxia, slurred speech, and tremor as late as 21 days after the rash, but usually within the first week. Meningoencephalitis is much more severe and presents with severe headache and progressive obtundation. In both cases, the CSF usually reveals lymphocytic pleocytosis and an elevated protein. EEGs in encephalopathic children are usually diffusely abnormal.

Varicella is associated with 10% to 20% of the cases of Reye's syndrome in the United States, generally when there was concomitant use of aspirin. The syndrome begins in the later stages of varicella with vomiting then irritability and progressive decrease of level of consciousness due to cerebral edema. An elevated serum ammonia level is a useful confirmatory finding.

Varicella is associated with more complications in adults than in children. The initial presentation is frequently more severe, with more pronounced malaise and a prolonged fever. In addition, adults are more likely to develop pneumonia, with 1 in 400 requiring hospitalization for it. Varicella pneumonia occurs in the vesicular stage of the disease, and chest x-ray findings of nodular opacifications and peribronchial infiltrates are usually more impressive than the clinical findings. In one study only 25% of those with radiological findings had associated symptoms of pneumonitis. Varicella pneumonia must be differentiated from a secondary bacterial pneumonia, which occurs later in the course of the infection and is generally caused by staphylococcus species.

Varicella in the immunocompromised host has a high incidence of serious complications. The acute illness is more severe, with higher fevers, a longer period of vesicle formation (10 to 14 days), and larger vesicles that often coalesce into bullae. There is a nearly 35% incidence of visceral dissemination. One fifth of these patients will die if they are not treated early with antiviral drugs. Life-threatening complications include pneumonia (varicella and bacterial), pancreatitis, bowel hemorrhage, perforation or obstruction, encephalopathy, and SIADH.

Herpes Zoster

Reactivation of VZV manifests as herpes zoster, commonly known as shingles. While this is rarely lifethreatening, its long-term sequelae are the source of significant morbidity. It begins as a unilateral sharp, burning, and well-localized pain, followed by the eruption of vesicles in a clearly defined dermatomal distribution. Thoracic dermatomes are the most commonly affected. About 10% of patients have involvement of the ophthalmic branch of the fifth cranial nerve; one fifth of these have ocular involvement. Involvement of the nasocilliary branch of the trigeminal nerve, as evidenced by lesions on the side and tip of the nose (Hutchinson's sign) mandates ophthalmologic consultation to exclude ocular involvement.

Herpes zoster lesions heal in two to three weeks, during which time the patient may experience, pain, low-grade fevers, nausea, and severe fatigue. After healing, 10% of patients have post-herpetic neuralgia, which can be disabling. It is more common in the elderly.

Complications of herpes zoster include bacterial superinfection and, rarely, dissemination. When there is ocular involvement, keratopathy can lead to corneal scarring and impairment of vision. From 1% to 5% of patients experience paralysis in the region affected by herpes zoster, due to involvement of anterior horn cells.

Herpes zoster can be severe, prolonged, and even fatal in the immunocompromised patient. Pain remains the usual presenting symptom, although the dermatomal rash may be confluent bullae. Dissemination occurs in one third of these patients. It is in itself not life threatening, but it may herald the development of visceral herpes zoster, which occurs in 10% of patients with dissemination.

Diagnosis

A diagnosis of varicella can usually be made based on clinical findings, coupled with the typical history of exposure. The differential diagnosis includes measles (which may have vesicles), group A coxsackieviruses (which usually occurs during the enteroviral season in late summer or early fall and has a more peripheral distribution), insect bites, scabies, and, theoretically, smallpox (which has all lesions at the same stage). Secondary impetigo can also make the diagnosis difficult. The variety of lesions in different stages of development, however, is usually diagnostic. Definitive diagnosis can be achieved by isolation of the VZV virus. A Tzanck smear can identify multinucleated giant cells which are found in all herpesvirus infections.

Treatment

Varicella

Varicella in the previously healthy child usually runs a benign five- to ten-day course. Treatment has been mainly symptomatic. Pruritus is treated with drying agents and occasionally antihistamines. Fever can be treated with acetaminophen, but aspirin is contraindicated. Aspirin should be avoided due to its association with Reye's syndrome. Complications such as varicella gangrenosa and bullous varicella require hospitalization. The use of acyclovir to treat varicella in the normal child remains controversial. While treatment reduces the duration of fever, lesion formation, and total number of lesions, the clinical significance and public health implications of this are unclear. Routine treatment with acyclovir is probably not warranted in the previously healthy child between 2 and 12 years of age. Secondary pediatric cases within one family tend to be more severe than the primary case and may benefit more from antiviral treatment.

Primary VZV infections in adolescents, adults, and the immunocompromised should be promptly treated with antiviral medication, ideally started within 24 hours of the appearance of the rash.

The immunocompromised patient with primary VZV infection requires intravenous antiviral therapy. Evidence of visceral dissemination in any patient should be aggressively treated. Antiviral therapy is probably not useful in the treatment of neurological complications, because these do not appear to be the result of viral replication in the CNS.

Treatment with acyclovir does not appear to prevent development of varicella in those who have been exposed to the virus, and there is no evidence that any antiviral treatment prevents the subsequent development of herpes zoster.

Herpes Zoster

Treatment of herpes zoster in the normal host consists mainly of pain reduction and the prevention of postherpetic neuralgia. Adequate hydration is important and may be difficult, especially in the debilitated elderly patient. High-dose oral acyclovir has been shown to shorten the course of the acute zoster if started early enough (within 2 to 3 days of the onset of the rash), and it decreases the rate of complications of trigeminal herpes zoster. Valacyclovir and famciclovir appear to be superior to acyclovir for acceleration of cutaneous healing and are at least as effective for resolution of pain. Topical acyclovir is not recommended for the treatment of herpes zoster. While steroids should not be used alone to treat herpes zoster, there is evidence that when added to acyclovir they decrease symptoms.

In the immunocompromised host, the goal of herpes zoster treatment is to reduce complications, especially dissemination and subsequent mortality. Since there is no way to identify who is at risk for dissemination, and since the occurrence rate ranges from 10% to 50%, all immunocompromised patients with herpes zoster require at least high-dose oral acyclovir, valacyclovir or famciclovir and close follow-up. Many will benefit from intravenous acyclovir.

Acute neuritis and post-herpetic neuralgia are managed with analgesics ranging from acetaminophen and NSAIDs to narcotic medications. Patients should be referred to their primary care providers for the ongoing management of post-herpetic pain.

Prevention

In the United States a vaccine was approved in 1995. Since 1996 it has been recommended that routine administration be carried out between 12 and 18 months of age. Immunization of older, varicella-susceptible persons is strongly encouraged. Elective vaccine administration is now recommended for healthy susceptible persons within 96 hours following an exposure to varicella. Routine screening of health care workers and elective vaccination of those susceptible has effectively prevented disease in this population. Exposed seronegative health care workers must be removed from patient areas from day 10 to day 21 after exposure.

While this live attenuated vaccine is both safe and effective in normal, healthy hosts, it is contraindicated for immunocompromised patients, pregnant women, anyone allergic to any of its components or anyone on chronic aspirin therapy. Varicella-zoster immune globulin (VZIG) should be given to persons with a significant exposure to varicella, if they are immunocompromised and not previously exposed to varicella; to women who are pregnant and known to be seronegative; or to newborns whose mothers have had the onset of varicella within five days before delivery or up to 48 hours postpartum.

Herpes Simplex Virus

Infections due to herpes simplex virus (HSV) are very common. Humans are considered the only natural reservoir for HSV, a DNA virus. The resultant infections vary from mild cases of oro-labial herpetic lesions (cold sores), to more serious genital ulcers or to devastating infections of the visceral organs and disseminated disease. Two identified serotypes of the virus are HSV-1 and HSV-2. HSV-1 is the main causative pathogen for labial and gingivostomatitis herpes and is transmitted predominantly through oral secretions. HSV-2 the causative pathogen for genital herpes and its main mode of transmission is by sexual contact. Each serotype possesses a distinctly unique and different glycoprotein G (gG) in its envelope protein. Most patients with genital herpes are not aware of their infection status, partly due to the disease presenting in a mild or atypical pattern. For the same reason, the misdiagnosis of genital herpes by health care providers is also a common occurrence.

Epidemiology

HSV has a variable distribution worldwide. Universally, the prevalence of HSV-1 has been estimated at a rate of 80.5%. The reported prevalence of HSV-2 in industrialized countries has been non-uniform, with a traditionally lower rate in Western Europe (5% to 10% sero-positivity in general population) and a higher rate in United States (22% sero-positivity in general population). Genital herpes is the most common sexually transmitted disease (STD) in this country. HVS-2 genital infections are at epidemic levels in the United States. In 1990, the CDC estimated that at least 25% of population over 20 years may be infected with HSV-2. This percentage has increased in the last 14 years. According to the recent National Health and Nutritional Examination Survey (NHANES III), 20% of white women, 15% of white men, 55% of African American women, and 35% of African American men were seropositive for HSV-2. More than a million new cases are diagnosed annually.

Although fairly common, HSV-1 can be encountered more frequently in specific occupations, including dentistry, oral hygienists, and respiratory therapists. Recent reports have identified participation in contact sports, specifically wrestling, as another risk factor for HSV-1 infections. The transmission rate for HSV-1 to a wrestling sparing partner is estimated to be about 40%. In these cases, the transmission is predominantly by direct skin-to-skin contact, and not through contact with the saliva on the wrestling mat. Risk factors for acquisition of HSV-2 infections have traditionally been considered female gender, African American race, individuals of lower socio-economic status, sexual history, and previous STD infections. However, recent findings have altered conventional stereotyping. Studies have identified high prevalence of HSV-2 seropositivity in relatively affluent suburban population (25%). Higher-level education or income, and marital status are not associated with lower risk for genital herpes. In is noteworthy that seropositivity has consistently been reported at a higher rate among women than men (28.3% versus 22.0%). Age is also an independent indicator for the prevalence of infection. The lowest rate of seropositivity has been reported in 18- to 29-year age group (13.4%) and the highest rate in 40- to 49-year age group (31.2%). In the past few years, various reports have suggested an increase in the incidence of HSV-1 as the causative virus for genital herpes. This epidemiological change has been attributed to the increase in practice of oro-genital sex in younger adults and

perhaps to a declining incidence of HSV-1 infection in childhood. Majority of the HSV-1 genital herpes occur in younger women, with 71% of the isolates being procured from females younger than 30 years of age, compared to only 5% in women older than 60 years of age. Bacterial vaginosis (BV) should also be considered as an independent predictor for the acquisition of genital herpes. In one study, 42% of patients with BV were sero-positive for HSV-2, compared to only 15% of patients without BV ($P < .001$). This link was more prominent in younger women and a new sexual partner.

HSV-2 should be considered as an independent risk factor for HIV infection. The risk of HIV acquisition is increased by 2 to 5 times in persons who are seropositive for HSV-2. Conversely, patients who are seropositive for both HIV and HSV transmit HIV more efficiently and have an increased rate of HIV replication.

A major contributing factor to propagation and universal spread of HVS infections is the often "invisible" nature of the disease. A large portion of the patients are not aware of their "chronic" infection. The "classic" ulcerative lesions are manifested in a relatively small number (less than 20%) of the patients. Majority of infections are either "atypical" or asymptomatic. In the National Health and Nutritional Examination Survey III (1988–1994), of the 22% who were seropositive for HSV-2, fewer than 10% reported a history of genital herpes. In another study, where a more than 40% HSV-2 seropositivity was identified, 90% of patients were never diagnosed to have genital herpes. Asymptomatic HSV shedding is a major contributor to the spread of the virus and most viral transmission occurs during these asymptomatic periods.

Pathology

HVS replicates locally and propagates intracellularly. Subsequently it results in cellular lysis and damage, multinucleated infected cells, and localized inflammatory process. Depending on the patient's immune status, the disease may be complicated by viremia, visceral organ involvement or by a disseminated viral infection. Once infected, the patient will remain infected for life. After the primary infection, HSV may become latent and dwell within the sensory nerve ganglion sites. The latency period may last for weeks or years. However, viral reactivations and secondary recurrences, specifically in HVS-2 infections, are common. Predisposing factors include physical or emotional stress, pregnancy, menstruation, excessive sunlight, local trauma, immunosuppression or fever. The frequency of recurrent episodes depends on gender, HSV serotype, and the titer of HSV neutralizing antibody.

Clinical Presentation

HSV infections predominantly affect the mucocutaneous tissues and resultant lesions may appear anywhere on the mucocutaneous area. The majority of lesions present on the oro-labial, ocular, and genital areas. HSV may also infect the CNS, and occasionally other visceral organs, i.e., liver. Disseminated forms of the disease can be encountered in immunosuppressed patients. Organ transplant patients, malnutrition, and AIDS are considered high risk for disseminated disease. In these situations, esophagitis, pneumonia or encephalitis may be the main manifestation of the infection.

HSV-1 Infections

The incubation period for *primary* HSV-1 infection is anywhere between 2 to 12 days. The symptoms generally start with a prodromal period, usually lasting less than 6 hours. The symptoms include localized tingling, burning, discomfort, or itching. Subsequently small tense vesicle(s) filled with clear fluid appear on an erythematous base on the lips, gingiva, tongue or oropharyngeal areas. The lesions can be isolated in single clusters, varying in size between 0.5 to 1.5 centimeters. Lesions may also coalesce. The infectious presentation may mimic an acute pharyngitis in adults or acute gingivostomatitis in infants and young children. In this group of patients the resultant ulceration of the gingiva and mouth is extremely painful. These patients may also manifest anorexia, irritability, and fever, and may be misdiagnosed as having sepsis. Vesicular lesions on the vermilion margin of the lips are highly suggestive of herpes labialis. Similar lesions may also appear on the skin. Lesions of the ear and nose are particularly painful. By means of finger sucking and nail biting, children may re-inoculate themselves and develop painful lesions on the distal phalanx of their finger(s). These lesions are known as herpetic whitlow. These same lesions may also be seen in health care workers. At this stage of primary disease, systemic signs, such as fever, chills, malaise, headache, and palpable tender cervical adenopathy, are also fairly common. The lesion(s) will eventually become flaccid and subsequently "un-roof." At this stage, a yellowish crust usually covers the lesions. In a matter of 8 to 14 days, the lesion(s) subsides spontaneously and the recovery will be complete and without any scarring.

Excluding the neonatal age, the majority of cases of herpetic encephalitis are caused by HSV-1. Encephalitis is a rare complication of HSV-1 infection. The transmission of the disease occurs through the direct spread of virus to the brain via the neural routes. The clinical presentation includes fever, headache, change in behavior and personality, and focal seizures. The temporal lobes are usually the primary sites of the infection. If undiagnosed or left untreated, the mortality can exceed 60%.

Recurrent labial and gingivostomatitis HSV-1 infections are due to reactivation of the virus and are usually milder in severity. The patient may initially feel either itching, burning, or a tingling sensation. The subsequent occurrence of the vesicles is not usually associated with any systemic symptoms. The duration of recurrent disease is approximately 8 to 10 days. Recovery is complete. However, frequent recurrent attacks may result in atrophy and scarring.

HSV-1 may also infect the eye. Dendritic keratitis is the hallmark of primary HSV-1 eye infection. Ocular involvement is usually unilateral and mainly affects the conjunctivae or the cornea. The patient with follicular conjunctivitis presents with "red eye," photophobia, and swelling and tenderness of the eyelids. Corneal infections manifest with corneal opacifications. In these patients, fluorescein staining will reveal dendritic ulcerations in the involved cornea. The symptoms and signs usually last for 2 to 3 weeks. With proper therapy, recovery is complete and without any expected sequelae. The use of steroid drops in these patients is contraindicated, may result in worsening of infection and potentially perforation of the involved eye.

Recurrent HSV-1 eye infections may manifest as uveitis, keratitis, blepharitis, or keratoconjunctivitis. It may also present with involvement of deeper eye tissues and proceed to scarring, neovascularization, corneal opacification, and blindness.

HSV-2 Infections

Seventy to 95% of all genital herpes are due to HSV-2 infections. The incubation period for primary HSV-2 infections is anywhere between 2 to 7 days. Patients may experience prodromal symptoms similar to HSV-1 infections. The "typical" presentation of HSV-2 infections can be classified into two groups. The first group, known as primary genital herpes, occurs in patients who do not have any antibody to HSV-1 or HSV-2. These patients experience a severe and relatively prolonged course of disease. The manifestations of the disease may exceed 3 weeks. In patients with primary genital herpes who have been previously infected with HSV-1 infection and are sero-positive for antibody to HSV-1, the presentation of primary HSV-2 infection is modified and the disease will manifest itself in a "milder" form. This second group, known as recurrent genital herpes, consists of secondary attacks that traditionally last for 7 to 10 days. In this group the symptoms are less severe and systemic signs are usually absent. In majority of cases, the recurrent episodes are preceded by symptoms such as itching, tingling, or pain hours to days before the eruption of the herpetic lesions. When compared to HSV-1, the recurrent episodes occur at a significantly higher rate in HSV-2.

The "typical" clear fluid filled vesicles are predominantly manifested, in a cluster format, on the vulva and cervix in women and on the prepoce and glans penis in men. These vesicles develop on an erythematous base and are extremely painful. The ano-rectal manifestations of the primary HSV-2 disease, in both heterosexual and homosexual patients, include vesicular lesions on the anus or perianal regions. These patients present with tenesmus, pain, itching, drainage, or anal leakage. They may develop ulcerative lesions of the anus or perianal area. Systemic signs, such as fever, chills, malaise, arthralgia, myalgia, photophobia, neck stiffness, and headache occur quite frequently in conjunction with the primary infections. Painful regional adenopathy is also fairly common and may become ulcerative. The disease may be complicated by hepatitis and by self-limiting aseptic meningitis. Autonomic neuropathy and involvement of sacral plexus (lumbosacral myeloradiculitis syndrome) is manifested with abnormalities of bowel and bladder emptying, such as urinary retention or incontinence and obstipation. Anesthesia of the region innervated by sacral nerve may also occur. In a small portion of cases, HSV-2 may be the causative agent for herpes labialis. In patients with AIDS or other immunocompromised states, HSV-2 infections can become very serious and may manifest as acute pneumonia, severe hepatitis, progressive esophagitis, colitis, perianal lesions, and various neurological syndromes.

A large percentage of either primary or recurrent genital herpes manifest themselves in an "atypical" form. These presentations may include skin splits and fissures, minor abrasions, non descript erythematous and painful lesions, "jock itch" or ill-defined discharge. These manifestations are the most common form and the predominant pattern of genital herpes presentation.

Pregnancy and Neonatal HSV Infection

In general the overall health of most immunocompetent patients, who acquire HSV during their pregnancy, is not significantly affected in an adverse manner. However, occurrence of life-threatening disseminated HSV infections in previously healthy pregnant women has been reported. Although rare, majority of these infections occur during the third trimester of the pregnancy. In most cases, the symptoms are nonspecific and mucocutaneous signs are absent. These patients are frequently febrile and reveal elevated serum transaminases without any elevation in bilirubin. If untreated, mortality rate may exceed 63%. Death usually occurs around 31 weeks' gestation. HSV-2 and HIV co-infection is also fairly common in pregnant patients. Additionally near delivery recurrent HSV infections occur at a higher rate in HIV positive patients. All HIV patients, who are HSV seronegative, must be closely monitored for acquisition of primary HSV infection.

The most dangerous and debilitating of HSV infections occur in neonatal form. HSV infected neonates suffer from significantly high morbidity and mortality. Annually in the United States, approximately 1,600 to 2,000 neonates develop neonatal HSV infection. The majority of the neonatal HSV infections are caused by HSV-2. In 30% of cases, HSV-1 is the responsible pathogen. The overall risk of acquisition of HSV-2 from a previously infected mother or with a case of recurrent genital herpes is relatively low (<1%). However, considering the prevalence of HSV-2 infections, even such a low transmission rate translates into a large number of neonatal HSV-2 infections. In pregnant women who acquire a primary HSV-2 infection, this risk increases precipitously. This risk increases even more if the infection happens during the third trimester of pregnancy, specifically if the occurrence of the infection is near the time of the delivery. The transmission rate in this subset of neonates may exceed 50%.

Pregnant women experience a higher incidence of recurrent genital herpes. Furthermore, the rate of asymptomatic viral shedding also increases with pregnancy, specifically during third trimester. The prominent site of this shedding is the vulva. The cervix is another site for viral shedding. The majority of neonatal HSV cases occur secondary to retrograde exposure to virus in asymptomatic women. In a minority of cases, contact with active herpetic lesions is the cause of this disease. About 4% of neonatal HVS infections result from intrauterine transmission of virus from the mother's blood to the fetus. These congenital cases may be complicated by jaundice, intrauterine growth retardation, low birth weight, chorioretinitis, vesicular skin lesions, hydrocephaly, and microcephaly. Vertical viral transmission may also occur through amniotic fluid, secondary to premature rupture of membranes (PRM). Coincidentally PRM may happen at a higher rate in HSV-2 infected pregnant patients.

Neonatal HSV infections can arrange from mild localized infections to fatal disseminated cases. Its incidence has been estimated to be 1 in 5,000 live births. Neonatal HSV infections are divided in the following three distinct categories: lesions of skin, eye, and mouth (SEM disease), CNS disease, and disseminated viral disease. In the past 20 years the epidemiology of neonatal HSV infections has changed. There has been an increase in the incidence of SEM disease and a decline in the number of cases of disseminated disease. The incidence of CNS disease has remained unchanged. SEM is the mildest form of the three categories and is manifested by conjunctivitis and lesions of skin and the mouth. With appropriate antiviral therapy a complete recovery should be expected. The morbidity rate in SEM disease is less than 5%. If untreated patients or if initiation of therapy is delayed, 75% of the SEM cases will progress to the CNS or disseminated diseases. CNS disease is predominantly manifested as encephalitis. Clinical presentation includes fever for 2 to 3 weeks followed by lethargy, cranial nerve palsies, poorly controllable focal seizures, and eventually coma. The CSF is bloody and has elevated white cells and protein. Even with proper therapy, patients with CNS disease will suffer from long-term morbidities such as spasticity, blindness, focal seizures, psychomotor retardation, and learning disabilities. In this patient population, the onset of seizures or infections caused by HSV-2 is independent indicators for a poor outcome. The disseminated disease is the most severe form of neonatal HVS infection and can involve various organs including the CNS, liver, lungs, adrenal glands, skin, mouth, and eyes. Patients are frequently febrile and present with hepatomegaly and concomitant abnormalities of liver function, pneumonia and respiratory distress. Skin lesions are also a common finding. These cases are often misdiagnosed as a bacterial sepsis. In spite of aggressive therapy, the mortality rate in CNS and disseminated diseases is high and has been reported as 15% and 57%, respectively.

Herpes Simplex-Associated Erythema Multiforme (HAEM)

A subset of erythema multiforme (EM) can be caused by HSV infections. It has been suggested that these lesions occur secondary to the autoreactive T-cells that are triggered by HSV.

Diagnosis Despite high prevalence, the diagnosis of HSV infections can be challenging. Studies have proven that diagnosis of HSV infection based on clinical findings has a very poor sensitivity, rarely exceeding 40%.

Laboratory diagnostic methods fall in the following categories:

Direct methods depend on direct acquisition of samples from the site of the infection. To be accurate, these samples should be obtained from a fresh crop of lesions and no later than the vesicular stage. In recurrent infections the sensitivity of these tests is further reduced.

Cytological methods: By scraping a potential herpetic lesion, a Tzanck smear can be obtained. In 50% of cases, the subsequent staining of this sample with Wright-Giesma stain will reveal multinucleated giant cells. This inexpensive, rapid, and simple method has a high rate of false negativity. In symptomatic patients, the Tzanck smear can be utilized to provide additional evidence for the presence of a herpetic lesion.

Currently, obtaining *viral cultures* is the principal method for the reliable and readily available diagnosis of heretic infections. The test can also be utilized, as a relatively easy tool, to differentiate between HVS-1 and HSV-2 infections. Its 100% specificity makes it an ideal test. However, its sensitivity hardly exceeds 75% in primary infections and 50% in recurrent infections. The culture should only be obtained from the active lesions. The sensitivity will further decline if cultures are obtained from healing lesions. The high prevalence of "atypical" presentation of HSV-2 infections also has a negative impact on the value of this test as a diagnostic tool. Furthermore, viral cultures can not be utilized in asymptomatic patients. Considering the specificity of the test and the relative ease of its procurement, cultures should always be obtained.

Indirect Serological Methods

Western Blot Assay is the gold standard for the identification of type-specific HSV antibodies. Its specificity and sensitivity is close to 100%. It is also the fastest commercially available test in detecting sero-conversion. Unfortunately, it is not performed in all laboratories. This test is relatively difficult to perform, is expensive, and usually takes 2 to 5 days to complete.

Enzyme immunoassays are based on crude antigenic preparations, so the tests lack type-specificity and cannot differentiate between a HSV-1 and HSV-2 infection.

Glycoprotein G-Based immunoassays are type-specific tests that detect the glycoprotein G in the envelope protein of the virus. The assays respond to the specific glycoproteins that are found in HSV-1 (gG1) and HSV-2 (gG2) and antigenically differentiate these two infections. These tests compare favorably with Western Blot Assay.

POCkit HSV-2 rapid test can identify the presence of HSV-2 infection within 10 minutes. In general, the test will detect HSV-2 antibodies within 2 weeks. However, its response time may vary, from 3 to 102 days. The test's specificity and sensitivity is 97% and 96%, respectively. Its ability to detect HSV-2 related IgM antibody makes it a valuable tool in detection of primary infections.

HSV-1 and HSV-2 PCR: Viral DNA detection by means of PCR is still very much considered as a research tool. However, its 100% specificity and very high sensitivity makes it a very attractive diagnostic tool. It can be a very valuable tool in diagnosis of neonatal HSV infections, specifically the CNS disease, and can eliminate the need for invasive brain biopsy. PCR is not yet standardized among different laboratories.

In accordance with the latest related guidelines, the symptomatic patients who are suspected of having a HSV infection should undergo a direct diagnostic test. Should this test reveal a negative result, these patients may further benefit from a type-specific antibody test for HSV-2. In the recent CDC treatment guideline for treatment of sexually transmitted diseases, the type-specific serologic tests are considered useful, "in confirming a diagnosis of genital herpes."

Treatment *Labial* and *gingivostomatitis herpes* lesions are best treated with in a palliative manner. Topical analgesics, such as viscous Xylocaine, can alleviate the initial painful episodes. Patients will also benefit from warm saline rinses and avoidance of caustic agents. Patients with severely painful oral lesions must be assessed for dehydration. Use of topical antiviral agents, such as acyclovir and penciclovir, is not recommended. Furthermore, the use of oral acyclovir in herpes labialis has not been extensively studied. Immunocompetent adults suffering from a primary attack however may be prescribed oral acyclovir (Zovirax) 200 mg 5 times per day for 5 to 7 days. Another alternative is oral valacyclovir (Valtrex) 2 g twice a day for 5 to 7 days. In children with primary HSV infection, oral acyclovir can be used (15 mg/kg 5 times per day for 5 to 7 days). Infrequently recurrent episodes of herpes labialis may respond to therapy with acyclovir. All patients with labial and gingivo-stomatitis herpes must be assessed for secondary bacterial infection. Superficial bacterial infections should be treated with topical antibiotics and more severe bacterial infections with systemic antibiotics.

In *genital herpes*, the recommended therapy for primary lesions is oral acyclovir 400 mg 3 times per day for 7 to 10 days. Other alternatives include oral valacyclovir 1 g twice per day for 7 to 10 days, or oral famciclovir (Famvir) 250 mg three times per day for 7 to 10 days. For recurrent episodes, the choices of antiviral medications are oral acyclovir 400 mg three times per day for 5 days; valacyclovir 500 mg twice per day for 3 days; or oral famciclovir 125 mg twice per day for 5 days. Although these abbreviated regimens will ameliorate the severity of the presentation of the diseases they do not affect the frequency or severity of the recurrent episodes. The best therapeutic response with oral acyclovir in recurrent herpes labialis is seen in immunocompromised patients. In this subset of patients, oral antiviral therapy can suppress the frequent recurrent episodes. The most recent CDC guidelines support the use of shorter and/or less frequent dosing regimens of valacyclovir therapy. However, with the persistent lesions or recurrence of new lesions, the therapy should be extended to 5 days. As a matter of convenience, valacyclovir can be dosed at 1,000 mg once a day, rather than 500 mg twice daily. A shorter course of therapy with acyclovir (800 mg three times daily for 2 days) has also been approved and is effective in shortening of the duration and severity of the clinical presentations.

The treatment of choice for *primary diffuse mucocutaneous, labial,* or *gingivostomatitis HSV*, specifically in immunocompromised hosts, includes intravenous acyclovir 5 mg/kg every 8 hours for 7 days; oral famciclovir 500 mg twice per day for 7 days; or valacyclovir 500 to 1,000 mg twice per day for 7 days. There is no requirement for dose adjustment of acyclovir, famciclovir, and valacyclovir in immunocompromised patients.

Under the direct supervision of an ophthalmologist, the treatment of *herpetic keratoconjunctivitis* lesions consist of topical 1% trifluridine (Viroptic) eye drops, 2 drops every one hour 9 times per day for 3 weeks. In afflicted children, the treatment of choice is vidarabine ointment 5 times per day for 3 weeks. If started within 72 hours of the eruption of vesicles, oral acyclovir (800 mg five times per day for 10 days) decreases the incidence of ocular complications in ophthalmic zoster. Reactivation of herpetic ocular infections, manifested with iritis and stromal keratitis, will mandate immediate ophthalmological referral. HSV retinal lesions and acute retinal necrosis must be treated with intravenous acyclovir 10 to 20 mg/kg every 8 hours for 5 to 7 days, followed by oral acyclovir 800 mg, 5 times per day for 6 weeks.

The recommended treatment for *herpetic encephalitis* is intravenous acyclovir 10 mg/kg every 8 hours for 14 to 21 days.

Herpetic perineal infections must be treated with intravenous acyclovir 10 mg/kg every 8 hours for 10 to 21 days.

Herpetic Whitlow is treated with oral acyclovir 400 mg three times per day for 10 days. Other alternatives include valacyclovir or famciclovir.

In patients with frequent recurrent episodes *herpetic suppression therapy* may include either oral acyclovir 400 mg twice a day; oral valacyclovir 500 to 1,000 mg once a day; or oral famciclovir 250 mg twice a day.

Although relatively rare, in the presence of either suspected or confirmed *acyclovir resistance* HSV, the antiviral therapy must be substituted with intravenous foscarnet 40 mg/kg every 8 to 12 hours for 2 to 3 weeks.

Prevention   Abstinence from sexual activity, when lesions are present, is the first line of defense toward acquisition of HSV infection. However, majority of viral transmission occur secondary to the asymptomatic shedding of the virus.

Vaccine   Development of various HSV vaccines are in the experimental phase and are currently undergoing clinical trials. The initial reports from these trials have demonstrated either no protection or only partial protection against HVS-2 infections. The available vaccine has proven to be immunogenic and induce high titers of neutralizing antibody response. However, its cell-mediated immune responses have been variable. The vaccine has been only effective in HSV-1 and HSV-2 seronegative women, with efficacy rates of about 70%. It has not revealed any benefit in HSV-1 seropositive women and men. The overall reduction in seroconversion has been reported as 40%. The protective effect of the vaccine is short-lived and lasts only for 5 months.

Antiviral Prophylactic Therapy   In clinical trials use of valacyclovir (500 mg PO daily for 8 months) in infected partner has significantly reduced the rate of HSV seroconversion (50%) and symptomatic genital herpes (77%) in the uninfected heterosexual monogamous part-

ner. The absolute rate of seroconversion was reported at 2% over 8 months. It is known that valacyclovir reduces the frequency of asymptomatic HSV-2 viral shedding and the viral load during the symptomatic presentation of the disease. Sixty percent of infected patients did not have any recurrent infection during the 8-month period. Prior to the initiation of prophylactic therapy, the "uninfected" sexual partner should undergo a type-specific serological testing to confirm susceptibility to HSV-2. An asymptomatic seropositivity status will obviate the need for prophylactic therapy. In persons with 10 or more annual symptomatic genital herpes outbreaks or in patients who experience symptomatic outbreaks on 500 mg daily dosage, the dosage of valacyclovir should be increased to 1 g per day. This medication is very safe and has been used continuously for 12 months. However, it may cause nausea, headache, or abdominal pain.

Managing Pregnant Women   Considering the potential for neonatal HSV infections' high morbidity and mortality, all pregnant women should be screened and counseled for acquisition of HSV-2 infection. Involved health care providers must be aware of the pregnant woman's HSV status by the beginning of the third trimester, preferentially before week 28. Careful examination of the pregnant patient for the presence of a herpetic lesion at the time of delivery should be considered a requirement. It should be mentioned that only 50% of patients who report a history of genital herpes actually are infected with HSV. Pending the commercial availability of inexpensive tests, universal type-specific serologic HSV testing has been proposed.

It is also important to differentiate between primary and recurrent genital herpes during pregnancy. This task can be accomplished by obtaining a type-specific serologic HSV test. At the time of occurrence of the herpetic lesions, this test will be negative in primary disease.

All efforts should be aimed toward the prevention of the transmission of HSV from mother to the infant. The current prevention strategies include serologic screening of pregnant women, use of antiviral prophylaxis, and cesarean section delivery. The two strategies most accepted by authorities are cesarean section delivery in pregnant women who are manifesting active herpetic lesions or prodromal symptoms, and use of prophylactic antiviral agents in pregnant women with gestational genital herpes.

Selected Readings

Allain JP, Laurian Y, Paul DA, et al. Serological markers in early stages of human immunodeficiency virus infection in haemophiliacs. *Lancet* 1986;2:1233–1236.

Anderson JP. Clinical aspects on Epstein-Barr virus infection. *Scand J Infect Dis Suppl* 1991;78:94–104.

Anderson LJ, Nicholson KG, et al. Human rabies in the United States, 1960 to 1979: epidemiology, diagnosis, and prevention. *Ann Intern Med* 1984;100: 728–735.

Aurelian L, Ono F, Burnett J. Herpes simplex virus (HSV)-associated erythema multiforme (HAEM): A viral disease with an autoimmune component. *Dermatol Online J* 2003;9:1.

Bailey RE. Diagnosis and treatment of infectious mononucleosis. *Am Fam Phys* 1994;49:879–885.

Bonthius, DJ. Meningitis and encephalitis in children. An update. *Neurol Clin* 2002;20:1013–1038.

Centers for Disease Control and Prevention. 1993 revised classification system for HIV infection and expanded surveillance case definition for AIDS among adolescents and adults. *Morb Mort Wkly Rep* 1992;41.

Centers for Disease Control and Prevention. Case definitions for infectious conditions under public health surveillance. *Morb Mort Wkly Rep* 1997;46:5–6.

Centers for Disease Control and Prevention. *HIV/AIDS Surveillance Report* 2002; 14:1–9.

Centers for Disease Control and Prevention. Management of possible sexual, injecting-drug use, or other nonoccupational exposure to HIV, including considerations related to antiretroviral therapy. Public Health Service statement. *Morb Mort Wkly Rep* 1998;47:1–14.

Centers for Disease Control and Prevention. Sexually transmitted diseases treatment guidelines. *Morb Mort Wkly Rep* 2002;51:26–27.

Centers for Disease Control and Prevention. Updated U.S. Public Health Service guidelines for the management of occupational exposures to HBV, HCV, and HIV and recommendations for postexposure prophylaxis. *Morb Mort Wkly Rep* 2001;50:1–42.

Centers for Disease Control and Prevention. U.S. Public Health Service guidelines for the prevention of opportunistic infection in persons infected with HIV. *Morb Mort Wkly Rep* 1995;44:1–44.

Cesario TC, Yousefi S. Viral infections. *Clin Geriatr Med* 1992;8:735–737.

Chen TM. Clinical manifestations of varicella-zoster virus infection. *Dermatol Clins* 2002;20.

Cherry JD. Contemporary infectious exanthems. *Clin Infect Dis* 1993;16:199–205.

Connelly KP, DeWitt LD. Neurological complications of infectious mononucleosis. *Pediatr Neurol* 1994;10:181–184.

Corey L, Langenberg AG, Ashley R, et al. Recombinant glycoprotein vaccine for the prevention of genital HSV-2 infection: two randomized controlled trials. *JAMA* 1999;282:331–340.

Corey L, Tyring S, Beutner K, et al. Once daily valacyclovir reduces transmission of genital herpes. Presented at the program and abstracts of 42nd Annual Interscience Conference on Antimicrobial Agents and Chemotherapy; September 27–30, 2002, San Diego, CA.

Cordes RJ, Ryan ME. Pitfalls in HIV testing: application and limitations of current tests. *Postgrad Med* 1995;98:177–180.

Dannemann B, McCutchan JA, et al. Treatment of toxoplasmic encephalitis in patients with AIDS. A randomized trial comparing pyrimethamine plus clindamycin to pyrimethamin plus sulfadiazine. *Ann Intern Med* 1992;116:33–43.

Darras-Joly C, Chevret S, Wolff M, et al. Cryptococcus neoformans infection in France: epidemiologic features of and early prognostic parameters for 76 patients who were infected with human immunodeficiency virus. *Clin Infect Dis* 1996:23: 369–376.

Fishbein DB, Baer GM. Animal rabies: implications for diagnosis and human treatment. *Ann Intern Med* 1988;109:935–937.

Fishbein DB, Robinson LE. Rabies. *N Engl J Med* 1993;329:1632–1638.

Flegg PJ, Laing RB, Lee C, et al. Disseminated disease due to Mycobacterium avium complex in AIDS. *Q J Med* 1995;88:617–626.

Freij BJ, South MA, Sever JL. Maternal Rubella and the congenital rubella syndrome. *Clin Perinatol* 1988;15:247–257.

Gable EK "Pediatric exanthems." *Prim Care* 2000;27:353–369

Gershon AA. Rubella virus (German measles). In: Mandell GL, Bennett JE, Dolin R, eds. *Principles and Practices of Infectious Diseases*, 5th ed. New York: Churchill Livingstone 2000:1708–1713.

Gold E. Almost extinct diseases: measles, mumps, rubella, and pertussis. *Pediatric Rev* 1996;17:120–127.

Gozlan M. Update on HIV transmission and pathogenesis. *Lancet* 1995;346:1290.

Gruden JF, Huang L, Turner J. High-resolution CT in evaluation of clinically suspected Pneumocystis carinii pneumonia in AIDS patients with normal, equivocal, or nonspecific radiographic findings. *Am J Roentgenol* 1997;169: 967–975.

Hattwick MAW, Rubin RH, Music S, et al. Postexposure rabies prophylaxis with human rabies immune globulin. *JAMA* 1974;227:407–410.

Hattwick MA, Hochberg FH, et al. Skunk-associated human rabies. *JAMA* 1972; 222:44–47.

Hayden GF, Preblud SR, et al. Current status of mumps and mumps vaccine in the United States. *Pediatrics* 1978;62:965–969.

Helmick CG. The epidemiology of human rabies postexposure prophylaxis, 1980-1981. *JAMA* 1983;250:1990–1996.

Hermans P, Clumeck M. Kaposi's sarcoma in patients infected with human virus (HIV): an overview. *Cell Mol Biol* 1995;41:357–364.

Herrmann KL. Rubella in the United States: toward a strategy for disease control and elimination. *Epidemiol Infect* 1991;107:55–61.

Houff SA, Burton RC, Wilson RW, et al. Human-to-human transmission of rabies virus by corneal transplant. *N Engl J Med* 1979;300:603–604.

Jacobson MA. Human immunodeficiency virus-associated immune reconstitution disease. *Am J Med* 2001;110:662–663.

Johnson RT. The pathogenesis of HIV infections in the brain. *Curr Top Microbiol Immunol* 1995;202:3–10.

Johnson RW. Treatment of herpes zoster and post herpetic neuralgia. *Brit Med J* 2003;326:748–750.

Kalama WC, De Wit S, O'Doherty E, et al. Pyrimethamin-clindamycin vs. pyrimethamine-sulfadiazine as acute and long-term therapy for toxoplasmic encephalitis in patients with AIDS. *Clin Infect Dis* 1996;22:268–275.

Kimberlin DW. Rubella Immunization. *Pediatr Ann* 1997;26:366–730.

Koch WC. Fifth (human parvovirus) and sixth (herpesvirus 6) diseases. *Curr Opin Infect Dis* 2001;14:343–356.

LaForce FM, et al. Influenza: virology, epidemiology, disease, and prevention. *Am J Prev Med* 1994;10:31–40.

LaRussa P. The success of varicella vaccine. *Pediatr Ann* 2002;31:710–715.

Lindegren ML, Fehrs LJ, et al. Update: rubella and congenital rubella syndrome. *Epidemiol Rev* 1991;13:341–348.

Loachim HL. Kaposi's sarcoma and KSHV. *Lancet* 1995;346:1360.

Luft BJ, Hafner R, Korzun AH, et al. Toxoplasmic encephalitis in patients with acquired immunodeficiency syndrome. *N Eng J Med* 1993;329:995–1000.

Lutwick LI. Post exposure prophylaxis. *Infect Dis Clin North Am* 1996;10:899–915.

MacGowan JR, Mahendra P, et al. Case report: thrombocytopenia and spontaneous rupture of the spleen associated with infectious mononucleosis. *Clin Lab Haematol* 1995;17:93–94.

Marcy SM, et al. In: Hoeprich PD, Jordan MC, Ronald AR, eds. *Infectious diseases*. 5th ed. Philadelphia: Lippincott 1994:903–911.

Martinez AJ, Sell M, Mitrovics T, et al. The neuropathology and epidemiology of AIDS. A Berlin experience. A review of 200 cases. *Pathol Res Pract* 1995;191: 427–443.

Martinez-Vazquez C, Bordon J, Rodriguez-Gonzalez A, et al. Cerebral tuberculoma—a comparative study in patients with and without HIV infection. *Infection* 1995;23:149–153.

McKinnon HD. Evaluating the febrile patient with a rash. *Am Fam Phys* 2000;62:804–816.

Mehta JB, Morris F. Impact of HIV infection on mycobacterial disease. *Am Fam Phys* 1992;45:2203–2211.

Memar O. Cutaneous viral infections. *J Am Acad Dermatol* 1995;33:279–287.

Moylett EH, Shearer WT. HIV: clinical manifestations (review). *J Allergy Clin Immunol* 2002;110:3–16.

Murray HW, Gellene RA, Libby DM, et al. Activation of tissue macrophages from AIDS patients: in vitro response of AIDS alveolar macrophages to lymphokines and interferon-gamma. *J Immunol* 1985;135:2374.

Murray, HW, Rubin, BY, et al. Impaired production of lymphokines and immune (gamma) interferon in the acquired immunodeficiency syndrome. *N Engl J Med* 1984;310:883.

Mylonakis E, Paliou M, Lally M, et al. Laboratory testing for infection with the human immunodeficiency virus: Established and novel approaches. *Am J Med* 2000;109:568–576.

Nussinovitch M, Volovitz B, Varsano I. Complications of mumps requiring hospitalization in children. *Eur J Pediatr* 1995;154:732–734.

O'Brien TR, George JR, Holmberg SD. Human immunodeficiency virus type 2 infection in the United States: Epidemiology, diagnosis, and public health implications. *JAMA* 1992;267:2775–2779.

Orenstein MS, Tavitian A, Yonk B, et al. Granulomatous involvement of the liver in patients with AIDS. *Gut* 1985;26:1220–1225.

Pauza CD, Streblow DN. Therapeutic approaches of HIV infection based on virus structure and the host pathogen interaction. *Curr Top Microbiol Immunol* 1995;202:117–132.

Peter G, ed. *Red Book: Report of the Committee on Infectious Diseases*. St. Louis, MO: American Academy of Pediatrics 1997.

Quion N, Dewitt TG. Diagnosis: mumps parotitis (case 3). *Pediatr Rev* 1995;16:351.

Ray MC, Gately LE 3rd. Dermatologic manifestations of HIV infection and AIDS. *Infect Dis Clin North Am* 1994;8:583–605.

Rayfield MA, Sullivan P, Bandera CI, et al. HIV-1 group O virus identified for the first time in the United States. *Emerg Infect Dis* 1996;2:209.

Rhame FS. *AIDS in Infectious Diseases*. 5th ed. Philadelphia: Lippincott 1994: 642.

Rhoda AM, Friedrich D. Inaccuracy of commercial enzyme immunoassays in diagnosing genial infections with herpes simplex virus types 1 or 2. *Am J Clin Pathol* 2003;120:839–844.

Ruzicka T, Kalka K, Diercks K, et al. Papular pruritic "gloves and socks" syndrome associated with human herpesvirus 6 infection. *Arch Dermatol* 1998;134:242–244.

Safrin S, Ashley R, Houlihan C, et al. Clinical and serologic features of herpes simplex virus infection in patients with AIDS. *AIDS* 1991;5:1107–1110.

Salomon N, Perlman DC, DePalo VA, et al. Drug-resistant tuberculosis: factors associated with rise in resistance in an HIV-infected urban population. *Mt Sinai J Med* 1994;61:341–348.

Sepkowitz KA, Raffalli J, Riley L, et al. Tuberculosis in the AIDS era. *Clin Microbiol Rev* 1995;8:180–199.

Simon HE. Infectious complications. In: Cohen PT, Volberding PA, Sande MA, eds. *The AIDS Knowledge Base*. 2nd ed. Boston: Little, Brown 1994.

Smith J, Robinson NJ. Age specific prevalence of infection with herpes simplex virus types 2 and 1: a global review. *J Infect Dis* 2002;186:S3–S28.

Stiver, G. The treatment of influenza with antiviral drugs. *Can Med Assoc J* 2003;168:49–57

Straus SE, Cohen JI, et al. Epstein-Barr virus infections: biology, pathogenesis, and management. *Ann Intern Med* 1993;18:45–58.

Sullivan JS. HIV and AIDS. *Nature* 1995;378:10.

Sullivan KM, Halpin TJ, et al. Mumps disease and its health impact: an outbreak-based report. *Pediatrics* 1985;76:533–536.

Sweet SP, Cookson S, Challacombe SJ. Candida albicans isolates from HIV-infected and AIDS patients exhibit enhanced adherence to epithelial cells. *J Med Microbiol* 1995;43:452–457.

Tintinalli JE, et al., eds. *Emergency Medicine: A Comprehensive Study Guide*. 2nd ed. New York: McGraw-Hill 1988:758–759.

Tyring SK. Natural history of varicella zoster virus. *Semin Dermatol* 1992;11: 211–217.

Uttley AH, Pozniak A. Resurgence of tuberculosis. *J Hosp Infect* 1993;23:249–253.

Villa A, Berman B. Genital herpes infection: Beyond a clinical diagnosis. *SKINmed* 2003;2:108–112.

Volk WA. *Essentials of Microbiology,* 2nd ed. Philadelphia: Lippincott 1982: 661–662, 668–671.

Wainberg MA, Gu Z. Targeting HIV reverse transcriptase in novel ways. *Nat Med* 1995;1:628–629.

Wald A, Zeh J, Selke S, et al. Reactivation of genital herpes simplex virus type 2 infection in asymptomatic seropositive persons. *N Engl J Med* 2000;342: 844–850.

Wald A, Link K. Human immunodeficiency virus infection in herpes simplex type 2 seropositive persons: a meta-analysis. *J Infect Dis* 2002;185:45–52.

Whitley RJ. Therapeutic approaches to varicella zoster infections. *J Infect Dis* 1992;166:s51–s57.

Whitley RJ. Varicella-zoster virus. In: Mandell GL, Douglas RG Jr, Bennett JE, eds. *Principles and Practice of Infectious Disease,* 4th ed. New York: Churchill Livingstone 2000:1580–1586.

Wiselka M. Influenza: diagnosis, management, and prophylaxis. *Br Med J* 1994;308: 1341–1345.

Woods CW, McRill C, Plikaytis BD, et al. Coccidioidomycosis in human immuno-deficiency virus-infected persons in Arizona, 1994–1997: Incidence, risk factors, and prevention. *J Infect Dis* 2000;181:1428–1434.

World Health Organization. Acquired immunodeficiency syndrome (AIDS): 1987 revision of CDC/WHO case definition for AIDS. *Wkly Epidem Rec* 1988: 63:1–8.

Yew WW. Drug-resistant tuberculosis in the 1990s. *Eur Respir J* 1995;8:1184–1192.

Zaman MK, White DA. Serum lactate dehydrogenase levels and Pneumocystis carinii pneumonia. Diagnostic and prognostic significance. *Am Rev Respir Dis* 1988;137:796–800.

Sepsis

Ronald J. DeBellis
Jason E. Cross

Sepsis is a clinical syndrome manifested by systemic inflammation in the setting of infection. The infection triggers an immune response that results in a localized inflammatory reaction, which in a small population of patients, a systemic spillover of inflammatory mediators triggers a more generalized reaction. The generalized systemic reaction is termed systemic inflammatory response syndrome (SIRS). The manifestations of SIRS include fever or hypothermia, leukocytosis or leukopenia, tachycardia, and tachypnea. SIRS may also be precipitated by trauma, pancreatitis, or other noninfectious etiologies but the end result is the same—a systemic inflammatory response that is manifested by multiple organ dysfunction and eventual vascular collapse. A patient may experience minimal or life-threatening complications as a result of SIRS. Sepsis should not be confused with bacteremia—the presence of bacteria within the blood stream. Bacteremia is not present in a significant percentage of sepsis cases. According to the study conducted by the Protein C Worldwide Evaluation in Severe Sepsis (PROWESS) Study Group, a recent landmark trial involving the use of activated protein C in the treatment of severe sepsis, only 33% of patients with severe sepsis (sepsis plus one or more organ dysfunctions) had a positive blood culture of bacteria. The end stage of sepsis, septic shock—a subgroup of severe sepsis—is global hypotension and hypoperfusion (cardiovascular dysfunction) of the body as a result of the inflammatory response to infection.

The patient with manifestations of sepsis represents a special challenge to emergency physicians from both a diagnostic and therapeutic standpoint. While many patients present with fever and an obvious source, in many others, particularly the elderly, very young, and immunocompromised, the true nature of the patient's symptoms may be far more difficult to elucidate. Supportive care, the initiation of a diagnostic plan, and the choice of empiric antibiotic therapy are specifically the responsibility of the emergency physician.

Epidemiology

Recent epidemiological studies indicate there are more than 750,000 new cases of sepsis and severe sepsis occurring each year. The incidence is believed to be greater than heart failure and the number of deaths per year similar to myocardial infarctions. There are more than 200,000 deaths due to sepsis and septic shock each year. Those who appear to be at greater risk for sepsis include immunosuppressed patients, those with significant comorbid conditions, infants under 1 year, and the elderly, particularly those older than 75 years. Additionally, patients with indwelling Foley catheters or indwelling intravenous lines are at greater risk for the development of sepsis as a result of these sources. Once the septic process has advanced to septic shock the associated mortality may be 50% or more.

Pathophysiology

The pathophysiology of sepsis involves two processes: inflammation and uncontrolled coagulation. The pathophysiology is considered to have a network of cascading events. Once the systemic inflammatory process occurs after an infectious process, uncontrolled coagulation can flourish and cause emboli in the microvasculature of organs and tissues. The formation of emboli in the microvasculature leads to organ dysfunction and worsening of outcomes.

The initial event in the downhill spiral from health to death in the patient with sepsis is an initial infectious focus. Common initial sources include the urinary tract, the lung, and the skin. Additionally, intra-abdominal infection and sinusitis are examples of more occult sources of sepsis. As noted above, bacteremia is not a prerequisite for sepsis. Pulmonary and abdominal sources are the most common sites of infection. Also, Gram-positive and Gram-negative infections occur at similar rates. It appears that sepsis may result from the direct invasion of the blood by bacteria or via the liberation of chemical mediators of inflammation. While some aspects of the inflammatory response have been well elucidated, it is safe to conclude that much more remains elusive.

One well-recognized trigger of the septic process is exposure of the immune system to certain chemical moieties produced by various strains of bacteria or other microbes. Bacterial exotoxins are inflammatory mediators that are secreted by viable organisms. Either gram-positive or gram-negative organisms may liberate such substances. Examples of exotoxins are the proteins secreted by certain strains of *Staphylococcus* and *Streptococcus* responsible for toxic shock syndromes observed in patients with these infections. These exotoxins are potent mediators of both the humeral and cellular components of the inflammatory response.

Similar to the response characterized by exotoxins is that which is caused by bacterial endotoxin. Endotoxin is different from exotoxin in that it is not secreted, but rather is intrinsic to the bacterial cell wall. Endotoxin has been identified as the lipopolysaccharide (LPS) found in Gram-negative cell walls. Numerous humeral mediators of the inflammatory response have been described and it is likely that many more have yet to be recognized. Of these mediators, several have been well-characterized. Tumor necrosis factor (TNF) is a protein produced by macrophages, monocytes, and other cells in response to exposure to endotoxin. TNF is currently recognized as one of the earliest and most potent mediators of the inflammatory cascade. TNF is believed to cause an amplified response of the inflammatory cascade with subsequent increased production of various mediators of inflammation such as interleukins, platelet activators, prostaglandins, and leukotrienes. Subsequent activation of the complement cascade, as well as degranulation of macrophages, results in vascular endothelial damage allowing fluid leakage from capillary beds. This occurrence, along with increased levels of circulating vasodilatory substances (e.g., nitrous oxide, serotonin, bradykinin, and histamine), results in systemic vasodilation, causing relative hypovolemia. This peripheral vasodilation, combined with a decreased responsiveness of arteriolar smooth muscle to catecholamines, depleted plasma levels of vasopressin and the third spacing (described above), results in a decrease in systemic vascular resistance and a decrease in venous return to the heart, with subsequent loss of cardiac output and blood pressure. This is poorly tolerated by the septic patient, especially if febrile, since these patients appear to have an increased overall cellular oxygen demand. The situation is made worse by myocardial suppression, which results directly from TNF and other inflammatory substances. Shock resistance to IV fluids and pharmacologic therapy may ensue as a preterminal event.

As described above, the first step in the pathophysiology of sepsis is an infectious process. In some persons, the initial localized inflammatory response develops into a systemic inflammatory response and the steps to sepsis have begun. If the process is not halted, the inflammatory response can progress and can begin to cause coagulopathies. Uncontrolled coagulation is thought to have a major role in organ dysfunction via the formation of emboli in the microvasculature of organs and tissues. Sepsis (infectious process plus SIRS) patients that develop acute organ dysfunction are defined as having severe sepsis.

Describing the pathophysiology of severe sepsis begins with understanding the definition of sepsis (infectious process plus SIRS) and then adding uncontrolled coagulation. After the development of systemic inflammation, endothelial injury occurs and triggers coagulation via the direct stimulation of tissue factor, the direct inhibition of plasminogen activator inhibitor-1 (PAI-1), and the indirect stimulation of thrombin. The stimulation of tissue factor promotes coagulation, which then, in turn, stimulates thrombin. Again, the direct stimulation of tissue factor results in coagulation. Yet, the direct inhibition of PAI-1 and the indirect stimulation of thrombin result in the inhibition of fibrinolysis. The final piece to the coagulopathy puzzle is the relationship of thrombomodulin and protein C. Thrombomodulin converts protein C to its activated form (activated protein C). Activated protein C has anti-inflammatory, anticoagulant, and profibrinolytic properties (**FIGURE 67.1**). In patients with severe sepsis, there is a downregulation of thrombomodulin which results in a lower concentration of activated protein C. The net effect of all of these processes results in uncontrolled coagulation, which sees its detrimental effects in the microvasculature of organs and tissues leading to organ dysfunction.

Diagnosis

The first step in diagnosing these syndromes is to be able to define sepsis, severe sepsis, and septic shock (a common subgroup of severe sepsis). Sepsis is defined as a patient having a known or suspected infection and two out of the four SIRS criteria. Suspected infection is proven with evidence by one or more of the following: white cells in a normally sterile body fluid, perforated viscus, radiographic evidence of pneumonia in association with the production of purulent sputum, or a syndrome associated with a high risk of infection. SIRS criteria are met when the patient meets two out of the four SIRS criteria as defined as fever or hypothermia, leukocytosis or leukopenia, tachycardia, and tachypnea.

Severe sepsis is defined as sepsis plus one or more acute organ or system dysfunction. Common sites of dysfunction include cardiovascular system dysfunction (hypotension despite adequate fluid resuscitation and use of vasopressors), kidney dysfunction (urine output < 0.5 mL/kg), respiratory system dysfunction (PaO_2 to $FiO_2 \leq 200$), hematologic dysfunction (platelet count < 80,000/mm^3 or a decrease by 50% within 3 days), and unexplained metabolic acidosis.

The most common type of severe sepsis is septic shock. Septic shock is defined as severe sepsis due to cardiovascular dysfunction. Septic shock was the most common type of severe sepsis found in the PROWESS study.

Sepsis in any given patient may be clinically obvious or notoriously occult. Emergency physicians must identify at-risk individuals and institute appropriate therapy early on since once the process becomes advanced the likelihood of a "good" outcome is considerably reduced. Historical clues to a probable difficult course in the setting of an infectious disease include patients at the extremes of age, patients with comorbid conditions such as heart disease or diabetes, those who are immunocompromised such as asplenic patients, HIV-infected individuals, patients undergoing chemotherapy for malignancy, and patients maintained on steroid therapy for a variety of

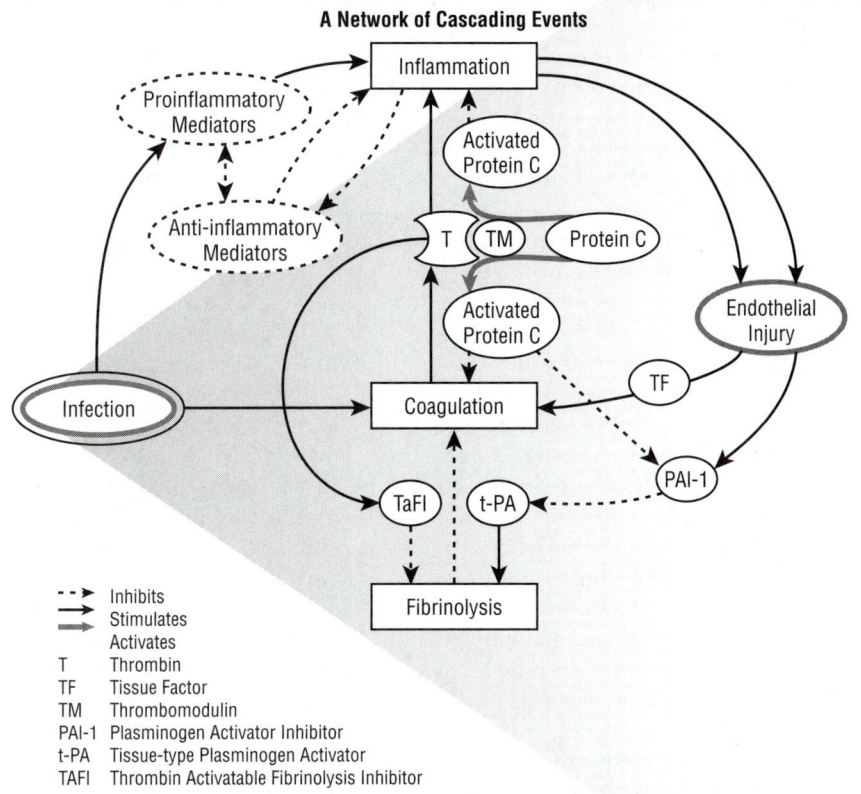

A Network of Cascading Events

Inflammation

Proinflammatory Mediators

Anti-inflammatory Mediators

Activated Protein C

T TM Protein C

Activated Protein C

Endothelial Injury

Infection

Coagulation

TF

PAI-1

TaFI t-PA

Fibrinolysis

- - ▸ Inhibits
——▸ Stimulates
       Activates
T   Thrombin
TF   Tissue Factor
TM   Thrombomodulin
PAI-1   Plasminogen Activator Inhibitor
t-PA   Tissue-type Plasminogen Activator
TAFI   Thrombin Activatable Fibrinolysis Inhibitor

FIGURE 67.1 Infection as a network of cascading events.

maladies. As noted above, patients with indwelling catheters, whether urinary or intravenous, have additional risks from these sources. Where valvular heart disease or intravenous drug use is suspected, endocarditis is a concern.

The presentation of the potentially septic patient varies widely from the straightforward (flank pain, dysuria, fever, and tachycardia in a young, previously healthy female) to the nonspecific (subtle alteration in mental status in an elderly patient with underlying dementia). In addition, the presentations of individuals who are either very young or old, as well as those who are immunosuppressed are frequently nonspecific.

A fundamental rule of emergency practice is to "know the vital signs." With respect to the evaluation and diagnosis of the potentially septic patient this is of critical importance. A rectal temperature is still the most important modality to find a fever. Most patients who are septic or bacteremic are febrile, but normothermia and hypothermia may occur, particularly in neonates, the immunosuppressed, and the elderly. Physicians should be wary of normothermic patients given antipyretics prior to emergency department (ED) presentation as well as infants whose parents report either documented or subjective fever. Tachypnea may result from acidosis, agitation, or pulmonary pathology such as pneumonia or ARDS. Tachycardia may result from fever alone, dehydration, or third space losses as a result of sepsis. Hypotension in the setting of an acute infectious process is a late and ominous sign and should be aggressively treated. Patients with sep-

tic shock are frequently warm and dry in the initial phases of their illness, unlike patients with hypovolemic or cardiogenic shock who are vasoconstricted.

Alterations of mental status may be subtle and difficult to recognize especially in patients with a history of dementia. Often, information regarding the patient's previous level of functioning is obtained by speaking with family members, nursing home staff, home health aides, or others who have frequent contact with the patient. A thorough neurologic examination helps to distinguish sepsis from intracranial pathology. Patients should be completely undressed unless the source of their problem is obvious. Skin findings of importance include areas of cellulitis, petechiae, purpura, or rash. Inspecting the feet is important especially in diabetic patients and in those with vascular disease or at risk for neuropathy, such as the alcoholic. The back should be examined for perirectal or pilonidal abscess as well as decubitus ulcer. Costovertebral angle percussion tenderness should be sought; when present, suggests pyelonephritis. Since pneumonia and intra-abdominal sources of sepsis are common, careful examination of the chest and abdomen is mandatory. Nuchal rigidity mandates lumbar puncture, although nuchal rigidity may be absent in the elderly or those under 24 months of age, even with meningitis. More occult sources of infection would include the sinuses or orthopedic foci in non-communicative patients.

Ancillary studies in the infected patient may provide clues to the source and severity of the initial focus of infection. A complete blood count should be obtained with an understanding that most but not all patients with a significant source of infection have an elevated WBC count. In adults and in pediatric patients there may be a crude association between the magnitude of the white count and the seriousness of its underlying cause. Patients with WBC counts lower than normal should be approached with extra caution. In the absence of DIC, sepsis should not cause anemia or thrombocytopenia. When the suspicion for DIC exists, laboratory confirmation should be carried out. Chemistry values of specific importance include BUN and creatinine, which may suggest renal failure, serum glucose to rule out either hypo- or hyperglycemia, which may suggest diabetic ketoacidosis (DKA) or hyperosmolar coma, as well as serum sodium and chloride, which when taken together with the renal functions may reveal dehydration. Additionally, serum bicarbonate may become depressed in the septic patient, which may be the result of systemic hypoperfusion, ischemia to an extremity or the bowel, or other metabolic derangements. Abnormalities may occur in the liver functions with elevation of transaminases. Abnormal coagulation parameters should be considered DIC until proven otherwise. Elevations of pancreatic amylase and lipase may also occur. Arterial blood gases may reveal hyperventilation as the result of agitation or sepsis or a high alveolar-arterial oxygen gradient in the setting of pneumonia or ARDS. Hypoxemia unresponsive to supplemental oxygen may result from ARDS. ECG and cardiac enzymes may identify patients with underlying heart disease or concomitant myocardial ischemia.

Blood cultures should be obtained from at least two peripheral sites. In the immunocompromised, viral and fungal cultures should be obtained. Gram stain and culture done on potential sources of infection such as sputum may also be of value. Urinalysis and culture should be performed on any patient where the urinary tract may be the source of infection. A chest x-ray is warranted unless the patient has a known source and is free of any pulmonary symptoms. Other radiology studies such as abdominal plain films or computed tomography (CT), ultrasound, or head CT should be employed under the correct clinical paradigms.

Treatment and Disposition

When considering advanced pharmacotherapy in the critically ill patient, there are five essentials of therapy: fluid resuscitation; pharmacologic vasopressors; antibiotic administration; consideration of activated protein C; and glycemic control and evaluation for adrenal insufficiency.

Fluids

Fluid management and resuscitation is the undisputed initial intervention in septic shock patients. There has been a lack of prospective studies to determine the preferred fluid for volume resuscitation in patients with septic shock. One meta-analysis compares colloid to crystalloid in non-septic surgical patients. The outcomes in patients using either colloids or crystalloids are equivocal. In general, colloids have been associated with the administration of less fluid at a higher expense than crystalloid, however crystalloids appear to be the favorite, due to ease of use and lower cost.

Some data demonstrate that in immediate life threatening situations, colloid administration may provide a slight benefit in that it provides a more rapid fluid correction, however the infusion may be rate limited.

Markers for adequate volume resuscitation are dependent upon whether or not a pulmonary artery (PA) catheter is placed or the patient is intubated. If a PA catheter is placed to address volume status, the following information should be useful in gauging adequate resuscitation:

- A patient is considered to be adequately volume resuscitated when the central venous pressure (CVP) is between 8 to 14 mm Hg.
- In the event the patient has a PA catheter placed, the pulmonary capillary wedge pressure (PCWP) signifying appropriate volume resuscitation should be maintained at 14 to 18 mm Hg.
- In the event the patient does not have an invasive monitoring device in place, clinical evaluation of the situation becomes critical. First and foremost the correction of the hypotensive state is an indicator of adequate volume resuscitation.
- In the event that hypotension may not be resolved, auscultated crackles in the lungs or a change in the oxyhemoglobin dissociation curve are clinical measures of adequate volume resuscitation. Crystalloid should be administered as 250 to 1,000 mL over 5 to 15 minutes. This should be repeated until hypotension resolves or adverse clinical events from overhydration are present.
- Non-intubated patients who may have a penchant for maintaining adequate oxygenation, as well as intubated, mechanically ventilated patients, can be more aggressively resuscitated with fluids.

Pharmacologic Vasopressors

In the event of falling blood pressure after adequate volume resuscitation, as described above, pharmacologic vasopressors may be in order. The mechanism of hypotension in sepsis is twofold. Increased intravascular nitric oxide and depleted plasma levels of vasopressin are responsible for the vasodilation associated with sepsis. Persistent hypotension after adequate volume resuscitation requires administration of pharmacologic vasopressor agents. The preferred agent to "buy time" in septic shock is norepinephrine (**Table 67.1**). Norepinephrine is nearly a pure alpha-adrenergic agonist. There truly is no need for other vasopressors in the setting of septic shock. Norepinephrine should be titrated to maintain systolic blood pressure greater than 90 mm Hg.

When considering vasopressor choice, examine the following information. Tyrosine is the parent compound for all pharmacologic vasopressors:

Tyrosine → Dopa → Dopamine → Norepinephrine → Epinephrine → Phenylephrine → Methoxamine

All of the compounds listed above are chemically related to each other and they all work at the same receptors. Dopamine requires that it be broken down by dopa-decarboxylase to get to norepinephrine. Since norepinephrine is the most potent and clinically useful of all the

Table 67.1

Pharmacologic Vasopressor Pharmacology and Rationale

Drug	Dose	α-1	β-1	β-2	VD	VC	INT	CHT
Dopamine	2–5 µg/kg/min	0	1	0	Renal	1	1	1
	5–10 µg/kg/min	1	2	0	Renal	2	2	2
	15–20 µg/kg/min	3	2	0	Renal	3	2	2
Norepinephrine	Titrate for BP	4	2	0	0	4	1	1
Phenylephrine	Titrate for BP	3	0	0	0	3	0	0

vasoconstrictors in septic shock, we should consider using it as not only the first-line choice, but the only choice in treating refractory hypotension. There is no benefit to adding another vasopressor that acts on α-1 adrenergic receptors. Two drugs would be competing for the same amount of receptors, add potential toxic effects in the form of both supraventricular and ventricular arrhythmias and furthermore, benefit from the addition of alternative catecholamines to norepinephrine through clinical studies has not been demonstrated. As the dose of catecholamine increases, the adrenergic receptors become down-regulated which may lead a patient toward requiring larger than normal doses of vasopressors. The maximum dose of norepinephrine is whatever is required to maintain a patient's systolic blood pressure greater than 90 mm Hg.

Norepinephrine is the vasopressor of choice in a situation where septic shock is present. It is nearly a pure α-1 drug that will maximize constriction of the peripheral vasculature, which is the desired effect. Be careful of dose creep to maintain blood pressure. Reports of doses up to 120 µg have been administered. Dose creep may be a clinical sign that plasma vasopressin levels are waning and down-regulation of catechol receptors is occurring. This would be an appropriate time to consider adding vasopressin to the regimen.

Vasopressin should be administered as a continuous infusion of 0.04 units per minute. This dose is generally adequate to maintain plasma vasopressin levels. Increasing the dose of vasopressin may result in profound vasoconstriction of splanchnic blood flow areas, compromising internal organ perfusion.

If cardiogenic shock is coupled with septic shock, the need for inotropic support such as dobutamine may be necessary to maximize forward flow of blood through the heart.

The best outcomes in patients with sepsis occur with early, goal directed therapy, including aggressive fluid resuscitation, vasopressor or dilator agents, red-cell transfusions, and inotropic medications to achieve a target CVP of 8 to 12 mm Hg. Other monitoring parameters targeted include a mean arterial pressure of 65 to 90 mmg Hg, urine output of at least 0.5 mL/kg per hour, and a central venous oxygen saturation of 70%.

Antimicrobial Therapy

There have been relatively few clinical studies that address appropriate antibiotic therapy for the septic patient. Current knowledge and practice is derived from patients who have bacteremia and is applied to the septic patient. To date there is little information regarding the treatment of gram positive or fungal infections in the septic patient. See **FIGURES 67.2, 67.3, and 67.4** for empiric antibiotic selection in septic patients.

Activated Protein C (Drotrecogin Alpha)

The PROWESS study was a randomized, placebo controlled, double blinded, multi-center trial that demonstrated a significant reduction in 28-day mortality in patients with sepsis. The study included 1,728 patients and had mortality rates of 30.8% in the placebo group and 24.7% in the drotrecogin alpha group that statistically demonstrated a relative risk reduction of mortality of 19.8%. The most common adverse effect is bleeding at 3.5%. The aPTT needs to be less than 100 seconds, the INR should be less than 3, and the platelets should be maintained at greater than 30,000. If any of these parameters is altered the medication should be discontinued. This drug is contraindicated if the patient has a history of clin-

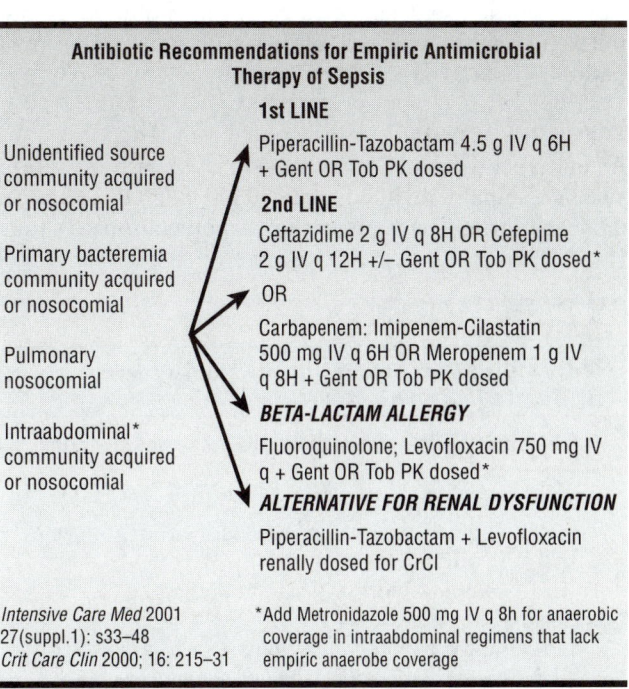

Antibiotic Recommendations for Empiric Antimicrobial Therapy of Sepsis

Unidentified source community acquired or nosocomial

Primary bacteremia community acquired or nosocomial

Pulmonary nosocomial

Intraabdominal* community acquired or nosocomial

1st LINE
Piperacillin-Tazobactam 4.5 g IV q 6H + Gent OR Tob PK dosed

2nd LINE
Ceftazidime 2 g IV q 8H OR Cefepime 2 g IV q 12H +/– Gent OR Tob PK dosed*
OR
Carbapenem: Imipenem-Cilastatin 500 mg IV q 6H OR Meropenem 1 g IV q 8H + Gent OR Tob PK dosed

BETA-LACTAM ALLERGY
Fluoroquinolone; Levofloxacin 750 mg IV q + Gent OR Tob PK dosed*

ALTERNATIVE FOR RENAL DYSFUNCTION
Piperacillin-Tazobactam + Levofloxacin renally dosed for CrCl

Intensive Care Med 2001 27(suppl.1): s33–48
Crit Care Clin 2000; 16: 215–31

*Add Metronidazole 500 mg IV q 8h for anaerobic coverage in intraabdominal regimens that lack empiric anaerobe coverage

FIGURE 67.2 Antibiotic recommendations for empiric antimicrobial therapy of sepsis of the following types: sepsis from an unidentified source, primary bacteremia, pulmonary nosocomial, or intra-abdominal infection.

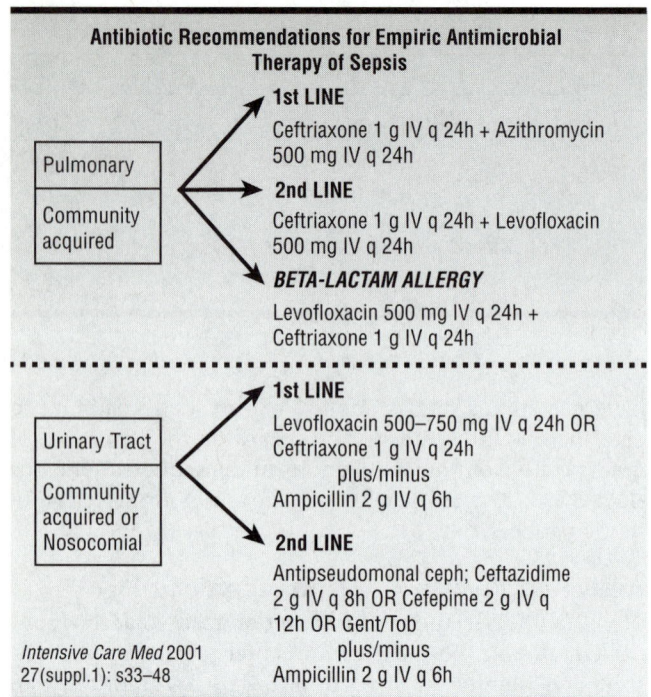

FIGURE 67.3 Antibiotic recommendations for empiric antimicrobial therapy of sepsis of the following types: pulmonary community-acquired or urinary tract infection.

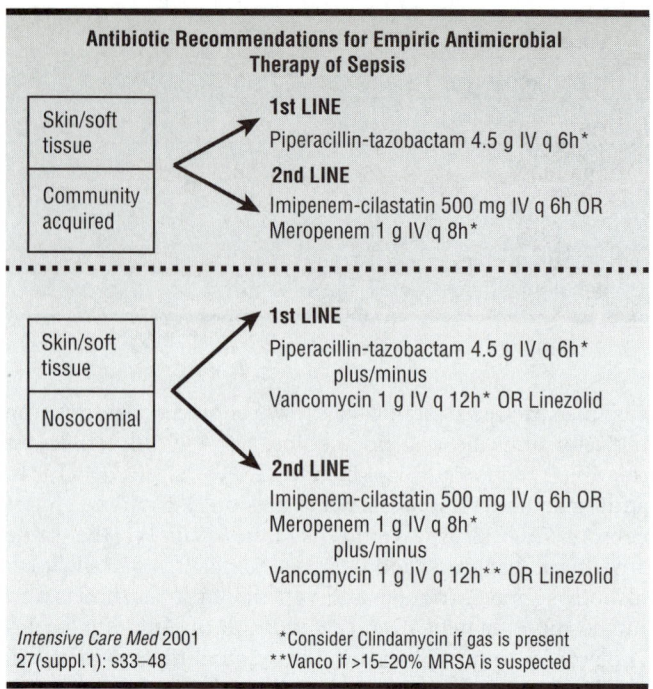

FIGURE 67.4 Antibiotic recommendations for empiric antimicrobial therapy of sepsis of the following types: skin/soft tissue community-acquired or nosocomial infection.

ically significant bleeding or in conjunction with other medications that may cause clinically significant bleeding.

Suggested criteria for administration and institutional use of this drug are listed in **Tables 67.2, 67.3, and 67.4**.

Drotrecogin alpha must be administered at 24 µg/kg per hour for 96 hours through a dedicated port with no other medications or solutions except 0.9% sodium chloride, 5% dextrose, lactated ringers, with up to 40 mEq of potassium chloride, in any of these solutions. Other compatibility data to date is non-existent.

Insulin Therapy

Acute hyperglycemia has been associated with insulin resistance, impaired white blood cell chemotaxis, end organ damage (particularly nephropathy), polyneuropathy, mus-

cle wasting and gastropathy, and an increased rate of mortality in patients with and without diabetes mellitus. A prospective, randomized controlled trial in mechanically ventilated surgical intensive care unit (SICU) patients was conducted by Van den Berghe et al. over a 12-month period with 1,548 patients. Patients were randomized for an intensive insulin therapy via continuous infusion targeting blood glucose values in the 80 to 110 mg/dL range. The control group received conventional insulin therapy targeting blood glucose at 180 to 200 mg/dL range. Patients in the control group received insulin infusion only if their blood glucose value exceeded 215 mg/dL.

Table 67.2

Infection Criteria Guidelines for the Use of Drotregcogin-α (Xigris®)

Infection Criteria—Patient should meet one or more of the following criteria
- Known infection
- Suspected infection as evidenced by one or more of the following:
  white cells in a normally sterile body fluid
  perforated viscus
  radiographic evidence of pneumonia in association with the production of purulent sputum
- A syndrome associated with a high risk of infection (e.g., ascending cholangitis)

Table 67.3

Modified SIRS Criteria Guidelines for the Use of Drotregcogin-α (Xigris®)

Modified SIRS Criteria—Patients should meet at least three of the following four criteria
- A core temperature of ≥38° C (100.4° F) or ≤36° C (96.8°F)
- A heart rate of ≥ 90 beats/min, except in patients with a medical condition known tincrease the heart rate or those receiving treatment that would prevent tachycardia
- A respiratory rate of ≥ 20 breaths/min or a $PaCO_2$ of ≤ 32 mm Hg or the use of mechanical ventilation for an acute respiratory process
- A white-cell count of ≥ 12,000/mm^3 or ≤ 4,000/mm^3 or a differential count showing >10 percent immature neutrophils

Table 67.4

Criteria for Dysfunctional Organ Guidelines for the Use of Drotrecogin-α (Xigris®)

Criteria for Dysfunctional Organs—Patients should meet at least one of the following five criteria

- Cardiovascular system dysfunction—arterial systolic blood pressure ≤90 mm Hg or mean arterial pressure ≤70 mm Hg for at least 1 hour despite adequate fluid resuscitation, adequate intravascular volume status or the use of vasopressors in an attempt to maintain a systolic blood pressure of ≥90 mm Hg or a mean arterial pressure of ≥70 mm Hg
- Kidney dysfunction—urine output < 0.5 mL/kg of body weight/hr for 1 hour, despite adequate fluid resuscitation
- Respiratory-system dysfunction—ratio of PaO_2 to FiO_2 ≤250 in the presence of other dysfunctional organ or ≤200 if the lung is the only dysfunctional organ
- Hematologic dysfunction—platelet count <80,000/mm^3 or a decrease by 50 percent within 3 days
- Unexplained metabolic acidosis—pH ≤ 7.30 or a base deficit of ≥5.0 mmol/L in association with a plasma lactate level >1.5 times the upper limit of normal

Overall SICU mortality decreased from 8% to 4.6% (P = <0.04) and mortality in the SICU for length of stays longer than 5 days decreased from 20.2% to 10.6% (P = 0.005). Additional trends though not statistically significant due to small numbers included deaths involving multiple organ failure with a proven septic focus demonstrated the greatest reduction in mortality; overall hospital mortality decreased by 34%; bloodstream infections decreased by 46%; acute renal failure requiring intervention by 41%; decreased red-cell transfusions by 50%; and decreased critical illness polyneuropathy by 44%. Consult your institutional critical care unit for an insulin protocol specific to your patient population and comfort level.

Steroids

Generally steroids are not part of the initial management of patients presenting with sepsis, however critically ill patients who remain in the ED for prolonged periods of time should be assessed for corticosteroid deficiency. There are some symptoms that are suggestive of corticosteroid deficiency in critically ill patients. The physical examination findings include postural hypotension, tachycardia and fever. Clinical problems that may co-exist include hemodynamic instability, ongoing inflammation with no obvious source, and multiple organ dysfunction. Laboratory findings may be marked by hyponatremia, hyperkalemia, hypoglycemia, and eosinophilia.

The following are guidelines for instituting corticosteroid therapy in acute illness. All critically ill patients should receive a random cortisol level particularly in the presence of corticosteroid deficiency. If the random cortisol level is less than 15 μg/dL, hypoadrenalism is likely and supplemental corticosteroids should be administered. If the random cortisol level is between 15 and 34 μg/dL, a cortisol stimulation test should be administered. A baseline cortisol level should be obtained, 250 μg of corticotropin should be administered to the patient, and a cortisol level should be obtained 60 minutes after the corticotropin was administered. If the increase in cortisol is greater than 9 μg/dL, supplemental corticosteroids should be initiated. If the increase in cortisol is greater than 9 μg/dL, functional hypoadrenalism is unlikely, and supplemental corticosteroids will not provide any benefit. Lastly, if the patient's baseline cortisol level is greater than 34 μg/dL, functional hypoadrenalism is not present, and there is no benefit from supplemental steroid administration.

Dosing corticosteroids in septic shock is as follows: hydrocortisone, 50 mg IV every 6 hours, and fludrocortisone, 50 μg daily for 7 days of therapy.

Summary of Therapy

- Fluid resuscitation
- Pharmacologic vasopressors
- Appropriate empiric antibiotic selection
- Activated protein C
- Glycemic control
- Steroids
- Transfer

Selected Readings

Angus DC, Linde-Zwirble WT, Lidicker J, et al. Epidemiology of severe sepsis in the United States: Analysis of incidence, outcome, and associated costs of care. *Crit Care Med* 2001;29:1303–1310.

Annane D, Sebille V, Charpentier C, et al. Effect of treatment with low doses of hydrocortisone and fludrocortisone on mortality in patients with septic shock. *JAMA* 2002;288:862–871.

Annane D, Sébille V, Troché G, et al. A 3-level prognostic classification in septic shock based on cortisol levels and cortisol response to corticotropin. *JAMA* 2000;283:1038–1045.

Bernard GR, Vincent JL, Laterre PF, et al. Efficacy and safety of recombinant activated protein C for severe sepsis. *N Engl J Med* 2001;344:699–709.

Dellinger RP, Carlet JM, Masur H, et al. Surviving sepsis campaign guidelines for management of severe sepsis and septic shock. *Crit Care Med* 2004; 32:858–873.

Dellinger RP. Cardiovascular management of septic shock. *Crit Care Med* 2003;31: 946–955.

Landry DW, Oliver JA. The pathogenesis of vasodilatory shock. *N Engl J Med* 2001;345:588–595.

Rivers E, Nguyen B, Havstad S, et al. Early goal directed therapy in the treatment of sepsis and septic shock. *N Engl J Med* 2001;345:1368–1377.

Van Den Berghe G, Wouters P, Weekers F, et al. Intensive insulin therapy in critically ill patients. *N Engl J Med* 2001;345:1359–1367.

Musculoskeletal Disorders (Non-Traumatic)

John C. Moorhead

Patients with non-traumatic musculoskeletal complaints frequently seek care in the emergency department. Symptoms may represent a first presentation or acute manifestation of an ongoing illnesses or injury. A careful occupational and recreational history is helpful in diagnosis and acute management. Seemingly minor conditions, if left unrecognized and untreated, can lead to significant morbidity and disability, particularly in high-risk patients. Appropriate pain management is often a challenge for the emergency physician. Consultation when indicated and arrangement of follow-up care is an important component of emergency department management.

Bony Abnormalities

Rania Habal

Bony Abnormalities

Diseases of the musculoskeletal system are frequently encountered in the emergency department (ED). Nontraumatic bony abnormalities result from a number of different conditions, including infectious, inflammatory, degenerative, endocrine, neoplastic, and genetic causes. Although they rarely result in an immediately life-threatening condition, acute problems such as osteomyelitis, hypercalcemia, pathologic fractures, and their complications require emergency treatment.

Bone's main constituents are type I collagen and mineral salts. Its structure is maintained by three types of cells: osteoblasts, osteocytes (both of which derive from the mesenchymal cell line), and osteoclasts (which originate from the hematopoietic cell line). Osteoblasts synthesize collagen and organize it into an intricate matrix called osteoid. When this matrix calcifies, osteoblasts become embedded into the matrix and are then called osteocytes. The mechanisms by which calcium salts are incorporated into bone continue to elude scientists, despite intensive research in this area. However, they are believed to be under the control of a number of different local, as well as by other systemic factors. Osteoclasts, on the other hand, ensure phagocytosis, lysis, and resorption of bone. Functionally, bone may be classified into two types: The metabolically active trabecular bone forms the inner layers and constitutes 25% of total bone mass; the compact outer layer of bone constitutes 75% of total bone mass and is less metabolically active. As the life of bone depends on the interplay among resorption, mineralization, and growth, failure in any aspect of bone remodeling leads to devastating and disabling disease.

Aseptic Necrosis of the Hip

Aseptic necrosis of bone, also known as avascular necrosis (AVN), is a relatively common condition that affects bones with poor collateral circulation. These include the scaphoid, the humeral head, and the femoral head. Because of its anatomical blood supply and the stress of weight bearing, the femoral head is, by far, the most commonly affected region.

AVN of the femoral head is most commonly encountered after fractures and dislocations, where there is complete disruption of the bone's blood supply. Other causes include external pressure on arterial walls (mass, infection, inflammation, fibrosis or edema), thromboembolic phenomena (caisson disease, hypercoagulable states, hyperlipidemia, vasculitis, hemoglobinopathies), or obstruction of venous outflow.

AVN is also commonly seen in alcoholics and in patients using glucocorticoids, where 5% to 20% of patients may be affected and in many cases both femurs are affected. It may also be encountered in patients with HIV infection, chronic renal disease, leukemia, interferon use, and radiation therapy. The underlying mechanism for bone necrosis in these instances is probably multifactorial and may involve fat microemboli, microfractures with abnormal healing and inhibition of angiogenesis. These result in extravascular edema, which, in the setting of a limited bony compartment, can lead to further ischemia and necrosis. In approximately 5% of cases, the condition is idiopathic.

The clinical picture depends on the underlying insult. Infarction of small areas of bone is usually asymptomatic; however, in the setting of sickle cell disease, dysbaric air embolus, or other large embolic phenomena, a large area of bone becomes acutely ischemic. Patients present with sudden onset of severe pain and are unable to bear weight or use the affected extremity. Laboratory tests are nonspecific, but may be helpful in diagnosing the underlying cause. As the initial radiographs are normal, further studies such as a bone scan or magnetic resonance imaging (MRI) must be obtained. Treatment should be aggressive and directed at the underlying cause of the infarction and immediate orthopedic referral for bone marrow decompression and other joint preservation therapy.

In the chronic form of the disease, patients present with worsening hip or groin pain. Initially, the pain is vague, occurs on ambulation and weight bearing, and is relieved by rest. Pain is worse with internal rotation. Laboratory tests are not helpful. In the early stages of disease, radiographs are not sensitive and are generally normal. In these cases, the study of choice is magnetic resonance imaging (MRI), as it is both sensitive and specific. When MRI is not available, a CT scan or a bone scan may be performed. CT scanning is more sensitive than radiographs in determining the presence of subchondral fractures and in the detection of articular collapse and may, therefore be useful in equivocal cases. Bone scans are also sensitive in determining the presence of necrosis, but they lack specificity. The most important factor affecting the outcome of disease at this stage is to limit the progression of the disease by withdrawing the inciting factor, encouraging non–weight bearing and referral to the orthopedic service. Treatment may include core decompression, bone grafts, and electrical stimulation.

In the advanced stages, pain may be constant and disabling. The physical examination reveals a decrease in the range of motion of the hip. Radiographs are useful in classifying the extent of the disease. These may show mottling of bone, bone cysts with sclerotic margins, increased density of the femoral head, crescent-shaped radiolucencies or collapse of the joint. Treatment consists of non–weight bearing and referral to the orthopedic service for total hip arthroplasty.

Osteogenesis Imperfecta

Osteogenesis imperfecta (OI) refers to a number of genetic diseases characterized by various abnormalities in the synthesis of type I collagen and resulting in defective bone matrix. The disease affects 1 out of 20,000 live births and is characterized by fragile bones. Associated findings include blue sclerae, hearing loss, and abnormalities in dentogenesis. Rarely, affected individuals also develop hydrocephalus, carotid cavernous fistulas, and pulmonary hypoplasia. OI is classified into four types depending on the clinical manifestations and its mode of inheritance. The most common type, Sillence type I, which accounts for 70% to 80% of all cases of OI, is characterized by mild to moderately severe disease and is inherited in an autosomal dominant manner with occasional sporadic mutations. Affected individuals appear normal at birth and during childhood, but have an increased incidence of fractures and mildly stunted growth. Once the growth period is completed, the risk of fractures decreases, only to rebound in the later years. The characteristic blue sclerae are prominent and are thought to be due to thinning of scleral collagen, thus allowing the choroid to be more apparent. Otosclerosis leading to sensorineural deafness occurs in most affected individuals and begins after adolescence. Sillence type II, also called lethal OI, accounts for 10% of OI cases and is characterized by absent ossification in the fetus, multiple intrauterine fractures, and severe fetal deformities that are incompatible with life. Death occurs in utero or soon after birth. Sillence type III is a progressively deforming disease characterized by severe osteopenia leading to multiple fractures that occur spontaneously or with minimal trauma. Abnormal healing of these fractures results in striking skeletal deformities, growth retardation, and severe kyphoscoliosis. Sillence type IV is also rare and is inherited as an autosomal dominant trait with variable manifestations. Although manifestations are similar to those in type I of OI, they are more severe. Marked osteopenia is usually present, but sclerae are usually white and dentogenesis is variably affected.

Prenatal diagnosis of severe forms of OI has been facilitated by the use of sonography, which may note in utero fractures and skeletal deformities. The mild form of OI, on the other hand, may go unrecognized for many years. Children with this form of the disease are at risk for multiple fractures in the absence of a clear mechanism for the injuries. These patients present a special challenge to the ED physician as the differential diagnosis rightfully includes inflicted nonaccidental trauma. Other conditions, such as glucocorticoid excess, malabsorption syndromes, and nutritional deficiencies have also been associated with an increased fragility of bone and should therefore be considered in the differential diagnosis. The presence of a family history of OI, blue sclerae, or abnormal dentogenesis, however, should guide the physician toward the diagnosis of OI. The ED management of OI rests in the diagnosis and treatment of immediately life-threatening complications, and in the appropriate splinting of fractures and referral/admission to the appropriate service. Children and adolescents with osteogenesis imperfecta type I, III, and IV may benefit from cyclic biphosphonate therapy. When the diagnosis is unclear, a multidisciplinary consultation, including social services, should be considered.

Osteomyelitis

Osteomyelitis refers to the suppurative infection of bone that may lead to extensive bone necrosis and significant morbidity and mortality.

Risk factors for the development of osteomyelitis include prosthetic devices and prior bone surgery, bone disease, malnutrition, intravenous drug use, and conditions associated with suppression of the immune system such as diabetes mellitus, corticosteroid use, chronic alcohol consumption, sickle cell disease, and the immunodeficiencies. Elderly diabetic patients with peripheral vascular disease may also develop osteomyelitis of the feet and toes due to inadequate blood flow to those regions.

Invasion of bone by bacteria may occur in three different ways: hematogenous, where seeding of bone occurs during a bacteremic episode, contiguous spread, where infection is spread through extension from an adjacent site or through direct inoculation (as occurs in open fractures, puncture wounds, or during septic surgical procedures). Whatever the mechanism, all may progress to the chronic form of the disease with its complications, including chronic pain and loss of function, draining sinuses, and bone necrosis. Early detection and treatment are, therefore, necessary in order to prevent these sequelae.

Hematogeneous osteomyelitis occurs most commonly in children (85%), adult intravenous drug users, hemodialysis patients, and the elderly. The sites involved in hematogeneous osteomyelitis may be predicted based on the age of the patient. Areas of bone with rich blood supply but with a sluggish or valveless venous system or sinusoids are at greatest risk for hematogeneous seeding by bacteria. Areas of bone with a relative lack of phagocytes are also at increased risk for osteomyelitis. These include the metaphysis of long bones in growing children and the vertebrae in adults. Infants younger than 18 months may also develop epiphyseal osteomyelitis, because the epiphysis receives its blood supply from the metaphyseal blood vessels until 18 months of age.

Microbiology

In the majority of cases of acute hematogeneous osteomyelitis, a single organism is isolated as the infecting pathogen. *Staphylococcus aureus* is the most commonly isolated pathogen in all age groups except the neonatal period. In addition to *S. aureus*, Gram-negative coliform bacteria are common pathogens in the elderly, where the genitourinary tract is a frequent source of bacteremia, and *Pseudomonas aeruginosa* is an important pathogen in intravenous drug users. Patients with sickle cell disease are at risk for salmonella osteomyelitis. Osteomyelitis following an upper respiratory infection may be due to *Streptococcus pneumoniae* or *Bacteroides fragilis*. Furthermore, with the resurgence of mycobacterial disease, tuberculosis of the spine is becoming an increasingly common cause of osteomyelitis. During the neonatal period, group B *Streptococci* spp. is the most important pathogen.

In contrast to hematogeneous bone infections, osteomyelitis resulting from contiguous spread or from direct inoculation, as well as osteomyelitis in diabetic patients are usually polymicrobial. These infections commonly become chronic and persistent. Commonly isolated organisms include different *Staphylococcal* species, *Pseudomonas aeruginosa*, *Escherichia coli*, and *Serratia marcescens*. *Pseudomonas aeruginosa* is an important pathogen in burn victims, in patients with prosthetic devices and in patients with puncture wounds to the feet. Dog or cat bites are associated with *Pasteurella multocida*, human bites (clenched fist injuries) with *Eikenella corrodens*.

Clinical Syndromes

Acute hematogeneous osteomyelitis in children usually presents acutely with fever, chills, and pain in the involved bone. Boys are affected more commonly than girls. As the tibia and femur are the most commonly affected bones, the child presents with a limp or inability to bear weight. Other symptoms such as abdominal pain, anorexia, and general malaise may be present. Physical examination may reveal an acutely ill child with fever and point tenderness of the involved area of bone. There may be accompanying erythema and edema of the soft tissues overlying the area.

Vertebral osteomyelitis, on the other hand, may be acute or subacute and mainly affects the cervical vertebrae in intravenous drug users or the lumbar vertebrae in older adults. In the latter group, the mean age is 60 to 70 years, and the source of infection is frequently traced to the genitourinary system. In the acute presentation of the disease, patients complain of fever, neck or back pain, and stiffness. The physical examination reveals tenderness to palpation and percussion of the involved area. There may be paraspinal muscle spasm, with splinting and kyphosis. Back motion is limited. Occasionally, the infection may

spread rapidly to involve adjacent vertebral bodies and the disk space between them, or inward to involve the spinal canal. When the latter occurs, patients present with neurologic deficits or signs of spinal cord compression. In about half of the cases, vertebral osteomyelitis is subacute. Patients may present with vague, dull pain over weeks to months. In these instances, fever is typically absent or low grade. Chronic osteomyelitis may present with persistent dull pain overlying the involved bone or any complication of chronic infection, most notably draining sinus tracts.

Diagnosis and Treatment

The diagnosis of osteomyelitis can often be made on the basis of history and physical examination, aided by laboratory and radiographic tests. The ESR is elevated in a great majority of patients with osteomyelitis. The WBC count is often normal. Blood cultures may identify the causative organism in acute hematogeneous osteomyelitis in children and occasionally in the adult. Radiographs may be helpful in staging the disease. The earliest radiographic findings of acute osteomyelitis, however, may lag 10 to 14 days behind the clinical syndrome, which roughly corresponds to the development of bone necrosis. Typical x-ray findings include cortical disruption, periosteal elevation, focal osteopenia, lytic lesions, and new bone formation. In advanced stages and chronic osteomyelitis, radiographs may demonstrate a characteristic periosteal reaction, as well as evidence of bone necrosis and sclerosis. When the diagnosis is suspected, but the x-ray is normal, as is common early in the course of disease, a triple phase technetium 99 bone scan is recommended. Bone scans are generally highly sensitive for osteomyelitis but are not specific. False-positive bone scans occur in healing fractures, heterotopic ossification, and bone tumors, and false-negative results occur in areas where the edema causes decreased vascular flow and ischemia of the affected area. Other radioisotope scans (gallium and indium) have also been used with good results. Recently, ultrasound was found useful in detecting periosteal elevation and periosteal abcesses and in localizing the osteomyelitic area for needle aspiration. This method is, however, operator-dependent, hence limiting its use. CT scan may be useful in the early diagnosis of osteomyelitis, as it may demonstrate increased density of the bone marrow and intramedullary gas, and may identify areas of necrotic bone. It is also useful in detecting foreign bodies and can help guide needle biopsies. MRI is a highly sensitive study that is useful in delineating the boundaries of the infection, especially when extension into the soft tissues is suspected. MRI, however, cannot differentiate between post-surgical changes, tumors, infections, and fractures.

Admission to the hospital and prompt antibiotic administration are advisable at least initially, until culture and sensitivity results are obtained. Failure to diagnose and treat acute osteomyelitis may lead to extensive bone necrosis, chronic osteomyelitis, and death. The choice of antibiotics must be guided by the patient's risk factors and based on etiologic considerations. Because *S. aureus* is the most commonly isolated pathogen, antibiotic treatment must include coverage for this organism. An antistaphylococcal penicillin, such as nafcillin, or a first generation cephalosporin, such as cefazolin, would be reasonable choices. Vancomycin may be used in individuals allergic to penicillin and cephalosporins. Vancomycin is also the drug of choice for osteomyelitis caused by methicillin-resistant *S. aureus* (MRSA). When MRSA is suspected, rifampin may be added as it provides synergistic antistaphylococcal activity. Treatment of immunosuppressed patients, those with hemoglobinopathies, chronic alcohol consumers, diabetics, and the elderly should also include coverage for Gram-negative organisms. A third generation cephalosporin such as ceftazidime or an aminoglycoside is recommended in such instances. An antipseudomonal penicillin and/or an aminoglycoside should be considered in burn victims, in intravenous drug users, and in those with puncture wounds to the feet. Indications for surgery in acute hematogeneous osteomyelitis include the presence of subperiosteal and subcutaneous abscesses, and the presence of devascularized bone fragments. Sequestrae (necrotic infected bone islands) also need to be surgically debrided.

Cases of chronic or contiguous osteomyelitis are generally resistant to antibiotics alone, and often require surgery in order to remove devitalized bone and to restore its structure and vascularity. In these cases, broad-spectrum antibiotics, such as piperacillin-tazobactam, ampicillin-sulbactam, and clindamycin are often prescribed.

Tumors

Bone tumors may be primary or metastatic. Except for multiple myeloma, primary bone tumors predominantly occur in children and adolescents, during maximal growth rates. They may be benign or malignant, and may arise from the hematopoietic, stromal, vascular, and neural cell lines. In adults, metastatic bone lesions from breast, lung, kidney, prostate, and thyroid tumors predominate. A detailed description of all tumors affecting bone is beyond the scope of this chapter; only the most common neoplasms are discussed.

Benign Bone Tumors

Most benign bone tumors do not cause pain and are found incidentally or when a fracture or compression of other structures occurs. Patients present with a history of a slowly growing bone mass or deformity over several weeks or months. Radiographically, benign tumors may be well circumscribed or expansile, septated or not, radiolucent or mixed with sclerotic lesions. Benign bone tumor may originate from cartilage (chondromas, chondroblastomas), bone (osteoma, osteoid osteoma, osteoblastoma), mixed bone and cartilage (osteochondroma), or giant cells.

Osteochondroma is probably a developmental malformation rather than a true neoplasm, but it is the most common benign tumor of bone. Usually nonpainful, it is an exostosis of well-differentiated bone covered by cartilage. It affects children and adolescents most commonly, and is generally a solitary lesion. When multiple lesions are found, the condition may be familial and may have a higher incidence of malignant degeneration.

Chondromas are relatively common benign lesions of cartilagenous origin. They are usually solitary; however, they may be multiple in the familial Ollier's disease. Chondromas most commonly affect the diaphysis of small bones of the hands and feet and are generally painless and found incidentally on x-ray. Pain may be a sign of malignant degeneration into chondrosarcoma as occurs in Ollier's disease.

Chondroblastoma is an uncommon benign neoplasm with a predilection for the epiphysis. It occurs most commonly in males younger than 20 years of age. Patients complain of progressive pain similar to that of chronic synovitis.

Osteoid osteoma, a benign tumor that is closely related to osteoblastoma, commonly presents during the second decade of life, predominantly in males. Although any bone may be affected, the most frequent sites are the femur and tibia. Patients typically present with progressively worsening pain of the involved bone, especially at night, and relieved by salicylates. The physical examination may disclose edema, erythema, induration, or tenderness of the involved area. Radiographically, this tumor is a well-circumscribed radiolucent area surrounded by a sclerotic margin. Referral for excision is indicated.

Osteomas are well-circumscribed benign collections of sclerotic bone that occur almost exclusively in the face and skull. They are rare, commonly affect young adults, and are very similar to osteoid osteoma, but are typically larger and lack the sclerotic margin on radiographic evaluation. These may be associated with the familial Gardner's syndrome.

Malignant Bone Tumors

In children and young adults, malignant bone tumors are highly aggressive, rapidly growing tumors that have a high propensity for metastatic spread. It is not uncommon for patients to have metastases at the time of presentation. The neoplasms may originate from bone (osteogenic sarcoma), cartilage (chondrosarcoma), neuroectodermal elements (Ewing's sarcoma), or lymphoid tissue (multiple myeloma, leukemia, etc.). Osteogenic sarcoma and Ewing's sarcoma occur primarily in children and young adults, whereas chondrosarcoma occurs primarily in middle age and multiple myeloma in the elderly.

Osteogenic sarcoma is the most common malignant bone tumor in children and young adults, where it is thought to have a genetic predisposition, whereas in older patients it may occur as a complication of Paget's disease or after exposure to radiation. It is highly aggressive, with a propensity for rapid hematogeneous spread to the lungs. The neoplasm most commonly affects the metaphysis of the distal femur and may exhibit skip areas histologically. Patients present with progressive pain of a few weeks' duration, associated with a limp or limited motion of the extremity. The physical examination may reveal a painful, tender mass associated with edema, increased warmth, and erythema. Radiographic evaluation may disclose a typical "sunburst" appearance, with a radiolucent intramedullary area, surrounded by sclerosis, and periosteal new bone formation, with extension of the calcification into the surrounding soft tissue. Multi-agent chemotherapy combined with wide radical amputation have greatly improved prognosis of this neoplasm.

Ewing's sarcoma is the second most common malignant bone neoplasm in patients younger than 30. It has recently been reclassified as a tumor of neuroectodermal origin. It is highly aggressive and, like osteogenic sarcoma, metastasizes rapidly through the bloodstream to the lungs.

Patients present with progressive pain and tenderness of the involved extremity. This may be accompanied by fever, leukocytosis, and elevated erythrocyte sedimentation rate and C-reactive protein, making it difficult to differentiate from osteomyelitis. Radiographically, Ewing's sarcoma is described as a radiolucent intramedullary area surrounded by eroded cortical bone and reactive new bone formation, which gives it the appearance of "onion layers." Metastases to the lungs are common at presentation, and, although aggressive chemotherapy and surgery have improved survival, prognosis remains poor.

Chondrosarcomas occur most commonly in adults and can be primary or may arise from malignant degeneration of a preexisting benign bone neoplasm. They most commonly affect the pelvis, ribs, and shoulders, but any bone may be affected. Patients present with a painful mass in bone, which is expansile and may become extensive, resulting in pathologic fractures. They metastasize slowly through the bloodstream to involve other bones and the lungs. Chondrosarcomas are both radioresistant and chemotherapy-resistant, making surgical excision the principal mode of treatment. Prognosis depends on the histologic grade of the disease, and ranges from excellent for grade I to poor for grade III.

ED management of bone tumors consists of obtaining a detailed history and physical examination and rapidly assessing patients for potentially immediately life-threatening complications. These include pathologic fractures, impingement on vital structures such as the central nervous system, and metabolic abnormalities. Once stabilized, the ED workup of bone tumors consists of x-rays of the involved bones and a chest x-ray searching for metastases. CT scanning is also an important tool as it is able to delineate the borders and the extent of the lesion; furthermore, it is more sensitive than the radiograph in detecting metastatic lesions of the lungs. Immediate referral to orthopedic and oncology services are indicated, since definitive diagnosis requires a biopsy.

Bone Cysts

Bone cysts are uncommon lesions of bone, which grow slowly and are thought to be secondary to developmental defects. They tend to present insidiously with a slowly growing mass, chronic pain, and often with a pathologic fracture. They may be classified into two categories.

Solitary or unicameral bone cysts occur most commonly in children and young adults and frequently affect the metaphysis of long bones. The cyst, which may vary in size, is of unknown etiology, and may contain hemosiderin and cholesterol deposits and have elevated levels of prostaglandin PGE2. Cysts commonly present as a pathologic fracture. Occasionally, patients may give a history of chronic pain or a slowly growing mass. Treatment is mainly supportive and preventative, unless the cyst is large, in which case, patients may require aspiration with instillation of methylprednisolone, internal fixation with nails and occasionally, bone grafting.

Aneurysmal bone cysts occur most commonly in the second decade of life and most frequently affect flat bones, although the metaphysis of any long bone may also be affected. These lesions are often sponge-like, multicystic, destructive, and expansile. They contain hemorrhagic fluid and cause pain and swelling in the involved bone. Radiographically, aneurysmal bone cysts appear as lytic bone lesions that are well-circumscribed and delimited by periosteum and that expand into the surrounding soft tissue. These lesions require wide surgical excision or aggressive curettage and cauterization. Radiation therapy, which was highly effective, is no longer recommended because of a high incidence of sarcomatous transformation of the cyst.

Osteoporosis

Osteoporosis is a term used to describe a decrease in bone mass. Both the collagenous matrix (osteoid) and bone mineralization are affected. The most important risk factors are gonadal senescence and advanced age. Other factors, such as diabetes and the use of glucocorticoids, chronic alcohol, and nicotine consumption, prolonged immobilization, and malabsorption syndromes, may also predispose to the development of osteoporosis.

Occasionally, it may be idiopathic. Osteoporosis is generally clinically silent until fractures occur. In the absence of fractures, chronic back pain is the most common presenting complaint.

When osteoporosis is associated with loss of gonadal function, both bone resorption and formation are increased but resorption occurs at a higher rate. This is characterized by an increase in osteoclastic activity and is most visible in areas where cancellous bone is prominent, such as the vertebrae, the ribs, and the pelvis. When fractures occur, they do so after seemingly trivial trauma. Rib fractures, for example, may result from coughing and sneezing. Patients present with pain and splinting of their respirations. Physical examination may reveal tenderness and crepitation over the fractured rib, or they may present with complications of rib fractures such as atelectasis, hypoxia, and pneumonia. Vertebral compression fractures may result from such mundane activities as bending or jumping. Patients present with back pain that begins suddenly and may radiate to the abdomen. It may be exacerbated by standing and valsalva maneuvers. The physical examination reveals tenderness over the spinous process, and radiographic evaluation will show anterior vertebral body collapse and wedging with decreased mineral bone density.

In contrast to postmenopausal events, osteoporosis of aging is associated with a decline in osteoblastic activity, especially noted in cortical areas of long bones. This form of osteoporosis most commonly affects patients older than 70 years. Patients may develop fractures of the femoral and humeral heads after minor mechanisms of trauma such as falls from a bed or tripping over a carpet. Pain and decreased range of motion of the involved extremity are common findings. As radiographic evaluation may yield negative results, a high index of suspicion should be kept in the elderly with falls, and further diagnostic workup with bone scans or CT scans should be pursued.

Treatment should focus on the stabilization of patients and immobilization of the injured bone. For compression fractures of the vertebrae, treatment is symptomatic with bed rest and adequate pain relief, and instructions should focus on the elimination of additional trauma. As these fractures may be complicated by paralytic ileus, patients must be given instructions to return for symptoms of bowel obstruction. Cautious mobilization should begin as pain resolves. Femoral head fractures require hospitalization and surgical fixation. They are associated with a high complication rate, including thromboembolic phenomena and death.

When decreased bone mass is an incidental radiographic finding, patients must be referred for workup. A number of therapeutic modalities have been suggested; however, none have proven to be beneficial when the disease is already established. These include pharmacologic and nonpharmacologic therapy. Nonpharmacologic therapy consists of exercise, diets rich in calcium, vitamin D and protein, and the cessation of smoking. Pharmacologic therapy consists of vitamin D, bisphosphonates, and calcitonin. Estrogen therapy is no longer recommended because of its risks, but estrogen-receptor modulators may be helpful in attenuating bone loss, without the increased risk of breast cancer. Other substances, such as androgens and HMG-CoA reductase inhibitors are currently being studied. ED instuctions must focus on preventative measures such as the avoidance of sudden movements and cautious back exercises.

Osteomalacia

Osteomalacia is a metabolic bone defect in the adult in which the mineralization of bone is defective. As mineralization of bone depends on an adequate supply of calcium, which in turn depends on vitamin D, any process that interferes with the function or quantity of vitamin D may result in osteomalacia (in adults) and rickets (in children). These include decreased vitamin D intake, decreased sunlight exposure, malabsorption syndromes, renal failure, and drug interactions. In the presence of normal vitamin D function, osteomalacia may also be caused by low levels of phosphate or by a decreased ability of bone to rapidly accumulate calcium (as occurs in aluminium toxicity). The clinical manifestations of osteomalacia include generalized bone pain and tenderness, which may be severe enough to restrict activity of the patient. Proximal muscle weakness may be a prominent finding. When the pelvic or hip girdle is affected, patients may present with an abnormal gait. Bone fractures may occur with minimal trauma. Radiographically, bone may be normal even in advanced disease or show a generalized decrease in mineralization. Occasionally, pseudofractures or looser's zones may be noted: these are bilateral, symmetrical linear radiolucencies that are perpendicular to the axis of bone and that in-

volve only one cortex. They are not tender and are not associated with any evidence of bone healing. They are thought to be secondary to the mechanical stress imposed by the nourishing arteries. A careful clinical history and physical examination will guide the physician toward the diagnosis. Often, the underlying disease may dominate the clinical picture, and treatment of these conditions, when they do present to the ED, may supersede the diagnosis of osteomalacia. The treatment of osteomalacia is therefore deferred until the underlying condition is stabilized and the exact mechanism of the disease established.

Bone Spurs

Bone spurs (osteophytes) are bony protrusions frequently noted in the middle aged and older patient and are thought to result from chronic stress on the involved bone. The exact mechanism of spur formation remains unclear. They may be incidental radiographic findings or may present with pain.

Bone spurs are common in the cervical and lumbar spines, and are usually associated with chronic degenerative disk disease of the spine. When symptoms occur, pain, paresthesias, and sensory or motor deficits secondary to nerve root compression are common complaints. Treatment is supportive, with soft collars, salicylates or other nonsteroidal anti-inflammatory drugs (NSAIDs).

Another frequent site for spur formation is at the plantar aspect of the calcaneum. They are generally asymptomatic and found incidentally. When they become symptomatic, patients complain of heel pain, which is worse in the morning, improves during the early part of the day, but intensifies at the end of the day. They may be associated with certain systemic diseases, such as ankylosing spondylitis, Reiter's syndrome, or rheumatoid arthritis. ED treatment consists of heel padding, NSAIDs, and referral for orthotic considerations. Surgery is needed if the spur is palpable.

Paget's Disease

Paget's disease is a disease of unknown etiology that may affect up to 3% of the population older than 40 years. It is characterized by an increased resorption of bone, with a rapid but disorganized deposition of new bone. The disease is usually localized to one area of the skeleton but occasionally may be widespread. Characteristically, patients are asymptomatic. The diagnosis is suspected based on the mosaic appearance of bone on the radiographs. When symptoms do occur, pain in the involved bone is the initial complaint. The patient may present with a complication of the disease, such as pathologic fractures, nerve root compression, hypercalcemia, calcific aortic stenosis, and high-output cardiac failure (owing to increased blood flow to affected bone). Rarely, the disease is complicated by the occurrence of osteogenic sarcoma. The ED diagnosis is made based on the radiographic appearance and the presence of elevated levels of alkaline phosphatase. Treatment is usually symptomatic. When pain occurs, mild analgesics are effective. Complications are treated accordingly, fractures need to be immobilized and referred to the orthopedic surgeon, adequate hydration must be ensured, and symptomatic hypercalcemia must be treated with intravenous fluids, furosemide, and corticosteroids. Cortico-steroids have also been found to alleviate the high cardiac outputs associated with Paget's disease. The use of agents that reduce excessive bone resorption (e.g., calcitonin and etidronate) are indicated when patients present with spinal or cranial nerve involvement and should only be given after consultation with the appropriate services.

Selected Readings

Assouline-Dayan Y. Pathogenesis and natural history of osteonecrosis. *Semin Arthritis Rheum* 2002;32:94–124.

Atsumi T, Kuroki Y. Role of impairment of blood supply of the femoral head in the pathogenesis of idiopathic osteonecrosis. *Clin Orthop* 1992;227:22–30.

Babbitt AM. Osteoporosis. *Orthopedics* 1994;10:935.

Bassett GS. Idiopathic and heritable disorders. In: Weinstein SL, Buckwalter JA, eds. *Turek's Orthopaedics. Principles and Their Application,* 5th ed. Philadelphia: Lippincott, Williams and Wilkins 1994:251–255.

Bone tumors: evaluation and treatment. *Orthop Clin North Am* 1989;20:273–518.

Carnesale PG. Benign tumors of bone. In: Canale ST, ed. *Campbell's Operative Orthopaedics.* 10th ed., St. Louis, MO: Mosby 2003:793–812.

Delaney MF, LeBoff MS. Metabolic bone disease. In: Kelley WN, Harris ED, Ruddy S, et al., eds. *Textbook of Rheumatology,* 6th ed. Philadelphia: Saunders 2001: 1635–1652.

Esterhai JL Jr. Orthopedic infection. *Orthop Clin North Am* 1991;22:363–549.

Falk MJ, Heeger S, Lynch KA, et al. Intravenous bisphosphonate therapy in children with osteogenesis imperfecta. *Pediatrics* 2003;111:573–578.

Heck RK Jr. Benign (occasionally aggressive tumors of bone) and malignant tumors of bone. In: Canale ST, ed. *Campbell's Operative Orthopaedics,* 10th ed. St. Louis, MO: Mosby 2003:813–858.

Lew DP, Waldvogel FA. Osteomyelitis. *N Engl J Med* 1997;336:999–1007.

Ma M, Hungerford DS. Nontraumatic avascular necrosis of the femoral head. *J Bone Joint Surg* 1995;77:459–474.

Mankin HJ. Nontraumatic necrosis of bone. *N Engl J Med* 1992;326:1473.

Manolagas SC, Jilka RL. Bone marrow, cytokines and bone remodelling: emerging insights into the pathophysiology of osteoporosis. *N Engl J Med* 1995;332:305.

McGuire MH. The pathogenesis of adult osteomyelitis. *Orthop Res* 1989;18:564.

Paluska SA. Osteomyelitis. *Clin Fam Pract* 2004;6;127.

Shapiro JR. Heritable disorders of structural proteins. In: Kelley WN, Harris ED, Ruddy S, et al, eds. *Textbook of Rheumatology,* 6th ed. Philadelphia: Saunders 2001:1433–1461.

Smith DWE. Is avascular necrosis of femoral head the result of inhibition of angiogenesis? *Med Hypotheses* 1997;49:497–500.

Watson RM. Avascular necrosis of bone and bone marrow edema syndrome. *Radiol Clin North Am* 2004;42:207–219.

69 Joint Disorders

Brian Sloan

Introduction

The patient that presents with the complaint of an injured or painful joint is common in the emergency department (ED) setting. The disorder must be thoroughly evaluated and treated promptly to avoid morbidity. A thoughtful workup must include a detailed history and physical examination, as well as the use of selected diagnostic tests to assist in making a diagnosis.

Joint disorders affect all age groups; however the prevalence of arthritides increases with advancing age. The focus of this chapter is directed toward non-traumatic causes of joint disorders.

The causes of joint disorders can be categorized into those that involve a single joint (monoarticular arthritis), those that involve more than one joint (polyarticular arthritis), and disorders outside the joint capsule (periarticular) disorders. The classification into mono- or polyarticular arthritis has overlap but it does serve as a method for diagnosis of the patient presenting with complaints of a painful joint.

Anatomy

Human joint work with an intricate arrangement of bones, tendons, muscles, ligaments, and cartilage. The efficient function of joint and all of the surrounding structures is imperative to ensure smooth function.[1] Synovial joints are classified according to shape as in ball and socket (hip), hinge (interphalangeal), saddle (first metacarpal), and plane (patellofemoral) joints.

Articular cartilage is a specialized avascular and neural connective tissue that provides covering for the osseous components of diarthrodial (synovial) joints.[1] Articular cartilage serves as load bearing material, absorbs impact, and is capable of withstanding shearing forces.[1]

The synovial membrane lines the joint space and lubricates joints by secreting fluid that is made in the synovial lining. Joint fluid has a high viscosity due to the presence of hyaluronic acid.

Joints can become inflamed by a variety of mechanism including trauma, infection, crystal deposition, and various other arthritides.

Monoarticular Arthritis

The most common diseases causing pain and swelling in a single joint are infection and the crystalline arthropathies.[2,3] The early evaluation and diagnosis of patients presenting with acute joint swelling is mandatory to preserve the articular cartilage and reduce the chance of long term sequelae.

Diagnostic studies such as radiographs, complete blood counts, erythrocyte sedimentation rates, C-reactive proteins, and serologic studies are occasionally useful in the initial workup of patients with joint disorders, however, the history and physical examination remain the keys to making the diagnosis in patients with joint complaints.

Infectious Arthritis

Infectious arthritis if untreated can lead to irreversible joint damage.[2-7] Therefore, a patient presenting with acute onset of monoarticular arthritis should be considered to have septic arthritis until proven otherwise.

Bacteria, fungi, and viruses can enter the joint via direct inoculation, hematogenous spread, an abscess, trauma, foreign body invasion, or during joint surgery.[5,6] Certain bacteria, such as *Neisseria gonorrhoeae,* are particularly likely to infect a joint during a bacteremic episode.

Systemic disorders that alter the bodies' immune system can predispose patients to infection involving the joints. Patients with diabetes mellitus, liver disease, chronic renal insufficiency, malignancy, recent prosthetic surgery, intravenous drug abuse, alcoholism, organ transplantation, acquired immune deficiency syndrome, and hypogammaglobulinemia all are more likely than the patient with a competent immune system to develop septic arthritis.[5,6] In addition, a thorough social history is warranted to uncover if the patient is using illicit intravenous drugs or alcohol.

Physical exam findings in patients with infectious arthritis in 80% to 90% of cases reveal a painful, hot swollen single joint. In 10% to 20% of cases a polyarticular pattern may occur. The knee is the most common site for septic arthritis, however, any joint can be infected.[2,3,5,6] Patients infected with the *Neisseria gonor-*

rhoeae can present with migratory polyarthritis, dermatis, and fever. Virtually any microorganism can cause septic arthritis.[2,5,6] The most common cause of septic arthritis is *Staphylococcus aureus*. *Staphylococcus epidermis* infection is much more commonly seen in prosthetic infection compared to native joint infection. Anaerobic infection is most commonly seen in prosthetic joint infections and in diabetics who develop septic arthritis.

Gram-negative bacilla and *Haemophilus influenzae* are the most common pathogens in children under the age of 5.[4] *N. gonorrhoeae* is the most common form of bacterial arthritis in the young, healthy, sexually active adult in the United States. It occurs in 1% to 3% of patients infected with *N. gonorrhoeae*.

The diagnostic modality of choice in patients who present with acute onset of monoarticular arthritis is arthrocentesis. Routine synovial fluid studies should include leukocyte count, Gram stain, culture with antibiotic sensitivities, crystal analysis, glucose, and lactate dehydrogenase. Synovial fluid aspirated from infected joints often yields a leukocyte count between 50,000 and 100,000 cell/mm[3]. Polymorphonuclear cells predominate in septic arthritis. Glucose levels are usually decreased and lactate dehydrogenase levels typically are elevated. Gram stains can be helpful when positive, however they are only positive between 60% to 80% of the time.[5]

Treatment for septic arthritis should be initiated once the leukocyte count or the Gram stain returns. The antibiotics that are selected should be targeted toward the fluid analysis and the clinical scenario. At the time diagnosis is made emergent orthopedic consultation should be made to arrange for admission and possible joint irrigation and drainage.

Crystal-Induced Arthritis

Acute Gout

Gout is a common disorder of urate metabolism that is characterized by the deposition of monosodium urate crystals in the joints and soft tissues and is currently the most common cause in inflammatory arthritis in men over the age of 40.[8] Gout has been described as a heterogenous disorder that can progress through four clinical phases if untreated: asymptomatic hyperuricemia, acute/recurrent gout, intercritical gout, and chronic tophaceous gout. For the purpose of this text, we will focus on the clinical presentation of acute gout.

The symptoms of an acute gout attack include sudden onset of severe pain that often prohibits even the lightest touch of the affected joint. Other symptoms include swelling, fever, warmth, and severe limitation of motion.[2,3,8-10] Fever, leukocytosis, elevation of the erythrocyte sedimentation rate, and an elevated C reactive protein may also be present. Approximately 90% of first attacks are monoarticular. Inflammation of the first metatarsophalangeal joint occurs in more than 50% of first attacks. Acute gout can occur in the presence or absence of precipitating factors such as stress, trauma, excess alcohol consumption, infection, surgery, initiation of uric

acid lowering drugs, or drugs that can cause increased urate levels.

The clinical triad of an acute gout attack is monoarticular arthritis, an elevated serum uric acid level, and a response to colchicine. However, many elderly patients will present to the ED in an atypical fashion. Atypical gout in elderly patients can be polyarticular and chronic. Serum acid levels can be high in asymptomatic patients and normal in those with an acute gout presentation.

In patients with an acute gout attack that the clinician is unsure of the disease process and septic arthritis is in the differential diagnosis one must perform an arthrocentesis. The presence of monosodium urate crystals in synovial fluid will confirm the diagnosis. The monosodium crystals are needle shaped under standard light microscopy and when examined under a polarizing light microscope the crystals are strongly negatively birefringent. Proper identification of MSU or other crystals in synovial fluid is highly dependent on the experience of the observer.

The synovial fluid in patients with an acute attack of gout can be confusing to the ED practitioner due to the elevation in white blood cells in the synovial fluid. Patients with acute gouty arthritis will have a white blood count in the range of 5,000 to 50,000/μL and are predominately neutrophils. For patients with elevated synovial white blood cell counts, the practitioner may want to initiate antibiotic therapy until crystal identification is performed because, in many laboratories, the crystal identification, Gram stain, and culture results may lag behind the white blood cell count report by several hours. This option will prevent delay in treatment for those with undifferentiated monoarticular arthritis that could still be infectious.

Treatment options for acute gout include nonsteroidal anti-inflammatory drugs, colchicine, corticosteroids, opioid analgesics, and corticotropin (adrenocorticotropin).[10]

Nonsteroidal anti-inflammatory drugs are considered first-line treatment for treating acute gout in the United States. A variety of nonsteroidal medications have been approved for the treatment of acute gout. The ED physician should decide on which to use based on side effects and availability. Shrestha et al suggested that intramuscularly administered ketorolac was comparable to indomethacin for improving pain associated with acute gout.[11] In general, high doses of NSAIDs are initially used for the treatment of acute gout in patients that can tolerate the medication. Newer cyclooxygenase-2 selective inhibitors have been tested for the acute treatment of gout. This data has suggested that these agents are as effective as traditional NSAIDs without the adverse events.[9]

Colchicine is effective treatment for an acute gout attack if initiated within the first 24 to 48 hours of symptoms. A randomized double blind, controlled trial of colchicine versus placebo did reveal a faster clinical response and superior pain relief in the group treated with colchicine compared to the placebo group.[12] Colchicine was given 1 mg initially followed by 0.5 mg every 2 hours until pain relief or the patient experiences toxicity. Colchicine however carries with it significant risk of side effects. Common side effects include nausea, diarrhea, vomiting, and stomach upset. Other important side effects include myopathy and neuropathy.

The use of intravenously administered colchicine should be initiated with great caution due to its potentially serious adverse events.[8-10] Tissue necrosis from IV infiltration of colchicine into the soft tissues, cytopenia, disseminated intravascular coagulation, and death has been reported.

Corticosteroids given intra-articular or systemically, ACTH, and opioid analgesics are all alternative therapies that can be used in the treatment of gout in selective patients.

Pseudogout

In middle-aged and elderly adults, acute monoarticular arthritis may also be induced by crystals of calcium pyrophosphate dihydrate (CPPD). In 1961 CPPD deposition was identified in synovial fluid of patients with acute gout like arthritis thus the term "pseudogout" was initiated.[13]

The knee is the most affected joint in patients with pseudogout.[14] In one study by Masuda, the knee was noted to be the primary joint involved in 51% of patients who tested positive by arthrocentesis.[14]

Attacks have also been known to affect more than one joint however, many polyarticular events occur after a systemic illness, surgery, or after an intraarticular injection of depot steroid.

Previous investigators have noted that pseudogout is often misdiagnosed as septic arthritis (**Table 69.1**). Patients with sudden onset of fever, acute joint pain, swelling, and redness of the affected joint will often prompt the ED physician to treat the patient as a case of septic arthritis until the crystal evaluation has been completed. The presence of rhomboid shaped positively birefringent crystals

Table 69.1

Clinical Characteristics Suggestive of Pseudogout in Differential Diagnosis of Septic Arthritis

1. More common in elderly patients.
2. A history of an acute arthritic attack or a subclinical (petite) arthritic attack.
3. No history of arthrocentesis before the onset of the attack.
4. Chondrocalcinosis of the affected joint or other joints.
5. Turbid and blood stained or whitish synovial fluid.
6. Intracellular or extracellular rhomboid crystals with a positive birefringence in synovial fluid.
7. Sterile culture in synovial fluid.
8. Acute arthritic attacks affecting more than one joint.
9. Neuropsychiatric disorders or mental confusion.
10. Symptomatic improvement following joint lavage and intraarticular injection of microcrystalline glucocorticoid.

in polarized light will confirm the diagnosis. Since it is not always practical to delay treatment in patients in whom CPPD deposition versus septic arthritis is being considered, Ishikawa suggested ten clinical characteristics. For the treatment of pseudogout attacks once the diagnosis has been made an arthrocentesis followed by lavage and injection of a long acting steroid has shown very promising results.[16]

Polyarticular Arthritis

Significant overlap exists between arthropathy causing monoarticular and polyarticular arthritis. Many of the polyarticular arthropathies will cause migratory symptoms and patients may exhibit other systemic signs such as fever, rash, or other organ involvement. Diseases such as rheumatoid arthritis, systemic lupus erythematosus, scleroderma, osteoarthritis, and other systemic illnesses do not infrequently cause polyarticular arthropathy. Several that deserve further mention are discussed here.

Infectious Arthritis

Although infectious arthritis commonly affects only one joint, there are exceptions that deserve mention. In up to 9% of confirmed cases of infectious arthritis more than one joint is involved/5 Gonococcal arthritis can be both migratory and polyarticular before seeing one joint. Tuberculosis in 10% to 15% of cases can cause a polyarticular infectious arthritis.[5]

Lyme Disease

Lyme disease is the most common tick-borne disorder in the United States.[17] Lyme disease is recognized in 47 states but occurs mostly in northeastern United States and on the west coast.[16,18,19] The disease is caused by the tick borne spirochete *Borrelia burgdorferi*.[18] The clinical features begin after a 3- to 32-day incubation period.[18] The characteristic large annular rash called erythema migrans occurs in 80% of patients. The arthritis that occurs due to Lyme disease is polyarticular in 37% of patients and the disease is noted to occur more frequently than adults. Lyme disease can often be mistaken for other forms of arthritis, therefore, the serologic confirmation of the disease by ELISA and a confirmatory immunoblot are necessary to initiate appropriate antimicrobial therapy. Patients testing positive for Lyme disease should be started on antibiotic therapy for four weeks. Current recommendations are doxycycline, tetracycline, amoxicillin, or penicillin V.

Rheumatic Fever

Rheumatic fever is an acute inflammatory condition that follows and infection caused by Group A beta-hemolytic streptococcus.[20] Rheumatic fever is uncommon in developed countries but remains a source of significant morbidity in underdeveloped countries. Rheumatic fever may develop at any age, but is infrequent in early infancy and after the age of 30.[20] The diagnosis of rheumatic fever is

Table 69.2

Jones Criteria for Diagnosing Rheumatic Fever

Major Manifestations	Minor Manifestations
Carditis	Clinical
Polyarthritis	Fever
Chorea	Arthralgia
Erythema marginatum	Previous rheumatic fever or rheumatic heart disease
Subcutaneous nodules	Plus: Supporting evidence of preceding streptococcal infection: Increased ASO or other streptococcal antibodies. Positive throat culture for group A *Streptococcus* spp. Recent scarlet fever.

based on clinical features plus evidence of an antecedent streptococcal infection. The Jones criteria for diagnosis of rheumatic fever were developed in 1944 which combine clinical and laboratory studies to confirm the diagnosis (**Table 69.2**).[21] The presence of two major and one minor, or one major and one minor, in addition to the evidence of prior streptococcal infection are highly suggestive of the disease. Acute polyarthritis is the most frequent initial symptom, occurring in 85% to 95% of patients.[20] Large joints are most commonly affected, and symptoms are usually severe, develop acutely, and have prominent periarticular inflammation.

Arthrocentesis

Arthrocentesis is a relatively common procedure in the emergency department.

Arthrocentesis is indicated in patients who present with an acutely swollen joint or in any patient where the diagnosis of septic arthritis is entertained.[6,22] In addition to diagnosing septic arthritis, arthrocentesis can be performed to diagnose crystal-induced arthropathies, and occult fractures. A therapeutic arthrocentesis can be performed to help alleviate symptoms in patients with acute hemarthrosis, crystal-induced arthropathy, and in patients with osteoarthritis.

Arthrocentesis is a relatively simple procedure. Knowledge of anatomic landmarks and patient positioning will aid in the successful completion of joint aspiration. Ultrasound has aided physicians when performing arthrocentesis in areas traditionally reserved for orthopedic surgeons or interventional radiologists.[23] Reports of ED physicians aspirated joints such as the hip have been described in the literature.[23,24]

The contraindications for performing an arthrocentesis are to be debated. Some experts feel that a joint should not be aspirated if cellulitis is present where the needle will be inserted. This has been debated and current recommenda-

tions are such that if you suspect a joint to be infected the ED physician should make every attempt to obtain fluid for diagnosis. There are no reported cases in the literature of physicians inoculating the join with bacteria due to an overlying skin infection.

The complications from arthrocentesis are rare. The reported incidence of complications varies but most likely lies between 0.01% and 0.1%. In one study the incidence of infection from the introduction of bacteria during arthrocentesis was reported as 0.0002%.[25] The most common complications that do occur are pain during the procedure, infection of the joint, arthritis flare, and re-accumulation of joint fluid.

Synovial Fluid Evaluation

The evaluation of synovial fluid once obtained is required for accurate diagnosis. A reasonable "routine" fluid analysis should include microbiologic culture, Gram stains, crystal analysis, cell count, and differential.[26] Obtaining chemistry analysis of synovial fluid is left to the discretion of the clinician.

References

1. Simkin P. The musculoskeletal system. In: Schumacher R, ed. *Primer on Rheumatic Diseases*. Atlanta: Arthritis Foundation 1993:349.
2. Sack K. Monoarthritis: differential diagnosis. *Am J Med* 1997;102:30s–34s.
3. Schumacher R. Arthritis of recent onset. *Postgrad Med* 1995;97:52–63.
4. Shetty A. Septic arthritis in children. *Rheum Dis Clin North Amer* 1998;24:287–304.
5. Torre IL. Advances in the management of septic arthritis. *Rheum Dis Clin North Am* 2003;29:61–75.
6. Mitchell M, Howard B, Haller J, et al. Septic arthritis. *Radiol Clin North Am* 1988;26:1295–1313.
7. Levine I MK, McGowan K, Flynn J. Assessment for the test characteristics of c-reactive protein for septic arthritis in children. *J Pediatr Orthoped* 2003:23:373–377.
8. Rott K, Agudelo CA. Gout. *JAMA* 2003;289:2857–2860.
9. Kim K, et al. A literature review of the epidemiology and treatment of acute gout. *Clin Therapeut* 2003:25:1593–1617.
10. Emmerson B. The management of gout. *N Engl J Med* 1996;334:445–451.
11. Shrestha M, Morgan DL, Moreden J, et al. Randomized double blind comparison of the analgesic efficacy of intramuscular ketorolac and oral indomethacin in the treatment of acute gouty arthritis. *Ann Emerg Med* 1995;26:682–686.
12. Ahern M, et al. Does colchicine work? The results of the first controlled study in acute gout. *Aust N Z J Med* 1987;17:301–304.
13. McCarty D, et al. Identification of urate crystals in gouty synovial fluid. *Ann Int Med* 1961;54:152.
14. Masuda-I IK. Clinical features of pseudogout attack: A survey of 50 cases. *Clin Orthoped Rel Res* 1988; 229:174–181.
15. K I. Osteoarthritis of the knee and articular chondrocalcinosis. *J Joint Surg (Japan)* 1985;4:725.
16. Simkin P. The musculoskeletal system. In: Schumacher R, ed. *Primer on Rheumatic Diseases*. Atlanta: Arthritis Foundation 1993:349.
17. Orloski KA, Hayes EB, Campbell JL. Surveillance for Lyme disease, United States, 1992-1998. *Morb Mort Wkly Rep* 2000:49:1–11.
18. Willis A, et al. Lyme arthritis presenting as acute septic arthritis in children. *J Pediatr Orthoped* 2003;23:114–118.
19. Gerber M, Zemel LS, Shapiro E. Lyme arthritis in children: clinical epidemiology and long-term outcomes. *Pediatrics* 1998;102:905–908.
20. L G. Rheumatic fever. In: Schumacher R, ed. *Primer on the Rheumatic Diseases*. Atlanta: Arthritis Foundation 1993:168–169.
21. Stollerman GMM, Taranta A, et al. Jones criteria (revised) for guidance in the diagnosis of rheumatic fever. *Circulation* 1965;32:664–668.
22. Johnson M. Acute knee effusions: a systematic approach to diagnosis. *Amer Fam Phys* 2000;61:2391–2400.
23. Smith S. Emergency physician-performed ultrasonography-guided hip arthrocentesis. *Acad Emerg Med* 1999;6:84–86.
24. Roy S, Dewitz A, Paul I. Ultrasound assisted ankle arthrocentesis. *Am J Emerg Med* 1999;17:300–301.
25. Gray R, Gottlieb N. Local corticosteroid injection treatment in rheumatic disorders. *Sem Arthritis Rheum* 1982;10:231–254.
26. Shmerling RH, Delbanco TL, Toteson AN, Trentham DE. Synovial fluid tests, what should be ordered. *JAMA* 1990;264:1009–1014.

70 Disorders of the Spine

Colleen N. Roche
Genevieve Bensinger

Anatomy of the Spine

The human spine consists of 33 vertebrae, separated by intervertebral disks. There are 7 cervical, 12 thoracic, 5 lumbar, 5 fused sacral, and 4 fused coccygeal vertebrae composing the axial skeleton. An intricate network of ligaments and musculature support the spine and contribute to its overall stability and flexibility.

The spinal column itself can be divided into 2 separate columns: the anterior and the posterior column. The anterior column is composed of the anterior longitudinal ligament, the vertebral body, and the posterior longitudinal ligament. The posterior column consists of the posterior bony structures (transverse processes, pedicles, laminae, facets, and transverse processes), the ligamentum flavum, the interspinous ligaments, and the supraspinous ligaments. The interspersed vertebral disks are composed of the outer annulus fibrosis and the inner nucleus pulposis. The annulus fibrosis is a network of concentric, interlaced fibrocartilagenous tissue, and is strongest anteriorly. The nucleus pulposus is a gelatinous substance that acts as the primary shock absorber of the spine.

The spinal cord is nestled between the anterior and posterior columns, extending from the midbrain to the conus medullaris, which terminates at L2, and forms the tethered bunch of nerves known as the cauda equina. There are 30 cervical nerves that exit the spinal column. The first cervical nerve exits above the level of the vertebrae, whereas all the other spinal nerves exit below the level of the associated vertebrae.

Evaluation of Spinal Disorders

The emergency department (ED) evaluation of disorders requires diligent history and physical skills. The examiner must understand the quality, location, and duration of the pain; associated symptoms, particularly paresthesias or weakness; alleviating and exacerbating factors; dysfunction of the bladder or bowels; presence of other systemic disease; and any potential external forces to the spine—the majority of injuries to the spine are caused by an acute flexion overload. Physical examination needs to focus on the musculoskeletal and neurologic examination, and should include evaluation of muscle strength, reflexes, gait, sensorium, and rectal tone.

The differential diagnosis for back pain is expansive, and careful evaluation can help narrow the differential, and avoid overlooking a catastrophic disease process. This chapter focuses on common disorders of the spine itself.

Ankylosing Spondylitis

Ankylosing spondylitis (AS) is a genetically predisposed chronic polyarticular inflammatory disease primarily involving the axial skeleton. Over 90% of patients with AS have been found to carry the HLA-B27 antigen, and is more commonly found in men than in women, although no linkage to the X-chromosome has been found.[1] The synovium of affected joints are infiltrated by leukocytes, which release cytokines, such as TNF-α. This creates a cascade of events involving progressive destruction of cartilaginous tissue and subchondral bone, formation of both granulation tissue, and new bone, ultimately resulting in joint ossification.

Patients with AS typically are young, since the disease typically manifests before the age of 40. AS patients present with a history of insidious onset of low back pain for more than 3 months, commonly located over the gluteal and sacroiliac (SI) region. As the disease progresses, back stiffness develops, particularly after periods of inactivity. This is what contributes to the classic symptom of "morning stiffness." The stiffness improves with activity throughout the day.

The first radiographic sign of AS is bilateral sacroiliitis. Spinal manifestations begin at either the thoracolumbar or lumbosacral junction, then progress. Initially, the margins of the vertebral bodies will appear to be squared off, secondary to new bone formation anteriorly, as well as periarticular osteopenia, which occurs secondary to inflammatory bone resorption. As the disease progresses, syndesmophytes are formed along the anterior fibers of the annulus fibrosis, and progressive ossification of the annulus fibrosis, facet joints, interspinous and supraspinous ligaments, and ligamentum flavum occurs. Once this degree of extensive ossification has occurred, spine radiographs will reveal the classic "bamboo spine," which is actually seen in relatively few patients with AS.

Although any joint in the body can theoretically be affected by AS, the most commonly affected joints outside the axial skeleton are the hips, shoulders, and knees. Involvement of the hips is often the most debilitating manifestation of this disease, and can lead to fusion of the hip in flexion. Joint replacement in these situations is warranted and has led to good results. Peripheral joint involvement is usually asymmetric, and rarely leads to chronic arthropathy.

Extra-articular organ systems may be affected by AS, primarily the eyes, cardiovascular system, and pulmonary system. Anterior uveitis is the most common extra-articular manifestation of the disease, and requires close follow-up with ophthalmology. Aortitis can develop, leading to fibrotic changes in the ascending aorta. This may then lead to a range of cardiac complications, including aortic insufficiency, cardiac conduction defects, and arrhythmias. Interstitial lung disease may also develop in this patient population. The most common pulmonary complication in AS is decreased chest expansion, and therefore, impaired pulmonary function testing, secondary to costosternal or costovertebral inflammation.

Complications of AS include slowly progressive cauda equina syndrome, as well as spinal fractures. Cauda equina syndrome can occur secondary to progressive sclerosis of the spinal canal, thus directly impinging on the nerves. Spinal fractures seen with AS are of two types: traumatic and stress fractures. Traumatic fractures occur with even minor trauma and are quite debilitating, and often missed on initial presentation, despite diligent clinical diagnostic skills and radiography. Fractures often present at the cervicothoracic junction, thoracolumbar junction, and mid-low cervical spine. Patients with stress fractures present with new pain in their spine and/or increased spinal range of motion from their norm. Radiographs may also be subtle initially. Therefore, if there is any suspicion that a patient with AS may have a spinal injury, advanced radiography, such as MRI or CT scan, is warranted in the initial workup.

The treatment of AS has centered around symptomatic pain relief, since no therapy has been shown to hasten the disease progression.[2] The hallmark of treatment for AS has included NSAIDs and physical therapy. Sulfasalazine has been shown to be effective in early disease, and a recent study by Gorman et al revealed some promise for anti-TNF-α injections improving outcomes in these patients.[2]

Spondylolysis/Spondylolisthesis

Spondylolysis is defined as a defect in the pars articularis, which is the bony isthmus between the superior and inferior facets. Spondylolysis may be congenital or acquired, and is most commonly seen in the lumbosacral spine. Spondylolisthesis is a progression of spondylolysis, and is defined as anterior displacement of a vertebral body on the one caudal to it. The incidence is equal among men and women, and the prevalence of spondylolisthesis is 5% to 6% in the general population. Genetic risk factors have been associated with this disease, including Alaskan Eskimo heritage, first-degree relative with the disease, presence of spina bifida occulta, and the presence of scoliosis.[3] Repetitive spinal forces, particularly with athletics such as football, gymnastics, and ballet, are the most common etiology of acquired spondylolysis.

Although radiographic evidence of congenitally acquired spondylolysis can be found in up to 75% of afflicted children by age 6,[4] children are often asymptomatic. Low back pain usually develops during the adolescent growth spurt, is insidious in nature, and is rarely associated with acute trauma. It is often exacerbated by hyperextension. Physical examination findings include antalgic gait, unilateral positive straight leg raise secondary to hamstring spasm, a flattened lumbar lordosis, and limitation of lumbar flexion and extension. In advanced disease, examination reveals a vertically oriented sacrum with visible step-off, and the buttocks may appear heart-shaped because of the sacral prominence. Neurologic findings are rarely observed, although a full neurologic examination should be performed when evaluating these patients.

Diagnostic evaluation of patients with possible spondylolisthesis includes AP, standing lateral, and supine oblique radiographs of the lumbar spine. The pars itself is best seen on the oblique films, and the full extent of spondylolisthesis can be evaluated with the standing lateral film. The Mayerding grading system is most commonly used to define the ratio of slippage between the cephalad and caudal vertebrae: grades I, < 25%; II, 25% to 50%; III, 50% to 75%; IV, > 75%.

For patients who present to the ED with diagnosed or suspected spondylysis or spondylolisthesis, treatment includes pain management, cessation of athletics, and follow-up with orthopaedics for immobilization and potential operative repair. Complications of this disease, if left unmanaged, include non-union of the pars defect and progressive disk disease, which can severely limit the patient's physical abilities.

Disk Disease

Herniated Lumbar Intervertebral Disk

The intervertebral discs are comprised of a gelatinous nucleus pulposus surrounded by a fibrous capsule, the annulus fibrosus. With repetitive movements, the annulus fibrosus may weaken, and the nucleus pulposus can protrude through the defect into the spinal canal. Disk herniation most commonly occurs in a posterolateral direction where the annulus is naturally the weakest. Ninety-five percent of herniated lumbar disks occur at the L4-5 or L5-S1 levels.[5] The nerve roots in the lumbar region exit the spinal canal below the level of their respective vertebral body, but above the intervertebral disk. Therefore, herniation of a lumbar disk does not affect the nerve roots exiting above it, but can impinge on the nerve roots exiting the canal below it.

Lumbar disk herniations most commonly occur in patients aged 30 to 40 years of age,[6] and these patients report a history of intermittent low back pain, which is often relieved with rest. Acutely, they experience sudden onset of low back and leg pain exacerbated by a flexion episode, although a history of trauma is rarely elicited. The pain is greater in the leg than in the back itself, and it is increased with Valsalva maneuvers or sitting. Physical examination reveals lumbar paraspinal spasm and findings consistent with sciatica. In fact, the likelihood of having a herniated lumbar disk in a patient who shows no evidence of sciatica has been estimated to be only one in 1,000.[7] A positive crossed-straight leg test is pathoneumonic for disk herniation. Radicular symptoms are localized unilaterally to the nerve root compressed, and full evaluation of motor strength, reflexes, and sensation can localize the level of the disk herniation. Upper lumbar or large disk herniations may compress the cauda equina, and these patients will present with lower extremity motor and sensory loss, perineal paresthesias, and decreased sphincter tone. Cauda equina syndrome is an acute emergency and is discussed later in this chapter.

Plain radiography is of limited use in the ED evaluation of disk herniation, unless there is suspicion of other disease processes, such as malignancy. MRI is warranted if there is evidence of cauda equina syndrome.

Patients with lumbar disk herniation should be treated conservatively with anti-inflammatory agents, and should be encouraged to immediately resume their daily activities. The majority of patients will recover with conservative management. Patients who present with cauda equina syndrome, progressive neurologic deficit, or sciatica persistent beyond 4 to 6 weeks may be candidates for surgical diskectomy, and a spine specialist should be involved in their care.[8]

Diskitis

Diskitis is a rare primary infection of the nucleus pulposus which may spread to adjacent vertebral bodies. It is acquired by hematogenous seeding, direct spread from vertebral osteomyelitis, and direct trauma, including surgery and spinal manipulation. Hematogenous spread is more likely to occur in the pediatric population because the intervertebral disks are highly vascularized in this age group; discitis is most commonly seen in children younger than six years of age. As patients age, their disks become more avascular, and adults are therefore less susceptible to this disease, although intravenous drug abusers, elderly patients, and the immunocompromised are at greater risk. In spontaneous cases, the infecting organisms are varied, including Gram-positives, Gram-negatives, and fungi; in postoperative patients, the infecting organism is usually *Staphylococcus aureus* or *Staphylococcus epidermidis.*[9]

The diagnosis of diskitis is primarily a clinical one. Patients present with malaise, irritability, and inability to walk or stand comfortably. On examination, the patients are often well-appearing, and they may have hamstring tightness or spinal tenderness on examination. Focal neurologic findings are rare. Fever is rarely present. Laboratory evaluation may reveal a mild leukocytosis and an elevated sedimentation rate.[10] The presence of both fever and leukocytosis are specific, but insensitive for the diagnosis of discitis. The causative organism has rarely been isolated from blood cultures. Plain radiographs may reveal

disk space narrowing, but cannot be seen for 4 to 6 weeks. Twenty-five percent of cases will progress to form spontaneous fusion of the two adjacent vertebral bodies. Definitive diagnosis primarily rests on fine needle aspiration of the disk space and culture.

Complications of diskitis include formation of epidural abscess, which would cause more discrete neurologic compromise, and vertebral osteomyelitis. Although administration of antibiotics has been somewhat controversial, patients should receive either antistaphylococcal antibiotic or antibiotics targeted at the isolated organism until the patients' symptoms improve and their sedimentation rate normalizes.[11]

Low Back Syndromes
Acute Lumbosacral Strain

Acute lumbosacral strain refers to muscular low back pain without neurologic involvement lasting less than 4 to 6 weeks in duration. Other names for this syndrome include mechanical back pain, low back sprain, and lumbago. Onset of pain may be abrupt, occurring immediately after an acute trauma or stress, or may occur gradually over a matter of hours. Patients report lumbar or sacral pain that may radiate to the buttocks or thighs, and are often unable to recall a particular event which may have precipitated the pain. Symptoms are exacerbated by movement and relieved with rest, especially lying still. If the pain radiates past the knees or if other neurologic symptoms are present, then the diagnosis of acute strain should be questioned.[5]

Physical examination commonly reveals lumbar muscular tenderness, accompanied by paravertebral muscle spasm. Point tenderness over the spine is not present and neurologic examination is normal. Plain radiographs are negative, as is further radiographic imaging, and are, therefore, unnecessary in the ED, unless an alternate diagnosis is expected.

Treatment should focus on pain control which is adequate to allow the patient to resume reasonable normal activity as soon as possible. Despite years of treating acute strain with varying durations of bed rest and back-mobilizing exercises, recent studies have shown that prompt return to daily activities will lead to a more rapid recovery than with bed rest or exercises.[12] Analgesic and anti-inflammatory medications should include acetaminophen, NSAIDs, and opioids, if necessary. The use of muscle relaxants and steroids for acute strain remains controversial.[5] Spontaneous resolution of symptoms within four weeks is seen in 90% of these patients.[13]

Sciatica

Sciatica refers to the symptoms of impingement of the sciatic nerve or the nerve roots which comprise it, namely the L4-S3 nerve roots. Although it is a common complaint, true sciatica is relatively uncommon, affecting only 2% to 3% of all patients complaining of low back pain.[5] The vast majority sciatica cases are secondary to a herniated nucleus pulposus at the L4-L5 or L5-S1 vertebral levels; but other causes include nerve root compression from foraminal stenosis, tumor, infection, hematoma, or lumbar spinal stenosis.

Patients with sciatica present with pain which radiates along the course of the sciatic nerve, down the posterolateral aspect of the leg, past the knee, and into the foot. Physical examination reveals a positive straight leg raise, which is a highly sensitive test for sciatica. This test has been found to be positive in 95% of cases of surgically proven herniated disks.[6] To perform the straight leg raise test, place the patient in the supine position and hold the affected leg by the ankle, keeping the knee extended. Begin to slowly lift the leg off the bed. If there is exacerbation of radicular pain when the leg is less than sixty degrees elevated, then the test is considered to be positive. A less sensitive but more specific test is the crossed straight leg raise test.[7] This test is performed by lifting the contralateral leg in a manner similar to the straight leg raise test. If pain is exacerbated in the originally affected leg, then the crossed straight leg raise test is considered to be positive. A focused neurologic exam can delineate the vertebral level of compression.

Plain radiographs of the lumbar spine should be obtained to rule out other causes of nerve root compression such as tumor, fracture, and spondylolisthesis. Further radiographic imaging should be reserved for those patients who have failed 3 to 4 weeks of conservative therapy.[6] Initial treatment is similar to that of acute lumbosacral strain. Analgesic and anti-inflammatory medications such as acetaminophen, NSAIDs, and opioids are typically used. The use of epidural steroid injections remains controversial.[5] Recent studies have shown no benefit of bed rest over prompt return to daily activities in the treatment of sciatica.[4] The majority of these patients will respond to conservative management within 4 to 6 weeks; only a small percentage will require surgical intervention for herniated lumbar intervertebral disks.[14]

Tumors

Tumors within the spine or spinal canal are a rare but a serious cause of low back pain. Only 1% of all cases of low back pain are attributable to malignant neoplasm, and greater than 80% of these patients are over 50 years of age.[7] Metastatic disease is the most common cause of the tumors; primary neoplasms are rare. If a patient has a history of cancer and is presenting with low back pain, then the diagnosis is presumed to be cancer until proven otherwise. However, only one third of patients with underlying malignant neoplasm carry the diagnosis.[7] The principal cancers which metastasize to bone are lung, prostate, breast, thyroid, and kidney. Other malignancies affecting the spine or spinal canal are malignant myeloma, lymphoma, leukemia, primary bone tumors, and primary cord or dural tumors.[14]

Patients with spinal malignancies often present with complaints of low back pain lasting greater than six weeks, pain which is worse at night, and recent weight loss. Physical examination must include evaluation of the organs typically involved in metastatic disease. Examination

of the spine may reveal point tenderness, but this is neither sensitive nor specific. Neurologic examination will vary depending on the specific area(s) of the spinal column involved. In patients exhibiting new or progressive neurologic deficits, high-dose dexamethasone must be administered before further evaluation.[5] Pain control is extremely important in the management of these patients. Plain radiographs are commonly negative; an MRI is needed for adequate evaluation. Further workup is centered on management of the malignant neoplasm.

Cauda Equina Syndrome

Cauda equina syndrome involves central epidural compression below the level of L1, where the spinal cord ends and becomes the collection of lumbar and sacral nerves known as the cauda equina. It is considered a neurosurgical emergency due to the potential for severe, permanent neurological sequelae. The most common cause of cauda equina syndrome is a significant midline herniation of an intervertebral disk.[5] Other etiologies include trauma, tumor, abscess, and hematoma. Patients usually present secondary to neurological symptoms; complaints of back pain are less common. A highly sensitive and specific symptom is urinary retention. In fact, a negative post-void residual has a negative predictive value of 99.99% for ruling out this diagnosis.[7] The patient may report urinary incontinence, not retention; this results from overflow of urine from a distended, denervated bladder. Anal sphincter tone is also decreased in the majority of cases. Lower extremity symptoms are bilateral, including sensory deficits over the buttocks, posterior thighs, and perineum and motor deficits ranging from weakness to complete paralysis.

If the diagnosis of cauda equina syndrome is being seriously considered, then the patient must receive systemic steroids prior to any further diagnostic testing. Dexamethasone is routinely used, though the dosing regimen remains controversial.[5] Although plain radiographs of the spine are an important initial exam, an MRI of the entire spine is the diagnostic test of choice. The MRI will delineate the extent of the cauda equina compression, as well as rule out any other site of spinal cord compression. The outcome for patients with cauda equina syndrome is related to the extent of their symptoms at presentation; those with earlier intervention have more extensive recovery.

Spinal Stenosis

Spinal stenosis is a chronic narrowing of the spinal canal at multiple vertebral levels most commonly due to degenerative hypertrophy of the ligamentum flavum. Hypertrophy of the intervertebral disks, vertebral bodies, and facets may also cause canal narrowing. Patients are usually in their 50s or 60s upon presentation, and report chronic low back pain without a history of trauma. The hallmark symptom is "pseudoclaudication."[7] Pseudoclaudication or neurogenic claudication is pain, weakness, and paresthesias in the lower extremities that occur with walking and are improved with rest in the face of adequate arterial flow.

Patients with spinal stenosis also report an improvement in their symptoms with low back flexion and exacerbation with extension: they will often state that it is more painful to walk downhill, when the back is naturally flexed, than uphill, when the back is naturally extended. The diagnosis is made by CT or MRI. Pain is usually controlled with NSAIDs or opioid analgesics. Persistent, debilitating pain or progressive neurologic symptoms may improve with laminectomy and/or spinal fusion.[8]

References

1. Bennett DL, Ohashi K, El-Koury G. Spondyloarthropathies: ankylosing spondylitis and psoriatic arthritis. *Radiol Clin North Amer* 2004;42:121–134.
2. Gorman JD, Sack KE, Davis JC. Treatment of ankylosing spondylitis by inhibition of tumor necrosis factor. *N Engl J Med* 2002;346:1349–1356.
3. Wimberly RL, Lauerman WC. Spondylolisthesis in the athlete. *Clin Sports Med* 2002;21:133–145, vii–viii.
4. Fredrickson BE, Baker D, McHolick WJ, et al: The natural history of spondylolysis and spondylolisthesis. *J Bone Joint Surg Am* 1984;66:699–707.
5. Della-Giustina DA. Orthopedic emergencies: emergency department evaluation and treatment of back pain. *Emerg Med Clin North Am* 1999;17:877–893.
6. Deyo RA, Loeser JD, Bigos, SJ. Herniated lumbar intervertebral disk. *Ann Intern Med* 1990;112:598–603.
7. Deyo RA, Rainville J, Kent DL. What can the history and physical examination tell us about low back pain? *JAMA* 1992;268:760–765.
8. Deyo RA, Weinstein JN. Primary care: low back pain. *N Engl J Med* 2001;344:363–370.
9. Honan M, White WG, Eisenberg GM. Spontaneous infectious discitis in adults. *Am J Med* 1996;100:85–89.
10. Crawford A, Kucharzyk D, et al. Diskitis in children. *Clin Orthop* 1991;266:70.
11. Gutierrez K. Discitis. In: Long SS, Pickering LK, Prober CG, eds. *Principles and Practice of Pediatric Infectious Diseases,* 2nd ed. New York: Churchill Livingstone, 2003.
12. Malmivaara A, Hakkinen UT, Heinrichs MJ, et al. The treatment of acute low back pain—bed rest, exercises, or ordinary activity. *N Engl J Med* 1995;332:351–355.
13. Bigos S, Bowyer O, Braen G, et al. Acute low back problems in adults. In: *Clinical Practice Guideline, Quick Reference Guide Number 14.* Rockville, MD: US Department of Health and Human Services, Public Health Service, Agency for Health Care Policy and Research 1994; AHCPR Pub. No. 95-0643.
14. Vroomen P, de Krom M, Wilmink JT, et al. Lack of effectiveness of bed rest for sciatica. *N Engl J Med* 1999;340:418–423.
15. Campana B. Soft tissue spine injuries and back pain. In: Marx JA, ed. *Rosen's Emergency Medicine,* 5th ed. St. Louis: Mosby 2002:606–625.

Overuse Syndromes

Lauren Pipas

Overuse Syndromes

Overuse syndromes, specifically tendonitis, bursitis, fibrositis, and carpal tunnel syndrome, develop as a result of repetitive strains and microtrauma. These injuries are seen commonly in patients whose occupations require repetitive movements, and in poorly conditioned people following overexertion. Initial treatment includes rest and a trial of nonsteroidal anti-inflammatory drugs (NSAIDs). There are specific therapies for primary treatment failures. Referral to orthopedic or occupational medicine specialist is frequently indicated.

Tendonitis

Tendonitis is inflammation of the tendon. In distinction, tenosynovitis includes inflammation of the tendon and tendon sheath. Tendonitis results from repetitive microtrauma sustained from forceful motions, vibration, and unusual postures. Infection and systemic diseases processes, such as rheumatoid arthritis or hypothyroidism, can be important predisposing conditions.

As inflammation progresses the normal structure of the tendon changes. There is thickening of the tendon and normal blood flow to the tendon is compromised by swelling which limits the ability of the tendon to heal.

On physical exam, the tendon will be tender to palpation, with swelling, crepitus, and erythema. An important physical finding is that active range of motion will elicit pain, whereas passive range of motion will not. This helps to distinguish tendonitis from intra-articular processes. Radiographs may be necessary to rule out fractures, mass lesions, and foreign bodies.

Therapy is initiated with NSAIDs. The patient should be instructed to discontinue or modify the activity that exacerbates the symptoms. Splinting for immobilization may also help. Corticosteroid injection is effective, but is more appropriately carried out in follow up as repeated injections can predispose to tendon rupture, dermatologic changes, and tenosynovitis. Physical therapy should be utilized for treatment failures.

Bursitis

A bursa is an extra-articular fluid-filled sac, lined with synovium. It functions to reduce friction associated with the movement of muscle and tendons over bony prominences near joints. Bursitis results when the bursae become inflamed. There is proliferation of the synovium, and infiltration by inflammatory cells into the sac. This can result from crystalline deposition, infection, rheumatologic diseases, and trauma.

The patient will have pain that can limit range of motion, with swelling, erythema, and tenderness. The physical exam should allow the clinician to differentiate periarticular from articular processes.

Aspiration of swollen bursae is indicated to rule out infective or crystalline causes for the bursitis and also for temporary relief of symptoms. Aspiration is important in patients with risk factors for infection, including local breaks in the skin, diabetes or immunosuppression. A white blood cell count of greater than $5,000/mm^3$ in bursal fluid is an indication of infection. Intravenous antibiotics and potentially operative irrigation is necessary.

Treatment includes pain relief with NSAIDs. Immobilization and local therapy (heat or ice) is helpful. A non-infected bursa can be injected with local anesthetic and corticosteroids. Physical therapy may be indicated.

Fibrositis

Fibrositis, also called fibromyalgia, is a syndrome of diffuse pain most commonly seen in women in their third to fifth decades of life. The pain is worse in the morning, and exacerbated by non-restorative sleep. There is subjective stiffness and swelling. On physical exam, no evidence for limitation of range of motion can be documented.

The American College of Rheumatology has given specific diagnostic criteria which include a history of widespread pain that persists for greater than three months on both sides of the body, above and below the waist. The pain is precipitated by applying pressure to trigger points. To meet diagnostic criteria, 11 out of 18 specific trigger points must be identified. These include the occiput, low cervical spine, trapezius, supraspinatus, anterior second rib, lateral epicondyle, gluteal muscle, and the greater trochanter at the hip and the knee, on both sides of the body.

Treatment includes analgesics (acetaminophen, NSAIDs). Amitriptyline has been shown to be effective in normalizing sleep patterns. Mild aerobic exercise programs also reduce symptoms.

This disease is rarely diagnosed in the emergency department. This is a chronic, but not progressive syndrome. It is important for patients to identify a primary care physician with whom to follow.

Carpal Tunnel Syndrome

Carpal tunnel syndrome results from entrapment of the median nerve as it passes beneath the transverse carpal ligament at the wrist. It results from any condition causing swelling of the tissues; manual labor or systemic conditions such as pregnancy, hypothyroidism, amyloidosis, and rheumatoid arthritis. Patients having sustained fractures to the carpal bones and distal forearm are at increased risk.

Patients will present complaining of pain or paresthesis along the distribution of the distal median nerve, into the thenar eminence, thumb, the index and middle fingers. Symptoms typically occur at night, awakening the patient from sleep. They may have temporary relief by shaking the hand. As the condition progresses, symptoms become more frequent; weakness and atrophy of the thenar eminence can result.

The clinician can elicit symptoms by performing Tinels test, in which tapping the wrist at the transverse carpal ligament elicits subjective symptoms. Phalens test exacerbates symptoms by having the patient hold the wrists together in flexion, pressing the dorsal surfaces of the hands together for a minute.

Treatment is initiated with NSAIDs. Immobilization with the wrist splinted in neutral position is first-line therapy. If this first-line therapy fails, injection of steroids or surgical carpal tunnel release is definitive therapy. Physical and occupational therapy can be beneficial.

Selected Readings

Antonelli MAS, Vawter RL. Nonarticular pain syndromes. *Postgrad Med* 1992;91:95–98.

Clain MR, Baxter DE. Achilles tendonitis. *Foot Ankle* 1992;13:482–487.

Curtis AS, Snyder SJ. Evaluation and treatment of biceps tendon pathology. *Orthop Clin North Am* 1993;24:33–43.

Nirschl RP. Elbow tendinosis/tennis elbow. *Clin Sports Med* 1992;11:851–870.

Pyne JI, Adams BD. Hand tendon injuries in athletics. *Clin Sports Med* 1992;11:833–850.

Thorson E, Szabo RM. Common tendonitis problems in the hand and forearm. *Orthop Clin North Am* 1992;23:65–74.

Muscle Abnormalities

Lauren Pipas

Muscle Abnormalities

This chapter covers four disease processes that involve skeletal muscles: muscular dystrophy, rhabdomyolysis, compartment syndromes, and myositis. Muscular dystrophy and myositis are rarely diagnosed in the emergency department (ED); however, rhabdomyolysis and compartment syndromes are not uncommonly diagnosed, and the emergency physician should maintain a high index of suspicion for these two disease processes.

Muscular Dystrophy

Many forms of muscular dystrophy have been described. The two most common are Duchenne muscular dystrophy and Becker's muscular dystrophy. Duchenne's affects one out of 3,000 boys. It results in progressive proximal muscle weakness and death in the early 20s. Becker's muscular dystrophy is a less severe disease and results in a much slower progression of muscle dysfunction.

Duchenne

A typical patient with Duchenne's presents around age 3 to 5 years, with difficulty running and jumping, and a history of frequent falls. They may have pseudohypertrophy, where muscle tissue is replaced by fat and connective tissue of many muscle groups, especially of the calves. A waddling gait, toe walking, and an exaggerated lumbar lordosis are common. About 30% of patients have mildly low IQs. Gowers' maneuver indicates severe proximal muscle weakness, where the child uses his arms to raise up the body from a crouched position.

There is progressive proximal muscle weakness. Functional abilities markedly deteriorate between the ages of 8 to 12 years. Patients develop contractures and a progressive scoliosis, which further impairs respiration. By 12 years of age, the patients are usually wheelchair-bound. Patients develop repeated pulmonary infections. They are prone to gastric dilatation and aspiration. Patient death in the late teens and early 20s usually occurs from progressive respiratory failure and infection. Myocardial fibrosis of the left ventricle is common and most often manifests as congestive heart failure during stresses such as respiratory infections.

Becker's

Becker's is a less severe form of muscular dystrophy where patients can continue to ambulate after age 15 and can survive into the 4th or 5th decade.

Presentation to the emergency department will occur after an acute decompensation. This most often will be secondary to pulmonary infection. Sepsis can occur after aspiration, urinary tract infection or decubitus ulcer formation. Therapy is aimed at respiratory support, hydration, correction of electrolyte abnormalities, and administration of appropriate antibiotics.

Rhabdomyolysis

Rhabdomyolysis is a syndrome of muscle tissue damage resulting in cell breakdown and release of cellular components systemically, ultimately resulting in acute renal failure. First described in victims of crush injuries in World War II, it is now known to result from a number of etiologies (**Table 72.1**).

Muscle cell injury results in violation of the cell membrane integrity, and subsequent leakage of cell contents into the extracellular space. These contents include myoglobin and cellular enzymes. Potassium and phosphate are released from damaged cells. Hyperphosphatemia results in calcium deposition in soft tissues and hypocalcemia. Hyperuricemia and lactic acidosis occur with muscle cell damage.

Patients with rhabdomyolysis will present with muscle pain and swelling, nausea, and dark urine. Studies have demonstrated that up to 50% of patients may lack complaints of muscle pain. Therefore, a high index of suspicion must be maintained in order to direct the physician toward appropriate laboratory evaluation in patients with risk factors.

A finding of positive urine dip for hemoglobin in the absence of red cells may be an indication of rhabdomyolysis. The diagnosis is confirmed by a finding of elevated serum creatinine phosphokinase (CPK) greater than five

Table 72.1
Etiologies of Rhabdomyolysis

Trauma
Burns
Hyper- and hypothermia
Drug use (cocaine, sympathomimetics, etc.)
Seizures
Sepsis
Exercise
Limb ischemia and reperfusion
Compartment syndrome
Surgery
Viral/bacterial infection
Genetic and immunologic disorders
Metabolic derangements

Table 72.2
Etiology of Compartment Syndrome

Fracture: closed or open
Soft tissue injury
Burns
Prolonged immobilization
Fracture management
Anticoagulation and hemorrhage
Vascular injury: arterial or venous
Systemic hypotension
MAST trouser application

times that of normal. Screening tests for urine myoglobin are available.

Therapy is aimed at restoration of hydration status, maintenance of urine output, and diuresis. Alkalinization of urine to prevent dissociation of myoglobin into nephrotoxic substances and prevent acidosis and hyperkalemia is the cornerstone of therapy. Disseminated intravascular coagulation is a known complication, and thrombocytopenia may be an early indicator of DIC.

Patients should be aggressively hydrated with as much as 11 liters of saline within the first 24 hours to prevent hypovolemic shock and acute tubular necrosis. Maintenance of urine output at greater than 100 cc per hour may be accomplished with mannitol, which increases intravascular volume and promotes renal blood flow. Loop diuretics should be avoided, as they tend to acidify the urine. The goal of therapy is to alkalinize the urine to a pH greater than 6.5, as myoglobin becomes nephrotoxic in acid urine. Sodium bicarbonate is the mainstay of therapy. It can be given as a bolus and as a constant infusion, with monitoring of urine pH to maintain it above 6.0.

Dialysis is indicated if there is progressive worsening of renal failure or uremia, uncorrectable electrolyte abnormalities (hyperkalemia) or fluid overload.

The most important complication of rhabdomyolysis, acute renal failure, has an incidence of 17% to 40%. Disseminated intravascular coagulation and compartment syndrome occur less frequently. Emergency department management is focused on hydration and electrolyte correction. It is important for the clinician to recognize precipitating factors.

Compartment Syndrome

The diagnosis of compartment syndrome requires a high index of suspicion, with treatment to prevent disability, amputation or death. The classic signs of compartment syndrome or the "5 Ps" may only become apparent late in the disease process, and include pain that is out of proportion to stimuli, and pain on passive stretch of the affected compartment; pallor; pulselessness; paresthesias; and pa-

ralysis. Compartment syndrome occurs when increased pressure within a closed facial space causes decreased perfusion pressure, resulting in tissue damage and, ultimately, tissue death.

Trauma and hemorrhage cause compartment syndrome most commonly. Specific causes are numerous (**Table 72.2**). The diagnosis is suspected in the patient with pain on passive movement of the affected compartment. Parasthesia, pallor, pulselessness, and paralysis are all late sequelae. Measurement of compartment pressure with a commercially available needle manometer system should be done based on clinical suspicion. A pressure above 30 mm Hg confirms the diagnosis. Irreversible tissue damage can occur as soon as within 4 to 6 hours.

Ultimately, the treatment is to decrease intercompartment pressure with fasciotomy of affected compartments.

Myositis

The term myositis is a general one, which includes polymyositis and dermatomyositis. These are rare inflammatory, autoimmune conditions in which skeletal muscle is infiltrated with lymphocytes. They should be part of the differential diagnosis for a patient complaining of weakness.

The etiology is unclear. Diagnosis is made by clinical picture, with elevated CPK and a characteristic EMG and muscle biopsy. A clinical suspicion may lead the ED physician to the appropriate referral, and therefore expedite diagnosis and care.

Patients presenting with polymyositis may complain of proximal muscle weakness. They may have progressive difficulty with activities of daily living, such as getting out of a car or chair, brushing their hair or difficulty swallowing. The weakness can be acute or insidious. It is rare to make the diagnosis in the emergency department.

Patients with dermatomyositis may present with a rash that consists of a purple discoloration around the eyelids, or a red rash on the knuckles, face, elbows, knees, or toes. The pattern of the rash can be nonspecific, but when associated with proximal muscle weakness, dermatomyositis should be entertained.

Patients may complain of shortness of breath that results from the interstitial lung disease that accompanies myositis.

Long-term treatment consists of steroid and immuno-suppressive therapy.

Selected Readings

Arrington ED, Miller MD. Skeletal muscle injuries. *Orthoped Clin North Am* 1995;26:411–422.

Elliott KG, Johnstone AJ. Diagnosing acute compartment syndrome. *J Bone Joint Surg* 2003;85:625–632.

Evans BK, Goyne C. Duchenne's muscular dystrophy: review of recent scientific findings. *Am J Med Sci* 1991;30:118–123.

Iannaccone ST. Current status of Duchenne muscular dystrophy. *Pediatr Clin North Am* 1992;39:879–894.

Line RL, et al. Acute exertional rhabdomyolysis. *Am Fam Phys* 1995;52 .

Lynn DJ, Woda RP, Mendall JR. Respiratory dysfunction in muscular dystrophy and other myopathies. *Clin Chest Med* 1994;15:661–674.

Pina EM, Mehlman CT. Rhabdomyolysis a primer for the orthopaedist. *Orthopaed Rev* 1994;23:28–32.

Plotz, PH. New understanding of myositis. *Hosp Pract* 1992:27:33–43.

Sinert R, et al. Exercise-induced rhabdomyolysis. *Ann Emerg Med* 1994;23: 1301–1306.

Tiwari A, Haq A. Acute compartment syndromes. *Brit J Surg* 2002;89:397–412.

Soft Tissue Infections

James Winslow III
David E. Manthey

Infections of the soft tissues are a common presenting complaint in emergency department patients. Soft tissue infections range from superficial cellulitis to necrotizing fasciitis, from paronychia to suppurative flexor tenosynovitis. Emergency department physicians must quickly identify the life- or limb-threatening diseases, as well as initiate treatment on the entire spectrum of disease. This monograph will review the more serious as well as the more common infections.

Cellulitis

Cellulitis is a superficial infection of the skin and subcutaneous tissue. The predisposing cause is usually a break in the protective layer of skin but is only found in 50% to 60% of cases. Lymphatic and hematogenous spread also occurs. *Staphylococcus aureus* and *Streptococcus pyogenes* are the most common culture results.

Cellulitis presents as a tender, erythematous area of dermis that is warm and often swollen. It usually blanches with pressure and the tenderness is confined to the area of erythema.

Fever or other systemic symptoms are uncommon. The white blood cell count is most often normal or mildly elevated. Lymphangitis and lymphadenopathy may be associated findings.

Haemophilus influenzae B may cause a facial (or extremity) cellulitis in children younger than 5 years of age where the skin appears red with a violaceous tinge. The patient is acutely ill with a high fever and elevated WBC count with a left shift.

Treatment of cellulitis is antibiotic coverage of the suspected organisms. First generation cephalosporins or penicillinase-resistant penicillins are good initial therapy for most cellulitis. *H. influenzae* cellulitis, due to the high incidence (80% to 90%) of positive blood cultures, is treated with parenteral antibiotics such as second- or third-generation cephalosporins.

Erysipelas

Erysipelas is a superficial infection of the dermis and lymphatics of the skin. Erysipelas starts via an area of skin disruption more commonly secondary to venous insufficiency or stasis ulcerations. An upper respiratory tract infection sometimes precedes the facial form of erysipelas. The organisms responsible for approximately 80% of cases are β-hemolytic streptococci. *S. aureus* is implicated in recurrent cases.

Erysipelas produces an intense erythematous rash with characteristically sharply demarcated palpable borders. The rash has a brilliant red color and shiny appearance. Lymphangitis and lymphadenopathy often occur with this infection. Eighty-five percent of cases occur on the lower extremities. The face is the next most commonly affected area.

Fever and sometimes chills occur. The white blood cell count can be elevated. Sepsis may occur in immunocompromised patients and should also be considered in anyone with systemic signs and symptoms of disease.

Erysipelas can be treated by either a macrolide or penicillin. If the treating physician is unable to differentiate between erysipelas and cellulitis, then it is best to utilize broader spectrum antibiotics that treat cellulitis.

Necrotizing Fasciitis

Necrotizing fasciitis is a rapidly progressive and destructive infection of the subcutaneous tissues and fascia. It can also involve the skin and muscle. This relatively rare group of infections has received a great deal of attention by the popular press because of "flesh-eating" properties. Before the introduction of antibiotics, the mortality was more than 50%. Today, the mortality of necrotizing fasciitis is between 25% and 50%. The most important determinant of survival is time to debridement.

This infection has two different etiologies. The first is a polymicrobial infection involving a combination of anaerobes (usually *Bacteroides* and *Peptostreptococcus* spp.) and a facultative anaerobe (such as streptococci non-group A and Enterobacteriaceae (i.e., *Escherichia coli, Enterobacter, Klebsiella* or *Proteus* spp.). The second type involves group A streptococci in combination with another organism, usually *S. aureus*. Fournier's gangrene is the eponym for necrotizing fasciitis affecting male genitalia. Necrotizing fasciitis appears to begin from a site of trauma (laceration, abrasion, burn, injection site, insect bite, surgical incision, perirectal abscess or decubitus ulcer). Clinical conditions that increase the risk for development of these infections include peripheral vascular disease, diabetes mellitus, chronic renal failure, malignancy, chronic alcoholism, and immunosuppressive medication use. Debilitated patients and those unable to provide a history should be completely disrobed so that all areas of skin can be evaluated.

The clinical presentation of early necrotizing fasciitis may be subtle and is often misdiagnosed as superficial cellulitis. In a series of 39 pediatric cases, the correct diagnosis was made at initial presentation in only 33%. Only 14.6% were correctly diagnosed at admission in Wong's series. Although both cellulitis and necrotizing fasciitis may present with erythema and skin warmth, necrotizing fasciitis may include additional signs and symptoms early in the clinical course. These include pain out of proportion to exam, poorly defined margins of erythema, shiny appearance to the skin as well as tenderness and edema outside the border of erythema. Systemic toxicity may not be present until late in the disease, but can occur abruptly. In the series by Wong and Chang, only 52% of patients with necrotizing fasciitis presented with fever. Lymphangitis and lymphadenitis are infrequent. In the intermediate stages, the skin color changes from red-violet to blue-gray. In the late stages, frank bullae appear filled with reddish-blue fluid. Cutaneous gangrene develops, and the area becomes anesthetic. The white blood cell count is often elevated; Gram stain and blood cultures are usually positive for the organisms and leukocytes.

Radiographic evaluation may include a CT scan which may show asymmetric thickening of the deep fascia associated with gas. Ultrasound can demonstrate thickening of the skin, underlying subcutaneous tissues, and deeper fascial planes. Fluid collections may also be seen in interlobular septa near the skin surface. Plain films, although they may sometimes show gas in the tissues, are often of little help when the diagnosis is in question.

Immediate intervention in the emergency department includes aggressive fluid resuscitation as dictated by the clinical situation. As necrotizing fasciitis can progress rapidly and the definitive treatment is surgical debridement, emergent surgical consultation should be made as soon as the diagnosis is entertained. A retrospective review by Wong of 89 patients with necrotizing fasciitis showed that the only factor associated with mortality was a delay of more than 24 hours to debridement. Operative debridement may be extensive and continues until areas of normal fascia are identified.

In the ED, antibiotics should be started immediately to attempt to limit the infection's spread until definitive debridement can be done. They should never be used as the definitive treatment without surgical debridement. Recommended antibiotics should empirically cover anaerobes (metronidazole or clindamycin), streptococcal spp. (synthetic penicillins), and Enterobacteriaceae (aminoglycosides). Two appropriate triple antibiotic regimens include ampicillin, gentamycin, and clindamycin, as well as vancomycin, ceftriaxone, and metronidazole. Tetanus pro-phylaxis is recommended. A systematic review by the Agency for Healthcare Research and Quality (AHRQ) found no clear evidence supporting the use of HBOT.

Gas Gangrene

Gas gangrene, also known as clostridial myonecrosis, is a life-threatening infection of the muscle tissue caused by clostridial species (usually *Clostridium perfringens,* and sometimes *C. novyi* or *C. septicum*). These species and their spores are ubiquitous in the environment and very resistant to environmental degradation. There are roughly 1,000 to 3,000 cases of gas gangrene a year. The disease usually begins as a result of trauma to the muscle tissue. Comorbid factors such as those listed for necrotizing fasciitis increase the risk of development of infection. Contaminated wounds caused by high speed missiles are especially prone to myonecrosis. This rapidly fatal condition can often be prevented by proper wound cleansing and consideration of delayed closure of severely contaminated wounds in the ED.

The incubation period is usually relatively short at 2 to 3 days, but can be as short as 6 to 12 hours. The symptoms begin with a sense of heaviness that quickly progresses to pain usually out of proportion to exam. Soon after onset of pain, the patient may develop signs of systemic toxicity to include tachycardia, clammy skin, diaphoresis, and altered mental status. Curiously, only a low-grade fever (100° F to 101° F) may be present. The wound characteristically has profound edema which may obscure the associated crepitus. The overlying skin quickly discolors after bullae filled with thin reddish-blue fluid develop.

Laboratory tests generally are not remarkable. Leukocytosis and mild anemia are the most common findings. A Gram stain of bullae fluid may show gram-positive rods as well as Gram-negative rods, but few leukocytes. In 15% of cases, a clostridial bacteremia may be present. Radiographic views of the affected area are suggested to look for osteomyelitis and subcutaneous gas. Ultrasound may show fluid collections around the muscle.

Subcutaneous gas is often apparent by the time the patient complains of severe pain. Surgical exploration of the infected area will reveal pale edematous muscle that does not bleed and loses contractility as infection progresses.

Immediate surgical consultation for debridement is the definitive treatment for infectious myonecrosis. The patient will also require rapid volume replacement because of third spacing of fluid into infected muscle tissue. Tetanus prophylaxis is recommended. Recommended antibiotics to limit the spread of infection include penicillin G (*Clostridium* spp.) and clindamycin (anaerobes). Penicillin-allergic patients may receive chloramphenicol. Aminoglycosides for possible Gram-negative rods and penicillinase-resistant synthetic penicillin for possible *S. aureus* may be given if the diagnosis is in doubt. Hyperbaric oxygen (HBO) therapy has been shown in animal models and in vitro studies to stop toxin production and limit reproduction of clostridial species. Surgery should only be delayed if the patient can receive HBO therapy in the first 1 to 2 hours. Some hyperbaric centers believe that HBO therapy can help define the infected tissue, therefore making wound debridement easier.

Anaerobic streptococcal myonecrosis is another type of infectious myonecrosis caused by a mixed group of organisms (anaerobic streptococci with group A strep or *S. aureus*). The clinical appearance of this infection is similar to clostridial myonecrosis, but some important differences should be noted. The incubation period is longer, generally 3 to 4 days. Infection presents with erythematous skin developing seropurulent bullae. Pain begins after significant skin changes and usually before the development of signs of systemic toxicity. The treatment still consists of penicillinase-resistant synthetic penicillin and surgical debridement.

Paronychia

A paronychia is a superficial cellulitis or abscess at the lateral skin fold of the nail that can be efficiently treated in the ED. An eponychia is a similar infection that involves the basal skin fold. These are usually caused by a polymicrobial infection, with anaerobes and *S. aureus* being the most frequently cultured microbes. This infection must be differentiated from a felon (discussed next) as the treatment and outcome changes dramatically.

The infection is caused by repeated trauma so the patient's history may include nail biting or aggressive manicures. The examination should be focused on the extent of the infection. The patient will have tenderness around the nail, but the finger pad should remain non-tender. Any tenderness of the pad of the finger should raise the suspicion that the infection has progressed to a felon. Chronic infections that last for longer than a few weeks can progress to osteomyelitis.

Treatment varies depending on the severity of the condition. In mild cases involving inflammation of the lateral skin fold and no areas of fluctuance, the patient may be discharged on a short 3- to 5-day course of antibiotics and with direction for hot water soaks, 6 to 8 times a day. Controversy exists about the class of antibiotic. Penicillinase-resistant penicillin is effective against most oral bacteria. Some sources suggest clindamycin or augmentin as they are effective against the polymicrobials cultured from these infections. The finger should also be immobilized and protected from further trauma.

More severe cases involving frank abscesses, however, require minor surgical drainage. Although the procedure can often be performed without anesthesia, a digital block may be required. Soak the finger in warm water first to aid in lifting the eponychium. A no. 11 scalpel blade, iris scissors, or an 18 g needle may be used to lift the eponychium from the nail and release the pus. The blade is placed under the eponychium parallel to the nail bed at the point of maximal swelling, then moved in both directions until all the pus is released. If a large amount of pus is removed, consider placing packing for 24 hours. Add antibiotics only if there are signs of surrounding cellulitis.

Rarely, if the abscess extends under the nail, treatment may require removal of or trephination of part of the nail. Take care to not damage the nail matrix. The eponychium

should be elevated with fine mesh dressing to improve normal development of the growing nail. All of these therapies should be checked in 24 to 48 hours and dressings removed and warm water soaks begun.

Complications of paronychia result from damage to the germinal matrix of the nail or osteomyelitis of the distal phalanx. Patients should be informed of the risk of abnormal nail growth from the infection and procedure.

Be aware that herpetic whitlow, an infection of the distal phalanx by herpes simplex virus, may be mistaken as a paronychia. Whitlow presents as localized pain, swelling and pruritus in a single digit that may progress to vesicles and ulcers. Treatment for herpetic whitlow does not include incision or antibiotics, but instead analgesia, splinting, and antivirals. Fungal paronychia is not addressed here. Interestingly, up to 9% of patients on indinavir (antiretroviral) develop paronychia.

Felon

A felon is a soft tissue abscess involving the distal volar aspect of the digit. The fingertip has tough, fibrous, longitudinally oriented septae that extend radially from the bone to the skin. These septae serve to stabilize the fingertips during pincer and grasping actions. This is a closed space infection that becomes loculated between the septae. The most common causative organisms are *Staphylococcus* or *Streptococcus* spp., but may include anaerobic and polymicrobial infections.

Although often caused by a splinter or progression from a paronychia, a traumatic injury may not be identified. The finger pad is swollen, erythematous, and exquisitely tender due to the compartment pressure. Pointing of the abscess may not occur due to the septae. Dependent positioning of the hand makes the pain worse.

Treatment involves incision and drainage of the felon. Many methods have been advocated, each with its own set of complications. A digital block with a long acting anesthetic and a finger tourniquet are recommended. A longitudinal incision over the area of maximal tenderness may be utilized as long as care is taken to prevent injury to the digital nerves and arteries as well as the flexor tendon. The position of the digital nerve and artery may be approximated by drawing a line along the edge of the flexor crease folds on either side of the finger. This approach will minimize septae disruption and its associated finger pad instability, but may cause a scar in a sensitive area. Recurrent or more severe infections may require more aggressive incisions such as the hockey stick, through and through, or fish-mouth incisions. These have a greater incidence of finger pad instability, postoperative anesthesia, and tissue sloughing.

A hemostat should be utilized to bluntly dissect loculations and promote adequate drainage. Necrotic tissue and interstitial fluid is more commonly encountered than frank pus. The wound should be packed with iodoform gauze, splinted, and elevated. The gauze can be removed in 2 days with a thorough re-examination for necrotic tissue. Begin warm water soaks three times a day. Most authorities recommend treating with a broad spectrum cephalosporin for five days and collecting wound cultures. If infection is left untreated, osteomyelitis, septic arthritis, or flexor tenosynovitis may develop. These infections should be followed up with a hand specialist.

Flexor Tenosynovitis

The tenosynovia are synovial membranes that encircle tendons providing lubrication to decrease friction. In the hand, only the flexor tendons are covered by tenosynovia. If an infection develops within this sheath, it quickly progresses along the length of the synovia. As this is a closed space infection, infection quickly leads to increased pressure which decreases circulation to the tendon leading to necrosis. The infection is most commonly caused by direct trauma to the area, but may occur from hematogenous spread.

The patient complains of a painful swollen finger that developed over 1 to 3 days. The four cardinal signs of flexor tenosynovitis are: (a) tenderness along the course of the flexor tendon, (b) symmetric swelling, (c) pain on passive extension of finger, and (d) a finger that is held in flexed position. Passively extend the involved finger by lifting on the nail without touching the flexor tendon.

Treatment consists of immediate consultation with an orthopedic surgeon or hand surgeon for operative incision and drainage, and parenteral antibiotics. If the infection presents early, conservative management may be attempted with parenteral antibiotics, immobilization, and elevation.

Selected Readings

Bessman AN, Wagner W. Nonclostridial gas gangrene. Report of 48 cases and review of the literature. *JAMA* 1978;233:958.

Bickels J, Ben-Sira L, et al. Primary pyomyositis. *J Bone Joint Surg Am* 2002;12:2277–2286.

Brenner EB. Necrotizing fasciitis. *Ann Am Med* 1982;11:384.

Canales FL, Newmeyer WL III, Kilgore ES Jr. The treatment of felons and paronychias. *Hand Clin* 1989;5:515–523.

Cardinal E, Bureau NJ, et al. Role of ultrasound in musculoskeletal infections. *Radiol Clin North Am* 2001;39:191–201.

Cline KA, Turnbull TL. Clostridial myonecrosis. *Ann Emerg Med* 1985;14:459.

Dunn F. Two cases of biceps injury in bodybuilders with initially misleading presentation. *Emerg Med J* 2002;19:461–462.

Elliott D, Kufera JA, et al. The microbiology of necrotizing soft tissue infections. *Am J Surg* 2000;179:361–366.

Freeman HP, Oluwole SF, et al. Necrotizing fasciitis. *Am J Surg* 1981;142:377–383.

Hart G, Lamb RC, Strauss MG. Gas gangrene: I. A collective review. *J Trauma* 1983;23:991.

Mabry RM, Harwood AL. Fournier's disease: necrotizing gangrene of the male genitalia. *J Emerg Med* 1983;1:133–136.

Rich RS, Salluzzo RF. Spontaneous clostridial myonecrosis with abdominal involvement in a nonimmunocompramized patient. *Ann Emerg Med* 1993;22:1477.

Rockwell, PG. Acute and chronic paronychia. *Am Fam Phys* 2001;63:1113–1116.

Stone HH, Martin JD. Synergistic necrotizing cellulitis. *Ann Surg* 1972;175:702–711.

Struk DW, Munk PL, et al. Imaging of soft tissue infections. *Radiol Clin North Am* 2001;39:277–303.

Tehrani MA, Ledingham IM. Necrotizing fasciitis. *Postgrad Med J* 1977;53:237–242.

Wang C, Schwaitzberg S, et al. Hyperbaric oxygen for treating wounds: a systematic review of the literature. *Arch Surg* 2003;138:272–280.

Wong CH, Chang HC, et al. Necrotizing fasciitis: clinical presentation, microbiology, and determinants of mortality. *J Bone Joint Surg Am* 2003;85A:1454–1460.

Nervous System Disorders

John C. Moorhead

Patients with acute nervous system complaints often present to the emergency department, may require timely interventions, and may present challenges for emergency physicians. Diagnosis and management are often performed as part of a team, utilizing predetermined guidelines. Identification of appropriate patients, and determining and differentiating new or changing signs and/or symptoms are essential contributions from emergency physicians in these protocols. A careful neurological exam remains an important aspect of the evaluation. Increasing utilization of sophisticated diagnostic imaging, including computer tomographic (CT) scan and magnetic resonance imaging/angiography (MRI/MRA), has enhanced specificity of diagnosis in the emergency department. Exciting research is underway to identify interventions, which may limit progression, improve recovery, and/or prevent secondary injury or illness.

Cerebrovascular Disorders

Jonathan M. Sullivan

Cerebral Aneurysm

Most intracerebral aneurysms (ICAs) are clinically silent, and have a benign clinical course. The cited prevalence of ICA ranges from 3.6% to 6%, and ICA is an incidental finding in up to 8.9% of autopsy cases. The most important clinical manifestation is rupture of the aneurysm, which results in intracranial hemorrhage (ICH), with potentially devastating results. The etiology of saccular ICA, the most common cause of aneurysm-related ICH, remains a matter of some controversy. Although the vast majority of aneurysms appear to be congenital, other risk factors such as uncontrolled hypertension, tobacco and alcohol use, and atherosclerosis appear to play a part in the natural history and risk of rupture of these lesions. Because most unruptured ICAs are asymptomatic, diagnosis and management are clinically challenging. Treatment options for ICA depend on location, size, and the condition and age of the patient, and include endovascular coiling or aneurysmal clipping to ablate the aneurysm.

Etiology/Anatomy/Pathophysiology

Saccular or "berry" aneurysms are the most common form of ICA, and account for over three-fourths of all cases of subarachnoid hemorrhage (SAH). The pathogenesis of these aneurysms remains unclear. A potentially confounding issue in understanding this debate is discriminating between factors that lead to the initial formation of the aneurysm and those that promote the development and eventual rupture of the aneurysm. Based on the available evidence, it seems clear that genetic factors predominate in the formation of saccular ICAs, while environmental and behavioral factors have a greater impact on development and risk of rupture. Risk factors invoked for the formation of saccular ICA include female sex and alterations in the genes for polycystin, fibrillin, collagen III, elastin, collagen IV, protease inhibitor or $\alpha 1$-antitrypsin and various cellular proteases. Recently, Farnham et al. reported a linkage of ICA with chromosomal region 7q11 in a genomic search of 85 Japanese nuclear families with at least two affected siblings (this chromosomal region includes the elastin gene). Risk factors that may contribute to the development and eventual rupture of ICAs include smoking, arterial hypertension, alcohol use, and increasing age.

The most common sites for saccular intracranial aneurysms are at bifurcations of the anastomotic network known as the Circle of Willis. Basilar artery ICAs, at the bifurcations to the vertebral or posterior communicating arteries, account for 5% to 10%. Anterior circulation aneurysms are more common, at bifurcations of the internal carotid (40%), middle cerebral (20%), and anterior communicating arteries (30%). This observation has led several authors to hypothesize that hemodynamic stress at the intimal cusp of the arterial bifurcation, combined with predisposing genetic factors, leads weakening of the media, with consequent aneurysm formation. Futami et al found no evidence for such an etiology. However, their experimental design incorporated an animal model and artificially induced medial defects, and should be interpreted with caution.

The International Study of Unruptured Intracranial Aneurysms was a multicenter investigation of natural history and clinical outcome in 4,060 patients with unruptured ICA. Their findings for the 5-year cumulative rupture rates for patients who did not have a history of SAH are summarized in **Table 74.1**. These results must be interpreted with some caution, as the population under study included both treated and untreated cohorts, limited follow-up for half the patients studied, and probably selection bias. The findings, nevertheless, emphasize that aneurysm size and location have a significant role in determining the risk of future rupture. The authors noted that in patients with unruptured intracranial aneurysms of less than 7 mm in diameter without a history of previous SAH from a different aneurysm, the annual rupture rate is approximately 0.1%, which makes it difficult to improve on the natural history of these lesions, given the morbidity and mortality associated with currently available techniques of invasive therapy.

Some unruptured ICAs will produce symptoms by compressing neural or vascular structures, leading to headache, visual field deficits or cranial nerve palsies. However, the vast majority of these lesions are clinically silent, unless and until rupture occurs.

Table 74.1

5-Year Cumulative Rupture Rates According to Size and Location of Unruptured ICA

	<7 mm		7 to 12 mm	13 to 24 mm	≥25 mm
	Gr 1	Gr 2			
Cavernous Carotid artery	0	0	0	3.0%	6.5%
AC/MC/IC	0	1.5%	2.6%	14.5%	40%
Post–P comm.	2.5%	3.4%	14.5%	18.4%	50%

Findings of the International Study of Unruptured Intracranial Aneurysms Investigators. Group 1 = patients without previous history of SAH. Group 2 = patients with history of previous SAH from a different aneurysm. AC, anterior communicating or anterior cerebral artery; IC, internal carotid artery (not cavernous carotid artery); MC, middle cerebral artery; Post-P comm., vertebrobasilar, posterior cerebral arterial system, or posterior communicating artery. Used by permission.

Emergency Department Evaluation

Although definitive data is lacking, it is probably safe to assume that a large percentage of ICAs diagnosed in the emergency department (ED) are incidental findings. The small number of patients who present with complaints related to unruptured ICA will usually have mild or vague symptoms, and clinical evaluation can be challenging. Although most aneurysms do not go on to rupture, those that do cause symptoms tend to be larger, with a higher risk of progressing to SAH. The emergency physician should maintain a high index of suspicion for intracranial pathology, including ICA, in patients presenting with headache and other neurological complaints.

Symptoms associated with ICA are wide-ranging and include headache, eye pain, diplopia or visual field deficits, blurry vision, facial pain, and cranial nerve palsies. Differential diagnosis can obviously be quite extensive for such presentations, including acute ischemic stroke, SAH or other intracranial hemorrhage, encephalitis, meningitis, Bell's palsy, carotid artery dissection, temporal arteritis, myasthenia gravis, multiple sclerosis, botulism, retinal artery occlusion, and intracranial neoplasm. Patient presentation, combined with a careful history and thorough physical examination, will help to clarify the differential. However, evaluation for suspected intracranial lesions, including ICA, will ultimately rest on diagnostic imaging.

History should include questions regarding the onset and duration symptoms; what the patient was doing when symptoms were first noticed; associated symptoms such as fever, nausea and vomiting, and visual changes; history of head trauma; history of previous neurological or cardiovascular disorders; a family history of cerebrovascular disease including ICA, and whether the patient uses tobacco, alcohol or illicit drugs, especially cocaine and other sympathomimetics.

Physical examination should obviously emphasize a search for neurological deficits, and in particular the physician suspecting unruptured ICA should be on the lookout for cranial nerve palsies. A careful evaluation of extraocular movements is mandatory, as this examination may indicate possible aneurysmal compression of CNs III, IV and VI. The physician should also perform visual field testing by confrontation to determine whether quadrantanopsia or hemianopsia are present; these conditions indicate possible compression of the optic chiasm or optic tract, respectively. All neurologic examinations should incorporate testing of muscle strength, deep tendon reflexes, cerebellar function (Romberg, rapid alternating movements), and gait.

All patients with suspected intracranial lesions, including ICA, require brain imaging. CT angiography can be performed in most EDs, with sensitivity ranging from 94% to 98% for ICAs larger than 5 mm in diameter. However, for lesions smaller than 5 mm, sensitivity drops to around 60%. Similar values hold for MR angiography. White et al. performed a systematic review to determine the accuracy of CT angiography, MR angiography and transcranial Doppler ultrasonography in depicting intracranial aneurysms. They found that CT angiography and MR angiography had overall accuracies per aneurysm of 89% and 90%, respectively, with similar accuracies for anterior and posterior circulation aneurysms. The authors went on to perform a clinical trial of CT angiography and MR angiography, using intra-arterial digital subtraction angiography as a gold standard, and found similar results.

Given this data, and with what is known about the natural history of ICA, it is reasonable to suggest that the clinical approach to patients with suspected ICA in the ED should incorporate CT angiography. CT is less expensive than MR and has comparable accuracy. Both studies will miss small aneurysms, but these lesions have much lower rates of rupture and available invasive interventional strategies are unlikely to positively impact upon their natural history. Stable patients with suspected unruptured ICA and negative CT angiography should be referred for further outpatient evaluation, which may include additional invasive or noninvasive imaging at the discretion of the neurologist or neurosurgeon.

Of those patients found to have ICA in the ED, many will not require hospitalization or urgent angiography. However, these decisions should be made in consultation with a neurosurgeon, and immediate referral is highly recommended.

Conventional therapy for unruptured ICA is occlusion of the aneurysm by means of vascular clipping at surgery. In the last decade, however, occlusion of ICA by percutaneous intravascular coiling has come into increasing use. The relative risks and benefits of these two procedures, and whether any invasive intervention should be used for aneurysms below a certain size, are subjects of ongoing debate and investigation.

Arteriovenous Malformation

Arteriovenous malformations (AVMs) are congenital vascular anomalies in which the arterial and venous systems are connected directly, without an intervening capillary bed. These abnormal vascular networks are characterized by dilated tortuous vessels and associated abnormal brain parenchyma. Most AVMs will hemorrhage, and most SAH arising from AVM occurs before the age of 40. As with unruptured ICA, the presentation of unruptured AVM can be subtle, and diagnosis of this lesion is clinically challenging.

Etiology/Anatomy/Pathophysiology

An AVM is an abnormal arteriovenous shunt through a plexus of dilated, tortuous vessels. Hypertrophic arterial feeding vessels connect directly to thickened, dilated veins without an intervening microvascular bed. Due in part to the inadequate perfusion in the territory of an AVM, the surrounding or underlying parenchyma is usually abnormal, with nonfunctional neurons and gliosis being prominent histological features. Both the abnormal parenchyma and the abnormal vascular morphology contribute to the spectrum of clinical effects produced by AVM, which include headache, neurological deficit, seizure, and hemorrhage.

The natural history of AVM differs considerably from that of ICA. Although most ICAs never rupture, the majority of AVMs will bleed, if untreated. Brown showed that the risk of hemorrhage from a previously unruptured AVM is approximately equal to 105 minus the patient's age. For example, the lifetime risk of rupture in a 20 year-old with a newly diagnosed AVM is 85%. Furthermore, although rupture of ICA is more common with advancing age, most patients experience the first hemorrhage from AVM between the ages of 20 and 40. Accordingly, older patients with SAH are more like to have an aneurysmal etiology for the event.

The etiology of AVM, like that of ICA, is a matter of some controversy, although it is generally agreed that these lesions are congenital. The exact embryological and genetic origins have not been identified, and AVM is rarely familial. It should be noted that Ehlers-Danlos IV syndrome is associated with direct AV fistula, and Rendu-Osler Weber's disease is associated with cavernoma, but these AV shunts are more uncommon than "true" AVM.

Emergency Department Evaluation

Unfortunately, primary presentation of unruptured AVM is uncommon. The most common revealing event for these lesions is SAH, which is discussed in the following section. AVM should be part of the differential diagnosis for any patient presenting with headache, unexplained seizure, or neurologic deficit. Many if not most unruptured AVMs diagnosed in the ED will be incidental findings on MRI or CT brain scanning performed for unrelated indications.

As always, the emergency physician will first direct attention to stabilization of the ABCs and the administration of supportive care. History and physical examination priorities are much as for ICA, although AVM is less likely than ICA to present with bulbar palsy. A thorough neurological examination is of course essential.

The ED evaluation of a suspected intracranial lesion hinges on diagnostic imaging. CT angiography and MRI angiography are both capable of identifying intracranial AVM, although MRI gives better vascular and parenchymal definition and may be more sensitive.

Prompt neurosurgical consultation should be obtained for all patients diagnosed with unruptured intracranial AVM. Most patients will require additional imaging with MRI and/or digital subtraction angiography. Treatment options include embolisation, surgery, and radiosurgical ablation.

Stroke Syndromes

Hemorrhagic Stroke

Hemorrhagic stroke accounts for about 20% of all acute cerebrovascular accidents, with SAH accounting for 3% to 5% and ICH for 15% to 18%. However, these catastrophes have a disproportionate impact on mortality, disability, and potential life-years lost. The vast majority of hemorrhagic strokes can be classified as intraparenchymal hemorrhage (IPH) or SAH. While both IPH and SAH reflect bleeding from intracranial vessels, the two entities are otherwise quite distinct in their etiology and pathophysiology. Patients with hemorrhagic stroke require rapid stabilization, diagnosis and referral for definitive neurosurgical management.

Spontaneous Subarachnoid Hemorrhage
Etiology/Anatomy/Pathophysiology

Spontaneous (as opposed to traumatic) intracranial SAH is a potentially devastating vascular catastrophe that almost always results from rupture of an ICA or AVM. The incidence rate of SAH has remained stable for decades, at about 5 to 10 cases per 100,000 patient years. Although SAH accounts for only 3% of all strokes, it accounts for 25% of potential life-years lost to stroke, and 5% of all stroke deaths. Most patients are under 60 years of age. Women are 1.6 times more likely to have an SAH than their male counterparts, and African Americans are more than twice as likely to suffer an SAH as whites.

A family history of SAH places one at a greater risk of cerebral hemorrhage. First-degree relatives of SAH victims have up to a sevenfold increased risk of SAH. Inherited connective tissue diseases such as autosomal dominant polycystic kidney disease, neurofibromatosis, and Ehlers-Danlos IV are also associated to varying degrees with increased risk of SAH. Modifiable risk factors include alcohol abuse, smoking, and hypertension. Evidence for increased risk of SAH from heavy coffee intake and oral contraceptives is mixed at best.

The vast majority (85%) of primary spontaneous SAH results from the rupture of a saccular ICA. AVM accounts for another 5% to 10% of cases, and the remaining 5% to 10% (including those with nonaneurysmal permisencephalic hemorrhage) have no demonstrable vascular abnormality at arteriography. These values do not incorporate data for secondary SAH, which results from the extension of a parenchymal hemorrhage of neoplastic, traumatic, hypertensive or coagulopathic etiology into the subarachnoid space. Furthermore, the values for AVM are potentially misleading, as many if not most cases of SAH associated with an AVM result from rupture of a saccular aneurysm on a feeding artery, rather than the AVM itself.

Emergency Department Evaluation

The diagnosis of SAH in the ED is fraught with peril. Misdiagnoses—and missed opportunities for patient salvage—are common. Up to one-third of all patients presenting with SAH are incorrectly diagnosed upon their first visit to a physician. Much of the traditional medical "wisdom" surrounding the evaluation of this condition is clearly wrong, and the emergency physician must maintain a high index of suspicion and low threshold for the performance of diagnostic testing to avoid misdiagnosis and inappropriate disposition.

Classically, patients with SAH present with headache of explosive, catastrophic onset during strenuous activity, associated with syncope, nausea, vomiting, stiff neck, and obtundation. Patients with such a "textbook" presentation are easily recognized; however, not all patients with SAH will present with such clear-cut findings.

The emergency physician must recognize that SAH encompasses a broad spectrum of clinical manifestations. Half of all patients with SAH present with atypical features. Although headache from SAH tends to be sudden in onset, the headache may not be severe, and may not be associated with strenuous activity. Headache from SAH may be relieved by non-narcotic analgesics, or may resolve spontaneously. Nuchal rigidity, focal neurologic signs, and ophthalmologic manifestations may be absent or so subtle as to escape cursory examination.

Furthermore, patients may present with the so-called "warning leak," rather than a catastrophic hemorrhage. Such "leaks" are in fact relatively mild episodes of SAH, and are harbingers of more serious events to follow. These patients typically have abrupt onset of headache, which may be self-limited, in the absence of acute neurologic findings, meningismus or ophthalmologic abnormalities. Early diagnosis and management of such patients may result in full preservation of neurologic function.

SAH must therefore be part of the differential diagnosis for any patient presenting to the ED with a history of abrupt onset of headache, regardless of the severity, location, duration, response to non-narcotic analgesia or presence or absence of associated findings, such as retinal hemorrhage or meningismus. Patients with chronic headaches who present with "worst" headaches or those presenting with atypical headaches also raise the suspicion of SAH. Finally, it must be emphasized that the emergency physician should never make a primary diagnosis of vascular or migraine headache. Not only does a first episode of severe headache fail to meet the criterion of the

International Headache Society for diagnosis of vascular headache, but its consideration in the differential practically invites misdiagnosis of SAH.

The emergency physician should first address the ABCs, patient stabilization, and supportive care. Obtunded or combative patients may require rapid sequence induction of anesthesia and tracheal intubation. IV access and cardiac monitoring are essential for all patients with a suspected stroke syndrome, including SAH. Seizure precautions and working suction at the bedside are highly recommended. The physician should obtain a careful medical history, including time of onset, duration, and location of the headache; associated activity; what analgesics may have been taken; family history of SAH or stroke; and use of tobacco, coffee, alcohol, and illicit drugs. Physical examination should include a search for subhyaloid retinal hemorrhage, papilledema, cranial nerve palsies, meningismus, temporal artery tenderness, carotid bruits, and focal neurological deficits. An electrocardiogram may reveal an associated tachyarrhythmia or myocardial infarction.

Diagnosis of SAH is made at non-contrast CT or with lumbar puncture. CT scanning is up to 98% sensitive for SAH, although small amounts of subarachnoid blood can be subtle and difficult to detect. It is important to recognize that CT is to some degree an operator-dependent test, and subtle hemorrhage may escape detection by all but the most capable radiologists.

CT fails to identify at least 2% to 3% of patients with SAH, and, therefore, the traditional diagnostic algorithm for patients with suspected SAH has been to follow a negative CT study with lumbar puncture. Misinformation and controversy abound, however, and misinterpretation of lumbar puncture results presents another potential pitfall in the diagnosis of SAH. Visual inspection of spinal fluid for either blood or xanthochromia is completely unreliable. Operators have long ruled out "traumatic taps" by comparing the erythrocyte count in the first tube to that in the third or fourth tube: If the first tube shows a high erythrocyte count but the later tube has a lower count, the tap is said to be "traumatic" and SAH is excluded. This ostensibly reassuring and persistent article of medical folklore has no solid evidentiary basis. Diagnosis of SAH by lumbar puncture is made by the finding of erythrocytes or of xanthochromia, which is the staining of CSF by bilirubin and oxyhemoglobin due to erythrocytolysis. The relative accuracy of these two findings remains an issue of contention.

Some authors have suggested that, contrary to traditional practice, lumbar puncture should be performed prior to CT imaging in the patient with lone acute sudden headache (LASH). Patients meeting LASH criteria have normal neurological examinations, normal vital signs including temperature, and no meningismus. Several advantages are cited for the LP-first strategy. Proponents note that, although a negative CT should be followed by lumbar puncture, physicians (and patients) will frequently take inappropriate reassurance from a negative study and defer the LP. Performing the LP first would bypass this potentially catastrophic lapse in judgment. A negative LP is said to obviate the need for further evaluation for SAH in patients without focal neurological findings or altered level of consciousness, with consequent improvements in resource utilization. Finally, LP-first proponents correctly point out that lumbar puncture is safe in LASH patients.

Critics of this approach argue that the vast majority of CT scans will be positive in patients with SAH, obviating the need for a painful, invasive procedure that could theoretically precipitate rebleeding from a ruptured aneurysm or catastrophic deterioration in a patient with cerebellar hemorrhage. Critics also point out that CT is not merely a screen to determine whether the patient can safely undergo lumbar puncture. CT will delineate the location of bleeding and the presence or absence of intraventricular hemorrhage, and may also identify alternative sources for the headache, such as intracerebral bleeding and mass lesions.

At the time of this writing, emergency medicine practice appears to be shifting increasingly to the LP-first strategy, although strong evidentiary support is limited. Several caveats should be borne in mind. The LP-first strategy may not be appropriate for patients presenting less than twelve hours after the onset of headache. Patients must meet LASH criteria: patients with altered consciousness, fever, and focal neurologic signs should undergo CT scanning as soon as possible. Finally, the emergency physician should be aware that in a small number of LASH patients, a potentially serious intracranial lesion other than SAH may be present and will be missed if CT scan is deferred.

Patients diagnosed with SAH should receive immediate neurosurgical consultation for additional evaluation, imaging, and management. The patient's vital signs and neurological status must be closely monitored, as deterioration can occur suddenly due to rebleeding, acute hydrocephalus, expanding subdural hematoma or intraparenchymal hemorrhage. Hypoxia must be avoided at all costs. Management of hypertensive patients is difficult, and should be conducted in close consultation with a neurosurgeon. Changes in cerebral autoregulation after intracranial hemorrhage render the brain more dependent on arterial pressure to maintain perfusion. Lowering blood pressure in the hypertensive patient with SAH therefore entails a very real risk of inducing or exacerbating cerebral ischemia, and should generally be avoided in all but the most extreme scenarios.

Neuroprotective strategies in SAH include treatment with calcium channel blockers and antioxidant compounds. Calcium channel blockers were first employed on the rationale that they would prevent the cerebral vasospasm and resultant ischemia complicating SAH. However, nimodipine, the calcium channel blocker that seems to have the greatest salutary impact on outcome, also appears to be the one with the least effect on vasospasm. The mechanism for the limited neuroprotective effect (if any) of nimodipine, therefore, remains in doubt.

Tirilazad, which prevents iron-mediated lipid peroxidation, performed poorly in clinical trials. Similarly, N-propylenedinicotinamide, a free radical scavenger, failed to significantly improve outcome at 3 months after SAH.

Surgical ablation of the ruptured aneurysm has been the mainstay of treatment for decades, but in the last 10 years endovascular coiling has come into increasing use. The International Subarachnoid Aneurysm Trial (ISAT) enrolled 2,143 patients with ruptured aneurysms and randomized them to coiling or clipping. The investigators found significantly better 1-year outcomes with endovascular coiling, but the long-term advantages of coiling, especially with respect to aneurysmal recanalization and bleeding, are still unclear.

Intracerebral Hemorrhage

Intraparenchymal cerebral hemorrhage (IPH) usually results from long-standing uncontrolled hypertension, and occurs most frequently in the basal ganglia. Presentation is highly variable, ranging from simple headache with or without neurological deficit to full-blown coma, quadriparesis, and cardiorespiratory depression. Emergency care emphasizes rapid stabilization and diagnosis, prompt neurosurgical consultation, and optimization of intracranial pressure, hemodynamics and metabolic parameters.

Etiology/Anatomy/Pathophysiology

The most common cause of nontraumatic IPH is long-standing uncontrolled hypertension. In this setting, small cerebral arteries and arterioles undergo degenerative changes that lead to the development of microscopic defects, called Charcot-Broussard aneurysms. These microaneurysms are most commonly found in the basal ganglia, thalamus, internal capsule, cerebral white matter, cerebellum and brainstem, and it is in these locations that IPH occurs with the greatest frequency, with basal ganglia hemorrhage predominating. In elderly patients, IPH may be due to cerebral amyloid angiopathy, in which deposition of proteinaceous material in the walls of leptomeningeal blood vessels leads to decreased vascular integrity. In younger patients and in those without chronic hypertension, arteriovenous malformation or abuse of sympathomimetic drugs (cocaine, methamphetamine) are more likely culprits. Other causes include iatrogenic coagulopathy, neoplasm, iatrogenic hemorrhage from stroke thrombolysis, and vasculitis.

Patients with intracerebral hemorrhage classically present with sudden headache, neurological deficit, syncope, vomiting, alteration of mental status, seizures or coma. As with SAH, however, the physician must beware of relying on such a "textbook" presentation, have a low index of suspicion for the diagnosis, and rely heavily on diagnostic imaging.

Neurological presentation of intracerebral hemorrhage is highly variable, depending on the location of hemorrhage, the structures affected, and the presence of edema or mass effect. Putamenal hemorrhage, which accounts for roughly 50% of IPH, presents with contralateral motor and sensory deficits, homonymous hemianopsia, aphasia, and ipsilateral gaze deviation (toward the lesion). This pattern can be difficult to distinguish from middle cerebral artery ischemic stroke. Pontine hemorrhage is a devastating injury that rapidly progresses to coma, pinpoint pupils, decerebrate posturing, loss of oculovestibular reflexes, and respiratory ataxia. Cerebellar hemorrhage manifests as vomiting, vertigo, dysequilibrium, and ataxia. Signs of pontine compression may also be present, such as facial weakness and CN VI palsy. The presentation of cerebellar hemorrhage may be subtle and difficult to differentiate from more benign causes of vertigo and ataxia. This is an important point, because patients with posterior fossa hemorrhage respond well to surgical evaluation, but will deteriorate rapidly due to brainstem compression and herniation if the condition is not recognized and treated early.

Emergency Department Evaluation

The emergency physician begins with a rapid primary survey of the ABCs in conjunction with patient stabilization. Many patients with IPH will be comatose and require immediate endotracheal intubation. IV access, supplemental oxygen, cardiac monitoring, seizure precautions, and working suction at the bedside are essential. Early evaluation should also include measurement of capillary blood glucose, pulse oximetry, assessment for trauma, a search for evidence of aspiration, and core body temperature. Rapid neurologic screening will include level of consciousness, pupillary examination, speech, motor function, and, if possible, gait.

Patients who require endotracheal intubation should be managed with rapid sequence induction of anesthesia, utilizing a protocol that incorporates intravenous lidocaine (1 mg/kg over 1 minute) to blunt the increase in intracranial pressure that accompanies manipulation of the airway. The use of lidocaine in this setting has been challenged recently, but this evidence is still preliminary and lidocaine remains appropriate for airway management in these patients.

Many patients with ICH will have delayed presentations, and may have been comatose or immobile for hours or even days. Dehydration should be treated with volume expansion, and the physician should search for evidence of trauma, limb ischemia due to compression, sepsis and rhabdomyolysis. Derangements in serum glucose should be corrected with dextrose or insulin, and every effort should be made to keep serum glucose levels below 200 mg/dL.

When the patient has been stabilized, a complete history and physical examination should be performed. History should focus on determining when the event occurred and under what circumstances, whether associated trauma occurred, pre-existing medical problems, medications taken, and use of illicit drugs such as cocaine or methamphetamine. Neurologic examination should include complete assessment of cranial nerves, pupillary reactivity, visual fields by confrontation, deep tendon reflexes, muscle strength, and sensation, including proprioception, fine touch, steriognosis, and pinprick. The physician should look for and document pronator drift, degenerate reflexes or posturing. A fundoscopic examination is mandatory. Special attention should be paid to assessing the patient's gait, if possible. A complete assessment of cerebellar function (including heel-shin maneuvers, rapid alternating movements, Rom-

berg, and gait testing), are extremely important and often overlooked.

Laboratory evaluation includes electrolytes, renal function, complete blood count, PT/PTT/INR, and serum glucose.

Diagnosis of acute ICH is made by nonenhanced CT, which will identify a well-circumscribed radiodense lesion that may be associated with edema, mass effect, hydrocephalus, or extension of the hemorrhage to the cerebral ventricles or subarachnoid space. Patients with suspected intracranial hemorrhage are at risk for sudden deterioration and must be accompanied to the CT suite by appropriate personnel and equipment for monitoring and resuscitation. Identification of ICH at CT mandates immediate neurosurgical referral.

Moderate hypertension is well tolerated in patients with acute ICH, and the emergency physician must be judicious in his use of antihypertensive agents. Lowering blood pressure in the setting of ICH may exacerbate abnormal autoregulatory parameters and result in brain ischemia. In patients with severe hypertension (MAP > 130 mm Hg or SBP > 220 mm Hg), in whom control of hypertension is deemed essential to prevent additional injury, cautious use of antihypertensive agents such as labetalol or esmolol may be warranted. Use of long-acting or oral agents is contraindicated.

Intracranial hypertension from mass effect and brain edema is the predominant threat to the patient with IPH. Cerebral perfusion pressure (CPP) is defined as the difference between MAP (normally about 90 mm Hg) and ICP (normally about 15 mm Hg). If CPP drops below 50 to 60 mm Hg, brain ischemia ensues, resulting in additional injury. Rising intracranial pressure may also result in transtentorial herniation. This catastrophe manifests as decreased level of consciousness, a dilated and unreactive pupil which is usually (but not always) ipsilateral to the lesion, and altered respiratory pattern or apnea. If not corrected immediately, transtentorial herniation will lead to irreversible brain damage and death. Patients with late or unrecognized cerebellar hemorrhage will also progress to brainstem compression, apnea and death.

Monitoring and treatment of elevated ICP should be aggressive and conducted in consultation with a neurosurgical specialist. Direct measurement via ICP monitor, which is usually placed ipsilateral to the lesion, is an indispensable guide to management. The goal of therapy is to maintain the patient's ICP in the range of 15 to 20 mm Hg. Options for the management of ICP include diuretic and osmotic therapy, fluid management, patient positioning, CSF drainage, and proper patient positioning. Of all these, elevating the patient's head 30° to 40° is the most benign, although the degree of benefit is questionable. The effectiveness and safety of osmotic therapy and hyperventilation have come under question in recent years, and should probably be used aggressively only in the most severe cases or where brain herniation is imminent, and in close consultation with a neurosurgeon. Hyperventilation to a $PaCO_2$ of 25 to 30 mm Hg has a direct vasoconstrictor effect on cerebral arterioles and lowers ICP, but may also exacerbate concomitant cerebral ischemia. Mannitol is administered intravenously in a dose 1 g/kg, and repeat doses of 0.25 mg/kg may be given every three to four hours for persistent elevations of ICP.

All patients with acute ICH require immediate neurosurgical consultation and intensive hemodynamic, neurological and ICP monitoring. Many patients, especially those with posterior fossa hemorrhages, will go to immediate craniotomy for evacuation. Indications for evacuation of lobar, putamenal, thalamic and brainstem hematomas are variable and controversial, and depend on the location, accessibility, and size of the lesion, as well as the presence of comorbidities, response of intracranial hypertension to medical management, and the threat of impending herniation. All patients with ICH require admission to an intensive care setting.

Ischemic Stroke

The brain has no long-term stores of oxidizable substrates, and undergoes rapid loss of high-energy phosphate in the setting of ischemia. Furthermore, neurons are terminally differentiated, nonmitotic cells, and cannot be replaced once lost. Brain tissue and brain function are therefore exquisitely sensitive to circulatory impairment. Cerebral ischemia is a complication of subarachnoid hemorrhage (secondary to vasospasm), traumatic brain injury or any condition that diminishes CPP, such as cerebral edema or rapidly expanding cerebral hematoma. Transient global brain ischemia is a devastating consequence of prolonged cardiac arrest. However, the following discussion focuses on focal ischemic stroke arising from either embolic or thrombotic occlusion of part of the brain's blood supply. Focal ischemic stroke affects at least 600,000 patients per year in the United States alone. The monetary cost of stroke exceeds $20 billion per year, and the human cost in disability and suffering is incalculable. Recent developments in the pharmacologic treatment of ischemic stroke have given the evaluation and management of this condition a new urgency, and emergency physicians have an increasingly central role in the acute care of focal cerebral ischemia. For most patients, however, supportive care continues to be the cornerstone of management, with special attention directed to the maintenance of cerebral perfusion and oxygenation, control of serum glucose, and the prevention of complications and recurrent injury. The distinction between thrombotic and embolic stroke is somewhat hazy, in terms of both pathophysiology and clinical evaluation and management. Much of the material covered in the following discussion of embolic stroke is therefore equally applicable to the setting of thrombotic stroke.

Embolic Stroke
Etiology/Anatomy/Pathophysiology
The brain's blood supply enters the skull as the anterior and posterior circulations. The anterior circulation is supplied by the internal carotid arteries, which enter the skull through the petrous portion of the temporal bone. The internal carotids give rise to the ophthalmic arteries and then branch into the anterior cerebral, middle cerebral and posterior communicating arteries. The posterior circulation arises from the vertebral arteries, which enter the cranial vault through the foramen magnum. The two vertebral arteries unite to form the basilar artery, which lies on the ventral surface of the pons. At the level of the midbrain, the basilar artery gives rise to the posterior cerebral arteries.

The anterior and posterior circulations are integrated into an anastomotic structure, the Circle of Willis, which lies on the ventral surface of the cerebrum, surrounding the pituitary gland and optic chiasm. The two circulations are joined by the posterior communicating arteries, which link the posterior cerebral arteries to the middle cerebral arteries. Moreover, the right and left anterior circulations are linked by the anterior communicating artery.

This anastomotic structure confers upon the brain a robust protection against injury arising from occlusion of the proximal arteries. In the presence of adequate collateral circulation, such an occlusion may result in minimal damage or even be clinically silent. On the other hand, anatomic variations of the Circle of Willis may leave the brain catastrophically vulnerable to a lesion that would be of little consequence in an individual with normal anatomy.

Embolization of thrombi to the cerebrovascular system accounts for roughly 15% to 25% of ischemic strokes. Cardiogenic emboli are the most frequent offenders, and may arise from diseased cardiac valves, prosthetic valves, atrial thrombi in the setting of atrial fibrillation, or ventricular thrombi in the setting of myocardial infarction. It is not unusual for acute ischemic stroke to be the presenting symptom of new-onset atrial fibrillation or "silent" myocardial infarction. Bacterial endocarditis, congenital heart disease, and cerebrovascular disease also place the patient at increased risk of embolic stroke.

Most focal ischemic strokes (as distinguished from the global cerebral ischemia that occurs during cardiac arrest) are characterized by a central "core" territory, in which ischemia is complete or near-complete, surrounded by a "penumbra" of tissue in which some collateral perfusion is preserved. Neurons in the ischemic core tend to die early and demonstrate frankly necrotic death phenotypes. In the penumbra, delayed neuronal death through apoptosis (programmed cell death or "cell suicide") is more predominant. This is important because, unlike necrosis, apoptosis is a highly regulated phenomenon, subject to modulation by growth factors, inhibition of proteases, and changes in genetic expression. Accordingly, therapeutic interventions of value in stroke must focus on limiting the size of the ischemic core, optimizing perfusion of the penumbra and promoting a biochemical milieu that favors survival signaling over programmed cell death processes.

The presentation of acute ischemic stroke depends on the vascular territory affected, and encompasses a broad spectrum of clinical syndromes. The reader is referred to **Table 74.2** for a summary of the most commonly encountered stroke scenarios and their corresponding vascular lesions. In patients who have "showered" emboli to multiple

Table 74.2

Stroke Syndromes and Corresponding Vascular Lesions

ANTERIOR CIRCULATION

Vascular Lesion	Clinical Features
Complete MCA occlusion	Global aphasia (dominant hemisphere), neglect (nondominant hemisphere), homonymous hemianopia.
Occlusion of lentriculo-striate branches of MCA	Lacunar Infarction. Internal Capsule: Hemiparesis or hemiplegia with sensory deficit, affecting contralateral face, arm and leg, without cortical deficit or visual loss.
Anterior MCA occlusion	Broca's aphasia (dominant hemisphere), contralateral weakness of the face and arm.
Posterior MCA occlusion	Wernicke's (fluent) aphasia (dominant hemisphere) and hemianopia without motor deficit.
ACA occlusion	Contralateral lower extremity weakness and sensory deficit; upper extremity "drift" on sustained extension, impairment of judgment and insight, confusion, gait apraxia, bowel and bladder incontinence.

POSTERIOR CIRCULATION

Vascular Lesion	Clinical Features
PICA or PICA branch occlusion	*Cerebellar infarction:* Ipsilateral ataxia, dysequilibrium, vertigo. Cerebellar edema at 2–4 days may be life threatening. *Lateral medullary infarction:* Ipsilateral ataxia, decreased pain/temperature sensation on contralateral arm, trunk or leg; vertigo, nystagmus, Horner's syndrome, hoarseness, hiccups, possible airway compromise.
Basilar artery occlusion	*Massive brainstem infarction:* Pontine and midbrain infarction results in coma, quadriparesis, meiosis, respiratory ataxia, apnea, death. *Locked-in syndrome:* Pontine infarction with midbrain sparing results in quadriparesis/quadriplegia, loss of horizontal gaze, facial paralysis and anarthria, with preservation of consciousness. *Anton's syndrome:* Embolus to distal BA occludes both PCAs, resulting in cortical blindness.
Penetrating branches of basilar artery	*Pontine lacunar infarction syndromes:* Pure motor hemiparesis, clumsy hand-dysarthria syndrome, ataxic hemiparesis.
Circumferential branches of basilar artery	*Pontine-midbrain infarction:* Crossed findings—contralateral extremity weakness, with ipsilateral facial weakness, bulbar palsy, ataxia, nystagmus, vertigo.
Posterior cerebral artery occlusion	*Occipital lobe infarction:* Contralateral homonymous hemianopia. Involvement of thalamogeniculate arteries produces an accompanying contralateral hemisensory deficit. *Alexia without agraphia:* Left PCA occlusion produces inability to read with preservation of writing ability.

cerebrovascular territories, the clinical picture will naturally be more complex.

Emergency Department Evaluation

As always, the emergency physician's first priority is to perform an expeditious primary survey and stabilize the patient. Critically ill patients with airway compromise will require prompt intubation, but a rapid neurological examination should be performed prior to sedation and paralysis whenever possible. Hypoglycemia, narcotic overdose, Todd's postictal paresis and other readily reversible causes of altered mental status and neurological deficit should also be considered prior to rapid sequence induction and intubation. All patients require cardiac monitoring, evaluation of pulse oximetry, vascular access, seizure precautions, and working suction at the bedside.

Administration of supplemental oxygen in patients without respiratory compromise or desaturation is an issue of some controversy. Some authorities worry that maintaining high cerebral oxygen concentrations will promote the elaboration of reactive oxygen species, which damage neuronal membranes, induce organelle stress responses, and promote the activation or maintenance of cell death processes. Ronning and Guldvog found that supplemental oxygen was of no benefit and might be slightly detrimental in acute ischemic stroke. However, patients in this study were given 100% oxygen. While cerebral hyperoxia presents certain theoretical concerns, hypoxia is indisputably an aggravating factor in the setting of stroke. At present, it seems reasonable to treat non-intubated stroke patients with low-flow supplemental oxygen, and to avoid excessively high oxygen fractions in intubated patients.

A thorough history and physical examination, with emphasis on cardiovascular and neurological findings, should be performed as soon as possible. It is important to determine, if possible, when symptom onset occurred, or when the patient was last observed to be functioning normally. The physician should search for meningismus, temporal artery tenderness, irregular pulses, carotid bruits, and cardiac murmurs, gallops or clicks that might suggest valvular disease or myocardial ischemia. Fundoscopic examination and a careful assessment of the cranial nerves are crucial. The neurological examination should also include an assessment of mental status, judgment, insight and language, visual fields by confrontation, cerebellar function, motor strength of all four extremities, deep tendon reflexes, sensation, and the presence of degenerate reflexes. Gait testing, if possible, can be extremely useful in localizing the putative ischemic lesion. A frequently neglected aspect of neurological assessment is repeated examination, which will often identify progression or resolution of deficits, clarify the presentation, and guide management and disposition.

Rapid imaging at CT is of paramount importance, especially in patients who present early, as the results of this study are crucial in identifying those patients who are suitable candidates for thrombolysis. CT will delineate subacute strokes and identify focal edema in many cases. CT may offer alternative diagnoses, such as intracranial mass or hemorrhage.

All patients should have blood drawn for basic laboratory studies, including complete blood count, electrolytes and creatinine, and coagulation profile. A 12-lead EKG is mandatory, to evaluate for arrhythmia or occult myocardial injury. Prompt neurological consultation is essential for all patients with suspected cerebral ischemia.

Unless a specific contraindication exists, aspirin should be administered early to all patients with suspected acute ischemic stroke, as this is the single most effective pharmacological intervention available for these patients. Administration of heparin and heparinoids to patients with acute ischemic stroke not known to be cardioembolic in origin does not improve outcome, presents considerable risk to the patient, and cannot be recommended. Patients with documented atrial fibrillation or other embolic source certainly may require anticoagulation to prevent additional injury; this intervention is ideally undertaken after early echocardiography, and in consultation with a neurologist and cardiologist.

A growing body of data underscores the importance of controlling serum glucose levels in the setting of acute ischemic stroke and other forms of brain injury. Elevated glucose levels are strongly associated with increased mortality and neurological deficit. Severe hyperglycemia in the stroke patient should be treated aggressively, and every effort should be made to maintain serum glucose levels below 200 mg/dL. The neuroprotective effect of serum glucose control in acute ischemic stroke may have less to do with brain glucose levels than with the intrinsic growth factor properties of insulin, which is a potent inhibitor of programmed cell death. Post-stroke hyperglycemia may therefore be a biomarker for decreased "insulin tone" that places vulnerable neurons in the penumbra at greater risk.

The physician must avoid the temptation to aggressively treat hypertension in the patient with acute ischemic stroke. Cerebral autoregulation may be impaired in the stroke patient, and lowering the blood pressure may disproportionately compromise collateral flow to salvageable neurons in the penumbra, needlessly expanding stroke volume and worsening outcome. Control of profound hypertension (MAP > 130 mm Hg or SBP > 220 mm Hg) in the patient with acute ischemic stroke should entail the use of agents that preserve cerebral autoregulation, such as labetalol, or agents that are subject to rapid titration, such as esmolol or nitroprusside. Oral antihypertensive agents are contraindicated.

Hypotension poses a dire threat to salvageable neurons in the penumbra, and should be corrected aggressively with volume expansion. Pressors should be used with great caution, and only when euvolemia has been established, because these agents can actually impair cerebral blood flow. Furthermore, vasopressors, such as dopamine and norepinephrine, probably "counter-signal" intrinsic growth-factor mediated cell survival processes, and may promote apoptosis in vulnerable neurons.

Until recently, ED treatment of ischemic stroke was nonspecific and largely limited to supportive care. The advent of thrombolytic therapy for acute ischemic stroke has had a tremendous impact on the emergency physician's approach to such patients, not least by imparting a new sense of urgency to their evaluation and management. Most protocols exclude patients from thrombolytic intervention if stroke symptoms have been present for more than three hours. It is therefore essential that patient evaluation, neurological consultation, and CT imaging be performed as expeditiously as possible in eligible patients if thrombolysis is contemplated.

It is important, however, to cast a judicious eye on the risks, benefits, and effectiveness of stroke thrombolysis. The landmark study conducted by the National Institutes of Neurological Disease and Stroke, published in 1995, demonstrated a 12% increase in the number of patients with minimal or no disability compared to placebo, but this effect was accompanied by a tenfold increase in the rate of symptomatic intracranial hemorrhage. All subsequent studies with rt-PA in the setting of acute ischemic stroke have demonstrated a similarly narrow therapeutic margin for this intervention. It is both instructive and sobering to compare the number-needed-to-treat (NNT) and the number-needed-to-harm (NNH) obtained from various clinical trials of stroke thrombolysis. In a meta-analysis of 6 studies of rt-PA for stroke, Lindbloom derived aggregate values for NNT and NNH at 17 and 19, respectively; the number-needed-to-kill (from iatrogenic intracranial hemorrhage) was 40. Furthermore, an objective evaluation of the clinical effectiveness of this therapy when administered in the community setting reveals that thrombolysis is unlikely to have a major impact on outcomes in stroke populations, primarily because most patients who present with acute ischemic stroke will fail to meet rigid inclusion criteria. An additional problem is the inappropriate administration of thrombolytics to patients who do not actually have a stroke. In one study, 19% of patients evaluated by a stroke team were misdiagnosed as having acute ischemic stroke. Finally, it is worth noting that a study by Shriger et al. suggests that many emergency physicians, neurologists, and radiologists will fail to detect subtle radiographic signs of pre-existing cerebral hemorrhage—an absolute contraindication to thrombolytic therapy—on a screening CT examination, which casts additional doubt on the safety of this intervention.

Both physician and patient must be aware of the profound risk associated with thrombolytic therapy. Indeed, the issue of informed consent is an important and often confounding factor to consider when contemplating thrombolysis for stroke. A patient suffering from acute ischemic stroke may not be competent to render informed consent, raising difficult ethical and medicolegal issues. Up to 20% of patients presenting to an emergency department with stroke may be unable to understand the relevant information sufficiently to render informed consent. Institutions using thrombolysis for acute ischemic stroke would be well-advised to have in place explicit protocols for dealing with these eventualities.

Multiple studies have confirmed that the risk of symptomatic intracranial hemorrhage from stroke thrombolysis is increased when deviations from established criteria for rt-PA administration occur. **Table 74.3** outlines generally accepted criteria for stroke thrombolysis, based on those utilized in the NINDS trial. If stroke thrombolysis is contemplated, it is absolutely imperative that the emergency physician insist on strict observation of these criteria, as any deviation from them is likely to place the patient in even greater jeopardy from an already risky therapy.

Consideration of potential medicolegal consequences has no part in the decision to use rt-PA for stroke or any other therapeutic or diagnostic modality. Not only do such considerations invite deviation from criteria for thrombolytic stroke therapy, but "thrombolitigation" may ensue whether thrombolysis is employed or not.

At least one study has suggested that emergency physicians are qualified to administer thrombolytics for acute ischemic stroke. In practice, however, the decision to use thrombolytics should almost always be made in consultation with a neurologist, who can assist in evaluation, patient selection and education, optimization of metabolic and hemodynamic parameters, and disposition.

Clinical trials with putative neuroprotective agents have been disappointing, and at present, no such agent can be recommended for routine clinical practice. For the time being, the best "neuroprotective" strategy is meticulous supportive care, with special attention directed to maintaining cerebral perfusion and oxygenation, controlling serum glucose levels, rigorous adherence to criteria for thrombolysis, prevention of recurrent stroke, and protecting the patient from comorbidities such as aspiration, infection, and thromboembolic events.

A large body of data confirms that patients with acute ischemic stroke are much more likely to enjoy a better outcome and early discharge when admitted to multidisciplinary "stroke units." These units, which ideally occupy a fixed location within the institution and a committed multidisciplinary staff, focus on early diagnostics, appropriate control of blood pressure and serum glucose, early mobilization and rehabilitation, and close follow-up and social support.

Table 74.3

Suggested Inclusion and Exclusion Criteria for Administration of rt-PA to Patients with Acute Ischemic Stroke

Inclusion Criteria

1. Patient or legal surrogate capable of giving informed consent.
2. Age $\geq$ 18 years.
3. Onset of symptoms of hemispheric stroke within the last 3 hours.
4. Clinically apparent hemispheric ischemic stroke with neurological deficit.
5. NIHSS stroke severity score $\geq$ 4.
6. CT scan complete prior to expiration of 3-hour limit.

Exclusion Criteria

1. Total anterior circulation syndrome: coma or severe obtundation with fixed gaze deviation and/or complete hemiplegia or NIHSS score > 22.
2. Evidence of rapid improvement or resolution of symptoms.
3. NIHSS score < 4.
4. Previous stroke within past 6 weeks.
5. Seizure with onset of stroke symptoms.
6. Any clinical evidence or suspicion of ICH, even in the face of a normal CT examination.
7. History of prior intracranial hemorrhage, AVM, aneurysm, or intracranial neoplasm.
8. SBP > 185 mm Hg or diastolic BP > 110 mm Hg despite acute antihypertensive therapy.
9. Known or suspected septic embolus.
10. Myocardial infarction within last 30 days.
11. History of moderate-severe trauma within last 30 days.
12. History of surgery within last 30 days.
13. Recent arterial puncture at a noncompressible site.
14. History of hemorrhagic diathesis or anticoagulant therapy with INR > 1.5.
15. Pregnancy, lactation or parturition within the last 30 days.
16. Thrombocytopenia (platelet count < 100×10^9/L).
17. Evidence of intracranial hemorrhage on CT.
18. CT evidence of infarction encompassing more than one third of MCA territory.

Thrombotic Stroke

Approximately half of all acute ischemic stroke events are due to atherothrombotic disease of the cerebrovascular system, primarily in the extracranial and large intracranial vessels. Atherosclerotic disease can result in brain ischemia either by complete or near-complete thrombotic occlusion of the vessel itself, or by embolization of thrombus fragments from the diseased vessel to the distal cerebral circulation. Patient presentation, management, and disposition are much the same as for embolic stroke, as discussed in the preceding section.

Etiology/Anatomy/Pathophysiology

Most thrombotic strokes arise from atherosclerotic disease, which can progress to the formation of luminal thrombus in a manner not unlike that known to occur in acute coronary thrombosis. The most common sites for atherosclerotic plaque formation are at the bifurcation of the common carotid artery, the bifurcation of the middle and anterior cerebral arteries, and in the vertebrobasilar system. Ischemic stroke may then result either from occlusion by the thrombus, or by embolization of thrombus fragments to the cerebral circulation. Less common causes of thrombotic stroke include vasculitis, syphilis, systemic lupus erythematosis, carotid or vertebral artery dissection, and hypercoagulable states such as those seen in polycythemia, sickle cell disease, or deficiency of antithrombin III, proteins C and protein S.

Presentation of thrombotic stroke will vary depending on the site of occlusion and resultant brain injury. The reader is referred to the foregoing discussion of embolic stroke and Table 74.2 for more information.

Emergency Department Evaluation

Evaluation and management of acute thrombotic stroke is essentially identical to that discussed in the preceding section on acute embolic stroke. Rapid assessment of ABCs, patient stabilization and supportive care, cardiac monitoring, careful history and physical examination, diagnostic imaging, and early neurological consultation are the cornerstones of care. All patients should receive aspirin unless a specific contraindication exists. Anticoagulation is not indicated. The use of thrombolytics may be considered in eligible patients, but the issue of informed consent must be explicitly addressed, and the emergency physician must insist on strict adherence to selection criteria and treatment protocols.

Transient Ischemic Attack

The emergency physician may usefully regard transient ischemic attack (TIA) as the cerebrovascular analogue of unstable angina: an indicator of advanced cerebrovascular disease and harbinger of acute ischemic stroke. TIA represents an opportunity to initiate preventive therapy before permanent damage occurs, and as such its identification, management and appropriate disposition are exceedingly important.

Etiology/Anatomy/Pathophysiology

A TIA is defined as a transient focal neurological deficit that resolves within 24 hours, although most resolve within 1 to 2 hours. Reversible deficits lasting longer than 24 hours are commonly referred to as RIND or reversible ischemic neurologic deficit. These two conditions represent one end of a spectrum that progresses from reversible deficit to complete ischemic stroke, and are probably more reflective of clinical presentation than actual pathophysiology. Many if not most TIAs and RINDs will result in some small, albeit clinically silent, loss of brain tissue.

Moreover, the definition of TIA seems to be undergoing a quiet evolution in the age of thrombolytic therapy: thrombolytics are not indicated for TIA, yet it is impossible to discriminate between TIA and stroke during the therapeutic window in which thrombolysis may be contemplated.

The overwhelming majority of TIAs arise from atherosclerotic lesions in the extracranial carotid vessels. TIA may occur either because of critical reversible thrombotic occlusion, or embolization of thrombus fragment from the atherosclerotic lumen to a distal vessel, with subsequent resolution due to distal displacement of the fragment or disintegration of the fragment by hemodynamic forces or intrinsic fibrinolytic processes. Neurological deficits arising from TIA correspond to those arising from complete ischemic stroke in the same vascular distribution (Table 74.2).

Amaurosis fugax (AF) is a painless, monocular visual loss, which may be partial or complete, lasting seconds to hours, with complete resolution. AF is usually thromboembolic in etiology, and generally occurs without other neurological deficits. AF is clinically equivalent to other TIAs: a sign of atherosclerotic cerebrovascular disease and a harbinger of acute ischemic stroke.

Emergency Department Evaluation

There is no way to determine which patients with acute focal neurological deficits will resolve. Therefore, all such patients should be evaluated and managed as for acute ischemic stroke. Patients who have resolved their deficits prior to presentation or who resolve during their clinical course will also require similar evaluation. Patient stabilization is, as usual, the first priority. All patients without contraindications should receive aspirin early in their ED course. IV access, cardiac monitoring, measurement of capillary blood glucose and pulse oximetry and, if necessary, supplemental oxygen should be instituted, and an EKG should be obtained early. History should focus on time of onset and duration of ischemic symptoms, associated symptoms such as nausea or vertigo, previous episodes if any, presence of vascular disease or atherosclerotic risk factors, medications, and use of tobacco, alcohol or illicit drugs. A thorough physical examination should be performed, including a complete neurological assessment, documenting the status of cranial nerves, presence or absence of carotid bruits, motor and sensory function, deep tendon reflexes, gait, and cerebellar testing. Fundoscopic exam should be performed in all patients, although visualization of retinal emboli in patients with AF is uncommon. Basic laboratory evaluation should be conducted as for acute ischemic stroke. All patients should undergo unenhanced CT imaging.

Patients with new TIA, those with crescendo TIA, and those with more than three episodes in 72 hours, require prompt neurological evaluation and hospitalization for observation and further evaluation. Although some authors have suggested that many patients with TIA can be managed on an outpatient basis, convincing data of the safety and cost-effectiveness of this approach is lacking. The risk of full-blown stroke after TIA is highest soon after the event, approaching 7% to 9% in the first week, and 10% to 12% in the first 90 days. Given these data, admitting virtually all patients with new or crescendo TIA seems not only justifiable, but medically prudent. Admission allows for rapid performance of ancillary studies such as carotid duplex and cardiac echocardiography, immediate institution of appropriate antiplatelet and cholesterol-lowering therapies, anticoagulant therapy when indicated, optimization of hemodynamics and metabolic parameters, careful monitoring during the early high-risk interval, and expeditious triage to definitive therapy such as carotid endarterectomy (CEA) for selected patients.

In patients with carotid stenosis of 70% or greater, CEA may be warranted, substantially lowering the risk of recurrent ipsilateral TIA or acute ischemic stroke. Patients with less severe stenosis are probably best managed medically, with blood pressure control, cholesterol-lowering drugs, and aspirin or other antiplatelet agents. Anticoagulant therapy may be of benefit in patients with TIA due to atrial fibrillation. The current evidence does not support anticoagulation of TIA patients without atrial fibrillation, however, and most patients should be treated with aspirin or another antiplatelet agent.

Selected Readings

Adams JG, Chisholm CD. SAEM Board of Directors. The Society for Academic Emergency Medicine position on optimizing care of the stroke patient. *Acad Emerg Med* 2003;10:805.

Ciccone A, Bonito V; Italian Neurological Society's Study Group for Bioethics and Palliative Care in Neurology. Thrombolysis for acute ischemic stroke: the problem of consent. *Neurol Sci* 2001;22:339–351.

Edlow JA, Caplan LR. Avoiding pitfalls in the diagnosis of subarachnoid hemorrhage. *N Engl J Med* 2000;342:29–36.

Fleetwood IG, Steinberg GK. Arteriovenous malformations. *Lancet* 2002;359: 863–873.

Gopal AK, Whitehouse JD, Simel DL, et al. Cranial computed tomography before lumbar puncture. *Arch Intern Med* 1999;159:2681–2685.

Hankey GJ. Heparin in acute ischaemic stroke: the t-wave is negative and it's time to stop. *Med J Australia* 1998;169:534–537.

Henneman PL, Lewis RJ. Is admission medically justified for all patients with acute stroke or transient ischemic attack? *Ann Emerg Med* 1995;25:458–463.

Isaksen J, Egge A, Waterloo K, et al. Risk factors for aneurysmal subarachnoid hemorrhage: the Tromsø study. *J Neurol Neurosurg Psych* 2002;73:185–187.

Molyneux A, Kerr R, Stratton I, et al. International subarachnoid aneurysm trial (ISAT) of neurosurgical clipping versus endovascular coiling in 2143 patients with ruptured intracranial aneurysms: a randomised trial. *Lancet* 2002;360: 1267–1274.

National Institute of Neurological Disorders and Stroke rt-PA Stroke Study Group. Tissue plasminogen activator for acute ischemic stroke. *N Engl J Med* 1995; 333:1581–1587.

Ronning OM, Guldvog B. Should stroke victims routinely receive supplemental oxygen? A quasi-randomized controlled trial. *Stroke* 1999;30:2033–2037.

White BC, Sullivan JM, DeGracia DJ, et al. Brain ischemia and reperfusion: molecular mechanisms of neuronal injury. *J Neurol Sci* 2000;179:1–33.

Wiebers DO, Whisnant JP, Huston J 3rd, et al. Unruptured intracranial aneurysms: natural history, clinical outcome, and risks of surgical and endovascular treatment. *Lancet* 2003;362:103–110.

Cranial Nerve Disorders

Sheila Webb

Introduction

Evaluation and treatment of the patient presenting with symptoms of cranial nerve disorder presents a unique challenge to the emergency physician. The potential etiologies of isolated cranial nerve disorders represent a wide spectrum of pathologies, ranging from benign to life-threatening in nature. The emergency physician must place a priority on the rapid evaluation for signs and symptoms that may be suggestive of life-threatening causes of cranial nerve dysfunction, particularly hemorrhage, mass lesion or inflammation with increased intracranial pressure, which may result in herniation and death. The simultaneous onset of dysfunction of multiple cranial nerves which is acute in nature is almost always secondary to an acute cerebrovascular accident (CVA). In contrast, patients who present with gradual onset and progression of symptoms should be considered to have a neoplastic lesion until proven otherwise. As always, initial evaluation should include assessment of the ABCs, with frequent reevaluation of all patients in whom a central lesion has not been excluded. In addition to the more common etiologies of intracranial hemorrhage, infarct, and neoplasm, other etiologies of toxic, metabolic, and infectious natures must be considered in the differential diagnosis and in a thorough evaluation of cranial nerve dysfunction. Consultation with a neurologist or neurosurgeon should occur based on clinical presentation and evaluation including appropriate neuroimaging.

While patients may present with dysfunction of any isolated cranial nerve, common presentations to the emergency department (ED) related to cranial nerve dysfunction fall within the following categories, which will be discussed below:

1. Facial palsy (including Bell's palsy) involving the facial nerve (VII).
2. Trigeminal neuralgia (tic douloureux) involving the trigeminal nerve (V).
3. Visual disturbance and disorders of eye movement due to dysfunction of optic (II), oculomotor (III), trochlear (IV), and abducens (VI) nerves.

Seventh Nerve Palsy/Bell's Palsy

First described in 1882 by Dr. Charles Bell, the diagnosis of Bell's palsy refers to a subset of patients with seventh nerve palsies. Specifically, Bell's palsy is the term used to identify a peripheral seventh nerve palsy that is of idiopathic etiology. The diagnosis of Bell's palsy may only be made after determination that the causative lesion of the seventh nerve palsy is peripheral in nature, and appropriate evaluation reveals no identifiable etiology. Features of the seventh nerve palsy are summarized in **Table 75.1**.

Etiology/Pathophysiology

Superior to the brain stem, the facial nerve is composed of both crossed and uncrossed fibers. The motor root is responsible for innervation of the facial muscles of expression. The nervus intermedius provides taste perception for the anterior two-thirds of the tongue in addition to providing parasympathetic fiber innervation to some salivary and lacrimal glands. Upper motor neuron ("central") lesions are defined as occurring superior to or within the brain stem. Lower motor neuron ("peripheral" or "complete") lesions are defined as occurring after the seventh nerve has exited the brain stem.

Seventh nerve dysfunction can result from a central or peripheral lesson. Identifiable etiologies of peripheral seventh nerve dysfunction are listed in **Table 75.2**.

Emergency Evaluation and Intervention

History and review of symptoms should focus on any significant past medical history and recent illnesses. A history of recent travel or exposures is crucial if etiologies such as Lyme disease are to be correctly diagnosed and treated. Physical examination should, as always, initially focus on the ABCs. Upper motor neuron lesions present with paralysis and facial droop of the lower facial muscles only, with sparing of the forehead musculature. Presentations of central seventh nerve dysfunction due to cerebrovascular accidents or compressive lesions (usually neoplastic) generally occur along with other symptoms of CNS dysfunction due to the widespread effect of hemor-

Table 75.1

Seventh Nerve Palsy

	Central	Peripheral
Historical Features	Presence of other neurological deficits	Absence of other neurological signs
Physical Exam Findings	Lower facial weakness (forehead spared)	Complete unilateral facial weakness (including forehead)
Etiologies	Vascular, neoplastic, infectious	Infectious, systemic illness, local inflammation

rhage or edema and the proximity of other sensitive structures in the brain stem. A thorough neurologic examination is necessary to identify any concurrent neurologic deficits.

Neuroimaging is indicated in any patient suspected of having a central seventh nerve lesion. MRI, if available and if no contraindications exist, may provide more definitive diagnosis due to brain stem imaging potential. Head CT allows for evaluation of acute intracranial hemorrhage and tumor or other mass lesions. Laboratory evaluation should be directed at any signs or symptoms that suggest underlying pathology or infection.

Patients with a peripheral seventh nerve palsy in whom there is no identifiable underlying etiology, may be tentatively ascribed the diagnosis of Bell's palsy. Although the treatment of Bell's palsy with corticosteroids is still controversial, if there are no contraindications, a short course of prednisone, 60 mg/day for 5 days, followed by gradual taper over 10 to 14 days is accepted therapy. Based on clinical and electrophysiologic follow-up evaluations, treatment with corticosteroids should be started within 3 days of the onset of symptoms. Antiviral medication such as valacyclovir may also be of some benefit, if herpes simplex virus is being considered as a possible etiology.

Artificial tear solution should be recommended for those patients who are unable to adequately lubricate the corneal surface as a result of lid dysfunction. These patients should also be instructed to tape the affected eyelid closed during sleep to prevent possible corneal ulceration. Consultation with a neurologist or ENT, depending on the institution, should occur prior to discharge from the ED, especially if corticosteroid therapy has been initiated.

Approximately 98% of patients with Bell's palsy will have some degree of spontaneous recovery. For those patients who have persistent severe symptoms, surgery to unroof the canal of the seventh nerve may be considered.

Trigeminal Neuralgia (Tic Douloureaux)

Trigeminal neuralgia is a condition characterized by recurrent and brief episodes of sharp facial pain. Occurring rarely before the fifth decade of life, and with a higher incidence in women, trigeminal neuralgia can produce marked disability due to the difficulty in obtaining adequate analgesia and preventing recurrences of the pain. Trigeminal neuralgia is nearly always unilateral, although a small percentage of patients experience bilateral symptoms.

Etiology/Pathophysiology

Trigeminal neuralgia is caused by an irritative process affecting one or more of the peripheral branches of the fifth cranial nerve. The fifth cranial nerve is responsible for facial sensation and control of the muscles of mastication through its three branches: ophthalmic (V1), maxillary (V2), and mandibular (V3). Isolated central fifth cranial nerve lesions are rare. A central mass at the cerebellopontine angle affecting the fifth cranial nerve would likely produce symptoms in the seventh or eighth cranial nerves as well as due to their anatomic proximity. Isolated involvement of the ophthalmic branch supplying the forehead is rarely seen. However, combination of forehead (V1) and midfacial (V2) episodes do occur. Midfacial (V2) and lower facial (V3) distributions of pain may be seen individually or in combination. Patients often describe "triggers," specific facial movements (eating, yawning, etc.) that consistently reproduce symptoms. There are no other disease processes identified as causes of trigeminal neuralgia.

Emergency Department Evaluation

History taking should focus on the presence of any other neurologic symptoms in addition to the complaint of fa-

Table 75.2

Etiologies of Peripheral Seventh Nerve Dysfunction

Infections	Systemic Illnesses	Local Irritative Conditions
Mumps	Mastoiditis	Lyme disease
Echovirus	Cholesteatoma	Lymphoma
Herpes simplex	Otitis media	
HIV		
Rubella		
Herpes zoster (Ramsay Hunt syndrome)		

cial pain. Any history indicative of involvement of cranial nerves other than an isolated fifth nerve is highly suggestive of a central etiology for the pain and warrants detailed evaluation. Similarly, symptoms extending clearly into all three branches of the fifth nerve are indicative of a significant mass lesion. Physical examination including neurologic evaluation is almost always normal in the presence of an isolated peripheral process. History or findings consistent with a central process requiring emergent neuroimaging, with MRI being the study of choice. The differential diagnosis of unilateral facial pain includes maxillary sinus disease, atypical migraine or cluster headaches, and odontogenic causes, which must be excluded prior to the initiation of therapy.

Emergency Department Intervention

Treatment of a central lesion identified during neuroimaging should be based on the patient's clinical status and the findings on MRI or head CT. Consultation with neurosurgery or neurology, as appropriate, should be obtained for patients with central lesions. For patients without evidence of a central lesion, treatment is aimed at providing adequate analgesia. Carbamazepine 400 to 1,200 mg/day is the mainstay of therapy, although phenytoin, baclofen, and gabapentin are occasionally utilized. Narcotic analgesics may be required to provide adequate analgesia. Patients who fail to improve with adequate oral therapy may consider neurosurgical treatment aimed at providing decompression of the affected fifth nerve.

Visual Disturbances Due to Cranial Nerve Disorders

Visual disturbance may occur due to disorders of the optic (II), oculomotor (III), trochlear (IV), or abducens (VI) cranial nerves. Dysfunction of an isolated optic nerve produces only unilateral complete loss of vision or field defect. In addition, changes in the perception of color and brightness may occur. The unilateral nature of symptoms produced by an optic nerve lesion is helpful in distinguishing lesions of the optic chiasm or deeper structures of the visual system that produce bilateral symptoms.

Disorders of the oculomotor, trochlear, and abducens nerves result in abnormal eye movements and pupillary responses without vision loss.

Etiology/Pathophysiology

The causes and resultant dysfunction caused by a visual nerve defect are outlined in **Table 75.3**. Optic neuritis is due to a demyelinating process and is a common presenting symptom for patients with an initial presentation of multiple sclerosis. Acute ischemia of the optic nerve presents with acute vision loss and may be accompanied by symptoms of headache, jaw claudication, anorexia, myalgias, and malaise when secondary to giant cell arteritis. Tumors may cause compression of the optic nerve due to intrinsic or extrinsic effects. Tumors that affect the optic nerve intrinsically are optic nerve sheath meningiomas and gliomas. Significantly increased intracranial pressure usually produces abnormalities of multiple cranial nerves and may be caused by trauma, mass lesions, or infection. Local extrinsic compression of the optic nerve may be due to tumors of the orbit, middle cranial fossa, or giant pituitary adenomas, or abnormally enlarged extraocular muscles in the setting of Graves' disease.

The oculomotor (III) nerve innervates the superior rectus, inferior rectus, medial rectus, and inferior oblique ocular muscles. In the absence of abnormal pupillary size and reflex (iridoplegia), the patient is said to have an "incomplete" third nerve palsy, which is more likely to be a result of vascular disease due to diabetes mellitus. The acute onset of a painful, isolated oculomotor palsy is usually due to aneurysm of the posterior communicating artery.

Emergency Department Evaluation

The goal of the ED evaluation of acute visual disturbances and disorders of eye movement should be to quickly determine the presence or absence of increased intracranial pressure due to hemorrhage or mass lesion. Recognition of the potential for life-threatening conditions and the necessity of immediate evaluation should be the goal of triage. Neuroimaging, utilizing MRI or CT, based on availability, should be promptly obtained.

Initial diagnosis of an oculomotor, trochlear or abducens nerve palsy should be straightforward, as visual inspection of the patient demonstrates an abnormal eye

Table 75.3

Visual Nerve Dysfunctions

Nerve	Symptoms of Dysfunction	Cause of Dysfunction
Optic Nerve (II)	Unilateral complete loss of vision or field defect.	Neuritis, ischemia, physical compression, infection, toxins, neoplasias
Oculomotor Nerve (III)	Pupillary dilatation and loss of pupillary reflex. Down and out gaze. Ptosis	Aneurysmal compression, vascular disease, trauma, neoplasias
Trochlear Nerve (IV)	Superior lateral gaze	Trauma, vascular compromise
Abducens (VI)	Inability to perform a lateral gaze	Increased intracranial pressure, vascular disease and infarct, multiple sclerosis, myasthenia gravis, and Wernicke's syndrome

position with or without iridoplegia. Funduscopic examination may reveal papilledema in the setting of optic nerve dysfunction, indicative of increased intracranial pressure. Pallor of the optic disk may be seen with chronic optic neuropathy.

Asymmetry of the pupil sizes may be due to increased intracranial pressure, a complete third nerve palsy, pharmacologic agents, parasympathetic dysfunction or due to an essential anisocoria. Patients with essential anisocoria have symmetrical responses to increases and decreases in illumination.

Pupil asymmetry that is augmented by increased or decreased illumination indicates an abnormal parasympathetic or sympathetic response in the pupil, respectively. Etiologies of an abnormal constriction response include pharmacologic (mydriatic) agents, oculomotor nerve palsy, Adie's pupil (denervation of the parasympathetic innervation of the iris sphincter), and traumatic mydriasis. Etiologies of an abnormal dilatation response include pharmacologic (miotic) agents, acute iritis, and Horner's pupil, in which there is no response to topical 4% cocaine.

Evaluation for myasthenia gravis is accomplished by the performance of Tensilon (edrophonium) testing. Patients are given a rapid intravenous initial test dose of 2 mg and then observed for any adverse effects. If none occur, the patient is then given up to an additional 8 mg of Tensilon. Patients with myasthenia gravis have a brief period of symptomatic improvement, indicating a positive test response.

After the completion of neuroimaging has ruled out an intracranial hemorrhage, mass lesion, or evidence of increased intracranial pressure, a lumbar puncture should be performed. Evaluation of the cerebrospinal fluid (CSF) for evidence of infection or for other conditions, such as multiple sclerosis, in which the CSF may provide diagnostic clues, should be performed.

Emergency Department Intervention

The treatment and disposition of patients with disorders of vision or eye movement is based on their overall clinical status. Patients may be obtunded and acutely ill in the setting of intracranial disease and may require immediate resuscitative care, including airway management. Frequently reevaluation for signs of clinical deterioration must be performed until life-threatening conditions are ruled out.

Patients with abnormalities of vision or eye movement with demonstrated intracranial mass lesion, hemorrhage or increased intracranial pressure during neuroimaging should be referred for emergent neurosurgical evaluation. In the setting of symptom onset after trauma, neurosurgical consultation should also be obtained, even in the absence of acute findings during initial neuroimaging.

Treatment of specific cranial nerve lesions is focused on identifiable causes. Therapy for underlying causes of vascular disease, including hypertension and diabetes mellitus, should be initiated in conjunction with the patient's primary care physician. Thiamine may be administered empirically in the setting of sixth nerve palsy for the treatment of Wernicke's syndrome.

In the absence of emergency neurosurgical conditions, patients with acute disorders of vision or eye movement should be referred to an ophthalmologist or neurologist for follow-up care based on clinical findings during the ED evaluation.

Selected Readings

Carlow TJ. Paresis of cranial nerves III, IV, and VI: clinical manifestation and differential diagnosis. *Bull Soc Belge Ophthalmol* 1989;237:285–301.

DeJong RN. *The Neurologic Examination,* 5th ed. New York: Harper & Row 1992.

Henry G, Little N. *Neurologic Emergencies: A Symptom Oriented Approach.* New York: McGraw-Hill 1985.

Shafshak TS, Essa AY, Bakey FA. The possible contributing factors for the success of steroid therapy in Bell's palsy: a clinical and electrophysiological study. *J Laryngol Otol* 1994;108:940–943.

Demyelinating Diseases of the Nervous System

Samuel H. Kim
John C. Moorhead

The demyelinating diseases are a group of heterogeneous nervous system disorders that are characterized by degeneration of axonal myelin sheaths. They include both central nervous system (CNS) and peripheral nervous system (PNS) disorders. In all these disorders, the proposed mechanism of action is thought to be autoimmune in nature. It is not known whether this is due to a primary insult with neuronal damage and subsequent sensitization to endogenous antigens, or through a mimicry type of mechanism whereby the immune system is sensitized to an exogenous antigen that is structurally similar to endogenous proteins. The prototypical CNS demyelinating disease is multiple sclerosis (MS). The PNS equivalent is Guillain-Barré syndrome, which is discussed in the section on neuromuscular disorders.

Multiple Sclerosis

Multiple sclerosis (MS) is an inflammatory disease that is characterized by CNS axonal myelin sheath degeneration with relative axonal sparing. The exact etiology is unknown although an autoimmune mechanism is proposed along with environmental factors. The presentation of MS is highly variable, but usually presents with multiple episodes of neurologic complaints that develop over several days and resolve over several weeks.

The myelin sheath destruction in MS results in discrete regions of demyelination, known as plaques. The location, size, and time of development of the plaques are highly variable, and are described as being spread throughout "time and space." Myelin sheathes are composed of tightly wrapped lipid bilayers with specialized protein constituents. They provide insulation of the axon and allow saltatory conduction, thus increasing nerve impulse speed tremendously. Loss of the myelin sheathes results in drastically reduced conduction velocities, and either slowed or blocked nerve impulses. Myelin sheathes are produced by oligodendrocytes in the CNS and by Schwann cells in the PNS, and are different in composition. MS preferentially affects the myelin sheathes produced by oligodendrocytes.

The prevalence of MS varies considerably with geographical location. There is a higher prevalence in the temperate climates of both the Northern and Southern hemispheres. In the United States, the prevalence among the Caucasian population is approximately 60 per 100,000, twice the rate for non-Caucasians. The annual incidence is approximately 12,000 in the United States. The variation with geographic location is suggestive of an environmental factor in the development of MS. This is supported by the fact that the risk of developing MS depends partially on where individuals live in the first 15 years of life. If an individual moves from an area of low incidence to high incidence within this time period, they tend to have the same incidence as the area to which they move, and vice versa. The male to female ratio is approximately 1:3, although men who develop MS tend to have more severe cases. Cases typically present between 18 and 45 years of age. There is also a genetic component, with a concordance rate of approximately 30% in identical twins. In first degree relatives the risk of developing MS is approximately 2% to 4%.

Emergency Department Evaluation

Multiple sclerosis, by its nature, may present in a highly variable manner, depending on the location of lesions and stage of disease. Patients sometimes present with a new onset of subtle, seemingly unrelated neurological symptoms or with an exacerbation of symptoms with a previously established diagnosis. Since the long-term disease course of MS can be significantly affected by early diagnosis and treatment, the emergency physician's role in detecting the disease and/or referring the patient to a neurologist in a timely manner cannot be overemphasized. There are no specific tests for MS, making diagnosis challenging. Often the diagnosis must be arrived at through clinical observation and exclusion of other possible causes. Although MS may present in many different ways, there are a few neurological presentations that are more strongly suggestive of the diagnosis than others.

A detailed history focusing on prior episodes of the development of neurological complaints should be obtained. A history of discrete episodes of symptoms followed by relapse is suggestive of the diagnosis. Symptoms of MS are varied and may include:

- Numbness and paresthesias.
- Visual disturbances: blurry vision, color desaturation, diplopia, visual field loss, and/or loss of vision.
- Weakness and fatigue.
- Spasms and spasticity.
- Tremors.
- Cranial nerve neuralgias (optic, trigeminal, glossopharyngeal).
- Cognitive complaints.
- Bowel and bladder dysfunction.
- Sexual dysfunction.

Symptoms exacerbated by elevations in body temperature caused by exercise, hot showers or baths, or high ambient temperatures or fever, known as the Uhthoff phenomenon, are also quite specific for MS. It should be recognized as a cause of recurrence of symptoms, as well, and may not represent a true exacerbation in patients with a prior diagnosis.

The most common initial presentations of MS include partial spinal cord syndromes (~50% of cases), optic neuritis (~25%), and brainstem syndromes (~15%). Spinal cord involvement usually involves some form of myelitis, which may present in the form of a peculiar band-like sensation, pressure, paresthesias or decreased sensation. With cervical spine involvement an electrical shock, sensation with neck flexion is sometimes seen (Lhermitte's sign). Optic neuritis is characterized by slowly progressive ocular pain, especially with extraocular movements, loss of visual acuity, loss of color perception, and usually an afferent papillary defect. Fundoscopic examination is usually normal.

Physical examination should include a thorough and well-documented neurological examination. Subtle abnormalities should be noted, even if they are not related to the presenting complaint. Documentation of these findings may prove relevant to demonstrating the progression of the disease, especially at follow-up with a neurologist.

The ophthalmologic examination should be done looking for signs of optic neuritis, but should also focus on extraocular movements. This may reveal pendular nystagmus or diplopia suggesting a brainstem lesion. In particular, a unilateral or bilateral internuclear ophthalmoplegia is suggestive of a medial longitudinal fasciculus lesion. This is the most common eye movement abnormality found in MS, and its presence is highly suggestive of the disease, although not completely pathognomonic. The physical exam finding in internuclear ophthalmoplegia is a slowing or complete lack of adduction of the affected eye with gaze toward the contralateral side, resulting in diplopia.

Diagnostic tests used to aid in the diagnosis of MS include MRI, evoked-potential studies, and CSF fluid analysis. There are two MRI modalities that are commonly used. T2-weighted head and spine MRIs are capable of showing the location and size of MS plaques, however, this imaging modality does not provide any information about the age of the plaques. With gadolinium-enhanced

T1-weighted images, newer plaques with active inflammatory processes are much brighter, presumably due to the disruption of the blood-brain barrier in active lesions. The sensitivity of MRI at detecting MS lesions has been estimated at up to 95%. Evoked-potential studies measure the speed of the cerebral response to stimuli. This modality can sometimes detect more subtle peripheral lesions that are missed by MRI, with sensitivity up to 90%. Finally, CSF analysis can be performed to detect cellular and chemical abnormalities. The leukocyte count may be elevated (usually with a lymphocyte predominance), as well as protein levels (especially myelin basic protein). The most characteristic finding on analysis is the presence of oligoclonal bands. All of these diagnostic tools are nonspecific and the clinical picture must be consistent in order to diagnose MS. In addition, other MS mimics must be considered and ruled out as well. In order to do this, additional laboratory testing needs to be performed, including ESR, Lyme titers, B_{12} levels, HIV Ab titers, VDRL test, Rf titers, and ANA titers.

In most cases of suspected MS, the diagnosis cannot be made readily in the emergency department (ED). MRI is often obtained in follow-up in cases without debilitating symptomatology. CSF analysis through the ED does not routinely include the studies necessary to detect oligoclonal banding. Evoked potential studies are almost always obtained as an outpatient study after referral to a neurologist. As a result, cases with minor complaints should be referred to a neurologist for outpatient follow-up, while more severe symptoms may necessitate emergent neurological consultation.

Emergency Department Management

The emergent management of multiple sclerosis, outside of referral in suspected cases, should focus on the treatment of exacerbations in patients with previously diagnosed disease. Long-term management usually involves immunomodulatory therapies managed in consultation with a neurologist, with the goal of slowing or halting the progression of the disease. Patients with MS are also susceptible to complications secondary to their neurological lesions. Examples include urinary tract infections secondary to incomplete bladder emptying.

The mainstay of therapy for acute exacerbations is intravenous and oral corticosteroids. Most exacerbations will eventually resolve on their own. However, steroid therapy has demonstrated a decrease in the duration of the exacerbation in 85% of cases. The standard protocol is the administration of 250 to 1,000 mg of methylprednisolone IV q12h, for 3 to 7 days. This is usually followed by an oral taper of prednisone or dexamethasone.

The options for long-term therapy are constantly evolving. The two most commonly used agents for long-term management include IVIG and glatiramer acetate. Other adjunctive immunosuppressive agents that are sometimes helpful include azathioprine, methotrexate, and mitoxantrone. Any changes in the patient's long-term regimen should be done in consultation with a neurologist. In the rare case of a newly diagnosed MS patient, glatiramer or

IVIG may be started. New evidence suggests that starting patients on these agents very early in the course of the disease will slow progression and make a significant impact on the patient's quality of life.

Complications related to MS include tremor, spasm, and bladder dysfunction. Sexual dysfunction is also a common complaint. Tremor is usually controlled with propranolol or a long-acting benzodiazepine. Spasm is usually managed with baclofen, delivered either orally or via intrathecal pump. Other medical options for spasm include tizanidine, dantrolene, or diazepam. Bladder dysfunction may result in retention and urinary tract infections, as mentioned above.

Selected Readings

Medical Advisory Board of the National Multiple Sclerosis Society. Disease Management Consensus Statement. New York: National Multiple Sclerosis Society 2002.

Noseworthy JH. Management of multiple sclerosis: current trials and future options. *Curr Opin Neurol* 2003;16:289–297.

Noseworthy JH. Treatment of multiple sclerosis and related disorders: what's new in the past 2 years? *Clin Neuropharmacol* 2003;26:28–37.

Owens T. The enigma of multiple sclerosis: inflammation and neurodegeneration cause heterogenous dysfunction and damage. *Curr Opin Neurol* 2003;16:259–265.

77 Neuromuscular Disorders

John C. Moorhead
Samuel H. Kim

Neuromuscular disorders include several diseases that are characterized by muscular weakness that is secondary to nervous system involvement. The exact location of the lesion in the nervous system that causes weakness varies among the different entities. Diseases which fall into this category include Guillain-Barré syndrome, Lambert-Eaton syndrome, and myasthenia gravis (Lambert-Eaton syndrome is discussed in this chapter within the section on myasthenia gravis).

These disorders should be considered in the differential for any patient presenting with a chief complaint of weakness. In addition, these disorders may present with more focal neurological findings. In more advanced cases, respiratory system involvement may also prompt complaints of shortness of breath.

Guillain-Barré Syndrome

The Guillain-Barré syndrome (GBS) is actually a constellation of entities that vary by their degree of motor and sensory involvement, the predominance of ophthalmoplegia and bulbar weakness, and the amount of axonal involvement. The most common and widely recognized entitiy is acute inflammatory demyelinating polyradiculopathy (AIDP), characterized by an acute autoimmune inflammatory process that destroys the myelin sheathes of the peripheral nervous system. This causes an interruption in saltatory conduction and slowed or blocked nerve conduction. As a result, the patient usually presents with paresthesias, followed by an ascending paralysis. Other subtypes of GBS include acute motor sensory axonal neuropathy (AMSAN), acute motor axonal neuropathy (AMAN), Fisher syndrome, and acute panautonomic neuropathy. All these variants share the following features:

- Acute onset
- Monophasic disease course
- Self-limited
- Elevated CSF protein without pleiocytosis

The exact etiology of the inflammatory process is unknown, but an autoimmune process has been proposed. Molecular mimicry has been implicated by multiple investigations. Many possible triggers for this immune-mediated response have been postulated and include antecedent infections, vaccinations, malignancies, and surgery. In about two-thirds of cases, an antecedent upper respiratory or gastrointestinal infection is reported. Many organisms have been associated with the development of GBS, but the most commonly implicated are *Campylobacter jejuni, Mycoplasma pneumoniae,* cytomegalovirus, Epstein-Barr virus, and HIV. The malignancies that are associated with GBS development are lymphomas and Hodgkin's disease. The most commonly associated vaccines are rabies and swine flu.

GBS is quite rare, with a reported incidence of 0.6 to 4.0 per 100,000. There have been no reported environmental factors, with a similar incidence globally. There are no reported ethnic group preferences. There seems to be a slight male preference, with a reported male to female ratio of 1.1:1 to 2:1. The clinical course of GBS seems to be influenced by the age at onset, with younger patients usually having a more severe course and prolonged residual disability. In most longitudinal studies, a bimodal population distribution is reported, with a major peak in the 60 to 69 age group and a smaller peak among young adults. The mortality rate is reported between 2.4% to 8.0%. In more severe cases requiring mechanical ventilation, the mortality rate may be as high as 30%.

Emergency Department Evaluation

The diagnosis of GBS is clinical and can be challenging if presenting early in the disease process. The emergency physician must attempt to make a presumptive diagnosis and provide supportive therapy. Depending on the severity of presentation, disposition to an intensive care setting may be necessary. AIDP is the most common variant of GBS and will be described here as the prototypical presentation.

Early in the AIDP disease process, patients present with paresthesias in distal extremities, usually starting in the digits of the upper and lower extremities. There may also be shoulder, thigh, and lumbar involvement. The paresthesias are usually described as decreased sensation, a "crawling skin" sensation, or more rarely, a deep, aching pain. As the disease progresses, an ascending symmetric weakness is observed. The patient may have both distal and proximal weakness, although it most commonly occurs in a distal to proximal progression. The weakness may progress to a profound paralysis. In 15% to 25% of patients, significant diaphragmatic weakness may result in respiratory failure requiring mechanical ventilation. The progression of the disease is fairly slow, with onset of maximal symptoms at about 2 to 3 weeks into the disease course.

The axonal variants of GBS include AMAN and AMSAN. These entities differ in their presence or lack of sensory axonal involvement. In both, significant axonal damage occurs in addition to demyelination. This results in a significant residual deficit. Most patients cannot walk one year after onset. Permanent disability requiring orthoses occurs in about 10% of cases. Patients with these variants usually reach maximal symptoms more quickly, often within 6 days. Otherwise, these variants are similar in presentation to AIDP and are difficult to distinguish from AIDP clinically.

In all variants of GBS some facial and bulbar involvement may be seen. Depending on the severity of the bulbar and facial involvement, dysarthria, drooling, and/or dysphagia may be seen. Advanced cases may present a significant risk of aspiration. The Fisher variant has a predominance of bulbar involvement along with ataxia.

Autonomic involvement may also be seen in all variants. Acute panautonomic neuropathy is the rarest variant of GBS and is characterized by a neuropathy of the autonomic system only. Usually both the sympathetic and parasympathetic systems are involved. Some degree of autonomic dysfunction can also be seen in the other variants as well, and may present with orthostatic hypotension, bradycardia, urinary retention, blurry vision, dry eyes, cardiac arrhythmias, and/or impotence.

The initial ED evaluation should include a thorough history, with attention to possible triggers. The physical exam should focus on documenting a thorough motor and sensory neurological examination as well as a cardiovascular evaluation. Continuous cardiac monitoring may be necessary in cases with significant autonomic instability. Close attention should be paid to respiratory and bulbar symptoms to assess for possible respiratory compromise and aspiration risk. Paradoxic movement of the diaphragm is one sign of impending respiratory failure. Another simple test to assess viability of respiratory strength is to have the patient lift his head off the bed. If the patient is unable to perform this action, the phrenic nerve is usually affected to the point that which respiratory effort is not sufficient to maintain adequate ventilation. In these cases endoctracheal intubation should be strongly considered. Serum electrolyte and hematology studies, in addition to imaging studies such as CT or MRI of the brain and spinal cord, may be useful in excluding other diagnoses.

An electrocardiogram, chest radiograph, and arterial blood gases should be obtained to assess cardiopulmonary status and to establish a baseline. CSF studies will often reveal albuminocytologic dissociation, with an elevated protein concentration in the absence of a pleiocytosis. There are no other studies specific for GBS.

Emergency Department Management

The ED physician's role in the management of cases of GBS should focus on diagnosis, neurological consultation, management of complications, and initiation of treatment.

In many cases of advanced GBS, the patient will need admission to the ICU to monitor for impending respiratory failure. Neurologic consultation will often facilitate diagnosis and admission. If symptoms are relatively mild, either admission to the hospital for observation or discharge with close follow-up may be appropriate.

In advanced cases of GBS, there are several life-threatening potential complications that should be addressed:

- Respiratory failure due to diaphragmatic weakness.
- Aspiration due to severe bulbar weakness.
- Deep venous thrombosis (DVT)/pulmonary embolism due to prolonged immobilization.
- Autonomic instability, including cardiac arrhythmias, labile blood pressures, urinary retention, neurogenic pulmonary edema, and colonic pseudoobstruction.

Respiratory function should be assessed, and endotracheal intubation for respiratory support should be performed as needed. Succinylcholine as a paralytic agent should be avoided or used with extreme caution as it may induce severe hyperkalemia. DVT prophylaxis including subcutaneous heparin and pressure stockings should be instituted. Continuous cardiac monitoring should be performed. Bradycardia should be treated with atropine and/or a temporary pacemaker. Hypotension should be treated with fluids and Trendelenberg positioning initially. Hypertension can be treated with short-acting beta blockers. Vasodilators should be used with extreme caution as they may cause a dramatic drop in blood pressure. Foley catheterization and a vigorous bowel regimen should be initiated.

Treatment options to consider in GBS include:

- Plasma exchange.
- Intravenous immunoglobulin.
- Corticosteroids.

Plasma exchange has been clinically proven to reduce the length of the disease. Time on the ventilator is reduced by about half and a higher percentage will have full recovery one year after therapy. Approximately 200 to 250 cc/kg of plasma is exchanged over 7 to 10 days. It is limited by the need for venous access (central access is often necessary), and high volume exchanges may potentially exacerbate blood pressure lability and deplete clotting factors.

Intravenous immunoglobulin (IVIG) has also demonstrated benefit. No difference in outcome is seen between IVIG and plasma exchange, and no additional benefit is seen by concurrent use. The appropriate dose of IVIG is 0.4 g/kg per day infused over 5 days. IVIG's main limitations are its side effects, which include fever, chills, and myalgias, or, more seriously, aseptic meningitis, acute renal tubular necrosis, and anaphylaxis. IVIG is also more expensive than plasma exchange.

Corticosteroids have not been demonstrated to be helpful in the treatment of GBS.

Election of the appropriate treatment option should take into account potential complications and should be done in conjunction with the consulting neurologist. Disposition should be to an appropriate setting.

Myasthenia Gravis

Myasthenia gravis (MG) is one of the best understood autoimmune diseases. It is characterized by diffuse weakness that is exacerbated with continued and repeated exertion. The disease is caused in most cases by an attack against the acetylcholine receptors (AChR) in the neuromuscular junction by autoantibodies. Approximately 15% of patients with MG demonstrate no detectable levels of antibodies against AChR. These cases of seronegative MG are clinically indistinguishable from typical MG, and the management in these cases is identical.

The exact etiology of the autoimmune response to AChR is unknown, but most evidence seems to indicate that the thymus gland is the site of initial autosensitization. The association of MG with thymus gland abnormalities has been noted for decades and was the basis for instituting surgical thymectomy as a therapeutic regimen for many patients. Up to 75% of cases have thymic abnormalities, and of these 70% to 85% have hyperplasia, 10% to 15% have thymomas, and the remainder experience atrophy. Two hypotheses have been proposed as the triggering event. The first is a viral infection of the thymus. However, there is no supportive evidence for this theory. More promising is a molecular mimicry mechanism by which a prior viral infection causes sensitization to antigens similar in structure to AChR.

Sensitization to AChR results in the production of autoantibodies directed against the nicotinic glycoprotein acetylcholine receptors. Autoantibodies causes reduction in functional AChR units by three different mechanisms. First, autoantibodies act as competitive inhibitors of the ACh receptor. Second, autoantibody binding to the receptors results in more rapid degradation of the receptors. Third, autoantibodies mediate complement driven damage to the neuromuscular end plate. The end result is a decrease in the end plate muscle fiber potentials, thus resulting in failure to trigger contraction in specific muscle fibers. When enough of these muscle fibers fail to respond, weakness is seen.

Myasthenia gravis is a relatively uncommon disease, with a reported incidence from 5 to 14 per 100,000. The incidence has a bimodal distribution, with an early peak in the second and third decades of life (mostly women), and a second peak later in the sixth and seventh decades of life (mostly men). There does seem to be a genetic component with an association with certain human leukocyte antigen (HLA) subtypes.

Emergency Department Evaluation

The ED physician's role in the evaluation of patients with established MG and suspected MG center around diagnosis of new cases, and assessing the severity of disease in known cases. The diagnosis of MG may be challenging in more subtle cases, and a neurologist should be consulted. Other possible diseases in the differential should also be considered and ruled out prior to making the final diagnosis. The differential for MG includes:

- Congenital myasthenia
- Drug-induced myasthenia
- Lambert-Eaton syndrome
- Hyperthyroidism
- Botulism
- Progressive external ophthalmoplegia
- Intracranial masses

MG may present with any number of symptoms. The most common presenting complaints include generalized weakness, ptosis, dysarthria, dysphagia, shortness of breath, respiratory distress, double vision, and fatigue. Muscle weakness is usually diffuse, with a more proximal distribution. Often, ptosis and diplopia are the earliest presenting symptoms. Weakness will remain localized to the periorbital and extraocular muscles in up to 15% of cases. The patient will often note that it is worse at night after a day of work, and improves with rest. There is no sensory loss or paresthesias noted with MG. Reflexes are preserved. Shortness of breath can be severe, progressing at times to respiratory failure. Orthopnea is sometimes noted, as the weakened diaphragm is more effective in a supine position, where the effect of gravity is minimized. In known cases of MG, a grading system is used to denote the severity of the disease (**Table 77.1**).

A thorough history describing exacerbating factors and chronicity of symptoms should be taken. Also, information about possible triggers for worsening myasthenic symptoms should also be elicited. Triggers include:

- Drugs (aminoglycosides, beta blockers, procainamide, quinidine, quinine, local anesthetics)
- Infections (especially upper respiratory infections)
- Surgery
- Rapid steroid tapers

The physical exam should include a neurological evaluation, including a careful cranial nerve exam. Baseline quantitative strength testing should be performed. Respiratory status should be evaluated carefully for any evidence of respiratory muscle weakness. The same techniques employed above for Guillain-Barré syndrome may be used. In undiagnosed cases, certain maneuvers may be used to elicit exam findings suggestive of the diagnosis. Rapid lid retraction on reaccommodation from a downward gaze may be seen (Cogan's sign). Ptosis when

Table 77.1	
Severity Grade of Myasthenia Gravis (Adapted from Osserman)	
Grade	**Characteristics**
I	Focal weakness
IIa	Mild generalized disease
IIb	Moderate generalized disease
III	Severe generalized disease
IV	Myasthenic crisis: Severe disease with respiratory involvement

present may be aggravated by direct sunlight and improved with cooling. Dysarthria that worsens as speech continues may be seen, indicating progressive pharyngeal muscle fatigue with use. An easy way to test this is to have the patient count to 100: As the weakness progresses, the speech may take on a nasal quality. Another common exam finding is strong jaw opening strength with diminished jaw closure.

Laboratory studies are not very helpful in the acute setting except to help rule out other disease entities in the differential. A chest radiograph should be ordered to assess the size of the thymus. Imaging studies of the brain via MRI or head CT should be obtained to help rule out intracranial abnormalities such as infarcts or mass lesions.

The diagnosis of MG in new cases requires a set of tests that are not usually performed in the ED. Usually, an anticholinesterase test (most commonly performed using edrophonium) is the first line of testing. This may be done in the ED in consultation with a neurologist. Care should be taken in individuals with severe obstructive lung disease and cardiac disease due to the excessive vagal tone that may be elicited from its administration. The test should be performed under continuous cardiac monitoring, and a test dose should be given beforehand. A positive test is one where a rapid but transient improvement in symptoms lasting about 5 minutes is seen.

Other tests that may be used in the diagnosis of MG includes repetitive nerve stimulation tests, serological assays for anti-AChR antibodies, and single fiber electromyography. These tests are not normally part of the ED physician evaluation.

Emergency Department Management

The management of myasthenia gravis in the emergency department centers around treatment of exacerbations, and supportive therapy for severe cases. There are several long-term therapies that are used to control symptoms. These include immunosuppressive treatments like corticosteroids, azathioprine, and cyclosporine, among others, as well as cholinesterase inhibitors. These medications should only be adjusted in consultation with the patient's neurologist. Plasma exchange and intravenous immunoglobulin are sometimes used for more immediate treatment of severe exacerbations and crises.

Corticosteroids are the starting point for most immunosuppressive regimens. They are often administered in the ED for exacerbations, but their effects take several days to become apparent. In cases of patients on chronic corticosteroids, some coordination of dosages should be attempted with the patient's neurologist. Azathioprine is also well-established as an alternative or adjunct to corticosteroids. When these agents fail, other treatments such as cyclosporine, methotrexate, cyclophosphamide, and mycophenolate mofetil might be considered. Usually, immunosuppressives are not started unless symptoms cannot be controlled with cholinesterase inhibitors alone.

Cholinesterase inhibitors are the mainstay of symptomatic management. They act by slowing the degradation of acetylcholine released into the neuromuscular junction.

Pyridostigmine bromide (Mestinon) is the most commonly used agent. It has a longer duration of action than neostigmine (Prostigmin). The usual starting dose is 30 mg of pyridostigmine, every 4 to 6 hours. Side effects include diarrhea, abdominal cramping, nausea and vomiting, bronchorrhea, bronchospasm, and bradycardia.

Plasma exchange and intravenous immunoglobulin have been used to achieve a more rapid clinical response in severe cases. Plasma exchange works by removal of antibodies and other immune system mediators from the circulation. IVIG has been shown to have a therapeutic benefit in severe cases, by down-modulating the immune response via several mechanisms of action.

In cases of myasthenic crisis, continuous cardiac monitoring should be instituted. If impending respiratory failure is noted, endotracheal tube intubation and ventilatory support may be necessary. It should be noted that depolarizing paralytic agents such as succinylcholine have a shorter duration of action in these patients. Also, nondepolarizing agents have a much longer duration of action.

Disposition of cases with significant respiratory involvement should be admitted to the ICU regardless of whether the patient is intubated or not, as these patients may decompensate rapidly. Admission or disposition of patients with known MG should be decided on the basis of their current clinical presentation and in conjunction with the treating neurologist.

Lambert-Eaton Syndrome

The Lambert-Eaton syndrome is a neuromuscular disorder that is similar in presentation to myasthenia gravis. However, unlike myasthenia gravis, it is caused by an inhibition of the release of acetylcholine at the neuromuscular end plate. The weakness seen in Lambert-Eaton syndrome is similar in distribution to MG, and fatigability may also be noted. However, patients with Lambert-Eaton syndrome may present with paresthesias and autonomic symptoms as well. Respiratory weakness is not commonly seen. Anticholinesterase testing will be negative, unlike MG.

Lambert-Eaton syndrome has an association with lung cancer. Treatment is otherwise similar to MG, except that guanidine hydrochloride is sometimes added to the regimen.

Selected Readings

Berrouschot J, Baumann I, Kalischewski P, et al. Therapy of myasthenic crisis. *Crit Care Med* 1997;25:1228–1235.

Chi O. Guillain-Barre syndrome. *Neurology* 2003;60:1146.

Drachman DB. Medical progress: myasthenia gravis. *N Engl J Med* 1994;330: 1797–1810.

Hopkins LC. Clinical features of myasthenia gravis. *Neurol Clin North Am* 1994; 12:243–261.

Hund EF, Borel CO, Cornblath DR, et al. Intensive management and treatment of severe Guillain-Barre syndrome. *Crit Care Med* 1993;21:433–446.

Lindenbaum Y, Kissel JT, Mendell JR. Treatment approaches for Guillain-Barre syndrome and chronic inflammatory demyelinating polyradiculopathy. *Neurol Clin North Am* 2001;19:187–204.

Maselli RA. Pathophysiology of myasthenia gravis and Lambert-Eaton syndrome. *Neurol Clin North Am* 1994;12:285–303.

Palace J, Vincent A, Beeson D. Myasthenia gravis: diagnostic and management dilemmas. *Curr Opin Neurol* 2001;14:583–589.

Rees J. Guillain-Barre syndrome: Clinical manifestations and directions for treatment. *Drugs* 1995;49:912–919.

Peripheral Neuropathies

Blaine C. White

Introduction

The peripheral nervous system serves sensory, motor, and autonomic functions; and neuropathic dysfunction may affect any of these activities at the levels of either peripheral nerves or the spinal cord. Sensory neuropathy can produce paresthesia, dysthesia, pain or ataxia due to loss of proprioception. Motor neuropathy can cause weakness, muscle wasting, or fasciculation. Autonomic neuropathy can produce hemodynamic instability involving orthostasis or arrhythmias, bowel or bladder problems, gastroparesis, sexual dysfunction, and regional anhydrosis of the skin.

In the emergency department (ED) the greatest acute concern with these diseases is ventilatory adequacy in the presence of a generalized weakness. Because several of these diseases are chronic, the primary diagnosis is often already solidly established with the ED presentation being that of exacerbated weaknesses. In all patients with real generalized weakness, examination and continuous monitoring of ventilatory status is the most urgent aspect of the emergency evaluation. Endotracheal intubation and mechanical ventilation are indicated for adult patients with a forced vital capacity of less than one liter due to a neuropathy: Arterial blood gasses should not guide the decision in this setting.

In the practice of emergency medicine, encounter with most of these diseases is relatively uncommon, and the discussion that follows is not intended to be exhaustive, but rather to provide a basic framework by which these problems may be approached. Anatomic localization of primary lesions provides a useful way of thinking about diseases producing such symptoms. Myopathies are diseases of muscles generally prominent in proximal extremity muscle groups; are commonly associated with increased ESR and serum CPK; do not produce sensory or autonomic disturbances; and have little effect on reflexes. Neuromuscular junction diseases produce weakness in cranial nerve ("bulbar") motor functions, as well as prominent weakness in proximal extremity muscle groups, but do not produce sensory loss, consistent autonomic dysfunction, or diagnostic alterations in reflexes. Generalized peripheral neuropathies that involve peripheral nerves between their targets and the spinal cord are associated with both motor and sensory dysfunction; do not display prominence of proximal muscle involvement; do cause substantial reduction of reflexes; and often cause autonomic dysfunction in the areas innervated. Focal peripheral neuropathies involve entrapment or inflammation of a single nerve. Spinal neuropathies not associated with trauma involve degenerative neuronal processes that may affect primarily motor function (i.e., amyotrophic lateral sclerosis) or specific sensory functions (i.e., loss of posterior column functions with tabes dorsalis).

Myopathies

Polymyositis[1,2] is an immunopathologic inflammatory myopathy usually seen in adults over 30 years old. Proximal symmetrical muscle weakness and tender muscles are predominant findings, and patients may have difficulty raising their arms over their heads. Sensation and deep tendon reflexes are typically intact. In laboratory studies, both ESR and CPK show substantial elevations. Dysphagia may be present and produce complications including aspiration and ventilatory failure. A new diagnosis or respiratory compromise warrants admission with close monitoring. The therapeutic approaches are those of immunosuppression.

Dermatomyositis[1,2] is an immunopathologic inflammatory myopathy similar to polymyositis, except that it can also be seen in children and is accompanied by a violaceous rash often present on the face and hands.

Toxic myopathies should be considered once the presence of myalgia, proximal muscle weakness, intact reflexes, and elevated ESR and CPK are appreciated. Major drug families implicated in toxic myopathies include (1) cholesterol lowering agents, (2) thiazides, (3) neuroleptics, (4) antineoplastic agents, such as adriamycin and vincristine, and (5) drugs of abuse such as amphetamines, phencyclidine, and ethanol. Such agents should be discontinued in any patient admitted to the hospital with myopathy.

Trichinellosis[3] is an infectious myositis caused by parasitic infection with *Trichinella* species, which are obligate intracellular parasites. Reservoirs for human-infecting species of these organisms are swine, wild boars, bears, and horses, and infection in families or communities results from consumption of undercooked meat. Freezing does not kill the organisms. USDA-mandated slaughterhouse surveillance is not as strict as that in Europe, and periodic outbreaks of trichinellosis occur in the United States and remain common in underdeveloped countries.

Ingested larvae invade intestinal epithelium, where maturation, mating, and production of approximately 1,500 new larvae per female worm occur within about 6 days. This "enteral" phase usually produces minimal symptoms. The "parenteral" phase begins when newborn larvae disseminate through lymph and blood into host muscle cells; here within approximately 20 days, "nurse cell" complexes develop, which contain many more larvae. The infection elicits an intense immune response, much of which is directed at the infected muscle cells.

The parenteral phase often involves myalgia, fever, skin edema and rash, insomnia, muscle weakness that may be profound, and may involve dysphagia and near paralysis of extraocular muscles. In severe cases CNS symptoms including seizures may develop as a consequence of endothelial inflammation and ischemia caused by large numbers of larvae obstructing microvascular perfusion. Laboratory studies characteristically identify elevated CPK and a marked increase in eosinophils, from 30% to 60% of all circulating leukocytes. Immunoassays for circulating anti-trichinella antibodies have excellent sensitivity and specificity in the parenteral phase when most patients present, and PCR amplification from a muscle biopsy is pathoneumonic.

In addition to supportive critical care and ventilatory management, high dose steroid treatment to alleviate the inflammatory process is mandated by seizures, respiratory failure, or acute congestive heart failure due to involvement of the myocardium. Anti-parasitic treatment utilizes benzimidazoles (mebendazole 200 mg per day for 5 days or albendazole 400 mg per day for 3 days) and must be initiated when steroids are utilized. Survival confers lifelong immunity.

Neuromuscular Junction Diseases

Molecular approaches are identifying a growing number of rare neuromuscular junction diseases whose molecular pathologies involve very diverse mechanisms including aberrant mitochondrial tRNAs, mutant calcium channels, and autoimmunity. Emergency physicians are most likely to confront myasthenia gravis or the Lambert-Eaton myasthenic-like syndrome (LEMS) seen in association with several malignancies.

Myasthenia gravis[4,5] is a non-Mendelian autoimmune disorder in which antibodies are directed against acetylcholine receptors. This leads to a deficiency of these receptors on postsynaptic membranes. Acetylcholine receptors are traditionally classified as either muscarinic receptors on postsynaptic parasympathetic neurons or nicotinic receptors at synapses on skeletal muscle. It is the loss of nicotinic receptors that produces myasthenic symptoms, and it is uncommon for anti-muscarinic agents, such as atropine, to aggravate myasthenic weakness.

The clinical presentation is that of diplopia, ptosis, and oral-pharyngeal weakness that may impair speech and/or airway maintenance. With prolonged disease proximal muscle weakness involving especially the shoulder girdle and respiratory muscles may be seen. Alleviation of the weakness is typically noted following rest. Muscle wasting is seldom seen, and symmetrical reflexes and sensory function are typically preserved. Hypertrophy of the thymus is found in approximately 75% of these patients, and thymectomy is established as a useful management adjunct. Chronic management often involves immunosuppression, plasma exchange, and anticholinesterase agents such as pyridostigmine.

In females the onset often occurs at 30 to 40 years of age, while in males the onset more often occurs at 60 to 80 years old. However, it is important to note that in both sexes the initial presentation can occur at a younger age in association with thyroid storm, and myasthenia should be considered when thyroid storm presents with respiratory muscle weakness that requires intubation and mechanical ventilation. Conversely, hypothyroidism can also exacerbate myasthenic weakness.

Myasthenia patients often present to the ED with an established diagnosis and a complaint of increasing weakness. If ventilation is adequate and stable, urgent consultation should be obtained with an experienced neurologist. With an established diagnosis of myasthenia gravis, emergency physicians are wise to avoid use of the edrophonium test, although this procedure is described by several emergency medicine texts. In fact, emergency physicians are unlikely to have adequate experience with this procedure and its potential significant complications, and this approach to evaluating under- versus over-treatment with cholinesterase inhibitors is better left to an experienced neurologist with the patient in a more controlled environment.

Patients may also come to the ED in myasthenic crisis. This presents as oropharyngeal weakness and marginal ventilation, which can rapidly progress to aspiration pneumonia, respiratory failure, and death. In this situation endotracheal intubation and mechanical ventilation are lifesaving. All neuromuscular blocking agents should be avoided when intubating these patients. Although management of myasthenic crisis may require 2 to 4 weeks of mechanical ventilation, most myasthenic patients who require intubation are successfully weaned.

Generalized Peripheral Neuropathies

Diabetic Neuropathy

Diabetic neuropathy commonly develops in patients with Type 1 (hypoinsulinemic) diabetes and involves distal sensory and often autonomic dysfunction. The electrophysiological hallmark of diabetic neuropathy is slowed nerve conduction, which is present in at least 50% of Type I diabetics.[6] Ultrastructurally, neuronal damage is seen in the intranodal spaces at the nodes of Ranvier, which normally accelerate action potential transmission by saltatory conduction. Numbness and tingling of the feet are frequent complaints. The sensory loss is often severe enough to cause loss of the Achilles tendon reflex, and these patients may display an ataxic gait or the need to look at their feet as they walk. The lack of sensation coupled with microvascular compromise can lead to pressure sores that may progress to deep and seriously infected foot ulcers.

Gastroparesis and impaired regulation of peripheral vascular resistance are consequences of autonomic neuropathy. Gastroparesis[7] is a problem of gastric emptying that must be differentiated from and is not related to obstruction or mesenteric ischemia. Significant delay in gastric emptying may occur as an autonomic peripheral neuropathy in approximately 50% of long-term Type I diabetic patients and also may occur in Type II diabetes. Diabetic gastroparesis is exacerbated by hyperglycemia, concurrent hypothyroidism, and use of anti-motility agents and can result in significant malnutrition and poor absorption of orally administered drugs. Its common symptoms include early satiation, epigastric pain and fullness, nausea and vomiting, and weight loss. Significant malnutrition associated with this syndrome may require hospitalization for hyperalimentation or jejunal feeding.

Good glycemic control is a primary therapeutic objective in management of diabetic gastroparesis because hyperglycemia itself delays gastric emptying. Metoclopramide (oral and parenteral $5\text{-}HT_4$ receptor agonist and dopamine D_2 receptor antagonist) is an approved prokinetic and antiemetic drug for gastroparesis but may be associated with extrapyramidal reactions. Domperidone (oral dopamine D_2 receptor antagonist) is also an effective prokinetic and antiemetic agent and doesn't cross the blood-brain barrier. Erythromycin (motilin receptor agonist) is the most potent parenteral prokinetic (approximately 2.5 mg/kg IV) and may be particularly useful in the initial management of significantly symptomatic gastroparesis after good glycemic control is achieved; hyperglycemia substantially attenuates the prokinetic effects of erythromycin. The use of cisapride (oral $5\text{-}HT_4$ receptor agonist) as a prokinetic is now generally to be avoided because of QT prolongation and an associated increase in sudden death.

Substantial progress has recently been made in the molecular understanding of diabetic neuropathy. Insulin itself, in addition to regulating glucose, is a critical signal-transduction hormone in counter-regulating cell-suicide mechanisms to which neurons are particularly sensitive.[8] In addition, there is some evidence that inappropriate protein glycosylation driven by elevated glucose levels damages neurons, and recent insulin protocols utilizing 70/30 NPH twice daily have provided diabetic patients with more physiologic insulin rhythms and improved glycemic control. Perhaps most importantly, it has very recently become clear that the C-peptide normally cleaved from proinsulin is itself an important signal transduction molecule for specific G-protein-coupled receptors, and utilization of C-peptide together with insulin prevents or reverses both ultrastructural and conduction diabetic neuropathy and also prevents the early glomerular abnormalities associated with development of diabetic nephropathy.[6] Thus, we are quite likely soon to see incorporation of C-peptide into insulin protocols specifically directed at the problem of diabetic neuropathy.

Guillain-Barré Syndrome

Guillain-Barré syndrome (GBS) is the most common cause of an acute general peripheral neuropathy and is an acute polyradiculopathy that occurs following a variety of infections. Infectious processes that have been particularly implicated include those caused by members of the herpesvirus family, upper respiratory infections involving *Haemophilus influenzae* or *Mycoplasma pneumoniae,* and gastroenteritis—particularly that caused by *Campylobacter jejuni.* There is considerable evidence that GBS is autoimmune and arises after uncommon idiosyncratic immune responses against infectious agents' oligosaccharide structures that are molecular mimics of our own glycolipids.[9] GBS neurological injury and the categories of glycolipids targeted by the autoimmune process reflect to some extent the antecedent infection. Demyelination affecting both sensory and motor neurological function is prominent in GBS following most antecedent infections, but GBS after *H. influenza* or *C. jejuni* infections tends to spare sensory function, involve direct motor neuron axonal injury at the nodes of Ranvier with little demyelination, and have a more difficult and prolonged course.[9]

GBS typically begins within 1 to 3 weeks after the antecedent infection, with numbness and tingling of the lower extremities, followed by rapidly evolving ascending symmetric flaccid paralysis, and areflexia progressing from weakness of the thighs to the legs, arms, and respiratory muscles. The diagnostic hallmark is symmetrical loss of deep tendon reflexes. Respiratory failure requiring mechanical ventilation is common, and autonomic instability may produce severe effects on vascular resistance and heart rate. Early plasma exchange is effective in retarding disease progression and accelerating recovery, and this is thought to reflect removal of IgG antibodies whose levels are not quickly restored. Fortunately, there is rapid decay of production of anti-glycolipid antibodies; thus, GBS is a monophasic acute neuropathy that characteristically does not reoccur. There is a generally favorable prognosis with good supportive care, although some patients with axonal damage go on to develop Wallerian degeneration and prolonged disability.

Tick Paralysis

Tick paralysis[10,11] is an ascending (legs → arms → bulbar muscles → respiratory muscles) flaccid paralysis caused by a toxin that several species of female ticks secrete while feeding. Sensory function is spared, but full areflexia may develop. In the United States, the two ticks most commonly involved are *Dermacentor andersoni* (a livestock tick in the Northwest) and *Dermacentor variabilis* (a dog tick in the South and Southeast). Tick paralysis is most often seen in children and favors females because the tick may go undetected in longer hair. Although the toxin has been identified, its molecular mode of action is unclear with some evidence for activity affecting both the neuromuscular junction and reduced action potential conduction velocity. Resolution of the paralysis occurs within a few days once the tick is removed. This disease has been commonly mistaken for GBS, and all patients with ascending paralysis must be diligently examined for the presence of a tick.

Porphyria

Acute intermittent porphyria[12-14] is among a group of porphyria diseases that result from deficient enzymatic activity in the heme biosynthetic pathway with consequent accumulation of various porphyrin precursors of heme. The genetic and clinical spectrum of the diseases is quite complex because the heme biosynthetic pathway involves seven catalytic enzymes beyond the formation of β-aminolevulinic acid by the condensation of succinyl-CoA and glycine. The genes for most of these heme-biosynthetic enzymes are present as a single copy in the haploid genome, and normal expression of these enzymes involves both variable mRNA splicing and tissue-specific isoform expression. There are porphyrias associated with genetic mutations and/or splicing errors for each of these seven enzymes, and typically the activity of the affected enzyme is reduced approximately 50% below normal because we carry a diploid genome.

Thus, the spectrum of presentation of porphyrias can range from photodynamic skin blistering to that of acute intermittent porphyria presenting as a neuropathy that may affect autonomic, sensory, motor, and CNS functions resulting in acute abdominal pain, features of peripheral neuropathy, confusion or psychosis, and even seizures. Although the causal mechanisms of the neuropathy are not completely understood, many of these patients are hyponatremic, and there is evidence supporting interaction of excess β-aminolevulinic acid with GABA receptors. The heme moiety is also an essential redox component of many enzymes, and there is evidence that intracellular metabolic derangements as a result of neuronal heme deficiency are also neurotoxic.

The overall incidence of porphyria is approximately 1:100,000, although the incidence in Scandinavians may reach 60:100,000. Children may show unusual photosensitivity, but presentation of full-blown acute intermittent porphyria before puberty is very rare, and indeed the residual enzymatic activity is often adequate to preclude presentation, unless acute disease is provoked by a variety of drugs including estrogens, barbiturates, and anticancer agents.

The presentation of acute abdominal pain with vomiting, hypertension, and neurological symptoms and/or acute psychosis should alert the emergency physician to include acute intermittent porphyria in the differential diagnosis. The presence of hyponatremia is suggestive, and increased urinary excretion of β-aminolevulinic acid and porphobilinogen is diagnostic. Increased urine porphyrins may cause pink-to-red urine or initially normal-appearing urine that develops a burgundy color if it is exposed to sunlight. Initial treatment includes saline volume expansion, correction of electrolyte abnormalities, and seizure control with benzodiazepines (phenobarbital is contraindicated). Very recently treatment with heme moieties directed at correction of heme deficiency for critical neuronal enzymes has become available, and urgent consultation with specialists in neurology and hematology should guide initiation of this treatment.

Focal Peripheral Neuropathies

Entrapment syndromes include carpal tunnel syndrome, ulnar nerve entrapment, and deep peroneal nerve entrapment. Carpal tunnel syndrome is commonly encountered by the emergency physician and presents often as nocturnal and bilateral pain and/or numbness in the distribution of the median nerve in the thumb and first two fingers. Conservative management includes wrist splints at night, and referral to a hand surgeon is appropriate for follow-up care. Ulnar nerve entrapment usually occurs at the elbow and presents as numbness and/or pain in the fifth finger. This presentation may also occur with C8 radiculopathy, and these patients should be referred to a neurologist for definitive diagnosis by electromyography. Deep peroneal nerve entrapment at the fibular head may present with foot drop and distal numbness in the dorsal medial foot and is often associated with leg crossing or rapid weight loss. Generally, these patients respond well to cessation of the underlying behaviors, but neurological follow-up is appropriate to ensure that disease at a lumbar root is ruled out.

Bell's palsy[15-17] is an acute unilateral facial paralysis involving peripheral CN7. It is characterized by forehead weakness, inability to close the eye, and mouth droop or even drooling on the affected side. Because CN7 has a small sensory component at the external acoustic meatus, numbness may be found in this area (Hitselberger's sign). It is essential that this focal peripheral neuropathy of CN7 be carefully differentiated from the central facial weakness and extremity motor weakness associated with stroke syndromes. A careful examination to rule out herpes zoster oticus (Ramsay-Hunt syndrome) is also important because of the potential threat to the eye.

Bell's palsy historically was considered to be an idiopathic, self-limited, and fairly benign syndrome. More careful studies during the last decade have revealed that as much as 30% of untreated patients experience some degree of permanent residual, and about 5% of patients develop substantial permanent dysfunction in facial nerve function. Studies also have provided a growing body of evidence that Bell's palsy is a manifestation of recrudescence of chronic HSV1 infection, and early (within the first 3 days) initiation of treatment (7 days with both acyclovir 400 mg every 4 hours while awake and prednisone 50 mg per day, followed by a 5 day steroid taper) produces faster recovery from the facial paresis and a substantially reduced incidence of permanent complications. Referral should be made to a neurologist for follow-up care.

Spinal Neuropathies

Posterior Column Syndrome

Posterior column syndrome involves loss of proprioception and vibratory sense, and these patients often present with a wide-based ataxic foot-slapping gait and staring at their feet and the ground as they walk in order to visually compensate for the loss of positional sense. Proprioception can be examined through comparing performance with eyes open versus closed in the upper extremities of finger-to-nose motion and in the lower extremities of the accuracy and smoothness of heel-to-knee motion, and then sliding the heel down the shin. Neurosyphillis (tabes dorsalis) and B_{12} deficiency are two important causes of posterior column degeneration.

Amyotrophic Lateral Sclerosis

Amyotrophic lateral sclerosis is a chronic neurodegenerative disease involving both upper and lower motor neurons and degeneration of lateral motor tracts in the spinal cord. The upper motor neuron component leads to spasticity, hyperreflexia, and positive Babinski's sign, while the lower motor neuron component produces weakness, muscle atrophy, and dysphagia. The initial presentation often has predominant upper extremity findings of muscle weakness, cramps, fasciculation, and atrophy, although primary presentation of this disease in the ED is unusual. Rather, emergency presentation more commonly results from disease progression to respiratory failure.

The current molecular understanding of this disease is that the neuronal injury is caused by failure of mechanisms that dispose of oxygen radicals. The very rare inherited form of the disease involves dysfunctional mutation of a gene for superoxide dismutase, and it is thought that the more common non-Mendelian sporadic form of the disease arises from toxin-induced damage to the systems for controlling radicals. Other than airway management and ventilatory support, there are no established treatments for this disease. Its molecular basis does make it one of the leading candidates for gene therapy as such technology emerges.

References

1. Dalakas, M. Polymyositis, dermatomyositis, and inclusion body myositis. *N Engl J Med* 1991;325:1487–1498.
2. Mantegazza R, Bernasconi P, Confalonieri P, et al. Inflamatory myopathies and systemic disorders: A review of immunopathogenetic mechanisms and clinical features. *J Neurol* 1997;244:277–287.
3. Capo V, Despommier DD. Clinical aspects of infection with Trichinella species. *Clin Microbiology Rev* 1996;9:47–54.
4. Victor M, Roper AH. *Adams and Victor's Principles of Neurology,* 7th edition. New York: McGraw-Hill 2001.
5. Thomas CE, Mayer SA, Gungor Y, et al. Myasthenic crisis: clinical features, mortality, complications and risk factors for prolonged intubation. *Neurology* 1997;48:1253–1260.
6. Johansson J, Ekberg K, Shafqat J, et al. Molecular effects of proinsulin C-peptide. *Biochem Biophys Res Comm* 2002;295:1035–1040.
7. O'Donovan D, Feinie-Bisset C, et al. Idiopathic and diabetic gastroparesis. *Curr Treat Options Gastroenterol* 2003;6:299–309.
8. White BC, Sullivan JM, DeGracia DJ, et al. Brain ischemia and reperfusion: Molecular mechanisms of neuronal injury (477 references). *J Neurological Sci* 2000;179:1–33.
9. Willison HJ, Yuki N. Peripheral neuropathies and anti-glycolipid antibodies. *Brain* 2002;125:2591–2625.
10. Vedanarayanan VV, Evans OB, Subramony SH. Tick paralysis in children: Electrophysiology and misdiagnosis. *Neurology* 2002;59:1088–1090.
11. Dworkin MS, Shoemaker PC, Anderson DE. Tick paralysis: 33 cases in Washington State, 1946-1996. *Clin Infectious Dis* 1999;29:1435–1439.
12. Sassa S, Kappas A. Molecular aspects of the inherited porphyrias. *J Internal Med* 2000;247:169–178.
13. Meyer UA, Schuurmans MM, Lindberg RL. Acute porphyria: Pathogenesis of neurological manifestations. *Sem Liver Dis* 1998;18:43–52.
14. Elder GH, Hift RJ. Treatment of acute porphyria. *Hosp Med* 2001;62:422–425.
15. Grogan PM, Gronseth GS. Practice parameter: Steroids, acyclovir, and surgery for Bell's palsy (an evidence-based review): Report of the Quality Standards Subcommittee of the American Academy of Neurology. *Neurology* 2001; 56:830–836.
16. Adour KK, Ruboyianes JM, Von Doersten PG, et al. Bell's palsy treatment with acyclovir and prednisone compared with prednisone alone: A double-blind, randomized, controlled trial. *Ann Otol Rhinol Laryngol* 1996;105:371–378.
17. Hato N, Matsumoto S, Kisaki H, et al. Efficacy of early treatment of Bell's Palsy with oral acyclovir and prednisone. *Otol Neurotol* 2003;24:948–951.

Acute Spinal Cord Compression

Eustacia Su

Spinal cord compression (SCC) and cauda equina compression are neurosurgical emergencies requiring a high index of suspicion, prompt diagnosis, and rapid referral for decompression. Any patient presenting with axial neurologic complaints of either acute onset or gradual progression should be suspected of having an SCC.

Acute SCC most commonly follows an injury that results in compromise of the spinal canal by bony or disk fragments or both. Nontraumatic herniation of a large disk fragment or collapse of a vertebra eroded by tumor or infection may also cause acute SCC.

Spinal cord compression may also occur more gradually. Disk herniation, spinal neoplasms, degenerative spinal disease, and infection are the common causes of nonacute, progressive SCC.

Pathophysiology

Complete neurologic deficits following traumatic spinal cord injury were thought to result from total disruption of the spinal cord (SC), spinal epidural hemorrhage, or both. Studies of several series of SC-injured patients have demonstrated that contusions of the cord are responsible for the majority of observed deficits and that the size of these contusions does not correlate with the observed neurologic deficits.

Like brain injury, SC injury may be thought of as having primary (direct compression and severing of axons) and secondary components (vascular damage with hemorrhage, microvascular ischemia, edema, and necrosis). Removal of the cause of compression is postulated to aid SC recovery, both by relieving the direct compression and by reversing the resultant vascular compromise.

Clinical Presentation

The "sensory level," defined as loss of sensation below a circumferential, horizontal line on the trunk and weakness of the extremities innervated by the corresponding corticospinous fibers, is the hallmark of complete SCC. Most acute, traumatic SCC presents with the history of the recent, causative injury and acute loss of function.

Nontraumatic SCC is more insidious and easily missed. Local back pain, exacerbated by direct percussion of the spinous processes involved, is often the first sign of nontraumatic SCC. The pain is usually exacerbated when the patient is in the recumbent position and it often awakens the patient from sleep. Neurologic signs may not become manifest for days or weeks. Progressive weakness, leading to paraparesis, and a sensory level, demarcating the area of sensory loss, herald the transverse myelopathy that accompanies SCC. False localizing signs may occur, especially in the upper cervical spine: lesions above C4 may present with proprioceptive loss, paresthesias and/or atrophy of the hands.

Neurologic deficit resulting from SCC is categorized as either a complete or a partial (incomplete) lesion.

Complete Spinal Cord Lesion: Loss of function of all three columns of the spinal cord (motor, sensory, and autonomic) below the level of injury occurs in a complete SC lesion. Sphincter tone is lost. Deep tendon reflexes may initially be absent.

Partial Spinal Cord Lesion: Most injuries do not fit the "pure" definition of the syndromes described below, but have a pattern that closely resembles one of these.

Anterior Cord Syndrome: Direct anterior pressure on the spinothalamic and corticospinous tracts in the anterior and lateral columns of the cord results in loss of motor and temperature sensation below the level of the injury. Vibratory and position sense (posterior columns) are more or less preserved.

Brown-Séquard Syndrome: A functional hemisection of the spinal cord results in loss of ipsilateral position sense and motor function and contralateral pain and temperature sensation.

Central Cord Syndrome: Weakness and numbness of the upper extremities with preservation of lower extremity function are the hallmark of this syndrome. The concept of compromised function of the central part of the spinal cord has been challenged. A similar syndrome is seen in high cervical (C1–C2) injuries and is called the cruciate paralysis of Bell.

Foramen Magnum Syndrome: Weakness of the shoulder and arm develops first, followed by weakness in the contralateral leg and then the contralateral arm. Suboccipital pain radiating to the neck and shoulders is the usual presenting symptom. Horner's syndrome can

Table 79.1

Differentiation Between Intramedullary and Extramedullary Spinal Cord Compression

Intramedullary	Extramedullary
Poorly localized burning pain	Radicular pain
Dissociated loss of pain	Brown-Séquard syndrome: sensation with sparing proprioception
Sparing of perineal and sacral sensation	Asymmetric lower motor neuron signs in 1 or 2 segments
Late, less prominent corticospinal signs	Early corticospinal signs
Normal or near-normal cerebrospinal fluid analysis	Early prominent cerebrospinal fluid abnormalities

be seen with this syndrome, indicating a high cervical lesion.

Cauda Equina Compression: Occurs with lesions inferior to L1 and results in flaccidity, areflexia, and asymmetric paraparesis, usually accompanied by bowel or bladder dysfunction. The sensory level is in a saddle distribution up to L1, corresponding to roots carried in the cauda equina. Achilles and patellar reflexes are diminished or absent. Pain is common and projects to the perineum or thighs.

Conus Medullaris Compression: Pain is a less prominent presenting symptom here, but bowel and bladder dysfunction occur early. Lesions may compress both the cauda equina and the conus medullaris, causing a combination of lower motor neuron signs and some hyperreflexia or a Babinski sign.

Table 79.1 contains a comparison of findings of intramedullary versus extramedullary lesions.

Etiology

Trauma, herniated nucleus pulposus, and tumor are the major causes of SCC. Infection is the next largest category: tuberculosis, osteomyelitis, parasites (e.g., echinococcus), gummas, and spinal epidural and intramedullary abscesses. Other diseases of the spine can also cause SCC: arthritides (especially rheumatoid arthritis, which destroys the atlantoaxial joint), ankylosing spondylitis (lumbar or cauda equina compression), ossified ligamenta flava or spinal stenosis. Congenital abnormalities and subsequent complications such as infection or hemorrhage occur less commonly. Rare causes include Cushing's syndrome (increased epidural fat thickness), extramedullary hematopoiesis, lymphomatoid granulomatosis, and mucopolysaccharidoses. Epidural hemorrhage and hematomyelia may also present as SCC. Anticoagulated patients are at risk for spontaneous spinal epidural hemorrhage.

Diagnosis

A careful history, with meticulous attention to determining the patient's ability to detect bladder fullness and to void or defecate at will, is crucial to the diagnosis of SCC. A high index of suspicion, in tandem with a very thorough overall physical examination and painstaking neurologic examination, generally helps the physician to detect SCC as early as possible. Special note should be made of dim-

ples and hairy patches in the low back or any other signs of possible spinal dysraphism or other congenital lesion. Acquired lesions such as melanoma, breast lumps, or furuncles must also be sought as the possible cause of SCC. Missing the diagnosis most often results from a cursory examination that fails to detect the muscle weakness, loss of sphincter tone, or associated sensory deficits.

Emergency Department Management

In the acutely injured patient, spinal immobilization, if not already performed by prehospital personnel, should be the first priority after determining that the airway is patent and stable. Any need for ventilatory assistance and fluid resuscitation should be determined and the appropriate interventions begun. A thorough, but rapid, assessment of the patient's neurologic status should be performed during the secondary survey and frequent, serial reexaminations must be done to monitor the progression of signs, especially in partial spinal cord injuries.

The patient whose symptoms have progressed gradually should have any unstable portions of the spine immobilized, if possible. Surgical decompression and stabilization of the spine are still the definitive treatment in most cases of SCC.

High-dose steroids (methylprednisolone, 30 mg/kg bolus then 5.4 mg/kg per hour for the next 23 hours) were indicated in acute traumatic lesions but are now controversial. Consult with the neurosurgeon before administering steroids. In tumor-related, epidural cord compression, steroids (dexamethasone 2 mg/kg, maximum 100 mg, then 1 to 2 mg/kg per day qid) still have a role.

Emergency computerized tomographic imaging of the spine and spinal cord has become standard in the management of acute SCC, especially in the context of trauma. Emergent magnetic resonance imaging after acute SCI provides more accurate prognostic information regarding neurological function, but the patient must be stable enough to tolerate the procedure. Intra-axial hematomas, spinal cord edema, and compression by extra-axial hematoma are clearly demonstrated and may direct further surgical decompression.

Selected Readings

Bohlman HH, Ducker TB. Spine and spinal cord injuries. In: Herkowitz HN, Garfin SR, Balderston RA, et al, eds. *The Spine.* Philadelphia: Saunders, 1992: 973–1103.

Dahlbeck S, Kagan AR. Spinal cord compression, infection and unknown primary cancers. *Am J Clin Oncol* 2001;24:315–318.

Johnston RA. The management of acute spinal cord compression. *J Neurol Neurosurg Psychiatry* 1993;56:1046–1054.

McCormack B, MacMillan M, Fessler RG. Management of thoracic, lumbar and sacral injuries. In: Tindall GT, Cooper PR, Barrow DL, eds. *The Practice of Neurosurgery.* Baltimore: Williams and Wilkins 1996:1730.

Packer RJ, Berman PH. Neurologic emergencies. In: Fleisher GR, Ludwig S, eds. *Textbook of Pediatric Emergency Medicine,* 3rd ed. Baltimore: Williams and Wilkins 1993:585–586.

Ropper AH, Martin JB. Diseases of the spinal cord. In: Wilson JD, Braunwald E, Isselbacher KJ, et al, eds. *Harrison's Principles of Internal Medicine,* 12th ed. New York: McGraw-Hill 1991:2081–2083.

Schmidt RD, Markovchick V. Nontraumatic spinal cord compression. *J Emerg Med* 1992;10:1898–1199.

Selden NR, Quint DJ, Patel N et al. Emergency magnetic resonance imaging of cervical spinal cord injuries: clinical correlation and prognosis. *Neurosurgery* 1999;44:785–792.

Sonstein WJ, LaSala PA, Michelsen WJ, et al. False localizing signs in upper cervical spinal cord compression. *Neurosurgery* 1996;38:445–449.

80 | Hydrocephalus

Eustacia Su
Jenna Timm

Definition

Hydrocephalus is the enlargement of the cerebral ventricles due to an imbalance between the production of cerebrospinal fluid (CSF) and its absorption; obstruction to CSF flow may also cause hydrocephalus.

Hydrocephalus ex-vacuo, due to primary cortical atrophy, is noted with prominent sulci and large ventricles on CT scan of the brain.

Ventriculomegaly is the presence of large cerebral ventricles that are not necessarily associated with increased intracranial pressure.

Physiology

CSF is secreted by the choroid plexus, mostly in the lateral ventricles; the choroid plexus responds to adrenergic and cholinergic stimulation, respectively, by decreasing and increasing CSF production. Total CSF volume is approximately 50 ml in an infant and 150 mL in an adult. Turnover time for CSF is approximately 5 to 7 hours.

Cerebrospinal fluid movement occurs as a result of the hydrostatic gradient between the ventricular system (180 mm H_2O) and the venous channels (90 mm H_2O in the superior sagittal sinus). Normal CSF flow starts from the lateral ventricles, through the foramina of Monro, into the third ventricle. CSF then traverses the aqueduct of Sylvius to the fourth ventricle and out of the lateral foramina of Luschka and the midline foramen of Magendie and into the basilar cisterns. Then CSF flows posteriorly over the cerebellum and cerebral cortex and anteriorly through the cistern system. Most of the CSF is absorbed when the hydrostatic pressure gradient forces it through the tight junctions of the arachnoid villous epithelium. A small proportion of CSF is absorbed by the lymphatic channels to the paranasal sinuses, along the nerve sleeves and by the choroid plexus itself.

Noncommunicating hydrocephalus results from obstruction to CSF flow in the ventricular system, proximal to the fourth ventricle, most commonly due to aqueductal stenosis, congenital or acquired, or fourth ventricle lesions (**Table 80.1**).

Communicating (nonobstructive) hydrocephalus results from blockage distal to the fourth ventricle. It most commonly results from subarachnoid hemorrhage due to intraventricular hemorrhage in the premature infant. The subarachnoid bleed obliterates the cisterns and the arachnoid villi, decreasing or eliminating CSF absorption. Pneumococcal and tuberculous meningitis produce a thick, tenacious exudate that obstructs the basal cisterns. Intrauterine infection and leukemia seeding the subarachnoid space may also produce communicating hydrocephalus.

Normal pressure hydrocephalus occurs in communicating hydrocephalus when intracranial hypertension is either absent or not recognized, due to lack of symptoms. The majority of these patients give no history of trauma or known central nervous system infection to account for the partial obliteration of the subarachnoid space, which is believed to result in defective CSF resorption through the arachnoid villi. Episodes of increased intracranial pressure (ICP) may occur during the course of this illness, since some fluctuations of pressure are seen in those patients with normal pressure hydrocephalus, and whose ICP is being continuously monitored.

The incidence of hydrocephalus is unknown. Most cases of hydrocephalus occur during or after parturition. With improved neonatal care, many extremely low birth weight neonates are surviving; 20% to 30% of them develop germinal matrix-intraventricular hemorrhage, and between 2% and 10% of very or extremely low birth weight neonates require ventricular shunt treatment for hydrocephalus. Other etiologies of acquired hydrocephalus include tumor, infection, trauma, and vitamin A intoxication. Congenital hydrocephalus is most often associated with spinal dysraphism and meningomyelocele: the incidence of the latter is 1 to 3 per 1,000 live births.

Clinical Presentation

Hydrocephalus in the infant rarely presents in the emergency department (ED). Rather, an accelerated rate of head enlargement detected by serial measurements during

Table 80.1
Noncommunication Hydrocephalus

Aqueductal Stenosis
  X-linked recessive:
  - Associated with minor neural tube closure defects (spina bifida occulta)
  Neurofibromatosis:
  - Glial scarring after neonatal meningitis or subarachnoid
  - Hemorrhage in the premature infant; may case complete obstruction
  Intrauterine infections
  Mumps meningoencephalitis
Vein of Galen Malformation (enlarged)
Fourth Ventricle
  Posterior fossa brain tumors:
  - Arnold-Chiari II malformations (hindbrain anomaly) (probably due to failure of pontine flexure during embryogenesis, causes elongation of the fourth ventricle, kinking of the brain stem, and displacement of the inferior vermis, pons, and medulla into the cervical canal)
  - Dandy-Walker malformation (cyst) (cystic expansion of the fourth ventricle in the posterior fossa, due to developmental failure of the roof during embryogenesis; associated anomalies include agenesis of the posterior vermis and corpus callosum)

scheduled well-child visits usually alerts the physician to this problem in infancy. An open, bulging anterior fontanelle and dilated scalp veins are helpful ancillary signs; downward deviation of the eyes (the "setting sun" sign), more noticeable in the broadened forehead, is almost pathognomonic.

Irritability, lethargy, poor appetite, and vomiting are the most common presenting signs in children. Headache becomes a more prominent complaint as the patient's age and verbal ability increase. Visual blurring, mental dullness, depression, difficulty walking, and urinary incontinence are more common presenting complaints in adults with hydrocephalus. Stretching and disruption of the cortical fibers originating from the leg region of the motor cortex produce long tract signs: hyperreflexia, spasticity, clonus, and Babinski's sign.

A much slower onset of mental and motor deterioration, particularly with gait abnormalities, is seen in adults with normal pressure hydrocephalus. No single gait disorder is pathognomonic: a broad-based stance with hesitancy in initiating walking is most common, and some patients show more ataxic features.

Papilledema, if present, is a helpful finding; its absence does not rule out hydrocephalus, especially in the young infant or child whose open fontanelles and sutures relieve the pressure on the optic nerve.

The neurologic examination is frequently non-focal or unchanged from baseline, except for some decrease in the level of intellectual function.

Differential Diagnosis

Macrocrania may result from cranial thickening due to primary or secondary bone disorders, or intracranial enlargement, both extracerebral (e.g., chronic subdural collections) or megalencephaly (e.g., lysosomal diseases, aminoacidurias or leukodystrophies).

Irritability, lethargy, and decreased mental status share the differential diagnosis of altered mental status in general, including toxic, metabolic, infectious, trauma, anatomic, and postictal conditions. In infancy, disorders such as intussusception and shaken baby syndrome must also be considered in this presentation.

Gait disorders may also be due to intrinsic or extrinsic spinal cord processes, muscle disorders, trauma, or neurologic diseases (e.g., Parkinsonism). Vomiting may result from intracranial processes, bowel problems (such as pyloric stenosis, bowel obstruction) or infections resulting in clinical gastroenteritis and metabolic presentations, such as diabetic ketoacidosis. Visual disturbances may result from strabismus, cranial nerve palsies, trauma or infection.

Treatment

To restore flow and to accommodate the continued CSF secretion, the imbalance between secretion and absorption must be corrected. This correction usually takes the form of a shunt, "the act or process of moving to an alternate course." Alternative treatment modalities include third ventriculostomy, cannulation of the aqueduct of Sylvius, and opening the ventricles to the CSF space.

There are three types of shunt commonly employed to treat hydrocephalus. The most commonly used is the ventriculoperitoneal (VP) shunt. The ventriculoatrial (VA) shunt used to be more commonly used but was associated with many cardiovascular complications. The lumboperitoneal shunt is mostly used for communicating hydrocephalus.

Anatomy of a Shunt

There are three portions of a shunt to be considered when evaluating a shunt that might not be functioning.
1. Proximal: ventricular or lumbar catheter
2. Intermediate: reservoir (optional), valve, and tubing
3. Distal atrial, peritoneal or lumbar catheter

Other Devices

On/off devices have a radiopaque button that turns the system on or off, when pressed. In-line shunt filters are sometimes included to prevent seeding of metastatic tumors. Antisiphon devices close when negative pressure exists in a system to prevent overdrainage. Telemetric pressure sensors allow continuous assessment of system function but are not frequently used. The exact combination of components and accessories varies considerably, but knowledge of the basic components allows adequate assessment of patients with CSF shunts.

The incidence of shunt malfunction is unknown. The patients who present to the ED are generally those whose shunts do malfunction. The frequency of shunt revisions is 1.7 to 7 times in 10 years.

CNS Shunt Malfunction

Etiology

Obstruction is the most common cause of CSF shunt malfunction, and generally mandates a revision of the shunt. Shunts may also malfunction due to obstruction or overdrainage.

Overdrainage can occur when patients with ventricular shunts assume an upright position, causing the pressure differential across the valve to increase and resulting in a siphon effect. Small hygromas and recurrent low-pressure headaches are the minor consequences of overdrainage. Aqueductal stenosis may also result from chronic overdrainage, converting a communicating hydrocephalus to a noncommunicating hydrocephalus.

Acute mild overdrainage, e.g., in the postoperative stage, leads to subdural hematomas, seen in 4% to 20% of all shunt patients. Sudden, rapid overdrainage is reported to cause "upward herniation" of the brain stem, resulting in apnea, bradycardia, syncope, hypotension, and laryngospasm, although there is controversy over whether upward herniation actually occurs. Lowering the patient's head usually suffices, if the problem is diagnosed early.

Chronic overdrainage may cause hyperpneumatization of the sinuses, pneumocranium, and tension pneumocranium: these conditions manifest themselves as recurrent severe headaches, malaise, focal neurologic findings, seizures, and even coma. Approximately 5% of children who are shunt-dependent develop slit ventricle syndrome from chronic overdrainage. The symptoms of episodic minor headaches and decreased performance with asymptomatic periods suggest intermittent elevated intracranial pressure from proximal obstruction. When the ventricles collapse around the catheter and intermittently occlude it, a more severe presentation occurs with severe headache, nausea, vomiting, and bradycardia progressing to obtundation. Decreased cerebral compliance, perhaps due to subependymal gliosis, may not allow the ventricles to reexpand when the intracranial pressure increases.

Obstruction occurs when any of the different elements malfunctions and no longer allows drainage.

Proximal Catheter

The proximal catheter, which is placed in one of the ventricles through a burr hole, is usually made of Silastic. The tip may be smooth, grooved, or flanged like a brush and has multiple perforations. The catheter may fail to conduct CSF, due to blockage by the choroid plexus, debris, calcification, breakage, disconnection or migration (the grooves and flanges of catheters were developed to try to minimize obstruction). The catheter can also become infected or it may erode through the skin. The ventricular catheter connects to a valve apparatus in the intermediate portion.

Intermediate Portion

Conduction of CSF may be hampered in the intermediate portion of the shunt by disconnection or blockage, the two most common causes.

Valves

The valve allows unidirectional flow of CSF and regulates the pressure at which flow occurs. Failure of the valve can occur due to improper pressure settings or due to collection of protein debris. Infection and erosion are the next most common causes of shunt revision. Incorrect valve mechanism can also result in recurrent hydrocephalus. There are four types of valve in use: slit valves, miter valves, ball valves, and diaphragm valves.

Slit valves contain a slit in the wall of tubing that has a closed end. As the pressure inside the tubing increases, the slit opens and allows flow. When the external pressure exceeds the internal pressure, the slit closes, preventing reverse flow.

Ball-in-cone valves have a sapphire ball held in place by a calibrated spring. Miter valves have silicone leaflets that are pushed apart by the built-up pressure of the CSF, which flows out until the external pressure exceeds the internal pressure, when the leaflets are pushed back together again, preventing flow.

Diaphragm valves open when the CSF pushes the diaphragm up off its seat; these valves are usually placed in the burr hole reservoir with the ventricular catheter directly attached to the valve.

Reservoirs and Flush Chambers

The reservoir provides access to the shunt system for fluid sampling, pressure measurement, and injection of medication or contrast materials. Flush chambers are usually found in shunts with a single distal valve and consist of either a single or a double bubble. The distal bubble can be compressed allowing access proximally to the system; conversely occluding the proximal bubble allows access to the distal part of the system.

Distal Portion

The peritoneal catheter has radiopaque markings to facilitate radiographic identification. The distal end may be open or have a slit valve attached. The catheter may fail allow CSF flow or require replacement (again because of disconnection), due to blockage, infection, valve failure.

Evaluation of Possible CSF Shunt Malfunction

In evaluating for possible CNS shunt malfunction, the following questions arise:

1. Is the clinical presentation consistent with CSF shunt malfunction?
2. Is CSF flow indeed restricted? If so, at which anatomic point?
3. What type of shunt system is in place?

Table 80.2

Unique Complications of Less Common Types of Shunts

Type of Shunt	Complications
Ventriculoatrial shunt	Pulmonary embolism, endocarditis, cor pulmonale, cardiac arrhythmias, septic emboli, migration of the catheter into the coronary sinus, shunt nephritis
Ventriculopleural shunt	Pleural effusion, excessive CSF drainage with inspiration (resulting in intracranial hypotension), bronchial fistula formation
Lumboperitoneal shunt	Arachnoiditis, back pain, nerve root irritation, tonsillar herniation from overdrainage

Table 80.2 details some possible complications that occur with less common shunt devices.

Clinical Presentation of CSF Shunt Malfunction

The patient with diagnosed and treated hydrocephalus most likely presents in the same manner as the initial presentation when the shunt fails to function. The risk of shunt malfunction is greatest in the first months following placement. Approximately 80% of patients will require revision of the shunt by 10 years.

Parents will often state that their child is not acting normally and will suspect a shunt malfunction from previous experience. This is an important piece of information that should not be ignored. Children may present with constant headaches, lethargy, irritability, poor feeding or regression of developmental milestones. Adults may present with problems with gait or concentration. If the intracranial hypertension is not treated, the patients will develop herniation, resulting in hypertension, bradycardia, irregular respiratory patterns and death or severe neurologic sequelae.

Other manifestations of shunt complications or malfunction are related to the type of shunt present. Ventriculoatrial shunts cause vascular system complications; ventriculoperitoneal shunts tend to cause abdominal problems (**Table 80.3**).

Table 80.3

Complications of Shunts

Ventriculoatrial shunts
- Glomerulonephritis (immune-complex)
- Septic pulmonary emboli
- Right atrial pseudotumor
- Cardiac perforation and tamponade
- Inferior and superior vena cava obstruction
- Tricuspid valvulitis
- Pulmonary artery mycotic aneurysm
- Perforated interatrial septum

Ventriculoperitoneal shunts
- Perionitis
- Bowel obstruction due to adhesions
- Peritoneal cyst
- Migration through hernia into scrotum

Shunt infections are the neurosurgeon's nightmare: they are responsible for up to 60% of the mortality associated with shunts. Fever is the most common presenting symptom of CSF shunt infection (although up to half of patients with infected CSF shunts are afebrile); other manifestations include nausea, vomiting, headache, lethargy, feeding problems, and shunt malfunction. Inflammation along the course of the shunt is very specific for shunt infection but not very sensitive. Only one-third of patients with shunt infections demonstrate meningeal signs.

History

In evaluation of the patient history, the following questions should be considered:
1. What is the underlying disorder that required shunting?
2. When was the first shunt inserted, where and by whom?
3. What type of shunt is in place?
4. What were the cause, signs/symptoms, and response to treatment of prior episodes of shunt malfunction?
5. How long has this shunt been in place?
6. What complications have already occurred with the present shunt?
7. How many revisions have already been done?

Examination

First assess the patient's level of function and risk of immediate lethality: Is the patient about to herniate? If the patient appears to be in immediate danger of herniation, intubation, hyperventilation to an end-tidal CO_2 of 30 to 35 mm Hg, and mannitol administration should be performed immediately while the neurosurgeon is being contacted. Acetazolamide 30 mg/day and dexamethasone 0.5 to 1.0 mg/kg may also help to keep the intracranial pressure down. Aspiration of CSF through the shunt to relieve intracranial hypertension may be needed as an immediately lifesaving measure. This should be performed by the neurosurgeon if at all possible.

If a neurosurgeon is not immediately available, insert a 23-gauge scalp vein needle ("butterfly") into the reservoir and hold the tubing upright. The level to which the fluid rises in the tubing corresponds to the ventricular pressure if the proximal end is not obstructed. High pressure suggests distal obstruction, while low pressure suggests either proximal obstruction or overdrainage. Shunt patency at the distal end is determined by holding up the tubing and observing the flow of CSF distally.

If the pressure is high, CSF should be withdrawn until a pressure of approximately 10 cm of water is reached. This is usually effective in distal end obstruction. If the proximal end of the shunt is obstructed so that no CSF can be withdrawn and the patient is deteriorating, the ventricle must be tapped through the fontanelle or the sutures, if open, or through the burr hole where the shunt is located. The latter maneuver is a temporizing measure, but it damages the shunt, which will need revision anyway.

If the patient is stable, and there are no other findings on physical examination to account for the presenting complaints or changes in mentation, assess the functioning of the shunt. Neurosurgeons disagree about the extent to which the emergency physician should manipulate the shunt. There is concern that too much pumping of the shunt will cause overdrainage. Other neurosurgeons would like to know whether the problem is proximal or distal to the reservoir or valve.

There are three types of shunt component arrangement:

Type A: The shunt valve is located in the cranial burr hole.
Type B: The shunt valve is positioned between the burr hole and the distal catheter.
Type C: The shunt valve is part of the distal catheter.

To determine the type of shunt, first inspect the components: bulges under the skin along the course of the shunt show the location of the components. Look for swelling and erythema along the tract and incisions. Next, palpate along the course of the shunt from proximal to distal. Locate the components, and feel for swelling, subcutaneous fluid collections, tenderness, and breaks in the system; and determine where the distal end terminates (atrial or peritoneal). Obtain a shunt series to determine the locations of the valve and the ventricular catheter and to see if the catheters are broken or disconnected.

A noninvasive method for determining shunt function is to first locate the valve by examination and x-ray. Depress the valve and note the ease with which it is depressed and its rate of refill. Normally the valve depresses and refills rapidly and easily. If there is a distal occlusion, the valve depresses either reluctantly or not at all. If there is a proximal occlusion, the valve depresses normally but refills very slowly or not at all. A click may indicate an incompetent valve. Normal compression and refill is observed in up to 40% of shunts with obstruction; difficulty on compression of the valve is therefore a very specific but not sensitive finding for CSF shunt obstruction.

Further evaluation usually includes a CT scan of the head. Only light sedation is needed for this procedure since small movement artifacts are unlikely to obscure crucial findings. A CT of the head, looking at ventricle and cistern size, is almost always requested. Previous CT scans, if available for comparison, are extremely helpful. However, intracranial pressure may be high despite unchanged ventricle size. Obliteration of the perimesen-

cephalic cisterns connotes possibly life-threatening shunt malfunction. In some cases, isotope flow study or MRI may be needed.

CSF Shunt Infections

Epidemiology

The mean frequency of shunt infections is 10% to 15% per procedure; 5% to 8% is considered an acceptable rate of infection, the major cause of the mortality associated with CSF shunts.

Most infections are caused by low virulence skin flora; 60% to 80% are *Staphylococcus* species, most commonly slime-producing *Staphylococcus epidermidis*. The slime helps to attach the organisms to the shunt surface while protecting them from host defenses and antibiotics. From 5% to 10% of shunt infections are caused by gram-negative and anaerobic organisms: *Klebsiella, Escherichia coli, Proteus, Pseudomonas,* etc. These cause the highest rates of morbidity and mortality. Diphtheroid organisms are becoming a more prevalent cause of shunt infection, usually presenting as delayed infection months after the procedure. The rising significance of diphtheroid infection is perhaps related to perioperative antibiotic treatment of both the patient and the shunt components. The organisms traditionally associated with meningitis (*Haemophilus influenzae, Streptococcus pneumoniae, Neisseria meningitidis*) cause only 5% of shunt infections. Fungal infections are rare. Mixed bacterial infections usually result from bowel perforation. No causative organism is isolated in 3% of infections; antibiotic therapy or the fastidiousness of the organisms probably accounts for the failure to culture the culprits.

Host Factors

The elderly, young infants (younger than 3 months of age) and premature (extremely low birth weight) infants are the groups with the highest infection rates. Skin condition at the time of insertion impacts the rate of infection, as does any concurrent infection (e.g., nose, ear, urinary tract, or respiratory). The presence of the shunt may allow organisms to bypass the blood-brain barrier, resulting in a higher incidence of meningitis.

Technical Factors

The incidence of infection increases exponentially with the number of connections in the system. Operative technique, the individual surgeon's experience, and the midsummer arrival of new housestaff are all debated factors in the rate of infection.

Pathogenesis

Cerebrospinal fluid shunts are infected by three main routes. Wound colonization at the time of surgery is the most common route, followed by hematogenous spread and retrograde contamination from the distal catheter. Some 70% of all infections occur within 2 months of surgery, and the most common pathogen is a low virulence organism, *S. epidermidis*. Hematogenous spread seems to result in more frequent meningitis in shunted patients, the common pathogens being *H. influenzae, S. pneumoniae,* and *N. meningitidis*. Blood cultures are frequently normal and these infections clear with antibiotic therapy alone, not requiring shunt removal. Retrograde spread usually occurs with lumboureteral shunts or when a peritoneal catheter encounters perforated bowel or pelvic inflammatory disease.

Diagnosis

The emergency physician must have a high index of suspicion for shunt infection in the shunted patient, since the presentation can be nonspecific and variable. CSF from lumbar puncture is rarely positive, even when the indwelling shunt is infected. Percutaneous aspiration of the shunt reservoir produces CSF specimens with the highest yield in positive cultures (60% to 100%) in patients who are not currently treated with antibiotics. The leukocyte count strongly predicts the culture results: 90% of cultures are positive when greater than 100 white blood cells/mm^3 are present in the CSF. Anaerobic and fungal cultures should be done if the routine bacterial cultures are repeatedly sterile in the face of a persistently elevated CSF white cell count. Hypoglycorrachia is seldom seen in shunt infections. The total protein level may be elevated. Gram's stain is usually positive if *Staphylococcus aureus* or Gram-negative bacilli are present. The peripheral white blood cell count may be normal or elevated and is of no diagnostic value in shunt infection.

Blood cultures are positive in 95% of ventriculoatrial shunt infections, but only in 20% of ventriculoperitoneal shunt infections. Cultures of subcutaneous aspirates obtained from the erythematous shunt tract are often positive.

Management

All patients with shunt malfunction or infection require neurosurgical consultation and ICU admission. If there are signs of imminent herniation, intubation, hyperventilation to an end-tidal CO_2 or 30 to 35 mm Hg should be rapidly accomplished, followed by administration of mannitol. Approximately 50% of patients with infected shunts require shunt removal; symptoms may disappear during antibiotic treatment but often recrudesce after discontinuing the drugs.

The antibiotics selected must be effective against the common pathogens, be able to penetrate the blood-brain barrier, and have low toxicity. Nafcillin has been the drug of choice for *S. epidermidis* infections. The increasing prevalence of methicillin-resistant *Staphylococcus* species has forced an increase in the use of vancomycin, which rarely achieves high CSF levels in the absence of significant meningeal inflammation and must therefore be given by intraventricular administration. Newer drugs are being studied as alternative solutions to the problem of methicillin-resistant staphylococcal shunt infections. Other regimens, including oral drugs given in combination with newer parenteral drugs, are also under investigation.

Gram-negative bacillary shunt infections usually require treatment with a third-generation cephalosporin, as do shunted patients with meningitis due to traditional organisms (e.g., *H. influenzae*). Pseudomonal infections are usually treated with an antipseudomonal β-lactam in combination with an aminoglycoside.

Selected Readings

Arriada N, Sotelo J. Review: treatment of hydrocephalus in adults. *Surg Neurol* 2002;58:377–384.

Beal MF, Richardson EP, Martin JB. Degenerative diseases of the nervous system. In: Wilson JD, Braunwald E, Isselbacher KJ, et al, eds. *Harrison's Principles of Internal Medicine*. 12th ed. New York: McGraw-Hill 1991:2068.

Bruce DA. Neurosurgical emergencies. In: Fleisher GR, Ludwig S, eds. *Textbook of Pediatric Emergency Medicine*, 3rd ed. Baltimore: Williams and Wilkins 1993:1412–1413.

Caviness VS. Neurocutaneous syndromes and other disorders of the central nervous system. In: Wilson JD, Braunwald E, Isselbacher KJ, et al., eds. *Harrison's Principles of Internal Medicine*, 12th ed. New York: McGraw-Hill 1991:2059.

Haslam R. Congenital anomalies of the central nervous system. In: Behrman RE, ed. *Nelson Textbook of Pediatrics*. 14th ed. Philadelphia: Saunders 1992:1487–1490.

Jordan KT. Cerebrospinal fluid shunts [review]. *Emerg Med Clin North Am* 1994;12: 779–786.

Key CB, Rothrock SG, Falk JL. Cerebrospinal fluid shunt complications: an emergency medicine perspective. *Pediatr Emerg Care* 1995;11:265–273.

Piatt JH. Physical examination of patients with cerebrospinal fluid shunts: Is there useful information in pumping the shunt? *Pediatrics* 1992;89:470–473.

Seizures

Robert C. Reiser

One in ten people will have at least one seizure in their lifetime and 2 to 4 million people in the United States have epilepsy. Seizure-related complaints challenge the emergency medicine clinician to differentiate the benign presentation from the immediately life threatening (**Table 81.1**).

Presentation

The most common seizure presentation in the emergency department (ED) is historical, i.e., the seizure is reported by a bystander, usually a family member or coworker. Typically, seizures are described as "spells," "fits," "falling out," and other imprecise terms. Because the historical trail rapidly grows cold, the conscientious emergency physician should seek out all witnesses and obtain and document the detailed history of the event from them. A grand mal tonic clonic seizure is characterized by a sudden loss of consciousness with a fall to the ground. This begins the tonic stage of the seizure, in which all the muscles of the body contract nearly simultaneously, with the stronger muscles (flexors versus extensors) of each pair dominating to produce a characteristic stereotypical posture. The neck is extended, the arms are flexed and abducted, and the hands pronated (hands up position). This is followed by snapping shut of the jaw as the masseter spasms (tongue may be bitten). There may be a piercing cry as the entire musculature spasms and air is forced through a closed glottis. The knees are held in extension with the feet in dorsiflexion, breathing is impossible, and after several seconds the patient becomes cyanotic. It is during this phase that the pupils may be unequal but dilated and unreactive to light. This tonic phase lasts 10 to 20 seconds. After that, a transition comes to the clonic phase, which at first is just a mild tremor that gradually becomes coarser, turning into violent muscular contractions in rhythmic salvos.

The eyes roll, the face grimaces and becomes violaceous, the pulse becomes rapid, and bloody froth may accumulate at the mouth. The clonic jerks then decrease in frequency and amplitude over 30 seconds or so, and the entire clonic phase usually lasts about 1 minute. The patient appears apneic during the entire period. A deep inspiration marks the end of the seizure, followed by a deep coma. As the patient is aroused, he is noted to be confused and agitated, and, if allowed to, often drops into a deep sleep. Upon awakening, he may complain of a headache, but is noted to have normal mental status.

Evaluation

The goal of the evaluation is to first elucidate whether the event was in fact a true seizure or one of the several events that may mimic a seizure such as syncope or pseudoseizure.

Questions to be answered by the history are:
1. Was the onset focal or generalized?
2. Did the patient suffer a loss of consciousness? Did anyone try to arouse patient?
3. Were there unusual respiratory patterns? (E.g., apnea, snoring respirations, foaming at the mouth.)
4. What was the pattern of shaking? (Have witnesses demonstrate.)
5. Was there postictal confusion, agitation, etc.? If so, how long did it last?

The seizure activity seen during syncopal episodes or arrhythmic episodes is very brief. Usually only several beats of clonic activity are noted with no postictal mental status changes when the patient recovers consciousness and reorients very quickly, with little confusion evident.

Psychogenic seizures are often difficult to differentiate from true seizures, but several clues are helpful:
1. A tonic phase is absent.
2. Clonic movements of the head are side to side, rather than flexion extension (a pathognomonic sign).
3. Pupils are reactive (patients often resist having their eyes opened, unlike in true seizures).
4. Gaze is not fixed. When the eyes are opened, patient appears to look briefly at the examiner.
5. Clonic movements are out of phase between upper extremities and lower extremities.
6. There is minimal or no postictal confusion.
7. Pelvic thrusting occurs, which should be regarded as inconsistent with generalized tonic clonic grand mal seizure activity.

Management

William Shakespeare made many of his characters epileptic, including Julius Caesar, Othello, and Macbeth. After

Table 81.1

Classifications of Seizures

  I. Partial (focal) seizures, beginning locally
    A. Simple (usually no loss of consciousness)
      1. Motor
      2. Sensory
      3. Autonomic
      4. Psychic
    B. Complex (with impaired consciousness)
    C. Partial becoming generalized
  II. Generalized, bilaterally symmetric without local onset (involve loss of consciousness)
    A. Tonic clonic (grand mal)
    B. Absence (petite mal)
    C. Myoclonic seizures
    D. Clonic seizures
    E. Tonic seizures
    F. Atonic seizures
  III. Unclassifiable (because of inadequate data)

Macbeth suffers a seizure at a banquet, Lady Macbeth offers this still relevant council (Act III, scene iv):

> "Sit worthy friends, my lord is often thus and hath been from his youth. Pray you, keep seat. The fit is momentary upon a thought. He will again be well, if much you note him, you shall offend him and extend his passion. Feed, and regard him not."

Shakespeare understood the brief and self-limited nature of seizures and the principle of doing no harm.

In the ED, the spirit of this sage advice can be followed while ensuring patients' safety, using a typical ED approach. First ensure the ABCs. Also put in place an IV, oxygen, monitor, and a pulse oximeter. Do a brief examination during the postictal period to screen for injuries caused by or causing the ictus. Possible injuries include craniofacial trauma, tongue lacerations, extremity injuries, including dislocations, and vertebral column injuries. Later, the detailed medical and neurologic examination can be done to answer specific questions.

Take a brief history to screen for emergent conditions and to direct the pace of the subsequent management:

- Does the patient have a history of a seizure disorder?
- Fever?
- Head trauma?
- Ingestion?
- Diabetes mellitus?

For treatment, a coma cocktail, such as D50, Narcan, thiamine, should be considered.

Therapeutics

Should a seizure occur in the ED, benzodiazepines are the first-line drug for stopping seizures. It is important to note that they will not work to prophylax against any further seizure with one exception, the seizures caused by acute alcohol withdrawal. The choice of benzodiazepine is hotly debated, but many are effective if given in the right doses. The clinician should become proficient with one or two, and know the dosage range. Reasonable starting doses are Valium (diazepam) 0.2 to 0.5 mg/kg (2 to 5 mg IV, average adult dose); Ativan (lorazepam) 0.05 to 0.1 mg/kg (1 to 2 mg IV average, adult dose). If these doses prove ineffective, higher dosages should be given until the seizure is controlled. Respiratory depression occurs only at high doses, but is easily managed in the ED and represents a lesser threat to the patient than continued seizure activity.

Status Epilepticus

Status epilepticus can be defined as a single seizure lasting greater than 30 minutes, or two or more seizures without return to baseline level of consciousness in between. The previous definition of status epilepticus—seizures lasting longer than 1 hour—has been amended with the recognition that neuronal damage occurs more rapidly than was believed. While there are case reports of patients in status epilepticus for longer than 24 hours without demonstrable brain damage, it is now a consensus opinion that neuronal damage may begin as early as 90 minutes into a seizure. Benzodiazepines should continue to be administered intravenously during status epilepticus, but other drugs may need to be added to control the seizure activity.

The first-line drug to add to benzodiazepines is phenytoin, 18 mg/kg IV at 50 mg per minute maximum infusion rate (average adult dose 1 g over 20 minutes). The major side effects of phenytoin are hypotension and bradycardia, which are secondary to the vehicle it is suspended in—propylene glycol. Phenytoin should be avoided in bradycardia, conduction blocks, and congestive heart failure.

A prodrug formula version of phenytoin, fosphenytoin, has recently been approved for use in epilepsy, including status epilepticus. The dosage of fosphenytoin in status epilepticus is 15 to 20 mg phenytoin equivalent (PE)/kg administered at a maximum rate of 150 mg per minute IV. Fosphenytoin may offer several advantages over phenytoin for parenteral administration in that it is water-soluble. Therefore, the vehicle does not cause the same number of side effects. In addition, fosphenytoin can be infused more rapidly. It is a more expensive drug than phenytoin.

The third-line drug for status epilepticus is phenobarbital (dosage 8 to 20 mg/kg at 60 mg per min IV). Phenobarbital is synergistic with benzodiazepines for respiratory depression, and caution should be exercised when combining parenteral benzodiazepines and parenteral phenobarbital.

If none of these drugs controls the seizure activity, paraldehyde and lidocaine are mentioned as drugs occasionally effective for status epilepticus.

Definitive management of refractory status epilepticus requires general anesthesia with an inhalational anesthetic such as halothane. Paralytic drugs, such as succinylcholine and vecuronium, should be avoided unless continuous EEG monitoring is available. Paralytic drugs eliminate the motor signs of status epilepticus without affecting the epileptic neuronal discharge within the central nervous system. It is this electrical activity within the central nervous system that causes brain damage in status epilepticus and not the motor activity, hyperpyrexia, and acidosis associated with continuous seizure activity.

Laboratory Evaluation

Anticonvulsant levels should be obtained on all patients maintained on these drugs. It is reasonable to get routine laboratories on new-onset seizure patients, such as CBC, serum chemistries, glucose, and calcium levels. Although it is recognized that the utility of such laboratory evaluations is low, these tests are relatively inexpensive, easy to do, and may detect significant abnormalities 2% to 7% of the time. Other laboratory tests may be more selectively ordered, including a toxicology screen and alcohol level.

Neuroimaging

All first-time seizure patients should receive an emergent (in the ED) or urgent (arranged for the next morning) noncontrast head CT. Patients with focal neurologic deficits or altered mental status, persistent headache, history of cancer, history of anticoagulation, fever, recent trauma, or suspicion of AIDS should receive an emergent noncontrast head CT. Patients with typical febrile seizures (described below) or patients with typical recurrent seizures related to previously treated epilepsy are unlikely to have life-threatening structural lesions. These patients do not require emergent or urgent neuroimaging.

Lumbar Puncture

Lumbar puncture is not required in all first-time seizure patients. Lumbar puncture should be performed if meningitis is suspected or in a new-onset seizure in an immunocompromised host after a negative CT scan is obtained. Lumbar puncture may occasionally be used when subarachnoid hemorrhage is highly suspected, despite a negative CT scan.

Disposition

The disposition of seizure patients depends on the etiology of the seizure. For patients with chronic, treated epilepsy, once their anticonvulsant levels are checked and normalized, there is little else to do, and discharge from the ED is appropriate.

In first-time seizure patients, the workup in the ED should direct the disposition. Patients in whom significant abnormalities are detected by the standard medical evaluation (including history, physical, CBC, Chem 7, calcium, magnesium, tox screen, and CT of the head) should be admitted. A recent study estimates up to half of all first-time seizure patients require admission for significant abnormalities detected on the standard medical examination. If no abnormalities are detected with laboratory evaluation, CT scan, and lumbar puncture if indicated, the patients can be safely discharged with follow-up arranged for a primary care provider or a neurologist. Antiepileptics should not be prescribed for first-time seizure episodes.

The risk of recurrent seizure within the next 2 years, for a patient with an idiopathic seizure, ranges from 24% to 50%. A diligent search should be made in the patient's history to determine if any seizure activity may have oc-

curred in the remote past, as this raises the recurrence rate to 50% to 60%. The choice in placing that patient on antiepileptics can be made in consultation with the patient and a neurologist. In all cases, patients should have follow-up, which ensures that an EEG is performed on an outpatient basis.

Febrile Seizures

Unlike adults, children are at risk for seizures provoked by temperature elevation alone, without an underlying epileptogenic focus. From 2% to 5% of all children suffer at least one febrile seizure. There is a 30% risk of recurrent febrile seizures with subsequent febrile illnesses.

To be classified as a simple febrile seizure, the patient must meet the following definitional criteria:

1. Age between 5 months and 5 years (with peak incidence from 8 to 20 months).
2. The seizure must be generalized, not focal, in onset.
3. The seizure must last less than 15 minutes.
4. There can only be one febrile seizure per illness, although occasionally two febrile seizures may be seen within the same disease course.
5. The temperature must be greater than 38.5° C (101.3° F).

Evaluation of the Febrile Seizure

The evaluation of the febrile seizure patient should focus on determining the etiology of the fever and determining whether or not the potential for a central nervous system infection exists. In one study of febrile seizures, 73% of the patients were found to have an identifiable source of a fever, most commonly otitis media, but also encompassing viral infections such as upper respiratory infections. Shigella gastroenteritis has been reported to produce febrile seizures in as many as 10% to 45% of children infected, usually before the onset of the diarrhea. Roseola infantum is associated with an 8% incidence of febrile seizures, virtually always before the diagnostic rash is present.

Laboratory and Radiographic Studies

The National Institutes of Health consensus conference on febrile seizures has concluded that studies such as a complete blood count, serum electrolytes, calcium and glucose, and CT of the brain are rarely useful in uncomplicated febrile seizures. Appropriate radiographic and laboratory studies should be used as indicated to determine the source of the fever, such as chest x-ray and blood cultures. The incidence of occult bacteremia in febrile seizures appears to be no higher than the incidence in other febrile children.

Lumbar Puncture

The need for lumbar puncture in the evaluation of febrile seizures remains controversial. Isolated case reports exist of pediatric meningitis presenting with fever and seizure, but with no additional signs and symptoms. However, these cases have to be viewed as quite rare. A rational approach suggests that lumbar puncture is not indicated in the routine evaluation of a simple febrile seizure if the child looks well and has a normal neurologic examination after the seizure. Lumbar puncture should be considered in patients with the following factors:

1. Age less than 12 months
2. Complex febrile seizures
3. Meningeal signs
4. Lethargy and irritability
5. An abnormal neurologic examination
6. Potential for partially treated meningitis, such as a patient on oral antibiotics or having received parenteral antibiotics within the last 72 hours.

Disposition

The disposition is based on the illness diagnosed in the ED. Febrile seizures in and of themselves do not require treatment with anticonvulsants. Parents should be advised that subsequent febrile seizures are possible and even likely. The parents may need to be reassured about the likelihood of future epilepsy. In the absence of other risk factors, febrile seizures do not significantly increase the likelihood that a child will develop idiopathic epilepsy.

Partial Seizures

Partial seizures represent electrical storm in an isolated section of the brain. Most often focal motor, they may also become generalized if the ictus spreads. Consciousness may be impaired during partial seizures depending on the region of the brain involved, and confusingly, consciousness may be only partly affected, with the patient still able to follow certain (usually simple) commands or even perform common activities of daily life.

Partial seizures in the ED respond to the same therapeutics as generalized seizures, including benzodiazepines. Suspected complex status epilepticus ("nonconvulsive status") usually requires emergent consultation with a neurologist for diagnosis and management.

Alcohol-Related Seizures

Chronic alcoholics are frequent visitors to the ED and occasionally present with one of the complications of alcoholism, that is, alcohol-related seizures.

The term "alcohol withdrawal seizure" is no longer thought to be appropriate, as it does not adequately define the spectrum of the disease. Alcohol-related seizures can occur anywhere in the course of a patient's intoxication, although most frequently they are seen during the withdrawal phase from alcohol.

The first-time suspected alcohol-related seizure should be treated as any new-onset seizure disorder, with the recommendations listed above. In patients with documented alcohol-related or alcohol-withdrawal seizures who present to the ED with another episode of alcohol-related seizure, the evaluation and the disposition are based on the medical status of the patient.

A prudent approach to the chronic alcoholic, who has suffered one or more new or recurrent alcohol-related seizures, is to observe the patient in the ED for signs of alcohol withdrawal over a period of at least 6 hours. If the patient exhibits the signs and symptoms of acute alcohol withdrawal, admission should be made to the hospital. If no signs or symptoms of alcohol withdrawal develop within the observation period and the patient has no further seizures, the patient may be safely discharged from the ED provided there is an adequate living situation with support for the patient's safety.

Antiepileptics

Antiepileptics have no role in the management of alcohol-related seizures, and may in fact be detrimental to the patient's health. Benzodiazepines should not be prescribed on an outpatient basis. If the patient is felt to warrant benzodiazepines to stave off alcohol-withdrawal syndrome or alcohol-withdrawal seizures, the patient should be admitted to the hospital to be medically managed. Alcoholic patients with abnormal neurologic examinations or in status epilepticus warrant emergent evaluation including emergent cranial non-contrast CT scanning followed by admission to the hospital for observation.

Summary

Seizures are a frequent presenting complaint to the ED, and they challenge the clinician on a daily basis. With careful consideration and knowledge we may become as sanguine as Lady Macbeth, assured that the fit is momentary and the patient will again be well.

Selected Readings

D'Onofrio G, Niels K, et al. Lorazepam for the prevention of recurrent seizures related to alcohol. *N Engl J Med* 1999;340:915–919.

James J, Riviello M Jr. Classification of seizures and epilepsy. *Curr Neuro Neurosci Rep* 2003;3:325–331.

National Institutes of Health. Febrile Seizures Fact Sheet. NIH Publication No. 95-3930. Bethesda, Maryland 20892–2540, 1995.

NIH Consensus statements: medical management of epilepsy. *Neurology* 1998;51: S39–S43.

Shakespeare, W. *Macbeth*. London: Oxford University Press 1914.

Steven Go

Introduction

Headache is a common presenting complaint in the emergency department (ED) and accounts for approximately 1% to 2% of all patient visits. Epidemiologic studies reveal that 70% to 90% of the general population experience at least one headache annually. Although most headaches are benign and require only supportive care, life-threatening causes of headache must be rapidly distinguished from the former to increase the chances of a favorable outcome. The causes of headache are legion. This chapter focuses on the most lethal and disabling causes.

Triage and Clinical Assessment

The initial triage evaluation should focus on the presence of high-risk factors such as fever, trauma, sudden or new-onset, ocular pain, prior neurosurgical procedure, or atypical headache. Vital signs, mental status and gross neurologic function should be noted. Any abnormality should increase the priority for rapid evaluation and treatment. The screening examination should consist of a more detailed history and physical examination, including thorough HEENT (head, ears, eyes, nose, and throat), ophthalmic, neck and neurologic examinations. Patients may require further testing such as laboratory studies, neuroimaging, and lumbar puncture (LP).

Radiologic Evaluation

The medical literature varies on which patients require neuroimaging in the ED. However, published indications for obtaining an emergent non-contrast head CT scan have included new-onset of headache (especially in patients at the extremes of age, immunocompromised, pregnant, or cancer patients), worst headache, headache of acute sudden-onset (including awakening from sleep), change in headache quality, severity, or pattern, neurologic symptoms lasting longer than one hour, headaches triggered by exertion, Valsalva, or sexual activity, or any abnormal findings on a neurologic examination (including changes in mental status). Response to therapy should not be used as the sole diagnostic indicator of the underlying etiology of an acute headache or whether or not a CT should be performed.

Meningitis

Meningitis presents classically with a fever, headache, and nuchal rigidity. Bacterial meningitis, if untreated, carries a 90% mortality rate, and its survivors may have severe developmental disabilities or neurologic sequelae. Even when treated, mortality is not infrequent. Risk factors include chronic disease and immunocompromised states.

The bacteriology of meningitis is influenced by age. While *Streptococcus pneumoniae* is now the most common cause of bacterial meningitis overall in the United States, *Neisseria meningitidis* predominates in children and adolescents. Group B *Streptococci* spp., *Listeria monocytogenes*, and enteric Gram-negative rods can cause newborn meningitis. Three epidemiological trends have been identified: *Haemophilus influenzae* meningitis in children has declined dramatically due to routine vaccination, bacterial meningitis is now a disease of adults rather than children, and β-lactam resistant strains of *Streptococcus pneumoniae* have emerged. Other causes of meningitis include herpes simplex, arboviruses, tuberculosis, cryptococcus, toxoplasmosis, and fungi.

Many patients have a history of 1 to 3 days of fever, headache, and neck stiffness, malaise, nausea, photophobia, and lethargy; however, classic triad of symptoms occurs in only two-thirds of cases. These symptoms may be difficult to assess in the very young and very old, and the physical examination may reveal only irritability or lethargy. Signs of meningeal irritation such as Kernig's or Brudzinski's sign should be elicited. An elevated white blood cell count is often present, but is neither sensitive nor specific.

Empiric parenteral antimicrobial therapy based on the patient's age group and comorbidities must be started as soon as possible, and should not be delayed for test results or ancillary studies. Typically, a third-generation cephalosporin is used, with ampicillin added in patients less than 3 years old or less than 50 years old. Immunocompromised patients require coverage for *Pseudomonas aeruginosa* and enhanced Gram-negative and listeria coverage. Vancomycin may be required for resistant *Streptococcus pneumoniae*, as well as in recent post-neurosurgical patients (who must also have Gram-negative coverage). Antibiotic therapy given one to two hours prior to LP will not decrease the sensitivity of the LP, as long as CSF cultures are done. In addition, prophylactic therapy for all exposed individuals, including health care workers, should be considered.

Recent studies suggest that dexamethasone (0.15 mg/kg every 6 hours) should be given with or just before antibiotics in children with meningitis to prevent unfavorable neurologic sequelae secondary to bacterial lysis. A recent landmark study strongly suggests that adults with meningitis should be given dexamethasone simultaneously with antibiotics, as well. An important caveat is that dexamethasone should probably be avoided in patients with septic shock, as this therapy may be deleterious in patients with inadequate adrenal function.

The diagnostic procedure of choice remains the LP. In bacterial meningitis, the LP may reveal CSF pleocytosis with a neutrophilic predominance, glucose less than 40% of the serum glucose, and elevated protein. Viral infection of the CNS tends to produce a lymphocytic predominance. Cerebrospinal fluid Gram staining and bacterial antigen detection is important to identify the pathogen and gauge therapy. The question of whether a head CT scan is required prior to LP has been studied in recent years. Preliminary data suggest that adults with signs of increased intracranial pressure, altered mental status, or focal neurological deficits should have a CT prior to LP; however, other criteria such as immunocompromised state and history of cancer have also been proposed. Clinical judgment must suffice until further studies can be done to definitively answer this question.

Subarachnoid Hemorrhage

The hallmark of subarachnoid hemorrhage (SAH) is the familiar sudden onset of the "worst headache of my life" (the aptly named "thunderclap" headache). The peak incidence occurs in the fourth decade of life, with females and blacks carrying a higher risk. Risk factors also include smoking, a family history of aneurysmal disease, and underlying collagen vascular disease. SAH is caused by aneurysm in 75% of cases (present in 0.5 to 6% of the general population), and by arteriovascular malformations in 10%. The remaining 15% are associated with trauma, vasculitis, and other etiologies.

The thunderclap headache may be associated with exertion, a transient loss of consciousness, nausea and vomiting, and altered level of consciousness. Vital signs may reveal hypertension and a low-grade fever. Ocular findings of papilledema, retinal hemorrhage, third and sixth nerve palsies, and nystagmus can occur, along with nuchal rigidity. Any or all of these associated symptoms and signs may be present or absent. Tachycardia and ST-T wave changes on the ECG are extremely common, and have sometimes led to the misdiagnosis of an acute coronary event.

The headache may represent a "warning" or "sentinel" leak—a severe headache that occurs a mean of 2 weeks before a more severe bleed. Roughly 50% of these headaches present with atypical traits. In addition, these warning headaches may last only hours and then resolve spontaneously or with mild analgesia, thus fooling clinicians into thinking they are benign. Sometimes SAH patients who fall due to syncope are mistakenly assumed to have bled from trauma. For all of these reasons, the initial presentation of SAH is misdiagnosed 23% to 53% of the time, with sometimes devastating results.

Due to its rapid availability, greater sensitivity than MRI, and cost-effectiveness, the non-contrast CT scan remains the imaging modality of choice to detect early SAH. With third generation CT scanners, the sensitivity of detection of SAH has been reported to be 98% to 100% in the first 12 hours after onset, 93% in the first 24 hours, 85% at three days, and 50% at seven days. "Real world" sensitivity may actually be lower than suggested by the literature. Unlike in many research studies, in a typical community hospital, expert neuroradiologists will not often be available to detect subtle CT findings of SAH. In addition, anemic (hematocrit less than 30%) patients may have false-negative CT scans. Therefore, in the event of a normal CT scan, an LP is mandatory to make the diagnosis, as it will detect virtually all SAH. A diagnostic strategy of performing an LP without CT in selected patients has been proposed, but its clinical validity has yet to be established.

The cerebrospinal fluid typically has several thousand red blood cells present in SAH. Xanthochromia is usually present as early as 4 hours, to as late as 12 hours after hemorrhage, but may resolve by 2 weeks. Visual inspection, while not very accurate, may detect xanthochromia earlier than more precise photometric methods. The opening pressure should be measured, as an elevation may indicate the presence of a cerebral venous sinus thrombosis or pseudotumor cerebri, as well as help differentiate a traumatic LP from a true SAH, 66% of which have an elevated opening pressure. Traumatic LP may also be distinguished from an actual SAH by repeating the LP in an interspace above the initial site. Unfortunately, traditional methods of distinguishing traumatic LPs such as diminishing erythrocyte count in subsequent tubes (where red blood cells are still present in the last tube), operator impression, presence of crenated erythrocytes, and elevated D-dimer levels have been shown to be unreliable.

Once the diagnosis of SAH is made, emergent neurosurgical consultation is indicated, and vascular imaging performed if the patient is stable. SAH patients may require rapid sequence intubation to maintain the airway. Measures should be taken to prevent increase in intracranial pressure. For example, premedication prior to intubation, elevation of the head of the bed, avoidance of constricting tapes or devices around the neck. Dexamethasone (0.1 mg/kg IV) or mannitol (0.5 to 1 g/kg IV) may be given if evidence of increased intracranial pressure (ICP) exists. For awake patients, antiemetics such as prochlorperazine (10 mg IV every 6 hours) should be used to prevent emesis. Recent data suggest that hyperventilation is to be avoided, and the CO_2 should be kept within normal limits in order to maintain cerebral perfusion. Further treatment should be directed toward the control of hypertension (nitroprusside), cerebral vasospasm (nimodipine 60 mg orally every 4 hours), and seizure (benzodiazepines or phenytoin). Such interventions should be performed in consultation with the neurosurgeon. Serial neurologic examinations are essential in monitoring for changes in mental or physical status, which may indicate vasospasm or rebleeding. ICP monitoring or acute surgical decompression may be required, although the timing is controversial.

Other Intracranial Hemorrhages

Epidural hematoma is usually secondary to trauma and subsequent rupture of epidural vessels, commonly the middle meningeal artery. Skull fracture along the middle meningeal groove secondary to a direct blow is commonly associated. Rapid progression of bleeding and uncal herniation can occur. Prompt neurosurgical intervention is essential in preventing morbidity and mortality.

Subdural hematoma may be acute or chronic. Patients present with a history of trauma or headache with depressed mental status out of proportion to findings. Rupture of bridging veins occurs more readily after minor trauma in patients with atrophy. Elderly patients or alcoholics with forgotten minor trauma or an atraumatic history may have a chronic subdural hematoma. Acute subdural hematomas are usually associated with significant trauma, and patients are often unable to give a history.

Acute Angle Closure Glaucoma

Acute angle closure glaucoma presents with headache, eye pain, cloudy vision, colored halos around lights, conjunctival injection, a fixed, mid-dilated pupil, and increased IOP of 40 to 70 mm Hg (normal range: 10 to 20 mm Hg), with nausea and vomiting. Sudden attacks in patients with narrow anterior chamber angles can be precipitated in movie theaters, while reading, and after use of dilatory agents or inhaled anticholinergics. Treatment is begun in a step-wise fashion to decrease the IOP and may include topical timolol, apraclonidine, prednisone, pilocarpine, and systemic acetazolamide or mannitol. Symptoms of pain and nausea should be treated, and the IOP monitored hourly. Immediate ophthalmologic consultation is required.

Temporal Arteritis (Giant Cell Arteritis)

Temporal arteritis is a systemic vasculitis that can present with temporal headache, jaw claudication, diplopia, scalp, and temporal artery tenderness. Patients are typically women younger than 55 years of age, often with a history of polymyalgia rheumatica, and nonspecific constitutional complaints. The physical exam is frequently unremarkable, but temporal artery abnormalities and evidence of ischemic optic neuropathy, retinal artery occlusion, or a visual field cut may be present. An erythrocyte sedimentation rate (ESR) and C-reactive protein are often elevated. The presence of jaw claudication and diplopia increase the likelihood of a positive biopsy. If the ESR is normal, temporal arteritis is unlikely. If there is strong suspicion of temporal arteritis or vision loss is present, the patient should be admitted for intravenous methylprednisolone. For less suspicious patients with no vision loss, they may be discharged with prednisone and close follow-up. Steroids should probably not be delayed pending results of a confirmatory biopsy.

Carbon Monoxide Poisoning

Carbon monoxide (CO) poisoning may present with number of symptoms, including headache, dizziness, weakness, nausea, shortness of breath, seizures, and coma. It occurs most commonly during cold weather and from occupational or intentional exposures. Classic findings of red lips and cyanosis occur rarely. Carboxyhemoglobin levels often do not correlate well with symptoms. Measurement of ambient CO at the scene by prehospital personnel may help in the diagnosis. Administration of 100% O_2 is the first-line therapy. Hyperbaric oxygen (HBO) therapy is the treatment of choice in severe poisoning. Patients with abnormal levels of consciousness, CO level greater than 40% (15% in pregnancy), evidence of cardiac or pulmonary dysfunction, significant acidosis or symptoms, despite 6 hours of 100% O_2, should be considered for HBO therapy.

Migraine Headaches

Migraines present frequently as episodic attacks of moderate to severe, unilateral, throbbing headaches, which typically get worse with movement. Nausea, vomiting, photophobia, and phonophobia are often present, and migraines can occur with or without an aura (usually visual). Untreated migraines generally last between 4 to 72 hours. Migraine attacks may be precipitated by stimuli such as odors, stress, fatigue, foods, alcohol, medications, and menstruation. In North America, more than 2.5 million persons have at least 1 day of migraine per week, with the highest incidence in young females. Most never present to the ED. Despite extensive study, the precise pathogenesis of migraines remains unclear.

Diagnosis is made primarily by history and physical exam, with careful attention to the presence or absence of typical features. In a first or atypical presentation, neuroimaging may be needed to rule out other etiologies. An LP may be needed to exclude subarachnoid hemorrhage, infection, or pseudotumor cerebri.

For many patients, prompt treatment with non-narcotic pain medications may relieve symptoms as long as the dose is adequate (e.g., 900 mg of aspirin, 1,000 mg of acetaminophen, 500 to 1,000 mg of naproxen). Parenteral phenothiazines such as chlorpromazine, prochlorperazine, and metoclopramide are effective in acute migraine. Combining 900 mg aspirin with 10 mg oral metoclopramide is as efficacious as 100 mg sumatriptan orally, when compared with placebo. Narcotics such as meperidine, morphine, or codeine may also be considered, but many experts caution against their use, citing their abuse potential.

Triptans have become the treatment of choice in many centers. Evidence based dosages and indications have been shown to be safe and effective, but triptans are expensive and are contraindicated in patients with uncontrolled hypertension, coronary artery disease, and cerebrovascular disease. Sumatriptan (50 to 100 mg orally or 6 mg subcutaneously) has been used extensively, but several studies indicate some of the newer triptans may be superior. In addition, recent studies have shown that patients who take triptans during the mild phase of an attack are more likely to have rapid relief of headache and lower rates of recurrence. Intranasal sumatriptan (20 mg) is the only triptan shown effective in adolescents.

Ergot derivatives have a venerable history, but are less commonly used today. They are cost effective, but have several important limitations, including the lack of evidence for effective doses, vasoconstrictor effects, tolerance, and rebound headaches. They should be used with caution in patients with coronary artery disease, peripheral vascular disease, hypertension, hepatic disease, renal failure, and pregnancy.

A recent study suggested that a stratified approach to treatment of acute migraines (with therapy tailored to severity of symptoms) resulted in improved headache response and reduced disability time compared to that of traditional step-wise care (escalating treatment if the first-line treatments fail). BIBN 4096 BS, one of a new class of drugs, calcitonin gene-related peptide (CGRP)-receptor antagonists, has recently shown efficacy similar to the triptans, without the untoward cardiovascular effects; however, its promise awaits confirmation with further studies.

Preventive therapies such as amitriptyline, divalproex sodium, and propranolol should be considered in consultation with the patient's primary physician. The patient should be educated with regards to lifestyle suggestions that may help prevent acute attacks (regulation of meals, exercise, and sleep, avoidance of triggers and migraine-inducing food and drugs).

Cluster Headaches

Cluster headaches typically present as unilateral periorbital pain that lasts a few minutes to hours. There may be a prodromal syndrome similar to other vascular headaches, as well as rhinorrhea, a feeling of nasal congestion, lacrimation, or miosis on the ipsilateral side of the face. Patients may have long intervals of time, months to years, between paroxysms of pain. However, attacks may occur several times per day, lasting for weeks to months. Stress, alcohol, and nitrates may be triggers. First-line treatment includes 100% oxygen at 7 to 12 L per minute. Sumatriptan (6 mg subcutaneously) is the only highly effective abortive agent, but parenteral dihydroergotamine, ipsilateral intranasal lidocaine, and intranasal sumatriptan may be useful. Ergotamine tartrate, corticosteroids, verapamil, methysergide, or lithium may be used as prophy-

laxis. Ablation of the trigeminal ganglia has been successful in selected resistant cases.

Tension Headache

Tension headache is typically described as a band-like, bilateral ache or pressure sensation. The headache is usually constant, but may vary in intensity, frequency, and duration. It rarely interferes with sleep, and associated depression may be present. Prodromal symptoms or focal neurologic findings are absent. Tension headaches are common in the general population, but recent research suggests that ED physicians markedly overdiagnose this entity. Treatment consists of oral analgesics to be used only 2 or 3 times a week. Muscle relaxants are not useful. Some patients with chronic tension headache may benefit from amitriptyline and stress management. Counseling and relaxation techniques may be effective.

Tumor

In general, tumors are an unusual cause of headaches in the ED. Headaches that are worse in the morning may indicate a tumor causing increased intracranial pressure (ICP). The initial evaluation may be nonfocal. ED neuroimaging of patients who present with evidence of increased ICP, new seizure, new onset headache in cancer patients or focal neurologic deficit is indicated. Neurosurgical consultation should be obtained when the diagnosis is made.

Brain or Parameningeal Abscess

Findings consistent with increased ICP may be the only evidence of intracranial abscess, since fever is present in only 50% of patients. Patients with sustained bacteremia (IV drug abusers, immunocompromised) or adjacent infections (sinusitis, otitis media, mastoiditis) are at higher risk. Signs of meningeal irritation are rare, and immunocompromised patients may look either well or ill. A CT scan with contrast is very sensitive. LP may be necessary if meningismus is present and CT is negative. Emergent neurosurgical consultation is warranted.

Pseudotumor Cerebri (Benign Intracranial Hypertension)

Pseudotumor cerebri presents as a headache with signs of increased ICP, diplopia, and transient vision obscurations, and is most common in middle aged, obese females. Headaches are typically worse in the morning, and exacerbated by Valsalva. Visual acuity may be preserved even with evidence of papilledema on funduscopic examination, but visual field defects may develop. The diagnosis is made with a normal CT scan and an elevated ICP on an LP. Treatment aimed at alleviating symptoms and preserving sight may include acetazolamide and prednisone (if severe papilledema and visual compromise are present). Consultation with a neurologist is indicated. Optic nerve sheath fenestration and lumboperitoneal shunting are options if maximal medical treatment fails. Repeated LPs are no longer the standard of care.

Acute Stroke

Headache is seen in 25% to 38% of all patients with acute stroke, more commonly in those patients with hemorrhagic events. Typically, transient ischemic attacks of the internal carotid system usually produce frontal headache, while the vertebrobasilar artery system causes occipital headache. An ipsilateral headache and focal neurologic deficit are common. CT scan is the diagnostic study of choice. Current controversies regarding acute stroke therapy are beyond the scope of this chapter, but thrombolysis in selected subsets of patients may be beneficial.

Trigeminal Neuralgia (Tic Douloureaux)

Trigeminal neuralgia is an idiopathic disorder, characterized by sharp, severe, stabbing pains along one or more of the branches of the trigeminal nerve. It typically affects patients over 50 years of age and women more than men. It is often triggered by seemingly innocuous factors such as wind exposure, touch, eating, brushing teeth or shaving. The diagnosis is made by excluding other causes of facial pain by history and physician examination. Carbamazepine (100 bid) or phenytoin (300 mg per day) has been shown to be effective. Baclofen (50 mg per day divided tid) may be used as a second-line treatment. Surgery may be useful for refractory cases, but the evidence for its effectiveness is largely anecdotal. Spontaneous remission may also occur.

Post-Lumbar Puncture Headache (PLPHA)

Thirty-two percent of patients who undergo lumbar puncture develop this complication. PLPHA typically occurs hours after the procedure and is due to low CSF pressure secondary to leakage of CSF into the epidural space. Standing exacerbates the pain, and nausea and vomiting are common. Using smaller needle sizes, keeping the flat part of the needle bevel parallel to the dural fibers, replacing the stylet before withdrawing the needle, and using atraumatic, non-cutting needles are all associated with a decreased incidence of PLPHA. Treatment includes analgesia and antiemetics. No firm evidence exists that withdrawing less spinal fluid, prolonged direct pressure on the site, post-procedural bed rest, increased hydration, or caffeine either reduce the incidence or are effective in the treatment of spinal headache. If first-line treatments fail, autologous epidural blood patching appears to be effective in many patients; however, adequately powered randomized trials supporting this procedure's efficacy are currently lacking.

Temporomandibular Joint Syndrome (TMJ)

Headache related to this disorder is usually unilateral, aching, and begins right after chewing. Joint noises, limitation of jaw opening, crepitus, and tenderness over the joint may be evident on physical examination. TMJ is regarded as a multifactoral syndrome, including physical, affective, and cognitive components. Treatment includes mild analgesia and referral to a qualified oral surgeon for evaluation.

Special Considerations

Headache in Pregnancy

Pregnancy has been associated with exacerbation and improvement of migraines and tension headaches through a variety of vascular, neuroregulatory, and hormonal mechanisms. Acute strokes, cerebral venous thrombosis, accelerated growth of meningiomas and pituitary adenomas, subarachnoid hemorrhage, and pseudotumor cerebri are associated with pregnancy. Preeclampsia is an important cause of headache and must be ruled out after the twentieth week of gestation. LPs can be performed safely during pregnancy, and normal values for CSF do not change. MRI without contrast is thought to be safer than CT during pregnancy, and special care should be taken to avoid medications contraindicated in pregnancy when treating these patients.

Geriatric Headache

Headaches in the elderly are less common but are more likely to be caused by serious illness than in younger adults. Therefore, it is important to aggressively seek serious etiologies in these patients, and refrain from defaulting to diagnoses of exclusion, such as tension headache. The emergency physician should have a low threshold for neuroimaging and LP in these patients.

Pediatric Headache

In one recent study, nearly half of headaches in children presenting to a pediatric ED were secondary to viral and respiratory illness and minor head trauma, and required minimal, if any, pharmacologic treatment. However, approximately 7% of children had serious etiologies, such as intracranial hemorrhages and infections. The authors suggested that CT be reserved for those patients with high-risk presentations, as mentioned previously in this chapter.

Selected Readings

American College of Emergency Physicians. Clinical policy for the initial approach to adolescents and adults presenting to the emergency department with a chief complaint of headache. *Ann Emerg Med* 2002;39:108–122.

Brazis PW. Pseudotumor cerebri. *Curr Neurol Neurosci Rep* 2004;4:1111–1116.

de Gans J, van de Beek D. Dexamethasone in adults with bacterial meningitis. *N Engl J Med* 2002;347:1549–1556.

Delzell JE, Greele AR. Trigeminal neuralgia. New treatment options for a well-known cause of facial pain. *Arch Fam Med* 1999;8:264–268.

Durham PL. CGRP-receptor antagonists—a fresh approach to migraine therapy? *N Engl J Med* 2004;350:1073–1075.

Edlow JA. Diagnosis of subarachnoid hemorrhage in the emergency department. *Emerg Med Clin N Am* 2003;21:73–87.

Ernst A, Zibrak JD. Carbon monoxide poisoning. *N Engl J Med* 1998;339:1603–1608.

Goadsby PJ, Lipton RB, Ferrari MD. Migraine—current understanding and treatment. *N Engl J Med* 2002;346:257–270.

Headache Classification Subcommittee of the International Headache Society. The international classification of headache disorders, 2d ed. *Cephalalgia* 2004; 24:1–151.

Kan L, Nagelberg J, Maytal J. Headaches in a pediatric emergency department: etiology, imaging and treatment. *Headache* 2000;40:25–29.

Kaniecki R. Headache assessment and management. *JAMA* 2003;289:1430–1433.

Lin W, Geiderman J. Myth: fluids, bed rest, and caffeine are effective in preventing and treating patients with post-lumbar puncture headache. *West J Med* 2002;176:69–70.

Lipton RB, Stewart WF, Stone AM, et al. Stratified care vs step care strategies for migraine. The disability in strategies of care (DISC) study: a randomized trial. *JAMA* 2000;284:2599–2605.

Marcus DA. Headache in pregnancy. *Curr Pain Head Rep* 2003;7:288–296.

Schull MJ. Lumbar puncture first: an alternative model for the investigation of lone acute sudden headache. *Acad Emerg Med* 1999;6:131–136.

Smetana GW, Shmerling RH. Does this patient have temporal arteritis? *JAMA* 2002;287:92–101.

Ward TN. Headache disorders in the elderly. *Curr Treat Opt Neuro* 2002;4:403–408.

83 Tumors of the Central Nervous System

James Winslow III

Tumors of the Central Nervous System

Cancer of the central nervous system (CNS) is a serious and complex disease. While some knowledge of the different type of tumors is important, emergency physicians must be able to identify the common presenting signs and symptoms of CNS tumors. They should also be able to recognize and manage the potentially serious sequelae of CNS tumors.

Epidemiology

Cancer in the CNS is a rare entity, representing 2% of all cancers. However, because of the aggressive nature of many CNS malignancies and their proximity to vital CNS structures, they are the fourth leading cause of cancer-related deaths in adults. CNS tumors are the most common type of solid tumor in children and rank second among all causes of childhood malignancy.[1] From 1992 to 1997 the annual incidence for all CNS tumors was 12.7 per 100,000 persons per year.[2] In individuals younger than 35 years of age, the incidence of metastatic tumors found in the brain is 1 : 100,000. That figure increases to 30 : 100,000 by the age of 60. The ages of those diagnosed with CNS tumors fall into a bimodal distribution. The first peak occurs in early childhood. The most common tumors in children are cerebellar astrocytomas and medulloblastomas. Fifty-five percent of CNS tumors in children are found below the tentorium.[1] The second peak is found in individuals in their 5th and 6th decades. Adults more commonly have CNS metastases, as well as gliomas and primary CNS lymphomas.[3]) Around 55% of tumors are in the posterior fossa or are infratentorial. The other 45% are supratentorial.[1] The American Cancer Society states that the lifetime risk of developing a CNS malignancy at 0.67% for men and 0.52% for women.[2]

Etiology and Pathophysiology

The cause of most CNS tumors is unknown. To date few tumors have been linked to heredity. The neurophakomatosis of von Recklinghausen neurofibromatosis, von Hippel–Lindau hemangioblastoma, and tuberous sclerosis are syndromes in which individuals have a higher incidence of CNS tumors than in the general population. Oncogenic viruses and chemical carcinogens can produce CNS tumors in animal models, but their role in humans is still speculative. Embryologic factors are responsible for the rare congenital pineoblastomas, teratomas, and germinomas. Some evidence exists for meningiomas forming along fracture lines in the cranium. Research into the associations between workers exposed to radiation in the fields of dentistry and medicine and CNS tumors is ongoing. No association has been shown between the frequent use of cellular phones and exposure to high-tension electrical lines. The only know risk factor for CNS tumors is exposure to ionizing radiation which increases the risk of nerve sheath tumors, meningiomas, and gliomas.[2] Many of the neurologic complications of CNS tumors result from increases in intracranial pressure (ICP). This may result directly from the tumor mass, or from cerebral edema due to altered capillary permeability. As the tumor infiltrates normal brain tissue, there can be obstruction of venous drainage in the brain or obstruction of cerebrospinal fluid (CSF) flow contributing to elevations in ICP. Necrosis and hemorrhage into the tumor may also elevate ICP. The nature and severity of symptoms resulting from an encroaching mass depends on the location of the tumor and the rate of its growth. Slowly growing tumors can often be accommodated initially. When masses grow larger than 3 cm, they compress the brain, its blood supply, and the adjacent neuronal pathways. The mass effect is exacerbated by vasogenic edema around the tumor. The severity of neurologic complications resulting from CNS tumors does not always correlate with the degree of malignancy found on histologic evaluation of the tumor. For example, some glial cell tumors that histologically are not malignant may grow to a large size, and although they do not invade surrounding tissue, they result in compression and displacement of crucial structures of the brain. These particular cases may have as poor a prognosis as a more invasive, malignant tumor. A relatively benign tumor may have lethal consequences if the risks of surgical excision are considered too high due to critical adjacent CNS structures. Signs of increased ICP can include headache, nausea, vomiting, drowsiness, and visual abnormalities.[3] Symptoms may be more prominent in the morning. Metastatic tumors are more likely than primary CNS tumors to produce symptoms evolving over days to weeks. Metastases from lung, melanoma, renal cell carcinoma, choriocarcinoma, and thyroid carcinoma can hemorrhage, causing rapid onset of neurologic symptoms. Oligodendrogliomas and malignant astrocytomas are the only two primary CNS tumors likely to cause hemorrhage. CNS malignancies can spread to the subarachnoid space but rarely metastasize outside the CNS. Neurologic complications can arise from cancer outside the CNS as well as from chemotherapy and radiation therapy for systemic cancer. Some systemic cancers cause cerebral vascular disease, leading to multiple cerebral infarcts. Disseminated intravascular coagulation, or consumptive coagulopathy, a complication of lymphoma and leukemia, can cause encephalopathy from multiple infarcts. Nonbacterial, thrombotic endocarditis can send emboli to the brain, resulting in focal neurologic findings. Thrombocytopenia and altered coagulation are complications of numerous cancers, which can lead to intracranial hemorrhage.

Natural History

The progression of symptoms of intracranial tumors and prognosis depends on the location in the brain as well as the growth characteristics of the specific tumor type. Slow growing tumors in relatively silent regions like the frontal lobes can reach large sizes before manifesting symptoms or signs. Conversely, any small mass near vital structures can produce profound neurologic signs and symptoms. It is for this reason that the distinction between benign and malignant tumors bears less importance than their location.

Signs and Symptoms

Headache

Headache results from compression or tension on pain-sensitive intracranial structures, the dura, blood vessels, and cranial nerves, due to increased intracranial pressure, edema, or hydrocephalus. The brain tissue itself has no pain receptors. Headache occurs in roughly half of all patients with intracranial neoplasms.[4] Headaches present as the initial symptom with or without signs of increased intracranial pressure 20% of the time. The location of headaches occurring as a result of intracranial tumors is usually diffuse, but is sometimes located over the hemisphere where the tumor is located.[4] The patient who presents with a headache due to a brain tumor describes the headache as recent in onset, or with a change in the usual character of previous headaches. Headaches resulting from intracranial tumors usually go away over a few hours even without treatment.[4] The character of headaches resulting from intracranial tumors may be throbbing, similar in character to migraines and cluster headaches.[4] Initially the headache may be mild and intermittent. As the tumor grows, the headache becomes more severe, frequent, and persistent. The headache more often occurs in the morning as the patient awakens. As the patient becomes upright, drainage from the cranium is promoted, decreasing the intracranial pressure. Additionally,

the ventilation rate increases, and there is CNS vasoconstriction which further lowers the intracranial pressure. There may be associated vomiting with or without nausea. The headache is often made worse by Valsalva, bending forward, coughing or with sudden head movements. Any headache associated with seizure activity, abnormal mental status, focal neurologic signs or papilledema must be considered a brain tumor until this possibility is appropriately ruled out.

Seizures

The seizures that are caused by brain tumors are usually focal, but may be generalized. Todd's paralysis can indicate the location of the tumor. The seizure threshold is lowered when brain tissue is infiltrated by tumor, or when it is mechanically compressed by tumor; 35% of CNS tumors are associated with seizures, and 15% to 19% of people with brain tumors present with seizures. The exact percentage depends on the location and type of tumor.[4] With patients who present with seizures and a focal neurologic finding, a tumor is responsible 50% of the time. When a patient presents in status epilepticus, 50% of patients without a prior history of seizures will be diagnosed with a CNS tumor. In patients younger than 20 years of age, seizures are very rare complications of tumors. The risk of seizure increases over the age of 20, especially when they are associated with a prolonged postictal period or Todd's paralysis. Seizures are associated with supratentorial tumors 50% of the time, but rarely with infratentorial lesions (<3%). New-onset seizures or a change in a previously documented seizure disorder suggests a brain tumor, especially when associated with focal motor, sensory, or psychomotor features. Certain patient groups with preexisting conditions are at high risk for a CNS lesion if they present with new-onset seizures. These include previously diagnosed systemic cancer, long-standing neurologic diseases including von Recklinghausen's disease and tuberous sclerosis, or patients presenting with acute or atypical psychiatric disorders. Certain seizure types can suggest the tumor location. Generalized, tonic-clonic seizures or focal motor seizures (known as Jacksonian march) occur with frontal tumors. A sensory march occurs with parietal lobe masses. Complex partial seizures can be caused by temporal lobe lesions. "Absence" seizures are usually not associated with CNS tumors.

Mental Status Changes

Behavioral changes caused by brain tumors can be subtle. Patients may be irritable, restless, apathetic, have difficulty sleeping or exhibit memory loss or loss of spontaneity. The symptoms can mimic psychiatric disorders including depression and Alzheimer's disease with a predominance of apathy. The patients themselves may be unaware of their behavior changes, and often they do not seek medical attention until focal neurologic deficits appear.

Vomiting

Vomiting occurs in 70% of patients with CNS tumors, but is the presenting complaint in only 10% of cases. Vomiting commonly occurs in the absence of nausea, without relation to food, and may be projectile in nature. When vomiting occurs together with headache, and papilledema, there is a high likelihood that the intracranial pressure is elevated.

Papilledema

Papilledema occurs in 10% of patients with CNS tumors. It is more common in children and young adults because in the elderly, brain atrophy results in greater accommodation of the mass effect and hydrocephalus before the intracranial pressure begins to rise.

Focal Neurologic Deficits

Focal neurologic deficits usually can be distinguished from transient ischemic episodes, strokes, and intraparenchymal bleeds by the slowness of symptom onset caused by tumors. Focal symptoms are caused by the intracranial location of the tumor. Patients may demonstrate aphasia, hemiparesis, sensory and visual deficits, and cranial nerve palsies. The sixth cranial nerve, which controls lateral gaze, has the longest intracranial course and is the nerve most commonly affected by increased intracranial pressure. Spinal cord lesions may present with sensory or motor findings, which correlate with the level of the lesion.

Presentation by Anatomic Location

The anatomic location of a CNS tumor determines whether signs are generalized or focal. The location of the tumor can also be neuroanatomically linked to focal neurologic symptoms and signs. Around 55% of tumors are in the posterior fossa or are infratentorial. The other 45% are supratentorial. Posterior fossa tumors can cause many different symptoms. Headaches, gait disturbances, ataxia, decreased coordination, head tilt, visual problems, cranial nerve problems, nerve deficits, vomiting when awakening in the morning, papilledema, hydrocephalus are some of the symptoms. Patients with supratentorial tumors will exhibit signs and symptoms consistent with the area of the brain affected. There can be seizures, hemiplegia, memory loss, impaired judgment, behavior changes, visual field cuts, hormonal insufficiency, handwriting problems, and hydrocephalus.[1]

Frontal Lobe

Tumors of the frontal lobe may grow to a large size and raise intracranial pressure before focal signs are present. Generalized phenomena like tonic-clonic seizures may occur. Slow changes, taking months to years, may occur. Dementia is an example. Personality changes may be manifested, especially in social behaviors such as inappropriate language, uninhibited behavior or actions without regard to the effect on other individuals. Patients may also show a decline in intellect and memory.

The parietal lobes house the postcentral gyrus, which is the seat of the somatosensory system. Left parietal masses can produce receptive aphasia and contralateral hemianopsia. Right parietal masses lead to spatial disorientation, constructional apraxia, and left homonymous hemianopsia.

Temporal Lobe

Seizures are often the initial presenting sign of temporal lobe masses. Complex partial seizures with gustatory, olfactory, auditory or visual hallucinations have occurred. Patients have also described a sensation of déjà vu with their temporal lobe seizures. Behavior changes associated with temporal lobe tumors differ from the frontal lobe presentation. Changes in affect more resemble psychosis rather than the dementia seen with frontal lobe masses. The personality changes may be subtle.

Occipital Lobe

Occipital lobe tumors are rare. They may cause visual hallucinations, flashing lights or colors, or contralateral visual loss.

Infratentorial Tumors

The infratentorial area is more difficult to visualize with CT and is better visualized with MRI. As with supratentorial tumors the symptoms of the tumor depends in the location of the tumor. Symptoms of midline tumors can cause headaches, nausea, vomiting, papilledema, nystagmus, visual field cuts, and difficultly with sense of smell.[1] Pons tumors can lead to facial movement problems, facial sensation deficit, ocular movement difficulty, and hearing deficits. Tumors of the medulla oblongata can affect taste and the gag reflex, lead to tongue fasciculations, cause changes in heart rate, and impair the spinal accessory muscles.[1]

Cerebellum

Cerebellar tumors are more commonly seen in the pediatric population than in adults. If the fourth ventricle is occluded, the ventricular system backs up and intracranial pressure increases. Medulloblastomas are typically midline cerebellar tumors, and they can cause ataxia. Astrocytomas of the cerebellum are frequently located laterally. They cause ataxia of the ipsilateral extremities, dysmetria, hypotonia, nystagmus, and intermittent decerebrate rigidity known as "cerebellar fits."

Cranial Nerves

Meningiomas may invade the olfactory groove causing a change in the sense of smell by invading cranial nerve I, the olfactory nerve. Supratentorial tumors of the frontal lobes can compress cranial nerve V. Patients may experience symptoms similar to trigeminal neuralgia. Cranial nerve VI has the longest path within the cranium and is the cranial nerve most frequently affected by a mass or increased intracranial pressure. The patient is unable to gaze laterally ipsilateral to the compressed nerve. Cranial nerve VIII lesions can occur in the presence of acoustic neuromas at the cerebellopontine angle. Patients present with neurosensory hearing loss and balance problems. Cranial nerves IX and X are compressed by infratentorial masses. They innervate cervical structures, and patients can experience cervical region pain.

Spinal Cord

Compression of the spinal cord takes place when tumor in the vertebrae compresses the dural sac. The most common presenting symptom is pain at the level of the lesion. The pain is sometimes radicular. Early detection of such lesions is critical in order to prevent permanent loss of neurologic function. Five percent of patients with lung cancer have extradural metastases.[5] The location of the metastases is usually the thoracic spine.[5] The next most common location is the lumbosacral spine. Cauda equina can result from spinal compression at this location. Breast and lung cancer are the most common malignancies leading to spinal cord compression. Prostate cancer is also a very common cause of spinal metastases. The main signs and symptoms are weakness, pain, autonomic deficits, ataxia, and sensory abnormalities. Autonomic deficits can include urinary retention. If a patient is suspected of having spinal cord compression a post void residual should be done. If the residual is greater than 150 cc, then a Foley catheter should be placed.[5] The emergency physician should have a very high index of suspicion for spinal cord compression secondary to metastases in any patient with back pain and a history of cancer. MRI is the best method of evaluation. High dose steroids and radiotherapy are the main treatments for metastatic lesions to the spinal cord. Surgery is usually not indicated unless there is collapse of bone or spinal instability.[6]

Leptomeningeal Metastasis (Meningeal Carcinomatosis)

Leptomeningeal metastasis (meningeal carcinomatosis is characterized by the spread of malignancy through the CSF. Meningiomas can also lead to meningeal carcinomatosis.[7] Multiple neurologic signs and symptoms, both generalized and focal, are possible depending on the region and extent of involvement of the neuro axis. Patients may exhibit headache, mental status changes, seizures, nuchal rigidity, and focal neurologic abnormalities. Cranial nerve abnormalities are seen in up to 50% of patients. The diagnosis is based on identifying positive cytology for malignant cells in the CSF. Multiple CSF examinations may be required to demonstrate malignant cells on cytology. MRI has a sensitivity of anywhere from 33% to 66%.[7] Treatment is focused on the entire leptomeningeal space and may include whole neuro axis radiation and intrathecal chemotherapy. The prognosis is poor.

Clinical Emergencies

Although slow, progressive clinical deterioration is most typically seen in patients with brain tumors, rapid deterioration can occur. The etiology of a rapid deterioration can be from intraneoplastic hemorrhage, herniation, increased ICP from hydrocephalus, or seizure activity.[8] Other causes of acute decompensation include abscess, and meningitis.

Hydrocephalus

Acute hydrocephalus is a rare complication that presents with severe headache leading to changes in mental status and even coma. It can remit and recur spontaneously and is thought to be due to a ball valve mechanism. This phenomenon is seen in children with tumors blocking the fourth ventricle and in adults with colloid cysts obstructing outflow of cerebrospinal fluid at the foramen of Monro.

Cerebral Herniation

Cerebral herniation occurs when the mass effect creates enough intracranial pressure to force the brain tissue through the rigid, noncompliant cranial vault. The brain tissue is forced caudally along the path of least resistance through structures such as the foramen magnum and the tentorium cerebelli. Three distinct herniation syndromes are described.

Uncal Herniation

Uncal herniation results from a lateral mass in one hemisphere displacing the medial temporal lobe (uncus) downward through the tentorial notch, compressing the upper brain stem and cranial nerve III. In the early stages, the parasympathetic fibers that run in the peripheral bundle of cranial nerve III are compressed and there is resultant unilateral fixed and dilated pupil. There may be progressive contralateral hemiparesis as the pyramidal motor column is compressed, contralateral Babinski sign, and spastic hypertonicity. In its late stages, both pupils become fixed and dilated, there is oculoparesis unresponsive to caloric testing, bilateral Babinski sign, and decerebration in response to pain. In the preterminal stage, as the midbrain is compressed, there is hyperventilation, which slows as death approaches. The pulse rises, and the blood pressure falls as the patient enters a syndrome of neurogenic shock.

Cerebellar Herniation

Cerebellar herniation results from a large posterior fossa mass that pushes the cerebellar tonsils through the foramen magnum, compressing the medulla and upper cervical spinal cord. The patient presents with rapidly decreasing level of consciousness, occipital headache, vomiting, hiccups, and meningismus. Preterminal signs of cardiovascular regulatory abnormalities include bradycardia, hypertension, and finally respiratory arrest.

Central Herniation

Central herniation results from a centrally located supratentorial lesion, which causes a downward and lateral shift of the diencephalon and upper pons. The patient presents with a slowly decreasing level of consciousness, small but equally reactive pupils, and Cheyne-Stokes respirations. Central herniation may present without focal signs and could be mistaken for toxic or metabolic encephalopathy.

Seizure Activity

Seizure activity is another emergent clinical entity with which the CNS tumor patient may present. The seizure threshold is lowered when brain tissue is infiltrated by tumor or when there is mechanical distortion of brain tissue by a mass. Seizures may, however, also occur due to infection, toxic-metabolic derangements like hyponatremia and uremia, and vascular problems including hemorrhage, all of which may be seen in the setting of a neoplasm. Seizure activity increases the brain's metabolic requirements, thereby increasing cerebral blood flow, which increases intracranial pressure. This places the seizing patient at risk for herniation. Besides herniation, the seizing patient is at risk for aspiration, anoxia, physical injury, acid-base disturbances, and metabolic derangements. The importance of maintaining the patient's airway, ensuring oxygenation, and supporting the patient's hemodynamic status can not be overstated. Insuring adequate blood glucose is also vital.

Infectious Complications

Patients with CNS tumors are at risk for developing serious infectious complications. There are many factors which put them at risk. Patients with intracranial tumors are often on immunosuppressive agents which make them vulnerable to infection. Such patients may also have had recent neurosurgical procedures, intracerebral devices, and long-term central venous catheters all of which place these patients at increased risk for CNS infections.[9] The different CNS infections include:

Meningitis

Patients with meningitis characteristically present with fever, headache, photophobia, meningismus, and altered mental status. In immunocompromised patients this fulminant picture my not develop and the symptoms may be more subtle.[9] Any patient with a fever and uncertain source should have a lumbar puncture performed. Altered mental status may be the only presenting symptom of meningitis. Steroids can complicate the clinical picture because they can blunt the immune response as well as the onset of fever. A CT to rule out increased intracranial pressure should be done prior to the spinal tap. *S. aureus*, *S. pneumoniae*, and *L. monocytogenes* are the most common microbes to cause meningitis. Patients who have had recent craniotomies may be more likely to develop meningitis from *S. aureus*, *S. epidermidis*, or *Propionibacterium acnes*.[9] Long-term venous catheters can increase the risk of meningitis from *Candida*, *Aspergillus*, and *Acinetobacter*. Cancer patients may also be coagulopathic or thrombocytopenic, which should be corrected before a lumbar puncture is done.

Brain Abscess

Up to 30% of CNS infections in cancer patients are brain abscesses. Symptoms of elevated intracranial pressure are seen, as well as lateralizing signs with fever. Neither CT or MRI can easily differentiate between a brain abscess or tumor.[9] Care must be taken if a lumbar puncture is to be performed since edema and mass effect are common. If mass effect is shown on CT or MRI then a lumbar puncture should not be done because there is a risk of herniation. Common organisms include Gram-negative rods, *Aspergillus*, *Phycomycetes* species, and *Toxoplasma gondii*.

Encephalitis

Encephalitis is rare, and may be difficult to distinguish from meningitis in the ED. Symptoms include headache, fever, and altered mental status. Encephalitis is associated with herpes zoster and *Toxoplasma gondii* infections. CT scan results range from normal to diffuse edema. Lumbar puncture shows pleocytosis, elevated protein, and no organisms. Polymerase chain reaction is the laboratory test that can be used to detect many possible causes of encephalitis including cytomegalovirus, enterovirus, herpes simplex virus, varicella-zoster virus, and others.[9] Chemotherapy may have toxic side effects that can mimic encephalitis. In addition to the infectious workup, if toxic metabolic causes are suspected, urine and serum toxic screen are required, as well as electrolytes, BUN, creatinine, glucose, calcium, arterial blood gas, and liver function tests.

Complications from Cranial Radiotherapy

Radiation, like most treatments for cancer, is cytotoxic to all cells. The incidence of complications from radiotherapy has decreased in incidence as the awareness of the danger of radiation has improved. The spectrum of complications includes acute radiation encephalopathy, delayed cerebral radionecrosis, the inducement of second primary tumors, and other non-neurologic side effects. Acute radiation induced encephalopathy can result in increased ICP that can cause death or permanent disability. Other symptoms may include seizure, headache, nausea, vomiting, fever, and progressive neurologic deficits. This syndrome usually begins within the first 24 hours. Later complications can include dementia, ataxia, personality changes, and personality change. Delayed symptoms due to radiation therapy may begin 6 to 24 months after finishing treatment. Non-neurological side-effects can include increased fatigue, loss of taste and appetite, decreased hearing, and loss of hair.[10]

Chemotherapy Complications

Antineoplastic chemotherapeutic agents may produce a wide variety of neurologic symptoms easily confused with CNS tumor recurrence, tumor progression, or other CNS disease processes. Nitrosourea can produce encephalopathy. Cisplatin can cause peripheral sensory neuropathy. Nitrogen mustard can produce confusion, lethargy, personality changes, and seizures. Methotrexate, if given IV or intrathecally, can result in aseptic meningitis, myelopathy, and seizures. Corticosteroids can cause myopathy with proximal weakness, depression, mania, and affective disease.[11]

Emergency Department Evaluation

The primary goal of the ED evaluation is to identify and treat the complications of increased intracranial pressure and brain compression. The patient may present with clinical entities ranging in severity from a herniation syndrome, seizures, or encephalopathy, or a simple headache.

Radiotherapy and chemotherapy can also cause many different signs and symptoms. If the patient is yet undiagnosed with CNS cancer, the differential should remain broad so as not to miss infectious, toxic-metabolic, endocrine, vascular, or traumatic causes of neurologic symptoms.

Triage Options and Initial Management

Patients who present comatose with the suggestion of neurologic deterioration should receive highest priority in triage. The physician should immediately see any patient presenting with a depressed level of consciousness and signs of acute deterioration from increased intracranial pressure such as a unilaterally dilated pupil and posturing. Standard cardiopulmonary resuscitation measures are instituted. Intubation using methods to minimize elevation of the intracranial pressure is performed. The patient is hyperventilated. The head of the bed may be elevated to 30 degrees, if the systolic pressure is above 100 mm Hg and there is no history of trauma to the spine.

Actively seizing patients require high priority triage and should be seen immediately in an acute care room. Standard cardiopulmonary resuscitation is undertaken. The airway is managed if necessary. Correction of reversible causes of seizures should commence immediately. Hypoxia, hypoglycemia, and toxic-metabolic causes can be quickly addressed with appropriate tests. Persistent seizures should be controlled with anticonvulsant medications.

Patients who are comatose, but not yet showing signs of neurologic deterioration secondary to increased intracranial pressure require urgent attention. The differential diagnosis includes trauma, vascular, toxic-metabolic, infectious, and endocrine disorders. Particular attention is paid to securing the airway. A trial of naloxone and thiamine may be given initially if the etiology of coma is unknown. Glucose should be given if the patient is hypoglycemic.

Patients who are stable but have complaints suggestive of intracranial neoplasm can be triaged to the patient treatment area for further evaluation. These complaints include headache with or without fever or nuchal rigidity, and headache with vomiting; other signs include new onset of a focal neurologic deficit, altered mental status in an alert patient, and a patient with a diagnosed CNS tumor.

History

The history should include information about the onset of symptoms, whether rapid or gradual. Patients presenting with new-onset headaches should be asked if the headaches occur in the early morning and improve upon rising, or whether the headaches are progressively worsening. Vomiting with or without nausea is common. Have there been any recent behavioral changes, generalized or focal neurologic symptoms? Has the patient had any seizures? What was the patient's premorbid level of function?

Physical Examination

Patients with acutely elevated intracranial pressure may present with headache, meningismus, bradycardia, hypertension, and changes in mental status. If the patient is herniating, the ipsilateral pupil is fixed and dilated, and there may be contralateral hemiparesis. The preterminal patient has bilateral fixed and dilated pupils, and decerebrate posturing, and may be hypotensive, tachycardiac, and hypoventilating. If a CNS tumor is suspected in an adult, there is a high probability that it is a metastasis. A thorough examination for evidence of a primary cancer should be undertaken.

The eye examination includes a close look at symmetry and reactivity of the pupils. Careful funduscopic examination often reveals papilledema. A close look for spontaneous venous pulsations is required. The presence of the pulsations rules out increased intracranial pressure, since increased intracranial pressure interferes with venous return of blood from the eye and inhibits the pulsations. The iris in neurofibromatosis may have hamartomatous elevations (Lisch nodules).

Examination of the neck may reveal nuchal rigidity. Brudzinski's sign is an involuntary flexion of the knee and hip with passive flexion of the neck and is a sign of increased intracranial pressure. Kernig's sign ("K" for "knee") is performed with the patient in a supine position while flexing the hip to 90°, then flexing the knee to 90°. If there is increased intracranial pressure, the patient will resist attempts to straighten the knee and will experience pain in the hamstrings.

Neurologic examination should include the mini–mental status examination to detect subtle attention, memory, or speech deficits. Any cranial nerve abnormality may be a result of edema adjacent to that nerve or compression of the nerve. Motor examination includes assessment for pronator drift, asterixis, tremor, tone, strength, and atrophy. On sensory examination, light touch fibers primarily use the dorsal columns, but some fibers ascend the spinothalamic tract. Thus, when testing sensation, pinprick should be used to assess the spinothalamic tract and proprioception or vibration should be used to assess the dorsal columns.

Differential Diagnosis

Numerous other entities can present with signs and symptoms similar to those seen with CNS tumors.

Brain Abscess

Patients who have brain abscesses may present with headache, papilledema, seizures, fever, leukocytosis, and often tachycardia and other signs of infection. There may be a history of head injury or rheumatic heart disease. Sometimes even contrast-enhanced CT or cerebral angiography does not discern obvious differences between brain tumors and brain abscesses.

Cerebrovascular Accident (CVA)

Brain tumors can present with sudden onset of focal neurologic findings similar to strokes, usually as a result of hemorrhagic complications. The symptoms caused by tumors worsen over time, whereas those caused by CVAs often improve over time.

Subdural Hematoma

Chronic subdural hematomas can present with headache, seizures or papilledema. Patients may have retrograde amnesia of the event and not give a history of trauma. CT and MRI differentiate a tumor from a hematoma.

Intracerebral Hemorrhage

Intracerebral hemorrhage from any source presents with similar symptoms, which may include headache, coma, stupor, hemiparesis, and bloody CSF. If an initial noncontrast CT is followed by a contrast CT, there may be contrast enhancement of the tumor surrounding the central clot.

Demyelination Syndromes

Demyelinating diseases, such as multiple sclerosis, can have slowly progressive symptoms, which mimic tumors. MRI is the imaging modality of choice.

Migraine Headache

Classical migraine headaches may present with aura, and scintillating scotomata, and can be unilateral with vomiting. Neurologic findings include visual field defects, hemiparesis, or hemiplegia. Migraines are generally self-limited, and symptoms tend not to progress. The headaches of tumors are dull, aching, worse in the morning, and intermittent. Tension headaches are typically dull, occipital, and have no associations with neurologic deficits or seizures.

New-Onset Seizures

In adults with new-onset seizures, a tumor must be ruled out. If the individual has a history of seizures, then a change in that patient's typical pattern of seizures should alert the clinician to the possibility of a new structural abnormality. New focal neurologic signs or a prolonged post-ictal state are worrisome for a mass.

Pseudotumor Cerebri

Pseudotumor cerebri, as its name implies, presents with symptoms of increased intracranial pressure much like a tumor would. Patients often complain of blurred vision or double vision, with nausea and vomiting. Signs include papilledema, nuchal rigidity, and diplopia. Diagnosis is made by a negative head CT with high opening pressure on the LP without signs of infection. LP is considered safe if the ventricular system appears normal or smaller sized. Although the etiology of this disorder is unknown, it has an association with endocrine abnormalities. Patients are typically obese women, young, with menstrual irregularities. There is an increased incidence in individuals with Addison's disease, ovarian dysfunction, hypoparathyroidism, pregnancy, menarche, and intracranial venous sinus thrombosis. Drugs that have been implicated include oral contraceptives, vitamin A abuse, tetracycline use in infancy, nalidixic acid, nitrofurantoin sulfa, lithium, indomethacin, and phenytoin. If an offending agent is recognized and removed, symptoms resolve spontaneously over several weeks. Refractory cases may respond to acetazolamide, furosemide, steroids, or lumboperitoneal shunting; 80% of cases respond to conservative therapy. Ten percent of patients experience recurrent or permanent visual defects.

Progressive Dementia

Dementing illnesses like Alzheimer's and Pick's disease may have a clinical prodrome indistinguishable from an intracranial mass. Patients present with progressive mental slowness and memory loss. Sometimes they will exhibit personality changes. All patients with gradual changes in mentation or personality should have a brain imaging study for diagnostic purposes. In contrast to the progressive deterioration in mental status of dementia, patients with delirium exhibit a waxing and waning mental status. Patients may be intermittently agitated and show impaired thought processes. The differential diagnosis is large and includes drug abuse, metabolic abnormalities, hypoxia, hypoglycemia, vitamin deficiencies, and endocrinopathies.

Psychosis

Psychosis is an unusual presenting sign of a brain tumor. Some temporal lobe masses may induce schizophrenic-like behaviors. A cautionary note is that these behaviors often improve on antipsychotic medications even when a tumor is the etiology of the problem. Therefore, resolution of signs of psychosis on antipsychotic medicines should not be used as a diagnostic challenge to rule out a mass in the psychotic patient. CT or MRI will show the tumor.

Hydrocephalus

Hydrocephalus caused by a tumor obstructing the CSF outflow tracts should be differentiated from subarachnoid hemorrhage, inflammatory changes in CSF absorption pathways, or neoplastic meningitis. CT or MRI will aid in the diagnosis.

Diagnostic Testing

Laboratory testing should include a complete blood count and differential to assess for infection, which is also helpful if the patient has newly presenting leukemia. Electrolytes, blood urea nitrogen, creatinine, glucose, calcium, magnesium, and phosphorus testing will reveal metabolic abnormalities. A patient who is seizing or has an acute change in mental status should have a fingerstick glucose taken immediately to rule out hypoglycemia. If hepatic encephalopathy is suspected, liver function tests may be done along with an ammonia level, which must be collected on ice. If neurosurgical intervention is a possibility, blood should be drawn for coagulation studies and a type and screen.

ECG is of limited value in diagnosing intracerebral masses. Diffuse T-wave widening and inversion may occur with large intracerebral hemorrhage from a mass. The QTc may be prolonged, and a bradyarrhythmia is associated with the Cushing's response to increased intracranial pressure.

A chest x-ray will reveal pneumonia or congestive heart failure, which can account for hypoxia and altered mental status. Pulmonary nodules associated with lung cancer can also be identified.

Computed tomography and MRI scanning of the head and spinal column are the primary imaging modalities used for evaluating CNS disease processes. Plain films offer little added value in the workup of the patient, although they may be useful in demonstrating facial fractures and sinus disease. CT is the most widely used test in the ED to image the brain. A spiral continuous time scanner can complete the study in only 5 to 10 minutes. CT scan can detect intracranial masses as small as 0.5 cm. Since most metastatic tumors are at least 1 cm in diameter, CT is usually an adequate test to find brain metastases. A noncontrast CT should always precede any contrast CT in the ED in order to identify intracranial blood, which is the same density as contrast. The anatomic location of the mass can accurately be found in 85% of noncontrast CTs and 95% of contrast-enhanced CTs. Some pathologic features of the mass can also be determined. A smooth homogeneous mass is usually benign. The use of intravenous contrast outlines the more vascular periphery of tumors. Meningiomas and other calcium-containing tumors like the oligodendrogliomas and pineal tumors are easily seen on CT. High-density tumors such as meningiomas, melanomas, primary lymphomas, and tumors with spontaneous hemorrhage may show up on CT without contrast. If the initial CT is negative, MRI should be performed as part of the workup for the patient but does not need to be arranged directly from the ED.

Magnetic resonance imaging has a greater resolution than CT, but is significantly slower than CT, taking 25 to 30 minutes for the study. There are more patients that have contraindications to the test, including surgically implanted pacemakers and other metallic prostheses. MRI is the best test for the subacute presentation of disease. It uses no ionizing radiation and has multiplanar imaging capabilities. A scan using gadolinium contrast is the most accurate test. Posterior fossa lesions and skull base, brain stem, cerebellum, and spinal cord tumors are seen more easily with MRI than CT due to the absence of bony artifact. Vascular malformations and aneurysms can be diagnosed because of the distinctive signal void features caused by blood flow. MRI also gives a sense of the tumor's vascularity.

Lumbar puncture should not be performed before an imaging study if a mass with edema is in the differential diagnosis. There is a risk that creating a low-pressure environment in the area of the spinal cord will create the conditions for transtentorial herniation and death. Leukocytosis on the LP suggests infectious meningitis. Xanthochromia or persistent red cells in the last collection tube indicate intracranial bleeding. If a tumor is suspected or seen on imaging, a sample of CSF should be sent for cytology to determine the etiology of the tumor, primary or metastasis.

Emergency Department Intervention

The focus of the ED workup is to distinguish tumors from other causes of neurologic dysfunction, institute early therapy to control cerebral edema, avoid seizure activity, and limit damage to CNS structures.

Pre-hospital interventions include intravenous access, oxygen, and airway management if required. Unless the patient is hypotensive, fluid rates should be kept to a minimum. Normal saline is the fluid of choice, since dextrose can exacerbate cerebral edema if it is present. Any associated symptoms requiring acute management should be addressed.

In the ED, the goals are to achieve cardiopulmonary stability, maintain adequate cerebral perfusion pressure, decrease cerebral edema, prevent seizures, and obtain appropriate neurology and neurosurgery consultation for the best disposition for the patient.

Patients with depressed levels of consciousness or exhibiting herniation syndromes should be intubated immediately. Orotracheal intubation is preferable. Pretreatment with 1.5 mg/kg of lidocaine IV 2 to 3 minutes prior to intubation is believed to help prevent a rise in intracranial pressure in response to intubation. Rapid sequence induction is the preferred method of intubation.

Controlled hyperventilation should be used in the situation where the patient is clinically herniating, or has new neurologic symptoms. Hyperventilation causes cerebral vasoconstriction by lowering CO_2 in the CSF. Chronic hyperventilation to a pCO_2 of 28 mm Hg predisposes the patient to cerebral ischemia. Hyperventilation should be performed to a pCO_2 of 35 mm Hg, but may be continued to a pCO_2 of 28 mm Hg in an acute deterioration as a temporizing measure before more definitive actions can be taken.

Osmotic diuretics include mannitol, urea, and glycerol. They should be reserved for acute deterioration either with new neurologic symptoms or signs of herniation. They are only a temporizing measure before definitive treatment can be initiated, usually neurosurgery. Mannitol is sold as a 20% solution and is administered as 1 g/kg IV over 20 to 30 minutes. There is a potential rebound phenomenon to the use of mannitol. The intracranial pressure may rise when mannitol is taken up by the cells of the CNS. Therefore, the smallest dose should be used to achieve the desired effect. The electrolytes, serum osmolality, blood pressure, urine output, and intracranial pressure when possible should be monitored. The serum osmolality should be kept at 310 mOsm. Mannitol can worsen intracranial bleeds, and should not be used if there are hemorrhagic complications with the tumor.

Corticosteroids reduce cerebral edema, but have a delayed onset of action. Dexamethasone is given as 10 mg IV push initially. In patients with epidural spinal cord compression, corticosteroid therapy is useful for reducing pain and occasionally reduces the amount of neurologic deficit. High-dose IV dexamethasone is used with taper over 2 to 3 weeks. Steroids in combination and radiation therapy are the treatment of choice for single or multiple epidural tumors. If spinal instability is present or if neurologic deterioration occurs, laminectomy may be considered.

Hypertension is more commonly seen in patients with intracranial hemorrhage. Hypertension may be a response to maintain cerebral perfusion pressure in the presence of increased intracranial pressure. Optimally, a measurement reflecting intracranial pressure would be used in the ED and cerebral perfusion pressure could be estimated by subtracting the ICP from the mean arterial pressure.

Cerebral perfusion pressures below 80 mm Hg are associated with poor survival and neurologic outcome. Since there is no standard tool used in EDs to derive these values, hypertension in a patient with an intracranial mass should be treated with caution. Hyperventilation and osmotic diuretics are the initial management choices. If these efforts fail, pressure should be lowered gradually using nitroprusside or labetalol. Serial neurologic examinations and cardiac monitoring are essential. Seizure activity in the setting of suspected increased intracranial pressure should be controlled promptly, as it increases cerebral metabolic requirements and cerebral blood flow, and it may precipitate herniation in the patient with preexisting intracranial mass effect. The patient is placed on oxygen, IV access is established, and the airway is secured. Common causes of seizures, including hypoglycemia, hypoxia, and toxic-metabolic abnormalities, are sought and addressed. The patient must be protected from injury. Bite blocks are usually difficult to insert and may be of limited value. The left lateral decubitus position helps to prevent aspiration if the patient is vomiting. Most seizures are short-lived and resolve spontaneously without any intervention. If the patient has had continuous seizure activity or has not regained consciousness within 30 minutes, then the patient is considered to be in status epilepticus and requires emergent treatment. Benzodiazepines are effective drugs in initial seizure management. Lorazepam at 0.5 mg/kg IV or diazepam at 1 to 1.5 mg/kg is typically used. The patient should then be loaded with fosphenytoin at 18 mg/kg over 5 to 10 minutes, or phenytoin at 18 mg/kg over 30 minutes.

Patient Disposition

Depending on the type of neoplasm, definitive therapy may include a surgical excision or debulking procedure with adjuvant chemotherapy and radiation therapy. When signs of increased intracranial pressure are present or if the patient is in status epilepticus in the context of presumed intracranial mass, immediate neurosurgical consultation is required. Patients requiring intubation and hyperventilation, and/or osmotic diuresis, should be admitted to the intensive care unit. Patients with stable vital signs and no signs of increased intracranial pressure can be admitted to a nonmonitored bed.

References

1. Kline NE, Sevier N. Solid tumors in children. *J Pediatr Nurs* 2003;18:96–102.
2. Gurney JG, Kadan-Lottick N. Brain and other central nervous system tumors: rates, trends, and epidemiology. *Curr Opin Oncol* 2001;13:160–166.
3. Behin A, Hoang-Xuan K, Carpentier AF, et al. Primary brain tumours in adults. *Lancet* 2003;361:323–331.
4. DeAngelis LM. Brain tumors. *N Engl J Med* 2001;344:114–123.
5. Flynn DF, Shipley WU. Management of spinal cord compression secondary to metastatic prostatic carcinoma. *Urol Clin North Am* 1991;18:145–152.
6. Kvale PA, Simoff M, Prakash UB. Lung cancer. Palliative care. *Chest* 2003;123:284S–311S.
7. Sze G. Diseases of the intracranial meninges: MR imaging features. *AJR Am J Roentgenol* 1993;160:727–733.
8. Eberhart CG, Morrison A, Gyure KA, et al. Decreasing incidence of sudden death due to undiagnosed primary central nervous system tumors. *Arch Pathol Lab Med* 2001;125:1024–1030.
9. Pruitt AA. Nervous system infections in patients with cancer. *Neurol Clin* 2003;21:193–219.
10. Cross NE, Glantz MJ. Neurologic complications of radiation therapy. *Neurol Clin* 2003;21:249–277.
11. Plotkin SR, Wen PY. Neurologic complications of cancer therapy. *Neurol Clin* 2003;21:279–318.

Selected Readings

Barr LC, Skene AI, Thomas JM. Metastasectomy. *Br J Surg* 1992;79:1268–1274.

Black PM. Solitary brain metastases. Radiation, resection, or radiosurgery? *Chest* 1993;103:s367–s369.

Cascino TL. Neurologic complications of systemic cancer. *Med Clin North Am* 1993;77:265–278.

Chong BW, Newton TH. Hypothalamic and pituitary pathology. *Radiol Clin North Am* 1993;31:1147–1153.

Duffner PK, Cohen ME. Changes in the approach to central nervous system tumors in childhood. *Pediatr Clin North Am* 1992;39:859–877.

Laperriere NJ, Bernstein M. Radiotherapy for brain tumors. *CA Cancer J Clin* 1994;44:96–108.

Laws ER Jr, Thapar K. Brain tumors. *CA Cancer J Clin* 1993;43:263–271.

Longstreth WT Jr, Dennis LK, McGuire VM, et al. Epidemiology of intracranial meningioma. *Cancer* 1993;72:639–648.

Lukens JN. Progress resulting from clinical trials. Solid tumors in childhood cancer. *Cancer* 1994;74:2710–2718.

McConachie NS, Worthington BS, Cornford EJ, et al. Review article: computed tomography and magnetic resonance in the diagnosis of intraventricular cerebral masses. *Br J Radiol* 1994;67:223–243.

Newton HB. Primary brain tumors: review of etiology, diagnosis and treatment. *Am Fam Phys* 1994;49:787–797.

O'Neill BP, Buckner JC, Coffey RJ, et al. Brain metastatic lesions. *Mayo Clin Proc* 1994;69:1062–1068.

Pollack IF. Brain tumors in children. *N Engl J Med* 1994;331:1500–1507.

Rorke LB. Experimental production of primitive neuroectodermal tumors and its relevance to human neuro-oncology. *Am J Pathol* 1994;144:444–448.

Watterson J, Toogood I, Nieder M, et al. Excessive spinal cord toxicity from intensive central nervous system-directed therapies. *Cancer* 1994;74:3034–3041.

Wronski M, Arbit E, et al. Survival after surgical treatment of brain metastases from lung cancer: a follow-up study of 231 patients treated between 1976 and 1991. *J Neurosurg* 1995;83:605–616.

Introduction to Obstetrical and Pregnancy Disorders

G. Richard Braen

Drs. Michalakes, Pundt, and Broderick are the authors of chapters in this section covering obstetrics and disorders of pregnancy, labor and delivery, and post partum complications.

Dr. Michalakes describes the current use of contraceptive methods: their complications and their failures. He also discusses the problems that can arise during pregnancy. Dr. Pundt describes both normal and abnormal labor and delivery, and Dr. Broderick describes complications that can arise following delivery.

Combined, the chapters in this section cover the broad spectrum of pregnancy, from before to after, and particularly describe the most important aspects of pregnancy concerning emergency medical practice.

Contraception, Uncomplicated Pregnancy, and Complicated Pregnancy

Chris J. Michalakes

The female menstrual cycle has two major purposes: The release of one mature ovum and the preparation of the uterine endometrium for implantation. It generally repeats every 22 to 35 days, from menarche to menopause, for an average of 35 years.

Ovarian changes during the cycle depend on gonadotropin secretion from the anterior pituitary gland. Secretion of follicle stimulating hormone (FSH) and luteinizing hormone (LH) generally begins at age 8. Puberty, or the initiation of monthly sexual cycles, typically begins between 11 and 15 years.

The monthly increase and decrease of FSH and LH stimulates ovarian cells via specific membrane receptors and cyclic AMP interactions. Each cycle starts at about the beginning of menstruation. Increasing FSH and LH secretion results in the growth of a few ovarian follicles. Stimulation of these follicles causes growth of granulosa and theca cells. Granulosa cells secrete follicular fluid rich in estrogen. This assists the development of several follicles. Eventually one dominates the mature or graffian follicle.

Ovulation involves the migration of the graffian follicle to the ovarian surface. Importantly LH production spikes preceding ovulation by 1 to 2 days. This LH surge is necessary for the final growth and ovulation of the follicle. LH also appears responsible for changing the theca and granulosa cells into lutein cells. Lutein cells are necessary for both estrogen and progesterone production.

The surface cells of the ovary continue to thin until a virtually transparent, essentially avascular central stigma results. Necrobiosis occurs and ovulation results. The released oocyte is then collected via the oviduct fimbriae.

Near the time of ovulation, approximately 25% of women experience lower abdominal discomfort. Classically termed "Mittelschmerz," this symptom complex is believed to be the result of released follicular fluid and the resulting peritoneal irritation that accompanies ovulation. It is usually a random event and not necessarily repetitive.

After follicular rupture, the granulosa cells undergo a rapid physiologic change, or "luteinization." The resulting structure, the corpus luteum, goes through four phases: proliferation, vascularization, maturity, and regression. Initially lutein cells secrete large amounts of progesterone

and lesser amounts of estrogen. Strands of theca cells, harbored within the developing corpus, continue to secrete and are believed to be the prime producers of estrogen.

The outcome of the corpus depends on potential fertilization and implantation of the ovum. In the absence of fertilization, regressive changes develop. This occurs at about the twenty-third day of the menstrual cycle and results in the short-lived corpus luteum of menstruation. If implantation occurs, trophoblastic human chorionic gonadotropin (HCG) production prevents the breakdown of the corpus, and the corpus luteum of pregnancy is maintained. The corpus luteum of pregnancy is most responsible for the stable production of progesterone during the first trimester of pregnancy.

The mature ovum is fertilizable for about 24 hours, but maximally so for only 8 to 12 hours. Sperm can remain viable in the female genital tract for 24 to 72 hours, but remain highly fertile for only 12 to 24 hours. Therefore, the prime period of fertility occurs if coitus overlaps these two periods.

Conception occurs upon penetration of the lattice structure of the ovum's zona pellucida by a single sperm. After this single penetration, the cellular structure rapidly changes, allowing no further complete sperm migration through the zona.

After fertilization, 3 days are normally required for transport throughout the fallopian tube to the uterus. Once in the uterus, implantation into the endometrium occurs within 4 to 5 days. Several cell divisions occur by this stage, the blastocyst stage.

Implantation occurs with the aid and action of surface trophoblastic cells residing on the blastocyst surface. After implantation trophoblastic and sublying cells continue to proliferate, ultimately forming the placenta and other membranes of pregnancy.

Contraception

If no contraception is used, approximately 90% of fertile couples will achieve pregnancy within one year. The majority of young women likely ovulate prior to their first menses. Thus, contraception is necessary to avoid pregnancy even prior to the achievement of puberty. As women become older, most ovulate with every cycle. As menopause approaches, even with the appearance of hot flashes and prolonged periods of amenorrhea, the guarantee of ovulatory demise does not exist. It is known that women rarely become pregnant after age 50. Usually, if an older woman has not menstruated for 2 consecutive years, the risk of pregnancy is minor.

Contraception is available via a variety of sources. These include oral steroid preparations, transdermal, subdermal, or injectable steroid preparations, intrauterine devices (IUDs), physical and/or chemical barrier methods, and withdrawal and/or abstinence techniques. The first four methods are the most commonly used.

The 1989 national survey by Trussell et al is the most commonly referenced survey on contraceptive use. The percentage of women who use do not use contraceptives and become pregnant within a year varies from 43% to 85%. With the use of steroidal preparations, regardless of type, rates of pregnancy within the first year of use ranges from 0.03% to 1.1%. The failure rates of mechanical contraceptive devices (i.e., condoms, diaphragms, etc.) range from 2% to 30% within the initial year of use. Methods involving carefully managed periodic abstinence (i.e., calendar or symptothermal techniques) have failure rates ranging from 10% to 20% over the initial year of use.

When looking at continued compliance with contraception, the chosen method is most important. Effectiveness, safety, ease of use, and "life fit" are all factors.

Oral Contraceptives

Oral contraceptives were introduced in the United States in late 1959. Untoward effects were initially not uncommon and were significantly dose-related. Today's preparations hold the lowest steroid doses at which reliable contraception remains. Combination estrogen and progesterone pills are highly effective, with theoretical rates at 99.1% and actual use effectiveness noted at 97% to 98%.

The primary estrogen used is ethinyl estradiol. Several 19-nor progestins are in use, each with varying degrees of androgenic, estrogenic, and antiestrogenic activities.

Combination oral contraceptives are prepared as monophasic, biphasic or triphasic preparations. They are usually presented in packs of 21 active or daily pills, along with seven inert tablets. The biphasic and triphasic tablets have two of three sets of tablets with varying dosing per set, taken at set phases of the 21-day cycle. These were developed to more accurately approximate natural steroid ratios during the menstrual cycle. Higher progestins tablets were the norm until the 1980s, when information regarding potential negative cardiovascular effects began to surface. Now most contain less than 1 mg of progestins. Estrogen content has likewise decreased. The lowest acceptable dose is governed by its ability to prevent unwanted breakthrough bleeding.

Combination oral contraceptives act by preventing ovulation. FSH and LH are suppressed, and no midcycle LH surge occurs. The combined action of an estrogen and progestins tablet synergistically suppresses ovulation more effectively than either alone.

Progesterone decreases the frequency of gonadotropin-releasing hormone (GnRH) pulsed releases from the hypothalamus. It affects LH similarly. LH pulsed release is a necessary factor for ovulation induction. Estrogen may assist in altering pulsed steroid release.

Estrogen affects the pituitary by suppressing FSH release during the follicular phase of the menstrual cycle. The resulting arrest of ovarian follicle development has been demonstrated in women using oral contraceptives. The sustained elevation of estrogen is also known to be a necessary trigger for the midcycle LH surge. Progesterone, as pharmacologically administered, is known to inhibit this effect.

Other mechanisms are believed to contribute to the high efficacy rate of oral contraceptives. A precise hormonal milieu must be present, creating the environment that allows tubal transport and endometrial preparation for implantation. Estrogens are known to accelerate tubal transport, and progestins to slow it. The combined effect is disruptive. Estrogen also inhibits blastocyst implantation in the endometrium. The properties of the cervical mucus, involving sperm motility and transportation, are similarly hormone-dependent. Progestins cause thick, scanty mucus, and inhibit sperm capitation.

When initiating oral contraceptives, it is recommended that women begin within the first 7 days of the menstrual cycle. This not only prevents ovulation induction, but also minimizes the risk of preexisting pregnancy.

Phasic pills were developed in an attempt to minimize progestin dosing and related side effects, without compromising birth control effect. Progestin dosing generally begins low and increases through the cycle. Estrogen dosing is usually kept stable or may increase somewhat toward cycle end.

Various drug interactions are known to occur with oral contraceptive use. Medications that stimulate hepatic enzymes (such as phenytoin, barbiturates, and sulfonamides) hasten the degradation of the hormones and decrease contraceptive usefulness. Other antibiotics, such as rifampin and ampicillin, are thought to alter the gut flora, either increasing oral contraceptive metabolism or decreasing their absorption. When any of these medications are in use or pondered, an alternative, nonhormone birth control method is recommended.

Shortly after the introduction of oral contraceptives, reports of adverse effects began. Most were dose-dependent, leading to the current regimens of low dose preparations. Overall, the side effect profiles fall within a few major categories: adverse cardiovascular effects, possible cancer risks, and endocrine/metabolic effects.

With high dose estrogen preparations, the risk of myocardial infarction and ischemic vascular disease were believed significant risks. For smokers, the risk is increased, particularly if older than 35 years. This smoking risk continues, even with today's low dose preparations. There is general agreement that low dose oral contraceptives do not increase the risk of ischemic vascular disease in non-smokers.

The incidence of deep venous thrombosis (DVT) is increased with oral contraceptives. The proposed mechanism is likely related to the induction of clotting factor production, along with platelet aggretory effects. It is known that the levels of fibrinogen, plus factors II, VII, IX, X, XII, and XIII are increased, while the activity of antithrombin III and endothelial plasminogen activator decrease. All seem directly related to the degree of estrogen dosing. The current dose combinations of oral contraceptives lower this risk. Associated vascular pathology unique to women that develop DVT while on hormone therapy is likely. These women also have a higher risk of DVT and pulmonary embolism during pregnancy and early puerperium.

Hypertension develops in 4% to 5% of previously normotensive women and increases in 10% to 15% of those previously hypertensive. Lower dose combinations minimize this effect and it is reversible with the cessation of therapy. An induced increase of angiotensinogen is likely the major contributor. Predicting which women are prone to hypertension is difficult. The incidence does increase with age and in smokers. Hypertension during pregnancy does not subsequently predict it, if oral contraceptives are chosen as a method of birth control.

The effects on lipids are even less uniform. Estrogens generally cause an increase in HDL and decrease in LDL. Progestins can cause the reverse. Precise effects are not predictable in the individual. Studies have shown no overall significant effect with the use of combination preparations. Overall, occasional serum monitoring to establish an individual profile is recommended.

Since estrogen has known growth-promoting effects, a concern of long standing duration involves the potential risk of developing breast, ovarian, endometrial, cervical, and other carcinomas while using steroidal contraceptives. Endometrial and ovarian cancers have been noted to have a decreased incidence in the oral contraceptive user. The relationship to the incidence of breast cancer has been more controversial. Current evidence supports that the incidence is not increased during the reproductive years for the majority of women. Likewise, there is no definitive evidence to implicate oral contraceptives as an independent cause of cervical cancer.

Oral contraceptives alter glucose tolerance. This appears to be minimized by lower dose contraceptive combinations, but even these lower doses cause a degree of peripheral insulin-resistance. Overall, their use is believed to intensify existing diabetes and perhaps unmask subclinical glucose intolerance in those susceptible. The effect of oral contraceptives in women with prior gestational diabetes is not clear. A reasonable recommendation is that the use of combination oral contraceptives in the setting of overt diabetes or glucose intolerance must be based on assessment of clinical risk-benefit.

Other less severe side effects of hormonal contraceptive use occur to varying degrees. Gallbladder disease increases two- or three-fold among those using oral contraceptives. This higher incidence likely results from estrogenic effect and the increased ratio of cholesterol to bile acids. Headaches, varying from relatively benign symptoms to the promotion of more severe migraine patterns, may occur. Weight gain, acne, and hirsutism are likely mediated via the androgenic activity of the 19-nor progestins. Cervical mucorrhea is thought related to the estrogen component and may cause vaginal irritation or an increase in the susceptibility to vaginal infections. Depression has been associated with the higher estrogen dosing of earlier generation preparations. It is believed not associated with the low dose preparations of today.

Combination preparations also have reported beneficial effects, such as fewer cases of dysmenorrhea, fewer ovarian cysts, episodes of salpingitis, and premenstrual symptoms. The incidence of iron deficiency anemia diminishes along with the incidence of benign breast disease and rheumatoid arthritis.

Subdermal, Injectable, and Transdermal Contraceptives

Implantable agents, long-acting injectable preparations, and transdermal agents rely on progestins and achieve contraceptive effectiveness comparable to oral contraceptives.

Progestin implants (the Norplant system) uses silastic tubes containing levonogestrel planted subdermally. The total dose is variably released over 5 years. Failure rates are comparable to oral contraceptives, e.g., 0.04 per 100 women years in the first year, then 0.2 to 1.1 over the remaining 4 years. The mode of action is analogous to progestin-only oral contraceptives. The advantages and disadvantages are similar to the progestin-only oral preparations. The most common disadvantage remains irregular uterine bleeding, which varies from total amenorrhea to spotting, variable breakthrough, or overt menorrhagia. The degree of symptomatology occasionally necessitates removal of the device and a change to another method of contraception. Normal fertility is rapidly restored once the implants are removed.

Injectable progestins (Depo-Provera or Norgest) are popular methods. They approximate oral contraceptives in their effectiveness and can be dosed every 2 to 3 months by deep intramuscular injection. Therapeutic levels are reached within a few days. The mechanisms of action, advantages, disadvantages and contraindications are again similar to the other progestational contraceptives. Prolonged amenorrhea and anovulation may occur after discontinuation. Return of fertility is variably delayed but not prevented.

Transdermal progestins are emerging as a popular method. When compared to oral contraceptives, they are equally effective with perhaps improved overall compliance. They generally need to be changed weekly. They have been associated with generally mild, irritation type skin reactions. Overall, they are well tolerated. During initial application cycles, they may have a slight increase in breakthrough bleeding.

Intrauterine Devices

Prior to the 1990s, IUDs enjoyed wide popularity in the United States. In the mid 1980s, the two most popular IUDs (Lippes Loop and Cu-7) were removed from the market due to liability defense concerns. IUDs remain available in the US market, but are not widely popular, due to cost and the devices' potential adverse effects.

The mechanism of action, although not precisely understood, is believed to involve an intense localized uterine inflammatory reaction that is ultimately spermicidal. This differs from the previously held concept that IUDs acted by preventing implantation. If fertilization does occur, this same inflammatory reaction is directed against the blastocyst. Copper is believed to intensify the inflammatory response. Some IUDs have a progestin component. This causes an atrophic endometrium and thus may compromise implantation. The overall effectiveness of IUDs is believed to be equivalent to that of oral contraceptives.

Numerous adverse effects for IUDs have been described. Serious effects, although uncommon, can be severe. Pelvic infection is more likely, presumptively due to the attached synthetic filament tail wicking pathogenic bacteria into the uterine cavity. Pelvic infection (e.g., salpingitis, pelvic peritonitis, pelvic abscess) and rare devastating complications, including death and sterility, have occurred with these devices. If these symptoms appear in conjunction with IUD use, the patient should be treated with an appropriate broad spectrum antibiotic and have the device promptly removed.

A common side effect is also menorrhagia, where typically blood loss is increased by a factor of two and may result in a iron deficient state. IUDs with a progestin may have a lower rate of blood loss secondary to endometrial atrophy.

Ectopic pregnancy concerns exist with these devices. IUDs are designed to prevent intrauterine pregnancies, but they offer little protection against extrauterine sources. If a pregnancy occurs with an IUD in place, the risk of ectopic pregnancy increases, along with a markedly increased risk of second trimester abortion and septic abortion. The likelihood of abortion approaches 50%. If sepsis occurs, it is often fulminate and complicated. Women becoming pregnant with an IUD in place are usually offered the option of pregnancy termination.

Uncomplicated Pregnancy

Normal Landmarks and Physiologic Parameters

Pregnancy should be considered a normal physiologic state. However, complex physiologic, anatomic, and functional changes often cause medical professionals to support the concept of pregnancy as a disease. Understanding the anatomic landmarks, physiologic changes, and standard terminology of a normal pregnancy is fundamental to dispelling this opinion.

The normal duration of pregnancy averages 280 days or 40 weeks. By convention, the standard measure is from the first day of the last menstrual period. Naegele's Rule defines the standard method of estimating the delivery date. Adding 7 days to the date of the first day of the last normal menstrual period and subtracting 3 months yields the EDC (estimated date of confinement). Be aware that these estimates represent a clinical quirk. This method of estimating the EDC actually places time 0 at 2 weeks be-

fore ovulation. Pregnancy "wheels" use the same methodology in an easy-to-use format. An erroneous delivery date of up to five days has been described. In spite of these inaccuracies, clinical methods for estimating gestational age persist as the norm. The more precise measure, ovulatory age, is 2 weeks shorter. Ovulatory age is generally only useful if developmental or fertility concerns are tantamount.

Terminology and Timeline

A basic terminology review is necessary in any discussion of uncomplicated pregnancy. By definition, a *primipara* is a woman who has been delivered only once or has achieved a viable fetus only once. Delivery of a fetus after the normal time of a spontaneous abortion, i.e. after 20 weeks gestation, defines parity. With the establishment of pregnancy, a women becomes a primigravida. A *multiparous* woman has achieved pregnancy to viability of 2 or more fetuses. Note that the achievement of pregnancy viability defines parity, not the number of delivered fetuses. For example, a twin birth represents one viable pregnancy, not two. *Gravida* refers only to the achievement of a pregnant state, irrespective of pregnancy outcome. The generally accepted numerical notation summarizing the above uses a single number to represent gravida and four numbers representing parity. For example, a woman who has been pregnant 5 times with 2 full term deliveries, 1 preterm delivery, 2 abortions, and 2 living children, would be numerically expressed as G5 P2-1-2-2.

The timeline of pregnancy is classically divided into trimesters. Historically these are blocked such that the first trimester represents conception through the 14th week, the second through the 28th week, and the third through week 42. Complications are clinically grouped during these periods. Representative examples of complications include spontaneous abortion during the initial trimester and pre-eclampsia/eclampsia occurring predominately through the third. The categorization of patient and possible complications by trimester is limited. The most clinically appropriate measure of gestation remains the estimated weeks completed.

Examination of the pregnant patient yields landmarks and milestones based on gestational age. Some of the earliest changes are subtle and not diagnostic. Breast tenderness is frequent and non-specific. Bluish-red hyperemia of the cervix occurs early in the first trimester and represents increased pelvic blood flow. Dilated cervical glands, Nabothian cysts, may be apparent in the exocervical area. They represent occluded, non-pathologic structures. Normally, a moderate amount of mucoid, white vaginal discharge is present. Discoloration or odor, if present, usually represents a vaginal infection. *Trichomonas* is most common. The uterus is palpable above the symphysis pubis at about 12 weeks of gestation. Twenty weeks finds the uterus at the level of the umbilicus. Until roughly 36 weeks the uterus can be sized, from the symphysis, on a centimeter-by-centimeter march superiorly. Each centimeter approximates one gestational week. To measure, a cloth tape is placed over the curve of the gravid abdomen with an empty urinary bladder. A simple linear measure is performed. A full bladder may add up to three weeks to this estimation. Fetal heart tones may be heard as early as 10 weeks with a Doppler fetoscope, but easy auscultation with a hand held Doppler fetoscope by 12 to 14 weeks is more usual.

As the normal pregnancy proceeds, the fetus is defined according to anatomic location within the uterine cavity. By convention, fetal position is described according to lie, presentation, attitude, and position. Establishment utilizes abdominal examination, vaginal examination, and auscultation. Ultrasound and/or x-ray exams are options for a more complete investigation.

Lie is the longitudinal relationship of the fetus to the mother. It is termed as either longitudinal, i.e., arranged according to the long axis of the mother, or transverse. By far the most common lie, at term, is longitudinal (>99%).

Fetal attitude is the posture or habitus occupied within the uterine cavity. Most often, the fetal head and neck are flexed, facing caudally, with the chin touching the chest. The legs and hips are hyperflexed with the feet resting on the anterior leg surface. The arms are usually tightly folded across the chest with the umbilical cord occupying the space between arms and legs.

Fetal position refers to the presenting part in the birth canal. The nomenclature utilized names the presentation according to right or left (the delivering provider's right or left), and whether it is anterior, posterior, or transverse. The most common presenting parts are occipital, mental, or sacral. Clinically, the diagnosis of presentation and position is performed utilizing Leopold's Maneuvers. Originally described by Leopold and Sporlin in 1894, these exam techniques allow a systematic, descriptive approach. Maneuvers number 1–3 require that the examiner stand to the side and facing the patient. Number 1 outlines the contour of the uterus and encroachment toward the mother's xyphoid. Using the palms of both hands, the examiner gently palpates the uterine fundus symmetrically to distinguish the smooth curves of a head down longitudinal lie versus the more irregular, hard sensation of a breech position. The second maneuver places the examiner's palmar hands on either side of the gravid abdomen to firmly distinguish the fetal back from the more nodular, anterior limb structures. Maneuver 3 uses the examiner's thumb and forefinger of one hand to determine engagement of the fetal head in the pelvis. An attempt to gently grasp the fetal head is made immediately above the symphysis. If freely moveable, the head is not engaged. If not engaged, the attitude and subsequent relation to the small body parts may assist in determining the likely presenting part. If engaged, the fourth maneuver is necessary. The fourth maneuver requires that the examiner face the woman's feet. Three-finger palpation by both examining hands over the pelvic inlet provides tactile information regarding the lie, attitude, and presenting part. These maneuvers are most valuable in the later stages of pregnancy. With experience it is possible to estimate accurate size of a fetus and map even a twin birth.

Physiologic Changes During Pregnancy

Weight Gain

Weight gain is the most visible physiologic change. An increase in total body water is the major factor. Expansion of the intracellular components and extracellular fluid of rapidly growing fetal organs plus the maternal products of conception are the direct causes. The average gained varies between 15 to 45 lbs with the mean of about 25 lbs. Little weight gain, approximately 3 lbs, occurs during the first trimester. After the first trimester, the gain is roughly linear and averages 1 lb per week. This weight gained during pregnancy, when compared to pre-pregnancy weight, is predictable of appropriate fetal growth and gestational-age adjusted birth weight.

Metabolic Changes

Metabolic changes during pregnancy involve three major components: carbohydrates, protein, and fat. Hormonal components, especially fluctuations in steroids, insulin, and insulin antagonists, are the most important proteins. Glucose metabolism during pregnancy and a "diabetogenic" tendency dominates any discussion of metabolic effects.

Fasting glucose levels are known to decrease toward the end of the first trimester by 5–10 mg/dL. Although exact mechanisms are unknown, multiple regulatory factors are believed involved. The uteroplacental-fetal unit is known to increase the uptake of both glucose and amino acids. This especially accelerates in the second half of pregnancy, leading to diminished hepatic glucose production, and increased lipolysis. In effect, a local "starvation" state occurs at the hepatic level. Increased substrate clearance is carried out via renal excretion of amino acids and glucose. Combined with lower amino acid levels secondary to hemodilution, the global effect is less substrate availability. Increasing estrogen and progesterone contribute by stimulating glycogenesis. Lipolysis increases as a result of the combination of the above interactions. Lipolytic hormones, including cortisol, ACTH, growth hormone, glucagon, and human placental lactogen are all stimulated via a variety of mechanisms. The combined effect on the fasting state is one of increased free fatty acids and early morning ketonuria. The appearance of urinary ketones need not be interpreted as pathologic, but rather is a secondary response to the inherent pregnant fasting state.

The characteristics of the fed state in pregnancy demonstrates altered glycemic and insulin responses. Pregnancy tends to induce a state of impaired tolerance to a carbohydrate load. Hyperglycemia occurs, associated with increased insulin release and decreased peripheral insulin effectiveness. A diabetogenic state can occur, especially in those felt susceptible pre-pregnancy. Indeed, those with latent diabetes or with some degree of glucose intolerance may be "unmasked" by the physiologic changes of pregnancy.

Hematologic Changes

Hematologic changes during pregnancy predominately involve an increase in blood volume and changes in coagulation factors. Blood volume increases for the likely teleological reason of maximal uteroplacental perfusion and overall maternal-fetal protection. It increases by almost 50% over the non-pregnant state. Seventy-five percent of this expansion is due to increased plasma volume and 25% secondary to increased red cell mass. Resulting hemodilution is referred to as the "physiologic anemia" of pregnancy. Leukocytes, especially PMNs, increase in number, a change attributed to higher estrogen levels. A peak occurs at roughly 30 weeks' gestation and averages 9,000/mm^3. Thirty percent of pregnant women may have a total white blood cell count exceeding 10,000 without evidence of illness or infection. During the later stages of labor, counts of 25,000–50,000 have been reported. PMNs predominate with a corresponding diminution of lymphocytes. The effect on the immune response is not clear, but is felt to be of minor significance. Normal values return within a few weeks of delivery. Platelets decrease slightly in number. The total rarely dips below 150,000 and usually is within the normal range. The physiologic reason for this decrease is not known. Some authorities simply ascribe it to hemodilution. Within several days of delivery, the count rebounds and is usually normal.

Coagulation factors do change significantly during pregnancy. The factors most increased are VII, VIII, IX, X, XII and fibrinogen. Fibrinogen has a marked increase, approximately double the non-pregnant state. It is probably the chief reason the erythrocyte sedimentation rate (ESR) increases so dramatically in pregnancy, rendering it of little use clinically. At the same time, antithrombin III, necessary as an endogenous anticoagulant, decreases. There is also a decrease in tissue plasminogen activator by the end of the first trimester. These coagulation system changes act in concert with the normal pregnancy associated lower extremity venous pooling. This combination of anatomic and physiologic factors contribute to the higher incidence of deep venous thrombosis and pulmonary embolus throughout pregnancy. DVT incidence approaches 5 per 1,000 deliveries and is further increased postpartum.

Cardiovascular Changes

The cardiovascular system undergoes extensive change during a normal pregnancy. Perhaps most significant is an increase in cardiac output of 30% to 50%. This increase begins early in the first trimester, peaks mid-second, and then remains relatively constant for the remainder. Initially this increase is presumed due to an increase in heart rate and ventricular performance combined with a progressive decrease in peripheral vascular resistance. The growing uterus can affect cardiac output dramatically. As the uterus increases in size, inferior vena cava (IVC) compression occurs, predominately in the supine position. Cardiac output may be decreased by 25% to 30% secondary to decreased venous return. Heart rate mildly increases during the second trimester, presumptively due to increased venous return. It increases by 10% to 20 % compared to prepregnancy values. A typical resting pulse in pregnancy is 80–90 beats per minute.

Blood pressure changes by a systolic and diastolic decrease. Systolic BP decreases 5–10 mm Hg throughout pregnancy. Diastolic BP tends to decrease to a somewhat greater extent, averaging about 10 to 15 mm Hg. In women that do not undergo this natural decrease in BP early in pregnancy, the risk of pregnancy related hypertension increases.

Postpartum, usually within two–three weeks, most cardiovascular changes revert to normal. Immediately however, the post delivery response is a 10-20% increase in cardiac output. Rapid decompression of the IVC by the gravid uterus is the presumptive cause. A relative bradycardia often occurs during this transition. Otherwise, the reversion to the prepregnancy cardiovascular norm occurs smoothly. Accompanying the 30% decline to baseline cardiac output is an approximate 15% to 20% decline in heart rate and left ventricular stroke volume.

Pulmonary physiologic change in pregnancy reflects the need for increased oxygen consumption during development. Oxygen consumption increases by 20–30% secondary to fetal and placental needs. This increase does not affect the partial pressure of oxygen (PaO$_2$). The PaO$_2$ remains above 90 mm Hg due to augmented ventilation. Ventilation is increased secondary to a baseline 40% increase in tidal volume. The respiratory rate does not change from the normal 16 per minute. Increased O$_2$ consumption leads directly to increased CO$_2$ production. This increase drives the increase in ventilation but is not the only factor involved. Progesterone is believed to contribute via direct stimulation of the respiratory center. The resulting minute ventilation is above that needed to excrete produced CO$_2$. The baseline PaCO$_2$ in pregnancy therefore approximates 30 mm Hg. A compensated, mild respiratory alkalosis is "normal" in pregnancy. The typical ABG has a pH between 7.40–7.45, pCO$_2$ of 30 mm Hg, and due to renal compensation, a HCO$_3$ of 18 to 21 mEq/L. The functional residual capacity, or the volume of air left in the lungs at the end of passive exhalation, decreases through pregnancy. This effect is secondary to the progressive increase in intraabdominal pressure from the gravid uterus. The diaphragm in effect is "pushed up" into the thoracic cavity thereby decreasing the ability of the chest wall to recoil properly. Since vital capacity does not change during pregnancy, the compensatory effect is a lower residual lung volume. Clinically, this decrease in FRC is only relevant if the pregnant women suddenly becomes apneic. Since less air remains after passive exhalation, the risk of hypoxia in the pregnant patient increases.

The renal system changes both anatomically and physiologically during pregnancy. Kidney size increases slightly, by 1–1.5 cm in length. As the uterus grows out of the pelvis, an obstructive pressure on the ureters is believed to occur. Mild hydronephrosis, more so on the right, results. The exact reasons for the asymmetry are not proven. The presumption is that the left renal system is "cushioned" by the presence of the sigmoid colon. The right ureter has the burden of the natural tendency of the pregnant uterus to dextrorotate, hence increasing direct pressure and physiologic obstruction. Kidney dilation decreases postpartum, but slowly. Mild hydronephrosis may persist for 3 to 4 months.

The urinalysis in pregnancy has subtle changes over the nonpregnant state. Protein excretion in nonpregnant women is less than 100 mg/day. In pregnancy, proteinuria is not considered abnormal until it exceeds 150–300 mg/day. Generally a doubling of prepregnancy values is acceptable. Glycosuria occurs to a mild degree. This results from the combination of increased GFR and decreased tubular glucose reabsorption.

Urinary sediment may have subtle changes during pregnancy. The excretion of red blood cells (RBCs) increases, presumptively due to the slight renal pelvis dilation and rupture of small venules. Only 1 to 2 RBCs/hpf are generally considered acceptable. The standard causes of hematuria must be considered in the same manner as in the nonpregnant state. If minimal hematuria appears without inciting cause, it generally resolves postpartum. The issue of leukocyturia is more controversial. Most authors believe any increase in leukocytes represent a pathologic condition. A urinary tract infection is the most common, and requires investigation.

Nausea and vomiting occur in up to 56% of pregnancies, usually beginning after the first missed menstrual period. Common in the morning and rare throughout the entire day, these symptoms usually abate near the fourth month of gestation. Symptoms are most often mild and do not impact on acid-base or electrolyte status. No specific physiologic disturbance has been identified.

Complicated Pregnancy

Hyperemesis Gravidarum

Hyperemesis gravidarum, or severe vomiting of pregnancy, is characterized by intractable vomiting. It causes fluid, electrolyte, acid/base, and nutritional deficiencies. It most commonly occurs during the first month of pregnancy and usually remits by the close of the first trimester. Less commonly, it is accompanied by increased salivation, elevated bilirubin, and increased transaminase levels. The precise pathogenesis is unknown. It is associated with multiparity, younger women, and obesity. Hormonal influences are likely, with rapidly rising chorionic gonadotropin and estrogens implicated. Treatment is based upon correction of the fluid, electrolyte, and acid/base abnormalities. Generous replacement of potassium, sodium, chloride, and water, with B vitamin supplementation, is recommended. Antiemetics may be given and are useful. Metoclopromide is the most useful and is a category B drug. In addition to the typical action of a central dopamine antagonist, it stimulates motility of the upper gastrointestinal tract. The other common antiemetics are useful, but act only as central dopamine antagonists. They include promethazine, prochlorperazine, and chlorpromazine, and are classified as category C drugs. Hospitalization for total parental nutrition is rarely necessary but remains an option in the most severe cases.

Ectopic Pregnancy

Ectopic pregnancy is the term applied to implantation of the fetus other than normally in the uterine endometrium. The most common site (approximately 90%) is in the distal ampullary region of a fallopian tube. Other sites are the ovaries, intra-abdominal cavity, and the intrauterine portion of the fallopian tube (cornual pregnancy). Ectopic pregnancy occurs in 1 out of 100–150 pregnancies and is the second leading cause of maternal mortality. Increased tubal infection rates, or sexually transmitted salpingitis, are likely a major contributor. Pelvic inflammatory disease (PID) is believed predisposing in 35% to 50% of patients. However, 50% of ectopics occur in tubes that by pathologic examination are normal. Other, less common predisposing factors include peritubal adhesions, tubal developmental abnormalities, prior tubal surgery (including sterilization), prior ectopics, intrauterine devices, and multiple induced abortions. After one ectopic pregnancy, the chance of another is 7% to 15%. If a pregnancy is discovered in the setting of a past tubal sterilization, the risk of an ectopic is overwhelming. Low dose progestational oral contraceptives may also be associated with a slight increase in ectopic pregnancy. Analogous to IUDs, they prevent intrauterine pregnancies, not extrauterine. Heterotopic pregnancies (coexisting ectopic and intrauterine gestation) were formerly considered rare. The incidence was estimated at 1:30,000 gestations. With available infertility corrective procedures now common, more recent incidence is estimated at 1:1,000.

Clinical manifestations of an ectopic pregnancy are diverse. In the "classic" presentation, a women presents with "slight' vaginal bleeding or "spotting," and the sudden onset of severe lower abdominal pain. Unfortunately, this presentation is neither sensitive nor specific to the final diagnosis. Pain may be constant, reflecting a peritoneal quality, may be intermittent, cramping, or absent. Up to 20% present without a history of a missed menses and 50% do not have identifiable risk factors.

The physical exam may be equally misleading. If the patient presents with a history of a missed menses, vaginal bleeding, and sudden abdominal pain, the diagnosis of ectopic is finalized in less than 20%. If a positive pregnancy test is associated, the rate increases to 60%. Localizing adenexal tenderness or mass is noted in 60% of cases. A contralateral corpus luteal cyst rupture may mimic the clinical picture of a ruptured ectopic and can add confusion to the diagnosis. The palpation of the corpus of pregnancy may lead to an erroneous physical exam with the opposite adenexa containing the ectopic. Free cystic fluid or blood can cause peritoneal irritation to the degree that an accurate physical exam is precluded. Unless products of conception or fetal tissue is demonstrated, ectopic may not be excluded. Even then, if in the setting of infertility therapy, the diagnosis may not be assured.

The previous "gold standard" for diagnostic evaluation was direct visualization by laparoscopy. This technique may fail in the setting of a small gestational sac and early pregnancy. Algorithms have been recently developed combining transvaginal ultrasound, uterine curettage, single measurements of serum progesterone and serial measures of the beta subunit of human chorionic gonadotropin.

Ultrasound is used to establish location of the gestation, estimate age, and assess viability. It is most optimal if performed transvaginally. Transabdominal scanning cannot generally visualize a yolk sac at less than 6 weeks' gestation and is indeterminate in 50% of subsequently proven ectopic pregnancies. Transvaginal scanning optimizes patient comfort and allows visualization of the gestational sac and other landmarks up to one week prior to the transabdominal technique. Eight possible sonographic categories of intrauterine and extrauterine findings in consideration of the diagnosis are possible in patients without a visible intrauterine pregnancy. These are confirmed ectopic pregnancy, highly likely ectopic pregnancy, very early normal pregnancy, occult unruptured ectopic pregnancy, complete or incomplete spontaneous abortion, dead embryo, embryonic resorption/blighted ovum, and hydatidiform mole/trophoblastic disease. A confirmed ectopic pregnancy is only visualized in 25% of transvaginal scans and 10% of those done transabdominally. In the highly likely category, reliance on ancillary findings is required. **Table 84.1** lists these findings and their overall accuracy in predicting ectopic pregnancies.

When combined with serum hormone testing and menstrual dating, an expected template of visualized intrauterine structures is created. The failure to visualize these structures implies the category of an occult unruptured ectopic pregnancy. Management must be individualized and may rely on repeat hormone testing, serial sonography, or laparoscopy. Inpatient versus outpatient care is based on an assessment of clinical risk–benefit. If a quantitative serum Hcg is present at a level of 1,800 MIU/mL, with an empty uterus by transvaginal scanning, the risk of an ectopic gestation is high. Further clinical evaluation must proceed along this course. In the hands of a skilled operator, a small unruptured ectopic may be visualized in select patients without severe symptoms. For recently developed medical treatment options, visualization of an unruptured gestational mass less then 4 cm is optimal.

Serial beta-Hcg occupies a predictable slope in most normal gestations. Production doubles at approximately 2 day intervals. In ectopic pregnancy, beta Hcg is produced by ectopic trophoblastic tissue and "drops off" the expected slope. The doubling time is prolonged. In a low risk, clinically stable patient, close follow-up of this slope change can provide valuable assistance in confirming the diagnosis. Pitfalls occur. Fifteen percent of normal pregnancies do not follow a predictable slope, and approximately 15% of ectopics do. Overall, serial beta-Hcg is valuable as an assessment of fetal viability, to clue the optimal time for ultrasound, and to document the effectiveness of uterine curettage.

The serum progesterone level reflects production of the corpus luteum by a viable pregnancy. During the first trimester, production is constant. If the pregnancy fails, production decreases. As a screening test, it is inexpensive and can assist in the identification of patients requiring further testing. If the level on one single test is greater than or equal to 25 ng/mL, it excludes ectopic pregnancy with 97% to 98% sensitivity. This may obviate the need for further testing. If a single level is less than or equal to 5 ng/mL, a nonviable pregnancy is established with 100% sensitivity. This low level does not establish the diagnosis of ectopic, but encourages a definitive study such as diagnostic uterine evacuation by uterine curettage. For a level between 5 to 25 ng/mL, ultrasound examination is usually the test of choice to assist in establishing viability.

Uterine curettage should be performed after the documentation of a nonviable fetus by a single progesterone level or plateauing of serial beta-Hcg with time. Intrauterine scrapings are examined for the appearance of villi. If present, they indicate the occurrence of a spontaneous intrauterine abortion. In the absence of villi, a decrease in the beta-Hcg of 15% over 8 to 12 hours is diagnostic of a completed abortion. If an ectopic gestation, the trophoblastic tissue will continue Hcg production causing a continued plateau or even rising hormone levels.

The role of culdocentesis in the early diagnosis of ectopic pregnancy has been severely curtailed by these recent diagnostic strategies. In the unstable patient, a role may persist where time does not permit ultrasonography or in the situation where it is not available. The procedure is performed by pulling the cervix anteriorly and inserting a 16–18 gauge needle via the posterior vaginal fornix into the peritoneal cavity. A return of non-clotting blood is considered diagnostic. Formerly a hemocrit >12% was considered significant for ectopic rupture. Less than 12% was considered more likely to imply a ruptured corpus luteum. More recently, the significance of this measure has been questioned. Eighty-five percent to 90% of patients with a ruptured ectopic will have a positive tap. Sixty-five percent to 70% of those with an unruptured ectopic will be positive. In the case of brisk bleeding, usually with hypovolemic shock, the blood may clot due to a lack of time for the natural activation of the fibrinolytic system. Blood will clot if a pelvic vein is entered erroneously. A negative culdocentesis, i.e., no fluid return, may result from a failure to enter the peritoneum. This may be due to a technical error or secondary to obliteration of the cul de sac from pelvic inflammatory disease and scar formation. The withdrawal of serous fluid implies a negative result. Occasionally, a ruptured corpus luteum may likewise present. In fewer than 5% of cases, unruptured ectopics present initially with a serous withdrawal.

The treatment of ectopic pregnancy has changed in the last few years with the onset of a medical option. Previously, multiple drugs were attempted with limited success. More recently, regimens utilizing methotrexate at relatively low doses have yielded success rates analogous to those of the

Table 84.1	
Ultrasound Findings and Ectopic Risk	
Ultrasound Findings	**% Ectopic**
Any free fluid	20
Echogenic mass	71
Moderate-large fluid	95
Echogenic mass + fluid	100
No ancillary findings	20

surgical standard, laparoscopic salpingostomy or salpingectomy. Systemic methotrexate, a folic acid antagonist, inhibits the spontaneous synthesis of purines and pyrimidines. The effect is the interference with DNA synthesis and cell division. Low doses and shorter courses minimize side effects and are further attenuated by leucovorin (citrovorum factor) rescue. In high doses, methrotrexate has been documented to cause bone marrow suppression, acute and chronic hepatotoxicity, stomatitis, pulmonary fibrosis, alopecia, and photosensitivity. With the extensive data now available from the treatment of trophoblastic disease, the risk of neoplasia, congenital anomalies, subsequent abortions, and fetal abnormalities is believed exceedingly low. Eligible patients for treatment are hemodynamically stable with ectopic pregnancies that are unruptured and measure less than 4 cm by ultrasound. If patients have any clinical evidence of rupture (acute abdomen), acute intra-abdominal bleedings (hypotension, decreasing hematocrit), ectopic mass greater than 4 cm, or fetal cardiac activity, they are ineligible for this treatment. Results compare well with laparoscopic techniques, comparing oviduct patency, subsequent pregnancies, and the future risk of ectopic pregnancy. Colicky abdominal pain is common in the days post procedure, especially in the time frame of days 3–7. The pain can be difficult to distinguish from that of a rupturing ectopic and is presumably due to a tubal abortion.

The surgical management of ectopic pregnancy has evolved over the last several years to emphasize the preservation of fertility, cost reduction, and allow a rapid recovery. Laparotomy is now only performed if the laparoscopic approach is difficult or the patient is hemodynamically unstable. Linear salpingostomy has become the standard laparoscopic operation. A longitudinal incision is made over the bulging antimesenteric border of the implantation site, the products of conception are removed, hemostasis is achieved, and the incision is left to heal by secondary intention. This procedure is successful in approximately 95% of ectopics, i.e., no further procedure is necessary. Greater than 85% of women are left with patent oviducts, 66% achieved subsequent pregnancy, and up to 23% had subsequent ectopics.

Post-operative bleeding, persistently elevated beta-Hcgs indicative of remaining trophoblastic tissue, or other associated symptoms occur in 5% to 20% of these conservatively managed surgical cases. Usually re-exploration and salpingectomy is necessary.

With either medical or surgical therapy, weekly quantitative beta-Hcgs are necessary until they are undetectable.

Abortion

Abortion is defined as the termination of pregnancy by any means before the fetus is sufficiently developed to allow survival. Spontaneous abortion is categorized as that which occurs prior to the 20th week of gestation as defined by the first day of the last menstrual period. Overall, 20% of all pregnancies end in abortion, 80% within the initial 12 weeks. First trimester bleeding occurs in 30% to 40% of pregnancies. Spontaneous abortion ultimately results in half of those pregnancies with bleeding. The incidence of spontaneous abortion increases with parity,

advancing maternal or paternal age, and if pregnancy occurs within 3 months of a prior birth.

The exact mechanisms causing abortions are not clear. Early pregnancy demise is presumptively caused by death of the fetus and subsequent expulsion. In later stages, other factors presumably cause failure and expulsion of an initially live fetus. Etiologically, the number one cause is fetal genetic abnormalities, responsible for approximately 50% of all spontaneous abortions.

The usual clinical presentation of a first trimester spontaneous abortion is one of a moderate amount of vaginal bleeding—bleeding often not substantially more than that a typical menses. Bleeding tends to begin prior to the onset of midline lower abdominal "cramping" pain; it can begin hours or days before the pain starts. This pain is generally described as similar in quality and character to the typical menses, but is usually more pronounced. If the abortion is actively progressing, bleeding becomes more profuse, often with visible clots or tissue, and the abdominal pain becomes more severe. If complete passage of the fetus occurs, signs and symptoms often quickly resolve.

Threatened abortion is loosely defined as any bleeding in pregnancy prior to 20 weeks. The cervix is closed without evidence of tissue extrusion. Abdominal pain, if present, is not a favorable sign. Most women with significant associated abdominal pain will abort. The physical exam is generally unrevealing with exception of blood being present in the vagina. Management in the ED is expectant. A CBC and quantitative beta-Hcg should be obtained. If blood loss is severe enough to cause a significant anemia, evacuation of the conceptus is usually recommended. Occasionally, slight hemorrhage continues for several weeks. Quantitative Hcg becomes important in establishing fetal viability during outpatient follow-up. Analogous to the outpatient evaluation of ectopic pregnancy, the use of ultrasound and quantitative Hcg measures, assist in establishing standard development templates. Management options during outpatient follow-up should be reviewed with the patient. On ED discharge, women should be prescribed bed rest with defined instructions to return if bleeding recurs or increases, abdominal pain returns, or if fever/chills develop. Women must also be instructed to refrain from sexual intercourse or inserting tampons.

Inevitable abortion is signaled by membrane rupture and cervical dilation. During the initial 20 weeks of gestation, this is usually noted as sudden bleeding without expulsion of the conceptus. If associated with abdominal pain or fever, emergent evacuation of the uterus should be recommended. During the later stages of the initial half of pregnancy, this event may occur without bleeding, i.e., only with a loss of amniotic fluid. This is believed secondary to a small loss of fluid which has accumulated between the amnion and the chorion. The rent in the chorion is not believed to extend through to the amnion, thus preventing complete fluid loss and pregnancy failure. In these cases, bed rest and re-evaluation in 48 hours is recommended. If no continuing fluid leak, bleeding, abdominal pain, or fever ensues, conservative management may be continued. The patient may resume regular activities, except that no vaginal penetration is permitted, and continue close outpatient follow-up.

Incomplete abortion occurs with the incomplete passage of fetal products. The fetus and placenta have a high likelihood of complete passage prior to the 10th week of gestation. After that, the likelihood of placental retention after the fetus has been expelled increases. If the placenta is only partially detached, it acts as a "wedge," not allowing local myometrial contraction. Denuded placental vessels bleed profusely without myometrial constriction. Hypovolemia may result. Emergent evacuation, usually via dilation and curettage, is indicated.

Complete abortion is defined by complete expulsion of both the fetus and associated placental structures. The uterus will contract and the cervix will close. Any abdominal pain that the patient presented with will resolve in a modest time. Complete abortion is sometimes difficult to confirm in the ED setting unless a complete gestational sac is available for examination. In doubtful cases, ultrasound examination should be obtained. If the uterus is sonographically empty, complete passage is assured. If the thickness of the uterine contents exceeds 5 mm, retained tissue is highly likely. A "uterine stripe," or non-dilated uterus cavity, will negate the need for further evaluation. If continued diagnostic doubt exists, especially in the setting of a tender uterus, dilation and curettage should be pursued. It will be both diagnostic and therapeutic. If complete expulsion is confirmed, management is supportive. Outpatient follow-up should be routinely available in approximately 2 weeks. Discharge instructions should suggest immediate return to the ED if excessive bleeding, foul smelling vaginal discharge, or fever.

Missed abortion is defined as the retention of dead conception products in utero, usually at less than 20 weeks gestation, for an extended period of time. The time frame is arbitrarily applied as several weeks. Typically, missed abortions occur in early pregnancy. Over time, it will become apparent that the pregnancy is not progressing. Maternal changes regress, and the uterus does not enlarge and may even contract. The woman may have no symptoms unless complications develop. Generally, the course remains an asymptomatic maternal state until signs and symptoms of a spontaneous abortion supersede. The expelled product, if retained for several weeks, may be macerated and shriveled. If complications occur, they are related to infection and coagulopathy. This is more likely if the fetus is more developed, especially if progressing through the second trimester. Treatment is based on the emergent evacuation of the fetus and blood product support. The consumptive coagulopathy stops once the products of conception are removed. Resolution of the clinical state resolves more slowly.

Septic abortion is defined as a uterine infection following an abortion at any stage. The bacteria flora is mixed originating from the bowel and vagina. Anaerobic bacteria occur in a greater percentage of cases with bacteremia (60%), with *Peptostreptococcus* species the most common. Aerobic organisms represent 40% of positive blood culture cases with *Escherichia coli, Pseudomonas* species, beta-hemolytic streptococci, and *Enterococcus faecalis* predominating. Metritis is typical, but parametritis, peritonitis, or generalized septicemia are not unusual. Even mild infec-

tions require vigorous treatment from the start including prompt conceptus evacuation and broad spectrum antibiotics.

Abruptio Placenta

Abruptio placenta is defined as the premature separation of the normally implanted placenta. It typically occurs in the second half of gestation and accounts for about 30% of mid to late pregnancy-related bleeding.

The source of the separation in abruption is believed secondary to the rupture of small, abnormal arterioles in the decidua basalis layer of the uterus. The bleeding "dissects" the normally adhered placental–uterine junction. This can be classified in a few ways. The bleeding may insinuate itself between the placental membranes and the uterus completely, escaping from the cervix, and causing signs of "external" hemorrhage. Less often the blood does not escape externally and is retained between the uterus and placenta, forming a "concealed" hemorrhage. Abruption may be "total," i.e., including the entire placenta, or may be "partial," involving a segmental separation of the junction. Concealed hemorrhage carries a higher risk of complications. The extent of hemorrhage is not as apparent and the risk of an induced coagulopathy increases.

The precise etiology of the inciting incident in abruption is not known, but associated conditions have been well described. The most common is hypertension, whether pregnancy induced or chronic. Associated subtle vascular disease is postulated as a factor. Cigarette smoking, chronic alcohol consumption, and cocaine abuse have all been linked. Placental abruption may complicate 5% to 6% of "minor" traumatic events and up to 50% of major injuries. The presence of uterine leiomyoma, especially if located behind the placental implantation site, is associated. Preterm, premature ruptured membranes are a known risk factor for the early separation of membranes leading to abruption.

Abruption occurs in approximately 1 out of 150–200 deliveries, typically in the middle trimester. The classic presentation is vaginal bleeding associated with abdominal pain. However, presentation is often subtle and quite variable. Description of the pain is described as relatively benign, to mimicking normal labor, to a severe, unremitting event. In one frequently cited study, 22% of cases of idiopathic preterm labor were considered the diagnosis until late in the course of abruption. Vaginal bleeding is present in 80%. Its presentation is similarly variable. The volume or color does not correlate with the maternal amount lost or the amount concealed around the uterus. Uterine tenderness or back pain is present in 66%. Like the associated abdominal pain, its presentation varies from subtle to severe. Uterine contractions also present as a spectrum, from hypertonic (17%), to high frequency (17%). Maternal shock occurs, sometimes out of proportion to the amount of hemorrhage. The presumptive mechanism is uterine–placental release of vasoactive and coagulation mediators causing DIC and hemodynamic compromise.

The main differential diagnosis is always placenta previa. Using pain as the distinguishing characteristic, although generally useful, does not always apply. Case studies mimicking each other with "classic" clinical descriptions have been recorded. Other diagnoses to be distinguished in the later stages of pregnancy include early labor, uterine rupture, degenerating leiomyomas, complications of pre-eclampsia, and ovarian torsion. Medical illnesses to be considered include pyelonephritis, biliary colic, other liver diseases, and appendicitis. Ultrasound has a relatively low sensitivity in discriminating the diagnosis of abruption. Acute bleeding is difficult to recognize, given the density of the placenta, and small collections may be easily missed. It is a useful tool to screen for associated differential diagnoses, especially placenta previa, and is warranted in that role.

The management of any bleeding in the later stages of pregnancy is based on rapid maternal stabilization and assessment. In severe cases, fluid resuscitation and the treatment of consumptive coagulopathy requires immediate institution. Patients require multiple large bore IVs, blood product availability, and laboratories studies including hematocrit, platelet count, PT, PTT, fibrinogen level, and a test of fibrin degradation products. Maternal Rh status must be assessed since fetomaternal hemorrhage occurs. Fetal monitoring should be applied in an emergent fashion. Patients with significant abruption and associated complications require emergency cesarean section. In milder degrees of abruption, admission and close observation is the rule. A more complete assessment of fetal maturity may then be undertaken.

Placenta Previa

Normal implantation and placental development takes place in the posterior, superior portion of the uterine fundus. Placenta previa is defined as implantation of the placenta over or near the cervical os. Four degrees of presentation are categorized: Total placenta previa has the cervical os completely covered by placenta. Partial placenta previa has the internal os incompletely covered. In marginal placenta previa, the edge of the placenta is at the cervical os. A low-lying placenta is implanted in the lower uterine segment such that the edge does not intrude upon the internal os, but is in close proximity. The extent of os coverage will depend on the degree of cervical dilation at the time of evaluation. As cervical dilation increases, the os may be more or less covered based on the original position of the placenta.

Placenta previa represents approximately 20% of the bleeding episodes in the later stages of pregnancy, but overall represents a relatively rare occurrence. Its frequency is roughly 1 of 200 to 300 pregnancies, or 0.3% to 0.5 %. Although the zygote does intermittently implant in the lower uterine segment, posterior-superior migration of the placenta usually occurs during pregnancy, resulting in a normal position by birth.

Increasing age and multiparity are known risk factors for placenta previa. The risk for women delivering after age 40 approximates 1 in 50. Other risk factors include prior cesarean section, induced abortion, and cigarette smoking. Prior cesarean increases a woman's risk by 25%.

The classic presentation of placenta previa is painless vaginal bleeding toward the end of the second or in the third trimester of pregnancy. The bleeding usually occurs without warning, often in an otherwise normal pregnancy. The rate varies from a moderate amount that may spontaneously remit to profuse and potentially fatal. If the placenta is not covering the os, but is close, bleeding may not begin until the onset of labor. Abdominal pain occurs (20%), based on the degree of uterine irritability. Abdominal pain may also result from induced active labor.

Pathologically, the bleeding results from the shearing of placental attachments as the uterus elongates or the os dilates. Since there is no underlying myometrium, the natural hemostatic mechanism of myometrial contraction does not exist. A consumptive coagulopathy does not usually occur in placenta previa. Since the mechanism of disease involves passage out the os exclusively, coagulation cascade and mediator activation is not as likely.

The diagnosis must be suspected and ruled out in any pregnant women presenting with bleeding in the later stages of pregnancy. Clinical exam is limited by the danger of inducing a potentially profound hemorrhage. Digital examination is contraindicated if the diagnosis is suspected. Pelvic examination should optimally be carried out in a setting where an emergent cesarean could be performed. If an ED exam is necessary, only an atraumatic, partial speculum insertion should be performed in order to determine cervical bleeding. Ultrasonography is the diagnostic procedure of choice for placental localization, and should be performed, if available, prior to pelvic exam in a highly suspect case. Transabdominally, a full urinary bladder may deform the lower uterine segment to give a false impression of a placenta previa. A repeat scan with a nearly empty bladder may resolve this issue. The scan may alternatively be safely performed transvaginally. Use of the transvaginal method has decreased the false positive results found via the transabdominal route.

The management of placenta previa is based on the acuity of the presenting episode and the maturity of the fetus. The ultrasound examination has demonstrated the high likelihood of placental migration if the placenta previa is discovered prior to 30 weeks' gestation on routine sonography. The incidence of placenta previa or hemorrhage at delivery is about 3% if the previa is noted between 20 to 25 weeks, 5% at 25 to 30 weeks, and approximately 24% if noted at 30–35 weeks. Asymptomatic placenta previa prior to 30 weeks does not require activity restriction. It is only required if the previa persists beyond 30 weeks or becomes symptomatic. If the bleeding is minor and the fetus premature, management tends to be conservative. Bed rest, tocolytics, and close observation are the key elements. Cesarean section is the delivery method of choice, in prime consideration of the welfare of the mother. Aggressive management with transfusion and cesarean section has markedly reduced maternal morbidity and mortality. Preterm delivery is the major cause of perinatal mortality. However, even with matched controls, the group with placenta previa remains with slightly higher mortality. The placenta previa group also has a slightly higher incidence of small for gestational age infants (5%).

Pregnancy-Induced Hypertension

Elevated blood pressure during pregnancy is a challenging clinical problem. In addition to the basic management of the chronic hypertensive, the spectrum of pregnancy-induced hypertension (PIH) must be considered. Termed pre-eclampsia/eclampsia, PIH entails substantially greater maternal and fetal risk than is typical of uncomplicated essential hypertension.

The most accurate method of measuring blood pressure in the pregnant women has been controversial. Blood pressure responds to a greater degree to position change during pregnancy. The current recommendation is for the sitting position in outpatients and left lateral recumbent for hospitalized patients. The measurement of the diastolic pressure has been debated in the literature. Typically phase V (disappearance of sound) of Korotkoff's sounds is used. In pregnancy, Korotkoff sounds may be audible to very low levels. Thus, some have advocated the measure of Korotkoff phase IV (muffling) instead. In various clinical trials, this has been significant in less than 10% of patients. Therefore, the current recommendation remains to focus on phase V or the disappearance of sound. This is accepted as an accurate measure of the diastolic pressure in the pregnant patient.

Pre-eclampsia is a disorder unique to the pregnant patient. It is characterized by hypertension, proteinuria, generalized edema, and frequently coagulation and liver function abnormalities. It is present in 5% to 10% of all pregnancies. It occurs predominately in primigravidas, after the 20th week of gestation, and often near term. Additional predisposing factors include diabetes, multiple gestation, extremes of age (especially less than 20 years), changing paternity in successive pregnancies, high body mass, African-American heritage, hydatiform mole, and fetal hydrops. Chronic hypertension prior to pregnancy may predispose if of a moderate to severe nature. Mild, uncomplicated, essential hypertension is not believed a risk factor. Pre-eclampsia may progress to the convulsive stage, termed eclampsia, that is potentially life-threatening. Overall, pregnancy induced hypertension is responsible for 70% of hypertension in pregnancy and complicates 2.6% of all births.

In the nonpregnant patient, hypertension is usually defined as blood pressure greater than 140/90. In pregnancy, a diastolic pressure greater than 85 is significant. In addition, any change in systolic greater than 30 mm Hg and in diastolic greater than 15 mm Hg over early pregnancy levels is considered ominous. Blood pressure does normally increase somewhat toward the end of gestation, and a rise of 10 mm during late third trimester can be normal. Total protein excretion in a normal pregnancy may double over nonpregnant levels. Levels above 300 mg in a 24-hour collection is considered abnormal in the pregnant patient. Dipstick urine testing does not necessarily provide an accurate reflection of a 24-hour collection and should be cautiously used as a screening tool. Edema is no longer felt a significant criterion by many authorities, but remains in the classification scheme. Most normal gravidas develop dependent edema. In 30%, edema may become generalized without other evidence of a pre-eclamptic state. Conversely, it is not unusual for an eclamptic patient to have no edema on initial presentation.

The severity of pregnancy-induced hypertension can not be universally categorized. A rough categorization uses multiple signs and symptoms. Typically, "mild" PIH assumes a diastolic BP < 100 mm Hg, and trace to 1+ proteinuria. It also has a normal creatinine and normal to minimally elevated liver enzymes. There is usually no headache, visual disturbances, upper abdominal pain, oliguria, thrombocytopenia, hyperbilirubinemia, fetal growth retardation, or pulmonary edema. "Severe" PIH generally is reported as having the diastolic measured consistently greater than 110 mm Hg or higher and 2+ or greater proteinuria. Severe PIH also has an elevated serum creatinine and markedly elevated liver enzymes. Headache, visual disturbances, hyperreflexia, upper abdominal pain, oliguria, thrombocytopenia, hyperbilirubinemia, and pulmonary edema are typically present. Fetal growth retardation is a given. The presence of seizures defines the eclamptic progression of PIH.

Eclamptic seizures are generalized motor convulsions that may be preceded by any of the above descriptors of severe PIH either alone or in combination. Most seizures occur antepartum, but may occur during labor or within 48 hours of delivery. Some controversy exists regarding "late" postpartum eclampsia. It is defined as eclampsia occurring greater than 48 hours post delivery and is believed to involve 4% to 10% of all cases. Although seizures are the most common neurologic complication of pre-eclampsia, coma, cortical blindness, and retinal detachment have also been described.

Hemolysis, elevated liver, and low platelet or HELLP syndrome is a further complication of severe PIH and occurs in 5–10% of pre-eclamptic cases. It is characterized by hemolytic anemia, elevated liver enzymes (transaminases), and low platelet counts (<100,000). PT, PTT, and fibrinogen are normal. The blood smear notes an intravascular hemolytic process (microangiopathic hemolytic anemia). Clinically the patient is similar to the pre-eclamptic, but with more severe acute liver symptoms (pain), and bleeding risk from multiple sites. Maternal mortality is increased as a result.

Vasospasm is inherent to a discussion of the pathophysiology of pre-eclampsia/eclampsia. It is believed to be the main ingredient necessary for arterial damage and subsequent vasculopathy. Angiotensin II is believed the main agent of vasoconstriction. Its target structures are endothelial cells and vessel wall integrity. As these cells and arterioles undergo cyclical contraction, damage occurs and blood constituents, such as platelets, and fibrinogen are deposited subendothelially. Progressive vascular changes ensue, with hemorrhage and cell necrosis contributing to the end organ dysfunction marking severe PIH. Prostaglandins likely have a significant supporting role in this vasospastic phenomenon. Although the exact pathologic basis remains elusive, it is known that prostacycline release is blunted while thromboxane A2 levels are markedly increased. Recent studies have demonstrated the ability of low dose aspirin to markedly alter morbidity and mortality, presumably via prostaglandin inhibition.

The basic management of the patient with pregnancy induced hypertension has three easily defined goals: termination of pregnancy with the least risk to mother and fetus, birth of a healthy infant, and a completely healthy mother post delivery. Reaching this involves ambulatory care, precise hospital care, and if necessary, the careful induction of labor. Women with predisposing factors must be monitored closely during the last trimester. Rapid weight gain or an upward diastolic pressure trend in the later stages of pregnancy is cause for concern. Women at risk should be followed as an outpatient with weekly checks during the last month and biweekly checks the preceding two months. They must be advised to report symptoms such as headache, visual disturbances, and edema of the hands or feet. Preventing pre-eclampsia by rigid salt restriction and diuretics has been attempted in the past without scientific evidence of success. It is not currently recommended. Low dose aspirin therapy has been advocated by some to lessen the risk of progression to pre-eclampsia by at risk women. There is little evidence of fetal risk utilizing this therapy and it may act to stem the outcome of fetal growth retardation in women affected by PIH. The presumptive mechanism involves thromboxane inhibition, likely interference with vasospasm, and altered platelet aggregation. Women with blood pressures less than 140/90 and no proteinuria may often be carefully managed at home. This requires close follow-up and biweekly visits to an outpatient setting. The women must be considered reliable enough to report symptoms and must spend the majority of time at bed rest. Minor elevations of blood pressure will often be quite responsive. Hospitalization should be considered for sustained blood pressures of 140 systolic or greater, and a diastolic of 90 or greater. The mainstay of therapy remains is bed rest with careful observation. Unless fetal immaturity is an overriding concern, any further progression of mild PIH would be an indication for cesarean section. The use of multiple antihypertensive regimens in the pool of women that have advancing symptoms of PIH and fetal immaturity have not demonstrated beneficial effect for either the mother or fetus. There is no evidence that the pregnancy may be prolonged or the mother's complications limited. In severe pre-eclampsia, i.e., with BP > 160/110 and end organ symptoms and signs, antihypertensive therapy is indicated as well as urgent delivery. This must occur regardless of fetal age. Treatment is identical to that of eclampsia.

Most facilities still base treatment on modifications of the original 1955 Parkland Hospital regimen. Magnesium sulfate is utilized to control seizures and works in most instances. It is not used as a strict antihypertensive. Generally the IV route is most commonly used. The initial rate is 6 g IV over 15 minutes, followed by 2 g per hour as a maintenance drip. An achieved serum level for magnesium of 5–8 mg/dL is adequate. Clinical observation for signs of toxicity is important. Observation for the loss of reflexes (patellar) and respiratory depression is key. Patellar reflexes are lost at serum magnesium concentrations 8.4–12 mg/dL. Respiratory depression can occur with levels greater than 12 mg/dL. Calcium gluconate given as a 1 g dose slowly IV is an effective reversal agent if respiratory depression occurs. Care must be taken as this reversal may be short lived. If necessary more aggressive airway management and respiratory support must be undertaken. Although magnesium is not a direct antihypertensive, blood pressure is often controlled in concert with the seizure control. Magnesium does seemingly act to relax arterial vasculature and decrease systemic vascular resistance.

Other antihypertensive treatment is generally indicated only if the blood pressure remains out of control, i.e., diastolic >110 mm Hg. Hydralazine is the classic choice due to the large base of experience, but regimens utilizing nitroprusside and labetalol have been utilized with success. The rapid lowering of blood pressure must be avoided. Uterine hypoperfusion and fetal distress may result.

Alternative anticonvulsants such as phenytoin and benzodiazepines have been used but are infrequently necessary. Magnesium has an effectiveness approaching 95% in initial seizure control. If phenytoin is used, a lower loading dose, i.e., 10 mg/kg is appropriate secondary to protein changes (hypoalbuminemia) in pregnancy. Benzodiazepines have the disadvantage of placental transfer and fetal depression.

Infant outcome after pregnancy-induced hypertension is generally thought favorable if no immediate hypoxic complications are present. A slight delay in growth rate has been documented to age 1.5 years. Long-term follow-up data are not available. Most women followed long term are not believed to have a higher rate of chronic hypertension versus age matched controls. Some studies differ with this view, especially for younger primigravidas, with severe PIH, and of African-American descent.

Hydatiform Mole (Molar Pregnancy)

Hydatiform moles are characterized by the growth of chorionic villi, usually occupying the uterine cavity. Rarely they present in the oviduct or ovary. The presence or absence of a fetus is used to classify the mole as partial or complete. They occur in 1 per 1,000 pregnancies, with the incidence highest in women at the beginning and end of the childbearing years. Recurrence is uncommon.

Clinically, early in pregnancy, there are few characteristics to distinguish it from any other. Late in the first to early in the second trimester, signs and symptoms begin to emerge. Uterine bleeding is the most common. It is generally intermittent and may be present for months. Profuse bleeding is less common. Uterine size often rapidly increases. In 50%, the appropriate size for gestational age will be rapidly exceeded. Corresponding fetal heart tones will not be heard. Pre-eclampsia often occurs prior to what is seen typically, i.e., before 20 to 24 weeks of gestation. Systemic venous embolization of chorionic material has been described and may mimic pulmonary embolism.

The diagnosis is usually made with ultrasound. The uterine contents are typically described as a "snowstorm." Uterine myomas and pregnancies with multiple fetuses may be confused with a somewhat similar appearance initially.

The treatment of hydatiform mole is evacuation of the mole and careful follow-up for detection of persistent proliferation or malignant change. Evaluation for metastatic disease must occur. This usually consists of a chest x-ray and a careful physical exam. A more extensive evaluation is reserved for those with some clinical indicator of spread. Prophylactic chemotherapy is not currently recommended. Most women will spontaneously regress after evacuation of the uterus. The mortality from this entity is practically zero.

Guidelines for Prescribing Drugs in Pregnancy

In the United States, prescription drugs are tested in non-pregnant populations prior to approval by the Food and Drug Administration (FDA). Extensive, well controlled clinical trials to examine the efficacy, safety, and pharmacokinetic profile in the pregnant population are rare. The FDA advocates use of its classification to categorize the potential fetal risk of drugs based on currently available information. This follows in **Table 84.2**.

Any drug or chemical substance administered to the mother crosses the placenta to some extent unless it is altered or destroyed during passage. Placental transport of maternal substrates is established at approximately the 5th week of pregnancy. Substances of low molecular weight are freely permeable across the placenta, driven solely by concentration gradients. The transport of all substances to the fetus is accepted. The issue is whether the rate and extent of this transport results in a fetal concentration sufficient to exert a physiologic change. Subtle effects have not been investigated in any extensive manner, e.g., in regard to neonatal adaptation, behavioral, psychological, and intellectual development.

Teratogenic effects of drugs are mostly frequently noted as anatomic malformations. These effects are dose related and are most important in the initial three months of gestation. Susceptibility during other times of the gestation is likely. This impact is often much more difficult to discern scientifically. Drugs may have maternal effects that indirectly affect the fetus. The impairment may occur on the cellular level, e.g., embryonic cell alteration, or on the cellular environment, e.g., the nutritional milieu of the fetus. Nutritional disruption may occur via the interruption in placental transport or metabolism. It is crucial that concerns be noted beyond the initial obvious teratogenic phase. The diethylstilbestrol (DES) saga and the delayed appearance of female adenocarcinoma and male reproductive abnormalities have been well described. This concept of long-term latency has likewise been well described in the lab environment.

The issue of drug transfer through breast milk and the postpartum period is significant. Human milk is a suspension of fat and protein in a carbohydrate-mineral solution. Transport modalities for maternal–infant drug delivery can operate with any of those components. Issues of protein binding, lipid solubility, direct membrane concentration gradients, and ionization structure are all significant. Much of the current available information in humans gives information only on milk concentration of a drug af-

Table 84.2

FDA Pregnancy Risk Classification for Pharmaceuticals

Category A
- Controlled trials in women fail to demonstrate a risk to the fetus in the first trimester.
- There is no evidence of risk in later trimesters.
- The possibility of fetal harm appears remote.

Category B
- Animal-reproduction studies have not demonstrated a fetal risk, but there are no controlled trials in pregnant women or
- Animal-reproduction studies have shown an adverse effect, other than a decrease in fertility, that was not confirmed in controlled studies in women in the first trimester and there is no risk in later trimesters

Category C
- Studies in animals have revealed adverse effect on the fetus, teratogenic/embryocidal effect or other, and there is no controlled trials in women, or
- Studies in women and animals are not available.
- Drugs should be given only if the potential benefit outweighs the potential risk to the fetus.

Category D
- There is positive evidence of human fetal risk.
- The benefits from use in pregnant women may be acceptable despite the risk, i.e., if the drug is to be used in a life threatening situation or for a serious disease where an alternative is not available.
- There will be an appropriate statement in the "warnings" section of the labeling

Category X
- Studies in animals or humans have demonstrated fetal abnormalities or there is evidence of fetal risk based on human experience, or both.
- The risk of use of the drug in pregnant women clearly outweighs any possible benefit.
- The drug is contraindicated in women who are or may become pregnant.
- There will be an appropriate statement in the "contraindications" section of the labeling.

ter a single measurement. Information such as maternal dose, frequency of administration, time of dose to sampling, frequency of nursing, and the length of lactation are not known. Therefore precise advice regarding a specific drug cannot be given. Animal studies provide some, but limited, assistance. The ultimate decision on drug use during lactation is analogous to drug use during pregnancy. A risk-benefit assessment must again occur. The important difference is that if the mother needs a drug as a therapeutic modality, the choice to not nurse can be recommended.

Most pharmaceuticals carry a "C" designation due to this lack of precise clinical information. Even "B" drugs are often classified utilizing insensitive markers of drug safety. All drug use in pregnancy and immediately post pregnancy must be gauged against a clear risk–benefit analysis. The respective FDA classification should be used as a guide with the limitations as described. In spite of this statement, studies have consistently demonstrated increasing drug utilization during pregnancy on a worldwide basis. This includes prescription medications and all forms of over-the-counter preparations. The World Health Organization conducted a recent survey of 15,000 pregnant women from 22 countries and found that 86% of these women took medication during their pregnancies, averaging 3 prescriptions per woman. Pregnancy, as a symptom-producing event, has the capacity to drive the increasing utilization of pharmaceuticals. Health care providers must be able to use all available scientific information in a cohesive fashion to provide accurate advice and information to patients.

Selected Readings

Audet MC, Moreau M, Koltun WD, et al. Evaluation of contraceptive efficacy and cycle control of a transdermal contraceptive patch vs an oral contraceptive. *JAMA* 2001;285:2347–2354.

Barron WM, Lindheimer MD, Davison JM (eds). *Medical Disorders During Pregnancy,* 2d ed. St. Louis: Mosby-Year Book, Inc., 1995.

Bracken MB, Belanger K. Calculation of delivery dates. *N Engl J Med* 1989; 321:1483.

Briggs GG, Freeman RK, Yaffe SJ. *Drugs in Pregnancy and Lactation,* 4th ed. Baltimore: Williams & Wilkens, 1994.

Burkman RT, Collins JA, Shulman LP, Williams JK. Current perspectives on oral contraceptive use. *Am J Obstet Gynecol* 2001;185(2 Suppl):s4–s12.

Carson SA, Buster JE. Ectopic pregnancy. *N Engl J Med* 1993;329:1174–1181.

Comeau J, Shaw L, Marcell CC, Lavery JP. Early placenta previa and delivery outcome. *Obstet Gynecol* 1983;61:577–580.

Cunningham FG, Gant NF, et al (eds). *Williams Obstetrics,* 21st ed. New York: McGraw-Hill 2001.

Elliot M, Riccio J, Abbott J. Serous culdocentesis in ectopic pregnancy: A report of two cases caused by coexistent corpus luteum cysts. *Ann Emerg Med* 1990;19: 407–410.

Gleicher N, Elkayam U, Galbraith RM, et al (eds). *Principles and Practice of Medical Therapy in Pregnancy,* 2d ed. New York: Appleton & Lange, 1992.

Hardman J, Limbird LE, Gilman AG, eds. *Goodman & Gilman's The Pharmacological Basis of Therapeutics,* 10th ed. New York: McGraw-Hill 2001.

Heller M, Jehle D. *Ultrasound in Emergency Medicine.* Philadelphia: W.B. Saunders Company, 1995.

Hurd WW, Miodovnik M, Hertzberg V, Lavin JP. Selective management of abruptio placentae: a prospective study. *Obstet Gynecol* 1983;61:467–473.

Klebanoff MA, Koslowe PA, Kaslow R, Rhoads GG. Epidemiology of vomiting in early pregnancy. *Obstet Gynecol* 1985;66:612–616.

Lubarsky SL, Barton JR, Friedman SA, et al. Late postpartum eclampsia revisited. *Obstet Gynecol* 1994;83:502–505.

Rosen P, Barkin RM, Braen GR, et al (eds). *Emergency Medicine Concepts and Clinical Practice,* 3rd ed. St. Louis: Mosby-Year Book, Inc., 1992.

Rosenberg L, Palmer JR, Rao RS, Shapiro S. Low-dose oral contraceptive use and the risk of myocardial infarction. *Arch Intern Med* 2001;161:1065–1070.

Sibai BM, McCubbin JH, Anderson GD, et al. Eclampsia. I. Observations from 67 recent cases. *Obstet Gynecol* 1981;58:609–613.

Trussell J, Hatcher RA, Cates W Jr, et al. Contraceptive failure in the United States: an update. *Stud Fam Plann* 1990;21:269–273.

Trussell J, Kost K. Contraceptive failure in the United States: a critical review of the literature. *Stud Fam Plann* 1987;18:237–283.

Walker GR, Schlesselman JJ, Ness RB. Family history of cancer, oral contraceptive use, and ovarian cancer risk. *Am J Obstet Gynecol* 2002;186:8–14.

Wolf EJ, Mallozzi A, Rodis JF, et al. Placenta previa is not an independent risk factor for small for gestational age infant. *Obstet Gynecol* 1991;77:707–709.

Labor and Delivery

Mark R. Pundt

Uncomplicated Labor

Delivery of a neonate in the emergency department is not a common occurrence. Usually the patient is evaluated by the emergency physician and triaged to labor and delivery. However, in hospitals where obstetrical back-up is nonexistent or limited, and in situations where patients present with imminent delivery, the emergency physician must be prepared to provide the obstetrical care. The perinatal mortality rate related to deliveries in the emergency department (ED) is between 8% and 10%.[1]

Precipitous labor may occur in the multiparous patient whose course of labor is shorter than previous pregnancies or in the young nulliparous patient who does not recognize her symptoms of back pain or abdominal pain as labor. Premature labor or mistaking the symptoms of labor as false labor may also lead to a presentation where delivery is imminent. With the increasing population of the uninsured in our country, fewer women can afford prenatal care and present to the ED at the time of delivery. It is important for the emergency physicians to be prepared to manage patients who present in active labor with delivery imminent.

Labor is divided into four stages. Stage I begins at the onset of labor and ends, when dilatation of the cervix is complete (10 cm). Labor begins when uterine contractions occur at regular intervals (every 3 to 5 minutes) and last 30 to 45 seconds, and results in the dilatation and effacement of the cervix. The first stage is the longest stage of labor, commonly lasting 8 to 12 hours in the primigravida and 6 to 8 hours in the multiparous women. The duration is dependent on the multiple factors including: maternal parity, fetal presentation and lie, contraction intensity, fetopelvic diameters, and the ability of the cervix to dilate.

Stage II begins with full dilatation of the cervix and ends with the birth of the child. This stage can last from a few minutes to 1 to 2 hours. The duration is affected by the fetal presentation and lie, fetopelvic relationships, intensity of uterine contractions, and the efficiency of maternal pushing. During this stage of labor the contractions last 1 to 2 minutes, recur every minute and are accompanied by the maternal urge to push. This results in the progression of the fetal station to +3 and crowning of the presenting part.

Stage III begins with the birth of the child and ends with the delivery of the placenta. Placental separation usually occurs within 5 to 10 minutes of fetal delivery.

Stage IV involves the first hour after delivery of the placenta. This is an important period of observation for post-partum hemorrhage. Post-partum hemorrhage is most likely to occur during this period.

When a pregnant patient presents to the ED with contractions, abdominal pain, abdominal cramping, or back pain, it is important to differentiate between true and false labor. True labor occurs when the patient experiences regular uterine contractions that become more forceful with time and result in dilatation and effacement of the cervix. "Effacement" is the term used to describe the thinning of the cervix. False labor, also referred to as Braxton Hicks contractions, presents as irregular, brief contractions that do not result in cervical change.

The evaluation of the pregnant patient begins with a pertinent history, including the LMP; estimated gestational age (EGA); expected date of confinement (EDC); onset, frequency, and duration of contractions; and the presence of a single or multiple gestations. It is also important to know if this is the first pregnancy, if there is vaginal bleeding or a loss of amniotic fluid, and if any complications occurred during the pregnancy. The maternal past medical history and timing of her last meal will also be helpful.

The physical examination should include vital signs and, if time allows, a brief general physical examination. The abdominal examination should include palpation of the uterus to note the position of the fetus. Leopold's maneuver includes examining the gravid uterus at the apex, along its lateral aspects and along the inferior aspects. The fetal part that is palpated is noted at each point, allowing the examiner to determine the fetal presentation, position, lie, and if the fetal head has engaged in the pelvis. The fetal presentation refers to the fetal part that is most dependent in the birth canal. "Cephalic" and "breech" are terms used to describe the fetal presentation. The position refers to the relationship between a specific reference point on the fetus to a specific point on the maternal pelvis. For example, a fetus with a cephalic presentation may be in an occipitoanterior position. In this case, the occipital aspect of the fetal head is directed toward the maternal pubic symphysis. The fetal lie refers to the relationship between the long axis of the fetus and the long axis of the uterus. The fetus may present in a vertical, transverse, or oblique lie. The station indicates the level of the presenting part in relation to the maternal ischial spines. It is described as a number from −3 to +3. Position −3 is the pelvic inlet, position 0 is the ischial spines, and position +3 is the perineum. The examiner should also note the frequency, intensity, duration, and regularity of contractions. The fetal heart rate should be determined.

A vaginal examination should be performed if there is no evidence of vaginal bleeding. If bleeding is present, the vaginal examination should be deferred until placenta previa and abruptio placenta are ruled out by ultrasound. The vaginal exam should be performed using sterile gloves and a sterile speculum to prevent the chorioamnionitis. When performing the vaginal examination, the physician should note the presence of amniotic fluid, the dilatation and effacement of the cervix, and the presentation, station, and lie of the fetus. The presence of amniotic fluid can be confirmed with the use of nitrazine paper. If amniotic fluid is present, the nitrazine paper will turn from yellow to blue-green. The presence of amniotic fluid can also be confirmed by the appearance of ferning on a microscopic slide of the vaginal discharge. The examiner should note the presence or absence of meconium if amniotic fluid is present.

The frequency, character, and duration of uterine contractions should be monitored by external tocodynomometry. Tocodynomometry is the monitoring of the strength and pattern of uterine contractions. Abnormal uterine contraction patterns can be detected by tocodynomometry. If the patient remains in the ED, vaginal examinations should be performed hourly and repeated more frequently as labor progresses.

The fetal heart rate should be monitored every 15 minutes. Continuous electronic fetal monitoring should be used in high-risk pregnancies and in pregnancies in which a com-plication has arisen. Fetal well-being is demonstrated by fetal heart rate accelerations of at least 15 beats per minute, lasting for at least 15 seconds, associated with uterine contractions or fetal movement. Persistent fetal tachycardia, bradycardia, variable decelerations, late decelerations, or a flattened heart rate tracing suggest fetal distress. Decreased heart rate variability denotes an inactive, poorly responsive fetus. This may be due to fetal hypoxia, fetal acidosis, or the effects of drugs or toxins. Medications known to cause decreased variability include analgesics, phenothiazines, and sedative-hypnotics. Alcohol use can also result in decreased variability. Variable decelerations are relatively common and represent the physiologic response to fetal head compression in the birth canal or intermittent cord compression. Late decelerations usually indicate fetal hypoxemia and acidosis resulting from uteroplacental insufficiency. The heart rate deceleration occurs after maximal uterine contraction. The later and longer the deceleration, the greater the fetal distress. Late decelerations accompanied by baseline fetal bradycardia or decreased variability denotes significant fetal distress necessitating immediate delivery.

Bedside ultrasonography can be helpful in assessing the patient in labor and plan for the need of consultants. Ultrasonography of the uterus by the emergency physician will provide information on the fetal presentation and lie as well as an assessment of fetal heart rate, fetal viability and the presence of multiple gestations.

If time permits, intravenous access should be established with lactated Ringer's solution or normal saline. Blood testing, including a CBC, blood type, hepatitis B surface antigen, and an extra tube for cross-match, should be drawn. A urine sample should be evaluated for glucose and protein. The patient's vulvar area should be cleansed with betadine, and surgical drapes should be applied. The physician should scrub and apply a mask, sterile gloves, and gown. An assistant should acquire the delivery cart containing the equipment, supplies, and medications required to manage the emergent labor and delivery (**Table 85.1**).

If time permits, the physician should consider performing an episiotomy using local anesthesia to permit easier

---

Table 85.1

Suggested Contents of the Labor and Delivery Cart

Equipment	Supplies	Medications
Ambu bag, adult	Angiocaths	Calcium gluconate
Ambu bag, neonatal	Betadine	Diazepam
Blood pressure cuff	D5W solution	Diphenhydramine
Bulb syringe	Gauze sponges	Epinephrine 1:1,000
Cord clamp	IV tubing	Hydralazine
Doppler stethoscope	Lactated Ringer's solution	Lidocaine
Elastic tourniquet	Needles	Magnesium sulfate
Hemostats	Normal saline solution	Methyl ergonovine
Neonatal ET tubes	Sterile gloves	Nalaxone
Neonatal laryngoscopes	Sponges	Oxytocin
Plastic airway	Syringes	Prochlorperazine
Surgical scissors	Tape	Terbutaline
Umbilical tape	Towels	

delivery of the fetus. An episiotomy may prevent perineal lacerations, relieve compression of the fetal head, and shorten the second stage of labor by allowing easier delivery of the fetus; and an episiotomy is easier to repair than a vaginal or perineal tear. However, episiotomies result in greater blood loss during delivery, increase the incidence of third and fourth degree extension, result in more postpartum discomfort, and more commonly result in postpartum dyspareunia. During controlled, uncomplicated labor routine use performance of an episiotomy is not indicated.[2]

An episiotomy is indicated:
- When a vaginal tear is imminent
- In a breech or forceps delivery
- To facilitate a difficult delivery related to shoulder dystocia.

An episiotomy should be considered when the presenting part begins to distend the perineum.

To perform an episiotomy, the physician should infiltrate the posterior vaginal wall with 1% lidocaine and incise the posterior vaginal wall, perineal skin and subcutaneous tissue, and perineal body with scissors. The mediolateral approach is recommended to avoid perineal and rectal tears. After delivery, the episiotomy should be repaired with absorbable sutures. The posterior vaginal wall should be closed first with a running suture. Next, the perineal muscle and fascia should be closed with three to four interrupted sutures. The superficial fascia of the perineum should then be closed with a continuous suture. Finally, the perineal skin should be closed with a subcuticular stitch.

The sequence of events occurring in labor with a vertex presentation includes:
- Fetal engagement
- Descent
- Flexion
- Internal rotation
- Extension
- External rotation

Engagement is the movement of the fetal head into the maternal pelvis. It occurs late in the third trimester of pregnancy, occurring in the last 2 weeks of pregnancy in the primigravida and commonly with the onset of labor in the multigravida patient. Descent and flexion of the fetal head occur due to uterine contractions. Proper head flexion aids further fetal descent. Descent is also affected by the:
- Maternal pelvic configuration
- Size and position of the presenting fetal part
- Thinning of the lower uterine segment

Internal rotation occurs as the presenting part approaches the pelvic floor. The presenting part rotates anteriorly due to the gutter effect of the pelvic musculature. As the fetal head reaches the pelvic outlet, it is delivered by extension of the fetal head under the pubic symphysis and pubic rami, which act as a fulcrum. After delivery of the fetal head, external rotation occurs as the shoulders align with the anteroposterior diameter of the pelvis. The anterior shoulder is delivered first under the pubic symphysis; the posterior shoulder follows as the pubic symphysis is used as a fulcrum. The body, arms, and legs are delivered immediately after the shoulders.

Delivery of the fetus begins as the fetal head crowns. Crowning occurs when the fetal head is visible at the vaginal introitus and does not recede between contractions. Delivery of the fetal head should be controlled to prevent sudden expulsion of the baby and prevent fetal and maternal injury. During the delivery of the fetal head, the mother should pant or breathe through the nose to prevent the urge to push. Place one hand over the fetal head to prevent sudden expulsion and assist with normal head extension by gently lifting the baby's chin posterior to the mother's anus. As the head delivers, check for the presence of a nuchal cord, which occurs in approximately 25% of deliveries. If a nuchal cord is present and is loose and pulsating, gently slip it over the baby's head. If it is tight, apply two clamps close together on the cord, cut the cord and slip it over the baby's head. Next, suction the baby's oral and nasal passages with a bulb syringe.

After delivery of the fetal head, external rotation occurs. Following external rotation, apply one hand on either side of the baby's head and apply gentle, downward traction. The anterior shoulder will deliver under the symphysis pubis. If resistance is met, have an assistant apply suprapubic pressure. When the anterior shoulder is visible, apply gentle upward traction to deliver the posterior shoulder. Preventing rapid expulsion of the posterior shoulder will minimize the risk of tearing the anus and rectum. Next, slide the posterior hand onto the posterior shoulder and behind the neck to support the head. Slide the anterior hand along the baby's back as the body spontaneously delivers and grasp the leg with the third finger and thumb and place the index finger between the legs. Hold the baby's head lower than the body and suction the nose and mouth. Apply two cord clamps ~1 cm from the umbilicus and cut the cord between the clamps with sterile scissors. If the neonate requires resuscitation leave a longer umbilical stump to allow for venous access. Dry the baby, wrap it in a warm towel, and place the baby in a radiant warmer or on the mother's chest if a warmer is not available.

Allow the placenta to separate spontaneously. This usually occurs within 5 to 10 minutes of fetal delivery. Signs of placental separation include a rush of blood from the vagina and lengthening of the umbilical cord. One should not pull on the cord, as this may result in cord rupture or an inverted uterus. As the placenta is expelled, twist it to assist in removal of the membranes. After delivery of the placenta, assist the uterine contraction by performing suprapubic uterine massage and administering oxytocin 20 to 40 U/L at 200 mL per hour IV. Lastly, explore the vagina, cervix, and perineum for lacerations. Repair any lacerations and the episiotomy if it was performed.

Complicated Labor

Premature Rupture of Membranes

Premature rupture of membranes (PROM) occurs in approximately 3% of pregnancies. PROM can occur at any time during pregnancy. The patient may present with a complaint of a rush of fluid from the vagina or a continuous leak of fluid from the vagina. Vaginal exam should be performed under sterile conditions and digital exam of the cervix should be avoided to decrease the risk of infection. The diagnosis can be confirmed on physical examination by the use of nitrazine paper. If amniotic fluid is present in vaginal discharge, the nitrazine paper will turn from yellow to blue-green. The presence of amniotic fluid can also be confirmed by demonstrating ferning on a microscopic slide of the vaginal fluid. An ultrasound of the uterus may reveal oligohydramnios in a patient with PROM. PROM may result in premature labor, prolapsed umbilical cord, or intrauterine infection. PROM is the leading cause of endometritis and puerperal sepsis.

Treatment of PROM is dependent on the fetal maturity. In pregnancies with a gestational age of more than 36 weeks, the mother should be admitted so that labor can be induced with oxytocin if spontaneous labor has not commenced within 8 to 12 hours. When the gestational age is between 34 and 36 weeks, labor may be induced with oxytocin; however, the patient may be observed for up to 48 hours prior to labor induction. If the gestational age is less than 34 weeks, the patient should be hospitalized with strict bed rest and treatment with steroids to hasten fetal lung maturation.

Preterm Labor

Premature labor is defined as coordinated uterine contractions, occurring between 20 and 37 weeks of gestation, which lead to uterine effacement and dilatation. Premature labor occurs in 8% to 10% of pregnancies, and premature births account for 75% of perinatal mortality. Premature labor may be due to pregnancy induced hypertension (PIH), abruptio placenta or previa, multiple gestations, urogenital infections, cocaine abuse, or cigarette smoking.[3] The woman in premature labor may present with new pain in the back, thighs, pelvis, or abdomen; pressure in the pelvis, rectum, or bladder; vaginal pain or bleeding or a change in the vaginal discharge. The physical examination may reveal uterine contractions, dilatation and effacement of the cervix, vaginal bleeding, or PROM.

Management options include allowing the labor to continue or arresting labor with tocolysis. One can allow labor to continue if:

- Cervical dilatation is greater than 4 cm
- Cervical effacement is greater than 80%
- There is evidence of maternal hemorrhage
  - fetal distress or demise
  - intrauterine infection
  - PROM
  - severe PIH

Suppression of premature labor is indicated when there is evidence of:

- A healthy fetus and mother
- The gestational age is 20 to 36 weeks
- The membranes are intact
- The cervical dilatation is less than 4 cm
- The cervical effacement is less than 80%

Hydration with D5 1/2NS and sedation with morphine sulfate (8 to 12 mg i.m.) may be successful in suppressing premature labor. Tocolysis with beta adrenergic agents and magnesium sulfate may be required to suppress premature labor. β-adrenergic agents act on the B2 receptors to relax the myometrium and uterine vessels. Terbutaline (0.01 to 0.08 mg per minute IV or 0.25 to 0.5 mg sq q, for 2 to 4 hours) or ritodrine (0.05 to 0.35 mg per minute IV) are β-adrenergic agents used for this purpose. Magnesium sulfate also results in myometrial relaxation. Magnesium sulfate should be administered as follows: 4 to 5 g over 30 minutes IV, followed by 2 to 4 g per hour IV. The patient should be monitored for signs of toxicity, which include diminished reflexes and depressed respirations. If signs of magnesium toxicity occur, one should administer calcium gluconate as the antidote.

Failure to Progress

Failure to progress is defined as labor that results in no cervical change for 2 to 3 hours. Failure to progress may be due to cephalopelvic disproportion or problems with the strength or pattern of uterine contractions. All possible precipitating factors must be addressed before this diagnosis is made. The treatment for labor that is not progressing appropriately is most commonly cesarean section, although in certain instances the use oxytocin may be attempted.

Fetal Distress

Fetal compromise is due to fetal hypoxia and/or acidosis. Acute fetal compromise is classified into possible compromise, probable compromise, and certain fetal compromise. Possible fetal compromise should be considered when there is evidence of transient accelerations of the fetal heart rate with contractions; however, there is normal fetal heart rate variability. Probable fetal compromise should be considered when there is a lack of short-term variability of the fetal heart rate, but fetal heart rate accelerations occur during uterine contractions. Certain fetal compromise is evident with the presence of fetal tachycardia, lack of short-term fetal heart rate variability, and late fetal heart rate decelerations. It is important to monitor the fetus during labor to determine if there are any late decelerations or episodes of fetal bradycardia. If one does not have fetal monitoring available, it is important to check the heart rate using a fetal heart tone Doppler during and immediately after uterine contractions to evaluate for possible fetal distress or compromise.

When fetal compromise is considered, the patient should be placed in the left lateral position to relieve pressure on the inferior vena cava and oxygen should be applied. Maternal hypotension should be treated with intravenous fluids and ephedrine if required. Oxytocin should be discontinued if in use. If fetal compromise persists, the fetus must be delivered.

Ruptured Uterus

Uterine rupture occurs in one of 1,500 deliveries. Maternal mortality secondary to uterine rupture is 10% to 20%, with fetal perinatal mortality of more than 50%. Causes of uterine rupture include:

- Motor vehicle accidents
- Improper administration of oxytocin

- Excessive fundal pressure or bearing down
- Uterine scar from a:
  - previous cesarean section
  - myomectomy
  - previous abortion

The incidence of uterine rupture occurring due to scar dehiscence during a vaginal birth after cesarean section is between 0.3% and 1.7%.[4] The incidence is greater after a classical cesarean section with a vertical scar or in mothers who have had three previous cesarean sections. The patient with a uterine rupture may present with a complaint of vaginal bleeding or suprapubic pain or tenderness. However, uterine rupture can present without pain or vaginal bleeding. On physical examination, one may find:

- Tachycardia
- Hypotension
- Recession of the presenting fetal part
- Disappearance of fetal heart tones
- Cessation of uterine contractions
- Vaginal bleeding

One must consider uterine rupture whenever there is persistent bleeding or shock after delivery.

The treatment of uterine rupture includes resuscitation with intravenous fluids, blood and blood products, and immediate cesarean section and delivery of the fetus. A uterine repair can be attempted if future childbearing is important and maternal condition allows; otherwise, a hysterectomy is indicated. Potential complications of a ruptured uterus include hemorrhage, shock, amniotic fluid embolism, disseminated intravascular coagulation, and death.

Complicated Delivery

Dystocia

Dystocia is defined as difficult labor. Pelvic dystocia is due to aberrations of the pelvic architecture and its relationship to the presenting fetal part. The bony pelvis may have an abnormal size or structure. There may be a reproductive tract mass or neoplasm obstructing the birth canal. The placenta may be partially obstructing the birth canal. Fetal dystocia may be due to excessive fetal size from gestational diabetes or congenital anomalies. The most common cause of fetal dystocia is fetal malpresentation, which occurs in 5% of all pregnancies. Fetal malpresentation is due to abnormal fetal presentation, position, or lie. Fetal dystocia may also be due to multiple gestations. Uterine dystocia is due to ineffective uterine contractions or lack of voluntary expulsive forces.

The treatment of dystocia is dependent on the cause. Pelvic dystocia is treated with delivery by cesarean section. Uterine dystocia can be treated with oxytocin if the uterine contractions are hypotonic, or with tocolysis if the uterine contractions are hypertonic but ineffective. Fetal dystocia is treated by fetal manipulation. If fetal manipulation fails, then a cesarean section should be performed.

Maternal and fetal manipulation may be especially helpful in shoulder dystocia. Shoulder dystocia is the inability to deliver the fetal shoulders after delivery of the head. It occurs in up to 1.7% of all deliveries.[5] Fetal complications include:

- Brachial plexus injuries
- Humeral fractures
- Clavicular fractures
- Fetal hypoxia
- Fetal demise

Risk factors include:

- Maternal obesity
- Maternal diabetes mellitus
- Gestational diabetes

Shoulder dystocia presents during delivery as inability to deliver the anterior shoulder with downward traction and retraction of the fetal head against the perineum, the "turtle sign."

The management of shoulder dystocia includes draining the mother's bladder to increase the space in the pelvis and the performing an episiotomy. The mother's legs should be flexed to a knee-chest position to disengage the anterior shoulder (McRobert's maneuver). If this is unsuccessful then applying suprapubic pressure and gentle downward pressure on the fetal head may result in delivery of the anterior shoulder. If the shoulder dystocia persists the physician should insert a hand along the fetal spine and rotate the fetal shoulders 180° in an attempt to "corkscrew" the fetus and deliver a shoulder (Wood's maneuver). If this maneuver fails the physician should reach into the birth canal and deliver the posterior shoulder first by flexing the elbow, sweeping the fetal arm over its chest, bringing the hand to its chin and delivering the arm and posterior shoulder.

Prolapsed Cord

Umbilical cord prolapse occurs in 0.5% of cephalic presentations, 5% of breech presentations, and 20% of transverse presentations. It is associated with perinatal mortality rates of 8.6% to 49%.[6] Occult cord prolapse occurs when the cord lies adjacent to the presenting part. It can be inferred if the fetal heart rate changes associated with intermittent cord compression are detected by fetal monitoring. Overt cord prolapse occurs when the cord lies below the presenting part. The cord can be visualized or palpated in the vaginal canal. Risk factors for umbilical cord prolapse include:

- Prematurity
- Abnormal presentations
- Placenta previa
- Multiple gestations
- PROM[7]
- Cephalopelvic disproportion

Malpresentation is the cause of 50% of the cases of umbilical cord prolapse.

Management of occult cord prolapse includes placing the patient in the lateral, or Trendelenburg position to relieve pressure on the cord and administering oxygen to the mother. If the fetal heart rate normalizes, one can allow labor to continue. If the cord compression pattern persists or recurs on the fetal monitor, then the fetus should be delivered by cesarean section. Management of overt cord prolapse includes administering oxygen to the mother, placing the mother in the Trendelenburg position, with her knees to her chest, and applying continuous upward pressure on the presenting part to relieve pressure on the cord. The upward pressure on the presenting part should be maintained until the fetus is delivered by cesarean section.

Uterine Inversion

The uterus may become externalized immediately post delivery, usually due to traction on the umbilical cord during delivery. This may be partial, with inversion of the uterus into the vaginal vault, or complete, with entire externalization of the uterus. A combination of factors may cause uterine inversion, including:

- Primiparity
- Implantation of the placenta at the uterine fundus
- Excessive traction on the umbilical cord which remains attached to the placenta
- Fundal pressure to a relaxed uterus, including the lower segment and cervix
- Oxytocin use
- Placenta accreta[9]

The incidence of this condition is from one in 2,100 to one in 6,400 deliveries.

In partial uterine inversion, abdominal palpation reveals a crater-like depression in the suprapubic region, and vaginal examination reveals the uterine fundal wall in the cervix and lower vaginal segment. Complete inversion is diagnosed when the uterus is visualized outside the body. It is associated with immediate hemorrhage and should be considered a life-threatening complication.

Management includes the immediate assistance of an anesthesiologist, establishment of large-bore intravenous lines with lactated Ringer's solution and contact of the blood bank. If the placenta is still attached, it should not be manually removed until the intravenous tubes are secured and anesthesia is being administered to the patient. Tocolytic drugs such as terbutaline (2.5 mg per minute IV to start, and increase by 2.5 mg per minute, up to 20 mg per minute), ritrodrine (50 mg per minute IV to start, and increase by 50 mg per minute, up to 350 mg per minute) and magnesium sulfate (2 to 6 g IV load, then 2 to 4 g per hour drip) can be used for relaxation of the uterus to allow manual reimplantation. To attempt to remove the placenta before these resuscitation efforts are achieved increases the risk of hemorrhage, although the prolapsed uterus may be replaced into the vagina as a temporizing measure. If possible, an attempt should be made to try to reimplant the uterus without removing the placenta. If this maneuver proves impossible, after the placenta is separated from the uterus, reimplantation of the uterus may be performed by placing the palm of the hand on the center of the fundus with the fingers extended to identify the margins of the cervix. Pressure is applied with the hand along the long axis of the vagina to push the fundus upwards through the cervix.

Once reimplantation is accomplished, the tocolytic therapy should be stopped and oxytocin and prostaglandin therapy initiated to contract the uterus while the operator manually maintains the uterus in position. Bimanual compression will aid in this as well as decrease uterine hemorrhage until the uterus is contracting well. Oxytocin is not given until the uterus is reimplanted into its normal configuration; otherwise, reimplantation will be impossible due to a hard and contracted uterus that will not fit through the cervix.

Occasionally, the uterus cannot be reimplanted to its normal configuration manually, in which case an emergent laparotomy is indicated. Broad-spectrum antibiotics should be started after manipulation is complete and the patient is stabilized.

Multiple Births

The incidence of multiple gestations is increasing due to the use of fertility-enhancing medications and procedures. Signs and symptoms of multiple gestations include:

- A uterus larger than is usual for the length of the pregnancy
- Increased fetal activity
- Maternal weight gain greater than anticipated

The diagnosis is confirmed by ultrasound. It is important to know of the presence of multiple gestations to anticipate complications and prepare for the possible resuscitation of multiple babies. Potential complications include:

- Spontaneous abortion of a fetus
- Premature labor
- PROM
- Pregnancy induced hypertension
- Placenta previa
- Abnormal presentation
- Postpartum uterine atony

Stillbirth

Neonatal mortality, excluding stillbirths, is approximately 10 deaths per 1,000 births in the United States. Causes of perinatal deaths include:

- Congenital anomalies
- Breech presentation
- Placenta previa
- Abruptio placenta
- Pregnancy induced hypertension
- Multiple gestation
- Polyhydramnios

Stillbirth is associated with massive maternal obesity, advanced maternal age, and a high antepartum risk score.

Emergency Cesarean Section

If and when to perform a cesarean section on a pregnant patient in cardiopulmonary arrest is a difficult medical and ethical decision. Performing a cesarean section may improve maternal venous return and cardiac output, thereby increasing the likelihood of fetal survival. Early thoracotomy and open cardiac massage may increase the likelihood of both maternal and fetal survival. Factors that may be useful in predicting the possibility of fetal survival include:

- Gestational age
- Cause of maternal demise
- Fetal status prior to maternal death
- The quality and duration of the maternal resuscitation

- The interval between maternal cardiac arrest and the delivery of the fetus.

Chances of fetal survival are improved if the gestational age is greater than 28 weeks and the mother has not experienced prolonged hypoxia prior to arrest. The interval between maternal death and delivery is a major predictor of fetal survival. If the fetus is delivered within 5 minutes of maternal cardiac arrest, there is an excellent chance for fetal survival. If the fetus is delivered greater than 15 minutes after maternal cardiac arrest, the chances for fetal survival are poor. The decision to perform a postmortem cesarean section must be made and performed as early as possible after maternal cardiac arrest to enhance the likelihood of fetal survival.

When performing a perimortem cesarean section, informed consent from the family should be obtained if possible. If family is not immediately available, implied consent can be assumed. The abdomen should be opened as quickly as possible using a vertical incision. The fetus should be delivered through a vertical (classical) uterine incision. If a neonatologist is available, he or she should be in attendance to assist in the neonatal assessment and resuscitation.

References

1. Brunette DD, Sterner SP. Prehospital and emergency department delivery: a review of eight years experience. *Ann Emerg Med* 1989;18:1116–1118.
2. Borgatta L, Peining SL, Choen WR. Association of episiotomy and delivery position with deep perineal laceration during spontaneous delivery in the nulliparous woman. *Am J Obstetr Gyn* 1989;160:294–297.
3. Gonik B, Creasy RK. Preterm labor: its diagnosis and management. *Am J Obstetr Gyn* 1986;154:3–8.
4. Leung AS, Leung EK, Paul RH. Uterine rupture after previous cesarean delivery: maternal and fetal consequences. *Am J Obstetr Gyn* 1993;169:945–950.
5. Carlan SJ, Angel JL, Knuppel RA. Shoulder dystocia. *Amer Fam Phys* 1991;43:1307–1311.
6. Critchlow CW, Leet TL, Benedetti TJ, et al. Risk factors and infant outcomes associated with umbilical prolapse: a population-based case-control study among births in Washington State. *Am J Obstetr Gyn* 1994;170:613–618.
7. Koonings PP, Paul RH, Campbell K. Umbilical cord prolapse. A contemporary look. *J Repro Med* 1991;36:13–14
8. Barnett WM. Umbilical cord prolapse: a true obstetrical emergency. *J Emerg Med* 1989;7:149–152.
9. Lago JD. Presentation of acute uterine inversion in the emergency department. *Amer J Emerg Med* 1991;9:239–242.

Selected Readings

Al-Azzawi F. *A Color Atlas of Childbirth and Obstetric Techniques.* Aylesbury, UK: Wolfe Publishing. 1990.

Decherrney AH, Pernoll MC, ed. *Current Obstetrics and Gynecologic Diagnosis And Treatment.* 8th ed. Norwalk, CT: Appleton and Lange 1994.

Deutchman ME, Sakornbut EL. Diagnostic ultrasound in labor and delivery. *Amer Fam Phys* 1995;51:145–154.

Smith MA, Ruffin MT, Green LA. The rational management of labor. *Amer Fam Phys* 1993;47:1471–1481.

Postpartum Complications

Kerry B. Broderick

Retained Placenta

Placental expulsion occurs during the third stage of labor approximately thirty minutes after birth. However, fragmentation of the placenta causes abnormal expulsion. Fragmentation may be noted at initial delivery or diagnosis may be delayed until postpartum hemorrhage occurs. A less common etiology of retained placenta is a retained succenturiate lobe of the placenta. A succenturiate lobe is a small accessory lobe that develops at a distance from the periphery of the main placenta, this occurs in approximately 3% of pregnancies.

Delayed diagnosis retained placenta most commonly presents with bleeding 7 to 14 days after delivery. Patients may present with a history of intermittent spotting, followed by sudden, brisk, painless bleeding. Complaints of foul-smelling lochia may indicate infection of retained fragments. Abdominal examination is usually positive for a boggy, large uterus that is painless unless infection is present. Visual examination reveals bleeding through the cervix, and bimanual examination confirms a soft uterus, with or without tenderness. Ultrasound showing hypoechoic debris in the uterus is useful in confirming the diagnosis of retained fragments. However, blood clots and retained products have similar sonographic qualities. Retained placenta is unlikely when the ultrasound shows a normal uterine stripe or hyperechoic foci in the uterus without an associated mass. Clinical assessment using criteria such as enlarged uterus, open cervical os, offensive lochia, uterine tenderness and pyrexia are important clinical indicators to be considered along with the ultrasound appearance of the uterus.

In most cases, the necrotic placental fragment is extruded with initiation of bleeding, and no further treatment, other than contracting the uterus, is required. Fluid resuscitation and initial laboratory studies should be initiated. Laboratory studies may include CBC, type and screen, possible cross-match, coagulation studies, and fibrinogen levels. Medical management consists of pharmacologic agents, which contract and vasoconstrict the uterus. Agents include oxytocin, methylergonovine, or ergonovine until bleeding is controlled. Antibiotics should be added to the medical regimen if infection is suspected. Uterine curettage is occasionally necessary.

Hemorrhage

There is primary and secondary postpartum hemorrhage, Primary is immediate within 6 hours of delivery and secondary hemorrhage occurs after 24 hours and up to 6 weeks. In primary hemorrhage an estimated blood loss of greater than 500 mL is indicative that dangerous hemorrhage may be imminent. Prepartum factors which increase the potential for postpartum hemorrhage include overdistended uterus (multiple fetuses, large fetus or polyhydramnios), prolonged labor, rapid labor, high parity, oxytocin-induced or augmented labors, chorioamnionitis, and a poorly perfused myometrium secondary to maternal hypotension or hemorrhage prior to delivery.

The two most frequent causes of immediate postpartum hemorrhage are uterine atony and lacerations of the cervix and/or vagina. Less common factors include; retention of all or part of the placenta, uterine hematoma, uterine rupture, uterine inversion, and coagulation abnormalities. Although episiotomy blood loss can average 200 mL, it is infrequent that episiotomy alone causes significant postpartum hemorrhage. A complete uterine inversion should be readily recognized.

With an estimated blood loss of greater than 500 mL measures should be taken to reduce bleeding. Manual or bimanual uterine massage should be initiated to slow or halt hemorrhage. Uterine contraction not induced by manual massage should raise suspicion of uterine rupture with intraperitoneal hemorrhage. A firm and contracted uterus with continued hemorrhage despite manual massage should prompt a gentle vaginal exam to assess for incomplete uterine inversion. If vaginal examination is normal, a visual inspection of the perineum, vagina, cervix, and uterus should be performed. Anesthesia may be required for this examination. Complete pelvic examination is necessary after vaginal delivery in a woman with a previous cesarean section, breech extraction, or forceps delivery, and in any woman with excessive bleeding during the second stage of labor (combined etiologies such as uterine atony and trauma may be present).

If uterine massage fails to abate the hemorrhage, intravenous fluid administration should be continued at a rapid rate. One may consider cross-matching blood or ordering type-specific blood in anticipation of possible transfusion.

Uterine Atony

Uterine atony requires both mechanical and medical management. Uterine massage should be performed initially with one hand over the top of the uterine fundus, massaging downward. If this manuver is not rapidly effective, bimanual compression should be performed. This technique consists of massaging the anterior aspect of the uterus with one hand as described above, while placing the second hand in the vaginal vault in a fisted position with the knuckles contacting the uterine wall. If the placenta has already been delivered, the following drug regimen may be given:

- Oxytocin: 10 to 20 units in 1 L of lactated Ringer's solution at a rate of 20 to 40 milliunits per minute
- Methylergonovine: 0.2 mg IM every 2 to 4 hours to control bleeding. May be given IV in severe emergencies at a fractionated dose of 0.06 mg each dose. Intravenous methylergonovine increases the risk of severe hypertension, particularly in preeclamptic women. Cases of myocardial and cardiac arrest have been reported with IV use.
- Carboprost (0.25 mg IM may be repeated every 15 to 90 minutes, total dose not to exceed 2 mg): the most clinically significant side effects are due to hypertension and vascular and pulmonary airway constriction, and include an arterial oxygen desaturation of approximately 10%.

Uterine atony due to uterine rupture will not respond to uterine fundal massage or medical management. Uterine rupture should be treated emergently with laparotomy, and in many cases hysterectomy is required.

Lacerations

Lacerations should be suspected in the setting of a firm, well-contracted uterus and continued brisk bleeding. The perineum, vagina, cervix, and uterus must be thoroughly inspected. Perineal lacerations should be easily identified. Perineal lacerations, unless very superficial, involve the lower portion of the vagina and should be repaired with either simple or figure-of-eight absorbable sutures in a 3.0 or 4.0 size. Vaginal lacerations are identified by inserting two retractors into the vagina and widely separating the vaginal walls. Ring forceps are applied on the anterior and posterior lips of the cervix for inspection of the lateral vaginal walls. Lacerations of the middle or upper third of the vagina are less common, usually longitudinal and often extend through the vaginal wall into the underlying tissues, causing significant hemorrhage. These frequently result from a forceps delivery or use of a vacuum tool. Lacerations of the anterior vaginal wall are relatively common. These are in close proximity to the urethra, are frequently superficial and infrequently require repair. If repair is required, a Foley catheter inserted into the urethra during the procedure will help protect against inadvertent suturing of the urethra. Urethral lacerations may be difficult to determine initially, and when diagnosed, should be repaired by an urologist as soon as possible.

Cervical lacerations should be suspected in cases of severe hemorrhage during and after the third stage of labor, especially if the uterus is firm. Cervical lacerations up to 2 cm should be considered part of the natural birth process. These heal rapidly and rarely cause significant problems. Cervical lacerations, which extend into the upper third of the vagina or into the lower third of the uterus, may involve the uterine artery and its branches. The depth of these lacerations may not be fully appreciated initially but become apparent at a later time, when excessive vaginal hemorrhage occurs. Rarely, the cervix may be partially or completely avulsed. Cervical injuries follow difficult forceps deliveries or deliveries through an incompletely dilated cervix with forceps blades placed over the cervix.

Hematomas

Hematomas are most frequently caused by birth trauma, although blood dyscrasias may also be an etiology. While episiotomy is the most common etiology of a puerperal hematoma, another cause is injury to a blood vessel without a visible mucosal laceration. These injuries may be classified as vulvar, vaginal, vulvovaginal, or retroperitoneal.

Vulvar Hematomas: Most often involve bleeding from branches of the pudendal artery. The presenting symptom is usually excruciating vulvar pain. Small to moderate sized hematomas may be resorbed, however the tissue overlying the hematoma may undergo pressure necrosis and profuse hemorrhage may occur. Conversely, contents of the hematoma may rupture externally without causing damage to overlying soft tissues.

Vulvovaginal Hematomas: Occasionally develop adjacent to the vagina and may not be diagnosed promptly. Symptoms of pain and pressure in the vulvovaginal area should prompt a complete pelvic examination. These hematomas may go undetected until the woman cannot void due to local pressure on the urethra. A subperitoneal variety of vulvar hematoma, due to extravasation of blood beneath the peritoneum, may be massive and occasionally fatal. Vulvar hematomas may rupture into the vagina, causing infection and occasionally fatal sepsis. Vaginal hematomas are commonly associated with a forceps delivery. The vagina is a closed space and blood loss is limited due to tamponade of the bleeding site. The patient may complain of severe rectal pressure.

Retroperitoneal Hematomas: The least common, but most dangerous type. The retroperitoneal space is large; therefore, a great deal of bleeding may occur before symptoms of shock are evident. This type of hematoma occurs when there is a laceration of one of the branches of the internal iliac artery, occurring most frequently during cesarean section or rupture of a previous cesarean section scar.

Small Vulvar Hematomas: May be treated with ice packs and pain control. If this fails to control symptoms, incision and drainage with evacuation of clots and ligation of bleeding sources may be necessary. This may be performed in the emergency department (ED), assuming anesthesia and proper equipment are available; otherwise these should be repaired in the operating suite.

Vaginal Hematomas: Should be adequately exposed, incised, and drained. The wound should be left open and vaginal packing should be placed (such as a tampon) for at least 12 hours. Subperitonal and anterior vaginal hematomas are more difficult to identify and treat. They can be treated by incision of the perineum, but, unless there is complete hemostasis, laparotomy is advised. Retroperitoneal hematomas usually prompt laparotomy with ligation or embolization of the internal iliac artery as soon as possible to minimize blood loss.

Uterine Rupture

Uterine rupture is defined as complete, in which the uterus communicates directly with the peritoneal cavity, and incomplete, in which the uterus is separated from the peritoneal cavity by the peritoneum or broad ligament. It is important to differentiate uterine rupture versus dehiscence of a cesarean section scar. Rupture is separation of the old scar with a rupture of the fetal membranes and communication of the uterus and peritoneal cavity with associated massive bleeding. In dehiscence, the fetal membranes are not ruptured and the fetus is not in the peritoneal cavity. Dehiscence occurs gradually, whereas rupture is sudden and severe.

Uterine rupture can result from preexisting injury, anomaly, iatrogenic (traumatic procedures), blunt trauma, uterine overdistention (hydramnios, multiple fetuses), and excessive uterine stimulation with oxytocin. Currently, the most common cause is a previous cesarean section. Uterine rupture is increasingly more common due to the increased incidence of vaginal delivery trial in women with previous cesarean sections. The incidence of uterine rupture has increased from less than 1% to 3% over the last decade due to the increased incidence of vaginal birth after cesarean section.

Diagnosis of uterine rupture may be difficult, and symptoms may be unusual. For example, a hemoperitoneum from a ruptured uterus may produce irritation in the diaphragm and cause referred pain to the chest, leading one to suspect pulmonary or amniotic fluid embolism. If rupture occurs during labor, it is usually at the peak of a contraction and the patient may complain of sudden and severe tearing pelvic pain. Many women are under some form of anesthesia during delivery, which may blunt the pain that would normally occur with rupture. In some cases, there is loss of the presenting fetal part as it enters into the peritoneum. Occasionally, a fetus may be felt adjacent to a firm, contracted uterus; often, fetal parts are more easily palpated than usual on abdominal examination. The woman may exhibit shock, and significant fetal distress should be noted. Ultrasound may be helpful in the identification of rupture, as well as confirming hemoperitoneum. Culdocentesis or abdominal paracentesis may also be used to detect a hemoperitoneum, however, ultrasound has virtually replaced these procedures.

The prognosis for the fetus is poor with fetal mortality rates of 50% to 75%, with death caused by hypoxia due to placental separation and maternal hemorrhage. Fetal death is imminent unless immediate delivery by cesarean section is performed.

Treatment of a ruptured uterus consists of hemodynamic resuscitation with large-bore intravenous lines and blood transfusions. Blood requirements may be high, requiring 10 U or more. A surgical team should be assembled and be prepared to perform an emergent hysterectomy in the operating suite. Pediatric personnel skilled in neonatal resuscitation should be present. It should be stressed that hypovolemic shock will not be reversed until the arterial bleeding is controlled; therefore, surgery should not be delayed for any reason. In extremis, the aorta may be manually compressed to aid in temporary reduction of the hemorrhage. Oxytocin may also be given as adjunctive therapy.

Placenta Accreta, Increta, and Percreta

Placenta accreta is a condition in which the placenta is implanted with abnormal firmness to the uterine wall. There is a definite link to previous cesarean section, placenta previa and placenta accreta. With placenta previa alone the risk is 1% to 5%. In a patient with previous cesarean section and placenta previa, the risk is 14% to 24%; in a patient with 3 prior cesarean sections, the risk increases 47%. In placenta accreta, the placental villi are attached to the myometrium. In placenta increta, the villi invade the myometrium. In placenta percreta, the villi penetrate through the myometrium. These conditions cause morbidity and mortality from severe hemorrhage, uterine perforation, and infection. The overall incidence of all these conditions is approximately 1 in 2,500 deliveries.

The clinical course of placenta accreta is characterized by antepartum bleeding. Diagnosis is made by the use of ultrasound with sensitivity and specificity of 85%. Other problems vary depending on the site and depth of implantation. With extensive involvement, such as placenta percreta, hemorrhage becomes profuse when delivery of the placenta is attempted. Blood products and appropriate personnel should all be activated when a woman presents to the ED with known placental accreta. Occasionally, the uterus can be inverted due to excessive traction on the umbilical cord used to delivery the placenta. Treatment is supportive and consists of volume resuscitation followed by emergent hysterectomy if excessive bleeding continues.

Infections

Approximately 4% to 8% of maternal deaths are caused by puerperal infections, with women undergoing cesarean sections presenting a greater risk. Puerperal infections are bacterial infections occurring from 2 to 14 days after delivery. Puerperal fever may be caused by genital or extragenital sources. Post-partal infections are most frequently of genital tract origin; however, a careful history and examination will help to assure that an extragenital infection is not overlooked. Group B *Streptococcus* is a common pathogen in puerperal infections and can be colonized bacteria in maternal genitourinary and gastrointestinal. Other pathogens include anerobes, *Escherichia coli, Chlamydia, Neisseria gonorrhoeae,* and *Ureaplasma urealyticum.*

Extragenital infections may arise from the respiratory tract, urinary tract, breast, or veins (thrombophlebitis). Respiratory causes of puerperal fever may present early in patients who underwent general anesthesia. These include atelectasis, aspiration pneumonia, or, infrequently, bacterial pneumonia.

Urinary tract infections may be slightly more delayed than respiratory causes and may be difficult to diagnose. The postpartum woman may have other physical discomforts masking her urinary pain and may present solely with a fever. The diagnosis is made by the presence of bacteriuria and a thorough examination to exclude pelvic infection. Many patients with pelvic infections have a vaginal discharge, which may contaminate the urine sample. This discharge may lead to a misdiagnosis unless both speculum and bimanual pelvic examinations are performed to exclude a pelvic infection. Breast engorgement ("milk fever") causes a fever in 9.5% of women, occurring in the first few postpartum days. Tender swollen breasts suggest a clinically obvious source of fever. The temperature does not usually exceed 39°C, and the fever typically lasts for approximately 24 hours. In contrast, bacterial mastitis usually develops later in the postpartum course. Thrombophlebitis may cause fever in puerperal women with diagnosis being suspected by the presence of a painful, swollen leg and a positive imaging study (duplex Doppler ultrasound or venogram). Septic pelvic thrombophlebitis is rare and occurs in 1 in 3,000 to 1.7 in 1,000 vaginal deliveries, with a 10- to 20-fold increase in post–cesarean section women. The thrombosed vein becomes infected and showers the body with bacteria-laden emboli that present as pulmonary emboli, metastatic abscesses, and fever of unknown origin with intermittent septicemia. Diagnosis can be made by magnetic resonance imaging, ultrasound, or a heparin challenge test. The heparin challenge test consists of defervesence of symptoms within 48 hours of beginning heparin therapy. Treatment consists of antibiotics and heparin for 7 to 10 days followed by at least 1 month of coumadin therapy. There is however, controversy surrounding the heparin approach to septic pelvic thrombophlebitis.

Endometritis

Endometritis is a genital source of puerperal fever. Endometritis is an infection that involves the decidua, myometrium, and parametrial tissues. This infection is relatively uncommon, with a 3% incidence following uncomplicated vaginal infection. Endometritis is the most common postpartum complication in cesarean delivered women, with reported rates of 15% to 35%. There is a strong association of untreated bacterial vaginosis and postpartum endometritis. Prophylactic use of extended broad-spectrum antibiotics in cesarean delivered women shortens hospital stay and reduces the frequency of endometritis and wound infections. Other risk factors include prolonged rupture of membranes, prolonged labor, and multiple cervical examinations during labor, internal fetal monitoring, and chorioamnionitis.

Patients' present with fever, abdominal pain and foul-smelling lochia. On pelvic examination, parametrial tenderness with or without discharge is noted. Infections caused by Group A β-hemolytic *Streptococcus* frequently have a thin, odorless lochia. The diagnosis is a clinical

one, and laboratory tests are not very helpful. Mixed aerobic and anaerobic organisms cause the majority of infections. Predominant anaerobes include Gram-positive cocci (*Peptostreptococcus* and *Peptococcus*), bacteroides, and clostridia. Common Gram-positive aerobic cocci include *Enterococcus* and Group B *Streptococcus*, and Gram-negative rods include *E. coli*. *Chlamydia trachomatis* is thought to be an etiologic agent in late onset, indolent endometritis. This may develop in up to one-third of women who have antepartum chlamydial infection.

Broad-spectrum intravenous antibiotics are required to treat endometritis since a single drug will not cover all the agents potentially causing endometritis. The β-lactam antimicrobials have been the most successful at treating this disease. Effective agents include some cephalosporines (cefoxitine and cefotaxime) and extended spectrum penicillins (piperacillin, ticarcillin, and mezlocillin). When used concurrently, the β-lactamase inhibitors, clavulinic acid and sulbactam have increased the efficacy of ticaricillin, ampicillin, and amoxicillin. A common combination for inpatient use is gentamicin and clindamycin. There is some evidence that once daily dosing with gentamycin at 5 mg/kg and clindamycin at 2,700 mg may be as effective as every 8-hour dosing. This regimen would allow the patient to return to home and receive home IV therapy or return to the ED for daily dosing. Metronidazole has very strong anaerobic antimicrobial activity and is recommended in combination with an aminoglycoside, especially if an abscess is suspected. Due to increasing antibiotic-resistant bacteria, carbapenam and its derivative, imipenam, are reserved for those cases in which the patient has overwhelming pelvic infection or where treatment with other antibiotics fails. Other regimens include aztreonam and clindamycin.

In the vast majority of patients with endometritis, there is a response to antibiotic therapy in the first 48 to 72 hours. In others, complications may arise, including wound infection, adnexal infection, parametrial phlegmon, and peritonitis.

Wound infections can be seen in approximately 7% of patients following cesarean sections. Administration of prophylactic antibiotics (at the time of cesarean incision) decreases the incidence to 2%. Fever usually occurs postpartum day four. Wound infections are usually preceded by a uterine infection and are differentiated by a persistent fever despite antimicrobial therapy. Incision and drainage is necessary, with careful inspection and palpation of the wound to ascertain that the underlying fascia is not involved. Wet to dry packing and oral out-patient antibiotics may suffice.

The most common adnexal infection is a perisalpingitis, where the fallopian tubes remain patent and functional. Ovarian abscesses develop rarely. Women with adnexal infection present approximately 1 to 2 weeks after delivery with fever and unilateral abdominal pain. Intravenous antibiotics are given initially, but surgical or percutaneous drainage is usually necessary.

Parametrial phlegmon develops when there is extensive parametrial cellulitis, which forms an area of induration within the broad ligament. This is the most common cause of persistent fever in postpartum women with pelvic infections after cesarean section.

Extensive cellulitis of the uterine incision may cause necrosis and dehiscence, causing purulent material to be expelled into the peritoneal cavity leading to peritonitis and an acute abdomen. Peritonitis may also occur by way of extension through the lymphatics. This has a presentation similar to surgical peritonitis; however, the abdomen is usually less rigid. Initial therapy varies with the proposed etiology. If the peritonitis is thought to be due to extension of a uterine infection via the lymphatics, then the initial therapy is medical treatment with antibiotics; however, if the cause is thought to be a perforation of a bowel loop, then surgery is indicated.

Mastitis

Mastitis symptoms seldom appear before the end of the first postpartum week, and usually not until the third or fourth postpartum week. The disease is almost exclusive to lactating women.

Mastitis is usually associated with a contaminated nursery. This has previously reached epidemic proportions, usually corresponding to methicillin-resistant *Staphylococcus aureus* (MRSA). *S. aureus* is the causative agent in approximately 40% of women with epidemic mastitis. Other agents include coagulase-negative staphylococcus and viridian streptococcus. The immediate source of the agent is usually the infant's mouth and nose, and the agent enters the breast during nursing through an abrasion or fissure in the nipple. Infection is unilateral, with marked engorgement preceding inflammation, chills, fever, and pain. The breast is red, indurated, and tender. Approximately 5% to 11% of these women will also develop an abscess and have severe concurrent constitutional symptoms. The organism can usually be cultured from the breast milk.

Breast-feeding may continue as long as the bacteria are not antibiotic-resistant. The usual treatment consists of warm compresses, analgesics, antibiotics, and continued breast-feeding. In cases where an abscess has formed, the breast-feeding should be discontinued until the infection has cleared. Complications are rare due to the excellent results achieved with the administration of antimicrobial agents. Abscess formation is the most common complication and presents as a discrete, fluctuant mass that will require surgical drainage, as well as antimicrobial therapy. The surgical drainage is typically quite extensive, very painful, and frequently requires either conscious sedation or general anesthesia. The drainage should probably not be attempted in the ED, since the wound dissection may need to be extensive.

In diagnosing puerperal fever, laboratory studies are generally not very useful, although urinalysis may be helpful in diagnosing a urinary tract infection. Puerperal fever is a clinical diagnosis based on fever, pain, and evident inflammation. Cultures (wound, urine, and blood) are occasionally useful in directing antibiotic treatment. Cultures may assist in tracking trends in infections; however, many times multiple agents are present. Culture results are not available until 24 to 72 hours after treatment is initiated and therefore lack a timely clinical benefit for the emergency provider.

Postpartum Pre-Eclampsia/Eclampsia

Postpartum eclampsia is an uncommon occurrence, but it is considered to be on the rise. Among those woman who develop eclampsia, the incidence in the subgroup of postpartum eclampsia ranges from 16% to 50%. Patients may present with seizure but most commonly present with complaints of a headache, swelling, or altered mental status. Diagnosis of pre-eclampsia pre-term is common, but not necessary. Treatment is the same as for pre-term eclampsia with magnesium sulfate and anti-hypertensive agents.

Postpartum Blues/Depression

Postpartum blues/depression (PPD) refers to a common condition immediately following delivery that is characterized by rapid mood swings, sadness, irritability, insomnia, and tearfulness. Forty to eighty percent of postpartum women develop these mood changes within the first 5 postpartum days, which usually resolves in 2 weeks. Conservative management and reassurance usually leads to improvement.

Postpartum psychosis is very rare, with a prevalence of 0.1% to 0.2%. Risk factors include previous psychiatric disease, history of puerperal psychosis, and family history of puerperal psychosis. Relapse rates are as high as 70%. Without prior history of psychiatric disease, a thorough medical work-up should be completed. Urine toxicological screen, thyroid studies, electrolytes, and a CT scan of the brain should be considered.

Selected Readings

Andrews WW, Hauth JC, Cliver SP, et al. Randomized clinical trial of extended spectrum antibiotic prophylaxis with coverage for ureaplasma urealyticum to reduce post-cesarean delivery endometritis. *Obstet Gynecol* 2003;101: 1183–1189.

Brown CE, Stettler RW, Twickler D, et al. Puerperal septic pelvic thrombophlebitis: Incidence and response to heparin therapy. *Am J Obstet Gynecol* 1999; 181:143–148.

Chaim W, Burstein W. Postpartum infection treatments: a review. *Expert Opin Pharmacother* 2003;4:1297–1313.

Chaim W, Horowitz S, David JB, et al. Ureaplasma urealyticum in the development of postpartum endometritis. *Eur J Obstet Gynecol Reprod Biol* 2003;109: 145–148.

Chames MC, Livingston JC, Ivester TS. Late postpartum eclampsia: a preventable disease? *Am J Obstet Gynecol* 2002;186:1174–1177.

Clark SL, Koonings P, Phelan JP. Placenta previa/accreta and prior cesarean section. *Obstet Gynecol* 1985;66:89–92.

Crochetiere C. Obstetric emergencies. *Anesth Clin North Am* 2003;21:111–125.

Cunningham FG, Macdonald PC, Gant NF. *Williams Obstetrics*, 19th ed. Norwalk, CT: Appleton and Lange 1993.

Finberg HJ, Williams JW. Placenta accreta: prospective sonographic diagnosis in patients with placenta previa and prior cesarean section. *J Ultrasound Med* 1992; 11:333.

Foxman B, D'Arcy H, Gillespie B, et al. Lactation mastitis: occurrence and medical management among 946 breastfeeding women in the United States. *Am J Epidemiol* 2002;155:103–114.

Gabbe SG, Niebyl JR, Simpson JL. *Obstetrics: Normal and Problem Pregnancies*, 2d ed. New York: Churchill and Livingstone 1991.

Hertzberg BS, Bowie JD. Ultrasound of the postpartum uterus: prediction of retained placental tissue. *J Ultrasound Med* 1991;10:451–456.

Isler CM, Rinehart BK, Terrone DA, et al. Septic pelvic thrombophlebitis and preeclampsia are related disorders. *Hypertens Pregnan* 2004;23:121–127.

Jacobsson B, Pernevi P, Chidekel L. Bacterial vaginosis in early pregnancy may predispose for preterm birth and postpartum endometritis. *Acta Obstet Gynecol Scand* 2002;81:1006–1010.

Levine D, Hulka CA, Ludmor J, et al. Placenta accreta: evaluation with color Doppler US, power Doppler US and MR imaging. *Radiology* 1997;205:773.

Livingston JC, Lata E, Rinehart, E. Gentamicin and clindamycin therapy in postpartum endometritis: The efficacy of daily dosing versus dosing every 8 hours. *Am J Obstet Gynecol* 2003;188:149–152.

Matthys LA, Coppage KH, Lambers DS, et al. Delayed postpartum preeclampsia: An experience of 151 cases. *Am J Obstet Gynecol* 2002;190:1464–1466.

Miller DA, Chollet JA, Goodwin TM. Clinical risk factors for placenta previa-placenta accreta. *Am J Obstet Gynecol* 1997;177:210–214.

O'Hara MW, Schlechte JA, Lewis DA. Prospective study of postpartum blues. Biologic and psychosocial factors. *Arch Gen Psych* 1991;48:801–806.

Prachniak GK. Common breastfeeding problems. *Obstet Gynecol Clin North Am* 2002;29:77–88.

Rageth JC, Juzi C, Grossenbacher H. Delivery after previous cesarean section: a rsik evaluation. *Obstet Gynecol* 1999;93:332–337.

Rivlin ME, Martin RW. *Manual of Clinical Problems in Obstetrics and Gynecology,* 4th ed. Boston: Little, Brown 1994.

Sachs B, Kobelin C, Castro M, et al. The risks of lowering the cesarean-delivery rate. *N Engl J Med* 1999;340:54–57.

Scott JR, Disain PJ, Hammond JB. *Danforth's Obstetrics and Gynecology,* 7th ed. Philadelphia: Lippincott 1994.

Steiner M. Postpartum psychiatric disorders. *Can J Psych* 1990;35:89–95.

Tsui BCH, Stewart B, Fitzmaurice A, et al. Cardiac arrest and myocardial infarction induced by postpartum intravenous ergonovine administration. *Anesthesiology* 2001;94:363–364.

Pediatric Disorders

Mariann M. Manno

Introduction

Clinical decision-making in infants and young children is based on a careful history and physical examination. In the Emergency Department this includes a focused accounting of the chief complaint, a review of symptoms, and past medical history including perinatal problems. In young infants, attention to changes in patterns of breathing, sleep, playfulness, and feeding may suggest serious conditions like sepsis, meningitis, or congestive heart failure, which may present in subtle or nonspecific ways.

The physical examination in children presents challenges throughout the pediatric age range. Young children frightened by strangers, an over-stimulating environment, and the prospect of painful procedures. The emergency physician needs patience and skill in order to perform an accurate assessment. In general, a calm and gentle approach begins with observation of the level of alertness and activity of the child and his/her interaction with the environment. This should be followed by evaluation of the least threatening parts of the exam. Distraction with books, videos, and involvement of parents is helpful.

Critically ill infants and children develop cardiopulmonary failure or arrest from a large number of etiologies.

The goal of the initial assessment is not to determine a specific diagnosis, but the severity of illness, which will in turn dictate management. The first step is determining the child's physiological state. Compensated physiological states include respiratory distress (increased work of breathing with adequate oxygenation and ventilation) or compensated shock (hypoperfusion with normal blood pressure). Decompensated states including respiratory failure (inadequate oxygenation and ventilation), decompensated shock (hypoperfusion with hypotension), and cardiopulmonary failure (global deficits in oxygenation, ventilation, and perfusion) require immediate intervention.

This section focuses on common clinical entities and presentations seen in infants and young children with special emphasis on conditions where rapid diagnosis and intervention are required. It is not meant to replace a comprehensive Pediatric Emergency Medicine textbook. In addition to textbooks, interactive training programs may be valuable to the emergency physician in developing pediatric-specific assessment, diagnostic, and management skills. These include PALS (Pediatric Advanced Life Support), APLS (Advanced Pediatric Life Support), and NRP (Neonatal Resuscitation Program).

Important Aspects in the Care of the Pediatric Patient

Mariann M. Manno

A General Approach to the Pediatric Patient

Arrival in the hospital with a child who has experienced an emergency following an illness or injury is a highly stressful event for children and families, no matter how routine and straightforward the circumstances may seem to health care providers. Most children who seek emergency care do so in general emergency departments (EDs) where advanced pediatric life support resuscitation is a rare event. A number of considerations in the care of young acutely ill and injured patients include: unique aspects of their anatomy and physiology, pediatric triage, management of pain in young children, family presence during resuscitation, injury prevention, and Emergency Department preparedness for pediatric emergencies.

Pediatric Anatomy and Physiology

Airway and Breathing

An appreciation of unique aspects of the pediatric airway is of central importance in pediatric emergency care. A large occiput allows flexion of the head and functional obstruction of the pharynx by the tongue, especially when the child is immobilized or supine. A small towel roll placed under the shoulders extends the head on the neck (sniffing position) and opens the airway.

Within the mouth and airway itself, the oral cavity is small, the tongue is relatively large and the epiglottis is large and floppy. To overcome this anatomy, straight (Miller) blades are used during intubation. The larynx is cephalad and anterior. The vocal cords are shorter, cartilaginous, and often not visible in their entirety during larnygoscopy. The cricoid ring is the narrowest point of the airway. Noncuffed endotracheal tubes are recommended in children less than 8 years old because the cricoid ring provides a physiologic cuff.

Shorter tracheal length makes intubation of main stem bronchus and accidental extubation common especially during transport. Narrow diameter and greater compliance of the trachea and bronchi predispose to obstruction. This resilience of the chest wall results in a lower incidence of rib fractures with trauma. However, increased compliance allows for transmission of kinetic energy to the lungs and heart, without injury to the chest wall itself.

Respiratory distress is characterized by increased work of breathing including: tachypnea, abnormal sounds (stridor, wheezing), retractions, and flaring. Respiratory distress coupled with other signs such as poor color, poor tone, and abnormal mental status indicate the possibility of respiratory failure, a decompensated state with inadequate oxygenation and ventilation.

Circulation

An assessment of circulatory compromise requires examination of the end organs of perfusion (skin, mental status, central and peripheral pulses, urine output) rather than reliance on vital signs (**Table 87.1**). Children compensate for a decrease in cardiac output primarily by increasing heart rate and increasing peripheral vascular resistance. Most children in shock will be tachycardia and normotensive. Hypotension, which characterizes decompensated shock, is a late and ominous sign.

Cervical Spine

The pediatric spine is elastic, so momentary displacements can cause a spinal cord injury without radiographic abnormality (SCIWORA). Children who have had transient paresthesias, clumsiness, tingling, or "total body paralysis" after experiencing flexion, extension, distraction, or compression forces are at risk for sustaining SCIWORA. They should be carefully evaluated even though normal cervical spine radiographs have been obtained.

Abdominal Organs

The relatively large size of the liver increases its susceptibility to injury after blunt trauma. A child's horizontally situated diaphragm displaces the liver and spleen into the abdomen. Abdominal organs are at greater risk of injury for blunt injury because they are protected by compliant ribs and a thin layer of muscle and fat.

Table 87.1		
Ranges for Vital Signs		
Age	**HR Awake**	**HR Mean**
Newborn–3 months	85–205	140
3 months–2 years	100–190	130
2–10 years	60–140	80
>10 years	60–100	75
Systolic BP		
Newborn	60–90	
6 months	87–105	
2 years	95–105	
7 years	97–112	
15 years	112–128	

Source: Used with permission from the American Heart Association, *AHA PALS 2000 Guidelines.*

Triage

Nursing staff should be trained to recognize high risk conditions and accurately assess seriously young ill children to ensure that care is expedited appropriately. Congenital cardiac anomalies, sickle cell disease, endocrine disorders (diabetes, congenital adrenal hyperplasia), neutropenia (including oncology patients), steroid dependent patients are among those at highest risk for decompensation. A useful schematic is outlined in **FIGURE 87.1**.

Triage is an opportunity for interventions that can shorten the child's stay in the ED. The triage nurse can generally predict the procedures (IV placement, phlebotomy, sutures) or tests (radiographs). Guidelines can be provided for the administration of antipyretics and topical anesthetics in triage.

Developmental Considerations

Development commonly is categorized into five areas: fine motor, gross motor, language, social, and cognitive. Milestones are acquired in a predictable fashion. Babies sit at 6 months, develop peak stranger anxiety at a year, have temper tantrums at 2 years, are curious and engageable at 5 years, and want to be directly involved in decision-making by the early teen years (**Table 87.2**).

Incorporating developmental behavior typical at a specific age span is very helpful in approaching the individual patient and allows the provider to anticipate the child's capabilities in the medical setting.

Communication with Children and Families

Parents have a strong need to know details of their child's illness and are dissatisfied when they feel that communication with providers has been scant or unclear. Often, the most memorable aspects of an ED experience involves the communication that flows (or should) between the medical staff, children-patients, and parents. This communication actually has two aspects: the content or the medical message and the

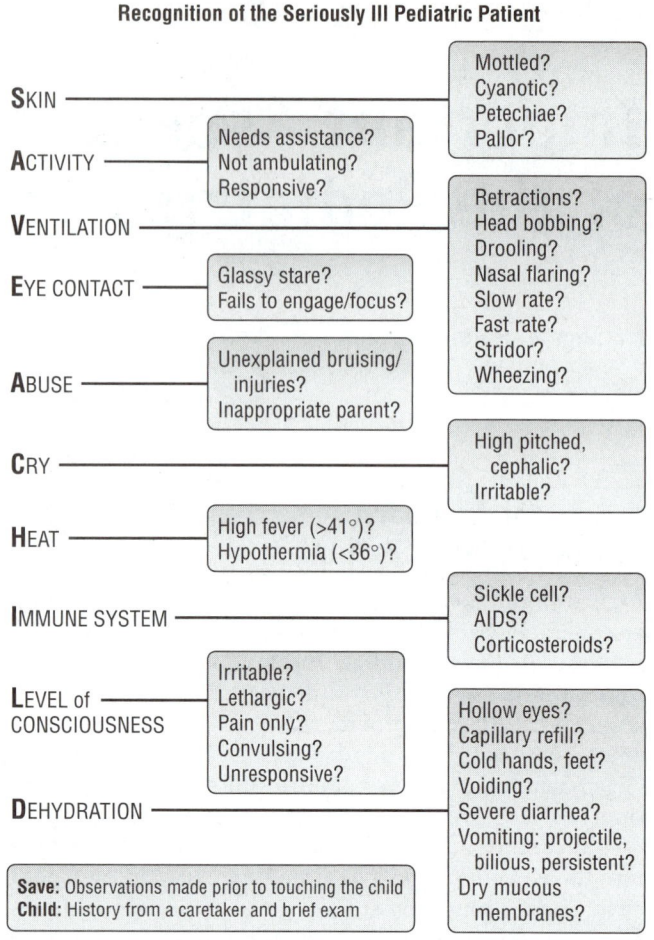

FIGURE 87.1 A schematic guide to triage of the seriously ill child. *Source:* Used with permission from Wiebe RA, Rosen LM. Triage in the emergency department. *Emerg Med Clin North Am* 1991;9:491–505.

process or how the message is delivered. Connecting with families in a busy emergency department is complicated. It involves the provider (doctor, nurse or medic) and the parent, the provider and the child, and the parent and the child. A thoughtful approach is required for all of this to go well. Understanding that the ED is an overcrowded, hectic clinical environment, the ideal for interactions with parents and children include:

1. *Honesty.* Be truthful about procedures. Children are not helped with statements such as, "this won't hurt." It would be more realistic to say "this will hurt like a bee sting."
2. *Respect.* Introduce yourself by name and role to families. Shake hands. Sit down. Speak in understandable, developmentally appropriate language to both the parent and child.
3. *Understanding.* Be patient with parents and children. Communicate that you realize that it is hard for certain children to hold still and cooperate. Avoid statements like, "be a good boy." Allow parents time to absorb and adjust to what is happening.
4. *Efficiency.* Realize that a child in the ED has a different perspective on time. Waits, even ones that are not

Table 87.2

Developmental Milestones in Children and Adolescents

Age	Gross and Fine Motor	Social and Cognitive	Language	Things That Help
Neonate	Flexed, head sags if unsupported	Fixates on face or light	Alerts to voice	Keep warm and comfortable. Pay attention to frightened parents.
2 mo	Raises head from prone position, head lag on pull to sit	Smiles on social contact, attracts to voice	Coos	
6 mo	Sits alone, rolls over, pivots, creeps, transfers hand to hand	Prefers mother, responds to emotion, imitates banging	Babbles, blows bubbles, laughs	
9 mo	Sits, crawls, pulls to stand, can get to sitting position	Plays peek-a-boo, waves "bye-bye"; cry at sight of unfamiliar person	Responds to "no"; imitates some sounds; uses "mama," "dada"	Peak stranger anxiety. Keep with parent.
12 mo	Cruises, stands alone, starts to walk, pincer grasp	Plays ball, drinks from a cup, imitates	1–2 true words, shakes head "no," points to indicate needs	
18 mo	Runs, walks up stairs with rail, tower of 4 cubes	Feeds self with utensils	10 words, "no," names pictures, points to 1 body part	Counteract stubbornness with distractions (picture book). Explain and then move quickly. Use parents to help with exam
2 yr	Runs, jumps, climbs, walks up and down stairs	Looks at picture book, parallel play	30–50 words, 2- or 3-word sentences	
3–5 yr	Pedals tricycle, throws ball overhand	Knows age, sex, full name. Thinks illness or pain are punishment and death is reversible	Complete sentences; speech intelligible to strangers. Interprets language literally ("draw blood")	Choose words carefully. Magical thinking translates to fears. Allow touching of equipment.
6–10 yr	Runs, bikes, plays sports	Group play/role playing, mastery of complex cognitive tasks, following rules	Understand true causality and permanency of death. Logical, cooperative, curious	Use curiosity to engage and distract. Include in discussion about their health. Offer choices.
Teens			Huge ranges in judgment and risk taking behaviors. Capable of abstract thinking and complex reasoning. Retain egocentric or dramatic tendencies. Quest for autonomy.	Deserve full and honest explanations. Encourage questions and participation in decisions. Maturity and privacy should be respected.

excess, can be excruciating and anxiety-provoking. Move quickly, for example, from the examination, to the discussion about sutures and to the procedure itself. Avoid having a child view equipment (needles, syringes) while they wait. Explain to families what they are waiting for and what the time course is likely to be.

Treatment of Pain

Control of pain in the prehospital setting or ED is a vital component of overall emergency care. A child of any age who suffers a painful injury or undergoes a painful procedure will experience pain. Myths that children do not feel pain the same way adults do still exist in the minds of some providers. There is ample evidence in the literature that children's pain is overlooked in the ED and prehospital setting. This appears to be especially true of younger and therefore less verbal children. Children's pain may be underestimated because of difficulty in interpreting behaviors at younger developmental stages. Pain is often undermedicated because of fears of oversedation, respiratory depression, addiction, and unfamiliarity with doses in children. Individual systems should identify and eliminate specific barriers that prevent appropriate and timely administration of analgesia to children.

Nonpharmacological measures to control stress and pain are useful strategies and adjuncts to analgesia. These include distraction (bubbles, music, counting) and guided imagery. A *child life specialist* is a trained, certified professional familiar with child development and children's responses to medical procedures and hospitalization. These individuals play an important role with procedures in the ED. They can initiate these activities, support the patient and parents, and educate the staff. Parents of children who receive child life support report a significantly higher degree of satisfaction with the overall care in the ED.

Topical anesthetics can be administered proactively. EMLA (eutectic mixture of local anesthetics) and LMX4 (topical liposomal 4% lidocaine) are applied to intact skin most commonly in anticipation of venipuncture or lumbar puncture. LET (lidocaine, epinephrine, tetracaine) can be prepared as a liquid or gel preparation to certain wounds that will require sutures. Tissue adhesives such as Dermabond (octyl cyanoacrylate) provide essentially painless closure of selected wounds.

Recent studies have reported the effectiveness of oral sucrose in decreasing the response to painful stimuli from heel sticks and injections in neonates. This effect seems to be strongest in the newborn infant and diminish over the first several months of life.

Involvement of Families in Resuscitation

Considerable controversy has surrounded family presence during invasive procedures and resuscitations. There is increasing evidence that patients, families, and health care providers believe that a supportive, structured environment for the presence of family members during resuscitation is desirable. In a retrospective study of 25 family members (who were not given the option to remain during the resuscitation) of 94 ED patients who died following traumatic injuries, almost all families voiced the belief that family members should be given the option to be present during resuscitation. Eighty percent stated that they would have remained with their family member.

Individual EDs should develop a multidisciplinary protocol that would allow family presence during procedures and resuscitation. It is important for all providers to have input into this policy and to create a system that ensures that families receive individualized attention from medical personnel not involved in patient care.

A Child's Death in the ED

After a child has died, doctors and nurses must shift their efforts from treating the patient to caring for parents and families. This is an enormously challenging task that hinges on many factors, including the circumstances surrounding the child's death, the experience of the providers, and the existing volume and complexity of other patients in the ED. Ideally, if the family is present in the ED, they have been present for part of the resuscitation or have been kept abreast of the child's medical condition.

Emergency physicians are in the difficult position of informing a family that their child has died without the benefit of a prior relationship with the family. Primary care providers and/or subspecialists who have an established rapport can fill an important role in the immediate aftermath of the child's death. Whenever possible, parents and other relatives should meet together with the medical team (doctor, nurse, medic). The grief response among parents ranges from passiveness to anger to blame. The staff should be prepared to support families through this very painful experience.

When actually speaking to parents, identify yourself by name. Have others who participated in the care of their child speak with the family with you. Nurses, social workers, or child life therapists may have already spent time with the family. Use a space where you can sit down with the parents and use words that are understandable. It is better to say the "your child died, even though the medics, doctors, and nurses did everything possible to save him," than to use euphemisms or phrases like "he passed on." A study of these parents whose children died in the ED reported that all of these parents would have liked a memento (lock of hair, handprint) to take from the ED. Almost all found that holding their child's body was helpful.

Injury Prevention

Childhood injuries cause significant morbidity and mortality. Injuries are responsible for more deaths than all other childhood diseases combined. Motor vehicle-related injury is the leading cause of death and disability for children and adolescents in the United States. Other important causes of pediatric injuries include pedestrians struck by motor vehicles, bicycles, firearms, drownings, and burns.

General Emergency Department Preparedness for Pediatric Emergencies

The majority of children who require emergency care do so in general emergency departments. Therefore, all EDs should have the capability to identify and manage acutely ill or injured children who require resuscitation.

The American College of Emergency Physicians and the American Academy of Pediatrics have jointly published guidelines on preparedness of EDs to care for children. These guidelines outline staff, policies, quality improvement, equipment, and supplies needed for the care of children in the ED. Information on these guidelines can be found at *http://www.acep.org* or *http://www.aap.org*.

Selected Readings

Ahrens W, Hart R, Maruyama N. Pediatric death: managing the aftermath in the emergency department. *J Emerg Med* 1997;15:601–603.

American Academy of Pediatrics, Committee on Pediatric Emergency Medicine; and American College of Emergency Physicians, Pediatric Committee. Care of children in the emergency department: guidelines for preparedness. *Pediatrics* 2001;107:777–781.

American Academy of Pediatrics, Committee on Pediatric Emergency Medicine; and American College of Emergency Physicians, Pediatric Committee. Care of children in the emergency department: guidelines for preparedness, *Ann Emerg Med* 2001;37:423–427.

Bagatell R, Meyer R. When children die: a seminar series for pediatric residents. *Pediatrics* 2002;110(2 Pt 1):348–353.

Beckman AW, Sloan BK. Should parents be present during emergency department procedures on children, and who should make that decision? A survey of emergency physician and nurse attitudes. *Acad Emerg Med* 2002;9:154–158. Erratum: 2002;9:287.

Boudreaux ED, Francis JL, Loyacano T. Family presence during invasive procedures and resuscitations in the emergency department: a critical review and suggestions for future research. *Ann Emerg Med* 2002;40:193–205.

Fordyce J, Blanks FS, Pekow P, et al. Errors in a busy emergency department. *Ann Emerg Med* 2003;42:324–333.

Goldberg RM, Kuhn G, Andrew LB, Thomas HA Jr. Coping with medical mistakes and errors in judgment. *Ann Emerg Med* 2002;39:287–292.

Meyers T, Eichhorn D, Guzzetta CE. Do families want to be present during CPR? A retrospective survey. *J Emerg Nurs* 1998;24:400–405.

Quintana EC. Parental presence during invasive procedures in children: what is the physician's perspective? *Ann Emerg Med* 2004;44:432–433.

Serwint JR, Rutherford LE. "I learned that no death is routine": description of a death and bereavement seminar for pediatrics residents. *Acad Med* 2002;77: 278–284.

Wears RL, Wu AW. Dealing with failure: the aftermath of errors and adverse events. *Ann Emerg Med* 2002;39:344–346.

Zempsky WT, Cravero JP. Relief of pain and anxiety in pediatric patients in emergency medical systems. Pediatrics 2004;114:1348–1356.

88 Respiratory Disorders

Susan Torrey
Mariann M. Manno

Apnea

Apnea is not unique to neonates and infants. In this age group, however, it may be caused by a number of pathophysiologic processes that do not affect older children and adults. Congenital anomalies in metabolism or anatomy, differences in maturity of the central nervous system, respiratory reserve, and susceptibility to infectious agents are among the factors that interact to make this age group unique. Since these young patients are the most challenging for the emergency physician, this discussion focuses on them.

Apnea is defined as a respiratory pause of greater than 20 seconds or of any duration if there is associated pallor or cyanosis and/or bradycardia. Periodic breathing is a common respiratory pattern in young infants characterized by cycles of a short respiratory pause followed by an increase in respiratory rate. Normal newborn infants display respiratory patterns that vary by sex and by conceptual age as well as by sleep state. Premature infants have more apneic episodes than do full-term infants. Normal full-term infants experience significantly more episodes of nonperiodic apnea during active sleep than during quiet sleep, although respiratory failure occurs more often during quiet sleep. Severe apnea may be accompanied by change in color or muscle tone, and choking. A clinically significant apneic episode is called an acute life-threatening event (ALTE).

Etiology

Many processes may cause apnea in newborns and young infants. Apnea may be the only physical manifestation of seizure activity. In this case, the emergency physician may be confronted with a baby who has an entirely normal neurologic examination. The only significant finding may be the history. Several infectious processes can cause apnea. Meningitis, for example, even in the absence of fever, must be included in the differential diagnosis. Respiratory syncytial virus is a frequent cause of bronchiolitis and may cause apnea in infants, especially those who were premature or have preexisting pulmonary or congenital heart disease. Infant botulism is a diagnosis that should be made before apnea occurs, and must be suspected on the basis of age, symptoms of hypotonia, weak cry, and geography. Recent data suggest that gastroesophageal reflux frequently occurs in infants with an ALTE despite the absence of a history of vomiting. Inborn errors of metabolism, cardiac conduction abnormalities, hypoglycemia, and anatomic abnormalities must always be considered in newborns and young infants. Apnea has occurred rarely in some infants in upright car seats.

Of great concern to parents and the physicians is the risk of sudden infant death in infants who have an unexplained ALTE. Although any of the diagnoses described above can result in an ALTE, no cause is identified in about half of patients. There is no clear relationship between an "idiopathic" ALTE and sudden infant death. Sudden infant death syndrome (SIDS) is implicated in approximately 1.5 to 2 deaths per 1,000 live births in the United States. This rate varies widely based on epidemiological variables such as socioeconomic status, ethnic origin, maternal drug addiction, discharge from a neonatal intensive care unit, season of the year (higher in winter), and vigor with which other diagnoses are pursued. Finally, the possibility of Munchausen's syndrome by proxy or some other form of child abuse must be considered.

Evaluation

The first priority of the emergency physician is to identify a life-threatening condition such as persistent or recurrent apnea, hypoxia, hypoventilation, septic shock, or hypoglycemia. In addition to assessment of the vital signs, including a rectal temperature, blood pressure, and pulse oximetry, the general appearance and mental status should be noted. Regardless of etiology, significant apnea (>20 seconds) is life-threatening. Therefore, even in the absence of abnormal physical findings, appropriate diagnostic studies should be performed to evaluate the child for several common etiologies.

The next phase of evaluation addresses two key questions: (1) Is this episode of clinical significance? (2) What is the risk of recurrence? Factors to consider include: (a) signs of an acute illness, (b) the age of the child, and (c) risk factors for clinically significant and/or recurrent apnea.

The history is the most useful part of the evaluation of apnea. Therefore, every effort should be made to obtain precise information from a first-hand observer. This may not be a simple task, considering the observer's recent stressful experience, but a clear initial history without the predictable influence of repeated questions is vital. The following details should be included: (1) where the event took place; (2) how long it lasted; (3) whether the infant was awake or asleep; (4) whether there was an associated color change and, if so, to what colors and in what order; (5) description of associated movements, posture, or changes in tone; (6) what resuscitative efforts were made and the infant's response to them; (7) when the infant was last fed; and (8) the position the baby was in when the event occurred. Attention to the response to these questions may provide the physician with a diagnosis. For example, an older sibling took a favorite toy away from an 11-month-old infant and the baby began to cry, turned red, then blue, and finally had several minutes of tonic-clonic motor activity. In this situation, the diagnosis of a breath-holding spell would be straightforward. In contrast, a story of 40 minutes of cyanosis and apnea in a now well-appearing child suggests that parts of the history are unreliable. Other recent events that should be documented are symptoms of other illnesses, including fever, changes in behavior, activity, and appetite as well as recent trauma and immunizations.

If the description of the event suggests that significant apnea did occur, hospitalization for further workup is warranted. A typical case might be the previously well 6-week-old child who became blue while sitting upright in a car seat and then became limp, pale, and "looked like he was dead." There was initially no response to tactile or verbal stimulation, but after about 15 to 20 seconds of mouth-to-mouth breathing, he coughed, gagged, and began to breathe. His color improved over the next 30 seconds, and the parents rushed him to the ED. Such a baby may look entirely normal on examination in the ED, yet be at grave risk for ALTE.

The medical history may also provide important information regarding infants at risk for significant and/or recurrent apnea. It is imperative to ask specifically about previous similar episodes. Information about perinatal events including gestational age (birth weight), labor and delivery, maternal health, and nursery course is helpful. A family history with specific reference to seizures, infant deaths, and serious illnesses in young family members should also be included. Finally, information regarding poisons available in the household may be important in treating an older child.

A careful physical examination identifies many treatable acute illnesses that can cause apnea; however, the likelihood of an underlying illness varies by age. Clues to serious systemic disease include presence of fever or hypothermia. Tachypnea suggests either a respiratory or metabolic problem, and shock may be secondary to sepsis, hypovolemia, or occult trauma. Evaluation of the nervous system should include notation of mental status, palpation of the fontanelles, and funduscopic examination. Dysmorphic features might suggest an underlying con-

genital abnormality. However, an entirely normal physical examination does not provide absolute reassurance that the described event was clinically insignificant and will not recur.

Laboratory evaluation should be guided by the history and physical examination. Tests to consider in the ED include CBC, and a measurement of blood glucose and serum electrolytes. Any indication that the infant could have a serious infection should be pursued with cultures of blood and urine and by examination of cerebrospinal fluid. Urine and blood for toxologic analysis should be obtained in patients for whom poisoning is suggested by the history. In the child with a normal oxygen saturation by pulse oximetry, an arterial blood gas is unnecessary. Venous pH may identify a significant metabolic acidosis as in, for example in carbon monoxide poisoning where the pO_2 may be normal, but there will be a metabolic acidosis. A significant apneic episode can occur, followed by recovery and a completely normal arterial blood gas determination. Therefore, the arterial or venous blood gas examination does not serve as a screening test for a serious event and should be obtained based on specific indications. Radiologic studies during the initial evaluation might include lateral neck, chest, abdomen, or head CT, again as indicated by the history and physical examination.

The tasks of the emergency physician faced with a young patient who has had an apneic episode are to identify patients who should be hospitalized and to treat underlying conditions. If a careful history and physical examination suggest that a significant apneic episode has not occurred, the diagnosis of periodic breathing or breath holding can be made and the patient discharged after appropriate counseling of the parents and arrangements for follow-up. However, the evaluation of a young child with apnea is rarely so straightforward. If historical information indicates that significant apnea has occurred, the infant is at risk for a recurrence of this life-threatening event. An aggressive search for an underlying cause is necessary and often includes laboratory studies, lumbar puncture, chest radiograph, and electrocardiogram. Hospital admission should be considered for observation and further diagnostic evaluation.

A significant apneic episode in the absence of systemic disease suggests a diagnosis of primary apnea. Since there may not be a satisfactory explanation for the event, it may be judicious to consider an inpatient evaluation to identify known causes of primary apnea. This might include observation with monitoring as well as an electroencephalogram, some type of sleep study, a chest radiograph, and electrocardiogram. Respiratory function is evaluated with a pneumogram, and a barium swallow and esophageal pH study may identify gastroesophageal reflux. An ultrasound or CT of the head should be considered if the child has a central cause for apnea. The decision to recommend home cardiorespiratory monitoring is complex and beyond the scope of emergency pediatric practice. It necessitates a level of continuity of care and follow-up best provided by the primary care provider.

In many instances, a thorough history and careful physical examination with appropriate laboratory studies suggest that a significant apneic event has not occurred and that there is no serious underlying illness. In this situation, the emergency physician should reassure and educate the family before discharging the patient. Parents should also be given specific instructions regarding indications for returning to the ED and follow-up with their primary care provider.

Stridor

Stridor, from the Latin *stridulus,* is a harsh or whistling vibratory sound caused by air movement through partial obstruction of any portion of the airway from the nares to the bronchi. Airflow through the upper respiratory tract and trachea is normally laminar. The Venturi and Bernoulli laws explain the phenomenon of turbulent airflow through a narrowed segment of the airway. On physical examination, this turbulence is appreciated as stridor.

Stridor itself is not a disease, but an important clinical finding requiring careful investigation. It is commonly seen in young patients and represents a large differential diagnosis ranging from a static congenital anomaly to a rapid progressing acute infection to an airway or esophageal foreign body. Age, onset, severity, progression, and associated features (feeding, fever) are all helpful historical variables in determining the cause of stridor. Observation of the degree of respiratory distress and timing of stridor with the respiratory cycle may further define its cause.

Pathophysiology

Unique aspects of infant and pediatric airway anatomy and physiology are important considerations in understanding and treating upper airway obstruction in young children (**FIGURE 88.1**). A prominent occiput allows flexion of the head and neck when the infant is supine. This causes the tongue to flop back on the posterior pharynx creating a functional obstruction. The tongue is a relative large structure in the child's small mouth and a difficult obstacle to overcome while performing bag-valve-mouth ventilation or intubation. The larynx is more anterior and cephalad and is funnel shaped (**FIGURE 88.2**). The

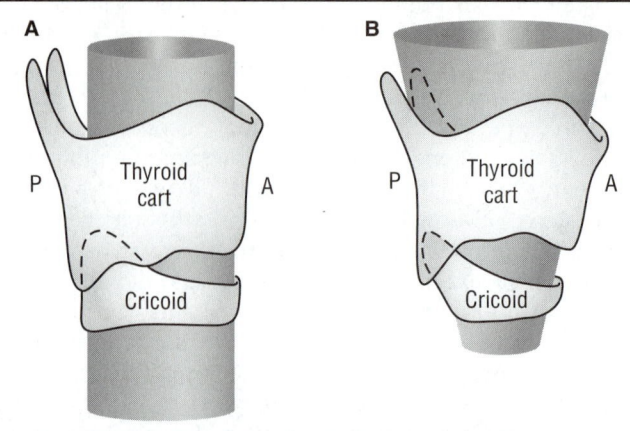

FIGURE 88.2 Configuration of the adult (A, cylindrically shaped) and the infant (B, funnel-shaped) larynx. *Source:* Reprinted with permission from W.B. Saunders. Wheeler M, Coté CJ, Todres ID. Pediatric airway. In: Cote CJ, Ryan JF, Todres ID, et al, eds. *A Practice of Anesthesia for Infants and Children,* 3rd edition. Philadelphia: WB Saunders; 2001:85.

cords themselves are short and concave. The epiglottis is U-shaped and horizontally situated, making a complete view of the cords difficult. The narrowest point in the infant's airway is at the level of the cricoid cartilage. The caliber of all airway structures is small. For example, the newborn tracheal length is 57 mm and laryngeal diameter is 4 mm. One millimeter of edema of the mucosal lining of the trachea can significantly reduce the cross sectional diameter of the airway. Special equipment is required to ventilate and/or intubate and child: a shoulder roll to overcome the occiput, a straight (Miller) blade to displace the tongue during intubation, appropriately sized endotracheal tubes (using the PALS rule of thumb for children > 2 years of age: ETT size = 4 + age/4), uncuffed tubes in children over 8 years of age because of the anatomic cuff at the narrow cricoid ring, and a properly sized mask to ensure a tight seal during assisted ventilation.

Cartilaginous supporting structures throughout the airway are soft and compliant, making them prone to dynamic narrowing or collapse with changes in intralumenal pressures during inspiration and expiration.

Evaluation

A careful history will provide many clues to the diagnosis in an infant or child with stridor. Items that are of particular importance include:

- *Acute or chronic duration:* Is this likely to be a congenital anomaly, an acute infectious process or foreign body?
- *Presence of fever:* Is this an infectious process or a congenital anomaly complicated by an upper airway infection? In the absence of fever, is this a congeniality anomaly, or trauma or a foreign body?
- *Progression of the stridor:* Is the stridor stable and the child at baseline? Is it rapidly progressing and associated with distress and toxicity?
- *Circumstances surrounding the onset:* Is stridor associated with trauma, feeding, playing with small toys, exposure to a caustic substance, coughing, or choking?

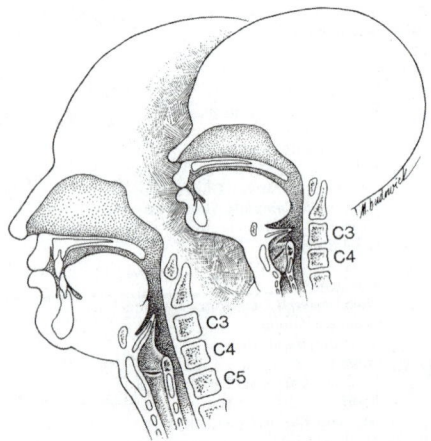

FIGURE 88.1 Comparison of pediatric and adult airway structures. Note differences in size of occiput, tongue, and mouth, and orientation of cords and epiglottitis. *Source:* Reprinted with permission from A. Davis Company. Finucane BT, Santora AH. *Principles of Airway Management.* 1988.

- *Sore throat, drooling, dysphagia:* How severe are these symptoms?
- *Age of the patient at the onset of stridor:* Has stridor or noisy breathing been present since birth? Does it worsen with feeding, viral infections, or positioning?
- *Feeding difficulties:* Does stridor worsen with feeding?
- *Position of maximal comfort:* Does the stridor improve when the infant is prone (laryngomalacia), in the decubitus position (vocal cord paralysis), or with a nasopharyngeal airway (micrognathia, macroglossia)? Does the patient maintain himself in a tripod position or refuse to lie down (epiglottitis, foreign body)?
- *The quality and pitch of voice or cry:* Is the cry normal? Does the voice seem hoarse?
- *Past medical history:* Is there a history of intubations, frequent respiratory infections, bouts of "recurrent croup," or cardiac disease?

The physical examination begins with careful observation of the *degree of respiratory distress* (respiratory rate, heart rate, nasal flaring, retractions), *presence of respiratory failure* (altered mental status, cyanosis, poor muscle tone, poor respiratory effort), the *position the patient assumes,* the *quality of stridor* (snorious, inspiratory, expiratory, biphasic), and the *timing with the respiratory cycle.*

The site of obstruction determines the quality of stridor (**FIGURE 88.3**). Obstruction at the level of the pharynx or nasopharynx (choanal atresia, polyps, tonsillar hypertrophy, macroglossia) has a loud, snorious quality. High pitched, inspiratory stridor is associated with obstruction of the supraglottic and immediate subglottic airway (croup, laryngomalacia). Biphasic stridor is heard with fixed lesions especially of the glottis (laryngeal web) and subglottic trachea/cricoid ring (subglottic stenosis, severe croup) because the size of the airway lumen does not change with the respiratory cycle. Tracheal obstruction (bacterial tracheitis, foreign body) typically results in expiratory stridor. In addition, it is important to auscultate the neck, to listen to the chest for ronchi or wheezes. The mouth and jaw should be noted for micrognathia or macroglossia. Abnormal muscle tone may be a sign of hypocalcemia. Cutaneous lesions would suggest the possibility of airway hemangioma. A cardiac murmur would suggest a vascular anomaly like a vascular ring.

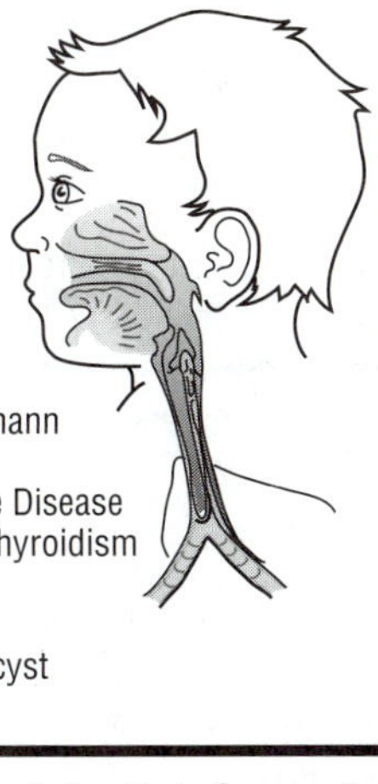

Radiographs of the neck and chest may be helpful to further pinpoint a diagnosis. Soft tissue lateral views of the neck should be examined for the contour of the vallecula, epiglottis, aryepiglottic folds, tracheal air column and retropharyngeal space. This radiograph should be taken with the head in extension. An anteroposterior (AP) of the airway provides an additional view of the trachea. An AP and lateral chest radiograph may be helpful in identifying a right-sided aortic arch (suggestive of a vascular ring), extrinsic tracheal compression, a radiopaque foreign body, atelectasis or hyperinflation.

A foreign body in a bronchus creates a ball-valve effect causing hyperlucency on the affected side. If this is suspected, right and left decubitus films may be helpful. Normally, the dependent lung is smaller and the mediastinum seems to fall to that side. With hyperinflation, the affected/obstructed lung looks bigger or more lucent than expected with less mediastinal compression. Direct observation of diaphragmatic movement with inspiration and exhalation with fluoroscopy may be helpful.

A barium swallow is useful to demonstrate tracheal compression by a mass including a vascular ring or an esophageal foreign body. Computed tomography or magnetic resonance imaging is usually required to further define many of these anomalies. Nasopharyngoscopy, bronchoscopy, and endoscopy are important diagnostic and therapeutic tools that are employed in an individualized fashion.

Stridor is a common and serious complaint in young children. A complete differential diagnosis should be entertained while assessing and managing a distressed child with stridor. Emergency management of the child with stridor depends on the cause of the obstruction.

Upper Airway Obstruction and Infection

The differential diagnosis of stridor in the pediatric patient requires a systematic approach. The patient should be carefully assessed for extreme distress that would mandate advanced airway management (**FIGURE 88.4**). In the less emergent setting, determination of the patient's age, the duration of stridor (acute, chronic), and associated symptoms (cough, fever) are most helpful.

Congenital Lesions

Congenital lesions present with stridor within the first weeks of life. In some cases, the diagnosis is unmasked when inflammation and edema from an upper respiratory infection exacerbate the infant's symptoms. *Laryngomalacia* is the most common form of stridor in infants. Collapse of the epiglottis, arytenoids, and aryepiglottic folds into the glottic opening results in harsh, high-pitched inspiratory stridor beginning within the first few months of age. Symptoms worsen with supine position, agitation, and respiratory infections. Most infants with laryngomalacia thrive with resolution of symptoms by 18 to 24 months of age.

Supraglottic
- Craniofacial
  Pierre Robin
  Treacher Collins
  Hallermann-Streiff
- Macroglossia
  Beckwith-Wiedemann
  Down Syndrome
  Glycogen Storage Disease
  Congential Hypothyroidism
- Choanal atresia
- Encephalocele
- Thyroglossal duct cyst
- Lingual thyroid

Laryngeal
- Laryngomalacia
- Vocal cord paralysis
- Congenital subglottic stenosis
- Laryngeal web
- Laryngeal cyst
- Subglottic hemangioma
- Laryngotracheoesophageal cleft

Intrathoracic
- Tracheomalacia
- Tracheal stenosis
- Vascular rings/slings
- Mediastinal masses

FIGURE 88.3 Anatomic location of congenital etiologies of stridor.
Source: Used with permission from *Clinical Pediatrics.* Simon, NP, Simon N. Evaluation and management of stridor in the newborn. *Clin Pediatr* 1991;30:211–216.

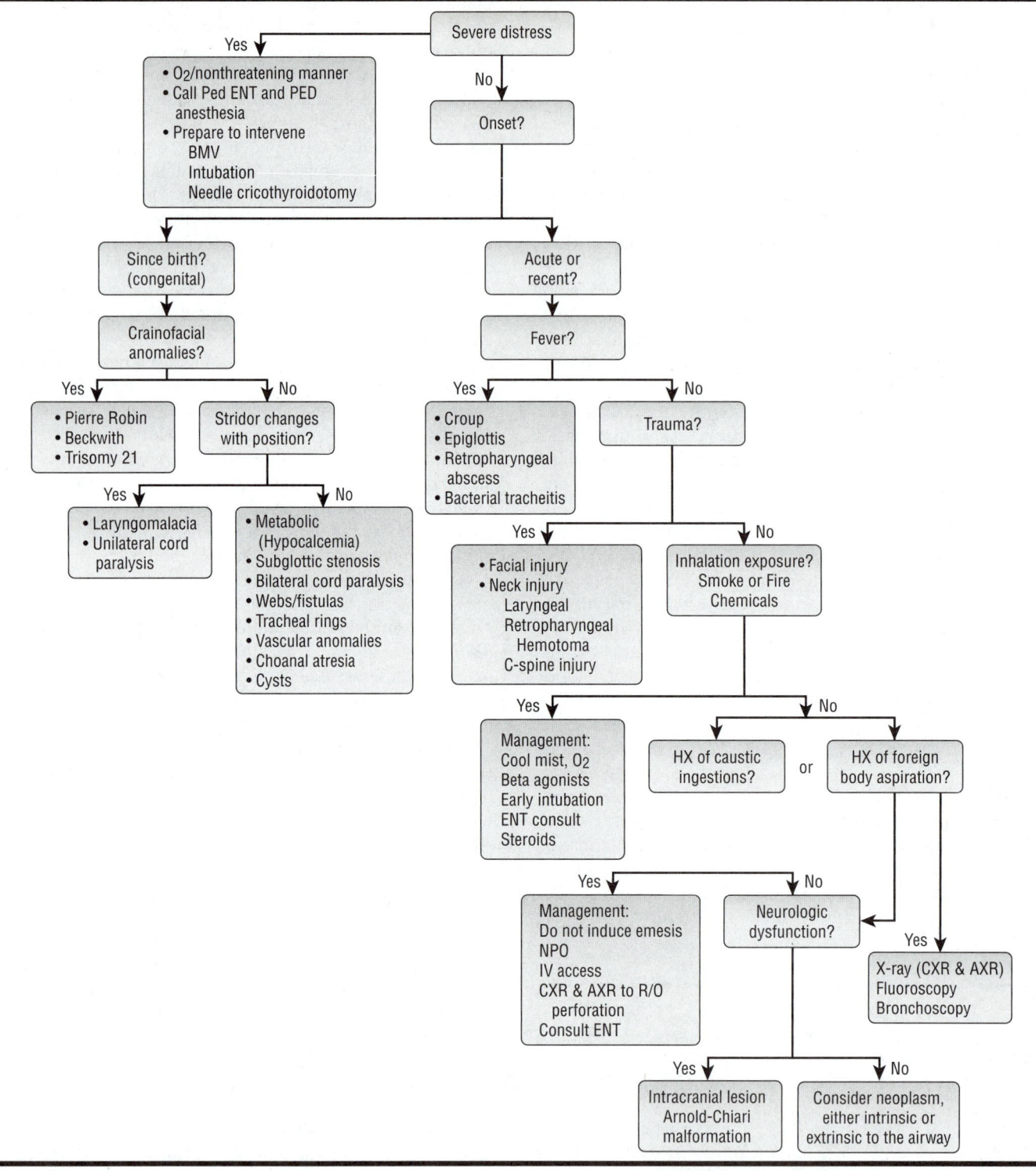

FIGURE 88.4 A systematic approach to the child with suspected upper airway obstruction. *Source:* Used with permission from Lippincott-Raven. Aghababian RH et al, eds. *Emergency Medicine: The Core Curriculum.* Philadelphia: Lippincott-Raven, 1998.

Vocal cord paralysis is the second most common cause of chronic stridor in infants. Bilateral vocal cord paralysis presents with severe respiratory distress and stridor, and can be associated with central nervous system abnormalities such as Arnold Chiari malformation. Unilateral vocal cord paralysis is most commonly left sided and related to traction to the left recurrent laryngeal nerve at birth or

compression from mediastinal structures. Infants with unilateral vocal cord paralysis have a hoarse, weak cry. Stridor often worsens with distress and improves with positioning of the affected side down.

A *laryngeal web* results from failure in complete canalization of the airway. Most webs lie between the cords and appear as a partial anterior fusion. The severity of symptoms reflects the size of the web. Small webs may cause a hoarse, weak cry and mild stridor. Larger, more complete webs are associated with aphonia and severe distress.

Congenital laryngotracheal ("subglottic") stenosis results from a congenital defect in canalization of the subglottic trachea. Deformity of the cricoid ring is usually seen. Severe cases present with stridor at birth. More mild lesions may be asymptomatic until additional obstruction from infection or inflammation occurs. Subglottic stenosis is also an acquired condition seen following prolonged intubation or blunt trauma to the neck.

A *subglottic hemangioma* is a less common cause of stridor in infants. The infant is usually asymptomatic at birth but develops stridor (which may be biphasic) and cough within the first few weeks to months of life. Symptoms generally peak at 6 months, reflecting the rapid growth of the infant as well as the hemangioma during the first months of life. Respiratory symptoms worsen with crying and agitation. Cutaneous hemangioma are seen in approximately half of cases. Hemangiomas of the airway may be seen on plain radiograph as an asymmetric lesion along the tracheal air column.

A *vascular ring* is an anomaly of the great vessels that form a ring encircling the trachea, esophagus, or both. Examples of these "vascular rings" include a double aortic arch, and right-sided aortic arch with persistent left ligament. These are rare and often present in infancy with symptoms related to breathing and feeding. However, the nonspecific nature of the infant's symptoms and low prevalence of these lesions often results in an initial incorrect diagnosis of croup or upper respiratory infection.

Acquired Infectious Lesions

The acute onset of stridor with fever and symptoms such as cough, hoarse voice, drooling, and sore throat suggests an infectious process. The most important in this group include croup, epiglottitis or supraglottitis, retropharyngeal abscess, and bacterial tracheitis.

Acute *laryngotracheobronchitis (viral croup)* is characterized by stridor, barky cough, and hoarseness. It is caused by obstruction due to inflammation of the subglottic area. Typically, croup presents episodically through the year. One peak occurs in the fall and a second peak occurring in early winter. Parainfluenza viruses are seen most frequently in the fall. Respiratory syncytial virus (RSV) typically occurs in the winter. Croup occurs in children between the ages of 6 months and 3 years, with a peak incidence in the second year of life. It is rare in children over 6. *Typical croup* is common, benign and self-limited which is associated with URI symptoms and fever. The symptoms are worse at night or when the child is agitated.

Clinical Presentation

Children with mild and moderate croup are able to speak and drink. These patients often have a hoarse voice and a loud, brassy, barking cough. They are not stridulous or distressed at rest and have normal oxygen saturations. The diagnosis of croup in these patients can usually determined by history and physical examination. Patients with severe or atypical croup may be in severe distress, have the sudden onset of symptoms without upper respiratory infection prodrome, have an oxygen requirement, or refuse to talk or swallow. They may have stridor at rest or biphasic stridor. Soft tissue views of the neck may be helpful to exclude other serious upper airway infections. Skilled medical personnel should carefully observe such patients while radiographs are being taken.

Diagnosis

Croup is largely a clinical diagnosis. Laboratory tests and radiographs are of value in excluding other possibilities when the diagnosis of croup is not clear or when symptoms are atypical or severe. The anteroposterior and lateral neck radiographs show subglottic narrowing, which is the classic "steeple" sign.

Treatment

Humidification has been the mainstay for treatment of croup at home and in the ED. Parents commonly observe an improvement in symptoms following exposure to the cool night air. Cool mist is postulated to moisten secretions in the throat and cause vasoconstriction of inflamed mucosa. However, there is no evidenced based literature to support cool mist.

Nebulized epinephrine is used in the treatment of moderate and severe croup. After administration of racemic or L-epinephrine (1:1,000) clinical improvement should be seen within 30 minutes. Nebulized epinephrine can be repeated, if needed, to treat more severe or recurrent symptoms. Patients receiving repeated does of nebulized epinephrine should be carefully monitored. Patients with moderate croup who receive nebulized epinephrine can be discharged from the ED after several hours of observation as long as they are asymptomatic: normal mental status, no stridor or retractions, and normal lung examination. Close follow-up should be arranged as part of discharge planning with parents.

Corticosteroids improve symptoms in patients with croup by anti-inflammatory effects that reduce mucosa edema of the subglottic space. Clinical improvement is typically delayed by 2 to 6 hours after administration. Dexamethasone is commonly used as an oral and IM agent for moderate to severe croup, in part, because of its long a half-life of 36 to 72 hours. Dexamethasone was initially studied in hospitalized patients who received an IM total dose of 0.6 mg/kg. These studies showed a dramatic decrease in length of stay in the hospital and ICU and rates of intubations. Subsequent studies demonstrated no difference in admitted patents who received 0.15 mg/kg, 0.3 mg/kg, and 0.6 mg/kg of dexamethasone syrup. In addition, nebulized budesonide has been shown to be effective in the treatment of hospitalized children with croup. Geelhoed demonstrated the effectiveness of a single oral dose of 0.15 mg/kg of dexamethasone in improvement of symptoms in outpatients with mild croup. Finally, Klassen et al. reported added improvement with budesonide in children with mild or moderate croup who had received oral dexamethasone.

Epiglottitis has become uncommon since the introduction of *Haemophilus influenzae* type B vaccine. Studies of patients with epiglottitis since 1990 reveal that the average age is older (80 months vs. 35 months) with a different profile of infectious agents. *Haemophilus influenzae* type B is seen in a small minority of patients. More likely organisms include Group A beta-hemolytic streptococcus, *Staphlococcus aureus,* and *Streptococcus pneumoniae.* Noninfectious causes are rare but include thermal injury from swallowing hot liquids.

Clinical Presentation

Classically described epiglottitis clinically presents as a toxic appearing, highly febrile child, typically 2 to 6 years old, with severe sore throat, dysphonia, and dysphagia. These children appear anxious and sit upright in the sniffing position to enhance airway patency. Symptoms are rapid in onset and progress rapidly.

Diagnosis

Epiglottitis is largely a clinical diagnosis based on typical presentation described above. Laboratory tests, blood gases and x-rays should be avoided unless the diagnosis is in doubt. Soft tissue lateral radiographs reveal an enlarged contour of the epiglottitis (the classic thumbprint), lack of air in the vallecula, and thickened aryepiglottic folds (**FIGURE 88.5**). Medical staff skill with advanced airway skill should remain with the patient during x-rays if they are needed.

Treatment

The treatment of epiglottitis is to secure the airway with intubation in a controlled (preferably OF) setting. With direct visualization at intubation, the epiglottis and surrounding structures are inflamed, edematous, and coated with exudate. Therapies including antibiotics and laboratory tests should be delayed until after the airway is secure. At that time, blood cultures can be obtained and antibiotics and fluids administered.

Retropharyngeal abscess has become more common than epiglottitis. It is commonly related to penetrating trauma to the pharynx (such as a fall with a sharp object in the mouth of a toddler, gagging on a chicken bone) but also occur spontaneously secondary to *Streptococcus pyogenes, Staphylococcus aureus,* or mouth anaerobes.

Clinical Presentation

Most commonly, retropharyngeal abscess presents in young children with a variety of symptoms including: fever, toxicity, respiratory distress, stridor, drooling, and meningismus or torticollis. The classic described physical examination finding is a bulging forward of the posterior pharyngeal wall, although this is a difficult assessment in a young child.

Diagnosis

Lateral neck radiographs are often helpful in establishing this diagnosis. They should be taken with the head in mild extension and reveal widening of the prevertebral soft tissues. A contrast CT is a helpful diagnostic test when the lateral neck is equivocal and to determine the extent of pathology (**FIGURE 88.6**).

Treatment

Patients with retropharyngeal abscess should be managed in consultation with an ENT specialist and require intravenous antibiotics and close observation in a setting when skilled personnel are on hand. Complications include airway obstruction, sepsis, mediastinitis, or vascular complications of the internal jugular vein or carotid artery.

Bacterial tracheitis is a bacterial infection of the lining of the tracheal. It is believed to be a bacterial suprainfection since respiratory viruses (parainfluenza, influenza, RSV) are typically cultured along with common bacterial agents (*S. aureus, M. catarrhalis, Streptococcus pneumoniae,* and Gram-negative organisms).

Clinical Presentation

Patients with bacterial tracheitis classically have a viral, often croup-like prodrome that acutely worsen and develop toxicity, high fever, productive cough, and stridor. Bacterial tracheitis should be suspected in patients with symptoms of severe, atypical croup with a normal epiglottis and retropharyngeal space on lateral neck radiographs.

Diagnosis

Radiographs of the airway and chest may reveal wavy, linear densities (the sloughed pseudomembrane) within the lumen of the trachea. Alternatively, the tracheal air column may have a shaggy appearance rather that a normally crisp border.

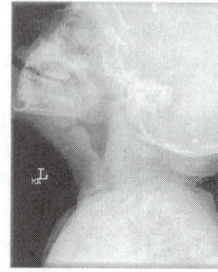

FIGURE 88.5 Epiglottitis. *Source:* Used with permission from W.B. Saunders Co., © 2002. Stevenson M. Upper Airway Obstruction: Infectious Cases. In: *Clinical Pediatric Emergency Medicine,* vol 3, no 3, St Louis, MO: W.B. Saunders Company, 2002.

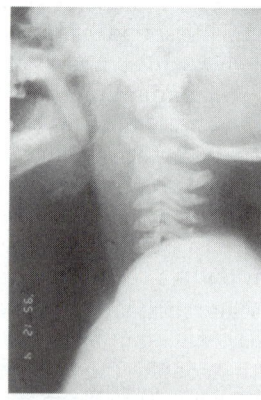

FIGURE 88.6 Retropharyngeal abscess. *Source:* Used with permission from W.B. Saunders Co., © 2002. Stevenson M. Upper Airway Obstruction: Infectious Cases. In: *Clinical Pediatric Emergency Medicine,* vol 3, no 3. St Louis, MO: W.B. Saunders Company, 2002.

Treatment

Bronchoscopy for suctioning and debridment of thick, purulent tracheal secretions, and establishment of an airway should be quickly accomplished in patients with severe distress. Antibiotic coverage for *S. aureus*, *S. pyogenes*, and *Streptococcus pneumoniae* should be administered promptly.

Acquired, Noninfectious Causes of Stridor

Foreign body within the airway or proximal esophagus, anaphylaxis, and trauma to the neck are important noninfectious causes of stridor.

An aspirated foreign body is most commonly seen in children less than 3 years of age. Round toys, food, and balloons are the most commonly aspirated objects. Symptoms of a centrally-located foreign body may be abrupt in onset and associated with coughing or choking and stridor. Foreign bodies can move within the airway converting a partial to complete obstruction. Many airway and esophageal foreign bodies (including food) are not radiopaque and cannot be seen on plain radiography. Bronchoscopy should be considered in any child in whom foreign body aspiration is suspected, even in the absence of radiographic evidence. Esophageal foreign bodies can present with stridor because of swelling and compression of the airway.

Upper airway edema with anaphylaxis occurs in small children following exposure to allergens. Symptoms may begin with sneezing, an itchy throat, or may progress rapidly with upper airway edema. Immediate management steps include: assessment of the degree of obstruction, presence of concomitant bronchospasm and shock, administration of oxygen, nebulized beta-agonists, subcutaneous epinephrine, H_1 and H_2 blocking agents, and steroids.

The onset of stridor following a fall or blow to the neck, especially in the presence of hoarse voice, sore throat, cough, or trouble swallowing, represents a potential airway emergency. External signs of injury may be absent. Physical examination may reveal crepitis or localized laryngeal tenderness. Radiographs of the neck and chest should be obtained, with attention to larynx and tracheal air column. Computed tomography is of value in further defining specific injuries. Additional considerations include consultation with an ENT specialist, orotracheal intubation, and corticosteriods.

Lower Respiratory Tract Infections

Pathophysiology

The clinical presentation and differential diagnosis of lower respiratory tract infections in infants and young children differ dramatically from adolescents and adults. Agents that cause upper respiratory tract illness in older children and adults may cause severe lower respiratory tract symptoms in young infants. The agents responsible for infection differ with age; the annual incidence of pneumonia in industrialized countries is higher from birth to 5 years than at any other time in life. The pathophysiology of bronchiolitis serves as an excellent example of the effect of viral infection on the lower respiratory tract. This infection causes inflammation, edema, and mucus production in small airways, resulting in narrowing of the intraluminal airway diameter. This small decrease in radius results in a dramatic increase in airway resistance manifested as the characteristic air trapping and wheezing seen in lower respiratory tract disease in small infants.

Vulnerability to respiratory failure occurs, in part, because mechanisms to improve respiratory function fail in the young infant. For example, hypoxia and hypercarbia are signals to increase minute ventilation. Although the respiratory rate will increase, attempts to increase tidal volume often fail because of increased chest wall compliance. An increase in negative intrathoracic pressure tends to cause the chest wall to collapse and, in fact, increases the work of breathing. Retractions and abdominal breathing are the manifestations of this process. The diaphragm, a key muscle for respiration in infants, is also prone to fatigue. Finally, hypoxia can inhibit respiratory drive in the very young rather than stimulate it (see **Apnea** section, above).

The differential diagnosis of lower respiratory tract symptoms such as tachypnea, cough, and wheezing is broad. The age of the child is a helpful consideration in limiting the diagnostic possibilities. In the neonate, a change in the respiratory pattern can be a symptom of cardiac or metabolic disease. Infection can be present without fever. In fact, hypothermia may indicate overwhelming infection. In toddlers, who are notorious for putting everything in their mouths, the same symptoms may be the result of an aspirated foreign body or a toxic ingestion.

Atypical Pneumonia Syndromes

Although atypical, or nonbacterial, pneumonia syndromes were initially described in adult patients, they occur in children as well. There are a number of organisms that cause atypical pneumonia. The agents most often associated with pediatric infection include *Mycoplasma pneumoniae*, *Chlamydia pneumoniae*, and *Chlamydia trachomatis*.

Chlamydia pneumoniae (or TWAR) can cause pneumonia in adults and children. This agent was first recognized as a respiratory pathogen in 1986. Infections are usually mild or asymptomatic. Severe illness is usually associated with a chronic underlying condition. *Chlamydia pneumoniae* is sensitive to erythromycin, azithromycin, and clarithromycin, but the optimal dose and length of treatment are uncertain, however. Erythromycin at a dose of 50 mg/kg/day for 21 days has been recommended to avoid relapse.

Chlamydia trachomatis is an important cause of afebrile pneumonia in infants from 4 to 11 weeks of age. The infection is acquired at birth. The infant develops tachypnea and cough without fever or wheezing. Some babies may have previously had chlamydial conjunctivitis. Treatment is with erythromycin at 50 mg/kg/day for 10 to 14 days.

Mycoplasma pneumoniae is the most frequent cause of nonbacterial pneumonia in children over 5 years of age. Although pneumonia from this agent also occurs in those younger than 5, it is rare under 2 years of age. The incubation period is about 3 weeks. The onset of symptoms occurs slowly, over days to weeks. Many children have pharyngitis as well. The cough generally worsens and becomes productive by the second week. The clinical presentation and radiographic findings of mycoplasma pneumonia are often nonspecific and share many features with *Chlamydia pneumoniae* infections. There is often a discrepancy between the clinical and radiologic findings. For example, a child may have impressive rales and a normal chest radiograph. There are no readily available techniques for identifying mycoplasma infection other than serology. Bedside cold agglutinins have been advocated as a specific test. Since cold agglutinins do not appear until late in the first week or early in the second week of the illness, a negative test does not exclude mycoplasma. Treatment with erythromycin, clarithromycin, or azithromycin may lead to more rapid resolution of symptoms when administered early in the course.

Bacterial Pneumonia

In the neonate, loosely identified to include the first 4 weeks of life, lower respiratory pathogens can be acquired transplacentally, during birth, or postnatally. Congenital infections are usually associated with other signs of a congenital process such as microcephaly, intrauterine growth retardation, or hepatosplenomegaly, and rarely cause pneumonia alone. Perinatal infection can involve organisms from either the maternal gastrointestinal or genitourinary tract. Specific organisms include group B streptococcus, Gram-negative enteric organisms, and *Listeria monocytogenes*. Infection with group B streptococcus that develops in the first week of life is associated with overwhelming multisystem disease including pneumonia. Likewise, the early clinical manifestation of infection with *Listeria* is sepsis and perhaps pneumonia. Infections with both group B streptococcus and *Listeria* tend to localize to the central nervous system after the first week of life. Enteric organisms infrequently cause pneumonia in the otherwise healthy neonate. Disease is more often manifested as sepsis and/or meningitis. The newborn is also susceptible to pneumonia caused by *S. aureus*.

Between the first month of life and 5 years of age, bacterial pneumonia is usually caused by *S. pneumoniae*, *H. influenzae*, group A streptococcus, or *S. aureus*.

Most children who develop staphylococcal pneumonia are under 1 year of age. Routine vaccination of young infants against *S. pneumoniae* and *H. influenzae* type B has resulted in a decline in the incidence of pneumonia caused by these organisms. Nevertheless, *S. pneumoniae* remains the most likely cause of bacterial pneumonia in school-age children. Nontypeable *Haemophilus* usually causes upper respiratory infection and otitis media, rather than pneumonia. Infection from *S. aureus* is always a concern in immunocompromised individuals or in children recovering from a prior viral lower respiratory tract infection.

The child with bacterial pneumonia often has the abrupt onset of severe symptoms including fever, malaise, cough, tachypnea, and dyspnea. Irritation of the pleura may result in localized pain. Basilar pneumonia may cause severe abdominal pain. In the infant, signs and symptoms may be less specific. Grunting respirations are of particular significance and indicate serious lower respiratory tract disease. Dehydration as the result of fever, tachypnea, and poor intake is often a feature in all age groups. Inspiratory rales may be localized to a specific lobe. However, absence of auscultatory findings in a patient with cough, fever, and tachypnea does not exclude the possibility of pneumonia. Conjunctivitis, otitis media, and diarrhea can occur with bacterial pneumonia in younger children. Evaluation should include vital signs with pulse oximetry if hypoxemia is suspected, since it may be particularly difficult to detect hypoxemia in the young infant. Observations of movement, consolability, attentiveness, color, and use of accessory muscles have been shown to be better predictors of hypoxemia than tachypnea and auscultatory findings. The chest radiograph may be normal early in the course of a bacterial pneumonia or with dehydration. Therefore, the diagnosis will be made on clinical grounds alone in some cases. A decision to hospitalize the patient is based on the following considerations: degree of respiratory distress, presence of hypoxemia, ability of the child to tolerate oral fluids and medications, underlying state of health, and reliability of the child's caregivers. In addition, young infants, especially younger than 3 months of age, have a greater likelihood of severe infection and are more susceptible to respiratory failure. Infants and more toxic-appearing children may require a more extensive evaluation including CBC, blood culture, and possible lumbar puncture, particularly in infants less than 8 weeks. Infants under 4 weeks of age should receive antibiotics, which will cover *E. coli,* group B streptococcus, and *Listeria* (such as ampicillin and gentamicin). Older infants and children who are well appearing should be treated with an antibiotic that will cover pneumococcus (such as amoxicillin). In sicker children, an antibiotic effective against penicilliase-producing Hib (e.g., amoxicillin-clavulinic acid) should be considered, although these infections are rare since the introduction of vaccination against this organism.

Viral Lower Respiratory Tract Infections

Most lower respiratory tract infections are viral in etiology. The nature and severity of these illnesses vary by age, the general health of the host, and etiologic agent. For example, although adenovirus occurs infrequently in the young infant, it can cause severe multisystem disease. Cytomegalovirus and herpes simplex occur more frequently in the very young infant. The frequency of measles has declined particularly since a booster dose of vaccine has been recommended in school-age children. However, when an infected individual develops measles pneumonia, it is a very serious infection. Finally, immunocompromised children and healthy adults who acquire varicella frequently develop pneumonia. Fortunately, viral pneumonia is usually a relatively mild illness. Respiratory syncytial virus, parainfluenza (particularly type 3), and influenza A and B cause most of these cases. The importance of human metapneumonia virus, an RNA virus related to respiratory syncytial virus, has been recently described.

The clinical characteristics of viral pneumonia vary with age. Onset of symptoms is more gradual than in bacterial illness. Initially upper respiratory tract symptoms and a low-grade fever predominate. Over several days, progressive cough and perhaps tachypnea may develop. Infants under 1 year of age may develop wheezing as well. Auscultatory findings are usually not localized to a specific lobar distribution as in bacterial disease. The characteristic radiographic finding in infants with lower respiratory tract infection is hyperinflation, a manifestation of air trapping. Interstitial infiltrates and atelectasis can be seen as well. Treatment is symptomatic and supportive. Because younger children may have associated fever and dehydration, a more extensive laboratory evaluation may be considered. Respiratory failure clearly develops more quickly in the young infant with viral pneumonia. Therefore, evaluation of respiratory effort, oxygenation, and ability to maintain oral hydration determines disposition.

Bronchiolitis/Respiratory Syncytial Virus

Bronchiolitis is an extremely common inflammatory disease of the small airways that is unique to young infants. Respiratory syncytial virus (RSV), parainfluenza, influenza, adenovirus, and human metapneumovirus all cause bronchiolitis. The incidence of RSV and influenza viruses peak in the winter months. Parainfluenza is more common in autumn and adenovirus occurs throughout the year.

As infection moves into the lower airways, peribronchiolar mononuclear infiltration occurs. Submucosal edema and mucus production also contribute to narrowing of the intraluminal airway and increased resistance to airflow. Bronchospasm may play a role as evidenced by increased concentrations of several mediators of bronchospasm (RSV-IgE, histamine, and leukotriene C4) in some patients. A response to bronchodilator therapy has also been described in some children.

The clinical features of bronchiolitis include rhinorrhea, fever, cough, and wheezing. Tachypnea, retractions, and grunting may develop as the illness becomes more severe. Young infants less than 8 weeks of age may develop apnea associated with RSV infection. Severe bronchiolitis with rapid progression to respiratory failure can occur in infants with pulmonary or cardiac disease. Clinical predictors of the severity of disease include ill appearance, respiratory rate >70, pulse oximetry <95%, and use of accessory muscles. Treatment of bronchiolitis is largely supportive. Some infants do respond to bronchodilators, so a trial of a nebulized β-agonist may be useful. Steroids have no proven efficacy.

Infants born prematurely, those with apnea of prematurity or infants with congenital heart disease may be at risk for developing severe RSV infection. These children are often treated with either RSV immune globulin or palivizumab, a humanized mouse monoclonal antibody, during the winter months to prevent RSV infection.

Pertussis

Although pertussis is often included in the discussion of afebrile pneumonia syndromes, it is not a lower respiratory tract infection. Infection with *Bordetella pertussis* typically evolves in three stages. The initial catarrhal symptoms are nonspecific and after 1 to 3 weeks a paroxysmal cough predominates. This cough is the distinguishing and persistent feature of pertussis. Any stimulation results in a prolonged paroxysm of cough. In stage two, between spells, the infant appears well. The final stage of the illness is the convalescent phase. Significant complications such as apnea and secondary bacterial pneumonia occur most often in infants younger than 3 months of age. It is therefore important to identify possible pertussis in this age group. The diagnosis must be initially made on clinical grounds. The history is suggestive. On examination, the infant appears well. Thorough assessment must include observation of a coughing paroxysm. An infant who becomes hypoxic or apneic, or experiences airway compromise during a spell, must be observed in the hospital. The CBC may show an elevated leukocyte count with an absolute lymphocytosis. Treatment with erythromycin at 50 mg/kg/day may be of clinical benefit and limits spread of infection. The patient with signs of lower respiratory tract disease such as tachypnea or rales may have developed a secondary bacterial pneumonia. This is a serious complication warranting admission to the hospital. Treatment of household and close contacts with erythromycin is an important control measure, which must be instituted as soon as possible.

Evaluation

The emergency physician must immediately identify the child with respiratory compromise. Any evidence of significant hypoventilation, hypoxemia, or airway compromise must be treated rapidly. All patients with symptoms suggesting a lower respiratory tract infection should have a full set of vital signs including pulse oximetry.

As the child's condition is being stabilized, consideration of a more detailed evaluation can begin. The history is sometimes helpful in differentiating a viral from a bacterial infection. If the child is highly febrile and younger than 3 years of age, a CBC and blood culture should be considered, particularly for the patient who may have bacterial pneumonia. In the child with fever and lower respiratory tract symptoms, a chest radiograph is useful. Other laboratory data such as arterial blood gas analysis, electrolytes, and urinalysis should be obtained as clinically indicated.

Management

Treatment of the patient with respiratory failure includes oxygenation and intubation. Seriously ill infants and children with respiratory tract disease often have had poor oral intake and have increased fluid requirements as the result of fever and tachypnea. Intravenous hydration is therefore usually indicated. Appropriate antibiotics should be given to the child with suspected bacterial disease as soon as cultures have been obtained. However, antibiotics should not be withheld in the unstable patient or if IV access is difficult to obtain. A trial of bronchodilator therapy, usually as albuterol at 0.01 cc/kg with 2.5 cc saline, is worthwhile in the infant who is wheezing, particularly if there is a family history of asthma or the child has underlying pulmonary disease. Racemic epinephrine has also been used with variable efficacy to treat wheezing from bronchiolitis.

Disposition

Most children with a lower respiratory tract infection can be managed at home. Successful outpatient treatment is dependent on good followup and adequate family resources. Follow-up with the primary care provider within 24 to 48 hours is important to reassess respiratory function and hydration.

Children with the following clinical features should be hospitalized:

1. Severe respiratory distress
2. Impending respiratory failure as indicated by hypoxia on a $pCO_2 > 40$ mm Hg
3. Rapidly deteriorating clinical course
4. An infant with an oxygen saturation <93% to 95% or desaturation to <93% to 95% during feeding
5. Inability to maintain adequate oral intake and/or to take indicated oral medications.

Other factors that favor a more conservative approach include:

1. Age younger than 3 months
2. Gestational age <36 weeks in an infant <1 year of age
3. Congenital heart disease or chronic lung disease
4. Immunocompromise
5. Limited family resources.

Selected Readings

American Academy of Pediatrics Task Force on Infant Sleep Position and Sudden Infant Death Syndrome. Changing concepts of sudden infant death syndrome: implications for infant sleeping environment and sleep position. *Pediatrics* 2000;105:650–656.

Bass J, Mehta KA. Oxygen desaturation of selected term infants in car seats. *Pediatrics* 1995;96:288–290.

Consuelos MJ, Osterhoudt K, Lavelle J. Infantile Stridor: An Important Factor to Consider. *Pediatr Ann* 2001;30:10633–10637.

Davies F, Gupta R. Apparent life threatening events in infants presenting to an emergency department. *Emerg Med J* 2002;19:11–16.

Geelhoed GC, Macdonald WBG. Oral dexamethasone in the treatment of croup: 0.15 mg/kg versus 0.3 mg/kg versus 0.6 mg/kg. *Pediatr Pulmonol* 1995;20: 362–368.

Geelhoed GC. Sixteen years of croup in a western Australian teaching hospital: effects of routine steroid treatment. *Ann Emerg Med* 1995;28:621–626.

Geelhoed GC, Macdonald WBG. Oral and inhaled steroids in croup: a randomized, placebo-controlled trial. *Pediatr Pulmonol* 1995;20:355.

Geelhoed GC, Turner J, Macdonald WBG. Efficacy of a small single dose of oral dexamethasone for outpatient croup: a double-blind placebo-controlled clinical trial. *BMJ* 1996;313:140–142.

Grpsz AB, Jacobs MD, Cho C, et al. Use of helium-oxygen mixtures relieve upper airway obstruction in a pediatric population. *Laryngoscope* 2001;111;1512–1514.

Hammerschlag MR. Atypical pneumonias in children. *Adv Pediatr Infect Dis* 1995;10:1–39.

Harrington C, Kirjavainen T, Teng A, Sullivan C. Altered autonomic function and reduced arousability in apparent life-threatening event infants with obstructive sleep apnea. *Am J Respir Crit Care Med* 2002;165:1048–1054.

Harris PG. Retropharyngeal abscess and acute torticollis. *J Laryngol Otol* 1997;111: 1183–1185.

Hoffman J, Lister G. The implications of a relationship between prolonged QT interval and the sudden infant death syndrome. *Pediatrics* 1999;103:815–817.

Jeffrey H, Megevand A, Page M. Why the prone position is a risk factor for sudden infant death syndrome. *Pediatrics* 1999;104:263–269.

Klassen TP, Rowe PC, Sutcliffe T, et al. Randomized trial of salbutamol in acute bronchiolitis. *J Pediatr* 1991;118:807–811.

Kemp J, Unger B, Wilkins D, et al. Unsafe sleep practices and analysis of bedsharing among infants dying suddenly and unexpectedly: results of a four-year population-based, death-scene investigation study of sudden infant death syndrome and related deaths. *Pediatrics* 2000;106;e41.

Kumar SR, Rosner IK, Rappaport I. Recurrent wheezing and stridor in a young infant. *Ann Allergy* 1987;59:334–335, 373–375.

Lee SS, Schwartz RH, Bahadori R. Retropharyngeal abscess: epiglottitis of the new millennium. *J Pediatr* 2001;138:435–437.

Long SS, Edwards K, Pertussis. In: Long S, Prober C, Pickering L, eds. *Principles and Practice of Pediatric Infectious Diseases,* 2nd ed. Philadelphia: Elsevier, 2003.

Margolis PA, Ferkol TW, Marsocci S, et al. Accuracy of the clinical examination in detecting hypoxemia in infants with respiratory illness. *J Pediatr* 1994;124: 552–560.

McIntosh KM. Community-acquired pneumonia in children. *N Engl J Med* 2002;346:429–437.

McIntosh KM, Harper M. Acute uncomplicated pneumonia. In: Long S, Prober C, Pickering L, eds. *Principles and Practice of Pediatric Infectious Diseases,* 2nd ed. Philadelphia: Elsevier, 2003.

Nichols DG, Rogers MC. Developmental physiology of the respiratory system. In: Rogers MC, ed. *Textbook of Pediatric Critical Care,* 3rd ed. Baltimore: Williams & Wilkins, 1996.

O'Keeffe LJ, Maw AR. The dangers of minor blunt laryngeal trauma. *J Laryngol Otolaryngol* 1992;106:372–373.

Qureshi S, Mink R. Aspiration of gel fruit snacks. *Pediatrics* 2003;111:687–689.

Prendergast M, Jones JS, Harman D. Racemic epinephrine in the treatment of laryngotracheitis: can we identify children for outpatient therapy? *Am J Emerg Med* 1994;12:613–616.

Rigatto H. Maturation of breathing. *Clin Perinat* 1992;19:739–755.

Rimell FL, Thome A Jr, Stool S, et al. Characteristics of objects that cause choking in children. *JAMA* 1995;274:1763–1766.

Ross DA, Ward PH. Central vocal cord paralysis and paresis presenting as laryngeal stridor in children. *Laryngoscope* 1990;100:10–13.

Ryckman F, Rogers BM. Obstructive airway disease in infants and children. *Surg Clin North Am* 1985;65:1663–1687.

Santamaria JP, Schafermeyer R. Stridor: a review. *Pediatr Emerg Care* 1991;7:61–62.

Simon NP. Evaluation and management of stridor in the newborn. *Clin Pediatr* 1991;30:211–216.

Southall DP, Plunkett CB, Banks MW, et al. Covert video recordings of life-threatening child abuse: lessons for child protection. *Pediatrics* 1997;100:735–760.

Stroud RH, Friedman N. UN updated on inflammatory disorders of the pediatric airway: epiglottitis, croup and tracheitis. *Am J Otolaryngol* 2001;22:268–275.

Williams JV, Harris PA, Tollefson SJ, et al. Human metapneumonia virus in lower respiratory tract disease in otherwise healthy infants and children. *N Engl J Med* 2004;350:443–450.

Gastrointestinal Disorders

Sig Karasch
John Alexander

Anthony Montoya
Gail Galletta

Gastrointestinal Bleeding

Gastrointestinal (GI) bleeding is a relatively common problem in pediatrics. The majority of infants and children who arrive in the ED with GI bleeding have an acute, self-limited episode and are hemodynamically stable. In such patients three important questions must be asked: (1) Is the patient really bleeding? (2) Is the blood coming from the GI tract? and (3) Is there more than a trivial amount of blood? Children with only a few drops or flecks of blood in the vomit or stool should not be considered "GI bleeders" if their history and physical examination are otherwise unremarkable. Likewise, many substances ingested by children may simulate fresh or chemically altered blood. Red food coloring (found in some cereals, antibiotics, and cough syrups, Jello, and Kool-Aid) as well as fruit juices and beets may resemble blood if vomited. Melena may be confused with dark or black colored stools due to iron supplementation, dark chocolate, bismuth, spinach, cranberries, blueberries, grapes, or licorice. In these cases, confirmation of the absence of blood with Gastroccult (vomitus) and Hematest or Hemoccult (stool) assays will allay parental anxiety and prevent unnecessary concern and workup. Gastroccult is a specific and sensitive assay, stable in an acid environment, that can detect as little as 300 mg/dL of hemoglobin. Other causes of presumed GI bleeding, such as recent epistaxis, dental work, and sore throat, should be carefully sought.

In most cases of upper and lower GI bleeding, the source of the bleeding is inflamed mucosa (infectious, allergic, drug induced, stress related, or idiopathic). The emergency physician needs to differentiate inflammatory conditions that are frequently self-limited from causes that may require emergent surgical or endoscopic intervention such as ischemic bowel (intussusception, volvulus), structural abnormalities (Meckel's diverticulum, angiodysplasia), and portal hypertension (esophageal varices).

Initial Assessment

The differential diagnosis of GI bleeding is broad. A systematic approach to all patients includes:

1. Assessment of the severity of the bleeding and institution of appropriate resuscitative measures.

2. Establishing the level of bleeding within the GI tract.
3. Pertinent history, physical examination, and laboratory tests based on knowledge of age-related etiologies.
4. Emergency treatment based on general categories of causes.

Estimation of blood loss (a few drops, a spoonful, a cupful, or more) should be obtained initially. Vomiting of coffee grounds material does not necessarily signify a specific quantity of blood, nor does the vomiting of bright red blood mean that major bleeding is taking place. Hemoglobin and hematocrit are unreliable estimates of acute blood loss because of the time required for hemodilution to occur. The estimated volume of blood loss should be correlated with the patient's clinical status. The presence of resting tachycardia, pallor, prolonged capillary refill time, and metabolic acidosis point to significant blood loss. An orthostatic decrease in systolic blood pressure of 10 mm Hg or more or an increase of 20 beats per minute in pulse suggests a 10% to 20% loss of intravascular volume. Hypotension is a late finding in young children and demands immediate resuscitative measures.

Establishing the Level of Bleeding

There are two general categories of GI bleeding: upper and lower. Upper GI bleeding refers to bleeding proximal to the ligament of Treitz, and lower GI bleeding is distal to the ligament. In most cases, the clinical findings, along with gastric lavage, delineate the site of bleeding within the GI tract. *Hematemesis* is defined as vomiting of blood that is either fresh and bright red or old with the appearance of coffee grounds. *Melena*, the passage of stool that is shiny, black, and sticky as a result of enzymatic or bacterial action on intraluminal blood, reflects bleeding from either the upper GI tract or the proximal small bowel. In general, the darker the blood in the stool, the higher it originates in the GI tract. *Hematochezia*, or the passage of bright red blood per rectum, is usually a manifestation of lower GI bleeding. Currant jelly-like stools indicate vascular congestion and hyperemia as seen with intussuception. Maroon colored stools occur with a large bleed anywhere proximal to the rectosigmoid area, such as seen with a Meckel's diverticulum.

All patients with a significant episode of bleeding should have a nasogastric tube placed for diagnostic purposes. In patients with hematemesis or melena, a nasogastric aspirate positive for blood confirms an upper source of GI bleeding, whereas a negative examination almost always excludes an active upper GI bleed. Occasionally, a postpyloric upper GI lesion, such as a duodenal ulcer, bleeds massively without reflux into the stomach, resulting in a negative gastric aspirate. An upper GI endoscopic study is the best method to detect such a lesion. Patients with hematochezia and massive rectal bleeding should likewise have a nasogastric tube placed. Because blood exerts a cathartic action, brisk bleeding from an upper GI lesion may induce rapid transit through the gut, thus preventing blood from becoming melanotic. In patients with hematochezia manifested as bloody diarrhea or minimally blood streak stools, a lower GI source should be investigated.

Upper Gastrointestinal Bleeding

Differential Diagnosis

As seen in **Table 89.1**, there is considerable overlap between age groups and etiologies of upper GI bleeding. Mucosal lesions, including esophagitis, gastritis, stress ulcers, peptic ulceration, and Mallory-Weiss tears, are the most common sources of GI bleeding in all age groups. Ninety-five percent of all cases of upper GI bleeding in children are related to mucosal lesions and esophageal varices.

Hematemesis in a healthy newborn is most likely due to swallowed maternal blood either at delivery or from breast-feeding (i.e., from cracked nipples). The Apt test can differentiate neonatal from maternal hemoglobin based on the conversion of oxyhemoglobin to hematin when mixed with alkali. To perform the Apt test, mix one part bloody stool or vomitus with five parts water, centrifuge at 2,000 rpm for 2 minutes, and mix the supernatant with 1 mL of 0.1 N sodium hydroxide. Fetal hemoglobin is more resistant to denaturing than adult hemoglobin and remains pink, while maternal hemoglobin becomes brown.

Hemorrhagic disease of the newborn, while rare, should be considered with prolongation of the prothrombin time, if vitamin K has not been administered.

Significant and sometimes massive upper GI hemorrhage in a newborn infant may occur with no demonstrative anatomic lesion or only "hemorrhagic gastritis" at endoscopy. This is usually a single, self-limited event that is benign if treated with appropriate blood replacement and supportive measures.

Critically ill children of any age are at risk for developing stress-related peptic ulcer disease. Such ulcers occur with life-threatening illnesses, including shock, respiratory failure, hypoglycemia, dehydration, burns (Curling ulcer), intracranial lesions or trauma (Cushing ulcer), renal failure, and vasculitis. These ulcers may develop within minutes to hours after the initial insult and are primarily due to ischemia. Hematemesis, melena, and perforation of a viscus may accompany stress-associated ulcers. Hematemesis secondary to gastroesophageal reflux and esophagitis is uncommon but should be considered in patients who are severely symptomatic with vomiting or aspiration. Hematemesis following the acute onset of vigorous vomiting or retching at any age suggests a Mallory-Weiss tear.

Idiopathic peptic ulcer disease is a common cause of GI bleeding in preschool and older children. Complications including obstruction and perforation may occur. Younger children have less characteristic symptoms than teenagers, as they frequently localize abdominal pain poorly and may have vomiting as a predominant symptom. Older children and adolescents describe epigastric pain in a pattern typical of adults. At least 40% of children with peptic ulcers have a positive family history of duodenal ulcer disease, usually in the father. *Helicobacter pylori* has emerged as a leading cause of secondary gastritis, particularly in older children. Similar to adults, pediatric patients with evidence of *H. pylori* infection are often treated with antibiotics, bismuth preparations, and H_2-antagonists or omeprazole (Prilosec).

In older children, the possibility of bleeding esophageal varices must be considered in the differential diagnosis of upper GI bleeding. Though variceal bleeding is rare in in-

---

Table 89.1

Etiology of Upper Gastrointestinal Bleeding Based on Age

Neonatal (<4 Weeks)	Infancy (<2 Years)	Preschool (2–5 Years)	School Age
Swallow maternal blood	Gastritis	Epistaxis	Gastritis
Hemorrhagic gastritis	Esophagitis	Gastritis	Mallory-Weiss tear
Stress ulcer	Stress uncer	Stress ulcer	Stress ulcer
Idiopathic	Mallory Weiss tear	Mallory Weiss tear	Peptic ulcer
Bleeding diathesis	Pyloric stenosis	Toxic ingestion	Toxic ingestion
Esophagitis	Vascular malformation	Esophagitis	Esophagitis
Duplication	Toxic ingestion	Foreign body	IBD
Vascular malformation	Duplication	Vascular malformation	Esophageal varices
		Esophageal varices	Vascular malformation
		Hemobilia	Hemobilia

fancy, esophageal and gastric varices associated with portal hypertension are the most common cause of severe upper GI hemorrhage in older children. One-half to two-thirds of these children have an extrahepatic presinusoidal obstruction, often due to portal vein thrombosis, as the cause of portal hypertension. Omphalitis with or without a history of umbilical vein cannulation, dehydration, and a number of other factors may contribute. Other children with portal hypertension have hepatic parenchymal disorders such as neonatal hepatitis, congenital hepatic fibrosis, cystic fibrosis, or biliary cirrhosis associated with biliary atresia. Two-thirds of patients with portal hypertension develop bleeding before 5 years of age, and 85% do so by 10 years of age.

Diagnosis

Pertinent historical elements to be sought include a history of umbilical catheterization or sepsis in the neonatal period, previous episodes of bleeding from the GI tract or other sites as well as past hematological disorders and liver disease. A family history of peptic ulcer disease can be found in up to 30% of patients with idiopathic peptic ulcer disease. Ingestions should be sought as a possible etiology. These include theophylline, aspirin, iron, nonsteroidal anti-inflammatory drugs (NSAIDs), alcohol, and steroids. Massive hemorrhage associated with right upper quadrant pain and jaundice in the posttrauma patient indicates bleeding into the biliary tract or hemobilia.

The physical examination should include visualization of the nares and pharynx to eliminate epistaxis as a source of bleeding. Signs of liver disease or portal hypertension may be subtle in a child. Icterus, abdominal distention, prominent abdominal venous pattern, hepatosplenomegaly, cutaneous spider nevi, or ascites suggest liver disease and/or portal hypertension with esophageal varices.

Laboratory tests are not useful for identifying a precise cause of upper GI bleeding. Mucosal lesions are more likely than esophageal varices to be associated with prior occult bleeding. A low mean corpuscular volume (MCV) and hypochromic microcytic anemia are suggestive of chronic mucosal bleeding. Initial low white blood cell and platelet counts may be seen in either hypersplenism from portal hypertension or sepsis with associated stress mucosal ulceration. Abnormal liver studies, including an elevation of serum bilirubin, transaminase, and prothrombin time, and a low serum albumin are suggestive of esophageal varices as an etiology of bleeding. A BUN/creatinine ratio greater than 30 may indicate blood resorption and an upper GI source of bleeding.

Once it has been determined that a significant upper GI bleed has occurred and hemodynamic stability is restored, identification of the specific disorder is the next step. If the bleeding is mild and self-limited or the gastric aspirate negative, a minor mucosal lesion is likely. Although mucosal lesions such as esophagitis, gastritis, or peptic ulcer disease can present with severe hemorrhage, most often bleeding from mucosal lesions is self-limiting and will respond to conservative medical management. In the patient with persistent or recurrent hemorrhage, emergent endoscopy may be necessary if the bleeding is considered to

be life-threatening (continued transfusion requirement, hemodynamic instability). In a small percentage of cases, where bleeding is too massive to make endoscopic visualization possible, angiography or radionuclide studies (technetium-sulfur colloid/Tc-labeled red blood cells) may be indicated.

From 80% to 85% of upper GI bleeding stops spontaneously, regardless of the source, prior to or early in the hospital course. In stable patients who have stopped bleeding, double contrast barium examination of the upper GI tract and/or endoscopy provide valuable and frequently complementary information. In this group of patients, endoscopy need not be performed on an emergent basis and may be performed electively in the first 12 to 24 hours after admission. Elective endoscopy should be performed in patients who stop bleeding spontaneously but who have required transfusion and/or have a history of previously unexplained upper GI bleeding episodes.

Lower Gastrointestinal Bleeding
Differential Diagnosis

Table 89.2 outlines the etiology of lower GI bleeding based on age.

Neonatal Period (0–1 Month) As is true for upper GI bleeding, a common cause of blood in the stool in well infants is the passage of maternal blood swallowed either at delivery or from a fissured maternal breast during feeding. While hemorrhagic disease of the newborn is uncommon after prophylactic administration of vitamin K at delivery, maternal drugs that cross the placenta, including aspirin, phenytoin, cephalothin, and phenobarbital, may interfere with clotting factors and cause hemorrhage. Infectious diarrhea can occur in very young infants and cause bloody, mucous stools. Common bacterial pathogens in this age group include *Campylobacter jejuni* and *Salmonella*.

In the ill-appearing infant with lower GI bleeding, midgut volvulus, necrotizing enterocolitis, and Hirschsprung's disease should be considered. Malrotation with midgut volvulus is most common during this period. Initially bilious vomiting, abdominal distention, and pain are present. Melena is present in 10% to 20% of cases and signifies vascular compromise. Ten percent of all cases of necrotizing enterocolitis occur in full-term infants. These patients can present with nonspecific signs of sepsis (temperature instability or apnea and bradycardia) as well as with specific GI tract findings, such as abdominal distention, pain, and abdominal wall erythema. GI bleeding can occur in the form of guaiac-positive or grossly bloody stools. Hirschsprung's disease with enterocolitis may present with GI bleeding in the newborn period. Enterocolitis has recently been shown to occur in up to 25% of children with Hirschsprung's disease. The risk of enterocolitis remains high until about 6 months of age. The diagnosis should be considered in any newborn who does not pass meconium in the first 24 to 48 hours of life.

Infancy (1 Month to 2 Years) In the first 2 years of life, anal fissures are the most common cause of rectal bleeding and are usually associated with hard stools or

Table 89.2

Etiologies of Lower Gastrointestinal Bleeding

Neonatal (<4 Weeks)	Infancy (<2 Years)	Preschool (2–5 Years)	School Age
Well infant	Anal fissure	Anal fissure	Infectious colitis
Swallowed maternal blood	Infectious colitis	Infectious colitis	Polyps
Infectious colitis	Milk allergy	Juvenile polyps	IBD
Milk allergy	Nonspecific colitis	Intussusception	Hemmorrhoids
Hemorrhagic disease	Juvenile polyps	HSP	Meckel's diverticulum
Duplication of bowel	Intussusception	Meckel's diverticulum	HUS
Meckel's diverticulum	Meckel's diverticulum	HUS	Pseudomemabaranous colitis
Sick infant	Duplication	IBD	Ischemic colitis
Infectious colitis	HUS	Peptic ulcer	Peptic ulcer
Midgut volvulus	IBD	Pseudomembranous enterocolitis	Angiodysplasia
Hirschprung's disease	Pseudomembranous enterocolitis	Ischemic colitis	
DIC		Angiodysplasia	
Necrotizing enterocolitis	Ischemic colitis		
Intussusception	Lymphonodular hyperplasia		
Congestive heart failure			

constipation. Treatment with stool softeners and sitz baths often resolves the problem rapidly. Milk or soy enterocolitis usually presents during the first month of life or shortly thereafter. These infants can present with chronic diarrhea, stools containing blood or mucus, or fulminant colitis and shock. Milk-protein allergy responds to a change in formula from cow milk or soy protein to a casein hydrolysate (Nutramigen, Alimentum, Pregestimil). Breast-fed infants whose mothers drink cow milk may develop an allergic colitis that responds to removal of cow milk from the mother's diet. Infectious enterocolitis as a cause of bloody diarrhea is common in all age groups. Bacterial etiologies (*Salmonella, Shigella, Campylobacter,* pathogenic *Escherichia coli,* and *Yersinia enterocolitica*) should be identified with stool cultures. In symptomatic infants and children, the presence of leukocytes in a stool smear for white cells may aid in preliminary diagnosis. Pseudomembranous colitis should be considered in any infant or child with bloody stools and a history of recent antibiotic therapy. "Nonspecific colitis" has recently been demonstrated to be a frequent cause of hematochezia in infants younger than 6 months of age. While the cause of nonspecific colitis is unknown, it may represent a variation in the colonic response to viral invasion.

Meckel's diverticulum should be suspected in an infant or young child who passes bright or dark red blood per rectum. Intermittent painless bleeding or massive GI hemorrhage can occur. Sixty percent of complications from Meckel's diverticulum (hemorrhage and intestinal obstruction) occur in patients younger than 2 years of age.

Idiopathic intussusception may occur in children at any age, with 80% occurring before 2 years of age. In patients older than 3 years, a lead point (polyp, Meckel's diverticulum, or hypertrophied lymphoid patch) is often found. Paroxysmal pain may be associated with guaiac-positive stools or hematochezia. Lethargy alone (without pain) has been increasingly recognized as a presenting symptom of

intussusception in young children. Lymphonodular hyperplasia is a common cause of rectal bleeding in this age group and may cause mild, painless hematochezia. The nodular lymphoid response is self-limited and does not require any specific therapy. Intestinal duplications are an uncommon cause of lower GI bleeding, and when diagnosed are usually found in children younger than 2 years of age. Duplications can be found anywhere in the GI tract but are most common in the distal ileum. These usually present with obstruction and lower GI bleeding.

Preschool (2 to 5 Years) The two conditions most likely to cause bleeding in this age group are juvenile polyps and infectious enterocolitis. Most polyps in childhood are inflammatory without significant malignant potential and are frequently multiple; 30% to 40% are palpable on rectal examination. Polyps may cause painless rectal bleeding in this age group. Significant bleeding is unusual. Infectious etiologies of colitis are similar to those discussed in younger age groups. Hematochezia is often a manifestation of systemic disease in infancy and throughout childhood. Hemolytic uremic syndrome is the most prevalent of these conditions reported in infants and children up to 3 years of age. Bloody diarrhea may precede the development of renal and hematological abnormalities. GI manifestations of Henoch-Schönlein purpura (HSP) occur in 50% of cases and include colicky abdominal pain, melena, and bloody diarrhea. These symptoms precede the characteristic rash in 20% of cases. GI complications of HSP include hemorrhage (5%), intussusception (3%), and, rarely, intestinal perforation.

Angiodysplasia is a rare cause of GI bleeding, but can be associated with massive hemorrhage. Vascular lesions of the GI tract probably have a congenital basis. Several recognized syndromes, including Rendu-Osler-Weber syndrome, blue rubber bleb syndrome, and Turner's syndrome, may be associated with intestinal telangiectasia.

School Age (5 Years Through Adolescence) For the most part, the diagnostic considerations relevant to the preschool child apply to school-age and adolescent children with the addition of inflammatory bowel disease. Although inflammatory bowel disease occurs in younger children, it is rare before the age of 10. Rectal bleeding is a common presentation of both ulcerative colitis and Crohn's disease. Massive lower GI bleeding occurs in 2% to 5% of children with Crohn's disease. Toxic megacolon is a life-threatening presentation of both ulcerative colitis and Crohn's disease.

Diagnosis

Symptoms of an acute abdominal process, including abdominal pain, distention, and vomiting, should be elicited. A history of bloody diarrhea may indicate infectious colitis, intussusception, or hemolytic-uremic syndrome. Extraintestinal manifestations of inflammatory bowel disease, including weight loss, anorexia, and arthralgias, may be the predominant symptoms in school-aged children. The dietary history may suggest features of a protein intolerance (cow's milk). Firm stool streaked with red blood characterizes anal fissures. A detailed family history (bleeding diathesis, familial polyposis) as well as drug history (NSAIDs, salicylates, iron) or antibiotics (pseudomembranous colitis) is important in patients with lower GI bleeding. Long-standing constipation with acute onset of bloody diarrhea is suggestive of enterocolitis associated with Hirschsprung's disease.

Physical examination to detect abdominal obstruction (abdominal tenderness, distention, palpable mass, peritoneal signs, hyperactive bowel sounds) is the most urgent task for the evaluating physician. Careful separation of the buttocks with eversion of the anal mucosa may reveal a fissure. Prominent or multiple perianal skin tags may raise suspicion of Crohn's disease. Rectal polyps may be palpable. Cutaneous lesions may provide important diagnostic clues in patients with GI bleeding. Eczema may be associated with milk allergy, while erythema nodosum is the most common skin manifestation of inflammatory bowel disease. Mucocutaneous pigmentation (Peutz-Jeghers syndrome) and cutaneous or subcutaneous tumors (Gardner's syndrome) indicate intestinal polyposis.

The urgency and extent of evaluation of patients with lower GI bleeding depend on the amount of bleeding, the patient's age, and associated physical findings. In a healthy infant with a few streaks of blood in the stool and a normal examination, stool culture and observation are reasonable. If hematochezia is found and nasogastric aspirate is negative, significant pathology must be sought. Flat and upright abdominal radiographs should be performed if an obstructive process (i.e., intussusception, volvulus) is suspected by history or physical examination. The absence of findings on radiological examination should not, however, deter the physician from pursuing further diagnostic evaluation. A barium or air enema examination is diagnostic and frequently therapeutic in children with intussusception. If obstruction is not considered likely, the decision to perform contrast enema examination or colonoscopy depends on the diagnosis suspected. Air contrast barium enema is ex-tremely valuable in the detection of polyps or inflammatory bowel disease. Indications for colonoscopy include severe bleeding, moderate but persistent bleeding with a negative double-contrast barium enema, and a lesion of unknown nature seen on barium enema. If undefined bleeding persists, radionuclide studies or angiography should be considered. A technetium scan may detect ectopic gastric mucosa as seen in Meckel's diverticulum, while angiography helps to identify bleeding vascular malformations in the GI tract. Ongoing, undiagnosed GI hemorrhage accounts for fewer than 10% of cases in infants and children. Exploratory laparotomy may be necessary and lifesaving in these circumstances.

Conclusion

Management of acute GI bleeding frequently requires a team approach including the emergency physician, surgeon, and gastroenterologist. The foremost goals of ED evaluation of the patient with GI bleeding are establishment of hemodynamic stability and determination of level of bleeding. All patients with nontrivial upper GI bleeding should be admitted for observation and further evaluation. If an acute abdominal process is suspected, surgical consultation and diagnostic workup should be instituted. If rectal bleeding is mild and self-limited, and the history and physical are unremarkable, further investigation with a gastroenterologist is recommended.

Pyloric Stenosis

Pyloric stenosis is one of the most common conditions requiring surgical intervention in infants, second only to inguinal hernias. The incidence ranges from 1 to 3 per 1,000 live births but is markedly lower in certain populations. There is a 4:1 male preponderance, and the presentation occurs between prior to 10 weeks of age, most commonly in the fourth week of life. The risks associated with pyloric stenosis relate to the development of dehydration, electrolyte abnormalities, and surgical intervention.

Pathophysiology

The etiology of pyloric stenosis has been researched extensively but remains elusive. A genetic predisposition does exist. There is a significantly increased incidence of pyloric stenosis in the offspring of affected parents: up to 20% in male infants born to affected mothers. Several studies have demonstrated an increased incidence in first-born children, especially males. In addition, Caucasian infants have a significantly higher incidence of pyloric stenosis when compared to Hispanic, African-American, and Asian children.

Environmental factors that have been explored include birth weight, maternal and neonatal antibiotic use, maternal tobacco use, and feeding patterns. There are limited data to support birth weight as an independent risk factor, although studies that have explored tobacco use—a recognized cause of intrauterine growth retardation—have found up to a twofold increased risk associated with maternal smoking. Several authors have described an increased incidence of pyloric stenosis in children treated with oral erythromycin for pertussis prophylaxis. One study reported an eightfold increase risk for infants treated in the first two weeks of life. Limited data exist to support the role of breastfeeding as a protective factor for the development of pyloric stenosis, although large population studies have shown a tendency for reduced incidence in infants nursed during the first week of life.

Although its cause remains unclear, the gross and microscopic pathology, and the physiological consequences of pyloric stenosis are well appreciated. The pylorus appears uniformly hypertrophied to an average size of 1.5 by 3 cm, with a firm, rubbery consistency. In long-standing cases, the stomach is dilated and the antrum hypertrophied. The circular muscle layer is both hypertrophied and hyperplastic, and can be up to four times thicker than normal.

As a result of the high level of gastric outlet obstruction that develops with pyloric stenosis, a hypochloremic hypokalemic metabolic alkalosis may develop due to the loss of hydrogen, sodium, and chloride ions, with a net gain of bicarbonate. The resultant depletion and alkalemia prompt the kidneys to conserve sodium and excrete bicarbonate. As gastric losses continue, severe chloride depletion occurs, directly limiting renal efforts to handle both sodium and bicarbonate at the tubular level. The kidneys must then excrete hydrogen ion in their efforts to conserve sodium. A systemic alkalosis and paradoxical aciduria develop. As a result, infants with advanced cases of pyloric stenosis may have significant electrolyte abnormalities ($Na^+ < 130$, $Cl^- < 85$, $HCO_3^- > 30$ mEq/L).

Evaluation

The causes of nonbilious vomiting during infancy are extensive and include both intra- and extra-intestinal etiologies (**Table 89.3**). The history and physical examination should address these alternative diagnoses in cases where the presentation is atypical.

Projectile, nonbilious vomiting in a young infant is the cardinal symptom of pyloric stenosis. Symptoms often first appear during the third week of life, although onset of symptoms as early as one week and as late as four months have been described. Vomiting typically begins as mild regurgitation 30 to 60 minutes after feeding, with progression to projectile vomiting within the first day. Prior to the development of dehydration and electrolyte abnormalities, the infant appears well and exhibits signs of postemesis hunger, such as increased fussiness and aggressive feeding. Hematemesis or coffee-ground emesis may ensue secondary to esophagitis and/or gastritis.

Other symptoms useful in differentiating pyloric stenosis from other causes of nonbilious vomiting include a history of constipation, poor weight gain, irritability, and decreased urine output. Any historical features concerning for dehydration should be addressed by a brief physical assessment and aggressive fluid management.

The physical examination should begin with an assessment of hydration status. A sunken fontanel, absent tearing, dry mucous membranes, and decreased skin turgor may point to significant dehydration. Irritability may reflect both hunger and dehydration. Jaundice may be present, reflective of a poorly understood indirect hyperbilirubinemia associated with pyloric stenosis and several other abnormalities that cause proximal bowel obstruction. The abdominal examination may reveal distention and hypoactive bowel sounds. With feeding, visible waves of peristalsis may occur in the epigastrium. The pathognomonic feature of pyloric stenosis is a palpable "olive"—representing the hypertrophied pylorus muscle—located in the epigastrium; however, this finding is present in a variable number (50%–90%) of cases.

Laboratory evaluation is often of limited use and is primarily a tool for assessment of hydration status and a means for ruling out alternative diagnoses. A complete blood count may reveal an elevated hemoglobin level if there is significant dehydration. Electrolytes may reveal a hypochloremic metabolic alkalosis in up to 50% of patients. Potassium levels may be elevated or decreased. A small percentage of infants will have a direct hyperbilirubinemia. Urinalysis may be obtained to assess the degree of dehydration and to rule out urinary tract infection.

The role of plain radiography in the diagnosis of pyloric stenosis has minimal utility. Supine and upright views of the abdomen will most often appear normal. Abnormal findings may include a dilated gastric bubble or a paucity of air in the small and large bowel.

Patients with suspected pyloric stenosis based on history or physical examination should undergo ultrasonographic evaluation. Ultrasound has the benefit of being quick, noninvasive, and safe. Studies have demonstrated high degrees of sensitivity and specificity (97% and 100%, respectively). The hypertrophied pylorus is visualized as a "doughnut" or "bull's eye" on transverse image. The criteria used for the diagnosis include: muscle thickness ≥ 3 mm, pyloric diameter ≥ 15 mm, and a pyloric length > 18 mm. Failure to demonstrate the typical findings by ultrasound should

Table 89.3
Differential Diagnosis for Vomiting in Infancy

Intestinal	Extra-Intestinal
Overfeeding	Pneumonia
Formula intolerance	Urinary tract infection
Gastroesophageal reflux	Sepsis
Gastroenteritis	Meningitis
Gastric or duodenal stenosis	Intracranial hypertension
Gastric or duodenal webs	Drug withdrawal
Duodenal atresia (within 1st week of life)	Adrenal insufficiency
Duodenal hematoma (due to trauma)	Inborn errors of metabolism
Midgut volvulus (early finding)	
Intussusception (early finding)	
Incarcerated inguinal hernia	
Appendicitis	

prompt an immediate upper-gastrointestinal series in suspected cases. Visualization of delayed gastric emptying and an elongated pyloric channel confirms the diagnosis.

Management

Emergency department management of a child with suspected pyloric stenosis includes prompt recognition and treatment of hydration and electrolyte abnormalities. An intravenous line should be placed. In cases where volume depletion is significant, central or intraosseous access should be sought, or a cutdown should be performed if peripheral sites are lacking. Fluid, sodium, chloride, and potassium deficits should be estimated using standard formulas, and appropriate replacement should be given.

Generally, an initial bolus of 20 mL/kg of normal saline or lactated Ringer's can be administered. Subsequent fluids should contain glucose. Chloride replacement is central to correction of an otherwise self-perpetuating metabolic alkalosis. In most cases, dextrose 5% in 0.45% normal saline or 0.23% normal saline can be administered after the initial bolus. The rate of maintenance fluids should be determined by a weight-based calculation.

Pediatric surgical consultation should be obtained as soon as the diagnosis is suspected. Once the diagnosis is confirmed, admission to the hospital for fluid and electrolyte replacement should occur; emergent surgical correction of pyloric stenosis is not necessary.

Since the first surgery performed by Ramstedt in 1917, the definitive treatment of pyloric stenosis has been pyloromyotomy. When performed under careful general anesthesia following correction of any fluid and electrolyte abnormalities, the procedure carries a mortality rate between 0.1 and 0.3%. Complications associated with surgical correction include wound infection, mucosal perforation, postoperative vomiting, and delayed oral feeding. Most infants resume feeding within 4 to 6 hours after operation and return home in 2 to 3 days.

Gastroenteritis and Dehydration

Gastroenteritis

Acute gastroenteritis in children is the leading cause of morbidity and mortality worldwide. In 2002, an estimated 1.5 to 2.5 million children under the age of 5 years died as a result of dehydration secondary to acute gastroenteritis. In the United States, the mortality associated with acute diarrheal illnesses is much less, accounting for only 300 deaths each year. Nevertheless, gastroenteritis results in significant morbidity and economic costs, resulting in 1.5 million outpatient visits, 200,000 hospitalizations, and one billion in total costs annually in the United States.

The organisms that commonly cause gastroenteritis in children are listed in **Table 89.4**. Viruses account for the majority of causative agents in infectious diarrhea. The organisms frequently isolated include rotavirus, Norwalk virus, enteric adenovirus, and astrovirus. The most common causes of bacterial gastroenteritis include *Salmonella*, *Shigella*, *Campylobacter*, *Yersinia*, and *E. coli*. Parasitic are more common in developing countries. *Giardia* and *Cryptosporidium* should be suspected in patients who attend day care centers. *Cryptosporidium* can cause protracted diarrhea in the immunocompromised patient.

Viral Pathogens

Rotavirus is the most common cause of severe diarrhea in young children in both developed and developing countries. Rotaviral infections affect patients between 3 and 15 months of age and by 24 months 90% of children have acquired serum antibody. The incidence of rotavirus diar-

Table 89.4
Common Causes of Acute Gastroenteritis

Bacterial	Viral	Parasitic
Enterotoxigenic	Adenovirus	*Blastocystis hominis*
Bacillus cereus	Astrovirus	*Cryptosporidium parvum*
Clostridium difficile	Calicivirus	*Cyclospora cayetanensis*
Clostridium perfringens	Coronavirus	*Entamoeba histolytica*
Escherichia coli	Norwalk virus	*Giardia lamblia*
Staphylococcus aureus	Rotavirus	*Isospora belli*
Vibrio cholerae		
Enteroinvasive		
Campylobacter jejuni		
Escherichia coli		
Salmonella sp.		
Shigella sp.		
Yersinia enterocolitica		
Other		
Aeromonas hydrophila		
Vibrio parahaemolyticus		

rhea peaks sharply in the winter. The primary mode of transmission is via the fecal-oral route although transmission via the respiratory route has been postulated. The incubation period is usually 1 to 3 days; diarrhea typically lasts 5 to 7 days. Rotavirus invades the villus epithelium causing abnormally low levels of disaccharidases, resulting in carbohydrate malabsorption and osmotic diarrhea. Rotavirus is shed in the stool prior to the onset of symptoms and resolves by the fifth to seventh day of the disease. Children who have been infected previously may experience asymptomatic infection with fecal viral excretion. Malnourished or immunocompromised patients may develop protracted diarrhea. Chronic diarrhea has also been reported in healthy infants.

The Norwalk virus produces an illness characterized predominantly by vomiting and affects school-aged children and adults. In contrast to rotavirus, which occurs endemically, Norwalk virus causes large epidemics. Transmission is by the fecal-oral route or by consumption of contaminated food or water. The incubation period is 1 to 2 days and the duration of disease is usually less than 2 days.

Enteric adenoviruses are the second most common organism isolated from children requiring hospitalization for viral gastroenteritis. Enteric adenovirus disease occurs endemically throughout the year, affects primarily children under 2 years of age. The incubation period (8 to 10 days) and duration of illness (5 to 12 days) are longer than those associated with other enteric viruses.

Other viral agents shown to cause gastroenteritis include astrovirus, calicivirus, and parvovirus. Viral enteropathogens have a common clinical presentation. They all produce watery diarrhea that is often accompanied by vomiting and fever. Blood and leukocytes are usually absent from the stool.

Bacterial Pathogens

Bacterial gastroenteritis can be classified according to pathogenesis. Enteroinvasive bacteria produce illness following invasion and inflammation of the intestinal mucosa. Enterotoxigenic pathogens cause disease by elaborating toxins. The symptoms and signs associated with each of these mechanisms is helpful in identifying the causative agent and appropriate treatment.

Salmonella is the most common cause of bacterial diarrhea in children. Infection rate is highest in infants younger than 6 months of age. Infection typically requires a large inoculum; 10^5 virulent organisms are necessary to induce disease in 30% of healthy adults. Person-to-person transmission is rare, and salmonellosis results from ingestion of contaminated meat, dairy, or poultry products. Iguanas and turtles are also common carriers of the organism.

Salmonella invades the distal ileum, and infection is generally limited to the gastrointestinal tract. However, the organism may enter the circulation and result in disseminated infections such as meningitis, osteomyelitis, and endocarditis. Patients with sickle cell hemoglobinopathies, reticuloendothelial dysfunction, and AIDS are prone to developing these life-threatening complications.

The clinical syndrome associated with *Salmonella* infection includes a short incubation period (24 to 36

hours) and a brief illness (2 to 3 days) characterized by abdominal cramps, fever, vomiting, and diarrhea. Stools are watery and may contain blood.

Enteric fever may be caused by several serotypes of *Salmonella*, particularly *S. typhi*. This causes fever, chills, constipation, abdominal pain, and lack of tachycardia relative to the height of the fever. Diarrhea, splenomegaly, and a macular rash (rose spots) may develop during the second week. The most prominent complications are intestinal hemorrhage, perforation, hepatitis, cholecystitis, and myocarditis. The frequency of these has been reduced with effective therapy. Asymptomatic chronic excretion occurs in 4% of patients with enteric fever and less than 1% of patients with nontyphoidal infection.

Shigella is the second most commonly isolated bacterial pathogen in children 6 months to 10 years. *Shigella* rarely causes infection in infants younger than 6 months of age, possibly because of the developmental absence of receptors for Shiga toxin. Unlike *Salmonella*, infection requires a small inoculum; 10 to 100 virulent *Shigella* can cause disease. The organism is transmitted easily from person to person via the fecal-oral route and is more common in crowded living conditions with poor sanitation. *S. sonnei* and *S. flexneri* account for most of the infections encountered in the United States. *S. dysenteriae* frequently causes epidemics in the developing world.

Shigella may cause asymptomatic infection, mild diarrhea, or bacillary dysentery. The incubation period is usually 2 days. Mild illness occurs in a significant proportion of infected individuals. These patients exhibit watery diarrhea without associated symptoms. *Shigella* also produces an exotoxin, Shiga toxin, which has cytotoxic, neurotoxic, and enterotoxic properties. Bacillary dysentery frequently begins with abdominal pain followed by fever and diarrhea. Stools are greenish in color and contain blood and mucus. Microscopic examination of the stool reveals sheets of leukocytes.

Shigellosis is usually a self-limited disease; most patients recover within a week. Complications include dehydration, seizures, perforation of the colon, and hemolytic uremic syndrome. *Shigella* rarely causes bacteremia and is not more common in immunocompromised hosts.

Campylobacter species are an important cause of gastroenteritis in the first year of life and in young adult years. Although *C. jejuni* is the most common species, *C. coli*, *C. laridis*, and *C. hyointestinalis* can also cause illness. The organism is transmitted primarily via the fecal-oral route. Outbreaks have been associated with ingestion of undercooked poultry or meat and unpasteurized dairy products. Approximately 10^4 organisms are required for clinical infection. After an incubation period of 1 to 7 days, the patient develops fever, headache, and myalgias. These symptoms are followed by an acute inflammatory enterocolitis with crampy abdominal pain and diarrhea. Stools may be watery or mucous, and blood is often present. *Campylobacter* can replicate in Peyer's patches, causing a mesenteric lymphadenitis. The inflammation leads to severe abdominal pain that mimics appendicitis.

Campylobacter gastroenteritis is a self-limited illness. However, diarrhea may persist for more than 1 week.

Children may shed the organism for up to 3 weeks. Prolonged carriage is uncommon. Complications include dehydration, toxic megacolon, and colonic hemorrhage.

Yersinia enterocolitica is seen primarily in developed, cool climate countries, particularly in Canada, northern Europe, and Japan. Transmission has been traced to contact with infected domestic animals or ingestion of contaminated food, milk, or water. After invading the intestinal epithelium, bacteria may extend to the mesenteric lymph nodes or disseminate to the liver and spleen. Common features of yersiniosis include headache, fever, abdominal pain, and in some, pharyngitis. The stools are watery or mucoid and may contain blood. Older children and adolescents may develop mesenteric adenitis or an autoimmune arthritis. The diarrhea is usually self-limited. Occasionally it can be prolonged, lasting more than 30 days. The organism can be excreted in the stool for 3 months. A chronic carrier state has not been described. Complications include appendicitis, intestinal perforation, intussusception, and peritonitis. Infants younger than 3 months may develop bacteremia.

Escherichia coli strains have been divided into five groups: enteropathogenic (EPEC), enterotoxigenic (ETEC), enteroinvasive (EIEC), enteroaggregative, and enterohemorrhagic (EHEC). In the United States, disease is primarily associated with EHEC, especially the *E. coli* serotype O157:H7, which causes hemorrhagic colitis and has been associated with hemolytic uremic syndrome (HUS). Infection with EHEC occurs most commonly after ingestion of contaminated milk or beef. Person to person transmission also occurs. EHEC produces Shiga-like cytotoxins that may have a role in bacterial virulence. Stools are bloody but contain very few leukocytes. Patients who develop HUS present with bloody diarrhea, thrombocytopenia, hemolytic anemia, and acute renal failure.

Enterotoxigenic *E. coli* is the most common cause of traveler's diarrhea. However, food-borne outbreaks have been reported in the United States in patients without any travel history. Enteroaggregative *E. coli* has been identified frequently in patients with persistent diarrhea.

Vibrio cholera is the classic example of enterotoxin-induced gastrointestinal disease. Endemic and epidemic areas of cholera are found in Southern Asia and Africa. In the United States endemic regions are located in the coastal areas of Texas and Louisiana. Infection is related to consumption of seafood. After inoculation, *Vibrio cholera* attaches to mucosal cells and multiplies. The organism produces a heat-labile enterotoxin that stimulates cellular adenylate cyclase, which in turn alters salt and water transport. Patients present with high-volume watery diarrhea, vomiting, and crampy abdominal pain. The illness usually resolves within a week. Potential complications are dehydration, electrolyte abnormalities, and hypoglycemia.

Staphylococcus aureus is the most common cause of toxin-induced food poisoning in the United States. The organism grows to high concentrations in inadequately refrigerated food such as potato salad, pastries, and ham. The heat-stable enterotoxin is ingested directly in contaminated food. A short incubation period of 1 to 6 hours is followed by vomiting, abdominal pain, and watery diarrhea. Symptoms resolve within 12 hours. Other bacterial toxin-related food poisonings include caused by *Bacillus cereus* and *Clostridium perfringens*.

Clostridium difficile is a major cause of iatrogenic diarrhea in patients who have been treated with antibiotics and spreads easily among hospitalized patients. Almost all antibiotics have been associated with *C. difficile* diarrhea. Cephalosporins and amoxicillin account for most cases, probably due to their widespread use in children. *C. difficile* produces two major toxins that cause mucosal inflammation, hemorrhage, and necrosis. The organism frequently colonizes the intestine of newborn infants without evidence of disease. The clinical presentation of *C. difficile* ranges from asymptomatic carriage to classic pseudomembranous colitis (PMC). PMC affects only 10% of infected individuals. Patients complain of abdominal cramping, fever, and diarrhea. Stools are watery without gross blood. Microscopic examination of the stool reveals leukocytes and erythrocytes. Discontinuation of antibiotics often results in spontaneous resolution of symptoms.

Parasitic Pathogens

Giardia lamblia is the most common cause of parasitic diarrheal disease in the United States. Ingestion of as few as 10 cysts may lead to infection. *Giardia* is spread from person to person via the fecal-oral route or through contaminated community water supplies. Campers may become infected after consuming water from mountain wilderness streams. *Giardia* has also been associated with foreign travel and day care attendance. Overall, the highest prevalence of infection is in infants and toddlers. Predisposing conditions include chronic pancreatitis, cystic fibrosis, achlorhydria, and agammaglobulinemia.

Giardiasis develops insidiously over 5 to 10 days. The disease is characterized by crampy abdominal pain, and frequent loose, foul-smelling stools. Blood and leukocytes are unusual in stool. Some children may develop chronic malabsorption with steatorrhea and failure to thrive. Infestation with *Giardia* may lead to an asymptomatic carrier state.

Cryptosporidium parvum is an important cause of pediatric diarrhea. Like *Giardia*, the cysts are transmitted through contaminated water. *Cryptosporidium* is 14 times more resistant to chlorination than *Giardia;* water filtration is required to ensure adequate removal. Person-to-person transmission is well documented, especially in day care center outbreaks. *Cryptosporidium* may spread from animals to children by fecal contamination.

Cryptosporidiosis has an incubation period of 5 to 21 days. The disease is characterized by watery diarrhea without blood or leukocytes. Systemic symptoms include anorexia, weight loss, crampy abdominal pain, and low-grade fever. In immunocompetent patients, cryptosporidiosis resolves within 2 weeks. In immunocompromised hosts, diarrhea may be protracted and may be debilitating. These patients are also at risk for biliary tract disease and pulmonary or systemic dissemination.

Entamoeba histolytica is uncommon in the United States but is the most common parasitic diarrhea worldwide. It is transmitted from person to person as well as through contaminated water. Boiling is the only effective method to eliminate cysts in water. Amebiasis should be suspected in children from institutions, immigrants, or foreign travelers.

Clinical Evaluation

The presence, frequency, and quantity of vomiting and diarrhea are important historical factors. Urinary output and oral intake are important in determining the risk for dehydration. The appearance of the stool may provide a clue to etiology, as enteroinvasive bacterial pathogens often cause mucous and/or bloody stools. Associated symptoms such as abdominal pain and fever should also be documented. The underlying etiology may be determined by obtaining a careful epidemiologic history including medication history, attendance at day care facilities, foreign travel, ill contacts, exposure to animals, and ingestion of food or water from unusual sources. The occurrence of seizures may indicate infection with *Shigella* or an electrolyte imbalance.

The physical examination should begin with the general appearance of the child. Vital signs, including a current measured weight, are important in determining hydration status. In addition, dehydration may be manifest by dry mucous membranes, sunken fontanel, prolonged capillary refill, decreased skin turgor, and altered mental status. The abdominal exam should include an assessment of distention, focal tenderness, peritoneal signs, hepatosplenomegaly, and masses. A rectal examination is indicated if the abdomen is distended, peristalsis is absent, or masses are identified. A complete physical examination helps identify extraintestinal infections, such as otitis media, pneumonia, or meningitis.

Laboratory Studies

A fresh stool specimen helps to corroborate the history of diarrhea and document the presence of occult or gross blood. Microscopic examination of the stool can be a useful screening tool. The presence of white blood cells (over five leukocytes/high power field) on a fecal smear suggests infection with an inflammatory bacterial pathogen such as *Salmonella, Shigella, Campylobacter,* or *Yersinia.* Neutrophils may also be associated with pseudomembranous colitis due to *C. difficile.* Leukocytes are typically absent from the stool when gastroenteritis is caused by noninvasive organisms such as ETEC, *V. cholera,* parasites, or viruses.

A stool culture should be obtained in the following settings: (1) presence of mucus, blood, or leukocytes in stool; (2) signs of inflammatory disease such as prolonged fever, myalgias, or arthralgias; (3) prolonged or recurrent diarrhea; and (4) epidemiological conditions make bacterial or unusual organisms likely.

Viral studies rarely lead to changes in management but can be important from an epidemiological standpoint. Rotavirus and enteric adenovirus can be detected by enzyme immunoassay with commercially available kits. Diagnosis of Norwalk virus and other enteric viruses requires electron microscopy.

Studies for ova and parasites should be considered when there is a history of day care attendance, ingestion of improperly chlorinated water, or prolonged (more than 7 days) diarrhea. Three stool specimens should be collected on different days to exclude parasitic infection.

A leukocyte count and differential should be obtained in patients who appear acutely ill. Patients with shigellosis often show an increase in band forms. Blood cultures are indicated in febrile, ill-appearing infants with suspected bacterial disease. Serum electrolytes and blood urea nitrogen should be obtained in patients who appear clinically dehydrated.

Management

Major elements in the management of acute gastroenteritis include: fluid and electrolyte therapy; dietary intake; antiemetic and antidiarrheal medications; and antimicrobial agents.

Fluid and electrolyte replacement is the first step in the management of infectious diarrhea of any etiology. Most children with acute gastroenteritis can be treated as outpatients. Oral rehydration therapy (ORT) has been the most important advance in the treatment of diarrhea in developing countries and has reduced the mortality from gastroenteritis by approximately to 2.5 million deaths annually since 1990.

Dehydration should be treated with an oral rehydration solution (ORS) containing 45 to 60 mmol/L sodium, 20 mmol/L potassium, 20% to 30% of anions as base (acetate, citrate, lactate, or bicarbonate), and the remainder as chloride and glucose 2% to 2.5% (110 to 140 mmol/L). A similar solution with a reduced sodium concentration has been recommended for maintenance replacement following initial rehydration.

Patients with mild diarrhea without signs of dehydration do not require specific therapy. Breast milk or standard formula should be offered. Supplementation with a maintenance oral electrolyte solution should prevent significant complications from ongoing fluid losses.

Children with mild to moderate dehydration should receive 50 mL/kg and 100 mL/kg, respectively, of ORS plus replacement of losses over a 4-hour period. Once rehydration has been completed, maintenance oral solution may be given.

Children who are vomiting generally respond to a brief cessation of oral intake. After 2 to 4 hours of fasting, ORS should be given in small volumes of 5 to 10 mL every 5 to 15 minutes. Volumes are gradually increased until the child can drink normally. ORS can also be administered as a continuous drip via nasogastric tube, and a recent study found nasogastric rehydration to be as effective as intravenous rehydration, with greater cost savings.

Oral rehydration therapy can be limited by the presence of severe dehydration, glucose intolerance, persistent vomiting, or high stool output. Intravenous fluid and hospitalization should be considered for the patient who is moderately dehydrated and is indicated for the child who is severely dehydrated with greater than 10% body weight loss.

Severe dehydration (10% to 12% of body weight loss) should be corrected with 20 to 60 cc/kg of isotonic fluid given as 20 cc/kg boluses until signs of hypoperfusion improve. The length of time for compete replacement and type of fluid used should be guided by the patient's acid-base status and electrolyte abnormalities.

Dietary therapy for children with acute gastroenteritis should consist of a gradual return to a usual diet. Infants receiving breast milk should be permitted to continue nursing during the acute illness. Infants receiving formula and cow's milk may resume their usual dietary intake once rehydration has occurred. Recent studies have demonstrated no advantage to most infants and small children receiving a lactose-reduced diet compared with lactose-containing products. Older children receiving semisolid and solid foods may continue their usual diet during an acute diarrheal illness. Early feeding prevents changes in the intestinal ability to absorb nutrients, shortens the duration of illness, and improves nutritional outcomes. Foods high in simple sugars should be avoided because of the potential for osmotic diarrhea.

Antidiarrheal compounds are of questionable value in young children. Drugs that alter intestinal motility may result in fluid retention in the intestine as well as worsening of diarrhea. Such drugs include atropine, loperamide, and diphenoxylate. Adsorbents such as kaolin and pectate may interfere with absorption of nutrients and antibiotics. Theoretical toxicity from salicylate absorption remains a concern with the use of bismuth subsalicylate. Physicians prescribing antiemetics for the treatment of acute gastroenteritis should carefully weigh side effects in young children. Prochlorperazine can cause extrapyramidal symptoms that may outlast the antiemetic effects of the drug. Promethazine has a low risk of extrapyramidal side effects but is not approved for use in children younger than 2 years. Ondansetron and other 5-hydroxytryptamine (5-HT) antagonists are effective antiemetics in children, and should be used in children with persistent vomiting who are unable to tolerate oral intake.

Gastroenteritis associated with certain organisms may require specific drug therapy (**Table 89.5**). Selection of antimicrobial agents can be complicated by several factors: delay in identifying the organism, poor correlation between in vitro susceptibility and clinical efficacy, antibiotic resistance of enteric pathogens, and limited use of some drugs in the pediatric population.

Good handwashing and exclusion of infected children from day care facilities may prevent the spread of some enteric pathogens. Studies suggest that breast-feeding provides protection against rotavirus. In the future, vaccines may be applied effectively to the prevention of gastrointestinal infections.

Dehydration

Dehydration is defined as a decrease in total body water and electrolytes. It is one of the most frequent causes of pediatric mortality worldwide, accounting for more than 2.2 million deaths each year. The high mortality associated with dehydration is due to the high prevalence of gastroenteritis, poor nutrition and hygiene, and lack of medical care in developing countries. Dehydration can represent a diagnostic challenge due to the numerous etiologies of fluid loss involving the gastrointestinal, renal, respiratory, and dermatologic systems (**Table 89.6**).

Pathophysiology

The clinical importance of a fluid deficit in the acute setting depends on a number of variables: (1) the amount of water and solute lost; (2) the length of time over which the fluid and solute is lost; (3) the amount of ongoing losses and maintenance requirements; (4) the child's ability to drink and retain fluids; and (5) the ability of compensatory mechanisms to preserve tissue perfusion, electrolyte homeostasis, and acid-base balance.

Total body water and solute is partitioned into intracellular fluid (ICF) (approximately 40% of body weight) and extracellular fluid (ECF; ~25% to 30% of body weight). Despite the fact that children have a greater percentage of body water than adults, they are more vulnerable to sudden losses in body fluids. Children have proportionately higher urine and stool losses, metabolic rates, and surface area-to-mass ratios. A higher surface area-to-mass ratio requires higher expenditure of calories and body water to maintain body temperature. As a result, children with fluid and solute losses are particularly susceptible to the following complications associated with dehydration:

1. Altered organ perfusion and function due to a depletion of intravascular volume.
2. Excess hydrogen ion production due to anaerobic glucose metabolism and lipolysis sometimes in the face of bicarbonate loss in stool.
3. Interruption of electrolyte, osmolar, and cell volume homeostasis.

Clinical Assessment

The clinical evaluation of dehydration involves a careful history and physical examination and evaluation of laboratory data. During assessment, the emergency physician should determine: (1) the severity of the fluid deficit; (2) the etiology of the fluid deficit (e.g., gastroenteritis, DKA, third spacing, bleeding); (3) the presence of complications associated with dehydration (e.g., metabolic acidosis, hyponatremia); and (4) the best method for rehydration.

Important historical elements include: an approximation of fluid intake and output (vomiting, diarrhea, urine, sweat) over the duration of the illness; the type of fluids taken (e.g., free water vs. electrolyte solution); the duration and height of fever (each 1° C of temperature elevation increases fluid losses by 12%); a recent premorbid weight; and a pertinent acute and past medical history. The physical examination should focus on the vital signs, weight, mucous membranes, skin (color, temperature, and texture), peripheral and central pulses, capillary refill, fontanel, activity level, and mental status. The degree of dehydration is typically graded as mild, moderate, or severe based on the physical findings (**Table 89.7**) based on the percentage of dehydration.

Laboratory testing is not necessary in all children with dehydration. However, in patients with a history suggestive of significant fluid losses and poor oral intake, and physical findings of moderate-to-severe dehydration,

Table 89.5

Laboratory Testing and Antimicrobial Therapy for Selected Pathogens

Pathogen	Blood Tests	Stool Tests	Treatment	Potential Complications
Campylobacter jejuni	None	Routine culture; fecal leukocytes	Only in severe cases—erythromycin or fluoroquinolone	Guillain-Barré syndrome
Escherichia coli (enterotoxigenic)	None	Specific culture (usually not indicated)	Only in severe cases—TMP-SMX or fluoroquinolone	None
Esherichia coli (enterohemorrhagic)	CBC, BUN, creatinine (if HUS is suspected)	Specific culture for O157:H7; fecal leukocytes	None	Hemolytic uremic syndrome (HUS)
Salmonella sp.	None	Routine culture; fecal leukocytes	Only for extra-intestinal spread—ampicillin, gentamicin, TMP-SMX, or fluoroquinolone	Disseminated infection including meningitis, osteomyelitis or endocarditis
Shigella sp.	None	Routine culture; fecal leukocytes	TMP-SMX or fluoroquinolone recommended	Seizures, colonic perforation, HUS
Yersinia enterocolitica	Routine blood culture; serology available	Specific culture; fecal leukocytes	Only for disseminated disease—gentamicin, cefotaxime, or fluoroquinolone	Appendicitis-like syndrome, bacteremia
Bacillus cereus	None	None	None	None
Clostridium difficile	None	Specific culture, assay for toxin; fecal leukocytes	Metronidazole or vancomycin	Toxic megacolon, chronic infection
Clostridium perfringens	None	Specific culture, assay for toxin	None	None
Staphylococcus aureus	None	None	None	None
Vibrio cholera	None	Specific culture	TMP-SMX, tetracycline or doxycycline	Severe dehydration, death
Entamoeba histolytica	Serology available	Ova and parasites	Metronidazole	Chronic infection
Giardia lamblia	None	Ova and parasites	Metronidazole	Chronic infection

serum electrolytes, glucose, BUN, and creatinine help to guide therapy. In patients with severe dehydration, obtaining a blood gas should be considered to assess acid-base status. In addition, urine testing for pH, glucose, and ketones may be helpful in monitoring hydration status as well as determining the etiology of the fluid deficit.

Treatment

Any child in the ED with historical or physical examination findings suggestive of a clinically significant fluid deficit requires either carefully supervised oral or intravenous rehydration.

Children with signs of circulatory failure need immediate intravenous resuscitation and often hospitalization. Early manifestations of circulatory insufficiency include persistent tachycardia, tachypnea, and evidence of poor peripheral perfusion (capillary refill >2 seconds, cool distal extremities, weak or absent pulses). Late findings of

circulatory insufficiency are altered mental status, hypotension, and oliguria. The goals of therapy in severe dehydration are: (1) to reverse of circulatory failure with isotonic fluids; and (2) subsequently provide fluid volumes and types needed to supply maintenance requirements, deficit replacement, and ongoing losses.

In most cases of mild or moderate dehydration, oral rehydration therapy is sufficient. In one study, children with mild to moderate dehydration were equally likely to be successfully resuscitated using oral rehydration therapy when compared with intravenous therapy (Issenman and Leung, 1993). Efforts at oral rehydration should use a commercially available electrolyte solution containing standard concentrations of sodium and glucose. Recent data suggest that electrolyte solutions containing 45 to 60 mEq/L of Na are effective in the rehydration phase of therapy (Pedialyte, Infalyte). Maintenance fluids also need to be provided as well as a 1:1 replacement of ongoing losses.

Table 89.6

Differential Diagnosis of Dehydration in Children

Gastrointestinal Losses
- Vomiting
  - Gastroenteritis (viral, bacterial, parasitic, toxin-mediated)
  - Toxic Ingestions (iron, lead, aspirin, theophylline, ipecac)
  - Intestinal Obstruction (pyloric stenosis, intussusception, volvulus)
  - Infection (pneumonia, urinary tract infection, sepsis, meningitis)
  - Increased Intracranial Pressure (tumor, infection, trauma)
- Diarrhea
  - Enterocolitis (viral, bacterial, parasitic)
  - Celiac Disease
  - Short Gut Syndrome
  - Dysmotility Syndromes (Hirschsprung's disease)
  - Laxative Use
- Malabsorption Syndromes

Renal Losses
- Osmotic Diuresis
  - Diabetes Mellitus
  - Diabetes Insipidus
- Drug-Induced Diuresis
  - Caffeine
  - Theophylline
  - Diuretics
- Glomerular Dysfunction
  - Membranoproliferative Glomerulonephritis
  - Post-Streptococcal Glomerulonephritis
  - Minimal Change Nephrosis
  - Focal Sclerosing Glomerulonephrosis
- Tubular Dysfunction
  - Acute Tubular Necrosis
  - Acute Interstitial Nephritis
- Hypoaldosteronism
  - Addison's Disease
  - Congenital Adrenal Hyperplasia

Pulmonary Losses (due to tachypnea)
- Asthma
- Bronchiolitis
- Pneumonia

Dermatologic Losses
- Cystic Fibrosis
- Heat Exposure
- Burns
- Toxic Epidermal Necrolysis
- Staphylococcal Scalded Skin Syndrome
- Stevens Johnson Syndrome

Children who are not able to tolerate oral therapy should be reassessed for the need for intravenous therapy.

Intravenous fluid replacement be should administered to children with significant physical findings of dehydration. Intravenous rehydration is usually given in 20 cc/kg bolus of isotonic fluid. Since a child's intravascular volume is approximately 80 cc/kg, a 20 cc/kg bolus replenishes 25% of a child's intravascular volume. Additional boluses of 10–20 cc/kg may be given until improvement in vital signs (especially heart rate), mental status, urine output, and skin perfusion are reached. Fluid boluses should be given rapidly and followed by repeated clinical assessments. Subsequent IV therapy should replace the remaining fluid deficit over a 24- to 48-hour period depending on the patient's electrolyte profile. Maintenance fluids and replacement of ongoing fluid losses must also be administered. Frequent reevaluation, especially of skin perfusion, heart rate, mental status and urine output are essential to gauge the effectiveness of therapy.

Complications

Metabolic Acidosis Metabolic acidosis is a common complication of moderate to severe dehydration. In diarrheal dehydration, most excess hydrogen ion is due to excessive bicarbonate loss in the stools, resulting in a non-anion gap metabolic acidosis. The initial, and generally only, therapy for metabolic acidosis from hypoperfusion is repletion of the intravascular volume with isotonic fluid bolus(es). Bicarbonate administration is generally contraindicated in the early resuscitation of most clinical situations. Patients with a significant metabolic acidosis that persists despite fluid resuscitation require frequent blood gas and electrolyte monitoring. Such patients may benefit from pediatric subspecialty consultation.

Careful attention is required in the setting of metabolic acidosis with normal or low potassium levels. Correction of the patient's acidosis with rehydration may cause hypokalemia. Frequent electrolyte monitoring and supplementation of intravenous fluids with potassium should be considered for those patients.

Hyponatremia Hyponatremia, defined as a sodium level <130 mEq/mL, is the most common electrolyte abnormality causing seizures with dehydration. Hyponatremic dehydration is commonly caused by replacement of excessive body fluid losses with hypotonic fluids. It can present with lethargy, muscle weakness, poor appetite, irritability, and seizures. This is most commonly seen with a serum sodium less than 120 mEq/L. Asymptomatic patients with a serum sodium of less than 120 mEq/kg can be treated with normal saline at 20 cc/kg bolus over 2 hours to raise the serum sodium by 5 mEq/L. Symptomatic patients with this degree of hyponatremia, particularly patients who are actively seizing, should be treated with a 5 to 10 cc/kg of 3% NS over 30 to 60 minutes. The remaining sodium deficit can be replaced over 16 to 24 hours using D5 one-half NS at 1.5 to 2 times the maintenance rate.

Hypernatremia Dehydration in the presence of hypernatremia (serum sodium level >150 mEq/mL) is decreasing in prevalence among patients admitted for dehydration, but nonetheless represents a true emergency and requires slower correction than iso- or hyponatremic dehydration. Hypernatremic dehydration may be clini-

Table 89.7

Signs and Symptoms Associated with Dehydration

Clinical Finding	Mild Dehydration (<5% Loss of BW)	Moderate Dehydration (5%–10% Loss of BW)	Severe Dehydration (>10% Loss of BW)
Mental status	Alert, well-appearing	Fatigued, irritable	Lethargic, apathetic, unresponsive
Thirst	Normal, may refuse liquids	Thirsty, eager to drink	Unable to drink
Heart rate	Normal	Normal to increased	Increased
Pulses	Normal	Normal to decreased	Decreased, thready or nonpalpable
Breathing	Normal	Normal to rapid	Rapid or deep
Eyes	Normal	Mildly sunken	Deeply sunken
Tears	Present	Decreased	Absent
Mucous membranes	Moist	Dry	Fissured
Skin turgor	Normal	Recoil <2 seconds	Recoil >2 seconds
Capillary refill	Normal	Prolonged <5 seconds	Prolonged >5 seconds
Extremities	Warm	Cool	Cool, mottled or cyanotic
Urine output	Normal to decreased	Decreased	Decreased to absent

cally less apparent. The hyperosmolar state preserves the intravascular volume despite a significant total body water deficit. Hypernatremic dehydration is associated with serious CNS complications including intracerebral hemorrhage and increased intracranial pressure during fluid and electrolyte correction. Bleeding from the bridging vessels of the subarachnoid and dural spaces is thought to occur when rapidly evolving hypernatremia results in volume contraction in the CNS. Thromboses of the dural sinus and other large vessels also have been described. During intravenous fluid therapy, however, problems of cellular swelling are the major concern. In the face of extracellular hypertonicity, cells of the CNS protect their cellular volumes by generating organic osmolytes. These intracellular osmotic particles can cause an intracellular fluid shift when rapid correction or a relatively hypotonic fluid is used. Additionally, two other metabolic complications associated with hypernatremia are hyperglycemia and hypocalcemia. The hypocalcemia is not usually clinically significant, but hyperglycemia can be severe and requires treatment.

As in other forms of dehydration, the immediate goal of therapy in hypernatremic dehydration is to reverse shock and improve tissue perfusion. Carefully administered boluses of 20 cc/kg of isotonic fluid should be given. A physical assessment of perfusion should follow each bolus. Subsequent therapy should be individualized and guided by the patient's electrolytes. In general, the remaining fluid deficit is replaced over a 48-hour period. The goal should be to lower serum sodium slowly at a rate of 0.5 to 1 mEq/L/h. Seizures during therapy are common and long-term neurological sequelae have been reported in approximately 10% of patients.

Hypoglycemia Hypoglycemia is a common complication associated with dehydration due to gastrointestinal losses and poor oral intake. Prompt recognition of hypo-

glycemia is essential to appropriate management as well as prevention of the potential complications including coma and seizure. Children presenting with altered mental status, hypotension, poor perfusion, or a history of limited oral intake should have bedside glucose testing performed. Children presenting with hypoglycemia, commonly defined as a level <60 mg/dL, should be treated with 0.5 to 1g/kg of dextrose. This can be given as a 10 to 20 cc/kg bolus of D5NS (to asymptomatic patients) or 2 to 4cc/kg of D25 (to patients with significant symptoms).

Intussusception Intussusception is the invagination, or telescoping inward of a portion of bowel into a more distal segment (intussusceptum) (**FIGURE 89.1**). It is the most common cause of acute intestinal obstruction in infants beyond the neonatal period. There is a male preponderance, and three quarters of intussusceptions occur in the first two years of life, with a peak incidence between 5 and 9 months of age. Most cases of intussusception, especially those in children under age 2 years, are idiopathic without an identifiable lead point. In only 5% to 10% of cases, a lead point is found.

Pathophysiology

With intussusception, the invaginating bowel is compressed within the layers of the intussusceptum, resulting in acute venous stasis and edema of the bowel wall. The goblet cells of the mucosa release mucus into the bowel lumen, which mixes with blood from the engorged intestine to form a "currant jelly" stool. Progressive venous compression, tissue edema, and compromised arterial blood flow result in intestinal obstruction, ischemic necrosis, perforation, and peritonitis.

Intussusceptions most commonly involve the ileocecal valve and are idiopathic. An etiology or identifiable lead point for intussusception is found in only 5% to 10% of cases in children less than 2 years of age (**Table 89.8**). The

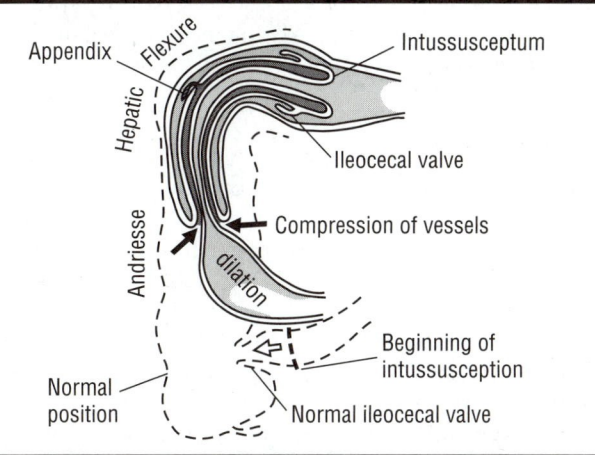

FIGURE 89.1 Schematic representation of an ileocolic intussusception. *Source:* Used with permission from Blickman H. Pediatric Radiology, The Requisites, 2d ed. St. Louis: Mosby, 1998.

cause of idiopathic, ileocolic intussusception in young children is believed to be related to viral infections, especially adenovirus, resulting in enlarged Peyer's patches and mesenteric adenitis.

A minority (10% to 15%) are ileoileal or colocolonic, and a smaller percentage involving the rectum, duodenum, and pylorus. Ileoileal intussusceptions are most commonly seen in postoperative patients. Pathological lead points that result in intussusception include inspissated meconium (cystic fibrosis), Meckel's diverticulum, polyps, duplications of the gastrointestinal tract, tumors, hemangiomas, and submucosal bleeding (Henoch-Schönlein purpura).

Table 89.8
Causes of Intussusception

Infectious
  Adenovirus
  Yersinia enterocolitica
Iatrogenic
  Rotavirus vaccination
  Recent antibiotic use
  Postoperative adhesions
Anatomic
  Appendicitis
  Appendiceal mucocele
  Meckel's diverticulum
  Colonic and intestinal polyps
  Small bowel duplication
  Inspissated meconium
  Intestinal bezoar
Neoplastic
  Adenomyoma
  Lymphosarcoma
  Lymphangioma
  Non-Hodgkin's lymphoma
Miscellaneous
  Henoch-Schönlein purpura
  Peutz-Jeghers syndrome

Lead points are typical in neonates and children over 2 years of age.

Clinical Presentation

The constellation of symptoms associated with intussusception includes vomiting, crampy abdominal pain, abdominal mass, and blood in the stool. These classically occur in a healthy infant with nonbilious vomiting and recurrent waves or paroxysms of colicky abdominal pain. Patient will typically present with periods of painful cry with legs drawn up to the abdomen that lasts several minutes. In between these episodes, the baby may appear comfortable or lethargic, ill or pale. Emesis is typically nonbilious in the early phases but may become bilious as symptoms progress. Loose stools may be reported and may be streaked with blood and/or mucus.

The pathognomonic currant jelly stool consists of mucus streaked with blood. Fever is not typical in the early stages of intussusception. An altered mental status is a well described presentation of intussusception, especially in infants. The diagnosis of intussusception can be difficult when lethargy or depressed mental status is the predominant or only complaint.

On physical examination, the child appears inconsolable during a paroxysm of pain and seems normal, quiet, lethargic, ill or pale between episodes. Evidence of dehydration may be present if vomiting or poor oral intake has been prolonged. The abdominal examination may reveal a mass, distention, or peritonitis. A sausage-shaped mass in the right upper quadrant can be palpated in up to 85% of cases early in the course of symptoms. Alternatively, emptiness in the right lower quadrant, known as Dance's sign, may be appreciated. The absence of abdominal findings on physical examination should not dissuade the examiner from pursuing the diagnosis of intussusception in the child with a suspicious history. Abdominal distention or signs of peritonitis suggest more advanced pathology. A rectal examination must be performed to test for occult or gross blood in the stool.

Laboratory Studies

Laboratory evaluation is generally not helpful in making the diagnosis of intussusception. The white blood cell count may be slightly elevated or normal. Hemoglobin is usually normal. Acid-base status and electrolyte abnormalities reflect the degree of dehydration and vomiting. In advanced stages with bowel compromise and sepsis, laboratory findings are more likely to be abnormal and helpful in guiding therapy.

Radiological Evaluation

Abdominal plain radiography should be obtained in patients with suspected intussusception looking for signs that support the diagnosis and contraindications to a contrast enema. Radiographic findings most suggestive of intussusception include: a soft tissue density in the right or mid abdomen; a paucity of right-sided intestinal gas; a double-lumen (target) sign; or crescent sign. Normal plain radiography, seen in up to 25% of cases, does not exclude an intussusception. Radiographic signs of complete small bowel obstruction or perforation should be identified, if they are present.

Abdominal ultrasound has become an increasingly important tool in the diagnosis of intussusception and identification of a lead point. The doughnut or target sign seen in the transverse view and the pseudokidney sign seen longitudinally are described as up to 97% sensitive for intussusception (Harrington et al., 1998). It may be useful in diagnosing intussusception in patients with contraindications to contrast enemas, including long-standing small bowel obstruction or suspected peritonitis or sepsis.

Abdominal computed tomography (CT) scanning has a limited role in the diagnosis of intussusception. The need for oral contrast mandates a prolonged wait time for the CT scan to be performed, increasing the risk of complications.

Management

The child with suspected intussusception should receive fluid resuscitation to reverse hypoperfusion and electrolyte abnormalities. Children with signs of bowel obstruction, peritonitis, or excessive vomiting may benefit form bowel decompression with a nasogastric tube. In the absence of peritoneal signs or radiographic evidence of significant bowel obstruction or perforation, a diagnostic and therapeutic contrast enema should be performed by an experienced radiologist. Surgical consultation at this point is generally advised.

Air, water, barium, and water-soluble contrast have all been used. Success rates with contrast enema reduction are reported are 50% to 90%. Air contrast, or hydrostatic, enemas have become increasingly popular because of high published success rates and lower complication rates compared with barium contrast enemas. The endpoint of a successful reduction is the free flow of barium into the small bowel.

For the child with evidence of small bowel obstruction, peritonitis, or the patient with failed hydrostatic reduction, surgery is necessary. Fluid resuscitation and intravenous antibiotics with broad gram-positive and gram-negative coverage should be undertaken. Intraoperatively, an attempt at manual reduction by the surgeon is attempted. If successful, intestinal resection is not needed. Bowel that cannot be reduced or appears compromised is resected.

Recurrent intussusception can occur following surgical or nonsurgical reduction in 4% and 6% of cases. The likelihood of a pathological lead point is higher in recurrent intussusception.

Disposition

For the patient in whom intussusception is clinically suspected, consultation with a surgeon should be obtained and radiographic imaging performed. The patient with a negative contrast enema and no signs of intestinal obstruction or dehydration should be followed carefully. Those with an intussusception that has been successfully reduced should be observed for 24 hours to ensure passage of contrast agent and stool. Patients undergoing exploratory laparotomy require hospitalization.

The emergency physician must maintain a high index of suspicion for the possibility of intussusception in children who present with suggestive gastrointestinal and neurological complaints. Early diagnosis and management may avoid surgery and a more complicated course.

Midgut Volvulus

Volvulus is a potentially life-threatening complication of the abnormal rotation and fixation of the midgut during embryologic development. Because it is one of the most serious causes of acute bowel obstruction in children under one year of age, it should be considered immediately in any child who presents with bilious vomiting (**Table 89.9**). In the acute setting, early recognition and timely surgical intervention is the only way to interrupt the natural course of this disease. Failure to recognize a volvulus can quickly result in bowel necrosis and may ultimately lead to the death of the patient.

The majority of patients that develop a volvulus are neonates. Up to three quarters of them present with signs of bowel obstruction during their first month of life. Ninety percent of those who develop a volvulus will do so at some point during the first year. The potential for volvulus persists in older children with malrotation, but this becomes more difficult to diagnose because symptoms of the older child may be more subtle or confused with other causes of vomiting. These children often present with chronic, intermittent, non-bilious vomiting, failure to thrive, and nonspecific abdominal pain.

Pathophysiology

Normal development of the midgut begins during the fifth week of gestation when the rapidly lengthening ileum exceeds the capacity of the primitive peritoneum (**FIGURE 89.2**). The expanding structure herniates into the umbilical cord forming a loop of bowel that continues to grow outside the abdominal cavity. This process continues for four weeks with the entire structure rotating counterclockwise around an axis formed by the omphalomesenteric vessels (precursor to superior mesenteric artery and vein). By the time the bowel returns the abdomen during the tenth week of gestation, it has rotated 270 degrees relative to its original orientation. Normal development is completed during the eleventh week when the mesentery condenses around the gut and fixes it to the posterior abdominal wall. The resulting broad base attachment allows the mobile small intestines to move freely about the abdomen without forming a volvulus. Under normal conditions, the cecum is fixed in the right lower quadrant and the duodenojejunal junction (ligament of Treitz) will be located to the left of the spine. These landmarks become important markers in the radiographic evaluation of any patient with suspected malrotation.

Abnormal rotation and failure of fixation can result in a spectrum of disease that ranges from early volvulus with bowel necrosis to partial small bowel obstruction presenting with chronic pain and intermittent vomiting. In the former case, the intestines are attached to the retroperitoneum by a narrow pedicle that contains the superior mesenteric artery and vein (**FIGURE 89.3**). Rotation around this stalk occludes the blood supply to the entire midgut

Table 89.9
Differential Diagnosis of Bilious Vomiting

Diagnosis	Common Age	Pain	Stool	Bowel Sounds	Tenderness	Masses	X-ray Findings Air/Fluid Levels	Non-Ca^{++} Opacities	Further Studies
Duodenal stenosis (webs)	Infant (young child)	Minimal	Normal–decreased	Normal–increased	No	No	±	±	UGI, endoscopy
Volvulus	Infant (any)	Severe	Hematochezia	Absent–increased	Yes	±	±	No	UGI/BE
Intussusception	10 mo–2 yr	Crampy	Currant jelly	Increased	Yes	Yes	±	Yes	BE
Meconium ileus equivalent	Infant (any)	Crampy	Obstipation	Increased	±	Yes	±	±	Water-soluble contrast enema
Hirschsprung's disease	Infant (any)	? Tenesmus	Obstipation/ diarrhea	Increased	No	Palpable stool	Yes	No	BE
Incarcerated inguinal hernia	Any	Moderate–severe	Obstipation/ diarrhea	Increased	Yes	Inguinal/ scrotal	Yes	No	None
Anal stenosis	Infant	? Tenesmus	Obstipation	Increased	No	Yes	Yes	No	BE

Source: Used with permission from Aghababian RH, ed. *Emergency Medicine, The Core Curriculum.* Philadelphia: Lippincott-Raven Press, 1998:680.

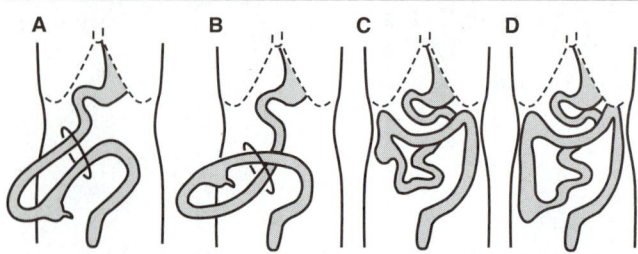

FIGURE 89.2 Normal fetal rotation of midgut. *Source:* Used with permission from Berrocal T, Lamas M, Guiterrez J, et al. Congenital anomalies of the small intestine, colon, and rectum. *Radiographics* 1999;19:1219–1236.

in the acute setting or results in vascular congestion and ischemia in the more chronic setting. Obstruction can be caused when aberrant Ladd's bands occlude the duodenum, or by volvulus as the entire mid-gut rotates around the vascular pedicle. When that rotation occludes the superior mesenteric artery, bowel necrosis can occur over the course of a few hours. Although more common in the first year this malformation can lead to necrosis, sepsis, and death at anytime during the patient's lifetime. Seventy-five percent of all patients with malrotation will eventually develop a volvulus.

Evaluation

The evaluation of a patient with malrotation and midgut volvulus can be complicated by the nonspecific nature of its early presentation. One of the first signs of acute volvulus is feeding intolerance that progresses to bilious vomiting in an infant under one year of age. The initial physical exam may be benign with little or no distention and abdominal tenderness. Heightened awareness and early intervention will help to prevent the development of the "classic" signs of volvulus such as a painful distended abdomen, fever, tachycardia, and other manifestations of impending cardiovascular collapse. By the time these more concerning signs materialize, ischemia and bowel infarction are well underway. It is important to remember that the presence of diarrhea does not rule out a volvulus and blood in the stool is an ominous sign.

Laboratory Studies

The use of laboratory testing has a limited role in the evaluation of volvulus. Abnormal values tend to be non-specific. As a result, they rarely lead to the diagnosis if volvulus is not already part of the differential diagnosis. When used to support a clinical suspicion of volvulus, laboratory tests can be useful in assessing the acuity of the patient at the time of presentation. For instance, an elevated lactate and evidence of acidosis indicate that the disease has progressed to the point that bowel ischemia and infarction are present. The presence of normal values such as white blood cell count should be interpreted cautiously because they do not exclude the diagnosis.

Radiology

Diagnostic imaging plays a vital role in the evaluation of malrotation in any child regardless of his presentation. The choice of a particular study is often dictated by both the acuity of the presenting symptoms and by the availability of the imaging to the emergency physician. The most commonly utilized are plain films, ultrasound, CT scan, and both upper and lower GI contrast studies.

Plain films are the typical starting point in the radiographic evaluation of a patient with suspected volvulus. Their utility in the setting of volvulus is often limited to the demonstration of the nonspecific signs of small bowel obstruction. The classically described "double bubble" sign is seen when an aberrant Ladd's band occludes the duodenum. The resulting distention causes the formation of a second "gas bubble" adjacent to the typical gastric air collection. The duodenal triangle is described as a triangular gas pattern in the right upper quadrant that is caused by the liver edge overlying a gas-filled duodenum. When these signs are seen, they are more common in patients who present at less than one month of age. Nonspecific findings such as distended bowel and air-fluid levels are more characteristic of the presentation in older children.

Ultrasound is able to identify nonspecific signs of necrosis and obstruction such as distended, fluid filled small bowel, or free fluid in the peritoneum, but can also diagnose malrotation by evaluating the relationship between the mesenteric vein and artery. During normal development, the superior mesenteric vein becomes fixed to the right of the artery. When malrotation occurs, the vein is usually found immediately posterior to the artery. A normal relationship between these vessels doesn't rule out malrotation, however. The pathognomonic counterclockwise "whirlpool" sign is another finding that is readily apparent by ultrasound (**FIGURE 89.4**). When it is visualized, it is highly specific for midgut volvulus. Unfortunately, ultrasound does have some disadvantages. It is highly operator-dependent, and bowel gas can easily obscure these essential findings.

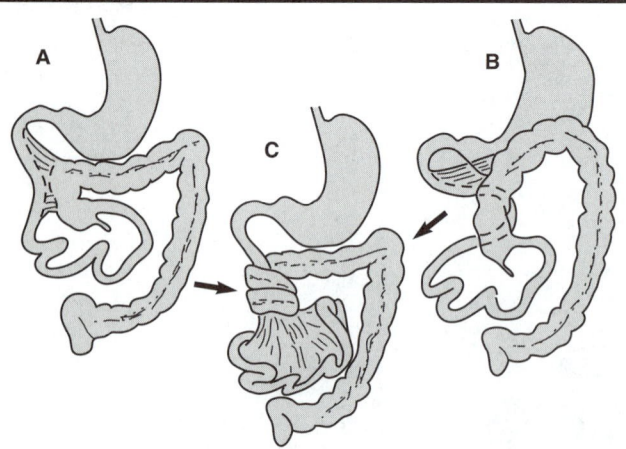

FIGURE 89.3 Malrotation (A, B) with development of volvulus (C). *Source:* Used with permission from Berrocal T, Lamas M, Guiterrez J, et al. Congenital anomalies of the small intestine, colon, and rectum. *Radiographics* 1999;19:1219–1236.

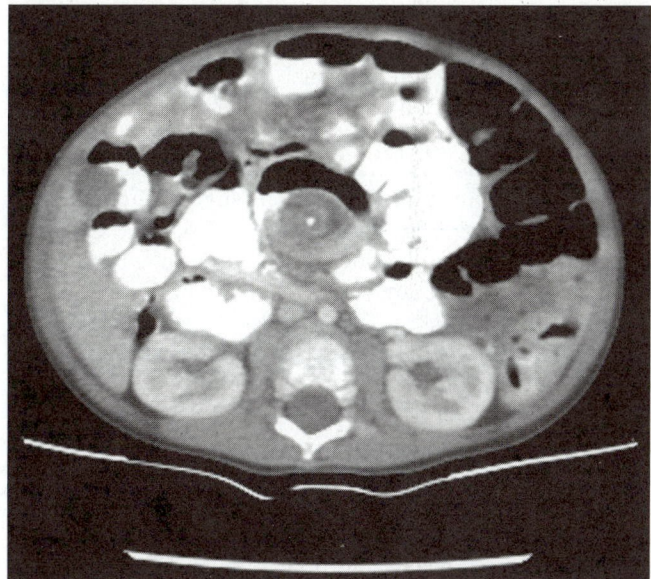

FIGURE 89.4 Whirlpool sign by computed tomography. *Source:* Used with permission from Patino MO, Munden MM. Utility of the sonographic whirlpool sign in diagnosing midgut volvulus in patients with atypical clinical presentations. *J Ultrasound Med* 2004;23:397–401.

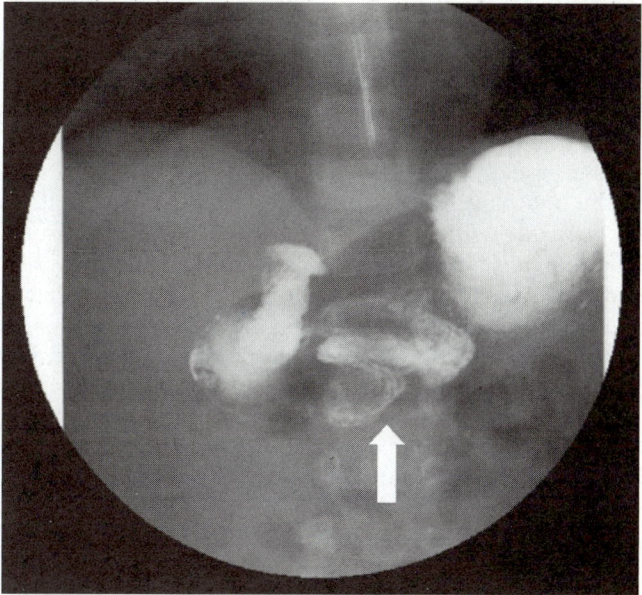

FIGURE 89.5 Barium swallow. Used with permission from Patino MO, Munden MM. Utility of the sonographic whirlpool sign in diagnosing midgut volvulus in patients with atypical clinical presentations. *J Ultrasound Med* 2004;23:397–401.

Computed tomography (CT) scanning is another diagnostic tool that is usually readily available to most emergency physicians. This accessibility makes it ideally suited for the rapid evaluation of all but the most unstable patients. The characteristic "whirlpool" sign caused by twisting of the bowel and mesentery around the vascular pedicle is easily visualized on CT. The abnormal relationship of the superior mesenteric artery to the vein that results from failure of normal rotation can be readily demonstrated on CT scan as well. CT is also capable of visualizing signs of vascular compromise caused by chronic malrotation such as thickened bowel, and tortuous, dilated mesenteric vessels.

The upper GI contrast study has traditionally been considered the gold standard for the evaluation of malrotation. The majority of patients with this disease will demonstrate an abnormality that is readily apparent with contrast study. In this case, diagnosis is based on the location and shape of the duodenum. A corkscrew or coiled distal duodenum located to the right of the midline is highly specific for malrotation. The lower GI or barium enema study is another popular modality, but again some authors consider it to be less reliable because it is dependent on the location of the cecum, which varies considerably in the volvulus (**FIGURE 89.5**).

Management

The role of the emergency physician in this disease process is to stabilize the patient and to expedite early surgical intervention. Initial management of acute volvulus includes volume resuscitation, gastric decompression, and broad-spectrum antibiotic coverage. Consultation with a pediatric surgeon should not be delayed by radiographic studies. Regardless of the severity of the presenting signs and symptoms, the definitive treatment for malrotation and volvulus is surgery.

Appendicitis in Children

Epidemiology

Appendicitis is the most common nontraumatic surgical emergency in children. All ages are affected, with the peak incidence in the pediatric population being six to ten years. Appendicitis is rare in children less than five years. The male to female ratio is approximately 2:1.

The mortality rate for children with appendicitis is 0.1% if unruptured and 3% to 5% if ruptured. The rate of perforation is approximately 17% to 40% at the time of diagnosis. Perforation rates are higher (50%–80%) in younger children and are greater than 90% in children less than two years due to the difficulty in diagnosis.

Pathophysiology

The appendix is a blind-ending sac that arises from the cecum. Appendicitis occurs when the lumen of the appendix becomes obstructed, usually by a fecalith. Hyperplasia of submucosal lymphoid follicles may also lead to obstruction. Gradually, the intraluminal pressure rises, leading to mucosal inflammation and edema, bacterial overgrowth, and eventually ischemia, infarction, and perforation. The appendiceal wall is thinner in children, which predisposes them to more rapid progression to perforation. Peritonitis occurs when the intestinal contents are released into the abdominal cavity. The omentum aids in walling off the infection thereby creating a focal abscess. Young children lack a fully developed omentum, which predisposes them to a more diffuse peritonitis.

Clinical Manifestations

The classic presentation of appendicitis begins with poorly localized periumbilical pain, caused by stretch receptors relaying pain via *visceral* fibers. This pain is constant, crampy, and of moderate severity. After a variable period (usually 1–12 hours), the pain becomes localized to the right lower quadrant. This is caused by stimulation of *parietal* nerve fibers of the surrounding tissues. Approximately one-third of patients will localize pain somewhere other than the right lower quadrant. A retrocecal appendix will produce back, flank, or testicular pain. A pelvic appendix may cause suprapubic pain. And patients with an unusually long appendix or with situ inversus may have pain in the left lower quadrant. Anorexia is the initial symptom in a vast majority of patients, but this history may be difficult to elicit from younger patients. Nausea and vomiting generally occur after the onset of pain (in contrast to gastroenteritis). Fever occurs later and may not be present upon the patient's initial exam. Approximately one third of patients will complain of mild diarrhea (frequent, small, soft stools), and a few may have constipation.

Begin the physical examination by observing the child. Patients with appendicitis prefer to lay still, possibly with their right hip flexed. If forced to move, they may walk slightly bent over with a limp. Rocking the bed or tapping the patient's heels will cause pain (as will bumps on the drive to the hospital). Tenderness is usually located at McBurney's point (midway between the anterior-superior iliac spine and the umbilicus). Patients may exhibit voluntary guarding early on, followed by involuntary guarding (rigid abdomen) as perforation occurs. Rebound tenderness is caused by rapidly moving the inflamed peritoneum, and can be elicited by gentle percussion of the abdomen. Rovsing's sign is pain felt in the right lower quadrant during palpation of the left lower quadrant. The psoas sign is caused by an inflamed appendix overlying the ileopsoas muscle. Stretching this muscle, by having the patient lay on his/her left side and slowly extending the right hip, will cause pain. The obturator sign is elicited by passive internal rotation of the flexed right thigh while the patient is supine. A testicular exam (or pelvic exam in adolescent females if indicated) should be performed to rule out other causes of lower abdominal pain when the diagnosis is in doubt. Finally, a rectal exam may localize tenderness in the right lower quadrant.

Laboratory Data

There is no diagnostic laboratory test for appendicitis. A suggestive history and physical exam is sufficient to warrant a surgical consultation. In patients with a less typical presentation, labs may aid in the diagnosis of appendicitis or reveal an alternative diagnosis. A complete blood count with differential is the most commonly ordered lab test in the evaluation of appendicitis. Approximately 96% of patients will have either a white blood count of greater than 10,000/mm or a left shift with greater than 75% neutrophils. An increased white blood cell count is not specific for appendicitis and a normal white blood cell count does not rule out the diagnosis.

A urinalysis is usually normal in appendicitis but may reveal a few (5–10) white or red blood cells per high powered field due to the close proximity of the appendix to the ureter. There should be an absence of bacteria. Greater than 20–30 white or red blood cells suggests an alternate diagnosis such as UTI, kidney stone, vasculitis, mass, or trauma. Glucose and ketones in the urine suggest diabetic ketoacidosis. A pregnancy test should be performed on all girls of childbearing age. Electrolytes, BUN, and creatinine may be useful if there is evidence of dehydration. Since strep throat may present with abdominal pain, a rapid strep test should be performed if there is any complaint of pharyngitis.

Diagnostic Imaging

Plain films are most useful in eliminating other causes of abdominal pain such as right lower lobe pneumonia, constipation, free air, or obstruction. A radiopaque fecalith in the right lower quadrant (present in 10%) is highly suggestive of acute appendicitis. In the vast majority of children with possible appendicitis, however, plain films do not aid in the diagnosis.

Ultrasound has become an important diagnostic imaging modality children with possible appendicitis. Appendiceal ultrasounds have an overall sensitivity and specificity of 90% to 95% with an experienced sonographer. Ultrasound findings consistent with appendicitis include a noncompressible, enlarged (greater than 6 mm in AP diameter) appendix, tenderness over the appendix, and a fecalith inside an enlarged appendix. Ultrasounds are limited by sonographer experience, a retrocecal appendix, bowel gas, obesity, and the nonvisualization of a normal appendix. Some clinicians will discharge home (with good follow-up instructions), children with a low clinical suspicion for appendicitis and a negative ultrasound.

When ultrasound is not available or nondiagnostic, a CT scan, optimally with oral or rectal contrast, may be helpful. The CT scan offers sensitivities and specificities in the range of 90% to 96% and may be a cost-effective screening tool compared to inpatient admission for observation. CT is also more likely than ultrasound to identify an alternative diagnosis such as mesenteric adenitis, inflammatory bowel disease.

Differential Diagnosis

Mesenteric adenitis is the condition most likely to mimic acute appendicitis. Children will usually be afebrile and without true peritoneal signs. Mesenteric adenitis usually follows a viral illness or strep pharyngitis, and is probably more common than appendicitis.

Gastroenteritis is the most common cause of abdominal pain in children and also the most common misdiagnosis in patients with missed appendicitis. Gastroenteritis involves vomiting and diarrhea, which generally precedes or is coexistent with abdominal pain. Fever may or may not be present. There are often sick contacts with similar symptoms. Acute gastroenteritis rarely causes localized abdominal tenderness.

Testicular or ovarian torsion usually causes severe lower abdominal pain which is sudden in onset. There may be a history of similar previous episodes. Intussusception typically presents with the clinical triad of colic, intermittent paroxysm of abdominal pain, vomiting, and current jelly or bloody stools. It may be diagnosed by ultrasound or barium edema.

Midgut volvulus is due to a congenital malrotation of the midgut and typically presents with bilious vomiting. Although it can present at any age, it is most commonly diagnosed in the newborn period. Meckel's diverticulum often presents with appendicitis-like abdominal pain. There is often associated rectal bleeding. Inflammatory bowel disease, in addition to abdominal pain, often presents with extraintestinal symptoms such as arthritis, conjunctivitis, and rash. Henoch-Schönlein purpura is often preceded by upper respiratory infection symptoms and accompanied by a rash, arthalgias, and hematuria but abdominal pain may be the first symptom. Constipation often presents with abdominal pain from distension of the cecum. Rectal exam may reveal impacted feces and a plain film will demonstrate a large amount of stool.

Urinary tract infection and pregnancy can easily be ruled out with a urinalysis and urine pregnancy test. Pelvic inflammatory disease in adolescent females may be confused with appendicitis. Diabetic ketoacidosis may present with abdominal pain, but these patients will generally not have localized tenderness. Diagnosis is made by laboratory findings of hyperglycemia, metabolic acidosis, and ketonuria.

Management

For patients with a high suspicion for appendicitis, a surgery consult should be obtained. These patients should have an IV established and be kept NPO in anticipation of surgery. Narcotic pain control should be administered if it is warranted and does not interfere with subsequent exams as previously believed. If the patient has a high fever, if perforation is suspected, or if there is a delay in getting the patient to the operating room, broad spectrum IV antibiotics to cover gram-negatives and anaerobes should be started.

Appendectomy is the definitive treatment for appendicitis. Approximately 10% to 20% of patients undergoing appendectomy will have a normal appendix on visual and histologic exam. This is directly due to the difficulty in diagnosis, especially in younger children. Laparoscopic appendectomy is becoming increasingly more common, especially in older children. Complication rates are similar to open appendectomy and hospital length of stay is usually shorter.

Children with a less clear diagnosis require further laboratory and radiological work-up as well as serial abdominal exams. Children with a low suspicion for appendicitis who have resolving symptoms, minimal tenderness, and are able to tolerate oral fluids may be discharged home with a responsible adult. Discharge instructions must require that the child return to the emergency department if symptoms recur or worsen, and parents must understand that the diagnosis of appendicitis cannot be definitively excluded.

Selected Readings

American Academy of Pediatrics. Practice parameter: the management of acute gastroenteritis in young children. *Pediatrics.* 1996;97:424–435.

Acute infectious gastroenteritis. *The Merck Manual,* ed 17. 1999. Available at http://www.merck.com/mrkshared/mmanual/home.jsp. Accessed May 2005.

Afghani B, Stutman HR. Toxin-related diarrheas. *Pediatr Ann.* 1994;23:549–555.

Ai VHG. CT appearance of midgut volvulus with malrotation in a young infant. *Clin Radiol* 1999;54:687–689.

Ament M. Diagnosis and management of upper gastrointestinal tract bleeding in the pediatric patient. *Pediatr Rev* 1990;12:107–115.

American Academy of Pediatrics. Practice parameter: the management of acute gastroenteritis in young children. *Pediatrics.* 1996;97:424–435.

Ang A. Pediatric appendicitis in "real-time": the value of sonography in diagnosis and treatment. *Pediatr Emerg Care* 2001;17:334–340.

Brandt M. Late presentations of midgut malrotation in children. *Am J Surg* 1985; 150:767–771.

Brender JD, Marcuse EK, Koepsell TD, Hatch E. Childhood appendicitis: factors associated with perforation, *Pediatrics* 1985;76:301–306.

Callahan MJ. CT of appendicitis in children. *Radiology* 2002;224:325–332.

Centers for Disease Control and Prevention. Managing acute gastroenteritis among children: oral rehydration, maintenance and nutritional therapy. *MMWR* 2003;52(RR-16):1–16.

Centers for Disease Control. Diagnosis and management of foodborne illnesses: a primer for physicians. *MMWR* 2001;50(RR02):1–69.

Cohen MB, Mezoff AG, Laney DW, et al. Use of a single solution for oral rehydration and maintenance therapy of infants with diarrhea and mild to moderate dehydration. *Pediatrics* 1995;95:639–645.

Conway EE. Central nervous system findings and intussusception: how are they related? *Pediatr Emerg Care* 1993;9:15–18.

Cooper WO, Griffin MR, Arbogast P, et al. Very early exposure to erythromycin and infantile hypertrophic pyloric stenosis. *Arch Pediatr Adolesc Med* 2002;156: 647–650.

Crystal P, Hertzanu Y, Farber B, et al. Sonographically guided hydrostatic reduction of intussusception in children. *J Clin Ultrasound* 2002;30:343–348.

D'Agostino J. Common abdominal emergencies in children. *Emerg Med Clin North Am* 2002;20:139–153.

Daneman A, Alton DJ. Intussusception: issues and controversies related to diagnosis and reduction. *Radiol Clin North Am* 1996;34:743–756.

Davenport M. ABC of general surgery in children: surgically correctable causes of vomiting in infancy. *Br Med J* 1996;312:236–239.

del-Pozo G, Albillos JC, Tejedor D, et al. Intussusception in children: current concepts in diagnosis and enema reduction. *Radiographics* 1999;19:299–319.

DiFiore JW. Intussusception. *Semin Pediatr Surg* 1999;8:214–220.

Doherty GM, Lewis FR Jr. Appendicitis: continuing diagnostic challenge. *Emerg Med Clin North Am* 1989;7:537–553.

Dueholm S, Bagi P, Bud M. Laboratory aid in the diagnosis of acute appendicitis. A blinded, prospective trial concerning diagnostic value of leukocyte count, neutrophil differential count, and C-reactive protein. *Dis Colon Rectum* 1989; October:855–859.

Dufour D. Midgut malrotation, the reliability of sonographic diagnosis. *Pediatr Radiol* 1992;22:21–23.

Duke T, Molyneux EM. Intravenous fluids for seriously ill children: time to reconsider. *Lancet* 2003;362:1320–1323.

Feldman M, Friedman LS, Sleisenger MH. *Sleisenger & Fordtran's Gastrointestinal and Liver Disease,* ed 7. New York: Saunders, 2002.

Felter RA. Nontraumatic surgical emergencies in children. *Emerg Med Clin North Am* 1991;9:589–610.

Garcia Peña BM, Cook EF, Mandl KD. Selective imaging strategies for the diagnosis of appendicitis in children. *Pediatrics* 2004;113:24–28.

Godbole P, Sprigg A, Dickson JA, Lin PC. Ultrasound compared with clinical examination in infantile hypertrophic pyloric stenosis. *Arch Dis Child* 1996;75: 335–337.

Gorelick MH, Shaw KN, Baker MD. Effect of ambient temperature on capillary refill in healthy children. *Pediatrics* 1993;92:699–702.

Harrington L, Connolly B, Hu Y, et al. Ultrasonographic and clinical predictors of intussusception. *J Pediatr* 1998;132:836–839.

Heller RM, Hernanz-Schulman M. Applications of new imaging modalities to the evaluation of common pediatric conditions. *J Pediatr* 1999;135:632–639.

Hernanz-Schulman M. Infantile hypertrophic pyloric stenosis. *Radiology* 2003;227: 319–331.

Hillemeier C, Gryboski J. Gastrointestinal bleeding in the pediatric patient. *Yale J Biol Med* 1984;57:135–147.

Hostetter M, Bracikowski A. Appendicitis. In: *Rosen's Emergency Medicine: Concepts and Clinical Practice,* ed 5. St. Louis, MO: C.V. Mosby, 2002.

Hulka F. Complications of pyloromyotomy for infantile hypertrophic pyloric stenosis. *Am J Surg* 1997;173:450–452.

Hyams J, Leichtner A, Schwartz A. Recent advances in diagnosis and treatment of gastrointestinal hemorrhage in infants and children. *J Pediatr* 1985; 106:1–9.

Issenman RM, Leung AK. Oral and intravenous rehydration in children. *Can Fam Physician* 1993;39:2129–2136.

Jones S. A clinical pathway for pediatric gastroenteritis. *Gastroenterol Nurs* 2003;26:7–18.

Kallen RJ. The management of diarrheal dehydration in infants using parenteral fluids. *Pediatr Clin North Am* 1990;37:265–286.

Kao SCS, Smith WL, Abu-Yousef MM, et al. Acute appendicitis in children: sonographic findings. *AJR Am J Roentgenol* 1989;153:375–379.

Kuppermann N, O'Dea T, Pinckney L, Hoecker C. Predictors of intussusception in young children. *Arch Pediatr Adolesc Med* 2000;154:250–255.

Kwon KT, Rudkin SE, Langdorf MI. Antiemetic use in pediatric gastroenteriits: a national survey of emergency physicians, pediatricians, and pediatric emergency physicians. *Clin Pediatr* 2002;41:641–652.

Letton RW. Pyloric stenosis. *Pediatr Ann* 2001;31:745–750.

Lieberman JM. Rotavirus and other viral causes of gastroenteritis. *Pediatr Ann* 1994;23:529–535.

Long FR. Radiographic patterns of intestinal malrotation in children. *RadioGraphics* 1996;16:547–556.

Losek JD. Intussusception: don't miss the diagnosis! *Pediatr Emerg Care* 1993;9:46–51.

Martin LP. Implementing a critical pathway for oral rehydration of mild to moderate dehydration in children. *J Emerg Nurs* 2001;27:597–601.

McCollough M. Abdominal surgery emergencies in infants and young children. *Emerg Med Clin North Am* 2003;21:909–935.

McManus ML, Churchwell KB, Strange K. Regulation of cell volume in health and disease. *N Engl J Med* 1995;333:1260–1266.

Meguerditchian AN. Laparoscopic appendectomy in children: a favorable alternative in simple and complicated appendicitis. *J Pediatr Surg* 2002;37:695–698.

Mezoff A, Preud'Homme D. How serious is that GI bleed? *Contemp Pediatr* 1994;11:60–92.

Millar AJW. Malrotation and volvulus in infancy and childhood. *Semin Pediatr Surg* 2003;12:229–236.

Murphy TV, Gargiullo PM, Massoudi MS, et al. Intussusception among infants given an oral rotavirus vaccine. *N Engl J Med* 2001;344:564–572.

Nager AL, Wang VJ. Comparison of nasogastric and intravenous methods of rehydration in pediatric patients with acute dehydration. *Pediatrics* 2002;109:566–572.

Neilson D, Hollman AS. The ultrasonic diagnosis of infantile hypertrophic pyloric stenosis: technique and accuracy. *Clin Radiol* 1994;49:246–247.

Okada T. Pulsed Doppler sonography for the diagnosis of strangulation in small bowel obstruction. *J Pediatr Surg* 2001;36:430–435.

Okada PJ. Pediatric surgical emergencies. *Clin Pediatr Emerg Med* 2002;3:3–13.

Oldham K, Lobe T. Gastrointestinal hemorrhage in children—a pragmatic update. *Pediatr Clin North Am* 1985;32:1247–1263.

Peña BM, Taylor GA, Lund DP, Mandl KD. Effect of computed tomography on patient management and costs in children with suspected appendicitis. *Pediatrics* 1999;104:440–446.

Pisacane A, de Luca U, Crisuolo L, et al. Breast feeding and hypertrophic pyloric stenosis: population based case-control study. *BMJ* 1996;312:745–746.

Pracros JP. Ultrasound diagnosis of midgut volvulus: the "whirlpool" sign. *Pediatr Radiol* 1992;22:18–20.

Rao PM, Rhea JT, Novelline Ra, et al. Effect of computed tomography of the appendix on the treatment of patients and use of hospital resources. *N Engl J Med* 1998;338:141–146.

Ramsook C, Sahagun-Carreon I, Kozinetz CA, Moro-Sutherland D. A randomized clinical trial comparing oral ondansetron with placebo in children with vomiting from acute gastroenteritis. *Ann Emerg Med* 2002;39:397–403.

Rosen P, Barkin RM, Hayden SR, et al. (eds.). *Rosen and Barkin's 5-Minute Emergency Medicine Consult*, ed 2. Philadelphia: Lippincott, Williams & Wilkins Inc., 2005.

Samuel M. Pediatric appendicitis score. *J Pediatr Surg* 2002;37:877–881.

Schwartz D, Connelly NR, Manikantan P, Nichols JH. Hyperkalemia and pyloric stenosis. *Anesth Analg* 2003;97:355–357.

Seashore JH. Midgut volvulus an ever-present threat. *Arch Pediatr Adolesc Med* 1994;148:43–46.

Silber G, Klish W. Hematochezia in infants less than 6 months of age. *Am J Dis Child* 1986;140:1097–1098.

Sorenson HT, Norgard B, Pederson L, et al. Maternal smoking and risk of hypertrophic infantile pyloric stenosis: 10 year population based cohort study. *BMJ* 2002;325:1011–1012.

Spigland N. Malrotation presenting beyond the neonatal period. *J Pediatr Surg* 1990;25:1139–1142.

Spiro DM, Arnold DH, Barbone F. Association between antibiotic use and primary idiopathic intussusception. *Arch Pediatr Adolesc Med* 2003;157:54–59.

Steffen R, Wyllie R, Sivak M, et al. Colonoscopy in the pediatric patient. *J Pediatr* 1989;115:507–513.

Stutman HR. *Salmonella, Shigella,* and *Campylobacter:* common bacterial causes of infectious diarrhea. *Pediatr Ann* 1994;23:538–543.

Torres AM. Malrotation of the intestine. *World J Surg* 1993;17:326–331.

Townsend CM, Beauchamp RD, Evers M, Mattox K. *Sabiston Textbook of Surgery, The Biological Basis of Modern Surgical Practice (Textbook of Surgery)*, ed 16. Philadelphia: W.B. Saunders Company, 2001.

Watkins BP. Midgut volvulus. *J Am Coll Surg* 2003;197:986.

Winslow BT, Westfall JM, Nicholas RA. Intussusception. *Am Fam Physician* 1996;54:213–217.

Congenital Heart Disease, Congestive Heart Failure, and Acquired Heart Disease

Michele VanderHeyden
Mariann M. Manno

Congenital Heart Disease in Infancy

Congestive Heart Failure

Congestive heart failure is the inability of the heart to maintain cardiac output, either due to a primary abnormality of cardiac function or excessive work requirement placed on the heart. Cardiac output is the product of heart rate and stroke volume $[CO = HR \times SV]$. Stroke volume is determined by preload, afterload, and contractility. The most common causes of congestive heart failure in the newborn period is congenital heart defects with large left to right shunts and left ventricular outflow tract (LVOT) obstruction.

Congestive heart failure in the older infant and child is predominantly from acquired heart disease and dysrhythmias. Undiagnosed congenital heart defects are responsible for a minority of cases of CHF in children beyond 6 months of age (**Table 90.1**).

Clinical Presentation

Common symptoms of congestive heart failure include poor feeding, failure to thrive, respiratory distress (tachypnea, increased work of breathing), poor color (cyanosis, pallor, mottled) and irritability. A careful physical examination should identify subtle signs of congestive failure and shock when they are present. Tachypnea with grunting, flaring, and retracting is common. Auscultation of the lung fields may reveal crackles or rales, although these signs are often absent in very young infants with congestive heart failure. Cardiac auscultation typically reveals an active precordium, abnormal splitting of S2, a gallop rhythm, and other murmurs indicative of an underlying heart defect. Poor skin perfusion may be present with a mottling or a gray appearance. The overall quality of the pulses may be poor, especially with forms of LVOT obstruction such as hypoplastic left heart syndrome (HLHS) and critical aortic stenosis. A difference in the intensity of the pulse between the upper and lower extremities is an important clinical finding, and suggests coarctation of the aorta or interrupted aortic arch. Hepatomegaly and edema is frequently present. Jugular venous distension is uncommonly appreciated in newborns.

Laboratory Findings

Arterial blood gas, electrolytes, BUN, and creatinine are all helpful in quantifying the degree of metabolic acidosis and renal insufficiency. Hypoglycemia is often present in critically ill neonates because of increased glucose utilization, decreased oral intake, and limited glycogen stores. Chest radiography is helpful to assess heart size and shape as well as lung fields. Heart size is often enlarged and with left sided heart failure, pulmonary vascular markings are increased. Some lesions such as total anomalous pulmonary venous return (TAPVR) will present with a normal size heart but markedly increased pulmonary vascularity. Electrocardiography may suggest a specific etiology, but often is nonspecific and most commonly demonstrates sinus tachycardia. Blood pressure taken in all four extremities will help identify patients with coarctation of the aorta and interrupted aortic arch. In any infant with suspected congenital heart defects, consultation with a pediatric cardiologist, and an echocardiogram should be obtained as soon as possible.

Management

Management of infants with signs of congestive heart failure begins with basic assessment and resuscitation. All patients should receive supplemental oxygen. Ventilation should be carefully assessed and supported. Temperature control and fever reduction is necessary. Diuretics are a mainstay for most types of congestive heart failure, especially those due to overcirculation or primary pump failure. Inotropes such as digoxin improve contractility and vasodilators such as captopril and enalopril provide afterload reduction. Importantly, when heart failure from a ductal dependent lesion is suspected, prostaglandin E_1 (PGE_1) infusion can be life-saving. Side effects of PGE_1 include apnea, seizures, hypotension, fever, and rash. It is important to anticipate and prepare for these life-threatening complications especially when the infant will require transport to a tertiary care facility.

Congenital Heart Defects

Congenital heart disease is a common pediatric emergency. It is critical that both undiagnosed congenital heart disease and the complications of these lesions are recognized and managed. Patients with congenital heart defects can present in varied and sometimes subtle ways: congestive heart failure, circulatory failure, respiratory distress, respiratory failure, and cyanosis. The overlap between the presentations of primary respiratory processes, congestive heat failure, and cardiogenic shock make it difficult to distinguish between respiratory and cardiac etiologies in a sick infant. A careful history and physical examination coupled with a high index of suspicion for congenital heart disease is critical when assessing distressed or acutely ill young infants.

The incidence of congenital heart disease is estimated to be between 6 and 10 per 1,000 live births. Many of these are life-threatening cyanotic lesions that present at birth and are diagnosed in the nursery. However, several physiological changes that occur as the neonate transitions from fetal to postnatal circulation and many lesions will be unapparent until the ductus arteriosus closes. Ductal dependent lesions are cardiac malformations that depend on blood flow through a patent ductus arteriosus either for pulmonary or systemic blood flow. Prompt initiation of an intravenous infusion of PGE_1 to maintain patency of the ductus arteriosus can be life-saving. Understanding the physiological changes that occur during the transition from fetal to neonatal circulation may help in the understanding, identification, and acute management of many congenital heart defects.

Fetal Circulation

Fetal circulation differs from that of a neonate in several regards. In the fetus, oxygenation occurs via the placenta; the lungs are not involved with gas exchange. Fetal circulation requires several shunts to bypass the lungs. Briefly, oxygenated blood from the placenta goes into the umbilical vein and is diverted past the liver via the ductus venosus. Blood then enters the inferior vena cava and the right atrium, where the oxygenated blood from the placenta mixes with deoxygenated venous return from the lower body. This mixed blood preferentially exits the right atrium via the patent foramen ovale and enters the left atrium, the left ventricle, and the ascending aorta, which supplies the upper part of the body and the myocardium. Blood from the upper body flows into the superior vena cava and preferentially flows from the right atrium into the right ventricle. Because pulmonary vascular resistance is high in utero, about 90% of the blood entering the pulmonary artery is diverted through the ductus arteriosus to the descending aorta and supplies the lower parts of the body (**FIGURE 90.1**).

Neonatal Circulation

When the infant is born and begins to breathe, oxygen tension increases, the lungs expand, and pulmonary vascular resistance decreases. Simultaneously, systemic vascular resistance increases because of the loss of the low resistance placental circulation. Because of the increase in systemic pressure, blood in the right atrium no longer passes through the foramen ovale, but enters the right ventricle and the pulmonary artery, bypassing the ductus arteriosus, and flows into the lungs. Functional closure of the ductus arteriosus usually occurs after about 48 hours; however full anatomic closure occurs weeks later. Closure is related to an increase in oxygen tension, an increase in pH and a decrease in endogenous prostaglandins.

Clinical Presentation

Signs of congenital heart defects are sometimes subtle and may be difficult to distinguish from primary pulmonary disease or sepsis. Cyanosis is often the first sign that a significant congenital heart defect is present. While the differential of cyanosis is broad and includes upper airway disease, primary pulmonary disease, and sepsis, the history and physical remains the most important way to make the diagnosis of congenital heart disease (**Table 90.2**). Critical congenital heart defects usually present in the first days or weeks of life. In general, the earlier symptoms appear, the more critical the lesion. A delayed pres-

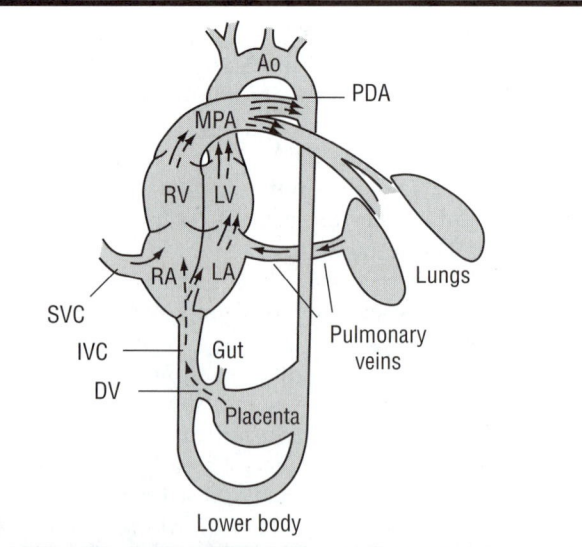

FIGURE 90.1 Fetal circulation, where oxygenated blood comes from the placenta. Two right → left shunts (PDA and PFO) allow blood to bypass the pulmonary circuit. *Source:* Used with permission from Saunders. Polin R, Yoder M, Berg F, eds. *Workbook in Practical Neonatology,* ed 2. Philadelphia: Saunders, 1993.

Table 90.2

Congenital Heart Lesions that Typically Present with Cyanosis

Pulmonary atresia
Transposition of the great arteries
Tetralogy of Fallot
Total anomalous pulmonary venous return
Truncus arteriosus
Tricuspid atresia

Table 90.3

Ductal Dependent Lesions

For Pulmonary Blood Flow	For Systemic Blood Flow
Pulmonary atresia with intact ventricular septum	Coarctation of the aorta
Tricuspid atresia	Interrupted aortic arch
Critical pulmonary stenosis	Hypoplastic left heart syndrome
Tetralogy of Fallot (newborn with cyanosis)	Critical aortic stenosis

entation is most often related to the closure of the ductus arteriosus.

Cyanosis is present when 5 grams of deoxygenated hemoglobin with oxygen saturation less than 80% to 85% is present in the blood. Cyanosis secondary to congenital heart defects is due to right to left shunting within the heart, blood bypassing the lungs, mixing of blood within the heart, or the existence of a parallel circulation. Murmurs represent turbulent flow through the heart. Murmurs are common in the first 24 to 48 hours after birth as many physiological changes in the circulation are occurring. Murmurs may indicate a congenital heart defect; however, many severe lesions are not characterized by a murmur. If cardiac output is severely diminished or if the obstruction is highly restrictive to flow, no murmur will be appreciated. Physical examination should auscultation of the heart and lungs, palpation of peripheral and central pulses, palpation for an enlarged liver, and measurement of blood pressures in all four extremities.

Management

The most urgent neonatal congenital cardiac defects include: transposition of the great arteries, tetralogy of Fallot, tricuspid atresia, truncus arteriosus, total anomalous pulmonary venous return, hypoplastic left heart syndrome, critical aortic stenosis, coarctation of the aorta, and pulmonary atresia with intact ventricular septum. Therapy always begins with evaluation of vital functions of airway, breathing, and circulation (the ABCs). All patients with suspected congenital heart defects should receive supplemental oxygen therapy. Many patients will need intubation and mechanical ventilation to both maximize oxygen delivery and to decrease the myocardial demands of the work of breathing. Consultation with a pediatric cardiologist and echocardiogram should be obtained as soon as possible. Determining the specific diagnosis is less important than identifying the presence of a ductal dependent lesion (**Table 90.3**). Once a ductal dependent lesion is suspected, a PGE_1 infusion can be life-saving. Side effects of PGE_1 include apnea, seizures, hypotension, fever, and rash. It is important to anticipate and prepare for these life-threatening complications especially when the infant will require transport to a tertiary care facility.

Cyanotic Congenital Heart Defects

Cyanotic lesions include pulmonary stenosis and the "5 Ts": truncus arteriosus, transposition of the great arteries,

tetralogy of Fallot, tricuspid atresia, and total anomalous venous return. While most of these lesions will present with profound cyanosis in the newborn nursery, many patients will present to the emergency department after the ductus arteriosus has closed.

Transposition of the Great Arteries

Anatomy and Pathophysiology Transposition of the great arteries (TGA) represents approximately 6% of all forms of congenital heart defects. In the simple, uncorrected type of this defect, the aorta rises from the right ventricle and the pulmonary artery arises from the left ventricle, leading to parallel circulation. There is usually, but not always, an associated defect or channel for mixing (ventricular septal defect [VSD], atrial septal defect [ASD], patent foramen ovale [PFO] or a patent ductus arteriosus [PDA]). The size and adequacy of the mixing lesion will determine the degree of cyanosis present.

Clinical Presentation Patients without an adequate mixing lesion, such as those with TGA and an intact ventricular septum, will have profound cyanosis that presents shortly after birth. In patients with TGA a large VSD may have delayed onset of symptoms when the ductus arteriosus closes. This latter group presents with mild cyanosis typically developing within the first week of life. TGA with a large, unrestrictive VSD may present with ventricular failure in the first month of life. On exam a pansystolic murmur with a loud pulmonic component of the second heart sound is typically present. A gallop can also be heard. Chest radiography classically shows an egg shaped heart with a narrow mediastinum, increased pulmonary vascular markings and cardiomegaly. ECG may be normal in the first few days but later right axis deviation is seen.

Management Oxygenation and ventilation should be supported. Patients with congestive heart failure may benefit from diuretic therapy (Table 90.3). If possible, consultation with a pediatric cardiologist should be obtained prior to starting a prostaglandin infusion. Treatment with prostaglandin should not be delayed if the clinical presentation is highly suggestive. Arrangements should be made as soon as possible to transfer the infant to a cardiac surgery center.

Tetralogy of Fallot

Anatomy and Pathophysiology   Tetralogy of Fallot is the most common form of cyanotic congenital heart disease (10% of all cyanotic heart disease). Anatomically, it consists of four anomalies: right ventricular outflow tract obstruction (pulmonary stenosis or atresia), dextroposition of the aorta, a VSD, and right ventricular hypertrophy.

Clinical Presentation and Laboratory Evaluation Patients have a right to left shunt and usually present with respiratory distress and cyanosis. The appearance of cyanosis depends on the degree of pulmonary stenosis but most patients usually present within the first few months of life. Some patients are cyanotic only with crying or feeding. Chest radiography classically reveals a boot-shaped heart and decreased pulmonary vascular markings. It is not uncommon to have a right-sided aortic arch. ECG reveals right ventricular hypertrophy with right axis deviation.

Management   Prostaglandin infusion is necessary if the patient presents in the newborn period. The older child with cyanotic episodes, called "Tet spells," should be treated with morphine and knee-chest position. Occasionally propranolol is necessary to control the episodes.

Total Anomalous Pulmonary Venous Return

Anatomy and Pathophysiology   With total anomalous pulmonary venous return (TAPVR), the pulmonary veins form a common vein that drains into the right side of the heart via the superior vena cava or coronary sinus. Venous return may be obstructed anywhere along this pathway. Patients with obstructed total anomalous venous return have significant pulmonary hypertension. In the unobstructed type, patients usually present with cyanosis and congestive heart failure due to significant left to right "shunting" because both systemic and pulmonary venous return enter the right side of the heart.

Clinical Presentation   Patients with obstructed pulmonary venous return are severely ill with significant cyanosis, respiratory distress, and present shortly after birth. They do not improve with oxygen administration or with mechanical ventilation. Patients with unobstructed venous return present slightly later, usually the first week, with respiratory distress, cyanosis, and signs of congestive heart failure.

Laboratory Findings   Chest radiography in patients with unobstructed pulmonary venous return shows an enlarged heart with increased pulmonary vascular markings. Classically, the heart is described to have the appearance of a snowman. In the obstructed form of the defect, the heart size will appear normal and there will be marked pulmonary venous congestion. Echocardiography usually will demonstrate the defect but, in rare cases, cardiac catheterization is necessary to visualize all anomalous connections.

Management   Obstructed total anomalous pulmonary venous return is a medical emergency with high morbidity and mortality. Prompt recognition of this defect is essential and referral for cardiac surgery is necessary. Oxygen therapy should be instituted and intubation should be considered. These patients will often remain profoundly cyanotic despite oxygen administration. Patients with unobstructed veins and signs of congestive heart failure, inotropic therapy with digoxin or dopamine as well as diuresis may lead to improvement until surgery can be performed.

Truncus Arteriosus

Anatomy and Pathophysiology   In truncus arteriosus, the aorta and main pulmonary artery arise from the heart as a single, common vessel. Patients always have an associated VSD. Pulmonary hypertension is present and related to pulmonary overcirculation.

Clinical Presentation   Newborns usually present within the first few days of life with significant cyanosis, respiratory distress, and signs of congestive heart failure. The precordium is hyperdynamic with a systolic murmur present at the upper sternal border with a loud, single S2. Pulses are usually bounding unless heart failure is advanced. Chest radiography will show an enlarged heart with increased pulmonary vascular markings, many patients will also have a right-sided aortic arch. ECG shows right axis deviation and biventricular hypertrophy.

Management   Management is supportive with attention to airway, breathing and circulation. Patients often have signs of significant congestive heart failure and will benefit from diuresis and inotropic support. This lesion is not dependent on flow through a patent ductus arteriosus and, therefore, PGE_1 is not indicated and could exacerbate pulmonary overcirculation. Consultation with a pediatric cardiologist and transfer to a cardiac surgery center should occur as soon as possible.

Tricuspid Atresia

Anatomy and Pathophysiology   In tricuspid atresia (TA), there is absence of the tricuspid valve. All venous return to the right atrium passes through a patent foramen ovale or ASD to the left atrium. Pulmonary blood flow is dependent on either the presence of a VSD defect or a PDA.

Clinical Presentation and Laboratory Evaluation Cyanosis is typically present from birth, but if the ventricular septal defect is large, cyanosis may be less pronounced. Cyanosis will increase as the ductus arteriosus closes. Auscultation will reveal a continuous murmur at the upper left sternal border from a PDA or a systolic murmur at the lower left sternal border from a VSD. Chest radiography will show a normal size heart with decreased pulmonary vascular markings. ECG will show left axis deviation and left ventricular hypertrophy.

Management Patients with TA are dependent on the ductus arteriosus for pulmonary blood flow. An infusion of PGE_1 is necessary to help maintain patency of the ductus arteriosus. Consultation with a pediatric cardiologist and transfer to a cardiac surgery center should occur as soon as possible.

Pulmonary Stenosis and Atresia

Anatomy and Pathophysiology Pulmonary stenosis and atresia are forms of right ventricular outflow tract obstruction (RVOT). This can be complete atresia of the pulmonary valve, subvalvar stenosis, or supravalular stenosis (branch pulmonary artery stenosis). RVOT is associated with syndromes such as William's syndrome and Noonan's syndrome. With RVOT obstruction, right ventricular hypertrophy, and increased right ventricular pressures correspond to the degree of obstruction. Pulmonary blood flow is diminished and with time right-sided heart failure is seen.

Clinical Presentation Initially, the infant with PS can usually accommodate the extra work placed on the RV because the right ventricle is the predominate ventricle in utero. However, some infants with critical pulmonary valve stenosis will develop congestive heart failure and cyanosis early. With time right ventricular failure ensues and patients develop cyanosis and dyspnea. Cardiac auscultation reveals a systolic ejection murmur at the upper left sternal border with a split second heart sound with a pulmonary click. On chest radiography, heart size is usually normal as are pulmonary vascular markings. ECG may show right ventricular hypertrophy related to the severity of obstruction.

Management Cyanotic patients with critical pulmonary valve stenosis are dependent on the ductus arteriosus for pulmonary blood flow; therefore, a PGE_1 infusion to maintain ductal patency is necessary. If congestive heart failure is present, diuresis and inotropic support may be beneficial. Consultation with a pediatric cardiologist and transfer to a cardiac surgery center should occur as soon as possible.

Acyanotic Congenital Heart Defects

Acyanotic congenital heart defects fall into two broad categories: those with left ventricular outflow tract obstruction and those with pulmonary overcirculation (left to right shunt). Although patients do not have cyanosis, they are often dependent on the ductus arteriosus for *systemic* blood flow. While many cyanotic heart defects present in the newborn nursery, the presentation of most acyanotic defects is delayed until the ductus arteriosus closes. Therefore, emergency physician must be able to identify

patients with these defects. These patients typically present within the first or two week of life with a clinical picture consistent with shock.

Hypoplastic Left Heart Syndrome

Hypoplastic left heart syndrome (HLHS) is the result of underdevelopment of the left sided heart structures. There is mitral and aortic valve atresia, the left ventricle is small, and there is a hypoplastic ascending aorta. Systemic blood flow is dependent on the ductus arteriosus and the right ventricle is responsible for both systemic and pulmonary output. Once the ductus arteriosus closes there is no pathway for systemic blood flow (**FIGURES 90.2** and **90.3**).

Clinical Presentation Infants with HLHS appear normal at birth. As the ductus arteriosus closes during the first week of life, patients develop respiratory distress and shock. Grey and mottled extremities, poor pulses, metabolic acidosis, and poor urine output are all features of HLHS, and it is difficult to distinguish from sepsis. Subtle cardiac findings that suggest a primary cardiac etiology include a hyperdynamic precordium deviated to the right and a single second heart sound. Chest radiography will show an enlarged heart with increased pulmonary vascular markings. ECG shows right axis deviation, with right ventricular hypertrophy and absent left sided forces.

Management Several decades ago, HLHS was incompatible with life and surgical repair did not improve outcomes. However, surgical advances have improved survival such that few infants die from HLHS. Prompt initiation of PGE_1 along with intubation, mechanical ventilation, and inotropic support for patients in shock, are critical in the early phases of resuscitation of these infants.

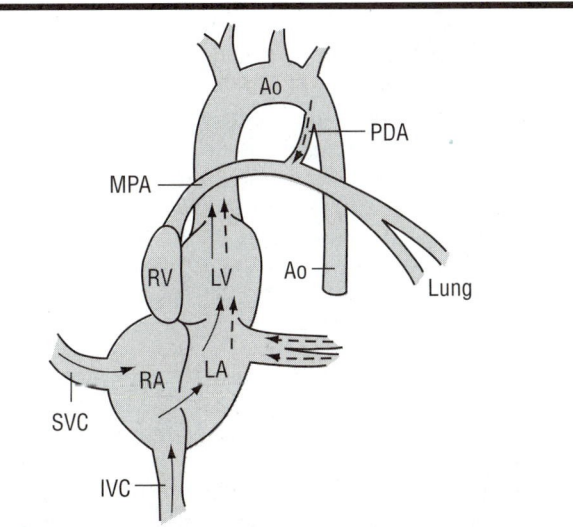

FIGURE 90.2 Hypoplastic right heart syndromes (pulmonary or tricuspid atresias) require patency of the ductus arteriosus for pulmonary perfusion. *Source:* Used with permission from Saunders. Polin R, Yoder M, Berg F, eds. *Workbook in Practical Neonatology,* ed 2. Philadelphia: Saunders, 1993.

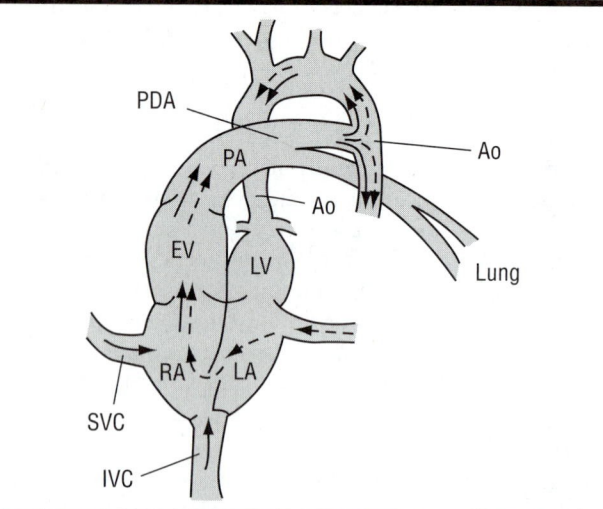

FIGURE 90.3 Hypoplastic left heart syndrome and left ventricular outflow tract obstruction requires patency of the ductus for systemic circulation. *Source:* Used with permission from Saunders. Polin R, Yoder M, Berg F, eds. *Workbook in Practical Neonatology*, ed 2. Philadelphia: Saunders, 1993.

Coarctation of the Aorta

Anatomy and Pathophysiology Coarctation of the aorta is obstruction of the aorta which commonly at the site where the ductus arteriosus meets the aortic arch (juxta-ductal) and just distal to the left subclavian artery. Coarctation leads to increase afterload of the left ventricle and decreased left ventricular output. The right ventricle compensates for this with increased output. Blood flows from the LV → RV → Ductus → descending aorta. Because there is increase work to both the right and left ventricle, neonates present with signs of congestive heart failure. Once the ductus arteriosus closes, systemic blood flow is drastically diminished and the infant develops signs of shock.

Clinical Presentation and Laboratory Evaluation Patients commonly present with congestive heart failure within the first week of life. Signs of shock develop as systemic blood flow becomes markedly diminished with closure of the ductus. Infants present with shock, respiratory distress and hepatomegaly. Systolic blood pressure will be significantly higher in the upper versus the lower extremities. Chest radiography will show cardiac enlargement with increase in pulmonary vascular markings. ECG will show right axis deviation and signs of right ventricular hypertrophy.

Management Infants with coarctation are critically ill and often require oxygenation, assisted ventilation, and inotropic support. Since systemic blood flow is dependent on the ductus arteriosus, prostaglandin infusion should be started as soon as the diagnosis is made. Pediatric cardiology consultation and arrangements to transfer the patient to a cardiac surgery center should occur as soon as possible.

Critical Aortic Stenosis

Anatomy and Pathophysiology Obstruction of left ventricular outflow with aortic stenosis is due to obstruction at the aortic valve leaflets or supravalvar stenosis at the level of the ascending aorta. In patients with aortic stenosis, left ventricular output is significantly diminished and systemic blood flow is dependent on left to right shunting at the atrial level with increased flow to the right ventricle and the ductus arteriosus. As pulmonary vascular resistance falls and the ductus closes, patients will present with congestive heart failure and shock.

Clinical Presentation Patients will have weak pulses, delayed capillary refill, respiratory distress, and hepatomegaly. If cardiac output is severely diminished, then a murmur may not be appreciated despite significant obstruction. Chest radiography will show an enlarged heart with an increase in pulmonary vascular markings. ECG will often show right ventricular hypertrophy.

Management The management of these critically ill infants includes oxygenation, assisted ventilation, and inotropic support. Because systemic blood flow is dependent on the ductus arteriosus, prostaglandin infusion should be started as soon as the diagnosis is made. Pediatric cardiology consultation and arrangements to transfer the patient to a cardiac surgery center should occur as soon as possible.

Ventricular Septal Defect

Anatomy and Pathophysiology An isolated ventricular septal defect (VSD) is the most common type of congenital heart defects accounting for approximately 30% of all patients with congenital heart disease. In the immediate newborn period, pulmonary vascular resistance is high and flow through the VSD is minimal. Murmurs are rarely appreciated even with large defects. As pulmonary vascular resistance decreases, L → R shunting through a large VSD results in pulmonary overcirculation. A murmur is typically easily heard and the infant will develop congestive heart failure.

Clinical Presentation and Laboratory Evaluation The diagnosis of a VSD is usually made in the first few weeks of life with a harsh systolic murmur at the lower left sternal border. Infants with large, undiagnosed VSDs typically develop congestive heart failure within the first month or two of life. Tachypnea, poor feeding, diaphoresis are all common presentations. The precordium is hyperdynamic with a systolic murmur at the lower left sternal border. A gallop rhythm may be present. Eisenmenger's syndrome is a rare complication of a large, untreated VSD with reversal of the left to right shut. Over time, an unrestricted left to right shunt across the VSD causes pulmonary hypertension. When right sided pressures exceed the left sided pressures, right to left shunting occurs and the patient will develop cyanosis.

Chest radiography will show an enlarged heart and increased pulmonary vascular markings. ECG findings in infants with large defects will show biventricular hypertrophy and left atrial enlargement secondary to the increased pulmonary blood flow.

Management   Infants with congestive heart failure secondary to moderate-to-large defects require oxygenation and assisted ventilation if respiratory compromise is present. Diuretics and inotropic support are the mainstays of early therapy. Consultation with a pediatric cardiologist should be sought as soon as possible.

Acquired Heart Disease

Three types of acquired heart disease affecting children will be discussed in this chapter: myocarditis, rheumatic heart disease, and Kawasaki disease. Because heart disease is uncommon in children, the emergency physician must maintain a high degree of suspicion, and be aware of clinical presentations that differ from the adult population. Respiratory and constitutional symptoms may predominate, especially in infants.

Myocarditis

Epidemiology
Myocarditis is a rare disorder, especially in the United States and other developed countries. However, because of its insidious nature, it is likely to be under-diagnosed, and therefore, the true incidence is unknown.

Pathophysiology
Myocarditis generally refers to the inflammation of the heart muscle. It may occur secondary to any of a number of childhood infections, including viral, bacterial, rickettsial, protozoan, fungal, and parasitic, or it may represent a drug hypersensitivity reaction. Of all the possible etiologies, viral is the most common, specifically Coxsackievirus A and B, and adenovirus.

Clinical Manifestations
The clinical presentation of myocarditis will vary depending on the age and immunocompetence of the child, and the severity of the disease. Newborns are more likely to be severely affected, and myocarditis may be an underlying factor in SIDS cases. There is no pathognomonic finding for myocarditis. The typical clinical presentation is one of vague complaints with a preceding viral prodrome. In the winter months, myocarditis may mimic bronchiolitis, so the clinician must maintain a high index of suspicion.

Fever is a common finding, but hypothermia can also occur. Tachycardia is often out of proportion to the fever. Lethargy or irritability may be noted as well as poor appetite. If the disease progresses to a dilated cardiomyopathy, signs of congestive heart failure will ensue. The child may appear anxious, tachypnic and exhibit grunting, nasal flaring and retractions. Rales and rhonchi may be heard, and heart sounds may be muffled, especially with co-existing pericarditis. An S3 gallop rhythm is also common. Finally, hepatomegaly is a much more common finding than is peripheral edema in children who develop congestive heart failure.

Myocarditis may also coexist with hepatitis or encephalitis in a more severe, generalized illness.

Laboratory Data
Initial laboratory studies should include a complete blood count, acute phase reactants (erythrocyte sedimentation rate and C-reactive protein), blood cultures, and pharyngeal and stool viral cultures. Cardiac enzymes (creatine kinase and troponin) may also be elevated.

EKG findings classically demonstrate low-voltage QRS complexes, with low amplitude or inverted T waves. Dysrhythmias may also be noted, especially sinus tachycardia, paroxysmal atrial tachycardia, and occasionally ventricular dysrhythmias.

Diagnostic Imaging
Chest radiograph may demonstrate cardiomegaly with vascular congestion. However, echocardiography is essential in establishing a diagnosis of myocarditis. It should show poor ventricular function with chamber dilation, and the absence of any structural abnormalities. Magnetic resonance angiography and nuclear imaging may be of diagnostic value in the future.

Endomyocardial biopsy has been considered the gold standard in diagnosis, but is invasive and gives controversial results.

Differential Diagnosis
The differential diagnosis of myocarditis is broad and includes: acute rheumatic fever, bronchiolitis, cardiac tumors, connective tissue disorders, coronary artery anomalies, drug toxicity, hyperthyroidism, idiopathic dilated cardiomyopathy, inborn errors of metabolism, Kawasaki disease, pericarditis, pneumonia, sepsis, structural heart disease, and systemic lupus erythematosus.

Management
Early recognition is paramount in the management of myocarditis. Supportive care is the mainstay of treatment and is aimed at improving myocardial function and reducing afterload.

Diuresis with furosemide (1 mg/kg) and digitalis (dosage varies with age) can improve venous congestion. Inotropic support can be achieved with dobutamine (5–20 μg/kg/min) or dopamine (5–10 μg/kg/min). Afterload can be decreased with nitroprusside (0.5–3 μg/kg/min) or milrinone (0.5–0.75 μg/kg/min). Angiotensin converting enzyme (ACE)-inhibitors such as enalapril and captopril may be used chronically for afterload reduction. Dysrhythmias should be aggressively treated. Immunosuppression with IV immunoglobulin is highly controversial.

The prognosis of myocarditis varies with age. Mortality can be as high as 75% in newborns, whereas older infants and children have an overall mortality of 10% to 25% in clinically diagnosed cases. Approximately one third of children will show chronic residual cardiac dysfunction. Severe dysfunction may require cardiac transplantation.

Rheumatic Heart Disease

Epidemiology

Worldwide, rheumatic heart disease (RHD) is the most common form of acquired heart disease. In the United States and other industrialized nations, the incidence of RHD has dropped sharply over the past century and currently the incidence is approximately 0.5/100,000 population. However, as recently as the 1980s, epidemics have occurred in the United States. Children are primarily affected and the median age is 10 years. The mortality rate is less than 10% and is primarily a function of the degree of cardiac involvement.

Pathophysiology

RHD is a delayed (average 3 weeks), inflammatory response to an upper respiratory infection with group A β-hemolytic streptococci. Approximately 1% to 5% of Group A streptococcal pharyngitis infections are followed by rheumatic fever. Approximately one third of patients with acute rheumatic fever will develop varying degrees of pancarditis (endocarditis, myocarditis, and pericarditis). Endocardial inflammation leads to valvular insufficiency, where the mitral valve is most commonly affected (65%), followed by the aortic (25%), tricuspid (10%), and rarely the pulmonary valve. Rheumatic heart disease is responsible for the vast majority of mitral valve stenosis in adults in the United States. In addition to the heart, acute rheumatic fever may affect the blood vessels, joints, subcutaneous tissue, and the central nervous system.

Clinical Manifestations

There is no single diagnostic test for acute rheumatic fever. The modified (1992) Jones criteria (**Table 90.4**) are used to establish the diagnosis.

Children with RHD may be relatively asymptomatic until they develop pericarditis or heart failure, at which time they may exhibit dyspnea, pleuritic chest pain, cough, orthopnea, and edema. A pericardial friction rub may be heard and pulsus paradoxus (a decrease in systolic blood pressure with inspiration) may indicate impending pericardial tamponade.

Tachycardia will often be out of proportion to the fever. A new or changing murmur may be heard, most often involving the mitral valve.

Laboratory Data

Initial laboratory studies should include a complete blood count, acute phase reactants (erythrocyte sedimentation rate and C-reactive protein), pharyngeal culture, and anti-streptolysin-O (ASO) titers. The clinical presentation of rheumatic fever occurs as the antistreptococcal antibody levels are at their peak.

An EKG should be done to assess the PR interval. Findings consistent with myocarditis or pericarditis may also be seen.

Diagnostic Imaging

Chest radiograph may reveal cardiomegaly, pulmonary congestion, and other findings consistent with heart failure. An echocardiogram can identify and quantify valve insufficiency and ventricular dysfunction.

Differential Diagnosis

Rheumatic fever should be differentiated from aortic stenosis, aortic insufficiency, congestive heart failure, dilated cardiomyopathy, endocarditis, innocent flow murmurs associated with fever, Kawasaki disease, mitral insufficiency or prolapse, pericarditis, and systemic lupus erythematosus.

Management

Children diagnosed with acute rheumatic fever require hospital admission and bed rest. Elimination of Group A streptococcal pharyngitis (after throat cultures are obtained) can be accomplished with oral penicillin G (25–50 mg/kg/day divided 4 times daily) for 10 days or a single dose of intramuscular benzathine penicillin (25,000 U/kg, up to 1.2 million units). Erythromycin (50 mg/kg/day divided 4 times daily) for 10 days can be used in the penicillin-allergic patient. The inflammatory response should be suppressed with aspirin and corticosteroids. While this will have little effect on the carditis, the improvement in the arthritic component should be profound.

Recurrent streptococcal pharyngitis is the most important predisposing factor in the occurrence and recurrence of rheumatic fever and, therefore, prophylaxis is para-

Table 90.4		
Modified Jones Criteria		
Diagnostic Requirements	**Major Criteria**	**Minor Criteria**
Recent Strep infection	Carditis	Prior history of rheumatic fever
Plus	Arthritis	Arthralgia
Two major criteria	Chorea	Fever
Or	Erythema marginatum	Elevated ESR or CRP
One major and two minor criteria	Subcutaneous nodules	Leukocytosis
		Prolonged PR interval

mount. Primary prophylaxis entails treating streptococcal pharyngitis in order to prevent subsequent acute rheumatic fever. Antibiotics are effective in preventing rheumatic fever up to nine days after the onset of pharyngitis. Secondary prophylaxis is aimed at preventing recurrences of rheumatic fever by continuous chemoprophylaxis. This can be accomplished with a monthly dose of intramuscular benzathine penicillin or oral penicillin G twice daily (erythromycin in the penicillin allergic patient). Recurrences decline with age, and are unlikely once the individual has been free of the disease for ten years.

Kawasaki Disease

Epidemiology

Kawasaki disease, also known as mucocutaneous lymph node syndrome, was first described by Tomisaku Kawasaki in 1967. It is an acute, self-limited vasculitis of childhood. The peak incidence is from 13 to 24 months of age. The disease is not seen in newborns and is rare after 12 years of age. Kawasaki is a global disease, but it is most prevalent in Japan. In the United States, approximately 3,000 cases are documented annually, and Kawasaki disease has surpassed acute rheumatic fever as the number one cause of acquired heart disease in children.

Pathophysiology

The etiology of Kawasaki disease is unknown, though it is strongly suspected to be infectious, perhaps requiring genetic predisposition. Its rarity in neonates suggests protection from maternal antibodies, and adults are probably immune from subclinical childhood infection. Other evidence supporting an infectious etiology include its winter–spring seasonality and cyclical epidemics.

Pathologically, Kawasaki disease produces a systemic vasculitis. In autopsy cases, the coronary arteries are virtually always involved and demonstrate saccular or fusiform aneurysms. Children with coronary arteritis progress from severe inflammation to scarring and stenosis, thus predisposing them to myocardial infarction.

Clinical Manifestations

Kawasaki disease is diagnosed based on specific criteria (**Table 90.5**).

The clinical course of Kawasaki disease may be divided into four phases. The first phase is characterized by high fever that frequently exceeds 40.6° C. Fever will persist for a mean duration of 12 days in the untreated child. The second phase begins about the fourth day of illness. At this point, the child may exhibit lymphadenopathy, conjunctivitis, mucosal involvement, and a rash. Around day 12, the third phase ensues, which is characterized by desquamation and resolution of the other symptoms. The fourth phase is variable and consists of persistent inflammation, subacute vasculitis, and increased risk of death from coronary artery involvement.

Laboratory Data

There is no specific diagnostic test for Kawasaki disease. Complete blood count will typically demonstrate leukocy-

Table 90.5
Diagnostic Criteria for Kawasaki Disease
Fever of 5 days duration plus four of the following five findings: 1. Bilateral conjunctival injection without exudate 2. Mucosal involvement (strawberry tongue, cracked lips, oral-pharyngeal erythema) 3. Polymorphic rash 4. Cervical adenopathy (>1.5 cm diameter), usually unilateral 5. Extremity involvement Acute: Erythema of the palms and soles, peripheral edema Subacute: Desquamation of the fingers and toes Exclusion of other diseases with similar clinical presentation.

tosis with a left shift. Thrombocytosis is common during the second week of illness. Mild anemia may also be present. Acute phase reactants (erythrocyte sedimentation rate and C-reactive protein) will be elevated. Transaminases (AST and ALT) may also be elevated, but generally not more that three times normal. Hypoalbuminemia, hyponatremia, hypophosphatemia, and proteinuria may also be seen.

An EKG may show PR and QT prolongation, ischemic changes, and dysrhythmias.

Diagnostic Imaging

A chest radiograph may show cardiomegaly and pulmonary infiltrates. Echocardiography should be performed as soon as the diagnosis is suspected in order to assess the coronary arteries and left ventricular function. Magnetic resonance angiography can also accurately diagnose coronary artery aneurysms.

Differential Diagnosis

Several conditions can mimic Kawasaki disease, especially Group A β-hemolytic streptococcal infection and measles. Other conditions to consider include: drug reactions, infectious mononucleosis, meningococcemia, mercury toxicity, Rocky Mountain spotted fever, roseola infantum, scarlet fever, toxic epidermal necrolysis, and toxic shock syndrome.

Management

Treatment of Kawasaki disease is aimed at reducing the inflammatory response and decreasing the severity of cardiac complications. Aspirin and IV immune globulin (IVIG) have been the mainstay of treatment. Aspirin is administered in high doses (80 to 100 mg/kg/day divided into 4 doses) during the acute phase of the illness. However, it does not appear to decrease the incidence of coronary abnormalities. Children treated with aspirin are at risk for Reye syndrome and should receive an annual influenza vaccine. Unlike aspirin, IVIG (2 g/kg as a single infusion) has been proven to reduce the prevalence of coronary artery abnormalities (from 20% to as little as 3%) when administered during the acute phase of the disease (first 10 days). IVIG redosing may be beneficial in children who have persistent or recurrent fever after the initial infusion. Pentoxifylline is an inhibitor of tumor necrosis factor-alpha (TNF-α; involved in the inflammatory cascade) and is currently being evaluated as adjunctive therapy.

The prognosis of Kawasaki disease largely depends on the severity of coronary involvement. Death occurs in approximately 1% of affected children in the United States, and is usually the result of coronary artery thrombosis.

Rhythm Disturbances

Dysrhythmias Life-threatening cardiac arrhythmias are uncommon in children. When they occur, however, they are frequently associated with a noncardiac condition. Primary cardiac arrhythmias are usually seen in children with complex congenital heart disease (septal defects, tetralogy of Fallot) both before and after surgical correction. Acquired cardiac conditions associated with rhythm disturbances include cardiomyopathy, myocarditis, rheumatic heart disease, cardiac tumors and thoracic trauma.

In some instances, children with a cardiac arrhythmia are hemodynamically stable. Patients who are clinically stable generally do not require emergent treatment of their arrhythmia prior to a full evaluation and, in some cases, cardiology consultation. However, these patients require continuous cardiac monitoring and frequent reevaluation. Common arrhythmias that usually do not require emergency treatment include: sinus arrhythmia, premature ectopic beats, sinus bradycardia, sinus tachycardia, and first-degree atrioventricular heart block.

Cardiac arrhythmias that compromise cardiac output are considered to be unstable rhythms and present with clinical conditions such as cardiopulmonary arrest, shock, syncope, altered mental status, or signs of congestive heart failure. Older children may describe palpitations, chest pain, or a decrease in their level of activity.

The American Heart Association has provides a practical approach to initial treatment of arrhythmias in children by classifying them into slow, fast, and collapse (no cardiac output) rhythms. This section focuses on the identification, evaluation, and management of the symptomatic patient with an abnormal cardiac rhythm.

Evaluation and Management The initial management of a child with a cardiac arrhythmia begins with rapid cardiopulmonary assessment of airway, breathing and circulation looking for deficits in oxygenation, ventilation and perfusion. The initial diagnosis of an arrhythmia may be based on a rhythm strip (fast, slow, absent/collapse). However, a 12-lead electrocardiogram is necessary to evaluate abnormalities in conduction, especially Wolff-Parkinson-White and prolonged QT syndromes, and voltage criteria for chamber hypertrophy. Identification of an abnormal rate requires knowledge of normal heart rates for a given age. Mean heart rates in infants and children decrease with age.

A chest radiograph is helpful to evaluate cardiac silhouette, heart size, pulmonary vascularity, and signs of congestive heart failure. Appropriate laboratory studies should be obtained to rule out other medical conditions as indicated. In the unstable patient, treatment should not be delayed while waiting for diagnostic studies. In the stable patient, further evaluation may include Holter monitoring or echocardiography after consultation with a pediatric cardiologist.

Slow Rhythms Sinus bradycardia (normal P waves and conduction) may be normal, particularly in a sleeping child or an athletic adolescent, and usually does not require any further evaluation or treatment. In the patient being treated for a known cardiac condition, a slower than normal heart rate may be secondary to the effects of medications (digoxin, beta blockers, calcium channel blockers). Sick sinus syndrome may also present with sinus bradycardia or a slow junctional rhythm. Principles of treatment are the same as with other bradyarrhythmias.

Clinically significant bradycardia is defined as a heart rate of <60 bpm associated with signs of poor perfusion. Sinus bradycardia in young children with cardiopulmonary failure is almost always due to prolonged hypoxia and not primary cardiac disease. It is important for the emergency physician to recognize that symptomatic bradycardia is a pre-arrest rhythm and requires immediate initiate resuscitation to correct the underlying pathology. Pharmacologic management consists of epinephrine and atropine, and rarely cardiac pacing (**FIGURE 90.4**).

Atrioventricular heart block (AVHB) is recognized by electrocardiographic abnormalities in conduction between the atria and ventricles. First-degree AVHB is represented by a prolonged PR interval for the patient's age and is usually of no particular consequence for the child unless associated with an abnormal underlying condition (digitalis toxicity). Second-degree heart block is of two varieties, Mobitz type I or Wenckebach phenomenon, and Mobitz type II. Second-degree AVHB may be seen in normal children, or in those with myocarditis, cardiomyopathy, myocardial infarction, congenital heart disease before and after operative repair, or digitalis toxicity. Therapy consists of treating the underlying cause, and may sometimes require the use of a pacemaker.

Third-degree AVHB, or complete heart block, results in complete dissociation between atrial and ventricular impulses. Ventricular rates are usually 40 to 60 beats per minute and have a regular rhythm. Third-degree blocks are commonly due to pathological cardiac defects, perinatal conditions (maternal systemic lupus erythematosus), or drug ingestion, and may or may not be associated with bradycardia. Postsurgical complete heart block may be transient or permanent and with current surgical advances accounts for <2% of these patients.

Treatment of third-degree AVHB is based on medical management of congestive heart failure and bradycardia. In the absence of structural defects and evidence of poor perfusion, and if the heart rates remain above approximately 55 to 60 bpm, most children do not require emergency intervention; however, all of these patients need

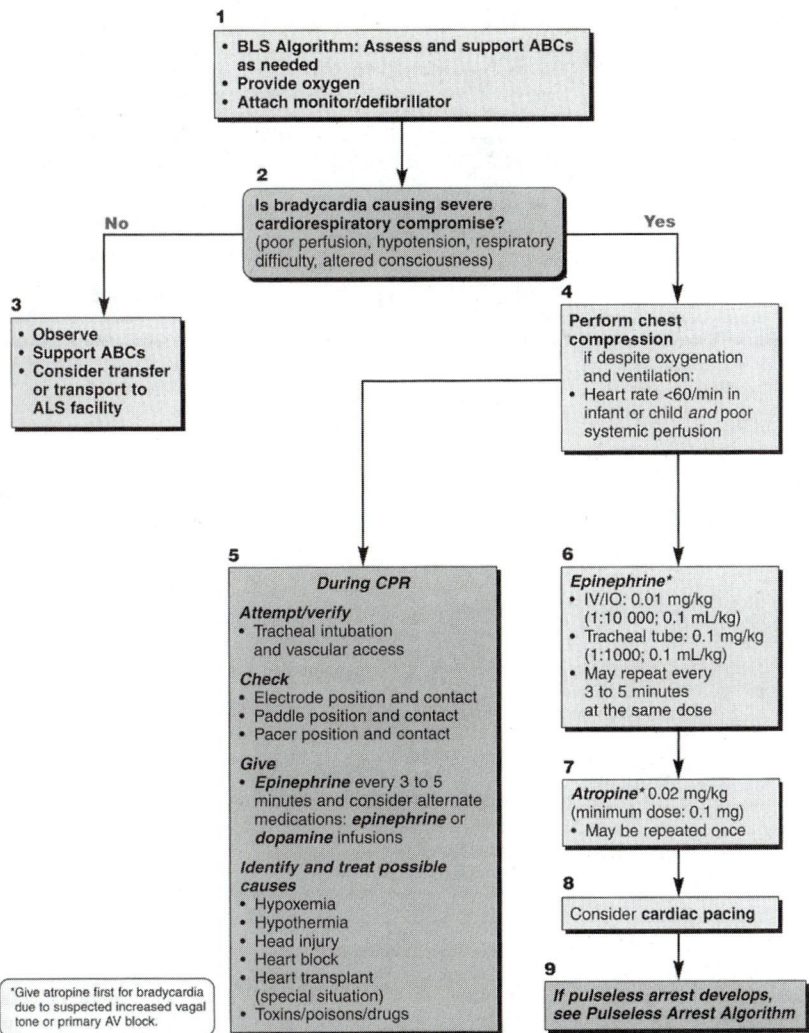

FIGURE 90.4 Treatment of symptomatic bradycardia. *Source:* Used with permission from the American Heart Association. Chameides L, Hazinski MF, eds. *American Heart Association: Pediatric Advanced Life Support.* Dallas: American Heart Association, 2000.

cardiology consultation and ultimately require permanent pacing.

For those children with bradyarrhythmias who fail medical intervention in the ED, transesophageal, transvenous, or transthoracic pacing may be performed by an experienced physician. Most emergency physicians find transcutaneous pacing to be a faster and easier procedure. Familiarity with the equipment is important. Of note, transcutaneous pacing, while easier to perform, can cause full-thickness burns in young children with prolonged use, and more permanent pacing should be sought as soon as possible.

Fast Rhythms The most common tachyarrhythmias seen in the pediatric population are sinus tachycardia and supraventricular tachycardia (SVT). Sinus tachycardia is an expected physiologic response to an alteration in hemodynamic status (dehydration, fever), and treatment is based on correction of the underlying cause. SVT usually represents AV nodal reentry above the bundle of His. It is the most common clinically significant arrhythmia in pediatrics and it is rarely lethal. In infants 50% of cases are

idiopathic, 20% are associated with underlying infection or drug exposure, 20% are with congenital heart disease, and 10% to 25% with Wolff-Parkinson-White syndrome. Features that may be helpful in distinguishing sinus tachycardia and supraventricular tachycardia are outlined in **Table 90.6.**

Traditionally, patients with stable supraventricular tachycardia can be treated with vagal maneuvers to induce the diving reflex, such as ice packs to the midface, facial submersion, or carotid massage. However, these maneuvers should be attempted only if the physician is prepared for potential deterioration of the patient. Valsalva and carotid massage are less effective in patients under the age of 4 years. Atropine should be available when attempting any of the various vagal maneuvers.

Adenosine is an endogenous nucleoside that exerts a suppressive effect on the sinus and atrioventricular nodes and can interrupt reentry pathways. Adenosine is considered the drug of choice for the treatment of SVT. While there are some transient side effects (facial flushing, nausea, chest pain, dyspnea, and brief asystole), adenosine has a very short half-life and is safe in all pediatric age

Table 90.6

Sinus Tachycardia versus Supraventricular Tachycardia (SVT)

	Sinus Tachycardia	SVT
History/physical examination	Fever, pain/anxiety, dehydration	Nonspecific history of poor feeding, anemia (blood loss), medications, lethargy. Signs of congestive heart failure may be present.
ECG	Heart rate usually <220 Variable heart rate Normal P wave	Heart rate usually >220; often higher Nonvarying heart rate ORS may be wide (resembling VT)

groups. The initial dose of adenosine is 0.1 mg/kg administered as a rapid intravenous bolus. If the initial dose is unsuccessful, a repeat dose of 0.2 to 0.3 mg/kg to a maximum adult dose of 12 mg should be given. Continuous cardiac monitoring is required during the administration of adenosine (or any cardiac medication), and the ability to record the rhythm during treatment is advised. Because

of its short half-life adenosine must be administered by a rapid IV push followed immediately by a rapid bolus of normal saline. Placement of as large bore and central IV is desirable.

Verapamil, a calcium channel blocker, is used in older children and adults for the medical management of SVT. Its use is contraindicated in younger children (particularly

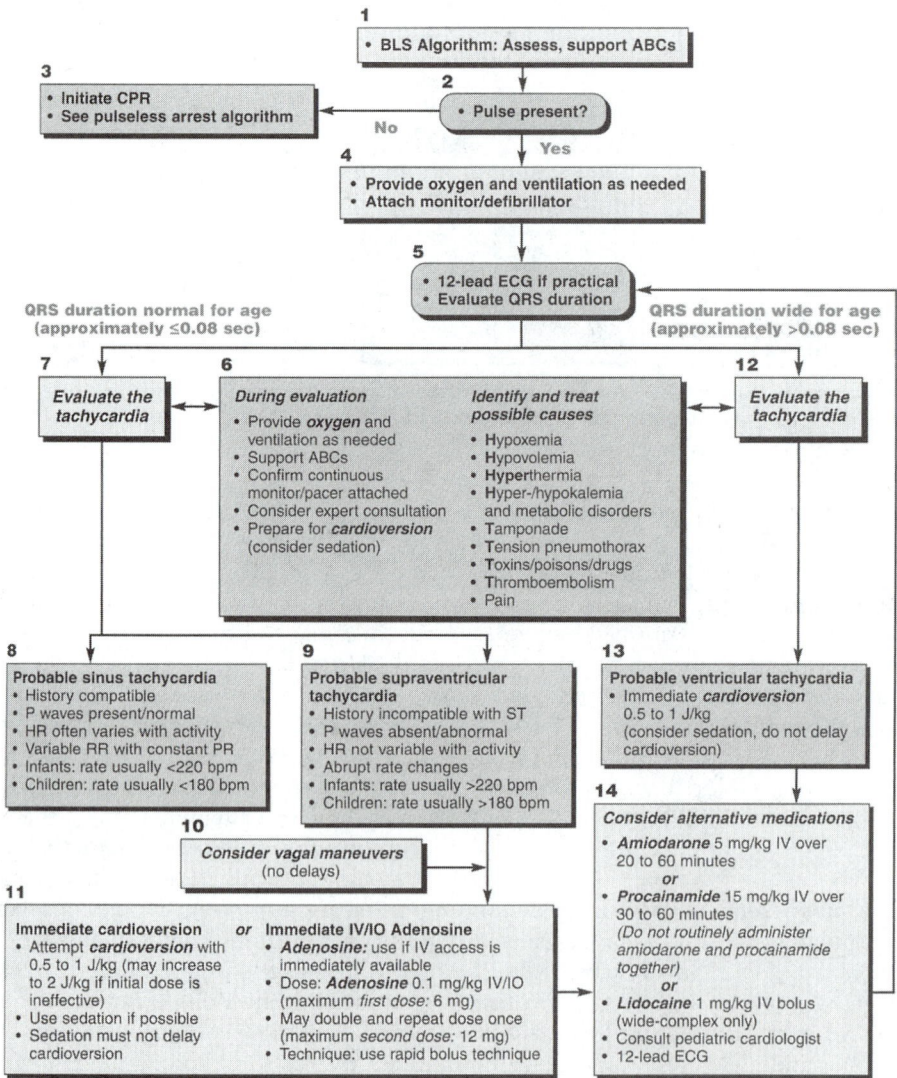

FIGURE 90.5 Treatment of tachycardia with poor perfusion: sinus tachycardia, supraventricular tachycardia, ventricular tachycardia with pulse. Used with permission from the American Heart Association. Chameides L, Hazinski MF, eds. *American Heart Association: Pediatric Advanced Life Support*. Dallas: American Heart Association, 2000.

younger than 1-year-old) because it can induce profound myocardial depression and circulatory collapse. Calcium should be available for intravenous administration. Other medications, including digoxin, propranolol, and procainamide are generally reserved for the long-term management of recurrent SVT and should only be administered following stabilization and cardiology consultation.

In the unstable patient with SVT, synchronized cardioversion should be performed without delay. Sedation should be considered in the conscious and alert child; however, this clinical situation is rare. Infant paddles (4.5 cm) should be used for the pediatric patient weighing less than 10 kg. Synchronized cardioversion is initiated at 0.5 J/kg and doubled (maximum 2–4 J/kg) until the rhythm converts. An experienced physician and necessary equipment must be available should the patient deteriorate. Overdrive pacing may be necessary if cardioversion and medical management fail. At this point it is generally helpful to have pediatric cardiology consultation.

Ventricular tachycardia (with a pulse) is unusual in the pediatric patient and is considered a potentially lethal arrhythmia. Sudden death occurs in approximately 30% of patients with congenital heart disease with ventricular tachycardia. VT in children with a normal heart carries a more favorable prognosis. Ventricular tachycardia may be seen in children with prolonged QT syndrome, cardiomyopathies, myocarditis, following cardiovascular surgery, and after ingestion of drugs. Treatment depends on hemodynamic stability. Management should be based on prevention of deterioration to ventricular fibrillation and avoiding recurrence.

Atrial fibrillation and flutter are rare in children and are usually associated with cardiac disease. In the patient with atrial flutter with 1:1 conduction, a fast ventricular rate may be seen. Atrial rates range from 200 to 350 beats per minute. Patients with atrial fibrillation have an irregularly irregular rhythm, without P waves on ECG. If signs of cardiogenic shock are present, synchronized cardioversion should be performed and overdrive cardiac pacing may

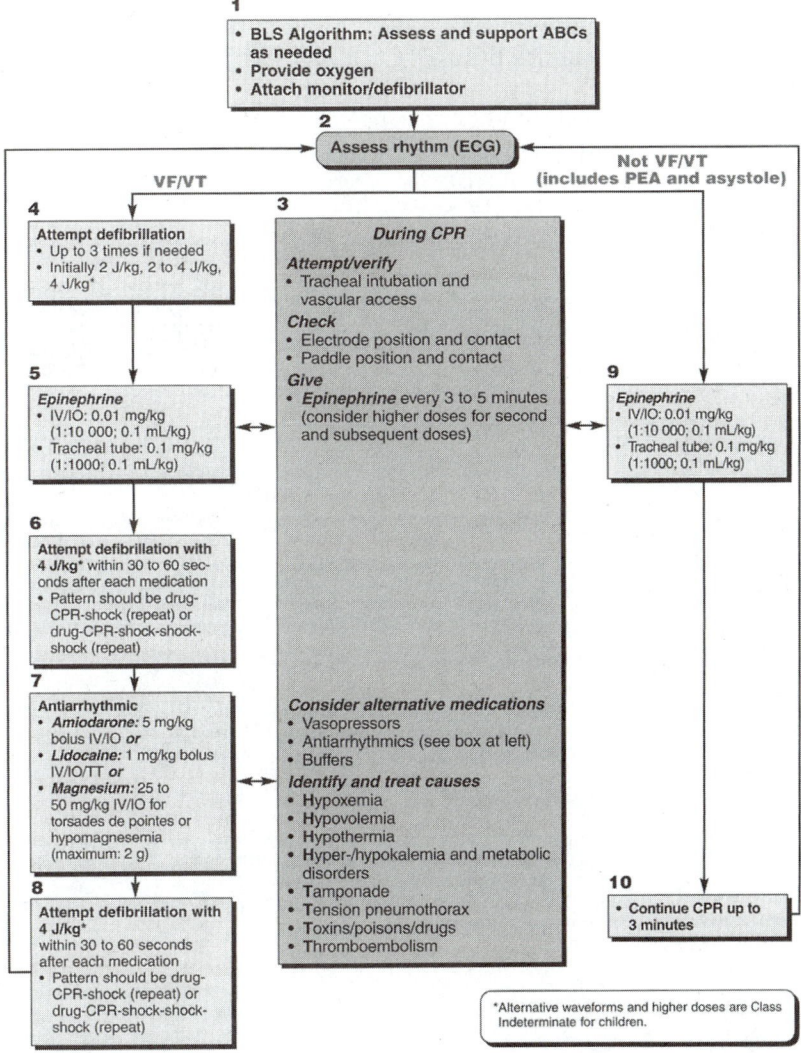

FIGURE 90.6 Treatment of collapse rhythms: asystole, VF, and VT without pulse. *Source:* Used with permission from the American Heart Association. Chameides L, Hazinski MF, eds. *American Heart Association: Pediatric Advanced Life Support.* Dallas: American Heart Association, 2000.

also be necessary. However, most cases of atrial fibrillation and flutter do not require emergent management. Consultation with a pediatric cardiologist is recommend if overdrive pacing is required and for further pharmacologic intervention (**FIGURE 90.5**).

Collapse Rhythms   Collapse rhythms are associated with no cardiac output. They include: asystole, ventricular fibrillation, ventricular tachycardia without pulse, and pulseless electrical activity (PEA). Asystole is the most common presenting rhythm in children who suffer an out-of-hospital cardiac arrest. The intact neurologic survival of children who present in the field or the ED in asystole is extremely low. Epinephrine (standard dose 0.01 mg/kg) drug is of primary value in the treatment of asystole. Transcutaneous pacing has not been found to be effective in pediatric patients presenting with asystole.

Pulseless electrical activity (PEA), formerly called electromechanical dissociation (EMD), is the presence of a rhythm on the ECG without a pulse or cardiac output. Treatment is the same as for asystole with aggressive evaluation for the cause of PEA. Causes of PEA are listed in **Table 90.7**.

Ventricular fibrillation is a relatively uncommon rhythm in healthy children. Treatment consists of electrical asynchronous defibrillation (2 J/kg then 4 J/kg) followed by antiarythmic infusion (**FIGURE 90.6**).

Prolonged QT syndrome is an inherited condition (Jervell and Lange-Nielsen or Romano-Ward syndromes). Affected children are at risk for syncope, seizures, dysrhythmias, and sudden death. A family history should be obtained from these patients with regard to syncopal episodes, congenital deafness, and sudden death. Syncope that is either recurrent or induced by exercise or stress is concerning and requires careful evaluation. Calculation of the corrected QT interval (QT interval in seconds/square root of RR interval in seconds) for heart rate during sinus rhythm should be performed on all patients with a suspicious history. Intervals >0.45 seconds considered to be significant. Death is due to ventricular arrhythmia and torsades de pointes, with degeneration to ventricular fibrillation and asystole. Prolonged QT is also seen with certain medications (antiarrhythmic agents, phenothiazines, tricyclic antidepressants, lithium) and metabolic abnormalities. Treatment includes lidocaine and cardioversion or temporary atrial or ventricular pacing, particularly if bradycardia is present.

Selected Readings

American Heart Association. Guidelines for the diagnosis of rheumatic fever. Jones Criteria, 1992 update. Committee on Rheumatic Fever, Endocarditis, and Kawasaki Disease of the Council on Cardiovascular Disease in the Young, the American Heart Association. *JAMA* 1992;268:2069–2073.

Chameides L, Hazinski MF, eds. *American Heart Association: Pediatric Advanced Life Support*. Dallas: American Heart Association, 2000.

Dimaio AM, Singh J. The infant with cyanosis in the emergency room. Pediatr Clin North Am. 1992;39:987–1006.

El-Said GM. Rheumatic fever. In: *Oski's Principles and Practices of Pediatrics*, ed 3. Philadelphia: Lippincott, 1999.

Epstein ML, Kiel EA, Victorica BE. Cardiac decompensation following verapamil therapy in infants with supraventricular tachycardia. *Pediatrics* 1985;75:737–740.

Feigin RD. Kawasaki disease. In: *Oski's Principles and Practices of Pediatrics*, ed 3. Philadelphia: Lippincott, 1999.

Friedman RA. Myocarditis. In: *Oski's Principles and Practices of Pediatrics*, ed 3. Philadelphia: Lippincott, 1999.

Gerber MA. Group A Strep. In: *Nelson Textbook of Pediatrics*, ed 17. Basel: Elsevier, 2004.

Gausche M, Persse DE, Sugarman T, et al. Adenosine for the prehospital treatment of paroxysmal supraventricular tachycardia. *Ann Emerg Med* 1994;24:183–189.

Gewitz MH, Vetter VL. Cardiac emergencies. In: Fleisher GR, Ludwig S, eds. *Textbook of Pediatric Emergency Medicine*, ed 3. Baltimore: Williams & Wilkins, 1993.

Kawasaki T. Acute febrile mucocutaneous syndrome with lymphoid involvement with specific desquamation of the fingers and toes in children. [in Japanese] *Arerugi* 1967;16:178–222.

Levin DL, Morriss FC. *Pediatric Intensive Care*. New York: Churchill Livingstone Inc., 1997.

Muta H. Early intravenous gamma-globulin treatment for Kawasaki disease: the nationwide surveys in Japan. *J Pediatr* 2004;144:496–499.

Newburger JW. Diagnosis, treatment, and long-term management of Kawasaki disease: a statement for health professionals from the Committee on Rheumatic Fever, Endocarditis, and Kawasaki Disease, Council on Cardiovascular Disease in the Young, American Heart Association. *Pediatrics* 2004;114:1708–1733.

Nichols DG, Cameron DE, Greeley WJ, et al. *Critical Heart Disease in Infants and Children*. St. Louis: Mosby-Year Book, Inc., 1995.

Park MK. *Pediatric Cardiology for Practitioners*, ed 2. Chicago: Year Book, 1988.

Park MK. *Pediatric Cardiology for Practitioners*, ed 4. St. Louis: Mosby, Inc., 2002.

Pfammatter JP, Paul T. Idiopathic ventricular tachycardia in infancy and childhood: a multicenter study on clinical profile and outcome. Electrophysiology of the Association for European Pediatric Cardiology. *J Am Coll Cardiol* 1999;33: 2067–2072.

Rasten-Almquist P, Eksborg S, Rajs J. Heart weight in infants: a comparison between sudden death infant syndrome and other causes of death. *Acta Paediatr* 2000;89:1032–1037.

Schamberger MS. Cardiac emergencies in children. *Pediatr Ann* 25:339–344, 1996.

Schulze-Bahr E, Monnig G, Eckardt L. The long QT syndrome: considerations in the athletic population. *Curr Sports Med Rep* 2003;2:72–78.

Sra J, Dhala A, Blanck Z. Sudden cardiac death. *Curr Probl Cardiol* 1999;24: 461–538.

Taubert KA, Rowley AH, Shulman ST. Nationwide survey of Kawasaki disease and acute rheumatic fever. *J Pediatr* 1991;119:279–282.

Tweddell JS, Hoffman GM, Mussatto KA, et al. Improved survival of patients undergoing palliation of hypoplastic left heart syndrome: lessons learned from 115 consecutive patients. *Circulation* 2002;106(Suppl 1):182–189.

Tworetzky W, McElhinney DB, Reddy VM, et al. Improved surgical outcome after fetal diagnosis of hypoplastic left heart syndrome. *Circulation* 2001;103:1269–1273.

Veasy LG, Wiedmeier SE, Orsmond GS, et al. Resurgence of acute rheumatic fever in the intermountain area of the United States. *N Engl J Med* 1987;316: 421–427.

Wheeler DS, Kooy NW. A formidable challenge: the diagnosis and treatment of viral myocarditis in children. *Crit Care Clin* 2003;19:365–391.

Table 90.7
Conditions Associated with Pulseless Electrical Activity
Tension pneumothorax
Pericardial tamponade
Hypovolemia
Acidosis
Pulmonary embolism
Hypoxemia
Profound hypothermia
Hyperkalemia
Drug overdose

Seizures

Douglas Nelson

Approximately 5% of children have a seizure before age 16. Priorities of initial management of this problem include: addressing airway, breathing and circulation; controlling ongoing seizure activity; and determining seizure etiology. Accomplishing these objectives is often difficult. Obtaining an accurate history may be time consuming. Neurological evaluation of the patient may be complicated by continued seizures, postictal state, or pharmacologic sedation. Obtaining vascular access in the actively seizuring young child is technically challenging. To help overcome these obstacles, this section summarizes seizure classification, reviews common etiologies of childhood seizures (**Table 91.1**), and details the evaluation and acute management of the pediatric seizure patient.

Seizure Terminology, Classification, and Pathophysiology

Seizures result from the abnormal hypersynchronous discharge of large numbers of CNS neurons. The location of these cells and the etiology of their abnormal activity determine the clinical appearance and duration of the seizure. Seizures may be preceded by a prodrome and followed by a postictal period. Epilepsy is a condition predisposing a patient to have recurrent seizures and synonymous with the term *seizure disorder*. The term *convulsion* is often used to indicate a seizure of any type, but properly signifies only those seizures with prominent motor manifestations.

Seizures are classified as partial or generalized. Partial (focal) seizures are due to abnormal neuronal activity in one locus of the brain, and may have primarily sensory or motor manifestations. Partial seizures are subclassified as simple if consciousness is not impaired or complex if it is impaired. Complex partial seizures, formerly called temporal lobe or psychomotor seizures, may involve repetitive motor acts (automatisms) preceded by an aura. A simple partial seizure may evolve into a complex one, and either type may become generalized.

Generalized seizures result from abnormal neuronal activity in both hemispheres of the brain, and impair consciousness by definition. Absence seizures, formerly known as petit mal seizures, produce brief interruptions

in consciousness lasting from seconds to a minute, without a postictal phase. Minor motor movements such as lip smacking or eye fluttering may occur. The majority of generalized seizures produce bilateral major muscle movements, consisting of contractions (tonic movements) or rapidly alternating contractions and relaxations (clonic movements). Atonic seizures are an exception; they are characterized by a sudden loss of motor tone. Generalized tonic-clonic seizures are the most common type seen in children, starting with a 5- to 30-second period of intense muscle contraction followed by jerking clonic movements of all extremities. Generalized seizures are typically followed by a postictal period lasting minutes to hours during which the patient has a diminished but slowly improving level of consciousness. Infantile spasms are myoclonic seizures that present in the young infant. Consisting of rapid flexion at the neck, hip, and knees with bilateral arm extension, this condition has a poor prognosis and is often refractory to medical management.

Febrile Seizures

Febrile seizures occur in 3% to 5% of children by their fifth birthday. They are the response of an immature central nervous system to rapid changes in body temperature. They usually occur within the first 24 hours of a febrile illness, in children between 6 months and 6 years of age. Their peak onset occurs during the second year of life. Parents may not suspect illness and may report finding the children febrile and seizing. A simple febrile seizure (**Table 91.2**) is a short, generalized seizure in a developmentally normal child who does not have evidence of an intracranial infection. The patient should quickly return to a normal mental status. Only one simple febrile seizure occurs per febrile illness. Complex febrile seizures are focal, prolonged, or multiple (more than one seizure per illness).

The diagnosis of febrile seizure is one of exclusion, especially in a child without prior history of such an event. Well-appearing children over 9 to 12 months of age who quickly return to a normal mental status following a simple febrile seizure often require only an evaluation for the source of fever. Occult urinary tract infection is common in this population.

Table 91.1
Etiology of Seizures

Febrile Seizures
- Simple[a] vs. complex

Underlying neurological disease
- Idiopathic[a]
- Congenital CNS abnormalities
- Neurodegenerative disease
- Post-CNS injury (trauma, infection, anoxia)
- Subtherapeutic anticonvulsant levels[a]

Infection
- Meningitis
- Intracranial abscess
- Encephalitis
- Parasitic (cysticercosis)
- Shigellosis
- Rotavirus

Neoplasms
- CNS primary
- Metastatic to CNS

Trauma
- Concussion[a]
- Intracranial hemorrhage
- Cerebral edema/contusion

Child abuse
- Shaken baby syndrome
- Drug administration
- Munchausen syndrome by proxy

Metabolic
- Hypoglycemia
- Hyponatremia
- Hypocalcemia
- Hypomagnesemia

Other causes
- Toxins
- Hypertensive encephalopathy
- Iatrogenic
- Pyridoxine dependency
- Thyrotoxicosis/hypothyroidism
- Inborn errors of metabolism
- Uremia

Paroxysmal disorders simulating seizures
- Breath-holding spells
- Syncope
- Night terrors

[a]Most common.

Table 91.2
Criteria for Diagnosis of a Simple Febrile Seizure

Patient is febrile (temperature usually $\geq 102°$ F)
Patient age between 6 months and 6 years
Generalized tonic-clonic type without focal onset
Seizure is self-limiting, no treatment required
Seizure occurs at onset of illness (first 24 hours)
Seizure duration <10 minutes
Minimal postictal symptoms
Previously neurologically normal child
No other etiology present (e.g., trauma)
Family history often present

The diagnosis of meningitis should be considered in children with febrile seizure who have had a complex febrile seizure (prolonged, focal, multiple); have been pretreated with antibiotics; have a prolonged abnormal mental status; and who are young (less than 9 to 12 months of age). These children usually require lumbar puncture for CSF analysis and culture. In children with a history of trauma, a history of focal seizure, or focality on exam, a head CT scan is recommended prior to lumbar puncture.

Febrile seizures have an overall recurrence rate of 30%. Risk factors for recurrence include: age <18 months, an initial febrile convulsion that was complex, and a positive family history. Care must be taken to educate the family about the risk of recurrence and to reassure them that the prognosis of simple febrile seizures is good. They must also be cautioned about leaving a febrile child unsupervised in a bathtub, where a seizure may lead to drowning.

The American Academy of Pediatrics has addressed the benefit of continuous or intermittent anticonvulsants in children with simple febrile seizures. After examining evidence for use of phenobarbital, valproic acid, or intermittent diazepam, they concluded that although effective in reducing the risk of seizure recurrence, the toxicities associated with their use outweighed any benefits.

CNS or Systemic Infections

Central nervous system infection should be suspected in any child with seizures, fever, and signs of toxicity. Seizures may be the result of infectious processes caused by viral, bacterial, or parasitic pathogens. Seizures are seen in 25% of children with bacterial meningitis, and are common in herpes meningoencephalitis during the first weeks of life. Nonmeningeal CNS foci such as intracerebral and epidural abscesses, as well as infections located outside the central nervous system may cause seizures. Gastrointestinal infection with toxin-producing *Shigella* may produce seizures before the onset of diarrhea. Rotavirus infection may also produce convulsions in infants and small children in the absence of electrolyte imbalance.

A lumbar puncture must be performed in children with fever, seizures, and any signs of CNS infection once they are clinically stable. Pretreatment with antibiotics for non-CNS infections (e.g., otitis media) may delay but not eliminate the onset of disease, and should therefore lower the clinician's threshold for performing a lumbar puncture. A CT scan prior to lumbar puncture should be considered in patients with focal seizures, a focal neurological examination, or signs of increased ICP (bulging fontanelle or blurred optic disk margins), to rule out intracranial hemorrhage, tumor, or abscess. Unstable or critically ill patients suspected of having bacterial meningitis should receive antibiotic therapy prior to lumbar puncture if obtaining CSF will be delayed, or deemed inadvisable.

Underlying Neurological Disease

Many chronic neurologic conditions predispose a child to seizures, including idiopathic epilepsy, congenital CNS abnormalities, neurodegenerative diseases, and residual CNS injury from trauma or anoxia. Convulsions due to these conditions are usually recurrent, with exacerbations sparked by intercurrent illnesses. Subtherapeutic anticonvulsant levels are a common treatable cause of convulsions in patients with seizure disorders. This may be caused by vomiting, poor compliance, or weight gain without corresponding dose adjustment.

Evaluation of the neurologically impaired child with a chronic seizure disorder may be complicated by an abnormal baseline neurologic examination and resulting communication difficulties. For this reason, the emergency physician must rely heavily on the child's caregivers' impressions and input from primary care and subspecialty providers. Subtherapeutic anticonvulsant levels and other medical problems are not mutually exclusive. Infections such as otitis media, aspiration pneumonia, and urinary tract infections occur at higher rates among neurologically impaired patients than the general population, and can exacerbate an underlying seizure disorder.

Accidental Trauma or Child Abuse

Posttraumatic seizures may occur immediately after an impact to the head, or at any time afterwards. Those occurring immediately after trauma are usually generalized and, if brief, do not require treatment. Seizures occurring within hours to the first several days after trauma may signal the presence of serious focal injury such as a cerebral contusion or hemorrhage. They are often focal in nature and typically require treatment for control. Approximately 20% of these patients have recurrent posttraumatic seizures. Those convulsions occurring more than 1 week after an episode of head trauma are thought to occur as a result of scar formation at the site of focal injury, and result in chronic seizures in up to 75% of patients. A head CT scan is indicated in the evaluation of a patient with new onset of seizures after head trauma to rule out focal lesions or bleeding.

Seizures may be the presentation of child abuse in infants. The infant with shaken baby syndrome (SBS) typically presents with seizures, depressed level of consciousness and shock. Intracranial bleeding in these infants results from a high-speed acceleration-deceleration mechanism produced by vigorous shaking. Physical examination may be unremarkable for external trauma. Retinal hemorrhages and unusual bruises are highly suggestive of inflicted injury. Signs of trauma including bruising and skull fracture are more likely to be present with direct impact to the skull. When nonaccidental trauma is suspected, a skeletal survey and pediatric ophthalmologic exam should be performed in conjunction with CNS imaging and appropriate protective services consultation.

Munchausen syndrome by proxy may present with actual observable seizures, or falsely reported ones. Actual seizures may be the result of intentional manipulation of anticonvulsant levels or the forced ingestion of seizurogenic substances. Falsely reported seizures should be suspected when parents claim that their otherwise well child has seizures that: (1) have never been witnessed by others; (2) are not accompanied by a post-ictal state; and (3) never produce signs of physical trauma, such as contusions or lacerations (see also Chapter 98, Child Maltreatment).

Metabolic Abnormalities

Abnormal concentrations of any compound used by neurons to generate energy (oxygen, glucose), transmit impulses (sodium, calcium), or maintain neuronal homeostasis (pyridoxine) may cause seizures. The most common metabolic disorders presenting with seizures in children are hypoglycemia, hyponatremia, and hypocalcemia.

Hypoglycemia may be the primary cause of seizures or the result of prolonged status epilepticus. Nonspecific neurological signs (irritability, headache, and confusion) commonly precede seizures due to hypoglycemia. Hypoglycemia can result from decreased oral intake or prolonged overnight fast in small children, sepsis, adrenal insufficiency, hypothyroidism, insulin overdose, or ingestion of medications (salicylates, ethanol, hypoglycemic drugs). American Heart Association Pediatric Life Support guidelines recommend IV administration of 0.5 to 1 g/kg of glucose for documented or suspected hypoglycemia (2–4 mL/kg of D25).

Hyponatremia is defined as a serum sodium <130 mEq/L, but seizures are rarely seen until this value falls below 120 mEq/L. The risk of seizure with hyponatremia also depends on the rate of fall of the serum sodium. The most common etiology for hyponatremia in young children is the consumption of hypotonic solutions such as plain water or overly-dilute formula, in a setting of excessive GI fluid losses.

Hypocalcemia is present when serum calcium values fall below 9.0 mg/dL. Common etiologies for this include hypoparathyroidism or disorders of vitamin D. Hypocalcemic seizures may be accompanied by vomiting, irritability, tetany, and positive Chvostek and Trousseau signs. Serum magnesium levels below 1.5 mEq/L may cause similar signs of neuromuscular irritability.

CNS and Metastatic Neoplasms

Intracranial neoplasms are the most common type of solid tumors in childhood. They may cause seizures due to abnormal neuronal function within the tumor itself, or in surrounding structures. The type and duration of seizure, as well as degree of illness on presentation, varies depending on tumor location, number, and size. Since pediatric (**Table 91.3**) are most commonly located infratentorially, a preexisting history of cerebellar dysfunction including vertigo or ataxia may be elicited, along with symptoms of increased intracranial pressure such as morning headache and/or vomiting. The primary tumors located outside the central nervous system most likely to metastasize to the

Table 91.3
Distribution of Common Brain Tumors in Children

Location and Type of Tumor	Percentage of All Brain Tumors
Infratentorial	45–60
PNET (medulloblastoma)	20–25
Low-grade astrocytoma, cerebellar	12–18
Ependymoma	4–8
Malignant glioma, brain stem	3–9
Supratentorial hemispheric	25–40
Low-grade astrocytoma	8–20
Malignant glioma	6–12
Ependymoma	2–5
Supratentorial midline	15–20
Craniopharyngioma	6–9
Low-grade glioma, chiasmatic-hypothalamic	4–8

Source: Adapted from Pollack IF. Brain tumors in children. *N Engl J Med* 1994;33:1500.

brain include rhabdomyosarcoma, Ewing's sarcoma, osteogenic sarcoma, and lymphoma.

Other Causes

A partial list of substances causing seizures is shown in **Table 91.4**. Pediatric intoxications may be unwitnessed, involve a high dose on a mg/kg basis, and be complicated by a young patient's inability to provide information regarding the quantity or identity of the substance ingested. The availability in the home of any of the substances listed in Table 91.4 should be thoroughly explored when taking a history in the case of a child with the new onset of afebrile seizures. Caregivers may be reluctant to reveal the presence in the home of illegal substances, such as cocaine.

Hypertensive encephalopathy may present with seizures, usually accompanied by headache, nausea, vomit-

Table 91.4
Compounds Causing Seizures

Amphetamines	Lindane
Belladonna alkaloids	Lithium
Caffeine	Methamphetamine
Camphor	Nicotine
Carbon monoxide	Organophosphates
Cocaine	Phencyclidine
Cyanide	Phenothiazines
Ethanol	Phenylpropanolamine
Hypoglycemics	Pseudoephedrine
Insulin	Salicylates
Isoniazid	Theophylline
Lead	Tricyclic antidepressants
Lidocaine	

ing, altered mental status, or visual disturbance. Seizures may result from iatrogenic causes. These include hyponatremia secondary to intravenous (IV) administration of hypotonic fluids. Lidocaine doses exceeding 4 mg/kg (7 mg/kg with epinephrine) resulting from the treatment of large wounds in small children may cause seizures as well.

In an infant under 6 months of age with new seizures, pyridoxine (vitamin B$_6$) deficiency should be suspected. This autosomal recessive metabolic disorder results in abnormal CNS γ-aminobutyric acid (GABA) metabolism. Seizures due to this condition stop shortly after IV administration of 100 mg of pyridoxine. In addition to the diseases described above, hepatic disease, hypothyroidism, hyperthyroidism, cerebrovascular accidents, uremia, and inborn errors of metabolism are rare causes of seizures in infants and children. The presentation of the majority of these conditions is accompanied by other signs and symptoms that guide the workup of the patient in the ED.

Nonconvulsive Paroxysmal Disorders

Several other common childhood conditions may produce "spells" of transiently depressed level of consciousness, without the occurrence of actual seizure activity. Breath-holding spells are seen during the first 2 years of life, produce short periods of unconsciousness and may be accompanied by tonic-clonic movements suggestive of seizures. Cyanotic breath-holding spells are often preceded by an event that upsets the child, who cries for 30 seconds or less and then holds his breath, becoming cyanotic. After a short period of rigid posturing, the child may have convulsive movements followed by a return to their baseline within minutes. Pallid breath-holding spells start in a less dramatic fashion. The child may or may not cry, then turns pale, and loses consciousness.

Syncope may be mistaken for seizures, as short periods of tonic or clonic movements may accompany the loss of consciousness caused by postural hypotension or fainting spells. Historical factors such as the sudden assumption of an upright posture, concurrent hair brushing, or a sudden painful stimulus help distinguish syncope from true seizures.

Night terrors (pavor nocturnus) present as recurrent episodes of abrupt awakenings from sleep accompanied by terrified crying and autonomic signs of intense fear. These occur in the school-aged child and may last from 1 to 10 minutes. The child may awaken tremulous, diaphoretic, unaware of their surroundings, and unresponsive to comfort. After going back to sleep, the child has no memory of the event. This disorder is rarely seen after early adolescence.

Diagnostic Evaluation of the Child with Seizures

History and Physical Examination

Details of seizure onset provide valuable clues to etiology. Focality, progression and duration of abnormal movements, eye position, mental status, skin color, and respiratory effort should all be determined. A history of fever, head trauma, or toxic ingestion must be elicited as well. Distraught caregivers may neglect to mention important information unless specifically asked.

A complete physical examination performed on a patient with seizures should focus on signs of trauma, toxic exposure, infection, or abuse. Vital signs may reveal the presence of fever or hypertension. Significant eye findings include anisocoria, pupil reactivity, papilledema, or retinal hemorrhage. Blood or pus behind the tympanic membrane may be noted, along with nuchal rigidity. The remainder of the physical examination is completed with particular emphasis on the patient's neurologic status. Focal neurologic deficits may follow a generalized seizure of any etiology, but must be presumed to indicate the presence of focal CNS lesions.

Laboratory Evaluation

When metabolic disturbances are suspected, electrolytes, glucose, calcium, magnesium, and phosphorus should be obtained. A blood culture is useful in young, unimmunized patients with fever without source, who are at risk for bacteremia. Drug levels should be measured in a patient who is taking anticonvulsants. White blood cell counts obtained after a seizure has occurred are of limited utility, because demargination of peripheral leukocytes may produce a dramatic rise in this value despite the absence of infection.

A toxicological screen should be considered in seizures of uncertain etiology. In a study of 1,680 consecutive toxicological screens at a children's hospital, 4.6% were positive for cocaine and/or its metabolites, and in 37% of those patients who tested positive, the cocaine exposure was unexpected. A toxicological screen may be important to perform in certain clinical situations even when parents assert that they saw what substance was ingested.

A lumbar puncture to diagnose meningitis should be performed in all children with fever, seizures, and lethargy or irritability, children less than 9 months of age with fever and seizures, and most patients with fever and the new onset of seizures. Pretreatment with antibiotics should raise the possibility of partially treated meningitis, characterized by a longer course, lower temperatures, and more vomiting than the classical presentation of this illness. Bacterial antigen detection panels should be ordered on CSF obtained in these cases.

Other Studies

Imaging studies to rule out tumors, hematomas, edema, and abscesses are indicated in all patients with seizures and signs of increased ICP (bulging fontanelle, blurred optic disk margins, protracted vomiting, severe headache) and those with posttraumatic seizures. CT scan is the modality of choice for these patients; MRI studies are rarely indicated on an emergent basis.

An electroencephalogram (EEG) remains the gold standard for the diagnosis of seizure disorders but is rarely indicated when evaluating a patient in the ED. The decisions to obtain an EEG and whether to perform the study on an inpatient or outpatient basis should be dis-

cussed with the patient's usual physician and/or a pediatric neurologist.

Status Epilepticus

Status epilepticus a generalized seizure of 30 minutes in duration, or a series of seizures lasting this long that occur without return of consciousness. During the first 30 minutes of seizure activity, catecholamine release causes an increase in heart rate, blood pressure, cerebral blood flow, and blood glucose. After 30 minutes, blood pressure and cerebral perfusion decrease, compromising oxygen and glucose delivery to the brain. Estimates of mortality of status epilepticus in children range from 3% to 11%. Status that continues for 60 minutes or more is called refractory status epilepticus. Children with status due to acute CNS injury, intoxication, or underlying neurological disease are more likely to suffer refractory status and/or permanent consequences than those with status secondary to fever or idiopathic causes.

Stabilization and Treatment

The treatment of seizures is outlined in **Table 91.5**. Assisted ventilation and supplemental oxygen are the mainstays of treatment in the prehospital setting. Attempts at IV access are usually not indicated for transport times of 15 minutes or less. Anticonvulsant administration via the IV route in the field is a mixed blessing because respiratory depression may place the patient at greater risk than several additional minutes of seizure activity. If anticonvulsant administration is desired in the absence of IV access, intramuscular (IM) or intranasal (IN) midazolam or rectal (PR) diazepam may be given.

The child arriving in the ED while actively seizing should be placed in an area where resuscitation supplies and intubation equipment are readily available. Airway patency should be preserved by placing the patient's head in a neutral or sniffing position, suctioning any accumulated secretions, and placing an oral or nasal airway as needed. Supplemental oxygen via face mask should be started, and venous access obtained. In young children the intraosseous (IO) route may be used. Blood samples obtained during IV or IO placement should be sent to the lab for serum glucose and other studies.

Drug therapy of status epilepticus is directed at stopping convulsive activity as quickly as possible and preventing its return, while avoiding exacerbating respiratory depression. To accomplish this, multiple benzodiazepine doses are used to stop seizure activity initially, accompanied by the slow administration of longer-acting medications such as phenytoin or phenobarbital. Loading with longer-acting medications may not be indicated for seizures caused by rapidly treatable problems such as hypoglycemia or hyperpyrexia. A careful, stepwise approach to drug administration decreases the risk of iatrogenic respiratory depression. Dosing guidelines are listed in **Table 91.6**.

Benzodiazepines commonly used as anticonvulsants include lorazepam, diazepam, and midazolam. All have a rapid onset of action and can cause respiratory depression. Lorazepam is favored by many authorities for the initial

Table 91.5

Management of Status Epilepticus

Prehospital Management

Airway: sniffing head position in midline, suction oral secretions

Breathing: supplemental oxygen, bag-mask ventilation, intubation

Circulation: IV access if transport time >15 minutes

Anticonvulsant treatment

Transport <15 minutes: medications not needed

Transport >15 minutes, IV access achieved: administer lorazepam IV

Transport >15 minutes, no IV access: diazepam PR or midazolam IN

Initial ED Stabilization

Airway, Breathing, Circulation as above

Monitoring: pulse oximetry, cardiorespiratory monitor

Labs: rapid glucose, drug levels (consider electrolytes, toxicologic screen)

Initial Treatment

Benzodiazepine: lorazepam 0.05–0.1 mg/kg IV; repeat as needed

Ongoing seizure activity

>2 years old: phenytoin 15–20 mg/kg IV (or phosphenytoin equivalent)

<2 years old: phenobarbital 10–20 mg/kg IV

Treat Specific Etiologies (see Table 91.1)

Treatment of Refractory Status Epilepticus

If previously loaded with phenobarbital, load with phenytoin

If previously loaded with phenytoin, load with phenobarbital

Endotracheal intubation (avoid use of prolonged paralytics)

Other medications: propofol, lidocaine

Critical care monitoring: midazolam infusion, general anesthesia, barbiturate coma

---

treatment of status epilepticus since it has the longest duration of action, lasting from several hours to a day. This facilitates the administration of longer-acting medications before seizures return. Midazolam becomes the preferred option when no venous access is available, as it is well absorbed when given IM or IN. Frequent doses may be required until status is brought under control due to its short (1 to 2 h) duration of action. Diazepam has an intermediate duration of action and may only be given IV or PR. The latter route is of limited utility due to variable absorption by rectal mucosa.

Phenytoin controls 70% to 90% of episodes of status epilepticus when given as an IV loading dose. Its efficacy is greatest for idiopathic generalized or posttraumatic seizures, and less for status due to absence of complex febrile seizures. Phenytoin is usually administered after benzodiazepines have been given, due to its slower onset of action and the need for a slow administration rate. Phenytoin must be administered in saline only, at a maximum rate of 1 mg/kg/min in children and 50 mg/min in adults, to avoid adverse effects such as hypotension and cardiac arrhythmias. Advantages of phenytoin use include its long duration of action (at least 24 h) and lack of mental status depression, allowing adequate seizure control while enabling evaluation of the patient's neurological status. Fosphenytoin is a prodrug of phenytoin which is considerably more expensive. It causes less tissue damage if extravasated and fewer cardiac side effects. Fosphenytoin can be mixed with any IV solution (including dextrose), and can be given IM, or infused more rapidly than phenytoin.

Phenobarbital is the other commonly used long-acting drug given to patients in status epilepticus. It is particularly effective in the treatment of neonatal or complex febrile seizures. Like phenytoin, it may be administered as an IV load, to provide 1 to 3 days of anticonvulsant effect. Unlike phenytoin, it depresses mental status and respiratory drive. For this reason rapid phenobarbital infusion following administration of benzodiazepines requires cau-

---

Table 91.6

Anticonvulsant Medications

	Route	Dose (mg/kg)	Dosing Information
Lorazepam	IV	0.05–0.1	
Midazolam	IV	0.1	
	IM	0.25	
	IN	0.2	
Diazepam	IV	0.1–0.3	Max dose 10 mg/dose
	PR	0.5	Max dose 20 mg/dose
Phenytoin	IV	15–20	Infuse @ 1 mg/kg/min, max 50 mg/min; max dose 1,000 mg
Phosphenytoin	IV or IM	15–20 PE	Phenytoin equivalent (PE)
Phenobarbital	IV or IM	10–20	Infuse @ 1 mg/kg/min, max 50 mg/min; max dose 1,000 mg
			Max dose 1,000 mg
Propofol	IV	1	May repeat several times
Lidocaine	IV	1–2	Follow initial bolus with infusion @ 6 mg/kg/hr (10 μg/kg/min)

Dosage recommendations are guidelines only. Scale back mg/kg doses for children >25 kg. Any anticonvulsant may cause respiratory depression. Multiple doses and combinations of medications are often required to control prolonged seizure activity.

Table 91.7
Treatment for Seizures of Specific Etiologies

Seizure Etiology	Treatment	Dose	Dosing Information
Hypoglycemia	Glucose	0.5 mg/kg	Use 2 mL/kg D25, or 5 mL/kg D10 in neonates
Hyponatremia	Sodium chloride	5–10 mL/kg	Use 3% NaCl over 10–20 min
Hypocalcemia	Calcium chloride	20 mg/kg	Central IV only, max dose 500 mg, infuse over 10 min
	Calcium gluconate	60 mg/kg	Peripheral or central IV over 10 min, max dose 1,000 mg
Hypomagnesemia	Magnesium sulfate	25–50 mg/kg	Infuse over 10–20 min
Isoniazid ingestion	Pyridoxine	1 g/g ingested	Give 5 g IV of 5–10% solution if amount ingested unknown
Hypertension	Hydralazine	0.1–0.2 mg/kg	Infuse over several min, monitor blood pressure
Pyridoxine dependency	Pyridoxine	100 mg	Give IV to infants with no previous history of seizures

tion, as it may lead to sufficient respiratory compromise to require intubation. IM dosing of phenobarbital is a possible but suboptimal therapy, because the time to peak activity may be delayed for 2 to 4 hours.

If multiple doses of benzodiazepines followed by a full loading dose of phenytoin or phenobarbital does not end seizure activity, administration of whichever long-acting medication has not been given (either phenobarbital or phenytoin) is indicated. Intubation should be considered at this point. Less frequently used medications to control status epilepticus, listed in Table 91.6, may then be indicated. Propofol is an excellent choice for the normotensive patient. Lidocaine is often effective as well, and is more available than propofol. Administration of neuromuscular blocking agents should be avoided whenever possible, as it ablates the motor responses resulting from seizures while allowing the abnormal CNS activity and resultant neuronal injury to continue invisibly.

Seizures unresponsive to the above measures require the administration of general anesthesia using isoflurane, or induction of a barbiturate coma. Continuous midazolam, consisting of a starting bolus dose of 0.2 mg/kg followed by infusion of from 0.75 to 11 μg/kg/min, is another recently described option. All patients receiving these therapies should have continuous cardiovascular and EEG monitoring in an intensive care unit setting. Drug therapy for specific seizure etiologies is listed in **Table 91.7**.

Disposition

Children whose seizures have stopped prior to arrival in the ED and who look well after their evaluation may be discharged with specified follow-up. This occurs in the majority of patients with febrile seizures. Children whose seizures required the acute administration of anticonvulsants often require admission to the hospital, to observe and treat additional seizures, or to facilitate their diagnostic evaluation. Observation or short-stay unit beds are becoming increasingly available for this purpose. Infants with new-onset seizures usually fall in this category. Patients who are intubated or who have complex etiologies for their seizure activity usually require admission to an intensive care unit, preferably one specializing in the care of pediatric patients.

Selected Readings

Baumann RJ, Duffner PK. Treatment of children with simple febrile seizures: the AAP practice parameter. *Pediatr Neurol* 2000;23:11–17.

Freedman S. Pediatric seizures and their management in the Emergency Department. *Clin Pediatr Emerg Med* 2003;4:195–201.

McBride M. Status epilepticus. *Pediatr Rev* 1995;16:386–389.

PALS Provider Manual. Dallas: American Heart Association, 2002.

Rosman NP. Evaluation of the child who convulses with fever. *Paediatr Drugs* 2003; 5:457–461.

Tunik MG, Young GM. Status epilepticus in children. *Pediatr Clin North Am* 1992; 39:1007–1030.

Working group on status epilepticus. Treatment of convulsive status epilepticus. *JAMA* 1993;270:854–859.

92 Infectious Diseases

Peter Murphy
Richard Bachur
Mariann M. Manno

Mary O'Neill
Alison Brent
Katherine Harrison

Bacteremia and Sepsis

Fever is a common presenting complaint in pediatric patients, accounting for as many as 25% of pediatric visits to an emergency department (ED). Generally, the evaluation and management of the febrile child focuses on infectious causes of fever. The ED approach to febrile children is to identify treatable infections and to recognize the characteristics of children at risk for occult infections.

Definitions

Both bacteremia and sepsis are defined by bacteria in the bloodstream. Their differentiation relies on the presence or absence of systemic symptoms and signs. Bacteremia and sepsis encompass a spectrum of disease with occult bacteremia at one end (the well-appearing child with fever and bacteremia) and sepsis at the other end (the child in septic shock with signs of toxicity and organ dysfunction). Additionally, blood infection can be a primary process or secondary to a focal infection. In this continuum, some patients with occult bacteremia progress to sepsis or develop secondary foci of infection including meningitis, pneumonia, arthritis, osteomyelitis, or cellulitis. The likelihood of spontaneous resolution of pneumococcal bacteremia is >90%, but the risk of a child with occult pneumococcal bacteremia later having meningitis is 3%.

Bacteriology

The pathogens responsible for occult bacteremia are changing. Prior to the introduction of a conjugate vaccine against *Haemophilus influenzae* type b (Hib), *H. influenzae* accounted for 13% of all cases of occult bacteremia and 40% of the complications. Now almost twenty years later, HIB consistently contributes only 1% of occult bacteremia. Prospective surveillance of invasive pneumococcal infections in children from 1994 through 2002 revealed a >75% decrease among children <24 months old, attributed to the 7-valent pneumococcal vaccine (PCV7) introduced in February of 2000. Continued surveillance will almost certainly influence the recommendations for the ED evaluation of the child with a fever without source (FWS). These new vaccines have not influenced the risk of occult bacteremia and serious bacterial infection (SBI) from other species, specifically *Salmonella* species, *Neisseria meningitidis*, or *Streptococcus pyogenes*. Also, the more vulnerable infant less than two months of age remains at risk for infection from group B *Streptococcus* (GBS), *Escherichia coli* (and other enteric Gram negatives), *Listeria monocytogenes* as well as *Pneumococcus* and *Meningococcus*.

Fever

Although temperature definitions are not standardized, a rectal temperature of 38.0° C (100.4° F) is the most widely accepted definition. Oral temperatures tend to be 0.6°C (1° F) lower than rectal and axillary temperatures are 1.2° C (2° F) less than rectal measurements. Infrared tympanometry is of variable reliability and reproducibility and should not be used for infants less than one year of age. Children who are afebrile but have a history of documented fever should be considered to be febrile.

Approach to the Febrile Child

Most febrile children have benign self-limited illnesses, so the evaluation and management of the febrile child should include detecting the early, often subtle signs of bacteremia or sepsis, recognizing those at risk for occult bacteremia as well as minimizing the trauma and unnecessary testing or use of antibiotics to which the child is exposed. Every febrile patient requires a careful history and physical examination.

The history of the present illness should include the symptoms of the present illness, illness exposure, details of input and output sufficient to evaluate risk for dehydration and exposure to antibiotics, steroids, antipyretics, and other medicines. The past medical history should include gestational and perinatal history, presence of chronic illness or immunodeficiency, pertinent family history and history of travel, and immunization history. Specific questions regarding previous urinary tract infection (UTI) or pneumonia may be helpful as well. The physical exam should include a complete set of vital signs including pulse oximetry, behavioral state, skin color and exanthems, and an assessment of the patient's state of hydration. Careful and complete scrutiny for petechiae will help to find children at risk for SBI, particularly *Neisseria meningitidis*.

Treatment of the fever itself is worthy of mention. Not only parents, but many medical professionals suffer from "fever phobia," a term coined to describe fear of the fever itself as a threat to the febrile patient. Although there is still much to learn about the role of the fever in the body's defense against infection, there are a few things than can be agreed upon:

- Fever often contributes to the discomfort experienced by the patient and caretakers.
- There is a growing body of indirect evidence that fever is part of the body's defense against infection.
- Treatment of fever has not been shown to prevent seizures with fever.

Therefore, it is reasonable to treat febrile children who appear to be uncomfortable with acetaminophen, 15 mg/kg/dose every four hours or ibuprofen 10 mg/kg/dose every eight hours as needed for discomfort. Combining these medicines fosters fever phobia in our patients' caretakers and risks medical errors by tired caretakers.

The Septic Child

Signs of poor perfusion (altered sensorium; cool, mottled or cyanotic skin; delayed capillary refill [>2 seconds]; weak peripheral pulses), tachypnea, tachycardia, hypotension, or evidence of coagulapathy in the febrile patient make a presumptive diagnosis of sepsis. The septic patient requires aggressive evaluation and resuscitation, focusing on the ABCs: *airway* (maintain a patent airway with supplemental oxygen; monitor pulse oximetry); *breathing* (be prepared to assist ventilation with bag-mask ventilation or endotracheal intubation as needed; monitor end-tidal CO_2 in intubated patients); *circulation* (intravenous or intraosseus infusion of isotonic crystalloid at 20–40 mL/kg should be immediate, and may need to be followed by additional fluids as well as dopamine or epinephrine infusions).

Drugs

Antibiotics should be given expeditiously, ideally after specimens for blood and urine culture are obtained; lumbar puncture may need to be deferred in the unstable patient. There may be a need to address hypoglycemia or metabolic acidosis. Patients need to be monitored for oxygenation, ventilation, arterial blood pressure, urine output and, therefore should be transported to a pediatric intensive care unit after stabilization.

Evaluation of the Febrile Infant Less than Three Months of Age

Younger infants are at greater risk of SBI because of their immature immune status. Also, a unique group of pathogens must be considered because of their recent birth. As mentioned, GBS, Gram-negative bacteria as well as *Listeria* cause SBI in this age group. Incidence of bacterial disease has been reported to be 13% in febrile infants in the first month and 10% in the second month of life,

with UTIs accounting for one third of bacterial disease in the first three months. Febrile infants in the first month of life have a 2% to 3% rate of bacteremia. While poor feeding, irritability, lethargy, vomiting, poor perfusion, and temperature instability are all signs of serious illness in children in the first three months of life, they are subtle and nonspecific. Clinical scales to identify the febrile child at low risk for SBI have no predictive value in children in the first three months of life. It cannot be overemphasized that any child with a fever in the first three months of life can have a serious infection regardless of appearance.

Management

Because it has been well established that well-appearing febrile infants may have SBI, laboratory evaluation is necessary. A number of researchers have developed screening tools that combine parts of the history and physical exam with laboratory data to identify infants at low risk (**Table 92.1**). When these screening tools have been applied to febrile patients in the first month of life, they consistently identify as "low-risk" 20% to 25% of febrile neonates eventually proven to have SBI. Therefore, for any febrile neonate 28 days of age or less, the management recommendations are conservative (**FIGURE 92.1**): complete laboratory evaluation ("sepsis work-up" includes: screening tests such as CBC, urinalysis, CSF cell count, CSF protein and glucose; and cultures of blood, urine, and CSF), admission to the hospital and administration of antibiotics pending culture results. Antibiotics include ampicillin (50 mg/kg/dose) and either gentamicin (2.5 mg/kg/dose) or cefotaxime (50 mg/kg/dose) (**Table 92.2**). Acyclovir should also be considered in any septic-appearing infant regardless of maternal history for herpes simplex.

The management of febrile infants one to three months of age is determined by their risk status. Low risk febrile infants are previously healthy (first illness in a full term baby) and well-appearing without focal infection on physical exam. Laboratory evaluation of infants who are identified as low risk include: a WBC between 5,000 and 15,000/mm^3, a band count less than 1,500/mm^3, a urinalysis with less than 5 WBC/hpf and, if diarrhea is present, microscopic examination of stool microscopic with less than

Table 92.1
Low-Risk Criteria for Infants 1 to 3 Months of Age

Clinical Criteria
  Previously healthy
  Nontoxic clinical appearance
  No focal bacterial infection (other than otitis media)
  Good social situation
Laboratory Criteria
  WBC count 5,000–20,000/mm^3
  Absolute band count <1,500/mm^3
  Normal urinalysis (<5 WBCs/high power field)
  If diarrhea present, <5 WBCs/hpf in stool

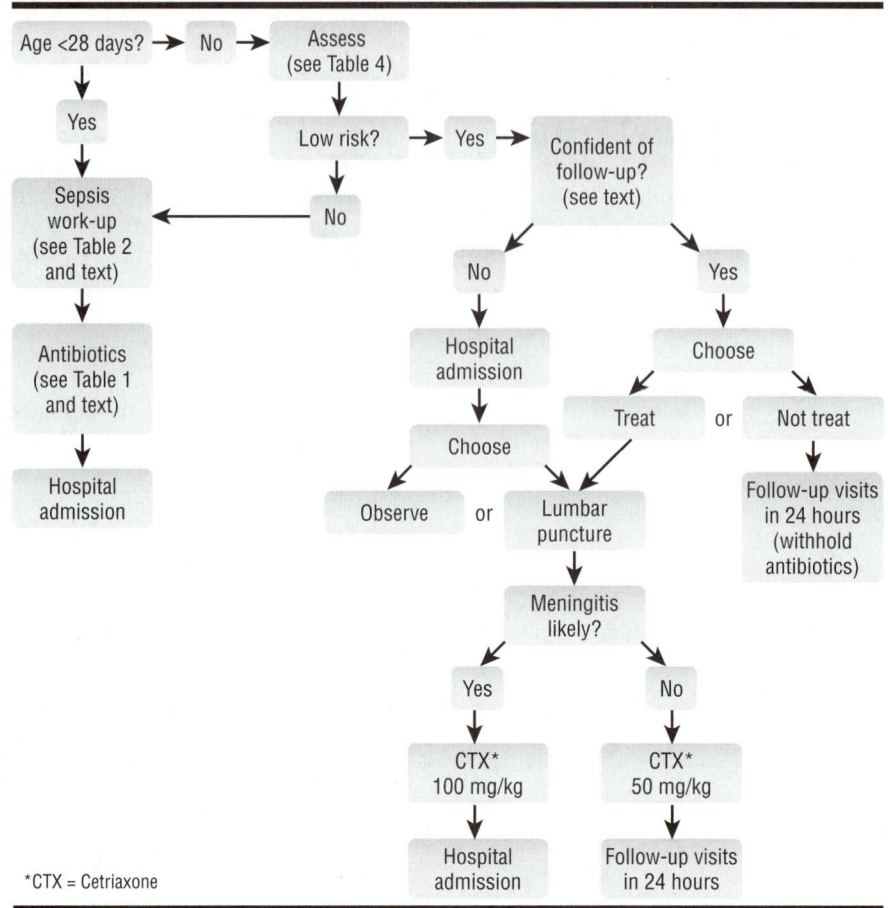

FIGURE 92.1 Algorithm for the management of the previously healthy infant age 0 to 90 days.

5 WBC/hpf (**Table 92.3**). If the family's social situation ensures follow-up (home telephone, transportation, parental maturity, and physician available to follow up), then these patients can be released and re-checked within 24 hours. If it is intended to treat prophylactically with antibiotics then a lumbar puncture must be performed and the CSF show no signs of meningitis (normal < 8 WBC/mm^3); this is the only way to avoid confounding treatment in a case of aseptic meningitis, which is not uncommon in febrile infants. Outpatient management of febrile one-to-three month olds who have been treated with antibiotics prophylactically (ceftriaxone 50 mg/kg/dose) also requires a social situation which ensures follow-up. Otherwise, treated or untreated, these children should be admitted and observed or treated pending culture results.

Any febrile infant one-to-three months of age who does not meet these low-risk criteria must have a complete sepsis work-up, be admitted to the hospital, and be treated with antibiotics pending culture results. Urinary tract infections are among the most common SBIs found in febrile neonates including those with symptoms of upper respiratory infection. They are more common in boys younger than six months, uncircumcised boys, and girls less than 12 months of age. The rate of UTI is higher in children whose fever is higher. Specimen collection should be by bladder catheterization or, if necessary, suprapubic bladder tap. A culture must be sent to determine if UTI is present as urinalysis is incompletely reliable. Absence of both white cells and bacteria on urine microscopy makes UTI unlikely. Presence of WBCs (>5 WBC/hpf) or bacteria on urinalysis, or positive leukocyte esterase or nitrate on urine dipstick, make UTI probable; more than one positive of these factors increases the specificity of the urine analysis as a screen for UTI.

Febrile infants who also show signs of respiratory disease should have chest radiographs. One of the most sensitive signs of pneumonia in the febrile infant is oxygen saturation less than 95%, but respiratory rate that is elevated out of proportion to the fever, cough, respiratory

Table 92.2	
Antibiotics for Sepsis	
Age	**Antibiotic**
<2 month	Ampicillin (200 mg/kg/day) plus either gentamicin (7.5 mg/kg/day) or cefotaxime (150 mg/kg/day)
≥2 months	Ceftriaxone (100 mg/kg/day) or cefotaxime (150 mg/kg/day); consider vancomycin[a]

[a]Vancomycin should be considered for life-threatening infections with resistant strains of *S. pneumoniae*.

Table 92.3

Laboratory Assessment of Sepsis

Blood
Complete blood count (CBC) with differential and platelets
Electrolytes, venous blood gas
Glucose (bedside measurement and serum)
Blood urea nitrogen (BUN) and creatinine
PT/PTT (consider fibrinogen level, D-dimer)
Urine
Urinalysis
Culture by catheterization or bladder aspiration
Cerebrospinal Fluid (CSF)
Cell count
Glucose and protein
Gram stain and culture
± bacterial antigen detection
Radiograph
Chest radiograph

distress, or lower respiratory tract signs (rales, wheezes, ronchi) are all indications for chest radiography.

Evaluation of the Febrile Child 3 to 36 Months of Age

Evaluation and management of the febrile child with no identifiable infection on physical exam (FWOS) between three months and three years of age has been the topic of great debate, research, and discussion because of the risk of occult bacteremia. Prior to initiation of immunization against HIB, this organism made a significant contribution to occult bacteremia and its serious complications, but is a rare occurrence now. A similar change is occurring in the incidence of invasive disease due to pneumococcus since the introduction of PCV7. The current prevalence of occult bacteremia in febrile children aged three to 36 months is probably between 1.5% and 2%, and preliminary studies indicate that 5% to 20% of these will develop SBI (sepsis, pneumonia, cellulitis, septic arthritis, osteomyelitis, or meningitis). Approximately 0.3% of previously healthy children aged 3 to 36 months who develop FWOS will develop significant sequelae, but only 0.03% will develop sepsis or meningitis. Recommendations regarding the evaluation of febrile well-appearing children three to 36 months of age have changed to reflect the impact of PCV7 immunization. As noted above, any febrile child who appears toxic should have a complete sepsis work-up and be admitted to the hospital for parenteral antibiotics. Risk for bacteremia in this age group increases with the fever. Children whose fever is less than 39° C (**FIGURE 92.2**), who do not appear toxic and for whom no bacterial source of infection can be found on physical exam require no diagnostic tests or antibiotics. These children can be treated with antipyretics as outlined above and instructed to return if their condition deteriorates or if the fever persists >48 hours. Children whose fever is greater than 39° C require selected laboratory evaluation.

Urine screening (leukocyte esterase [LE] and nitrite or urinalysis) and urine culture should be performed on all females ≤2 years and males ≤6 months with FWOS. All children with a positive urine screen should be treated with outpatient antibiotics (oral third-generation cephalosporin). For children who have not received all three doses of PCV7 (which, by definition, includes all children less than 6 months of age), laboratory evaluation for occult bacteremia is indicated if their fever is greater than 39° C. If WBC is found to be >15,000, then they should have a blood culture sent and be treated with ceftriaxone (50 mg/kg up to 1 g) pending culture results. Also, if their WBC > 20,000, then a chest radiograph is indicated even in the absence of respiratory symptoms; as many as 26% of non-PVC7 immunized children with higher fever and leukocytosis have been found to have radiographic evidence of pneumonia. Febrile children treated as outpatients require follow-up. Caretakers should be instructed to return if the child's condition deteriorates or if fever persists >48 hours. If either blood or urine cultures are positive and the child is still febrile or ill-appearing at recheck, the child should be admitted to the hospital for repeat cultures, LP if blood culture positive, and parenteral antibiotics. The child whose culture (blood or urine) is positive and is afebrile and well-appearing at recheck may continue to be treated as an outpatient with oral antibiotics.

Children older than three years of age are not considered to be at significant risk for occult bacteremia and a thorough history and physical is usually adequate to identify any bacterial infection. At any age, the febrile patient who appears to be toxic or whose fever lasts longer than expected from a viral syndrome requires laboratory evaluation as part of a complete consultation (**Table 92.4**).

Fever and Petechial Rash

The febrile patient with petechiae requires urgent evaluation. Petechiae can be a sign of infection with *Neisseria meningitidis* or other invasive bacterial disease, so these patients should be considered candidates for laboratory evaluation including lumbar puncture and parenteral antibiotics unless it can be determined sufficiently that the petechiae are from coughing or vomiting (in which case they are primarily on the face) or part of a streptococcal pharyngitis rash. This requires a CBC, throat culture, PT/PTT, possibly an LP and several hours of observation before a patient can be managed safely as an outpatient. The patient with normal laboratory values and no progression of illness or petechiae may be a candidate for outpatient management, but the child who gets sicker, whose rash worsens, becomes purpuric, or who has laboratory evidence of SBI should be admitted to to a setting with close monitoring. The notoriously rapid progression of meningococcal disease dictates that it is always better to err on the side of caution in the febrile child with petechiae.

Fever and Erythrodema

Streptococcus pyogenes and *Staphylococcus aureus* have the ability to produce toxins causing fever and erythroderma.

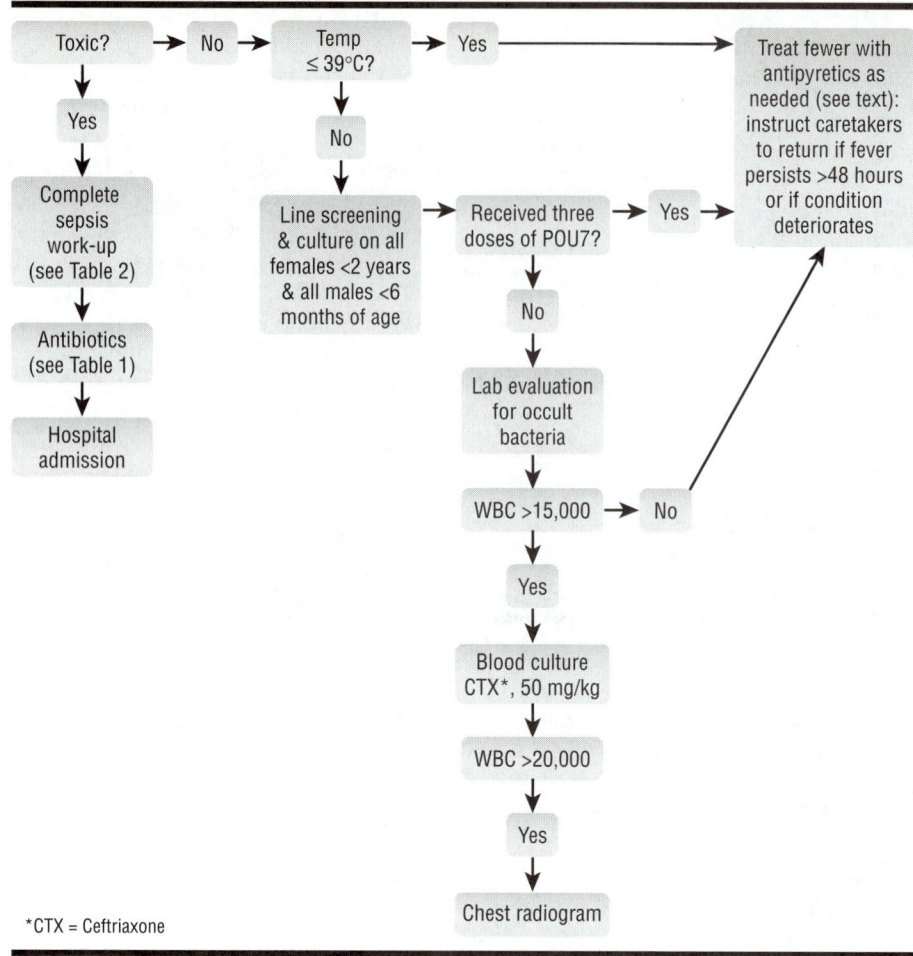

FIGURE 92.2 Algorithm for the management of the previously healthy child age 3 to 36 months.

Ill-appearing children with scarletiniform rash or erythroderma require aggressive management as they may be exhibiting the first signs of toxic shock syndrome. Careful evaluation for focal infection is appropriate but may not be fruitful.

Meningitis

Meningitis is caused by inflammation of the pia and arachnoid, the meninges that surround the brain and spinal cord. These form the subarachnoid space that contains spinal fluid. Meningoencephalitis occurs when infection involves the brain parenchyma as well as the meninges. Meningitis is a variable clinical condition with distinguishing characteristics depending on etiology (aseptic, viral, bacterial), the age of the patient, and chronicity (acute, chronic, recurrent).

Bacterial Meningitis

Epidemiology

The overall incidence of bacterial meningitis has decreased dramatically since the mid 1980s and the introduction of immunizations for *H. influenzae* and *Streptococcus pneumoniae*. There has also been a decline in cases of meningitis caused by *Neisseria meningitidis* and *group B streptococcus*.

As a result, the median age of meningitis is 25 years as opposed to 15 months in 1985. *Group B streptococcus* (GBS) is the most common organism in the neonatal period. From 1 to 2 years of age, *S. pneumoniae* and *N. meningitides* are the most common organisms. From 2 through 18 years of age, in immunized populations, the most common organisms are *N. meningitides* or *S. pneumoniae*. Newborns and those with immunodeficiency are at highest risk of meningitis. Immunodeficient states in children include sickle cell disease, AIDS, asplenia, renal disease, hepatic disease, diabetes mellitus, dysgammaglobulinemia, and immunosuppressive therapies including corticosteroids (**Table 92.5**).

Clinical Presentation

Fever, headache, and stiff neck are classic signs of meningitis seen in older children. Other findings include Brudzinski sign (flexion of the hips with flexion of the neck), Kernig sign (pain with knee extension when the hip is flexed), photophobia, nausea, vomiting, lethargy, and a diminished mental status. *N. meningitides* may be associated with a petechial or purpuric rash. These highly suggestive findings are absent in infants and young children who present in a nonspecific manner: irritability, lethargy, poor feeding, vomiting, apnea, seizure, hypothermia or fever.

Table 92.4

Differential Diagnosis of the Septic-Appearing Infant

Infection
  Sepsis (viral or bacterial)
  Meningitis
  Urinary tract infection
Cardiac Disorders
  Congenital heart disease
  Dysrhythmias
  Myocarditis/cardiomyopathy
  Pericarditis
Hematological Disorders
  Severe anemia from hemorrhage or hemolysis
  Methemoglobinemia
Metabolic Disorders
  Inborn errors of metabolism
  Hypohypernatremia
  Hypoglycemia
  Hyperammonemia
  Acidosis
  Renal dysfunction
Endocrine Disorders
  Congenital adrenal hyperplasia
Gastrointestinal Disorders
  Severe dehydration from gastroenteritis or pyloric
    stenosis
  Necrotizing enterocolitis
  Volvulus
  Intussusception
Neurological Disorders
  Infant botulism
  Intracranial hemorrhage

Table 92.5

High Risk Groups for Invasive Pneumococcal Infections

Sickle cell disease, asplenia, splenic dysfunction
HIV
Congenital immune deficiency
Chronic cardiac disease (including cyanotic congenital
  heart disease)
Chronic pulmonary disease (including asthma treated
  with steroids)
Chronic renal disease (including nephritic syndrome)
CNS abnormalities (including neurosurgery, skull
  fractures)
Immunosuppressive and radiation therapy
Diabetes mellitus

Source: Used with permission from the American Academy of Pediatrics *AAP Red Book.*

Diagnosis

The definitive diagnosis of meningitis is made by examination of spinal fluid. A CSF specimen should be obtained as soon as the patient's clinical stability allows. When signs of increased intracranial pressure (abnormal papillary response, papilledema, focal neurologic findings, profoundly abnormal mental status) are present, computed tomography should be emergently performed before a lumbar puncture is performed to rule out mass lesion, sinus thrombosis, or parameningeal focus. CT need not routinely be performed in children who clinically appear to have meningitis without increased intracranial pressure. CTs should be performed emergently when the patient evidences elevated ICP. The decision to defer the LP because of patient stability, the need to obtain a CT, or decision to transport the patient must not delay administration of empiric antibiotics. Bacterial meningitis can be confirmed with delayed lumbar puncture because cellular changes in the CSF remain for several days after antibiotics are begun.

Findings in the cerebral spinal fluid (CSF) that are characteristic for bacterial meningitis include a low glucose, an elevated protein, an elevated white blood cell count (commonly $>1,000/mm^3$). However, these values vary with age (**Table 92.6**). Gram stain of the CSF identifies an organism in 80% of culture-positive cases and about 10% in culture-negative cases. Blood cultures are positive in about half of patients with bacterial meningitis. Technically, the CSF glucose concentration is interpreted in relation to the serum glucose value. Hypoglycorrhachia, a CSF serum glucose ratio less than 0.4, is characteristically found in bacterial meningitis. There is a wide range of normal CSF protein in infants. Higher protein levels are seen in bacterial meningitis. A traumatic LP makes the interpretation of the CSF protein difficult. Normal CSF cellularity varies with age. Typically, the WBC count ranges from 1,000 to 20,000 in bacterial meningitis. In the first month of life, up to 60% of the cells in the normal CSF may be polymorphonuclear leukocytes (PMNs). Beyond 1 month in the normal state, not more than 3 PMNs per mm^3 should be seen.

The probability of visualizing bacteria on a stain depends on the number of bacterial organisms present at the time of LP. One fourth of the smears are positive with $\geq 10^3$ colony forming units (CFU) per mL; 97% are positive with 10^6 CFU/mL.

Partially Treated Meningitis

The partial treatment or pretreatment of a patient with antibiotics before the diagnosis of meningitis is made may delay the child's presentation to hospital and result in a diagnostic dilemma. The CSF findings may be altered. The Gram stain and culture may be negative, however, abnormal CSF protein, glucose and cellularity may persist. Because prior antibiotic therapy may impair bacterial growth from the CSF, a CSF bacterial antigen detection test (BAD) should be performed in the patient who has received prior antibiotics. The antigens are typically present at high levels in the CSF for several days, even after parenteral antibiotics have been initiated. The presence of a positive CSF assay provides reliable bacteriologic diagnosis. A negative antigen test cannot exclude the diagnosis of ABM.

Table 92.6

Normal Cerebrospinal Fluid Values

Age	WBC (mean% PMN)	Glucose	Protein
Preterm	0–25 WBC/mm³ (57%)	24–63 mg/dL	65–150 mg/dL
Term	0–22 WBC/mm³ (61%)	34–119 mg/dL	20–170 mg/dL
Child	0–7 WBC/mm³ (5%)	40–80mg/dL	5–40mg/dL

Source: Used with permission from *Harriett Lane Handbook,* ed 16. Philadelphia: Mosby, 2002:557.

Treatment

There has been worldwide increase in with penicillin- and cephalosporin-resistant strains of *S. pneumoniae.* The American Academy of Pediatrics recommends an initial treatment with vancomycin and cefotaxime or ceftriaxone for patients one month of age or older who have proven or probable bacterial meningitis. Vancomycin should be discontinued when the organism is proven susceptible to penicillin, cefotaxime, or ceftriaxone. Gram-negative meningitis is treated with cefotaxime or ceftriaxone. Aminoglycosides are sometimes added. Ampicillin should be added in young infants (less than 2 months old) to cover *Listeria monocytogenes.*

The duration of antibiotic therapy depends on the organism. *S. pneumoniae* and *H. influenzae* are treated for 10 to 14 days. *N. meningitidis* is treated for seven days. *L. monocytogenes* and group B streptococcal meningitis are treated for 14 to 21 days. For gram-negative bacilli, a minimum of three weeks is needed. Antibiotic therapy may be altered once a CSF culture results and antibiotic susceptibility are known.

Patients who are immunocompromised or have neurosurgical concerns (VP shunts, recent neurosurgery, recent head trauma) benefit form broad-spectrum gram-positive and gram-negative coverage with a combination of antibiotics such as vancomycin and ceftazidime. In the newborn, no single antibiotic has bactericidal activity against all of the possible organisms commonly encountered. The most widely used combination therapy is ampicillin with an aminoglycoside; ampicillin plus cefotaxime is equally effective. For an infant in the first 3 months of life, in the absence of evidence that suggests the presence of unusual organisms, conventional therapy is ampicillin and a third-generation cephalosporin. Beyond the third month of life, monotherapy with a third-generation cephalosporin provides adequate coverage, except where there are resistant strains of *S. pneumoniae.* When Gram-positive cocci are identified on the CSF Gram's stain, the combination of a broad-spectrum cephalosporin and vancomycin is suggested.

Corticosteroids are believed to be beneficial in the treatment of bacterial meningitis as it blunts the inflammatory response elaborated by cytokines, which decreases intracranial pressure and minimizes the sequelae of meningitis, including hearing loss. The best evidence for the use of dexamethasone is in *H. influenzae* type b meningitis. The benefit in pneumococcal meningitis is less certain. The Committee on Infectious Diseases of the American Academy of Pediatrics recommends dexamethasone therapy in the treatment of infants and children with *H. influenzae* type b meningitis, and suggests that it should be considered in pneumococcal meningitis in infants and children 6 weeks of age and older. Dexamethasone should not administered in cases of aseptic or "partially treated" meningitis, or in infants with bacterial meningitis who are less than 6 weeks of age. When dexamethasone is used, it should be administered as soon as possible in the course of treatment, preferable before or at the time of antibiotic administration. Different dosing regimens have been reported: 0.15 mg/kg every 6 hours for 4 days or 0.4 mg/kg every 12 hours for 2 days. The most commonly reported adverse effect of dexamethasone is gastrointestinal bleeding. Reduced penetration of vancomycin with dexamethasone therapy has been described. Prophylaxis for meningococcal and *Haemophilus meningitis* is described in **Tables 92.7** and **92.8**.

Meningitis with Febrile Seizures The suspicion of meningitis and decision to perform a lumbar puncture is a critical decision in the management of a child with febrile seizure. The American Academy of Pediatrics has recommended a lumbar puncture be strongly considered in children less than 12 months of age with a first febrile seizure and considered in patients 12 to 18 months. Findings that should raise the emergency physician's suspicion for meningitis in a child with a febrile seizure include: (1) concerning preseizure symptoms such as lethargy, irritability or poor feeding; (2) markedly prolonged postictal phase and/or abnormal postictal mental status; (3) specific physical signs of meningitis; (4) pretreatment with antibiotics; and (5) a complex febrile seizure which is prolonged, focal or multiple within 24 hours.

Neonatal Meningitis Bacterial meningitis is more common in the first month of life than at any other age. Newborn infants, particularly premature, are at greatest risk for bacteria meningitis because of immunologic immaturity. Early onset sepsis/meningitis presents within the first days of life and is associated with infections acquired during labor and delivery. Infants who develop early-onset sepsis/meningitis have risk factors that include prematurity, maternal colonization with Group B streptococcus (GBS), prolonged or premature rupture of membranes and chorioamnionitis. Late-onset sepsis presents after the first week of life with meningitis and results from bacterial colonization during the intrapartum period or transmission from a family member.

Table 92.7

Prophylaxis for High Risk Exposure to Invasive Meningococcal Disease

Medication	Age Group	Dose	Duration
Rifampin	≤1 month	5 mg/kg PO every 12 h	2 days
	>1 month	10 mg/kg PO, max 600, q 12 h	2 days
Ceftriaxone	≤15 years	125 mg IM	Single dose
	≥15 years	250 mg IM	Single dose
Ciprofloxacin	≥18 years, nonpregnant	500 mg PO	Single dose

Source: Used with permission from the American Academy of Pediatrics *AAP Red Book.*

Group B streptococcus is the major pathogen associated with meningitis in neonates and is seen in both early and late-onset disease. There has been a decline in the incidence of GBS due increased administration of maternal prophylaxis. Gram-negative enteric organisms account for another 30% of neonatal meningitis. *Escherichia coli* followed by *Klebsiella* are the most common organisms. *Listeria monocytogenes* accounts for approximately 5% to 20% of cases of neonatal meningitis and is associated with both early and late-onset disease.

Parameters of CSF in neonates are different from values beyond the neonatal period. CSF abnormalities are typically most pronounced with Gram-negative meningitis. Gram stains are frequently negative with *L. monocytogenes* because of the low number of bacteria in the CSF.

Empiric antibiotics for infants with suspected meningitis must cover Gram-positive and Gram-negative enteric organisms. Typically this includes ampicillin and an aminoglycoside (gentamicin) or a third generation cephalosporin (cefotaxime). Because there is synergy for ampicillin and gentamycin in the GBS, combined therapy is recommended until the CSF is sterilized.

Mortality from neonatal meningitis is in the range of 20%, greatest in preterm infants, and is related to the pathogen and timeliness of diagnosis. Significant sequelae (hydrocephalus, seizures, cerebral palsy, developmental delay, hearing loss) are seen in 25% to 50% of children, greatest in cases of Gram-negative meningitis, followed by GBS.

Aseptic Meningitis Enteroviruses (echovirus, coxsackie A and B viruses, polioviruses) account for more than half of cases of aseptic meningitis in children. Enteroviral infections occur year round, but also in outbreaks during summer and fall months. Rarely, aseptic meningitis is caused by nonviral agents (parasites, rickettsiae, mycoplasma) or noninfectious entities (drugs, autoimmune diseases, Kawasaki disease). Herpes is a particular concern in the newborn period.

Symptoms of aseptic meningitis overlap those seen with bacterial meningitis and in older children include, headache, fever, nausea, vomiting, photophobia, meningismus, and lethargy. Infants and young children will present in a nonspecific manner. The CSF typically shows a modest increase of WBC (<250 cells/mm^3) with a lymphocyte predominance, a mild elevation of protein and a normal glucose. A polymerase chain reaction (PCR) on CSF is the most useful test in making the diagnosis of viral encephalitis or meningitis.

Table 92.8

Categories of Risk for Contacts of Patients with Meningococcal Disease

High Risk: Prophylaxis Recommended
Household contact, especially young children
Child care, nursery school contact during 7 days before onset
Direct exposure to patient's oral secretions during 7 days before onset
Mouth to mouth resuscitation, exposure to endotracheal tube
Frequently slept/ate in same dwelling as patient during 7 days before onset

Low risk: Prophylaxis Not Recommended
Casual contact, not exposure to secretions
Indirect contact, only contact with high-risk contact, not with index patient
Health care professional without direct exposure to patient's oral secretions

Source: Used with permission from the American Academy of Pediatrics *AAP Red Book.*

Herpes Simplex Meningitis Neonatal herpes simplex virus (HSV) infection can be cutaneous with skin, eye, and mouth involvement, involve the CNS, or be disseminated involving multiple organs. The later two forms of neonatal herpes may occur in the absence of skin lesions. If HSV infection is suspected, CSF should be obtained for PCR detection as well as routine examination. Red cells in an atraumatic lumbar puncture are highly suggestive of HSV CNS infection. Laboratory tests should include liver function tests, complete blood cell count, and chest radiograph, if respiratory abnormalities are present. Swabs of the oropharynx, conjunctiva, and rectum should be obtained for viral culture. Neonates with suspected HSV infection should be treated with intravenous acyclovir (20 mg/kg) every 8 h for 21 days.

Ear, Eye, and Throat Infections in Children

Acute Otitis Media

Acute otitis media (AOM), defined as infected fluid in the middle ear associated with other signs of acute illness, is the most frequent diagnosis of children visiting physicians offices. The recent increase in antibiotic resistance has created new challenges for the physician diagnosing and treating otitis media.

Epidemiology

The highest incidence of AOM occurs in children between 6 months and 24 months of age. Two thirds of children in the United States are reported to have had an episode of otitis media by the time they are 1 year old. Children who attend day care facilities, particularly in centers with four or more children, have a higher incidence of otitis media than those cared for at home. Other identifiable risk factors include household smoking, pacifier use, season, and altered host defenses. The best protective factor appears to be breastfeeding in the first three months of life.

Pathogenesis

Most commonly, an antecedent upper respiratory infection or allergic rhinitis results in congestion of the nose, nasopharynx, which subsequently obstructs the isthmus of the eustachian tube. The middle ear accumulates secretions, which is conducive to microbial growth and suppuration. These middle ear effusions may persist for weeks to months following antimicrobial treatment and sterilization of middle ear fluid.

Microbiology

Three types of bacteria are responsible for middle ear disease in children. *Streptococcus pneumoniae* causes 30% of disease. Pneumococcal disease is the pathogen that will least likely resolve spontaneously without antibiotics. The conjugate pneumoccocal vaccine in one study decreased the number of cultured confirmed episodes of pneumococcal AOM by 34%.

Nontypable strains of *Haemophilus influenzae* cause 15% to 30% of cases of otitis media. One third to one half of *H. influenzae* strains produce beta-lactamase. The conjugate HIB vaccine has had relatively little impact on the incidence of otitis media since very few cases of *Haemophilus influenzae* type B have been isolated. *Moraxella catarrhalis* causes 5% to 15% of disease and most strains are beta lactamase producers. *Mycoplasma pneumonia* is a rare isolate from middle ear fluids, but has the distinct finding of bullous myringitis. *Chlamydia trachomatis* has been associated with otitis media in infants younger than 6 months of age.

Viruses comprise a large percentage of cases of acute otitis media, with respiratory syncytial virus isolate in 74% in one study. Parainfluenza virus and influenza virus were also isolated.

Clinical Manifestations

Symptoms of AOM include otalgia, fever, irritability, anorexia, hearing loss, and vertigo. Otorrhea or swelling behind the ear (suggesting mastoid extension of disease) are more specific findings.

Because many of the clinical symptoms are nonspecific, the diagnoses of AOM require a history of acute onset, signs of middle ear effusion and the presence of middle ear inflammation. The clinical practice guideline published by the American Academy of Pediatarics (AAP) and the American Academy of Family Practitioners (AAFP) in 2004 describes evidence of middle ear effusion as bulging of the tympanic membrane, limited mobility of tympanic membrane, air fluid level behind tympanic membrane, or otorrhea. Signs or symptoms of middle ear inflammation include distinct erythema of the tympanic membrane or distinct otalgia (**FIGURE 92.3**).

Treatment

The AAP currently recommends that the treatment of AOM includes an adequate assessment and pain control with benzocaine containing ear drops, acetaminophen, or ibuprofen. In addition, it recommends observation (with symptomatic relief) for 48 to 72 hours without antibiotic treatment in select populations:

- Children 6 months to 2 years of age who are otherwise healthy with mild disease (mild otalgia and fever <39) and an uncertain diagnosis (i.e., lack of physical findings such as bulging of the tympanic membrane, limited mobility of the tympanic membrane, air fluid level behind tympanic membrane, or otorrhea).
- Children over 2 years of age without severe symptoms or with uncertain diagnosis. Observation should only be considered if follow up can be assured and antimicrobial agents will be started if signs or symptoms worsen.

If the decision is made to treat with antibiotics, amoxicillin (80–90 mg/kg/day) is the initial choice in order to provide effective coverage against susceptible and intermediate resistant pneumococci. For patients with severe illness (fever >39° C) and for those who may need additional coverage for beta lactamase resistant organisms, amoxicillin-clavulanate (90 mg/kg of amoxicillin component) should be used. In the penicillin-allergic child with a previous mild reaction (not associated with urticaria or anaphylaxis), a cephalosporin such as cefpodoxime (10 mg/kg/day once daily) or cefuroxime (30 mg/kg/day in 2 divided doses) can be used. In those whom a penicillin allergy is considered severe, alternative options are azithromycin (10 mg/kg/day on day 1 and 5 mg/kg/day on days 2–5 in a single daily dose) or clarithromycin (15 mg/kg/day in two divided doses). In the patient who is vomiting or who cannot tolerate antibiotics for another reason, a single dose of ceftriaxone (50 mg/kg) has been shown to be effective treatment (**Tables 92.9 and 92.10**).

Conjunctivitis

Conjunctivitis, or inflammation of the conjunctiva, is the most common diagnosis in the patient with a red eye and

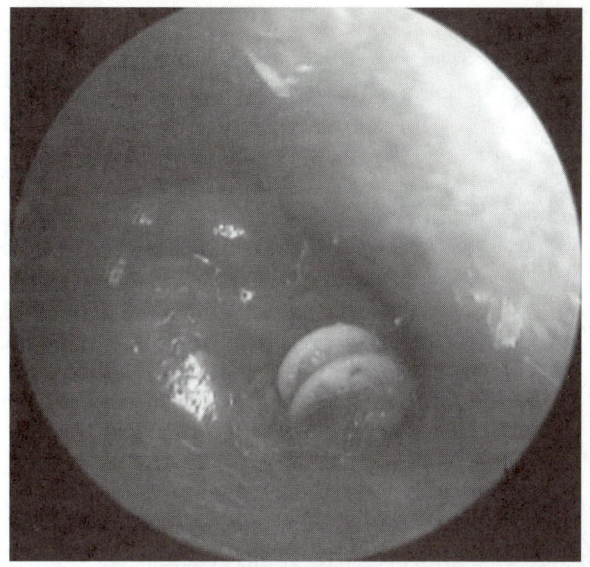
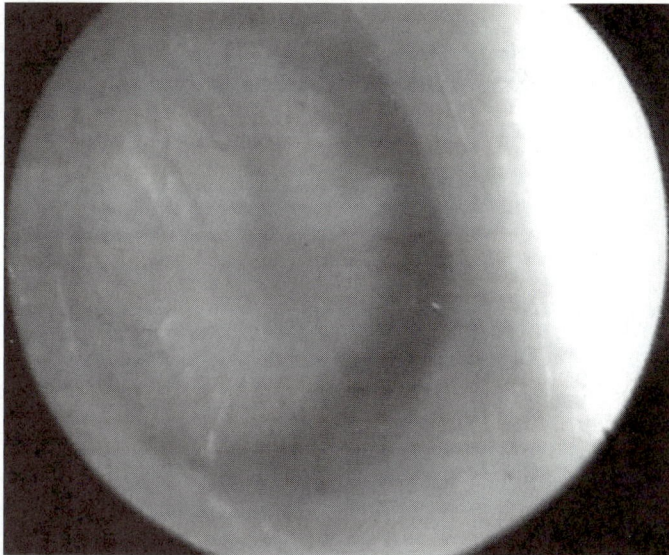
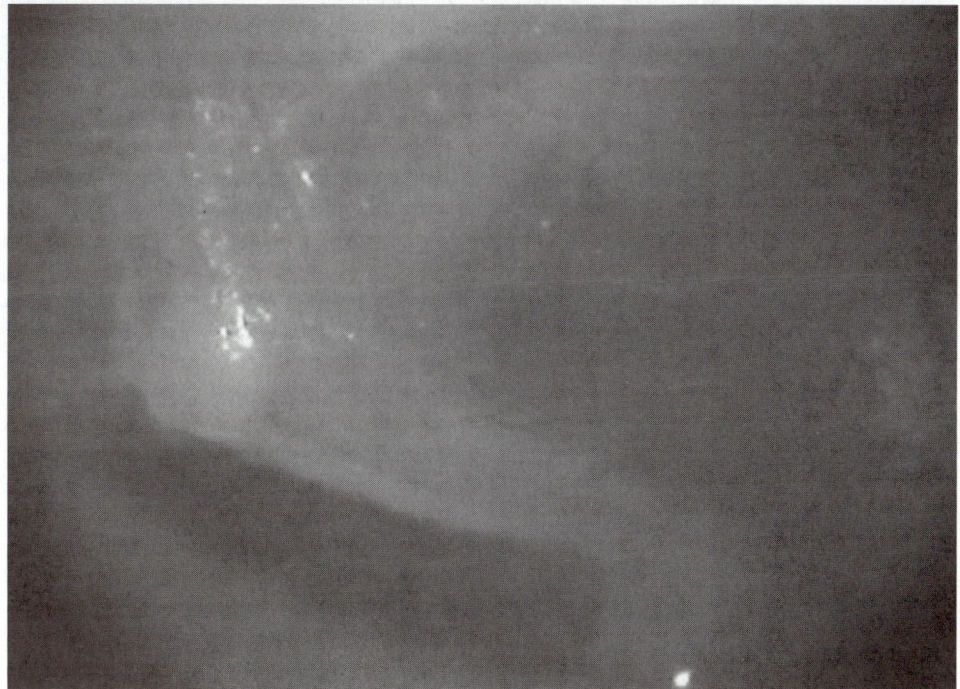

FIGURE 92.3 Photographs of the tympanic membrane.

discharge. The conjunctiva is normally clear and when inflamed looks red or pink and has the appearance of congested blood vessels. Causes of conjunctivitis are numerous and can be divided into infectious (bacterial or viral) or noninfectious (allergic, toxic). Bacterial conjunctivitis is more commonly found in children than adults, although most infectious conjunctivitis is viral.

Clinical Manifestations

Viral conjunctivitis is typically caused by adenovirus and begins with a viral prodrome followed by adenopathy, fever, and watery or mucoserous discharge in one eye. Discomfort is often described as gritty or sandy. Progression to the other eye often occurs in 24 to 48 hours. The drainage is

usually not purulent although patients describe crusting particularly after sleeping.

Bacterial conjunctivitis in children is commonly caused by the pathogens associated with otitis media: *Streptococcus pneumoniae,* non-typable *H. influenzae,* and *Moraxella catarrhalis. Staphylococcus aureus* may be encountered in older children and adolescents. *Neisseria gonorrhoeae* should be considered in the sexually active adolescent presenting with severe acute profuse purulent discharge associated with red conjunctiva. Gonococcal conjunctivitis is a serious infection that requires hospitalization for systemic and topical therapy. Bacterial conjunctivitis usually presents with redness or discharge in one eye, although bilateral disease does not rule out a bacterial etiology. The discharge is

Table 92.9

APP 2004 Recommendations for the Treatment of AOM

Age	Certain Diagnosis	Uncertain Diagnosis
<6 months	Antibacterial therapy	Antibacterial therapy
6 months–2 years	Antibacterial therapy	Antibacterial therapy if severe illness; Observation option* if nonsevere illness
>2 years	Antibacterial therapy if severe illness; Observation option* if nonsevere illness	Observation option*

*Observation is an appropriate option only when appropriate follow-up can be assured and antibacterial agents started if symptoms persist or worsen. Non severe illness is mild otalgia and fever <39° C.
Source: Used with permission from the American Academy of Pediatrics. AAP Clinical Guidelines: diagnosis and management of acute otitis media. *Pediatrics* 2004;113:1451.

thick and globular, and may be yellow, white or green. This thick discharge will continue throughout the day. The purulent discharge will be present at the lid margins. Allergic conjunctivitis typically presents with bilateral symptoms of itching, watery discharge and conjunctival injection.

Conjunctivitis in the newborn (ophthalmia neonatorum) is a form of conjunctivitis usually caused by *N. gonorrhea* or *Chlamydia trachomatis*. Gonococcal conjunctivitis may onset as soon as 12 hours after birth, and may cause severe conjunctivitis and corneal scarring. Because of the severe potential of this infection all children are treated prophylactically with erythromycin, Neosporin, or tobramycin ointment. If gonococcal infection is suspected in the neonate, topical as well as systemic treatment with ceftriaxone is indicated.

Management

Both viral and bacterial causes of conjunctivitis are extremely contagious, and can be spread by direct contact with infected secretions or through contact with contaminated surfaces such as household linens. Most cases of conjunctivitis are viral and resolve spontaneously within 3 to 5 days, although, similar to the accompanying viral upper respiratory infection, symptoms may persist up to two weeks. Some patients get symptomatic relief from topical antihistamine/decongestants.

Bacterial conjunctivitis can be treated topically with agents likely to cover the most common pathogens. Oint-

ments may be preferred in younger children, or those with difficulty accepting eye medications. These agents may blur vision for 15 to 20 minutes after application, but have the benefit of staying on the lid, even if the initial dose was not applied directly on the conjunctiva. Appropriate choices include erythromycin ointment or sulfa ophthalmic drops, bacitracin ointment or flouroquinolone drops.

Periorbital and Orbital Cellulitis

Periorbital or preseptal cellulitis is defined as an infection in the orbital space anterior to the orbital septum. The orbital septum acts as a protective barrier that prevents the spread of infection. If infection penetrates the septum, orbital cellulitis, a much more serious infection and an ophthalmological emergency, results. Periorbital cellulitis can present at any age, but is more common under the age of 5. Predisposing factors include: localized trauma (including insect bites and scratches); localized eyelid infections (hordeola, chalazia, dacrocystitis); upper respiratory infections; and sinusitis. *H. influenzae* type B, once responsible for a large number of cases, has virtually been eliminated with the extensive use of conjugated Hib vaccine. *S. aureus* and *S. pneumoniae* now predominate as pathogens causing periorbital cellulitis. *M. catarrhalis* has also been described. Orbital celluliltis may result from progression of periorbital cellulitis, but more commonly results from extension of severe sinusitis. Orbital trauma and orbital fractures are also significant causes of orbital

Table 92.10

1999 CDC Algorithm

First-Line Therapy	High risk for drug resistant *S. pneumoniae* (DRSP) (<2 years old, day care, antibiotics Rx in last 3 mo)	Amoxicillin 80–90 mg/kg/d
	Low risk for DRSP (none of the above factors present)	Amoxicillin 40–45 mg/kg/d
Treatment Failure	Consider tympanocentesis	Amoxicillin-Clavulanate Cefuroxime Axetil Ceftriaxone (IM)

Source: Used with permission from *Pediatric Infectious Disease Journal*. Acute otitis media: management and surveillance in an era of pneumococococcal resistance. *Pediatr Infect Dis J* 1999;18:1–9.

cellulitis, and may begin to develop 48 to 72 hours after trauma.

Clinical Manifestations

Patients with periorbital cellulitis present with eyelid hyperemia and distention of the surrounding soft tissue. They may also have fever, pain, nasal discharge, conjunctivitis, or chemosis.

Ocular movement need to be carefully examined in all directions, and any patient exhibiting limited ocular mobility or visual loss should be considered at risk for posterior extension of infection and orbital cellulitis. The presence of proptosis is also suggestive of orbital infection. A high index of suspicion is needed due to the severe nature of this infection. If there is any suspicion for orbital involvement a thin cut, contrast enhanced orbital CT or MRI is indicated to fully evaluate the orbit.

Management

Treatment of periorbital cellulitis depends on the age of the patient and severity of disease. Limited disease in those that appear nontoxic may be candidates for outpatient management with cephalexin or dicloxacillin, assuming good follow-up can be assured. Otherwise, inpatient management is with parenteral cefuroxime (150 mg/kg/day divided TID) or ceftriaxone 50–100 mg/kg/day).

Suspected cases of orbital cellulits demand early ophthalmological consultation, in anticipation of prompt surgical drainage of the paranasal sinuses or the orbital abscess if present. Parenteral antibiotics should be initiated early with broad coverage for against *S. aureus, S. pneumonia, S. pyogenes,* and anaerobic organisms. Cefuroxime (150 mg/kg/day divided tid) or ampicillin-sulbactam (200 mg/kg/day divided bid) should be considered. Anaerobic coverage with clindamycin (40 mg/kg/day divided 4 qid) or metronidazole (30 mg/kg/day divided bid) should be considered.

Acute Pharyngitis

Pharyngitis is defined as infection of the pharynx and the tonsils, and is one of the leading causes for children and young adults to seek medical care. Pharyngitis is caused by many different microorganisms, both viral and bacterial. Viral etiologies are the most common cause of pharyngitis and include: infectious mononucleosis, influenza, adenovirus, HSV, and primary HIV (adolescents). Bacterial causes of acute pharyngitis include non-group A streptococci, *Mycoplasma pneumoniae,* and *Neisseria gonorrhoeae* (in sexually active adolescents). Group A *Streptococcus* (GAS) is the most common bacterial cause of acute pharyngitis, causing approximately 25% of cases in children. The peak of streptococcal cases occurs in the winter and early spring. Because of its association with acute rheumatic disease, it is important to diagnose and treat cases of GAS. In addition, early treatment results in earlier symptomatic relief by approximately 24 hours.

Clinical Manifestations

Differentiating GAS from other causes of acute pharyngitis depends on several clinical factors. Acute onset of fever with an exudative pharyngitis associated with tender anterior cervical nodes increase the likelihood that the infection is due to GAS. Fever, headache, and abdominal pain may be present. Factors that decrease the likelihood of GAS include: the absence of fever (without antipyretic use), absence of pharyngeal erythema, and presence of other manifestations of upper respiratory infection such as rhinorrhea, conjunctivitis, and cough.

Clinical examination is notoriously unreliable, particularly in children less than 3 years of age. All patients in whom GAS pharyngitis is suspected should have rapid antigen testing as an initial screening test and for those in whom the rapid antigen screening is negative, a throat culture. Overall sensitivity of rapid testing is between 80% to 90%, but is highly specific for GAS infection.

Management

The goal in appropriately identifying and treating GAS is to prevent suppurative complication (peritonsillar or retropharyngeal abscess), decrease the likelihood of ARF, shorten the clinical course of the disease, and limit infectivity.

Penicillin remains the treatment of choice for GAS. A full 10-day course is necessary to eradicate the organism. Recently it has been shown that bid dosing is as efficacious as tid dosing (250 mg bid for children or 500 mg bid for adults). For those who are penicillin allergic, erythromycin is the first choice (20–40 mg/kg divided bid). Azithromycin has been shown to be effective in 5 day courses and may be better tolerated than erythromycin in the penicillin-allergic patient. However, care must be taken to avoid the use of this macrolide for first line treatment in those who can tolerate penicillin, as streptococcal resistance to macrolides develops rapidly with extensive use of these drugs.

Urinary Tract Infections

A urinary tract infection (UTI) is a significant cause of bacterial illness in the pediatric population. While often considered a trivial infection, UTIs can have significant associated morbidity resulting in chronic renal failure.

Epidemiology

The prevalence of UTIs varies with age and sex. UTIs are estimated to occur in 1% to 2% of neonates with males (usually uncircumcised) to females affected in a 3:1 ratio. Circumcision is associated with a tenfold decrease in the incidence of UTIs in males under the age of 1 year. In infancy and childhood, females are affected preferentially in a 10:1 ratio. UTIs occur in 1% to 3% of infants and 3% to 5% of the school-aged population. By adolescence, there is a further increase in female incidence associated with sexual activity.

Risk factors for UTIs in both males and females include urological anomalies, neurogenic bladder, indwelling urethral catheter, and a medical history of ureteral reflux in a sibling. For females, risk factors include sexual activity, sexual abuse, constipation, pinworms, infrequent or incomplete voiding, and use of bubble bath.

Pathogenesis

A UTI is a bacterial infection of the bladder, ureters, or collecting system of the kidney. This definition can be further specified by anatomic location. Infection or inflammation localized to the urethra without involvement of bladder or kidney is termed urethritis. Infection confined to the bladder is considered cystitis, and when it extends to involve the renal parenchyma, it is termed pyelonephritis. Reflux is defined as backflow of urine from the bladder to the ureters with potential extension to the renal parenchyma.

Although cystitis can be caused by adenovirus, the vast majority of UTIs are bacterial in origin. For all ages and sexes, *E. coli* is the most common etiologic agent. Some strains of *E. coli* have cell surface adherence factors that promote attachment to bladder mucosa. In neonates, common organisms responsible for UTIs include *E. coli* (74%), *Klebsiella* (7%), and *Proteus* (4%). In preschool and school-aged children, the most common organisms are the *Enterobacteriaceae*, where Gram-negative enterics such as *E. coli* are responsible for up to 90% of acute infections and 80% of recurrent infections. In adolescent females, *group D streptococci* (enterococci), *Staphylococcus aureus*, *Streptococcus viridans*, and *Staphylococcus saprophyticus* have been identified as causative agents in up to 40% of UTIs. In children with recurrent UTIs as well as hospitalized patients and males, infection with *Proteus* and *Pseudomonas* occurs more frequently. Aerobic Gram-positive cocci, previously thought to be contaminants, have recently been identified as true pathogens (**Table 92.11**).

The majority of UTIs are caused by the ascension of bacteria from the perineal area. Any anatomical or functional obstruction of the urinary tract predisposes a patient to a UTI and makes it more difficult to eradicate. A tight foreskin may promote backflow of contaminated urine. Once cystitis occurs, vesicourethral reflux permits infected urine to reach the kidney, which can result in permanent renal damage and scarring with eventual progression to chronic renal failure. UTIs in newborns, young infants, and immunocompromised patients often result in bacteremia.

Table 92.11

Bacteria Commonly Associated with Urinary Tract Infection

Infants
  Escherichia coli
  Klebsiella
  Proteus
Preschool to school age
  Escherichia coli
Adolescents
  Escherichia coli
  Group D streptococci (enterococci)
  Staphylococcus aureus
  Streptococcus viridans
  Staphylococcus saprophyticus

Clinical Presentation by Age

The clinical presentation of a UTI in an infant is vague and nonspecific including fever, hypothermia, irritability, and jaundice. Gastrointestinal symptoms such as vomiting, poor feeding, failure to thrive, and abdominal distention are common and may lead to misdiagnosis.

In older children, acute UTIs present with complaints specific to the urinary tract: dysuria, frequency, urgency, hematuria, malodorous, enuresis, and vomiting. Chronic UTIs and occasionally acute UTIs may present with relatively few symptoms.

The history should always include questions about a family history of UTI or reflux. A voiding history is crucial as children with infrequent or incomplete voiding are predisposed to develop a UTI. Specifically, a history of daytime enuresis, urinary dribbling, or weak stream should be obtained. In children with fever without a source, occult UTIs occurs in 3% to 4% of males under 12 months and 8% to 9% of females under the age of 5 years.

The physical examination should include growth parameters. Children with chronic or frequent UTIs may have a decreased rate of growth or failure to thrive. Blood pressure must be documented, as systemic hypertension occurs with renal failure. The abdominal examination may indicate the presence of a mass (e.g., enlarged bladder). The genitalia may reveal such findings as labial adhesions, phimosis, or evidence of sexual abuse. Infant males need to be evaluated for presence or absence of circumcised. A rectal examination may indicate pinworms or altered sphincter tone associated with sexual abuse or neurogenic compromise.

Diagnosis

The diagnosis of a UTI in children should be confirmed by culture rather than be based on the urinalysis or clinical grounds alone. A urinalysis revealing pyuria does not always correlate with bacteriuria, nor does bacteriuria always present with pyuria. Urine from the bladder and upper urinary tract should be sterile. A Gram stain of unspun urine that demonstrates bacteria is more likely to be diagnostic of a UTI; however, it is not possible to determine if a single bacterium is present or if there are multiple bacteria suggesting a contaminated specimen. The precise colony count required for diagnosis is dependent on the method of obtaining the urine specimen. A cleanly voided midstream specimen is useful in children who are toilet trained and in adolescents. For a cleanly voided midstream specimen, the definition of a UTI is based on the statistical concept that "significant bacteriuria" ($>10^5$ organisms per milliliter of one colony type) correlates with an 80% chance of true infection. Demonstrating two consecutive cultures with $>10^5$ organisms per milliliter of one colony type increases the likelihood of infection to 96%. Less than 10^4 organisms per milliliter or multiple organisms is suggestive of an absence of infection or specimen contamination. In adolescents who are symptomatic, any growth $\geq10^2$ colonies per milliliter is suggestive of a UTI. A catheterized specimen is suspicious if any organisms are found, while a pure growth of greater than 10^3

colonies per milliliter is diagnostic. In an infant, the urine specimen may be obtained by suprapubic bladder tap or bladder catheterization, where any growth in a urine culture is significant. Bagged urine specimens are unreliable and are only useful if the culture reveals no growth. In general, a bagged specimen should not be used to obtain a specimen for culture in an ED.

Management

To diminish renal morbidity, antibiotic treatment should begin as soon as an adequate urine specimen has been obtained for culture. Criteria for antibiotic therapy include a positive urine culture, clinical toxicity, or a febrile child in whom the urinalysis (pyuria) or Gram stain is suggestive of a UTI. If these criteria are not met, it is prudent to withhold antibiotics pending culture results.

The nontoxic child or adolescent can be treated as an outpatient with oral antibiotics. IV antibiotics and hospital admission are appropriate in infants younger than 6 months of age; toxic-appearing children and adolescents; any age with vomiting, immunocompromise, prior history, or UTI; or if a resistant pathogen is suspected (**Table 92.12**). Uncomplicated cystitis is adequately treated with 1 to 3 days of antibiotics. A child with a congenital anomaly or a history of UTI with incomplete radiographic evaluation should be given a 10-day course of treatment. If the culture is negative, the antibiotics may be stopped. The urine culture should be repeated in 48 hours to confirm urine

Table 92.12
Antimicrobials Options Treatment of UTI

Antimicrobial	Daily Dosage
Parenteral Treatment	
Ceftriaxone	75 mg/kg every 24 h
Cefotaxime	150 mg/kg/d divided every 6 h
Ceftazidime	150 mg/kg/d divided every 6 h
Cefazolin	50 mg/kg/d divided every 8 h
Gentamicin	7.5 mg/kg/d divided every 8 h
Tobramycin	5 mg/kg/d divided every 8 h
Ticarcillin	300 mg/kg/d divided every 6 h
Ampicillin	100 mg/kg/d divided every 6 h
Oral Treatment of UTI	
Amoxicillin*	20–40 mg/kg/d in 3 doses
TMP with SMX	6–12 mg TMP/30–60 mg SMX/kg/d in 2 doses
Sulfisoxazole	120–150 mg/kg/d in 4 doses
Cefixime	8 mg/kg/d in 2 doses
Cefpodixime	10 mg/kg/d in 2 doses
Cefprozil	30 mg/kg/d in 2 doses
Cephalexin	50–100 mg/kg/d in 4 doses
Loracarbef	15–30 mg/kg/d in 2 doses

*Note: Increasing E. coli resistance to ampicillin makes ampicillin and amoxicillin less effective than alternative agents.
Adapted from: Practice parameter: The diagnosis, treatment, and evaluation of the initial urinary tract infection in febrile infants and young children, American Academy of Pediatrics Committee on Quality Improvement. Subcommittee on Urinary Tract Infection. *Pediatrics* 1999;103;843–852.

sterilization. Suppressive doses of antibiotics, usually one third to one half of the regular dose given in one bedtime dose, are indicated for children with a documented UTI pending radiographic evaluation or in children with frequent episodes of uncomplicated cystitis.

Useful adjuncts to antibiotics include acidification of the urine with juices high in citric acid content or supplemental vitamin C to inhibit bacterial growth. Increased fluid intake promotes frequent voiding and bladder washout of bacteria. Bubble baths should be avoided since irritation of the urethral meatus may promote bacterial ascent. Appropriate wiping procedures should be reviewed with young females and their parents to prevent back to front wiping and consequent spread of bacteria.

Since approximately 50% of infants and 30% of older children have an anatomical anomaly of their renal system in conjunction with a UTI, radiographic evaluation is a crucial part of the overall management. Radiographic studies, including a voiding cystourethrogram (VCUG) and an ultrasound of the kidneys and bladder, are recommended after the first UTI in both male and female infants and toddlers. These studies are normally done 2 to 4 weeks after resolution of the UTI. In the case of a child who does not respond to antibiotic therapy, studies should be done sooner to rule out urinary tract obstruction.

Common Pediatric Rashes

Impetigo

Impetigo, a superficial skin infection caused by *Staphylococcus aureus* or *Streptococcus pyogenes*, is recognized by a honey-colored crusted appearance. Bullous impetigo is usually caused by *Strep. pyogenes*; impetigo contagiosa is caused by *S. aureus*.

Epidemiology and Pathophysiology

Impetigo primarily affects school-age children and young adults and has been associated with crowded living conditions, poor hygiene, and colonization of the patient's nares and/or skin. Skin biopsy shows a cleft in the stratum granulosum.

Clinical Features

Skin lesions begin as well demarcated reddened macules that progress to fluid filled bullae, which rupture and form a honey colored crust. Lesions are typically grouped, are highly contagious and recur until properly treated. They may form around an area of minor trauma. Bullous impetigo is a less common presentation characterized by larger areas of involvement as well as bullae that coalesce before rupture and crusting occurs. Because they may be clinically indistinguishable, management is aimed at both common pathogens for this disease.

Management

Mild, acute, and localized infections are treated with good hygiene with antibacterial soap, topical application of mupirocin to lesions and nares and treatment of household members for asymptomatic carriage. More severe or recurrent infections can be treated with oral dicloxacillin, cephalexin, or erythromycin.

Complications

Acute glomerulonephritis or scarlet fever may rarely present as complications of impetigo.

Ecthyma

Described as "deep impetigo," this infection is characterized by punctate tender lesions on the lower extremities and buttocks.

Epidemiology and Pathophysiology

A common skin finding following minor trauma, which becomes infected with skin flora, ecthyma occurs in young children as well as the elderly. Infection occurs deep to the stratum granulosum. It is caused by *Group A streptococcus* (GAS) and *S. aureus,* is slower to heal, and often leaves scars.

Clinical Presentation and Management

The lesions of ecthyma begin as excoriations or as evidence of minor trauma. They become infected with local skin flora, develop raised margins, pruritus, and may be associated with drainage. Fever and/or lymphadenopathy are rarely seen.

Staphyloccal Scalded Skin Syndrome

Staphylococcal scalded skin syndrome (SSSS) includes a number of a toxin-mediated diseases caused by *S. aureus.* The clinical manifestations of SSSS are generally age related and include Ritter's disease (in newborns) and Lyell's syndrome (in children). Milder forms include pemphigus neonatorum and bullous impetigo.

Epidemiology

Widespread, sheet-like desquamation typical of SSSS is seen predominantly in infants and children less than five years old. Transmission is through direct person-to-person contact.

Pathophysiology

Destruction of the stratum granulosum is thought to affect children under five due to the lack of antibody formation. Several strains of *S. aureus* produce an exfoliative toxin, which provokes a massive T cell stimulation as well as proliferation of the exotoxin. The toxin causes acantholysis and cleavage within the stratum granulosum.

Clinical Features

SSSS begins with a non-specific prodrome followed by a generalized erythematous, tender rash beginning in periorbital and perioral areas of the face. This rash spreads to the trunk and centrifugally to the limbs. It is followed by wrinkling and sloughing of the epidermis within hours to days. Nikolsky's sign, defined as sloughing of the skin with gentle lateral pressure, may be positive in areas of the skin, which appear uninvolved. Exfoliation may continue for hours to days, necessitating hospital admission in severe cases.

Management

During the acute phase of desquamation, newborns and young children with diffuse disease usually require hospitalization, monitoring of fluid and electrolyte balance, fluid resuscitation and parenteral antibiotic treatment. Topical therapy includes mupirocin ointment as well as treatment with a penicillinase-resistant agent. Patients should have contact isolation.

Toxic Shock Syndrome (TSS)

TSS is an acute toxin-mediated illness caused by *S. aureus* and characterized by fever, rash and hypotension.

Epidemiology

TSS is seen most commonly in young adults and in females. In the United States, up to 95% of cases of TSS are associated with highly absorptive tampon use.

Pathophysiology

S. aureus-mediated TSS is most often caused by toxic-shock syndrome toxin-1 (TSST-1), a "superantigen" that binds directly to major histocompatibility class II molecules causing direct, causing widespread stimulation of T cells and release of cytokines. Streptococcal TSS is also characterized by multisystem organ failure, but associated with a local GAS infection. TSS usually originates from the patient's own flora, and person-to-person transmission is rare. *Strep. pyogenes* TSS is seen in young children and is associated with varicella. The incubation period for both processes is poorly defined, but may be as short as 12 hours.

Clinical Findings

An acute illness characterized by the sudden onset of high fever, vomiting, and diarrhea. Generalized symptoms of headache and myalgias are reported. This disease progresses rapidly to hypotension, renal failure, and multisystem organ dysfunction. A generalized erythroderma develops with involvement of the hands and feet. Facial involvement includes erythema and hyperemia of mucous membranes and conjunctival injection. Shedding of the hair and nails can occur several months after the illness.

Four of the five the CDC criteria must be satisfied for the diagnosis of TSS to be made. They are:

- Fever 39.8° C or higher
- Diffuse macular erythroderma
- Desquamation of rash (1 to 2 weeks after beginning of illness, particularly if palms and soles are affected)
- Involvement of three or more organs (including gastrointestinal, muscular, mucous membrane, renal, hepatic, hematologic or central nervous system)
- Hypotension

Management

Aggressive fluid resuscitation, blood pressure support, and empiric antibiotics are important in the management of TSS. Both a β-lactamase–resistant antistaphylococcal agent and a protein synthesis-inhibiting antimicrobial, such as clindamycin, should be used early in the presentation. A thorough exam (including pelvic to remove tampon) for suspicious wounds or foreign bodies should be performed early in the course of the illness, and any suspected cause should be removed or drained.

Scarlet Fever

Scarlet fever is the characteristic diffuse erythematous (looks like a sunburn, feels like sandpaper) rash associated with Group A *Streptococcus* infection of the nasopharynx or skin.

Epidemiology

Scarlet fever is most commonly associated with streptococcal pharyngitis. Infection may be transmitted by respiratory secretions, or less commonly from impetiginous skin lesions. Scarlet fever is most common in school-age children.

Pathophysiology

Scarlet fever is caused by pyrogenic exotoxin A, B, and C produced by certain strains of Group A β-hemolytic streptococcus.

Clinical Features

This exanthem begins with punctuate erythema on the upper trunk and spreads to the extremities, sparing the palms and soles. Streptococcal pharyngitis is associated with a "strawberry tongue," fiery red edematous tonsils, petechiae on the soft palate, and circumoral pallor. It is usually preceded by a prodrome of fever, sore throat, headache, and tender lymphadenopathy. The "sandpaper" rash of scarlet fever is fine erythematous, rough, and blanches with pressure. It may be accentuated in the skin folds (Pastia's lines). This generalized exanthem may be followed by desquamation about a week after onset, and may continue for one to two months.

Management

Scarlet fever is treated with systemic antibiotics for the prevention of rheumatic fever and acute glomerulonephritis. Penicillin is the drug of choice, and may be administered as an intramuscular dose when compliance may be difficult. Alternatives include amoxicillin and first generation cephalosporins. Erythromycin, azithromycin, or clindamycin are alternatives in the penicillin allergic patient.

Erysipelas

Erysipelas is a less common, tender, rapidly spreading cellulites. It has a predilection for the face and nose and is caused by *Strep. pyogenes*. It may occur in any age group. Treatment is the same as for other strep infections, including penicillin, cephalexin or erythromycin (**Table 92.13**).

Erythema Infectiosium (Fifth Disease)

Erythema infectiosum, also known as Fifth disease, is an acute childhood viral exanthem caused by human parvovirus (HPV) B19.

Epidemiology and Pathophysiology

Although Parvovirus affects patients of all ages, the classic presentation of Fifth's disease is seen in children ages 3 to

12. Approximately 60% of the general population is seropositive for anti-HPV B19 by age 20 years. More prevalent in the late winter and early spring, this infection is common and transmitted by respiratory droplets during early illness. Parvovirus B19 is associated with several significant complications, including aplastic crisis, especially in patients with chronic hemolytic anemia, neurological conditions, and polyarthropathy thought to stem from deposition of antigen-antibody complexes. Transplacental transmission has been documented and can result in hydrops fetalis.

Clinical Features

After an incubation period of 4 to 14 days, fever, malaise, arthralgias, myalgias, and headache are present and represent acute viremia. Patients may be asymptomatic for about a week before the exanthem develops. This is characterized by "slapped cheek" rash, which appears in association with a lacy reticular rash on the trunk. The rash may start as erythematous macules and papules that coalesce to form larger plaque-like lesions and may persist for weeks to months. Patients are no longer infectious once the rash appears.

Management

Treatment of EI is supportive including NSAIDs, antipruritics, and avoidance of heat and sunlight. Patients with sickle cell disease are at risk for aplastic crisis and immunocompromised patients can develop chronic infection and require specific management.

Roseola Infantum (Exanthem Subitum, Sixth Disease)

Roseola infantum, caused by Human herpes virus 6 (HHV6), is characterized by high fever with rash that appears after defervescence. It may also occur without the classic rash as an acute febrile illness associated with gastrointestinal or respiratory symptoms.

Epidemiology

Roseola is a common, acute febrile illness of childhood. By age one, over 80% of children are seropositive for HHV6 with almost 100% positive by age four. Peak occurrence is between 6 and 14 months. Transmission of the virus is thought to be through respiratory secretions.

Clinical Features

This illness is characterized by an acute high fever and otherwise benign presentation. Because of the height of fever, roseola is also associated with febrile seizures. The maculopapular rash appears with defervescence and recedes within several days. An associated exanthem of pink papules on the soft palate may also be seen with this disease.

Management

Roseola is a self-limited, benign illness. Treatment is supportive.

Measles (Rubeola)

Characterized by fever, cough, coryza, conjunctivitis, and Koplik's spots, rubeola is an uncommon infection in the

Table 92.13

Common Infectious Rashes

Rash	Agent	Clinical Presentation	Treatment
Bullous impetigo	*Staph aureus* predominates, also strep species	Superficial tense clear bullae Preschool children, young adults Red skin lesions progress to bullae, rupture then crust	Dicloxacillin, cephalosporin, erythromycin, mupirocin ointment
Impetigo contagiosa	A β-hemolytic *Strep* predominates, also staph species	Painless honey crusted lesions	As for bullous impetigo—also, nephritogenic strains associated with post strep GN
Ecthyma	*Staph* or *Strep*	Punched out ulcers on the lower extremities; "deep impetigo"	As for bullous impetigo
Staphylococcal scalded skin syndrome	*Staph aureus* toxin-mediated	Scarlatiniform rash follows fever Nikolsky's sign may be present Predominantly children <5	β-lactamase resistant β-lactam antimicrobial agent
Toxic shock syndrome	Toxin producing *Staphylococcus aureus* or *Streptococcus pyogenes* (GAS)	Fever >38.9 C Diffuse macular erythroderma Rapid onset hypotension, multi-organ system failure	Parenteral β-lacatamase resistant antistaphylococcal antimicrobial agent, IVIG
Scarlet fever	Group A β-hemolytic streptococcus toxin	Sandpaper rash spreads from trunk to extremities Punctuate erythema Circumoral sparing Pastia's lines	Penicillin V IM Penicillin G benzathine Erythromycin in PCN allergic patients
Erysipelas	*Strep pyogenes*	Well demarcated, tender, red plaque, may surround a wound Rapidly advancing leading edge Predilection for facial area	Penicillin V, cephalexin, erythromycin

United States. However, it remains a major cause of morbidity and mortality of children in underdeveloped countries. It is caused by an RNA virus in the Paramyxo family.

Epidemiology

Rubeola is transmitted between humans, the only natural host of the disease, via respiratory droplets. Due to the MMR vaccine, the incidence has dropped dramatically, with fewer than 1,000 cases reported per year. The incubation period is between 8 and 12 days, with contagion being highest in the pre-rash stage. This is a highly contagious virus, with 90% to 100% of susceptible contacts becoming infected.

Clinical Features

Measles is characterized by a prodrome of coryza, cough, malaise, and fever. The enanthem (Koplik's spots) appears one to two days prior to the classic maculopapular rash. These are small blue-white lesions on the buccal mucosa. Three to four days later, the exanthema begins at the hairline and spreads downwards. Conjunctivitis improves rapidly with the appearance of the rash. The rash fades within 4 to 5 days, and may be followed by a fine desquamation.

Management

Complications of rubeola include pneumonia, laryngitis, myocarditis, encephalitis, and/or pericarditis. Acute encephalitis occurs in 1 of every 1000 cases. Subacute sclerosing panencephalitis (SSPE) is a very rare degenerative CNS disease that results from persistent measles infection.

There is no specific antiviral treatment for rubeola, although immunoglobulins may attenuate symptoms and lessen the severity of disease, especially in immunocompromised patients. Exposed nonimmune individuals should receive live measles vaccine within 72 hours of exposure unless contraindicated by pregnancy or immunocompromised status. Patients should be isolated for 4 days following the appearance of the rash.

Rubella (German Measles)

Rubella is a generally benign disease characterized by an erythematous maculopapular rash, fever, arthralgias, and lymphadenopathy. However, the major morbidity associated with rubella is congenital rubella syndrome, which consists of miscarriage, fetal death, or congenital anomalies associated with maternal rubella infection, especially during pregnancy.

Epidemiology

Rubella is an RNA virus in the Togaviridae family found only in humans and transmitted through direct or droplet contact. Peak incidence is winter through spring. Up to 50% of infections may be asymptomatic and a patient is most contagious several days before until about a week after the eruption of the rash. Infants with congenital rubella may shed virus for up to one year.

Clinical Features

Rubella in children is a self-limited illness, with a mild prodrome of fever, headache, malaise, lymphadenopathy, and cough. The enanthem of rubella is fine pinpoint macules on the palate (Forcheimer's sign). The rash that follows starts as discrete, red macules that spread from the face and rapidly down the trunk, and to the arms and legs. It is generally not associated with desquamation and resolves completely within days. Unlike rubeola, lesions of rubella do not tend to coalesce. Additional complications, including arthritis and encephalitis, are rare.

Congenital rubella syndrome causes a wide range of anomalies including cardiac (PDA, peripheral pulmonary artery stenosis), neurological (behavioral, meningoencephalitis, MR), bone disease, thrombocytopenia, and purpuric skin lesions ("blueberry muffin" appearance).

Management

School-age children should be isolated for 7 days after the appearance of the rash. Pregnant women with exposure should be evaluated serologic immunity. Treatment is supportive.

Hand-Foot-Mouth Disease

Hand-foot-mouth disease is a common pediatric illness characterized by shallow ulcers in the mouth and a papularvesicular eruption of the hands and feet. Hepangina is also a Coxsackie A16 infection with ulcers in the pharynx only.

Clinical Features

Hand-foot-mouth disease is caused by Coxsackie A16, A5, and A10 enteroviruses. Patients generally are under the age of ten years, with seasonal outbreaks in summer and early fall. Spread is person-to-person and fecal-oral and is highly contagious. The enterovirus infects the GI tracts, from which it produces a generalized viremia, associated with low-grade fever and general malaise, and generally is closely associated with the appearance of the rash. Oral lesions occur on the tongue, hard palate, and buccal mucosa. Lesions on the hands and feet are palpable pink or red lesions, which may appear vesicular. Symptoms are self-limited and benign, usually resolving within one week.

Management

Supportive care including adequate hydration, antipyretics, and analgesia is indicated for patients with acute HFMD and herpangina. However, Coxsackie virus has been associated with more serious systemic illnesses including myocarditis, meningitis, and encephalitis.

Varicella (Chickenpox)

Varicella zoster virus causes chickenpox during a primary infection and zoster (shingles) upon reactivation of the latent virus. It is a member or the herpesvirus family and is highly contagious.

Epidemiology

Varicella is transmitted through direct person-to-person contact, by airborne spread, and rarely from zoster lesions. The varicella vaccine is a live attenuated vaccine administered to healthy patients 12 months of age or older. Immunocompromised patients, including those with chronic corticosteroid use, are at increased risk of more severe disease and serious complications including pneumonia, disseminated disease, and even death. Incubation is 14 to 16 days and patients are contagious from 1 to 2 days before the onset of the rash until the lesions are crusted over. Fetal infection by varicella during the first or second trimester may result in congenital abnormalities such as limb atrophy, scarring of the skin, and mental retardation.

Clinical Features

The generalized pruritic vesicular rash of varicella is preceded by a mild prodrome of fever, headache, and malaise. It is generally distributed over the trunk, face, and proximal extremities. Varicella is generally more severe in older patients, and may be complicated by thrombocytopenia, encephalitis, meningitis, or glomerulonephritis. In immunocompromised hosts, varicella may become chronic and life-threatening. Reye syndrome was known to follow chickenpox cases.

During active infection, herpesvirus establishes latency in the dorsal root ganglia, which may become reactivated during times of stress or illness causing herpes zoster or shingles. Pain and paresthesia may precede the rash, which consists of grouped vesicular lesions distributed along the sensory dermatomes. Post-herpetic neuralgia is the painful sensation that remains after resolution of the rash, and may persist for months to years. The most serious complications of zoster are corneal involvement.

Management

For immunocompetent patients, varicella is usually a benign, self-limited disease. High-risk groups, including neonates, those with immunosuppression, or those with chronic skin conditions, should be considered for treat-

Table 92.14

Viral Exanthems

Rash	Agent	Clinical Presentation	Treatment
Erythema Infectiosum (slapped cheek disease)	Parvovirus B19	Fever, myalgias, diarrhea Slapped cheek appearance Lacey erythematous rash on limbs, trunk Complications include arthritis, aplastic anemia	NSAIDs
Roseola Infantum (roseala)	Human herpes virus 6	High fever with rash after defervescence Faint red macules on neck, trunk, arms 5%–15% febrile seizures	Supportive
Rubeola (measles)	Paramyxovirus	Fever, cough, conjunctivitis, coryza, Koplik spots Morbilliform rash spreads from head to feet	Prevention: Live attenuated vaccine
Rubella (German measles)	Togavirus	Posterior cervical lymphadenopathy URI, headache, N/V Congenital anomalies	Prevention: Live attenuated vaccine
Herpangina	Coxsackie virus, Echovirus	Fever, dysphagia, drooling, vomiting, headache	
Hand Foot and Mouth Disease	Coxsackie virus A16	Fecal oral transmission Fever, sore throat, malaise Anterior buccal mucosa vesicles/ulcers—"halo of erythema"	No antibiotics
Varicella-Zoster	Herpes zoster	Fever malaise, URI Concurrent macules—papules to vesicles—"dewdrop on a rose petal"	Avoid salicylates Acyclovir, immune globulin for immunocompromised.

ment with varicella zoster immunoglobulin (VZIG) and antiviral medication. Patients with shingles may benefit from treatment with antivirals if this is started within one to two days of rash outbreak. Aspirin products should be avoided because of association with Reye's syndrome. Secondary bacterial infection of varicella lesions may require treatment with antibiotics (**Table 92.14**).

Selected Readings

ACEP Clinical Policies Committee Clinical Policies Subcommittee on Pediatric Fever. Clinical policy for children younger than three years presenting to the emergency department with fever. *Ann Emerg Med.* 2003;42:530–545.

Agency for Healthcare Research and Quality. Diagnosis and treatment of uncomplicated acute sinusitis in children. *Summary, Evidence Report/Technology Assessment,* Number 9, Supplement. Rockville, MD: Agency for Health Care Policy and Research, October 2000.

American Academy of Pediatrics. Group A Streptococcal infections. In: Pickering LK (ed). *2000 Red Book: Report of the Committee on Infectious Diseases,* ed 25. Elk Grove Village, IL, American Academy of Pediatrics, 2000:526–530.

American Academy of Pediatrics Subcommittee on the Management of Acute Otitis Media. Clinical Practice Guidelines: diagnosis and management of acute otitis media. *Pediatrics* 2004;113:1451–1465.

Avner JR. Management of fever in infants and children. *Emerg Med Clin North Am* 2002;20:49–67.

Baraff L. Editorial: clinical policy for children younger than three years presenting to the emergency department with fever. *Ann Emerg Med* 2003;42:546–549.

Baraff L. Management of fever without source in infants and children. *Ann Emerg Med* 2000;36:602–614.

Baraff LJ, Lee SI, Schriger DL. Outcomes of bacterial meningitis in children. *Pediatr Infect Dis J* 1993;12:389–394.

Barkin RM. Facial and periorbital cellulitis in children. *J Emerg Med* 1984;1:195–199.

Berman S. Otitis media in children. *N Engl J Med* 1995;332:1560–1565.

Bhisitkul DM, Hogan AE. The role of bacterial antigen detection tests in the diagnosis of bacterial meningitis. *Pediatr Emerg Care* 1994;10:67–71.

Bisno AL, Gerber MA, Gwaltney JM Jr, et al. Practice guidelines for the diagnosis and management of group A streptococcal pharyngitis. *Clin Infect Dis* 2002;35:113–125.

Bluestone CD, Stephenson JS, Martin LM. Ten-year review of otitis media pathogens. *Pediatr Infect Dis J* 1992;11(8 suppl):S7–S11.

Bonsu BK, Harper MB. A low peripheral blood white blood cell count in infants younger than 90 days increases the odds of acute bacterial meningitis relative to bacteremia. *Acad Emerg Med* 2004;11:1297–1301.

Daly KA, Giebing GS. Clinical epidemiology of otitis media. *Pediatr Infect Dis J* 2000;19(Suppl 5):S31–S36.

Dayan PS, Bennet J. Test characteristics of the urine Gram stain in infants ≤60 days of age with fever. *Pediatr Emerg Care* 2000;18:12–14.

David P, Losh MD. Central nervous system infections. In: *Clinics in Family Practice,* vol 6, no 1. Philadelphia: W.B. Saunders Company, 2004.

Dewey C, Midgeley E, Maw R. The relationship between otitis media with effusion and contact with other children in British cohort studied from 8 months to 3½ years. The ALSPAC Study Team. Avon Longitudinal Study of Pregnancy and Childhood. *Int J Pediatr Otorhinolaryngol* 2000;55:33–45.

El Bashir H, Laundy M. Diagnosis and treatment of bacterial meningitis. *Arch Dis Child* 2003;88:615–620.

Fauci AS, Braunwald E. *Harrison's Principles of Internal Medicine,* ed 14. New York: McGraw-Hill, 1998.

Feigin RD. Use of corticosteroids in bacterial meningitis. *Pediatr Infect Dis J* 2004;23:355–357.

Garbutt JM, Goldstein M, Gellman E, et al. A randomized, placebo-controlled trial of antimicrobial treatment for children with clinically diagnosed acute sinusitis. *Pediatrics* 2001;107:619–625.

Giver LB. Periorbital versus orbital cellulitis. *Pediatr Infect Dis J* 2002;21:1157–1158.

Gopal AK, Whitehouse JD. Cranial computed tomography before lumbar puncture: a prospective clinical evaluation. *Arch Intern Med* 1999;159:2681–2685.

Heikkinen T, Thint M, Chonmaitree T. Prevalence of various respiratory viruses in the middle ear during acute otitis media. *N Engl J Med* 1999;340:260–264.

Honkinen O. Bacteremic urinary tract infection in children. *Pediatr Infect Dis J* 2000;19:630–634.

Kane KS, Ryder JB, Johnson RA. *Color Atlas and Synopsis of Pediatric Dermatology.* New York: McGraw-Hill, 2002.

Kaplan S. Decrease of invasive pneumococcal infections in children among 8 children's hospitals in the United States after the introduction of the 7-valent pneumococcal conjugate vaccine. *Pediatrics* 2004;113:443–449.

Klein JO. Microbiologic efficacy of antibacterial drugs for otitis media. *Pediatr Infect Dis J* 1993;12:973–975.

Kneen R, Appleton R. Status epilepticus with fever: how common is meningitis? *Arch Dis Child* 2005;90:3–4.

Kwon KT. Pediatrics, Fifth disease or erythema infectiousum. Available at http://www.EMedicine.com. Accessed May 2005.

Lan AJ, Colford JM Jr. The impact of dosing frequency of the efficacy of 10 day penicillin or amoxicillin therapy for streptococcal tonsillopharyngitis: a meta-analysis. *Pediatrics* 2000;105:E19.

Lewis LS. Pediatrics, Roseola Infantum. Available at http://www.EMedicine.com. Accessed May 2005.

McIssac WJ, Kellner JD, Aufricht, P et al. Empirical validation of guidelines for the management of pharyngitis in children and adults. *JAMA* 2004;291:1587–1595.

Nash DR, Wald ER. Sinusitis. *Pediatr Rev* 2001;22:111–117.

Polin R. Neonatal bacterial meningitis. *Semin Neonatol* 2001;6:157–172.

Nigrovic L, Malley R. Evaluation of the febrile child 3 to 36 months old in the era of pneumococcal conjugate vaccine: focus on occult bacteremia. *Clin Ped Emerg Med* 2004;5:13.

O'Hara MA. Ophthalmia neonatorum. *Pediatr Clin North Am* 1993;40:715–725.

Pasternak A, Irish B. Ophthalmologic infections in primary care. *Clin Fam Pract* 2004;6:19–33.

Pelton SI, Yogev R. Improving the outcome of pneumococcal meningitis. *Arch Dis Child* 2005;90:333–334.

Piccirrillo JF. Acute bacterial sinusits. *N Engl J Med* 204;351:902–910.

Pickering LK. Committee on Infectious Diseases. In: *The Red Book, 2003 Report of the Committee on Infectious Diseases,* 26th ed. 2003.

Rovers MM, Zielhuis GA, Ingels K van der Wilt GJ. Day-care and otitis media in young children: a critical overview. *Eur J Pediatr* 1999;158:1–6.

Schuchat A, Robinson K, Wenger JD, et al. Bacterial meningitis in the United States in 1995 Active Surveillance Team. *N Engl J Med* 1997;337:970–976.

Sheikh A, Hurwitz B, Cave J. Antibiotics for acute bacterial conjunctivitis. *Cochrane Database Syst Rev* 2000;001211.

Steere M, Sharieff GQ, Stenklyft PH. Fever in children less than 36 months of age-questions and strategies for management in the emergency department. *J Emerg Med* 2003;25:149–157.

Uhari M, Mantysaari K, Niemela M. A meta-analytic review of the risk factors for acute otitis media. *Clin Infect Dis* 1996;22:1079–1083.

Wald ER. Sinusitis in children. *N Engl J Med* 1992;326:319–323.

Weiss A, Brinser JH, Nazar-Stewart V. Acute conjunctivits in childhood. *J Pediatr* 1993;122:10–14.

Chapter 92: Infectious Diseases   569

CHAPTER

93 Sickle Cell Disease

Barbara M. Walsh

Sickle cell disease is an inherited hemoglobinopathy that carries significant morbidity and mortality. Children presenting to emergency departments (EDs) with this disease are at risk for complications from profound anemia, infectious issues, and sequestration or vaso-occulsive crises. It is characteristically seen in the African-American population but also affects people of Caribbean, Central and South American, and East Indian descent. It is important to entertain the diagnosis of sickle cell disease in any ill child from these ethnic backgrounds, with unexplained pain and swelling, infections, changes in mental status, and anemia.

Pathophysiologoy

Sickle cell disease is an autosomal, recessive, genetic disease that occurs in about 1:375 to 1:500 live African-American births. The beta hemoglobin chain has substitution of one amino acid, which makes the chain hydrophobic, predisposing it to polymerize into a sickle shape when exposed to low oxygen states. As a consequence, the cell becomes rigid and obstructs in the microcirculation, which leads to further hypoxia and more sickling.

Clinical Presentation and Management of Fever

Children with sickle cell disease have functional asplenia, low serum immunoglobulin levels, and abnormal opsonization, and complement activation. This places them at high risk for serious infections with encapsulated bacteria such as Streptococcus pneumoniae, Haemophilus influenzae, Salmonella, Staphylococcus aureus, and Escherichia coli. The risk of serious bacterial infection in a child 6 months to 3 years of age is increased several hundredfold over that of a normal child of the same age. These infections include sepsis, meningitis, pneumonia, osteomyelitis, and septic arthritis. In children with sickle cell disease the incidence of serious bacterial infection in the first 3 years of life is 7.98/100 patient-years compared to 3.54/100 in normal children. The mortality of bacterial infection in children with sickle cell disease is 20%.

Vaccination for H. flu and S. pneumoniae has helped prevent these serious infections but does completely eliminate them as a concern in the setting of an acutely ill, febrile patient with sickle cell anemia.

In the ED, a toxic-appearing child with sickle cell disease represents a true emergency. These patients require careful and immediate evaluation, monitoring, fluid resuscitation, and antibiotics. Cultures of blood, urine, and, if indicated, spinal fluid should be obtained but obtaining labs or performing procedures should not delay the administration of antibiotics. A type and cross should be sent. In areas with resistant Strep. pneumo strains, vancomycin should be considered in addition to a third generation cephalosporin. In the severely ill patient with sepsis and hypoxia, transfusion of packed red blood cells (pRBCs) should be considered to decrease sickling.

The nontoxic, febrile child with sickle cell disease requires a thorough physical exam and detailed history focusing on length, duration, and height of fever, associated symptoms such as cough, respiratory distress, abdominal pain, immunization status, and compliance with prophylactic antibiotics. Laboratory assessment should include a complete blood count, reticulocyte count, urine analysis with culture, blood culture, CXR, and KUB, if indicated. Prompt initiation of antibiotics is key even before laboratory results are known. Ceftriaxone is typically used as it will cover these patients for 24 hours while cultures are pending.

All children with sickle cell disease and fever need to be followed closely. Depending on the family's resources and abilities, selected, nontoxic patients with sickle cell disease may be discharged with follow-up within 24 hours. Any concern about the family's ability to assess a change in the child's status or comply with plans for follow-up requires admission. Criteria suggesting that a well-appearing febrile child with sickle cell disease can be safely discharged include the following: WBC between 5 and 30,000 thousand, fever <40° C, presence of the child's baseline hematocrit, absence of a significant percentage of bands, and absence of an elevated reticulocyte count. Younger children and those with previous sepsis generally warrant admission. It must be emphasized to the parents that if the symptoms worsen, then the child should return immediately for reevaluation.

The incidence of pneumococcal sepsis has been reduced with the institution of oral penicillin prophylaxis or erythromycin for those who are penicillin allergic. Prophylaxis is begun as soon as the diagnosis is made and continued until age 5 years. However, this does not completely protect the child from serious infection and parents should be educated about the need for prompt assessment of any fever.

Acute Chest Syndrome

Acute chest syndrome is a serious complication of sickle cell disease indicative of pneumonia or pulmonary infarction, and is one of the most common reasons for hospital admission is these patients. The patient usually presents with fever, tachypnea, chest pain, rales, and hypoxia. In a dehydrated patient, the initial physical examination findings may be minimal. Any child who presents with symptoms suggestive of acute chest syndrome requires immediate assessment, monitoring, and treatment including: IV access, fluids and antibiotics, oxygen administration, laboratory tests and cultures, and CXR (**Table 93.1**). Ceftriaxone or another third generation is recommended as part of empiric antibiotic treatment. Transfusion should be considered if severe anemia is present. The distinction between pneumonia and a vaso-occlusive crisis can be a difficult determination in the ED. Consultation with pediatric hematology subspecialists and admission to the hospital is generally needed.

Bone and Joint Complaints

Septic arthritis and osteomyelitis are difficult to distinguish from a vaso-occlusive crisis in patients with sickle cell disease because pain, erythema, and swelling at the afflicted site and fever are seen in all of these entities. A detailed physical exam and careful use of laboratory studies can assist in elucidating the correct diagnosis. If symptoms are present for three days or less, a bone scan (using ^{99m}Tc-diphosphonate to tag inflamed bone) and bone marrow scan (using ^{99m}Tc-sulfur colloid to tag infarcted marrow) may help discern osteomyelitis from bone infarction. A positive bone scan will show uptake solely in the bone while the bone marrow scan will be positive if uptake is only seen in the bone. Nevertheless, a closed or open bone aspirate should be pursued, optimally prior to the initiation of antibiotics, in patients who are highly suspect for osteomyelitis. If septic arthritis is strongly suspected, an arthrocentesis should be performed and joint fluid analyzed accordingly. Of note, the cell count and differential may be similar in septic arthritis and infarction and, thus, the Gram-stain and culture are very important in guiding management. In many instances, the patient reports that this is typical bone pain from a sickle cell crisis and in a recurrent location. In this case, prompt institution of fluids and analgesia, and an adequate observation period may identify the case as a sickle crisis.

Vaso-occlusive Crisis

Vaso-occlusion is another serious, frequently encountered emergency condition that presents in patients with sickle cell disease. The hemoglobin in sickle cell disease is hydrophobic. Under certain conditions, such as deoxygenation, the hemoglobin chain will polymerize and form a sickle shape, which is less flexible than normal hemoglobin. Sickled cells obstruct flow within blood vessels, causing ischemia and further sickling. Damage to the vessel wall disturbs that balance of vasoactive peptides that control vascular tone. This cycle worsens with dehydration.

The sickle crisis involves infarction of bone and other organs. Patients present with pain, swelling, and redness at the involved site. Dactylitis, infarction of the metacarpals and metatarsals, resulting in swelling of the hands and feet is a common presentation in children between 6 months and 2 years. The approach to a painful crisis depends on the severity of the symptoms. Patients with mild to moderate pain should have 1.5 maintenance fluids started either as PO or IV. Pain should be controlled with Tylenol, NSAIDs, codeine, or a combination of these. If the pain is not controlled, IV narcotics should be administered and the patient admitted. Patients with multiple visits to the ED or inadequate oral intake should be considered for admission. A severe painful crisis requires immediate and aggressive hydration and pain control. Morphine, ketorolac, and nonsteroidals should be used until the pain has improved. These patients usually require admission for ongoing hydration and pain control (**Table 93.2**).

Infarction of abdominal organs may produce symptoms similar to other disease processes that are of nonhematologic origin. In the child with sickle cell disease and right upper quadrant abdominal pain, the differential diagnosis includes liver infarction from sickling in the vascular

Table 93.1
Acute Chest Syndrome

Signs and Symptoms	Management
Tachypnea	IVF bolus
Hypoxia	IVF at 1.5 maintenance
Crackles	Oxygen
Chest pain	pRBC transfusion
+/− Fever	Pain control (narcotics and NSAIDs)
Tachycardia	Antibiotics (cephalosporin)

Studies	Disposition
ABG	Admit to hospital
CXR	ICU if severe anemia/ hypoxemia
CBC with differential/ smear	Floor if VS stable
Type and screen	

Table 93.2

Acute Painful Crisis

	Mild/Moderate Painful Sickle Crisis	Severe Painful Sickle Crisis
Fluids	NS IVF bolus 20 cc/kg D5 1/4 or 1/2 NS at 1.5 × maintenance	NS IVF bolus 20 cc/kg D5 1/4 or 1/2 NS at 1.5 × maintenance
Pain Control	NSAIDs: oral ibuprofen Narcotics: Tylenol with codeine	NSAIDs: IV ketorolac Narcotics: IV morphine
No relief with above	NSAIDS: IV ketorolac Narcotics: IV morphine	
Disposition	Discharge if control with PO meds & Discharge if adequate PO intake Follow-up in 24 hours Reliable parents Admit if poor pain control, inadequate PO intake	Admit

beds, cholecystitis from chronic hemolysis and stones that result from this entity, hepatitis from infectious causes, pancreatitis, peptic ulcer disease (PUD), and biliary obstruction. If the patient states that this is typical pain of a crisis and in a recurrent location, it is reasonable to start fluids, give analgesia, and observe the patient for hours for improvement. Elevated aspartate aminotransferase (AST) and hyperbilirubinemia may be present in infarction as well as biliary disease. Abdominal ultrasound is helpful to assess the anatomy of the liver and the biliary tree.

Priapism is a painful vaso-occlusive crisis causing a tender and engorged penis. Treatment is similar to other painful crises with hydration and analgesia; however, prolonged symptomatology may require aspiration of the corpora, transfusion of pRBCs, and exchange transfusion. Consultation with pediatric hematology and urology should be considered in selected patients.

An infarct involving the central nervous system presents with neurological signs ranging from headache, transient symptoms (TIA), seizures, hemiparesis, and coma. When these are recognized, aggressive treatment is required. Neuroimaging, subspecialty consultation, and exchange transfusion should be initiated immediately.

Aplastic Crisis

Patients with an aplastic crisis present with severe anemia, fatigue, pallor, and tachycardia in the absence of acute hemolysis and jaundice. Symptomatology depends on the acuity of the process. Patients with severe symptoms such as altered mental status, impaired oxygen delivery, and significant tachycardia should receive a transfusion of pRBCs. Reticulocyte count should be followed for signs of bone marrow recovery. Bone marrow aspirate is occasionally needed to evaluate recovery.

Splenic Sequestration

Splenic sequestration is a life-threatening event that presents in children younger than 5 years of age before the spleen has completely autoinfarcted. In this process, the spleen becomes acutely engorged with a significant portion of the blood volume. Patients will present with acute onset of left upper quadrant abdominal pain and progressively develop pallor, increasing tachycardia, and lethargy over several hours. The spleen is palpable and tender. Hypotension and cardiovascular collapse can occur. The mainstay of treatment is replenishment of the intravascular volume. Albumin or NS should be started immediately while pRBCs or whole blood is being prepared for transfusion.

Hemolytic Crisis

Viral or bacterial infection can trigger hemolysis and worsening of hemolytic anemia. Patients will present with fatigue, scleral icterus, and jaundice. Laboratory studies will demonstrate a fall in the hematocrit (HCT) from baseline, and an elevated reticulocyte count and bilirubin. Markers of hemolysis, such as lactate dehydrogenase (LDH), will also be elevated from increased destruction of RBCs. This is often a self-limited process and once the infection clears, the patient recovers. It is rare that these patients will need transfusion; supportive care only is generally indicated.

Conclusion

Sickle cell disease is a complex clinical entity that includes a variety of serious presentations that must be rapidly recognized and treated. The emergency physician must be able to identify these and swiftly intervene. Anticipation of the acute deterioration that these patients can develop should include empiric treatment of fever/infection, transfusion for aplastic/sequestration crisis, and consultation with pediatric hematology and critical care subspecialists. Close follow-up and parent education regarding hydration, analgesia, and prophylaxis for the young patient, in particular, should be emphasized. Follow up within 24 hours should be assured before discharge from the ED. As improvements in health care and long term management continue, patients with sickle cell disease are living well into their 30s and will continue to challenge the emergency medicine physician.

Selected Readings

Bunn HF. Pathogenesis and treatment of sickle cell disease. *N Engl J Med* 1997;337: 762–769.

Chesney PJ, Williams JA, Presbury G, et al., Penicillin- and Cephalosporin-resistant strains of streptococcus pneumoniae causing sepsis and meningitis in children with sickle cell disease. *J Pediatr* 1995;127:526–532.

Embury DH, Hebbel RP, Mohandas N, et al. *Sickle Cell Disease: Basic Principles and Clinical Practice*. New York: Raven Press, 1994.

Gaston MH, Verter JL, Woods G, et al. Prophylaxis with oral penicillin in children with sickle cell anemia. *N Engl J Med* 1986;14:1593–1599.

Gill FM, Sleeper LA, Weiner SJ, et al. Clinical events in the first decade in a cohort of infants with sickle cell disease. *Blood* 1995;86:776–783.

Lane PA. Sickle cell disease. *Pediatr Clin North Am* 1996;43:639–664.

Ohene-Frempong O. Stroke in sickle cell disease: demographic, clinical, and therapeutic considerations. *Semin Hematol* 1991;28:213–219.

Pollack CV Jr. Emergencies in sickle cell disease. *Emerg Med Clin North Am* 1993;11:365–378.

Rogers ZR, Morrison RA, Vedro DA, Buchanan GR. Outpatient management of febrile illness in infants and young children with sickle cell anemia. *J Pediatr* 1990;117:736–739.

Steen RG, Emudianughe T, Hankins GM, et al. Brain imaging findings in pediatric patients with sickle cell disease. *Radiology* 2003;228:216–225.

Vichinsky EP, Styles LA, Colangelo LH, et al. Acute chest syndrome in sickle cell disease: clinical presentation and course. Cooperative Study of Sickle Cell Disease. *Blood* 1997;89:1787–1792.

Vichinsky EP. Comprehensive care in sickle cell disease: its impact on morbidity and mortality. *Semin Hematol* 1991;28:220–226.

94 Renal Disorders

Alison Brent
Mary O'Neill

Genitourinary Disorders

Genital complaints are concerning to patients and families. Rapidity of diagnosis and intervention may be critical for some conditions such as testicular torsion, paraphimosis, and priaprism, while other diagnoses are less time sensitive but require thoroughness and careful explanation. Emergency physicians should be familiar with the penile and testicular problems reviewed in this chapter.

Penile Problems

Penile swelling can be caused by local trauma, infection, inflammation, disorders of the foreskin, or lymphatic or venous obstruction, and is usually accompanied by pain. Pain and perceived inability to urinate are often concerning to the patient or parent, but usually is not serious or life-threatening, with the exception of spinal cord compression. Nontender or mildly uncomfortable penile edema can occur with an insect bite or generalized allergic reaction. Penile swelling may represent a general edematous state associated with other organ system diseases such as renal, hepatic, or cardiac disease. The diagnosis of the primary disease dictates the therapy for resolution of the penile swelling.

An infection of the glans (balanitis) may extend to the foreskin (posthitis) and usually involves both areas concurrently (balanoposthitis). Balinitis usually results from a break in the skin and evolution to a cellulitis. It may also occur in the setting of local trauma or poor hygiene. Therapy for balanitis includes warm soaks and topical antibiotic therapy, whereas more severe cases may require oral amoxicillin or IV ampicillin. Soaking in a tub of warm water may promote urination. Inability to void is unusual. Follow-up care includes reexamination to ensure that true phimosis has not occurred due to scarring and inflammation. Recurrent infections or phimosis resulting from acute balanitis may be indications for circumcision.

Paraphimosis and Phimosis

Paraphimosis occurs when the foreskin is retracted behind the glans. The foreskin becomes edematous due to venous congestion and cannot be easily reduced to a normal position.

Treatment of paraphimosis includes ice and manual reduction. The discomfort of manual reduction can be decreased with a dorsal nerve block or the use of sedation and analgesia. By applying continuous gentle pressure on the glans while stabilizing the foreskin is usually successful in reducing the foreskin, and has been likened to turning a sock inside out. In the rare instance when manual reduction is unsuccessful, surgical reduction is required plus a subsequent elective circumcision. Paraphimosis can be prevented with good hygiene. At an early age, the foreskin should not be retracted since abrupt lysis of adhesions by aggressive retraction can lead to inflammation and pain. By school age, boys can be instructed how to gently retract the foreskin and cleanse this area.

Phimosis is a rare condition caused by tightness of the distal foreskin that prevents it from being withdrawn to expose the glans. This may result in obstruction to urine flow and urine retention. The cause is inflammation usually secondary to chronic rashes or infection. Corrections consist of dilation of the meatus or a dorsal slit procedure. In contrast to phimosis, penile adhesions are fairly common and lyse spontaneously by age 4 years in 90% of cases.

Priaprism

Priaprism is a painful prolonged erection not associated with sexual stimulation. The most common cause in children is a vaso-occlusive episode associated with sickle cell disease and may be the sole manifestation of sickling event. Less common causes include trauma or tumor infiltration. Therapy is based on etiology. In sickle cell disease, hydration, analgesia, and transfusion are used reduce the percentage of hemoglobin B (HgB) SS to 30% or less. Symptomatic relief includes heat, cold, local nerve blocks, spinal anesthesia, and appropriate sedation and analgesia. Erection that does not resolve despite hydration, and transfusion may warrant urologic consultation for the placement of a cavernosus to spongiosum shunt or irrigation of the corpus cavernosus with vasoactive substances. Long-term consequences of recurrent priaprism include fibrosis and impotence.

Penile Trauma

Trauma to the penis usually involves blunt trauma from toilet seats, lacerations, zipper injuries, or hair tourniquets. All genitourinary trauma requires a high index of suspicion for sexual abuse.

Blunt trauma is most often seen in toddlers in a scenario where the toilet seat lands on the penile shaft. Uncomplicated cases require warm sitz baths, analgesia, and observation of urination. Blood at the urethral meatus represents urethral damage until proven otherwise and warrants urology consultation. Follow-up should focus on the development of adhesions. Superficial penile shaft lacerations are repaired with absorbable sutures following appropriate sedation and analgesia.

Zipper injuries entrap the penis or foreskin in the zipper. Following adequate sedation and analgesia, a wire cutter to cut the median bar of the zipper will separate the two sides of the zipper and release skin caught in the teeth of the zipper. Children can be discharged home with local care to reduce swelling and pain.

A hair wound multiple times about the penile shaft results in a hair tourniquet. This constricting ring that can result in strangulation may be hidden by edema misdiagnosed as balanitis. Following appropriate sedation and analgesia, the hair can be removed by unwinding the hair or cutting it. If the removal is complex, consider urologic consultation, since rare complications include urethrocutaneous fistulas or penile loss.

Testicular Problems

Acute scrotal pain or swelling or a history of testicular trauma may represent a urologic emergency. A thorough history regarding trauma, urinary tract infections, instrumentation, and systemic diseases, such as mumps, may aid in the diagnosis. The onset, nature, and duration of pain and/or swelling as well as a thorough physical examination, standing and supine, is necessary.

Diagnostic imaging studies include radionuclide scintigraphy and color Doppler ultrasound. Radionuclide scintigraphy has a sensitivity of 90% or greater for detecting decreased or absent perfusion to a torsed testis. The specificity is estimated at 60%. In the neonate and very young child, it may be inaccurate due to inadequate magnification. False negatives can occur from technical errors and incomplete torsion with spontaneous detorsion. Ultrasonography offers a rapid noninvasive method for evaluating scrotal pathology and testicular perfusion but is operator dependent. False negatives are due to technique, spontaneous detorsion, or late torsion with increased flow from inflammation. False positives are due to technique or overlying hydroceles. If testicular torsion cannot be excluded, urologic consultation is indicated.

Hydrocele

A hydrocele is a nontender accumulation of fluid within the tunica vaginalis surrounding the testis. Fluid may remain in this space as the process vaginalis closes during development. A simple hydrocele, commonly seen in infants, is consistent in size and typically reabsorbs by age 8 to 12 months. Transillumination helps to confirm the diagnosis.

Occasionally, a hydrocele may be associated with underlying pathology including testicular torsion, torsion of the appendix of the testis, epididymitis, trauma, or tumor. In addition to a careful examination of all hydroceles, ultrasound and radionuclide testicular scans can be used to evaluate underlying structures when the diagnosis is uncertain. If the hydrocele has changed size, or if there is thickening of cord structures, the process vaginalis may still be patent, creating a communicating hydrocele. There is a risk of enlargement of the patent process vaginalis and development of a hernia. Surgical exploration is necessary to ligate the process vaginalis and decompress the hydrocele.

Hernia

Most inguinal hernias present as groin masses that may extend into the scrotum. Inguinal hernias are most common in children, resulting from an intact process vaginalis. There may be a complete hernia from the internal ring to the scrotum, or a segmental obliteration creating a hydrocele of the tunica vaginalis or spermatic cord. The distinction between a hydrocele of the spermatic cord and associated communicating hernia and an incarcerated hernia is often a difficult one to make. Palpation of an empty sac above the swelling indicates a hydrocele. Ultrasound can be helpful in identifying these structures.

An incarcerated hernia should be suspected if an empty sac above the hydrocele cannot be felt and there is pain or color change. Reduction of an incarcerated hernia requires appropriate sedation and analgesia. With the patient in Trendelenburg position, two fingers are used to stabilize the internal ring while gas or fluid is milked from the incarcerated bowel to facilitate reduction of the entrapped loop back into the abdominal cavity. Reduction with sedation is successful in 95% of cases. If successful, follow-up care includes herniorrhaphy once the edema has resolved. If reduction is not successful, urgent surgical intervention is required.

Testicular Torsion

Testicular torsion is a time sensitive urologic emergency. Torsion of the spermatic cord is characterized by acute testicular pain and swelling of the involved testicle, but may develop gradually in as many as one-fourth of cases. The twisting usually occurs in a lateral to medial direction. On examination the affected testicle appears elevated in the scrotum and is exquisitely tender. The loss of the cremasteric reflex represents complete torsion. Without intervention, the torsed testicle will infarct in 6 to 8 hours, although salvage may occur up to 24 hours after the onset of symptoms.

Rapid differentiation of testicular torsion from other causes of scrotal pain is crucial and can often be made based on history and physical examination. Non-torsion tends to present insidiously, or is suggested by a history of trauma or prior mass or swelling. Age is an important consideration in the differential of scrotal pain. Testicular torsion may occur in the 5- to 15-year-old age group, with two thirds of cases presenting between the ages of 12 and 18, representing a peak at puberty. In contrast, most cases of epididymitis are postpubertal, although some cases are associated with genitourinary anomalies in the prepubertal child. Torsion of the appendix testis occurs throughout childhood and adolescence, with a peak incidence between the ages of 10 and 14.

Doppler flow ultrasound to assess perfusion or radionuclide testicular flow scanning to demonstrate absent blood supply in the torsed testicle may facilitate the diagnosis. Treatment is immediate surgical exploration, detorsion, and fixation of the involved and contralateral testicle. In a few cases, manual detorsion may resolve the acute problem, but fixation is still indicated. Detorsion is performed in a medial to lateral orientation while observing for improvement in discomfort.

Torsion of the Appendix Testis

Torsion of the appendix testis may present as scrotal pain and swelling. The onset of pain is usually more gradual and less severe than with testicular torsion. True differentiation between torsion of the testis and torsion of the appendix testis must be ascertained by physical examination. Torsion of the appendix testis results in congestion, necrosis, and inflammation that gradually cause more diffuse swelling. There may be an associated hydrocele formation and, with time, a less distinct localization of the pain. Initial examination may identify by palpation a localized area of tenderness of the superior pole of the testis with an infrequently visualized "blue dot" sign of the necrotic appendage best seen with transillumination.

Differential diagnosis may be aided by scrotal ultrasound with Doppler flow and/or radionuclide testicular scanning. Suspicion of testicular torsion requires surgical exploration. Confirmed cases of torsion of an appendage are treated symptomatically with rest, ice, scrotal support, and anti-inflammatory medication. Rarely, the severely symptomatic child with nausea or vomiting and extreme pain may warrant surgical excision of the necrotic appendage.

Epididymitis

Infection and inflammation of the epididymis typically presents with a gradual onset of scrotal pain. In some there is a history of urinary tract infections, sexual activity, sexually transmitted disease, prior instrumentation, or genitourinary surgery. Initially there is a focal tenderness without a mass, and a slightly indurated or tender nodule may be palpated in the inferior or dependent portion of the epididymis. With time, the entire epididymis becomes inflamed and may have an associated hydrocele. With more diffuse swelling and tenderness, the differentiation between epididymitis, torsion of an appendix, and testicular torsion becomes difficult. The lack of relief of pain with testicular elevation (Prehn's sign) is unreliable in differentiating epididymitis from testicular torsion. Diagnosis of epididymitis may be supported by pyuria or a scrotal ultrasound demonstrating normal or increased flow to the affected area. In the adolescent with a history of sexual activity, an examination typical for epididymitis

(normal-size testis, normal lie, intact cremasteric), and pyuria, no further diagnostic testing may be needed. Treatment is supportive with rest, ice, scrotal support, NSAIDs medications, and antibiotics. Antibiotic choice is dictated by the likely organism. In general, sexually active patients should be treated for *Chlamydia trachomatis* and *Neisseria gonorrhoeae* with ceftriaxone 250 mg IM followed by at least 10 days of doxycycline or ceftriaxone 250 mg IM and 1,000 mg of azithromycin as a single dose. Prepubescent boys with associated genitourinary anomalies frequently have cultures positive for *E. coli, Aerobacter aerogenes, Pseudomonas,* and Gram-positive cocci, and thus should be covered for these organisms pending urine cultures. In the febrile patient with a tender fluctuant fluid-filled mass, intravenously administered antibiotics, and rarely, surgical drainage may be indicated.

Orchitis

A rare cause of scrotal pain or swelling associated with epididymitis or viral infection is orchitis. Mumps orchitis is the most common infectious etiology and presents as sudden unilateral pain with testicular enlargement. The overlying scrotum is often erythematous and edematous. The associated presence of parotitis is helpful in making the diagnosis. Microhematuria and proteinuria may be present as well. Treatment involves pain relief with rest, analgesics, and ice.

Other Scrotal Masses

Varicoceles are chronic, ill-defined asymptomatic scrotal masses located along the cord above the testis and epididymis. They usually occur on the left side. Varicoceles may be associated with heaviness or discomfort on the affected side. An obstructive mass should be considered if the varicocele remains after the patient is supine, if it is right sided, if it is diagnosed in a young boy, or if the onset is acute or associated with significant pain. An abdominal/pelvic ultrasound helps to define a retroperitoneal mass causing vena cava obstruction. Such a mass may obstruct the spermatic vein on the right, or a perinephric mass may obstruct the left renal vein, thus blocking drainage of the left spermatic vein. Occasionally, persistent pain or swelling can be relieved by spermatic vein ligation at the internal ring. All patients diagnosed with a varicocele should be referred to and followed by an urologist.

Testicular Trauma

Scrotal or testicular trauma may occur as the result of sporting events, motor vehicle accidents, or straddle injuries. A minor mechanism in association with significant pain or swelling raises the suspicion of primary testicular or scrotal pathology, such as testicular torsion, appendage torsion, epididymitis, or tumor.

Minor scrotal, testicular, or epididymal contusions, usually sports-related, heal in a few days. More severe injuries such as a testicular rupture, hematoma, or dislocation, resulting from greater forces such as motor vehicle collisions, need urological evaluation. Inspection of the scrotum and its contents may be difficult due to swelling or pain after injury. In cases where testicular rupture is suspected by severe pain associated with a tense and ecchymotic scrotum, the testicle needs to be palpated carefully. An enlarged, ill-defined, irregular testicle suggests rupture. If tenderness and swelling prohibit palpation of the testicle, or the sac appears empty suggesting testicular dislocation, an ultrasound may help define the testicle as well as identify hematoceles that suggest rupture. Radionuclide testicular scanning may provide information about function. Ultrasound may be particularly helpful in distinguishing a tense hematocele versus testicular torsion in cases of minor trauma. All scrotal lacerations require careful exploration to define the extent or risk of underlying injury. Superficial lacerations of the scrotum may be repaired with chromic catgut using local anesthesia. Intrascrotal hematomas, skin ecchymosis, and injuries limited to the dartos layer may be managed conservatively with ice and support.

Minor testicular contusions and hematomas may also be treated conservatively, whereas some large hematomas require surgical management to avoid necrosis, secondary infections, or disruption of testicular function. The presence of a traumatic hematocele suggests rupture. Testicular rupture, tearing the tunica albuginea with extravasation of the testis into the scrotum, requires surgical repair. Better salvage following rupture occurs with exploration and repair within the first 24 hours.

Urological consultation is recommended for all penetrating injuries through the dartos, degloving injuries of the scrotum, and traumatic hematoceles.

Sexually Transmitted Diseases

Sexually transmitted diseases (STDs) constitute a major health problem among sexually active adolescents, with more than a million cases reported annually.

Chlamydia Trachomatis

Chlamydia trachomatis is an obligate intracellular parasite that frequently accompanies gonorrheal infections and occurs alone. *Chlamydia* is the most common sexually transmitted disease in the United States. Prevalence rates may be higher than the reported 10% to 30% among sexually active teenage and adult women, since many cases of *Chlamydia* are asymptomatic. Risk factors for *Chlamydia* include multiple sexual partners.

Clinical syndromes produced by *Chlamydia* include: (1) asymptomatic disease; (2) cervicitis; (3) salpingitis; (4) urethritis; (5) perihepatitis (Fitz-Hugh-Curtis); (6) pelvic inflammatory disease (PID); (7) conjunctivitis; and (8) bartholinitis. Sequelae of *Chlamydia* infections include an increased risk of ectopic pregnancy and sterility.

Clinical Presentation

Clinical symptoms include vaginal discharge, dysuria, urinary frequency, and pelvic pain. Clinical findings include cervical erythema and friability, and a yellow, odoriferous, mucopurulent discharge.

Diagnostic analysis of endocervical secretions can be done by a variety of methods. The most reliable is culture (McCoy cell culture). However, this is expensive and la-

bor intensive, and results are not available for 2 to 3 days. Antigen detection assays, including ELISA (Chlamydiazyme) and monoclonal antibodies (Microtrack) are inexpensive, rapid, and convenient, although not as reliable as culture. All patients with suspected *Chlamydia* should also be tested for gonorrhea and syphilis. Consideration should be given to testing for HIV.

Uncomplicated *Chlamydia trachomatis* in nonpregnant patients can be treated with 1 g of azithromycin as a single dose or doxycycline 100 mg bid for 7 days. In patients who are pregnant or allergic to doxycycline, erythromycin can be used at a dose of 500 mg qid for 7 days. In addition, consideration should be given to treating patients for gonorrhea. All sexual partners need to be treated as well. Test of cure is only indicated if there is no improvement in symptoms.

Gonorrhea

Epidemiology

Gonorrhea is a genital infection caused by *Neisseria gonorrhoeae,* a gram-negative, intracellular diplococcus. Gonococcal infections occur relatively frequently in sexually active adolescent girls. Risk factors include multiple and new sexual partners as well as use of oral contraceptives. There are approximately 1 million cases reported annually in the United States, while the prevalence is estimated to be at least twice that number.

Pathophysiology

Children contract gonorrhea by direct contact with infected secretions. *N. gonorrhoeae* adheres to columnar epithelium and then penetrates to subepithelial tissues, where it induces an inflammatory response. Subsequent spread is hematogenous or lymphatic.

Clinical Presentation

While many patients are symptomatic, an equal number are asymptomatic. Clinical symptoms may occur 3 to 8 days following intercourse with an infected partner. Females may develop a yellow vaginal discharge, dysuria, urgency, vulvar pruritus, urinary frequency, lower abdominal pain, and abnormal vaginal bleeding. Findings may include a yellow discharge at the introitus as well as an exudate that can be expressed from the Bartholin or Skene's glands. The cervix may be normal, erythematous, or friable with a yellow, odoriferous, mucopurulent discharge from the os. Additional findings include fever (usually low grade) and lower abdominal tenderness. In severe cases, high fever and systemic symptoms occur. Males tend to develop a urethral discharge and occasionally may present with swelling of the penile shaft or urinary retention.

Untreated *N. gonorrhoeae* may lead to local infections of the Bartholin gland or periurethral duct abscess, tuboovarian abscess, or disseminated infections such as gonococcal arthritis-dermatitis syndrome.

Differential Diagnosis

Differential diagnosis includes *Chlamydia trachomatis, Trichomonas vaginitis,* bacterial vaginosis, and urinary tract infection.

Diagnosis and Treatment

Diagnosis is highly suggested by a Gram stain in males (urethral) and prepubertal females (endocervical) that reveals intracellular Gram-negative diplococci and white blood cells. In postpubertal females, the Gram stain may not be helpful. Culture is mandatory in children and alleged rape victims for medicolegal reasons to confirm the diagnosis. The role of enzyme immunoassays has yet to be determined.

Ceftriaxone 125 mg IM or IV is the treatment of choice for uncomplicated gonorrhea and is effective against strains resistant to penicillins and tetracycline. For patients allergic to cephalosporins and penicillins, alternative choices include parenteral spectinomycin 2 g IV or oral ciprofloxacin. All patients treated for gonorrhea should also be treated for *Chlamydia* (see above). Pregnant adolescents may be given oral erythromycin 500 mg qid for 7 days. At present, test of cure is not indicated because these regimens fail so rarely. Consideration should be given to testing for syphilis, *Chlamydia*, and HIV. Sexual partners should be evaluated and tested or treated presumptively.

Any infant younger than 1 month of age who presents to the ED with purulent conjunctivitis must have a Gram stain and culture obtained for GC. A Gram stain revealing Gram-negative diplococci warrants immediate treatment. While hospital admission and IV antibiotics has long been the standard of care, recent articles suggest single-dose IM ceftriaxone may be sufficient for neonatal conjunctivitis.

Herpes Genitalis

Epidemiology

Herpes genitalis is caused by the herpes simplex virus (HSV), including HSV-1 and HSV-2. HSV-1 primarily causes ocular (keratitis) and oral lesions (cold sores), and is responsible for only 10% of the herpetic genital lesions. In the prepubertal child, HSV-1 may cause genital infection either by autoinoculation by the hand or mouth, or by contact (hand, oral, or sexual) with an infected person. HSV-2 infection is responsible for the majority of herpetic genital lesions. It is extremely contagious and transmitted by sexual contact. The highest incidence occurs in 15- to 19-year-old adolescents. HSV-1 infections of the genitals have recently become more common in adolescents, perhaps related to changing sexual practices. Because carriers may be asymptomatic, a history of contact with an infected person is not routinely obtained.

Clinical Presentation

Clinical symptoms begin within 2 to 7 days from initial contact and may include dysuria, vulvar pruritus and burning, discomfort with ambulation, and paresthesias. In severe cases, patients may be unable to urinate or defecate due to pain. Symptoms consistent with viremia occur in primary HSV infection and include malaise, fever, headache, and myalgias. Within 48 hours, the pathognomonic primary lesions occur: multiple clusters of erythematous macules that progress to papules and then to vesicles on an erythematous base. These lesions cause intense pain, pruritus, and burning, and are often associated with significant lymphadenopathy. In prepubertal children, lesions are limited to the vulvar and perianal area, while in adolescents, lesions may also occur on the vaginal and cervical mucosa. Subsequently the vesicles rupture, ulcerate, and then progress though healing within 7 to 14 days.

A sequela of HSV in young children is secondary bacterial infection of lesions. In adolescents, complications include recurrence, systemic involvement, risk of fetal infection during pregnancy and delivery, and a long-term increased risk of genital malignancies. Recurrences occur in 60% to 90% of patients and are usually less severe than the primary infection. Symptoms that herald recurrence include paresthesias, pain, and pruritus. Systemic symptoms are usually absent in a recurrence and the lesions heal within 2 to 3 weeks.

Differential Diagnosis

Differential diagnosis includes varicella and inflicted burns. Ulcerated lesions may be confused with syphilis or chancroid.

Diagnosis and Treatment

In adolescents, a visual diagnosis of typical lesions is sufficient. In all other cases, a Wright stain, Tzanck prep, or Pap smears of HSV lesions may reveal pathognomonic multinucleate giant cells or intranuclear inclusion bodies. Diagnosis is confirmed by viral cultures of lesions. Culture and serology are useful adjuncts to differentiate HSV-1 and HSV-2. This differentiation may be crucial in prepubertal children when the diagnosis of sexual abuse is considered.

In prepubertal children, because of the high association of sexual abuse, it is prudent to involve child protective services as part of a multidisciplinary team. Treatment in this age group consists of local hygiene and antipruritic and pain medications, with consideration given to the use of acyclovir. Sitz baths are a useful adjunct for urinary retention.

In the adolescents with primary HSV infection, acyclovir is indicated to shorten the symptomatic period and reduce the number and healing times of lesions as well as diminish pain and systemic symptoms. Topical acyclovir is less effective than oral and has no additional benefits. For primary infections, acyclovir is recommended. For recurrent infections, acyclovir may be of benefit. Acyclovir is contraindicated during pregnancy. Inpatient treatment with IV acyclovir should be considered for patients with immunocompromised states or severe illness. These patients should be evaluated for other sexually transmitted diseases including *Chlamydia*, gonorrhea, syphilis, and HIV.

Protection

Despite adequate treatment and resolution of lesions, viral shedding continues for weeks to months following an infection. Sexual partners should be made aware of the infection and condoms should be used. All patients with HSV infections need regular gynecologic follow-up.

Syphilis

Syphilis is caused by the motile spirochete *Treponema pallidum,* and is spread by sexual contact or congenital infection. There has been a recent increase in syphilis in the United States in the adolescent population. The highest prevalence of syphilis occurs in urban settings, particularly among drug addicts, prostitutes, and HIV-positive patients.

Clinical Presentation

Clinical symptoms for primary syphilis begin 10 to 90 days after initial contact. The pathognomonic lesion is the chancre, appearing 3 to 4 weeks following clinical exposure. This lesion may be solitary or multiple. In males, the chancre is often easily visible on the penis, scrotum, anus, or oral mucosa, while in females it is more difficult to visualize; frequently it is located on the vulva, vagina, cervix, urethra, or oral mucosa. The chancre is notable as a painless ulcer with a smooth base, raised margins, and scant yellow discharge. The untreated chancre heals spontaneously within a few weeks, followed by the development of inguinal adenopathy in 70% to 80% of patients within 6 to 8 weeks.

Secondary syphilis causes pathognomonic skin and mucous membrane eruptions 6 to 20 weeks after exposure. The classic skin rash consists of brawny, nonpruritic maculopapular rash symmetrically located on trunk and extremities, including palms and soles. Classic mucous membrane involvement is seen as condylomata lata, consisting of pink, flat, moist papules seen in moist intertriginous areas. Fever, generalized nontender lymphadenopathy, headache, sore throat, malaise, weight loss, arthralgias, myalgias, splenomegaly, and "moth-eaten" alopecia may be present.

Differential Diagnosis

All genital lesions should be included in the differential diagnosis for syphilis.

Differential diagnosis for primary syphilis includes chancroid (exquisitely tender adjacent adenopathy with multiple soft and sensitive ulcers), lymphogranuloma inguinale (enlarged, tender adenopathy with fleeting vesicular ulceration), lichen planus (annular level-surfaced papular lesions), granuloma inguinale (painless, granulomatous, soft, and smooth-surfaced lesions), herpes (multiple tender papulovesicular lesions), molluscum contagiosum (umbilicated, flesh covered, painless papules occurring in groups and at distant body sites), pyogenic granuloma (painful, solitary, erythematous lesion following history of surgery or local trauma), and condyloma acuminata (verrucous lesions).

Differential diagnosis for secondary syphilis includes psoriasis and pityriasis rosea (lack of maculopapular lesions on the palms and soles are exclusionary).

Diagnosis and Treatment

Venereal Disease Research Laboratory (VDRL) or RPR serology may be negative during primary syphilis (e.g., chancre) but is usually positive at the time of secondary syphilis. Of note, false-positive VDRLs may be seen with hepatitis, mononucleosis, collagen vascular disorders, tuberculosis, viral pneumonitis, varicella, measles, and malaria. Dark-field microscopic examination of lesions scraping or fluid usually demonstrates the spirochete during primary syphilis.

Treatment should begin in the ED for all suspected or known cases of primary or secondary syphilis. Treatment for primary syphilis or secondary disease of less than 1 year's duration consists of benzathine penicillin G 2.4 million units IM as a single dose; for penicillin-allergic nonpregnant patients, doxycycline 100 mg PO bid for 2 weeks or tetracycline 500 mg PO qid for 2 weeks. Treatment for secondary syphilis of greater than 1 year's duration or tertiary syphilis is benzathine penicillin G 2.4×106 U IM $\times$ three doses.

Protection

Patients with known or suspected syphilis should be evaluated for other sexually transmitted diseases. The Centers for Disease Control (CDC) states that the combination of ceftriaxone and doxycycline for pelvic inflammatory disease (PID) is probably efficacious against incubating syphilis. Follow-up serology should be obtained in 3 to 6 months. Due to the close association between syphilis and HIV, consideration should be given to HIV testing.

Pelvic Inflammatory Disease

One of the most damaging sequelae of sexual activity in the adolescent population is pelvic inflammatory disease (PID). Factors known to escalate the risk for PID include nonwhite race, young age, multiple sexual partners, utilization of intrauterine devices (IUDs), and the immaturity of the adolescent cervix (columnar endothelium).

The pathogenesis of PID is complex and thought to result from the combination of an immature host and certain pathologic organisms that facilitate the ascension of organisms through the cervix to the uterus, fallopian tubes, and potentially to the abdominal cavity. Responsible organisms include *C. trachomatis* and *N. gonorrhoeae* as well as facultative aerobes and anaerobes. There may also be a role played by *Mycoplasma hominis* and *Gardnerella vaginalis.*

Sequelae include recurrent PID, chronic abdominal pain, infertility, chronic pelvic pain, tubo-ovarian abscess, ectopic pregnancy, perihepatitis (Fitz-Hugh-Curtis syndrome), and sacroileitis as well as acute and chronic changes to the pelvic organs.

Clinical Presentation

Clinical symptoms begin shortly after completion of menses and include fever, irregular vaginal bleeding, vaginal discharge, and abdominal pain. Diagnostic indicators include adnexal tenderness, cervical motion tenderness, lower abdominal pain, temperature $> 38°$ C, WBC $> 10,500/mm^3$, ESR > 15 mm/h, pelvic abscess on bimanual examination or sonogram, and purulent material from the peritoneal cavity on culdocentesis or laparoscopy. Definitive diagnosis is established by laparoscopy, which is impractical in the ED due to its expense, discomfort, risks, and time required.

Differential Diagnosis

Differential diagnosis includes appendicitis, cholecystitis, UTI, ectopic pregnancy, inflammatory bowel disease, ovarian torsion, and spontaneous or septic abortion.

Diagnosis and Treatment

Pelvic evaluation must include endocervical cultures for *N. gonorrhea* and *C. trachomatous*, a wet mount for *Trichomonas,* and a KOH preparation for *Candida.* Additional studies include VDRL or RPR serology, β-human chorionic gonadotropin (β-HCG), HIV test, and urinalysis. A pelvic ultrasound should be performed if ectopic pregnancy or tubo-ovarian abscess is suspected.

Patients with known or suspected PID should receive treatment in the ED, as early treatment has been shown to preserve tubal patency.

One outpatient treatment for PID consists of a single parenteral dose of ceftriaxone plus doxycycline, tetracycline, or erythromycin for 14 days. An alternative outpatient regimen consists of cefoxitin IM plus probenecid orally.

Inpatient treatment should be strongly considered for all adolescents. One regimen consists of cefoxitin 2 g IV q 6 hr plus doxycycline 100 mg PO or IV q 12 h followed by doxycycline 100 mg bid to finish a total of 14 days. An alternative regimen consists of clindamycin 900 mg IV q 8 h plus gentamicin 2 mg/kg load IM/IV, followed by gentamicin 1.5 mg/kg IV q 8 hours followed by doxycycline 100 mg bid for a total of 14 days.

All patients must be followed up within 24 to 48 hours to document clinical improvement. The protection of sexually transmitted diseases is summarized in **Table 94.1**.

Protection

Sexual abstinence should continue for 2 to 3 weeks following treatment for PID, followed by a test of cure. All sexual partners should be treated.

Acute Renal Failure

Acute renal failure (ARF) is defined as a precipitous decline in kidney function and glomerular filtration rate. There is an accumulation of nitrogenous end products causing azotemia, fluid electrolyte imbalances, and disturbances in blood pressure and in solute excretion. ARF occurs in as many as 2% to 3% of children admitted to tertiary care centers. The causes of ARF are divided into pre-renal (decreased renal blood flow), renal (parenchymal disorders), or post-renal (obstruction of urine flow). Pre-renal ARF results from decreased kidney perfusion from vomiting, diarrhea, poor fluid intake, fever, use of diuretics, and heart failure. NSAIDs can precipitate pre-renal failure in those with baseline diminished renal perfusion. Renal disorders causing ARF include acute tubular necrosis, nephrotoxic injuries from medications, and glomerular disease such as hemolytic uremic syndrome, poststreptococcal glomerulonephritis, and pyelonephritis. Of these, hemolytic uremic syndrome and acute glomerulonephritis are the leading causes of this form of ARF in children. Post-renal ARF is caused by obstruction from posterior urethral valves, nephrolithiasis, or intraabdominal and pelvic tumors. These are a relatively rare causes of ARF in children.

Clinical Findings

Clinical findings in patients who present with ARF are related to the specific underlying disorders. Urine output is often decreased to less than 1 mL/kg/h. The ED approach to ARF should occur in an organized fashion. First, correctable causes should be identified and addressed: hypotension, hemorrhage, dehydration, sepsis, and heart failure. Life-threatening complications should be anticipated: encephalopathy and seizures from hypertension, cardiac arrhythmia from hyperkalemia, and pulmonary edema from volume overload and CHF. Ultrasonography, CT, and cystourethrography should be considered to evaluate obstruction.

Laboratory

Laboratory evaluation should include a CBC, electrolytes, BUN, and creatinine calcium and phosphorus. Antistreptolysin O (ASO) titers can aid in the evaluation of poststreptococcal glomerulonephritis. C3 complement can point to lupus as an underlying cause. A creatine phosphokinase test (CPK) should be sent in cases of suspected rhabdomyolysis. Evaluation of the urine is critical. Patients with acute glomerulonephritis will have RBC casts and hematuria. Heme positive urine in the absence of erythrocytes suggests the presence of myoglobin and rhabdomyolysis. WBCs point to infection and WBC casts suggest interstitial nephritis. Urine culture should be obtained in all patients. Oxalate crystals are seen in cases of ethylene glycol ingestion. Hyaline casts are present in dehydration and acute tubular necrosis (ATN). Urine specific gravity may be helpful in differentiating pre-renal failure from ATN. Typically patients with pre-renal failure have an elevated specific gravity (>1.025) where patients with ATN have specific gravity in the range of 1.005 to 1.015. Urine indices, which measure urine osmolality, urine sodium and fractional excretion of sodium help, further differentiate pre-renal causes from tubular necrosis.

Because one of the earliest defects of tubular necrosis is urine concentrating ability, the urine osmolality measurements are helpful. Patient with pre-renal azotemia tend to have urine osmolality greater than 500 mOsm/kg, a urinary sodium concentration below 20 mmol/L, and a fractional excretion of sodium less than 1%. In contrast, patients with tubular damage have a urine osmolality less than 350 mOsm/kg, the urinary sodium excretion exceeds 40 mmol/L, and the fractional excretion of sodium exceeds 1%.

Management

One of the decision points is determining whether the cause of ARF is pre-renal and whether fluid resuscitation is appropriate. If the history and physical examination suggest pre-renal failure, isotonic fluid should be administered until signs of hypoperfusion are reversed. If no urine is produced in response to IV fluids, furosemide (1–2 mg/kg) should be administered. If myoglobinuria or he-

Table 94.1

Treatment of Sexually Transmitted Diseases

Disease	Treatment
Chlamydia trachomatis	Azithromycin 1 g PO × 1 dose
	or
	Doxycycline 100 g PO bid × 7 days (≥8 years)
	or
	Erythromycin 500 mg PO qid × 7 days (if pregnant)
Trichomonas/bacterial vaginosis	Metronidazole 2 g PO × 1 dose
Gonorrhea	
Outpatient	Ceftriaxone 125 mg IM *or* IV × 1 *or*
	Spectinomycin 2 g IM × 1 (40 mg/kg IM if <45 lbs) *or*
	Ciprofloxacin po 500 mg PO × 1
Herpes	
Primary infection	Treat within 6 days:
	Acyclovir 200 mg PO 5×/day × 5 days
	or
	Acyclovir 400 mg PO tid × 7–10 days
	or
	Famciclovir 250 mg, PO tid × 7–10 days
	or
	Valacyclovir 1 g PO bid × 7–10 days
Recurrent	Acyclovir 200 mg PO 5×/day × 5 days
Immunocompromised	Acyclovir IV
Syphilis	
Primary or secondary or latent <1 year	Benzathine penicillin 50,000 U/kg IM (G 2.4 × 10^6 U) × 1 *or*
	Doxycycline 100 mg PO bid × 14 days *or*
	Tetracycline 500 mg PO qid × 14 days
Secondary >1 year or tertiary	Benzathine penicillin G 2.4 × 10^6 U × 3 doses at 1 week intervals
Outpatient	Ceftriaxone 250 mg IM once *or* Ceftriaxone 2 g IM probenecid 1 g PO
	plus
	Doxycycline 100 mg PO bid × 14 days
	with or without
	Metronidazole 500 mg bid × 14 days
Inpatient	Cefotetan 2 g IV q 12 h *or*
	Cefoxitin 2 g IV q 6 h
	plus
	Doxycycline 100 mg po or IV q 12 h *or*
	Clindamycin 900 mg IV q 8 h
	plus
	Gentamicin: loading dose IV or IM (2 mg/kg) followed by maintenance dose (1.5 mg/kg) q 8 h (single daily dosing may be substituted)

moglobinuria is present, then furosemide (1 mg/kg) followed by 0.5 g mannitol/kg of mannitol is necessary to clear pigmenturia and prevent tubular damage.

Complications such as hyperkalemia must be recognized and addressed with binding resins, glucose and insulin, correction of acidosis, and hemodialysis.

If potassium is greater than 5.5 mEq/L, eliminate potassium intake; Kayexalate can be given orally or rectally. If the K^+ is greater than 6.5 mEq/L and there are EKG changes, Ca gluconate 10 % is cardioprotective. Intravenous fluids and improved perfusion may improve metabolic acidosis and drive K^+ intracellularly. In the setting of persistently low bicarbonate, consider the administration of sodium bicarbonate. If dysrhythmia persists, the patient can be started on an insulin glucose drip (0.5 g/kg glucose as D25

with 1 unit of insulin for every 4 g of glucose given). Dialysis may be required if above measures do not decrease the potassium. Consultation with a pediatric critical care specialist is advantageous at this juncture.

Seizures may be a complication of ARF, either due to severe hypertension or hyponatremia. A hypertensive emergency may be a result of volume overload and should be addressed with fluid restriction and furosemide (1–2 mg/kg). Nitroprusside (0.5–8 μg/kg/min) infusion or labetalol (0.2–1.0 mg/kg/dose) are effective in controlling the blood pressure. Blood pressure reduction should be cautious with the goal of 1/3 of the total reduction in the first 6 hours. Seizures resulting from hyponatremia may necessitate the use of hypertonic saline (3%).

Indications for dialysis include uremia with a BUN greater than 100 mg/dL, persistent hyperkalemia >6.5 mEqL, persistent metabolic acidosis ($HCO_3 < 10$ mEq/L), persistent CHF, oliguric renal failure due to HUS, or rhabdomyolysis with myoglobinuria.

Acute Glomerulonephritis

Glomerulonephritis (GN) is an acute clinical syndrome characterized by hematuria, edema, hypertension, and renal insufficiency. The most common clinical feature is edema, followed by hypertension. The urine can appear grossly bloody, tea-colored, or smoky.

Glomerulonephritis can occur as a primary process in which only the kidney is usually affected, including: postinfectious, familial, drug induced, Berger's disease (IgA nephropathy) and membroproliferative GN. Secondary forms include: Henoch-Schönlein purpura, hemolytic uremic syndrome, systemic lupus erythematosus, subacute bacterial endocarditis, and Goodpasture's syndrome.

By far the most common cause in children is poststreptococcal glomerulonephritis (PSGN), which may follow streptococcal infections of the skin or pharynx. PSGN commonly affects children between the ages of 2 and 10 with a slight male predominance. Only certain strains of streptococci have been found to be nephritogenic.

Pathophysiology

Immune complexes formed in response to streptococcal infection are planted in the glomerulus during acute infection. The complement system is subsequently activated which triggers the release of further inflammatory mediators in the basement membrane.

Clinical Findings

Typically gross hematuria or tea colored urine develops 1 to 3 weeks after streptococcal infection pharyngitis. Peripheral edema, especially around the eyes is seen in approximately 75% of cases. Oliguria and hypertension are present less frequently. Rarely, hypertensive encephalopathy and congestive heart failure occur at initial presentation.

Laboratory Data

Urinalysis is most helpful in establishing the diagnosis of PSGN and reveals gross or microscopic hematuria, RBC casts, hyaline or granular casts, and WBCs. A urine culture is helpful to rule out infection. BUN and creatinine may be elevated. Hyponatremia and/or hyperkalemia may be related to water retention and azotemia. Levels of total complement and C3 are decreased early in the disease. Antibodies to streptolysin O may provide evidence of recent streptococcal infection, although certain strains do not produce streptolysin, limiting the diagnostic utility of this test. The throat or skin should be cultured. A CXR should be obtained in those presenting with hypertension.

Management

The role of the emergency physician is the timely diagnosis of PSGN and treatment of the complications of CHF and hypertension. If CHF is present, supplemental oxygen and furosemide (0.5–1 mg/kg) should be considered. In mild cases, patient may be discharged on a salt restricted diet, limited activity, and close follow-up. Treatment of streptococcal infection in the patient and symptomatic contacts should be initiated after a throat culture is obtained. Most patients recover completely, although hypertension, persistent proteinuria and chronic renal insufficiency develop in a small percentage.

Hemolytic Uremic Syndrome

Hemolytic uremic syndrome (HUS) is the most common cause of acute renal failure in healthy infants and children. The triad of hemolytic anemia, thrombocytopenia, and acute renal failure characterizes HUS. Two subtypes are described in children: diarrhea associated (D+) and nondiarrhea associated (D−). Most cases are diarrhea associated (D+) and occur primarily in infants and children. Nondiarrhea associated cases result from nonenteric pathogens such as Coxsakie, influenza and RSV, malignancies, transplantation, and drugs. Nondiarrheal associated HUS also occurs as an inherited disorder. Incidence is similar in males and females; white children are affected more often than blacks.

Pathophysiology

Viral and/or bacterial organisms and their toxins cause damage to the renal capillary endothelium resulting in edema, thrombin deposition, platelet trapping, and microangiopathic hemolytic anemia. Platelets, fibrin, and complement deposit in the glomeruli, resulting in decreased glomeruli filtration rate and renal failure. E. coli, especially serotype O157:H7, has emerged as the most commonly isolated organism in North America associated with D+ HUS. The most common routes of infection are ingestion of contaminated meat or milk. During outbreaks of E. coli O157:H7, 10% of children develop HUS.

Clinical Findings

In D+ HUS, diarrhea and cramping abdominal pain precede the illness by one to two weeks. These symptoms may be associated with blood in the stool, vomiting, and fever. Patients then develop the acute symptoms of pallor, listlessness, irritability, and oliguria or anuria. Patients may have petechiae, GI bleeding, hypertension, hepatomegaly, edema, and CNS involvement, including seizures and coma.

Laboratory Studies

The classic laboratory findings seen in HUS include a nonimmune hemolytic anemia, thrombocytopenia, and abnormal renal function tests. The hematocrit and hemoglobin are markedly low and fall rapidly as a result of the brisk hemolysis that is occurring. Helmet cells, burr cells, and fragmented RBCs are present on the peripheral blood smear. The reticulocyte count is mildly elevated and the Coombs test is negative. The platelets are decreased, usually to less than 50,000/mm^3. WBC is usually increased with a left shift. The BUN and creatinine are elevated and hyponatremia, hyperkalemia, and acidosis may be seen.

The urinalysis reveals hematuria, with variable amounts of protein and leukocytes. Granular and hyaline casts can be seen in the urine sediment.

Differential Diagnosis

When typical, the history, clinical, and laboratory findings of D+ HUS are generally sufficiently characteristic to suggest the diagnoses. In some cases, the physical exam may reveal abdominal tenderness. When associated with hematochezia, this presentation may suggest an intussusception. The clinical presentation of D− HUS is often more confusing. Other causes of causes of renal failure such as poststreptococcal glomerulonephritis and sepsis with multiorgan failure should be considered.

Management

The treatment or HUS relies on early recognition and resuscitation. Particular attention must be given to fluid administration and balance. Specific treatment of hyperkalemia, acidosis, and hypocalcemia is indicated. Early consultation with a nephrologist is recommended. Indications for dialysis include: BUN more than 100 mg/dL, CHF, encephalopathy, and severe hyperkalemia. Severe anemia (hemoglobin <5 g/dL) warrants a slow transfusion with 5 to 10 mL/kg of packed red blood cells (pRBC). Platelet transfusion is indicated for symptomatic bleeding and plasma transfusion for hereditary, prolonged or recurrent HUS. Acute mortality has been reported as high as 25%, but recent estimates are closer to 5%. CNS involvement is associated with increased mortality.

Henoch-Schönlein Pupura

Henoch-Schönlein purpura (HSP) is a multisystem disorder involving skin, joints, abdomen, and kidneys. It presents with purpura, arthralgias, abdominal pain, and renal abnormalities to varying degrees. Renal involvement occurs in approximately one half of patients, usually after the onset of skin and joint findings. Children between the ages of 2 and 11 are most commonly affected and the incidence is greater in males.

Pathophysiology

HSP is thought to be a vasculitis with immunoglobulin A (IgA) deposition in the skin and glomeruli. Renal biopsy appearance is similar to IgA nephropathy (Berger's disease), but other clinical manifestations point to HSP.

Clinical Findings

The typical skin rash provides the key to diagnosis. These lesions begin as round pink papules on the extensor surface of the limbs, buttocks, and lower back. After 24 hours, they progress to palpable purpura. Arthralgia and joint swelling occur frequently, often in the knees and ankles. Abdominal pain with melena occurs in a significant percent of patients. In approximately 5% of these patients, these symptoms may represent an intussusception. Hematuria may be present, but is usually microscopic in nature. Rarely, a nephritic picture may develop with edema, hypertension, and azotemia, and is associated with a worse prognosis.

Laboratory Data

The laboratory is useful in excluding out other possibilities. WBC, platelet count, and coagulation tests are normal. Urinalysis often reveals hematuria and is should be monitored throughout the illness. BUN and creatinine may be elevated if renal involvement is significant.

Differential Diagnosis

Other causes of purpuric rashes should be considered including: Rocky Mountain spotted fever, meningococcemica, ITP. As noted above, intussusception should be carefully considered in the ill appearing child with HSP and abdominal pain.

Management

Treatment is supportive. The risk of intussusception provides the diagnostic greatest challenge to the emergency physician. Steroids continue to be utilized in the hopes of reducing intestinal edema and abdominal pain, although the supporting data for this are limited. Patients may be discharged if significant renal involvement is not present and if abdominal or joint pain is not severe. Close follow-up must be assured to monitor urinalysis to detect the development of glomerulonephritis. Overall prognosis is excellent with only 1% to 2 % progressing to serious renal sequelae.

Nephrotic Syndrome

Nephrotic syndrome (NS) is an uncommon clinical condition characterized by hypoproteinemia (serum albumin <3.0 g/dL), severe proteinuria (>40 mg/m^2/day), hypoalbuminemia (<2.5 g/dL), edema, and hypercholesterolemia (>250 mg/dL). The reported annual incidence is 2 to 5/100,000 children. Most cases of childhood nephrotic syndrome are *primary nephrotic syndrome*, which is disease limited to the kidney. Of these, the majority of cases are minimal change disease (76%). Other causes are focal segmental glomerulosclerosis, membranous glomerulonephritis, or membroproliferative nephritis. *Secondary nephrotic syndrome* is associated with other systemic diseases such as HIV, anaphylactoid purpura, lupus erythematosus, diabetes mellitus, sickle cell disease, and neoplasm (Wilms' tumor, lymphoma).

Pathophysiology

Plasma proteins, reaching the glomeruli, are restricted by a charge selective and size selective barrier. Normally only .03% of plasma proteins reach the tubules. A small increase in permeability in these barriers can overwhelm the resorptive capacity of the tubules, leading to proteinuria. This loss of protein contributes directly or through compensatory mechanism to the other clinical conditions that characterize nephrotic syndrome.

Edema (periorbital, peripheral, and scrotal) is classically described as being the result of a low serum albumin causing a decreased oncotic pressure with extravasation of water into the interstitial space. This decreased plasma volume was thought to lead to a decreased renal perfusion and a stimulation of the renin-angiotensin system. This combined with the release of antidiuretic hormone, enhances the reabsorption of sodium and water in the distal nephrons. However, in some cases, plasma volume is increased and there is no elevation of renin, angiotensin, or aldosterone. The precise mechanism of edema formation and persistence remains uncertain.

In addition to albumin, other proteins are excreted in the urine, leading to hypoimmunoglobulinemia and increased susceptibility to infections. Hepatic protein production is increased in a response to hypoalbuminemia and can lead to a hypercoagulable state and thrombotic complications.

Clinical Findings

Most children are asymptomatic except for the insidious development of edema. In the early stages, edema may be intermittent and primarily involve areas of low tissue resistance (periorbital, scrotal, and labia). As fluid retention becomes severe, it can progress to pleural effusions and respiratory distress. Ascites and bowel wall edema result in anorexia, nausea, vomiting, and diarrhea. Hypertension, hematuria, and oliguria may be present.

Complications

Bacterial infections are the most common complications in patients with new onset nephrotic syndrome and those already diagnosed and treated with steroids. A relative hypogammaglobulinemia predisposes patients to cellulitis, peritonitis, pneumonia, sepsis, and meningitis. Hypovolemia from intravascular depletion of salt and water, despite the presence of edema, may progress to shock. The hypercoagulable state predisposes to thrombosis in peripheral and internal vessels. Flank pain, hematuria, and worsening renal function should raise the suspicion of renal vein thrombosis.

Laboratory Data

Hypoalbuminemia is a cardinal feature of the NS. The serum albumin is less than 2.5 g/dL, with values as low as 0.5 g/dL. Urine protein is elevated (>2+ on urine dip or >40 mg/m^2/d). Hematuria may be present in those with primary NS as well as those with secondary NS. Renal function is typically normal at the onset of the syndrome. If the plasma volume is contracted and elevated, hematocrit may be seen. WBC may be elevated even in the absence of infection and may be normal in the infected patient on steroids.

Differential Diagnosis

Facial edema may be caused by an allergic reaction. Other causes of generalized edema to be considered are conges-

tive heart failure. Other conditions producing hypoalbuminemia include cirrhosis and the protein losing enteropathy of cystic fibrosis. The urinalysis with proteinuria will help further define NS.

Management

The most important role of the emergency physician is supportive treatment of complications. Symptomatic hypovolemia and shock are treated in the usual way with isotonic boluses until perfusion is restored. If the patient is adequately hydrated but has symptomatic edema, furosemide should be administered. Hypovolemia and hemoconcentration should be avoided because of the risk of thrombotic complications. If edema is severe and serum albumin is less than 1.5 g/dL, then albumin (0.5–1.0 g/kg of 25% salt deficient albumin) followed by furosemide (0.5–1.0 mg/kg) may be useful. After an aggressive search for infection (including a negative tuberculin test) and in consultation with a nephrologist, some patients benefit from corticosteroids. Prednisone, 2 mg/kg/day is the typical dose in newly diagnosed patients.

Selected Readings

AAP Red Book. 2003 Report of the Committee on Infectious Diseases. ed 25. Dallas: American Academy of Pediatrics, 2004.

Andreoli SP. Acute renal failure. Curr Opin Pediatr 2001;14:183–188.

Centers for Disease Control and Prevention. Sexually transmitted disease treatment guidelines—2002. MMWR Recomm Rep 2002;51(RR-6):1–80.

Clark A, Barratt T. Steroid-responsive nephrotic syndrome. In: Barratt T, ed. Pediatric Nephrology, 4th ed. Baltimore: Lippincott Williams and Wilkins, 1999: 731–747.

Edelsberg J, Surh Y. The acute scrotum. Emerg Med Clin North Am 1988:6:521–546.

Hricik D, Chung-Park M, Sedor J. Glomerulonephritis. N Engl J Med 1998;339: 888–899.

Kelsch R, Sedman A. Nephrotic syndrome. Pediatr Rev 1993;14:30–38.

Klauber GT, Sant GR. Disorders of the male external genitalia. In: Kelalis PP, King LR, Belman AB, eds. Clinical Pediatric Urology, 2d ed. Philadelphia: Saunders, 1985.

Lanzkowsky S, Lanzkowsky L, Lanzkowsky P. Henoch-Schönlein purpura. Pediatr Rev 1992;13:130–137.

Middleton RG, Matlack ME, Nixon GW, et al. Genitourinary injuries in children. In: Mayer TA, ed. Emergency Management of Pediatric Trauma. Philadelphia: Saunders, 1985:341–352.

Oosterlinck W. Unbloody management of penile zipper injury. Eur Urol 1981; 7:365.

Orth SR, Ritz E. The nephrotic syndrome. N Engl J Med 1998;338:1202–1211.

Robson W, Leung A. Henoch-Schönlein purpura. Adv Pediatr 1994;41:163–194.

Sehic A, Chesney RW. Acute renal failure: diagnosis. Pediatr Rev 1995;164: 101–106.

Sehic A, Chesney RW. Acute renal failure: therapy. Pediatr Rev 1995;16:137–141.

Stewart C, Tina L. Hemolytic uremic syndrome. Pediatr Rev 1993;14:218–224.

Thadhani R, Pascual M, Bonventre JV. Acute renal failure. N Engl J Med 1996;334: 1448–1460.

Tumeh S, Benson C, Richie J. Acute diseases of the scrotum. Semin Ultrasound CT MR 1991;12:115–130.

Vogt B, Avner E. Renal failure. In: Behrman RE, Kliegman RM, Jenson HB, eds. Nelson's Textbook of Pediatrics, ed 17. Philadelphia: Saunders, 2004:1768–1775.

Endocrine Disorders

Mariann M. Manno

Emergency Management of Diabetic Ketoacidosis

Definition

Diabetic ketoacidosis (DKA) is a serious complication of diabetes generally defined as a blood sugar greater than 300 mL/dL and a serum bicarbonate concentration less than 15 mEq/L or an arterial pH less than 7.30. Severe DKA has been defined as a serum bicarbonate value less than 10 or a pH less than 7.10. DKA is commonly encountered by the emergency physician and should be respected as a complex, potentially fatal metabolic emergency. Thirty percent of children with new-onset diabetes are in DKA. DKA at the time of diagnosis of diabetes is increased in very young children, indicative of the fact that recognition of symptoms of diabetes is difficult in this age group. Risk factors for DKA in children with known diabetes include poverty, lack of health insurance, poor compliance with insulin regimen, and mental health conditions. In children, DKA is more commonly seen with poor compliance than with infection, in contrast with adult populations were infections and illness are common precipitating reasons for DKA.

Mortality from DKA during the 30-year span from 1930 to 1960 is recorded to be approximately 40%. During the subsequent 18 years from 1960 to 1978, mortality from DKA decreased to 9%. Despite advances in pediatric critical care and diabetes research, DKA has a mortality of <5% and accounts for half of all diabetes-associated deaths in children and adolescents, largely from cerebral edema.

Pathogenesis (Biochemistry)

Insulin-dependent diabetes mellitus (IDDM), also known as juvenile onset or type I diabetes, is characterized by insulin deficiency. Produced by the pancreatic islet cells, insulin is the premiere anabolic hormone. In the nonfasted state, it enables glucose to enter cells and stimulates the formation of glucagon, protein, and adipose tissue. In the normal, fasted state (with low serum glucose) or in the insulin-deficient state, substrate is mobilized: glycogen is broken down to glucose (glycogenolysis), protein is catab-

olized to amino acid and then to glucose (gluconeogenesis), and lipid is converted to fatty acids (ketogenesis). The anabolic properties of insulin are opposed by counterregulatory hormones (growth hormone, cortisol, catecholamines, glucagon). They are produced by the body in response to stress (dehydration, fever, fasting), and act to increase glucose and fatty acid production.

A delicately orchestrated balance exists between the glucose-lowering, energy-storing properties of insulin and the glucose-elevating, energy-mobilizing properties of the counterregulatory hormones. The pathophysiological state of DKA results from the combined effects of insulin deficiency and the unopposed action of counterregulatory hormones. The final common pathway of these metabolic abnormalities is a clinical state characterized by hyperglycemia, dehydration, acidosis, electrolyte abnormalities, and hyperosmolality.

Hyperglycemia

Hyperglycemia contributes directly to dehydration. When the renal threshold for glucose reabsorption by the proximal tubule is exceeded, glucose draws free water and electrolytes into the urine, producing an osmotic diuresis. Increased serum glucose creates a gradient between the intracellular and extracellular fluids. Water shifts from the intracellular to the extracellular space, transiently augmenting intravascular volume and masking the actual degree of dehydration. A patient with vomiting, altered mental status, or very young age cannot compensate by drinking in this early state of hyperglycemia/dehydration and is at risk for more severe metabolic abnormalities. As dehydration and renal perfusion worsen, diminished urine output limits the excretion of glucose, ketones, and other organic acids. The result is a dramatic increase in blood sugar, BUN, and serum osmolality. Generally, the degree of hyperglycemia can serve as a gauge of the degree of volume depletion. Severe hyperglycemia suggests severe dehydration and diminished renal function with the attendant metabolic complications already mentioned.

Electrolyte Abnormality

Serum sodium concentrations are typically low. Urinary sodium losses are typically in the range of 5 to 13 mEq/kg or 40 to 100 mEq/L, approximating one-half normal saline. In addition, the dilutional effect of intracellular fluid shift into the extracellular space lowers the serum sodium. Hypertriglyceridemia interferes with the measurement of the serum sodium, resulting in artificially low measured values. The corrected serum sodium can be calculated once the serum glucose is known (**FIGURE 95.1**).

Abnormalities of potassium homeostasis are of major importance in DKA. Total body stores of potassium are profoundly depleted through urinary loss (typically 5–10 mEq/kg) and vomiting. Initially, acidosis shifts potassium into the extracellular space, typically resulting in normal or elevated initial serum levels. With hydration and correction of acidosis, potassium shifts intracellularly and serum potassium decreases, potentially leading to hypokalemia. Potassium levels must be monitored carefully throughout all phases of treatment as both hyperkalemia (peaked T waves, widened QRS) initially and hypokalemia (U waves), especially with therapy, predispose the patient to cardiac arrhythmia.

Serum phosphate levels may be normal despite significantly depleted stores but are of less clinical significance. Elevation in the serum BUN is a result of prerenal dysfunction and protein breakdown. Ketones interfere with creatinine measurement in some laboratories, resulting in artificially elevated creatinine levels.

Osmolality

Elevation of the serum sodium, glucose, and BUN all contribute to increased serum osmolality (Figure 95.1). Hyperosmolality promotes the formation of osmotically active substances within the brain. These "idiogenic osmoles" protect the cellular structure of the brain from fluid loss, or shrinking, as the osmolar gradient increases between the intracellular and systemic intravascular spaces. They are produced and metabolized gradually. Large changes in serum osmolality, such as rapid correction of the blood sugar and BUN, potentially reverse this osmotic gradient. Until idiogenic osmoles are cleared, the CNS will be relatively hyperosmolar and the patient is at risk for cerebral edema.

Acidosis

Organic acids are metabolized by the liver into acetone, acetoacetate, and β-hydroxybutyric acid. Acetoacetate (AcAc), a ketone, is reduced to β-hydroxybutyric acid (BHB) to varying degrees depending on the state of tissue perfusion. The ratio of BHB to AcAc increases with worsening acidosis and may be as high as 15:1 in severe DKA. Acetoacetate is also converted to acetone and CO_2. Acetone is excreted in the breath and urine. The usual method of serum ketone measurement by nitroprusside reaction primarily reflects AcAc and very small quantities of acetone. Because BHB, the ketoacid present in much greater quantities, is unmeasured, routine analysis of serum ketones may be helpful in diagnosing DKA but not useful in evaluating therapy. Likewise, urine ketones, largely acetone, may persist despite improving acidosis. Generally, measurement of the venous pH and calculation of the anion gap (reflective of lactate, AcAc and BHB) provides the most accurate assessment of acidemia. This tremendous load of organic acid as well as lactic acid elaborated by poorly perfused tissues causes a profound metabolic acidosis. The most serious effects of this are depression of arterial muscular tone and myocardial contractility.

Diagnosis

The diagnosis of DKA is straightforward when classic signs are present: polyuria, polydipsia, polyphagia, fruity breath, dehydration, and weight loss. Most children with new-onset diabetes are symptomatic to some degree for several weeks before the diagnosis is made and in some cases DKA develops. However, classic findings may be subtle or difficult to detect, particularly in the very young, and a timely diagnosis depends on a high index of suspicion. New-onset diabetes and DKA in a toddler or infant may present with listlessness, rapid breathing, or vomiting. Gastroenteritis, URI, or bacterial sepsis may be incorrectly presumed to be the underlying problem.

Rapidly available laboratory tests, including a blood sugar, serum electrolytes, BUN, creatinine, calcium, phosphate, venous blood gas, and urine analysis, confirms the diagnosis of DKA in almost all cases.

A careful physical examination is of critical importance. The degree of dehydration should be determined by assessing vital signs, mental status, skin turgor and temperature, and capillary refill. Patients presenting with shock require more aggressive fluid resuscitation. The actual degree of dehydration may be underestimated because the intravascular volume is maintained at the expense of the intracelluar dehydration. Urine output continues because of glucose diuresis until severe volume depletion is present, making it an unreliable tool in gauging dehydration. The quality of breathing should be evaluated for hyperpnea, or Kussmaul breathing, a sign of respiratory compensation for metabolic acidosis. A fruity odor of the breath may be present. A neurologic examination with particular attention to the child's mental status, level of alertness, developmentally appropriate responses, lethargy, combativeness, pupillary reactivity, and the presence of papilledema. Approximately 10% of children with DKA present with profoundly abnormal mental status. Children with an altered mental status should be presumed to be at risk for cerebral edema and should be carefully followed. The abdominal examination may reveal guarding and diffuse tenderness as paralytic ilius and gastric distention are common. Unless intraabdominal pathol-

---

Serum Osmolality (mOsm/L) = 2(Na + K) + glucose/18 + BUN/2/8

Correction of "pseudohyponatremia"

Corrected Na = Measured Na + (glucose − 100)/100

FIGURE 95.1 Calculation of serum osmolality.

ogy is strongly suspected, treatment of DKA should supersede the investigation of abdominal pain. A complete examination is important to exclude the possibility of an infectious etiology precipitating DKA. Repeated evaluations are critical in the careful management of these patients (**Table 95.1**).

Initial Resuscitation

The initial resuscitation of a patient in DKA must include an evaluation of the patient's airway patency, ventilatory effort, perfusion, and mental status. Specific management priorities are treatment of circulatory compromise, correction of life-threatening electrolyte abnormalities, institution of insulin therapy, and correction of acidosis.

Fluid resuscitation requires meticulous care. Most patients in DKA are 5% to 10% dehydrated. Physical examination (skin turgor, tears, sunken eyes, capillary refill), vital signs, and weight are all important for an accurate estimate of the degree of dehydration. The goal of initial fluid resuscitation is to restore the circulating blood volume and reestablish renal perfusion. An initial bolus of 10 to 20 cc/kg (depending on the child's age and degree of dehydration) isotonic fluid is generally recommended. In general, 10 cc/kg boluses should be administered to adolescents and 20 cc/kg boluses should be used for younger children and severely dehydrated patients. Volume expansion dilutes serum electrolytes and blood glucose and improves renal function, allowing glucose excretion in the urine. A repeat blood glucose, sodium, and potassium should be obtained shortly after the initial IV fluid bolus. Perfusion should be reassessed by physical examination to determine if a second bolus of isotonic saline is needed. Once hemodynamically stable, the total fluid requirement (maintenance, remaining deficit, and ongoing losses), the time frame for rehydration (generally over 48 hours), and type of fluid (usually half NS) should be determined.

Replacement of fluid and sodium deficit (~10 mEq/kg) can usually be accomplished with half normal saline. With treatment, the serum sodium should rise. Failure of the

sodium to increase may be a sign of excess free water and should prompt reevaluation of the tonicity and rate of fluid administration. Since the exact mechanism of cerebral edema remains unclear, the following issues are important to consider:

1. A fluid bolus may not be needed in a child without signs of dehydration on physical assessment.
2. Repeated fluid boluses should be given only in response to clinical signs of persistent hypoperfusion.
3. Fluid replacement should be gradual with correction over 48 hours in the setting of hyperosmolality and/or signs of altered mental status.

Despite normal or elevated initial potassium, all patients in DKA have lost significant amounts of potassium through urinary diuresis. As acidosis and dehydration resolve, potassium shifts intracellularly and hypokalemia may develop or worsen. Potassium should be added to IV fluids once urine is produced. Generally, 40 mEq/L of potassium (in equal amounts of KCl and KPhos) is given if the initial potassium is normal. If the initial potassium is low, more than 40 mEq/L and more careful monitoring may be needed. When the initial potassium is high, less potassium should be administered and potassium levels should be closely followed.

Routine administration of bicarbonate is not recommended because acidosis can be corrected with fluids and insulin alone. Several studies have demonstrated little benefit with bicarbonate in the rate of correction of acidosis. In addition, one study of children with DKA reported that bicarbonate administration was associated with an increased risk of cerebral edema (Glaser et al.). Bicarbonate should be reserved for severely acidotic patients with compromised cardiopulmonary function.

Insulin should be given as soon as initial fluid resuscitation is complete and laboratory values have confirmed the diagnosis of DKA. A continuous insulin infusion at 0.05 to 0.1 U/kg/h should be established with the goal of lowering the blood glucose at a rate of 100 mg/dL/h. An insulin bolus before the drip is not recommended. As the blood glucose and acidosis normalize, the concentration of the insulin infusion may be decreased. However, the serum glucose concentration will frequently decrease significantly with hydration alone because of improved renal perfusion and may normalize before ketosis and acidosis have resolved. When blood glucose corrects (250 to 300 mg/dL) *without* improvement in acidosis, insulin should be maintained (usually at at 0.1 U/kg/hr) and supplemental glucose (D5% to D10%) infused until ketosis improves and the serum bicarbonate is greater than 15 mEq/dL.

Careful monitoring of the patient's clinical condition (vital signs, mental status, perfusion), laboratory values (blood glucose, pH, bicarbonate, serum sodium, and potassium), and fluid status (fluids infused and ongoing losses) is the cornerstone of good care. All patients should have a flow sheet carefully maintained.

Complications

Clinical signs of cerebral edema occur in 1% of children in DKA. It is associated with mortality in the range of 20% to 25% and has similar rates of permanent neuro-

---

Table 95.1

Pitfalls in the Diagnosis and Management of Diabetic Ketoacidosis

- Failure to make the diagnosis in infants and young children with nonspecific presentation.
- Failure to include ongoing losses (especially urine) in replacement fluid.
- Failure to weigh the patient.
- Repeated fluid boluses without clinical reassessment of dehydration.
- Failure to measure laboratory values after initial hydration.
- Failure to establish a flow sheet with vital signs, laboratory values, and fluid status.
- Delay in instituting insulin.
- Discontinuation of insulin in response to decreasing blood glucose but before acidosis clears.

logical disability. Some data suggest that subclinical cerebral edema may exist in many patients with DKA, but only 1% fewer develop clinically significant signs of increased intracranial pressure. Cerebral edema present somewhat unpredictably, often after treatment has been established and laboratory parameters are improving. In one study, the median time to neurologic deterioration after commencement of treatment of DKA was 7 hours. The pathophysiology and predictors or this devastating complication remain unclear. Many etiologies have been suggested: a rapid decrease in blood sugar, the administration of excessive fluids, administration of hypotonic fluids, the administration of bicarbonate, failure of the serum sodium to increase with therapy, and the inappropriate release of vasopressin. Clinical reviews have failed to reveal a particular treatment modality or set of laboratory parameters that either contributes to or signals the development of cerebral edema except that children younger than 5 years and those with new-onset disease are at increased risk. The treatment of cerebral edema is one of watchful waiting for signs of increased ICP (complaint of headache, altered sensorium, fluctuations in blood pressure, decreased heart rate, sluggish pupils, seizures) and rapid intervention.

The ED phase of diagnosis, assessment, and resuscitation of DKA should not be unduly prolonged. Definitive management of these patients is best performed in a critical care environment where continued hemodynamic and neurologic monitoring can be ensured.

Congenital Adrenal Hyperplasia

Congenital adrenal hyperplasia (CAH), the most common disorder of the adrenal gland in the pediatric age group, results from an enzyme deficiency in one of the five pathways required for steroidogenesis. The incidence of CAH is approximately 1/15,000 births. It is inherited as an autosomal recessive trait and can be detected by newborn screening. The spectrum of clinical manifestations of CAH in infants includes ambiguous genitalia in females and severe electrolyte abnormalities in both sexes, leading to cardiac arrhythmias and shock in undiagnosed, untreated patients. Older males may present with precocious puberty alone.

Biochemistry

The adrenal cortex synthesizes three groups of hormones from cholesterol: glucocorticoids (cortisol), mineralocorticoids (aldosterone), and sex steroids (androgens) (**FIGURE 95.2**). Cortisol production occurs in the zona fasciculata and is modulated through negative feedback by adrenocorticotropic hormones (ACTH) secreted by the anterior pituitary and corticotropin-releasing factor (CRF) from the hypothalamus. Aldosterone is produced in the zona glomerulosa under the control of the renin-angiotensin system and ACTH stimulation. Low levels of cortisol and aldosterone result in high levels of ACTH. The term *congenital adrenal hyperplasia* describes morphological changes in the adrenal gland from chronic excess ACTH stimulation in response to low hormone levels.

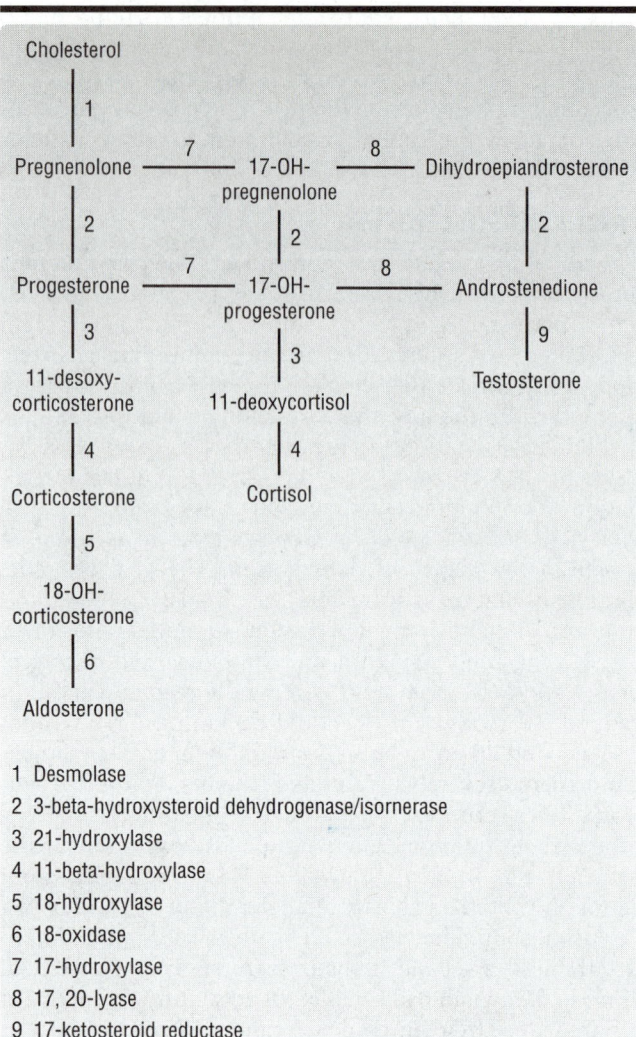

FIGURE 95.2 Metabolism of cholesterol to glucocorticoids, mineralcorticoids, and androgens in the adrenal cortex.

As seen in CAH, deficiency of a given enzyme results in the accumulation of precursors proximal to the block. Excess proximal intermediates are diverted to the other metabolic open pathways. The imbalance between deficient (cortisol, aldosterone) and excess (androgen) hormone production is responsible for the clinical manifestations of this disorder (Figure 95.2).

21-Hydroxylase Deficiency

Almost all (>90%) cases of CAH are caused by 21-hydroxylase (21-OH) deficiency. Absence of 21-hydroxylase blocks the production of deoxycorticosterone from progesterone and 11-deoxycortisol from 17-hydroxyprogesterone. Aldosterone and cortisol are not synthesized in normal quantities. Metabolites proximal to the defect (pregnenolone, progesterone, 17-hydroxypregnenolone, and 17-hydroxyprogesterone) are shunted to the androgen pathway, which does not require 21-OH for biosynthesis. Large amounts of androstenedione are produced and converted peripherally to testosterone.

Diagnosis/Clinical Presentation

Because fetal development of external genitalia is controlled by androgens, females with 21-OH deficiency are virilized at birth and present with variable abnormalities on physical examination: isolated clitoromegaly, fusion of the labioscrotal folds or, in the extreme, bilateral cryptorchidism (female pseudohermaphrodite). The virilizing effects of excess ACTH and androgens in male newborns are subtle; a slightly enlarged phallus and increased scrotal pigmentation and rugae are inconsistent findings on physical examination and often unrecognized at birth. Untreated male and female children who do not succumb to electrolyte disturbances develop rapid growth, advanced bone age, and precocious puberty.

Aldosterone synthesis is presumed to be abnormal in most patients with 21-OH deficiency. However, one third of these have clinically adequate mineralocorticoid synthesis and are described as having *simple virilizing disease*. Females with simple virilizing disease are masculinized at birth; genetic sex and internal genital anatomy are female. Males present with precocious puberty, which may become apparent within the first year of life.

Two thirds of patients with 21-OH deficiency have frank *salt-losing disease*. These patients with inadequate mineralocorticoid control of renal function are at risk for developing electrolyte abnormalities and even death from circulatory collapse and cardiac arrhythmia. Because most females are diagnosed shortly after birth with ambiguous genitalia, males are typically at greater risk for a salt-losing crisis as their disease is unrecognized until symptoms of electrolyte abnormalities become clinically apparent. In the ED, the usual patient with CAH is a male infant in the second week of life with vomiting, failure to regain birth weight, progressive weight loss, lethargy or irritability, poor feeding, and/or prolonged jaundice. The initial presentation may be fairly nonspecific and incorrectly diagnosed as dehydration, gastroenteritis, formula intolerance, pyloric stenosis, physiologic jaundice, or sepsis. The initial history on any such patient should include questioning about family history of renal or endocrine diseases as well as infant (especially male) deaths.

Routine laboratory data are usually helpful in distinguishing CAH from most other clinical entities. The classic electrolyte abnormalities associated with CAH include hyponatremia, hyperkalemia, and a hypochloremic metabolic acidosis. As the clinical condition worsens, azotemia, worsening acidosis, and hypoglycemia may develop. The initial rhythm may provide a clue to the diagnosis as peaked T waves or widened QRS complexes may be seen secondary to hyperkalemia. Potassium levels in the range of 8 to 12 mEq/L are frequently encountered, although the potassium rise may actually be blunted by electrolyte loss from vomiting.

Differential Diagnosis

In an afebrile infant of approximately 2 weeks of age with lethargy and vomiting, consider dehydration, overwhelming sepsis, malrotation with volvulus, and inborn errors of metabolism including galactosemia. Pyloric stenosis occurs in slightly older infants.

Treatment

Rapid IV access must be obtained and normal saline in 20 cc/kg boluses should be repeated until hemodynamic stability is achieved. Since urinary sodium losses approximate normal saline, isotonic fluid should be used during the resuscitative phase. Glucose (0.25–0.5 g/kg) should be considered if hypoglycemia is detected or suspected. Treatment of hyperkalemia is of particular concern in these patients because of the potential for cardiac arrhythmias including intraventricular conduction defect and ventricular fibrillation. An ECG is a helpful rapid diagnostic tool to determine or confirm hyperkalemia. Infants with CAH are better able to tolerate impressively high potassium than older children and adults. Volume expansion is usually the only measure needed to correct hyperkalemia. If arrhythmia is present, 10% calcium gluconate should be considered for its rapid, membrane stabilizing properties. Because of the risk of induced hypoglycemia, glucose and insulin infusions should be used with extreme caution in these small, sick infants.

In addition to serum electrolytes, BUN, creatinine, and blood sugar, plasma 17-hydroxyprogesterone, and urinary 17-ketosteroids are diagnostic especially if obtained before steroids are given. However, hydrocortisone stress doses (in the range of 25 mg IV) should be given urgently if signs of circulatory collapse are present. Long-term treatment for CAH is replacement of deficient steroid hormones. Physiologic doses of glucocorticoids (hydrocortisone 10 to 20 mg/m^2/d) are administered to suppress excess androgen production. Mineralocorticoids (fludrocortisone 0.1 to 0.2 mg/d) are administered in replacement doses and should normalize plasma renin levels. Patients require replacement therapy throughout life. Increased steroid doses (generally 3 to 4 times physiological dose) are indicated during periods of physiologic stress such as infection and surgery. In addition, most infants require oral sodium supplements in the first months of life.

11-Hydroxylase Deficiency

11-Hydroxylase deficiency accounts for approximately 5% of all patients with CAH. As with 21-hydroxylase deficiency, females are born virilized and males are usually diagnosed in infancy or childhood with precocious puberty. Deoxycorticosterone, a potent mineralocorticoid, accumulates proximal to the 11-hydroxylase enzyme defect. Therefore, hypertension, not salt-losing, is a feature of 11-hydroxylase deficiency. Hypertension is an inconsistent finding and may not be present at birth.

Inborn Errors of Metabolism

Inborn errors of metabolism (IEM) in their severe form manifest in infancy; however, presentation can occur at any time throughout childhood. Diagnosis requires a high index of suspicion and an understanding of the broad clinical manifestations of IEM, but not extensive knowledge of the biochemistry of individual metabolic diseases.

Pathophysiology

Inborn errors of metabolism are single gene defects resulting in abnormalities in synthesis or catabolism of proteins, carbohydrates, or fats. Most are due to a defect in an enzyme or transport protein that results in a block in a metabolic pathway. Effects are due to toxic accumulations of substrates before the block, intermediates from alternative metabolic pathways, and/or defects in energy production and utilization caused by a deficiency of products beyond the block. The diseases that result in toxic accumulations of substances include disorders of protein metabolism (i.e., amino acidopathies, organic acidopathies, urea cycle defects), disorders of carbohydrate metabolism (e.g., carbohydrate intolerance disorders, glycogen storage disorders), and lysosomal storage disorders. Diseases that result in a deficiency of energy production or utilization include defects of carbohydrate metabolism (i.e., gluconeogenesis and glycogenolysis), fatty acid oxidation, and mitochondrial and peroxisomal function.

History

Clues to an inborn error of metabolism can often be obtained by history. Developmental delay, particularly with loss of milestones, suggests the possibility of an inborn error of metabolism. Onset of symptoms with change in diet and unusual dietary preferences, particularly protein or carbohydrate aversion, is concerning. With intercurrent infection, decompensation out of proportion to the illness may occur. Also suggestive is a history of similar findings, or of unexplained neonatal or sudden infant deaths in siblings or maternal male relatives. Parental consanguinity increases the likelihood of autosomal recessively inherited metabolic disorders. Negative family history does not rule out an inborn error of metabolism.

A negative newborn screen does not exclude diagnosis of metabolic disease. Tests performed on neonatal screen vary by state. Most states screen for hypothyroidism, phenylketonuria, and galactosemia. Other metabolic disorders screened for in at least some states include congenital adrenal hyperplasia, biotinidase deficiency, maple syrup urine disease, and homocystinuria. False negatives can result from screening too early, medications, and transfusions.

Clinical Manifestations

Clinical manifestations of inborn errors of metabolism vary from those of acute life-threatening decompensation to subacute progressive degenerative disease. Progression of disease may be unrelenting with rapid life-threatening deterioration over hours, episodic with intermittent decompensations and asymptomatic intervals, or insidious with slow degeneration over decades. Nearly every metabolic disease has several forms that vary in age of onset and clinical severity. Life-threatening diseases tend to become clinically apparent by infancy, while those with intermittent or insidious manifestations tend to appear later. Onset and severity may be exacerbated by environmental factors, such as diet and intercurrent illness. Inborn errors of metabolism can affect any organ system and usually affect multiple organ systems. Physical examination often provides important diagnostic information.

Neonatal

Inborn errors of metabolism should be considered in a neonate who is critically ill. Clinical features of inborn errors of metabolism in the neonatal period are nonspecific. Manifestations may include poor feeding, vomiting, diarrhea, dehydration, temperature instability, tachypnea or apnea, bradycardia, poor perfusion, irritability, involuntary movements or posturing, abnormal tone, seizures, and altered level of consciousness. The same symptoms occur with sepsis, respiratory illness, cardiac disease, gastrointestinal obstruction, renal disease, and central nervous system problems. Presence of these conditions does not rule out the possibility of an inborn error of metabolism. In term infants without risk for sepsis who develop the symptoms of sepsis, metabolic disease may be nearly as common as sepsis. Additionally, certain metabolic diseases, including galactosemia during the newborn period, certain organic acidopathies, and CAH may be associated with an increased risk of sepsis.

Frequently, the most important clue to an inborn error of metabolism in the neonate is a history of deterioration after an initial period of apparent good health ranging from hours to weeks, usually following an uncomplicated pregnancy and delivery in a term infant. For inborn errors of substrate and intermediary metabolism, the timing of symptoms depends on significant accumulation of toxic metabolites following the initiation of feeding. Neonates with inborn errors that result in defects in energy production and utilization usually develop symptoms within the first 24 hours of life and are often symptomatic at birth. These neonates are less likely to have coma as an early manifestation and are more likely to have dysmorphic features, skeletal malformations, cardiopulmonary compromise, organomegaly, and severe generalized hypotonia.

Infant, Young Child (1 Month to 5 Years)

Infants or children with inborn errors of metabolism may develop recurrent episodes of vomiting, ataxia, seizures, lethargy, coma, and/or fulminant (Reye's syndrome-like) hepatoencephalopathy. More subtle findings include dysmorphic or coarse features, skeletal abnormalities, poor feeding, failure to thrive, dilated or hypertrophic cardiomyopathy, hepatomegaly, liver dysfunction, and developmental delay sometimes with loss of milestones, hypotonia, and vision and hearing dysfunction. With routine illnesses, these patients may become more severely symptomatic, develop symptoms more rapidly, or require longer recovery than unaffected children.

Older Child, Adolescent or Adult (Beyond 5 Years)

In the older child, adolescent, or even adult, undiagnosed metabolic disease should be considered in individuals with subtle neurological or psychiatric abnormalities. Many have diagnoses of birth injury or of atypical forms of psychiatric disorders or of medical diseases such as multiple sclerosis, migraines, or stroke. Among the more common findings are mild to profound mental retardation, autism, learning disorders, behavioral disturbances, hallucinations, delirium, aggressiveness, agitation, anxiety, panic attacks, seizures, dizziness, ataxia, exercise intolerance, muscle weakness, and paraparesis. Some manifestations may be intermittent, precipitated by the stress of illness, or progressive, with worsening over time. While most inborn errors diagnosed in this age group are not immediately life-threatening, partial ornithine transcarbamylase deficiency can manifest at this time as a life-threatening metabolic catastrophe. This is seen particularly in adolescent females with a history of protein aversion, abdominal pain, and migraine-like headaches.

Laboratory Tests

For diagnosis of inborn errors of metabolism, initial laboratory evaluation in the acutely ill patient should include a complete blood count to screen for neutropenia, anemia, and thrombocytopenia; serum electrolytes, bicarbonate, and blood gas analysis to detect electrolyte imbalances and evaluate anion gap and acid/base status; BUN and creatinine to evaluate renal function; bilirubin, transaminases, prothrombin time, partial thromboplastin time, and ammonia, as measures of hepatic function; blood glucose and urine pH, glucose, reducing substances, and ketones. In patients with evidence of neuromyopathy, lactate dehydrogenase, aldolase, creatinine kinase, and urine myoglobin should be evaluated.

If a metabolic disease is suspected, plasma should be collected and, based on results of initial studies, evaluated for lactate, pyruvate, albumin, triglycerides, uric acid, amino acids, organic acids, quantitative carnitine, and qualitative carnitines. Urine should be collected for potential analysis of amino acids, organic acids, orotic acid, and/or acylglycine. In selected cases, cerebral spinal fluid, collected at the same time as plasma, should be frozen for possible measurement of lactate, pyruvate, and/or glycine. Laboratory abnormalities can be transient; therefore, normal values do not rule out an inborn error of metabolism. Studies may need to be repeated during other episodes of illness or during provocative testing in a clinical research center.

Specialized tests are required for the diagnosis of many metabolic diseases. These tests include: detection of abnormal metabolites in plasma, urine, or cerebral spinal fluid; histological evaluation of affected tissues such as liver, brain, heart, kidney, and skeletal muscle; and enzyme assay or DNA analysis in leukocytes, erythrocytes, skin fibroblasts, liver, or other tissues.

In the child who has died, it is still important to attempt to diagnose a metabolic disease because of the possibility that presently asymptomatic siblings are affected or that future children will be affected. Plasma, serum, urine, and possibly CSF, skin, and selected organ specimens should be collected and frozen.

A metabolic specialist may be helpful in directing the evaluation of patients with suspected metabolic disease.

Most inborn errors of metabolism can be categorized based on findings of initial laboratory evaluations. Most patients with acute life-threatening presentation of metabolic disease have metabolic acidosis, hyperammonemia, and/or hypoglycemia. These initial findings guide immediate treatment and further evaluation. Exceptions include CAH characterized by hyponatremia and hyperkalemia in a child presenting with apparent sepsis; nonketotic hyperglycinemia, which presents with lethargy, coma, seizures, hypotonia, spasticity, hiccups, apnea, agenesis of the corpus collosum, and an EEG with burst suppression or hypsarrhythmia; and pyridoxine deficiency, which presents with encephalopathy and intractable seizures.

Metabolic Acidosis

Inborn errors of metabolism must be considered in patients with primary metabolic acidosis. Clinical manifestations of acidosis are vomiting and tachypnea. Primary metabolic acidosis is diagnosed by a low pH, low HCO_3, and a compensatory low pCO_2. Measurement of electrolytes and calculation of the anion gap are useful because acute inborn errors of metabolism are generally associated with increased anion gap metabolic acidosis. In any patient with a low serum bicarbonate, particularly out of proportion to the clinical presentation, the anion gap should be determined. An elevated anion gap with a normal chloride suggests excess acid production, usually of lactate, ketone bodies, or other unmeasured organic acids. Lactic acidosis (>2 mM) may be primarily due to a defect in energy metabolism, but far more commonly is secondary to poor perfusion or ischemia. In the absence of poor perfusion, an increased lactate/pyruvate ratio (>25; normal $10–20:1$) suggest certain mitochondrial disorders. In most organic acidopathies, disorders of carbohydrate metabolism, and fatty acid oxidation defects, serum levels of pyruvate are elevated in proportion to lactate. The metabolic diseases in which primary lactic acidosis is a feature include disorders of gluconeogenesis and mitochondrial disorders. Serum ammonia, glucose, urine ketones, and reducing substances should also be evaluated in patients with metabolic acidosis to help direct further metabolic workup.

Hyperammonemia

Hyperammonemia may cause an altered level of consciousness and/or persistent vomiting. Anorexia and irritability are early manifestations of hyperammonemia. Older individuals may report headache, abdominal pain, and fatigue. Progression to vomiting, lethargy, seizures, coma, and death may occur within hours. Ammonia is an intermediary in the catabolism of nitrogen-containing compounds, particularly amino acids. Normally, ammonia is converted in the liver to either urea by the urea cycle or, when production is rapid, to glutamine by glutamine synthetase. Primary respiratory alkalosis (pH > 7.4) with secondary metabolic acidosis may be seen in urea cycle defects and transient tachypnea of the newborn because hyperammonemia directly stimulates the respiratory center, resulting in tachypnea. Proper collection and handling of blood for ammonia determination is critical to prevent falsely elevated values. In patients with hyperammonemia, liver function should be evaluated. Hepatomegaly and mild elevation of transaminases may be seen in many metabolic disorders during acute periods of decompensation. Plasma should be evaluated for amino acids, and urine for ketones, reducing substances, amino acids, organic acids, and orotic acid to diagnose the specific metabolic defect in patients with hyperammonemia. For many disorders, leukocytes, fibroblasts, or liver is required for confirmatory enzyme assay.

Hypoglycemia

A serum glucose of less than 40 mg/dL should be considered abnormally low at all ages. Hypoglycemia is manifested by decreased level of consciousness ranging from lethargy to coma, confusion, irritability, and seizures. Newborns, in addition, may have a high-pitched cry, hypothermia, cyanosis, and poor feeding. In the older child or adult, symptoms may include headache, blurred vision, repeated yawning, diaphoresis, pallor, and nervousness. In patients with hypoglycemia, urine ketones, and reducing substances, acid/base status and ammonia should be measured. Normally, hypoglycemia is associated with significant ketonuria except in neonates who have higher capacity for ketone utilization. Beyond the neonatal period, inappropriately low ketones or absent ketones in the patient with hypoglycemia is always abnormal and suggests a hyperinsulinemic state, a glycogen storage disorder, or fatty acid oxidation defect. Patients with organic acidopathies or mitochondrial disorders may have ketonuria with normal glucose. In neonates, significant ketonuria may be a manifestation of an acutely presenting inborn error of metabolism.

Treatment

Initial treatment of inborn errors of metabolism is aimed at correcting metabolic abnormalities. Even the apparently stable patient with mild symptoms may deteriorate rapidly with progression to death within hours. With appropriate therapy, patients may recover completely without sequelae. As always, airway, breathing, and circulation must be addressed first. Hydration is critical not only to restore intravascular volume but also because urinary excretion is frequently the only way to eliminate toxic metabolites.

Treatment for a potential inborn error of metabolism should be started empirically as soon as the diagnosis is considered. All oral intake should be stopped to prevent the introduction of potentially harmful protein or sugars. Hypoglycemia, if present, should be corrected by intravenous dextrose bolus and followed by continuous administration of dextrose. All patients in whom an inborn error of metabolism cannot be ruled out should be given dextrose at a rate high enough to prevent catabolism (D_{10-15} with electrolytes as needed at a rate of 1 to 1.5 times maintenance). This improves most conditions. For the immediate treatment of acidosis, pH < 7.2, HCO_3 < 14, with CNS compromise, bicarbonate and/or potassium acetate (if hypokalemic) may be administered (as much as 1.0 mEq/kg/h). Rapid correction or overcorrection of acidosis may have paradoxical effects on the central nervous system.

Definitive treatment of inborn errors of metabolism requires removal of the abnormal metabolites by either restricting intake of the offending substrate, promoting renal excretion of toxic metabolites, or, in severe cases, dialysis, preferably hemodialysis. Significant hyperammonemia is life-threatening and must be treated immediately upon diagnosis. To reduce ammonia, sodium phenylacetate (250 mg/kg/d) and sodium benzoate (250 mg/kg/d) can be administered to augment nitrogen excretion. (These medications are currently investigational [Ucyclyd Pharma].) Arginine (210 mg/kg/d) also enhances clearance of ammonia in patients with most urea cycle defects. For ammonia levels >500 μg/dL, hemodialysis should be initiated. If hemodialysis is not readily available, peritoneal dialysis, which is less than 10% as effective as hemodialysis, or double-volume exchange transfusion, which is even less effective, can be performed while arrangements are made to transport the patient to a center where hemodialysis is available, as long as this does not delay the transfer. Two to three days of therapy are usually necessary. L-carnitine may be administered empirically in life-threatening situations associated with primary metabolic acidosis or hyperammonemia (e.g., organic acidopathies). Administration of carnitine to patients with fatty acid oxidation defects is controversial. Pyridoxine should be given to neonates with seizures unresponsive to conventional anticonvulsants.

Summary

Collectively, metabolic diseases are not rare. Clinical manifestations are often nonspecific and a high index of suspicion is therefore essential for diagnosis. A few screening tests are informative for most metabolic diseases. Rapid treatment may not only be lifesaving but often results in full recovery. Treatment for metabolic disease rarely if ever interferes with treatment of nonmetabolic diseases, and therefore should be initiated in all patients in whom an inborn error of metabolism cannot be ruled out.

Selected Readings

Edge J, Ford-Adams M, Dunger D. Causes of death in children with insulin-dependent diabetes 1990–96. *Arch Dis Child* 1999;81:318–323.

Fearon DM, Steele MD. End-tidal carbon dioxide predict the presence and severity of acidosis in children with diabetes. *Acad Emerg Med* 2002;9:1373–1378.

Felner EI, White PC. Improving management of diabetic ketoacidosis in children. *Pediatrics* 2001;108:735–740.

Glaser N, Barnett P, McCaslin I, et al. Risk factors for cerebral edema in children with diabetic ketoacidosis. *N Engl J Med* 2001;344:264–269.

Glaser N, Kuppermann N. The evaluation and management of children with diabetic ketoacidosis in the emergency department. *Pediatr Emerg Care* 2004;20:477–481.

Green S, Rothrock S, Ho J, et al. Failure of adjunctive bicarbonate to improve outcome in severe pediatric diabetic ketoacidosis. *Ann Emerg Med* 1998; 31:41–48.

Hoffman W, Steinhart C, El Gammal T, et al. Cranial CT in children and adolescents with diabetic ketoacidosis. *AJNR Am J Neuroradiol* 1988;9:733–739.

Krane E. Cerebral edema in diabetic ketoacidosis. *J Pediatr* 1989;114:166–168.

Lever E, Jaspan J. Sodium bicarbonate therapy in severe diabetic ketoacidosis. *Am J Med* 1983;75:263–268.

Mallare JT, Cordice CC. Identifying risk factors for the development of diabetic ketoacidosis in new onset type I diabetes mellitus. *Clin Pediatr* 2003;42:591–597.

Morris L, Murphy M, Kitabchi A. Bicarbonate therapy in severe diabetic ketoacidosis. *Ann Intern Med* 1986;105:836–840.

96 Orthopedic Disorders

Mariann M. Manno
Katie M. Hamblett

Limp

The complaint of limp is a clinical challenge in the emergency department (ED). Obtaining an accurate history, identifying the source of limp, the physical examination of an uncooperative young child, and the lack of definitive diagnostic tests often makes this evaluation difficult. The goal of the emergency department evaluation is the identification of emergent conditions, to determine the cause of the limp and arrange for consultation with appropriate subspecialists.

Gait consists of a stance and a swing portion. The stance portion begins when the heel hits the floor and ends when the foot leaves the floor. The swing portion occurs while the leg and foot move forward and the other leg is in the stance portion of the gait cycle. Normally, gait is a smooth and rhythmic process. Children will have a normal gait by three years of age. The stages of the development of a normal gait are described in **Table 96.1**.

Limp is an abnormal gait caused by pain (antalgic gait) resulting in decreased ability to bear weight (shortened stance) on the affected side and is seen with musculoskeletal injuries. Weakness of the hip abductors causes a Trendelenburg gait where the pelvis tilts away from the affected side during the stance phase. This is seen in patients with Legg-Calvé-Perthes disease, slipped capital femoral epiphysis, or a dislocated hip (**Table 96.2**).

Emergency Department Evaluation

History

Age, gender, presence and location of pain, and associated findings such as fever or trauma are important clues in determining the etiology limp. The presence and character of pain is also helpful. Limp in the absence of pain may be the result of a chronic or anatomic anomaly such as leg length discrepancy or hip dysplasia. Fever heightens the possibility of infectious processes such as transient synovitis of the hip, septic arthritis, and osteomyelitis. Fever with weight loss and malaise suggests a rheumatoid or malignant condition. Trauma is the most common cause of limp and is an important consideration even without a history of it.

Physical Examination

Initial examination of infants and toddlers begins with observation of the patient in the parent's lap. Distraction with toys and involvement of the parent may facilitate the examination. Begin with the uninvolved extremity and progress to the area where pain and pathology is expected.

Patients are optimally examined on an exam table. Important elements of the examination include inspection symmetry, resting position, deformity, swelling, and skin lesions. The involved extremity should be examined for focal tenderness, swelling, warmth, range of motion, muscle mass and tone, joint laxity, strength, and neurovascular integrity.

In patients who are able to stand and/or walk, observing the patient's posture and gait during walking and running are critical parts of the evaluation. This should be done without shoes.

Hip pathology is a common cause of limp. Important elements of the hip examination include: *internal rotation* (prone position, knees bent at 90 degrees, swing the foot out laterally), *external rotation* (prone position, knees bent at 90 degrees, swing the foot medially), *log roll* (supine position, legs fully extended, log roll the entire leg medially and laterally), *Faber test* (supine, the ankle placed on top of the opposite knee, downward pressure is applied to the ipsilateral knee), *Trendelenburg test* (assess the level of the hips while standing on one leg), and *psoas sign* (patient on side with affected sided up, hip extended).

The skin should be inspected for lesions seen with conditions associated with joint pain such as Henoch-Schönlein purpura or Lyme disease. The abdomen and genitourinary system must be examined to exclude psoas abscess, appendicitis, testicular torsion, pelvic inflammatory disease, or inguinal hernia.

Table 96.1

Developmental Stages of Gait

Age	Developmental Stage
10–12 months	Cruises while holding onto objects
12–14 months	Walks short distances and stands unassisted
17–21 months	Stands on one foot long enough to walk up steps
2.5–3 years	Balances on one foot for more than one second
3 years	Develops sufficient balance to attain a normal gait

Source: Used with permission from Elsevier, Basel. Buchmann RD, Jaramillo D. Imaging of articular disorders in children. *Radiol Clin North Am* 42:151–168.

Pediatric Orthopedics: Traumatic and Nontraumatic Conditions

Nontraumatic Pediatic Orthopedic Conditions

Toxic Synovitis

Toxic synovitis, also known as transient synovitis, is a self-limited, nonpyogenic inflammatory process of the synovial lining of the hip. It is the most common cause of nontraumatic hip pain in children. The precise etiology of toxic synovitis remains a mystery. Some postulate that it is the sequelae of a viral illness and others have suggested trauma or allergic hypersensitivity. There is a slight male predominance; children typically present at 5 to 10 years of age. A child with toxic synovitis typically presents with acute hip pain, stiffness, and limp or refusal to walk. Patients my also have a low grade fever and malaise. In a small number of cases, estimated to be less than 5%, the disease is bilateral. Children usually protect the affected hip in a flexed, abducted, and externally rotated position. Internal rotation (log rolling the femur) elicits pain.

The diagnosis of toxic synovitis is one of exclusion. The possibility of more serious hip pathology must be eliminated through a careful history, physical examination, and supportive laboratory tests and radiographs. Laboratory evaluation may help differentiate toxic synovitis from septic arthritis. In toxic synovitis, laboratory values are generally normal or may reveal mild elevations in the WBC or ESR, consistent with a nonspecific inflammatory process. Radiographs of the hips in transient synovitis are also usually normal. Ultrasonography is commonly required to exclude the presence of an effusion. Unless the diagnosis of toxic synovitis is certain, the urgent involvement of an orthopedist is important.

Toxic synovitis is a self-limited process that is often managed on an outpatient basis with close follow-up. Treatment consists of symptomatic relief including rest, non-weight bearing, and the use of NSAIDs to reduce the synovial inflammation. Activity may be gradually resumed as the symptoms are resolved with full return to physical activity when the child is pain-free. Toxic synovitis has an excellent prognosis for recovery; up to 75% of children have complete resolution of pain within 2 weeks and 88% resolve within a period of 4 weeks. For most patients, this is an isolated incident; very rarely do relapses occur.

Septic Arthritis

Septic arthritis is a true orthopedic emergency that requires rapid diagnosis and treatment. It is critical that this diagnosis is carefully considered and eliminated in all children who present with hip pain. The distinction between a septic hip and toxic synovitis is a common clinical challenge. Four specific criteria have been identified as predictive of septic arthritis rather than toxic synovitis: (1) severe hip pain and spasm; (2) tenderness on palpation; (3) a temperature greater than 38° C; and (4) an ESR greater than 20 mm/h. Failure to recognize the presence of a septic joint can result in significant morbidity as the articular cartilage is destroyed by this process. Bacterial pathogens account for the acute presentation of septic arthritis, compared to fungal and mycobacterial pathogens that result in a more chronic course. Seventy percent of cases of septic arthritis

Table 96.2

Causes of Limp by Age

	1–3 years	4–10 years	11–16 years
Most common	Fractures	Fractures	Fractures
	Soft tissue injury	Soft tissue injury	Soft tissue injury
	Toxic synovitis	Toxic synovitis	Overuse
		LCP	Osgood-Schlatter
Urgent/emergent	Osteomyelitis	Osteomyelitis	Osteomyelitis
	Septic arthritis	Septic arthritis	Septic arthritis
	Child abuse	Appendicitis	SCFE
	Hip dysplasia	Neoplasm	AVN hip
	Neoplasm	Testicular torsion	Appendicitis
	Testicular torsion	Inguinal hernia	Testicular torsion
	Inguinal hernia	Inguinal hernia	Neoplasm

occur in children less than four years of age, with a peak incidence in the 6-month to 24-month age group. Boys are affected twice as often as girls. Predisposing factors include: preceding viral infection, trauma, immunodeficiency, hemoglobinopathy, hemarthroses from hemophilia, IV drug abuse and intra-articular manipulations. More common in the lower extremities, the knee is most commonly affected followed by the hip.

The involved joint is usually painful with periarticular soft tissue swelling, warmth, and edema. Range of motion, both passive and active, is severely limited due to pain. The clinical presentation varies with the age of the child. Infants tend to present with fever, feeding difficulties, lethargy, refusing to move the affected limb, and pain with diaper changes. Older children may also present with fever, malaise, poor appetite, irritability, with localized symptoms of pain, limp, or refusal to walk. The leg is commonly held in flexion, abduction, and external rotation with pain on passive movement of the joint.

Septic arthritis is thought to occur through different mechanisms: hematogenous spread, direct spread of adjacent osteomyelitis, or direct penetration following trauma. Hematogenous spread across the highly vascular synovial membrane is most common. Lytic enzymes found in infected joint fluid leads to destruction of articular and epiphyseal cartilage. Destruction is caused by proteolytic enzymes and pressure necrosis caused by the accumulation of purulent synovial fluid. Epiphyseal ischemia and infarction may occur, with dislocation, deformity, and destruction of the femoral head. The most common pathogens in children include *Staphylococcus aureus*, *Streptococcus* species, and previously *Haemophilus influenza* type B. Group B beta hemolytic streptococcus and gram-negative rods are seen in infants. *Neisseria gonorrhoeae* can be found in neonates and sexually active adolescents. *Pseudomonas aeruginosa* and *Candida* sp. can be seen in IV drug abusers. *Salmonella* is common in children with sickle cell disease (**Table 96.3**).

Laboratory evaluation and radiographic imaging may support the diagnosis of a septic hip. Laboratory studies helpful in diagnosing septic arthritis include an elevated WBC, erythrocyte sedimentation rate (ESR), C-reactive protein (CRP), and joint fluid evaluation. Blood cultures should be obtained and are positive in about 40% of patients with septic arthritis. The peripheral WBC alone is not a predictor of septic arthritis. The mean WBCs for septic hip and toxic synovitis are similar although some studies suggest that band counts are higher in patients with septic arthritis. The ESR and CRP are also elevated in septic arthritis, and the CRP rises more quickly than the ESR. The CRP is typically elevated at the time of initial presentation and with appropriate therapy will normalize within a week, whereas the ESR often normalizes after several weeks. In one study, a CRP greater than 20 mg/L and a temperature greater than 38°5 C were found to be independent predictors for septic arthritis with a sensitivity of 100% and a specificity of 87%.

Plain radiographs of the hips and ultrasound are useful in establishing the diagnosis of a septic hip. Area postrema (AP) and frog's leg views of the hips may be helpful to exclude other causes of hip pain such as fracture or tumor and may demonstrate a joint effusion with asymmetry of the joint spaces. If the radiographs are normal or equivocal and the clinical suspicion of septic arthritis exists, an ultrasound to demonstrate a joint effusion is warranted. Increased Doppler blood flow suggests infection, but a normal blood flow cannot exclude septic arthritis. If the ultrasound is normal, further imaging should be considered to identify other serious pathology such as osteomyelitis or a psoas abscess.

The definitive diagnosis of septic arthritis is made by examination of joint fluid and orthopedic consultation should occur promptly. The evaluation of joint fluid should include: Gram stain, aerobic and anaerobic cultures, cell count with differential, glucose, and mucin clot. The mucin clot tests for the integrity of hyaluronic acid, which becomes degraded in the presence of bacteria. Synovial fluid of septic arthritis tends to be turbid or grossly purulent with a WBC > 40,000 with a predominance of neutrophils. Synovial glucose may be low with an elevated protein and lactate. A positive joint fluid culture provides the definitive diagnosis of septic arthritis. However, cultures of joint fluid are positive in approximately 50% of patients with septic arthritis.

Empiric antibiotic therapy for septic arthritis is directed against the most likely organisms based on patient age and should begin immediately after joint fluid is obtained. However, if joint aspiration is delayed and a strong clinical suspicion of septic arthritis is present, presumptive treatment with antibiotics should be considered. Treatment may be changed based on the results of blood and joint fluid cultures. Typically, for infants from birth to 2 months, treatment consists of nafcillin and gentamicin; for ages greater than 2 months, treatment consists of nafcillin and ceftriaxone with consideration of vancomycin. Response to therapy can be followed by monitoring clinical improvement, acute phase reactants including ESR and CRP and blood cultures. Morbidity includes leg-length discrepancy, persistent pain, limited range of motion, persistent limp, and aseptic necrosis of the femoral head.

Table 96.3

Pathogens Causing Septic Arthritis

Age	Organism
Birth to 2 months	Group B *Streptococcus*
	Staphylococcus aureus
	Gram-negative rods
2 months to 3 years	*Staphylococcus aureus*
	Streptococcus pneumoniae
	Haemophilus influenzae
3 years to 12 years	*Staphylococcus aureus*
	Streptococcus pneumoniae
	Streptococcus pyogenes
>12 years	*Staphylococcus aureus*
	Staphylococcus aureus
	Neisseria gonorrhoeae

Legg-Calvé-Perthes Disease

Legg-Calvé-Perthes Disease (LCP), also known as avascular necrosis of the proximal femoral epiphysis, is characterized by ischemic necrosis, collapse, and subsequent remodeling of the femoral head. This process occurs most frequently in males between the ages of 4 to 9 years. LCP has a familial predilection in approximately 10% of cases. The majority of cases are unilateral, but in approximately 20% of cases, both hips are affected. LCP has been associated with breech deliveries, later born children, lower socioeconomic groups, older parental age, lower birth weight, attention deficit hyperactivity disorder (ADHD), delayed bone age, and short stature. There is often a link between trauma and the onset of symptoms, but a direct relationship has not been established.

Children with LCP present with the insidious onset of limp, often with pain in the knee or hip, shortened limb, with or without limited range of motion of the hip. The pain is usually related to activity and is relieved by rest. Mild hip pain and limp may have existed for weeks to months before the diagnosis is entertained. The pain tends to be localized to the groin or referred to the anteromedial thigh or knee. LCP should be considered in the differential diagnosis for knee pain. Children with LCP will have a positive Trendelenburg test and may have thigh, calf, and buttock atrophy related to disuse. Limb length discrepancy is associated with advanced disease as the femoral head collapses.

The exact etiology of LCP remains unknown. Some suggest that it is a local manifestation of a transient, generalized disorder of the epiphyseal cartilage. As the growth plate thickens and becomes disorganized, blood vessels are unable to supply the femoral epiphysis and it becomes avascular. Some theories suggest an increase in the viscosity of the blood due to an irregularity within the vascular anastomotic network of the femoral epiphysis causing an infarction. Others suggest that growth hormones alter the vasculature causing infarction and thus necrosis. Symptoms may often become more noticeable after suffering minor trauma.

LCP is an important consideration in the differential diagnosis of limp in the young child. Diagnosis is often made with plain radiographs taken in the AP and frog-leg positions. These films show the extent of epiphyseal involvement and the stage of disease (**FIGURE 96.1**). In the early phase of disease, the joint space may appear widened due to the increased cartilage or joint effusion. The intermediate phase may show granular, fragmented appearance of the femoral epiphysis due to calcification of avascular cartilage, lateralization of ossification center, demineralization cysts, or dense appearance of the femoral head because of new bone formation. As the disease progresses, reossification occurs, normal bone density returns, and the femoral head appears flattened and distorted.

Compared to plain radiographs, CT and MRI provide earlier and more reliable information regarding the extant of femoral head necrosis.

Long-term studies of patients with LCP have identified patient age at presentation and degree of hip joint deformity to be the primary factors predicting outcome. The greater deformity of the femoral head is associated with the worst long term outcome. Most studies conclude that a worse long term prognosis is associated with presentations in children greater than 8-years-old.

Operative versus nonoperative treatment remains controversial. Treatment often is based on age at presentation. For those less than 5-years-old, treatment often consists of observation with anti-inflammatory medications and limited activity. Children in the 5- to 8-year age group are often treated with an abduction brace or osteotomy. Children older than 9 years of age fall into a poorer prognostic category and orthopedic operative treatment are least likely to be successful.

Slipped Capital Femoral Epiphysis

Slipped capital femoral epiphysis (SCFE) is a disorder in which the femoral epiphysis is displaced posteriorly and inferiorly from the metaphysic. It is a Salter-Harris type 1 fracture through the proximal femoral physis and the most common hip disorder in adolescent patients. It occurs more commonly in males, obese children, and African Americans. Typically, children present with SCFE during growth spurts; for males this occurs between the ages of 13 and 15, and for females between the ages of 11 to 13.

Pain and limp are the most common complaints in patients with SCFE. Typically, this pain is unilateral, but slippage occurs bilaterally in approximately 25% of patients. The pain is often referred to the anteromedial thigh or knee. Pain is usually weeks to months in duration, and may acutely worsen after trauma. Those with significant slippage may present with limb shortening.

SCFE is classified in four clinical categories: preslip, acute, acute on chronic, and chronic. An acute slip is the abrupt displacement through the proximal physeal cartilaginous plate in which there was a preexisting epiphyseolysis and usually presents with symptoms of less than 2 weeks' duration. Some describe a mild prodromal period in which there are minor symptoms in the few weeks leading up to the acute slip, considered the preslip. Patients with chronic SCFE have a history of chronic pain for several months to years. Most of them complain of knee or lower thigh pain.

SCFE can also be classified as stable versus unstable classification based on the patient's ability to weight bear. With a stable hip, weight bearing is possible with or without crutches. With an unstable hip, the pain is so severe

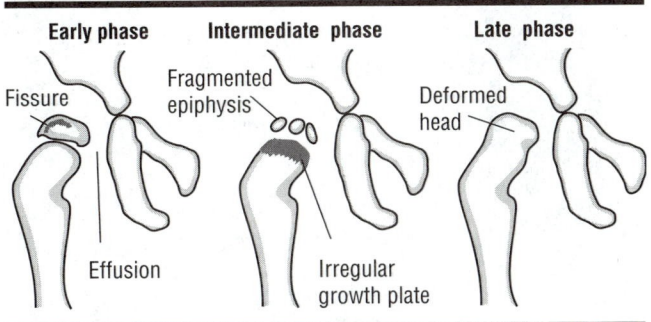

FIGURE 96.1 Radiographic features of Legg-Calvé-Perthes (LCP) disease.

that weight bearing is impossible even with crutches. An unstable SCFE has a poorer prognosis due to the increased risk of avascular necrosis.

SCFE can often be diagnosed by plain radiographs; AP and frog leg lateral views should be obtained. On the AP view, widening of the epiphysis may be seen even if the displacement is difficult to see. The epiphysis is almost always posteriorly displaced and this is best seen on the frog leg view as a decreased height of the epiphysis. The Klein line is a useful diagnostic tool. Klein's line, a line drawn along the superior surface of the femoral neck, should intersect a piece of the epiphysis. The epiphysis is not intersected by Klein's line when slippage of the epiphysis has occurred (**FIGURE 96.2**).

Patients with SCFE should be made non-weight bearing and referred to an orthopedic surgeon. The surgical treatment for SCFE is open reduction with internal fixation to prevent further slippage. Prognosis remains good for the child with stable SCFE. Conservative treatments, such as non-weight bearing or a hip spica cast, have been associated with poorer outcomes. There is an increased risk of degenerative hip arthritis in patients who have has a SCFE, especially those who have avascular necrosis.

Fractures in Children

Physiological and anatomical differences such as growth, bone remodeling potential, elastic bone, open physes, thick periosteum, and smaller anatomic structures distinguish pediatric from adult orthopedic trauma management. Because of structural differences, pediatric fractures tend to occur at lower energies than adult fractures. The pattern of fractures in the pediatric population depends on the age of the child and their stage of development. The physis (growth plate) is a cartilaginous structure that varies in thickness depending on age and location. It is frequently weaker than bone when subjected to torsion, shearing and bending forces. Approximately 10% to 30% of fractures in children involve the physis. The hypertrophic zone of the physis is the most vulnerable portion due to its limited collagenous matrix and the lack of calcification. Ligaments in children are functionally stronger than their bones. Therefore, injuries that would typically produce sprains in adults result in fractures in children. Growth plate disruption and bone avulsion are more common.

Salter-Harris Classification

The Salter-Harris Classification of physeal fractures uses radiographic evidence to determine the type of growth plate fracture, each having specific prognostic and treatment implications. Clinically, Types I to V are commonly used (**FIGURES 96.3** and **96.4**).

Type I injuries account for 5% of physeal injuries and consist of a complete fracture through the hypertrophic and calcified zones of the physis, completely separating the epiphysis from the metaphysis. These factures may be displaced or nondisplaced. A Salter I fracture usually has an excellent prognosis, although with displaced fractures there is the potential for growth arrest. The diagnosis of a nondisplaced Salter I fracture relies on the clinical detection of tenderness over the growth plate since they will appear radiographically normal due to the normally radiolucent physis (**FIGURE 96.5**).

Type II injuries are the most common physeal injury, accounting for 75% or growth plate fractures and consists of disruption through a portion of the growth plate with extension into the metaphysis. Type II fractures consist of a Type I fracture that exits the metaphysis with a metaphyseal spike attached to the epiphyseal fragment on the compression side of the fracture. The appearance of the metaphyseal spike is referred to as the Thurston-Holland fragment. Prognosis is excellent, although complete or partial growth arrest may occur with displaced fractures (**FIGURE 96.6**).

Type III fractures account for 10% of physeal fractures and are transphyseal, exiting the epiphysis causing intraarticular disruption. They often occur in children with a partially closed physis. This type of fracture typically requires reduction and fixation. The prognosis is less favorable than Type I or II fractures as partial growth arrest and angular deformity can be occur.

Type IV fractures also account for 10% of physeal fractures and transverse the metaphysis, physis, and epiphysis with intraarticular disruption. This type of fracture requires reduction and fixation. Once again, partial growth

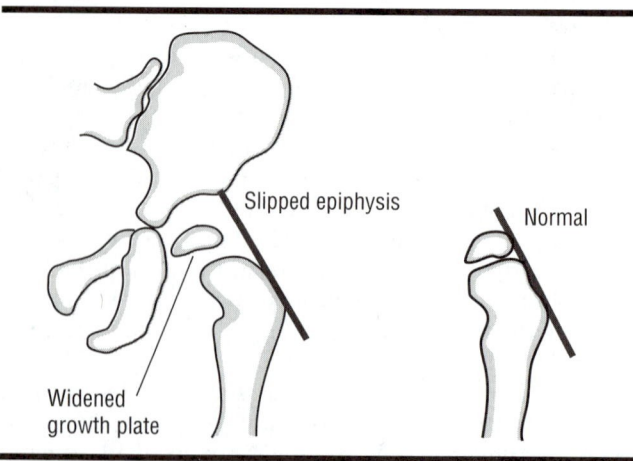

FIGURE 96.2 Klein's line.

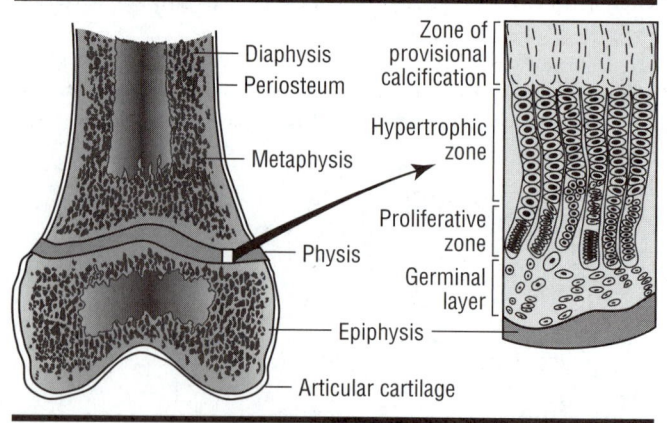

FIGURE 96.3 Diagram of the physis.

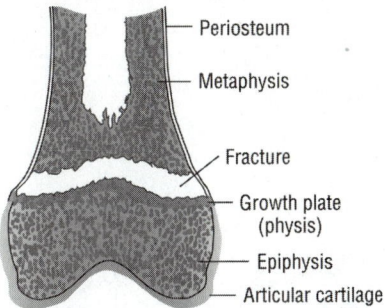
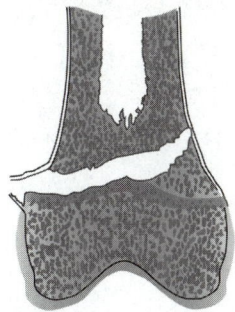

Type I. Complete separation of epiphysis from shaft through calcified (growth zone) of growth plate. No bone actually fractures; periosteum may remain intact. Most common in newborns and young children.

Type II. Most common. Line of separation extends partially across deep layer of growth plate and extends through metaphysis, leaving triangular portion of metaphysis attached to epiphyseal fragment.

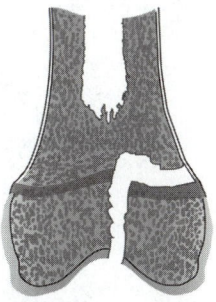
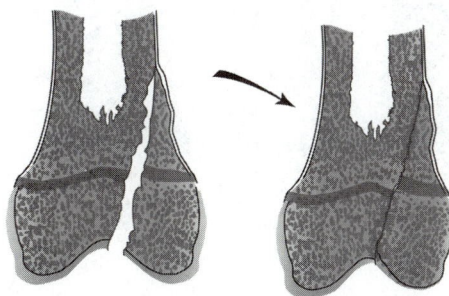

Type III. Uncommon. Intra-articular fracture through epiphysis, across deep zone of growth plate to periphery. Open reduction and fixation often necessary.

Type IV. Fracture line extends from articular surface through epiphysis, growth plate, and metaphysis. If fractured segment not perfectly realigned with openreduction, osseous bridge across growth plate may occur, resulting in partial growth arrest and joint angulation.

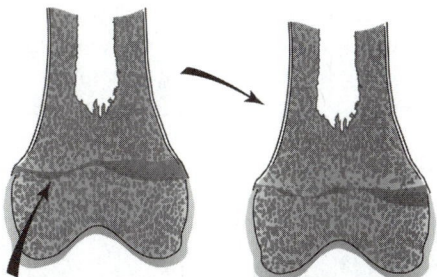
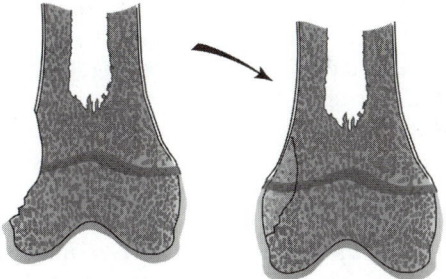

Type V. Severe crushing force transmitted across epiphysis to portion of growth plate by abduction or adduction stress or axial load. Minimal or no displacement makes radiographic duagnosis difficult; growth plate may nevertheless be damaged resulting in partial growth arrest or shortening and angular deformity.

Type VI. Portion of growth plate sheared or cut off. Raw surface heals by forming bone bridge across growth plate, limiting growth on injured side and resulting in angular deformity.

FIGURE 96.4 Salter-Harris Classification of fractures.

arrest and angular deformity are frequent complications (**FIGURE 96.7**).

Salter-Harris Type V accounts for only 1% of physeal fractures and has the highest rate of growth disturbance. This fracture results in a compression or torus fracture involving only the physis. These fractures are often diagnosed retrospectively when a growth disturbance is recognized in a patient with a history of trauma. Type V carries the least favorable prognosis because growth

arrest and partial physeal closure commonly result. Distinction between Type I and Type IV injuries are sometimes not apparent until resulting growth abnormalities occur.

Common Fracture Patterns in Children

Fracture patterns depend upon a child's age and stage of bone development. Nonphyseal fractures are complete and incomplete (**FIGURE 96.8**). Examples of complete fractures

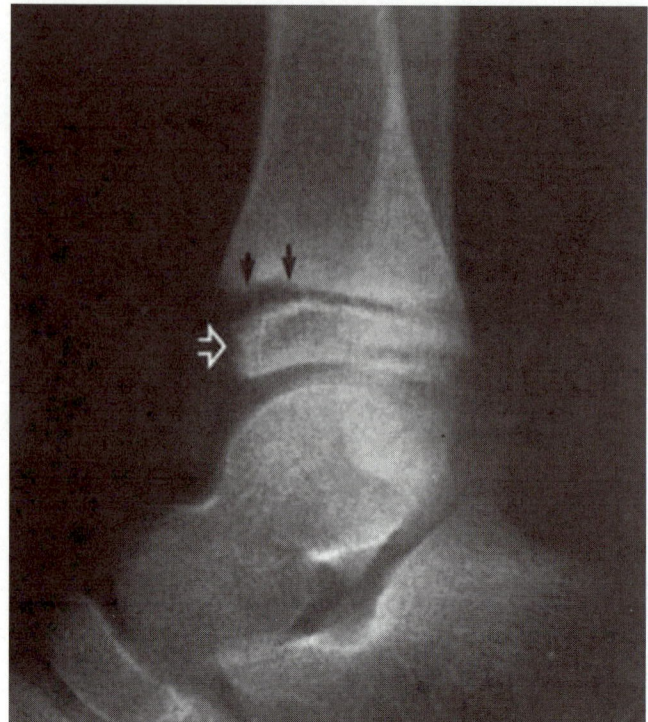

FIGURE 96.5 Radiograph of Salter-Harris type I.

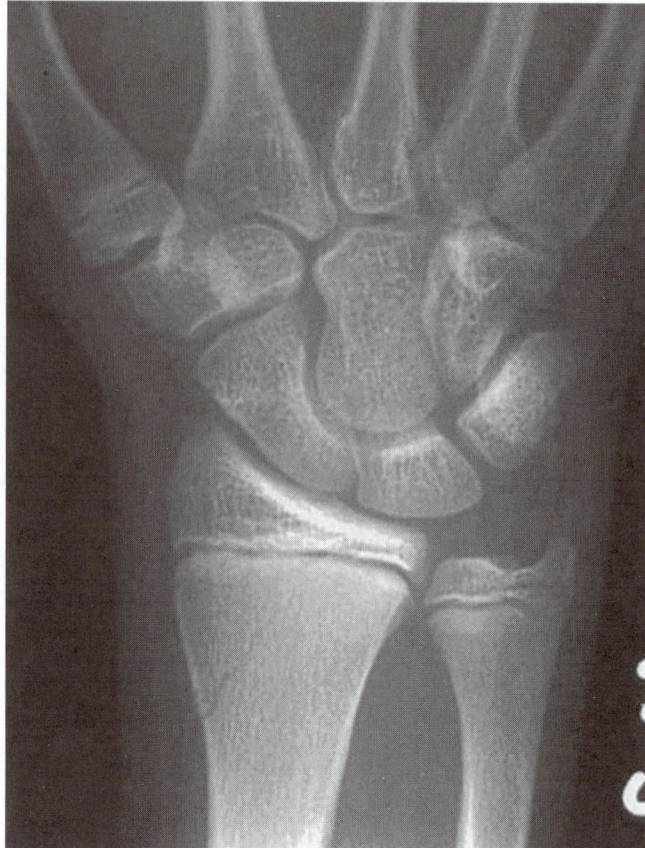

FIGURE 96.6 Radiograph of Salter-Harris type II.

include longitudinal, transverse, oblique, spiral, impacted, and comminuted. Incomplete fractures are common in children because of the flexibility of the developing bones. These fractures include greenstick, torus, and bowing fractures. Greenstick fractures are common in children 6 to 12 year of age and involve only the convex part of the cortex where tension is increased while the concave cortex remains intact. The distal radius is the most common site of a greenstick fracture following a fall on an outstretched hand. Bowing fractures are caused by forces that cause the bone to bend to a point of plastic deformation. It is not always clearly evident on radiographic images and may require comparison views of the unaffected extremity. Torus (meaning "little hill") fractures are buckle type fractures in which the concave cortex buckles while the convex side remains intact. Prognosis for complete recovery is excellent.

Toddler's Fracture

A toddler's fracture is an oblique spiral nondisplaced fractures of the distal tibia. This fracture results from low energy torsional forces typically associated with simple falls while one foot is planted and twists. These often occur with an insignificant or absent history of trauma, and the child will present with leg pain, limp or refusal to walk. Typically, toddler's fractures occur in the 1 to 3 year-old age group. Examination may reveal only mild swelling of the leg, point tenderness, or a slight increase in warmth over the affected area. AP and lateral radiographs may reveal a spiral or oblique fracture the distal third of the tibia. Oblique radiographs may be helpful in detecting the fracture. Some toddler's fractures may not be visible on initial

radiographs. If radiographs appear normal, but a fracture is clinically suspected, the child should be immobilized. Radiographs obtained in follow-up may show evidence of a healing fracture at about 10 days. Significant tibial fractures in nonambulating children should raise suspicion for abuse.

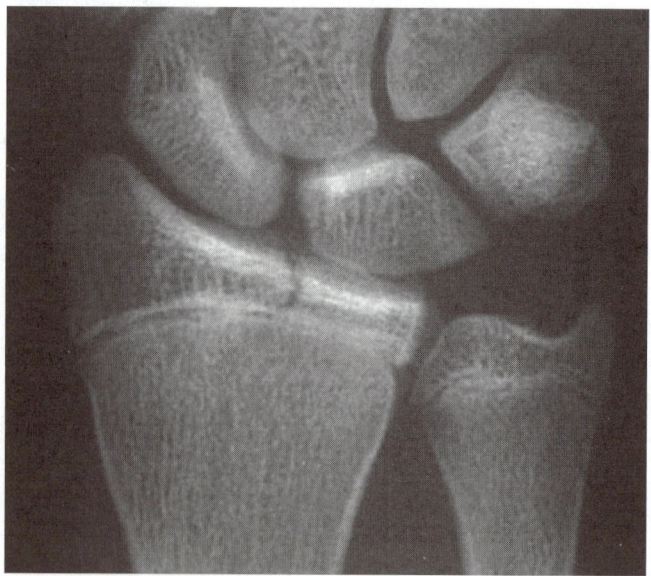

FIGURE 96.7 Radiograph of Salter-Harris type III.

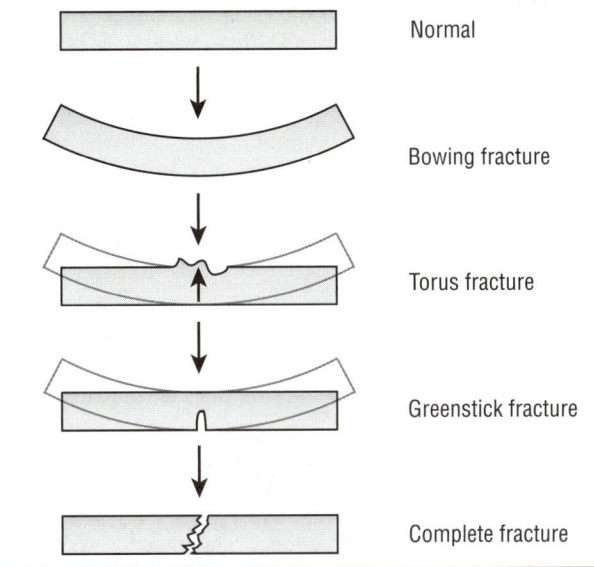

FIGURE 96.8 Complete and incomplete types of fractures.

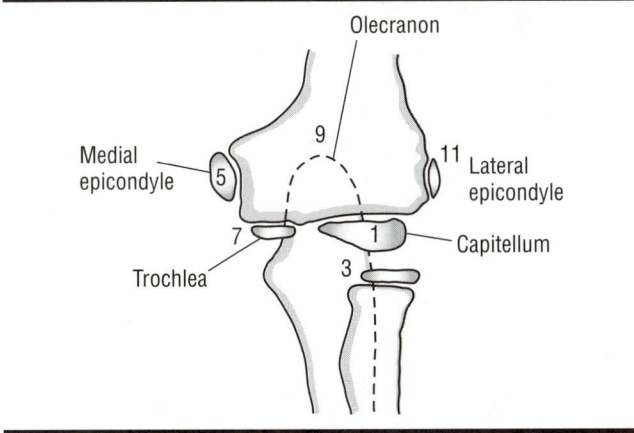

FIGURE 96.9 Ossification centers of the elbow.

Supracondylar Fractures

Upper extremity fractures are very common in young children who fall on outstretched hands. Supracondylar fractures of the elbow are the most common upper extremity fracture in children in the first decade of life and account for approximately 60% of elbow fractures. This FOOSH (fall on out stretched hand) mechanism with the elbow in extension transmits forces onto the distal humerus. In the extended position, the elbow extensor muscles are unopposed, resulting in hyperextension. The supracondyle fractures with force exerted by the olecranon.

Physical exam varies depending on the extent of displacement of the fracture fragment ranging from mild swelling and tenderness to a gross deformity. The brachial artery may become compromised with posterolateral displacement. Radial pulse and capillary refill should always be assessed. Compartment syndrome can result from the increased swelling of the fractured elbow. Nerve impairment is associated with approximately 5% to 10% of supracondylar fractures, although most are neuropraxias requiring no treatment. Median nerve is the most commonly affected nerve accounting for most nerve injuries, followed by injuries to the radial and then ulnar nerve.

The ossification centers of the pediatric elbow make radiographic evaluation difficult. Knowing the sequence of ossification centers will help make radiographic determination of a fracture possible. A recent fracture fragment will have an edge of irregularity and is not well corticated. These ossification centers have well corticated margins that are round and smooth, becoming fused as the growth plates close (**Table 96.4** and **FIGURE 96.9**).

The identification of non-displaced fractures can be difficult. An organized approach that looks at boney landmarks on a true lateral x-ray is helpful. On the lateral radiograph, there should be an hourglass configuration of the distal humerus, often referred to as a figure-of-eight. The appearance of an elbow joint effusion is characterized by displacement of the anterior and posterior humeral fat pads and is highly suggestive of an intracapsular fracture. In a child with no other radiographic evidence of trauma, a positive posterior fat pad sign is predictive of an occult fracture in approximately 75% of children with elbow injuries. Also on the lateral radiograph, the anterior humeral line, a line drawn along the anterior surface the distal humeral shaft, should intersect the middle third of the capitellum. With a fracture this line is abnormal. In an extension type injury the anterior humeral line will pass anterior to the middle third of the capitellum. To determine the articulation between the radial head and capitellum, a line drawn through the long axis of the radius should intersect the capitellum on all views (**FIGURE 96.10**).

The Gartland Classification classifies the degrees of displacement of supracondylar fractures into types I, II, and III. Type I fractures have minimal or no displacement. Nondisplaced fractures may be occult, relying on the presence of a abnormal fat pads (any posterior fat pad, elevated anterior fat pad or "sail" sign) for detection. These fractures are typically treated with a posterior splint or a long arm cast for approximately 2 to 3 weeks. Type II fractures are angulated with a partially intact posterior cortex but without complete displacement these require closed reduc-

Table 96.4	
Ossification Centers of the Elbow: CRITOE	
Ossification Center	**Approximate Age of Appearance**
Capitellum	1 year
Radial head	3 years
Internal (medial) epicondyle	5 years
Trochlea	7 years
Olecranon	9 years
External (lateral) epicondyle	11 years

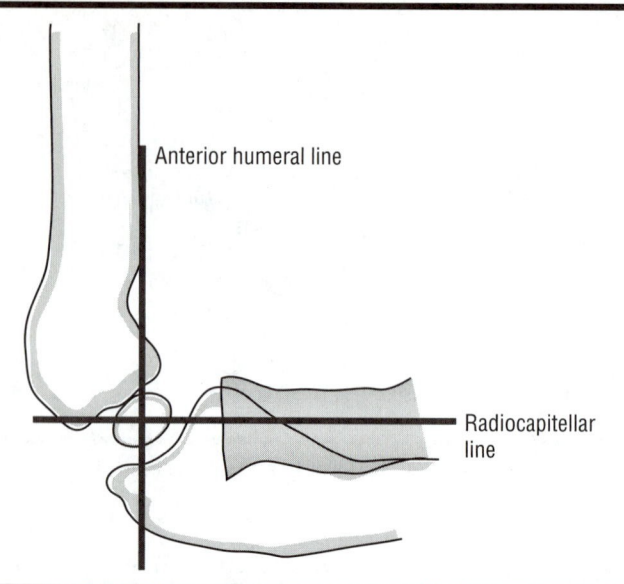

Anterior humeral line

Radiocapitellar line

FIGURE 96.10 Radiologic lines in pediatric elbow injuries.

tion and casting. Completely displaced, type III fractures have the worst prognosis and the most complications. Approximately 50% of completely displaced fractures involve a neurovascular injury or compartment syndrome. Type III fractures require closed reduction, pinning, and or internal fixation.

Selected Readings

Barkin RM, Barkin SZ, Barkin AZ. The limping child. *J Emerg Med* 1999;18:331–339.

Buchmann RD, Jaramillo D. Imaging of articular disorders in children. *Radiol Clin North Am* 2004;42:151–168.

Clinical Pediatric Emergency Medicine, vol 3, no 2. June 2002.

Herring JA, Kim HT, Browne R. Legg-Calve-Perthes disease: part I: classification of radiographs with use of the modified lateral pillar and Stullberg classifications. *J Bone Joint Surg American Volume* 2004;86-A:2103–2120.

Herring JA, Kim HT, Browne R. Legg-Calve-Perthes disease: part II: prospective multicenter study of the effect of treatment on outcome. *J Bone Joint Surg* 2004;86-A:2121–2134.

Kim MK, Karpas A. The limping child. *Clin Ped Emerg Med* 2002;3:129–137.

Kocher MS, Mandiga R, Zurakowski D, et al. Validation of a clinical prediction rule for the differentiation between septic arthritis and transient synovitis of the hip in children. *J Bone Joint Surg* 2004;86-A:1629–1635.

Koval KJ, Zuckerman JD. *Handbook of Fractures,* 2nd ed. Philadelphia: Lippincott Williams & Wilkins, 2002:314–316.

Lawrence LL. The limping child. *Emerg Med Clin North Am* 16:911–929, 1998.

Molczan KA. MSN, RN-CS, CRNP, CPN, CEN Triaging pediatric orthopedic injuries. *J Emerg Nurs* 2001;27:297–300.

Musgrave DS, Mendelson SA. Pediatric orthopedic trauma: principles in management. *Crit Care Med* 2002;30(Suppl):S431–S443.

Myers MT, Thompson GH. Imaging the child with a limp. *Pediatr Clin North Am* 1997;44:637–658.

Overly F, Steele DW. Common pediatric fractures and dislocations.*Clin Ped Emerg Med* 2002;3:106–117.

Perron AD, Miller MD, Brady WJ, et al. Orthopedic pitfalls in the ED: pediatric growth plate injuries. *Am J Emerg Med* 2002;20:50–51.

Perron AD, Miller MD, Brady WJ, et al. Orthopedic pitfalls in the ED: slipped capital femoral epiphysis. *Am J Emerg Med* 2002;20:484–487.

Salzbach R. Pediatric septic arthritis. AORN J 1999;70:986,988,991–992,994–998, 1000,1002–1004,1006,1009–1010.

Thompson JC. *Netter's Concise Atlas of Orthopaedic Anatomy.* Teterboro, NJ: ICON Learning Systems, 2004:288.

Weinstein SL. Natural history and treatment outcomes of childhood hip disorders. *Clin Orthop Related Res* 1997;344:227–242.

Weissleder R, et al. *Primer of Diagnostic Imaging,* 2nd ed. St. Louis: Mosby, 1997: 780–787.

White N, Sty J. Radiological evaluation and classification of pediatric fractures.*Clin Ped Emerg Med* 2002;3:94–105.

Wu J, Perron AD, Miller MD, et al. Orthopedic pitfalls in the ED: pediatric supracondylar humerus fractures. *Am J Emerg Med* 2002;2:544–550.

Pediatric Procedural Sedation and Analgesia

Baruch Krauss

The field of pediatric procedural sedation and analgesia (PSA) has undergone a rapid evolution in the last 10 years and is now recognized as a central element in for the practice of emergency medicine. Emergency procedures that once required patients to be taken to the operating room are now done on a routine basis in the ED. This section presents a practical approach to pediatric PSA (including definitions, general principles, factors used to determine when to use sedation, presedation preparation, and titration principles), and discusses individual sedation agents, management of complications encountered during PSA, and discharge guidelines.

Presedation Decision Making

The first set of pediatric PSA guidelines were issued in 1985, and they were revised in 1992 by the American Academy of Pediatrics (AAP) in response to the increasing use of general anesthetic agents in the ambulatory setting. Three levels of sedation were differentiated: conscious sedation, deep sedation, and general anesthesia. The AAP guidelines were developed for use in a wide range of ambulatory settings including dental practices, subspecialty suites, imaging centers, and office-based practice. These guidelines did not distinguish categories for analgesia (relief of pain without sedation), anxiolysis (relief of anxiety and apprehension without sedation), or ketamine dissociative sedation, and included preprocedural fasting guidelines that were not applicable to the ED. In 1991, in accordance with the Joint Commission on Accreditation of Healthcare Organizations mandates, hospital-wide and department-specific guidelines for the use of PSA were developed. In 1998, ACEP published evidence-based guidelines for ED PSA. Practitioners using pediatric PSA should be familiar with these guidelines.

General Principles

A risk-benefit analysis should be performed prior to every sedation. The benefits of controlling pain and anxiety must be carefully weighed against the risks associated with the use of sedative agents. Sedation use is a decision that must be made on a case-by-case basis by the treating physician. A complex set of variables determines the need for sedation, especially in children.

Age

Age is an important factor in determining the need for sedation. Most children over the age of 5 years will not require sedation for laceration repair. Age is also an important consideration in selecting the appropriate sedative, as some agents have age limitations.

Location of Injury

The location of an injury can be a significant factor in determining the need for sedation. For example, facial lacerations require the patient's cooperation. Lacerations of the nose, oral cavity (mouth, lips, tongue), and periorbital areas (eyelid, eyebrow, infraorbital) often require a high degree of control of agitation for safety.

Time of Day

Time of day is a critical factor in assessing the need for and extent of pharmacological intervention. An active, alert, toddler seen at midday who has just napped generally requires larger drug doses than the child seen at 11 PM, who is tired and sleepy. Young children (<5 years old) can be extremely difficult and uncooperative when they are tired and/or hungry. Many are kept NPO from the time they register in the ED, in anticipation of PSA. Creative solutions to these circumstances are numerous. Children who are tired and hungry may actually need minimal pharmacological intervention or may be managed by nonpharmacological means. In cases of children presenting late at night with facial lacerations, application of topical anesthesia in a quiet, dark, room for 20 to 30 minutes can result in a painless laceration repair while the child sleeps.

Need for Agitation Control

The degree of agitation control required for a procedure determines, to a large extent, whether sedation is needed and the level of sedation required. Selected procedures (fracture and dislocation reductions, facial laceration repair) require a higher degree of agitation control than other procedures. Procedures can be further divided into those

Table 97.1

Drug Dosing Recommendations for Pediatric Procedural Sedation & Analgesia*

Drug	Clinical Effects	Indications	Dose†	Onset (minutes)	Duration (minutes)	Comments
Sedative/Hypnotics						
Chloral Hydrate (Noctec)	Sedation, motion control, anxiolysis. No analgesia. Not reversible.	Diagnostic imaging (age < 3 years)	PO: 25–100 mg/kg, after 30 min may repeat 25–50 mg/kg. Maximum total dose: 2 g or 100 mg/kg (whichever is less). Single use only in neonates.	PO: 15–30	PO: 60–120	Effects unreliable if age > 3 years. Avoid in patients with significant cardiac, hepatic, renal disease. Rectal absorption erratic. May produce paradoxical excitement. Since drugs cannot be titrated with the oral route, monitor closely for oversedation.
Midazolam‡ (Versed)	Sedation, motion control, anxiolysis. No analgesia. Reversible with Flumazenil.	Procedures requiring sedation and/or anxiolysis	IV (0.5–5 yrs): Initial 0.05–0.1 mg/kg, then titrated to max 0.6 mg/kg IV (6–12 yrs): Initial 0.025–0.05 mg/kg, then titrated to max 0.4 mg/kg IM: 0.1–0.15 mg/kg PO: 0.5–0.75 mg/kg IN: 0.2–0.5 mg/kg PR: 0.25–0.5 mg/kg	IV: 2–3 IM: 10–20 PO: 15–30 IN: 10–15 PR: 10–30	IV: 45–60 IM: 60–120 PO: 60–90 IN: 60 PR: 60–90	Reduce dose when used in combination with opioids. May produce paradoxical excitement. Since drugs cannot be titrated with the oral/rectal/intranasal routes, monitor closely for oversedation.
Pentobarbital (Nembutal)	Sedation, motion control, anxiolysis. No analgesia. Not reversible.	Diagnostic imaging	IV: 1–6 mg/kg, titrated in increments of 1–2 mg/kg to desired effect IM: 2–6 mg/kg, max 100 mg PO/PR (<4 yrs): 3–6 mg/kg, max 100 mg PO/PR (>4 yrs): 1.5–3 mg/kg, max 100 mg	IV: 3–5 IM: 10–15 PO/PR: 15–60	IV: 15–45 IM: 60–120 PO/PR: 60–240	May produce paradoxical excitement. Avoid in patients with porphyria. Since drugs cannot be titrated with the oral/rectal routes, monitor closely for oversedation.
Methohexital (Brevital)	Sedation, motion control, anxiolysis. No analgesia. Not reversible.	Diagnostic imaging	PR: 25 mg/kg	PR: 10–15	PR: 60	Avoid in patients with temporal lobe epilepsy or porphyria. Since drugs cannot be titrated with the rectal route, monitor closely for oversedation.
Thiopental (Pentothal)	Sedation, motion control, anxiolysis. No analgesia. Not reversible.	Diagnostic imaging	PR: 25 mg/kg	PR: 10–15	PR: 60–120	Avoid in patients with porphyria. Since drugs cannot be titrated with the rectal route, monitor closely for oversedation.

Analgesic§						
Fentanyl (Sublimaze)	Analgesia. Reversible with Naloxone	Procedures of moderate to severe pain	IV: 1.0 µg/kg/dose, may repeat q3 min, titrate to effect	IV: 3–5	IV: 30–60	Reduce dosing when combined with midazolam
Ketamine						
Ketamine (Ketalar)	Analgesia, dissociation, amnesia, motion control. Not reversible.	Procedures of moderate to severe pain or requiring immobilization	IV: 1–1.5 mg/kg slowly over 1–2 min, may repeat ½ dose after 10 min IM: 4–5 mg/kg, may repeat after 10 min	IV: 1 IM: 3–5	IV: dissociation 15; recovery 60 IM: dissociation 15–30; recovery 90–150	Multiple contraindications.¶ Risk of unpleasant hallucinations/dreams if age > 15 years (rare if younger) which may be blunted with midazolam. Hypersalivation can be minimized with concurrent atropine 0.01 mg/kg IM/IV (min 0.1 mg, max 0.5 mg).
Nitrous Oxide						
Nitrous oxide (Nitronox)	Anxiolysis, analgesia, sedation, amnesia (all mild).	Procedures requiring mild analgesia or sedation (age > 4 years)	Preset mixture with minimum 40% O_2 self-administered by demand valve mask (requires cooperative child)	<5	<5 min following discontinuation	Requires specialized apparatus and gas scavenger capability. Several contraindications.‖ Synergistic effect with recent opioids or sedative/hypnotics—use with caution in this setting.
Reversa; Agents (Antagonists)						
Naloxone (Narcan)	Opioid reversal	Opioid toxicity	IV/IM: 0.1 mg/kg/dose up to max of 2 mg/dose, may repeat q2 min prn	IV: 2	IV: 20–40 IM: 60–90	If shorter acting than the reversed drug, serial doses may be required.
Flumazenil (Romazicon)	Benzodiazepine reversal	Benzodiazepine toxicity	IV: 0.02 mg/kg/dose, may repeat q1 min up to 1 mg	IV: 1–2	IV: 30–60	If shorter acting than the reversed drug, serial doses may be required. Do not use in patients receiving chronic benzodiazepines, cyclosporine, isoniazid, lithium, propoxyphene, theophylline, tricyclic antidepressants.

*Intravenous agents should be carefully titrated to the desired effect. Alterations in dosing may be indicated based upon the clinical situation and the practitioner's experience with these agents. Individual dosages may vary when used in combination with other agents, especially when benzodiazepines are combined with opioids.

†IV = intravenous; IM = intramuscular; PO = oral; IN = intranasal; PR = rectal

‡Midazolam is preferred to other benzodiazepines (e.g., diazepam, lorazepam) due to its shorter duration of action and multiple routes of administration.

§Fentanyl is preferred to other opioids (e.g., morphine, meperidine) due to its faster onset, shorter recovery, and lack of histamine release. There is insufficient published procedural sedation and analgesia experience with intranasal sufentanil to recommend its use.

¶Generally accepted contraindications to ketamine: Age < 3 months; history of airway instability, tracheal surgery, or tracheal stenosis; procedures involving stimulation of the posterior pharynx; active pulmonary infection or disease (including active upper respiratory infection); cardiovascular disease including angina, heart failure, or hypertension; significant head injury, CNS masses, hydrocephalus; glaucoma or acute globe injury; psychosis; porphyria; thyroid disorder or thyroid medication.

‖Generally accepted contraindications to nitrous oxide: Pregnancy (patient or personnel); preexisting nausea/vomiting; trapped gas pockets (e.g., middle ear infection, pneumothorax, bowel obstruction).

requiring sedation alone (laceration repair) and those requiring a combination of sedation and systemic analgesia (orthopedic procedures, burn debridement, incision and drainage of large abscess, bone marrow aspiration).

Previous Experience

Children's previous experience in hospitals can greatly affect their response to the current situation. Direct experience is not the only way to create anxious, frightened, and uncooperative patients. Images from television, stories from members of their peer group, or having watched a sibling be forcefully immobilized for a laceration repair can leave a powerful and lasting impression. Eliciting from the parents a history of a previous difficult experience in the ED can be a decisive factor in determining the degree of sedation required. Children who have had a recent (within 6 to 12 months) unpleasant laceration repair, and who now present with a new laceration, may well require moderate conscious sedation as opposed to simple anxiolysis (either pharmacological or nonpharmacological) had there been no previous trauma.

Behavior at Routine Primary Care Visits

Inquiring how children normally behave at their routine primary care visits may yield important information in deciding whether to use sedation. Children who cry but hold still when vaccinated may be more compliant than children who are described by their parents as being afraid of doctors or wild during visits to the primary care physician.

Level of Anxiety

The level of anxiety of both the child and accompanying adult(s) must be accurately assessed. Patients in the ED manifest anxiety in many different ways, and emergency physicians must be facile at recognizing expressions of anxiety in children. A child with a facial laceration quietly sitting on the stretcher during the initial examination will not necessarily be a calm and cooperative patient during laceration repair.

Physicians, when confronted by an extremely anxious child, must ascertain what the parents have told the child about the upcoming procedure. Many parents, in the hope of lessening their child's anxiety, tell the child that he/she will be getting a small needle and the procedure will only hurt for a minute. This type of preparation often results in an increase in anxiety, especially if the child has had a previous procedure in the ED.

It is also important to assess the parent's level of anxiety as this will determine the degree to which they can assist during the procedure. An extremely anxious parent or a parent who must take care of other siblings during the procedure will find it difficult to assist in distracting the patient or otherwise helping him/her cope with the procedure.

Parental and Primary Care Physician Input

Input from parents and referring primary care physicians is an important component in the decision-making process for sedation. They may be firmly for or against sedation. Some parents need to be convinced that a procedure can be done safely without sedation, while others need to be convinced of the need for sedation.

Last Meal

In the ED, every patient is assumed to have a full stomach and appropriate precautions are taken. The strict NPO guidelines for patients going to the operating room for general anesthesia are modified to accommodate the requirements of the ED PSA. On the other hand, if a teenager with a displaced fracture of the forearm who needs a reduction just finished a large meal at McDonald's, postponing the sedation and providing analgesia in the meantime may be the most prudent course.

Previous Medications

An accurate history about previous medications is especially important when patients are referred from other hospitals. Physicians at the accepting facility should determine whether patients received any medications prior to or during transport, as this will affect the type of sedation that can be given. Patients may also have received sedation prior to transfer and still be sedated on arrival, necessitating an adjustment in the sedation regimen to be used.

Presedation Preparation

Once the decision to use sedation has been made, meticulous presedation preparations must be taken. The room in which the sedation takes place must be equipped with monitoring equipment (pulse oximetry, capnography, blood pressure, and ECG monitoring), oxygen, properly sized face masks and ventilatory bags, suction apparatus with Yankauer tip, and reversal agents (flumazenil, naloxone). Physicians must make every effort to personally check all equipment before beginning a sedation. If the patient has an IV, it should be tested to make sure that it is free-flowing prior to infusion of any medications. Drug doses should be double checked prior to administration. Intubation and resuscitation equipment should be readily at hand. Physicians should know the doses of reversal agents as well as laryngoscope blade and endotracheal tube size for patients receiving IV sedation. Communicating this information to the nurse prior to the procedure allows for optimal management should a problem with the airway develop.

A full presedation evaluation should be performed, including relevant history and physical examination with emphasis on drug allergies, current medications, and significant family and past medical history, and a thorough airway evaluation including an assessment of the relative degree of difficulty required to intubate the patient.

Titration Principles

Understanding pharmacological titration principles is essential to providing safe and effective sedation. Physicians must be familiar with the pharmacokinetics, dosing, administration, and potential complications of the agents that they use (**Table 97.1**). Onset times (the time from injection to observed effect) of sedation agents must be understood especially when using drugs in combination. Failure to appreciate the time required to observe a drug effect can lead to stacking of drug doses, resulting in oversedation. Caution must also be taken when administering drugs in combination, most notably opioids and benzodiazepines, as the risks of hypoxemia and apnea are significantly greater than when either drug is given alone.

Emergency physicians must avoid being pressured by consultants to cut corners or rush a sedation. Incorporating into the presedation preparation a discussion with the consultant about the sedation plan and the length of time required to safely prepare and sedate the patient can avoid the risks associated with a hurried sedation.

It is particularly important for pediatric emergency physicians to know the adult doses of the sedation agents that they use. Understanding that the initial dose of midazolam in a 100-kg football player is far less than 0.1 mg/kg is essential to avoid unexpected mishaps in drug dosing. Appreciating the maximum doses of individual sedation agents, especially oral and intranasal agents, is also necessary for safe sedation.

Management of Adverse Effects

Although ED PSA has proven to be safe and effective when used properly, adverse effects do infrequently occur and can be life-threatening. Physicians should familiarize themselves with the sedation agents they will be using and the adverse effects associated with these drugs. Thinking through all adverse scenarios that could potentially occur with a particular drug and formulating a plan for each pre-

pares the physician to act quickly and decisively if and when they occur.

Discharge Instructions

When the procedure is completed the nurse and physician should assess the patient's readiness for discharge. All EDs using pediatric PSA should have written discharge criteria for patients receiving sedation and a mechanism for documenting recovery. Sedation discharge scoring should include vital signs with oxygen saturation, level of consciousness, and level of age-appropriate motor activity. Written sedation discharge instructions, with special emphasis on postsedation diet, sleep, and activity restrictions, should be reviewed with the patient and their family. Pediatric patients, especially young children, must be closely supervised by an adult in the postsedation period after discharge from the ED.

Selected Readings

Agrawal D, Manzi S, Krauss B. NPO status and adverse events in children undergoing procedural sedation and analgesia in a pediatric emergency department. *Ann Emerg Med* 2003;42:636–646.

Garcia Pena BM, Krauss B. Complications of procedural sedation and analgesia in a pediatric emergency department. *Ann Emerg Med* 1999;34:483–491.

Green SM, Krauss B. Pulmonary aspiration risk during ED procedural sedation—an examination of the role of fasting and sedation depth. *Acad Emerg Med* 2002; 9:35–42.

Green SM, Krauss B. Procedural sedation terminology: moving beyond "conscious sedation." [Editorial] *Ann Emerg Med* 2002;39:433–435.

Krauss B. Management of acute pain and anxiety in children undergoing procedures in the emergency department. *Pediatr Emerg Care* 2001;17:115–125.

Krauss B, Brustowicz R, eds. *Pediatric Procedural Sedation and Analgesia*. Philadelphia: Lippincott Williams & Wilkins, 1999.

Krauss B, Green SM. Procedural sedation and analgesia in children. *N Engl J Med* 2000;342:948–956.

Krauss B, Shannon MW, Damian FJ, Fleisher GR. *Guidelines for Pediatric Sedation 1995*. Irving, TX: American College of Emergency Physicians. (2nd edition published in 1998).

98 Child Maltreatment

Christine Barron

Scope of the Problem

Child maltreatment is a recognized national problem that impacts our entire society, and clinicians that work with children face this reality on a regular basis. The clinician's ability to correctly identify abusive and nonabusive injuries can have life-long impact on children and their families.

National statistics reveal that an estimated 3 million reports are made to child welfare system for concerns of child maltreatment annually, with nearly 1 million children identified to be victims of at least one form of child maltreatment during child welfare agencies' investigations. The rate of victimization for 2003 was 12.4 victims per 1,000 children. Among the child victims in 2003, 60.9% are from neglect, 18.9% physical abuse, 9.9% sexual abuse, 4.9% emotional or psychological abuse, and 2.3% medical neglect. In addition, it is not unusual for an individual child to suffer from more than one form of child maltreatment.[1] An estimated 1,500 child fatalities occur yearly, which is equivalent to 4 children dying each day as a result of child abuse and neglect. The majority of these fatalities occur in children younger than 4 years of age.

Physical Abuse

Emergency medicine clinicians are often faced with cases of potential child maltreatment. Although the interaction with any one child is brief in comparison to the time a child interacts with others such as primary care physicians, day care providers, and teachers, the correct identification of child physical abuse during that emergency department evaluation has tremendous potential impact on the safety and well-being of that child. Missed abuse may result in continued and possibly escalating abuse for the child victim, while misdiagnosing abuse could result in a child being removed from a home environment unnecessarily.

Mandatory reporting laws require clinicians to report when they have a reasonable suspicion of child abuse; therefore clinicians are not required to make a definitive diagnosis of child abuse prior to reporting. Clinicians are responsible for evaluating and treating child victims, and are not responsible for the identification of the person(s) responsible for injuring a child.

Definition

Physical abuse is present when any child younger than 18 years of age has experienced an injury as a result of having been hit with a hand or other object, or having been kicked, shaken, thrown, burned, stabbed, or choked by a parent or parent-surrogate.[2]

Etiology

Many risk factors have been identified for child physical abuse (**Table 98.1**). However, these risk factors are general and child abuse is not confined to only families with identified risk factors. Therefore, all evaluations for possible physical abuse should be completed in a uniform manner and the diagnosis of child maltreatment should not be dismissed due to lack of identified risk factors.

Components of Possible Physical Abuse Evaluations

Medical evaluations for possible physical abuse contain the same core components necessary in all other medical evaluations along with a few additional components:

Core Components
- History
- Past medical history
- Review of systems
- Developmental history
- Family history
- Social history
- Physical examination
- Complementary studies and laboratory data as necessary

Additional components
- Interviewing patient
- Mechanism of injury

Utilizing these components will ensure a uniform approach to all cases, and improve a clinician's ability to identify accidental injuries and abuse.

History

As with all medical conditions, history is the key to making a diagnosis of physical abuse. A detailed history should be

Table 98.1
Risk Factors for Child Maltreatment
Child Characteristics
Premature birth, multiple births
Multiple siblings
Developmental delay, chronic illness
Acute illness
Excessive crying in children
Difficult temperament
Caregiver Characteristics
History of abuse
Lack of appropriate parenting models
Unrealistic expectations
Mental illness
Substance abuse
Domestic violence
Family stressors
Poverty
Limited support system
Isolation
Young parent(s)
Single parent

obtained from caregivers separately in a nonjudgmental manner, and should include direct quotes when appropriate. A special criterion to obtaining histories of potential child abuse is identifying additional information from anyone who may have witnessed the incident, including verbal children. Since the perception of changing histories may identify concerns, it is imperative that open-ended questions are asked, allowing the caregiver to provide details, particularly noting if the history is provided as fact, or a theory that the caregiver is offering. Changing history in an attempt to conceal an inflicted injury is of significant concern. When obtaining a history the clinician needs to address any delay in seeking medical care including the caregivers' explanation for the delay.

Past Medical History

Identify if the child has past injuries, prior concerns for abuse, or identification of medical condition that may be mistaken for physical abuse (**Table 98.2**).

Review of Systems

Ascertain when the child was last noted to have normal behaviors and interactions including normal sleeping, eating, and activity level.

Developmental History

The developmental abilities of each child need to be identified to determine if the child is able to engage in the activity that is reportedly resulted in the injury. Concern for possible child maltreatment would be raised if the history provided were not in accordance with the child's developmental abilities. The developmental abilities of the child should be considered in the context of the type of injury and the mechanism required that would result in the injury.

For instance, a spiral femur fracture is not uncommon in mobile children due to the mechanism, which includes a force that includes a torsion being applied to the shaft of long bones. This mechanism is often seen in accidental injuries of older mobile children with the developmental abilities to engage in activities such as running and bicycling. However, this same injury in a nonmobile infant would be of great concern without an appropriate accidental history that included the necessary mechanism. Therefore a 4-year-old with a spiral femur fracture sustained from a fall would not raise concerns while a 4-month-old who sustains a spiral femur fracture would raise significant concern that required further evaluation and investigation for possible physical abuse.

Family History

Identify any family history of medical conditions that may be mistaken for physical abuse, including blood dyscrasias and metabolic bone disorders.

Social History

Identify all adults who reside in the home as well as any other caregivers. Identify other children that are in the same environment who may be at risk for abuse as well. Address any prior involvement with child welfare system and any concerns for domestic violence.

Physical Examination

Focal examination limited to the site of obvious injury is inadequate as additional injuries may be missed. All examinations should include a complete skin inspection. In addition, obtaining and plotting growth parameters is essential.

Interviewing the Patient

The patient should be interviewed when the clinician has identified suspicious injury. It is important to ask *only* open-ended questions such as, "How did it happen?" If the child has other clearly accidental injuries, it can be helpful to ask the patient the same open-ended question about the accidental injuries first, and then ask about the suspicious injuries.

Mechanism of Injuries

Understanding the mechanisms required for injuries will aid the clinician in determining if the history provided is plausible explanation for the injuries sustained. Skilled clinicians will often immediately recognize when the history is incongruent with the injury.

Physical Examination Findings

Physical examination findings that should be noted for possible physical abuse:
- Traction alopecia
- Subconjunctival hemorrhages or petechiae
- Pinnae injuries

Table 98.2

Hasbro Children's Hospital HIV Post-exposure Prophylaxis (PEP) After Sexual Assault

Recommend HIV PEP	1. Child *able* to give a disclosure of mucosal contact and the offender is known to be HIV or at higher* risk 2. Child *unable* to give a clear disclosure of mucosal contact but has acute evidence of sexual penetration** and the potential offender is known to be HIV infected or at higher risk* 3. Child *unable* to give a clear disclosure of mucosal contact but has acute evidence of sexual penetration,** and the potential offender is unknown	If patient $>$ 40 kg Combivir If patient $<$ 40 kg Retrovir (50 mg/mL) 180 mg/m^2/dose PO bid × 28d Maximum 300 mg/dose PO bid and Epivir (10 mg/mL) 4 mg/kg/dose PO bid × 28d Maximum 150 mg/dose bid $$m^2 = \frac{height\ (cm) \times weight\ (kg)}{3600}$$ If the assailant is known to be HIV infected and his/her drug regimen is known, consult a pediatric HIV specialist to tailor the patient's prophylaxis, and to possibly add a third medication
Consider PEP	Child *unable* to give a clear disclosure of mucosal contact, does *not* have evidence of sexual penetration,*** but the parent/guardian has significant concern around circumstances of the alleged assault	If patient $>$ 40 kg Combivir If patient $<$ 40 kg Retrovir (50 mg/mL) 180 mg/m^2/dose PO bid × 28d Maximum 300 mg/dose PO bid and Epivir (10 mg/mL) 4 mg/kg/dose PO bid × 28d Maximum 150 mg/dose bid

*History of incarceration, intravenous drug use, multiple sexual partners or prostitution, and/or male-male sex.
**Some signs of acute sexual penetration include vaginal bleeding, rectal bleeding, hymenal transection without evidence of healing, hymenal bruising, peri-anal bruising, frenulum tear, etc.
***In a child who cannot make a clear disclosure of sexual assault, the absence of physical findings does not exclude the possibility of penetration or the exchange of body fluids. For example, oral penetration will most often not leave mucosal damage. For the purpose of determining exposure to HIV and other STDs, prepubertal children will most likely have physical findings.

- Frenulum injuries
- Dental injuries or dental impression on inner aspect of mucosal membrane
- Pattern bruising
- Symmetric injuries
- Circumferential injuries
- Healing injuries that were not previously brought to medical attention
- Specific cutaneous injuries

Cutaneous injuries are the most frequent manifestation of physical abuse and clinicians must distinguish between accidental and nonaccidental trauma. As children become mobile their rate of cutaneous injuries increases.[3] Accidental and nonaccidental injuries will vary from minor to more severe. Reviewing components including child's developmental abilities, location and pattern of injury will aid the clinician in determining if the injury is consistent with physical abuse or not.

Bruises

Expect bruises and other soft tissue injuries of mobile children on areas of skin that overly bony prominence.

Concerns of possible physical abuse are identified for children who are nonmobile, injuries in less frequently injured area (ears, face, neck, chest, buttocks, and genitals), bilateral injuries, and pattern injuries (silhouette of objects or linear imprint from slap). Although concerns may be raised for these categories, it does not automatically indicate abuse. As stated above, the components of the history need to be obtained and linked to the physical exam findings to determine if there are indications of physical abuse. All injuries concerning for possible physical abuse must be documented (**Table 98.3**). Documentation of injuries should include measurement, physical description accompanied by a drawing, or photographs. Bruises cannot be aged based on their color; however, acute injuries may be observed to change during the evaluation, such as increased swelling and erythema, which should be documented to denote an acute injury. Document acute injuries as well as healed and/or faded injuries to establish a minimum of two separate incidents of trauma.

Bruises that are patterned marks due to an implement should be described and photographed. Photograph the implement if available as well.

Table 98.3

Photographic Documentation of Suspicious Injuries

- Describe injuries
- Describe any changes during examination
- Photograph with measurement tool
- If camera is not available complete drawings with size, color, and patterns
- Photograph implement if available at time of examination

Bites

Human bites are vastly different from animal bites because of the mechanism of infliction and resulting skin injuries. Human bites result in arched bruises, while animal bites result in puncturing and tearing of the tissue. Bites may be self-inflicted or due to another child or an adult. Children with dentition can bite themselves in areas reachable by their own mouth. Differentiating between child and adult bites requires measuring the intercanine distance, that is, the distance across the mouth between the third tooth on each side. A distance less than 3.0 cm corresponds to a young child with primary teeth, while a distance greater than 3.0 cm corresponds to an adult or an older child with permanent teeth. Bite marks should be photographed, measured, and may be swabbed with sterile water to collect genetic markers (ABO Group). If additional identification of a human bite mark is needed, a forensic dentist can be consulted.

Burns

The patterns of burned skin and spared skin are important in determining accidental from nonaccidental burn injuries. Contact burns and hot liquid burns are the most frequent causes.

Additional history elements that should be obtained:
- Time of exposure to the hot element or fluid.
- Temperature of the hot element or fluid.
- What was the child wearing at the time of the incident, as clothing may change the appearance of a burn, or in the case of a diaper it can be protective.
- Was there any delay in seeking medical care?

On physical examination determine if this is a burn; consider other possible etiologies in the differential diagnosis such as photophytodermatitis, infectious processes (for example impetigo, epidermolysis bullosa), fixed drug reactions, and hypersensitivity reactions.

A pattern burn mark could occur accidentally with a brief time of exposure if the object is very hot, while a lower temperature object would have to be held against the skin for a longer period of time to result in a pattern burn mark. Inflicted cigarette burns are well-circumscribed with an ulcerated center. Accidental cigarette burns are often oblong in shape with uniform depth and no ulcerated center.

Abdominal Trauma

Significant intra-abdominal injuries can occur without bruising or injuries noted on external abdominal wall examination. Blunt force trauma is transmitted to the internal organs and may result in duodenal, liver, spleen, pancreatic, adrenal, and renal injuries. Additional studies should be completed when abdominal trauma is suspected including:
- Urinalysis
- Liver function tests
- Amylase
- Lipase
- Abdominal ultrasound
- Abdominal CT

Head Injury Abusive Head Trauma

Head injury abusive head trauma (AHT), also known as shaken baby syndrome (SBS), is the most common cause of morbidity and mortality in physically abused infants. Presenting symptoms occur along a diverse continuum ranging from decreased responsiveness, irritability, and lethargy to convulsions, unresponsiveness, and death. The classic findings include: subdural hemorrhages, retinal hemorrhage, and fractures of long bones or ribs.[4–7]

Although there may be no external signs of trauma, it is important to remember that the majority of fatal AHT cases will have no external signs and, therefore, maintaining AHT within the differential diagnosis of infants who present to the emergency department is necessary.

Head CT is the imaging modality to identify acute intracranial injuries, and a head MRI should be completed approximately 5 days later. Head MRI is also recommended if the patient has no neurologic changes but has been identified to have other inflicted injuries (**Table 98.4**).

Table 98.4

Radiological Testing

Type	Purpose
Head CT	Utilized as initial imaging study for possible acute intracranial trauma.
MRI	Utilized as a second imaging study for possible acute intracranial trauma; completed 3–5 days after the initial head CT. MRI may also be utilized for children with nonacute abusive injuries and normal neurologic findings. MRI can identify deep structure injuries and aid in determining the age of intracranial hemorrhages.
SS	Utilized to identify occult fractures. Images are completed of the entire skeleton including American College of Radiology described technique.
Bone scintigraphy	May be used as an adjunct to skeletal survey but has lower specificity and often requires sedation.

Funduscopic examination needs to be completed for possible retinal hemorrhages.

Fractures

Accidental and nonaccidental fractures commonly occur in children. Both accidental and nonaccidental fractures may occur without any changes of the soft tissue overlying the fracture area.

Skeletal surveys should be completed according to the American College of Radiology Standards (**Table 98.5**).

Fractures considered high specificity for physical abuse include classic metaphyseal lesions, posterior rib fractures, scapular fractures, spinous process fractures, and sternal fractures. Fractures that are considered moderate specificity for abuse include, multiple fractures, fractures of different ages, vertebral body fractures, digital fractures, and complex skull fractures. Fractures that have low specificity for abuse include: subperiosteal new bone formation, clavicular fractures, long bone shaft fracture, linear skull fractures, and supracondylar fractures.[8]

Hospitalization

American Academy of Pediatrics (AAP) recommends that evaluations for possible child maltreatment must be completed while children are in a safe environment and, therefore, hospitalization of children during the evaluation and treatment should be viewed as medically necessary (**Table 98.6**).[9]

Munchausen's Syndrome by Proxy

Concerns may originate during an emergency department evaluation due to recognition of multiple evaluations, false history, and presentation of false or induced symptomatology. The diagnosis of this form of medical abuse will require a multidisciplinary team approach and careful record review that will not occur during the emergency department evaluation.

Neglect

Neglect accounts for the majority of child maltreatment, and yet its diagnosis is complicated due to lack of universal definitions and various presentations. Any concerns for neglect, including identified unmet basic needs, su-

Table 98.6

Laboratory Data

Physical Exam Finding	Laboratory Tests
Bruises	Complete blood count
	Physical therapy
	Partial thrombosplastin time
	von Willebrand factor
Fractures	Calcium
	Magnesium
	Phosphorus
	Alkaline phosphatase
	Vitamin D
	Metabolic studies (if clinically indicated)
	Skin biopsy (if clinically indicated)
Intracranial Injuries	Physical therapy
	Partial thrombospondin time
	Metabolic studies (if clinically indicated)

pervisional neglect, and dental neglect, should be documented and reported.

Treatment

Reporting

Although individual states have various definitions for mandated reporters, all states have mandatory reporting laws and all clinicians are mandated reporters. Mandatory reporters should familiarize themselves with their particular state statues to ensure they understand each state's reporting requirements, as often both a verbal and written report will be required.

When concerns for child physical abuse are identified, in addition to reporting to the state's child welfare system, it is important to identify if siblings or other children may be within the same environment and therefore potential victims that need to be evaluated and their safety ensured.

Consultation

Referral or consultation of programs that specialize in evaluations for suspected child maltreatment should be made when such a program is available. It is important for clinicians to remember that referral does not absolve them of their continued legal responsibility to report suspected child abuse and neglect. In addition, additional community resources will be valuable for the patients and their families.

References

1. U.S. Department of Health & Human Services, Children's Bureau. *Child Maltreatment 2003: Reports From the States to the National Child Abuse and Neglect Data System.* Washington, DC: U.S. Government Printing Office, 2005.
2. *The APSAC Handbook on Child Maltreatment*, ed 2. London: Sage Publications, 2002.

Table 98.5

Indications for Skeletal Survey

- Children < 2 years of age with suspicious bruises, burns, fracture, or intracranial injury.
- Children between 2 and 5 years of age; completed only if indicated, such as nonverbal or limited mobility due to other etiologies.
- If acute injuries are noted at the time of the initial skeletal survey, a repeat skeletal survey in 2 weeks is recommended.

3. Sugar N, Taylor J, et al. Bruises in infants and toddlers: those who don't cruise rarely bruise. *Arch Pediatr Adolesc Med* 1999;153:399–403.
4. Levitt CJ, Smith WL, Alexander RC. Abusive head trauma. In: Reece RM, ed. *Child Abuse: Medical Diagnosis and Management*. Philadelphia, PA: Lea & Febiger, 1994:1–22.
5. Billmire ME, Meyers PA. Serious head injury in infants: accident or abuse? *Pediatrics* 1985;75:340–342.
6. Hadley MD, Sonntag VKH, et al. The infant whiplash-shake injury syndrome: a clinical and pathological study. *Neurosurg* 1989;24:536–540.
7. Jenny C, Hymel K, et al. Analysis of missed cases of abusive head trauma, *JAMA* 1999;281:7.
8. Kleinman P. *Diagnostic Imaging of Child Abuse*, ed 2. St. Louis: Mosby, 1998.
9. American Academy of Pediatrics. Committee on Hospital Care and Committee on Child Abuse and Neglect. Medical necessity for hospitalization of the abused and neglected child. *Pediatrics* 1998;101:715–716.

Psychobehavioral Disorders

Patrick Smallwood
Heidi S. Vermette
Ralph J. Seymour

Introduction

With an estimated four million children and eight million adults in the United States suffering from serious and debilitating mental illness, there is little doubt that psychiatric disorders are prevalent in the general population. As in all areas of health care, however, access to treatment for these disorders is subject to the law of supply and demand; while the demand for psychiatric services continues to increase, access to these services has been sharply reduced by managed health care companies and budget cuts to federal, state, and local agencies that offer psychiatric services. This combination of restricted access and limited supply is further complicated by psychosocial variables common to patients with psychiatric illnesses, including being unemployed, having no insurance, lacking primary care services, and inadequately attending to their primary mental and comorbid medical illnesses until a crisis occurs. As a result, psychiatric patients are increasingly utilizing the emergency room for all facets of care, making it necessary that emergency physicians become more familiar with the presentations and treatments of psychiatric disorders. This chapter begins with a brief overview of the *Diagnostic and Statistical Manual* (DSM), followed by discussions of crisis theory, emergent presentations of psychiatric illness, acute exacerbations of chronic psychiatric illness, and the medico-legal aspects of mental illness.

The DSM

Historically, the classification of mental disorders arose from the need to collect statistical data about the frequency of mental illness in the general population. In the United States, such an attempt occurred during the 1840 census, with mentally ill persons being pigeonholed into one category: "idiocy/insanity." By the time of the 1880 census, the classification system had expanded to include seven categories: "mania, monomania, dipsomania, melancholia, paresis, dementia, epilepsy." No further improvements were made until 1952, at which time the American Psychiatric Association published a variant of the *International Classification of Diseases* (ICD-6) that was geared toward mental health professionals. That manual, known as the *Diagnostic and Statistical Manual: Mental Disorders* (DSM-I), was the first official classification system to provide useful and uniform descriptions of mental illness, thereby permitting key advances in both research and treatment of psychiatric disorders. Since its inception, the DSM-I has undergone five revisions, the most recent being the *Diagnostic and Statistical Manual of Mental Disorders, Fourth Edition, Text Revision* (DSM-IV-TR), the current official classification system for mental disorders in the world. The purpose of the DSM-IV-TR is to establish clear definitions of mental disorders in order to provide consistent diagnoses among and across professions as well as to act as guidelines for clinical practice, treatment planning, and future research. It utilizes a multiaxial system comprised of five information domains for reporting all relevant psychiatric, medical, psychosocial, and functional issues affecting an individual patient. These domains, or *axes,* are as follows:

Axis I:	Clinical disorders/other conditions that may be the focus of clinical attention
Axis II:	Personality disorder and mental retardation
Axis III:	General medical conditions
Axis IV:	Psychosocial and environmental problems
Axis V:	Global assessment of function

For the purpose of this chapter, all disorders and conditions are in agreement with DSM-IV-TR diagnostic criteria, unless otherwise specified.

Crisis Intervention

Patrick Smallwood

Crisis is any event or situation that impairs a person's ability to cope. It is often unexpected, quickly overwhelms one's coping skills, and disrupts emotional homeostasis. Should the crisis be greater than an individual can manage, he or she may present to an emergency room requesting assistance with its management and resolution. Emergency physicians have little difficulty in managing a crisis when based solely on the medical emergency that precipitated the visit. Often, however, an individual presents to the emergency department due to a crisis based entirely on psychosocial or psychiatric etiologies. In those situations, most emergency departments provide assistance through emergency mental health services (EMHS), programs that vary from a staff of a few social workers to a 24-hour comprehensive multidisciplinary team comprised of emergency psychiatrists, psychiatric nurses, crisis intervention specialists, and counseling social workers. The mission of EMHS is to provide those experiencing crisis rapid assessment and stabilization in a safe and caring environment that preserves their dignity. This is accomplished through a process known as *crisis intervention*. By understanding crisis intervention, emergency physicians are able to become valuable members of an EMHS team. Before discussing crisis intervention, however, it will be necessary to understand crisis in the context of crisis theory.

Modern crisis theory views crisis as a multi-step process that evolves gradually or instantaneously. The key elements leading to a crisis include an *initial stressor,* a *precipitating event*, and *individual factors*. An *initial stressor* is any anticipated or unanticipated event that places psychological strain on an individual's emotional homeostasis, and as such, is situationally and individually based; what is a stressor for one person may not be for another. Anticipated stressors are common and often planned for, such as *normal developmental phases* (e.g., childhood, adolescence, early adulthood) and *transitional points* (e.g., graduation, marriage, promotions). While placing some load on emotional homeostasis, these types of stressors are often insufficient to overwhelm a person's coping mechanisms. Unanticipated stressors, however, are the ones that most rapidly overwhelm the individual's coping mechanisms and can often bring him or her into the emergency room in crisis. These stressors can be divided into five major categories: (1) loss, real or perceived (e.g.,

death of a loved one, termination of a relationship); (2) gain, real or perceived (e.g., unplanned pregnancy, unwanted house guests); (3) individual trauma (e.g., assault, rape, car accident); (4) community disaster (e.g., natural disasters, stock market collapse, war); (5) chronic illness with associated medication noncompliance or self-medication (e.g., a patient with schizophrenia who is noncomplaint with neuroleptics and is abusing alcohol). Once the initial stressor occurs, a *precipitating event,* an environmental element that poses a barrier for successful maintenance of homeostasis, establishes the acuity. Examples of precipitating events include poverty, lack of transportation, inadequate housing, and limited access to health care. After experiencing an initial stressor and associated precipitating events, an individual begins using available coping skills in a less predictable and mature fashion. If successful coping skills are discovered, the situation stabilizes without progression to crisis. However, if *individual factors* such as limited psychosocial supports, ineffective coping skill, and a distorted perception of the outcome are encountered, a full-blown crisis ensues. At this point, the individual presents to the emergency room requesting intervention.

Crisis intervention is neither a band-aid for a current problem nor a substitute for a complete psychiatric evaluation. Rather, its major goals are to help the person in crisis stabilize the current situation, regain emotional homeostasis to a level prior to the crisis event, and reduce the potential long-term harmful effects that the situation may have on his or her life. The first step toward accomplishing these goals is the *crisis interview,* an active process involving the person in crisis and a mental health specialist. This interview is conducted in such a way as to establish rapport, gain the person's perspective, and obtain a rapid but thorough history that helps to identify the key elements leading to the present crisis. Once completed, the next step is the *negotiated problem*, an agreement between the mental health specialist and the person in crisis as to what is the nature of the problem. This step is crucial for successful crisis stabilization, as a lack of agreement may lead to an ineffective or unaccepted intervention, causing further prolongation and worsening of the crisis. Once the problem is successfully negotiated, the final step is the *negotiated intervention*, which involves connecting the patient to the necessary resource in the community to maintain stabilization and facilitate continued growth and change. To be successful, this intervention should be targeted and simple, as the more elaborate and detailed it is, the less likely the individual is to follow through. The most common negotiated interventions include: (1) inpatient psychiatric hospitalization (voluntary/involuntary); (2) outpatient psychiatric referrals (crisis stabilization units, outpatient mental health clinics, support groups); (3) substance dependence/abuse referrals (detoxification and rehabilitation programs, support groups); (4) family and parenting referrals (prenatal, general health, parenting resources, social services); (5) emergency shelter. Once selecting, offering, and accepting the appropriate intervention, emotional homeostasis often returns to pre-crisis level, and the person begins the early stages of healing.

Selected Reading

Hyman SE, Tesar GE (eds): *Manual of Psychiatric Emergencies*, 3rd ed. Boston, New York, Toronto, London: Little, Brown and Company, 1994.

Psychotic Disorders

Patrick Smallwood

Psychosis refers to a state of cognition in which the ability to accurately evaluate and measure one's perceptions and thoughts against external reality is grossly impaired. Common presentations include *delusions* (fixed false beliefs that are incongruent with the person's cultural background), *hallucinations* (false sensory perceptions not associated with actual external stimuli), *thought disorders* (disturbances in the content, form, or organization of expressed thought), and *disorganized* or *bizarre behaviors*. Like fever, psychosis is a nonspecific symptom seen in a whole host of medical and primary psychiatric conditions, and as such, has an underlying etiology that must be appropriately evaluated before initiation of definitive treatment. The following section is devoted primarily to the emergency presentation, diagnosis, and management of psychiatric and medical conditions encountered in the ED in which psychosis is the presenting symptom. Because schizophrenia is the most common primary psychotic disorder encountered in the ED, it will be the focus of discussion, followed by a brief review of other primary and secondary psychotic disorders.

Schizophrenia

Schizophrenia is a chronic, disabling mental illness that requires a thorough medical and psychiatric evaluation to ensure proper diagnosis and treatment. To assist in this process, the DSM-IV-TR has outlined specific criteria that must be met in order to confirm the diagnosis. These criteria include the presence of *positive* or *negative symptoms* that occur most of the time during a one month period, persist for at least six months, cause marked social and occupational dysfunction, and are not the result of other primary psychotic, mood, medical, or substance-related disorders. Positive symptoms are those symptoms that are either an excess or distortion of normal cognitive functions, and include delusions (e.g., paranoia, thought insertion, thought withdrawal, religiosity, control), hallucinations (e.g., auditory, visual, tactile), disorganized thought and speech (e.g., tangential, looseness of association, incoherence), and disorganized behaviors (e.g., inappropriate dress, public masturbation, catatonic posturing). Negative

symptoms are those symptoms that are a diminution of normal cognitive functions, and include *affective flattening* (restriction in the range and intensity of emotional expression), *alogia* (restriction in the fluency and production of thought and speech), and *avolition* (reduction in the initiation of goal-directed behavior). In contrast to positive symptoms, negative symptoms are associated with greater morbidity.

The DSM-IV-TR divides schizophrenia into five subtypes, based on the predominant symptomatology at the time of evaluation. Of the five, only the paranoid, disorganized, and catatonic subtypes have clinical relevance in the ED. Patients with *paranoid schizophrenia* present with either prominent delusions or frequent auditory hallucinations. These delusions are often persecutory or grandiose in nature, and auditory hallucinations are often congruent with organized delusional themes. The patient with *disorganized schizophrenia* displays grossly disorganized speech, behavior, or inappropriate affect. Delusions and hallucinations are often lacking, but when present, are not well organized. Finally, patient with *catatonic schizophrenia* exhibits gross psychomotor disturbances that may include *catalepsy* (waxy flexibility), stupor, motoric immobility, *catatonic excitement* (excessive nonpurposeful motor activity), *negativism* (motiveless resistance to all instructions for movement), posturing, *echolalia* (senseless repetition of words spoken by others), or *echopraxia* (repetitive imitation of movements made by others). Of the three subtypes, catatonic schizophrenia has the greatest medical morbidity, as patients exhibiting catatonic excitement may suffer self-injury, and patients exhibiting catatonic stupor may suffer from dehydration, malnutrition, hyperpyrexia, and rhabdomyolysis.

Schizophrenia is a global health problem, affecting approximately 1% of the general population. In the United States, this translates to over 2 million people, with a total cost for direct care, medication, and social issues exceeding twenty billion dollars annually, making it one of this country's most serious public health issues. Men and women are equally affected, yet the age of onset differs significantly: 18 to 25 years of age for men and 26 to 45 for women. The reason for this difference is poorly understood. With respect to age, over 80% of all cases have symptom onset prior to the age of 40, which is an important point to remember when differentiating a primary from a secondary psychotic disorder. Stress is known to have an impact the age of onset, as 44% of all cases diagnosed in college students occur during the first semester, and there is an eightfold increase in first-break psychotic episodes during the first few months of military service. Substance abuse is a significant problem in this patient population, with over 50% of patients suffering from co-morbid substance use. Sadly, this illness is not without morbidity, as 20% to 40% of these individuals will make at least one suicide, and 10% to 13% will succeed. The risk factors for patients who complete suicide include: being male, under 45 years of age, unemployed, current depressive symptoms, and recent discharge from the hospital.

The exact etiology of schizophrenia is unknown, but a growing body of scientific evidence suggests that it is an organic brain disease with complex genetic and environmental interactions. Heritability studies demonstrate a strong genetic component to this disorder, as the risk of developing schizophrenia is 15% if a dizygotic twin is affected, and 45% to 50% if a monozygotic twin is affected. The lack of 100% concordance rate between monozygotic twins, however, supports the idea that environmental factors also play a crucial role. These proposed environmental factors include: perinatal hypoxia, poor nutrition, seasonality of birth, and influenza infection. On a structural level, neuroimaging consistently shows reduced volumes of gray and white matter, enlarged third and lateral ventricles, and cortical sulci widening in patients suffering from schizophrenia. Functional imaging demonstrates hypoperfusion in the dorsolateral prefrontal cortex, which may explain several of the cognitive deficits seen in this patient population.

The prognosis for schizophrenia is poor. Approximately 50% of patients will maintain a moderate level of functioning with occasional psychotic episodes, while up to 30% will experience a chronic declining course ending in long-term institutionalization. Surprisingly, up to 10% recover completely, but the basis for this is currently unknown. The best prognostic indicators include acute onset, later age of onset, early treatment, compliance, good insight, good premorbid adjustment, being female, and having no family history of schizophrenia. The worst prognostic indicators include early age of onset, lower education, greater brain abnormalities, a preponderance of negative symptoms, and being male. Violence is an unfortunate outcome in this patient population, with a homicide rate being ten times greater than the general population; the paranoid subtype with persecutory delusions and command auditory hallucinations related to those delusions pose the greatest risk. As noted earlier, 10% to 13% end their lives by suicide.

Before the twentieth century, no effective treatment existed for schizophrenia. This changed, however, in 1952 with the introduction of chlorpromazine (Thorazine®), the first in a large group of medications known as *conventional antipsychotic agents* that revolutionized the field of psychopharmacology. While their exact mechanism of action is unknown, current evidence suggests that these agents are postsynaptic dopamine receptor antagonists working mainly on the mesolimbic and mesocortical pathways. Based on their affinity for dopamine receptors, they are divided into low, medium, and high potency agents. Unfortunately, the affinity is nonspecific, and while the higher potency agents are more effective as antipsychotics, they carry the greatest risk of *extrapyramidal syndromes* (EPS), which include dystonia, akathisia, akinesia, parkinsonism, and tardive dyskinesia.

In 1990, the United States saw the release of clozapine (Clozaril®), the first of a new class of agents known as *atypical antipsychotic agents*. Unlike conventional agents, the atypicals, which include aripiprazole (Abilify®), olanzapine (Zyprexa®), quetiapine (Seroquel®), risperidone (Risperdal®), and ziprasidone (Geodon®), are highly specific antagonist of the dopamine type two (D_2) and serotonin type two (5-HT_2) receptors, resulting in very low rates of EPS and a greater effect on negative symptoms. Today, atypical agents are the first line of treatment for schizophrenia, with conventional antipsychotic agents being reserved for those who are currently maintained on them or are nonresponsive to atypical agents. **Table 100.1** provides a list of common conventional and atypical antipsychotic agents, including initial dosages, maximum daily dosages, and important side effects.

In addition to pharmacology, patients with schizophrenia benefit greatly from psychosocial interventions, including supportive therapy, individual psychotherapy, cognitive-behavioral therapy, and group therapy. Family education aimed at stress reduction, early symptom recognition, treatment compliance, and relapse prevention is an equally important treatment strategy. For patients requiring more aggressive treatment, assertive community treatment (ACT) teams that provide outreach services have proven invaluable in maintaining patients in the community and preventing hospitalization. From time to time, acute hospitalization becomes necessary, and should focus on medication stabilization and reintegration into the outside community. For patients in whom psychopharmacology and psychosocial interventions have failed, long-term hospitalization may become an unavoidable reality.

Other Primary Psychotic Disorders

Other primary psychotic disorders that may present to the ED include:

1. *Schizophreniform disorder*—A primary psychotic disorder essentially identical to schizophrenia, except symptom duration is less than six months and psychosocial functioning is often preserved.
2. *Schizoaffective disorder*—A disorder in which a psychotic episode and mood episode occur concomitantly, and during the episode, psychotic symptoms persist for at least two weeks in the absence of prominent mood symptoms. Overall, it carries a better prognosis than schizophrenia but a worse prognosis than a primary mood disorder.

Table 100.1

Common Conventional and Atypical Antipsychotic Agents

Agent	Trade Name	Starting Dose	Average Daily Dose	Potential Side Effects
High potency conventional				akathisia, dystonia, neuroleptic malignant syndrome, parkinsonism, tardive dyskinesia
Fluphenazine	Prolixin	2.5–10 mg	2.5–30 mg	
Haloperidol	Haldol	0.5–5 mg	5–20 mg	
Pimozide	Orap	1–2 mg	1–10 mg	
Thiothixine	Navane	2–10 mg	5–30 mg	
Trifluoperazine	Stelazine	2–10 mg	5–20 mg	
Mid potency conventional				hypotension, neuroleptic malignant syndrome, QT prolongation, sedation, tardive dyskinesia, weight gain
Loxapine	Loxitane	10–50 mg	20–100 mg	
Molindone	Moban	50–75 mg	5–150 mg	
Perphenazine	Trilafon	4–24 mg	8–64 mg	
Low potency conventional				hypotension, lowered seizure threshold, neuroleptic malignant syndrome, QT prolongation, sedation, tardive dyskinesia, weight gain
Chlorpromazine	Thorazine	100–200 mg	100–800 mg	
Mesoridazine	Serentil	50–150 mg	100–300 mg	
Thioridazine	Mellaril	50–200 mg	100–400 mg	
Atypical				
Aripiprazole	Abilify	10–15 mg	10–30 mg	akathisia, extrapyramidal syndrome, gastrointestinal side effects, somnolence, tachycardia, weight gain
Clozapine	Clozaril	12.5 mg	25–900 mg	agranulocytosis, anticholinergic syndromes
Olanzapine	Zyprexa	2.5–10 mg	5–30 mg	constipation, dizziness, dry mouth, elevated SGPT, new onset diabetes, sedation, weight gain
Quetiapine	Seroquel	25–50 mg	25–500 mg	decreased T_3 & T_4, headache, increased LFTs, sedation, weight gain, cataracts
Risperidone	Risperdal	0.5–1 mg	0.5–12 mg	dizziness, hypotension, increased prolactin
Ziprasidone	Geodon	20–40 mg	40–160 mg	dizziness, nausea, QT prolongation, sedation

3. *Delusional disorder*—A primary psychotic disorder in which there is the presence of one or more well encapsulated, nonbizarre delusions about situations that could occur in real life. These delusions frequently involve fears of being followed, poisoned, cheated upon by a significant other, or having a terrible disease. Most areas of psychosocial functioning are preserved, except those that directly involve the delusion.

4. *Brief reactive psychosis*—A psychotic episode that arises suddenly, often after a significant stressor, and resolves completely in less than one month. This disorder is most often seen in severe personality disordered patients.

5. *Mood disorders with psychotic features*—A mood disorder, most often mania or depression, in which psychotic symptoms are present.

Treatment interventions are essentially the same as for schizophrenia, with the addition of mood stabilizers and antidepressants for schizoaffective disorders and mood disorders with psychotic features. Mood disorders as well as common medications used for treating them are discussed later in this chapter.

Secondary Psychotic Disorders

Secondary psychotic disorders are those that are directly caused by the physiological effect of a medical condition or substance, as evidenced by objective findings from the history, physical, or laboratory data. In addition, the symptoms are not better explained by another mental illness, or they arise exclusively during a course of delirium. Factors that should lead the ED physician to suspect secondary psychosis include: (1) a medical disorder requiring medication; (2) recent initiation or change in a medication; (3) history of substance abuse; (4) onset of symptoms in a person 40-years-old or older without a prior psychiatric history; (5) abrupt changes in behaviors; (6) visual hallucinations; (7) abnormal vital signs; and (8) disorientation or poor performance on cognitive testing. Definitive treatment consists of correcting the underlying medical condition or discontinuing the offending substance, which often leads to prompt resolution of psychotic symptoms, although symptoms can, on rare occasion, persist long after the primary process has reversed. Antipsychotic agents are used adjunctively to control dangerous behaviors and help ameliorate psychotic symptoms. **Table 100.2** provides a list of common substances and medical conditions that are known to cause psychosis.

Approach to the Psychotic Patient in the ED

When evaluating psychotic patients in the ED, a thorough history and physical exam is essential. Obtaining one, however, can prove problematic because these patients are notoriously poor historians and ED personnel are reluctant to approach patients who are uncooperative, agitated, and carry a risk of violence. As a result, psychotic patients may be prematurely restrained, tranquilized, and receive cursory examinations aimed at expediting transfers to psychiatric facilities. A rush to a psychiatric disposition unfortunately can result in misdiagnosis, significant morbidity, and inappropriate admissions to psychiatric units that are unable to manage medically compromised patients. To prevent this as well as provide a more comprehensive assessment, the ED physician must work collaboratively with the emergency mental health team.

The diagnostic interview is the first step in the evaluation process. It should be performed in a nonconfrontative manner, taking care to avoid any challenges to the patient's delusional system, as this may lead to agitation and increase the risk of assault. Questions must be simple and direct because the patient's attention and comprehension may be severely impaired by hallucinations or thought disorders. Key areas to explore include: the history of present illness, past medical history, family

---

Table 100.2
Organic Causes of Psychosis

Endocrine conditions
- hyper- and hypoadrenocorticism (e.g., Cushing's syndrome and Addison's disease)
- hyper- and hypoparathyroidism
- hyper- and hypothyroidism

Industrial exposures
- carbon monoxide/disulfide
- heavy metals
- nerve gases
- organophosphate insecticides
- volatile substances (e.g., fuel or paint)

Medications
- anticholinergic agents
- antihistamines
- antihypertensive and cardiovascular medications
  - digitalis
  - procainamide
  - prazosin
  - captopril
- antidepressant medication (esp. tricyclics)
- antiparkinsonian medications (both anticholinergic and dopaminergic agents)
- chemotherapeutic agents (e.g., cyclosporine and procarbazine)
- corticosteroids
- muscle relaxants
- nonsteroidal anti-inflammatory medications
- other over-the-counter
  - cold and flu preparations
  - decongestants
  - diet pills (esp. ephedra-containing stimulants)
  - sleeping aids

Metabolic conditions
- acute intermittent porphyria
- hyper- and hypocalcemia
- hypercarbia
- hypoxia
- hypoglycemia

Neurological conditions
- auditory or visual nerve injury/impairment
- central nervous system infections
- cerebrovascular disease
- complex partial seizures
- dementia (e.g., Alzheimer's dementia and AIDS dementia complex)
- encephalitis
- epilepsy
- Huntington's disease
- lupus cerebritis
- migraine
- multiple sclerosis
- neoplasms
- neurosyphilis
- paraneoplastic syndromes
- Wilson's disease

Nutritional deficiencies
- B_{12} deficiency
- niacin deficiency (pellagra)
- thiamine deficiency (Korsakoff's psychosis)

Substances
- substance intoxication
  - alcohol
  - amphetamine and related substances
  - cannabis
  - cocaine
  - inhalants
  - opioids (esp. meperidine)
  - PCP and hallucinogens
- substance withdrawal
  - alcohol
  - sedative-hypnotics (e.g., benzodiazepines)

Other
- hepatic encephalopathy

---

history, past psychiatric history (including presentation and any exacerbation of chronic psychotic disorders), substance use history, and current medications. If the patient is uncooperative or deemed unreliable, this information must be obtained from collateral sources, such as family members, outpatient treaters, police officers, firemen, emergency medical service personnel, and medical records from prior visits. Should the patient become too agitated to participate, medication should be offered. The preferred agent is lorazepam 1–2 mg PO or IM every 30 to 60 minutes until calm, taking care to avoid sedation, as this will prevent completion of the assessment and cloud the diagnostic picture. Unless the patient is severely agitated or combative, neuroleptics should be considered agents of second choice. If the clinical picture warrants, both chemical and physical restraints may become necessary to prevent harm to self and others; specific management recommendations for this situation are covered later in this chapter.

The crucial step in assessing a psychotic patient is the mental status examination (MSE), a two-part examination that includes a descriptive component, known by the acronym AMMSIT (appearance, motor activity, mood/affect, speech, intelligence, thought process and content), and a quantifiable cognitive examination, most often the Folstein Mini-Mental State Examination. The MSE, in conjunction with vital signs and a physical examination, should guide the medical workup. For patients with known primary psychotic disorders whose symptoms are consistent with prior exacerbations, extensive laboratory examination is often unnecessary. For psychotic patient who are unknown to the ED, or patients with known primary psychotic disorders whose symptoms are inconsistent with prior exacerbations, more extensive laboratory examination is indicated. This should include electrolytes, BUN, creatinine, glucose, liver function test, CBC, calcium, TSH, urinalysis, and toxicology screens for substances of abuse. If the clinical picture warrants, a chest radiograph and electrocardiogram may be included. For any patient presenting with new onset psychosis, lumbar puncture, CT/MRI, and an EEG should be considered, in addition to the aforementioned labs, if indicated by the presenting signs and symptoms.

Management of the Psychotic Patient in the ER

Agitation is a warning sign for impending aggression and as such, should be immediately addressed. The first step is to find the source of the agitation and if possible, eliminate it. Common sources of agitation in this patient population include involuntary admission to the ED, lengthy waiting times before assessment, inability to smoke, and frank paranoia. When possible, these sources should be addressed with behavioral interventions, such as offering food and beverages, allowing the patient to pace in an open area, seeing the patient immediately, or allowing the patient to smoke. If behavior interventions are ineffective or inadvisable due to the level of agitation, medication

should be offered. If the patient has prior experience with a medication that has been useful in alleviating agitation in the past, it should be considered. Otherwise, lorazepam 1–2 mg PO every 30–60 minutes until calm is the preferred management strategy. Oral atypical antipsychotic agents such as risperidone, olanzapine, and quetiapine may also be useful, but are considered second-line agents. If the patient remains severely agitated despite lesser restrictive interventions, or is so agitated upon presentation that they pose a significant risk of harm to self or others, physical restraint, followed by chemical restraint, is clearly indicated. If physical restraints are used, they must be applied safely, quickly, and in compliance with federal, state, and hospital guidelines. While in restraints, the patient must be monitored frequently for comfort and safety, and then released when calm and cooperative. The preferred agents for chemical restraint are a combination of a high potency typical antipsychotic and a benzodiazepine, usually haloperidol 2.5–10 mg IM and lorazepam 0.5–2 mg IM mixed in the same syringe, and repeated every 30–60 minutes until calm.

Treatment and Disposition

Once the evaluation has been completed and the type of psychosis established, the next step is to begin treatment. If the psychotic episode is secondary to a medical condition or substance, the definitive treatment is to correct the underlying cause. Should this require medical hospitalization, consultation with a hospital psychiatrist would be prudent. Antipsychotic agents are useful in the treatment of secondary psychosis but generally play an adjunctive role only. If the current psychotic episode is due to a psychiatric disorder, however, the definitive treatment will depend on the patient's presentation. For those patients who are severely psychotic and pose a significant risk of harm to self or others, or who are so disorganized that they are unable to care for themselves or respond appropriately to potentially life-threatening situations, inpatient psychiatric hospitalization is necessary. This may be on a voluntary or involuntary basis, with the primary goal being symptom stabilization through psychopharmacology. For those patients who are less psychotic and pose no significant risk of harm to self or others, treatment consists of a combination of outpatient pharmacological management and various psychosocial services.

The long-term management of all primary psychotic disorders is pharmacotherapy combined with adjunctive psychosocial interventions that include groups, cognitive behavioral therapy, and aggressive community treatment. When considering antipsychotic agents, atypicals are preferred over conventional agents, because of their increased effectiveness in treating both negative and positive symptoms as well as their lower risk of extrapyramidal side effects. Conventional agents are reserved for those patients who are refractory to atypicals, or who have had prior success with them. For non-compliant patients, long-acting depot forms of antipsychotic agents, given biweekly or monthly, should be considered.

Selected Readings

American Psychiatric Association. *Diagnostic and Statistical Manual of Mental Disorders, Fourth Edition, Text Revision.* Washington, DC: American Psychiatric Association, 2000.

Cancro R, Lehmann HE. Schizophrenia: clinical features. In: Sadock BJ, Sadock VA, eds. *Kaplan and Sadock's Comprehensive Textbook of Psychiatry,* ed 7. Philadelphia: Lippincott, Williams, and Wilkins, 2000:1169–1199.

Folstein MF, Folstein SD, McHugh PR. "Mini-mental state." A practical method for grading the cognitive state of patients for the clinician. *J Psychiatry Res* 1975;12:189–198.

Thaker GK, Tamminga CA. Treatment targets in schizophrenia and schizophrenia spectrum disorders. In: Gabbard GO, et al., eds. *Treatment of Psychiatric Disorders,* ed 3. Washington, DC: American Psychiatric Press, Inc., 2001: 1001–1025.

Suicide

Heidi S. Vermette

Given the time constraints of a busy ED, it is not surprising that many emergency physicians feel overwhelmed by the seemingly daunting task of evaluating distraught or agitated patients who are contemplating suicide. In the United States, suicide results in 29,350 deaths annually, and is ranked the eleventh most common cause of death across all age groups; in children and young adults, it is the third leading cause of death. Because of the low base rate, however, suicide is quite difficult to predict, making it important to focus on risk factors rather than probability of attempt or completion. The goals of suicide risk management are to assess the immediate degree of intent to commit suicide, project the risk over the next 24 hours, and identify strategies to decrease the risk. It is essential, therefore, that emergency physicians have a structure for evaluating suicide risk and a plan for managing suicidal patients who present to the ED.

Presentation in the Emergency Department

Patients with suicidal ideation can present to the ED in a number of ways. Common presentations include surviving an attempt, complaining of suicidal ideation, presenting with another chief complaint only to reveal suicidal ideation during the evaluation, demonstrating high-risk parasuicidal behaviors, or being brought in by family members who notice changes in behaviors. Overdose is by far the most common type of suicide attempt, accounting for 1% to 2% of all emergency room admissions and 70% of all suicide attempts. Other methods include self-inflicted wounds (e.g., cutting or stabbing), jumping, hanging, and motor vehicle crashes. Shooting is the most successful method for suicide completion.

Suicide Risk Assessment

While physicians are not expected to predict whether a suicide will occur, they are expected to do a thorough assessment of the risk. It is therefore crucial that they become familiar with the risk factors associated with suicide (**Table 101.1**). Risk factors can be divided into static factors, dynamic factors, and protective factors. *Static risk factors* are immutable characteristics of a patient's history that that

predispose them to suicide. Examples include parental loss during childhood and a family history of suicide. While useful in estimating the level of risk, static risk factors are not clinically useful, as they cannot be modified. *Dynamic risk factors,* on the other hand, are characteristics of the patient's history and presentation that do have the potential for change, and as such, become the focus of clinical attention. Examples include substance abuse, delirium, symptoms of mental illness, and social isolation (**Table 101.2**). *Protective factors* are factors that, if present, decrease the risk of suicide. Examples include the ability to form a good alliance with the evaluating physician and the availability of social supports. Contrary to popular belief, both the absence of previous suicide attempts and the ability to contract for safety are not considered protective factors. Once the static, dynamic, and protective factors are identified, the physician should clearly document them as well as the plan for addressing the dynamic risk factors, and the rationale behind any recommendations.

Assessment in the Emergency Department

All patients with histories of psychiatric disorders, frequent accidents, or excessive risk-taking behaviors should be screened for suicidal ideation. Any threat to commit suicide should be taken seriously, even if it seems trivial or manipulative. If a potentially suicidal patient requests to leave prior to an evaluation, he or she must be detained until an evaluation has been completed. Should the patient elope, hospital security and the local police should be alerted, and the patient returned to the ED to complete the evaluation (see Chapter 108, Legal Issues).

Prior to initiating an evaluation, an appropriate level of environmental and personal safety must be secured. This may be accomplished through frequent checks, video monitoring, direct observation by trained personnel, and by interviewing patients in rooms with limited access to objects that can be used for self-harm, such as sharp objects, medications, items with asphyxiation potential, or windows. Restraint devices should be kept close at hand for those patients who are actively attempting to hurt themselves. ED security should be alerted for those patients who pose an increased risk of self-harm.

Table 101.1

Suicide Risk Factors

	Static Risk Factors	Dynamic Risk Factors
Psychiatric	History of suicide attempts Family history of suicide Personal history of abuse	Major depressive disorder Alcohol or drug abuse/dependence Personality disorder Schizophrenia Posttraumatic stress disorder
Medical	Chronic illness Terminal illness	Psychosis secondary to medical condition Ostomy Delirium Pain Shortness of breath
Social	Recent loss Parental loss during childhood	Anniversary of important date Family instability Social isolation
Sex	Suicide completion: Male:female, 3:1 Suicide attempts: Female:male, 3:1	
Race	Higher risk for Caucasian and Native American	
Age		Males at highest risk in adolescence and late adulthood Females at highest risk in mid-life

Because patients are often reluctant to talk about suicidal ideation, careful attention must be paid to establishing good rapport. This may be accomplished by asking general questions first and then progressing to specific questions. For example, it may be best to ask questions in the following manner: "Have you ever wished you were dead?" "Have you ever thought about killing yourself?" "Are you thinking of killing yourself now?" "How are you thinking of killing yourself?"

In addition to a general psychiatric history and determination of suicide risk factors, the evaluation of a patient with suicidal ideation should include specifics about current suicidal ideas or wishes, the actual suicide plan (including amount of detail, degree of planning, lethality, and availability of means), potential for rescue, intent to act on wishes or plans (e.g., acquisition of firearms, settling of affairs, or a suicide note), future orientation, and any prior history of suicide attempts. When evaluating a patient who has just survived a suicide attempt, importance is placed on the lethality of the attempt, whether the attempt was impulsive or planned, the intent to die, the potential for rescue, the manner in which help was obtained, feelings about being saved, and whether the stressors that led to the attempt have changed.

Treatment and Disposition

There are three possible dispositions for the patient who presents with suicidal ideation: (1) home with outpatient follow-up; (2) admission to a general medical hospital; and (3) admission to a psychiatric hospital. Characteristics of patients who are good candidates for outpatient follow-up include nonsevere suicidal ideation, good impulse control, solid social supports, strong capacity to establish rapport during the interview, low risk for immediate decompensation, and no evidence of psychosis, intoxication, specific plan, and available means of access. If outpatient follow-up is selected, a friend or family member should stay with the patient to ensure that the means for suicide are inaccessible. In addition, the patient should be provided with an early follow-up appointment with outpatient providers and access to 24-hour emergency psychiatric services should the need arise.

Table 101.2

Common Deliriogenic Substances

Alcohol	Ergotamines
Anesthetics	Hallucinogens
Antiarrhythmics	Heavy metals
Antiasthmatics	Immunosuppressants
Antibiotics	Inhalants
Anticholinergics	Lithium
Anticonvulsants	MAOIs
Antihistamines	Muscle relaxants
Antihypertensives	Narcotics
Antivirals	NSAIDs
Antiparkinsonians	Organophosphates
Beta-blockers	Petrochemicals/solvents
Cannabis	Phencyclidine
Carbon monoxide	Sedative/hypnotics
Digitalis-like drugs	Steroids
Disulfiram	Sympathomimetics
Dopamine antagonists	TCAs

Admission to a general medical ward is appropriate for patients who, because of the suicide attempt, suffer a medical condition that requires treatment. Once admitted, psychiatric consultation should be arranged and the level of monitoring necessary to ensure the patient's safety ascertained. Depending on the presentation, monitoring may include constant observation, frequent checks (e.g., 5- to 30-minute intervals), or placement near the nursing station. If a patient is actively attempting to hurt him or herself, chemical and physical restraint may be necessary.

Admission to a psychiatric hospital is indicated for those patients who are severely suicidal with a high risk of immediate worsening. If the patient is willing to be hospitalized and is at low risk for leaving treatment, he or she may be placed in an unlocked or open unit. If, however, the patient is unwilling to be hospitalized or is at risk for leaving treatment, placement in a locked unit is indicated. If the patient is unwilling to sign in to the hospital voluntarily, the physician must make an application for involuntary admission according to state laws.

Selected Readings

American Psychiatric Association: *Diagnostic and Statistical Manual of Mental Disorders, Fourth Edition, Text Revision.* Washington, DC: American Psychiatric Association, 2000.

Anderson RN. Deaths: leading causes for 2000. *National Vital Statistics Reports vol. 50 no. 16.* Hyattsville, MD: National Center for Health Statistic, 2002.

Kleespies PM, Dettmer EL. An evidence-based approach to evaluating and managing suicidal emergencies. *J Clin Psychol* 2000;56:1109–1130.

National Institute of Mental Health. The numbers count: mental disorders in America. Washington, DC: NIMH Publication No. 01-4584, May 2003.

Thienhaus OJ, Piasecki M. Assessment of suicide risk. *Psychiatr Serv* 1997;48: 293–294.

Way BB, Banks S. Clinical factors related to admission and release decisions in psychiatric emergency services. *Psychiatr Serv* 2001;52:214–218.

Substance Intoxication and Withdrawal

Ralph J. Seymour

Intoxication and withdrawal from psychoactive substances can present in a variety of contexts in the ED. For example, patients or those who bring them in may complain specifically of one or the other. Others may come requesting a referral for detoxification or rehabilitation. Intoxication may be the precipitating factor in falls, fights, motor vehicle accidents, and deliberate self-injury, including suicide attempts, or they may present as an occult condition in unconscious, confused, or uncooperative patients. Symptoms of intoxication or withdrawal may be unmasked or develop during the evaluation of another medical condition.

The presentation of intoxication or withdrawal can vary widely, depending on severity, circumstance, and comorbid conditions (medical and psychological) as well as the type and combination of substances. Intoxication can present with no obvious disturbance or with complete unresponsiveness, while withdrawal can present as mild anxiety or irritability to frank delirium or status epilepticus. Patients in either state may be referred for psychiatric evaluation for their anxiety, disagreeable behavior, questionable judgment, or disturbed cognitive state. Because alcohol, opiates, sedative-hypnotics, and stimulants are the most common substances encountered in the ED, they will be the focus of this discussion.

Alcohol

Patients intoxicated from alcohol present in the ED with the odor of alcohol, behavioral disinhibition, emotional lability, impaired judgment, ataxic gait, poorly articulated speech, and if extremely intoxicated, may be obtunded or even comatose. Patients in alcohol withdrawal may present with or develop coarse tremor, nausea, autonomic instability, fever, anxiety, irritability, insomnia, disorientation, agitation, dilated pupils, and both visual and tactile hallucinations.

The DSM-IV-TR lists formal diagnostic criteria for alcohol intoxication withdrawal. For intoxication, it requires evidence of recent alcohol ingestion, maladaptive behaviors or psychological changes occurring during or shortly after ingestion, and at least one of the following: slurred speech, incoordination, unsteady gait, nystagmus, impairment in attention or memory, and stupor or coma. The cri-

teria for withdrawal includes cessation or reduction in prolonged heavy alcohol use, and two or more of the following: autonomic hyperactivity, increased hand tremor, insomnia, nausea or vomiting, transient visual, tactile, or auditory hallucinations, psychomotor agitation, anxiety, and generalized seizures. In both intoxication and withdrawal, one must exclude general medical condition and mental disorder as causes of the disturbances.

The intoxicated patient should be placed in a quiet area for observation. If alert, the patient may do well with the offer of food and drink. Prophylaxis against Wernicke's encephalopathy, including thiamine, folate, and multivitamins, should be administered promptly. Belligerent patients may respond well to lorazepam or haloperidol, but may also require the presence of security staff and either chemical or mechanical restraints if nonresponsive to other interventions. It is important to note that agitation may reflect withdrawal, indicating the need to institute a withdrawal protocol.

Management of withdrawal begins by taking the patient's blood pressure, heart rate, and temperature at intervals to assess autonomic stability. As noted earlier, the patient should receive thiamine, folate, and multivitamins for Wernicke's prophylaxis. Careful attention must be paid to the patient's fluids, electrolytes, and nutrition. Patients whose withdrawal is in tenuous control or who may have history of seizures should be placed on seizure precautions. The core of withdrawal management consists of pharmacologic treatment, typically with benzodiazepines, either in standing doses, gradually tapering doses, or doses based on a hospital-based protocol that uses vital signs and target symptoms. Beta-blockers may be used to counter the autonomic hyperactivity of withdrawal, but not as a single agent to prevent withdrawal.

Once stabilized, the patient should be referred for follow-up. Patients with uncomplicated alcohol abuse can be encouraged to participate in Alcoholics Anonymous or given information about local substance abuse clinics. Patients with alcohol dependence may need immediate transfer to a detoxification/rehabilitation facility. Some patients will present with comorbid psychiatric illness and may require an on-site psychiatric evaluation to facilitate transfer to a dual-diagnosis facility. When a patient cannot be medically stabilized in the emergency unit, admission to a medical unit for more aggressive withdrawal treatment is necessary.

Opiates

Patients intoxicated from opiates commonly present with apathy, dysphoria, euphoria, sedation (possibly to the point of coma), poorly articulated speech, pinpoint pupils, respiratory depression, and perhaps cardiopulmonary arrest. Patients in withdrawal, however, commonly present with drug cravings, irritability, insomnia, dilated pupils, piloerection, rhinorrhea, fever, cramping, and hypertension. The DSM-IV-TR criteria for opioid intoxication include recent use of an opioid, significantly maladaptive behavior or psychological changes developing during or shortly after opioid use, pupillary constriction (or dilation in the case of anoxia from severe overdose), along with one of the following: drowsiness or coma, slurred speech, and impaired attention or memory. The DSM-IV-TR criteria for opioid withdrawal include cessation of (or reduction in) opioid use that has been heavy and prolonged, along with three of the following: dysphoria, nausea/vomiting, lacrimation or rhinorrhea, dilated pupils, piloerection, diaphoresis, diarrhea, yawning, fever, or insomnia. The symptoms must also cause significant distress or impairment, and cannot be due to a medical condition or to a mental disorder.

Management in the emergency unit consists largely of observation, with supportive care as needed. The patient may require naloxone for respiratory depression. Severe intoxication may require intubation, ventilation, and even full cardiopulmonary resuscitation. Withdrawal symptoms can be ameliorated with clonidine. Following a test dose of 0.025 mg to 0.05 mg, clonidine can be given at 0.15 mg to 0.3 mg per day divided into three doses. If clonidine is used, the patient should be monitored for hypotension. Methadone is usually not initiated in the ED, although patients in methadone maintenance programs may have their outpatient regimens maintained while in the united, after confirmation from the program. Anxiolytics and antipsychotics can be used for anxiety and agitation.

Once stabilized, the patient should be referred for follow-up, which may include outpatient programs like Narcotics Anonymous and walk-in substance abuse clinics, or more intensive detoxification and rehabilitation facilities. As with alcohol abusers, patients with identified comorbid psychiatric issues may require on-site psychiatric evaluation for consideration to a dual-diagnosis facility. Patients with severe respiratory depression or with medical complications (injuries, aspiration, etc.) will require medical admission.

Sedatives, Hypnotics, and Anxiolytics

Patients presenting with sedative, hypnotic, or anxiolytic intoxication may present with disinhibition, emotionally lability, poor speech articulation, ataxia, hyporeflexia, and nystagmus. Their consciousness may range from mild sedation, or obtundation and unresponsiveness. Those in withdrawal may exhibit nausea, tremor, hyperreflexia, hyperphagia, tachycardia, dilated pupils, diaphoresis, irri-

tability, insomnia, restlessness, anxiety, delirium, and seizures.

The DSM-IV-TR diagnostic criteria for intoxication from these substances include recent use, significantly maladaptive behavior or psychological changes, and one or more of the following: slurred speech, incoordination, unsteady gait, nystagmus, impairment in attention or memory, and stupor or coma. Criteria for withdrawal from these substances include cessation or reduction in sedative, hypnotic, or anxiolytic use, with two or more of the following: autonomic hyperactivity, increased hand tremor, insomnia, nausea or vomiting, transient visual, tactile, or auditory hallucinations, psychomotor agitation, anxiety, and generalized seizures. These symptoms must cause significant distress or impairment, and cannot be due to another general medical condition or mental disorder.

Management of intoxication consists of observation for both safety and for signs of withdrawal. Patients with stupor, hypoxia, or unresponsiveness may require transfer to an intensive care unit. Agitation can be treated with lorazepam if there is no significant respiratory depression. An antipsychotic agent, such as haloperidol can also be used safely and effectively for severe agitation.

As with alcohol withdrawal, management of sedative, hypnotic, or anxiolytic withdrawal requires frequent monitoring of vital signs, seizure precautions, and use of a cross-reactive medication that can be titrated and gradually tapered to control withdrawal symptoms. Of note, gradual taper of the cross-reacting medication (e.g., 10% per day), while necessary, is often not feasible in the ED. Depending on the severity of withdrawal, the patient may require a medical admission for continued supervised detoxification.

Once the patient has been stabilized, he or she should be referred to an appropriate program, such as Narcotics Anonymous or outpatient substance abuse clinics that specialize in sedative, hypnotic, or anxiolytic abuse. In some cases, patients can undergo ambulatory detoxification by switching to a longer-acting agent and prescribing enough medication for a slow taper. Patients with severe or treatment-refractory substance abuse or dependence as well as those who require continuing detoxification may require transfer to a detoxification/rehabilitation facility. Patients with significant psychiatric complications may require admission to dual-diagnosis facility. For those whose withdrawal cannot be controlled in the ED, medical admission is required.

Stimulants

Patients intoxicated from central nervous system stimulants such as cocaine and amphetamines can present with euphoria, excessive self-esteem or grandiosity, suspiciousness, hypervigilance, paranoia, delusions, anxiety, diaphoresis, dilated pupils, hypertension, tachycardia, nausea, and agitation. The DSM-IV-TR diagnostic criteria for cocaine and amphetamine intoxication includes the recent use of amphetamine, cocaine, or related substances, significant maladaptive behavior or psychological changes, and two or more of the following: tachycardia or bradycardia, dilated pupils, elevated or lowered blood pressure, diaphoresis or chills, nausea/vomiting, weight loss, psychomotor agitation or retardation, muscular weakness, respiratory depression, chest pain, cardiac arrhythmia, confusion, seizures, dyskinesias, dystonia, or coma. General medical condition and mental disorders must be ruled out as causative factors. The DSM-IV-TR criteria for withdrawal includes the cessation or reduction in amphetamine, cocaine, or related substance use after heavy and prolonged use, resulting in dysphoria and two or more of the following: fatigue, vivid and unpleasant dreams, insomnia or hypersomnia, increased appetite, and either psychomotor agitation or retardation. As with intoxication, the symptoms cannot be due to a general medical condition and mental disorder. An electrocardiogram and/or cardiac telemetry should be obtained for all patients presenting with stimulant intoxication, because cardiac arrhythmias and myocardial may occur. In addition, these patients must be observed for aggressive or suicidal behavior, and provided regular verbal contact for reassurance. Anxiety and agitation respond well to lorazepam (1–3 mg PO/h). Severe agitation and psychotic symptoms can be treated with a high potency antipsychotic agent, such as haloperidol 1–5 mg PO or IV every 30 minutes until calm. Patients withdrawing from stimulants should be observed for abrupt onset of depressive symptoms. Anxiety and agitation associated with withdrawal can be treated with lorazepam 1–2 mg PO every 2–5 hours as needed.

Uncomplicated cases of stimulant abuse can be referred to self-help groups (e.g., Narcotics Anonymous) or to walk-in outpatient substance abuse clinics. Detoxification is unnecessary for stimulants, but treatment-refractory cases can be referred to outpatient rehabilitation programs. Patients with comorbid psychiatric illness may require referral to a dual-diagnosis program.

Other Substances

Patients presenting with hallucinogen intoxication are often mistaken as suffering from a new-onset psychotic disorder, as users are often within the age range associated with first-break psychosis and hallucinogens are rarely included in drug-of-abuse toxicology panels. The DSM-IV-TR diagnostic criteria for hallucinogen intoxication include a recent use of a hallucinogen, with subsequent significant maladaptive behavior or psychological changes. In addition, perceptual changes must occur in full wakefulness and alertness, and two or more of the following symptoms must be present: pupillary dilation, tachycardia, diaphoresis, palpitations, blurring of vision, tremors, and incoordination. Patient who abuse hallucinogens may also suffer from *hallucinogen persisting perception disorder,* also known as "flash-

backs," which involves the reexperiencing of perceptual disturbances, such as hallucinations, false perception of movement, flashes of color, intensified color, image trails, afterimages, macropsia, micropsia, all following cessation of hallucinogen use. In the ED, the patient will require close observation due to the potential for erratic, unpredictable behavior, which may be disruptive and even dangerous. Verbal reassurance as well as an anxiolytic, such as lorazepam, should be given for anxiety. Low potency antipsychotic agents and anticholinergic medications must be avoided, as they can worsen hallucinations. Physical restraint may be necessary for severe agitation. With respect to longer-term treatment, detoxification is unnecessary. Unfortunately, flashbacks may persist for years, but generally require no treatment, beyond reassurance.

Phencyclidine (PCP) intoxication often presents to the emergency unit as a true psychiatric emergency. Often, the patient is accompanied by the police after exhibiting aggressive, psychotic behavior that has placed others and himself in danger. Symptoms of PCP intoxication include nystagmus, hypertension, drooling, ataxia, poorly articulated speech, hyperreflexia, psychotic posturing, auditory/visual hallucinations, paranoia, delusions, agitation, and assaultiveness. The DSM-IV-TR diagnostic criteria for PCP intoxication include recent use of PCP followed by significantly maladaptive behavior. In addition, two or more of the following must be present: vertical or horizontal nystagmus, hypertension or tachycardia, numbness or reduced response to pain, ataxia dysarthria, muscle rigidity, seizure, coma, and hyperacusis. There is no known withdrawal syndrome. The patients presenting with PCP intoxication should be placed in a quiet area for observation, with readily available security staff. Reassurance and "talking down" the patient is not advisable, as this may result in further agitation. Anxiety and agitation should be treated with benzodiazepines, and psychotic symptoms treated with a high potency antipsychotic agent, such as haloperidol at 5 mg. IV every 30 minutes until calm. Ammonium chloride can be administered as a means to increase drug excretion. Most symptoms improve over a period of several hours, but medical admission may be required for severe, persistent symptoms. A small portion of patients can experience symptoms that persist for weeks or months, requiring transfer to an inpatient psychiatric facility for continued management and safety.

Selected Readings

American Psychiatric Association: *Diagnostic and Statistical Manual of Mental Disorders, Fourth Edition, Text Revision.* Washington, DC: American Psychiatric Association, 2000.

Hyman SE, Tesar GE, eds. *Manual of Psychiatric Emergencies,* 3rd ed. Boston, New York, Toronto, London: Little, Brown and Company, 1994.

Psychiatric Presentation of Delirium

Ralph J. Seymour

Delirium is a derangement of physiology that directly or indirectly insults the central nervous system (CNS). Its impact ranges from mild confusion—often undiscovered—to gross alteration of emotions, perceptions, cognition, and behavior. Delirium is known by many names, including *acute confusional state, organic brain syndrome, ICU psychosis,* and *encephalopathy.* Delirium has many medical, traumatic, toxic, and iatrogenic causes (see Tables 101.2 and 103.1). Predisposing factors for developing delirium include advanced age, chronic illness, history of CNS insult, postoperative state, and burns. Misinterpretation of the symptoms of delirium for primary psychiatric disorders, such as schizophrenia, major depression, or bipolar disorder, can result in delays or limitations in the evaluation of an acute medical illness.

Delirious patients present to the ED with abrupt onset of confusion, disorientation, and fluctuation between obtundation and agitation. They may voice delusional material and exhibit hallucinosis that is often auditory, visual, and tactile in nature. Those persons accompanying the patient may describe a prodrome of restlessness, anxiety, sleep disturbance, and irritability.

To make the diagnosis of delirium, the DSM-IV-TR requires the following: (1) a disturbance of consciousness (i.e., reduced clarity of awareness of the environment) with reduced ability to focus, sustain, or shift attention; (2) a change in cognition (such as memory deficit, disorientation, language disturbance), or the development of a perceptual disturbance that is not better accounted for by a preexisting, established, or evolving dementia; (3) development over a short period of time (usually hours to days) with fluctuation of symptoms over the course of the day; and (4) evidence from the history, physical examination, or laboratory findings that the disturbance is caused by the direct physiological consequences of a general medical condition.

Delirium is a syndrome, rather than a specific diagnosis. Once delirium has been identified, the next step is to identify the particular medical condition or conditions that are causing it. The mnemonic I WATCH DEATH (**Table 103.1**) is useful in forming a differential diagnosis.

Evaluation begins by obtaining the history of present illness and past medical history from the patient and those accompanying him. Medical records, if available, will prove invaluable. Particular attention must be paid to the time frame of the mental symptoms. A thorough physical examination, including vital signs, must also be performed, which may reveal signs of trauma, stigmata of acute and chronic illness, and neurologic deficits. All delirious patients must have a mental status examination that evaluates the level of arousal, psychomotor activity, appearance, speech form, affect, mood, intellectual function, thought process, and perception. Formal cognitive testing is included as part of the mental status examination, and may identify deficits that are not readily apparent by observation alone. If formal cognitive testing is not feasible, a useful bedside screening tool is to have the patient draw a clock face that includes a circle, the numerals, and then set the hands to a stated time (such as ten minutes past eleven). Patients in no obvious distress may reveal significant deficits in performing this simple test.

All delirious patients must have the following laboratory screens: electrolytes, glucose, BUN, creatinine, liver enzymes, thyroid function, B_{12} level, ammonia, sed rate, complete blood count with differential, urinalysis, and toxicology screening for basic substances of abuse. The clinical presentation will dictate the need for any additional studies, including a lumbar puncture, arterial blood gases, chest radiographs, and EKG. Neurodiagnostic testing, such as an EEG, CT, and MRI can help to identify and locate sources of mental status change with accompanying neurological findings as well as to distinguish functional from organic mental state changes.

The first concern for ED management of the delirious patient is that of safety. Agitation is a common manifestation in delirium, placing the patient as well as his caregivers at risk. Pharmacologic management reduces risk of injury and prevents disruption of treatment. High potency antipsychotic agents are a safe and well-tolerated first line treatment. Intravenous haloperidol is the treatment of choice, because it does not suppress respiratory drive, does not cause hypotension, is unlikely to worsen delirium, has a low risk of EPS, can be given in high doses, and if necessary, administered as an IV drip. In young adult patients, it should be administered at 0.5–2.0 mg for mild agitation, 2.0–5.0 mg for moderate agitation, and 5.0–10.0 mg for se-

Table 103.1

Differential Diagnosis for Delirium: I WATCH DEATH

Category	Example
Infection	encephalitis, meningitis, HIV, syphilis, urinary tract infections
Withdrawal	alcohol, benzodiazepines, babiturates
Acute	acidosis, alkalosis, electrolyte imbalance, renal and hepatic disease
Trauma	burns, closed head injury, postoperative state
CNS insult	abscess, hemorrhage, hydrocephalus, stroke, seizure, neoplasm
Hypoxia	anemia, carbon monoxide, hypotension, pulmonary failure, cardiac failure
Deficiencies	Wernicke-Korsakoff encephalopathy
Endocrinopathies	Cushing's disease, hyper- and hypothyroidism
Acute vascular	stroke, hypertension
Toxins or drugs	prescribed and unprescribed medication, drugs of abuse, pesticides, solvents
Heavy metals	lead, mercury

vere agitation. Elderly patients should be given a starting dose of 0.5–1.0 mg. When using the IV route, one should check the patient's serum potassium, magnesium, calcium, and phosphorous. One should also perform an EKG, noting the QTc interval; IV haloperidol should not be administered for QTc intervals >450. Prior to IV administration, the line must be cleared with normal saline, as heparin can precipitate the haloperidol solution. One should allow 30 minutes between doses, checking the QTc interval before repeating the dose. If the patient does not improve, the dose should be doubled. If there is no improvement after three doses, 0.5–1.0 mg of lorazepam can be administered either concurrently with the haloperidol or alternating with the haloperidol every 30 minutes. Once the patient is calm, the total milligrams of haloperidol are added and administered over the next 24 hours, in divided doses. If the patient remains in good control, the dose can be reduced by 50% every 24 hours. When converting to oral dosing, double the dose required and divide by bid to tid. Atypical antipsychotic medications are also used for agitated patients, though as of this writing, none are available in an IV formulation. Droperidol, a cousin to haloperidol, is another medication available for IV use. While having the advantage of a more rapid onset, it is much more sedating and hypotensive than haloperidol. Benzodiazepines, the treatment of choice for alcohol withdrawal delirium, should be used with caution for other causes of delirium because of their potential for sedation, suppression of respiratory drive, and occasional disinhibition.

Treatment of delirium begins and ends with supportive care, and requires an aggressive workup for and treatment of reversible medical conditions, which contribute to the altered mental state. It is important to note that delirium predisposes patients to other deliriogenic complications, such as dehydration, nosocomial infections, skin breakdown, and aspiration. While undergoing definitive treatment for the cause of delirium, patients should be kept in a quiet, adequately lit room (even at night). A clock and information board can help them reorient themselves. They should remain under close observation, including frequent vital signs and serial mental status examinations. The presence of a family member or sitter can have a calming influence, and may reduce the need for medication and restraint.

Though some patients will stabilize over a period of hours and be able to be discharged from the emergency department, many will require transfer to a medical floor for more extensive evaluation, treatment, and observation. The course of delirium is typically one of acute onset, followed by gradual resolution of symptoms over a period of days to weeks. Symptoms often resolve with supportive care, at times without identification of a specific cause. Rarely, delirium progresses to stupor, coma, seizures, chronic organic brain syndrome, and even death. Delirium is associated with a high mortality, depending on etiology and age; up to 50% of patients will die within six months to one year after suffering an episode of delirium.

Selected Readings

American Psychiatric Association. *Diagnostic and Statistical Manual of Mental Disorders, Fourth Edition, Text Revision.* Washington, DC: American Psychiatric Association, 2000.

Cassem NH, Murray GB. Delirious patients. In: Cassem NH, Stern TA, Rosenbaum JF, Jellinek MS, eds. *Massachusetts General Hospital Handbook of General Hospital Psychiatry,* 4th ed. St. Louis: Mosby, 1997:101–122.

Folstein MF, Folstein SD, McHugh PR. "Mini-mental state." A practical method for grading the cognitive state of patients for the clinician. *J Psychiatry Res* 1975;12:189–198.

Wise MG, Hilty DM, Cerda GM, Trzepacz PT. Delirium (confusional states). In: Rundell JR, Wise MG, eds. *The American Psychiatric Press Textbook of Consultation-Liaison Psychiatry.* Washington, DC: APA, 1996:257–272.

Mood Disorders

Heidi S. Vermette

Mood disorders include depressive disorders, bipolar disorders, and the combination of both mood states, and are more severe than the normal fluctuations that most people experience. Depressive disorders affect 18.8 million adults, or 9.5% of the U.S. population over the age of 18, and bipolar disorders affect 2.3 million adults, or 1.2% of the U.S. population. Major depressive disorder (MDD) and bipolar disorder Type I (BD-I) are two of the ten leading causes of disability in the United States, yet 59% of depressed individuals in the community receive no treatment, and bipolar disorders often go unrecognized and untreated for many years. Nearly twice as many women as men suffer from MDD, but men and women are equally likely to develop BD. Depression is common in the medically ill, with a point prevalence of 10 to 36% for inpatients, and 9 to 16% for outpatients.

Presentation in the Emergency Room

Most patients with depressive disorders can be managed on an outpatient basis. However, depression with suicidal ideation, inability to maintain adequate nutrition, or inability to maintain adequate hydration requires urgent evaluation. Some patients may not complain of depression, but present to the ED with unexplained weight loss, insomnia, fatigue, sad affect, or multiple ill-defined medical complaints. In patients with chronic medical illness, depression may present as refusal of care, withdrawal, or irritability. Patients with a known history of bipolar disorder typically present after stopping or switching medication, relapsing on drugs or alcohol, or following personal stressors. Some patients with mania are brought to the ED by the police because of disruptive behavior, or by family members who become concerned about poor judgment or unusual behavior.

Diagnosis

Mood disorder diagnoses are based upon depressive episodes, manic episodes, and hypomanic episodes. The mnemonic, SIG E CAPS ("prescribe energy capsules"), is a useful tool for remembering the neurovegetative symptoms of a depressive episode (**Table 104.1**). A depressive episode is a two-week period of depressed mood or loss of interest, accompanied by four additional SIG E CAPS symptoms. The mnemonic, DIG FAST, is a helpful way to remember the symptoms of a manic episode (Table 104.1). A manic episode is defined as a one-week period (less if hospitalized) of expansive mood, plus three DIG FAST symptoms, or irritable mood plus four DIG FAST symptoms. A hypomanic episode is defined as a four-day period of expansive mood, plus three DIG FAST symptoms, or irritable mood plus four DIG FAST symptoms representing a change in functioning that is not marked.

Before diagnosing a primary depressive disorder, it is important to rule out secondary conditions that present with similar symptoms. For example, alcohol intoxication, cocaine withdrawal, and heroin intoxication can present with symptoms that can be confused for major depression. Likewise, medical conditions such as hypothyroidism, anemia, stroke, early dementia, and influenza can mimic primary depressive disorders. Adjustment disorder and bereavement are important psychiatric disorders whose symptoms overlap with primary depressive disorders, but the etiologies and treatments are significantly different. As a rule, an adjustment disorder is diagnosed when depressive symptoms arise in the context of a clearly identifiable stressor that interferes with functioning; the full criteria for MDD are not met, and symptoms improve when the stressor resolves. Bereavement is a normal process of grieving that has some depressive symptoms, yet, like adjustment disorder, does not meet criteria for MDD.

The primary depressive disorders include MDD and dysthymia. The diagnosis of MDD requires that the patient meet the criteria for a depressive episode, and have no history of manic or hypomanic episodes. As part of its presentation, it may also have associated psychotic features, such as auditory hallucinations or paranoia. The diagnosis of dysthymia follows the rule of twos: two years of depressed mood, with two neurovegetative symptoms, and no more than two months without symptoms.

Before diagnosing a primary bipolar disorder, mania and hypomania secondary to substance use, medical dis-

Table 104.1

Mood Episode Symptoms

Depressive Episode Symptoms (SIG E CAPS)	Manic Episode Symptoms (DIG FAST)
Sleep: Decreased or increased **I**nterest: Decreased pleasure in activities **G**uilt: Feeling worthless or hopeless **E**nergy: Fatigue, loss of energy **C**oncentration: Decreased **A**ppetite: Decreased or increased **P**sychomotor: Retardation or agitation **S**uicidality: Ideation, plan, intent, attempt	**D**istractibility: Poorly focused **I**nsomnia **G**randiosity: Inflated self-esteem **F**light of Ideas: Racing thoughts **A**ctivities: Increased goal-directed activities **S**peech: Pressured **T**houghtlessness: Pleasure-seeking with high potential for painful consequences

orders, and other psychiatric disorders must be ruled out. For example, cocaine intoxication, marijuana intoxication, alcohol withdrawal, and amphetamine intoxication can present with symptoms that are indistinguishable from mania or hypomania. Medications such as antidepressants, psychostimulants, and steroids can likewise induce manic or hypomanic states. Hyperthyroidism, brain tumors, multiple sclerosis, encephalitis, and hyponatremia are examples of medical conditions that can present with symptoms similar to primary bipolar illness. Finally, mood instability arising from personality disorders may mimic or overlap with true mania or hypomania.

The primary bipolar disorders include bipolar disorder type I (BD-I), bipolar disorder type II (BD-II), and cyclothymia. BD-I is defined by the presence of a single manic episode, and may have associated psychotic symptoms, such as grandiose or religious delusions. BD-II requires one or more hypomanic episodes, one or more depressive episodes, but no history of mania. Like dysthymia, cyclothymia follows the rule of twos: two years of depressive symptoms that do not meet criteria for a depressive episode, hypomanic symptoms that do not meet criteria for a manic episode, and no more than two months without symptoms.

Treatment in the Emergency Room

This section will focus on the treatment of severe MDD and BD-I, as other mood disorders can usually be referred for outpatient management. Medication is the primary treatment modality for all mood disorders. With respect to MDD, the following must be considered prior to initiation of an antidepressant. First, antidepressants have a four to six week delayed onset of action, which limits their use in the ED. Second, antidepressants can trigger hypomania or mania in vulnerable patients, and therefore should not be given to any patient with a history of hypomania or mania. Finally, because emergency physicians are unable to follow patients over time, a physician in the community who will agree to follow the patient must be identified.

Because all antidepressant medications are equally efficacious, the choice of medication should be based on the patient's prior response to treatment, the side effect profile, and the family history of response to medications. Classes of antidepressant medications include selective serotonin reuptake inhibitors (SSRIs), tricyclic antidepressants (TCAs), monoamine oxidase inhibitors (MAOIs), and multimechanism antidepressants. Because of the potential for serious side effects and lethality in overdose, TCAs and monoamine oxidase inhibitors should not be started in the ED. **Table 104.2** lists starting and therapeutic doses for the SSRI and multimechanism antidepressants.

SSRIs are the first-line of treatment for MDD. Because they are well tolerated and less lethal than older generation antidepressants in overdose situations, they can be initiated in the ED. Common side effects include headache, nausea, decreased appetite, insomnia, weight loss, jitteriness, and sexual dysfunction. Multimechanism anti-depressants, such as bupropion, venlafaxine, nefazodone, and mirtazapine, are also well tolerated and safe, and like SSRIs, can be started in ED. Common side effects for bupropion include agitation, insomnia, nausea, and lowered seizure threshold; because of the seizure risk, it should not be started in patients with a history of seizures or bulimia. Common side effects of venlafaxine include sedation, headache, nausea, and dizziness. It also has the potential to raise blood pressure and should be used cautiously in patients with histories of hypertension. Common side effects of nefazodone include sedation, nausea, dizziness, dry mouth, and headache. It is also a potent cytochrome P-450 3A4 inhibitor, and can therefore interact with drugs that utilize this pathway. Mirtazapine's side effects of increased appetite, sedation, and weight gain make it a good medication for those patients who have insomnia and weight loss as part of their depression.

In severe cases of depression, an antidepressant alone may prove inadequate. Examples of this include patients suffering from MDD with psychotic features, who will require both an antidepressant and an antipsychotic agent (see Table 100.1), and patients whose depressive symptoms have a seasonal component, who may benefit from an antidepressant and light therapy. For patients whose symptoms of depression include severe malnourishment, dehydration, mutism, catatonia, or refractory

Table 104.2

Medications Used to Treat Mood Disorders

Antidepressants

Generic Name (Brand Name)	Starting Dose	Usual Dose	Dose Range
SSRIs (Selective Serotonin Reuptake Inhibitors)			
Fluoxetine (Prozac)	20 mg qd, 5–10 mg for elderly	20 mg qd	10–80 mg qd
Fluvoxamine (Luvox)	25–50 mg qhs, 25 mg qhs for elderly. Increase to 50 mg bid after 4–7 days	50 mg bid	50–150 mg bid
Citalopram (Celexa)	20 mg qd, 10 mg qd for elderly	20 mg qd	10–60 mg qd
Escitalopram (Lexapro)	10 mg qd	10 mg qd	10–20 qd
Paroxetine (Paxil)	10–20 mg qd, 5–10 mg qd for elderly	20 mg qd	10–50 mg qd
Sertraline (Zoloft)	50 mg qd, 25 mg qd for elderly	100 mg qd	50–200 mg qd
Multiple Mechanism and Atypicals			
Bupropion SR (Zyban, Wellbutrin SR)	100–150 mg qd. Increase to 100–150 mg bid after 4–7 days	100–150 mg bid	150–200 mg bid
Bupropion (Wellbutrin)	75 mg bid. Increase to 75 mg tid after 4–7 days and 100 mg tid after 1–2 weeks	100 mg tid	50–150 mg tid
Mirtazapine (Remeron)	15 mg qhs, 7.5 mg qhs (elderly)	30 mg qhs	15–45 mg qhs
Nefazodone (Serzone)	50 mg bid. Increase to 100 mg bid	200 mg bid	100–300 mg bid
Venlafaxine (Effexor)	37.5 mg bid, 12.5 mg bid elderly. Increase to 75 mg bid after 4 days	37.5–75 mg bid/tid	75–375 mg/day (divided)
Venlafaxine XR (Effexor XR)	37.5–75 mg qd. Increase to 75 mg qd after 1 week	75–150 mg qd	75–225 mg qd

Mood Stabilizers

Generic Name (Brand Name)	Starting Dose	Effective Dose	Dose Range	Recommended Labs/Monitoring
Lithium (Eskalith, Lithobid)	300 mg bid. Check trough level in 3 days, increase dose to achieve therapeutic level	Titrate to level of 0.8–1.2 mEq/L	900–1,200 mg/day divided bid/tid	Electrolytes, BUN, CR, TSH
Valproic acid (Depakote)	250 mg tid. Check trough level in 3 days, increase dose to achieve level of 50–100 μg/mL	Titrate to level of 50–100 μg/mL	15–60 mg/kg/d divided bid/tid	LFTs, CBC
Olanzapine (Zyprexa)	5–10 mg qhs, 2.5–5 mg qhs for elderly	10 mg qhs	5–20 mg qhs	Fasting glucose, triglycerides
Carbamazepine (Tegretol)	200 mg bid. Check trough level in 3 days, increase 200 mg every 3 days to achieve therapeutic level	Titrate to level of 4–12 μg/mL	800–1,200 mg/day divided bid/tid	LFTs, CBC, electrolytes
Lamotrigine (Lamictal)	25 mg qd. Increase by 25 mg every 2 weeks	200 mg qd	200 mg qd	Monitor for rash

suicidality, electroconvulsive therapy (ECT) may be required. Although there are no absolute contraindications for ECT, caution should be used in those patients who have a history of seizures, cardiac conditions, or space-occupying lesions in the brain.

When a patient with bipolar disorder presents to the ER in a manic state, the first priority is to calm the patient while ensuring the safety of others. The patient should be placed in a quiet room to decrease stimulation. If agitation persists, chemical and/or physical restraint may be necessary. Once calmed and the patient is able to participate in assessment, the etiology of the episode must be ascertained. Common reasons for a manic presentation include new onset of bipolar disorder, breakthrough symptoms despite adequate medication blood levels, addition or increase of an antidepressant medication, and noncompliance with treatment.

Mood stabilizers are used primarily to prevent manic episodes, although some newer agents are proving useful in preventing recurrent depressive episodes. Mood stabilizers that the emergency physician is likely to encounter, and which will be the focus of discussion, include lithium (Lithobid®), valproic acid (Depakote®), olanzapine (Zyprexa®), carbamazepine (Tegretol®), and lamotrigine (Lamictal®). Although mood stabilizers should not be started in the ED without consultation with a psychiatrist, it is helpful to be familiar with the side effects, therapeutic blood levels, and recommended laboratory studies (see Table 104.2).

Lithium is the mood stabilizer that most people associate with bipolar disorder. It is highly effective in the treatment of classic BD-I mania, but has a narrow therapeutic window that can quickly be exceeded during states of dehydration, resulting in severe neurotoxicity. Common side effects include dry mouth, nausea, fatigue, and tremor. It can also suppress thyroid function, and long-term use may lead to impairment of renal function. Prior to starting, and every six months thereafter, electrolytes, blood urea nitrogen, creatinine, thyroid function should be checked.

Valproic acid is an anticonvulsant that has gained popularity as a mood stabilizer. Common side effects include nausea, diarrhea, fatigue, and weight gain. It can also elevate liver function tests, suppress platelets, and rarely can cause fulminant liver failure or acute hemorrhagic pancreatitis. Prior to initiation, and every six months thereafter, a CBC and liver function tests should be checked.

Olanzapine, a medication originally approved for the treatment of psychosis, has recently been approved for the treatment of mania. It does not require blood level monitoring, and appears to be effective in patients with both mania and psychosis. Common side effects include weight gain, drowsiness, dizziness, and dry mouth. Because it has been associated with elevated blood glucose and triglycerides, patients taking olanzapine should receive regular blood glucose and triglycerides monitoring.

Carbamazepine, like valproic acid, is an anticonvulsant that is also an effective mood stabilizer. Common side effects include dizziness, drowsiness, nausea, and elevated liver enzymes. It can also cause hyponatremia, agranulocytosis, leukopenia, and thrombocytopenia, requiring that liver function tests, CBC, and electrolytes be checked before initiation and every six months thereafter.

Lamotrigine has recently been approved for use in bipolar disorder. Unlike other mood stabilizers that help to prevent mania, lamotrigine is most effective in preventing bipolar depression. It does not require blood level monitoring, but must be started slowly because of the risk of rash and Stevens-Johnson syndrome. Common side effects include fatigue, dizziness, headache, and rash.

Disposition

Because a depressive episode takes weeks to resolve, treatment planning beyond the initial ER visit is necessary. Inpatient hospitalization is indicated for those patients who have a high risk of suicide, are psychotic, unable to manage symptoms on an outpatient basis, have no social support, are medically compromised secondary to malnutrition, or cannot meet basic needs. If inpatient hospitalization is not indicated, outpatient follow-up must be arranged. If the patient is already engaged in psychiatric treatment, early follow-up appointments should be made. If the patient does not have psychiatric treatment providers, they should be referred to a psychiatrist and/or therapist prior to discharge. The patient and family should also be given instructions to return to the ER if suicidal thoughts intensify or if depressive symptoms worsen.

Patients with bipolar disorder may require hospitalization for a first-break episode, high risk of harm to self or others, severe psychotic symptoms, poor impulse control, high potential for ruining personal affairs, inability to maintain adequate nutrition, or an inability to manage symptoms on an outpatient basis. If the patient can be safely followed on an outpatient basis, follow-up appointments with outpatient treaters should be arranged. If the patient is not already taking a mood stabilizer, it may be useful to check baseline CBC, electrolytes, BUN, creatinine, liver function tests, and thyroid stimulating hormone in anticipation of starting one. If the decision is made to discharge the patient, the patient's family or friends should be asked to monitor symptoms and compliance. Likewise, the patient should be instructed not to return to work or make financial decisions until the symptoms resolve.

Prognosis

Mood disorders are chronic and relapsing. Patients hospitalized for a first episode of MDD have a 50% chance of recovery in the first year. Early treatment is important, as an untreated depressive episode can last 6 to 13 months, while a treated episode can last an average of 3 months. Factors associated with a good prognosis include mild episodes, no psychosis, short hospital stay, and an absence of co-morbid disorders. Bipolar disorders have a worse prognosis than depressive disorders. For patients with BD-I, 40% to 50% will have a second manic episode within two years of the first episode, 45% will have more than one episode, and 40% develop a chronic disorder. Factors associated with a good prognosis include short duration of mania, few suicidal thoughts, and absence of concurrent psychiatric or medical problems. Factors associated with a poor prognosis, however, include poor premorbid occupational achievement, alcohol dependence, psychotic features, inter-episode depression, and male gender.

Selected Reading

American Psychiatric Association. *Diagnostic and Statistical Manual of Mental Disorders, Fourth Edition, Text Revision.* Washington, DC: American Psychiatric Association, 2000.

CHAPTER

105 Anxiety Disorders

Ralph J. Seymour

Because anxiety is strongly associated with physical symptoms, the ED is often the first point of contact for patients with primary anxiety disorders. While some patients may present with frank complaints of anxiety, others may present with the sequelae of substance abuse for which an untreated or undertreated anxiety disorder has predisposed them, or with a predominance of somatic symptoms that they have interpreted as a heart attack or stroke. However, anxiety is also a normal consequence of many medical conditions, and should therefore be viewed as both a modifier of illness as well as a primary psychiatric illness. Hyman and Tesar and Rosenbaum et al. identified four dimensions of anxiety common to all anxious patients who present to the ED. These dimensions, which may be seen individually or in combination, include: (1) cognitive manifestations, including worry, obsession, and self-consciousness; (2) affective manifestations, such as uneasiness and dysphoria; (3) behavioral aspects, that is, avoidance, flight, and compulsion (repetitive, purposeless behaviors); and (4) physical manifestations, including musculoskeletal pain, gastrointestinal distress, urinary urgency and frequency, sensory disturbances (pain, numbness, tingling), and respiratory symptoms, such as dyspnea.

In the ED, the most common manifestation of an anxiety disorder is a panic attack, which may present with such dramatic somatic symptomatology that patients experiencing them often undergo an aggressive medical workup to rule out a major medical condition, most often a myocardial infarction. The DSM-IV-TR describes a panic attack as a discrete period of intense fear or discomfort, in which four or more of the following symptoms develop abruptly, and peak within 10 minutes: (1) palpitations, pounding heart, or accelerated heart rate; (2) sweating; (3) trembling or shaking; (4) shortness of breath or smothering; (5) feeling of choking; (6) chest pain or discomfort; (7) nausea or abdominal distress; (8) dizziness, lightheadedness, or faint; (9) derealization (feelings of unreality) or depersonalization (feeling detached from oneself); (10) fear of losing control or "going crazy"; (11) fear of dying; (12) paresthesias (numbness or tingling sensations); and (13) chills or hot flushes. It is important to note that panic attacks are symptoms, not a diagnosis, and

that they may occur in both primary and secondary anxiety disorders.

Differential Diagnosis

The DSM-IV-TR divides anxiety disorders into those that are primarily psychiatric, and those that are secondary to other causes. The primary anxiety disorders include the following:

1. *Panic disorder with or without agoraphobia*—Recurrent panic attacks with at least one-month duration of worry about additional attacks, or with resultant change in behaviors. When accompanied by fear of being in places from which escape is difficult or embarrassing, the provision "with agoraphobia" is added.

2. *Agoraphobia without panic disorder*—Fear of being in places from which escape is difficult or embarrassing exists, but there is an absence of panic attacks.

3. *Generalized anxiety disorder (GAD)*—Anxiety and worry of at least six months' duration that is associated with three or more somatic and cognitive symptoms, in the absence of a mood or psychotic disorder.

4. *Social phobia*—Anxiety triggered by the fear of public humiliation or embarrassment in social or performance situations.

5. *Specific phobia*—Anxiety triggered by specific objects or situations.

6. *Acute stress disorder*—Anxiety in response to a severe traumatic event, with intrusive reexperience, hyperarousal, and avoidance of associated stimuli. Onset of symptoms is less than one month duration.

7. *Posttraumatic stress disorder (PTSD)*—Anxiety in response to a severe traumatic event, with intrusive reexperience, hyperarousal, and avoidance of associated stimuli. Onset of symptoms is greater than one month duration.

8. *Obsessive-compulsive disorder (OCD)*—Anxiety related to obsessions (recurrent, persistent thoughts, impulses, or images) or compulsions (repetitive behaviors, including mental acts).

9. *Anxiety disorder not otherwise specified (NOS)*—Clinically significant anxiety symptoms that do not satisfy criteria for any specific anxiety disorder, but are not related to medical conditions or substances.

The secondary anxiety disorders include:

1. *Anxiety disorder due to a general medical condition*—Anxiety, fear, avoidance, or increased arousal due to the direct physiological effect of a medical condition.

2. *Substance induced anxiety disorder*—Anxiety, fear, avoidance, or increased arousal due to the direct physiological effect of a substance, including drugs of abuse, medications, or toxic exposure.

Management in the Emergency Room

Patients presenting to the ED with anxiety should be evaluated and treated for any acute medical illness or substance related cause of anxiety; this is especially important for any who has no prior history of panic attacks. Most symptoms of acute anxiety can be treated with benzodiazepines, such as diazepam 2–10 mg or lorazepam 1–2 mg. Benzodiazepines have rapid onset, are safe, well tolerated, and have low risk for abuse and dependence in short-term use. Antipsychotic medications are useful for anxiety symptoms that are related to a psychotic disorder or in situations where benzodiazepines are contraindicated. For acute management of severe anxiety with agitation, a high potency conventional antipsychotic agent (e.g., haloperidol) can be safely combined with combined with a benzodiazepine (e.g., lorazepam).

Treatment and Disposition

Patients should undergo psychiatric evaluation prior to discharge if their condition places them at risk for suicide or an inability to care for themselves. Inpatient psychiatric hospitalization is rarely indicated, and most patients can be referred for outpatient psychiatric treatment. The optimal treatment for anxiety disorder is the combination of psychotherapy and pharmacotherapy.

There are several modes of psychotherapy for the treatment of anxiety disorders. *Insight-oriented psychotherapy* helps a patient gain awareness of how unresolved issues of the past have pervasive and detrimental influences on current relationships. *Cognitive-behavioral therapy (CBT)* helps the patient to become aware of self-defeating patterns of thinking and responding to stress. *Exposure and response prevention therapies* systematically extinguish fear and patterns of avoidance by combining gradual exposure to the feared object or situation with relaxation and response prevention techniques. *Stress reduction* involves the use of imaging, exercise, breathing, and systematic relaxation to reduce levels of stress in an ongoing, prophylactic manner.

With respect to pharmacotherapy, antidepressant medications, particularly the selective serotonin reuptake inhibitors (SSRIs) and serotonin/norepinephrine reuptake inhibitors (SNRIs), have replaced benzodiazepines as the first-line therapy for the long-term treatment of anxiety disorders. The titration and dosages of these medications are similar to those used in the treatment of depression (see Table 104.2). Because antidepressant medications often require titration over several weeks, and are likely to increase anxiety and somatic symptoms in the short-term, they should not be initiated in an emergency setting. Buspirone is effective in treatment for generalized anxiety disorder, but here is little support for its use in more severe anxiety disorders, such as panic disorder. Antipsychotic agents are useful in treating anxiety-related symptoms of PTSD, steroid use, or for patients who cannot tolerate sedation or suppression of respiratory drive. Beta-blockers can be helpful in controlling sympathetically-mediated symptoms of anxiety, but must be used cautiously, as they may induce bradycardia and hypotension.

Prognosis

Most patients experience significant improvement with psychotherapy, pharmacotherapy, or a combination of both. Even with treatment, however, these patients often carry a significant, yet manageable residual of symptoms. Some will experience a loss in the efficacy of their medication regimen despite compliance, while others may have a satisfactory response to treatment, only to relapse later under medical or psychosocial crisis. A few patients can be tapered off their regimens without apparent difficulty, but many others will experience a high rate of symptom relapse or recurrence upon treatment discontinuation. Untreated anxiety disorders exhibit substantial morbidity and mortality, as these patients have a higher utilization of medical resources, are at greater risk for developing substance abuse, and carry a 15% to 20% risk for suicide completion.

Selected Readings

American Psychiatric Association. *Diagnostic and Statistical Manual of Mental Disorders, Fourth Edition, Text Revision.* Washington, DC: American Psychiatric Association, 2000.

Hyman SE, Tesar GE, eds. *Manual of Psychiatric Emergencies,* ed 3. Boston, New York, Toronto, London: Little, Brown and Company, 1994.

Rosenbaum JF, Pollack MH, Otto MW, Bernstein JG. Anxious patients. In: Cassem NH, Stern TA, Rosenbaum JF, Jellinek MS, eds. *Massachusetts General Hospital Handbook of General Hospital Psychiatry,* 4th ed. St. Louis: Mosby, 1996: 173–210.

106 Somatoform Disorders

Ralph J. Seymour

Most people experience somatic symptoms during any given week. When these symptoms persist or become severe, many will consult their primary care physician or, in some cases, present to the ED. Often, the emergency physician is unable to identify a specific cause, and the symptoms resolve as mysteriously as they arose. However, some patients will present repeatedly to the ED, often expressing distress that is incongruent with objective findings, and then undergo one negative medical workup after another. These patients often raise strong feelings of frustration and suspicion in the ED staff, especially when the complaints are also made in the context of seeking benefits or medications with abuse potential.

Many psychiatric conditions have prominent somatic symptoms. For example, panic disorder can mimic a heart attack, and certain psychotic disorders can include delusional beliefs about the body that remain unshaken by even the most compelling medical findings. Somatoform disorders, the focus of this discussion, are a group of disorders reserved for those individuals who perceive or express mental distress in the form of physical symptoms that lack significant objective findings, and are not the result of another psychiatric condition. While varying widely in presentation, these disorders share a common feature of being unconsciously produced.

Presentation in the Emergency Room

Patients with somatoform disorders often present to the ED with direct complaints of physical symptoms and, sometimes, specific and sophisticated diagnoses. There may be a history of multiple negative workups within a specific institution, or repeated visits to various local emergency rooms for the same physical symptomatology. Often, their complaints are inconsistent or at odds with known signs and symptoms of medical illness. Some may display mortal fear over seemingly trivial signs and symptoms, as is seen in those suffering from hypochondriasis, or have an acute onset of profound loss of function with marked indifference, as occurs with those suffering from a conversion disorder. It is important to remember, however, that somatoform disorders are diagnoses of exclusion, as patients suffering from primary psychiatric illnesses often

have a higher rate of untreated medical disorders. As a rule, somatic complaints initially should be taken at face value. In addition, a thorough medical history, augmented with available medical records, and corroborated by caregivers, will prove invaluable. Then, when the medical evaluation fails to find a physiological basis for the somatic complaints, or the evaluation uncovers frank psychiatric symptoms, the diagnosis of a somatoform disorder should be entertained, and a psychiatric consultation requested.

Differential Diagnosis

When differentiating somatoform disorders from other psychiatric disorders, it is important to know if the patient's symptoms are supported by objective physical findings, whether the symptoms are intentionally or unintentionally produced, and what may be the motivation behind the symptoms. The somatoform disorders are a group of disorders in which objective physical findings are lacking or in gross disproportion to the patient's symptoms, and the symptoms are unintentionally produced. There are essentially five major somatoform disorders:

1. *Somatization disorder*—A disorder in which there is long history of multiple physical complaints beginning before the age of thirty, and for which the patient is significantly distressed and seeks treatment. To make this diagnosis, there must be at least four pain symptoms, two gastrointestinal symptoms, one sexual symptom, and one pseudoneurological symptom.
2. *Conversion disorder*—A disorder in which motor or sensory deficits are associated with psychological stressors, are unconsciously produced, and not caused by a medical condition, substance, or religious/cultural belief.
3. *Pain disorder*—A disorder in which pain is the focus of clinical attention, causes significant distress and impairment, and is strongly associated with psychological factors. Pain disorders are acute if the duration is less than six months and chronic if greater than six months.
4. *Hypochondriasis*—A disorder based on the misinterpretation of bodily symptoms, in which an individual is a preoccupied with the fear or belief of having

a serious disease, despite medical evaluation and reassurance.

5. *Body dysmorphic disorder*—A disorder in which there is a preoccupation with an imagined defect in appearance, or an excessive concern over a slight abnormality, resulting in significant distress or impairment.

Two important disorders to differentiate from the somatoform disorders are *factitious disorder* and *malingering*. Patients suffering from a factitious disorder (formerly known as *Munchausen syndrome*) intentionally produce symptoms for the primary purpose of assuming the patient role. Patients presenting with malingering, however, intentionally produce symptoms to obtain identifiable external goals (e.g., financial benefits, avoidance of work or legal responsibility).

Management in the Emergency Department

The management of somatization disorder in the ED consists of doing a reasonable medical evaluation, minimizing medical procedures, and arranging regular time-limited visits with the patient's primary care physician. In addition, the patient may benefit from supportive psychiatric follow-up, which, through treatment of depressive and anxiety symptoms, may reduce the intensity of the somatic complaints. The condition is likely, however, to be chronic.

Symptoms of conversion disorder generally resolve quickly and spontaneously. The recovery can be hastened through suggestion and reassurance. Confrontation is seldom useful and may in fact backfire, as up to 30% of these patients are later found to have an objective neurological condition. At times, the patient may respond better to face-saving interventions, such as gradual recovery of function with physical therapy. Referral for psychotherapeutic intervention to reduce the impact of the psychosocial stressors that triggered the symptoms should be offered. Though most patients recover, some may have prolonged symptomatic periods or experience recurrences.

Pain disorder is a diagnosis of exclusion and as such, should be treated with the usual range of analgesic agents, unless a physiological cause has been definitively ruled out. Because of the psychological impact of pain, patients should be screened carefully and treated for any existing mood disorders. Whenever possible, patients with complicated pain disorders should be referred to multidisciplinary pain clinics for more comprehensive care as well as to reduce the risk narcotic and other substance abuse.

Patients with hypochondriasis respond poorly to emergency room interventions, as they are seldom reassured by negative findings and rational medical arguments. They can benefit from supportive psychotherapy, however, as their symptoms often wax and wane with psychosocial stress. Given the high rate of comorbid mood and anxiety disorders encountered with this disorder, these patients should also be encouraged to follow-up with psychiatric treatment.

Patients with body dysmorphic disorder present more commonly to primary care, dermatology, and plastic surgery clinics rather than an ED. When they do present, however, it is often after misguided and sometime disastrous attempts to alter their appearance. Referral to psychiatry is appropriate to identify and treat any comorbid mood and anxiety disorder. The course of this illness is chronic and unremitting.

Selected Readings

Abbey SE. Somatization and somatoform disorders. In: Rundell JR, Wise MG, eds. *The American Psychiatric Press Textbook of Consultation-Liaison Psychiatry.* Washington, DC: American Psychiatric Association, 1996:361–392.

American Psychiatric Association. *Diagnostic and Statistical Manual of Mental Disorders, Fourth Edition, Text Revision.* Washington, DC: American Psychiatric Association, 2000.

Barsky AJ, Stern TA, Greenberg DB, Cassem NH. Functional somatic symptoms and somatoform disorders. In: Cassem NH, Stern TA, Rosenbaum JF, Jellinek MS, eds. *Massachusetts General Hospital Handbook of General Hospital Psychiatry,* 4th ed. St. Louis: Mosby, 1996:305–336.

CHAPTER 107

Personality Disorders

Patrick Smallwood

No other population stirs such strong emotion among emergency room personnel than patients with severe personality disorders who are in crisis. While demanding constant attention on one hand, they often devalue the quality of their care on the other, placing staff in emotional double binds that are virtually impossible to resolve. If paid immediate attention, these patients consume a great deal of time, causing resentment from busy emergency room staff who may view these patients' presentation as purely psychiatric. If ignored or addressed negatively, these patients can quickly cause a scene with such brilliant displays of emotional firework that the normal flow of the emergency room comes to an immediate halt. With these ideas in mind, the following section explores personality disorders, paying special attention to presentation and management in the emergency room setting.

Personality is defined as an enduring pattern of perceiving, relating, and thinking about the environment and oneself that is seen in a wide range of social and personal situations. As such, it is relatively stable and predictable, characterizing an individual in ordinary situations. When normal, it is flexible and adaptable, with less mature coping strategies being kept in check. When disordered, it is maladaptive and implacable, with immature and primitive coping strategies rising to the surface and being used in such an inflexible manner as to cause significant distress for the patient and others. Because each of us has a unique personality comprised of these mature, immature, and primitive coping mechanisms, any one of which may be used in a crisis, each of us has the capacity to appear personality-disordered. It is therefore crucial that a definitive diagnosis of personality disorder not be made in the ED. Just as the diagnosis of essential hypertension cannot be confirmed with one blood pressure reading or without collateral data from the patient's primary care physician, neither can the diagnosis of a personality disorder be made based on one evaluation in the ED or without collateral data from the patient's therapist. However, once a definitive diagnosis of personality disorder is confirmed, clinicians must not ignore it out of a misguided sense of protecting the patient from a label, as this often lays the groundwork for inadequate or inappropriate treatment.

Who is the personality-disordered patient in an ED setting? Contrary to popular belief, men and women are equally represented. He or she is most likely to be young to middle aged, unmarried (divorced or single), have limited social supports, and present with a chief complaint of suicidal ideation or an actual attempt. With respect to specific epidemiology, 25% of patients presenting to the ED with a psychiatric complaint will have a diagnosable personality disorder, with 50% of those already engaged in psychotherapy. Not surprising, virtually 100% of chronic ED "repeaters" have a diagnosable personality disorder. For patient presenting to the ED with an anxiety or substance abuse/dependence disorder, 34% will meet criteria for a personality disorder. For patients who present with recurrent suicidal gestures and acts, the prevalence for personality disorders is between 48% and 68%.

The DSM-IV-TR recognizes ten major personality disorders, which are organized into three clusters based on shared diagnostic features: (1) cluster A personality disorders, which share the common features of being odd and eccentric (paranoid, schizoid, and schizotypal personality disorders); (2) cluster B personality disorders, which share the common features of being dramatic, emotional, and erratic (antisocial, borderline, histrionic, and narcissistic personality disorders); and (3) cluster C personality disorders, which share the common features of being anxious and fearful (avoidant, dependent, and obsessive-compulsive personality disorders). As a rule, patients often display traits of more than one personality disorder, and if they meet diagnostic criteria for another one, it should be diagnosed along with the primary one. The most commonly encountered personality disorders in the emergency department are the cluster B disorders, particularly the borderline personality disorder, which will be the primary focus of this discussion. For the sake of brevity, this section will highlight only the salient features of the remaining disorders.

Cluster B Disorders

Of the three personality clusters, cluster B personality disorders, particularly borderline personality disorder (BPD), are the most common ones to present to the ED. Known as the "dramatic" cluster, these disorders share the common features of being highly emotional, chaotic, unpredictable, and have low frustration tolerance (these patients are "now" oriented). In periods of great distress, it is not uncommon for these patients to experience brief reactive or transient psychotic episodes that quickly resolve once the crisis is stabilized. Patients with cluster B personality disorders frequently suffer from comorbid mood disorders, particularly bipolar disorders, as well as substance abuse/dependence disorders.

Borderline Personality Disorder

BPD is a common disorder, affecting up to 3% of the general population, with women three times more likely than men to suffer from it. The etiology, like all personality disorders, is unknown, but is most likely the result of a combined interaction between genetic and environmental factors. The hallmark of this disorder is a pervasive instability in relationships with others, with associated features that include intense affect instability with rapid mood swings, impulsivity, identity disturbance, feelings of chronic boredom or emptiness, and recurrent manipulative suicidal/parasuicidal behaviors (e.g., self-mutilation). The classic defense mechanism used by these patients is "splitting," a phenomenon in which people and objects are viewed as all good or all bad, with rapid oscillations between the two extremes.

The precipitant that generally leads to an ED visit is a real or perceived abandonment, particularly by a romantic partner, family member, or therapist. Because a borderline patient's sense of self is entwined with the significant other, this real or perceived separation often overwhelms them to the point that he or she may disorganize, regress, and present to the ED acutely agitated, psychotic, dissociative, or, more commonly, suicidal. When suicide is the presenting picture, it often takes the form of ingestions, overdoses, and self-induced lacerations, all of which may be planned consciously or unconsciously in such a way as to fail (i.e., low risk/high rescue). These threats or gestures must be taken seriously, however, as up to 10% of patients with BPD eventually complete suicide.

Evaluating the patient with BPD in the ED can be a difficult proposition. While the ED is an ideal place to receive emergency care, the waiting time for evaluation of non-imminently life-threatening situations can be intolerable, especially for borderline patients, who, by their very nature, have little or no frustration tolerance. Once the hurdle for waiting has passed, the next problem may arise when the actual evaluation begins. Like a genie who has been left in a bottle too long, the borderline patient, by now agitated and pacing, often greets the evaluating clinician with a litany of complaints for making them wait, which serves only to create an uncomfortable tension that may end in therapeutic failure. The actual evaluation may also prove to be difficult, as the borderline patient may give erroneous information, prevent collection of collateral information, become verbally abusive, or make a suicide gesture that culminates in physical or chemical restraint. If the clinician can successfully navigate the evaluation process, the final problem may arise when the final disposition is offered to the patient. At this point, the borderline patient,

whose expectations did not meet the reality of available resources, may refuse to accept it, escalate behaviors, and complain that the process was not only poorly done, it was much too brief. While all or none of these things may transpire, the following techniques may prove useful when evaluating these patients in the ED.

- See the patient as quickly as possible, as patients with BPD have low frustration tolerance. Additionally, they may view the delay as an avoidance of them personally, confirming their worst fears about their internal deficiencies and promoting self-mutilation. If unable to attend to them quickly, explain briefly the reason and how long of a waiting period may be expected.

- Evaluate the patient in a quiet place away from the main ED. Patients with BPD may become overly stimulated and begin to agitate. Additionally, they sometimes crave the attention of a large audience or seek to embarrass those who are trying to help them.

- Try to create a positive alliance with the patient. This should begin by placing them at ease and taking a nonconfrontative approach. Other techniques include offering food or beverages, allowing them to speak first, and permitting them to use their own transition objects, such as blanket, pictures, or stuffed animals.

- Establish the patient's expectations and goals for the evaluation. With the patient's assistance, set realistic goals and expectations, with a particularly focus on stabilization. Cure is not possible and long-term psychotherapy issues (e.g., sexual abuse, trauma work) should not be discussed.

- Provide a thorough but rapid evaluation that preserves their dignity and presents regression. Lengthy evaluations may prove regressive and harmful to the patient, who may look to the evaluator as all-powerful, only to be angry and disappointed when evaluation is completed.

- Elicit the initial stressor and acute precipitant, which are most often real or perceived abandonment by a significant other.

- Obtain a complete and focused evaluation, including a review of neurovegetative symptoms for depression and mania, a suicide risk assessment, and substance abuse/dependence assessment. It is important to remember that patients with BPD often suffer major mental illness, most commonly from bipolar-type disorders and substance dependence. With respect to safety, borderline patients may hide medications or sharp objects on their person, only to later overdose or cut themselves during the evaluation process.

- Obtain collateral information, as the patient is often in active treatment. If the therapist or treating psychiatrist can be contacted, there may be an established safety plan for times when the patient arrives in the ED in crisis.

Successful management of the borderline patient in the ED requires one to remain calm and professional at all times. Negative affect from the ED staff may be met with an even greater negative affect from these patients. Additionally, ignoring them completely serves as an invitation for "acting out," a rapid escalation in behavior that is often followed by severe agitation, aggression, complete decompensation, or brief reactive psychotic states. Below are helpful strategies for managing the two most dangerous situations that can arise while evaluating the BPD patient in the ED. These strategies are also useful in managing other patients who present similarly.

- *Agitation:* Just as chest pain can be a warning sign for an impending heart attack, agitation can be a warning sign for an impending physical attack. As such, agitation should be attended to as quickly as possible, rather than ignored. The first and most definitive step is to elicit the source of agitation, and if possible, eliminate it. Behavioral techniques are the interventions of first choice. They include distracting the patient from the source of agitation, offering food and beverages, enlisting the help of family members and significant others, or directing the patient to a quiet area. If behavioral techniques are ineffective, offer the patient medication. If the patient has prior experience using medication for agitation, ask him or her which one works best, and if it a reasonable choice, offer it. Otherwise, the medication of choice is lorazepam, given at 1–2 mg PO or IM every 30 to 60 minutes until calm. Alternative medications include orally administered low doses of either a high potency conventional antipsychotic agent, such as haloperidol, or an atypical antipsychotic agent, such as risperidone, olanzapine, or quetiapine.
- *Aggression toward self or others:* Aggressive behavior toward self or others is a true psychiatric emergency that can occur without warning or after numerous interventions have failed. If the patient gives sufficient warning prior to the commission of an aggressive act, he or she should be informed that all reasonable steps, including physical restraint, will be taken to ensure their safety and the safety of others. If necessary, this statement can be made in conjunction with or followed by a "show of force," a multidisciplinary team that includes hospital security. If successful, this intervention may be sufficient to thwart the act. If unsuccessful, however, or the situation is too dangerous, restraint becomes necessary. Once the decision to restrain has been made, it is unequivocal and non-negotiable; clinical experience demonstrates that when negotiation is permitted, the patient briefly de-escalates, only to rapidly escalate into a more volatile state than was present when the initial decision to restrain was made. Physical restraints must always be carried out safely, quickly, and in compliance with federal, state, and hospital guidelines. Once in restraints, the patient must be monitored frequently to ensure comfort and safety. If calm immediately, no other interventions may be necessary. However, if the patient continues to be agitated and violent while in restraints, parenteral medication should be administered. The medication of choice is lorazepam 1–2 mg IM every 30 minutes until sedated, or alternatively a combination of lorazepam and haloperidol.

Once the evaluation process has been completed, the final step in the ED treatment of the borderline patient is to arrange a disposition. Quite often, this is met with great resistance, because many of these patients prefer to remain in a highly structured environment filled with people who can meet their needs, prevent them from feeling lonely, and allay their fears of abandonment. Hospitalization should be avoided, but may prove necessary when crisis intervention techniques, including the use of medication, fail, and the patient remains acutely suicidal, homicidal, psychotic, or has such severe deficits in reality testing that he or she is unable to attend to or respond appropriately to potentially life-threatening situations. Once hospitalized, the goals must be simple and the length of stay brief to prevent significant regression and unrealistic fantasies of complete cure. Surprisingly, most borderline patients do not require hospitalization, even after such dramatic presentations such as suicide gestures, attempts, or being restrained. Often, the mere opportunity to speak or ventilate to a health care profession is sufficient for the patient to calm down, stabilize, and reorganizes to the point that they are no longer agitated or suicidal. If this should occur, and the patient contracts for safety, he or she should be discharged home, preferably under the supervision of another person, with an outpatient appointment to occur within the next 12 to 24 hours. Other possible disposition options include: (a) partial-hospitalization programs, which are programs associated with an inpatient psychiatric units that permit patients to attend structured treatment during the day, yet remain at their own home at night; (b) day treatment programs, programs associated with a local community health care facilities that provide daily structured treatment in a group setting; and (3) crisis stabilization units, community-based programs that promote crisis stabilization over a 24- to 72-hour period through the use of shelter, supportive therapy, medication supervision, and referral to vital community resources.

The long-term treatment of BPD is primarily psychotherapy, with pharmacology being reserved for the treatment of agitation, aggression, affective dysregulation, and any active comorbid major mental illness. Depending on the level of personality organization, patients with BPD can engage in several forms of psychotherapy, with dialectical behavioral therapy (DBT) being the most effective and preferred modality. DBT is a modified form of cognitive-behavioral therapy that focuses on opposing statements and views for almost every subject, with the primary point being that for every subject there is an opposing view. Patients must work with individual dialectical clinicians to help them achieve synthesis rather than validation of opposite views, and engage in highly structured DBT skills training groups designed to enhance coping with identity diffusion, affect dysregulation, low distress tolerance, interpersonal relationships, and crisis. The long-term prognosis for BPD is variable, with up to 10% of these patients eventually committing suicide, while others improve in middle age only to revisit core symptoms during periods of significant stress.

Antisocial Personality Disorder

Antisocial personality disorder (ASPD) is common in the general population, with a prevalence of 3% for men and 1% for women. Its essential feature is repetitive commission of unlawful and socially irresponsible acts without remorse or concern for the feelings and rights of others, beginning prior to the age of 15-years-old. Cloaked in facades of charm and pleasantry, these patients live complex lives fraught with illegal activity, promiscuity, substance abuse, and assaultive behavior. It is therefore not surprising that up to 75% of the prison population carry this diagnosis.

When these patients present to the ED, it is invariably for one of three reasons: to avoid incarceration; to avoid retaliation from others; or to obtain controlled substances. They are quite skilled at manipulating people to achieve these goals, initially using charm and deceit when things are going favorably for them, but intimidation, hostility, and threats when challenged or denied their requests. When evaluating and managing them, interventions similar to those discussed for BPD can be helpful. However, because of the criminal nature of this disorder, a few precautions are in order. First, clinicians should have a low threshold for having security present, if they feel threatened or unsafe in any way. Second, whenever possible, clinicians should collect collateral data from people who know the patient's history, given that these patients have a great propensity toward lying. Third, controlled substances should only be dispensed for objective findings, not merely complaints. Finally, to avoid incarceration, patients with ASPD may feign major mental illness or threaten suicide in order to be hospitalized. It is important to remember, however, that jails and prisons provide both suicide watch and mental health services for those who are incarcerated.

Because patients with ASPD are indifferent to how their actions impact others, they are the most treatment-resistant of all the personality disorders. The most effective form of treatment for this disorder is confined settings or sustained incarceration, such as prison, where external constraints act as a substitute for their moral deficits. Pharmacotherapy is reserved for the treatment of comorbid Axis I disorders or dangerous behaviors toward self and others. The prognosis is variable, with some patients burning out during middle age as they realize that society will no longer tolerate their behavior, while others end up in prison, succumb to the complications of drug dependency, or suffer violent deaths from injury, homicide, or suicide.

Histrionic Personality Disorder

The essential features of histrionic personality disorder (HPD) are pervasive overconcern with appearance, need for attention, exaggerated emotional response, poor frustration tolerance that ends in outbursts, and impressionistic speech that lacks detail. Physical attractiveness is the core of their existence, and as such, they often dress provocatively, display flamboyant mannerisms, and engage in inappropriately seductive behaviors. Like other cluster B personality disorders, patients with HPD are of-

ten loud and demanding of immediate attention when in the ED. Unlike BPD and ASPD patients, who often present suicidal or at risk of harm to others, the HPD patient most often presents with somatic complaints that have little or no objective findings. As a result, management generally consists of reassurance, avoidance of unnecessary tests, and firm limits on inappropriate behaviors. For overly seductive patients, it may be wise for the ED clinician to have another individual accompany them during the interview and examination. It is important to note that during times of great stress, these patients may experience panic attacks and transient psychotic states that require acute psychopharmacological management with small doses of benzodiazepines and antipsychotic agents.

Narcissistic Personality Disorder

The core feature of narcissistic personality disorder (NPD) is an overwhelming and pathological self-absorption. They exhibit a grandiose sense of self-importance and feel others with whom they associate must also be special and unique. When presenting to the ED, they are often entitled and demanding, feeling that they deserve immediate attention for even minor medical problems. In addition, they may request that the top physician in the ED care for them, and will frequently ask about the credentials and level of expertise of those who do care for them. Like other cluster B personality disorders, patients with NPD have little frustration tolerance, and are prone to emotional outbursts when their requests are not met or they are not seen immediately. Like HPD, they often do not present suicidal or at risk of harm to others, and management usually consists of setting limits on constant attention and entitled/demanding behaviors. Also, NPD patients, like HPD patients, may experience transient psychotic states under periods of great stress, and the use of an antipsychotic agent in the ED may become necessary.

Cluster A and C Disorders

Cluster A personality disorders, which include paranoid, schizoid, and schizotypal personality disorders, infrequently present to the ED. Known as the "odd/eccentric" cluster, this group of disorders share the common features of appearing paranoid, reclusive, and mistrustful of people. They may be inappropriately dressed, unkempt, and even talk to themselves, but are often not grossly psychotic or have the level of formal thought disorder encountered in patients with major psychotic disorders. These patients do not like being around people and will only present to an ED when experiencing a true medical emergency or on an involuntarily hold when someone has become concerned about their odd behaviors in public. When in the ED, they do not pose significant management problems with respect to the safety of self or others. General management consists of a nonthreatening, brief, and thorough examination by one clinician, preferably in a quiet area away from the public. Psychopharmacological interventions are rarely indicated, but because these patients occasionally suffer major psychotic illnesses, antipsychotic agents may prove useful.

Cluster C personality disorders, which include dependent, avoidant, and obsessive-compulsive personality disorders, occasionally present to the ED in crisis, but rarely, if ever, pose significant management issues. Known as the anxious/neurotic cluster, these disorders display pervasive anxiety, and struggle with issues of autonomy and control. In the ED, the greatest problem in caring for them is the time it requires, as they are quite indecisive and need a lot of reassurance to make even basic decisions. Management strategies consist of clear explanations, reinforcement of active coping mechanisms, and reasonable time limits for the encounter. Judicial use of anxiolytics may be warranted, as many of these patients suffer from comorbid anxiety disorders.

Suggested Readings

American Psychiatric Association. *Diagnostic and Statistical Manual of Mental Disorders, Fourth Edition, Text Revision.* Washington, DC: American Psychiatric Association, 2000.

Bender DS, Dolan RT, Skodol AE, et al. Treatment utilization by patients with personality disorders. *Am J Psychiatry* 2001;158:295–302.

Cloninger RC, Svrakic DM. Personality disorders. In: Sadock BJ, Sadock VA, eds. *Kaplan and Sadock's Comprehensive Textbook of Psychiatry,* 7th ed. Baltimore: Lippincott, Williams and Wilkins, 2000:1723–1764.

Phillips KA, Gunderson JG. Personality disorders. In: Hales RE, Yudofsky SC, Talbott JA, eds. *The American Psychiatric Press Textbook of Psychiatry,* 3rd ed. Washington, DC: American Psychiatric Press, 1999:795–823.

Tyrer P, Casey P, Ferguson B. Personality disorder in perspective. *Br J Psychiatry* 1991;159:463–471.

Legal Issues

Heidi S. Vermette

Becoming familiar with basic legal concepts can help the emergency physician become more efficient and less anxious about the medicolegal issues surrounding the management of psychiatric patients. Confidentiality, informed consent, right to refuse treatment, competence to consent to treatment, civil commitment, and restraint and seclusion are the medicolegal issues most likely to be encountered in the emergency room setting. Because laws vary from state to state and are subject to change, it is important to become familiar with the pertinent laws of the state within which one is practicing. In situations where medical and legal responsibilities seem in conflict, consultation with an attorney who understands medical practice is invaluable. If an attorney is not available, it is best to use good clinical judgment, solicit input from other members of the emergency care team, and thoroughly document the reasoning behind all decisions.

Confidentiality

Confidentiality, or the physician's obligation to keep information private, is an integral aspect of the physician-patient relationship. However, it is not absolute. For example, most states require physicians to report suspected abuse of children, elders, and disabled persons. In court, exceptions to confidentiality include court-mandated examinations, patient as litigant, and involuntary commitment. Confidentiality is also limited in situations where it is determined that the patient is at high risk of harming themselves or others. Every effort should be made to maintain confidentiality, but if deemed necessary to breach it, the physician should try to obtain the patient's permission, or have the patient convey the information him or herself, if not contraindicated. If the patient will not give permission, and there is a high likelihood that the patient or someone else will be harmed, it is important to divulge only the information necessary to carry out one's legal obligation.

Informed Consent

Informed consent is the foundation for the capacity to make medical decisions. In fact, procedures performed without it can be considered malpractice or even battery, a criminal offense. To qualify as informed consent, a patient must have enough information to make the decision, the capacity to make the decision, and the freedom to make the decision without coercion. Information provided to the patient should include the nature of the condition requiring treatment, the proposed treatment, the risks and benefits of the proposed treatment, and the alternatives to treatment, including no treatment. Exceptions to informed consent include emergency situations, incapacity, therapeutic privilege, and therapeutic waiver. In an emergency situation where the patient or others are endangered, and it is not possible to obtain the patient's consent or the consent of someone authorized on behalf of the patient, informed consent is not required. If a patient lacks the capacity to make an informed decision, a substitute decision-maker should be sought. *Therapeutic privilege* is a situation in which full disclosure of a condition or procedure would have a deleterious effect on the patient's health, whereas *therapeutic waiver* is a situation wherein the patient waives the right to informed consent. When using either of these exceptions to informed consent, extreme caution must be exercised, a second-opinion obtained, and clear reasoning behind the decision thoroughly documented in the chart.

Medical Decision-Making Capacity

Prior to an explanation on the assessment of capacity, it is important to keep a few basic facts in mind. First, a finding of competence or incompetence is a legal determination; while physicians are able to assess decision-making capacity and come to an opinion about what a court would likely find, only a court can make a finding of incompetence. Second, all adults are presumed to have the capacity to make medical decisions, and all competent adults have the right to refuse treatment. Third, decisional capacity is task-specific. For example, different skills are required to make a decision regarding a low-risk, high-benefit treatment, such as a blood draw, than to make a decision about a high-risk, potentially low-benefit treatment, such as experimental chemotherapy. Finally, decisional capacity can change with time or medical status, making it important to re-assess capacity frequently.

Assessment of medical decision-making capacity can be divided into four tasks. Deficits in the ability to perform any one of the four capacity tasks may lead to impairment of medical decision-making capacity.

1. *Expression of choice*—The patient must be able to both express a choice and maintain it long enough for treatment to be implemented. Patients who are unconscious or unable to come to a consistent decision may have impairment in this area.

2. *Understanding of the nature of the illness and proposed treatment*—Before a patient can understand their illness and the proposed treatment, the physician must explain the nature of the illness, the risks and benefits of the proposed treatment, and the alternatives to treatment, including no treatment. The best way to assess whether the patient understood this is to ask them to repeat the information in their own words.

3. *Appreciation of the consequences of accepting or rejecting treatment*—A good way to assess whether or not the patient appreciates the consequences of their decision is to ask what she thinks the likely outcome of her decision will be, and what impact it will have on her life. For example, if a mother of young children wants to refuse treatment, which is likely to result in her death, does she appreciate that her children will grow up without a mother?

4. *Useful manipulation of the information provided to come to a rational and logical decision*—The ability to use information to come to a rational and logical decision can be assessed by asking the patient to explain the reasons for his or her decision. The reasoning must follow a logical pattern, and not be influenced by depression or psychosis.

If it is determined that the patient does not appear to have the capacity to make medical decisions, the exam does not end there. It is important to identify the causes of the deficits and attempt to treat them. In the interim, a substitute decision-maker, generally the legal next of kin, should be identified. Guardianship should be pursued if the cause of the incapacity is unlikely to resolve, or the proposed treatment is invasive or high-risk.

Civil Commitment

The right to liberty is one of the most basic tenets of American society. Committing a person to a hospital for treatment against his will is a deprivation of that fundamental right, and therefore requires proper procedural protection. While laws vary from state to state, they generally require two elements for commitment; mental illness and dangerousness to self or others. Mental illness is defined by the state, and does not necessarily adhere to DSM-IV-TR diagnostic criteria. For example, in Massachusetts, mental illness is defined as "a substantial disorder of thought, mood, perception, orientation, or memory, which grossly impairs judgment, behavior, capacity to recognize reality, or ability to meet the ordinary demands of life." Like mental illness, dangerousness to self and others is also defined by the state. In most states, this is divided into suicidality and severe impairment of judgment that prevents an individual from living safely in the community. Prior to committing a patient to a hospital for treatment, less restrictive means of treatment, such as partial hospitalization or living in the community with support of family or friends, should be considered.

Restraint and Seclusion

Although every effort should be made to avoid restraint and seclusion, it is sometimes necessary for the protection of the patient and others who may be harmed by the patient's behavior. *Seclusion* is defined as the confinement of a patient in an area for the purpose of containing a clinical situation that may result in an emergency. Types of seclusion include opened-door and closed-door. *Restraints* are measures designed to confine a patient's bodily movements for the purpose of containing a clinical situation that may result in an emergency. Types of restraints include mechanical restraints (vest, 2-point, 4-point, etc.) and chemical restraints (antipsychotics, benzodiazepines, etc.). In most states, patients may be restrained for the purpose of examination, pending commitment, determination of medical decision-making capacity, or behavior that is likely to result in harm to the patient or others.

Prior to initiating a restraint or seclusion, alternative techniques must be attempted. These may include asking the patient to stop the dangerous behavior, reducing the stimulation in the environment, or offering medication to help the patient calm down. If alternatives fail and restraint becomes necessary, the least restrictive method that contains the dangerous behavior should be used. Once a patient is restrained, a physician is required to examine the patient within one hour of restrain initiation, and document the restraint alternatives attempted, the symptoms and behaviors that led to the restraint, and the type of restraint used. In addition, the physician is required to write an order that includes the reason for restraint, the type of restraint used, and the maximum amount of time the patient may be restrained before renewing the order. Although times vary by state and institution, restraints are generally valid up to four hours for adults, two hours for children aged 7 to 17 years, and one hour for children younger than age 7 years.

Selected Readings

American Psychiatric Association: *Diagnostic and Statistical Manual of Mental Disorders, Fourth Edition, Text Revision.* Washington, DC: American Psychiatric Association, 2000.

Kaplan HI, Sadock BJ. *Synopsis of Psychiatry,* 8th ed. Baltimore, MD: Lippincott Williams & Wilkins, 1998:1305–1320.

Renal Diseases

G. Richard Braen

Introduction

In this section on renal diseases, our authors describe the normal functioning of the renal system along with the problems that may present in an emergent fashion for our evaluation.

Patients may present with previously diagnosed renal disease but with complications of dialysis with or without problems of fluid overload or electrolyte imbalance. Patients with undiagnosed renal diseases may present with back or abdominal pain, dysuria, fever, electrolyte imbalances, edema, etc., and the emergency physician must be familiar with the protean presentations of renal disease, its appropriate ED evaluation, and its diagnosis.

With an increase in the number of elderly and nursing home patients that come to the ED for evaluation, the emergency physician should consider occult renal and urinary tract diseases when presented with a confused or febrile geriatric patient, who in many cases has no complaints specific to the GU tract.

The contributors from Jefferson Medical College describe structural renal disorders while those from the University of Buffalo describe the problems that arise with pyelonephritis, glomerular disorders, acute interstitial nephritis, acute renal failure, chronic renal failure and interstitial tubular necrosis. Our contributor from the University of Massachusetts discusses the complications of dialysis.

Combined, these authors have described the principles by which emergency physicians can recognize, treat, and appropriately refer patients who have developed some form of renal disease or have a continuation of a prior condition that now presents in an emergent fashion.

Structural Renal Disorders

Leonard G. Gomella
Juraj Letko

Acute Glomerulonephritis

Glomerulonephritis is an acute clinical syndrome characterized by hematuria, edema, hypertension, and renal insufficiency. The most common clinical feature is edema, followed by hypertension. The urine can appear grossly bloody, tea colored, or smoky.

Glomerulonephritis (GN) can occur as a primary process in which only the kidney is usually affected. These are: postinfectious, familial, drug induced, Berger's disease (IgA nephropathy), and membroproliferative GN. Secondary forms include: Henoch-Schönlein purpura, hemolytic uremic syndrome, systemic lupus erythematosus, subacute bacterial endocarditis, and Goodpasture's syndrome.

By far the most common cause in children is poststreptococcal glomerulonephritis (PSGN), which may follow streptococcal infections of the skin or pharynx. PSGN commonly affects children between the ages of 2 and 10 with a slight male predominance. Only certain strains of streptococci have been found to be nephritogenic.

Pathophysiology

Immune complexes formed in response to streptococcal infection are planted in the glomerulus during acute infection. The complement system is subsequently activated and this triggers the release of further inflammatory mediators in the basement membrane.

Clinical Findings

Typically gross hematuria or tea colored urine develops one to three weeks after streptococcal infection pharyngitis. Peripheral edema, especially around the eyes, is seen in approximately 75% of cases. Oliguria and hypertension are present less frequently. Rarely, hypertensive encephalopathy and congestive heart failure occur at initial presentation.

Laboratory Data

Urinalysis is most helpful in establishing the diagnosis of PSGN and reveals gross or microscopic hematuria, RBC casts, hyaline or granular casts, and WBCs. A urine culture is helpful to rule out infection. BUN and creatinine may be elevated. Hyponatremia and/or hyperkalemia may be related to water retention and azotemia. Levels of total complement and C3 are decreased early in the disease. Antibodies to streptolysin O may provide evidence of recent streptococcal infection, although certain strains do not produce streptolysin, limiting the diagnostic utility of this test. The throat or skin should be cultured. A CXR should be obtained in those presenting with hypertension.

Management

The role of the emergency physician is the timely diagnosis of PSGN and treatment of the complications of CHF and hypertension. If CHF is present supplemental oxygen, and furosemide (0.5–1 mg/kg) should be considered. In mild cases, patient may be discharged on a salt restricted diet, limited activity, and close follow-up. Streptococcal infection in the patient and symptomatic contacts should be initiated after a throat culture is obtained. Most patients recover completely, although hypertension, persistent proteinuria, and chronic renal insufficiency develop in a small percentage.

Hemolytic Uremic Syndrome

Hemolytic uremic syndrome (HUS) is the most common cause of acute renal failure in healthy infants and children. The triad of hemolytic anemia, thrombocytopenia, and acute renal failure characterizes HUS. Two subtypes are described in children: diarrhea associated (D+) and nondiarrhea associated (D–). Most cases are diarrhea associated and occur primarily in infants and children. Nondiarrhea associated cases result from: nonenteric pathogens such as Coxsakie, influenza, and RSV; malignancies; transplantation; and drugs. Nondiarrheal associated HUS also occurs as an inherited disorder. Incidence is similar in males and females; white children are affected more often than blacks.

Pathophysiology

Viral and/or bacterial organisms and their toxins cause damage to the renal capillary endothelium resulting in edema, thrombin deposition, platelet trapping, and microangiopathic hemolytic anemia. Platelets, fibrin, and complement deposit in the glomeruli, resulting in decreased glomeruli filtration rate and renal failure. *Escherichia coli,* especially serotype O157:H7, has emerged as the most commonly isolated organism in North America associated with D+ HUS. The most common routes of infection are ingestion of contaminated meat or milk. During outbreaks of *E. coli* O157:H7, 10% of children develop HUS.

Clinical Findings

In D+ HUS, diarrhea and cramping abdominal pain precede the illness by one to two weeks. These may be associated with blood in the stool, vomiting, and fever. Patients develop the acute symptoms of pallor, listlessness, irritability, and oliguria or anuria. Patients may have petechiae, GI bleeding, hypertension, hepatomegaly, edema, and CNS involvement, including seizures and coma.

Laboratory Studies

The classic laboratory findings seen in HUS include anemia, nonimmune hemolysis, thrombocytopenia, and abnormal renal function tests. The hematocrit and hemoglobin are markedly low and fall rapidly a result of the brisk hemolysis that is occurring. Helmet cells, burr cells, and fragmented RBCs are present on the peripheral blood smear. The reticulocyte count is mildly elevated and the Coombs test is negative. The platelets are decreased, usually to less than $50,000/mm^3$. WBC is usually increased with a left shift. The BUN and creatinine are elevated and hyponatremia, hyperkalemia, and acidosis may be seen. The urinalysis reveals hematuria, with variable amounts of protein and leukocytes. Granular and hyaline casts can be seen in the urine sediment.

Differential Diagnosis

When typical, the history, clinical, and laboratory findings of diarrhea associated HUS are present this is generally sufficiently to allow a clear diagnosis. In some cases, the physical exam may reveal abdominal tenderness. When associated with hematochezia, the presentation may suggest an intussusception. The clinical presentation of D–HUS is often more confusing. Other causes of causes of renal failure such as poststreptococcal glomerulonephritis and sepsis with multiorgan failure should be considered.

Management

The treatment or HUS relies on early recognition and resuscitation. Particular attention must be given to fluid administration and balance. Specific treatment of hyperkalemia, acidosis, and hypocalcemia is indicated. Early consultation with a nephrologist is recommended. Indications for dialysis include: BUN more than 100 mg/dL, CHF, encephalopathy, and severe hyperkalemia. Severe anemia (hemoglobin < 5 g/dL) warrants a slow transfusion with 5–10 mL/kg of packed red blood cells. Platelet transfusion is indicated for symptomatic bleeding and plasma transfusion for hereditary, prolonged or recurrent HUS. Acute mortality has been reported as high as

25%, but recent estimates are closer to 5%. CNS involvement is associated with increased mortality.

Henoch-Schönlein Purpura

Henoch-Schönlein purpura (HSP) is a multisystem disorder involving skin, joints, abdomen, and kidneys. It presents with purpura, arthralgias, abdominal pain, and renal abnormalities to varying degrees. Renal involvement occurs in approximately one half of patients, usually after the onset of skin and joint findings. Children between the ages of 2 and 11 are most commonly affected and the incidence is greater in males.

Pathophysiology

HSP is thought to be a vasculitis with immunoglobulin A deposition in the skin and glomeruli. Renal biopsy appearance is similar to IgA nephropathy (Berger's disease), but other clinical manifestations point to HSP.

Clinical Findings

The typical skin rash provides the key to diagnosis. These lesions begin as round pink papules on the extensor surface of the limbs, buttocks, and lower back. After 24 hours, they progress to palpable purpura. Arthralgia and joint swelling occur frequently, often in the knees and ankles. Abdominal pain with melena occurs in a significant percent of patients. In approximately 5% of these patients, these symptoms may represent an intussusception. Hematuria may be present, but is usually microscopic in nature. Rarely, a nephritic picture may develop with edema, hypertension, and azotemia, and is associated with a worse prognosis.

Laboratory Data

The laboratory is useful in excluding out other possibilities. WBC, platelet count, and coagulation tests are normal. Urinalysis often reveals hematuria and is should be monitored throughout the illness. BUN and creatinine may be elevated if renal involvement is significant.

Differential Diagnosis

Other causes of purpuric rashes should be considered including: Rocky Mountain spotted fever, meningococcemia, and ITP. As noted above, intussusception should be carefully considered in the ill appearing child with HSP and abdominal pain.

Management

Treatment is supportive. The risk of intussusception provides the greatest diagnostic challenge to the emergency physician. Steroids continue to be utilized in the hopes of reducing intestinal edema and abdominal pain, although the supporting data for this are limited. Patients may be discharged if significant renal involvement is not present and if abdominal or joint pain is not severe. Close follow-up must be assured to monitor urinalysis to detect the development of glomerulonephritis. Overall prognosis is excellent with only 1% to 2% progressing to serious renal sequelae.

Nephrotic Syndrome

Nephrotic syndrome (NS) is an uncommon clinical condition characterized by hypoproteinemia (serum albumin < 3.0 g/dL), severe proteinuria (>40 mg/m^2/day), hypoalbuminemia (<2.5 g/dL), edema, and hypercholesterolemia (>250 mg/dL). The reported annual incidence is 2–5/100,000 children. Most cases of childhood nephrotic syndrome are *primary nephrotic syndrome,* which is disease limited to the kidney. Of these, the majority of cases are minimal change disease (76%). Other causes are focal segmental glomerulosclerosis, membranous glomerulonephritis, or membranoproliferative nephritis. *Secondary nephrotic syndrome* is associated with other systemic diseases such as HIV, anaphylactoid purpura, lupus erythematosus, diabetes mellitus, sickle cell disease, and neoplasm (Wilms' tumor, lymphoma).

Pathophysiology

Plasma proteins, reaching the glomeruli, are restricted by a charge-selective and size-selective barrier. Normally only .03 % of plasma proteins reach the tubules. A small increase in permeability in these barriers can overwhelm the resorptive capacity of the tubules, leading to proteinuria. This loss of protein contributes directly or through compensatory mechanism to the other clinical conditions that characterize nephrotic syndrome.

Edema (periorbital, peripheral, and scrotal) is classically described as being the result of a low serum albumin causing a decreased oncotic pressure with extravasation of water into the interstitial space. This decreased plasma volume was thought to lead to a decreased renal perfusion and a stimulation of the renin-angiotensin system. This, combined with the release of antidiuretic hormone, enhances the reabsorption of sodium and water in the distal nephrons. However, in some cases, plasma volume is increased and there is no elevation of renin, angioensin, or aldosterone. The precise mechanism of edema formation and persistence remains uncertain.

In addition to albumin, other proteins are excreted in the urine, leading to hypoimmunoglobulinemia and increased susceptibility to infections. Hepatic protein production is increased in a response to hypoalbumemia and can lead to a hypercoagulable state and thrombotic complications.

Clinical Findings

Most children are asymptomatic except for the insidious development of edema. In the early stages, edema may be intermittent and primarily involve areas of low tissue resistance (periorbital, scrotal, and labia). As fluid retention becomes severe, it can progress to pleural effusions and respiratory distress. Ascites and bowel wall edema result in anorexia, nausea, vomiting, and diarrhea. Hypertension, hematuria, and oliguria may be present.

Complications

Bacterial infections are the most common complications in patients with new onset nephrotic syndrome and those already diagnosed and treated with steroids. A relative hypogammaglobulinemia predisposes patients to cellulitis, peritonitis, pneumonia, sepsis, and meningitis. Hypovolemia from intravascular depletion of salt and water, despite the presence of edema, may progress to shock. The hypercoagulable state predisposes to thrombosis in peripheral and internal vessels. Flank pain, hematuria, and worsening renal function should raise the suspicion of renal vein thrombosis.

Laboratory Data

Hypoalbuminemia is a cardinal feature of the NS. The serum albumin is less than 2.5 g/dL, with values as low as 0.5 g/dL. Urine protein is elevated (>2+ on urine dipstick or >40 mg/m^2/d). Hematuria may be present in those with primary NS as well as those with secondary NS. Renal function is typically normal at the onset of the syndrome. If the plasma volume is contracted and elevated hematocrit may be seen. WBC may be elevated even in the absence of infection and may normal in the infected patient on steroids.

Differential Diagnosis

Facial edema may be caused by an allergic reaction. Other causes of generalized edema to be considered are congestive heart failure. Other conditions producing hypoalbuminemia include cirrhosis and the protein losing enteropathy of cystic fibrosis. The urinalysis with proteinuria will help further define NS.

Management

The most important role of the emergency physician is supportive treatment of complications. Symptomatic hypovolemia and shock are treated in the usual way with isotonic boluses until perfusion is restored. If the patient is adequately hydrated, but has symptomatic edema, furosemide should be administered. Hypovolemia and hemoconcentration should be avoided because of the risk of thrombotic complications. If edema is severe and serum albumin is less than 1.5 g/dL, then albumin (0.5–1.0 g per kg of 25% salt-deficient albumin) followed by furosemide (0.5–1.0 mg/kg) may be useful. After an aggressive search for infection (including a negative tuberculin test) and in consultation with a nephrologist, some patients benefit from corticosteroids. Prednisone (2 mg/kg/d) is the typical dose in newly diagnosed patients.

Acute Renal Failure

Acute renal failure (ARF) is defined as a precipitous decline in kidney function and glomerular filtration rate. There is an accumulation of nitrogenous end products causing azotemia, fluid electrolyte imbalances, and disturbances in blood pressure and in solute excretion. ARF occurs in as many as 2% to 3% of children admitted to tertiary care centers.

The causes of ARF are divided into pre-renal (decreased renal blood flow), renal (parenchymal disorders), or post-renal (obstruction of urine flow).

Pre-renal renal failure results from decreased kidney perfusion from vomiting, diarrhea, poor fluid intake, fever, use of diuretics, and heart failure. NSAIDs can precipitate prerenal failure in those with baseline diminished renal perfusion. Renal disorders causing ARF include acute tubular necrosis, nephrotoxic injuries from medications, and glomerular disease such as HUS, PSGN, and pyelonephritis. Of these, HUS and acute GN are the leading causes of this form of ARF in children. Post-renal renal failure is caused by obstruction from posterior urethral valves, nephrolithiasis, or intraabdominal and pelvic tumors. These are a relatively rare cause of ARF in children.

Clinical Findings

Clinical findings in patients who present with ARF are related to the specific underlying disorders. Urine output is often decreased to less than 1 mL/kg/h. The ED approach to ARF should occur in an organized fashion. First, correctable causes should be identified and addressed: hypotension, hemorrhage, dehydration, sepsis, and heart failure. Life-threatening complications should be anticipated: encephalopathy and seizures from hypertension, cardiac arrhythmia from hyperkalemia, and pulmonary edema from volume overload and CHF. Ultrasonography, CT, and cystourethrography should be considered to evaluate obstruction.

Laboratory Data

Laboratory evaluation should include a CBC, electrolytes, BUN, and creatinine calcium and phosphorus. ASO titers can aid in the evaluation of post streptococcal glomerulonephritis. C3 complement can point to lupus as an underlying cause. CPK should be sent in cases of suspected rhabdomyolysis.

Evaluation of the urine is critical. Patients with acute glomerulonephritis will have RBC casts and hematuria. Heme positive urine in the absence of erythrocytes suggests the presence of myoglobin and rhabdomyolysis. WBCs point to infection and WBC casts suggest interstitial nephritis. Urine culture should be obtained in all patients. Oxalate crystals are seen in cases of ethylene glycol ingestion. Hyaline casts are present in dehydration and acute tubular necrosis (ATN). Urine specific gravity may be helpful in differentiating pre-renal failure from ATN. Typically patients with pre-renal failure have an elevated specific gravity (>1.025) whereas patients with ATN have specific gravity in the range of 1.005 to 1.015. Urine indices, which measure urine osmolality, urine sodium, and fractional excretion of sodium, help to further differentiate prerenal causes from tubular necrosis.

Because one of the earliest defects of tubular necrosis is urine concentrating ability, the urine osmolality measurements are helpful. Patient with pre-renal azotemia tend to have urine osmolality greater than 500 mOsm/kg, a urinary sodium concentration below 20 mmol/L and a fractional excretion of sodium less than 1%. In contrast, patients with tubular damage have a urine osmolality less than 350 mOsm/kg, the urinary sodium excretion exceeds 40 mmol/L and the fractional excretion of sodium exceeds 1%.

Management

Two of the decision points are to determine whether the cause of ARF is pre-renal and whether fluid resuscitation is appropriate. If the history and physical examination suggest pre-renal failure, isotonic fluid should be administered until signs of hypoperfusion are reversed. If no urine is produced in response to IV fluids, furosemide (1–2 mg/kg) should be administered. If myoglobinuria or hemoglobinuria is present, furosemide (1 mg/kg) followed by 0.5 g mannitol/kg of mannitol is necessary to clear pigmenturia and prevent tubular damage.

Complications such as hyperkalemia must be recognized and addressed with binding resins, glucose, and insulin, correction of acidosis, and possibly hemodialysis.

If potassium is greater than 5.5 mEq/L, eliminate potassium intake, kayexelate can be given orally or rectally. If the K^+ is greater than 6.5 mEq/L and there are EKG changes, Ca gluconate 10% is cardioprotective. Intravenous fluids and improved perfusion may improve metabolic acidosis and drive K^+ intracellularly. In the setting of persistently low bicarbonate, consider the administration of sodium bicarbonate. If dysrhythmia persists, the patient can be started on an insulin glucose drip (0.5 g/kg glucose as D25 with 1 unit of insulin for every 4 g of glucose given). Dialysis may be required if the above measures do not decrease the potassium. Consultation with a pediatric critical care specialist is advantageous at this juncture.

Seizures may be a complication of ARF, either because of severe hypertension or hyponatremia. A hypertensive emergency may be a result of volume overload and should be addressed with fluid restriction and furosemide (1–2 mg/kg). Nitroprusside (0.5–8 μg/kg/min) infusion or labetolol (0.2–1.0 mg/kg/dose) are effective in controlling the blood pressure. Blood pressure reduction should be cautious with the goal of $1/3$ of the total reduction in the first six hours. Seizures resulting from hyponatremia may necessitate the use of hypertonic saline (3%).

Indications for dialysis include uremia with a BUN greater than 100 mg/dL, persistent hyperkalemia >6.5 mEqL, persistent metabolic acidosis ($HCO_3 < 10$ mEq/L), persistent CHF, oliguric renal failure due to HUS, or rhabdomyolysis with myoglobinuria.

Selected Readings

Andreoli SP. Acute renal failure. *Curr Opin Pediatr* 2001;14:183–188.

Clark A, Barratt T. Steroid-responsive nephrotic syndrome. In Barratt T, ed. *Pediatric Nephrology*, ed 4. Baltimore: Lippincott, Williams and Wilkins, 1999: 731–747.

Hricik D, Chung-Park M, Sedor J. Glomerulonephritis. *N Engl J Med* 1998;339: 888–899.

Kelsch R, Sedman A. Nephrotic syndrome. *Pediatr Rev* 1993;14:30–38.

Lanzkowsky S, Lanzkowsky L, Lanzkowsky P. Henoch-Schönlein purpura. *Pediatr Rev* 1992;13:130–137.

Orth SR, Ritz E. The nephrotic syndrome. *N Engl J Med* 1998;338:1202–1211.

Robson W, Leung A. Henoch-Schönlein purpura. *Adv Pediatr* 1994;41:163–194.

Sehic A, Chesney RW. Acute renal failure: diagnosis. *Pediatr Rev* 1995;164: 101–106.

Sehic A, Chesney RW. Acute renal failure: therapy. *Pediatr Rev* 1995;16:137–141.

Stewart C, Tina L. Hemolytic uremic syndrome. *Pediatr Rev* 1993;14:218–224.

Thadhani R, Pascual M, Bonventre JV. Acute renal failure. *N Engl J Med* 1996;334: 1448–1460.

Vogt B, Avner E. Renal failure. In: Behrman RE, Kliegman RM, Jenson HB, eds. *Nelson's Textbook of Pediatrics*, 17th ed. Philadelphia: Saunders, 2004:1768–1775.

Pyelonephritis

Jennifer L. Brown

Urinary tract infection (UTI) is one of the most common infections seen in the Emergency Department. Pyelonephritis is a specific form of upper urinary tract infection that has increased morbidity and mortality compared to simple cystitis or lower urinary tract infection. According to data from the Hospitalization and In-Hospital Mortality study of Acute Pyelonephritis in U.S. Hospitals from 1997, there are approximately 250,000 cases of uncomplicated acute pyelonephritis in the United States each year. A total of 191,566 (76%) of these patients were hospitalized in the year studied. The annual death rate from infections of the kidney is 0.3/100,000, and case fatality rate is approximately 3.3/1000. The diagnosis of pyelonephritis is an important one to make in order to administer proper treatment and to decrease the associated morbidity and mortality.

The distribution of pyelonephritis among specific patient populations varies with age and sex. Pyelonephritis is most common in young women of reproductive age, and in patients at the extremes of age. The female to male ratio of UTI is approximately 30:1 in children after infancy and in adult patients of reproductive age younger than age 50; this ratio approaches 1:1 after age 50.

Definitions

The term UTI is often used to describe many different types of infections that can occur anywhere along the entire urinary system. Listed below are some specific definitions to aid in a better understanding of pyelonephritis.

- *Urinary tract infection (UTI)*—A general term used to describe the inflammatory response of the urothelium to invasion by microorganisms. This term does not distinguish upper tract (kidney/pyelonephritis) from lower tract (bladder/cystitis) infection.
- *Bacteriuria*—Describes the presence of bacteria in the urine, but does not necessarily indicate infection.
- *Pyuria*—Describes the presence of white blood cells in the urine; usually indicates an inflammatory response or UTI.
- *Pyelonephritis*—Infection of the "upper" urinary tract involving the renal parenchyma and collecting system (calyces and pelvis).

- *Uncomplicated pyelonephritis*—Upper (kidney) UTI in a urinary tract with normal structure and function.
- *Complicated pyelonephritis*—Upper urinary tract infection in a patient with underlying structural, neurological, or medical problems.

Signs and Symptoms

Suprapubic pain and tenderness, urgency, dysuria, and frequency are most often associated with cystitis or lower UTI. Acute onset of flank or back pain with costovertebral angle tenderness, fever, rigors, nausea, vomiting, body aches, and malaise are associated with pyelonephritis. However, correlation between clinical symptoms and the severity of infection is variable. Most patients with pyelonephritis will have a fever, but some may only have a few or even none of the typical "upper" UTI symptoms. Patients who are at the extremes of age, are immunocompromised, or have other comorbid diseases may not manifest any of the typical symptoms.

The differential diagnosis of acute pyelonephritis should include lower tract UTI, pelvic inflammatory disease, prostatitis, epididymitis, urethritis, nephrolithiasis, acute cholecystitis, diverticulitis, acute appendicitis, perforated viscus, herpes zoster, and lower lobe pneumonia.

Pathophysiology

The urine is usually sterile as it travels proximally from the glomerulus distally to the bladder. The major mechanism maintaining this sterility is the unobstructed forward flow of urine from the kidney, down the urethra to the bladder, followed by complete evacuation of urine from the bladder through the urethra. Obstruction to the flow of urine occurring anywhere along the urinary tract with resulting urinary stasis can increase susceptibility to UTI. Abnormal urinary tract anatomy, physiology, or the presence of a foreign body (calculi, stents, catheters, etc.) may also increase the risk of developing a UTI by causing obstruction or by compromising host defense mechanisms.

Most urinary tract bacterial pathogens arise from the perineal and GI tract flora. These organisms enter the urinary tract by ascending through the urethra to the bladder, and may extend proximally through the ureter to the kidney. Approximately 95% of all UTIs arise from "ascending" infection. Since the female urethra is shorter and located close to the rectum in the perineal area, female patients are at increased risk of infection due to the ease of bacterial colonization of the vaginal introitus and urethra. Bacterial pathogens can then spread from the perineum and utethra in an ascending fashion to cause UTI.

Much less commonly (in 5% of cases), pyelonephritis may result from hematogenous spread of bacteria to the kidney in a patient with bacteremia from an infectious source elsewhere in the body. Patients who have indwelling IV catheters, infectious endocarditis, or those who use IV drugs are at increased risk for pyelonephritis from bacteremia.

Patients with significant underlying medical problems, urinary tract structural disorders (i.e., hypospadias, ureteral ectopia, bifid ureter), or neurological diseases such as neurogenic bladder or spinal cord injury, are at risk for developing a complicated UTI. These patients also have higher rates of sepsis and are more susceptible to infection with uncommon bacterial pathogens. **Table 110.1** is a list of risk factors associated with an increased incidence of complicated UTI.

Possible complications of pyelonephritis include treatment failure, abscess formation, hydronephrosis, renal stone formation, disseminated intravascular coagulation, acute respiratory distress syndrome, sepsis, and the development of chronic renal failure.

Bacteriology

Understanding the most common pathogenic organisms in pyelonephritis is important to guide the choice of appropriate empiric antibiotic therapy. Fecal contamination of the urinary tract and ascending infection is responsible for most cases of UTI and pyelonephritis as described above. *Escherichia coli* is responsible for approximately 80% of all uncomplicated UTIs. *Proteus mirabilis, Klebsiella sp, Enterobacter sp,* and *Pseudomonas* are causative in 5% to 20%, and the remaining <5% are caused by *Staphylococcus saprophyticus,* group D streptococci, *Staphylococcus aureus,* and other atypicals (*Ureaplasma urealyticum, Mycoplasma hominis*). Yeast, anaerobic bacteria

---

Table 110.1

Risk Factors Linked to an Increased Incidence of Complicated UTI

- Extremes of age (<15, >55)
- Male sex
- History of prior UTI
- Structural or functional urinary tract abnormality
- Immunosuppression (HIV, diabetes mellitus, solid organ transplant, steroid use)
- Pregnancy
- Recent urologic procedures or instrumentation

---

or *Mycobacterium tuberculosis* infections should be considered in patients with negative or inconclusive urine culture results and clinical findings consistent with pyelonephritis.

Laboratory Testing

Urine Sample Collection

The value of the urinalysis is dependent on the quality of the specimen obtained. All samples should be sent fresh for immediate analysis. In children less than 12 months of age, urethral catheterization or suprapubic aspiration provides the best sample and has a very low complication rate. Urine collected by using a perineal "bag" usually has high contamination rates, and is only useful if the urine culture result is negative. In adult men, urine specimens are not significantly affected by specific cleansing techniques or by the timing of the sample in the urine stream. The most accurate and timely method of urine sample collection from women is a sterile catheterization. There have been several studies that show there are significant (up to 50%) contamination rates in urine obtained from a midstream "clean-catch" voided specimen. However, if the urine is obtained from a "clean catch" sample, the lower the ratio of leukocytes to vaginal epithelial cells on the microscopic examination, the more likely it is that the leukocytes are contaminants from the vagina.

Urine Dipstick

The urine dipstick is a common tool used to screen the urine for pyuria and nitrite-reducing bacteria. The leukocyte esterase reaction has an 88% sensitivity to detect >10 WBC/hpf. The combined negative predictive value for UTI is >95% when the leukocyte esterase and the nitrite tests are both negative from a properly collected urine specimen.

Urinalysis

Urinary sediment is typically examined microscopically under high power (400×), to determine the number of cells per high power field (hpf). If seen, white blood cell casts localize the infection to the kidney. The most accepted microscopic diagnostic threshold for UTI is 10 WBC/hpf because 96% of infected urine specimens contain more than 10 WBC/hpf. The most useful test for diagnosis of UTI is the presence of bacteria on microscopic examination of the urine. One bacterium per high power field corresponds to >100,000 colony forming units per mL of urine in culture. However, the absence of bacteria does not exclude the diagnosis. A false-negative result can occur due to the limited volume of urine examined on the individual high-power microscopic field.

Urine Culture

Urine cultures are indicated in patients with a suspected diagnosis of pyelonephritis with a positive leukocyte esterase reaction on urine dipstick or bacteria present on microscopy, and in those patients who are at risk for complications of UTI or bacteremia. In a study by Thanassi, results from urine cultures led to a change in antibiotic therapy in 5% of patients studied due to resistant organisms. The urine culture is considered positive or in the "significant" range if there are $>10^5$ bacterial colony forming units (CFU)/mL. Colony counts of 10^2 to 10^4 are considered to be in the "suspicious range" and can be considered positive in early infection, a urine sample obtained from a catheter or suprapubic aspiration, male patients, or in a patient who has clinical findings consistent with UTI.

Blood Cultures

Blood cultures for patients diagnosed with pyelonephritis are rarely clinically useful and when positive, usually produce the same results as the urine culture. In addition, positive blood cultures do not correlate with more severe disease, and the pathogenic bacteria responsible for the pyelonephritis are more readily identified from the urine culture.

Imaging Studies

According to the American College of Radiology Appropriateness Criteria for Imaging in Acute Pyelonephritis, imaging studies are not generally indicated for acute uncomplicated pyelonephritis. Diagnostic imaging should be considered for patients with suspected obstruction or calculi, renal insufficiency, persistent fever lasting longer than 48 to 72 hours after initiation of treatment, or diabetes mellitus (or other immunocompromised state). For patients with pyelonephritis who have suspected calculi, obstruction or underlying anatomic abnormalities, intravenous pyelogram (IVP) or excretory urography is the best overall screening study. CT of the abdomen and pelvis with and without contrast is less effective for demonstrating obstruction, but is useful for showing parenchymal complications.

For patients diagnosed with uncomplicated pyelonephritis that do not respond to therapy within 72 hours, imaging should be strongly considered. The most appropriate and cost-effective initial study is excretory urography or IVP. Excretory urography can help to identify an underlying anatomic abnormality (which may have pre-

disposed the patient to development of pyelonephritis), a calculus, or other obstruction that may prevent a rapid therapeutic response.

Precontrast and postcontrast CT should be considered within 24 to 48 hours for patients with diabetes mellitus or other immunocompromised states to exclude the associated complications of pyelonephrosis or perirenal abscess. Ultrasound should be reserved for pregnant patients and other patients for whom exposure to contrast or radiation is dangerous or contraindicated (i.e., those with azotemia or contrast sensitivity).

The first episode of UTI in certain patients, such as young children or adult men under the age of 50, usually requires a radiological evaluation after resolution of the infection because these patients are at a higher risk of having underlying urinary tract structural abnormalities. If these abnormalities go unrecognized and untreated these patients may develop recurrent UTIs or significant complications such as hydronephrosis, renal scarring, chronic pyelonephritis, and ultimately, renal failure. Imaging choices include intravenous pyelogram, ultrasound, voiding cystourethrogram, or CT.

Treatment Options

ED management includes clinical examination and diagnostic testing as described above as well as exclusion of other diagnoses in the differential. This may include pelvic examination in females to exclude vaginitis, cervicitis, and pelvic inflammatory disease. Once the diagnosis of pyelonephritis is made, early administration of empiric antibiotics is important to decrease the associated morbidity and mortality, and to decrease the likelihood of developing chronic pyelonephritis or other serious complications such as perinephric abscess, emphysematous pyelonephritis, or infection stones.

Antibiotics

The best empiric antibiotic therapy choice is a broad spectrum bactericidal antibiotic with good penetration into the renal tissue and high concentration levels in the urine. Whenever possible, the drug choice should be tailored to the results of a urine Gram stain or to the urine culture

Table 110.2

Antibiotic Therapy for Pyelonephritis

Drug Name	Dose	Route of Administration	Frequency
Fluoroquinolone			
Ciprofloxacin	500 mg	PO	q12h
Levofloxacin	250 mg	PO	q24h
Trimethoprim/sulfamethoxazole	DS 160/800 mg	PO	q12h
Cefpodoxime	200 mg	PO	q12h
Ceftriaxone	1 g	IV	q24h
Gentamicin	3–5 mg/kg/d	IV/IM	divided tid
Ampicillin	1–2 g	IV	q6h
and gentamicin	3–5 mg/kg/day	IV/IM	divided tid
Aztreonam	1 g	IV	q8h

Table 110.3

Admission and Discharge Criteria

Indications for Admission
- Inability to maintain adequate oral intake
- Inability to take oral medications
- Pregnancy
- Extremes of age
- Indwelling catheter
- Unstable vital signs or toxic appearance
- Comorbid disease
- Known urinary tract abnormality, obstruction or stone disease
- Recent urinary tract instrumentation
- Sickle cell anemia
- Concerns about compliance or follow-up
- Diagnostic uncertainty
- Failure of outpatient treatment

ED Discharge Criteria
- Pain controlled with oral analgesics
- Ability to maintain oral intake (fluids and medications)
- Able to arrange 48–72 hour follow-up

when specific organisms and sensitivities are known. Often, antibiotic therapy must be chosen empirically by the emergency physician if Gram stain and/or culture results are not available at the time of diagnosis. Some clinicians provide the first dose of antibiotic therapy intravenously, even for those patients who meet criteria for outpatient therapy. There is no conclusive evidence to support or refute this practice. Current recommendations for the treatment of pyelonephritis in adults are for 14 days of treatment and include the drugs listed in **Table 110.2**.

The Infectious Diseases Society of America recommends a two-week treatment course with an oral fluoroquinolone as the first-line agent for empiric treatment in adult women with mild uncomplicated pyelonephritis. However, newer studies indicate the possibility of successful outpatient treatment regimens with oral antibiotics for shorter durations than previously recommended. Talan et al. performed a prospective randomized trial in adult premenopausal women with acute uncomplicated pyelonephritis. The study results showed a 96% (109 of 113 patients) clinical cure rate in patients treated with a seven-day course of oral ciprofloxacin (500 mg bid) compared to 83% (92 of 111 patients) clinical cure rate in the group treated with a 14-day course of oral double strength trimethoprim-sulfamethoxazole (160/800 mg bid). Also, there appeared to be no difference in cure rates for patients that were given the first dose of antibiotics intravenously.

Disposition

Once the diagnosis of pyelonephritis has been made, the next step is for a decision about the patient's disposition. Otherwise healthy patients with uncomplicated infections who are able to take oral medications and maintain adequate oral hydration may be considered for outpatient treatment with oral antibiotics. Medications as necessary for fever, nausea/vomiting, and analgesia should also be provided. **Table 110.3** is a list of indications for admission and discharge criteria.

Treatment of Pyelonephritis in Pregnancy

Acute pyelonephritis is a common complication of pregnancy and is one of the leading causes of nonobstetric antepartum hospitalization. The conventional and conservative treatment recommendation for pyelonephritis in pregnant females is to admit all pregnant patients beyond 24 weeks gestation for IV fluids and parenteral antibiotics. Outpatient treatment for pregnant patients prior to 24 weeks gestation can be considered in carefully selected patients and in consultation with the patient's obstetrician. Usual therapy for these patients is started in the emergency department with parenteral ceftriaxone, and then continued with oral cephalexin 500 mg four times per day for 10 to 14 days. Further treatment can be modified according to the urine culture results. Patients being considered for outpatient treatment should be healthy and able to tolerate oral medications and fluids, have no signs of preterm labor or sepsis, have minimal or no fever, and able to comply with early follow-up evaluation within 24 hours. **Table 110.4** lists the parenteral antibiotics that are effective for treatment of pyelonephritis and safe for use in pregnancy.

Summary

Pyelonephritis is a fairly common and potentially serious infection seen in the emergency department patient population. The emergency physician should be familiar with

Table 110.4

Antimicrobials for Treatment of Pyelonephritis in Pregnancy

Drug Name	Dose	Route of Administration	Frequency
Ampicillin/sulbactam	3 g	IV	q6h
Cefazolin	1 g	IV	q8h
Ceftriaxone	1–2 g	IV/IM	q24h
Ampicillin	1–2 g	IV	q6h
and gentamicin	3–5 mg/kg/day	IV/IM	divided tid
Piperacillin	4 g	IV	q8h

diagnostic strategies and treatment regimens for pyelonephritis. Emergency department evaluation and treatment should be tailored to the individual patient's risk of complications. Patients at risk for developing complicated pyelonephritis should be treated conservatively because they are at a higher risk of developing sepsis and other complications associated with pyelonephritis.

Selected Readings

Bacheller CD, Bernstein J. Urinary tract infections. *Med Clin North Am* 1997;81: 719–730.

Chernow B, Zaloga G, Soldane S, et al. Measurement of urinary leukocyte esterase activity: a screening test for urinary tract infection. *Ann Emerg Med* 1984;13: 150–154.

Foxman B, Klemstein KL, Brown PD. Acute pyelonephritis in U.S. hospitals in 1997: hospitalization and in-hospital mortality. *Ann Epidemiol* 2003;13: 144–150.

McMurray BR, Wrenn KD, Wright SW. Usefulness of blood cultures in pyelonephritis. Am J Emerg Med 1997;15:137–140.

Miller O 2nd, Hemphill R. Urinary tract infection and pyelonephritis. Emerg Med Clin North Am 2001;19:655–674.

Roe EJ. Renal testing. In: Cantrill SV, Karas S Jr, eds. *Cost-Effective Diagnostic Testing in Emergency Medicine. Guidelines for Appropriate Utilization of Clinical Laboratory and Radiology Studies.* Dallas, TX: American College of Emergency Physicians, 2000;117–120.

Sandler CM, Amis ES, Bigongiari LR. *American College of Radiology ACR Appropriateness Criteria™ for Imaging in Acute Pyelonephritis.* National Guideline Clearinghouse, 2001. Available at http://www.guideline.gov/summary/summary.aspx?view_id=1&doc_id=3265. Accessed May 2005.

Talan DA, Stamm WE, Hooton TM, et al. Comparison of ciprofloxacin (7 days) and trimethoprim-sulfamethoxazole (14 days) for acute uncomplicated pyelonephritis in women: a randomized trial. *JAMA* 2000;283:1583–1590.

Thanassi M. Utility of urine and blood cultures in pyelonephritis. *Acad Emerg Med* 1997;4:797–800.

Warren JW, Abrutyne E, Hebel JR, et al. Guidelines for antimicrobial treatment of uncomplicated acute bacterial cystitis and acute pyelonephritis in women. Clin Infect Dis 1999;29:745–758.

Wing DA. Pyelonephritis in pregnancy. *Drugs* 2001;61:2087–2096.

111 Glomerular Disorders

Gerald P. Igoe

Approximately 400,000 people in the United States suffer from end-stage renal disease, requiring some form of dialysis or transplantation, and about two thirds of these people have renal failure due to some form of glomerular disease. The clinical sequelae of these glomerular disorders are azotemia, hypertension, and volume overload. The challenge to the clinician is to recognize those glomerular disorder injuries that are amenable to early intervention, thus obviating the suffering and cost imposed by end-stage renal disease.

Glomerulonephritis

Pathogenesis of Glomerulonephritis

Most cases of glomerulonephritis are thought to be caused by immunologically-mediated glomerular injury. The mechanisms of injury are believed to include the deposition of soluble antigen-antibody complexes on the glomerular basement membrane, the formation of antibodies directed against the glomerular basement membrane, and the activation of complement. Antigen-antibody complex deposition is a major mechanism of injury leading to glomerulonephritis. Immunofluorescence studies and electron microscopy of renal biopsies have demonstrated the presence of soluble antigen-antibody complexes lodged within the glomerulus, antibodies directed against the glomerular basement membrane and complement components 3 and 4. When glomerular injury is a result of soluble antigen-antibody complexes or antiglomerular basement membrane antibodies, IgG, IgM, IgA, C3, and C4 have been found within the glomerulus. In biopsies containing only C3 within the glomerulus, it is believed that the alternate complement pathway is directly activated, leading to the glomerular injury. In most biopsies containing immunoglobulin, C3, and C4, injury ultimately results from activation of the classic complement pathway.

Once complement activation occurs by either pathway, a cascade of events follows that results in glomerular injury. Biologically active fragments are generated with chemotactic, permeability-promoting, and vasoactive properties. Polymorphic neucleocytes, macrophages, and monocytes are attracted, causing direct tissue damage. Localized platelet aggregation with fibrin formation causes focal disruption of glomerular function, and the glomerular filtration rate (GFR) is affected by altered flow rates in the microvasculature of the nephron.

The majority of cases of glomerulonephritis are caused by soluble antigen-antibody complexes that form or deposit upon the glomerular basement membrane. The antigen that elicits this immune response may come from a variety of sources, including infections, systemic diseases, and medications.

Group A beta-hemolytic streptococcus causing poststreptococcal glomerulonephritis is the prototypical example of acute glomerulonephritis. In the northern United States, streptococcal pharyngitis is the most common antecedent event leading to poststreptococcal glomerulonephritis. In the southern United States, streptococcal pyoderma and impetigo are more common.

Subacute bacterial endocarditis is associated with acute glomerulonephritis in a small percentage of cases. A variety of organisms have been implicated in this process, with *Staphylococcus aureus* and *Streptococcus viridans* being the most common offenders.

Ventriculoatrial shunts employed in the treatment of hydrocephalus become infected by a variety of organisms in ~20% of cases, and a small percentage of those are associated with acute glomerulonephritis. *Staphylococcus albus* is the most commonly cited organism.

Visceral abscesses associated with acute glomerulonephritis are more common in Europe than the United States and present as acute renal failure (ARF) set within a clinical picture of pyogenic visceral abscess. Hematuria, red blood cell casts, and proteinuria with the abrupt onset of ARF define this entity.

Many other types of infections have been targeted as the initiating cause of acute glomerulonephritis, including viral infections, bacterial infections of all types, and protozoan infections. In other parts of the world, malaria, syphilis, and hepatitis B are common infectious causes of acute glomerulonephritis.

Wegener's granulomatosis is a classic example of a group of small vessel vasculitides that cause rapidly progressive glomerulonephritis and are associated with antineutrophil cytoplasmic antibodies. Wegener's granulomatosis is a multisystem small vessel vasculitis that predominately affects the upper airways, lungs, and kidneys, causing granulomatous lesions that lead to epistaxis, nasal discharge, otitis media, sinus disease, and cavitating pulmonary granulomas that may be associated with hemorrhage, hemoptysis, and rapidly progressive glomerulonephritis. Other vasculitides included in this group are microscopic polyarteritis, idiopathic rapidly progressing glomerulonephritis, and the Churg-Strauss syndrome.

Henoch-Schönlein purpura and IgA-IgG nephropathy are two entities that may be considered as a continuum, with IgA-IgG nephropathy targeting the kidneys alone and Henoch-Schönlein purpura having true multisystem manifestations. IgA-IgG nephropathy is a common cause of glomerulonephritis in Europe, Australia, and Japan. It is manifested by a viral prodrome, gross hematuria, onset before age 35, and intermittently elevated serum levels of IgA. Henoch-Schönlein purpura has similar renal manifestations but also includes thrombocytopenic purpura, arthralgias, and colicky abdominal pain associated with gastral intestinal bleeding. Both lead to rapidly progressive glomerulonephritis in 15% to 25% of the cases.

Antiglomerular basement membrane disease is an autoimmune disorder in which circulating antibodies directed against the glomerular basement membrane attach, causing rapidly progressive glomerulonephritis. These antibodies may selectively attack the glomerular basement membrane or may also target the lung basement membrane causing hemoptysis (Goodpasture's syndrome). In either case, the antibodies are detectable in the serum and are removable by plasmapheresis. Recovery from this entity is rare, with almost all patients requiring chronic dialysis at some point.

Systemic lupus erythematosus is often associated with glomerulonephritis. Glomerular involvement can range from mild microscopic hematuria with no derangement of renal function to rapidly progressive glomerulonephritis, nephrotic syndrome, and ARF. Serologic markers include high titers of anti–double-stranded DNA and low serum complement.

Several medications have been implicated in the development of glomerular injury. Gold, penicillamine, angiotensin-converting enzyme inhibitors, and NSAIDs have all been associated with glomerular injury and glomerulonephritis.

Once the immune system and complement cascade have been activated, leading to inflammatory glomerular injury, a series of events follows that cause impairment of renal function. The primary event is a decrease in the GFR, which is the direct result of inflammatory changes within the capillaries of the glomerular tuft. This results in decreased delivery of filtrate to the distal nephron in the face of unchanged distal sodium and water reabsorption. The end result is increased reabsorption of sodium and water, with subsequent expansion of the extracellular fluid compartment. Elevation of blood pressure is felt to be the result of extracellular fluid expansion. Plasma volume, cardiac output, and peripheral vascular resistance will all be increased in most patients suffering from acute glomerulonephritis.

Hematuria occurs because the inflammatory process causes structural gaps in the capillary walls that allow red blood cells to pass into the urinary space. Red cell casts are formed when red blood cells become embedded in the concentrated tubular fluid.

Proteinuria in the setting of glomerulonephritis is caused by a combination of factors, including a generalized increase in permeability of the capillary wall, altered glomerular hemodynamics, and mechanical disruptions in the capillary wall structure. The protein loss is usually <2 g per day.

More than half of the patients suffering acute glomerulonephritis will experience a combination of fatigue, malaise, anorexia, crampy abdominal pain, nausea, and emesis. Some patients experience a dull flank or lumbar pain, but this is not a common symptom. Edema is the chief presenting complaint in two thirds of patients and is usually noted in nondependent areas such as the face, eyelids, and hands. Although less common, edema can become generalized, causing anasarca, pulmonary congestion, and, rarely, ascites.

Elevations in blood pressure are felt to be volume dependent and occur in ~80% of cases. These elevations occasionally present as malignant hypertension, resulting in hypertensive encephalopathy, lethargy, somnolence, and coma. Papilledema and elevated cerebral spinal fluid opening pressures are not always present. Advanced cases of extracellular fluid volume expansion can result in pulmonary edema with dyspnea. Ascites may also cause dyspnea and orthopnea secondary to mechanical restriction of diaphragmatic excursion. In cases of Wegner's granulomatous and Goodpasture's diseases, hemoptysis secondary to pulmonary hemorrhage may also occur.

Half of patients will note upon presentation a decrease in the volume of urine produced on a daily basis. This is a direct result of a decrease in GFR, which initiates the pathophysiological changes in glomerulonephritis.

Acute glomerulonephritis refers to the abrupt onset of hematuria and proteinuria associated with some degree of renal impairment, edema, and hypertension. About 30% of patients with acute glomerulonephritis will have gross hematuria, which is described as tea-colored or smoky in appearance. All patients will have microscopic hematuria with red blood cell casts and dysmorphic red blood cells. Proteinuria is present in 80% of patients, with 10% of those having in excess of 2 g per day protein loss (normal urinary protein loss is <150 mg in 24 h). Four percent of children with acute glomerulonephritis will have nephrotic range proteinuria of >3.5 g of protein per day in their urine.

The presence of persistent hematuria with >5 red blood cells per high-power field without red blood cell casts, significant proteinuria, impaired renal function, or evidence of systemic disease is a common problem that may or may not be the result of glomerular disease. Nonglomerular urinary tract lesions that may cause similar findings include infection, prostatism, papillary necrosis, polycystic disease, renal or urinary tract tumors, arteriovenous malformations, renal calculi, blood dyscrasias, hemoglobinopathies, and gynecological sources of blood. The flank pain/hematuria syndrome is seen in young women on oral contraceptives who develop gross hematuria accompanied by flank pain and mild hypertension without proteinuria or decrease in renal function. This entity resolves with cessation of oral contraceptives and is felt to be benign.

Management and Disposition

Patients with acute glomerulonephritis may be managed as inpatients or as closely followed outpatients. Treatment is based in part upon managing the underlying process that incited the acute glomerulonephritis. A biopsy may demonstrate the histological type of glomerulonephritis, but a discussion of immunofluorescence studies and electron microscopies is beyond the scope of this text.

If there is a known precipitating event that has resulted in acute glomerulonephritis, that entity must first be controlled. Infections are treated by appropriate antibiotic therapy, and niduses of infection not immune to antibiotic therapy must be surgically removed, toxic agents must be withdrawn, and systemic disease must be contained if there is any hope of stemming the destructive progression of acute glomerulonephritis.

In the majority of cases, however, there is no known entity precipitating the acute glomerulonephritis. In these cases, the histology of the glomerular lesion as proven by biopsy dictates management. Immunosuppressive agents are a great part of the treatment and work by directly targeting the glomerular pathology. Corticosteroids, cyclophosphamide, cyclosporin, and plasmapheresis work by quieting the inflammatory process that is causing glomerular damage.

In several types of glomerulonephritis, only supportive measures are all that is indicated and management is directed at controlling the clinical sequelae of acute glomerulonephritis. Angiotensin-converting enzyme inhibitors are often employed in controlling hypertension because of their ability to decrease glomerular capillary pressure as well as to lower blood pressure. Renal function must be closely followed when these agents are used to alert the clinician to an unsuspected renal or intrarenal artery stenosis. Loop diuretics are used in cases of clinically significant edema to enhance urinary loss of salt and water.

Chronic Glomerulonephritis

Chronic glomerulonephritis represents the progressive stage of any primary or secondary glomerulonephritis that leads to end-stage renal disease. It is characterized by continued loss of renal function, hematuria, proteinuria, and diminishing kidney size. About 50% of patients will present with advanced renal insufficiency without a history of prior kidney disease.

Outside of the previously noted mechanisms of glomerular injury in acute glomerulonephrosis, the primary mechanism of progressive loss of function in chronic glomerulonephrosis appears to be hemodynamic in nature. Blood flow is shifted from nonfunctioning to functioning glomeruli in an effort to maintain a GFR. This results in increased glomerular capillary flow rates and transcapillary pressure gradients, which translates into glomerular hyperfiltration. Sustained above a certain level over a period of time, hyperfiltration leads to glomerular sclerosis and further loss of renal function, which eventually spirals into end-stage renal failure.

Nephrotic Syndrome

Nephrotic syndrome is defined by proteinuria of >3.5 g per day associated with hypoalbuminemia, edema, hyperlipidemia, and lipiduria. It is not a disease, but a collection of signs and symptoms usually seen in patients with noninflammatory glomerular disease and increased capillary wall permeability. Protein loss is often selective albuminuria only, but not necessarily so. Nephrotic syndrome primarily targets children under the age of 6 years but can occur later in childhood, adolescence, and/or during adulthood. Onset in patients after age 45 years may be associated with acute malignancy. In the majority of cases, nephrotic syndrome has no identifiable cause, although it is generally thought to be immunologically mediated.

Many entities have been associated with nephrotic syndrome, including drugs (gold, penicillamine, ampicillin, and NSAIDs), atopy, tumors, including Hodgkin's disease, lymphoma, and tumors of the lung, breast, and gastrointestinal (GI) tract, viral infections, immunizations, obesity, and dermatitis herpetiformis. Systemic diseases that may incite glomerulonephritis with a nephrotic syndrome include systemic lupus erythematosus, diabetes, and amyloidosis.

The ramifications of the nephrotic syndrome and proteinuria are wide ranging. As a result of the decrease in intravascular oncotic pressure that accompanies loss of circulating proteins, fluid causes edema by moving from the vascular space into the interstitium. Loss of intravascular volume signals the sympathetic nervous system to activate the renin-angiotensin-aldosterone axis to increase distal nephron absorption of sodium and water, which further promotes the accumulation of edema. Facial edema is often the first symptom of nephrotic syndrome. Edema becomes generalized and may accumulate in the pleural and intraperitoneal spaces. Dyspnea encountered in those suffering with nephrotic syndrome is usually a result of ascites or pleural fluid and not pulmonary edema, because the pulmonary capillary wedge pressure is not increased by this process.

Because of the significant decrease in oncotic pressure brought about by marked loss of albumin in the urine, the liver is stimulated to increase synthesis of all proteins, including lipoproteins. This results in a marked increase in all lipid components but especially of low density lipoprotein (LDL) and very low density lipoprotein (VLDL). This results in an acceleration of atherosclerotic vascular disease in these patients.

The association between nephrotic syndrome and intravascular coagulation is long established. Deep venous thrombosis (DVT), arterial thrombosis in children, and renal vein thrombosis are well recognized in nephrotic syndrome. Urinary loss of smaller sized proteins that promote fibrinosis and hepatic overproduction of clotting factors associated with fibrinolysis result in the balance being tipped in favor of coagulation. Platelets exhibit increased aggregability and degranulation during the nephrotic syndrome, and blood viscosity is increased. All of these factors contribute to a hypercoagulable state in the nephrotic patient.

Susceptibility to infection is significantly increased during the nephrotic syndrome. Urinary immunoglobulin loss, circulating immuncomplexes, defective opsonization, abnormal immunoglobulin production, altered cellular immunity, abnormalities of humeral immunity, immunosuppressive therapy, and the accumulation of pleural and peritoneal fluid that provides an excellent breeding ground for bacteria all contribute to this increased susceptibility to infection.

Edema, often facial, and normal or slightly elevated blood pressure are the most consistent physical findings at presentation of nephrotic syndrome.

The urinalysis is characterized by a high specific gravity and 3 to 4+ proteinuria on urine dipstick. The sediment usually reveals oval fat bodies (maltese crosses on a polarized microscope) but may have microscopic hematuria. Gross hematuria can occur in the nephrotic syndrome when incited by glomerulonephritis.

Laboratory Evaluation

Below-normal total serum protein, an albumin of <2 g/dL, hyperlipidemia, electrolyte preservation with the possible exemption of hyponatremia secondary to hyperlipidemia, BUN and creatinine within the normal range, and a normal or slightly elevated hemoglobin are the typical findings at presentation in primary nephrotic syndrome. Exceptions would include nephrotic syndrome secondary to glomerulonephritis, where laboratory findings would include features of both glomerulonephritis and nephrotic syndrome, which must be addressed by the clinician once the diagnosis of nephrotic syndrome has been made.

Management and Disposition

Patients suffering from nephrotic syndrome are best managed by specialists as inpatients initially and then as closely followed outpatients. Biopsy plays an important role in managing these patients as the histology of the glomerular lesion will direct treatment and give clues to prognosis, but such considerations are beyond the scope of this text. If there is an identifiable and treatable cause of nephrotic syndrome, treatment of that entity should cause a remission of the nephrotic syndrome. Beyond those rare instances, corticosteroids are the mainstay of therapy.

Cyclosporin and cyclophosphamide are used in cases of steroid-resistant, steroid-dependent (especially those with marked steroid side effects), and frequently relapsing nephrotics. Treatment response is defined as diuresis and protein-free urine for three consecutive days.

Symptomatic relief may play an important role in management of nephrotic syndrome. Edema may be controlled by sodium restriction to 2 to 3 g per day, and if this fails, the addition of diuretics—usually furosemide or metolazone in combination with spironobictene—is most effective. Water restriction should only be employed in cases of hyponatremia with hypoosmolality. Angiotensin-converting-enzyme inhibitors are first-line management of hypertension and have also been shown the decrease urinary protein loss. In general, these symptom-driven interventions have little use during the acute phase of nephrotic syndrome and play more of a role in chronic cases not responding to steroids or immunosuppressives. Diuretics have limited indications in children with nephrotic syndrome and are most useful in cases involving anasarca, respiratory compromise, scrotal edema threatening perforation, and massive ascites.

The complications of nephrotic syndrome bear reiteration because the prompt recognition and treatment of these entities will favorably affect morbidity and mortality in these patients. The complications include: increased susceptibility to infection, especially subacute bacterial peritonitis; hypercoagulability causing renal vein thrombosis, DVT, and arterial thrombosis in children; premature atherosclerosis; protein malnutrition; osteomalacia and secondary hyperparathyroidism due to loss of vitamin D and its metabolites in the urine; and, rarely, progression to ARF (especially in cases with associated glomerulonephritis).

Selected Readings

Brenner BM, ed. *The Kidney*, 5th ed. Philadelphia: Saunders, 1996.

Davidson AM, et al., eds. *Oxford Textbook of Clinical Nephrology*, 2nd ed. New York: Oxford University Press, 1998.

Issewlbacher KJ, Braunwald E, Wilson JD, et al., eds. *Harrison's Principles of Internal Medicine*, 13th ed. New York: McGraw-Hill, 1994.

Massry SG, Glassock RJ, eds. *Textbook of Nephrology*, 4th ed. Philadelphia: Lippincott, Williams Wilkins, 2001.

Roberts S, Isles C, Moro I. Glomerular diseases made easier. I. *Br J Hosp Med* 1995; 53:261–266.

Roberts S, Isles C, Moro I. Glomerular diseases made easier. II. *Br J Hosp Med* 1995;53:323–326.

Roberts S, Isles C, Moro I. Glomerular diseases made easier. III. *Br J Hosp Med* 1995; 53:379–386.

Schrier RW, Gottschalk CW, eds. *Diseases of the Kidney*, 5th ed. Boston: Little, Brown, 1993.

Schrier RW, ed. *Diseases of the Kidney and Urinary Tract*, 7th ed. Philadelphia: Lippincott, Williams & Wilkins, 2001.

Wyngaarden JB, Smith LH Jr, Bennett JC, eds. *Cecil's Textbook of Medicine*, 19th ed. Philadelphia: Saunders, 1992.

CHAPTER

112 Acute Interstitial Nephritis

Ronald Moscati

Acute interstitial nephritis (AIN) is an inflammatory process involving the renal tubules and interstitium. If not recognized promptly, AIN may result in acute renal failure. Onset of symptoms is abrupt and usually reversible. Although symptoms sometimes mimic glomerulonephritis, the glomeruli and renal vasculature are not involved. The presence of permanent changes, such as fibrosis in the tubular interstitium, is characteristic of chronic interstitial nephritis.

The major etiologies for AIN include immune mediated mechanisms, infection-related causes, and idiopathic causes. Immune mediated mechanisms include those associated with medication use as well as those in which patients have underlying immune disorders. Medication related cases are the most common cause of AIN in Western society. Infection-related cases include renal and systemic infections. In patients with acute renal failure who undergo biopsy, AIN is reported in 1% to 14% of cases.

Pathophysiology

Many features of AIN, such as fever, rash, and eosinophilia, suggest an immune mediated mechanism. The mechanism begins with the development of antibodies either to an inciting substance, such as a medication, or to antigens on the tubular basement membrane (TBM). The immune complexes formed by antibody binding then deposit in the renal tissue initiating an inflammatory response. Cell-mediated tissue injury occurs with infiltration by T-lymphocytes, monocytes, and macrophages.

The reason that certain drugs can lead to AIN or why certain individuals develop it is not known. Because many medications and their metabolites are excreted renally, the renal tubules are exposed to higher concentrations of these substances, which may lead to the medication binding to proteins on the TBM. There does not seem to be a clear relationship between either the dose or duration of medication and the development of AIN. The four main drug groups implicated are antibiotics, anti-inflammatory agents, diuretics and anticonvulsants. With infection-related AIN, it is thought that antigens from the infectious agent or immune complexes formed from the infection are deposited in the kidney eliciting the initial immune reaction.

Clinical Presentation

The clinical presentation in AIN varies from cases with mildly abnormal urinary sediment to cases with acute renal failure. Findings of hypersensitivity may be present. Patients on drug therapy who present with these symptoms should be suspected of having AIN.

Drug induced AIN appears to be a hypersensitivity reaction with abrupt onset of renal dysfunction along with fever, erythematous rash, and peripheral eosinophilia. Patients may also experience arthralgias, flank pain, lymphadenopathy, and other extrarenal signs of hypersensitivity. While most patients who develop AIN while on antibiotics are on high doses for severe infections, it can occur in patients on any dose for any time period. The time of onset has been reported to vary from the second to sixtieth day after starting a medication. In this form of AIN, proteinuria and either microscopic or macroscopic hematuria are universally present. Methicillin is the most commonly associated antibiotic, but other penicillins, cephalosporins, sulfonamides, and rifampin have occasionally been reported to cause a similar clinical picture.

Nonsteroidal anti-inflammatory drugs (NSAIDs) are also capable of inducing AIN. This is different from NSAID-related renal failure in which renal arterial blood flow is decreased. The clinical picture in NSAID-related AIN may not involve signs of hypersensitivity. Most of these patients have heavy proteinuria consistent with a nephrotic syndrome as well as hematuria, hyperkalemia, hyperchloremia, metabolic acidosis, and renal failure. Generally, this occurs in elderly patients with long-term NSAID use. Removal of the drug usually results in return of renal function.

Diuretics such as thiazide and furosemide and anticonvulsants, such as phenytoin, phenobarbital, and carbamazepine have rarely been reported to cause AIN. Symptoms are similar to methicillin-induced AIN. Almost all of these causes of drug-induced AIN resolve with removal of the offending agent.

AIN as a complication of infection can be seen with viral, bacterial, rickettsial, mycoplasmal, and parasitic pathogens. The primary source of infection is septicemia. Streptococcal infections are the most common of the infectious causes in the pediatric population. There is a 30% mortality with AIN and uncontrolled infection, but if infection is controlled rapidly, renal function usually returns to baseline.

Some patients with AIN have existing immune disorders such as lupus, uveitis, vasculitis, Sjögren's syndrome, or sarcoidosis. Additionally, idiopathic cases may result from hypersensitivity reactions to unidentified environmental agents.

Diagnosis

Patients taking the medications discussed above or those with renal or generalized infections who develop urine abnormalities or acute renal failure may have AIN. Fever, skin rash, eosinophilia, or hemolytic anemia help to establish the diagnosis. The diagnosis of AIN can be proven by renal biopsy. Patients with a suggestive history may have laboratory testing performed in the ED to try to confirm the diagnosis. The most common electrolyte abnormalities seen are hyperkalemia, hyperchloremia, and a metabolic acidosis with, in most cases, a normal anion gap. Creatinine and BUN can be elevated or normal. Serum sodium may be elevated if urine concentrating ability is impaired. A CBC may reveal eosinophilia. This is seen more commonly when there are clinical signs of hypersensitivity. If present, eosinophilia ranges between 10% and 30%; however, the absence of eosinophilia does not rule out AIN. Anemia may be present, particularly in those patients who have developed acute renal failure. Urinalysis usually demonstrates hematuria, proteinuria, and pyuria. Eosinophiluria is reported to be present in 50% to 90% of cases of drug-related AIN and, if present is strongly suggestive of AIN. Gallium renal scans have intense radionuclide uptake in AIN that decreases when AIN resolves. Plain radiographs and sonography may demonstrate kidney enlargement.

The differential diagnosis in AIN includes vasculitis, acute tubular necrosis, rapidly progressive glomerulonephritis, and thromboembolic disease. While differentiation on clinical grounds is difficult, the presence of associated hypersensitivity symptoms argues strongly for AIN. Resolution of renal failure upon discontinuing the offending agent is also more suggestive of AIN.

Management and Disposition

In medication related AIN, patients usually recover most of their baseline renal function when the agent is discontinued, with the time to recovery varying from days to weeks. Failure to recognize the disease and withdraw the agent can lead to prolonged renal impairment and death.

The administration of corticosteroids for treatment of AIN is controversial. Corticosteroids are reported to result in more rapid resolution of symptoms. However, objective trials are lacking.

Management of the renal abnormalities is dependent upon the degree of renal impairment. Those patients with abnormalities of urinary sediment or minor electrolyte abnormalities may be managed with supportive care after withdrawing the medication. Patients with oliguric renal failure frequently require hemodialysis until their renal function improves. Approximately one third of patients with AIN require hemodialysis.

Selected Readings

Cameron JS. Allergic interstitial nephritis: clinical features and pathogenesis. *Q J Med* 1988;66:97–115.

Gruenfeld JP, Kleinknecht D, Droz D. Acute interstitial nephritis. In: Schrier RW, Gottschalk CW, eds. *Diseases of the Kidney,* 5th ed, Boston: Little, Brown and Company, 1992:1331–1353.

Kodner C, Kudrimoti A. Diagnosis and management of acute interstitial nephritis. *Am Fam Phys* 2003;67:2527–2534.

Michel D, Kelly C. Acute interstitial nephritis. *J Am Soc Nephrol* 1998;9:506-515.

Toto RD. Review: acute tubulointerstitial nephritis. *Am J Med Sci* 1990;299: 392–410.

Acute and Chronic Renal Failure and Interstitial Tubular Necrosis

Richard S. Krause

Acute Renal Failure

The kidneys excrete end products of metabolism and regulate the concentration of many of the chemical constituents of the body. In normally functioning adult kidneys, approximately 20% of the resting cardiac output is filtered at the glomerulus. The glomerular filtration rate (GFR) averages 125 mL/min in adults. Approximately 99% of the water in the glomerular filtrate is reabsorbed in the renal tubules, along with electrolytes and other small molecules such as uric acid and glucose, and the resulting fluid is excreted as urine.

The clinical features of acute renal failure (ARF) are due to a rapid decline in renal function. Disturbances of volume regulation, acid-base balance, and electrolyte metabolism are responsible for the clinical features of ARF. Acute tubular necrosis (ATN) is a subset of ARF in which reversible renal failure is caused by renal ischemia (or other conditions) and that often results in the histologic pattern of interstitial tubular necrosis.

ARF may be described as oliguric, nonoliguric, and polyuric. In oliguric renal failure, the urine volume is <400 mL/m^2/d. The urine volume exceeds 400 mL/m^2/day in nonoliguric renal failure, and exceeds 3 L per day in polyuric renal failure. The expected decrease in urine output resulting from a decrease in the GFR is not always seen early in the course of ARF, and polyuria may occur early as the ability of the kidney to concentrate urine is lost.

Prerenal azotemia accounts for approximately 55% of cases of ARF. When renal hypoperfusion of any cause is sufficiently severe to cause a decrease in the GFR, a rise in the serum BUN concentration (azotemia) results. The azotemia is rapidly reversible if renal perfusion is promptly restored by volume resuscitation or discontinuation of an offending agent. Reversibility is thus one of the hallmarks of prerenal azotemia. If the hypoperfusion is sufficiently prolonged or severe, hypoxic renal parenchymal injury may result in ATN and irreversible renal failure. The most common causes of acute prerenal azotemia are conditions that cause volume loss. These include GI losses, diuretic use, hemorrhage, and dehydration due to environmental factors. In prerenal azotemia, the ratio of BUN to creatinine is increased above the normal ratio of 10:1, urine

specific gravity is increased, and urine sodium is <10 mEq/dL.

Renal blood flow is mediated in part by prostaglandins that act as vasodilators. NSAIDs inhibit vasodilator prostaglandin synthesis and decrease renal blood flow, leading to a condition similar to prerenal azotemia but with normal circulating volume and renal blood flow. NSAIDs are especially likely to precipitate ARF in patients with preexisting renal insufficiency, congestive heart failure (CHF), or cirrhosis. Diabetes, diuretic use, and advanced age are also risk factors for the development of NSAID-induced ARF. NSAIDs should be used in patients at increased risk at low doses for short periods. ARF secondary to NSAIDs is usually reversible if the drug is promptly discontinued. ACE inhibitors also decrease renal blood flow and may precipitate ARF.

Renal parenchymal injuries account for 40% of cases of ARF in adults. In children, intrinsic renal disease accounts for approximately 50% of the cases of ARF. Most cases are secondary to renal ischemia or exposure to nephrotoxins. Other causes include vasculitis, glomerulonephritis, interstitial nephritis, and scleroderma.

Acute glomerulonephritis due to an immunologic mechanism may present as a manifestation of a primary renal process or a number of systemic illnesses, including vasculitis, Henoch-Schönlein purpura, systemic lupus erythematosus, and endocarditis. Primary renal causes of acute glomerulonephritis include poststreptococcal glomerulonephritis or other postinfectious glomerulonephritides, and rapidly progressive glomerulonephritis.

Acute interstitial nephritis (AIN) is a consequence of exposure to a nephrotoxin, infection, or infiltration. Allergic reactions to certain drugs are commonly implicated. Causes include beta-lactam antibiotics, sulfonamides, diuretics, captopril, and NSAIDs. Bacterial, viral, and fungal infections may all cause AIN. Infiltration from lymphoma, leukemia, and sarcoidosis are additional causes of AIN.

Renovascular disease may cause renal failure. Both the large extrarenal and the smaller intrarenal vessels may be affected. Unless there is only one functioning kidney, the process must be bilateral to produce ARF. Embolism to the renal arteries may occur in the setting of renal arteriography, endocarditis, or chronic atrial fibrillation. While the process is often subclinical, renal artery embolism may present with acute symptoms of pain, nausea, vomiting, and hematuria. The diagnosis is made by renal arteriography. Renal vein thrombosis is a relatively common complication of the nephrotic syndrome and may also occur in the setting of pregnancy or oral contraceptive use. Renal vein compression and invasion by tumor are other causes of renal vein thrombosis. The diagnosis is made by renal venography. Anticoagulation is usually indicated to prevent pulmonary embolism. If recannulation occurs, there may be an improvement in renal function.

Disease of the smaller intrarenal vessels may also cause ARF. Malignant hypertension associated with ARF is most often seen in previously hypertensive individuals, particularly African-American males. The syndrome usually begins with neurologic symptoms and progresses to cardiac decompensation and ARF with hematuria and proteinuria. A microangiopathic hemolytic anemia with schistocytes on peripheral blood smear is usually present. Histologic examination of the kidneys shows changes in both the arterioles and interlobar arteries. Rapid control of hypertension often allows recovery of renal function. A syndrome known as scleroderma renal crisis may occur in patients with known or previously undiagnosed scleroderma. The renal manifestations are similar to those seen in malignant hypertension. ACE inhibitors have been reported to be helpful in treating this condition.

Acute tubular necrosis (ATN) refers to a type of intrinsic renal parenchymal damage due to toxic or ischemic injury. ATN is the most common cause of reversible, intrinsic renal failure. In ATN, the underlying renal histology usually reveals significant tubular cell death. In ischemic ATN, a complex set of intrarenal interactions between various hormonal systems occurs, with the end result of tubular cell injury and possible tubular obstruction from cellular debris. In toxic ATN, a nephrotoxin directly affects tubular cells.

Ischemic ATN is similar to prerenal azotemia but does not resolve rapidly upon restoration of renal perfusion. Any cause of severe renal hypoperfusion may lead to ischemic ATN. Common causes include trauma, cardiovascular or aortic surgery, severe dehydration, sepsis, and hemorrhage. Renal hypoperfusion leads to cellular ischemia, particularly in the region of the outer renal medulla and corticomedullary junction, which are relatively hypoxic compared to the rest of the renal cortex. Cellular necrosis of tubular epithelium leads to back-leak of filtered solutes, effectively reducing the GFR. Sloughing of tubular cells may obstruct the tubular lumen and further reduce the GFR.

Toxic ATN may be caused by exogenous nephrotoxins or the endogenous pigments hemoglobin and myoglobin. Commonly implicated exogenous nephrotoxins include intravenous contrast material, aminoglycoside antibiotics, cyclosporine, cisplatin, and ethylene glycol. Rhabdomyolysis is seen in crush injuries, severe hypokalemia, seizures, cocaine use, hyperthermia, muscle ischemia from arterial occlusion, or severe exercise, and is often associated with alcoholism. Transfusion reactions are the most common cause of ARF from hemolysis. The exact mechanism by which rhabdomyolysis and hemolysis cause ARF has not been determined, but both direct toxic effects of erythrocyte and myocyte components on the tubular epithelium and intrarenal obstruction from tubular cast formation are felt to contribute.

Radiocontrast-induced renal injury is a common cause of ARF. Many patients show asymptomatic increases in serum creatinine 1 to 3 days after exposure, with a decline to normal levels within 2 weeks. Severe, symptomatic ARF requiring dialysis also occurs. Several risk factors for the development of significant contrast-induced ARF have been identified. The most important is preexisting renal insufficiency. Less than 2% of patients with normal renal function experience a significant increase in serum creatinine. Up to one third of patients with a baseline serum creatinine over 2.5 mg/dL experience a significant increase in serum creatinine. Other identified risk factors include diabetes, multiple myeloma, advanced age, dehydration, and higher doses of intravenous radiocontrast material.

Urinary tract obstruction due to urethral or bilateral ureteral obstruction is the cause of approximately 5% of the cases of ARF (see section entitled Obstructive Uropathy above).

Diagnosis

The diagnosis of ARF rests on the laboratory demonstration of increases in serum urea (azotemia) and creatinine. Often, this occurs when blood tests are sent to screen patients with nonspecific signs and symptoms. At other times, patients present with signs and symptoms specifically related to the metabolic and physiological disturbances that are the consequences of decreased renal function. Alternatively, a patient may present with flank pain, hematuria, or some other symptom specifically referable to the urinary tract. Rarely, a patient may present with the specific complaint of absent or decreased urine output, leading both the patient and physician to suspect renal disease.

Early in the course of ARF, the only symptoms present may be those of a primary, nonrenal disorder. As GFR decreases, the ability to excrete dietary water is diminished and fluid overload results. Mild volume overload may cause peripheral edema or increased body weight and girth, but frank pulmonary edema may occur with severe volume expansion. Most patients are hypertensive. Inability to excrete water may cause hyponatremia, with changes in mental status, lethargy, or seizures.

When GFR falls to less than 50% of normal, the ability to excrete hydrogen ion decreases. Unmeasured anions, including phosphate and sulfate, are retained, and metabolic acidosis, with an increased anion gap, occurs. Metabolic acidosis thus often complicates ARF. Compensatory hyperpnea occurs and may cause dyspnea independent of pulmonary congestion.

Potassium homeostasis is preserved early in the course of ARF. Potassium is filtered at the glomerulus and reabsorbed in the renal tubule. Potassium is also secreted in the terminal portion of the nephron. As the mass of functioning nephrons is reduced, decreased potassium absorption and increased secretion initially compensate and the serum potassium concentration remains normal. As compensatory mechanisms fail, serum potassium rises. Acidosis also contributes to elevated serum potassium levels. Serum potassium levels of <6.0 mEq/L are often asymptomatic. At higher levels, the nervous system is affected, with symptoms of weakness, parasthesias, and paralysis occurring. Electrocardiogram (EKG) abnormalities progress from peaked T waves and prolonged P-R intervals to QRS widening, ventricular tachycardia or fibrillation, and asystole as hyperkalemia progresses.

Once azotemia is noted, it is important to determine if renal failure is acute or chronic. In the setting of a previously healthy patient with signs and symptoms of ARF, especially when a precipitating cause is present, the differentiation of acute versus chronic renal failure (CRF) may be obvious. At other times, additional history must be sought from previously documented laboratory tests or other health care providers. Clues to the presence of CRF include anemia, hypocalcemia, and hyperphosphatemia. In many cases, patients with preexisting mild renal impairment will present with worsening azotemia. The approach to these patients should be similar to that taken with patients who present with new onset renal failure. A medication history, including nonprescription drugs, is part of the workup. Drugs may precipitate either prerenal azotemia (diuretics, ACE inhibitors, NSAIDs), obstruction (tricyclics, other anticholinergics), or direct parenchymal injury (intravenous contrast, aminoglycosides). Environmental exposures to nephrotoxins (glycols, organic solvents, heavy metals) should also be considered. At times, patients without previously recognized renal disease may present with full blown uremia. Most major organ systems can be affected, including the CNS (lethargy, coma, seizures), immune system (sepsis), cardiovascular system (pericarditis, pericardial effusion or tamponade), integument (pruritus), GI system (nausea, vomiting), and the hematological system (anemia). These symptoms may be present individually or in any combination; renal failure should be considered whenever they are encountered.

After the diagnosis of ARF is established, steps should be taken to diagnose reversible causes. Prerenal azotemia is suspected when there is evidence of volume loss from bleeding, excessive GI losses, cutaneous losses such as burns, and in patients with restricted access to fluids or increased environmental losses. Diuretics predispose patients to develop prerenal azotemia and are most often used in patients with CHF, which may itself cause prerenal azotemia. Volume depletion may be suspected when there is weakness, postural dizziness or hypotension, excessive thirst, vomiting or diarrhea, GI bleeding, tachycardia, or dry mucous membranes. The hepatorenal syndrome should be suspected in patients with liver disease and ARF.

Obstructive uropathy may be painless if obstruction develops slowly. Acute obstruction is very likely to cause colicky pain in the suprapubic area or flank. Prostatic disease is suggested by hesitancy, frequency, or nocturia. Lower tract symptoms in females may represent infection or pelvic tumor. Pelvic and rectal exams are therefore recommended in cases of ARF.

Intrarenal causes of ARF should be considered after obvious cases of obstruction and prerenal azotemia have been excluded. These may be caused by nephrotoxins or be associated with infectious processes. A history of exposure to intravenous contrast material, prescription and nonprescription medications, or other toxins (e.g., ethylene glycol) should be sought. Signs and symptoms of acute glomerulonephritis include pharyngitis, hypertension, facial edema, and dark-colored urine. Hemolytic-uremic syndrome is a cause of renal failure in children and may also occur in adults. It usually follows an episode of gastroenteritis with crampy abdominal pain, vomiting, and bloody stools. Hypertension, petechiae, edema, and hepatosplenomegaly with irritability or lethargy are seen. If renal failure occurs after cancer chemotherapy, acute tumor lysis syndrome with resulting urate nephropathy should be suspected.

Chemical and microscopic examination of the urine is useful in the workup of ARF. An active urine sediment with many red cell casts suggests an inflammatory etiology such as glomerulonephritis, whereas urine sediment with few formed elements or only hyaline casts suggests prerenal azotemia or obstructive uropathy. Brownish pigmented cellular casts and renal tubular epithelial cells are often noted in ATN. Oxalate crystals suggest ethylene glycol toxicity, and large numbers of urate crystals may be seen in acute uric acid nephropathy. Large numbers of polymorphonuclear leukocytes and bacteria suggest infection. A positive dipstick test for blood in the absence of microscopic hematuria suggests either hemolysis with hemoglobinuria or myoglobinuria. High levels of proteinuria are most often seen in glomerular disease. In confusing cases, measurement of urine sodium may be useful in differentiating prerenal from intrarenal pathology. In prerenal azotemia, sodium is avidly reabsorbed in an attempt to maintain intravascular volume. Intrinsic renal failure causes tubular dysfunction and inability to reabsorb sodium. As a result, the urine sodium concentration is low (<10 mEq/L) in prerenal azotemia and higher (>40 mEq/L) in intrarenal disease.

The main use for imaging studies in the ED evaluation of ARF is in the diagnosis of urinary tract obstruction. A plain abdominal film may suggest stone disease and will help evaluate renal size. Retrograde pyelography does not lead to contrast-induced nephrotoxicity and provides definitive information about the presence and location of obstruction. Intravenous pyelography should be avoided due to the nephrotoxic effects of intravenous contrast material. Renal ultrasound is both sensitive (98%) and moderately specific (80%) in the detection of hydronephrosis. Ultrasound also provides measurements of the kidneys; bilateral small kidneys suggest CRF. Noncontrast CT scanning provides similar information and may also reveal the site of obstruction and suggest an etiology. **Table 113.1** lists diagnostic tests that should be considered in the evaluation of a patient with ARF.

Evaluation and Management

Management and evaluation frequently overlap in the ED management of ARF. As with all patients, potentially life-

Table 113.1

Diagnostic Tests in Acute Renal Failure

Test	Rationale[a]
CXR	Possible pulmonary congestion
Other imaging studies	See text
EKG	Possible changes secondary to hyperkalemia
Electrolytes	Hyperkalemia, hyper/hyponatremia
Bicarbonate	Acid-base status
BUN, creatinine	Diagnosis and differential diagnosis of ARF
Glucose	Detection of hyper/hypoglycemia
CBC	Diagnosis of CRF, evidence of bleeding or infection
Liver function tests	Diagnosis of hepatorenal syndrome
Calcium	Hypocalcemia
Phosphate	Hyperphosphatemia
Urinalysis	Differential diagnosis of ARF
Urate	Hyperuricemia
Magnesium	Hypermagnesemia
Urine sodium[b]	Differential diagnosis of ARF
Urine creatinine[b]	Differential diagnosis of ARF

[a]Based on the clinical condition of the patient.
[b]Simultaneous with serum tests.

threatening complications of ARF must be addressed first. Hyperkalemia is the most immediately life-threatening complication of ARF. Hyperkalemia primarily affects the cardiovascular system and is essentially asymptomatic until potentially life-threatening dysrhythmias occur. In addition to measurements of serum potassium, an EKG should be obtained when hyperkalemia is suspected. EKG signs of hyperkalemia develop progressively as serum potassium rises above 5.5 to 6.0 mEq/L. Tall, peaked T waves are seen initially and are followed by PR and QT interval prolongation. At a potassium concentration of 6.5 to 7.0 mEq/L, diminished P waves and ST depression or

elevation are seen. As potassium levels rise above 7.0 mEq/L, AV conduction is impaired and bundle branch block or an idioventricular rhythm may be seen. At levels of >7.5 to 8.0 mEq/L, P waves are no longer seen and QRS prolongation is progressive. Eventually, the QRS complex and the T wave merge and a sine wave pattern is seen. Ventricular fibrillation or cardiac standstill are terminal events. If there are EKG signs of hyperkalemia in a patient with known or suspected renal failure, treatment should be initiated prior to laboratory confirmation of hyperkalemia. ED treatment of hyperkalemia is outlined in **Table 113.2**. Pericarditis with pericardial effusion and tamponade are also associated with CRF. The presentation and ED treatment do not differ from that in the patient with normal renal function. Table 113.2 describes the ED treatment of hyperkalemia.

Pulmonary edema may be treated with oxygen, upright positioning of the patient, nitrates, and diuretics. Dialysis is often needed for refractory pulmonary edema or severe hyperkalemia. In the case of less severe volume overload, intravenous fluids and salt intake should be avoided. Diuretics may be effective.

In cases of acute hypertensive emergency, nitrates or nitroprusside may be used. Drug dosages may require adjustment, and the ototoxicity of loop diuretics is increased in renal failure.

After beginning treatment for potentially life-threatening complications of ARF, reversible causes of renal dysfunction may be sought and corrected. If prerenal azotemia due to volume depletion is suspected, intravascular volume must be restored with either crystalloid or blood. When prerenal azotemia occurs in the presence of normal or increased total body water and sodium (e.g., CHF, ACE inhibitors), the underlying disorder must be corrected. In most cases of ARF, the bladder should be catheterized. This procedure will be both therapeutic and diagnostic for lower tract obstruction. If the bladder cannot be catheterized and obstruction is suspected, urologic consultation should be considered. After relief of obstruction, a postobstructive diuresis may occur with significant fluid loss and hypovolemia. Close monitoring of fluid balance and electrolyte concentration is needed. After correction of prerenal factors

Table 113.2

Emergency Treatment of Hyperkalemia

Agent	Dose/Route (for Adults)	Time to Onset	Notes
Calcium chloride or calcium gluconate	10 cc of 10% solution (IV)	1 min	Slow IV push
Sodium bicarbonate	50 mg (IV)	5 min	May cause Na or volume overload
Furosemide	40–400 mg (IV)	15 min	Effective only in nonoliguric patients; may cause ototoxicity
Glucose and insulin	Glucose, 50 g (IV); followed by regular insulin, 10 U (IV)	30 min	May cause hyper- or hypoglycemia
Albuterol	10 mg (nebulized inhalation)	30 min	
Ion exchange resin (Kayexalate)	25 g (PO) or 50 g (IV)	Hours	May cause Na overload

and relief of obstruction, it is common practice to administer potent loop diuretics (e.g., furosemide) or mannitol to patients with oliguric ARF. The rationale for this treatment is the observation of lower morbidity and mortality of nonoliguric ARF compared with the oliguric variety. Low-dose dopamine (1 to 3 μg/kg/min) increases renal blood flow and may enhance the response to diuretics.

Patients with ARF should be considered for hospital admission and early consultation with a nephrologist. One notable exception is the patient with prerenal azotemia due to an easily correctable cause such as diuretic use or GI losses. If the primary process can be corrected and the volume deficit replaced, such patients may be considered for discharge with close follow-up.

Prevention of ARF is important due to the high morbidity and mortality of the condition. Early and aggressive fluid resuscitation of hypovolemic trauma patients may prevent or minimize the severity of ARF. Maintenance of high urine output in cases of hemolysis (e.g., transfusion reaction), rhabdomyolysis, or other exposures to nephrotoxins is also preventative. Avoidance of nephrotoxins, especially in high-risk patients, will minimize iatrogenic ARF. Intravenous contrast material should be administered cautiously to high-risk patients and only when clearly needed. The risk of contrast-induced ARF is minimized when patients are well hydrated prior to contrast administration.

Chronic Renal Failure

Seventy-five percent of cases of CRF in adults in the United States are caused by diabetic nephropathy, hypertension, or glomerulonephritis. In certain geographic areas, HIV-related renal failure may be common. Reflux nephropathy is the most common cause of CRF in children. Irrespective of the cause of CRF, as renal function progressively declines, a uremic syndrome eventually develops. Early in the course of CRF, when the GFR is greater than 35% to 50% of normal, patients are asymptomatic and serum levels of urea and creatinine are normal. When renal function declines to less than approximately 35% of normal, serum urea and creatinine levels begin to rise (azotemia) and symptoms begin to occur. As GFR decreases to less than 20% to 25% of normal, overt uremia occurs.

The physiological and metabolic derangements of uremia are thought to be due to the accumulation of the products of amino acid metabolism in the serum. Both decreased renal excretion of metabolic products and decreased renal catabolism of circulating peptide hormones contribute to toxin accumulation. Urea itself is the most abundant product of nitrogen metabolism and is responsible for only some of the toxicity of uremia. Other metabolic products are present in smaller amounts, but probably are more responsible than urea for uremic symptoms. Loss of active vitamin D production with increased plasma levels of parathyroid hormone has adverse effects on calcium and phosphate metabolism. These metabolic abnormalities are major contributors to the uremic syndrome. Volume overload occurs when water and salt are ingested in excess of losses and excretion. Excess free water intake causes hyponatremia. Except in cases of dietary excess or administration of potassium-containing or antikaliuretic drugs, potassium homeostasis is usually maintained until GFR drops to <5 mL/min. When renal function declines to this point, hyperkalemia with attendant cardiac toxicity may develop suddenly. Metabolic acidosis is a result of the inability to excrete acid and decreased production of endogenous buffers.

All major organ systems are affected by CRF, and patients with CRF suffer from malaise, weakness, and fatigue. Fluid overload often results in CHF or pulmonary edema secondary to increased alveolar capillary permeability. Pulmonary edema responds to dialysis. If pulmonary congestion is severe, arrangements for early dialysis should be made. Temporizing measures prior to dialysis may be effective and should be initiated promptly. These include application of oxygen and maintenance of an upright position. Topical, sublingual or intravenous nitrates may be beneficial due to decreases in preload and afterload. Nitroprusside is appropriate when there is severe hypertension. In patients who have residual urine output, high doses of loop diuretics may be effective.

GI disturbances are common in uremic patients. Anorexia, nausea, hiccups, and vomiting are chronic problems that may respond to conventional symptomatic treatment and usually improve with dialysis. Constipation is commonly seen in CRF. Sorbitol, bulk-forming laxatives, and stool softeners may be used. Magnesium-containing cathartics and phosphate or saline enemas should be avoided due to the risk of precipitating metabolic abnormalities. Peptic ulceration and diverticulosis are more prevalent in patients with CRF.

Early in the development of uremia, subtle neurological disturbances are common and include fatigue, difficulty concentrating, memory loss, and sleep disturbances. In advanced uremia, there may be delusions, hallucinations, seizures, stupor, and coma. These abnormalities are usually responsive to dialysis. Peripheral neuropathy is common in CRF and tends to affect the lower extremities more than the upper. Uremic neuropathy begins with sensory changes, followed by motor involvement and loss of reflexes. Foot drop (peroneal nerve palsy) and the restless legs syndrome are disturbing complications of CRF. In the restless legs syndrome, there is a sensation of discomfort and the need to frequently move the feet and legs. It is especially disturbing at night and may respond to benzodiazepines given before bed. Permanent neuropathy may be preventable with early institution of dialysis.

Anemia is an almost inevitable problem in CRF. It is normochromic and normocytic, and is due to decreased erythropoiesis. The anemia of CRF may be treated effectively with recombinant human erythropoietin. Uremia causes derangements in leukocyte chemotaxis. Patients with CRF therefore have an increased susceptibility to infection and may have a less pronounced febrile response to infection when compared to healthy individuals. Abnormal hemostasis may cause a tendency to abnormal bleeding and bruising in CRF.

The most disturbing dermatological consequence of uremia is pruritus. It is often severe and unresponsive to conventional systemic and topical therapies. Pruritus does not respond well to dialysis. Abnormal skin coloration is also common. Many patients have a sallow, yellow cast due to retention of pigments known as urochromes.

In general terms, the liver is the primary organ involved in the biotransformation of drugs into metabolites (which may be active or inactive). The kidney is the primary route of excretion for most parent drugs and metabolites. The two primary mechanisms that affect the choice and dose of drugs in renal failure are altered excretion and changes in protein binding. Excretion of drugs by the kidney depends upon glomerular filtration and to a lesser extent on tubular secretion and absorption. As these processes are impaired when renal function declines, the half life of many drugs increases and toxic concentrations may develop.

Choice of antibiotics in renal failure is based on standard indications. Penicillins and cephalosporins are excreted by the kidney, with some agents subject to hepatic metabolism. All drugs in these two classes may cause allergic interstitial nephritis. Some agents contain significant amounts of sodium (ampicillin, carbenicillin, moxalactam). Penicillin V potassium contains 2.7 mEq of potassium per gram. Usual doses of most penicillins and cephalosporins are appropriate, but the dosage interval should be increased. Supplemental doses may be needed after dialysis to maintain serum levels. Macrolide antibiotics undergo hepatic metabolism. Azithromycin is given in usual doses, but a decreased dose of clarithromycin or erythromycin is recommended. Aminoglycoside antibiotics are nephrotoxic and ototoxic. Usual initial doses are given, but subsequent doses and dosing intervals are altered. Formulas exist for dosage calculations, but therapy should be guided by serum levels. Vancomycin may be given as a single dose after each hemodialysis treatment. Fluoroquinolone antibiotics are excreted by the kidney. Fluoroquinolone dosage should be decreased in renal failure. Metronidazole is metabolized by the liver and excreted by the kidney. Usual doses are given at increased intervals in renal failure. Acyclovir is excreted by the kidney. It may cause CNS toxicity in CRF and can cause ARF when given rapidly intravenously. A decreased dose at increased intervals is recommended for patients with renal failure. TMP/SMX is excreted by the kidney and undergoes hepatic metabolism. An increased dosage interval with usual doses is recommended.

All NSAIDs are potentially nephrotoxic and should be given cautiously to patients with decreased renal function. Aspirin is metabolized in the liver and excreted by the kidney. The metabolic byproducts are active, and the drug should be used cautiously or not at all in patients with renal failure. Ibuprofen is metabolized in the liver and may be used in decreased doses. Acetaminophen is metabolized in the liver. It may be given in usual doses at increased intervals to patients with renal failure. A regimen of 650 mg of acetaminophen every 8 hours is a reasonable starting dose. Codeine and morphine are primarily metabolized in the liver, and usual regimens may be given to patients with renal failure. A decreased dose is suggested with prolonged usage. Meperidine may also be given in usual doses, but active metabolites accumulate in renal failure, making this drug useful primarily for acute usage only. Corticosteroids are metabolized in the liver and may cause salt and water retention in patients with diminished renal function. Acute dosages are unchanged, but decreased doses are used chronically.

Drugs used as sedatives and anticonvulsants include barbiturates, phenytoin, and benzodiazepines. Benzodiazepines and most of the commonly used barbiturates are primarily metabolized by the liver, but certain agents are also subject to renal excretion. Normal doses are used acutely, with decreased doses when use is chronic. Phenytoin is metabolized in the liver and excreted by the kidney. Haloperidol and phenothiazine antipsychotics are metabolized in the liver. For phenytoin, haloperidol, and the phenothiazines, acute doses are unchanged in renal failure. Decreased doses are employed when they are used on a chronic basis.

The calcium channel blockers and most beta-blockers (propranolol, labetalol, and metoprolol) are all metabolized in the liver. Acute doses are unchanged in renal failure patients, but dosage may need to be decreased when used chronically. Lidocaine and procainamide are also given in the usual acute dosages, with adjustments only for chronic dosing. Bretylium is excreted by the kidney and reported to be poorly tolerated in patients with renal failure and should be avoided when possible. Angiotensin-converting enzymes inhibitors are subject to both hepatic metabolism and renal excretion. They may precipitate renal failure by decreasing renal blood flow. Dosage is determined by the response observed. Nitrates are metabolized in the liver and may be used in the usual acute dosage. Sodium nitroprusside is metabolized in the periphery to cyanide and thiocyanate, both of which are toxic. Thiocyanate is excreted by the kidney, and the half life is prolonged in renal failure. Acute dosages of nitroprusside are adjusted according to the response, but thiocyanate levels must be used to guide chronic treatment. The half life of digoxin increases with decreasing creatinine clearance, and serum levels increase with chronic dosing. When used acutely, the usual doses are employed, with subsequent doses adjusted using serum levels and therapeutic response.

Doses of Coumadin® and heparin are adjusted according to the response of clotting parameters. Slightly lower doses of heparin may be needed in CRF due to increased half life. Streptokinase and tissue plasminogen activator (t-PA) are used in the usual doses.

The paralytic agent of choice for renal failure patients is vecuronium. It is metabolized by the liver, but a prolonged effect may be seen in renal failure. Succinylcholine and other depolarizing agents should be avoided in renal failure due to the risk of hyperkalemia.

Selected Readings

Anderson RJ, Linas SL, Berns AS, et al. Nonoliguric acute renal failure. *N Engl J Med* 1977;296:1134–1138.

Brady HR, Brenner BM. Acute renal failure. In: Fauci AS, Braunwald E, Isselbacher KJ, et al., eds. *Harrison's Principles of Internal Medicine,* 14th ed. New York: McGraw-Hill, 1998:1504–1513.

Brenner BM, Hostetter TH, Hebert SC. Disturbances of renal function. In: Wilson JD, et al., eds. *Harrison's Principles of Internal Medicine,* ed 12. New York: McGraw-Hill, 1991.

Corwin HL, Bonventure JV. Acute renal failure. *Med Clin North Am* 1986;70: 1037–1058.

Finn WF. Diagnosis and management of acute tubular necrosis. *Med Clin North Am* 1990;75:873–891.

Geyer SJ. Urinalysis and urinary sediment in patients with renal disease. *Clin Lab Med* 1993;13:13–20.

Gordillo-Paniagua G, Velasquez-Jones L. Acute renal failure. *Pediatr Clin North Am* 1976;23:817–828.

Harkonen S, Kjellstrand C. Contrast nephropathy. *Am J Nephrol* 1981;1:69–77.

Lazarus JM, Brenner BM. Chronic renal failure. In: Fauci AS, Braunwald E, Isselbacher KJ, et al., eds. *Harrison's Principles of Internal Medicine,* ed 14. New York: McGraw-Hill, 1998:1513–1520.

Schreiner GE, Maher JF. Toxic nephropathy. *Am J Med* 1965;38:409–449.

Schrier RW, Gottschalk CW, eds. *Diseases of the Kidneys,* 4th ed. Boston: Little, Brown, 1991.

Complications of Dialysis

Constance G. Nichols

A growing number of people in the United States have end-stage renal disease requiring some form of dialysis. When these patients experience problems during or after dialysis, the ED is a frequently utilized source of rapidly accessible medical care. ED physicians should be aware of the emergent complications of dialysis and their rapid assessment and treatment.

Hemodialysis Complications

Hemodialysis patients rely on vascular access for their thrice weekly dialysis. Thus, it is critical that dialysis access sites be treated with care.

Vascular access sites include temporary percutaneous central venous catheters, surgical native fistulas, and arteriovenous (AV) grafts. Generally, care involves not using the vascular access for blood sampling and intravenous fluid administration, and avoiding procedures, including blood pressure measurement, on the arm with the vascular access site. A present thrill or bruit over the site should be documented on arrival and departure from the ED. Branham's sign, reflex bradycardia with compression of the fistula, may also be elicited.

Access

In cases of dire necessity, the vascular access may be used. If temporary central venous catheters are present, they may be utilized like any other central venous catheter, but site contamination must be avoided. The native fistula or AV graft may be used with great care. Recommendations include strict aseptic technique, puncture sites 1 to 2 cm away from the graft anastomoses, and total avoidance of puncturing the back wall of the vein or graft. Aneurysmal sites should not be accessed.

Hemorrhage

Hemorrhage from a vascular access site is a common complication of hemodialysis. The use of heparin, large dialysis catheters, and uremic platelet dysfunction renders dialysis patients more susceptible to puncture site hemorrhage. Additional heparin is required prior to dialysis for patients taking erythropoietin, making hemorrhage a more frequent occurrence.

Infection

Infection most commonly occurs at the vascular access site in dialysis patients. Infected sites may be relatively asymptomatic, and the only findings may be vague symptoms such as fever, elevated white blood cell counts (WBC), and relative hypotension. AV grafts are much more commonly infected than endogenous grafts. With endogenous fistulae, the infected area is generally at the puncture site and is often found to be infected with the patient's own staphylococcus. This infection responds well to local care and aggressive antibiotic therapy. Infected AV grafts usually need to be excised. Clotted grafts may form a source of future infections, and removal must be considered.

Thrombosis

Clotting or thrombosis is the most common vascular access problem. The widespread use of erythropoietin therapy produces an increase in the occurrence of thrombosis, but the mechanism is not clearly understood. Stenosis of arteries causes 17% of thromboses, and stenosis of veins causes 35%. In 13% of cases, no anatomic cause can be located. Intragraft thrombosis at the site of repeated needle punctures is reported to be composed of stratified thrombus as opposed to stenosis caused by smooth muscle intimal proliferation.

Treatment of Complications

Treatment of hemorrhage involves direct pressure over the site for 5 to 10 minutes, which will stop most bleeding. If bleeding persists, reversal of heparin with protamine sulfate (0.01 mg/unit of protamine per unit of heparin) should be considered. If the graft has back wall puncture bleeding, it will be difficult to control, and a vascular surgeon should be consulted for management.

Treatment of infection in the dialysis patient includes immediate culturing followed by antibiotic treatment in consultation with the patient's nephrologist. Patients usually require hospitalization, but they may be treated as outpatients when the patient is reliable and close follow-up is available. *Staphylococcus aureus* is the leading cause of infection, followed by *Staphylococcus epidermidis* and then Gram-negative organisms. Most patients are treated with vancomycin, with the addition of aminoglycosides for Gram-negative coverage.

Treatment of clotting of a vascular access site must begin quickly if the graft's bruit or thrill is absent or markedly decreased. Salvage of graft sites may be possible if early diagnosis occurs; a vascular surgeon must be consulted early. Duplex ultrasound and color Doppler ultrasound are being studied as a way to detect stenoses.

When the graft is thrombosed, thrombectomy with graft revision is needed. The use of thrombolytics and angioplasty opens more avenues for graft salvage. Streptokinase and urokinase are agents of choice. Use of a crossed catheter technique delivering lytic agent throughout the clot has resulted in lysis rates as high as 90%. Lysis may be complicated by hematoma and frank bleeding through the dialysis puncture sites. The use of percutaneous balloon angioplasty with or without concomitant thrombectomy is being used with reasonable results. The advantage of outpatient thrombolysis with angioplasty over surgical thrombectomy or revision is the ability to resume dialysis.

Peritoneal Dialysis

Peritoneal access is most commonly obtained with the Tenckhoff catheter, which consists of a perforated plastic catheter with a Dacron felt cuff that prevents migration of bacteria into the peritoneum. Development of this catheter in 1968 led to the advent of safer peritoneal dialysis. Continuous ambulatory peritoneal dialysis (CAPD) was developed in 1976 and is the most common method of peritoneal dialysis used today.

Flow Problems

Flow problems with access include an inadequate return of dialysate. This is best dealt with by the peritoneal dialysis staff, and patients rarely present to the ED with this problem. It is a wise course to avoid catheter manipulation since it could result in peritonitis, catheter site infection, catheter migration, or obstruction or loss of function of the dialysis catheter. Leaks around the catheter require surgical consultation. These leaks are a significant source of contamination, and all fluid should be cultured, and bags and tubing discarded.

Infection

Infection is also a problem with CAPD, and peritonitis is the most common complication of CAPD. Organisms can reach the peritoneum by contiguous spread down the catheter tract or by contamination through the catheter and dialysis fluids.

Peritonitis must be ruled out in any peritoneal dialysis patient with abdominal pain and tenderness, nausea, or vomiting. Cloudy dialysate often occurs prior to the other symptoms and may be noticed during the drainage phase in the ED. The diagnosis of peritonitis is made if the dialysate had >100 WBC per mm^3. Gram staining of the dialysate may help to guide therapy.

Staphylococcus aureus and *S. epidermidis* are the most common infecting organisms, at 50% to 70%, and are of-

ten carried by the patient on skin or in nares. Some studies show a decrease in CAPD peritonitis with treatment of the nasal carrier state. Twenty percent of peritonitis is due to Gram-negative organisms, *Pseudomonas*, Enterobacteriaceae, or *Acinetobacter*. Less than 5% are fungal, and the remaining 10% to 20% are culture negative.

Management of peritonitis on an outpatient basis is typical, with hospitalization reserved for the severely ill or debilitated. Therapy should be instituted in consultation with the patient's nephrologist. Vancomycin is the most commonly used drug for gram-positive organisms, with a 1-g loading dose followed by 30 to 50 mg/kg intraperitoneally per 2-L exchange. Aminoglycosides are used for gram-negative coverage. Heparin and rapid exchanges may be used to clear inflammatory debris and prevent catheter clogging.

Special Considerations in Dialysis Patients

Infection

Infection is common in dialysis patients because their immune system is suppressed. Activation of complement results in a leukopenia within minutes of the start of hemodialysis. There is also an impairment of chemotaxis and phagocytosis. Lymphocytes are decreased, and the immune response to antigen challenges is variably impaired. CAPD patients also suffer from leukopenia, and their cellular immunity is depressed but to a lesser degree than hemodialysis patients.

Bacterial infections can take several forms in hemodialysis patients. The vascular access is a nidus for infection and an entry for organisms that can cause bacteremia and bacterial endocarditis. Bacterial endocarditis secondary to *Staphylococcus aureus* bacteremia is the most common, but it can also be caused by *Streptococcus viridans* and enterococci. Septic pulmonary emboli present with cough, fever, and pleuritic chest pain. Osteomyelitis and septic arthritis are also caused by *Staphylococcus aureus*. Respiratory infections may present with vague constitutional symptoms lacking fever or cough. UTIs can occur in anuric patients, and polycystic kidney patients are especially prone to these infections. If a source for infection in a renal failure patient is not found, one should consider the urine.

Infections spread by blood products are of special importance in the renal dialysis patient. Prior to the use of erythropoietin, frequent transfusions were a standard part of the therapy for renal failure. Hepatitis B and C have a large reservoir in the dialysis population, and although many have a chronic antigenemia, liver failure is an infrequent cause of death in the dialysis patient. The prevalence of HIV seropositivity in the dialysis population is not currently known. Pyrogens from contaminated or damaged dialysis equipment may produce fever in the dialysis patient, but these must be treated as septic events until negative culture results are obtained.

Malnutrition

Malnutrition must not be overlooked as a source of immune suppression in dialysis patients. Most have a relative protein calorie malnutrition, and enhancement of nutrition has been shown to improve immune status.

Volume Overload

Volume overload may result from dietary indiscretion, increased fluid intake, missed dialysis, or cardiac dysfunction. Underfiltration during a previous dialysis session may result in volume overload prior to the next scheduled session. Volume overload usually manifests itself as hypertension and or congestive failure/pulmonary edema. Intravenous nitrates and furosemide help to increase venous capacitance and decrease pre- and afterload. Use of bilevel positive airway pressure (BIPAP) oxygen delivery may allow emergent ultrafiltration to occur without need for intubation. Other less effective but potentially temporizing measures include oral sorbitol to shift fluid into the GI tract and morphine sulfate for an additional increase in venous capacitance.

The arteriovenous shunt may produce a rare form of high-output cardiac failure. This occurs when flow rates through the fistula, normally 200 to 400 cc per min, exceed 1 L per min. This may be corrected by placing a constricting band on the fistula.

Electrolyte Problems

Electrolyte imbalance occurs due to the significant role of the kidney in maintaining this balance. Dialysis patients are therefore at significant risk for hyperkalemia, hypernatremia, hypermagnesemia, and calcium/phosphorus imbalances.

Hyperkalemia is affected by dietary intake. Many patients have high levels of potassium between dialysis sessions due to dietary intake. Hyperkalemia alone can lead to cardiac rhythm disturbances, but its first symptom is often weakness. Any patient on dialysis presenting with weakness or cardiac rhythm abnormalities must be assumed to be hyperkalemic. The presence of tall peaked T waves is diagnostic for hyperkalemia. The subsequent changes are PR prolongation, ST depression, and QRS widening. This may then progress to a sine wave rhythm, ventricular fibrillation, and asystole. If a dialysis patient presents in cardiac arrest, one should assume hyperkalemia.

Repeated EKGs are effective for assessing the need for and results of treating hyperkalemia. Calcium is effective in antagonizing the effect of potassium on the heart. Calcium gluconate 10% IV, 10 to 30 cc over 10 to 20 minutes, or calcium chloride 10% IV, 2.5 to 10 cc over 10 to 15 min, may be used. If a patient is digoxin toxic, the toxic effects may be increased by calcium. Bicarbonate promotes potassium migration into cells, but its administration results in sodium and fluid overload. Insulin and glucose cause potassium to move intracellularly. After the patient is stabilized with intravenous therapy, potassium is best removed by GI excretion or dialysis. Kayexalate resin, 25 to 50 g orally or as an enema, will cause potassium to be eliminated in the stool. Dialysis is the definitive therapy.

Hypermagnesemia occurs secondary to excessive intake of magnesium containing phosphate binders. CNS or cardiac effects are noted. Muscle weakness and hyporeflexia are hallmarks of hypermagnesemia, which may progress to flaccid paralysis. Cardiac effects include conduction abnormalities, hypotension due to peripheral vasodilatation, bradydysrhythmias, and asystole. These are enhanced by hypocalcemia, hyperkalemia, and acidosis. Treatment is with intravenous calcium and emergency hemodialysis.

Calcium and phosphorus problems are common because dialysis does not adequately remove the phosphorus retained due to renal failure. Phosphate binders are administered to attempt to maintain balance. Hyperphosphatemia results in hypocalcemia, best remedied by decreasing phosphorus. Dietary sources of phosphorus are to be avoided, including beans, chocolate, and dairy products. Calcium-containing antacids are most commonly used, both to bind phosphorus and to enhance calcium intake.

Calcium uptake is diminished due to abnormal vitamin D activation. This is improved with intravenous calcitriol given at the end of dialysis. Hypercalcemia can occur in patients due to calcium supplementation, intravenous calcitriol, and hyperparathyroidism. Hypercalcemia is manifested by nausea, vomiting, weakness, hypertension, and neurological abnormalities, including disorientation, dysarthria, seizures, and coma. The EKG shows shortening of the Q-T interval and an abrupt slope of the proximal limb of the T wave. Severe elevations with acute neurological or cardiovascular symptoms require emergent hemodialysis. Intravenous calcitonin (5 mm/kg IV) may lower serum calcium within 2 hours.

Hypotension

Hypotension results from many causes in the dialysis patient. These include acute intravascular volume reduction, hemorrhage, sepsis, dysrhythmias, or cardiogenic shock. Less common etiologies include vascular instability secondary to autonomic neuropathy, overmedication, pericardial tamponade, and, during dialysis, anaphylactoid reaction or air embolism.

Hypovolemia can, like in all patients, be due to vomiting, diarrhea, hemorrhage, or decreased fluid intake. Dialysis-specific causes include removal of excessive fluid and would be more profound in a patient with preexisting autonomic neuropathy and or vascular instability.

Fluid replacement may require as little as 200 to 300 cc, and frequent reevaluation is necessary to prevent fluid overload. Causes of cardiogenic hypotension, including dysrhythmias, failure, and tamponade, must be evaluated. Dysrhythmias are due to a combination of atherosclerotic heart disease and a rapidly changing fluid and electrolyte status.

In this confusing scenario, it is important to stabilize the patient first by treating the dysrhythmia, then to determine the etiology of the dysrhythmia. Myocardial infarction may be difficult to diagnose by enzymes in the renal patient because many patients have elevated creatine phosphokinase, although the MM form predominates. A thorough laboratory evaluation, including CBC, electrolytes, calcium and magnesium, arterial blood gas, and levels of any drugs the patient is taking chronically, will help to evaluate the patient.

Pericardial Effusion

Pericardial effusion is present in up to 70% of patients when they begin dialysis, and uremic pericarditis is rarely symptomatic prior to dialysis. Dialysis-associated pericarditis, however, is more severe and has a worse prognosis. Symptoms include fever, weight loss, malaise, dyspnea, and chest pain, which are complicated by hypotension and dysrhythmias. Sixty percent to 70% of these patients with pericarditis have chest pain. ECG signs include ST elevation without reciprocal changes, and a physical examination may reveal a friction rub. Dialysis-associated pericarditis is treated by increasing the frequency or duration of dialysis. If fever, elevated WBC count, or a left shift is present, dialysis alone may fail. Pericardial drainage may be indicated at this time. Twenty percent of patients with dialysis-induced pericarditis will have tamponade. The signs and symptoms include tachycardia, hypotension, jugular venous distention, narrow pulse pressure, and pulsus paradoxus of >10 mm Hg. Increased heart size on radiograph, ECG changes, and echocardiography demonstrating the effusion may help, but Swan-Ganz catheterization revealing equalization of right ventricular end diastolic pressure, pulmonary artery diastolic pressure, and pulmonary capillary wedge pressure is diagnostic. If precipitated by volume depletion, intravenous saline or colloid will temporize by increasing the right ventricular filling pressure and temporarily increasing the cardiac output. Definitive treatment is surgical, with a pericardial window or pericardiectomy.

Miscellaneous Problems

Disequilibrium Syndrome

Other problems less easily recognized as related to dialysis may occur in this population. The disequilibrium syndrome was formerly a common cause of acute neurological dysfunction in hemodialysis patients. Symptoms include headache, muscle cramps, nausea, restlessness, confusion, seizures, or coma. The rapid decrease in osmolality during dialysis leaves the brain hyperosmolar and leads to cerebral edema. Modern protocols of more frequent and shorter dialysis sessions have reduced the incidence of this problem.

Intracranial Hemorrhage

Intracranial hemorrhage (ICH) occurs in patients in renal failure at a higher incidence than in the general population. Any patient with persistent headache, confusion, meningeal irritation, or focal neurologic signs must be evaluated for ICH. If increased intracranial pressure is present, intubation and hyperventilation are indicated.

Electrolyte imbalances may lead to seizure activity in the hemodialysis patient. Evaluation of the metabolic state by laboratory testing after control of seizures with benzodiazepines is the treatment of choice. Alterations in mental status may occur due to hypotension, electrolyte abnormalities, or intracranial processes. Fever should point toward a septic workup, although lack of fever is not reliable in ruling out infectious etiologies of altered mental status.

Chest Pain

Chest pain in the dialysis patient may have the same causes as in any patient, such as cardiovascular disease, pulmonary embolus, musculoskeletal chest wall pain, and pneumothorax. In the dialysis patient, septic emboli and pericardial tamponade must also be considered. Changes in bone density due to osteomalacia may result in rib fractures with minimal trauma, including coughing.

Aneurysm and Pseudoaneurysm

Other problems, such as aneurysm and pseudoaneurysm with frequently punctured grafts, are common. These manifest themselves as pain, skin changes, or distal neurological dysfunction. Vascular surgery should be consulted for symptomatic aneurysm. Most aneurysms are asymptomatic and can be observed. Pseudoaneurysm is a pulsating extravascular hematoma from dialysis puncture sites.

Air Embolism

Air embolism is a rare but devastating complication of hemodialysis. It should be considered for any patient with cardiovascular or neurological deterioration during hemodialysis. Access lines should be clamped and the patient placed left side down with feet above the head. One should give 100% oxygen. Hyperbaric oxygen (HBO) therapy is emergently indicated. Several case reports demonstrate that patients may have complete recovery within minutes of HBO therapy. Even patients with prolonged times to treatment have shown improvement with HBO therapy.

Selected Readings

Butterly DW, Schwab SJ. Dialysis access infections. *Curr Opin Nephrol Hypertens* 2000;9:631–635.

Eyrich H, Walton T, Macon EJ, et al. Alteplase versus urokinase in restoring blood flow in hemodialysis-catheter thrombosis. *Am J Health-Syst Pharm* 2002;59:1437–1440.

Gokal R, Mallick NP. Peritoneal dialysis. *Lancet* 1999;353:823–828.

Khosla N, Ahya SN. Improving dialysis access management. *Semin Nephrol* 2002;22:507–514.

Nassar GM, Ayus JC. Infectious complications of the hemodialysis access. *Kidney Int* 2001;60:1–13.

Vogel KM, Martino MA, O'Brien SP. Complications of lower extremity arteriovenous grafts in patients with end-stage renal disease. *South Med J* 2000;93:593–595.

Thoracic Respiratory Disorders

E. Jackson Allison, Jr.

Introduction

Thoracic-respiratory disorders, especially those dealing with acute respiratory distress, require immediate attention, including facile, expert management by the emergency physician.

Patients in acute respiratory distress present to the emergency department (ED) with a myriad of potential diagnoses such as pneumothorax, hemothorax, pulmonary edema, ARDS, asthma, COPD, pulmonary embolism, pneumonia, obstructing tumors, physical and chemical irritants, to name a few. The emergency physician must recognize and treat these patients promptly in order to avert potential catastrophe.

The following sections discuss the most common presentations and disorders encountered in emergency medicine, including management and treatment.

Asthma

Rita Manfredi

Acute asthma exacerbation represents one of the most common complaints seen in the ED. Asthma is a chronic inflammatory disease of the airways characterized by recurrent episodes of wheezing, breathlessness, chest tightness, and coughing. These symptoms are caused by a complex response involving eosinophils, mast cells, macrophages, neutrophils, epithelial cells, T lymphocytes, and mast cells. The ability to properly manage the asthmatic in acute respiratory distress is a skill that is crucial in the practice of emergency medicine. An emergency physician must be able to quickly assess the severity of the disease, initiate treatment, and determine the need for further therapy, airway intervention, and hospital admission.

Epidemiology

In the United States, 4 to 5% of the population is affected by asthma. Although the majority of patients have mild disease and are managed as outpatients, there is a subset of patients with potentially life-threatening disease. Asthma is the most common chronic childhood disease. There is a 2:1 male-to-female preponderance of asthma in childhood until age 30.

Pathophysiology

Asthma is a chronic disorder characterized by airway obstruction, airway inflammation, and increased airway responsiveness to many stimuli. A decrease in airway diameter caused by smooth muscle contraction, vascular congestion, mucosal edema, and mucus plugging is the pathophysiological hallmark of asthma. This airway hyperreactivity is characteristic of asthma and correlates with disease severity and treatment necessity.

Inflammatory cells are now believed to be responsible for both acute and chronic asthma. The acute response occurs when antigens react with mast cells in the submucosal, releasing mediators such as leukotrienes, tryptase, interleukins, histamine, cytokines, and chemokines. These mediators attract and activate neutrophils, platelets, and eosinophils, causing changes in epithelial integrity, autonomic control of airway tone, mucociliary function, and smooth muscle responsiveness. Chronic inflammation is manifested by persistent cell damage and a continuous re-

pair process where epithelial cells and fibroblasts proliferate and deposit collagen, causing thickening of the basement membrane.

The complex interaction of events resulting in airway inflammation may be triggered by a variety of factors. Immunologic stimuli include pollen, dust mites, molds, animal dander, and other environmental allergens. Nonimmunologic stimuli include viral upper respiratory infections, occupational chemicals, tobacco smoke, atmospheric pollutants, cold air, exercise, menstruation, emotional stress, and medications such as aspirin, NSAIDs and beta-blockers.

The clinical severity of asthma is related to the degree of bronchoconstriction, inflammation, mucosal edema, and mucus plugging causing airway obstruction and greater expiratory resistance. The work of breathing increases with the use of accessory muscles in order to maintain alveolar ventilation. Increased expiratory resistance results in air trapping, increased dead space, and hyperinflation (**Table 115.1**).

Emergency Department Evaluation— Clinical Features

Asthmatics usually present to triage with a triad of symptoms: wheezing, dyspnea, and cough. The patient may be familiar with symptoms suggesting an asthma exacerbation or may be uncertain as to the etiology of the shortness of breath. The emergency physician's highest priorities are to assess the degree of respiratory distress and determine the need for urgent medical intervention. After triage, the asthmatic patient should be admitted into the ED for medical evaluation and should not be triaged back into the waiting room.

In the initial evaluation, the severe asthmatic patient appears uncomfortable, sitting erect or leaning forward, using accessory muscles to assist in the respiratory effort. The patient is tachypneic, breathing quickly in order to increase air exchange. Confusion and lethargy may be present and are indicative of hypoxia and should be recognized as significant respiratory distress. The ability to speak in full sentences correlates with good air movement and the ability to speak only a few words between breaths correlates with poor air movement and severe disease (**Table 115.2**).

Table 115.1

Effects of Impaired Airflow

Increased airway resistance
Stiffness of airways due to hyperinflation
Air trapping
Flattened and contracted diaphragm
Increased airway pressures
Hypoxemia
Increased CO_2 production
Increased dead space
Barotrauma
Respiratory failure due to muscle fatigue
Negative hemodynamic effects

Table 115.2

Essential Elements in History and Physical Exam

History
Symptoms
    Cough, wheezing, breathlessness
    Chest tightness
    Fragmented speech
    Fever
    Sputum production
Occurrence
    Seasonal
    Episodic vs. continuous
    Onset, duration, and frequency
    Aggravating factors
Chronology
    Age of onset
    How initially diagnosed
    Medications
    Other diseases
    Visits to ED
    Steroid use
Family History
Social History
    Allergen exposure
    Tobacco use
Best Peak Expiratory Flow Rate (PEFR)
Risk Factors for Death
    Prior hospitalizations
    Intubations/ICU admission
    Treatment in ED in past month
    Comorbidity: COPD or cardiovascular disease
    Recent or chronic use of corticosteroids
    Failure of outpatient treatment
    Lack of access to medical care
    Inadequate medical management/follow-up
    Multiple ED visits/hospitalizations
    Psychiatric illness
    Use of more than 2 canisters/month of inhaled
    short-acting beta-agonist
Physical Exam
Signs
    Respiratory rate increased
    Prolonged expiratory phase
    Tachycardia
    Accessory muscle use
    Diaphoresis
    Unable to lie supine
    Paradoxical pulse (greater than 12 mm Hg)
Expiratory Flow
    PEFR
    Repeat PEFR after initial treatment
Oxygenation
    Room air PO_2 or O_2 saturation (pulse oximetry)
Ventilation
    PCO_2

The lung examination of the asthmatic often reveals wheezing. In mild to moderate exacerbations, wheezes are not always auscultated initially, and may present only after treatment is initiated. There are several conditions that present with wheezing and may mimic asthma, including congestive heart failure, upper airway obstruction, aspiration of gastric acid or a foreign body, carcinoma with endobronchial obstruction, and vocal cord dysfunction. The quiet, non-wheezing chest in the asthmatic, accompanied by paradoxical respirations, may represent impending respiratory failure.

Ancillary Tests

If the patient is able, lung function is assessed by measuring a Peak Expiratory Flow Rate (PEFR). In general, a PEFR greater than 300 (80% of predicted or personal best) reflects mild exacerbation. PEFR between 100 and 300 (between 50 and 80% of predicted or personal best) represents moderate airflow obstruction. PEFR less than 100 (less than 50% of predicted or personal best) is considered severe and associated with potential respiratory failure. Serial peak flows are necessary to assess clinical improvement. The degree of wheezing does not correlate with the degree of airflow obstruction.

Most asthmatics with mild to moderate disease can be managed without an arterial blood gas. A pulse oximetry reading of less than 91% is indicative of severe respiratory distress. The prime indication for an arterial blood gas is to assess for hypoventilation with carbon dioxide retention and respiratory acidosis. In an acute asthmatic exacerbation, ventilation is stimulated, the patient exhales more, and the $PaCO_2$ decreases. A normal or slightly elevated $PaCO_2$ (>41 mm Hg) indicates patient fatigue, extreme airway obstruction, and imminent respiratory failure. Blood gas analysis alone does not determine if endotracheal intubation is to be performed. Often it is obvious that the patient requires intubation based on clinical criteria: respiratory distress, poor air exchange, and obtundation. Arterial blood gas measurements may be useful only after the initiation of therapy, when the decision to intubate, based on clinical criteria alone, remains unclear. In this setting one can follow pH and $PaCO_2$ as ob-

Adapted from the *National Asthma Education and Prevention Program, Expert Panel Report II: Guidelines for the Diagnosis and Management of Asthma.* Publication 97-4051. Bethesda, MD: National Institutes of Health, 1997. Available at http://www.nhlbi.nih.gov/guidelines/asthma/asthgdln.pdf. Accessed May 2005.

jective indicators of respiratory failure within a clinical context.

A selective approach in obtaining a chest radiograph during an asthma exacerbation should be considered. Chest radiographs should be obtained if there is clinical suspicion of pneumonia, fever, foreign body aspiration, pneumothorax, or pneumomediastinum. In patients admitted with asthma exacerbations, about 33% will have an abnormality on chest radiograph.

An electrocardiogram is indicated if the diagnosis of asthma is uncertain, especially in older persons with coronary risk factors, or if pulmonary embolus is a consideration. Right ventricular strain or abnormal T waves may be present but will resolve with treatment. A white blood count is likely to be elevated in the setting of pneumonia, chronic steroid use, or beta-agonist therapy, but is not routinely indicated. A serum theophylline level should be obtained in every patient taking a theophylline preparation.

Emergency Department Intervention

The National Asthma Education and Prevention Program Expert Panel has developed a useful algorithm for the emergency treatment of asthma (**FIGURE 115.1**). *Beta-adrenergic agonists* are first-line therapy in the management of asthmatic exacerbations. There are two types of beta-adrenergic receptors: beta-1 and beta-2. Activated beta-2 receptors increase bronchodilation, vasodilation, uterine relaxation, and skeletal muscle tremor, while beta-1 receptors increase heart rate and strength of cardiac contractions and decrease small intestine activity and tone. Beta agonists increase the levels of adenosine $3',5'$-cyclic monophosphate (cAMP), which causes smooth muscle dilation in the bronchial walls, resulting in bronchodilation. Some beta-agonists are nonselective (metaproterenol) and may cause a greater incidence of tachycardia and tremors, whereas others are beta-2 selective (albuterol) and are associated with fewer side effects.

Albuterol is the primary beta-2 agonist used in the ED for acute exacerbations. The most commonly used form of albuterol is a racemic mixture of equal parts of R and S isomers. Some studies suggest that the S isomer, which has no bronchodilator activity, may cause bronchial hyperreactivity and contribute to the adverse effects of using albuterol excessively or on a long-term basis. The most common side effect of albuterol is skeletal muscle tremor. Despite earlier concerns regarding cardiotoxicity, clinical evidence has not demonstrated this when albuterol is used.

Beta-adrenergic agonists, when aerosolized, produce optimal bronchodilation (**Table 115.3**). Aerosol delivery is preferred over oral and parenteral routes. Nebulizers or metered dose inhalers (MDI) with a spacing device can be used to administer albuterol every 20 minutes. Nebulized albuterol treatments given on a continuous basis to *severe* asthmatics may play a role in determining the need for hospital admission. Salmeterol, a beta-2 agonist with greater affinity than albuterol for the beta-2 receptor site, is not for use in acute exacerbations and should be used only for stable, nocturnal, long-term control.

The use of subcutaneous *terbutaline* or *epinephrine* may be considered in severe exacerbations when there is poor air exchange, limited inhalation of aerosolized medications, and lack of success with inhaled beta-2 agonists. Intravenous epinephrine has been used in refractory asthma as well, although cardiac side effects limit its utility, especially in patients at risk for coronary disease.

Corticosteroids, along with beta-agonists, are considered first-line therapy in the acute management of asthma exacerbations. The mechanism of action of steroids in asthma is not clearly understood, but many believe that steroids decrease inflammation and increase the responsiveness of beta-receptors, thus improving bronchodilation with beta-agonists.

Steroids may be administered intravenously, orally, or by inhalation. Optimal doses are disputed by many, but an initial oral dose of 40 to 60 mg of prednisone or 60 to 125 mg IV of methylprednisolone is satisfactory. The dose should be repeated every 4 to 6 hours until improvement is noted. After treatment in the ED, if a patient is discharged home with a PEFR of less than 70% predicted, a 3- to-10 day nontapering course of oral steroids (40 to 60 mg prednisone) should be prescribed. Additionally, inhaled corticosteroids are recommended when discharging patients with mild persistent or more severe asthma.

Low flow oxygen should be administered to asthmatics in order to maintain oxygen saturation above 90%. High flow oxygen is required if hypoxemia is present. Oxygen administration may buffer the reduction in $PaCO_2$ due to increased ventilation/perfusion mismatch seen after initiation of bronchodilator therapy.

Anticholinergic agents are potent bronchodilators and are used as second-line therapy in the acute setting. They act by blocking vagally-mediated bronchoconstriction and by decreasing levels of guanosine $3',5'$-cyclic monophosphate (cGMP) in airway smooth muscle, which causes further bronchodilation. Although atropine sulfate may improve airflow obstruction, its side effects have made it obsolete and it has been replaced with ipratropium bromide. Aerosolized ipratropium, 0.5 mg, available as a nebulized solution or MDI, should be used in conjunction with beta-agonists in the treatment of severe exacerbations.

The use of intravenous magnesium sulfate (1 to 2 g IV over 20 min) is indicated in patients with the most compromised airways. Magnesium appears to inhibit bronchial smooth muscle contraction, potentially producing an effect within minutes to hours that may reduce the need for intubation.

Heliox, a combination of helium and oxygen, is available in different mixture ratios (80:20, 70:30, and 60:40). It is currently under investigation as to its role in the treatment of asthma exacerbations and is presently not recommended for routine use.

Leukotrienes are proinflammatory mediators that cause bronchospasm and edema in acute asthma. Blocking leukotrienes with *leukotriene-modifying agents* improves pulmonary function, decreases the need for rescue beta-agonists, and inhibits bronchoconstriction caused by leukotrienes. Leukotriene-modifying agents montelukast,

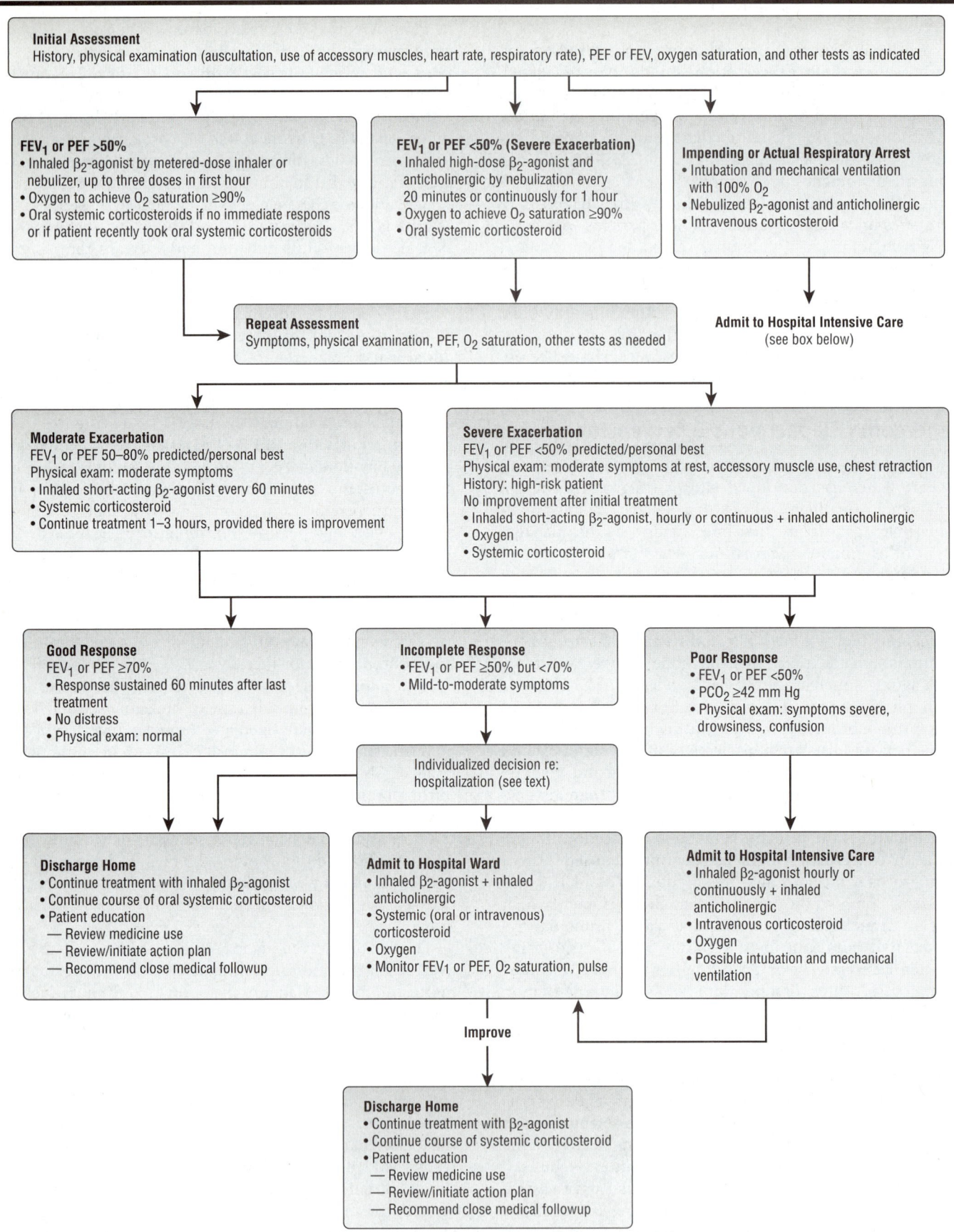

Initial Assessment
History, physical examination (auscultation, use of accessory muscles, heart rate, respiratory rate), PEF or FEV, oxygen saturation, and other tests as indicated

FEV$_1$ or PEF >50%
- Inhaled β$_2$-agonist by metered-dose inhaler or nebulizer, up to three doses in first hour
- Oxygen to achieve O$_2$ saturation ≥90%
- Oral systemic corticosteroids if no immediate respons or if patient recently took oral systemic corticosteroids

FEV$_1$ or PEF <50% (Severe Exacerbation)
- Inhaled high-dose β$_2$-agonist and anticholinergic by nebulization every 20 minutes or continuously for 1 hour
- Oxygen to achieve O$_2$ saturation ≥90%
- Oral systemic corticosteroid

Impending or Actual Respiratory Arrest
- Intubation and mechanical ventilation with 100% O$_2$
- Nebulized β$_2$-agonist and anticholinergic
- Intravenous corticosteroid

Repeat Assessment
Symptoms, physical examination, PEF, O$_2$ saturation, other tests as needed

Admit to Hospital Intensive Care
(see box below)

Moderate Exacerbation
FEV$_1$ or PEF 50–80% predicted/personal best
Physical exam: moderate symptoms
- Inhaled short-acting β$_2$-agonist every 60 minutes
- Systemic corticosteroid
- Continue treatment 1–3 hours, provided there is improvement

Severe Exacerbation
FEV$_1$ or PEF <50% predicted/personal best
Physical exam: moderate symptoms at rest, accessory muscle use, chest retraction
History: high-risk patient
No improvement after initial treatment
- Inhaled short-acting β$_2$-agonist, hourly or continuous + inhaled anticholinergic
- Oxygen
- Systemic corticosteroid

Good Response
FEV$_1$ or PEF ≥70%
- Response sustained 60 minutes after last treatment
- No distress
- Physical exam: normal

Incomplete Response
- FEV$_1$ or PEF ≥50% but <70%
- Mild-to-moderate symptoms

Poor Response
- FEV$_1$ or PEF <50%
- PCO$_2$ ≥42 mm Hg
- Physical exam: symptoms severe, drowsiness, confusion

Individualized decision re: hospitalization (see text)

Discharge Home
- Continue treatment with inhaled β$_2$-agonist
- Continue course of oral systemic corticosteroid
- Patient education
  — Review medicine use
  — Review/initiate action plan
  — Recommend close medical followup

Admit to Hospital Ward
- Inhaled β$_2$-agonist + inhaled anticholinergic
- Systemic (oral or intravenous) corticosteroid
- Oxygen
- Monitor FEV$_1$ or PEF, O$_2$ saturation, pulse

Admit to Hospital Intensive Care
- Inhaled β$_2$-agonist hourly or continuously + inhaled anticholinergic
- Intravenous corticosteroid
- Oxygen
- Possible intubation and mechanical ventilation

Improve

Discharge Home
- Continue treatment with β$_2$-agonist
- Continue course of systemic corticosteroid
- Patient education
  — Review medicine use
  — Review/initiate action plan
  — Recommend close medical followup

FIGURE 115.1 Management of asthma exacerbations in the emergency department. Adapted from the *National Asthma Education and Prevention Program, Expert Panel Report II: Guidelines for the Diagnosis and Management of Asthma*. Publication 97-4051. Bethesda, MD: National Institutes of Health, 1997. Available at http://www.nhlbi.nih.gov/guidelines/asthma/asthgdln.pdf. Accessed May 2005.

Table 115.3

Dosages of Drugs for Asthma Exacerbations in the Emergency Department

Medication	Dosages		Comments
	Adult Dose	Child Dose	
Inhaled Short-acting β_2 Agonists			
Albuterol			
Nebulizer solution, 5 mg/mL	2.5–5.0 mg every 20 min for 3 doses, then 2.5–10 mg every 1–4 h as needed, or 10–15 mg/h continuously	0.15 mg/kg (minimum dose 2.5 mg) every 20 min for 3 doses, then 0.15–0.3 mg/kg up to 0 mg every 1–4 hours as needed, or 0.5 mg/kg/h by continuous nebulization	Only selective β_2 agonists are recommended. For optimal delivery, dilute aerosols to minimum of 4 mL at gas flow of 6–8 L/min
MDI, 90 µg/puff	4–8 puffs every 20 min up to 4 h, then every 1–4 h as needed	4–8 puffs every 20 min for 3 doses, then every 1–4 h inhalation maneuver; use spacer/holding chamber	As effective as nebulized therapy if patient is able to coordinate
Bitolterol			
Nebulizer solution, 2 mg/mL	See albuterol dose	See albuterol dose; thought to be half as potent as albuterol on a per mg basis	Has not been studied in severe asthma exacerbations; do not mix with other drugs
MDI, 370 µg/puff	See albuterol dose	See albuterol dose	Has not been studied in severe asthma exacerbations
Pirbuterol			
MDI, 200 µg/puff	See albuterol dose	See albuterol dose; thought to be half as potent as albuterol on a per mg basis	Has not been studied in severe asthma exacerbations
Systemic (Injected) β_2 Agonists			
Epinephrine, 1:1000 (1 mg/mL)	0.3–0.5 mg every 20 min for 3 doses sq	0.01 mg/kg up to 0.3–0.5 mg every 20 min for 3 doses sq	No proven advantage of systemic therapy over aerosol
Terbutaline (1 mg/mL)	0.25 mg every 20 min for 3 doses sq	0.01 mg/kg every 20 min for 3 doses, then every 2–6 hours as needed sq	No proven advantage of systemic therapy over aerosol
Anticholinergics			
Ipratropium bromide			
Nebulizer solution (0.25 mg/mL)	0.5 mg every 30 min for 3 doses, then every 2–4 h as needed	0.25 mg every 20 min for 3 doses, then every 2–4 h	May mix in same nebulizer with albuterol. Should not be used as first-line therapy; should be added to β_2 agonist therapy
MDI, 18 µg/puff	4–8 puffs as needed	4–8 puffs as needed	Dose delivered from MDI is low and has not been studied in asthma exacerbations
Corticosteroids			
Prednisone Methylprednisolone Prednisolone	120–180 mg/d in 3 or 4 divided doses for 48 h, then 60–80 mg/d until PEF reaches 70% of predicted or personal best	1 mg/kg every 6 h for 48 h, then 1–2 mg/kg/d (max = 60 mg/d) in 2 divided doses until PEF reaches 70% of predicted or personal best	For outpatient "burst," use 40–60 mg in single or 2 divided doses for adults (children: 1–2 mg/kg/d, max 60 mg/d) for 3–10 days

Adapted from *The National Asthma Education and Prevention Program, Expert Panel Report II: Guidelines for the Diagnosis and Management of Asthma.* Publication 97-4051. Bethesda, MD, National Institutes of Health, 1997.

zafirlukast, and zileutron, are taken orally and may be used as alternatives to inhaled steroids in stable, persistent asthmatics. Recent data suggest that leukotriene-modifiers may have a role in the treatment of acute asthma in the ED. One study has shown rapid bronchodilator response to intravenous montelukast in acute exacerbations. Leukotriene modifiers may prevent subsequent relapse after ED discharge, but currently there is no recommendation for their routine use in the acutely compromised asthmatic.

Theophylline is not indicated in the treatment of acute asthma. There appears to be increased toxicity when theophylline is used concurrently with beta-agonist inhalers. Patients taking oral theophylline should have serum levels measured. Theophylline is metabolized by the liver, and at levels greater than 30 μg /mL, can cause seizures cardiac arrhythmias.

Antibiotics do not appear to have a role in the treatment of acute asthma unless the patient is febrile, has a focal infiltrate on lung examination, and has increased sputum production. *Sedatives* are contraindicated in the treatment of acute asthma unless the patient is intubated.

Mast cell modifiers such as cromolyn sodium and nedocromil inhibit the response to allergens and exercise, and are not recommended for use in the acute asthmatic exacerbation.

Intubation and mechanical ventilation of the asthmatic patient are indicated if there is progressive hypercarbia, acidosis, exhaustion, or confusion. Rapid sequence intubation should be modified for the asthmatic. Lidocaine (1–1.5 mg/kg) may be given as premedication to attenuate adverse airway reflexes. Ketamine, at doses of 1 to 1.5 mg/kg, is an anesthetic as well as a potent bronchodilator, and may be particularly useful when intubating the asthmatic. A large endotracheal tube greater than 7 mm should be used to facilitate ventilation. The use of noninvasive positive-pressure ventilation (Bi-PAP) in patients with status asthmaticus is controversial and cannot be recommended at this time.

Hypotension and barotrauma are complications of intubation and are both related to high peak airway pressures and lung hyperinflation. Due to the prolonged expiratory phase, the respiratory rate should be decreased to 11 to 14 per minute to allow for sufficient ventilation of CO_2 as long as the patient continues to have adequate oxygen saturation. This type of permissive hypoventilation will accomplish ventilatory support in the asthmatic patient without significant concern for correcting the hypercarbia.

Inhalational anesthetics such as halothane and enflurane are potent bronchodilators and may be used when other treatment modalities have failed.

Disposition

An asthmatic may be discharged from the ED if the following criteria are met: (1) subjective improvement, when the patient feels sufficient symptomatic relief; (2) clinical evidence of adequate ventilation based on clear lungs with good air movement; and (3) PEFR greater than 70% pre-dicted. In the average patient, peak flow should be greater than 300. Adequate follow-up should occur within 7 days.

Metered dose inhalers for beta-agonists and corticosteroids should be provided along with a spacer/holding chamber. Additionally, the patient should have a peak flow meter at home where an AM and PM PEFR can be recorded. The patient should be taught the purpose and technique of using these medications and the flow meter, and then should demonstrate the ability to do so before discharge home.

Patients with continued wheezing, diminished air movement, PEFR less than 40% of predicted levels, and no subjective improvement should be admitted to the hospital for continued inhaled beta-agonists and intravenous steroids. Patients with persistent respiratory distress, use of accessory muscles, PEFR less than 100, and minimal air movement warrant ICU admission and possible intubation.

Most asthmatics seen in the ED have a moderate response to therapy with some persistent symptoms and a PEFR between 40% and 70% of predicted values. If these patients have no risk factors for death from asthma (Table 115.1), they may be discharged home. Patients in the late phase of their exacerbation who demonstrate little improvement after several hours of treatment and who are at risk of death from asthma need admission to an observation unit or to the hospital.

Asthma in Pregnancy

Approximately 1% to 7% of all pregnancies are complicated by asthma. Hyperventilation, occurring normally in pregnancy, causes a higher PaO_2 and a lower $PaCO_2$. Respiratory alkalosis is a common finding with a $PaCO_2$ of 30 to 35. Therefore, a PaO_2 of less than 70 mm Hg and a $PaCO_2$ greater than 35 mm Hg signifies respiratory failure in a pregnant patient.

Inhaled beta-agonists and corticosteroids can be safely administered in pregnancy. In severe asthma exacerbations, given the maternal and fetal consequences, the use of systemic corticosteroids remains clinically indicated in pregnancy and must not be withheld if current medications are inadequate.

Selected Readings

Ducharme FM, Hicks GC. Anti-leukotriene agents compared to inhaled corticosteroids in the management of recurrent and/or chronic asthma in adults and children. *Cochrane Database Syst Rev 4.* Chichester, UK: John Wiley and Sons, Ltd, 2003.

Key Clinical Activities for Quality Asthma Care: Recommendations of the National Asthma Education and Prevention Program. *Morbid Mortal Wk Rep* March 28, 2003;52:RR-6.

National Heart, Lung, and Blood Institute, National Asthma Education and Prevention Program. Quick reference for the NAEPP Expert Panel Report: guides for the diagnosis and management of asthma—update on selected topics 2002. Bethesda, MD: US Department of Health and Human Services, National Institutes of Health, 2002; publication no. 02-5075. Available at http://www.nhlbi.nih.gov/guidelines/asthma/index.htm. Accessed May 2005.

Ram F, Wellington S, Rowe B, et al. Non-invasive positive pressure ventilation for treatment of respiratory failure due to severe acute exacerbations of asthma. *Cochrane Database Syst Rev* 2005;1:CD004360.

Rowe BH, Spooner C, Ducharme FA, et al: Early emergency department treatment of acute asthma with systemic corticosteroids. *Cochrane Database Syst Rev* 2003;4. Chichester, UK: John Wiley and Sons, Ltd.

Bronchitis

Gregory A. Volturo

Acute Bronchitis

Acute bronchitis is a common presenting complaint in the ED. Patients chiefly present with a productive cough. Often the illness begins as part of a common upper respiratory infection with associated rhinorrhea, sore throat, and sneezing. As the illness progresses, cough becomes the predominant symptom. These patients may have associated sputum production and fever. Physical examination may reveal normal lungs, diffuse rhonchi, or wheezing. Generally, in patients presenting with cough of less than two weeks duration, with or without sputum production, no further workup is necessary. Patients with fever should receive a chest radiograph to exclude pneumonia.

Etiology

Most acute bronchitis is of viral origin, Adenovirus, influenza, parainfluenza, respiratory syncytial virus, and rhinovirus being most common. When a bacterial infection is responsible for symptoms, *Streptococcus pneumoniae*, *Haemophilus influenzae*, *Mycoplasma*, and *Chlamydia pneumoniae* are most common. During community outbreaks, pertussis may also cause acute bronchitis.

Treatment

Acute bronchitis is usually a self-limited illness. Initial management should include symptomatic relief of symptoms. An albuterol metered dose inhaler will assist in decreasing bronchospasm and resultant cough. Cough suppressants may be a useful sleep aid. For patients in whom cough has persisted for greater than two weeks, the likelihood of infection with an atypical agent is increased, and empiric treatment with a macrolide antibiotic may help to shorten the course of the illness in this group. When outbreaks of pertussis occur in the community, consideration must be given for early administration of macrolide antibiotics in suspected patients.

Chronic Bronchitis

Chronic bronchitis is part of the spectrum of respiratory diseases that contribute to chronic obstructive pulmonary disease (COPD). Cigarette smoking is the major predisposing risk factor for developing chronic bronchitis, although pollution and industrial exposures also contribute to the development of this disease. Chronic bronchitis is defined as a persistent cough for more than three months per year for two or more consecutive years. Smoke and other irritants which enter the airways irritate the endobronchial surface, leading to mucosal swelling, impaired mucociliary function, hypersecretion of mucous from inflamed small and large bronchioles, and hypertrophied submucosal glands and mucous secreting cells. Obstruction occurs when mucous plugs airways that are narrowed from inflammation, trapping bacteria and contributing to ventilatory obstruction. Compensatory changes include increased cardiac output, polycythemia, and *cor pulmonale*. It is difficult to determine if exacerbations of chronic bronchitis are due to bacterial or viral infections.

Emergency Department Evaluation/Diagnosis

The triad of worsening cough, increasing mucopurulent sputum production, and shortness of breath is the hallmark of exacerbation of chronic bronchitis. Upon presentation to the ED, vital signs and assessment of oxygenation with pulse oximetry should be expedited. Oxygen and the early use of β-adrenergic agents should be considered. Some patients with a history of carbon dioxide retention may be dependent upon their hypoxic drive to stimulate respiration; caution must be used when administering oxygen to these patients. History should be obtained from the patient or family with particular regard to baseline respiratory function, recent changes in symptoms including worsening shortness of breath, presence of fever or chills, and changes in color, quality and quantity of sputum. Other historical information, including current medications, past or present steroid use, recent infectious exposures, prior hospitalizations, including the need for admission to an intensive care unit or the need for mechanical ventilation, all will assist in determining the severity of the patient's underlying disease as well as the need for admission to the hospital.

Physical Examination

Patient positioning and respiratory effort should be observed. The skin should be assessed for cyanosis, and use of accessory muscles of respiration, pursed lip breathing and ability to speak should be noted. Course crackles or bronchospasm with audible wheezing may be present upon auscultation of the chest. In more severe cases or symptoms of *cor pulmonale,* such as jugular venous distention, hepatomegaly, and peripheral edema may also be present. Complications such as pneumothorax and underlying infection should be considered in all decompensated patients.

Ancillary Tests

Bedside spirometry is a quick and inexpensive tool to assist with quantification of respiratory function and obstruction to airflow. Pre- and post-bronchodilator measurements should be obtained to give an objective measurement of treatment response. Although patients generally will require a peak expiratory flow of greater than 150 cc, it is not the absolute number that is as important, but rather the patient's response to therapy and trending improvement; often patients with higher peak flows may still need admission to the hospital because their response to therapy is minimal.

Chest radiography is mandatory in patients with chronic bronchitis with unexplained respiratory decompensation or fever. Underlying pneumonia and pneumothorax must be excluded. Chest radiographs will often demonstrate flattened diaphragms and hyperinflation, indicating increased lung volume. Mucous plugging may cause areas of atelectasis.

Pulse oximetry should be part of the initial evaluation of the patient; however, it may be difficult to obtain pulse oximetry readings in some hypoxic, peripherally vasoconstricted patient. In patients who are severely ill or in those where accurate readings cannot be obtained, the arterial blood gas remains the "gold standard" for documenting hypoxia. Additionally, blood gas analysis provides information about hypercapnia and acidosis, and thus may be a useful tool in guiding therapy in severely ill patients. In patients with severe polycythemia (who are prone to clot formation) and hypoxia, pulmonary embolism must be considered as part of the differential diagnosis.

An electrocardiogram will assist with identifying arrhythmias associated with COPD, such as atrial fibrillation or multifocal atrial tachycardia. The electrocardiogram may also demonstrate evidence of *cor pulmonale* with right ventricular hypertrophy.

Sputum examination has little utility in the acute management of chronic bronchitis. It is often difficult to obtain a good sputum sample in the emergency setting, and gram stain analysis is a poor predictor of response to antibiotics. Frequently, patients with chronic bronchitis are colonized with organisms that may not necessarily be responsible for the current illness. For severely ill patients who are being admitted to the hospital, if they can provide a good sputum specimen, it may have some value; however, therapy should not be delayed to obtain sputum samples.

Other laboratory tests, such as complete blood count, electrolytes, and liver function tests, are frequently ordered in the evaluation of patients with chronic bronchitis. These tests, however, have limited value in the initial diagnosis and treatment of chronic bronchitis patients in the ED setting.

Emergency Department Intervention

When patients with chronic bronchitis arrive in the ED in respiratory distress, oxygen should be administered immediately. The patients should be allowed to position themselves to allow optimization of respiratory effort, usually sitting upright. Nebulized, inhaled bronchodilators such as the β-adrenergic albuterol (2.5–5 mg every 20 min × 3) and inhaled anticholinergic agents such as ipratropium bromide (500 μg every 6–8 h) can be used. In the past anticholinergic agents were first-line therapy; however, current practice is to use both classes of agents initially. The effects of these agents are felt to be additive when used in combination; β-adrenergic agents act primarily on small airways, while anticholinergic agents affect large airways. Methylxanthines, such as theophylline or aminophylline, are believed to not be as effective as inhaled bronchodilators, and tend to have more side effects.

Steroids have been shown to decrease the incidence of relapse and should be used early in the management of decompensated chronic bronchitis. Intravenous methylprednisolone is preferred: 1–1.5 mg/kg followed by 40–60 mg every six hours until improvement. Oral administration of 40–80 mg of prednisone may be an effective alternative particularly, in the patient being managed outside the hospital. The greatest benefit from steroid use is achieved within the first two weeks following the initial ED visit. There does not appear to be a benefit in most patients to continue use of steroids beyond two weeks when treating an acute exacerbation.

Underlying infection may precipitate some exacerbations of chronic bronchitis. Bacterial infections most commonly involve *Haemophilus* species, *Moraxella catarrhalis,* and *Streptococcus pneumoniae.* Administration of broad-spectrum antibiotics, such as expanded spectrum macrolides (azithromycin, clarithromycin), telithromycin, or respiratory fluoroquinolones (levofloxacin, moxifloxacin, or gatifloxacin) are also recommended as part of initial therapy. As an alternative erythromycin and amoxicillin clavulanate may be used. Oral or intravenous hydration aids in secretion mobilization. While treatment of hypoxia remains the mainstay of therapy, it may also be necessary to treat tachyarrhythmias and right ventricular failure.

Patient Disposition

While some patients with mild decompensated chronic bronchitis may be managed in the outpatient environment, patients in whom symptomatic relief and correction of hypoxia cannot be achieved in the ED will require hospital admission. Additionally, patients who are unable to clear their own secretions or maintain oral hydration and those with multiple comorbid conditions will require admission. Patients who are severely hypoxic, hypercarbic, or acidotic will require endotracheal intubation and mechanical ventilation.

Selected Readings

Aaron SD, Vandemheen KL, Hebert P, et al. Outpatient oral prednisone after emergency treatment of chronic obstructive pulmonary disease. *N Engl J Med* 2003;348:2618–2625.

Barr RG, Rowe BH, Camargo CA. Methylxanthines for exacerbations of chronic obstructive pulmonary disease: meta-analysis of randomized trials. *BMJ* 2003; 327:1–6.

Sethi S, Evans N, Grant BB, et al. New strains of bacteria and exacerbations of chronic obstructive pulmonary disease. *N Engl J Med* 2002;347:465–471.

Schermer TR, Jacobs JE, Chavannes NH, et al. Validity of spirometric testing in a general practice population of patients with chronic obstructive pulmonary disease (COPD). *Thorax* 2003;58:861–866.

117 Chronic Obstructive Pulmonary Disease

Rita Manfredi

Chronic obstructive pulmonary disease (COPD) causes morbidity and mortality in more than 10% of the people in this country. It is a frequent underlying condition in patients presenting to the ED and is difficult to treat due to its refractory nature. There are numerous definitions of COPD, and multiple guidelines aimed at the evaluation and treatment of COPD. Historically, COPD has been defined as a combination of airway collapse, airway inflammation, and/or bronchospasm. The American Thoracic Society's definition has two components: emphysema, dramatized by the "pink puffer," and chronic bronchitis, dramatized by the "blue bloater." The World Health Organization defines A patient with COPD is one who complains of chronic cough and sputum, dyspnea, and exposure to certain risk factors. Spirometric evaluation will confirm the diagnosis. Of those patients with COPD, 15% have primarily emphysematous complaints, while 85% exhibit mostly chronic bronchitic symptoms. More often than not, patients have some combination of the two. COPD is airflow restriction that is not totally reversible and does not distinguish between chronic bronchitis and emphysema.

Epidemiology

In the United States, COPD is now the fourth leading cause of death (behind cancer, heart disease, and cerebrovascular disease). The mortality rate of COPD is increasing and is expected to be the third leading cause of death by 2020. The disease has doubled in women over the past decades as a result of increased smoking behavior but is still more common in men. COPD is most prevalent in those countries where cigarette use is common.

Pathophysiology

Cigarette smoking is known to be the most important cause of COPD. Other risk factors include: environmental pollution, industrial exposures, passive smoke, and α_1-antitrypsin deficiency.

Impedance to expiratory airflow fundamentally defines the dysfunction in COPD. This is a result of increased resistance, bronchospasm, and smaller airway diameters throughout the lesser bronchi and bronchioles due to mu-cosal edema and hypersecretion. Patients may develop emphysematous and/or bronchitic patterns, although one often predominates.

In the emphysematous pattern, the air spaces distal to the terminal bronchiole become enlarged and the alveolar walls are permanently destroyed. When alveolar walls collapse, the small bronchi and bronchioles are obliterated, causing significant expiratory airflow obstruction and ventilation-perfusion mismatching. As alveolar hypoventilation occurs, the pulmonary capillary bed is destroyed, leading to further hypoxemia. Patients with this emphysematous component compensate by hyperventilating, while maintaining a low cardiac output. They often breathe through pursed lips in a puffing fashion that increases expiratory intraluminal pressure and maintains airway structure by preventing bronchial collapse. These patients typically experience air hunger, utilize accessory muscles, and have an increased anterior-posterior chest wall diameter due to hyperinflation of the lungs. They often tend to be lean due to higher calorie expenditure from increased work of breathing.

The bronchitic pattern of COPD demonstrates inflammation of the small and large bronchi with mucus hypersecretion. Goblet cells and submucosal glands hypertrophy, contributing to increased mucus secretion and inflammation. Ultimately, this causes airway obstruction and these patients often progress to right-sided heart failure. This *cor pulmonale,* together with ventilatory inadequacy, leads to polycythemia and hypoxemia. The cyanotic appearance of these patients may be coupled with signs of congestive heart failure such as jugular venous distention and peripheral edema.

Emergency Department Evaluation: Clinical Features

The slow insidious nature of COPD makes it difficult to identify patients with early disease; therefore, most of the patients who present to the ED with COPD complaints are those with advanced pathology. Dyspnea on exertion and cough are the hallmarks of COPD (**Table 117.1**). Hypoxemia, where arterial saturation drops below 90%, is the most life-threatening feature of severe COPD exacerbations. Increased

Table 117.1

Essential Elements in History and Physical Exam

History
- *Symptoms*
  - Worsening shortness of breath
  - Change in sputum production or color
  - Fever or chills
  - New onset hemoptysis
  - Confusion or somnolence
  - Orthopnea
- *Social History*
  - Continuation of smoking
- *Comorbidity*
  - Cardiac disease
  - Noncompliance with medications
  - Noxious environmental exposures
  - Weight loss

Physical Exam
- *Signs*
  - Use of accessory muscles
  - Tachypnea
  - Tachycardia
  - Cyanosis
  - Sitting-up-and-forward position
  - Pursed-lip exhalation
  - Diaphoresis
  - Pulsus paradoxus
  - Nicotine stains on fingers
- *Expiratory Flow*
  - PEFR or FEV1
- *Oxygenation*
  - Arterial blood gas (PaO_2) if SaO_2 is less than 90%
- *Ventilation*
  - $PaCO_2$

work of breathing causes a rise in carbon dioxide, but alveolar ventilation is often unable to prevent carbon dioxide retention, so the patient becomes acidotic.

On physical exam, in the predominantly bronchitic patient, uncleared secretions present as coarse crackles and rhonchi, whereas in the emphysematous patient, diminished breath sounds are a common finding due to the increased anterior-posterior diameter of the thorax.

Diseases that mimic COPD exacerbations are congestive heart failure, pneumonia, asthma, pulmonary embolism, tuberculosis, lung carcinoma, ischemic heart disease, and metabolic abnormalities.

Ancillary Tests

Evaluating the patient's ability to oxygenate is critical. Pulse oximetry can identify hypoxemia but not hypercapnia or acid-base disorders. Carbon dioxide levels are variable depending on current alveolar ventilatory function. An arterial blood gas measurement with a PaO_2 of 60 mm Hg, correlating with a SaO_2 of 90%, indicates respiratory failure. If the patient is hypercapneic or has a pH of 7.3,

ventilatory failure is imminent and the patient requires critical care management in the ED and intensive care unit.

Bedside spirometry is a quick and inexpensive tool that helps to characterize current respiratory function. A peak expiratory flow rate (PEFR) of less than 100 L per min or a forced expiratory volume in 1 second (FEV1) of less than 1 L indicates a severe exacerbation. Pre- and post-bronchodilator measurements can be obtained to give an objective measure of treatment response. Peak flow rate trends, rather than absolute numbers, are most beneficial in patient management and disposition.

Chest radiographs commonly demonstrate abnormalities in COPD exacerbations and may reveal the underlying cause of the decompensation, such as pneumonia or congestive heart failure.

Electrocardiograms can identify arrhythmias associated with COPD such as multifocal atrial tachycardia and can indicate the extent of *cor pulmonale* by showing changes consistent with right ventricular hypertrophy. Findings of low QRS voltage and poor R-wave progression are often seen in COPD patients, but are considered nonspecific.

Sputum culture may be helpful in diagnosing acute bacterial infections, such as *Legionella*, tuberculosis, and fungal and pneumocystis pneumonias. An increase in sputum purulence, color, or volume may be an indication for antibiotic therapy. Obtaining a valid sputum specimen in a decompensated COPD patient is often difficult and guidelines for doing so vary widely.

Patients who take theophylline preparations should have their theophylline level measured. A complete blood count may reflect polycythemia or leukocytosis. Elevated hepatic enzymes are secondary to increased central venous pressure from *cor pulmonale*. D-dimers and spiral computed tomography are indicated if pulmonary embolism is in question. Emergency department bedside ultrasound can demonstrate ventricular dysfunction and is useful in the diagnosis and management of the decompensated patient. In the patient where it is unclear if the diagnosis is congestive heart failure or COPD exacerbation, measuring a β-natriuretic peptide level appears to be useful in sorting out this diagnostic dilemma.

Emergency Department Intervention

Because COPD is a disorder of oxygenation and ventilation, both problems need to be addressed in the management of the acutely decompensated patient. *Oxygen* should be administered to maintain a PaO_2 above 60 mm Hg or an SaO_2 greater than 90%. Care should be taken not to suppress the hypoxic ventilatory drive and produce hypercapnia, so arterial blood gas measurements of PaO_2 and $PaCO_2$ are imperative.

Bronchodilator therapy with *β-agonists* and *anticholinergics* are considered first-line therapy in acute COPD exacerbations. β-agonists activate β_2 adrenergic receptors by relaxation of smooth muscle and subsequent bronchodilation. Anticholinergics inhibit the action of acetylcholine on the muscarinic receptors and block bronchoconstriction in the larger central airways. Albuterol and ipratropium, nebulized or administered via metered dose inhalers with spacers, are synergistic when used together. Short-acting β-agonists may be given every 30 to 60 minutes if tolerated by the patient. Palpitations, tremor, and anxiety are side effects. Patients with cardiovascular disease should have cardiac monitoring when receiving β-agonists. The use of long-acting β-agonists, such as salmeterol and formoterol, is not indicated in acute COPD exacerbations, but should be employed in the management of chronic compensated COPD patients. Studies have shown that these agents enhance health and decrease typical COPD symptoms.

Nebulized anticholinergic agents, such as ipratropium and glycopyrrolate, are as effective as β-agonists in COPD and show synergism when used together. Ipratropium, given by metered dose inhaler with spacer or as a nebulized solution, is administered at 0.5 mg or 2.5 mL of the 0.02% solution and glycopyrrolate (2 mg) is aerosolized in 10 mL saline. Repeat doses of anticholinergic agents have not been well studied, although many physicians use the beta-agonist/anticholinergic combination initially and repeat the anticholinergic nebulization if the response to β-agonists is poor.

The beneficial anti-inflammatory effects of *corticosteroids* provide a strong rationale for their use in COPD exacerbations. In severely compromised patients requiring admission, intravenous methylprednisolone is indicated, whereas a 7- to 14-day course of oral corticosteroids is appropriate for discharged patients. Research validates significant benefit from long-term inhaled corticosteroids.

Antibiotic therapy may benefit COPD patients who have increased sputum purulence, volume, color change, and dyspnea. The most common pathogens associated with COPD exacerbations are *Streptococcus pneumoniae, Haemophilus influenzae,* and *Moraxella catarrhalis.* Treatment duration with antibiotics ranges from 3 to 14 days (**Table 117.2**).

The use of *methylxanthines*, theophylline and aminophylline, for COPD exacerbations is in question. Routine use is not supported, but administration of theophylline in severe exacerbations when all other treatments have failed is an option. If a patient is not currently using a theophylline preparation, then the loading dose is 5 to 6 mg/kg to obtain a serum level between 8 to 12 μg/mL. For patients who take theophylline on a regular basis, the measured serum concentration should be between 10 and 15 μg/mL. The intravenous maintenance dose is 0.2 to 0.8 mg/kg per hour. Methylxanthine toxicity is common, so it is important to lower maintenance dosages in patients with congestive heart failure or hepatic disease who have decreased clearance rates. Smokers have increased clearance rates, so the maintenance dose of theophylline will have to be adjusted upward.

Sedatives are not indicated in COPD exacerbations unless the patient is intubated. Currently, the use of magnesium, as well as *heliox,* is also not recommended.

A trial of noninvasive positive pressure ventilation may prevent endotracheal intubation in patients demonstrating respiratory muscle fatigue, worsening hypoxemia and acidosis, and a deterioration in mental status. Two of these techniques are nasal continuous positive airway pressure (CPAP), and bilevel positive airway pressure (BiPAP).

Indications for mechanical ventilation are as follows: (1) hypoxemia with PaO_2 less than 50 mm Hg; (2) severe acidosis with pH < 7.25; (3) hypercapnia with $PaCO_2$ greater than 60 mm Hg; (4) respiratory rate greater than 35 breaths per minute; (5) severe dyspnea with accessory muscle use and paradoxical abdominal breathing; (6) impaired mental status or somnolence; (7) hypotension or heart failure; (8) respiratory arrest; (9) failure of noninvasive continuous positive airway pressure ventilation.

Disposition

In contrast to asthma patients, COPD patients with an acute exacerbation often require hospital admission, recover slowly, and do not exhibit striking improvement after treatment. All patients with COPD need a primary care provider to treat and monitor their disease. Encouraging the patient to stop smoking and to avoid exposure to second-hand smoke is vital. Patients should also receive vaccines for pneumococcal pneumonia and influenza. In addition, these patients must be educated about their disease and its treatment, particularly in the use of inhalers and spacers. Provisions for follow-up outpatient care, vaccinations, and patient education should be made prior to the patient's discharge from the ED.

Selected Readings

The Asia Pacific COPD Roundtable Group. Global initiative for chronic obstructive lung disease strategy for the diagnosis, management, and prevention of chronic obstructive pulmonary disease: an Asia-Pacific perspective. *Respirology* 2005;10:9–17.

Brunton S, Carmichael BP, Colgan R, et al. Acute exacerbation of chronic bronchitis: a primary care consensus guideline. *Am J Manage Care* 2004;10:689–696.

Morrison LK, Harrison A, Krishnaswamy P, et al. Utility of a rapid β-natriuretic peptide assay in differentiating congestive heart failure from lung disease in patients presenting with dyspnea. *J Am Coll Cardiol* 2002;39:202–209.

Sethi S, Murphy TF. Acute exacerbations of chronic bronchitis: new developments concerning microbiology and pathophysiology—impact on approaches to risk stratification and therapy. *Infect Dis Clin North Am* 2004;18:861–882.

Snow V, Lascher S, Mottur-Pilson C. Evidence base of management of acute exacerbations of chronic obstructive pulmonary disease. *Ann Intern Med* 2001;134:595–599.

Wood-Baker R, Gibson P, Hannay M, et al. Systemic corticosteroids for acute exacerbations of chronic obstructive pulmonary disease. *Cochrane Database Syst Rev* 2005;1:CD001288.

Table 117.2	
Antibiotic Therapy in COPD Exacerbations	
Outpatient Therapy	Macrolide[a] *OR* Fluoroquinolone[b] *OR* Doxycycline
Inpatient Therapy	Beta-lactam ± Macrolide[a] *OR* Fluoroquinolone[b] alone
ICU Therapy	Azithromycin *OR* Fluoroquinolone[b] *PLUS* Ceftriaxone or Cefotaxime or β-lactam/β-lactamase[c] inhibitor

Modified from Bartlett JG, et al: Community-acquired pneumonia in adults: guidelines for management. The Infectious Diseases Society of America, *Clin Infect Dis* 1998;26:811–838.
[a]Azithromycin, clarithromycin, or erythromycin.
[b]Levofloxacin, sparfloxacin, or grepafloxacin.
[c]Ampicillin/sulbactam, ticarcillin/clavulanate, or piperacillin/tazobactam.

Pneumonia

Gregory A. Volturo
Ronald J. DeBellis

Community Acquired Pneumonia

Community acquired pneumonia (CAP) is a common and potentially serious infection. More than 75% of patients with community acquired pneumonia are initially managed in the emergency department. CAP is the most common infectious cause of deaths in adults, and the sixth leading cause of death in adults. Mortality in the outpatient setting is generally less than 1%; however, the inpatient setting averages 12% to 14%. Patients who are over 65 and those with comorbid conditions are at greatest risk of death and complications from CAP.

The lower respiratory tract is generally a sterile environment. Infection occurs due to inhalation of aerosols that contain infective microorganisms, or aspiration of oropharyngeal flora. Aspiration of small quantities of oropharyngeal material may occur in normal individuals during sleep, resulting in infection or colonization; however, it does not occur unless the body's natural defenses are overcome. Pneumonia may also occur from hematogenous seeding from a remote focus of infection. Impaired level of consciousness, neurologic disease, HIV, and smoking (which impairs mucociliary transport) are all considered risk factors for the development of CAP. The most common organisms associated with CAP are *Staphylococcus pneumoniae, Haemophilus influenzae, Moraxella catarrhalis, Mycoplasma pneumoniae, Legionella pneumoniae,* and *Chlamydia pneumoniae. S. pneumoniae* is responsible for 30% to 50% of the cases of CAP where a bacteriological diagnosis is made. An actual bacteriological diagnosis, however, is made in less than 50% of cases. The atypical agents, *Mycoplasma pneumoniae, Legionella pneumoniae,* and *Chlamydia pneumoniae,* appear to be responsible for 15% to 25% of cases of CAP. While it has been traditionally thought that elderly patients were not at risk for atypical infections, it is now clear that these organisms infect patients of all ages and are not more likely in any one age group. Several other organisms may also be responsible for CAP and these less common agents are listed in **Table 118.1**. The incidence of these less common etiologies varies throughout different regions of the country, as some organisms are endemic to particular areas.

Clinical Presentation

Classic bacterial pneumonia is described as presenting with the abrupt onset of fever, chills, cough productive of purulent, perhaps blood-tinged sputum, shortness of breath, signs of lobar consolidation, and of course rales on physical examination, with fever and tachycardia. Atypical pneumonia has been described as being of more insidious onset, with dry non-productive cough, myalgia, headache, and diffuse crackles or wheezing on physical exam. Unfortunately, history and physical examination are not adequate to make the diagnosis of pneumonia as there is no grouping of signs or symptoms that accurately predict the presence of a pulmonary infiltrate on chest radiography. Additionally, the overlap in clinical presentation between bacterial and atypical organisms makes it impossible to distinguish the infecting organism based on clinical presentation. Abnormal vital signs are the best predictor of the presence of a pulmonary infiltrate on chest x-ray. Therefore, initial therapy in the ED generally needs to be empiric, yet to provide adequate antibiotic coverage for the six most common organisms: *S. pneumoniae, H. influenzae, M. catarrhalis, Mycoplasma pneumoniae, Legionella pneumoniae,* and *Chlamydia pneumoniae.*

Diagnosis

The diagnosis of pneumonia begins with obtaining vital signs, including oxygenation. In most patients, pulse oximetry is acceptable; however, for patients in whom pending respiratory failure is suspected, arterial blood gas analysis should be performed. A detailed history should be taken, including recent travel (particularly to areas where unusual organisms may be endemic), potential infectious exposures, industrial exposures, HIV risk factors, smoking, alcohol or drug use, and recent antibiotic use (within four months). Past history should focus on any previous pulmonary infections, chronic comorbid conditions such as COPD, diabetes, CHF, malignancy, cerebrovascular disease, cardiovascular disease, and liver or renal disease.

In order to make an accurate diagnosis of pneumonia a chest radiograph must be done. The initial CXR may re-

Table 118.1

Less Common Etiologies of CAP

Cytomegalovirus
Varicella zoster
Plague
Tularemia
Pertussis
Fungal infections
Rickettsial infections
Hantavirus
Psittacosis
Diphtheroids

veal diffuse infiltrates, lobar or multilobar involvement, cavitation, or may be normal. An initial normal CXR should not preclude treatment in patients in whom there is a high clinical suspicion, as a small number of patients may initially present with a negative chest radiograph. A negative CXR, however, should prompt consideration of alternative etiologies, such as tumor, pulmonary embolism, CHF, etc. High resolution computed tomography is more accurate a plain radiography in detecting small infiltrates, but it is considerably more costly. In most patients <50 years of age who are otherwise healthy, additional diagnostic studies offer little to the decision analysis and treatment of CAP. For patients who are >50 years of age, or those with multiple comorbidities, additional diagnostic testing such as CBC, electrolyte analysis, serum glucose, renal function studies, etc., may be useful in managing comorbid conditions as well as to risk stratify the patient. Blood cultures are indicated for any patient being admitted to the hospital. While overall they change therapy only about 1% of the time, blood cultures continue to be useful in tracking the microbiology of CAP. Sputum Gram stain and culture have little utility in the initial management of CAP. If a patient is capable of providing a good sputum sample, it may be useful later if the patient is not responding to therapy; however, treatment should not be delayed to obtain these samples or their results. For patients with severe pneumonia, *Legionella* urinary antigen studies should be part of the initial diagnostic studies. Recently, urinary antigen testing for *S. pneumoniae* has become available. As compared to conventional methods, sensitivity ranges from 50% to 80% and the specificity is approximately 90%. The clinical significance for the initial management of CAP is not clear at this time, however. Most current studies suggest patient outcomes and overall treatment cost are reduced when using antibiotics that cover both classic bacterial pathogens as well as atypical agents, and there is the potential for co-infection with both pneumococcus and atypical bacteria. Therefore, knowledge that *S. pneumoniae* is present will not necessarily change the initial antibiotic regimen.

Treatment

The treatment of CAP should begin with a three-part assessment of risk to determine the site of treatment, either in the inpatient setting or as an outpatient. First is to assess the patient's overall health status, living conditions, and their ability to care for themselves. Second, calculation of the PORT pneumonia severity index (**Table 118.2**) may be helpful for the assessment of mortality risk. Third, clinical judgment must integrate and synthesize all available information. Patients with hypoxia should receive high flow oxygen, and endotracheal intubation/mechanical ventilation if necessary. Patients who are dehydrated should receive intravenous fluids. Patients with severe pneumonia and hemodynamic instability should be managed aggressively with intravenous fluids and vasopressors using an early goal directed approach.

The cornerstone of management for CAP is administration of antimicrobial therapy. Selection of appropriate antibiotic therapy involves consideration of multiple patient-related factors such as allergies, comorbid conditions, and renal or liver disease as well as a variety of non-patient related factors, such as cost, dosing schedule, and local antimicrobial resistance patterns. There are multiple potential antibiotics from which to choose. Most initial management of CAP is empiric, since it is unusual for the emergency physician to have microbiological data available when assessing these patients. Regardless of the agent chosen, it is mandatory to select empiric antibiotic therapy that has activity against *S. pneumoniae*, *H. influenzae*, *M. catarrhalis*, *Mycoplasma pneumoniae*, *Legionella pneumoniae*, and *Chlamydia pneumoniae* in all patients. **Table 118.3** lists several clinical scenarios with associated suggested antibiotic choices. All patients with severe pneumonia and those with suspected bacteremic pneumonia should receive combination therapy with two agents covering the most common organisms associated with CAP. Consideration for the additional antibiotics must also be given in areas where particular organisms may be endemic (e.g., tularemia, plague). Timing of antibiotic delivery is also important in CAP. Patients being admitted to the hospital with CAP should receive their initial dose of antibiotics within four hours of diagnosis. Multiple studies have demonstrated increases in morbidity and mortality with delay in antibiotic delivery: mortality starts to rise if antibiotics are delayed more than four hours; and increases by 15% if the delay is more than 8 hours. There are no comparison data for patients being treated in the outpatient setting; however, most experts agree that patients should be encouraged to purchase and take their antibiotics as soon as possible, ideally within 8 hours.

Emerging bacterial resistance to antibiotics is becoming a larger problem in most communities. Local resistance patterns should be considered when choosing appropriate empiric antibiotic therapy. Resistance to β-lactam antibiotics and macrolides has led to increased utilization of newer respiratory fluoroquinolones and ketolides as the initial therapy for CAP. Recent emergence of resistance to newer respiratory fluoroquinolones, however, has raised concern about this approach. Both the Centers for Disease Control and the recent Infectious Disease Society of America Clinical Guidelines for CAP suggest that fluoroquinolones should be reserved for patients who are more likely to have resistant infections, or those who have aller-

Table 118.2

PORT Severity Index

Patient Characteristics	Points	Physical exam	Points
Demographic		**Physical exam**	
Age: Males	In years	Respiratory rate > 30/min	+20
Age Females	In years (−10)	Systolic blood pressure < 90	+20
Nursing home residence	+10	Altered mental status	+20
Co-morbid conditions		Temperature < 35° C or > 40° C	+15
Neoplastic disease	+30	Pulse > 125 BPM	+10
Liver disease	+20	**Lab findings**	
CHF	+10	pH < 7.35	+3
Cerebrovascular disease	+10	BUN > 30 mg/dL	+20
Renal disease	+10	Sodium < 130 mEq/L	+20
		Glucose > 250 mg/dL	+10
		Hematocrit < 30%	+10
		PO_2 < 60 mm Hg	+10
		Pleural effusion	+10

Risk Class	No. of Points	Mortality (%)	Recommendations for Site of Care
I	No predictors	0.1	Outpatient
II	<70	0.6	Outpatient
III	71–90	2.8	Inpatient (briefly)
IV	91–130	8.2	Inpatient
V	>130	29.2	Inpatient (ICU)

Table 118.3

Empiric Antibiotic Therapy

Patient Variable	Preferred Antibiotic Choice
Outpatient	
Otherwise healthy	Doxycycline, erythromycin, azithromycin, telithromycin, clarithromycin[a]
Antibiotic therapy within 3 months	Advanced macrolide, telithromycin or respiratory quinolone[b]
Nursing home residence	A respiratory fluoroquinolone alone or amoxicillin-clavulanate plus an advanced macrolide
Comorbidities (COPD, diabetes, renal failure, CHF, or malignancy)	
No recent antibiotics	Advanced macrolide, telithromycin, or respiratory fluoroquinolone
Antibiotics within 3 months	Respiratory fluoroquinolone or advanced macrolide plus a β-lactam (amoxicillin-clavulanate, cefpodoxime, cefuroxime)
Suspected aspiration	Amoxicillin-clavulanate or clindamycin
Inpatient	
Medical ward	
No recent antibiotic therapy	Advanced generation macrolide plus a β-lactam,[c] or a respiratory fluoroquinolone
Recent antibiotic therapy	Same as above, selection will be dependent upon the nature of recent therapy-selection should be of a different class
ICU	A β-lactam plus either an advanced macrolide or a respiratory fluoroquinolone
Potential for pseudomonas infection	Antipseudomonal agent (piperacillin-tazobactam, imipenem, meropenem, and cefepime plus ciprofloxacin, or plus an aminoglycoside; plus a respiratory fluoroquinolone or a macrolide
Suspected aspiration	Ceftriaxone IV plus azithromycin IV, levofloxacin IV plus clindamycin IV *OR* levofloxacin IV plus metronidazole IV *OR* gatifloxacin IV plus clindamycin IV

[a]Expanded spectrum macrolides such as azithromycin and clarithromycin may be preferred over erythromycin because of better patient tolerability.
[b]Switch class of antibiotic, respiratory fluoroquinolones include: moxifloxacin, gatifloxacin, levofloxacin, or gemifloxacin.
[c]Ceftriaxone, cefotaxime, ampicillin-sulbactam, or ertapenem.

gies or failed therapy with other agents. In general, it is recommended that if patients have failed therapy with one class of antibiotics, subsequent treatment should be with an entirely different class of agents.

Most experts agree that antibiotics should be administered for 7 to 10 days; however, there are few studies validating this duration of therapy. Recent studies supporting the use of shorter course, and with some agents, a higher dose therapy have suggested an equivalent efficacy, particularly in the outpatient setting with expanded spectrum macrolides (azithromycin for 5 days) or advanced generation fluoroquinolones (levofloxacin for 5 days).

Disposition

Patients who are hypoxic with oxygen saturation <90%, who have multiple comorbid conditions, PORT scores >90, multilobar involvement, cannot be managed safely at home, or have poor living environments, and those patients who cannot take oral medications, in most instances will require admission to the hospital. Patients with severe pneumonia may require admission to an intensive care setting (see **Table 118.4**).

All patients who are being treated in the outpatient setting should have follow-up care arranged, ideally within 72 hours. Patients who fail to respond or worsen while on initial therapy should be reevaluated thoroughly with particular attention to alternative diagnoses or complications of CAP (**Table 118.5**) such as pleural effusion or empyema.

Nosocomial Pneumonia

Nosocomial pneumonia refers to the development of a new episode of pneumonia more than two days after the patient has been admitted to the hospital. Nosocomial pneumonia is second only to urinary tract infection as the most common nosocomial infection. Nosocomial pneumonia occurs in approximately 0.5% to 2% of patients who are hospitalized. Risk factors for the development of nosocomial pneumonia include: age >65 years, immunosuppression, COPD, depressed level of consciousness, surgery, conditions favoring aspiration (endotracheal intubation, nasogastric tubes, neuromuscular disorders, sedative therapy, supine position), conditions that enhance bacterial colonization of the oropharynx and stomach (antibiotic administration, malnutrition, antacid or H_2 blocker therapy, ICU

Table 118.4	
Criteria for ICU Admission	
Minor Criteria	**Major Criteria**
RR > 30 BPM @ admission	Needs mechanical ventilation
Respiratory failure: PaO_2/ FiO_2 ratio < 250 mm Hg	Vasopressors for > 4 hours
Systolic BP < 90 mm Hg	Urine output < 20 cc/h or acute renal failure requiring hemodialysis
Diastolic BP < 60 mm Hg	
Multilobar involvement	

Table 118.5
Differential Diagnosis of Failure of Initial Treatment
Incorrect Diagnosis
CHF
Embolus
Neoplasm
Sarcoidosis
Drug reaction
Hemorrhage
Host Issues
Local factors, e.g., obstruction, foreign body
Inadequate host response
Complication
Pulmonary
Superinfection
Empyema
Drug
Error in dose route
Error in drug selection
Compliance
Adverse drug reaction
Adverse drug interaction
Pathogen Issues
Mycobacteria
Nocardia
Fungal infection
Viral infection

admission), and mechanical ventilation. The most common source of infection is thought to be aspiration of oropharyngeal flora; however, it may also develop due to contamination of respiratory equipment, transfer from patient-to-patient from staff contact, or because of hematogenous spread from infected invasive devices.

Nosocomial, or hospital acquired pneumonia (HAP), is frequently more severe than CAP, and in general has a worse prognosis. Patients generally have more significant comorbid illness, and organisms are often resistant. HAP may be difficult to diagnose. Frequently patients are colonized with organisms that have the potential to cause infection, or they are already on antibiotics, making a bacteriological diagnosis difficult. Similarly, pulmonary infiltrates initially may or may not be present in patients with HAP; if they are present, infiltrates may be due to other conditions, such as pulmonary infarction, ARDS, or pulmonary hemorrhage, and not from pneumonia. Only approximately $1/3$ of the patients who are mechanically ventilated and develop pulmonary infiltrates will actually have pneumonia. As a result the presence of a superimposed pneumonia may not be recognized until the disease is advanced.

HAP can be divided into two distinct groups, microbiologically. Those patients who develop early-onset HAP, defined as less than five days after admission to the hospital, generally will have community acquired pathogens similar to CAP, with *S. pneumoniae, H. influenzae, M. catarrhalis,* methicillin sensitive *Staph aureus,* and *Legionella pneumoniae* being the most common organisms. Patients who develop late onset HAP, defined as more than five days after admission to the hospital, have a higher incidence of methicillin-resistant *Staph aureus* and gram-negative infections, including *Pseudomonas aeruginosa.* The microbiology of late-onset HAP will vary considerably, based on patient demographics and interhospital colonization variations.

Mortality from HAP ranges from 30% to 70%. Several studies have demonstrated that early, appropriate and adequate antibiotic therapy reduces mortality twofold, and if initial antibiotic therapy is not adequate, yet is subsequently altered based on microbiologic data, mortality is not impacted. Thus, prompt and adequate antibiotic therapy covering all of the suspected organisms is essential to optimize outcomes in patients with HAP. Often the offending organism is not known when HAP is suspected; therefore, similar to CAP, the initial management of HAP is empiric, providing antimicrobial coverage for the most likely organisms based on the patient's presentation. **Table 118.6** provides a clinical-based classification of hospital acquired pneumonia, indicates the most likely organism, and lists suggested therapy for each group. There is considerable controversy whether treatment with antibiotic monotherapy is adequate, or if patients with HAP should receive antibiotic combination therapy. It is agreed that patients with suspected or known infection with *Pseudomonas aeruginosa* should receive therapy with two agents known to be effective against this organism.

Empyema

Empyema is a collection of purulent material in the interpleural space. This may be as a result of an extension of pneumonia, spread from adjacent foci of infection, direct inoculation through the thoracic wall, or as a result of hematogenous spreading from a distant focus of infection. While small parapneumonic effusions are commonly seen in association with pneumococcal pneumonia, empyema is a rare finding.

Small collections of pleural fluid may be obscured by pneumonic infiltrates. Empyema should be considered in patients who remain febrile or do not respond to antibiotic therapy. Pleural effusions may be difficult to find on clinical examination, particularly if small. Most fluid collections, however, can readily be delineated with a CT scan or thoracic ultrasound. Diagnosis of empyema is confirmed with thoracentesis returning purulent material. In the early

---

Table 118.6

Antibiotic Therapy for Hospital Acquired Pneumonia

First Line Therapy
Piperacillin/tazobactam 4.5 g IV q6h
+
Gentamicin or tobramycin 5–7 mg/kg (IBW) daily pharmacokinetically dosed
+/−
Vancomycin[a] or linezolid 600 mg IV/PO q12hs (if institutional incidence of MRSA exceeds 20%)

Second Line Therapy
Ceftazidime 2 g IV q 8 hours *OR* Cefepime 2 g IV q12h
+
Gentamicin or tobramycin 5–7 mg/kg (IBW) daily pharmacokinetically dosed
+/−
Vancomycin[a] or linezolid 600 mg IV/PO q12h (if institutional incidence of MRSA exceeds 20%)
OR
Imipenem/cilastatin 500 mg IV q6h or Meropenem 1 g IV q8h
+
Gentamicin or tobramycin 5–7 mg/kg (IBW) daily pharmacokinetically dosed
+/−
Vancomycin[a] or linezolid 600 mg IV/PO q12h (if institutional incidence of MRSA exceeds 20%)

Patients with a Beta-Lactam Allergy
Levofloxacin 750 mg IV daily
+
Gentamicin or tobramycin 5–7 mg/kg (IBW) daily pharmacokinetically dosed

Alternatives for Patients with Renal Dysfunction
Piperacillin/tazobactam dosed for creatinine clearance
+
Levofloxacin dosed for creatinine clearance

[a]Vancomycin dosing on actual body weight in patients with normal creatinine clearance:
50–69 kg, 750 mg IV q 12 h
70–90 kg, 1 g IV q 12 h
90–110 kg, 1.25 g IV q 12 h
>110 kg, 1.5 g IV q 12 h

stages, the aspirated fluid may not be frankly purulent on gross examination; however, microscopic analysis will reveal organisms and leukocytes. Any plural fluid should be cultured and analyzed for cell count and chemistry. Pleural fluid acidosis is associated with severe pleural inflammation. A pH of less than 7.3 may be associated with parapneumonic effusions, malignancies, rheumatoid pleurisy, tuberculosis, and systemic acidosis, empyema or esophageal rupture. Some have used this value as a therapeutic guideline, in that parapneumonic effusions with a pH less than 7.3 are said to behave as empyemas and require chest tube drainage, whereas those with a higher pH resolve with antibiotic treatment alone. A pH of less than 7.0 is usually found only with empyema or esophageal rupture. Adequate treatment of empyema requires drainage of the infected pleural space by tube thoracostomy.

Selected Readings

American College of Emergency Physicians. Clinical policy for the management and risk stratification of community-acquired pneumonia in adults in the emergency department. *Ann Emerg Med* 2001;38:107–113.

Battleman DS, Calahan M, Thaler HT. Rapid antibiotic delivery and appropriate antibiotic selection reduce length of hospital stay with community acquired pneumonia: link between quality of care and resource utilization. *Arch Intern Med* 2002;162:682–688.

File TM, Mandell LA. What is optimal antimicrobial therapy for bacterial pneumococcal pneumonia. *Clin Infect Dis* 2003;36:396–398.

Gleason PP, Meehan TP, Fine JM, et al. Association between initial antimicrobial therapy and medical outcomes for hospitalized elderly patients with pneumonia. *Arch Intern Med* 1999;159:2562–2572.

Halm EA, Teirstein AS. Management of community-acquired pneumonia. *N Engl J Med* 2002;347:2039–2045.

Heffelfinger JD, Dowel SF, Jorgensen JH, et al. Management of community acquired pneumonia in the era of pneumococcal resistance: a report from the Drug-Resistant *Streptococcus pneumoniae* Therapeutic Working Group. *Arch Intern Med* 2000;160:1399–1408.

Lynch JP, Martinez FJ. Clinical relevance of macrolide-resistant *Streptococcus pneumoniae* for community-acquired pneumonia. *Clin Infect Dis* 2002;34(Suppl): S27–S46.

Malcolm C, Marrie TJ. Antibiotic therapy for ambulatory patients with community-acquired pneumonia in an emergency department setting. *Arch Intern Med* 2003;163:109–118.

Mandell LA, Bartlett JG, Dowell SF, et al. Update of practice guidelines for the management of community acquired pneumonia in immunocompetent adults. *Clin Infect Dis* 2003;37:1405–1433.

Marston BJ, Plouffe JF, File TM, et al. Incidence of community acquired pneumonia requiring hospitalizations: results of a population-based active surveillance study in Ohio. Community-Based Pneumonia Incidence Study Group. *Arch Intern Med* 1997;157:1709–1718.

Metlay JP, Fine MJ. Testing strategies in the initial management of patients with community-acquired pneumonia. *Ann Intern Med* 2003;138:109–118.

Niederman MS, Mandell LA, Anzueto A, et al. Guidelines for the management of adults with community-acquired pneumonia: diagnosis, assessment of severity, antimicrobial therapy, and prevention. *Am J Respir Crit Care Med* 2001;163: 1730–1754.

Stahl JE, Barza M, DesJardin J, et al. Effect of macrolides as part of initial empiric therapy on length of stay in patients hospitalized with community-acquired pneumonia. *Arch Intern Med* 1999;159:2576–2580.

Waterer GW, Somes GW, Wunderink RG. Monotherapy may be suboptimal for severe bacteremic pneumococcal pneumonia. *Arch Intern Med* 2001;161: 1837–1842.

Pulmonary Embolism

James Ducharme

Pulmonary thromboembolism (PE) is a common clinical problem associated with considerable morbidity and mortality. Between 200,000 and 300,000 are hospitalized with PE each year in the United States, with as many as 50 to 100,000 people dying annually. Mortality rates have decreased almost 30% since the late 1970s with the introduction of preventative measures as well as better identification and management. Identification is key: the three-month mortality rate directly attributable to PE after identification is 1.5%, whereas mortality rates are as high as 30% in patients who fail to have their PE recognized.

Risk Factors

Identifying risk factors allows not only the recognition of the possibility, but also may help establish the relative probability of PE. It is now accepted that almost no PE occurs in the absence of predisposing factors, with the chance of PE increasing in proportion to the number of factors present. Even so, the predictive value of any one factor is not necessarily equal to another.

Stasis, endothelial injury, and hypercoagulability are considered the three pathophysiological cornerstones behind all risk factors. For example, bed rest is a cause of stasis, and so places a patient at risk. The risk of PE in admitted medical patients is comparable with that seen after major general surgery. Up to 65% of patients over age 65 diagnosed with PE have been at bed rest for >4 days. At autopsy, 15% of patients in bed for the final week before death had venous thrombosis. **Table 119.1** lists the risk factors for PE.

Many patients, especially if younger than age 40, present with no obvious risk factors. Investigations to identify hypercoagulable states are required in such patients. In more than 50% of those with "idiopathic" thrombosis, an inherited thrombophilic condition can be identified. Such conditions include protein C and protein S deficiencies, and activated protein C resistance. Other patients will have antiphospholipid antibodies, such as lupus anticoagulant or IgG idiotype anticardiolipin antibodies. These may be found in patients with cancer, infection, severe atherosclerosis and even leg ulcers.

Recognition of risk factors may be as important in prophylaxis as it is in diagnosing and managing acute PE. Patients with one of the weak or moderate risk factors (Table 119.1) do not require prophylaxis, whereas most patients with multiple risk factors or with a strong risk factor should be considered for prophylaxis per national guidelines established by the American College of Chest Physicians.

Symptoms and Signs

Not all thrombosis is symptomatic, and much is of uncertain clinical importance. Tibial fractures are associated with a venous thromboembolism rate of 45%, but only $\frac{1}{3}$ are symptomatic. Up to 80% of hemiplegic patients have venous thrombosis in the affected limbs without embolic events. Similarly, more than 45% of trauma patients have been found to have deep vein thrombosis, with 12% being proximal. Consideration of both symptoms *and* epidemiologic risk is required to establish need for treatment.

The Prospective Investigation of Pulmonary Embolism Diagnosis (PIOPED) study identified the most frequent symptoms (dyspnea, pleuritic chest pain, cough, palpitations, anxiety, hemoptysis) and signs (tachypnea, tachycardia, leg swelling) of acute PE. Contrary to previous literature, these signs and symptoms were consistent irrespective of the age of the patient. Although pleuritic chest pain is more common, nonpleuritic pain is not infrequent.

The PIOPED study showed that proper interpretation of nuclear lung (V/Q) scans could only be achieved with *a priori* establishment of probability (low, moderate, or high). Risk stratification tools of varying complexity have been described, with the one produced by Wells et al. being the most validated. Establishing clinical probability is not meant to rule out PE, but to better interpret imaging results. The inherent assumption of all scoring systems is that the patient has *some* chance of having PE, and not *no* chance. Patients should usually have unexplained dys-

Table 119.1

Risk Factors for PE

Strong Risk Factors (odds ratio > 10)
Fracture (hip or leg)
Hip or knee replacement
Major general surgery
Major trauma
Spinal cord injury

Moderate Risk Factors (odds ratio 2–9)
Arthroscopic knee surgery
Central venous lines
Chemotherapy
Congestive heart or respiratory failure
Hormone replacement therapy
Oral contraception therapy
Malignancy
Paralytic stroke
Pregnancy, postpartum
Previous venous thromboembolism
Thrombophilia

Weak Risk Factors (odds ratio < 2)
Bed rest > 3 days
Immobility due to sitting (e.g., prolonged car or air travel)
Increasing age
Laparoscopic surgery
Obesity
Pregnancy, antepartum
Varicose veins

Used with permission from the American Heart Association. Anderson AF, Spencer AF. Risk factors for venous thromboembolism. *Circulation* 2003; 107:I10.

pnea or chest pain of sudden onset unrelated to trauma. Use of the Wells criteria allows for a rapid scoring system, allowing easy stratification of probability (**Table 119.2**):

1. Low probability: Score < 2.0 (1.3% rate of PE)
2. Moderate probability: Score 2.0–6.0 (16.2% rate of PE)
3. High probability: Score > 6.0 (40.1% rate of PE)

Table 119.2

Well's Clinical Parameters for VTE

Clinical findings of DVT	3.0
Absence of another diagnosis	3.0
Cardiac rate > 100	1.5
Immobilization or surgery within 4 weeks	1.5
Past DVT or VTE	1.5
Active cancer within previous 6 months	1.0
Hemoptysis	1.0

Used with permission from The International Society of Thrombosis and Haemostasis. Wells PS, Anderson DR, Rodger M, et al. Derivation of a simple clinical model to categorize patient's probability of pulmonary embolism. *Thromb Haemost* 2000;83:416–420.

Investigations

Lab testing is of limited value as it is essentially restricted to measurement of D-dimer. Clinical probability should be established prior to D-dimer testing. Use of a whole blood bedside qualitative test or an ELISA quantitative test allows elimination of PE in low clinical probability patients. Initially thought to be a sensitive screening tool for all potential PE patients, D-dimer can be falsely negative in up to 15% of angiographically proven PE in those with moderate or high clinical probability. A negative D-dimer in a low clinical probability patient does reduce the risk of PE to approximately 1% (when followed for 3 months), allowing such patients to be discharged without further investigation.

No arterial blood gas measurement is necessary because A-a gradient or pulse oximetry is able to rule in or rule out PE. Similarly, while classic ECG findings have been described, no finding is specific enough to aid in ruling in the diagnosis.

The CXR remains a very important test not only for interpretation of V/Q scans (matched vs. unmatched defects, parenchymal disease abnormalities in areas of abnormal ventilation or perfusion) but also in considering other diagnoses. Most studies that have quoted greater than 75% positive chest radiographic findings in patients with PE do not stress adequately two points. First, most findings are nonspecific or rare. Two, and more important, this percentage of positive films is found only when all radiography up to 72 hours after admission are included.

Nuclear Lung Scan

Despite its limitations, the V/Q scan continues to be a first line noninvasive test to diagnose PE. V/Q scans are also graded as low, moderate and high probability. The V/Q scan can be of diagnostic aid in only 2 scenarios:

1. In a low clinical probability patient (and a positive D-dimer), the risk of PTE is 1%–2% if the scan is normal or of low probability, allowing the patient to be discharged.
2. In a high clinical probability patient, a high probability V/Q scan is considered diagnostic of PE, with no further investigation required.

The majority of patients being considered for PE will not fall into one of the two diagnostic categories, and thus will require further investigation. Due to its inability to be diagnostic in patients with COPD or other pulmonary disease, the V/Q scan should not be considered a first-line test in such patients.

Venous Doppler

In patients with a nondiagnostic V/Q scan or in those who cannot benefit from a V/Q scan, venous Doppler studies of the extremities should be the next investigation. Greater than 80% of PE originates in the lower extremities. With regard to PE, these tests are only of value in ruling in the presence of significant venous thrombosis. A positive study allows diagnosis of PE, while a negative study mandates further investigation. Studies from Europe suggest that up to 10% of patients with PE will have a positive Doppler study. It must be reiterated that a negative Doppler study mandates further imaging studies in a patient considered to possibly have PE.

Pulmonary Angiography

This is considered the gold standard investigation, and should be performed if previous non-invasive studies have been non-diagnostic. It carries a low morbidity/mortality rate, related more to the severity of the clinical presentation than the test itself. Its limitations are:

1. Moderate to poor interobserver reliability (even if digital angiography is used)
2. Risk of renal injury from contrast load
3. Missing subsegmental emboli

Despite it still being the established gold standard, it is rarely performed.

CT Scan

Spiral CT with contrast is becoming *the* first-line investigation for PE. Concerns about sensitivity persist. CT has been found to miss up to 15% of smaller emboli when compared to angiography, but recent studies have demonstrated better interobserver agreement than that found with angiography. Therefore, it is likely that the rate of missed PE is much lower. Recent European data have reflected sensitivity rates of greater than 98%, using 3-month patient follow-up as the standard. More promising is contrast enhanced chest CT with immediate CT venography as part of the protocol. In one study, 18% of all diagnosed PE was discovered with the venous portion alone. At present, if a high clinical probability patient has a negative spiral CT, he/she should be heparinized, admitted, and after 24 hours of hydration, undergo angiography.

Similar concerns with contrast as seen with angiography exist; patients should not undergo both diagnostic modalities within the same 24-hour period. The study may be technically inadequate, with insufficient dye in the vasculature to allow proper visualization.

Treatment

Heparinization is still the treatment of choice. Use of unfractionated heparin (UH) requires weight-based algorithms, and close attention to PTT testing, for mortality is higher when therapeutic PTT levels are not attained within 24 hours. Many advocate baseline PTT testing to identify antiphospholipid antibodies, for their presence will prevent attaining therapeutic levels with normal protocols. Low molecular weight heparin (LMWH), the first choice for DVT, appears as effective as UH. Some studies suggest that LMWH prevents propagation of clot better than UH. LMWH requires less testing, yet at a higher cost.

Thrombolysis should be reserved for hemodynamically unstable patients demonstrating evidence of acute right-sided failure.

Oral warfarin should be initiated immediately, with heparin being stopped after three days of therapeutic INR levels. Direct thrombin inhibitors, such as ximelagatran, are being evaluated in clinical trials. These agents would replace warfarin and not require ongoing monitoring of INR. Fondaparinux inhibits thrombin generation, and appears to be effective in preventing DVT in patients at high risk such as those undergoing hip or knee surgery.

Fat Embolism Syndrome

Fat embolism syndrome (FES) is primarily associated with fractures and orthopedic procedures (**Table 119.3**). The true incidence of FES is not known but has been reported to be present in 1% to 20% of long bone fractures. The most widely accepted definition of FES is: (1) respiratory insufficiency meeting criteria for ARDS or mechanical ventilation (100%); (2) global neurologic deficits (85%); and (3) petechial rash (20% to 50%) and fever. It is known that fat particles can be found in the lungs or systemic circulation in up to 90% of patients with long bone or pelvic fractures and in 100% of patients receiving hip prostheses. FES usually occurs 24 to 72 hours after an event (usually trauma with a fracture), but late presentation (2 weeks) can occur. The symptoms and signs are usually dramatic and abrupt.

Treatment

Treatment is supportive with mechanical ventilation as necessary in conjunction with intensive care monitoring and definitive fracture management. To date no other therapy, including steroids or other agents, has been demonstrated to improve outcome over those achieved with supportive measures only. The incidence of FES is decreased when unstable long bone or pelvic fractures are surgically stabilized within 24 hours. Those patients who develop ARDS as a result of their injuries are the most likely to die.

Table 119.3

Fat Embolism Syndrome (FES): Associated Clinical Situations

Fractures of marrow containing bones	Nontraumatic orthopedic procedures	Soft tissue injuries
Burns	Osteomyelitis	Diabetes mellitus
Pancreatitis	Sickle cell	Hemoglobinopathies
Steroid therapy	Alcoholic liver disease	Lipid infusion
Bone marrow harvesting and transplant	Liposuction	Bone tumor lysis
Cyclosporin A solvent		

Septic

Suspect septic embolism in patients who display fever, rigors, or a toxic appearance in addition to the signs and symptoms seen with PE. Intravenous drug use, immune compromised states, a history of rheumatic fever, and indwelling catheters of any type (central venous catheters, shunts, or fistulae) are all clinical situations that increase the likelihood of septic embolism.

Investigations are essentially the same as for other causes of PE except for echocardiography (transthoracic, transesophageal) and blood cultures.

Treatment

Removal of the source of infection and broad-spectrum antibiotic coverage pending cultures are indicated. The choice in antimicrobial therapy should be individualized to the clinical situation: some immunocompromised individuals may require antiviral, antifungal, or tuberculosis therapy. Previous history, travel, social history (e.g., high-risk behavior), severity of signs (e.g., heart murmur, sepsis syndrome), and results of investigations (CXR, echocardiography, CBC, electrolytes, liver function, renal function) help in the choice of treatment.

Amniotic Fluid

The incidence of amniotic fluid embolism (AFE) is unknown. In those cases where the diagnosis is made, the mortality rate is high (85%) with half dying in the first hour. The clinical situations associated with fatal AFE are summarized in **Table 119.4**. The onset of symptoms is dramatic: acute dyspnea and hypotension, with rapid progression to cardiovascular collapse and arrest. Forty percent have disseminated intravascular coagulation (DIC). Signs or symptoms of CNS dysfunction (anxiety, confusion, seizures) are common. Pulmonary edema is frequent.

Treatment

Treatment is largely supportive, guided by invasive hemodynamic monitoring. Surgical delivery of the fetus is advocated by some physicians. The use of pressor agents, PEEP, and transfusion of fresh frozen plasma and blood products can all be expected in these patients.

Selected Readings

Anderson FA Jr, Spencer FA. Risk factors for venous thromboembolism. *Circulation* 2003;107(Suppl 1):I9–I16.

Francis CW, Berkowitz SD, Comp PC, et al. Comparison of ximelagatran with warfarin for the prevention of venous thromboembolism after total knee replacement. *N Engl J Med* 2003;349:1703–1712.

Horlander KT, Mannino DM, Leeper KV. Pulmonary embolism mortality in the United States, 1979-1998: an analysis using multiple-cause mortality data. *Arch Intern Med* 2003;163:1711–1717.

PIOPED Investigators. Value of the ventilation perfusion scan in acute pulmonary embolism. Results of the prospective investigation of pulmonary embolism diagnosis (PIOPED). *JAMA* 1990;263:2753–2759.

Richman PB, Wood J, Kasper DM, et al. Contribution of indirect computed tomography venography to computed tomography angiography of the chest for the diagnosis of thromboembolic disease in two United States emergency departments. *J Thromb Haemost* 2003;1:652–657.

Wells PS, Anderson DR, Rodger M, et al. Excluding pulmonary embolism at the bedside without diagnostic imaging: management of patients with suspected pulmonary embolism presenting to the emergency department by using a simple clinical model and d-dimer. *Ann Intern Med* 2001;135:98–107.

Wells PS, Anderson DR, Rodger M, et al. Derivation of a simple clinical model to categorize patients' probability of pulmonary embolism: increasing the models utility with the SimpliRED D-dimer. *Thromb Haemost* 2000;83:416–420.

Table 119.4

Amniotic Fluid Embolism (AFE): Associated Clinical Situations

Clinical Situations	Predisposing Factors
First trimester curettage abortion	Multiparity
Second trimester abortion with saline, urea, and hysterectomy	Premature rupture of membranes
	Increased maternal age
	Large gestational size
Uncomplicated second trimester pregnancy	Prolonged gestation
Abdominal trauma	Tumultuous or hypertonic labor
Amniocentesis	Intrauterine fetal distress and demise
Labor and vaginal delivery of prior cesarean section	Meconium staining of the AF
Postpartum	

Aspiration of Gastric Contents and Foreign Bodies

Bret P. Nelson
Stephen H. Thomas

Aspiration of Gastric Contents

Aspiration of gastric contents may be seen in the ED patient who has an unprotected airway from any cause, and is especially likely to occur in patients with a history of poor gastroesophageal sphincter tone or diminished airway protection reflexes from a variety of causes. Patients may be at increased risk for aspiration in the setting of:

- Dysphagia
- Acute stroke
- Trauma
- Altered sensorium (dementia, delirium, intoxication, ingestion)

Of note, placement of a nasogastric tube does not obviate the risk of aspiration of gastric contents. Nasogastric evacuation is often incomplete because of the presence of large particles, and the placement of the tube may be associated with failure of the lower esophageal sphincter to prevent reflux.

As is the case with other chemical aspirations, the extent of pneumonitis seen with gastric acid aspiration depends on both the volume and the pH of the aspirated material. Aspiration of as little as 1 mL/kg of gastric contents has been shown to cause diffuse lung parenchymal damage. The *pathophysiology of gastric acid aspiration* begins with direct caustic injury to lung parenchyma, causing:

- Neutrophil migration into alveoli
- Complement activation
- Increased protease and inflammatory cytokine activity
- Microvascular permeability defects
- Pulmonary edema

Decreased lung compliance and respiratory failure may occur in patients with gastric acid aspiration. Such deterioration is not uncommon, especially in patients with significant aspirate volumes. Aspiration of gastric contents has been singled out as a significant risk factor for development of ARDS.

Histological resolution begins 72 hours after initial development of pneumonitis, and in patients who heal, normal parenchyma may be seen within 3 to 4 weeks. Patients with significant or repeated episodes may develop pulmonary hypertension due to irreversible lung damage. Granuloma formation may be seen in patients who aspirate food particles. *Chronic sequelae* of gastric acid aspiration include:

- empyema
- lung abscess
- necrotizing pneumonia
- pulmonary fibrosis
- pulmonary hypertension

Emergency Department Evaluation

The ED evaluation of patients with chemical or physical pulmonary insult begins with careful initial assessment at triage and continues with a thorough history and physical examination. Assessment of oxygenation and radiographic evaluation represent the most important laboratory and ancillary tests in these patients. Treatment is based on:

- airway protection
- removal of the offending agent
- treatment of the pathophysiology of aspiration
- maintenance of adequate oxygenation and ventilation

Most patients with significant events will require hospitalization.

Chemical Agents

The screening examination at triage should identify the majority of patients with chemical aspiration, as the diagnosis and often the involved agent are known to the patient or those who arrive with him. After vital sign assessment, the most important triage action is immediate placement of the patient with chemical agent aspiration into an ED treatment room. These patients, even if asymptomatic at presentation, are capable of rapid deterioration and should receive high triage priority.

Triage vital signs are most relevant for respiratory rate, as tachypnea can be the first clue to pulmonary injury. By the time patients become hypotensive from chemical aspiration, respiratory distress is pronounced and collapse is imminent. Fever is present in almost a third of patients with hydrocarbon aspiration, and may represent direct tissue toxicity rather than infection. The timing of the fever relative to the aspiration event, as well as the presence of rigors, aids the clinician in deciding on the need for antibiotics.

Initial interventions after triage should include:

- pulse oximetry
- cardiac monitoring
- oxygen supplementation
- intravenous access for fluid resuscitation and drug administration

As the history usually makes the diagnosis and can thus guide specific therapy, pertinent questions should be asked during initial stabilization and supportive therapy. A careful history rarely misses the diagnosis of chemical aspiration. In relevant cases, drowning or ingestion may be reported to the clinician. Patients may relate sudden onset of symptoms while eating. There can also be a history of frothy, bloody sputum. Patients with known aspiration may be asymptomatic, or there may be respiratory distress with dyspnea, coughing, choking, or wheezing. In some cases, symptoms may not develop for up to a day, although most patients who aspirate develop symptoms within an hour. Patients aspirating hydrocarbons report respiratory tract irritation, burning, coughing, and choking. Particular attention should be given to the agent aspirated, as specific therapy is indicated for exposure to certain agents (e.g., treatment for methemoglobinemia in cases of aniline or nitrobenzene toxicity).

The physical examination of patients with suspected chemical aspiration is of paramount importance, as radiographic findings in aspiration cases may not reflect the patient's true condition. Vital signs may reveal tachypnea or fever. In addition to dyspnea, general inspection may reveal cyanosis due to hypoxia or methemoglobinemia. Chest inspection may reveal accessory muscle utilization. Auscultation is likely to reveal wheezes or rales in cases of significant injury. In hydrocarbon aspiration, early bronchospasm occurs as hydrocarbons are spread to the lower respiratory tract. Physical examination findings in hydrocarbon aspiration are similar to those of other chemical aspiration, and include wheezes, rales, rhonchi, and accessory muscle utilization.

Ancillary testing is directed at determining the degree of physical and functional damage incurred by chemical aspiration. Pulse oximetry is especially useful to document adequate hemoglobin saturation, except in cases of dyshemoglobinemia, which is particularly likely in patients exposed to combustion. Arterial blood gas abnormalities may be significant, with respiratory alkalosis and hypoxia. The decision to intubate is usually based on hypoxia or hypercapnia identified by arterial blood gas analysis.

Carboxyhemoglobin levels and methemoglobin analysis (in patients with cyanosis unresponsive to oxygen) are indicated in some clinical circumstances. Other laboratory testing indicated in patients with significant pulmonary injury includes baseline assessment of electrolytes and liver function. While results of these tests are expected to be normal, they provide important baseline information

for patients who are destined for lengthy hospitalization and systemic organ dysfunction. The complete blood count, especially the leukocyte count, is an important indicator in the decision to administer antibiotics to patients with delayed presentation and possible pneumonia. Toxicological analysis is rarely available or helpful in cases of chemical or hydrocarbon aspiration.

Other than assessment of oxygenation, the chest radiograph is the most important ancillary test in patients with chemical aspiration. Patients who are asymptomatic are safe to travel to the radiography suite for a chest radiograph, but should not have a prolonged wait in an uncontrolled setting. In symptomatic patients, it is prudent to order a portable chest x-ray. Radiographic abnormalities due to chemical aspiration may develop as soon as 30 minutes after the insult, and the extent of chest radiograph abnormality usually accurately reflects the distribution and severity of injury. In some cases, the radiographic appearance may be worse than that of the patient, who can be expected to worsen over time. The chest radiography findings are not pathognomonic, but are characteristic for aspiration, and include bilateral perihilar or basilar patchy or mottled areas of increased density. In severe cases, densities may obscure entire lobes. In patients with normal body positioning, the courses of the bronchi dictate that the right lower lobe and left upper lobe are affected most and least commonly, respectively.

Radiographic abnormalities may be present as early as 20 minutes or as late as 24 hours after aspiration of liquid hydrocarbons. Increased bronchovasicular markings and bibasilar infiltrates as well as perihilar infiltrates are most commonly seen. Lobar consolidation is unusual. Rapid evolution of radiographic abnormalities is associated with severe clinical courses. The clinical picture 6 hours after ED presentation has been shown to be more predictive of outcome than radiography, which can be positive in patients who have become asymptomatic.

ED therapy of patients with chemical aspiration is primarily supportive, although in some instances (e.g., methemoglobinemia, cyanide toxicity) specific measures may be required to treat extrapulmonary effects of aspirated substances. The most important therapy in the ED is oxygen. Utilization of sufficient oxygen to maintain SaO_2 in the 98% to 100% range (with corresponding confirmation of adequate oxygenation by blood gas analysis) is indicated in all patients. Bronchodilators are indicated in any patient with wheezing due to chemical aspiration.

Patients at risk for continuing airway compromise or respiratory deterioration, as indicated by PaO_2 less than 55 mm Hg, require endotracheal intubation. Proper cuff sizes are important for prevention of gastric acid aspiration in pediatric patients; adults undergoing endotracheal intubation should have low-pressure, high-volume cuffs inflated. Where possible, orotracheal intubation is recommended. This route allows direct visualization of laryngeal structures, which may be inflamed and subject to trauma from nasotracheal intubation attempts. In addition, the orotracheal approach allows placement of a larger endotracheal tube that will facilitate subsequent bronchoscopy. Finally, patients who require intubation for chemical aspiration may have prolonged critical care unit stays; orotracheal intubation in such patients minimizes infectious or bleeding complications.

In most respects, treatment of aspirated hydrocarbons is similar to that of other chemical aspirates. Suctioning of secretions is particularly important in patients with hydrocarbon aspiration. In addition, since aspirated hydrocarbons solubilize surfactant, the use of continuous positive airway pressure (CPAP) or positive end-expiratory pressure (PEEP) may be particularly effective. Epinephrine or isoproterenol may cause life-threatening dysrhythmias in patients with hydrocarbon-sensitized myocardium, so the use of these agents should be avoided.

Patients with significant chemical or inhalational exposure may develop serious symptoms, including ARDS. All symptomatic patients should be admitted, and those with significant toxicity may benefit from early pulmonary consultation for aid in ventilator management. Asymptomatic patients with significant exposure should be monitored for at least 6 hours in the ED for signs of respiratory deterioration. In most cases patients who are symptom-free may be safely discharged with precautions to return to the ED for any relapse. Uncommonly, precautionary admission may be prudent for patients (e.g., phosgene exposures) who have significant risk for development of delayed toxicity.

Patients with respiratory failure due to chemical exposure usually require critical care unit admission. Not infrequently pulmonary damage in such patients culminates in development of ARDS. A hallmark of ARDS is failure of adequate oxygenation despite increasing levels of inspired oxygen. While increasing the FIO_2 will suffice for a limited period of time, ARDS requires intensive respiratory and ventilator therapy. Intubation and mechanical ventilation are indicated when the PaO_2 falls below 55 mm Hg or when the FIO_2 required for adequate tissue oxygenation rises above 0.5; arterial cannulation is recommended to facilitate periodic blood gas analysis. Use of PEEP may decrease required FIO_2; optimal PEEP for individual patients is best determined by hemodynamic parameters of the particular case. New ventilation strategies that may prove therapeutic in cases of ARDS include inverse-ratio ventilation, high-frequency jet ventilation, permissive hypercapnia, and extracorporeal membrane oxygenation. Steroids are not beneficial in the treatment of ARDS due to chemical aspiration. Surfactant and immunologic therapies are currently under investigation for possible role in ARDS management.

Aspiration of Foreign Bodies

The course of initial evaluation of patients with aspirated foreign bodies depends in part on whether the patient or historian (e.g., parent) suspects aspiration. In some cases, patients may present with signs of airway obstruction after a known aspiration event. Patients with *lower airway foreign body aspiration* may demonstrate:

- Dyspnea
- Tachypnea
- Cough
- Wheezing

As these patients have significant chance for deterioration and respiratory collapse, triage and initiation of definitive therapy should be expedited. In other cases, however, patients may present with symptoms of pneumonia that have developed secondary to aspiration occurring days before ED presentation. Patients with unknown aspiration may also present with intermittent airway symptoms due to intermittent lodging of the foreign object. In cases where the historians are unable to recall an aspiration event, triage assessment of risk factors for aspiration (age, neurologic condition) may provide clues to possible aspiration-related pathology.

Initial triage interventions should include oxygen supplementation for all symptomatic patients, and expedited transport to an ED treatment area for all patients. Given the potential for deterioration, triage to an acute ED treatment area is prudent.

The history obtained in the ED treatment area should build on that begun in the triage area. For known aspirations, the time and nature of the aspiration event should be recorded. Immediate and subsequently occurring symptoms should also be sought. In patients with pneumonia or intermittent airway symptoms, risk factors for aspiration should be considered. These include age extremes and acute or chronic neurologic conditions. The diagnosis of foreign body aspiration should be suspected in patients who report loss of teeth, usually from trauma, and also in patients with oral instrumentation (e.g., bridgework) that could be aspirated.

Physical examination findings in aspiration depend on the level of the foreign body and on the time elapsed since the aspiration event. Foreign bodies lodged proximally result in increased symptoms due to proximal airway obstruction. Upper airway obstruction, occurring above the level of the vocal cords, is discussed in the first section of this chapter. Obstruction inferior to the level of the cords may also produce life-threatening airway compromise with concomitant symptoms of respiratory collapse. Stridor, coughing, and wheezing, or the lack of any air movement at all may be detected on physical examination. Patients with aspiration of foreign bodies into the lower respiratory tract may be febrile, especially if they present days after the aspiration event with development of pneumonia. Examination may also reveal unilateral wheezing, coughing, choking, decreased breath sounds, hyperresonance, or asymmetric chest excursion.

Ancillary testing in patients with foreign body aspiration is primarily focused on radiographic identification of the object, or at least delineation of the level of obstruction. In some patients who present with delayed presentation after unknown aspiration, a chest radiograph may provide the clue to aspiration by demonstrating a foreign body nidus around which a pneumonia or lung abscess has formed. In patients in whom aspiration is the primary suspected diagnosis, the chest radiograph remains the test of choice. Very often portable x-rays are indicated because of the patient's status or potential for catastrophic deterioration in the radiology suite. In cases where the patient is transported to radiology for better imaging (or in the unusual circumstances where computed tomography is performed), a physician skilled in airway management should be in attendance.

The desired radiographic finding in cases of foreign body aspiration is identification of the object on chest radiograph. In many cases, however, this is impossible, and radiographic diagnosis of foreign body aspiration must rely on changes in the thorax secondary to the presence of the foreign body. An expiratory chest radiograph may demonstrate a shift of mediastinal structures away from a hyperlucent hemithorax in cases of air trapping due to an occluding foreign body. Decubitus radiography may help demonstrate this ball-valve effect of expiratory hyperlucency. The expected physiological partial atelectasis of the dependent lung decubitus radiographs may be absent in cases of hyperlucency due to endobronchial obstruction and air trapping.

Therapy for any intrapulmonary foreign body is prompt bronchoscopic removal. Uncommonly, tracheotomy or thoracotomy may be required. Attempts at postural drainage with percussion may be appropriate in some nonurgent cases, but the risk of mobilization of foreign bodies into positions of complete airway obstruction argues against performance of this maneuver by emergency physicians.

Long-term complications from pulmonary aspiration include bronchiectasis, hemoptysis, emphysema, or infectious complications. In some cases, the diagnosis of aspiration may be made only after clinicians begin to investigate pneumonia refractory to antibiotics. Complications of foreign body aspiration can be expected to persist as long as the foreign body is in place.

Selected Readings

Anas N, Namasonthi V, Ginsburg CM. Criteria for hospitalizing children who have ingested products containing hydrocarbons. *JAMA* 1981;246:840–843.

Bernard GR, Luce JM, Sprung CL, et al. High-dose corticosteroids in patients with ARDS. *N Engl J Med* 1987;317:1565–1570.

Grimbert FA, Parker JC, Taylor AE. Increased pulmonary vascular permeability following acid aspiration. *J Appl Physiol* 1981;51:335–345.

Litovitz TL, Felberg L, Soloway RA, et al. 1994 Annual report of the American Association of Poison Control Centers toxic exposure surveillance system. *Am J Emerg Med* 1995;13:551–596.

Marik PE. Aspiration pneumonitis and aspiration pneumonia. *NEJM* 2001;344:665–671.

Marik PE, Kaplan D. Aspiration pneumonia and dysphagia in the elderly. *Chest* 2003;124:328–336.

Moss M, Goodman PL, Heinig M, et al. Establishing the relative accuracy of three new definitions of the adult respiratory distress syndrome. *Crit Care Med* 1995;23:1629–1637.

Rabinovici R, Neville LF, Abdullah F, et al. Aspiration-induced lung injury: role of complement. *Crit Care Med* 1995;23:1405–1411.

St. John RC, Dorinsky PM. Immunologic therapy for ARDS, septic shock, and multiple organ failure. *Chest* 1993;103:932–943.

Strain JD, Moore EE, Markovchick VJ. Cimetidine for the prophylaxis of potential gastric aspiration in trauma patients. *J Trauma* 1981;21:49–51.

Acute Respiratory Distress Syndrome

Sandeep K. Johar
E. Jackson Allison, Jr.

Acute respiratory distress syndrome (ARDS) is a diffuse pulmonary parenchymal injury associated with noncardiogenic pulmonary edema that results in severe respiratory distress and hypoxemic respiratory failure. Petty and Ashbaugh (1967) described a syndrome characterized by refractory hypoxemia, diffuse lung infiltrates on chest radiograph, and decreased lung compliance in a group of 12 patients suffering from severe respiratory failure. Originally, this condition was named by the authors as the *Acute Respiratory Distress Syndrome of Adults*. However, in 1971 the same authors renamed the syndrome to what we now know as the Adult Respiratory Distress Syndrome or Acute Respiratory Distress Syndrome (ARDS).

Diagnosis

Certain criteria are used for the clinical diagnosis of ARDS:
1. Clinical evidence of respiratory distress.
2. Presence of bilateral pulmonary infiltrates on chest radiograph.
3. A ratio of the partial pressure of arterial oxygen to the fraction of inspired oxygen (PaO_2/FIO_2) ratio less than 200.
4. Pulmonary artery wedge pressure less than 18 mm Hg (or no clinical signs of congestive heart failure).

Pathophysiology

The diffuse alveolar damage seen in ARDS results in loss of the integrity of the alveolar-capillary barrier, transudation of protein-rich fluid across the barrier into the alveolar space and disruption of pulmonary surfactant function, pulmonary edema, and hypoxemia from intrapulmonary shunting (due to ventilation/perfusion mismatch with shunting of blood through unventilated alveoli).

Three phases in the pathogenesis of ARDS have been described:
1. Exudative phase: injury to the endothelium and epithelium with diffuse alveolar damage, inflammation, and fluid exudation.
2. Fibroproliferative phase: proliferation of type 2 alveolar cells, squamous metaplasia, interstitial infiltration by myofibroblasts, and early deposition of collagen.
3. Fibrous phase: obliteration of normal lung architecture, diffuse fibrosis, and cyst formation (only seen in some patients).

Epidemiology

In the United States, there are about 150,000 to 200,000 cases of ARDS per year. Approximately 10% to 15% of patients admitted to an intensive care unit and up to 20% of mechanically ventilated patients meet the criteria for ARDS. The mortality rate is about 60%, with most patients dying of multiorgan system failure rather than isolated respiratory insufficiency. Factors influencing mortality rate include cigarette smoking, age greater than 65, and coexisting organ failure.

Causes

Sepsis

Sepsis is the most common cause of ARDS. This should be considered in any patient who develops unexplained ARDS with a new fever, hypotension, or a known source of infection. It may result from indirect toxic effects of neutrophil-derived inflammatory mediators of the lungs. There is also a correlation between alcoholic patients and sepsis resulting in ARDS. Alcoholism results in decreased concentrations of glutathione in the epithelial lining fluid, and thus predisposes to oxidative injury.

Aspirations of Gastric Contents

Approximately $1/3$ of hospitalized patients who experience a clinically recognized episode of gastric aspiration develop ARDS. This may be due to gastric enzymes and small food particles causing lung injury.

Infectious Pneumonia

Pneumonia may be the most common cause of ARDS developing outside the hospital. Common pathogens include *Streptococcus pneumoniae*, *Legionella pneumophila*,

Staphylococcus aureus, Pneumocystis carinii, enteric Gram-negative organisms, and a variety of respiratory viruses.

Severe Trauma

Bilateral lung contusion after blunt trauma to the chest can lead to ARDS. Long bone fractures can give rise to ARDS through fat embolism, which usually appears 12 to 48 hours after the injury. Head injury can cause ARDS from the sudden discharge of the sympathetic nervous system, resulting in acute pulmonary hypertension and injury to the pulmonary capillary bed.

Multiple Blood Transfusions

The incidence of ARDS increases with the number of units transfused. Preexisting liver disease and coagulation abnormalities further contribute to this risk.

Nearly Drowned Victims

This is due to aspiration with the development of infiltrates and hypoxia within 12 to 24 hours of the initial accident. Aspiration leads to an osmotic gradient that favors movement of water into airspaces of the lung and in turn damage to the lung.

Drugs

Overdoses with tricyclic antidepressants (most common), aspirin, cocaine, opioids, phenothiazines, and other sedatives have been associated with the development of ARDS.

Other, less common causes of ARDS are burns, lung and bone marrow transplantation, leukoagglutinin reactions, cardiopulmonary bypass, acute pancreatitis, neurogenic pulmonary edema, bronchiolitis obliterans with organizing pneumonia (BOOP), and miliary tuberculosis.

Signs and Symptoms

- shortness of breath/labored breathing
- tachypnea
- cyanosis with moist skin
- tachycardia
- hypotension
- shock
- diffuse rales in the chest

Lab Studies

- Arterial blood gas (ABG); hypoxia; respiratory alkalosis early in the course of the disease due to hyperventilation. Hypercarbia and respiratory acidosis may be evident as the disease progresses.
- Complete blood count (CBC), serúm electrolytes, blood urea nitrogen (BUN) and creatinine, blood cultures, and sputum for Gram stain and cultures.
- Chest radiograph: bilateral diffuse alveolar-interstitial infiltrates with prominent air bronchograms (may not be seen on an early CXR).

Management and Treatment

- Essential to start with the ABCs (Airway, Breathing, and Circulation)
- Cardiac monitor, pulse oximetry, and blood pressure
- IV fluids if the patient is hypotensive; monitor hydration status via urine output
- Manage hypoxemia with supplemental oxygen to maintain oxygen saturation at 90%. Endotracheal intubation may be necessary for patients who cannot maintain adequate oxygen saturation or if the patient develops fatigue or hypercarbia.
- Mechanical ventilation to maintain oxygenation and ventilation, while minimizing the effects of barotraumas on the lung. (If oxygen saturation cannot be kept above 90%, add positive end-expiratory pressure (PEEP) in small increments (e.g., 2–3 cm of water).

Selected Readings

Esteban A, Anzueto A, Frutos F, et al. Characteristics and outcomes in adult patients receiving mechanical ventilation: a 28-day international study. *JAMA* 2002;287:345–355.

Estenssoro E, Dubin A, Laffaire E, et al. Incidence, clinical course, and outcome in 217 patients with acute respiratory distress syndrome. *Crit Care Med* 2002;30:2450–2456.

Foreman MG, Hoor TT, Brown LA, Moss M. Effects of chronic hepatic dysfunction on pulmonary glutathione homeostasis. *Alcohol Clin Exp Res* 2002;26:1840–1845.

Frutos-Vivar F, Nin N, Esteban A. Epidemiology of acute lung injury and acute respiratory distress syndrome. *Curr Opin Crit Care* 2004;10:1–6.

Moss M, Parsons PE, Steinberg KP, et al. Chronic alcohol abuse is associated with an increased incidence of acute respiratory distress syndrome and severity of multiple organ dysfunction in patients with septic shock. *Crit Care Med* 2003;31:869–877.

Petty TL, Ashbaugh DG. The adult respiratory distress syndrome. Clinical features, factors influencing prognosis and principles of management. *Chest* 1971;60:233–239.

Severe Acute Respiratory Syndrome

Sandeep K. Johar
E. Jackson Allison, Jr.

Severe acute respiratory syndrome (SARS) is a serious, potentially life-threatening viral infection caused by the SARS-associated coronavirus (SARS-CoV). The first known cases of SARS occurred in Guangdong province, China, in November 2002.[1,2] The SARS-CoV is believed to be of zoonotic origin, and crossed the species barrier to humans recently when ecological changes or changes in human behavior increased opportunities for human exposure to the virus and virus adaptation, enabling human-to-human transmission.[3] By August 2003, there were 8,422 reported SARS cases in 30 countries, with more than 900 resulting deaths.[4]

Etiology

A novel coronavirus has been isolated from patients with the clinical syndrome of SARS.[5] This SARS-CoV has been identified from cell culture by electron microscopy, and by demonstration of specific genomic sequences by polymerase chain reaction (PCR) as well as indirect immunofluorescent antibody tests.[6–8] The coronaviruses, a group of enveloped positive-sense RNA viruses, synthesize a 3′ coterminal set of subgenomic mRNAs in infected cells.[9] Coronaviruses are known to cause respiratory and gastrointestinal diseases in humans and domestic animals.[10,11] The natural reservoir of SARS-CoV is believed to be from a group of rodents: the Himalayan masked palm civet (*Paguma larvata*), the Chinese ferret badger (*Melogale moschata*), and the raccoon dog (*Nyctereutes procyonoides*), which are consumed as delicacies in southern China.[12]

Epidemiology

The first documented epidemic spread of SARS took place in Hong Kong. A SARS-CoV-infected 64-year-old physician from Southern China, who had symptoms of a respiratory tract infection almost one week before arriving, checked into a hotel on February 21, 2003. The physician died ten days later of severe pneumonia; in the hotel, the infection spread to eight people who had been hotel guests or who had visited people at the hotel.[13] It is believed that these eight people carried the virus to other countries. By July 2003, the international spread of SARS-CoV resulted in 8,098 cases in 26 countries, with 774 deaths and 7,324 recoveries.[14] As of April 2004, there were 5,327 cases with 349 deaths in mainland China; 1,755 cases with 299 deaths in Hong Kong; 346 cases and 37 deaths in Taiwan; 251 cases with 43 deaths in Canada; and 8 cases with no deaths in the United States. The overall mortality rate for SARS has been about 10%, and the death rate exceeds 50% in individuals older than 65 years.[15]

Transmission

Droplets from the respiratory secretions of infected patients predominantly spread the SARS coronavirus. It may also have a fecal or airborne transmission, which is much less frequent.[16] Sequential quantitative PCR analysis of nasopharyngeal aspirates suggests that the viral load peaks at day 10 after the onset of symptoms. In the stool, the virus appears to peak at days 13 to 14.[17] Those at high risk of SARS-CoV infection are health care workers, family members, caregivers, or any other individual in close personal contact (e.g., kissing, embracing, the sharing of eating or drinking utensils, close conversation [<3 feet], physical examination) with a known or suspected SARS patient within ten days of onset of symptoms.[18]

Clinical Presentation

The incubation period for SARS is generally reported as 2 to 10 days.[19] During stage 1, the patient may have a flu-like prodrome, that begins 2 to 7 days after incubation and is characterized by fever >100.4° F (38° C), fatigue, headaches, chills, myalgias, malaise, anorexia, and diarrhea. This stage usually lasts for 3 to 7 days. Stage 2 is the lower respiratory tract phase which begins 3 or more days after incubation and is characterized by dry cough, dyspnea, and progressive hypoxemia.[15] Nearly half the patients develop radiographic abnormalities, which may be focal interstitial infiltrates that may progress to patchy, generalized distribution. About 20% of patients progress to stage 3, which is characterized by pulmonary injury and acute respiratory distress syndrome (ARDS), necessitating ventilatory support.[20]

Diagnosis

The diagnostic criteria of SARS have been proposed by the Centers for Disease Control and Prevention (CDC). These criteria follow clinical, epidemiological, and laboratory, and radiographic features.[21]

Clinical

Patients suspected of having the SARS must have: (1) asymptomatic or mild respiratory illness; (2) fever > 100.4° F (38° C) and at least one more clinical finding of respiratory illness (e.g., cough, hypoxia, dyspnea); (3) severe respiratory illness with clinical features of cough, hypoxia, or dyspnea, and respiratory distress syndrome or radiographic evidence of pneumonia that require hospitalization; or the patient is part of a cluster of cases of atypical pneumonia without an alternative diagnosis; or autopsy findings consistent with pneumonia; or the presence of respiratory distress syndrome without an identifiable cause.[21]

Epidemiology

Epidemiological criteria include: (1) within 10 days of symptom onset, the patient has a history of recent travel to mainland China, Hong Kong, or Taiwan, or close contact (defined as having cared for or lived with someone with SARS or having a high likelihood of direct contact with the respiratory secretions and/or body fluids of a patient known to have SARS) with ill persons with a history of recent travel to such areas; or (2) persons employed in an occupation at particular risk for SARS-CoV exposure, including a health care worker with direct patient contact or a worker in a laboratory that contains live SARS-CoV.[21]

Laboratory

Conformation of SARS CoV infection in the lab is based on: (1) serum antibodies to SARS-CoV in a single serum specimen detected by an enzyme immunoassay (EIA) or immunofluorescence assay (IFA); (2) a fourfold or greater increase in SARS-CoV antibody titer between acute- and convalescent-phase serum specimens tested by EIA or IFA in parallel; (3) negative SARS-CoV antibody test result on acute-phase serum and positive SARS-CoV antibody test result on convalescent-phase serum tested by EIA or IFA in parallel; (4) detection of SARS-CoV RNA by reverse transcription-polymerase chain reaction (RT-PCR) assay from two clinical specimens from different sources or from two clinical specimens collected from the same source on two different days; or (5) cell culture techniques for the identification of live virus.[21]

Other hematological findings in patients with SARS may be neutrophilia, lymphopenia, leucopenia, prolonged activated partial thromboplastin time, disseminated intravascular coagulation, and thrombocytopenia, which may lead to thrombocytosis.[22]

Metabolic abnormalities may include hyponatremia and hypokalemia. Hepatic involvement is reflected in elevated lactate dehydrogenase, alanine aminotransferase, and hepatic transaminase levels; similarly, cardiac involvement by elevated creatine kinase levels.

Assessment

Chest Radiograph

The first images to obtain are posteroanterior and lateral chest radiographs. These may be abnormal in up to 78% of patients at presentation. Initially small, unilateral, patchy infiltrates may be seen on chest radiograph. These may progress over 2 to 7 days to become multifocal or bilateral, and the distribution is usually peripheral with lower lobe predominance.[23] Pleural effusions, cavitation, and hilar lymphadenopathy are rarely present.

Computed Tomography

CT studies demonstrate areas of subpleural focal consolidation with air bronchograms or ground-glass opacities.

Management and Treatment

Until the diagnosis is confirmed, both suspect and probable cases of SARS should be in isolation from other patients. Notify the health department and evaluate for alternative diagnoses. Initial workup should include complete blood count (CBC) with differential, pulse oximetry, blood cultures, sputum Gram stain and culture, test for viral respiratory pathogens (influenza A, B, and respiratory syncytial virus, and specimens for legionella and pneumococcal urinary antigen).

Even though broad-spectrum antibiotics (e.g., fluoroquinolone or macrolide) have been used in many trials as part of the treatment regimen of SARS, they are not indicated. SARS is a viral infection; therefore antibiotics are not effective to combat this disease.

Steroid therapy (methylprednisone 3 mg/kg/d or oral prednisone 50 mg/d) for the management of patients with SARS, particularly in the patients with progressive pulmonary infiltrates and hypoxemia, has shown some promising results. A retrospective study of 72 patients suggests that an early pulse steroid (methylprednisone > 500 mg/d) is more efficacious and as safe as lower dose regimens.[24]

Antiviral agents (e.g., ribavirin and oseltamivir) have also been used for the management of SARS. These agents should not be used to combat SARS because they have not been proven to be efficacious against the coronavirus and may cause many adverse effects. The adverse effects of ribavirin include hemolytic anemia and teratogenic effects.

If the patient becomes hemodynamically unstable, respiratory care may be required. Respiratory support, including oxygen therapy and mechanical ventilation (avoidance of excessive pressure and volume, and adequate lung recruitment), is carried out according to the usual management principles for pneumonia and ARDS.

Nebulization therapy should be avoided because it has been suggested to increase aerosolization of virus and the risk of droplet spread.[25]

References

1. He J-F, Peng G-W, Zheng H-Z, et al. An epidemiological study on the index cases of severe acute respiratory syndrome which occurred in different cities in Guangdong province (English Abstract). In: *Collection of papers on SARS published in CMA Journals*. Beijing: Chinese Medical Association, 27 May 2003:44.
2. Guan Y, Zheng BJ, He YQ, et al. Isolation and characterization of viruses related to the SARS coronavirus from animals in southern China. *Science* 2003; 302:276–278.
3. Xu RH, He JF, Evans MR, et al. Epidemiologic clues to SARS origin in China. *Emerg Infect Dis* 2004;10:1030–1037.
4. World Health Organization. Summary table of SARS cases by country, 1 November 2002-7 August 2003. Available at http://www.who.int/csr/sars/country/2003_08_15/en/. Accessed May 2005.
5. Lapinsky SE, Granton JT. Critical care lessons from severe acute respiratory syndrome. *Curr Opin Crit Care* 2004,10:53–58.
6. Ksiazek TG, Erdman D, Goldsmith CS, et al.: A novel coronavirus associated with severe acute respiratory syndrome. *N Engl J Med* 2003;348:1953–1966 (Note: This is one of two papers identifying a novel coronavirus from clinical specimens of patients with SARS and demonstrating a lack of antibodies in a sample of control subjects from the United States.)
7. Drosten C, Gunther S, Preiser W, et al. Identification of a novel coronavirus in patients with severe acute respiratory syndrome. *N Engl J Med* 2003;348: 1967–1976. (Note: This is one of two initial publications identifying a novel coronavirus from clinical specimens of SARS patients.)
8. Peiris JS, Lai ST, Poon LL, et al. Coronavirus as a possible cause of severe acute respiratory syndrome. *Lancet* 2003;361:1319–1325. (Note: This study analyzed 50 patients with a clinical diagnosis of SARS and demonstrated evidence of infection with a novel coronavirus in clinical specimens of 45 patients.)
9. Cavanagh D. Nidovirales: a new order comprising *Coronaviridae* and *Arteriviridae*. *Arch Virol* 1997;142:629–633.
10. Siddell S, Wege H, ter Meulen V. The structure and replication of coronaviruses. *Curr Top Microbiol Immunol* 1982;99:131–163.
11. Wege H, Siddell S, ter Meulen V. The biology and pathogenesis of coronaviruses. *Curr Top Microbiol Immunol* 1982;99:165–200.
12. Cyranoski D, Abbott A. Virus detectives seek source of SARS in China's wild animals. *Nature* 2003;423:467.
13. Groneberg DA, Shang L, Welte T, Zabel P, Chung K.F. Severe acute respiratory syndrome: global initiatives for disease diagnosis. QJM 2003,96:845–852.
14. World Health Organization. *Summary of probable SARS cases with onset of illness from 1 November 2002 to 31 July 2003.* Available at http://www.who.int/csr/sars/country/table2004_04_21/en/. Accessed May 2005.
15. Oehler RL. *Severe Acute Respiratory Syndrome (SARS).* Available at http://www.emedicine.com/med/topic3662.htm. Accessed May 2005.
16. Severe acute respiratory syndrome: Singapore, 2003. *MMWR Morb Mortal Wkly Rep* 2003;52:405–411.
17. Peiris JSM, Chu CM, Cheng VCC, et al. Clinical progression and viral load in a community outbreak of coronavirus-associated SARS pneumonia: a prospective study. *Lancet* 2003;361:1767–1772. (Note: A very valuable study from Hong Kong that prospectively followed 75 patients for 3 weeks, describing the pattern of viral shedding, usefulness of viral testing, and prognostic factors for poor outcome.)
18. Oehler, Richard L. Severe Acute Respiratory Syndrome (SARS). http://www.emedicine.com/med/topic3662.htm. *Accessed* December 19, 2004.
19. Booth CM, Matukas LM, Tomlinson GA, et al.: Clinical features and short-term outcomes of 144 patients with SARS in the greater Toronto area. JAMA 2003, 289:2801–2809.
20. Updated Interim U.S. Case Definition for Severe Acute Respiratory Syndrome (SARS). Available at http://www.cdc.gov/ncidod/sars/casedefinition.htm. Accessed May 2005.
21. Lapinsky SE, Granton JT. Critical care lessons from severe acute respiratory syndrome. *Curr Opin Crit Care* 2004;10:53–58.
22. Wong RSM, Wu A, To KF, et al.: Hematological manifestations of patients with severe acute respiratory syndrome: retrospective analysis. *Br Med J* 2003;326: 1358–1362. (Note: Excellent article reporting the demographic, clinical, and laboratory characteristics of patients with SARS. Depletion of T lymphocyte subsets is associated with adverse outcomes.)
23. Wong KT, Antonio GE, Hui DS, et al. Severe acute respiratory syndrome: radiographic appearances and pattern of progression in 138 patients. *Radiology* 2003;228:401–406. (Note: This paper describes the chest radiographic appearance and evolution in 138 patients with SARS.)
24. Ho JC, Ooi GC, Mok TY, et al. High dose pulse versus non-pulse corticosteroid regimens in severe acute respiratory syndrome. *Am J Respir Crit Care Med* 2003;168:1449–1456. (Note: One of the first studies to compare treatment options in SARS, this paper demonstrates that high-dose pulse corticosteroids are as safe as, and probably more effective than, lower dose regimens.)
25. Cluster of severe acute respiratory syndrome cases among protected healthcare workers: Toronto, Canada, April 2003. *MMWR Morb Mortal Wkly Rep* 2003;52:433–436.

Urogenital/Gynecological Disorders

G. Richard Braen

Introduction

In this section problems of the female genital tract are discussed separately from those of the male genital tract with the exception of genital lesions, which are lumped into one chapter. Many of these problems present for the first time in emergency practice, and proper evaluation, treatment, and referral are necessary. Drugs cited for the treatment of these diseases are currently recommended, but it should be noted that many of the antibiotic regimens change at a faster rate than do editions of a textbook such as this. When in question, the provider should consult the recommendations of the day before beginning treatment.

Chapter 125 in this section deals with sexual assault. It is recommended that this chapter be reviewed in advance of a victim actually presenting to the emergency department, preferably during a quiet time or during time away from the department. The psychological needs, physical needs, legal needs, medical needs, and follow-up are discussed in a fashion that meets the needs of today's patients, departments, and courts.

Female Genital Tract

Katherine Brinsfield

Women frequently present to the emergency department (ED) with gynecological emergencies that can range from trivial problems to life-threatening hemorrhages and hidden cancers. Although many gynecological complaints present with similar symptoms, they can usually be differentiated based on a history and physical evaluation, including careful speculum and bimanual pelvic examinations.

Ovarian Disorders

Ovarian Cyst

Physiological or pathological enlargement of an ovary is the most common cause of adnexal tenderness. Follicular cysts occur during the first 2 weeks of the menstrual cycle and are considered to be normal. They are usually less than 5 cm in diameter and may last for more than 3 months. Luteal cysts occur during the last 2 weeks of the menstrual cycle and are rarely seen in women taking oral contraception. Both are almost always asymptomatic unless complicated by rupture, torsion, or hemorrhage. Endometrial cysts, also known as "chocolate cysts," occur in the ovaries, uterosacral ligaments, or posterior cul-de-sac, and represent the extrauterine growth of endometrial tissue.

The presentation and symptoms depend on the type of cyst. All may present with abdominal or pelvic pain, and vomiting. They may be associated with irregular menstrual bleeding and referred thigh pain. Rupture is often associated with recent sexual intercourse or exercise, and causes sharp unilateral abdominal pain. Teratomas and endometrial cysts commonly present in this way. Once ruptured, they spill material into the peritoneal cavity, causing a chemical peritonitis. Pain occurring around the time of ovulation and accompanied by withdrawal bleeding suggests follicular cysts, which usually resolve spontaneously. Luteal cysts usually occur shortly before the onset of menses, and may be accompanied with menstrual abnormalities because the cyst can interfere with normal ovarian function. Hemorrhagic complications occur if an ovarian vessel is torn. Intraovarian hemorrhage tends to cause more localized symptoms, whereas extraovarian hemorrhage, in which the ovarian capsule ruptures, is more often associated with bilateral pain and peritoneal

symptoms. Patients with severe ovarian hemorrhage may present with signs and symptoms of shock.

A history and examination, including rectal and pelvic examinations are mandatory. Tachycardia is often secondary to pain but may be a sign of hypovolemia. Cervical motion tenderness is a common finding and is indicative of adjacent pelvic irritation. Since this tenderness is also found in appendicitis, pelvic inflammatory disease, ectopic pregnancy, and tubo-ovarian abscess, each of these conditions is part of the differential diagnosis. A serum or urine pregnancy test should be obtained, because the presentation of ruptured ovarian cysts closely mimics that of an ectopic pregnancy. Complete blood count, type, and screen are indicated when hemorrhage is suspected. When the diagnosis is in doubt, transabdominal and endovaginal ultrasound help differentiate the conditions. Culdocentesis is rarely performed, but may be helpful when ultrasound is unavailable if there is the need to rapidly diagnose hemoperitoneum. Normal fluid is straw colored on culdocentesis, but is purulent if infection is present. If the fluid obtained is frankly bloody, the diagnosis of abdominal or pelvic bleeding is made and surgical exploration is necessary. A dry tap is nondiagnostic. Laparoscopy is required if the diagnosis remains unclear.

Management depends on the severity of findings. Frank shock is treated with aggressive fluid resuscitation and early surgical exploration. Patients with an unclear diagnosis or in whom a surgical cause of their pain cannot be excluded should be admitted and observed. Stable patients with good follow-up may be discharged with instructions to return if their symptoms worsen or do not abate. The unavailability of appropriate follow-up for a woman with unexplained pelvic pain may itself be an indication for admission.

Ovarian and Adnexal Torsion

Torsion of the adnexa or ovary occurs when the ovary or fallopian tube twists on its pedicle. This occludes venous supply but leaves arterial supply patent, causing ovarian edema, distention, and hemorrhage. Should the arterial supply become occluded, ischemic infarction and necrosis will become manifest in a short period of time. Adnexal torsion is therefore a true gynecologic emergency.

Torsion may occur at any age, with 20% occurring in premenarchy and 5% in infants. A case report has described the entity in a neonate. In over 95% of cases, torsion is associated with a structural or pathological process such as cysts and tumors. Rarely, the fallopian tube itself may undergo torsion due to an underlying cause such as previous tubal ligation, neoplasm, adhesions of the tube, or abdominal trauma. Torsion of the adnexa may accompany the ovarian hyperstimulation syndrome (OHSS), which results from the use of fertility drugs.

Patients present with severe abdominal pain often associated with nausea and vomiting. The pain is usually constant, unilateral, and dull with radiation into the inner thigh or flank. Up to 10% of patients report previous similar, intermittent, short-lived episodes with spontaneous resolution. This represents twisting and untwisting of the ovary on its pedicle. Patients are not usually febrile, and vaginal bleeding is uncommon. A review of 44 patients presenting with torsion described the following symptoms: pain (100%), nausea and vomiting (66%), abdominal fullness (16%), menstrual dysfunction (9%), diarrhea (7%), constipation (5%), rectal pressure (2%), and syncope (2%).

In ovarian torsion, abdominal examination reveals unilateral pain and tenderness. Guarding, rebound tenderness, and pain on tapping the heels or coughing are suggestive of peritonitis. Pelvic examination may reveal an enlarged, exquisitely tender adnexal mass. The torsion is more likely to involve the right adnexa (3:2). Patients should have a complete blood count in which a slight leukocytosis is common. A pregnancy test is obtained to rule out ectopic pregnancy. Abdominal and chest radiographs may be helpful in the early evaluation by ruling out free air or obstruction as possible etiologies for the pain. The test of choice, other than laparoscopy, is transvaginal ultrasound in which torsion may be represented as an enlarged adnexal mass. Doppler studies of the adenexa help delineate blood flow. Because up to 20% of patients with ovarian torsion have concomitant intrauterine pregnancy, it is important to carefully evaluate the adnexa with ultrasound despite the finding of an intrauterine pregnancy (IUP). Magnetic resonance imaging (MRI) may reveal deviation of the uterus to the twisted side, engorgement of the ovarian vessels, and complete absence of enhancement.

Important clinical entities to be considered in the differential diagnosis are appendicitis, pelvic inflammatory disease, ruptured ovarian cysts, ectopic pregnancy, endometrioma, and renal calculi. A laparotomy is needed to treat the torsion, although there is now increasing use of management of torsion by laparoscopy alone, and if diagnosed early on, untwisting may be possible. Patients with OHSS appear to recover well when the ovary is untwisted, even when it appears necrotic. In advanced cases, oophorectomy or salpingo-oophorectomy are the treatment options.

Ovarian Tumors

Ovarian carcinoma is the second most common gynecological malignancy but has the highest mortality. There are 17,000 new cases diagnosed each year in the United States and 11,000 deaths.

Most ovarian carcinomas present with abdominal distention. This may be associated with other features, such as pelvic pressure, increased urinary frequency, rectal fullness, leg swelling, nausea, and vomiting. Ascites may be massive enough to cause respiratory compromise.

There may be a history of weight loss or weight gain, the latter usually due to ascites. Pelvic examination may reveal a fixed unilateral mass. The erythrocythe sedimentation rate (ESR) and leukocyte counts are usually elevated, and a pregnancy test may exclude a concomitant uterine pregnancy. A pelvic ultrasound is helpful both in evaluating the ovarian mass and in differentiating a neoplasm from a functional ovarian cyst or endometrial cancer. Outpatient referral to a gynecologist may be appropriate, but emergency consultation may be preferable, especially if the woman does not have good access to health care or is unlikely to follow up.

Vagina and Vulva

Foreign Bodies

Vaginal foreign bodies are rare but should be considered in any women presenting with a foul-smelling vaginal discharge. In children, toys such as marbles or crayons are common foreign bodies, whereas in the reproductive years intrauterine devices (IUDs), tampons, cervical caps, and sexual aids are more common. Elderly patients may retain pessaries. Although a child may insert a foreign body into her vagina out of curiosity, child abuse should be suspected and the clinician should conduct a careful search for other signs of abuse.

Removal of vaginal foreign bodies is usually straightforward, and in most cases the odor and discharge rapidly resolve. Sedation or general anesthesia may be required to properly examine a child, although a cooperative child may be examined with a nasal speculum inserted into the vagina. Preexisting vaginal infection may be exacerbated by the presence of a foreign body and should be evaluated and treated, especially if the symptoms fail to improve after removal of that foreign body. After removal, the vagina should be carefully inspected for evidence of residual fragments, perforation, or infection. Close follow-up is important if perforation or infection is suspected.

Imperforate Hymen

An imperforate hymen is the result of the vaginal plate failing to perforate during the sixteenth to twentieth weeks of gestation. The incidence is reported as 0.1% in full-term female neonates. It is often missed during initial examination of the neonate, and may go undetected until late puberty. Presentation to the ED is associated with lower abdominal pain and a history of primary amenorrhea. If sufficient menstrual blood has accumulated, it may produce symptoms of frequency, hesitancy, or dysuria. On examination, the introitus is found to be covered by a bulging membrane with a bluish tinge. If the patient presents with urinary symptoms, electrolytes and urine should be tested to rule out renal dysfunction. Patients with acute urinary retention or severe abdominal pain should be admitted for surgical correction; outpatient follow-up and treatment may be appropriate for those with only mild symptoms.

Uterus

The uterus is situated deep in the true pelvis between the bladder and the rectum. (**FIGURE 123.1**) The nonpregnant uterus is approximately 8 cm long by 4 cm at its widest point, and is usually directed forward at almost a right angle to the long axis of the vagina (though 30% of women have a retroverted uterus). It is lined by endometrium, which proliferates, desquamates (bleeds), and regenerates cyclically when under hormonal control. Afferent pain impulses are carried by nerves that reach the spinal cord at T10 to L1.

Endometriosis

Endometriosis is the extrauterine occurrence of endometrium. It can involve the ovaries, fallopian tubes, posterior uterine surface, anterior surface of the rectum, appendix, and bladder. It is theorized that endometriosis originates as the result of partial occlusion of the cervix, causing menstrual flow to pass through the tubes into the abdominal cavity where it implants and comes under the influence of cyclic hormonal stimulation. Seventy-five percent of patients with endometriosis are 30- to 40-years-old. It is more common in nulliparous women and the ratio of Caucasian to African-American patients is 2:1. The characteristic symptom is constant pelvic pain beginning a few days prior to menses and increasing in severity until flow has ceased. Pain is due to local engorgement and bleeding and may be referred to the inguinal region, hips, or toward the rectum, depending on the location of the endometriosis. Defecation may be painful if the lower intestines are involved and there may be dyspareunia. Hypermenorrhea and shortening of the menstrual interval may occur, and there may be bleeding from the rectum or bladder during menses. Infertility is a frequent presentation of otherwise asymptomatic endometriosis.

Physical findings can include an adherent, retroverted uterus, "shotty" nodulation in the cul de sac, adnexal induration, and increased pelvic tenderness prior to and during menses. Obstruction of the fallopian tubes, bowels, and ureters are reported complications of endometriosis. Rupture of large intraabdominal endometrial cysts may lead to a chemical peritonitis.

Differential diagnosis includes salpingitis/pelvic inflammatory disease (PID), ovarian cancer, ovarian cysts, urinary tract infection (UTI), gastrointestinal bleeding, cancer, bowel perforation, diverticulitis, and appendicitis. Ultimately, endometriosis requires laparoscopic tissue sampling for definitive diagnosis.

Treatment in the immediate premenstrual interval should include nonsteroidal anti-inflammatory agents and narcotic analgesics. Long-term management usually requires hormonal therapy. Surgery is reserved for cases that fail to respond to medical management.

Dysfunctional Uterine Bleeding

Dysfunctional uterine bleeding (DUB) is always a diagnosis of exclusion made after ruling out other pathologic entities. The American College of Obstetrics and Gynecology has defined DUB as abnormal bleeding from the uterine endometrium unrelated to anatomic lesions of the uterus (**Table 123.1**). Nonuterine pathological entities (**Table 123.2**) are properly termed "pseudo-DUB." True DUB represents a disturbance in the delicate estrogen-progesterone balance, which maintains endometrial integrity. Over 80% of DUB is anovulatory, and 20% is due to dysfunction of the corpus luteum or an atrophic endometrium. Anovulatory DUB is most common in the postmenarcheal and premenopausal periods, and is characteristically painless and unpredictable (acyclic) in duration and amount of bleeding. In contrast, ovulatory DUB is regular and associated with premenstrual symptoms such as breast tenderness and dysmenorrhea.

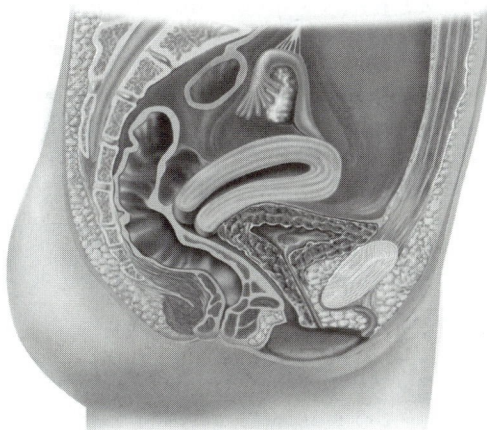

FIGURE 123.1 Anatomy of the female pelvis.

Table 123.1
Causes of Abnormal Uterine Bleeding

Dysfunctional uterine bleeding
   Anovulatory bleeding
   Corpus luteum dysfunction (inadequate or persistent)
   Atrophic endometrium
Intrauterine lesions
   Submucous fibroids (leiomyoma)
   Endometrial polyp
   Endometritus
   Intrauterine contraceptive device
   Endometrial carcinoma
Leiomyomas of the uterus
Pelvic inflammatory disease
Adenomyosis
Early pregnancy complications
   Abortion
   Ectopic pregnancy
   Hydatidiform mole

Table 123.2

Pseudodysfunctional Uterine Bleeding (DUB)

Pelvic diseases not detected clinically
  Uterine lesions (see Table 123.1)
  Pelvic inflammatory disease
  Endometriosis
  Ovarian neoplasm (granulose/theca cell)
Various endocrinopathy
  Hypothalamic/psychogenic
  Polycystic ovary syndrome
  Hyperprolactinemia
  Thyroid dysfunction
  Adrenal dysfunction
Systemic diseases
  Blood dyscrasia
  Thrombocytopenic purpura
  von Willebrand disease
  Leukemia
  Increased fibrinolysin (endrometrium)
Hepatic disease
  Impaired synthesis of coagulation factors
  Impaired metabolism of sex steroids (i.e., estrogen)
  Impaired synthesis of sex hormone-binding globulin
Renal disease
  Impaired excretion of estrogens
  Obesity
Iatrogenic causes
  Anticoagulants, digitalis, oral contraceptives
  (breakthrough bleeding), acetylsalicylic acid

Clinical evaluation includes a careful history to rule out nonuterine bleeding and an inquiry about systemic diseases, bleeding tendencies, and use of medications such as hormones and anticoagulants. Physical examination begins with an inspection of the perineum, vulva, urethra, and rectum to exclude bleeding from these sources. Speculum examination can confirm uterine bleeding by excluding lesions of the vagina and cervix. A bimanual examination is performed to rule out adnexal pathology and to assess uterine size, shape, and consistency. Laboratory evaluation should include a pregnancy test for all premenopausal women. A hematocrit is needed only if the patient has evidence of significant blood loss (prolonged and/or heavy bleeding, postural vital signs). Coagulation and platelet studies are warranted only if there is evidence of a bleeding disorder. Treatment is usually supportive, although oral contraceptive therapy may be given to nonsmoking, healthy women. Four pills a day of a combination oral contraceptive are taken for 7 days. The patient should be warned that heavy withdrawal bleeding will follow the cessation of therapy. Occasionally, in young women with life-threatening DUB, it may be necessary to give intravenous conjugated estrogen. It is difficult to fully exclude all pathologic entities in the ED, so all patients should be referred back to their primary care doctor or gynecologist. This is particularly true for postmenopausal women, since abnormal bleeding is considered to be carcinoma of the endometrium or cervix until proven otherwise.

Uterine Tumors (Leiomyoma, Adenomyosis, Polyps, Endometrial Carcinoma)

Uterine tumors can present with abnormal uterine bleeding, pain, or feelings of pressure or fullness, or can be an incidental finding on routine examination.

Leiomyoma (fibroid, myoma) is a benign tumor made up of smooth muscle and connective tissue. It is the most common uterine tumor, and is present to some degree in 40% of women over 40 years old. Leiomyomas are dependent on estrogenic stimulation and therefore can grow during pregnancy and involute postmenopausally. Such tumors are most often multiple and can occupy sites beneath the endometrium, within the muscular uterine wall, and under the serosal surface on the outside of the uterus. Less than 50% of patients have symptoms, 33% experience abnormal uterine bleeding, and 5% have ureteral compression. Intestinal compression and obstruction have also been reported. Dysmenorrhea and dyspareunia are common. Patients who become pregnant may experience acute pain, fever, uterine tenderness, and leukocytosis secondary to "red degeneration" of the fibroid, which can mimic acute infection. Pregnant patients are also at increased risk of miscarriage.

Emergencies associated with leiomyoma may require fluid resuscitation for heavy bleeding, and surgery should be considered for intestinal/ureteral obstruction or torsion of a pedunculated tumor.

Adenomyosis (internal endometriosis) is the invasion of endometrial tissue into the myometrium. As with endometriosis, the patient's pain and tenderness is maximal during menses and there may be abnormal uterine bleeding. Similarly, symptoms regress at menopause.

Endometrial polyps are highly vascular masses coated with endometrial tissue. They are usually finger-like tumors projecting above the endometrial surface. Patients most commonly present with abnormal bleeding. Occasionally, the polyp prolapses through the cervix and is visible on speculum examination. Malignant transformation of polyps is a rare event.

The most common malignancy of the uterus is *endometrial carcinoma*, which is most prevalent in women between 60 and 70 years of age. Risk factors include continuous estrogen therapy, obesity, diabetes, and hypertension. All women presenting with abnormal bleeding or painless enlargement of the uterus in the perimenopausal or postmenopausal period should be referred for evaluation for a gynecologist as soon as possible for a fractional dilation and curettage (D&C). Some centers are performing the uterine biopsy in the ED, with referral to GYN for follow-up of the pathology. A Pap smear detects only 20% of endometrial carcinomas and a recent negative Pap smear in no way excludes this diagnosis.

Uterine Prolapse

Uterine prolapse is a result of herniation of the uterus through the pelvic floor into the vagina. The principal components of the basin-like pelvic floor are the pelvic bones, levator musculature, and the endopelvic fascia. The weak zone of the pelvic floor is the slot-like aperture through which pass the urethra, vagina, and rectum. Normally, the pelvic floor supports and contains the pelvic viscera and withstands increased pressure during straining, lifting, and coughing. Prolapse occurs most commonly in postmenopausal, multiparous women as a gradually progressive and delayed result of childbirth, congenital anomaly, musculofascial weakness, pelvic tumor, or sacral nerve disorders such as spina bifida. Ascites, obesity, and asthma/chronic obstructive pulmonary disease (COPD) can accelerate the development of prolapse as well.

The clinical presentation can include a sense of heaviness or "dragging" in the low back, pelvis, or inguinal regions, which is related to traction on the uterine or cervical ligaments. However, symptoms may be minimal even with significant prolapse. A firm, mobile mass is palpable in the lower vagina, and with complete prolapse the entire cervix and uterus protrude beyond the introitus and the vagina is inverted. In premenopausal women, leukorrhea or abnormal uterine bleeding can develop. Compression, distortion, or herniation of the bladder into the vagina by the displaced uterus (a cystocele) may lead to residual urine, frequency, urgency, and urinary tract infection. Constipation and tenesmus can occur as a result of pressure on the rectum that can progress to form a rectocele. Crampy abdominal pain may follow intestinal constriction within a large enterocele (intestinal herniation into the vagina). Both ureteral and bowel obstruction can occur. Careful rectovaginal examination for tumors, rectocele, cystocele, enterocele, and bleeding should be performed as well as an abdominal examination.

Slow progression of the prolapse occurs unless corrected surgically. Temporizing measures include an avoidance of straining through the use of stool softeners, weight loss, and the use of pessaries. Patients with evidence of intestinal or ureteral obstruction, pyelonephritis, or obstructive uropathy should be further evaluated and considered for hospital admission.

Cervix

The cervix is a specialized portion of the uterus composed primarily of collagen with only 10% muscle. In nulliparous women it is about one-third the size of the uterus and connects to the uterus at the internal os, which lies at the peritoneal reflection of the bladder. The external os is visible on pelvic examination. Periovulation, the cervix produces mucus that allows for greater sperm transport, but the mucus also allows the passage of microorganisms. The os softens and becomes cyanotic during pregnancy. The main function of the cervix during pregnancy is to protect and support the fetus.

Carcinoma

The incidence of cervical tissue dysplasia is 25.7/1,000 women, and the incidence of carcinoma in situ is 4.7/1,000 except in pregnancy, during which it is 1.3/1,000. Cervical cancer is still common despite the advent of the Pap smear. A Pap smear is obtained by first inserting a cotton swab into the cervix and turning 360 degrees, then smear-

ing the cells onto a slide and immediately spraying with a fixative. The endocervix is scraped in a circle with a spatula; this is also smeared on a slide and is fixed immediately. The result classification system is as follows:

- Class I: normal
- Class II: atypical, inflammatory, or reactive; no evidence of malignancy
- Class III: cervical intraepithelial neoplasia; no conclusive evidence of malignancy
- Class IV: carcinoma in situ; strongly suggestive of malignancy
- Class V: invasive carcinoma; conclusive for malignancy

Any carcinoma visible on speculum examination is most likely class V and should be referred immediately. Class II is either followed by colposcopy or by a repeat Pap and a DNA test for human papilloma virus (HPV), which is potentially oncogenic. Higher classes are often cone biopsied. All abnormal Pap smears need to be referred to a gynecologist urgently. *Nabothian cysts* are cervical abnormalities that might be mistaken for carcinoma. They are formed by plugged mucus glands beneath the epithelial layer.

Infectious Disorders

Bartholin Gland Abscess

The Bartholin gland is located in the posterior part of the labia minora. It drains via ducts into the vestibule, exterior to the hymenal ring, and produces secretions that aid in lubrication during intercourse. Obstruction of these ducts is a common problem and causes cyst and abscess formation. Cyst formation is more likely after an episode of vaginitis and almost always develops into an abscess. The abscess may present with pain that interferes with walking or sitting. Rarely, the only complaint may be pain at the time of sexual arousal.

Definitive therapy usually involves surgical excision of the gland under general anesthesia. Emergency incision and drainage may be indicated for relief of pain and discomfort. Conscious sedation should be considered for analgesia. A posterior-medial incision is made close to the vaginal introitus at the area of maximal pointing, and the abscess packed to ensure drainage and epithelialization. A Word catheter is recommended in place of gauze packing. It is inserted through a stab wound on the vaginal side of the abscess. It is easier to insert the catheter before the abscess is fully drained; it may be difficult to fully insert into a collapsed cavity. The catheter should remain in place for 4 to 6 weeks, during which time the patient should take twice daily sitz baths. Antibiotics are not usually needed, but adequate analgesia should be prescribed to the patient. The problem often recurs, and gynecological referral is needed for definitive treatment, which usually involves excision of the entire gland.

Cervicitis and Urethritis

Cervicitis and urethritis are manifestations of the same etiologic agents, usually gonorrhea or chlamydia. Other pathogens such as *Mycoplasma hominis* and *Ureaplasma urealyticum* are less common. Often the only symptom is a purulent odorless vaginal discharge, but gonococcal and chlamydial cervicitis may be entirely asymptomatic. On gross examination, it is not possible to distinguish between chlamydial and gonococcal cervicitis, although studies show that chlamydial cervicitis is about five times more common.

Examination of the cervix reveals an erythema, ulceration, or friability with a purulent odorless discharge. Gram stain shows gram-negative diplococci in the case of gonococcal cervicitis, but this finding alone does not confirm the diagnosis since nonpathogenic *Neisseria* species are commensural flora in the female genital tract. Cervical Gram stain is only 50% sensitive, and cultures should therefore be obtained using a calcium alginate endocervical swab. The swab is placed in the cervical os for 40 seconds and is then plated on Thayer-Martin medium.

Laboratory tests for chlamydia include culture, but this is expensive and the results are not available for 2 or 3 days. Because of the problems associated with live culture, special laboratory expertise is required. These problems can be avoided by using a rapid fluorescent slide for the detection of chlamydial antigen, although the number of false-positive results is high. Overall, a high index of clinical suspicion is extremely important. A yellow mucopurulent secretion containing 10 or more polymorphonuclear leukocytes per high-powered field, in the absence of gram-negative intracellular diplococci, should strongly suggest chlamydial cervicitis.

Urethritis should be considered in any woman complaining of dysuria with white blood cells in the urine. Studies of patients have shown that many have less than the traditional count of 10^5 bacteria per milliliter, but nonetheless have symptoms of cystitis. Chlamydia, gonorrhea, and *Escherichia coli* are common pathogens. In about 15% of cases, no etiology is demonstrated. In all cases in which the history and physical examination is suspicious of gonorrheal or chlamydial urethritis, treatment should follow the outlines listed below.

Studies have shown that 20% to 50% of patients with gonorrhea have concomitant chlamydial infection. Therefore, any patient with a diagnosis of gonorrhea should be treated for presumed chlamydial infection. Many experts recommend concomitant treatment for gonorrhea with a positive chlamydia test; however, this remains controversial. A number of options for single dose therapy exist for the treatment of gonorrhea and the Centers for Disease Control (CDC) has approved azithromycin as a single-dose treatment for uncomplicated chlamydia. Current therapy is outlined in **Table 123.3** Any of the options should be followed by treatment of presumed or diagnosed concomitant chlamydia as outlined in **Table 123.4**.

Gonorrhea is reportable in all states and chlamydia in most. All sexual contacts within 30 days of the onset of symptoms must be traced and treated. Unless symptoms persist, a test of cure is not needed once the patient has taken her single-dose therapy. However, she should also be tested for syphilis in the ED. Chlamydial infection increases the risk of HIV transmission, and these patients should therefore be advised to seek follow-up care and possible HIV testing where clinically indicated. All patients with sexually transmitted diseases (STDs) should receive counseling in the ED regarding safe sex practices.

Pelvic Inflammatory Disease

Pelvic inflammatory disease (PID) describes bacterial infection of the uterine adnexa, occurring in young, sexually active women. It is responsible for 2.5 million outpatient visits and over 200,000 hospitalizations each year. In the year 2000 it is projected that the health care costs associated with PID will be $10 billion. Although *Neisseria gonorrhoeae* has long been identified as a causative agent, it is now thought to be responsible for only 50% of cases, although it is still the major cause in urban areas. *Chlamydia trachomatis* is responsible for 25% to 50% of cases, and is more common than gonococcal infection among college students. Other pathogens such as mycoplasma, aerobic bacteria (*E. coli, Streptococcus,* and *Haemophilus influenzae*), and anaerobic bacteria (*Bacteroides, Peptostreptococcus,* and *Lactobacillus*) are responsible for the remainder. Tuberculous PID is a remote consideration in immunocompromised patients or those from endemic areas. Polymicrobial infection is thought to

Table 123.3

Single Dose Therapy for Uncomplicated Gonorrhea

Antibiotic	Dosage
Cefixime	400 mg orally, once or
Ceftriaxone	125 mg intramuscularly, once or
Ciprofloxacin[a]	500 mg orally, once, or
Ofloxacin[a]	400 mg orally, once or
Levofloxacin	250 mg orally

[a]*Do not use on pregnant females.*
Cefixime 400 mg has been studied in pregnancy (efficacy: 96.2%).
For patients allergic to cefixime, ceftriaxone, ciprofloxacin, orfloxacin, or levofloxacin use azithromycin 2 g orally, once.

Table 123.4

Treatment of Uncomplicated Chlamydia

Antibiotic	Dosage
Azithromycin	1 g orally, once *or*
Doxycycline[a]	100 mg orally, twice daily for 7 days, *or*
Erythromycin base	500 mg orally four times daily for 7 days, *or*
Erythromycin ethylsuccinate	800 mg orally four times daily for 7 days *or*
Ofloxacin[a]	300 mg orally, twice daily for 7 days, *or*
Levofloxacin	500 mg orally for 7 days

[a]*Do not use in pregnant females.*

be very common. The method of ascending infection is unclear, but involves organisms seeding from the lower vaginal tract during sexual intercourse, and upward into the fallopian tubes and peritoneum. Risk factors include multiple sexual partners, IUD use, douching, smoking, engaging in intercourse near the time of menses, and young age. The end result of infection is destruction of the fallopian tubes and widespread inflammation within the peritoneal cavity. Complications of PID include chronic pelvic pain, perihepatitis, infertility, ectopic pregnancy, pelvic adhesions, and tubo-ovarian abscess.

PID should be considered in any woman of childbearing age with pelvic pain. In its classical presentation, the chief complaints are bilateral lower abdominal pain, abnormal vaginal discharge, vaginal bleeding, or fever. However, PID is notoriously difficult to diagnose on clinical grounds (**Table 123.5**). PID is clinically silent in some women, and only 33% of those with laparoscopically confirmed PID have the five classic signs of fever, adnexal tenderness, vaginal discharge, a pelvic mass, and a raised ESR. PID should enter into the differential diagnosis in a woman with signs and symptoms suggestive of urinary tract and gastrointestinal disease, appendicitis, ectopic pregnancy, or ovarian cyst.

A full sexual history is vital, including past and recent menstruation, the number of sexual partners, present sexual activity, the use of contraceptives, and previously treated sexually transmitted diseases. Vital signs including a temperature and orthostatics are essential. Physical examination should focus on the abdomen and pelvis, and the presence of cervical motion tenderness and adnexal tenderness should be noted. Cervical and urethral cultures should be sent for *N. gonorrhoeae*, *Chlamydia trachomatis*, anaerobes, and aerobes. Cultures should also be obtained from the rectum and anus depending on the sexual history. Serologic testing for syphilis is encouraged.

The diagnosis of PID can be challenging. Although not yet substantiated through clinical trials, the diagnosis is based on the presence of the three major criteria and one of the minor criteria.

Major criteria—all three should be present:
1. Lower abdominal tenderness
2. Cervical or uterine tenderness
3. Adnexal tenderness

Minor criteria—at least one should be present:
1. Temperature > 38° C
2. WBC > 10,500
3. ESR > 15 mm/h
4. Gram stain of endocervical discharge demonstrating Gram-negative diplococci
5. Positive monoclonal antibody test for *C. trachomatis* from endocervical discharge
6. Purulent material on culdocentesis
7. Adnexal mass consistent with tubo-ovarian abscess

Some investigators have criticized these criteria, noting that patients with mild PID may present without significant abdominal tenderness. In practice, PID may therefore be presumptively diagnosed and treated in the ED on the basis of adnexal tenderness and cervical motion tenderness, together with the presence of one of the minor criteria. One study of patients presenting with signs and symptoms of PID who underwent laparoscopy found that 65% had that diagnosis confirmed, 23% had normal pelvic anatomy, and 12% had other pathology such as appendicitis or endometriosis.

An additional test that may be helpful is culdocentesis, which is performed to identify the presence of pus or intraperitoneal bleeding and to obtain material for culture. Ultrasound should be performed if there is a suspicion of a tubo-ovarian abscess. It is also helpful in women who are difficult to examine either because of obesity, pain, or inability to cooperate. Computed tomography (CT) scanning may also be useful in delineating abscess formation. If there remains significant clinical doubt as to the pathology, diagnostic laparoscopy is required.

Once the diagnosis of PID has been made, the emergency physician must decide on the need for hospitalization. Opinion is divided as to the ideal disposition, and some physicians hospitalize even mild cases of PID, justifying this position with the need for close patient follow-up and the potential for complications. A group of patients exists in whom such a course of action is justified, but this decision should reflect the following generally accepted guidelines for inpatient therapy: (1) an uncertain diagnosis; (2) a nulliparous patient; (3) failed outpatient therapy; (4) pregnancy; (5) an adnexal mass consistent with tubo-ovarian abscess; (6) the presence of an IUD; (7) significant peritoneal signs, so that a surgical emergency such as appendicitis or ectopic pregnancy cannot be safely ruled out; (8) failure to take oral medicines; and (9) poor likelihood of adequate follow-up. Therapy for inpatients and outpatients is two-pronged, with the first part aimed at treating gonococci, anaerobes, and aerobes, and the second part aiming to eradicate *C. trachomatis* and genital mycoplasma. Examples of current recommendations for antibiotic therapy are shown in **Table 123.6**.

The removal of an IUD is controversial. Some consider it imperative, claiming it acts as a nidus of infection, while others have found little change in outcome if the IUD is removed. We recommend that it be removed by a gynecologist within 48 hours of the start of antibiotic therapy. If the patient refuses hospitalization, the IUD should be removed within 3 days of the commencement of therapy.

Table 123.5		
Sensitivity and Specificity of Signs and Symptoms of Pelvic Inflammatory Disease (PID)		
Symptom	**Sensitivity (%)**	**Specificity (%)**
Fever and chills	1	80
Temperature > 38° C	24–40	79–91
Palpable mass	24–49	74–79
ESR > 25 mm/h	55	84

Table 123.6

Outpatient Therapy for PID (Examples)

Use one of the three following regimens:
1. Ofloxacin 400 mg orally twice daily plus metronidazole 500 mg orally twice daily, both for 14 days
2. Cefoxitin 2 g intramuscularly once with 1 g probenecid orally once
3. Ceftriaxone 250 mg intramuscularly once plus doxycycline 100 mg orally twice daily for 14 days

Should the emergency physician feel that follow-up is very unlikely, the IUD should be removed after a dose of antibiotics has been given, and with written consent by the patient. Other important recommendations to the patient include abstinence from sexual intercourse for 14 days. Male sexual partners, both symptomatic and asymptomatic, should be examined and treated as necessary. Close follow-up is mandatory. No woman should be discharged unless it is clear that she will follow up within 48 to 72 hours. Failure to improve within this time frame is itself an indication for admission. Patients in the ED should also be counseled about the serious complications of PID and the need always to use barrier protection.

Tubo-ovarian abscess (TOA) is a common and potentially fatal complication of PID. It is caused by the trapping of purulent material within an occluded fallopian tube or from pus leaking from the distal end of the tube, causing abscess formation in the ovary or peritoneal cavity. It should be suspected if an adnexal mass is palpated in a woman with PID. Ultrasound is the confirming test of choice, and has been shown to diagnose TOA with a high degree of accuracy, although it is not always possible to distinguish an abscess from an inflammatory mass. The patient with a TOA should be admitted, closely observed, and treated with intravenous antibiotics as outlined for inpatient PID therapy. Up to 50% have no response within 72 hours and may require surgical drainage or a unilateral salpingo-oophorectomy. A ruptured TOA carries a 15% mortality rate. Patients with a ruptured TOA initially present with "warm shock," namely decreased systemic resistance and increased cardiac output. This rapidly progresses to end-organ hypoperfusion and marked acidosis. The diagnosis of a ruptured TOA should be presumptively made in a woman with a history suggestive of PID, hypotension, tachycardia, and peritonitis. The surgical team should be notified as early on as possible, and the patient should have two large-bore intravenous catheters placed. Blood should be sent for cross-match, clotting studies, and an arterial blood gas. Aggressive management includes large-volume colloid infusion, dopamine, broad-spectrum antibiotics, and rapid transfer to an intensive care unit or operating suite. Pharmacologic treatment is supportive only. The definitive therapy is surgery involving a total abdominal hysterectomy with bilateral salpingo-oophorectomy. Conservative surgery is occasionally possible.

Fitz-Hugh-Curtis syndrome, or perihepatitis, was originally thought to be a consequence of gonococcal infection, but it is now established that in 60% to 90% of women with the syndrome, *C. trachomatis* is the causative organism. Organisms are thought to ascend from the fallopian tubes into the paracolic gutters and into the subphrenic spaces, causing inflammation of the liver capsule. Perihepatitis is clinically evident in about 8% of women with PID and up to 20% show that pathology on laparoscopy. The onset of symptoms is usually sudden and the pain is pleuritic in quality. There is often referred pain to the right shoulder. Examination may reveal right upper quadrant tenderness, and Murphy's sign may be present. Because the symptoms overlap with the presentation of acute cholecystitis, pneumonia, or occasionally pyelonephritis, a high index of suspicion is required, and pelvic examination is needed to make the diagnosis. Clinical and laboratory findings are similar to those found in PID, but fever and a raised ESR are less common. Liver function tests may be mildly elevated in up to 50% of patients. Occasionally, isolation of *N. gonorrhoeae* is the only clue to the underlying pathology. Ultrasound examination is recommended to ensure that the gallbladder is not obstructed, and laparoscopy is needed if the diagnosis is in doubt. The classic anatomical finding of perihepatitis is "violin string" adhesions between the surface of the liver and surrounding structures. Management is the same as outlined for the inpatient treatment of PID, and the response is usually prompt.

Vulvovaginitis

The vaginal environment is a dynamic and easily disturbed system. The disruption of this system causes a change in vaginal pH from the normal range of 3.8 to 4.2, and allows pathogens to multiply. There are three common infections of the vagina. The most common is a bacterial vaginitis caused by a synergistic bacterial infection, in which the normal vaginal bacterial flora are displaced by predominantly anaerobic bacteria. The second most frequent cause is fungal infection, most commonly candidiasis, and the third is a protozoal infection caused by *Trichomonas*. All cause an abnormal vaginal discharge, itching and odor, dysuria, and dyspareunia. Vaginitis is a very common complaint and its etiology can usually be determined by the emergency physician. The characteristics of vaginal discharges are listed in **Table 123.7**.

Bacterial vaginitis usually presents with a profuse foul-smelling discharge, often gray in color and frothy. Patients often describe the odor as "musty" or "fishy," and this smell is often most apparent after intercourse, when the presence of alkaline semen results in the release of aromatic amines. The incubation is 5 to 10 days following exposure and most experts consider it a sexually transmitted disease. Although when first described it was thought to be caused by a single organism, it is now thought to be caused by the conversion of the normal mixed vaginal flora to a predominantly anaerobic organism. The cause of this change is not well understood. Speculum examination reveals a discharge that is mildly adherent to the vaginal walls, in contrast to a normal discharge, which is seen

Table 123.7

Characteristics of Vaginal Discharges

Clinical Parameter	Normal	*Candida albicans*	Trichomonas vaginalis	Bacterial vaginosis
Pruritus	None	Marked	Common	Less common
Discharge				
Amount	Variable, usually scant	Scant to moderate	Profuse	Moderate
Color	Clear or white	White	White or off-white	Clear or milky
Consistency	Nonhomogenous, flocculent	Cheesy with musty odor	Purulent, thin frothy	Homogeneous thin coating on vaginal walls; occasionally frothy with foul odor
Associated inflammatory signs	None	Erythema or friability of vaginal mucosa and introitus; vulvar dermatitis common	Strawberry lesions on vaginal mucosa: vulvae often involved	None
PH of secretions	<4.5	<4.5	>5.0	>5.0
Amine (fishy) odor with 10% KOH	None	None	Present	Present
Onset with menses		Last half of cycle	Yes	No
Wet amount	Lactobacilli predominate	Pseudohyphae or budding yeast in 50–80%	Motile forms seen in about 75%	Clue cells present PMNs rare. Lack of lactobacilli

in the most dependent part of the vagina. Vulvar irritation is rare. Diagnosis of bacterial vaginitis should be made if four criteria are present: (1) a thin homogeneous vaginal discharge; (2) a vaginal pH greater than 4.7; (3) the presence of an amine-like odor when vaginal secretions are mixed with potassium hydroxide; and (4) a wet smear of the vaginal discharge demonstrating clue cells. The amine "whiff" test is performed by adding a few drops of 10% KOH to a slide of the discharge. Release of diamines and their characteristic fishy smell indicates a positive test. Clue cells are vaginal epithelial cells with bacteria attached to their surface, and are seen in the wet mount under 40× magnification.

The preferred therapy for bacterial vaginitis is metronidazole, 250 mg orally three times a day for 7 days. It may also be given as a 500 mg twice daily dose. A single-dose regimen of 2 g orally has a cure rate of approximately 80%. Alternative therapy is clindamycin 300 mg orally twice a day for 7 days. Most physicians do not treat the male partner of affected patients, although this is controversial. Proponents of treatment claim lower rates of recurrence if the male partner is treated. If the patient is pregnant, metronidazole should not be used because of possible mutagenic potential. Alternatives are clindamycin or amoxicillin/clavulanic acid 500 mg three times a day for 7 days.

Candidiasis is the second most common cause of vaginitis. The majority of cases are caused by *Candida albicans*, which rapidly overgrows in the vagina when the relative concentration of lactobacilli declines. Predisposing factors include diabetes mellitus, pregnancy, steroid use, antibiotic therapy, and menstruation. It is not usually found in mixed infections with bacterial or *Trichomonas* vaginitis, and is not associated with other sexually transmitted diseases. Patients complain of a thick, white, curdy discharge associated with pruritus, vaginal itching, and irritation. The discharge does not have an odor. The diagnosis is made by noting the characteristics of the discharge of pelvic examination, and obtaining a smear of the vaginal secretions, which is mixed with 10% KOH. Spores, hyphae, or pseudohyphae are seen, but the sensitivity of microscopic detection is only about 65%, so that a negative smear does not exclude the diagnosis. A culture on Sabouraud medium may be sent, but is usually not necessary for a simple, uncomplicated infection.

The treatment of choice for candidal vaginitis is topical application of imidazoles, such as clotrimazole or miconazole. A 100 mg vaginal suppository should be used for 3 to 7 days. Studies have shown that the cure rates of the 3- and 7-day therapies are equal. A single oral dose of 150 mg of fluconazole is also effective. Recurrent candidiasis affects between 20% and 80% of patients. In these cases, cultures should be obtained from the mouth, rectum, ejaculate, and vagina of sexual partners, and treatment should be directed to the appropriate area of colonization. The urine should be screened for glycosuria. Recurrence also suggests a defect in cell-mediated immunity and the patient should be tested for HIV. A woman with a history of recurrence should have close follow-up with a gynecologist, and oral therapy with ketoconazole is usually required.

Trichomoniasis affects some 3 million American women each year, but its incidence and prevalence are declining. *Trichomonas vaginalis* is a flagellated protozoan that inhabits the lower urinary tract and vagina, and is sexually transmitted. The common presenting symptoms are vaginal itching and a green, frothy discharge. Vulvar pruritus is common. Examination reveals erythema and edema of the vagina and vulva, but the classic finding of reddened punctate spots on the cervix, the so-called strawberry cervix, is found in only 10% of women. Vaginal pH is usually greater than 5.0. A wet mount of the vaginal secretions may show flagellate motile trichomonads, slightly larger than a white blood cell. Numerous polymorphonuclear neutrophils are also seen. Although it is possible to culture for *Trichomonas,* this is rarely done. If the diagnosis is in doubt, the usual treatment is an empirical trial of metranidazole.

Single-dose therapy with 2 g of oral metronidazole is effective in curing *Trichomonas,* but should not be used in males. The emergency physician should encourage the patient to contact all her sexual partners, who should be followed and treated. Metronidazole is contraindicated in the first trimester of pregnancy, during which time clotrimazole vaginal suppositories should be used. It should be remembered that up to 15% of women infected with *Trichomonas* are asymptomatic, but when *Trichomonas* is found incidentally it should be treated. Patients should be warned of the possibility of a disulfiram-like reaction if ethanol is consumed while taking metronidazole and for 72 hours following the last dose.

Selected Readings

Benrubi GI, ed. *Obstetric and Gynecologic Emergencies.* Philadelphia: Lippincott, 1994.

Copeland LJ, ed. *Textbook of Gynecology.* Philadelphia: Saunders, 1993.

Dunnihoo DR, ed. *Fundamentals of Gynecology and Obstetrics,* 2nd ed. Philadelphia: Lippincott, 1992.

Farrell RG, ed. *OB/GYN Emergencies: The First 60 Minutes.* Rockville, MD: Aspen Systems, 1986.

[No authors listed]. Obstetric and gynecologic emergencies. *Emerg Med Clin North Am* 1987;5:399–647.

Scott JR, DiSaia PJ, Hammond CB, et al., eds. *Danforth's Obstetrics and Gynecology,* 7th ed. Philadelphia: Lippincott, 1994.

Male Genital Tract

Michael David DiBella

Congenital Disorders

Hydrocele

A hydrocele is an accumulation of clear serous fluid within the tunica vaginalis, a serosa-lined sac that surrounds the testes and epididymis. Congenital hydroceles occur following failure of the sac to fuse, allowing fluid to move back and forth between the peritoneal cavity and scrotum. Primary idiopathic hydrocele is the most common use of chronic intrascrotal swelling in adult males. Secondary causes usually present acutely from infections (epididymitis, mumps, tuberculosis), trauma, or tumor.

Upon examination, the hydrocele is usually a pear shaped, resilient smooth mass that may inhibit palpation of the testes and epididymis. Seven percent of males have an anteverted testes and epididymis, and in these patients a hydrocele presents as a posterior mass instead of its usual presentation as an anterior mass. The spermatic cord generally is palpable proximal to the hydrocele, unless the hydrocele extends to the external canal. Transillumination may reveal the hydrocele as a translucent mass.

Approximately 10% of testicular tumors are associated with a reactive hydrocele. If a tumor is suspected, the hydrocele should not be aspirated. Ultrasound can differentiate between a hydrocele, hematocele, or tumor. Acute hydrocele should have an urgent urologic consultation, while chronic hydrocele needs outpatient referral.

Hypospadias

Hypospadias is a congenital abnormality in which the opening of the urethral meatus is located on the ventral surface of the penis anywhere between the coronal sulcus and the perineum instead of its normal position at the tip of the glans penis. This condition occurs in 0.3% of male births and is associated with an increased incidence of cryptorchism.

In 70% of patients, the urethral meatus is distally located. This presents no major problems to the patient except an abnormal urinary stream and concern about cosmetic appearance. Patients with perineal or penoscrotal hypospadias have to micturate in the sitting position, and in adult life, fertility is impaired since semen is deposited outside the vagina. Cystitis is more common in males with hypospadias. Urological referral is needed for all patients with hypospadias.

Phimosis

Phimosis is a condition of uncircumcised males in which the narrowing of the meatus of prepuce prevents the foreskin from being retracted behind the glans penis. In children under the age of 2 the foreskin is normally unretractable. Anomalous development and inflammatory scarring are the usual etiologies of a small orifice that prevents the retraction of foreskin in older children and adults. Complications of phimosis include ballooning of the foreskin during micturition, urinary retention, balanitis, and carcinoma. If the patient is unable to void, dilation of the small orifice of the foreskin with a hemostate may be helpful. In some patients, circumcision may be needed if preventative measures such as cleaning the glans are unsuccessful.

Varicocele

A varicocele is a collection of enlarged tortuous veins resulting from either incompetent valves or obstruction of the testicular pampiniform venous plexus. It occurs in 4% to 20% of males. Left-sided varicoceles are more common because the left spermatic vein drains into the left renal vein, whereas the right spermatic vein drains directly into the inferior vena cava. Patients commonly present with a chronic, asymptomatic soft mass or swelling above the testes with the characteristic appearance and feeling of a "bag of worms" when the patient stands or strains. In the supine position the varicocele usually decreases in size or may collapse completely. If the varicocele is acute, occurs after the age of 40, is right-sided, or does not reduce in the supine position, a retroperitoneal neoplasm, renal cell carcinoma, or renal vein thrombosis should be suspected and evaluated with either sonogram or CT scanning.

Cryptorchidism

Cryptorchidism is the failure of the intraabdominal testes to complete its normal pattern of descent into the scrotal sac. Patients are asymptomatic and the cause is either hormonal or mechanical. This abnormality occurs in 4% of premature male infants, with the incidence decreasing to 3% in full-term infants and to 0.8% at 1 year of age.

Cryptorchidism must be differentiated from a retractable testes, which can be brought in the scrotum, and from an ectopic testes, which may be found in perineum or inner aspect of the thigh following migration beyond the external ring. Indirect inguinal hernias and testicular malignancy are associated with undescended testes. If cryptorchidism is bilateral and lasts beyond 1 year of age, it may be treated with gonadotropins. Sterility may occur if the disorder remains unresolved.

Structural Disorders

Paraphimosis

Paraphimosis occurs when the foreskin has been retracted over the glans penis and is unable to be replaced to its natural position. Unlike phimosis, which is neither painful nor an emergency, paraphimosis is extremely painful and is a true emergency. The constricting foreskin results in vascular engorgement, edema, and, if left untreated, arterial insufficiency, which may lead to gangrene of the glans penis.

Cases may be iatrogenic when health care providers, following physical examination or insertion of urethral catheter, forget to reposition the foreskin to its normal position and, rarely, from vigorous sexual activity. The emergency practitioner should attempt manual reduction to reduce the edema and to allow the foreskin to return to its normal position. Manual reduction is attempted by applying constant traction to the foreskin as the thumbs exert pressure on the glans, while the index and middle fingers apply pressure medially. Other techniques of reduction included elastic wrap compression, puncture technique, emergency dorsal slit, or circumcision.

Peyronie's Disease

This common disorder of unknown etiology occurs in middle to older aged males from fibrosis of the tunica albuginea, which envelops each corpus cavernosum. This fibrosis is similar microscopically to Dupuytren contractures of the hand. Patients complain of curvature of the penis during erection that may be painful. This curvature may not be visible if the penis is flaccid, but fibrous plaques usually are palpable on the midline dorsal surface. Spontaneous remissions may occur in up to 50% of the patients. Patients should be referred to a urologist. Most medications, techniques, and procedures have been unsatisfactory for correcting this disorder.

Priaprism

Priaprism is a rare condition in which an erection is pathological, prolonged, and involuntary. During erection the corpus spongiosum is engorged with blood while both corpus cavernosa remain soft. In priapism this is reversed. Self-administered intracavernous injections for the treatment of impotence (prostaglandin E_1) are now the most common cause of priaprism. Other causes include sickle cell disease, leukemia, metastatic carcinoma, spinal cord lesions, alcohol, medications (especially antihypertensives and psychotropic agents), and trauma to the perineum, genitalia, or spinal cord.

Most patients present after having had an erection for several hours. These erections are usually painful. Complications of priapism include infection, urinary retention, fibrosis of the corpora, and impotence. Initial workup may include a complete blood count, coagulation studies, and urinalysis. Supportive measures include intravenous hydration, supplemental oxygen, sedation, analgesia, and bladder catheterization if urinary retention is present. Ice-cold saline enemas are usually not effective.

Priaprism, regardless of the etiology, may be treated with terbutaline 0.25 to 0.50 mg in the deltoid muscle. Pseudoephedrine, 60 to 120 mg PO may be effective if given within 4 hours. If this treatment is unsuccessful or the priapism has lasted more than 4 hours, a dilute intracavernous injection with neosynephrine may be necessary (10 mg of 1% neosynephrine diluted in 1 L of normal saline). Patients receiving this treatment should be on a cardiac monitor because of rare instances of cardiac arrhythmias. If the patient's priaprism is unresponsive to medical treatment, a urologist should be consulted, since a corpora cavernosa shunt may be necessary.

Testicular Torsion

Testicular torsion is the rotation of the testes on the spermatic cord. If detorsion does not occur spontaneously, manually, or surgically, the strangulation of arterial blood flow may lead to infarction of the testes. Twisting of the spermatic cord initially causes occlusion of the venous system of the testes, and resultant edema leads to ischemia by impairment of the arterial blood flow.

Precipitating causes include physical trauma and conditions that give rise to abnormal mobility of the testes within the tunica vaginalis. Such conditions include incomplete descent, testicular atrophy, and absence of scrotal ligaments. Also, testes without the normal posterior fixation to the tunica vaginalis are especially prone to torsion.

Torsion usually occurs around puberty and most commonly presents between the ages of 10 and 20, with an incidence of 1 in 4,000 males. About 5% of patients with torsion are over 30 years of age. Patients with testicular torsion complain of pain, of which the intensity and onset can vary greatly. In half of the patients, there is either a history of a prior similar event or an onset that occurs during sleep. Patients complain of nausea, vomiting, and pain, which initially may be either in the abdominal or scrotal region. Upon examination, the axis of the affected testes will have changed from a horizontal to a transverse plane. This results in the affected hemiscrotum to be higher riding than the nonaffected testes. Prehn's sign (see below) is unreliable and should not be used to differentiate torsion from epididymitis. The loss of the ipsilateral cremasteric reflex is a frequent finding in torsion.

Unfortunately, many classical findings are absent because intrascrotal structures may not be identified on palpation due to swelling of the scrotum. Differential diagnosis includes epididymitis, torsion of the appendix testes, orchitis, tumor, hernia, and hydrocele. Acute epididymitis usually has more gradual onset, fever and leukocytosis. Urinalysis and white blood cell count are normal in torsion. Color flow Doppler ultrasound and radionuclide scanning are helpful aids, but should never delay the patient from going to the operating room to confirm or exclude the diagnosis of torsion. Therefore, once the history and physical examination is consistent with torsion, an emergent urology consultation for surgical exploration is indicated. Manual detorsion may be attempted in the ED if there is any surgical delay. If surgical detorsion occurs less than 6 hours after complete interruption of arterial blood flow, the salvage rate is close to 100%.

Urethral Strictures

Urethral strictures are fibrotic narrowings in the urethra that restrict urinary flow and produce obstructive symptoms and complications. Almost all urethral strictures in males are acquired, usually from infection or trauma. Infectious etiologies include urethritis from sexually transmitted diseases in younger males and from long-term indwelling catheters of instrumentation in older males.

Most patients complain of a decrease in their urinary stream. Other symptoms include double stream, postvoiding dribbling, dysuria, and frequency. Differential diagnosis of urethral strictures includes voluntary external sphincter spasm, urethral carcinoma, benign prostatic hypertrophy, prostatic cancer, and bladder neck contractures.

Patients requiring relief from urinary retention or needing residual urinary measurements may have a well-lubricated 14F Foley or Coude catheter gently inserted into the meatus. If passage is unsuccessful, a urological consultation should be obtained. Complications of multiple attempts include creation of a false passage, hemorrhage, Gram-negative bacteremia, and periurethral abscesses. All patients with residual urine or acute urinary retention should have a urinalysis and urine culture sent in addition to serum creatinine. Urinary tract infections should be treated, and patients should be referred to a urologist.

Urethral Foreign Bodies

Urethral foreign bodies, although uncommon, may be found in patients of all ages. Most urethral foreign bodies are found in young pediatric patients, usually from self-experimentation. Older patients may insert a variety of objects into the urethra in an attempt to heighten sexual pleasure. A history of decreased urinary flow with bloody infected urine should make the practitioner suspicious of a foreign body located in the lower genitourinary tract. A plain roentgenogram of the bladder and urethral area may reveal a foreign body.

If the foreign body is expelled spontaneously or removed manually, a retrograde urethrography or endoscopic examination is needed to determine any urethral damage. Urethral foreign bodies may need endoscopy or open cystotomy for removal.

Prostatic Hypertrophy

Prostatic hypertrophy is an enlargement of the prostate gland usually from benign prostatic hyperplasia (BPH).

Although patients with BPH do not have an increased incidence of prostatic cancer, both diseases are common and frequently occur together. Therefore, it is important to rule out cancer in patients with BPH. All such patients seen in the ED should have referral to a primary care physician or urologist.

Patients present to the ED seeking help for obstructive symptoms, such as a progressive weakened urinary stream, hesitancy, intermittency, dribbling, urinary retention, nocturia, or frequency. Urinary incontinence rarely is a symptom of BPH. Psychotropic, α-andrenergics, and anticholinergic medications as well as alcohol can precipitate acute urinary retention in patients with BPH.

Physical findings of BPD can range from an enlarged prostate on digital rectal examination to a distended bladder when there is outlet obstruction and signs of uremia, as occurs in patients with advanced BPH who develop renal failure. In patients with BPH, the prostate gland feels smooth and may have asymptomatic lobes of either a soft or firm consistency, whereas nodules, induration, or a stone-hard consistency are suggestive of prostatic cancer on digital rectal examination.

Initial laboratory evaluation of patients with BPD includes both urinalysis and serum creatinine. Patients presenting with mild symptoms of BPH who do not have urinary tract infections may be treated initially with an alpha-blocker and referred to a urologist. BPH patients with urinary retention and no evidence of urinary tract infection or renal failure may be discharged with a bladder catheter and bag, and urological follow-up in 1 to 2 days.

Inflammation/Infection

Epididymitis and Orchitis

Epididymitis usually started as an inflammatory process in the vas deferens and extends to the lower pole of the epididymis. The majority of cases of epididymitis are bacterial, and if the inflammation also affects the testes, it is termed epididymo-orchitis. This disease is rare before puberty. In adults, it results either from sexually transmitted diseases that are associated with urethritis in younger males or from recent genitourinary procedures, indwelling catheters, or obstructive urinary processes such as prostatitis in older males. Patients with acute epididymitis complain of scrotal pain that usually has a more gradual onset than of testicular torsion. Other complaints include fever, dysuria, frequency, and abdominal pain. Upon examination, the epididymis early in the infection is enlarged, indurated, and tender. Later, this may progress to a singular swollen scrotal mass in which the intrascrotal contents are indistinguishable. If the inflammatory process has been present for several days, a reactive hydrocele may be found. Prehn's sign (pain from epididymitis may be relieved when the scrotum is manually elevated, whereas in torsion the pain may be worsened) should not be used as a reliable indicator of epididymitis. Urethral discharge is occasionally found and should be Gram-stained and cultured.

Testicular torsion frequently is misdiagnosed as epididymitis. Color Doppler ultrasound may assist in the diagnosis but it is imperative not to delay an emergent urologic consult if torsion is suspected. Other differential diagnoses include testicular tumor, orchitis, and hernia.

Initial laboratory evaluation includes a CBC, urinalysis, and urine culture. Blood cultures should be obtained in patients suspected of sepsis. Leukocytosis is more elevated in epididymitis than in torsion, and urinalysis shows pyuria in up to 50% of the patients. Mild cases of epididymitis can be treated as an outpatient with antibiotics, analgesics, and scrotal support. Sexually active males under 35 should receive treatment outlined in **Table 124.1** for gonorrhea and *Chlamydia trachomatis*.

Males over age 35 are usually infected with Gram-negative enteric organisms; treatment is outlined in Table 124.1. Urologic follow-up should be within several days. Patients with severe inflection, epididymal abscess, or sepsis require admission, urgent urologic consultation, and intravenous antibiotics.

Orchitis is an inflammation of the testicle and usually the diagnosis is easily made if signs of systemic illness such as mumps are present. If there are no signs of systemic illness, urinalysis is helpful to determine if pyuria is present from an initial epididymal focus that has spread to the testes causing epididymo-orchitis; if present, this should be treated with appropriate antibiotics. If urinalysis is negative in patients without systemic signs of infection, testicular torsion should be considered in the differential diagnosis.

Balanitis

Balanitis is an inflammation of either the space between the glans penis and prepuce or of the glans penis itself. If the inflammation also involves the prepuce it is termed balanoposthitis. Most cases of balanitis occur in patients with phimosis or a redundant prepuce that predisposes to bacterial infection if proper hygiene is not maintained. Retraction of the foreskin reveals inflammation, purulent exudate, and occasionally small superficial ulcers of the mucosal covering of the glans. Gram stain and KOH preparations of the exudate help differentiate between bacterial and fungal infections. Besides local cleansing by sitz baths, bacterial infection requires treatment with a broad spectrum of antibiotics, while monilial balanitis can be treated with either Lotrimin 1% or miconazole 2% cream. Adults with new-onset balanitis or recurrent monilial balanitis should have serum glucose checked to rule out diabetes mellitus. Patients with recurrent balanitis need elective circumcision once the infection is resolved. Biopsy may be indicated in patients refractive to treatment to rule out a misdiagnosis of squamous cell carcinoma.

Gangrene of the Scrotum (Fournier's Gangrene)

Fournier's gangrene is a type of necrotizing fasciitis of the scrotum that may also involve the penis, perineum, and abdominal wall. Predisposing factors include immunocompromised males (especially diabetics), paraphimosis, perirectal infection, recent genital surgery, and local trauma.

Initially, the infection may be mistaken for cellulitis, since the patients present with fever, pain, scrotal swelling, and erythema. Later, marked edema, crepitus, and gangrene of the scrotal sac develop. Gas from subcutaneous emphysema may be found on either roentgenograms or ultrasound of the involved area. This necrotizing fasciitis is life-threatening with a mortality rate between 13% and 22%, prompting emergent urologic consultation once the diagnosis is considered.

Antimicrobial therapy with ampicillin, gentamicin, and clindamycin or metronidazole is begun immediately to cover anaerobes, gram-negative rods, and various streptococci. Alternatively, ampicillin-sulbactam with gentamicin may be substituted. If antibiotic treatment is unsuccessful or is widespread, wide surgical excision and debridement may be necessary.

Prostatitis

Acute bacterial prostatitis is usually associated with systemic signs of infection and, occasionally, urinary retention. Patients usually complain of fever, back pain, and lower urinary tract infection symptoms. Physical examination may reveal a febrile, toxic-appearing patient in which the prostate on digital rectal examination (DRE) is impressively tender. Overzealous manipulation of the prostate gland on DRE may lead to bacteremia.

Initial evaluation in the ED should include complete blood cell count with differential, electrolytes, renal function studies, blood culture, urine culture, and urinalysis (which will show evidence of pyuria). Parenteral antibiotics for patients in toxic condition (ampicillin 2 g IVq6h and gentamicin 3–5 g/kg/d) should be instituted early to provide coverage for Gram-negative organisms. Nontoxic patients may be treated as an out patient with either

Table 124.1		
Treatment of Epididymitis		
Etiology	**Primary Regimen**	**Alternative Regimen**
Males < 35-years-old (gonococcal and *C. trachomatis*)	Ceftriaxone 250 mg IM × 1 **plus** Doxycycline 100 mg PO bid × 10 d	Ofloxacin[a] 300 mg bid × 10 d *or* Levofloxacin[a]
Males > 35-years-old (Gram-negative enteric organisms)	Ofloxacin 300 mg bid × 10 d Levofloxacin 500 mg qd × 10 d	

[a]For patients allergic to cephalosporins and/or tetracyclines.

Table 124.2

Treatment of Urethritis

Etiology	Primary Regimen	Alternative Regimen
Uncomplicated urethritis (gonococcal and *C. trachomatis*)	Ceftriaxone 125 mg IM × 1 *plus* Azithromycin 1 g PO × 1	Cefixime 400 mg PO × 1 *or* Cipro 500 mg PO × 1 *or* Ofloxacin 400 mg PO × 1 *or* Levofloxacin 250 mg PO × 1 *plus* Doxycycline 100 mg bid × 7 d
Postgonococcal urethritis	Doxycycline 100 mg PO bid × 7 d Azithromycin 1 g PO × 1	
Trichomonias vaginalis	Metronidazole 2 g PO ×1	Metronidazole 500 mg bid × 7 d
Pregnant partners	Erythromycin base 500 mg PO qid 7 d Azithromycin 1 g PO × 1	

trimethoprim-sulfamethoxazole (TMP-SMX) or a fluoro-quinolone for 30 days. Strains of *E. coli* account for 80% of the cases. Urinary retention is best treated with suprapubic cystotomy. Patients with urinary retention have a septic condition and need admission for parental antibiotics.

In chronic bacterial prostatitis, patients usually present with nonspecific symptoms (spasm or discomfort in the perinal area) and the physical examination, DRE, and urinalysis are usually normal. Treatment consists of TMP-SMX for 4 to 16 weeks or a fluoroquinolone for 6 weeks.

Urethritis

Urethritis is the leading infectious urological disorder in males. Although it is usual practice to classify urethritis as either gonococcal urethritis (GU) or nongonococcal urethritis (NGU), the diagnosis cannot be made on clinical grounds alone because the symptoms of both entities overlap and frequently coexist. Urethral discharge is a common complaint and can range from clear, scanty discharge without dysuria to a purulent discharge with severe painful micturition.

The entire male genital area should be examined for evidence of other sexually transmitted diseases besides urethritis. In patients found to have gonococcal urethritis, the pharynx and rectal areas should also be inspected for signs of STDs. If urethral discharge cannot be expressed manually, a thin cotton swab should be gently inserted 1 to 2 cm into the urethra for Gram staining and culturing. On Gram stain, the presence of more than four polymorphonuclear neutrophils (PMNs) per oil immersion field confirms the diagnosis of urethritis.

Gonococcal urethritis is caused by the Gram-negative diplococcus *Neisseria gonorrhoeae* (GC) and is confirmed on Gram staining by seeing gram-negative diplococci within PMNs. GC has an incubation period of 3 to 7 days and usually presents with a more abrupt onset than NGU. Complications include urethral strictures, epididymitis, disseminated bacteremia causing tenosynovitis, arteritis, endocarditis, and meningitis. All patients found to have gonococcal urethritis should also be treated for NGU,

which coexists in up to 50% of patients; this treatment will help to prevent postgonococcal urethritis.

Chlamydia trachomatis, an obligate intracellular parasite with an intubation period of usually 7 to 14 days, is the most common sexually transmitted disease. This organism is also the most common cause of NGU in men. Up to 25% of infected males have no symptoms. Urethral discharge, when present, is usually less purulent than in gonococcal urethritis. *C. trachomatis* urethritis is more prevalent in blacks, males under 20, and heterosexuals. This infection may be difficult to diagnose since the Gram stain may not reveal PMNs on urethral smears. Complications include epididymitis, epididymo-orchitis, and procitis. Table 124.1 lists treatment recommendations. Another infectious cause of NGU is *U. urealyticum*, which usually responds to treatment for *C. trachomatis* and *T. vaginalis*. In *T. vaginalis* urethritis, the first morning voiding may reveal mobile trichomonads on saline solution slide preparations. Overall, in 30% of cases of urethritis no etiology is found. Reiter's syndrome, believed to be caused by NGU, may present initially as urethritis in 80% of the cases. Other manifestations of Reiter's syndrome include uveitis, arthritis, mucocutaneous lesions, and conjunctivitis.

Recurrent urethritis is either from reinfection, noncompliance, or treatment failures. Sexual partners of patients with urethritis should be treated. Both partners should be referred to an STD clinic for follow-up, HIV testing, and counseling. In pregnant partners, doxycycline and flouroquinones are contraindicated (**Table 124.2** contains treatment guidelines).

Selected Readings

Adimora AA. Treatment of uncomplicated genital Chlamydia trachomatis infection in adults. *Clin Infect Dis* 2002;35(suppl 2):S183–S186.

Burstein GR, Berman SM, Blumer JL, Moran JS. Ciprofloxacin for the treatment of uncomplicated gonorrhea infection in adolescents: Does the benefit outweigh the risks? *Clin Infect Dis* 2002;35(suppl 2):S191–S199.

Epidemiology Program Office, CDC. Sexually transmitted diseases treatment guidelines 2002. *Morbid Mortal Wkly Rep* 2002;51:36–37, 52–53.

Marx J. *Rosen's Emergency Medicine: Concepts and Clinical Practice,* 5th ed. St. Louis: Mosby, 2002:1413–1414, 1422–1426.

Tintinall J. *Emergency Medicine: A Comprehensive Study Guide,* 6th ed. New York: McGraw-Hill, 2004:613–620.

125 Sexual Assault

Mary K. Bennett
G. Richard Braen

Rape represents a profound emotional crisis for virtually all who are attacked. As with any traumatized patient, survivors of sexual assault often require simultaneous evaluation and treatment on multiple levels. Emotional, psychological, medical, and legal needs must be explored and cared for. Sexual assault includes rape, marital rape, incest, child molestation, sexual harassment, sexual abuse, voyeurism, indecent exposure, and forced sodomy. Although this discussion refers generally to females, the same procedural rules apply to males.

Rape traditionally has been defined as forcible carnal knowledge of a female by a male against her will. Carnal knowledge is any penetration of the female genitalia by the penis. Many laws now define rape as any carnal knowledge of an adolescent or adult by physical force, by threat of harm, or when the victim is not capable of giving consent because of mental illness, mental retardation, or intoxication.

Emotional and Psychological Care

Serious physical injury can occur, but in most patients emotional and psychological injuries are initially and ultimately more disabling. Sexual assaults are acts of violence committed with sex as a weapon primarily out of a need for control and power. Care should begin when the patient arrives in the emergency department (ED) with the early and frequent reassurance that she or he is in a safe and compassionate environment, and is no longer in danger. The patient should be assured of the confidentiality of her name and all records. One staff member should escort the patient to a quiet and comfortable private room, and stay with the patient throughout the examination and process of collecting evidence. Sympathetic nonjudgmental listening without pressing for details can allow the patient to share her feelings at her own pace. She may then begin the process of healing the emotional trauma and the transition from victim to survivor. A skilled rape crisis counselor should ideally meet with the patient in the ED prior to discharge to for ongoing support. Counselors may be from social services, nursing, psychiatry, or a rape counseling crisis service.

A positive interaction with hospital staff also enhances the likelihood that the patient will report the crime. Patients should be informed of all available services and encouraged to allow a full examination, treatment, and evidence collection, because patients may later change their minds and elect to prosecute. However, the patient has the right to decide if she will accept rape crisis counseling, allow physical or forensic examinations, receive medical treatment, or press legal charges. Her right to choose aspects of care should be at all times supported and respected. In some states, emergency medical personnel are required to report sexual assault to the police.

To maximize forensic evidence, the patient should be instructed to avoid changing clothes, urinating, defecating, and washing. Oral intake should be avoided if oral penetration may have occurred.

Consent

The patient must sign written consent for each aspect of the evaluation. Separate consent may be required in some states for the history, physical examination, any testing or treatment, collection of physical evidence, notification of the police, and the release of evidence to the police. Consent fulfills legal requirements and also allows the patient a sense of control over the examination. Parents or guardians must sign for dependent minors alleging rape. All necessary consent forms are often in kits available in the EDs. While patients may choose not to prosecute and so decline forensic examination, the medical and psychological evaluation and treatment is of course still offered.

History

Inform the patient of the reason for each question asked. The patient will be more likely to proceed if she understands the process and knows how it can help her. It may be helpful to start with the general aspects of the history, and then to ask more specific and sensitive questions about the assault.

The history of the assault can help the physician correlate the victim's allegations with the physical findings. For example, the time of last voluntary intercourse may be important. Sperm remain motile in the vagina only a few hours, but can remain motile in the cervix for up to days. Immotile sperm can be found in both locations for longer time periods. Time, date, and place of assault may help correlate debris such as sand or grass with the location. Knowing the specific use of force or restraints may help correlate marks on the skin that may have resulted from the assault. The physician should ask the victim whether ejaculation occurred, and if so, where. A question about whether a condom was used should also be asked.

A history of amnesia, particularly after consuming only one or two alcoholic beverages, can be the hallmark of intoxication with Rohypnol, a powerful sedative also known as the "date rape" drug for its role in increasing numbers of sexual assaults. It is ten times more potent than diazepam, and causes disinhibition, euphoria, and its sine qua non amnesia within about fifteen minutes; its effects can last up to eight hours. For the victim, the inability to reconstruct a sexual assault committed while under the influence of such hypnotic medications can be especially devastating, because it is committed not only without her consent, but also without her knowledge.

Basic History for the Sexual Assault Patient

Medical History
- Current medical problems
- Current medications; when last taken?
- Allergies
- Tetanus immunization status
- Recent use of drugs or alcohol

Gynecological History
- Use of contraceptives before assault. Any missed pills?
- Last normal menstrual period; are periods regular?
- Last voluntary intercourse (within a week)
- Gravity, parity, current pregnancy
- Recent gynecological surgery or sexually transmitted disease
- HIV status

History of Assault
- When and where did the assault occur?
  - Who was the assailant?
  - More than one assailant?
  - Known or unknown assailant; intimate partner or non-intimate partner, if known?
- Force or threats of force
  - Does the patient believe that the threat of force was used to coerce or intimidate?
  - Type of force; use of restraints?
  - Were drugs or alcohol used? Any amnesia that may indicate drugs were used?
  - Was the patient unconscious or intellectually impaired in any way prior to or during the incident?

- Type of assault
  - Fondling
  - Oral, anal, or vaginal penetration
  - Penetration or attempted penetration by what specifically (penis, foreign body)
  - Ejaculation by assailant? Where?
  - Was a condom used?
  - Last voluntary intercourse, or negative history of intercourse
- Drugs or alcohol taken voluntarily before or after the attack
- Douching, bathing, urination, defecation, clothing change, or oral hygiene following the assault?

Physical Examination

The physical examination should be conducted gently and with compassion. Less threatening aspects of the exam should precede more invasive aspects such as the pelvic examination. Four main questions should be addressed by the physical examination as described below.

First, are there significant physical or emotional injuries, or any medical or surgical problems that require emergency evaluation or treatment?

Second, is the patient capable of consent or was she capable of consent at the time of the assault? Minor children below the age of consent are by definition unable to consent. Rape of a minor is called statutory rape. Does the patient have an abnormal mental status? Whether due to voluntary or coerced alcohol or drug ingestion, mental retardation, or mental illness, the patient with altered mental status is unable to give consent. A formal psychiatric evaluation is recommended if mental retardation or mental illness is thought to limit the patient's ability to give consent for voluntary intercourse. With written consent, blood and urine can be sent for detection of drugs and alcohol that may have impaired the patient's ability to give voluntary consent.

Third, is there physical evidence that corroborates the history of alleged assault and the use of force?

Fourth, is there evidence of recent sexual contact?

Sequence of the Physical Examination

1. Evaluate for significant medical or surgical problems for immediate evaluation and treatment.
2. General appearance and demeanor. Photographs of the patient before she undresses may be taken with her written permission, and may document lacerations, bite marks, or torn or stained clothing.
3. Mental status. Any evidence that the patient wasn't capable of consent at the time of the assault? Drug or alcohol intoxication, mental retardation or mental illness, or any altered mental status can limit the patient's ability to give voluntary consent for intercourse.
4. Oral examination includes searching for signs of trauma. Sterile swabs moistened with sterile saline are used to collect sublingual and buccal secretions, and then air dried. Saliva samples are collected on filter paper held in the mouth until

moistened, and then air dried. Oral intake should be withheld for 30 minutes before this test. Allow the patient to rinse her mouth.

5. Collect nail scrapings from underneath nails for tissue such as blood, hair, or skin.

6. Patient should disrobe standing on a piece of examination table paper to catch any debris to include as evidence. Torn or stained clothing including underwear should be placed in paper bags. Only the patient should touch the clothing to prevent cross contamination with blood group antigens present in perspiration. Paper bags breathe and allow less molding of blood and secretions that may interfere with analysis of semen and blood antigens.

7. Physical evidence of force to corroborate the history of assault including bites, bruises, lacerations, and abrasions. Evaluate carefully the face and neck, breasts and torso, buttocks and thighs, wrists and ankles, for trauma and tenderness. Using diagrams, document areas of injury.

8. Search the skin and hair for dried secretions and signs of debris that can be collected for evidence. Use a Wood's fluorescent lamp to highlight dried semen for collection with moistened sterile cotton tipped swabs. Air-dry and submit for acid phosphatase analysis. Urine, semen, and other substances fluoresce. Dried semen appears as slightly crusted flaking areas.

9. Perform the pelvic examination. Flashbacks to the assault are common during this examination. Be empathetic and gentle while informing the patient of each step. Examine the perineum for trauma and document using diagrams. Use a Wood's lamp to search for stains that fluoresce; these may be semen, so collect samples using moistened swabs Toluidine blue can be used to locate small vulvar lacerations from intercourse. Collect semen samples first as toluidine blue has spermicidal activity. For the speculum examination, use only water as lubricant. Collect any foreign bodies such as tampons or condoms. Note the presence and condition of the hymen and note any trauma to the vaginal walls. Colposcopy if available can increase the visibility of genital injuries. Aspirate secretions from the posterior fornix for analysis for sperm and acid phosphatase. Five to ten milliliters (mL) of nonbacteriostatic normal saline can be first instilled. A swab from the posterior fornix can be placed in 1 or 2 mL of saline and examined for motile sperm. Send cultures for gonorrhea and chlamydia to the hospital lab. Perform a bimanual examination noting uterine size, adnexal masses, and tenderness.

10. Rectal examination should be performed if rectal penetration occurred. Swab and retain any lubricant used by the assailant. Use saline rinses or swabs to collect possible semen or sperm samples. Note any lacerations or abrasions.

11. Male victims may also require oral or rectal examinations as the history indicates. Evaluate the penis, scrotum, and perineum for signs of trauma. Swabs of the victim's penis should be taken if the history indicates oral contact.

Laboratory Testing

1. Cervical, oral, and rectal swabs for gonorrhea and chlamydia.
2. Blood tests for syphilis.
3. Baseline tests for hepatitis B.
4. Testing for baseline HIV status (may be referred to a clinic where counseling can be given about the test). Testing is recommended within 2 weeks for baseline HIV status, and again at 3 and 6 months to detect seroconversion.
5. Quantitative serum human chorionic gonadotropin (HCG) for the determination of preexisting pregnancy.
6. Blood and urine for evaluation for alcohol, drugs and toxins.

Sexual Assault Forensic Evidence Kit and the Chain of Evidence

Protocol varies by state and even locality. The kit usually contains:

- Consent forms appropriate to the jurisdiction.
- Evidence of force or coercion, including documentation of injuries, fingernail scrapings, urine or blood for alcohol, drugs and other toxins, as well as all clothing that may be torn, or contain
- Evidence of semen including swabs for collection of vaginal, oral, and anal semen, acid phosphatase, and p30 prostate specific antigen. Swab the sublingual and buccal surfaces if oral penetration is suspected. Wet mounts of vaginal, oral, and anal areas may yield sperm. Skin areas that highlight with a Wood's lamp should also be swabbed for semen.
- Evidence that may identify the assailant include: fingernail scrapings, pubic hair combings, and swabbing from bites that may contain saliva.
- Samples to identify the victim, including head and pubic hair, blood and saliva samples.

When the evidentiary exam is complete:

1. Label the specimens and completed forensic kit with time, date, patient's hospital number, the name of the staff member who collected it, and the area from which the evidence was taken.
2. Package properly all physical evidence from the examination.
3. Retain in the chart consent forms and notation of the samples taken.
4. Custody of the packet must be documented at each transferal. The chain of evidence is a written form documenting the transferal of information and physical forensic evidence. Breaks in the chain of evidence procedure can lead to rejection of this material by the courts.

Medical Treatment

Pregnancy Prevention

Obtain a negative serum HCG before offering postcoital contraception. Patients presenting within 24 to 48 hours of the assault with positive serum HCGs were pregnant before the assault. **Table 125.1** lists the postcoital contraception protocols.

Prevention of Sexually Transmitted Diseases

Currently, the Center for Disease Control (CDC) recommends prophylactic antibiotic treatment for gonorrhea, chlamydia, trichomonas, and bacterial vaginosis. The CDC also recommends postexposure vaccination for hepatitis B.

HIV Testing and Postexposure Prophylaxis (PEP)

Sexually assaulted patients should be tested of HIV status within 2 weeks of the assault, and again at 3 and 6 months. Antiretroviral agents have known toxicities and unknown efficacy, but PEP may be indicated for high risk exposures such as exposures to known HIV positive assailant or assailants from high risk populations. Unprotected receptive anal intercourse is higher than unprotected vaginal intercourse. PEP can be recommended for high risk exposures, and considered for low to moderate risk exposures.

Examination of the Assailant

EDs are sometimes asked to conduct examinations of an accused rapist. Treat the patient with respect and dignity whether guilty or not. Obtain a formal signed consent for each phase of the examination. A formal court order may be sufficient if written consent cannot be obtained.

Document past and present medical or surgical problems, medications, allergies, and tetanus status. Avoid questions about the assault. Law enforcement officer's role is to ask these questions. Confusion about the facts may weaken the case for the prosecution. Focus physical examination on general appearance, degree of sexual maturity, signs of trauma, especially trauma of the genitals. Look for scars from a prior vasectomy. Collect physical evidence including fingernail scrapings, foreign debris on body, saliva for secretor status, penile swabs for semen and acid phosphatase, and pubic hair. If STDs are suspected, culture for gonorrhea and chlamydia, and blood tests for syphilis and HIV as indicated.

Follow-up Care

Give the patient discharge instructions that discuss facts about sexual assault, possible pregnancy and infections, expected emotional responses to rape, and the names and numbers of the follow-up counselor and the treating physician to call if questions arise. Ask permission to place a follow-up call to the patient. Refer the patient for ongoing rape crisis counseling and psychological support, as first contact is best initiated in the ED prior to discharge.

Referral to a clinic for ongoing care includes:
- HIV testing within 2 weeks, and again at 3 and 6 months
- Repeat RPR or VDRL for patients
- Repeat gonorrhea and chlamydia culture if symptoms arise
- Completion of immunization for hepatitis B
- Gynecological follow-up in case of pregnancy after postcoital contraception

Selected Reading

Braen GR. Physical assessment and emergency medical management for adult victims of sexual assault. In: Warner CG, ed. *Rape and Sexual Assault: Management and Intervention.* Rockville, MD: Aspen Systems, 1980.

Table 125.1

Prevention of Pregnancy

1. Patients presenting within 24 to 48 hours of assault with serum HCG-positive were pregnant before the rape. Postcoital contraception requires formal written consent.
2. All protocols for pregnancy prevention can cause nausea. An antiemetic should be prescribed.
3. The following protocols for postcoital contraception should be given within 72 hours of the assault.
   - Plan B (levonorgestrel), 1 tab initially and 1 in 12 hours
   - Preven (ethinyl estradiol and levonorgestrel), 2 tabs initially and 2 in 12 hours
   - Ovral (ethinyl estradiol and norgestrel), 2 tabs initially and 2 in 12 hours

Genital Lesions

David Pierce
Dietrich V. K. Jehle

The skin of the genitalia is subject to many of the same diseases that involve the skin in other locations. The etiology of genital lesions may be due to a generalized disease process (e.g., psoriasis, or Behçet's syndrome), trauma, sexually transmitted infections, and infestations or nonvenereal infections. This discussion excludes or only briefly mentions gonorrhea, chlamydia, syphilis, chancroid, granuloma inguinale, mumps, herpes simplex (see Chapter 66), and generalized diseases that are covered more extensively in other sections.

Primary Genital Lesions

Pediculosis Pubis

There are two species of blood-sucking lice—*Phthirus pubis* and *Pediculus humanus* (var. corporis)—that tend to involve the genital region. Lice infestation occurs more commonly at times of overcrowding and during wars when there is less attention to personal hygiene. In addition to the cutaneous manifestations, lice are important vectors for other infectious diseases (epidemic typhus, trench fever, and relapsing fever).

Phthirus pubis is the "crab louse" that preferentially inhabits the genital region while *Pediculus humanus* is the "body louse"; however, either may involve any hair-bearing portion of the body.

The life span of the adult female is approximately 1 month, during which time she lays up to 10 eggs per day. The ova are firmly attached as nits to the hairs (crab louse) or clothing (body louse), hatch in 1 week, and reach maturity in another week. The lice inject fecal material and digested secretions into the skin, leading to intense pruritus. Confirmation of lice infestation is based on the observation of lice, nits, or miniscule red marks on the hair-bearing portion of the involved skin (excreta).

Permethrin (1% in Nix or 5% in ELIMITE) is currently the preferred topical therapy, Lindane (Kwell) is a second treatment option, but has been associated with seizures when applied to broad areas or ingested. Therefore, it is contraindicated in pregnancy and for children under 2 years of age.

Any drug treatment should be followed by fine-tooth combing to remove nits. Clothing, linen, and towels need to be washed in hot water or dry cleaned. Sexual partners and those sharing the same quarters need to be treated. Patients who remain symptomatic 1 week after completing treatment should be retreated if lice or nits are still present. Eyelash involvement should only be treated with petrolatum (Vaseline) bid for 8 days. Symptomatic treatment of pruritus may be provided with oral antihistamines or topical steroids. If secondary bacterial infection of the bite wounds is present, systemic antibiotic therapy with *Staphylococcus aureus* coverage is recommended.

Scabies

The human mite, *Sarcoptes scabiei*, is one of the most frequent causes of pruritic skin rashes in the world. Transfer of the fertilized female mite occurs as the result of close personal contact with an infected individual. Outbreaks are common in nursing homes, mental institutions, and similar settings where there is crowding and where hygiene is compromised.

Gravid females burrow under the superficial layers of the skin where they deposit two to three eggs per day. Larvae emerge from the skin in 2 weeks. The mites mate and the males die shortly thereafter. The fertilized female then tunnels into the epidermis of the same or another host.

Patients with scabies complain of a pruritic eruption that is usually worse at night and after bathing. Erythematous papules, nodules, and excoriations are commonly seen in the digital web spaces, wrists, elbows, genital region, and skin folds, and vesicles are occasionally present. Linear burrows (dark lines measuring 3 to 15 mm) may be detected; however, these can be difficult to visualize when obscured by excoriations.

Treatment for scabies is similar to the therapy for lice infestation. Permethrin 5% cream (ELIMITE) is the preferred medication. After appropriate treatment, scabies generally becomes noninfectious within 24 hours.

Ulcer-Node Syndrome

Genital ulcers are defined as defects in the epithelium of skin or mucosa of the genital region. Lymphadenopathy generally occurs in association with the genital lesions; however, it may occur independently, as seen with lymphogranuloma venereum. Open genital lesions enhance the transmission of the HIV virus and, therefore, HIV testing is recommended for all patients undergoing treatment for genital ulcers. The approach to ulcers of the genitalia with and without lymph node enlargement is discussed below.

Diagnosis

Sexually transmitted diseases are the most frequent cause of genital ulcers in adults; however, noninfectious diseases may also involve the genital area. The incubation period, travel history, presence of pain or pruritus, history of STD in a sexual partner, history of recurrence, and morphologic appearance of lesions are helpful in narrowing the differential diagnosis. A very short incubation period of minutes to hours suggests trauma or an allergic component, 2 to 7 days is more consistent with chancroid or herpes, and longer incubation periods are seen with syphilis (1 to 3 weeks), lice or scabies (4 weeks), and condyloma acuminata (4 to 12 weeks). Chancroid (Africa), lymphogranuloma venereum (Africa and Far East), and granuloma inguinale (India, New Guinea, West Indies, Africa, and South America) are much more common in other parts of the world than in the United States. Moderate to severe pain is frequently present with herpes and chancroid, while syphilis is usually pain-free unless secondarily infected with bacteria. Marked pruritus suggests scabies, lice infestation, or herpes. Recurrent eruptions with resolution between flare-ups are typical of herpes infections. The specific appearance (ulcerative, vesicular, papular, or verrucous) and number of the genital lesions are probably the most important final clues in making the correct diagnosis.

Causes

Genital Herpes

Herpes simplex virus type I and II can cause venereal disease. Approximately 60% to 80% of the genital lesions are type II. It is estimated that greater than 30 million people in the United States have had genital herpes infections. Recurrent infections are predominantly of the herpes type II subgroup.

The typical course consists of an incubation period of 4 days, followed by painful vesicles or shallow ulcers involving the external genitalia or cervix. The primary infection is often associated with fever and inguinal adenopathy, which is absent in recurrent infections. The skin lesions eventually dry up and form a crust. Skin lesions last for approximately 3 weeks during the primary infections versus approximately 12 days in the secondary infection. Duration of pain and viral shedding is approximately 10 days for a primary disease and approximately 4 days for secondary disease. Erythema multiforme and carcinoma of the cervix appear to be associated with herpes simplex genital infections.

Definitive diagnosis is made with viral or immunofluorescent staining of fluid and/or scrapings from the base of the vesicle. Giemsa or Wright stain may show multinucleated giant cells (consistent with herpes simplex virus or varicella-zoster virus infection).

Acyclovir may increase the rate of healing in acute episodic recurrences, and suppress recurrences if used chronically.

Syphilis

Treponema pallidum is the causative agent in syphilis. The disease has several stages. Early syphilis includes primary and secondary syphilis. During this time, the lesions are infectious and diagnosis can be made by dark field examination of fluid from these lesions (organisms cannot be grown on artificial media). Late syphilis is a disease of more than 1 year's duration and includes cardiovascular involvement, gummas, or central nervous system disease. Late syphilis develops in approximately one-third of all untreated cases of early syphilis. Secondary syphilis recurs in 25% of untreated cases and this usually occurs within the first year of infection. The placental barrier prevents transfer to the fetus for the first 16 to 20 weeks of pregnancy. Congenital syphilis rarely leads to first trimester abortion, yet it frequently leads to stillbirth later in pregnancy.

There are two types of tests available for the serologic diagnosis of syphilis. The first type is the nontreponemal test, which includes the Venereal Disease Research Laboratory test (VDRL) and the rapid plasma reagin (RPR). These are fairly nonspecific tests in comparison to the treponemal tests, the prototype of which is the (quite specific) fluorescent treponemal antibody absorption test (FTA-ABS). **Table 126.1** displays the percentage reactivity in untreated syphilis at various stages.

The role of the FTA-ABS test is as a confirmatory test after a positive VDRL (RPR) test is obtained. The VDRL generally responds to a course of therapy, while the FTA-ABS usually remains unchanged. Certain patients should have serological testing of their cerebral spinal fluid, such as patients with syphilis of more than 1 year's duration *and* neurological symptoms, aortitis, gummas, failure of treatment, FTA titer >1:16, or HIV disease. Penicillin remains the drug of choice for treating syphilis. Serological tests are unreliable during the early incubating stage; thus, all contacts should be treated as if they have early syphilis. In

Table 126.1		
Percentage of Reactivity in Untreated Syphilis at Various Stages		
Stage	**VDRL (RPR)**	**FTA-ABS**
Primary	75%	85%
Secondary	99%	99%
Latent	70%	97%
Late	65%	94%

addition, HIV testing should be offered to all patients with confirmed syphilis.

Lymphogranuloma Venereum

Lymphogranuloma venereum (LGV) is caused by several serotypes of *Chlamydia trachomatis* (trachoma group). One to three weeks after exposure, a small painless papule or herpetiform vesicle develops that heals without scarring. These lesions frequently go unnoticed. The nodes become matted and fluctuant, and in untreated disease these nodes (buboes) frequently suppurate and rupture. The nodes are unilateral in 70% of the cases of this disease. Systemic symptoms of fever, chills, and myalgias can be frequently seen at this stage. Occasionally, the disease progresses to lymphatic obstruction and rectal stricture. Diagnosis can be confirmed by complement fixation titers ($\geq 1:64$ or fourfold rise in titer), skin testing, or isolation of the organism from buboes. However, biopsy is contraindicated due to sinus tract development. Treatment is with either doxycycline or erythromycin, but usually yields poor results.

Chancroid

Chancroid is a venereal disease caused by *Haemophilus ducreyi* that is extremely common in Western Africa and seen more commonly in persons with poor hygiene and in uncircumcised men. Only 10% of symptomatic cases are seen in women. The incubation period is usually 2 to 5 days, after which single or multiple vesiculopustular lesions appear that develop into soft, painful, single or multiple (up to 10) ulcers. Tender adenopathy is seen in 30% to 60% of cases. This adenopathy appears 7 to 10 days after the ulcerated genital lesions and is usually unilateral. The diagnosis is usually made clinically because the organism may be difficult to isolate, yet occasionally the organism may be seen on Gram stain of material aspirated from a lesion. Treatment of choice is with erythromycin for 7 days, a single injection of ceftriaxone 250 mg IM, or a single oral dose of azithromycin 1 g.

Granuloma Inguinale

Granuloma inguinale (donovanosis) is caused by a gram-negative, encapsulated bacillus known as *Calymmatobacterium granulomatis*. After an incubation period of 8 to 80 days, a "beefy red," "heaped-up" friable region appears. The diagnosis can be confirmed by a crush preparation of the granulation tissue. Wright or Giemsa stains demonstrate mononuclear cells with intracytoplasmic bipolar rods (Donovan bodies). Doxycycline or TMP-SMX-DS are considered first-line therapy.

Condyloma Acuminata

Condyloma acuminata, epidermal manifestations or the human papilloma virus, are found on the penis, vagina, labia, urethra meatus, and the perianal region. They often develop into soft, vegetating clusters and can be transmitted sexually. Half of the lesions spontaneously involute with 1 year and 66% within 2 years. Cervical and vulvar warts (HPV types 16, 18, and others) have been linked with cervical and vulvar dysplasia and carcinoma.

A variety of treatment regimens are used for condyloma acuminata, the majority of which (liquid nitrogen, electrocurettage, laser surgery) should not be carried out in the emergency department. Patients should be referred to a dermatologist for further management.

Other Genital Lesions

Traumatic

Profound bruising of the penile shaft may occur as a result of prolonged intercourse or repetitive masturbation. Although the initial injury may appear significant, the vast majority of these injuries heal without residual damage. Another common traumatic injury to the penis is a tear of a tight frenulum in the uncircumcised male. If the frenal artery is involved, there may be notable bleeding. This can be a recurrent problem requiring circumcision or frenoplasty.

Vaginal tears may also occur during intercourse. These occur most commonly at the labial frenulum, which is located at the junction of the posterior/inferior aspects of the labia minora. This may cause marked dyspareunia if recurrent injury prevents healing. Surgical repair of vaginal lacerations may be required for some victims of sexual assault.

Bites to the external genitalia are seen more frequently with the greater acceptance of oral sex, and should receive antibiotic prophylaxis effective against mouth flora. Serious zipper injuries are surprisingly uncommon despite the daily risk to most men. There have been a variety of unusual injuries reported as complications of "sex toys."

Behçet's Syndrome

Hippocrates first described a syndrome of genital ulcers, oral ulcers, and iridocyclitis in the fifth century B.C. In the late 1930s, Behçet's syndrome was coined after the Turkish dermatologist who described the disease in detail. Other manifestations of Behçet's include arthritis, vascular lesions, skin lesions, gastrointestinal tract ulceration, and central nervous system involvement.

Tetracycline mouthwash, local and systemic steroids, intramuscular penicillin, colchicine, and immunosuppressives have been reported to be of some value in this disease.

Selected Readings

Benedetti J, Corey L, Ashley R. Recurrence rates in genital herpes after symptomatic first-episode infection. *Ann Intern Med* 1994;121:847–854.

Brown S, Becher J, Brady W. Treatment of ectoparasitic infections: review of the English-language literature, 1982–1992. *Clin Infect Dis* 1995;20(suppl 1): s104–s109.

Hart G, Donovanosis. In: Holmes KK, et al., eds. *Sexually Transmitted Diseases*, 2d ed. New York: McGraw-Hill, 1990:273–277.

Johnson RE, Nahmias AJ, Magder LS, et al. A seroepidemiologic survey of the prevalence of herpes simplex virus type 2 infection in the United States. *N Engl J Med* 1989;321:7–12.

Marrazzo JM, Handsfield HH. Chancroid: new developments in an old disease. *Curr Clin Top Infect Dis* 1995;15:129–152.

Rein MF. Genital skin and mucous membrane lesions. In: Mandell GL, Bennett JE, Dolin R, eds. *Principles and Practice of Infectious Diseases,* 4th ed. New York: Churchill Livingstone, 1995:1055.

Rolfs RT. Treatment of syphilis, 1993. *Clin Infect Dis* 1995;20(suppl 1):s23–s28.

Simonsen JN, Cameron DW, Gankinya MN, et al. Human immunodeficiency virus infection in men with sexually transmitted diseases. *N Engl J Med* 1988;319: 274–278.

Sturm AW, Stolting GJ, Cormane RH. Clinical and microbiological evaluation of 46 episodes of genital ulceration. *Genitourin Med* 1987;63:98–101.

Environmental Disorders

Richard V. Aghababian

Introduction

Patients who experience an unhealthy encounter with a threatening environment often end up seeking care in an emergency department. Exposure to extremes of temperature can result in minor injury or even be life-threatening. In addition, many organisms from insects to mammals have developed protective weapons that can do harm to humans through bites and stings. Electrical injuries can occur from exposure to sources of power or as a result of lightening strikes. Finally, recreational activities such as scuba diving, mountain climbing, or skiing can cause a wide variety of pathophysiological changes that can result in catastrophic bodily injury if unrecognized and untreated. Appreciating the dangers posed by Mother Nature and the medical consequences when humans are exposed to these threats add to the challenges of practicing emergency medicine.

Temperature-Related Disorders

Walter C. Robey III
Kevin J. Corcoran

Heat-Related Disorders

Heat illness develops when thermoregulatory mechanisms are overwhelmed or have failed when confronted with a large internal or environmental heat stress. This may result in a life-threatening elevation of body temperature with mental status changes as in heatstroke, or in less severe heat-related syndromes such as heat exhaustion, heat syncope, heat tetany, or heat cramps. Heat emergencies are most commonly seen during summer heat waves but can occur in more moderate temperatures in certain patient populations. The physiological response to heat stress occurs through behavioral mechanisms, peripheral vasodilatation, sweating, and decreased heat production. Excess exogenous heat, excess endogenous heat production, and decreased heat dissipation lead to heat illness (**Table 127.1**).

Initial Evaluation

The index of suspicion for severe heat illness is based on history, symptoms, and clinical signs of exogenous heat exposure, and predisposing factors. Initial evaluation consists of a primary evaluation of the airway, ventilation, circulation, and mental status. It must be recognized that comorbid conditions or injuries may complicate the clinical presentation. The initial evaluation must include vital signs with an accurate core temperature. The degree of hyperthermia, mental status changes, and hemodynamic stability determine the severity of heat illness and guide therapy.

History

A complete history including allergies, medications, predisposing medical history, the patient's activity, and events preceding presentation must be obtained. Input from prehospital personnel assists in identifying environmental conditions, extent of exposure, associated injury, initial mental status, and vital signs. A social history including alcohol use and availability of air-conditioning is helpful. The patient's response to prehospital therapy, including fluids, dextrose, thiamine, narcan, and cooling measures should be noted.

Physical Examination

Excessive clothing, disheveled appearance, perspiration-soaked clothing, remnants of an athletic uniform, or occupation-related accessories suggest heat-related illness. Characteristic odors of alcohol or other substances may assist in identifying predisposing conditions or toxins.

Primary evaluation of the airway, ventilation, circulation, and mental status should take precedence. The physiological response to heat illness is tachycardia and tachypnea. The stability of vital signs may vary. Hypotension indicates cardiovascular collapse secondary to organ failure or hypovolemia. Tachypnea may be a manifestation of heat syndromes as well as cardiopulmonary compromise or shock. An accurate core temperature must be obtained on all patients with a history of environmental or toxic exposure, altered mental status, cardiovascular instability, in the acutely psychotic patient, and the elderly. Options are an esophageal or rectal thermistor probe.

The secondary evaluation assists in determining the clinical severity of heat illness, the extent of multisystem involvement, and the presence of predisposing conditions, associated injuries, and related complications. Mental status abnormalities may indicate severe heat-related illness. Skin turgor may vary. Evidence of trauma, track marks, or dermatological disease should be noted. Oozing of blood from mucous membranes or petechiae indicate a developing coagulopathy. The presence of bite or sting lesions expands the differential diagnosis. The head should be examined for evidence of subtle injury. Cervical spine precautions should be maintained and the neck examined for evidence of trauma or thyromegaly.

Pulmonary examination is nonspecific in heat illness but may reveal findings consistent with pulmonary edema secondary to heat-related pulmonary capillary endothelial damage, myocardial insufficiency, or resuscitation-related volume overload. Aspiration-related findings may also be present in the obtunded or comatose patient.

In the absence of trauma the abdominal examination is usually nonspecific. A nasogastric tube may aid in diagnosing and monitoring gastrointestinal bleeding as well as decreasing the risk of aspiration. The placement of an indwelling urinary catheter may detect decreased urinary

Table 127.1
Heat Illness: Predisposing Factors
Behavioral
Overexertion (occupational, recreational, military recruits)
Impermeable/restrictive garments (fire protective gear)
Lack of acclimatization
Inadequate fluid repletion
Poor adaptive response (psychiatric, mental disability, intoxication)
Lack of awareness of prevention
Fatigue/lack of sleep
Poor physical conditioning
Neglect/criminal intent
Prior heatstroke
Exogenous
High ambient temperature
High relative humidity
Low wind velocity
Hot confined space
Lack of air-conditioning
Medical Conditions
Extremes of age
Dehydration
Cardiovascular disease
Febrile illness/infection
Autonomic neuropathies
Thyrotoxicosis
Skin disorders
Increased muscular activity (seizures, psychosis)
Obesity
Chronic illness/debilitation
Pharmacologic Agents
Sympathomimetics
Anticholinergics/antihistamines
Myocardial depressants (beta-blockers, calcium channel blockers)
Hallucinogens
Ethanol
Phenothiazines
Drug withdrawal
Salicylates
Lithium
MAO inhibitor

output or myoglobinuria and help monitor fluid resuscitation. The musculoskeletal examination may identify muscle rigidity, flaccidity, dystonia, involuntary spasmodic muscular constructions, carpopedal spasm, or compartment syndrome. Injury contributing to blood or fluid losses should be detected.

Ancillary Tests

Ancillary tests assist in determining the type and severity of heat illness, the extent of multiorgan damage in heatstroke, and assist in identifying predisposing or concurrent conditions.

Differential Diagnosis

Differentiating heatstroke from other heat-related and non–heat-related entities may be difficult initially. Heatstroke should be suspected in the context of a history of heat exposure, central nervous system dysfunction, and elevated core temperature. The classic definition of heatstroke cannot be relied on. Subtle presentations may exist with irritability or minor confusion and at a lower core temperature. A normal core temperature on presentation to the ED does not preclude the diagnosis. Heatstroke may coexist with heat exhaustion, and with predisposing conditions of various degrees of clinical expression. Heatstroke may be confused with any pathologic condition presenting with altered mental status and neurologic dysfunction (**Table 127.2**).

Initial Management

Field treatment of heat-related illness starts with removing the victim from the exposure, discontinuing physical activity, removing garments, and providing cooling measures based on resources. Wet sheets or a water mist should be applied. Fanning or opening windows improves cooling. Prehospital transport should be expeditious with resuscitation, monitoring, and cooling measures continuing as indicated.

The goals of ED intervention are to stabilize the patient, rapidly cool to a desired temperature end point, manage predisposing or concurrent medical conditions, and minimize complications of severe heat illness. Intervention is based on the type and severity of heat-related illness and resource availability. When the diagnosis of heatstroke is in doubt, the patient should be cooled aggressively, while continuing the assessment.

The patient with heat syncope, severe heat tetany, or heat cramps may require immediate attention due to their occasional impressive clinical presentations.

Initiate high-flow oxygen therapy, continuous pulse oximetry, peripheral intravenous lines, and cardiac monitoring while a core temperature is being obtained. The indications for endotracheal intubation include airway compromise, respiratory failure, or coma. Patients are commonly volume-depleted; therefore, normal saline vol-

Table 127.2
Heatstroke: Differential Diagnosis
CNS infection
CNS disorders (stroke, hemorrhage, trauma)
Sepsis/septic shock with coagulopathy
Neuroleptic malignant syndrome
Malignant hyperthermia
Toxins (anticholinergics, sympathomimetics, antidopaminergics, salicylates, lithium)
Status epilepticus
Withdrawal (alcohol, narcotic)
Agitation/increased muscular activity or tone
Thyrotoxicosis/DKA with sepsis/pheochromocytoma
Tetanus/malaria/typhoid fever

ume expansion is begun in the form of monitored fluid boluses. Monitoring fluid status and the response to hydration may necessitate central venous pressure or Swan-Ganz catheter placement in patients with underlying cardiac disease. If pressor agents are required, alpha-agonists should be avoided because of resulting vasoconstriction. Blood specimens should be obtained and dextrose, thiamine, and narcan administered as indicated.

Specific Heat-Related Disorders

Heatstroke

Heatstroke is a life-threatening heat-related illness defined clinically as a core temperature equal to or exceeding 40.5° C (105° F) with associated mental status changes. It is associated with high morbidity and mortality, and therefore should be considered in the differential diagnosis of any patient with hyperpyrexia and central nervous system dysfunction.

Heatstroke results when thermoregulatory mechanisms are unable to overcome exogenous heat stress. *Classic or nonexertional* heatstroke usually occurs in the elderly or debilitated patient who is passively exposed to thermal stress over a period of hours to days. *Exertional* heatstroke commonly occurs in young, healthy individuals whose thermoregulatory mechanisms are rapidly overwhelmed. The pathological effects of heatstroke are the result of the direct effect of heat upon cellular integrity and function. As temperature increases, proteins denature, and widespread necrosis leads to multisystem organ dysfunction and failure. The central nervous system, the cardiovascular system, and the liver are the predominant organ systems affected. The end organ effects are directly related to the height and duration of the elevated core temperature. Heatstroke may exist in a pathophysiological continuum following other heat-related syndromes.

History Classic heatstroke should be suspected in any infant, elderly, or debilitated patient who is exposed passively, over many hours to days, to a significant heatstress, usually during regional heat waves. The presence of cardiovascular disease, drugs, or alcohol should suggest a compromised patient from a thermoregulatory standpoint. A young, healthy individual involved in exertional activity in a hot, humid environment should suggest exertional heatstroke. CNS dysfunction is of historical importance in making the diagnosis.

Physical Examination In heatstroke, the patient may present with nonspecific bizarre behavior or be irritable, agitated, confused, combative, hallucinating, seizing, or comatose. The presence or absence of sweating cannot be used to distinguish between heatstroke and heat exhaustion. Heatstroke is described as anhidrotic; however, sweating may be present as an early manifestation. Hot flushed skin classically present in heatstroke may be altered by cooling that occurs prior to ED presentation. A hyperdynamic circulatory state with tachycardia is commonly seen in young healthy adults who are able to maintain increased cardiac output in response to the circulatory

demand. Pupillary response is variable. Focal neurologic findings or posturing may be present. Ataxia may also be an early finding. Any neurologic sign or symptom may be seen.

Laboratory Abnormalities Ancillary testing may reflect the initial and delayed multiorgan effects of heat stress. Hemoconcentration and leukocytosis may be present as a result of associated dehydration. Fluid and electrolyte abnormalities may exist. Hypoglycemia, hypokalemia, and hypocalcemia are commonly seen. Free calcium is released from injured muscle in 2 to 3 days, resulting in hypercalcemia. Respiratory alkalosis results from stimulation of the respiratory centers and resulting hyperventilation. Lactic acidosis may occur secondary to severe hypoperfusion from hypovolemia or cardiac dysfunction. Direct thermal injury to the liver manifests as centrilobular necrosis, which results in an elevation of liver enzymes over a period of 48 hours. Urinalysis may suggest myoglobinuria and evidence of acute tubular necrosis. Rhabdomyolysis with an elevated creatine phosphokinase is more common in exertional than in classic heatstroke. Coagulation abnormalities manifest as disseminated intravascular coagulation and thrombocytopenia. Additional laboratory tests such as toxicological screening, lactate, thyroid function tests, serum ammonia, cardiac enzymes, and bacteriologic culturing may be indicated. Cerebrospinal fluid results show nonspecific pleocytosis in heatstroke. The electrocardiogram (ECG) usually reveals a sinus tachycardia with nonspecific S-T changes. However, the ECG is important in identifying coexisting disease and heat-related cardiac injury.

Treatment Morbidity and mortality are directly related to the magnitude and duration of core temperature elevation; therefore, rapid, aggressive cooling measures should begin immediately (**Table 127.3**). There is some controversy as to which modality is most effective in that there is variation in cooling rates. It appears that combining various modalities based on local resources is a practical and effective approach.

The patient's core temperature should be rapidly lowered to 38.4 to 39° C (101.2° to 102.2° F), preferably within 30 to 60 minutes of the start of therapy. Core temperature

Table 127.3
Cooling Modalities
Passive cooling
Ice water immersion bath
Water-soaked sheets/towels, and ice chips
External evaporative
Water spray/fans
Body cooling unit
Iced peritoneal lavage
Cardiopulmonary bypass
Cold humidified oxygen
Cold intravenous fluids
Iced gastric lavage

must be closely monitored and cooling measures stopped when this temperature range is attained in order to avoid "overshoot hypothermia."

A simple cooling modality consists of thermostatic control of the resuscitation area's ambient temperature. Evaporative cooling is a well tolerated, safe, rapid, and clinically effective noninvasive cooling technique. This consists of placing the disrobed patient on a suspended support structure or stretcher, and spraying with tepid (15° C) water while room temperature air is passed across the skin surface using large fans. This technique maintains vasodilation and minimizes shivering. There are specifically designed mesh net "body cooling units" (BCU) constructed for this purpose.

Ice packs, plastic bags of crushed ice, or an ice-water mixture can be selectively placed over the neck, axillae, and the groin. These can be used in conjunction with evaporative techniques. The disadvantage is patient discomfort and shivering.

Whole-body ice packing consists of placing plastic cloths or bags under the undressed patient, and covering the torso and extremities with crushed ice. This, however, can be difficult for personnel, poorly tolerated by the patient, and a technique that promotes shivering.

Ice water immersion is a very effective method of rapidly lowering the core temperature. This consists of placing the patient in a cold or ice water bath using the high thermal conductivity of water to dissipate heat. Using cold water instead of ice water baths is nearly as effective in lowering temperature and decreases shivering, and is more comfortable for the patient. Monitoring and performing resuscitation techniques are difficult. There is minimal morbidity and mortality associated with this method.

Invasive core cooling techniques are described. Cardiopulmonary bypass provides perfusion, oxygenation, and rapid cooling; however, its use necessitates technical availability, and requires heparinization. Cold peritoneal lavage has been shown to have a more rapid cooling rate than noninvasive modalities and may be considered in heatstroke refractory to external cooling measures. Cooled humidified oxygen, intravenous fluids, and iced gastric lavage contribute minimally to heat exchange and cooling when utilized individually, but may have a cumulative cooling effect when combined.

Additional Therapeutic Considerations Benzodiazepines are used to treat acute agitation and seizures. Antipyretics are ineffective in controlling temperature. Phenothiazines such as thorazine may be titrated to control shivering; however, these may aggravate hypotension, cause dystonia, and lower the seizure threshold. Complications such as rhabdomyolysis, acute renal failure, hyperkalemia, coagulopathy, and acidosis should be treated aggressively. A poor response to cooling measures may indicate the presence of underlying infection or disease. Treatment of any predisposing conditions should take place during the resuscitation and cooling process. The role of inflammation and the stress response to heat is being investigated. There may be a future role for anti-inflammatory medications as adjunctive therapy.

Heat Exhaustion

Heat exhaustion is a syndrome of heat-related volume depletion caused by excessive loss of body water and salt depletion. It is a diagnosis of exclusion once life-threatening heatstroke has been ruled out. In heat exhaustion, there is absence of multiorgan dysfunction.

The patient may present with subtle, nonspecific symptoms such as thirst, malaise, weakness, light-headedness, nausea, vomiting, headache, and myalgias that mimic viral illnesses. Core temperature is usually less than 40°C (104° F). The patient may appear sedate, weak, and fatigued. Signs of dehydration are usually present. The patient may appear acutely ill with tachycardia and hypotension. Causes of hypovolemia such as gastrointestinal bleeding and trauma must be considered. Mental status is usually intact; however, mental response may be slowed in the patient with severe volume depletion and hypotension. The skin may be flushed and is commonly diaphoretic. Diaphoresis may accompany other conditions such as hypoglycemia. Hymenoptera anaphylaxis should be considered when a patient having been outdoors presents with cutaneous erythema and cardiovascular collapse.

There may be hemoconcentration with fluid and electrolyte abnormalities depending on the degree of salt and water depletion and intake. Hypernatremia predominates when there is little fluid intake. Isotonic dehydration may exist when the patient has been partially rehydrated with salt-containing solution. Potassium levels are variable. Severe and prolonged hypoperfusion may cause a metabolic acidosis.

Severe heat exhaustion may be difficult to differentiate from heatstroke so aggressive treatment is required initially. The treatment of heat exhaustion focuses on lowering a significantly elevated temperature and rehydration. Evaporative cooling methods usually suffice. The route and extent of fluid repletion depend on the degree of volume depletion. The majority of ED patients benefit from intravenous normal saline but the oral route may be considered in the alert, mildly symptomatic patient. Patients may require gradual rehydration over several hours.

Heat Syncope

Heat syncope is a loss of consciousness resulting from heat-related vasodilation, venous pooling, and volume depletion causing a transient decrease in cerebral perfusion. Commonly seen in the elderly, it may be preceded by malaise, weakness, and nausea. Postural symptoms should reinforce a suspicion of heat syncope. Syncope appearing to be associated with heat exposure may be secondary to life threatening non–heat-related causes. Cardiovascular, neurologic, and metabolic etiologies must be excluded. Fluid and electrolyte abnormalities are variable. Heat syncope is usually transient and self-correcting but may indicate the need for fluid repletion and monitoring.

Heat Tetany

Heat tetany results from a hyperventilation-induced respiratory alkalosis secondary to intense, transient heat stress. It presents as a hyperventilation syndrome with malaise, lightheadedness, paresthesias, carpopedal spasm, and tetany. It can be a manifestation of heatstroke or heat exhaustion and may be confused with respiratory or psychogenic causes of hyperventilation or an acute intoxication. Tetany is differentiated from heat cramps by the presence of paresthesias and lack of pain in muscle compartments. This syndrome is usually self-limited and responds to removal of the heat stress, reassurance, relief of hyperventilation, and treatment of co-existing heat exhaustion or heatstroke.

Heat Cramps

Heat cramps are painful, spasmodic muscular contractions that occur during or shortly after work or strenuous exercise in a hot environment. They typically occur during the first few days of work in a hot environment. They result from intense sweating with a disproportionate loss of water and salt. Frequently they are caused by replacement of water without adequate salt repletion. Cramping is due to severe painful contractions of large muscle groups, usually the calves. Hyponatremia is common. Rhabdomyolysis is rare. Treatment consists of removal of the heat stress, decreasing muscular activity, and fluid and salt replacement. Intravenous hydration with isotonic saline rapidly reverses the symptoms.

Heat Edema

Heat edema is characterized by mild swelling of the distal extremities attributed to vasodilation and orthostatic pooling of interstitial fluid. It is commonly found in nonacclimatized individuals, especially the elderly, upon initial exposure to a hot environment. Other causes of edema need to be considered. Treatment consists of removing heat stress, decreasing prolonged standing, and elevation of the extremity. The swelling resolves spontaneously over several days. Diuretics are not indicated.

Prickly Heat

Prickly heat, also known as heat rash, lichen tropicus, or miliaria rubra, is a heat-related rash caused by the acute inflammation of sweat ducts. It presents as intensely pruritic vesicles on an erythematous base that are confined to clothed areas. The effected skin is usually anhydrotic. Treatment includes wearing loose clothing, avoiding heat stress, and topical hydrocortisone cream or chlorhexidine.

Prognosis

Mortality in heatstroke has been reported to range from 30% to 80% in cases involving serious injury or comorbid conditions; however, survival may approach 90% in cases of exertional heatstroke in the young, healthy athlete or military recruit, with aggressive therapy. The elderly are at higher risk for morbidity and mortality. Morbidity and mortality is related to the duration and magnitude of hyperthermia, and comorbid conditions. It has been suggested that mortality is reduced in patients who are rapidly cooled to the desired temperature end point within the first hour of treatment. Clinical indicators of poor prognosis include prolonged hyperthermia, prolonged coma, a core temperature above 42° C (108° F), and hypotension. Laboratory indicators include elevated serum transaminases, hyperkalemia, acute

renal failure, and coagulopathy. Additionally, lactic acidosis with an elevated serum lactate correlates with poor prognosis in classic heatstroke. Permanent organ damage may occur as a result of heatstroke. Heat exhaustion, heat syncope, heat tetany, and heat cramps are usually less severe and do not result in significant morbidity or mortality.

Disposition

Patients with heatstroke should be admitted to the intensive care unit after ED stabilization and after having decreased core temperature by aggressive cooling. Heat exhaustion necessitates admission if there has been a poor response to fluid therapy with unstable vital signs, if heatstroke is suspected, or if comorbid conditions or complications are present. Patients with heat syncope, heat tetany, or heat cramps, may be discharged if associated heatstroke has been ruled out, and they have responded to therapy and are asymptomatic. Prophylactic measures must be emphasized to patients who are discharged as well as to the general population during heat waves. Preventive measures include avoidance of predisposing conditions; increasing fluid intake prior to exposure; frequent water intake; breaks from activity while functioning in a hot, humid environment; wearing cool clothing; performing activities during the coolest, least humid time of the day; use of air conditioning and recognizing the importance of physical conditioning and gradual acclimatization.

Cold-Related Disorders

Hypothermia

Hypothermia is defined as a core temperature less than 35° C (95° F). This condition can occur in any climate and present with subtle signs and symptoms. *Primary accidental hypothermia* is caused by direct exposure to cold and is defined as acute or chronic. Acute or "rural" hypothermia occurs after a sudden, usually outdoor cold exposure. Chronic or "urban" hypothermia results from a gradual indoor exposure commonly associated with substandard heating and comorbid conditions. Immersion cold exposure is unique in that it results from rapid cold exposure accompanied by asphyxia. *Secondary hypothermia* is the result of a disease process or a pharmacological agent. The severity of hypothermia may be classified according to the patient's core temperature as mild (32° to 35° C, 90° to 95° F), moderate (28° to 32° C, 82° to 90° F), severe (28° C to 20° C, 82° F to 68° F), and profound hypothermia (less than 20° C, 68° F).

Patients susceptible to hypothermia are those in substandard living conditions and those of lower socioeconomic status. Patients most commonly at risk are the intoxicated, psychiatric, and mentally disabled in that they have poor adaptive and behavioral responses to the cold. The elderly are frequent victims of chronic indoor hypothermia because of their inability to sense the cold, altered compensatory mechanisms, and coexisting diseases. Neonates and small infants have a decreased ability to produce and conserve heat, and readily dissipate heat from their large surface area.

In general, unacclimated individuals have increased susceptibility. Recreational sports, outdoor activities, and military exercises frequently expose young, healthy individuals to cold and wet climates, thus increasing the risk of primary accidental hypothermia. Hypothermia is common during and after resuscitation attempts.

The anterior hypothalamus maintains a core temperature within a narrow range between 36° C (96.8° F) and 38° C (100.4° F). This is accomplished by maintaining a balance between heat production and heat loss. When an individual's compensatory response to heat loss is overwhelmed, hypothermia develops. The clinical effects of hypothermia relate to depressant effects on cell membranes that result in abnormal cellular integrity and function. Organ-specific physiologic changes are temperature dependent. These physiological derangements occur in a progressive manner along a temperature continuum from mild to severe hypothermia where compensatory responses for conserving heat have become ineffective. A stimulatory, excitation phase occurs initially in mild hypothermia with progression toward a depression of metabolism (adynamic phase) with moderate to profound hypothermia. Any process that impairs or overwhelms the normal thermoregulatory response may result in hypothermia. The causes and predisposing factors of hypothermia may be categorized according to thermoregulatory mechanisms (**Table 127.4**).

Emergency Department Evaluation

Initial Presentation   Initial presentation of hypothermia may be very subtle, presenting with nonspecific clinical signs and symptoms. Prehospital providers, triage nurses, and emergency physicians must maintain a high index of suspicion for hypothermia in patients presenting with a predisposing exposure, altered mental status, coma or cardiopulmonary arrest. Hypothermia may occur without a significant history of cold exposure. The initial temperature, mental status, and cardiovascular stability at triage determine the urgency of resuscitation and rewarming. Moderate to profound hypothermia necessitates rapid, aggressive intervention.

History   A complete history should be obtained using all available sources. An initial history should identify allergies, medications, medical history, and events preceding presentation to the ED. The history is then directed toward environmental exposure and predisposing factors. The type, duration, and severity of exposure aid in differentiating primary from secondary hypothermia. Trauma patients are at high risk for hypothermia depending on age, injury type, transfusion requirements, presence of intoxication, time in field, time in the emergency department and operating room. The prehospital course of events, including presentation, associated injury, and response to dextrose or narcan, and rewarming therapy, should be emphasized in the history.

Physical Examination   The presence of wet garments, a disheveled appearance, malnourishment, or hypothyroid facies should be noted. Odors of alcohol,

Table 127.4
Hypothermia: Predisposing Factors

Impaired Thermoregulation
  Central nervous system/hypothalamic dysfunction
  Structural
  Hemorrhage/infarction
    Trauma
    Tumor
    Infection/sepsis
    Degenerative processes
  Metabolic
    Anoxia
    Acidosis
  Encephalopathy
  Toxic
    Pharmacologic
Decreased Heat Production
  Age extremes/lack of adaptation
  Hypoendocrine states/hypoglycemia
  Malnutrition/acute incapacitating illness
  Inactivity/immobilization
  CNS depression
Increased Heat Loss
  Environmental exposure/immersion
  Burns
  Exfoliative skin disease
  Vasodilation/impaired vasoconstriction
    Drugs/alcohol
    Shock
    Spinal cord injury/neuropathies
    Sepsis
Iatrogenic Factors
  Lack of recognition of hypothermic potential
  Lack of active external rewarming in acutely ill/
    injured patients
  Fluid resuscitation
  Overtreatment of hyperthermia

acetone, or other toxins may be present. A primary evaluation of the patient's airway, ventilation, circulation, and mental status takes precedence, and resuscitation should begin immediately. Vital signs may be severely depressed and appear to be absent in severe hypothermia. A pulse may not be palpable due to vasoconstriction and profound bradycardia. It may take 30 to 60 seconds for detection of a pulse or depressed respirations. A blood pressure may not be detectable by auscultation; therefore, Doppler determination may be useful. Bedside ultrasound may assist in detecting the presence or absence of cardiac contractions and vascular flow. An accurate core temperature must be determined in the presence of an altered mental status, in psychotic-appearing patients, the elderly, and when resuscitation is not improving patient status.

Standard electronic thermometers will not record temperatures below 34° C (94° F); therefore, a rectal thermistor probe is necessary. The probe should be inserted approximately 15 cm into the rectum. A falsely low reading may be obtained if inserted into cold stool. Rectal probe temperature readings do lag behind core temperatures. There is debate about the accuracy of infrared tympanic thermometers. Esophageal probes are useful to monitor myocardial and mediastinal temperature in the intubated patient. Bladder probes may be useful. Any immediate life-threats to the patient must be identified upon completion of the initial history and primary evaluation.

A secondary evaluation is performed in an attempt to determine the clinical severity of hypothermia and to identify predisposing or concurrent conditions. The skin and mucous membranes are evaluated for signs of cold-related vasoconstriction. Pallor caused by acute anemia or shock, as well as an ashen color, cyanosis, or mottling may be present. Skin temperature should be noted as well as evidence of trauma, track marks, dermatologic disease, or local cold-related injury. Oozing blood from needle sticks or lacerations may indicate coagulopathy. The scalp and skin folds must be examined closely for subtle signs of trauma. Cervical spine precautions should be maintained and the neck inspected for a thyroidectomy scar. The musculoskeletal examination may identify injury that could contribute to blood and fluid loss. The patient must be log-rolled, and the dorsal aspect inspected and palpated including inspection of creases. A rectal examination may detect blood, provide an indication of sphincter tone, and identify impaction that could hinder rectal core temperature monitoring.

Clinical presentations depend on the degree of hypothermia. In *mild* (32° to 35° C, 90° to 95° F) hypothermia, there may be vague symptoms of subjective coldness, chills, hunger, nausea, or fatigue. The patient may be pale from vasoconstriction, shivering, anxious, agitated, or apathetic. Metabolic rate increases. Central nervous system manifestations begin at 34° C (93° F) with an increase in muscle tone, mild incoordination, loss of fine motor control, some dysarthria, and ataxia. Impaired judgment, maladaptive behavior, mild confusion, lethargy, and amnesia of precipitous events may be present. The patient may be hyperreflexic. There is increased vascular resistance and cardiac output with tachycardia and elevated blood pressure. The patient is tachypneic.

In *moderate* (28° to 32° C, 82.4° to 90° F) hypothermia, metabolic rate and oxygen consumption decrease. The patient becomes poikilothermic. A sedate, slowly responding patient who is no longer shivering may indicate a core temperature below 30° C (86° F). CNS signs progress to confusion, delirium, lethargy, stupor, and light coma proportional to the degree of hypothermia. Confusion may manifest by "paradoxical undressing" in response to cold exposure and may indicate impending thermoregulatory failure. Pupillary function becomes sluggish. There is a progressive bradycardia, decreased cardiac output and blood pressure, with soft or even undetectable heart sounds. The patient is hypotensive. A characteristic Osborn (J) wave, which is a wide positive deflection at the end of the QRS complex, is seen at core temperatures below 32° C (90° F). Electrocardiographic abnormalities are indicative of a generalized, progressive, depression of myocardial conduction. Conduction intervals become prolonged and dysrhythmias such as sinus bradycardia,

atrial flutter and fibrillation with a slow ventricular response, or junctional rhythms appear. A fine baseline artifact reflecting a hypothermia-related muscle tremor may be present on the ECG. At temperatures below 30° C (86° F), ventricular irritability increases. Tachypnea progresses to hypoventilation with decreased oxygen consumption and CO_2 production at 30° C (86° F). Cough and gag reflexes are depressed then lost, which increases the risk of aspiration. There may be a cold-induced bronchorrhea with thick, copious secretions. Noncardiac pulmonary edema may occur. An intestinal ileus and cold diuresis are common. There is muscle rigidity and voluntary movement is minimal and difficult to recognize.

Severe (28° to 20° C, 82° to 68° F) hypothermia may present as an ashen, unresponsive, severely hypotensive, bradycardic or asystolic, areflexic patient appearing to be clinically dead. Below 25° C (77° F) the patient loses corneal and oculocephalic reflexes, however pupillary pathways are relatively resistant to metabolic insult. Magnification may have to be needed to detect pupillary reactivity, which may be absent. Fixed and dilated pupils may not be indicative of brain death. Cardiac output continues to decline, therefore blood pressure and pulse are difficult or impossible to obtain. Spontaneous ventricular fibrillation may occur at 28° C (82° F) and amplitude diminishes as the core temperature declines. Rhythms progress to asystole at temperatures toward 20° C (68° F). Pulmonary edema and oliguria may occur. Decreased esophageal, gastric, and intestinal motility leads to abdominal distention. Cold-induced rectus muscle spasm and ileus may mimic an acute abdominal process. Voluntary motion stops and muscular rigidity may resemble rigor mortis.

Profound (less than 20° C, 68° F) hypothermia mimics death with lividity, coma, fixed and dilated unreactive pupils, areflexia, and flaccid. The patient is apneic, pulseless, and asystolic.

Ancillary Tests

In the hypothermic patient ancillary tests are performed to determine the extent of multiorgan involvement. They also help to detect precipitating or concurrent conditions, and assist with clinical decision making.

Laboratory abnormalities are common in moderate to severe hypothermia; however, abnormalities occurring during rewarming cannot be predicted clinically. A decrease in plasma volume and resulting hemoconcentration leads to an increased hematocrit. The white blood count may be decreased due to white blood cell sequestration. Platelets are low in number and defective, resulting in a prolonged bleeding time. Platelet dysfunction, sludging of cold red blood cells with an increase in blood viscosity, and suppression of cascade enzyme function may result in intravascular thrombosis. Coagulopathy may exist clinically despite normal appearing prothrombin and partial thromboplastin time values.

Initial hyperglycemia is secondary to increased catecholamines and glycogenolysis. Hypoglycemia may occur with rewarming. Hypokalemia is common; however, hyperkalemia may signify rhabdomyolysis. Blood urea nitrogen and creatinine values are variable. An increase in amylase and lipase may indicate cold-induced pancreatitis. Urine characteristic of cold-induced diuresis is dilute.

Additional laboratory tests such as toxicological screening, lactate, cortisol and thyroid function tests, liver function tests and serum ammonia, cardiac enzymes, and bacteriological cultures may be indicated, especially when rewarming is ineffective.

The interpretation of arterial blood gas values in hypothermia is controversial. Blood gas specimens are normally rewarmed to 37° C in a blood gas analyzer; therefore, the pH and pCO_2 values reported are uncorrected for the patient's actual temperature. These values should be interpreted as in the normothermic patient to guide resuscitation. In hypothermia, there is a leftward shift of the oxyhemoglobin-dissociation curve with decreased release of oxygen to the tissues. A respiratory alkalosis is often initially present with progression toward a mixed metabolic and respiratory acidosis. Core temperature is not a predictor of a victim's acid-base status.

Peritoneal lavage may detect hemoperitoneum and provide access for active core rewarming. Diagnostic imaging may contribute to an underlying diagnosis. A cervical spine x-ray may indicate a fracture having resulted in a spinal cord injury contributing to hypothermia. A chest radiograph may indicate aspiration pneumonia, pneumothorax, or hemothorax. A radiograph of the pelvis may be indicated when acute traumatic blood loss is suspected. Computed tomography of the head may be useful in identifying structural etiology when there is failure to rewarm.

Differential Diagnosis

Hypothermia may be confused with any infectious, metabolic, toxicological, traumatic, neurological, or psychiatric condition causing altered mental status or coma. Central nervous system depression is proportional to the degree of hypothermia. Therefore, other causes should be suspected if a change in mental status is disproportionate to the degree of hypothermia or if there are focal neurological findings. A disproportionate heart rate may indicate other conditions such as hypovolemia, toxic exposure, or hypoglycemia. Hyperventilation may indicate mild hypothermia, a structural central nervous system lesion, or acidosis. Primary and secondary hypothermia may coexist.

Predisposing factors, concurrent conditions, and the extent of resulting multiorgan effects must be determined. Gathering additional historical information from family, caregivers, and medical records assists in identifying secondary hypothermia. Performing repeated physical examinations and noting the response to therapy are of diagnostic importance as well.

Emergency Department Intervention

The goals of ED intervention are to stabilize the patient, rewarm until normthermic, and manage predisposing or complicating conditions. Cardiovascular stability and severity of hypothermia determine therapy. Invasive monitoring of intraarterial pressure and core temperature during intervention assists in determining the success of resuscitation.

Rewarming does not take precedence over immediate resuscitation and stabilization. Therefore, airway, ventilation, and cardiovascular status are assessed and stabilized. This includes the initiation of high flow oxygen, intravenous line, and cardiac monitor placement. Prehospital treatment includes removing the patient from exposure, which frequently involves prolonged extrication and rescue. The patient is placed in a horizontal position to decrease orthostatic hypotension, wet garments are removed, and the patient protected from further heat loss by providing insulating blankets or garments. Manipulation, rough movement, and excess activity place the fragile hypothermic patient at risk for cardiovascular instability and should be avoided. Extremities should be protected from further local tissue injury. Transport should be gentle but expeditious, with monitoring and resuscitation continuing as indicated.

Resuscitation proceeds according to presence or absence of pulse and respirations, central nervous system responsiveness, and core temperature. Airway management with warmed high-flow 100% oxygen should be undertaken. Gentle initial ventilatory support with a bag-valve-mask may be indicated. The indications for endotracheal intubation in the hypothermic patient are the same as those in normothermia. The hypothermic patient with altered consciousness and inadequate respirations requires intubation and assisted ventilation. However, because of the risk of precipitating ventricular fibrillation with manipulation of the airway, preoxygenation and gentle intubation are the rule while observing cervical spine precautions. Intubation may be difficult due to rigidity of the jaw and necessitate blind nasotracheal or fiberoptic intubation. Hyperventilation should be avoided as this may induce respiratory alkalosis and resulting ventricular fibrillation.

When an emergency responder begins cardiopulmonary resuscitation (CPR) in the field, hypothermia may or may not be suspected. Due to the inability to obtain a core temperature, inaccuracy in determining depressed vital signs, the lack of monitor availability, and artifact, severe hypothermia is often initially treated as a normothermic prehospital arrest. If the patient is unresponsive, no pulse is detected, and there is a monitored rhythm such as sinus bradycardia, atrial fibrillation with a slow ventricular response, or pulseless electrical activity, it is generally recommended to perform CPR. However, the absence of a palpable pulse and blood pressure may be due to intense vasoconstriction and bradycardia in the case of an organized rhythm. The presence of respiratory efforts indicates brain stem perfusion from flow even in the absence of a palpable peripheral pulse. The performance of chest compressions may precipitate ventricular fibrillation and other dysrhythmias including asystole, and this risk must be weighed against the risk of decreased cerebral perfusion without performing CPR. The optimal rate and depth of cardiac compressions and the exact mechanism of flow generation during chest compression has not been determined. A gas-powered chest compressor device may be used if prolonged resuscitation efforts are needed. If ventricular fibrillation or pulseless ventricular tachycardia is identified, and the core temperature is below 30° C (86° F), it is recommended to defibrillate up to a total of three shocks. If there is no response, CPR is performed and aggressive rewarming is initiated. Upon achieving a core temperature of 30° C (86° F), repeat defibrillation should be attempted because of increased cardiovascular responsiveness at this temperature. Below this temperature, defibrillation is rarely successful. If a pulse is present or the patient is responsive, CPR should not be performed.

Many hypothermic patients are volume depleted due to prolonged exposure, poor oral intake, fluid sequestration, increased vascular permeability, and cold diuresis. A peripheral intravenous line of normal saline should be established, and volume expansion begun to correct hypovolemia. The use of dextrose in normal saline has been advocated by some authors. Lactated Ringers should be avoided because lactic acid clearance may be decreased secondary to decreased hepatic flow and metabolism. Volume must be expanded to assure perfusion to tissue threatened by vasoconstriction and to compensate for rewarming vasodilatation. Blood specimens are drawn to assess for comorbid conditions and precipitating events. Consciousness and thermoregulation may return on initiation of intravenous dextrose, naloxone, or thiamine.

Collapse of the cardiovascular system in severe hypothermia may not respond to pacemaker stimulation and cardioactive drugs until the patient is rewarmed to 30° C (86° F). However, drug metabolism is depressed; therefore, the initial response is unpredictable and accumulation resulting in toxic drug effects may occur as the patient is rewarmed. It has been suggested that medications should be given at longer dosing intervals. Bradycardia may be physiologic in hypothermia and revert to a normal rhythm with rewarming. If the blood pressure is disproportionately low for the degree of hypothermia, and unresponsive to volume repletion and rewarming, low-dose dopamine and dobutamine should be considered. Acid-base disturbances should be gradually corrected during rewarming based on actual arterial blood gas values.

Secondary causes of hypothermia such as sepsis, myxedema, and adrenal crisis need to be treated if these conditions are suspected based on history, physical examination, and when there is failure to rewarm.

A nasogastric tube should be inserted to relieve distention and diagnose hemorrhage, and can be used in rewarming. An indwelling urinary catheter should be placed to monitor urine output and for rewarming purposes.

The type of rewarming intervention often depends on local resources. The process of limiting heat loss and transferring heat to the body using various rewarming modalities is based on the principles of heat loss and transfer involving conduction, radiation, convection, and evaporation.

Rewarming modalities consist of passive external, active external, and active core rewarming (**Table 126.5**).

Passive external rewarming (PER) limits further heat loss and allows patients to rewarm by way of their own endogenous heat production. Sufficient metabolic activity must therefore be present. Metabolic heat production de-

Table 127.5
Rewarming Techniques

Passive External Rewarming
   Remove from cold environment
   Remove wet garments
   Provide insulation and warmth
Active External Rewarming
   Increase room temperature
   Warm blankets
   Heated objects (warm IV infusion bags, heating pads)
   Radiant heat sources/overhead heater lights
   Hypothermia heating blankets
   Forced-air rewarming systems
   Plumbed garments circulating warm water
   Warm whole-body water immersion
   Arteriovenous rewarming (distal extremities)
Active Core Rewarming
   Inhalation of warm humidified oxygen
   Heated IV fluids (via microwave oven, blood/fluid
      warmers)
   Heated lavage
      Gastric, colonic
      Bladder
      Peritoneal
      Pleural
   Extracorporeal blood rewarming
      Cardiac bypass
      Femoral bypass circuit
      Hemodialysis
   Mediastinal irrigation via open thoracotomy

clines and shivering becomes suppressed at temperatures less than 30° C (86° F); therefore, PER is recommended only for mild hypothermia. This provides slow, progressive rewarming that avoids rapid changes in cardiovascular status or complications. This modality involves removing the patient from the cold environment, removal of wet garments, and providing insulation and warmth.

Active external rewarming (AER) consists of the application of an exogenous heat source to the body surface. It has been recommended to apply heated objects to truncal areas. This avoids the influx of cold, acidotic, peripheral blood from rewarmed, vasoconstricted extremities to a depressed core cardiovascular system. Peripheral vasodilation and venous pooling may lead to rewarming shock, which is a relative hypovolemia with hypotension. Peripheral release of lactic acid may lead to a rewarming acidosis with resulting myocardial depression and dysrhythmias.

Rewarming the periphery may increase metabolic demand before the cardiovascular system can compensate. The core temperature may decrease during initial rewarming from the central cooling effect of cold peripheral blood, a phenomenon known as core temperature afterdrop.

Active external rewarming therapy begins with the heated ambulance compartment and thermostatic control of the ED resuscitation area. Blankets and intravenous infusion bags should be heated. Pediatric overhead heater lights and warm water-filled heat exchange blankets (Blanketrol) should be available. Forced-air rewarming systems (Bair Hugger) provide convective heat transfer and decrease radiant heat loss by utilizing a heat source and cover that circulates warm air directly onto the patient's skin. The technique of warm whole body water immersion may be utilized but is impractical in the case of an ongoing need for monitoring, CPR, and the performance of resuscitation procedures. Arteriovenous anastomoses rewarming involve immersing the distal extremities in 42° to 45° C temperature water. Warming blankets, commercial hot packs, and hot water bottles can place the patient at risk for cutaneous thermal injury.

Active internal or core rewarming (ACR) is utilized in moderate to severe hypothermia to deliver heat directly to the anatomic core, preferentially rewarming the heart, lungs, and central nervous system prior to the extremities. This decreases the shunting of cold peripheral blood to the core. These techniques are of variable invasiveness and have varying rewarming rates.

Warm humidified oxygen heated to 42° to 45° C (108° to 113° F) via heated cascade nebulizer may be administered to the airways by mask or endotracheal tube. Heat gain by this route is small, averaging 1° to 2° C per hour, but this technique minimizes respiratory heat loss. Intravenous fluids are warmed in a microwave oven, commercial fluid warmers, or countercurrent heat exchange devices and administered at a temperature of 40° to 42° C (104° to 108° F). The rate of rewarming depends on the volume infused. Gastric, colonic, and bladder lavage with aliquots of heated water or normal saline transfer minimal heat individually but may have a cumulative rewarming effect.

Severe hypothermia may necessitate using heated peritoneal and/or pleural lavages. Heated peritoneal lavage consists of instilling potassium-free isotonic dialysate heated from 40° to 45° C (104° to 113° F) into the peritoneal cavity in a dose of 10 to 20 mL/kg body weight. The fluid is exchanged every 20 to 30 minutes via a double catheter system. Rewarming occurs at approximately 2° to 4° C per hour. Physical impingement upon ventilation by infused fluid must be monitored. Heated pleural or thoracostomy tube lavage is accomplished by inserting two chest tubes into the thoracic cavity providing an anterior inflow and a more posterior axillary outflow tract. Normal saline heated to 40° C (104° F) is instilled by continuous infusion using a high flow infuser system (Level-1 Fluid Warmer). Fluid infused is collected with an autotransfusion thoracostomy drainage set (Pleur-evac) and the effects of increasing intrathoracic pressure monitored. It must be recognized that manipulation of a chest tube near the heart increases the risk of inducing ventricular fibrillation in the reperfusing patient. Open thoracotomy with continuous mediastinal irrigation with normal saline heated to 40° to 41° C (104° to 106° F) has been described in profound hypothermia with cardiac arrest. This permits direct rewarming and defibrillation.

Extracorporeal techniques are reserved for those patients with severe hypothermia and in the case of severe hemodynamic instability. These employ devices that reroute cold blood through external blood warming equipment via femoral arteriovenous or venovenous shunt. Countercurrent heat exchangers can be interposed between femoral vessels to provide continuous arteriovenous rewarming. Heated hemodialysis using percutaneous, two-way flow catheters is an effective means of rewarming. Dialysis can correct electrolyte abnormalities associated with hypothermia or concurrent drug overdose. Flow is blood pressure driven with these techniques and therefore would be ineffective in the event of hypotension or cardiac arrest.

Complete cardiac bypass or partial, femoral-to-femoral cardiopulmonary bypass provides rapid rewarming, oxygenation, and circulatory support. This modality can raise the core temperature 1° to 2° C every 3 to 5 minutes. Disadvantages include the need for heparinization as well as the need for specialized equipment and personnel. Modalities such as high-temperature intravenous fluids, and microwave diathermy techniques are not of practical use at this time.

Approach to Rewarming The approach to rewarming is controversial due to the lack of prospective controlled studies. Knowledge of the patient's core temperature, cardiovascular stability, and central nervous system responsiveness assists in guiding therapy. In general, the greater the hemodynamic instability and the more severe the degree of hypothermia below 32° C (90° F), the more aggressive and rapid the rewarming modality employed. Combining rewarming techniques, while considering the advantages and disadvantages of each, is patient-specific and appears to be the safest approach. The use of preexisting protocols, combined with clinical judgment and experience, should determine therapy.

Mild primary hypothermia with a core temperature above 32° C (90° F) commonly responds to PER techniques. In cases of decreased metabolic efficiency or in mild secondary hypothermia, selected AER techniques may be combined with these methods.

In the patient with a nonarrest rhythm, a central pulse, and moderate hypothermia, truncal AER is combined with noninvasive ACR techniques such as warm humidified oxygen, heated intravenous fluids, and selective heated lavage.

A temperature less than 30° C (86° F) with hemodynamic instability or the inability to rapidly rewarm using the above techniques may be an indication for heated peritoneal or pleural lavage. Extracorporeal rewarming should also be considered. Severe hypothermia with no central pulse or cardiopulmonary arrest (ventricular fibrillation, pulseless ventricular tachycardia, PEA or asystole) necessitates prolonged CPR and use of all available ACR techniques, including pleural lavage and/or extracorporeal rewarming. If neurological and cardiovascular status do not improve as expected with rewarming in primary hypothermia, comorbid pathological processes such as intracranial lesions, trauma, endocrine diseases or sepsis must be considered.

Prognosis

The long-term prognosis can be most closely associated with the presence or absence of comorbid conditions. In young, healthy patients with primary accidental hypothermia without complicating medical conditions, mortality is relatively low. However, when there is coexisting underlying illness, common in the elderly, mortality may be as high as 90%. Prognosis appears to be more favorable in children than in adults. The hypometabolic state induced by hypothermia not only imitates death but also protects against cerebral hypoxic injury. Therefore, standard brain death criteria do not apply. The lowest recorded infant core temperature with intact neurological recovery from accidental hypothermia is 15° C (59° F). In the adult it is reported as 13.7° C (56.6° F). The lowest reported core temperature for survival from therapeutic hypothermia is 9° C (48.2° F). There is no evidence of a direct correlation between core temperature and outcome. Patients who appear dead after prolonged exposure to cold temperature should not be considered dead until rewarmed to 32° C (90° F), and found to be unresponsive to resuscitation efforts. This may involve hours of resuscitative efforts in the emergency department or intensive care unit.

Disposition

Most patients with mild accidental hypothermia are rewarmed to normothermia, observed in the ED, and discharged if asymptomatic to a warm environment. Moderate to severe hypothermia patients are admitted to the intensive care unit for further rewarming and diagnosis and treatment of underlying conditions and complications. Whether the management of hypothermia falls under the auspices of trauma surgery or medical intensivists is institution specific.

Cold-Related Injuries

Unprotected exposure to a cold and/or wet environment may result in freezing or nonfreezing soft tissue injury. Freezing cold-induced injury includes frostnip and frostbite. Nonfreezing injury includes trenchfoot and chilblains.

Frostnip

Frostnip is a mild, superficial cold induced injury of the skin. It is characterized by discomfort such as the sensation of cold, numbness, and tingling that is transient. There is coolness to touch and pallor from intense vasoconstriction. There is no associated tissue destruction, and symptoms and signs resolve spontaneously upon rewarming.

Frostbite

Frostbite is tissue injury that results from freezing and is classified as superficial or deep according to severity. Frostbite injury occurs in phases, progressing from an initial prefreeze phase to ischemic injury of the involved

body part whenever the tissue temperature falls below 0° C (32° F). It results in tissue destruction, which is secondary to freezing within the skin and underlying structures. On exposure to cold, sympathetic microvascular vasoconstriction shunts blood away from ears, nose, and hands. Cold injury occurs in these acral structures that have abundant arteriovenous anastomoses that facilitate shunting and therefore decreased flow. This results in an increase in local heat loss, as well as stasis, sludging, and thrombosis resulting in local tissue ischemia. As tissue freezes, ice crystals form in the extracellular space, thereby increasing osmotic pressure. As a result, water is withdrawn from the intracellular compartment, which leads to intracellular dehydration and cell death. Intracellular ice crystal formation may contribute. These effects are associated with the release of vasoactive metabolites of arachidonic acid, thromboxane, and prostaglandin from damaged tissue. The effect of these substances on tissues results in vasoconstriction, inflammation, platelet aggregation, and further progressive dermal ischemia and necrosis. Tissue injury evolves over 2 to 3 days postthawing with worsening edema and blistering. The appearance of hemorrhagic blebs indicates damage to the deeper subdermal vascular plexuses. If nonviable tissue is present, there is gradual demarcation of the injured area, followed by dry gangrene or mummification. Final necrotic demarcation may be delayed 30 to 90 days. Sloughing of superficial necrotic tissue can leave a viable extremity beneath an eschar.

Predisposing Factors

There are many conditions that contribute to an individual's susceptibility to sustaining cold-related injury. Ambient temperature and duration of tissue exposure to the cold are the most important factors in determining the extent of tissue damage (**Table 127.6**). Particularly suscepti-

Table 127.6
Frostbite: Predisposing Factors
Acclimatization
Previous cold injury
Dehydration
Fatigue and exhaustion
Inadequate, constricting, or wet clothing
Immobility
Impaired judgment (intoxicants, psychiatric, mental disability)
Environmental (ambient temperature, duration exposure, wind chill, altitude)
Contact with good thermal conductors (metal, water, volatiles)
Aerosol propellants (propane, freon)
Comorbidities (cardiovascular, diabetes, vasoactive medications, trauma, dermatologic)
Toxic substances (ethanol, sympathomimetics, nicotine)

ble to cold-induced injury are military personnel subjected to inclement weather conditions and civilians such as the homeless, outdoor laborers, those involved in winter recreational or sporting activities, and survivors of natural disasters.

Emergency Department Evaluation

Initial Evaluation

The initial presentation may be misleading because tissues may already be thawed or partially thawed on presentation to the ED, and initial physical findings can be deceptively benign. It should be remembered that even the mildest forms of frostbite involve some measure of tissue destruction.

History

The diagnosis of cold-related injury and, specifically, freezing versus nonfreezing injury can usually be made based on a history of environmental conditions. Emphasis is placed on type and duration of exposure, the potential for systemic hypothermia, the extent of rewarming and thawing, associated trauma, and on any medical or other risk factors.

Cold-induced symptoms are most commonly localized to the distal appendages. Cold-related corneal injury should be suspected in patients presenting with eye complaints after winter recreational activities. Initially, the patient may have local discomfort with stinging, burning, throbbing, or aching as the tissues begin to freeze. The patient may complain of distal sensory deficits and a sensation of cold. Light touch, pain, and temperature perception are commonly affected. Hyperhidrosis may be present. Numbness is the most common complaint and may progress to a "block of wood" sensation in deep frostbite followed by varying degrees of pain. Deep, aching joint pain may be present in severe full-thickness injury.

Physical Examination

Frostbite can be clinically classified into degrees of severity based on extent of tissue injury. First- and second-degree frostbite are superficial injuries and less severe. Third and fourth degree injuries involve deeper structures and result in tissue loss.

First-degree frostbite is partial skin freezing that manifests as an anesthetic, hyperemic, edematous body part. The skin may desquamate several days later.

Second-degree frostbite is a full thickness injury of the skin characterized by clear, superficial blisters typically surrounded by erythema and edema. Desquamation occurs with the formation of blackened eschars over a period of several days. Subcutaneous tissue is still soft and pliable when manipulated.

Third-degree frostbite indicates freezing of the skin and subcutaneous tissues with deeper violaceous or hemorrhagic vesicles. The skin may take on a blue-gray discoloration and is insensate.

Fourth-degree frostbite is characterized by the initial signs of mottling or deep red color, and then followed by cyanosis, necrosis, and gangrene. In fourth-degree injury there may be tendon, muscle, and bone involvement.

Ancillary Tests

Ancillary studies are usually not indicated unless the patient has significant comorbidity or other injuries. If there is concern about vascular compromise to an affected extremity, a Doppler device may be used to detect peripheral pulses. There are a number of radiographic studies, such as angiography and radioisotope scanning, that have been utilized to assess the extent of tissue injury but these are considered only once the patient has been stabilized and thawing completed.

Emergency Department Diagnosis

Local cold-related injury must be differentiated from a number of other conditions. These include other causes of distal ischemia, iatrogenic thermal burns from rewarming attempts, chemical burns, soft tissue trauma, compartment syndrome, cellulitis, cold urticaria, inflammatory bites and stings, dermatitis, cryoglobulinemia, and Raynaud's phenomenon.

Emergency Department Intervention

The patient's airway, ventilation, and cardiovascular status are assessed and resuscitation initiated before local cold injury is addressed. This includes recognizing systemic hypothermia, associated trauma, or medical conditions, and initiating systemic rewarming therapy as necessary. Systemic hypothermia and volume depletion must be corrected. The patient should be removed from the cold environment and have constricting garments atraumatically removed. Local rewarming of the frozen part should not be attempted if there is any possibility of refreezing before definitive rewarming therapy can be started. Refreezing a thawed or partially thawed extremity or rubbing the affected area can result in increased injury. The goal of therapy is to prevent or decrease the amount of tissue loss by rapidly reversing ice crystal formation within the tissues.

Frostbite is treated by rapid rewarming. The affected part is immersed in gentle, circulating water heated to and maintained at 40° C (104° F). Strict aseptic techniques should be employed during rewarming and subsequent wound care. The bath should be large enough so that the frostbitten part avoids contact with the container and so that it does not rapidly decrease the temperature of the water. Dry heat is to be avoided because it may desiccate tissue. Higher rewarming temperatures may burn. Rewarming is continued until evidence that circulation is reestablished and thawing is complete. This is characterized by hyperemia in an increasingly pliable extremity within approximately 30 minutes of rewarming. Edema and vesicles may not appear for 24 hours. Rewarming and resulting reperfusion is painful and therefore parenteral narcotics may be necessary. Tissue should be handled gently after thawing to avoid further trauma and the extremity elevated to decrease edema. Constricting or compressive dressings should be avoided.

The clear or whitish blisters of superficial frostbite can be left intact or debrided; however, debridement is favored in order to decrease contact of toxic blister components with the underlying tissue. Topical aloe vera cream is applied for its thromboxane inhibitor effect. The hemorrhagic blisters of deep injury are left intact or aspirated to avoid tissue desiccation and to keep from converting the wound to a full-thickness injury. Aloe vera is then applied. The injured part is loosely wrapped with sterile gauze, splinted as necessary, and elevated. The antiprostaglandin, ibuprofen, is prescribed to minimize accumulation of arachidonic acid breakdown products. After admission, daily hydrotherapy is recommended with active movement of joints to maintain range of motion. Suppurative or necrotic debris is gently removed from the wounds. The use of tobacco or alcohol should be avoided. Compartment pressures may need to be monitored.

Because of the difficulty in determining the depth of tissue destruction at initial presentation, a conservative approach is favored. Subsequent to blister formation, dry eschars may evolve in severe frostbite. Generally, surgical debridement and amputation are delayed for several weeks unless severe infection or sepsis develops. Amputation is indicated when there is clear demarcation, mummification, and sloughing. Emergency surgery is occasionally required for constricting eschars or associated severe infection.

A number of ancillary treatment modalities have been described including medical and surgical vasodilatory sympathectomies, dextran, heparin, ascorbic acid, and hyperbaric oxygen. Recent experimental evidence suggests that thrombolytic agents may be of value in limiting tissue loss. Appropriate tetanus prophylaxis must be instituted. Intravenous antibiotics are recommended during the initial 48 to 72 hours or until edema resolves due to an increased susceptibility to streptococcal infection.

Disposition

The majority of patients who present to the ED after sustaining a cold injury require admission for wound care and observation after rewarming has been initiated. This is particularly true for frostbite injury. Surgical consultation should also be obtained. The patient with a limited area of superficial injury that has been completely thawed and appears clinically uncompromised may be discharged with close, prearranged follow-up care. The patient should also be instructed to apply aloe vera cream, take ibuprofen, and elevate and protect the affected extremity or body part. This includes wearing protective clothing and avoiding reexposure to the cold. The patient should be reevaluated within 24 hours if discharged from the ED.

Prognosis

Superficial and deep frostbite result in various degrees of tissue destruction that increases with the length of time frozen. However, freezing itself is not absolutely destructive if rapid thawing takes place and prognosis may be good. Favorable signs include normal color, sensation, and warmth after thawing. Conversely, tissue that remains cold, anesthetic, pale or violaceous after rewarming usually indicates an unfavorable prognosis. Early clear bleb formation is more favorable than delayed hemorrhagic blebs. Lack of edema after thawing may indicate major tissue damage. Slow, incomplete rewarming can lead to increased tissue loss. Recovery from frostbite is often incomplete, and neuronal injury and abnormal sympa-

thetic tone may result in throbbing pain for several weeks and sequelae such as thermal misperception, paresthesias, and hyperhidrosis. Decreased nail and hair growth and a residual Raynaud's phenomenon may persist.

Trench Foot

Trench foot (immersion foot) is tissue injury sustained during prolonged exposure of a distal extremity to wet cold at above freezing temperatures. Neurovascular damage and tissue maceration occurs slowly over a period of hours to days without actual tissue freezing.

The patient presents with the complaint of pruritus, pain, tingling, and numbness and a cool, swollen, macerated, dusky distal extremity. Initially the extremity is erythematous, and becomes cool, pale, and wrinkled with decreased sensation, then swollen, mottled, and immobile within hours to days. Leg cramps may be present. The initial presentation may be difficult to distinguish from frostbite in that vesiculation may develop. A hyperemic reperfusion phase can last up to 6 weeks during which time skin changes occur with a return to normal or to progressive tissue loss.

The prognosis in trench foot tends to be better than in frostbite injury. The limb usually returns to normal with increased cold sensitivity but may progress to liquefaction gangrene if severe. The therapeutic approach involves gentle rewarming and local wound care.

Chilblains

Chilblains (or pernio) is a nonfreezing injury occurring after repetitive exposure to dry cold. The skin lesions manifest within 24 hours of exposure and are more common in young women. The patient commonly presents with complaints of redness, swelling, and pruritus of the face, and burning paresthesias of the dorsum of the hands, lower legs, and feet. Localized areas of erythema, edema, nodules, or plaques are common manifestations. Vesicles, bullae, and ulcerations are rare. Upon rewarming, tender, blue nodules may appear and persist for several days to 2 to 3 weeks.

Lesions associated with chilblains are usually less severe than other cold-related lesions and usually heal, but patients are at risk for recurrence with less significant exposures. The therapeutic approach to chilblains involves gentle rewarming and supportive therapy. This includes daily cleansing, topical antibiotics, dry, soft, sterile dressings, and elevation in order to avoid tissue maceration, bacterial or fungal infection, and further injury. Nifedipine and topical corticosteroids have been used in the treatment of chilblains.

Acknowledgments

The authors wish to thank Hervy Kornegey, M.D., Michael Seim, M.D., and Raffi Terzian, M.D. for their invaluable contributions and authorship of the previous chapter edition.

Selected Readings: Heat-Related Disorders

Backer HD, Shopes E, Collins SL, Barkan H. Exertional heat illness and hyponatremia in hikers, *Am J Emerg Med* 1999;17:532–539.
Bouchama A, Knochel JP. Heat stroke. *N Engl J Med* 2002;345:1978–1988.

Delaney KA, Vassallo SU. Thermoregulatory principles. In: Goldfrank LR, et al., ed. *Toxicology Emergencies*, 6th ed. Norwalk, CT: Appleton & Lange, 1998:287.

Falk B. Effect of thermal stress during rest and exercise in the pediatric population. *Sports Med* 1998;25:221–240.

Gaffin SL, Gardner JW, Flinn S. Cooling methods for heatstroke victims. *Ann Intern Med* 2000;132:678.

Gaffin SL, Moran DS. Pathophysiology of heat-related illnesses. In Auerbach PS, ed. *Wilderness Medicine,* 4th ed. St. Louis: Mosby, 2001:240.

Graham B. Features and outcomes of classic heat stroke. *Ann Intern Med* 1999;130:613–614, discussion 614–615.

Leads from the MMWR. Heat-related mortality, Chicago, July 1995. *MMWR* 1995;44:577.

Rajek A, Greif R, Sessler DI, et al. Core cooling by central venous infusion of ice-cold (4° C and 20° C) fluid: isolation of core and peripheral thermal compartments. *Anesthesiology* 2000;93:629–637.

Tek D, Olshaker JS. Heat illness. *Emerg Med Clin North Am* 1992;10:299–310.

Vicario S, Okabajue R, Haltom T. Rapid cooling in classical heatstroke: effect on mortality rates. *Am J Emerg Med* 1989;4:394.

White JD, Kamath R, Nucci R, et al. Evaporation versus iced peritoneal lavage treatment of heatstroke: comparative efficacy in canine model. *Am J Emerg Med* 1993;11:1–3.

Wolfe MI, Kaiser R, Naughton MP, et al. Heat-related mortality in selected United States cities, summer 1999. *Am J Forensic Med Pathol* 2001;22:352–357.

Selected Readings: Cold-Related Disorders

ACLS for Experienced Providers in ACLS—The Reference Textbook. American Heart Association: 2003;83.

Bernardo LM, Gardner MJ, Lucke J, et al. The effects of core and peripheral warming methods on temperature and physiologic variables in injured children. *Pediatr Emerg Care* 2001;17:138–142.

Bolgiano E, Sykes L, Barish RA, et al. Accidental hypothermia with cardiac arrest: recovery following rewarming by cardiopulmonary bypass. *J Emerg Med* 1992;10:427–433.

Brunette D, McVaney K. Hypothermic cardiac arrest: an 11 year review of ED management and outcome. *Am J Emerg Med* 2000;18:418–422.

Danzl DF. Accidental hypothermia. In Auerbach PS, ed. *Wilderness Medicine,* 4th ed. St. Louis: Mosby, 2001;135.

Danzl DF, Hedges JR, Pozos RS, Auerbach PS. Multicenter hypothermia survey. *Ann Emerg Med* 1987;16:1042–1055.

Farstad M, Andersen KS, Koller MC, et al. Rewarming from accidental hypothermia by extracorporeal circulation. A retrospective study. *Eur J Cardiothorac Surg* 2001;20:58–64.

Gentilello LM, Cobean RA, Offber PJ, et al. Continuous arteriovenous rewarming. Rapid reversal of hypothermia in critically ill patients. *J Trauma* 1992;32:316–325; discussion 325–327.

Muszkat M, Durst RM, Ben-Yehuda A. Factors associated with mortality among elderly patients with hypothermia. *Am J Med* 2002;113:234–237.

Owda A, Osama S. Hemodialysis in the management of hypothermia. *Am J Kidney Dis* 200;138:E8.

Papadimos TJ, Fowler E. Hypothermia and rapid cold, peritoneal crystalloid infusion. *Anesthesia* 2001;56:805.

Steele MT, Nelson MJ, Sessler DI, et al. Forced air speeds rewarming in accidental hypothermia. *Ann Emerg Med* 1996;27:479–484.

Thomas R, Cahill CJ. Successful defibrillation in profound hypothermia (core body temperature 25.6 degrees C). *Resuscitation* 2000;47:317–320.

Vassallo SU, Delaney KA. Thermoregulatory principles. In: Goldfrank LR, et al., eds. *Toxicologic Emergencies,* 6th ed. Norwalk, CT: Appleton & Lange, 1998:285.

Vassallo SU, Delaney KA, Hoffman RS, et al. A prospective evaluation of the electrocardiographic manifestations of hypothermia. *Acad Emerg Med* 1999;6:1121–1126.

Walpoth BH, Walpoth-Aslan BN, Mattle HP, et al. Outcome of survivors of accidental deep hypothermia and circulatory arrest treated with extracorporeal blood warming. *N Engl J Med* 1997;337:1500–1505.

Selected Readings: Cold Injury

Cauchy E, Chetaille E, Marchand V, Marsigny B: Retrospective study of 70 cases of severe frostbite: A proposed new classification scheme. *Wilderness Environ Med* 2001;12:248–255.

Heggers JP, Robson MC, Manavalen K, et al. Experimental and clinical observations on frostbite. *Ann Emerg Med* 1987;16:1056–1062.

McCaulay RL, Smith DJ, Robson MC, Heggers, JP. Frostbite. In: Auerbach PS, ed. *Wilderness Medicine,* 4th ed. St. Louis: Mosby, 2001;178.

Murphy JV, Banwell PE, Roberts AH, McGrouther DA. Frostbite: pathogenesis and treatment. *J Trauma* 2000;48:171–178.

Oumeish OY, Parish LC. Marching in the army: common cutaneous disorders of the feet. *Clin Dermatol* 2002;20:445–451.

Stewart C. Local cold injuries in children: diagnosis, management, and prevention. *Pediatr EM Rep* 1999;4:1.

Diving Emergencies/Dysbarism

Eunice M. Singletary

Pathophysiology

SCUBA (Self-Contained Underwater Breathing Apparatus) diving is a popular sport that through advances in equipment and education has become safer over the past 10 years. Nonetheless, approximately 1,000 injuries occur annually as a result of SCUBA diving, and approximately 100 deaths.[1] Injuries may present up to 24 hours following a dive, making it not unusual for divers to present for emergency care at inland facilities. Most diving-related injuries and many fatalities are related to changes in ambient pressure occurring during ascent or descent. High blood pressure and heart disease are the most commonly reported chronic health problems reported in diving fatalities.[1]

Barotrauma occurs when a closed, gas-filled body space, such as the lungs, fails to equalize its internal pressure to correspond to changes in ambient pressure. Any gas-filled space is subject to barotrauma, and examples of such injury include barotitis media (ear squeeze), barosinusitis (sinus squeeze), and pulmonary overpressurization syndrome (POPS). Dysbarism refers to the spectrum of injuries that result from changes in environmental pressure and includes barotrauma, nitrogen narcosis, decompression sickness, and blast injuries. Many of these injuries occur in recreational divers, but may also be seen in aviators or industrial workers exposed to abrupt changes in ambient pressure or while working with compressed air.

Barotrauma injuries are most commonly associated with diving. As a diver descends, ambient pressure increases from 14.7 psi or 1 atmosphere absolute (ATM) at the surface to 2 ATM at 33 feet of sea water (fsw). Pressure increases by 1 ATM for each additional 33 feet of depth. Most body organs and tissues have high water content, making them less susceptible to compression than hollow, air-filled organs or cavities. Since gases are compressible, gas-filled organs and cavities—such as the sinuses, lungs, and middle and inner ear—are subject to injury from changes in pressure. Boyle's law states that the volume of a given mass of a gas is inversely proportional to the absolute (total) pressure. Thus, volume of a gas bubble is halved as the absolute pressure is doubled. At 2 ATM, or 33 fsw, gas bubble volume is one-half its volume on the surface. At 4 ATM, or 99 fsw, the volume is one-fourth its

surface volume. Large changes in volume of a gas will accompany small fluctuations in depth, with the greatest proportionate change near the surface. Thus, diving injuries frequently occur in relatively shallow water.

Mask Squeeze

Face masks used for diving form a seal, creating an air-filled space. If a diver fails to equalize the pressure in this space during descent, a negative pressure develops within the mask and can lead to facial or ocular barotrauma. Physical findings may include subconjunctival hemorrhages, periorbital and facial ecchymosis in a mask-like pattern, and facial edema, all of which resolves spontaneously. ED evaluation includes documentation of visual acuity, extraocular movements, and fundoscopic examination. Orbital hemorrhage is a rare finding that may present with proptosis and limitation of extraocular movement.[2,3] CT of the orbits is diagnostic.

Barotitis Media

Barotrauma of the middle ear usually occurs during a dive descent and results from compression of the tympanic membrane (ear "squeeze") as ambient pressure increases. By performing a gentle Valsalva maneuver, divers can force additional air into the middle ear through the eustachian tubes and equalize the pressure. If the eustachian tubes are blocked, such as from allergy or infection, pressure on the tympanic membrane continues to increase with descent, causing a feeling of fullness or pain. This pressure imbalance may lead to rupture of the tympanic membrane, hemorrhage, or serous transudation into the middle ear. Occasionally middle ear barotrauma occurs during ascent if the diver is unable to equalize the pressure of the expanding gas within the middle ear ("reverse squeeze"). Mild middle ear squeeze is very common in recreational SCUBA divers, reported in over 52% of experienced divers in one survey.[4]

Emergency Department Evaluation and Management

Symptoms of middle ear barotrauma may include pressure sensation, ear pain, hearing loss, vertigo, and bloody drainage from the ear. There is usually a history of difficulty clearing the ears during a change in altitude either flying or diving. Sudden onset of vertigo while attempting to equalize ear pressure suggests tympanic membrane rupture and cold-water caloric stimulation. Patients with tympanic membrane (TM) rupture present with serosanguineous drainage from the involved ear and decreased hearing. Pain is less severe than preceding perforation. A conductive hearing loss is usually present to some degree. Classic, progressive categories of physical finding of middle ear squeeze have been described (**Table 128.1**).[5]

ED intervention includes carefully cleaning the external auditory canal, if possible using an otic microscope and Frazier suction catheter. Management of this condition is with use of topical nasal and systemic decongestants, such as oxymetazoline and pseudoephedrine. Systemic antibiotics are not recommended except in the case of membrane perforation or preexisting infection.[6] If infection is controlled and eustachian tube function restored, most membrane perforations will heal spontaneously. Patients should avoid further diving or flying until the condition has resolved, generally in 3 to 7 days without membrane perforation. The use of pseudoephedrine prior to diving may decrease the incidence and severity of middle ear squeeze.[7]

Barosinusitis

Barosinusitis is an acute or chronic inflammation of the paranasal sinuses resulting from a pressure difference between the air inside the sinuses and that of the surrounding atmosphere or water. It is frequently associated with a preexisting upper respiratory infection with subsequent blockage of the sinus duct or ostium and inability to equalize pressure in the sinuses. The maxillary and frontal sinuses are most commonly involved. The mechanism of injury is similar to that for barotitis media: squeeze or reverse squeeze. Sinus squeeze is produced with increasing ambient pressure, such as by descent from altitude or rapid underwater descent in a person with a blocked sinus ostium, resulting in a negative

intrasinus pressure relative to the ambient pressure. This causes sharp pain over the affected sinus(es), mucosal edema, mucosal or submucosal hemorrhage, or transudation of serosanguineous fluid. Accumulation of fluid within the sinus partially relieves the negative pressure (and associated discomfort). Less commonly, reverse squeeze occurs when increasing pressure within the sinus cavity relative to the ambient pressure cannot be relieved spontaneously by passive flow of air into the nasal cavity. Pain associated with sinus squeeze may masquerade as acute toothache.[8]

Emergency Department Evaluation and Management

Physical findings may include tenderness over the affected sinus, serosanguineous or purulent nasal secretions, mucosal edema, polyps, or preexisting septal deviation. Barotrauma-induced changes of the tympanic membranes may coincide. Rarely, neurological manifestations occur and include fifth or seventh cranial nerve dysfunction or dysesthesia in the distribution of the infraorbital nerve.[9,10]

The diagnosis is primarily clinical. Helpful ancillary studies when needed include routine radiographs, CT or MRI of the sinuses, which will show mucosal thickening, sinus opacification, air-fluid levels, or a polypoid mass within the sinus, representing submucosal hematoma formation (**FIGURE 128.1**).[11-13]

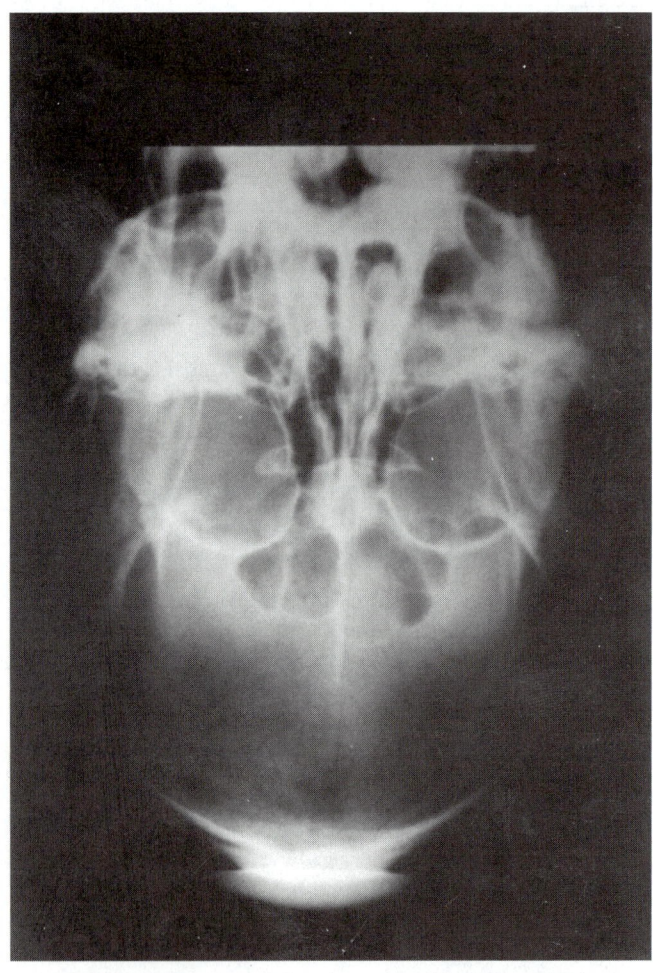

FIGURE 128.1 Frontal sinus hematoma. (Photo by author.)

Table 128.1

Categories of Middle Ear Squeeze

Category	Description
0	Normal tympanic membrane appearance (symptoms only)
1	Vascular congestion of pars flacida, umbo, anulus
2	Vascular congestion of entire membrane, spotty hemorrhage
3	Hemorrhage throughout tympanic membrane
4	Hemorrhage into middle ear with or without membrane rupture
5	Hemorrhage fills middle ear, perforation of tympanic membrane

Reprinted with permission from Australian Medical Publishing, Glebe, New South Wales, Australia. Edmonds C, Freeman P, Thomas R. *Otologic Aspects of Diving*, 1973.

Management of barosinusitis includes application of topical decongestants such as Afrin (oxymetazoline hydrochloride) or Neosynephrine (phenylephrine hydrochloride), systemic decongestants, and analgesics. Antibiotics are not necessary unless preexisting or subsequent infection occurs. Flying or diving should be discontinued until signs and symptoms have resolved. Patients with persistent symptoms should be referred to an otolaryngologist for evaluation for surgical intervention.

Barodontalgia

Dental barotrauma can occur in patients with caries or poorly filled caries. Change in ambient pressure causes severe tooth pain, and in some cases results in implosion of the tooth during descent or explosion during ascent. Upper tooth pain associated with pressure change should also raise consideration for maxillary sinus barotrauma and, if necessary, be ruled out by imaging. Physical findings include pain with percussion of the involved tooth and possible submucosal emphysema of the gums. ED intervention includes administering analgesics and/or a dental nerve block for severe odontalgia. Patients should be discharged on an oral antibiotic (such as penicillin), analgesics, and referred to a dentist for definitive therapy.

Inner Ear

Etiology

Inner ear barotrauma (IEBT) is primarily associated with shallow water diving or use of hyperbaric chambers and results from forceful efforts to equalize middle ear pressure when the eustachian tube is blocked. This results in rupture of the round window and/or oval window rupture and possible perilymph fistulae. Although much less common than middle ear barotrauma, IEBT is potentially more disabling because of possible injury to the cochleovestibular system and persistent deafness or vertigo. The classic triad of symptoms of IEBT includes a roaring tinnitus, vertigo, and sensorineural hearing loss. Additional symptoms may include a feeling of fullness in the affected ear, nausea, vomiting, diaphoresis, or ataxia. These symptoms can develop acutely or be delayed several hours postinjury. Onset of symptoms during or after a decompression dive, and without a history of difficulty with ear clearing on descent, suggests decompression sickness rather than inner ear barotrauma.[6,14,15]

Emergency Department Evaluation and Management

Patients present with intractable vomiting, pallor, diaphoresis, and nystagmus. On physical examination, the tympanic membrane may appear normal with a perilymph fistula, although sensorineural hearing loss is present and frequently accompanied by cochleovestibular dysfunction. Since IEBT often results from forceful attempts to equalize middle ear pressure, findings of barotitis media may be present.

ED intervention includes maintaining the patient's head elevated to 30 degrees and parenteral antiemetics for nausea or vomiting. Upon discharge from the ED, patients should be maintained on bed rest with the head of the bed elevated until symptoms resolve, and treated with decongestants and antiemetics as needed. Refer patients for prompt otolaryngologic follow-up. Further diving, flying, or strenuous activity is to be avoided. Hearing usually recovers with inner ear hemorrhage within 3 to 12 weeks. Persistent, fluctuating, or worsening sensorineural hearing loss 2 to 4 weeks postinjury indicates the need for surgical exploration and repair. Recompression treatment in a hyperbaric chamber is contraindicated with inner ear barotrauma because of potential further barotrauma, but should be considered for the rare case in which symptoms are believed to be due to decompression sickness.[14]

Alternobaric Vertigo

Alternobaric vertigo is a brief, transient, sudden onset of vertigo that occurs more frequently on ascent than descent. It is thought to be due to a unilateral pressure differential between the middle and inner ear. Vertigo and disorientation may be preceded by a feeling of fullness in the ear. Symptoms usually last less than a minute, although they occasionally persist for hours. A history of otitis media, eustachian tube dysfunction, or difficulty in clearing ears during diving may be important risk factors for development of alternobaric vertigo in SCUBA divers.[16] The disorientation of alternobaric vertigo can be particularly hazardous in the underwater environment, leading to a panic response with rapid or uncontrolled ascent and pulmonary barotraumas with air embolism or near drowning. Occasionally vertigo is accompanied by nausea, vomiting, and nystagmus without tinnitus. Patients presenting with persistent symptoms should be evaluated for inner ear barotrauma, treated with decongestants, and referred to ENT for further evaluation.

Pulmonary Overpressurization Syndrome

Etiology

Pulmonary overpressurization syndrome (POPS), or burst lung, can occur when the alveolar pressure exceeds ambient pressure by 50 to 100 mm Hg. This is the most severe form of barotrauma and is frequently associated with breath holding during ascent or rapid buoyancy ascent, even from depths as shallow as 6 feet. Other activities associated with POPS include use of inhaled drugs of abuse, mechanical ventilation with positive end-expiratory pressure, transtracheal jet insufflation, and virtually any activity that increases intraalveolar pressure.[17] Pulmonary overpressurization causes microtears or rupture of the alveolar membranes and escape of air, leading to subcutaneous or mediastinal emphysema, pneumothorax, and/or arterial gas embolism (AGE). Arterial gas embolism can coexist with the other forms of POPS. Rarely, alveolar membrane tears cause hemorrhage without other signs of pulmonary barotrauma.

Evaluation and Management

Obtain an immediate chest radiograph on all patients with suspected pulmonary overpressurization to rule out pneumothorax. Patients with alveolar hemorrhage without other forms of pulmonary barotrauma present with hemoptysis, pleuritic chest pain, dyspnea, and cyanosis. Chest radiographs show interstitial infiltrates. Patients with pneumomediastinum may experience substernal pain, a sensation of fullness in the neck, dyspnea, dysphagia, a change in voice timbre, and, in extreme cases, cardiac compression with near-syncope. Physical manifestations include anterior cervical and supraclavicular edema, crepitus, or a Hamman's (substernal) crunch. Chest radiograph will demonstrate interstitial air in the supraclavicular region, mediastinum, or both. Place patients with suspected POPS on supplemental oxygen until radiographs are obtained and perform a thorough neurological examination to search for signs of arterial gas embolism (AGE). Isolated mediastinal and subcutaneous emphysema generally resolve spontaneously, and following observation for signs of AGE these patients may be discharged home with arrangements for follow-up.

Pneumothorax is surprisingly the rarest of pulmonary overpressurization syndrome injuries.[18] Patients present with pleuritic chest pain, splinting, dyspnea, and possible tracheal deviation or jugular venous distention. Patients have typical findings of pneumothorax, including diminished breath sounds on the affected side, tachypnea, and possible tachycardia or hypotension. Individuals should be immediately placed on supplemental oxygen, pulse oximetry, and a cardiac monitor while awaiting stat chest radiograph. Emergent needle thoracostomy followed by chest tube insertion is indicated for signs of tension with cardiac decompensation. Recompression therapy is not indicated for pulmonary barotrauma without signs of AGE. Should a pneumothorax be present in a patient with AGE, insert a chest tube on the affected side prior to or during recompression therapy to prevent tension from developing on ascent.

Arterial Gas Embolism

Etiology

When pulmonary overpressurization results in alveolar rupture, the pulmonary veins around the alveoli are also subject to damage. Air then can pass from the alveoli into the pulmonary circulation and embolize systemically. Bubbles are also commonly found in the venous circulation after diving and may pass to the arterial circulation through a right to left shunt. Embolization can occur in any part of the body, although since divers are most frequently upright, embolization is typically to the brain. Arterial gas embolism is the third leading cause of death among scuba divers following drowning and cardiac arrest.[1] Onset of symptoms occurs abruptly during or within 15 minutes of ascent, although they may be delayed for up to 1 hour. Most commonly, divers develop a sudden loss of consciousness within minutes of surfacing from a relatively shallow dive, or experience stroke-like symptoms.

Air can embolize to multiple cerebral vessels simultaneously, causing various and potentially bilateral neurological symptoms. The rapidity of onset and cerebral nature of neurological symptoms are useful indicators when trying to differentiate between AGE and decompression sickness. Coronary artery and vertebral artery gas embolization may result in dysrhythmias or cardiopulmonary arrest from brain stem or cardiac ischemia, although complete occlusion of the central circulation is also hypothesized as a cause of death due to arterial gas embolism.[19]

Emergency Department Evaluation and Management

Neurological manifestations of AGE depend on the site(s) of vascular occlusion, and can be variable and confusing to the examiner. Asymmetric multiplegia, monoplegia, focal paralysis, paresthesias, hypesthesias, aphasia, visual disturbances, confusion, vertigo, headache, focal or generalized seizures, and even mood disturbances are all potential manifestations. Physical findings also vary with the site(s) of occlusion. Occlusion of regional brain blood flow by larger columns of gas may be transient, with a period of apparent recovery that is followed by a relapse. The relapse is believed to be due to failure of reperfusion, and of ominous prognostic significance. Patients with CNS symptoms are to be maintained on oxygen despite any spontaneous resolution of symptoms. Recompression is recommended for all patients regardless of ongoing symptoms. Effects of recompression therapy are attributed to its ability to antagonize leukocyte-mediated reperfusion injury, aid in resolution of cerebral edema, limited potential re-embolization or further embolization, and diminished likelihood of late brain infarction in patients with clinical recovery.[20]

Emergency treatment of all forms of AGE mandates immediate recompression therapy in a hyperbaric chamber. The Divers Alert Network (DAN), located at Duke University Medical Center (Durham, NC), can assist with locating a hyperbaric facility, and with the management of diving accidents. The 24-hour phone number for DAN is (919) 684-4326.

While arranging hyperbaric therapy, assess the patient's airway and ventilatory and circulatory status, intubating if necessary. Administer 100% oxygen for all patients to help reduce the bubble size by diffusion. Establish an IV of isotonic crystalloid solution and maintain urine output at 1 to 2 mL/kg/h. Obtain an EKG, looking for ischemia or dysrhythmias. Should dysrhythmias or cardiac arrest occur, follow standard advanced cardiac life support guidelines. Dysrhythmias from coronary artery embolism are usually refractory to treatment until bubble size is reduced with recompression therapy. Patients requiring cardiopulmonary resuscitation will need a multiplace chamber for recompression to allow for external cardiac compression, although it is recommended that patients in asystole not undergo recompression therapy until cardiac activity is restored.[21]

Transport patients in the supine position with the head in neutral to allow unrestricted arterial and venous blood flow. Fill endotracheal tube and Foley catheter tube cuffs with water to avoid volume changes and cuff breakage during recompression therapy. Imaging of the central nervous system (CNS) should be deferred after recompression therapy. In cases of subtle neurological symptoms or when symptoms have resolved prior to presentation, magnetic resonance imaging (MRI) of the brain may be useful in detecting and characterizing foci of cerebral ischemia caused by air embolism, and help differentiate ischemia of cerebral air embolism from spinal cord decompression sickness. Creatine kinase is thought to be a marker for size and severity of arterial gas embolism.[22]

Hyperbaric therapy involves compression with air following Navy diving table guidelines, followed by gradual decompression while breathing 100% oxygen alternating with air. Multiple hyperbaric sessions may be required until complete neurological recovery. Hyperbaric therapy initially reduces the volume of the offending bubble to enhance passage through the capillary circulation, and provides a large diffusion gradient to aid bubble absorption. It improves tissue oxygenation, reducing brain edema and intracranial pressure. Recompression therapy is recommended for all patients with suspected arterial gas embolism, even if neurological symptoms have resolved by the time of presentation.[20]

Decompression Sickness

Etiology and Pathophysiology

Once known as Caisson's disease, decompression sickness (or the "bends") is a multisystem disorder that results when dissolved inert tissue gases such as nitrogen come out of solution by rapid reduction in ambient pressure, with subsequent release of inert gas bubbles into the tissues and venous blood. Bubbles can form in either the venous circulation or arterial side, and thus lead to the consequences of AGE. It can be difficult to differentiate if symptoms are due to DCS or AGE, and in some cases they may occur concurrently.[23] Bubbles may also interact with blood vessel endothelium, creating an inflammatory reaction and pathology similar to reperfusion injury.[21] Signs and symptoms vary according to the size and location of nitrogen bubbles, but typically do not occur until 1 to 12 hours following the dive. Unlike classic AGE, decompres-

sion sickness usually occurs with dives to depths greater than 33 feet, and is seldom fatal. Predisposing factors include obesity, poor physical conditioning, age, dehydration, and flying after a decompression dive.[1] **Table 128.2** compares general characteristics of arterial gas embolism and decompression sickness.

Emergency Department Evaluation

Diagnosis is clinical, based on the history of diving with compressed air and the subsequent development of typical signs and symptoms. Decompression sickness is traditionally divided into two types. Type I DCS is considered a mild form of illness, and includes musculoskeletal and cutaneous symptoms. Type II DCS is severe, and includes the cardiopulmonary and neurological forms of illness.

"Pain-only" (Type I) decompression sickness is the most common form, occurring in up to 80% of cases and usually confined to an extremity. Pain is typically periarticular, steady, and most frequently involves the shoulder or elbow. Movement tends to aggravate the pain, and the involved joint is usually held in a flexed (bent) position. The extremity is normal in appearance and nontender to palpation. Paresthesias and numbness may accompany the extremity pain. Cutaneous forms of decompression sickness are considered mild, and usually include pruritus, transient rashes, or purplish marbling of the skin (cutis marmorata). Skin manifestations may be a harbinger of more severe DCS.[24] Type II DCS with pulmonary involvement, known as "the chokes," is characterized by chest pain on deep inspiration, dyspnea, cyanosis, and occasional cough. This form of DCS is thought to be due to massive pulmonary nitrogen gas embolism with obstruction of the pulmonary bed. Physical findings may include tachypnea, tachycardia, wheezing, and cyanosis.

CNS bends is the most serious form of Type II DCS and is primarily because of spinal cord lesions, particularly of the lower segments. Symptoms may include weakness of the legs, bladder paralysis with urinary retention, fecal incontinence, paresthesias or hypesthesias of the legs, and back pain with radiation to the abdomen. The etiology is thought to be due to venous bubbles in the epidural venous plexus with subsequent venous stasis and spinal cord ischemia or infarction. Cerebral DCS is rare, and may present with seizures, visual disturbances, or hemiplegia.

Table 128.2

General Characteristics of Arterial Gas Embolism and Decompression Sickness

Arterial Gas Embolism	Decompression Sickness
Pulmonary overpressurization	Nitrogen desaturation
Rapid ascent, breath holding	Recompression dive
Shallow water	Failure to recompress
Symptoms immediate/within 10 min	Symptoms 1–>12 h post-dive
Unconsciousness, seizure, confusion, headache, hemoptysis, hemi- or monoplegia, focal motor or sensory deficits, asymmetric monoplegia	Rash, joint or back pain, paresthesias, weakness, urinary retention, confusion, headache, chest pain, cough, vertigo

Table 128.3
Treatment of Decompression Sickness (DCS)

- Arrange recompression with hyperbaric oxygen (DAN: 1-[919] 684-4326)
- 100% oxygen via nonrebreather face mask
- IV NS at 250–500 mL/hr (normotensive), oral fluids if alert
- Ancillary studies: Chest radiograph, EKG, lab to include CPK
- Foley catheter (water in balloon) for spinal cord involvement
- Methylprednisolone 125 mg or hydrocortisone 1 g IV for neurological symptoms
- Consider antiplatelet or anti-inflammatory therapy

Emergency Department Management

MRI may be useful in diagnosis and management of DCS of the spinal cord.[25,26] Treatment of decompression sickness is by recompression in a hyperbaric chamber. If treated rapidly, symptoms frequently resolve completely and without neurologic residual. Permanent sequelae may result if treatment is delayed. Patients with transient symptoms that completely resolve while breathing oxygen with a nonrebreather face mask should undergo a "washout" recompression. This is recommended because of concerns about recurrent symptoms and possible occult injuries from bubbling to silent areas of the brain and spinal cord.[21] Additional care while arranging for transport to a hyperbaric facility is outlined in **Table 128.3**. Obtain a chest radiograph to rule out pneumothorax prior to recompression therapy. Hydration treats the associated fluid loss, hemoconcentration, and increased viscosity, which promotes vascular occlusion in DCS.

References

1. Vann RD DP, Dovenbarger JA, et al. *Report on Decompression Illness, Diving Fatalities and Project Dive Exploration. The Divers Alert Network Annual Review of Recreational Scuba Diving Injuries and Fatalities.* Based on 2002 data. Durham, NC: Divers Alert Network, 2004:1–152.
2. Butler FK, Gurney N. Orbital hemorrhage following face-mask barotrauma. *Undersea Hyperb Med* 2001;28:31–34.
3. Andenmatten R, Piguet B, Klainguti G. Orbital hemorrhage induced by barotrauma. *Am J Ophthalmol* 1994;118:536–537.
4. Taylor DM, O'Toole KS, Ryan CM. Experienced scuba divers in Australia and the United States suffer considerable injury and morbidity. *Wilderness Environ Med* 2003;14:83–88.
5. Edmonds C, Freeman P, Thomas R. *Otologic Aspects of Diving.* Glebe, New South Wales, Australia: Australian Medical Publishing, 1973.
6. Kizer KW. Diving Medicine. In: PS Auerbach, ed. *Wilderness Medicine.* St. Louis, MO: Mosby, 2001:1366–1401.
7. Brown M, Jones J, Krohmer J. Pseudoephedrine for the prevention of barotitis media: a controlled clinical trial in underwater divers. *Ann Emerg Med* 1992;21:849–852.
8. Kieser J. Sinus barotrauma presenting as acute dental pain. *S Afr Med J* 1997:87:184.
9. Butler FK, Bove AA. Infraorbital hypesthesia after maxillary sinus barotrauma. *Undersea Hyperb Med* 1999;26:257–259.
10. Murrison AW, Smith DJ, Francis TJ, Counter RT. Maxillary sinus barotrauma with fifth cranial nerve involvement. *J Laryngol Otol* 1991;105:217–219.
11. Singletary EM, Reilly JF Jr. Acute frontal sinus barotrauma. *Am J Emerg Med* 1990;8:329–331.
12. Segev Y, Landsberg R, Fliss DM. MR imaging appearance of frontal sinus barotrauma. *AJNR Am J Neuroradiol* 2003;24:346–347.
13. Parris C, Frenkiel S. Effects and management of barometric change on cavities in the head and neck. *J Otolaryngol* 1995;24:46–50.
14. Shupak A, Doweck I, Greenberg E, et al. Diving-related inner ear injuries. *Laryngoscope* 1991;101:173–179.
15. Reissman P, Shupak A, Nachum Z, Melamed Y. Inner ear decompression sickness following a shallow scuba dive. *Aviat Space Environ Med* 1990;61:563–566.
16. Uzun C, Yagiz R, Tas A, et al. Alternobaric vertigo in sport SCUBA divers and the risk factors. *J Laryngol Otol* 2003;117:854–860.
17. Seaman ME. Barotrauma related to inhalational drug abuse. *J Emerg Med* 1990;8:141–9.
18. Neuman TS. 1987. Diving medicine. *Clin Sports Med* 6: 647–61.
19. Neuman TS, Jacoby I, Bove AA. Fatal pulmonary barotrauma due to obstruction of the central circulation with air. *J Emerg Med* 1998;16:413–417.
20. Clarke D, Gerard W, Norris T. Pulmonary barotrauma-induced cerebral arterial gas embolism with spontaneous recovery: commentary on the rationale for therapeutic compression. *Aviat Space Environ Med* 2002;73:139–146.
21. Strauss MB, Borer RC Jr. Diving medicine: contemporary topics and their controversies. *Am J Emerg Med* 2001;19:232–238.
22. Smith RM, Neuman TS. Elevation of serum creatine kinase in divers with arterial gas embolization. *N Engl J Med* 1994;330:19–24.
23. Ikeda M. Delayed onset pulmonary barotrauma or decompression sickness? A case report of decompression-related disorder. *Aviat Space Environ Med* 2000;71:849–850.
24. Buttolph TB, Dick EJ Jr, Toner CB, et al. Cutaneous lesions in swine after decompression: histopathology and ultrastructure. *Undersea Hyperb Med* 1998;25:115–121.
25. Kimbro T, Tom T, Neuman T. A case of spinal cord decompression sickness presenting as partial Brown-Sequard syndrome. *Neurology* 1997;48:1454–1456.
26. Sipinen SA, Ahovuo J, Halonen JP. Electroencephalography and magnetic resonance imaging after diving and decompression incidents: a controlled study. *Undersea Hyperb Med* 1999;26:61–65.

High-Altitude Illness

Eric M. Kardon

Rapid air travel allows unacclimatized sea-level residents to ascend to high altitude within hours. Each year, an increasing number of people travel to high-altitude destinations. Millions of people travel to western U.S. ski resorts annually, with destination altitudes greater than 8,000 feet. Hundreds of thousands of trekkers and climbers visit the Himalayas and Andes yearly, with many peaks greater than 12,000 feet. High altitude illness encompasses central nervous system symptoms (CNS) in the forms of acute mountain sickness (AMS) and high altitude cerebral edema (HACE), and pulmonary symptoms in the form of high altitude pulmonary edema (HAPE). Acute mountain sickness in its mild form is benign and self-limiting; however, HAPE and HACE are lethal if not recognized promptly and aggressively treated.

Etiology/Pathophysiology

Acclimatization

Conditions at High Altitude

The term *high altitude* generally refers to elevations greater than 8,000 feet. It is rare for a person to become ill at altitudes less than this. The majority of persons traveling to altitudes greater than 14,000 feet display some symptoms of altitude illness. The partial pressure of atmospheric oxygen is directly related to the atmospheric pressure, and therefore inversely related to altitude, which results in a decreased concentration of oxygen delivered to the alveoli, and thus a lower arterial PO_2 as the altitude is increased. As the elevation increases to greater than 8,000 feet, the hemoglobin saturation becomes less than 90%. The PO_2 on the summit of Mt. Everest (29,029 feet) is about 30 mm Hg. The bodily response to this hypoxic stress is the major factor in the pathogenesis of high-altitude illness.

Acclimatization is the mechanism by which a person normally adapts to hypoxic stress. Some variability exists between individuals. High-altitude illness may be thought of as the failure of the body to acclimate properly.

There are natural limits to the body's ability to acclimate. At elevations greater than 17,000 feet, most humans are unable to fully acclimate. Prolonged stays at this altitude cause continued deterioration with weakness, weight loss, and increasing lethargy.

Hypoxic Ventilatory Response

The initial physiologic response to hypoxic stress is an increase in minute ventilation in order to increase the PO_2. This increase is termed the hypoxic ventilatory response (HVR), and is mediated by the carotid body. The HVR occurs at elevations as low as 5,000 feet, and begins within a few hours following arrival. Individual variation in the degree of HVR exists, and those with a diminished HVR have a greater tendency to develop high-altitude illness. This process is limited by the development of a respiratory alkalosis, which inhibits the medullary center from continuing to increase the respiratory rate.

Renal Response

After 24 to 48 hours, a compensatory bicarbonate diuresis occurs that lowers the pH, allowing the ventilatory response to further increase. This diuresis is mediated through hypoxia-induced antidiuretic hormone inhibition, alterations in the rennin-angiotensin-aldosterone system, atrial natriuretic hormone, or some combination of these factors. The importance of this compensatory response is underscored by the fact that those who do not diurese are prone to AMS, and that clinical improvement in patients with AMS is usually preceded by diuresis.

Cardiovascular Response

Hypoxia induces a release of catecholamines, which results in an increased heart rate. This maintains cardiac output despite the diuresis-mediated hypovolemia. Catecholamine release also results in an increased sympathetic tone, which increases blood pressure and shifts the circulating blood volume to the central circulation.

Pulmonary Response

Hypoxia leads to pulmonary vasoconstriction, which results in pulmonary hypertension. Pulmonary vasoconstriction is accentuated by strenuous exercise and by cold temperatures. In extreme cases, pulmonary pressures may approach systemic pressures during exertion. There is a significant degree of individual response, and those prone to AMS and HAPE generate higher pulmonary artery pressures in response to hypoxia than do controls. Other mechanisms in addition to hypoxia are probably at work, because supplemental oxygen improves, but does not completely reverse, the pulmonary hypertension.

Periodic respirations occur in almost all persons sleeping at high altitude. Periodic breathing is defined as alternating periods of hyperpnea and apnea, mediated by the central respiratory center's response to fluctuating pCO_2. This process is associated with insomnia, restlessness, and frequent arousals. It is lessened but does not disappear with acclimatization. Periodic breathing is more pronounced in those individuals with a high HVR, and these individuals have a relatively stable SaO_2. Those with a low HVR tend to have more regular respirations during sleep, but have episodes of profound desaturation. Periodic breathing is diminished by the use of ethanol, sedatives, and antihistamines, resulting in worsened hypoxia.

Cerebral Circulation

Cerebral vascular tone is very sensitive to changes in oxygenation and ventilation. Hypoxia causes cerebral vasodilation, whereas hypocapnia causes cerebral vasoconstriction. These opposing forces help to maintain an adequate cerebral blood flow. When the pO_2 falls below 60 mm Hg, hypoxic vasodilation overwhelms hypocapnic vasoconstriction. This causes cerebral blood flow to initially increase by 20% to 25%, which may be a causative factor in the formation of cerebral edema. Cerebral blood flow returns to baseline after 5 to 7 days.

Acute Mountain Sickness (AMS)

Incidence

The incidence of AMS depends on the altitude obtained. Twenty-four percent of Colorado skiers at 7,900 to 9,200 feet are affected, while greater than 50% develop symptoms at 15,000 feet. The incidence is equal between males and females, and all ages are affected equally. The risk of AMS is higher with increasing altitude, especially sleeping altitude, increasing degrees of exertion, increased speed of ascent, and previous episodes of AMS. There is also some individual susceptibility, including those with a decreased HVR, and those with increased hypoxic pulmonary vasoconstriction. AMS is usually self-limiting; however, the clinical importance lies in the fact that it may portend the development of potentially fatal HACE or HAPE.

The symptoms of AMS usually begin between 6 to 12 hours after arrival. The symptoms continue, peaking in 2 to 3 days. After a duration of 3 to 5 days, the symptoms gradually resolve. In over 90% of patients, the symptoms are self-limiting and resolve within 3 days. A few patients go on to develop HACE.

Pathophysiology

The symptoms of AMS are caused by hypoxia. Hypoxic cerebral vasodilation is responsible for the majority of symptoms that occur in AMS. Cerebral edema has also been shown to occur in this setting and is probably responsible for the increased symptoms seen in severe AMS. The role of cerebral edema in the setting of mild AMS is not clear.

Emergency Department Evaluation

Initial Presentation and Assessment

In the majority of cases of AMS, the initial screening examination reveals nonspecific symptoms and physical findings. The presence of ataxia, mental status changes, or respiratory distress implies HACE or HAPE, and therefore should place the patient in a more emergent category, demanding immediate assessment and treatment.

Triage Options and Initial Interventions

As soon as possible, the patient suspected of having AMS should be placed on supplemental oxygen, especially if the symptoms are severe. In the presence of ataxia, mental status changes, or respiratory distress, plans for descent should be made as soon as possible.

History, and Relevant Positives and Negatives

The history is the most important factor in making the proper diagnosis. The most common presenting complaint is that of headache, usually described as being moderate to severe, located in the bifrontal or occipital location. It is noted to be worse in the supine position, in the morning, and with strenuous activity. There is a significant variability in the characteristics of the headache that make it impossible to exclude the diagnosis based on the presentation.

Insomnia with frequent arousals associated with feelings of suffocation is also commonly reported. The patient may complain of fatigue, which may be disabling. Dyspnea on exertion is common. Nausea and vomiting is also common, especially in children. Other nonspecific symptoms include generalized malaise, dizziness, anorexia, irritability, reduced concentration, and auditory and visual disturbances. Somnolence is frequent in children.

Concomitant HAPE can occur with AMS and the provider needs to ask about the presence of dyspnea at rest and cough.

Physical Examination, and Relevant Positives and Negatives

There are no reliable signs to diagnose AMS, as most findings are nonspecific. They include postural hypotension, tachycardia, rales, peripheral edema, retinal hemorrhages, and mental slowness. Ataxia and mental status changes are the most sensitive indicators of the progression to severe AMS or HACE and should be thoroughly investigated. The presence or absence of signs of HAPE should be noted.

Ancillary Tests

For uncomplicated mountain illness, an adequate history and physical examination should be sufficient to make the diagnosis. There are no specific laboratory tests to confirm the diagnosis.

Development of an Emergency Department Diagnosis

The diagnosis of AMS should be considered in any patient complaining of headache along with other nonspecific symptoms, in the setting of an arrival to an elevation greater than 8,000 feet within the past few days. The differential diagnosis to be considered includes viral illnesses, dehydration, exhaustion, hypothermia, hangover, migraine, and other structural or vascular CNS abnormalities. Carbon monoxide poisoning should be considered in those who have been cooking food inside of tents. A focused history and physical examination should help to differentiate the diagnosis.

Emergency Department Intervention

Prevention

Staging, defined as remaining at an intermediate altitude before continuing ascent, is recommended to allow the acclimatization process to proceed. Traditionally, it has been recommended to stay 1 to 2 nights at or below 8,000 feet before beginning any further climbs. The ascent should be made gradually, going no more than 1,000 feet per day for altitudes at or below 14,000 feet, and no more than 500 feet per day for altitudes over 14,000 feet. These recommendations are not practical for many travelers. Recent recommendations have been more relaxed, requiring the change in sleeping altitude not to exceed 2,000 feet per day while ascending. The adage "climb high, sleep low" is used to remind hikers that the sleeping altitude is more important than the maximum altitude achieved. The use of substances such as ethanol, sedatives, or antihistamines should be avoided, especially in those with a history of AMS.

Acetazolamide, a carbonic anhydrase inhibitor, has been used in the prevention of AMS. It induces a bicarbonate diuresis by reducing renal resorption of bicarbonate. This results in a hyperchloremic metabolic acidosis that allows increased ventilation to occur. Acetazolamide is indicated in patients with a past history of recurrent AMS, or when a slow ascent is not possible. It should not be used in patients allergic to sulfonamides, in pregnant females, and in those with preexisting renal disease. The recommended oral dosage for prophylaxis is 250 mg taken two to three times a day starting 24 to 48 hours before ascent and continued for 3 to 4 days after ascent. Side effects include paresthesias, gastrointestinal upset, polyuria, transient myopia, photosensitivity, altered taste, somnolence, and cramping of the hands and feet.

Dexamethasone has also been shown to be effective in the prevention of AMS, with fewer side effects than acetazolamide. The mechanism of action is thought to be related to the control of vasogenic cerebral edema. In addition, dexamethasone's ability to produce a mood-enhancing effect may make the symptoms of AMS tolerable. The major drawback is that a rebound phenomenon exists when the drug is stopped, making long-term pro-

phylaxis necessary. The combination of dexamethasone and acetazolamide appears to be more effective than either drug used alone. Due to the potential serious side effects of corticosteroids, they are probably best used in those unable to take acetazolamide. The recommended dosage of dexamethasone is 8 to 12 mg PO per day in divided doses beginning on the day of ascent, continuing for 3 days, and tapered over the next 5 days.

Treatment

Patients suffering with mild AMS should rest, discontinuing any further planned ascent until their symptoms have resolved. Continued ascent when symptomatic is dangerous and should be discouraged. The patient should be at bed rest, and the oral intake of fluids should be encouraged. Supplemental oxygen if available, especially during sleep, may relieve insomnia and headache. Ethanol, tobacco, and sedatives should be avoided. Symptomatic treatment with acetaminophen or aspirin for headaches, and anti-emetics may increase the patient's level of comfort.

Acetazolamide is useful in the treatment of AMS along with the above measures. The oral dosage for treatment is 250-mg two to three times a day. In more severe cases, 500-mg two to three times a day may be given. Acetazolamide should never take the place of descent in severe cases of AMS, or allow further ascent in any symptomatic patient.

Dexamethasone 4-mg every 6 hours PO or IM has also been shown to be effective in the treatment of established AMS. In some cases, the symptoms may recur following cessation of the drug. In severe cases, dexamethasone may be used as an adjunct, if descent to a lower altitude is not immediately possible.

Descent is the most important component of therapy for patients with severe AMS, especially those with ataxia, mental status changes, and evidence of pulmonary edema. In addition, descent should be undertaken for patients with mild or moderate AMS who are not improving, or worsening, with more conservative treatment in the wilderness, the majority of patients should be able to descend on their own power with supervision. Assistance or evacuation may be necessary in extreme cases. A descent of only 1,000 to 2,000 feet is usually sufficient. Supplemental oxygen should be provided if available.

In some cases, descent may not be possible, due to inclement weather, avalanche, or inadequate transport gear. In these cases, bed rest, oxygen, acetazolamide, and dexamethasone should be used until descent is feasible. In addition, a portable hyperbaric chamber may be used. These devices weigh between 10 and 15 pounds are inflated by a manual pump. They work by simulating a descent of 5,000 feet.

Disposition

Most patients with uncomplicated mountain sickness may be discharged, as long as they have access to emergency care, are felt to be reliable, and are not alone. Patients with evidence of severe mountain sickness require immediate descent or evacuation to a lower altitude.

High-Altitude Cerebral Edema (HACE)

HACE may be thought of as a continuation of the cerebral aspect of AMS. Unlike AMS, however, permanent central nervous system injury has been reported with HACE. The incidence depends on the altitude achieved, and in one large study were 1.2% of soldiers between 11,000 and 15,000 feet. Men and women are affected equally, and the condition is preceded by an average of 5 days of being at high altitude. The overall mortality is 13%.

Pathophysiology

The cerebral edema that characterizes HACE is felt to be largely due to a vasogenic etiology. There are several pathophysiological factors that may contribute to the development of cerebral edema. These include impaired cerebral autoregulation; hypoxia mediated changes in the blood-brain barrier as a result of the effects of vasoactive mediators, and increased cerebral capillary pressure resulting in mechanical stress. The net result is the extravasation of protein and fluid in to the interstitial space. The vasogenic mechanism is supported by clinical date, CNS imaging studies and animal studies.

A cytotoxic mechanism for cerebral edema is also considered. Hypoxia causes loss of function of the adenosine triphosphate dependent sodium-potassium pump, causing a leakage of sodium and water into cells. Cell dysfunction and eventual cell death occur. Cytotoxic edema is most likely a late phase development in the pathogenesis of HACE.

The degree to which the cerebrospinal fluid (CSF) can accommodate the cerebral edema has been postulated to be responsible for some of the individual susceptibility to develop HACE. Those with smaller cranial CSF to brain volume ratios may be less able to displace enough CSF to accommodate the swollen brain than those with higher ratios.

Emergency Department Evaluation

Initial Presentation and Assessment

HACE should be suspected in patients presenting with typical symptoms, who give a history of travel to an altitude greater than 10,000 feet for 3 or more days. Headache, difficulty concentrating, ataxia, altered mental status, and overwhelming fatigue are common presenting symptoms.

Triage Options and Initial Interventions

In all patients suspected of suffering from HACE, supplemental oxygen should be provided if available. Plans for immediate descent should be made. Bed rest should be instituted while waiting for descent. In a health care facility continuous cardiac monitoring, pulse oximetry monitoring, and intravenous access should be initiated.

History, and Relevant Positives and Negatives

The majority of patients suffering from HACE are alert, complain of a severe headache, nausea and vomiting, fa-

tigue, weakness, loss of coordination, and poor concentration. There are no complaints that are specific to HACE.

Physical Examination, and Relevant Positives and Negatives

The most common physical findings in the patient suffering from HACE are extreme lassitude and altered mental status. Mental status changes include disorientation, hallucinations, bizarre behavior, obtundation, and coma. Ataxia is an ominous sign, and most ataxic patients usually become comatose within 12 to 24 hours. Papilledema and retinal hemorrhages are seen in up to 70% of cases. Less common findings are focal neurologic signs such as cranial nerve palsies and hemiparesis. Seizures rarely occur.

Many patients also have evidence of concomitant HAPE with respiratory distress, cyanosis, and rales.

Ancillary Tests

In most cases, an adequate history and physical examination should be sufficient to determine the cause of the patient's symptoms. There are no tests that are specific for the diagnosis of HACE. A complete blood count may help if an infectious cause is suspected. Rapid bedside glucose testing and an arterial blood gas with co-oximetry identify hypoglycemia and carbon monoxide toxicity in suspected cases. Unenhanced CT scan of the brain may help to exclude other etiologies of altered mental status, and in HACE shows evidence of cerebral edema. A chest radiograph should be obtained since HAPE occurs commonly in patients with HACE.

Development of an Emergency Department Diagnosis

The diagnosis of HACE should be considered in any patient with an altered mental status or ataxia, with or without evidence of AMS, in the setting of arrival to high altitude within the past few days. The differential diagnosis in the patient experiencing headache or mental status changes at high altitude includes hypoglycemia, toxic ingestion, carbon monoxide poisoning, head trauma, mass, and intracranial hemorrhage.

Emergency Department Intervention

Prevention

Prevention of HACE is similar to that for prevention of AMS. Staging and gradual ascent allow better acclimatization to occur. Persons with AMS should not ascend to higher elevations until the symptoms of AMS have resolved. It would be wise for individuals who have developed HACE in the past to avoid exposure to high altitudes. If, however, exposure is unavoidable, then acetazolamide and dexamethasone should be administered as prophylaxis.

Treatment

In the field, descent is the only definitive treatment for HACE and is mandatory at the first sign of ataxia or altered mental status. Descending 2,000 to 3,000 feet is usually associated with clinical improvement.

Adjuncts to descent may be helpful, particularly if it is not possible to evacuate the patient due to inclement weather or technical difficulties. Strict rest should be enforced with the patient in a sitting position. Supplemental oxygen should be supplied if available. If the patient is comatose, endotracheal intubation may be necessary. Dexamethasone 8 mg given PO, IM, or IV may also be helpful, followed by 4 mg every 6 hours. A portable hyperbaric chamber may be used, if available, as an adjunct if descent is not possible, but its use should not delay descent. There is no evidence showing benefit for the use of acetazolamide in this situation.

Patient Disposition
After arrival at the receiving hospital bed rest and oxygen should be continued. Once the patients are stabilized, they should be admitted to a critical care unit until a sustained improvement in their mental status is demonstrated. Coma may persist for several days following descent.

Further Considerations
Long-Term Effects
Deterioration of fine motor coordination, short-term and long-term memory, and language abilities have been shown to occur at high altitude and may persist after descent. Many subjects still have some significant cognitive and personality changes for more than 1 year after descent.

High-Altitude Pulmonary Edema (HAPE)

HAPE is a form of noncardiogenic pulmonary edema. Although not common, it is the most common cause of high-altitude death. The untreated mortality is 50%. The incidence depends on the altitude obtained, the rate of the ascent, physical exertion, and the individual's susceptibility. The incidence in Colorado skiers is about 0.01%. At higher elevations of 12,000 to 14,000 feet, the incidence increases to 2% to 3%. Patients with prior histories of HAPE may have an incidence as high as 60%. Males are affected more often than females, and it is more common in those less than 20 years of age.

Pathophysiology

HAPE is a noncardiogenic pulmonary edema. The inciting cause of HAPE is alveolar hypoxia, caused by low atmospheric oxygen and worsened by sleep disordered breathing, and a low HVR. This results in pulmonary artery vasoconstriction, pulmonary hypertension, and ultimately pulmonary edema. Individual predisposition is likely, since persons who develop HAPE tend to have a more pronounced elevation of pulmonary artery pressure in response to hypoxia or exertion, than those who do not.

Several theories have been proposed to explain the pathogenesis of HAPE. Uneven hypoxic pulmonary vasoconstriction may be responsible for causing an increased pulmonary vascular resistance and segmental overperfusion of vascular beds that are not vasoconstricted. This results in an increase in pulmonary capillary pressure regionally, resulting in stress failure of the pulmonary capillary membranes. Endothelial cell dysfunction also may have a significant role in the development of HAPE. This would include an impaired release of endothelial relaxing factors and an enhanced release of vasodilating factors. There is also evidence that impaired clearance of fluid from the alveolus, due to hypoxia induced decreased sodium transport across the epithelial cells, further compounds the problem.

Emergency Department Evaluation
Initial Presentation and Assessment
Most patients with HAPE have a history of travel to altitudes greater than 9,000 feet, although it may occur at lower altitudes. The symptoms usually begin 2 to 5 days after the ascent. Prompt attention should be given to the presence of any dyspnea at rest, rales, cyanosis, and mental status changes, all of which are indicative of severe HAPE.

Triage Options and Initial Interventions
Plans for immediate descent should be undertaken as soon as the patient presenting with advanced HAPE is identified. Supplemental oxygen, if available, should be provided. Continuous cardiac monitoring, intravenous access, and continuous pulse oximetry should be used, when available.

History, and Relevant Positives and Negatives
Most, but not all patients suffering with HAPE often have some degree of AMS, and therefore exhibit the nonspecific symptoms of headache, fatigue, and weakness. Early pulmonary-specific symptoms seen in HAPE include a nonproductive cough, dyspnea on exertion, and decreased exercise tolerance. As the disease process continues, more severe pulmonary symptoms develop, including dyspnea at rest, cough productive of pink frothy sputum, confusion, and coma. Symptoms often take a dramatic turn for the worse overnight, possibly due to worsened hypoxia as a result of sleep-disordered breathing.

Physical Examination, and Relevant Positives and Negatives
The patient suffering from HAPE appears to be in some degree of respiratory distress, depending on the stage of the disease. Vital sign abnormalities include tachycardia, tachypnea, and fevers up to 38.5° C. The patient may appear cyanotic. Rales are heard upon auscultation of the lungs. These may be localized to the mid-lung fields at first, becoming more diffuse as the process worsens.

As the patient becomes more hypoxic, the ability to concentrate is affected, and the patient develops an altered level of consciousness ranging from delirium to coma. It is important to differentiate these CNS symptoms from signs of concomitant HACE, which include altered sensorium, ataxia, and retinal hemorrhages.

Ancillary Tests

Chest radiography demonstrates noncardiogenic pulmonary edema. Pulmonary infiltrates are typically seen. In early or mild disease, a fluffy or patchy interstitial pattern occurs, often in the right middle lobe. As the disease progresses, the infiltrates become more diffuse and may take on an alveolar pattern. The cardiac silhouette appears to be of normal size. Kerley's lines are not present.

In cases of suspected pulmonary infection, a complete blood count may be useful. If arterial blood gasses are obtained, they usually demonstrate a degree of hypoxia worse than expected from the clinical appearance of the patient. Arterial pO_2 is typically 30 mm Hg in mild HAPE and 23 mm Hg in advanced HAPE at 15,000 feet. Respiratory alkalosis will also be present.

The electrocardiogram often demonstrates sinus tachycardia with evidence of right axis deviation, right atrial enlargement, and right ventricular strain.

Development of an Emergency Department Diagnosis

The diagnosis of HAPE should be considered in any patient complaining of dyspnea, cough, and decreasing exercise tolerance along with the findings of tachycardia, tachypnea, and rales, in the setting of an arrival to an elevation greater than 9,000 feet within the past few days.

The differential diagnosis for the patient with dyspnea and rales include pneumonia, aspiration, cardiogenic pulmonary edema, and adult respiratory distress syndrome. A carefully directed history and physical examination along with a complete blood count, electrocardiogram, and chest radiograph help differentiate the cause.

Emergency Department Intervention

Prevention

Persons with AMS should not ascend to higher elevations until the symptoms of AMS have resolved. Those with AMS, those with a history of HAPE, and anyone rapidly ascending to elevations greater than 11,000 feet should abstain from rigorous physical activity.

Prevention of HAPE by staging and grading the ascent are the same as that for AMS. Physical conditioning prior to ascent does not provide any protective role in the development of HAPE. No studies have shown acetazolamide to be suitable for prophylaxis or treatment of HAPE. Nifedipine may be used in those with a history of HAPE when a slow ascent is not possible. Twenty milligrams of a slow-release preparation given every eight hours while ascending and continued for three days at altitude prevented HAPE in susceptible persons in one study. The proposed method of action involves vasodilation of the pulmonary arteries, thereby improving pulmonary hemodynamics.

Treatment of Mild Disease

In patients suffering with mild HAPE, treatment depends on the patient's location. If oxygen, medical equipment, and personnel are available, and descent is not technically difficult, then strict bed rest and close observation is appropriate. Resolution of symptoms usually occurs in two to three days. If the patient does not improve, continues to worsen, or if oxygen saturations cannot be maintained above 90% with low flow oxygen, then descent is indicated. In situations where oxygen and medical equipment and personnel are unavailable, or in situations in which descent would be difficult should the patient's condition worsen, then descent or evacuation should be undertaken. In mild cases in the field, the patient may descend under his/her own power. In either case, supplemental oxygen, especially during sleep, should be provided.

Treatment of Severe Disease

In patients suffering from severe disease, descent is mandatory. It is usually necessary to descend 1,000 to 2,000 feet. In the field, the patient may descend under his or her own power if possible, if adequate supervision is available. If this is not possible, then the patient will need to be carried or arrangements for evacuation will need to be made. While plans to evacuate the patient to a lower altitude are under way, supplemental oxygen should be provided if available, which will reduce the pulmonary artery pressure, heart rate, and respiratory rate. The patient should be kept warm because cold air increases the pulmonary artery pressure. Bed rest should be enforced.

The portable hyperbaric chamber has been shown to be effective in temporarily improving the patient's symptoms. If patients are unable to descend on their own power, and evacuation is not possible, then one or more hours in a portable hyperbaric chamber may improve the patient's symptoms enough to allow them to descend on their own. This device should never be used in place of descent or to delay descent in a severely symptomatic patient.

Nifedipine may be used as an adjunct to descent and oxygen, but its use should never replace or delay descent. Twenty milligrams of a slow release form given every 6 hours may decrease pulmonary artery pressure and improve symptoms. Other medications, including furosemide, morphine, and phentolamine have all been shown to have some benefit in the treatment of HAPE, but their usefulness has become less clear since nifedipine seems to be more effective and associated with less side effects.

Antibiotics are useful for documented infection, but are not necessary for routine use.

Patients with altered mental status may be suffering from concomitant HACE, and may benefit from the use of dexamethasone.

Patient Disposition

Once the patient is at a sufficient altitude, bed rest and supplemental oxygen should be continued. This may be done in an outpatient setting in the mildest cases, as long as the patient is not alone and has access to medical care. In more severe cases, the patient should be admitted until clinical improvement is ensured. The patient may be discharged when the pO_2 has returned to normal and the patient's symptoms resolve. Antibiotics should be used in the presence of pneumonia.

Reentry Pulmonary Edema

The incidence of HAPE in high-altitude residents who descend to sea level and then return to high altitude may be higher than sea-level residents who develop HAPE. This is seen primarily in those persons less than 20 years of age, affects males and females equally, and has occurred after as few as 10 days of descent. The proposed mechanism is the development of hypertrophy of the muscular layer of the pulmonary arterioles in those chronically exposed to high altitude. This causes a much higher pulmonary artery pressure upon reascent.

Selected Readings

Bärtsch P, Mairbäurl H. Swenson ER, et al. High altitude pulmonary oedema. *Swiss Med Wkly* 2003;133:377–384.

Bärtsch P, Maggiorini M, Ritter M, et al. Prevention of high-altitude pulmonary edema by nifedipine. *N Engl J Med* 1991;325:1284–1289.

Basnyat B, Murdoch DR. High-altitude illness. *Lancet* 2003;361:1967–1974.

Bernhard WN, Schalick LM, Delaney PA, et al. Acetazolamide plus low-dose dexamethasone is better than acetazolamide alone to ameliorate symptoms of acute mountain sickness. *Aviat Space Environ Med* 1998;69:883–886.

Dumont L, Mardirosoff C, Tramèr MR. Efficacy and harm of pharmacological prevention of acute mountain sickness: quantitative systematic review. *Br Med J* 2000;321:267–272.

Hackett PH, Roach RC. High-altitude illness. *N Engl J Med* 2001;345:107–114.

Keller HR, Maggiorini M, Bärtsch P. Simulated descent v dexamethasone in treatment of acute mountain sickness: a randomized trial. *Br Med J* 1995;310:1232–1235.

Krasney JA. A neurogenic basis for acute altitude illness. *Med Sci Sports Exerc* 1994;26:195–208.

Peacock AJ. ABC of oxygen: Oxygen at high altitude. *Br Med J* 1998;317:1063–1066.

CHAPTER

130 Electrical Injuries

Taryn Kennedy

Electrical injuries are not uncommonly observed in the emergency department. The clinical spectrum may range from the absence of any physical signs to severe, multiple trauma with high morbidity and mortality.

Most electrical injuries, in addition, are occupational exposures causing more than 500 deaths per year in the United States. The United States Department of Labor statistics report 4,000 nondisabling and 3,000 disabling electrical-work-related injuries annually. Electrical injuries are the second most common cause of death in the construction industry, following only falls from a height. Ninety percent of electrical injuries occur in males with four-to-eight years of on-the-job experience. The high frequency of permanent disability, coupled with the relative youth and potential productivity of the victim, leads to the significant cost of these injuries to victims, families, and employers.

Electrocutions at home cause about 200 deaths each year in the United States, usually resulting from malfunctioning or misused consumer products. Two-to-five percent of burns in children that require emergency department care are electrical in nature. For children, the vast majority occur in the home and are associated with electrical and extension cords and wall outlets. Toddlers may experience burns to the oral commissure due to sucking or biting on electrical cords.

The severity of the injury depends on the intensity of the electrical current, the pathway throughout the victim's body, and the duration of contact with the source.

Etiology and Pathophysiology

Electricity is the flow of electrons (negatively charged outer particles of an atom) through a conductor. The electrons flow from higher to lower potential, creating a current, which is measured in amperes. The force that causes the flow is the voltage and is measured in volts. Anything that impedes the flow through a conductor creates resistance, which is measured in ohms. An electrical injury occurs when a person makes contact with the current produced by the source. The National Electrical Code defines low voltage as less than 600 volts. Most domestic voltage in the United States is 110 volts with 240 in Europe, Australia, and Asia. High voltage injuries involve

greater than 600 volts and are usually caused by alternating current (AC).

Electrical current exists as AC and direct current (DC). In AC the electrons cycle back and forth at a standardized frequency of 60 cycles/second (60 Hz). This is the more efficient form of electricity but is about three times more dangerous than DC as it causes tetanic muscle contraction; prolonging the length of time the victim is in contact with the electrical source. In direct current, the flow is in only one direction. This is used in certain medical equipment, such as defibrillators, pacemakers, and electrical scalpels.

Injuries result from both direct and indirect mechanisms. Direct damage results from the effect of the electrical current on various body tissues or by burns, which occur when, electrical energy is converted to thermal energy or by burns caused by combustion of clothing and/or surrounding materials. Indirect injuries may result from severe muscle contractions caused by the electrical injury, associated blast injuries, or resulting falls.

Tissue damage results from a number of variables including tissue resistance, voltage, type of current, amperage, duration of contact, current pathways, and the surface area of contact. The damage resulting is directly proportional to the intensity of the current that passes through the body. This is dependent on Ohm's Law:

$$\text{current (amps)} = \frac{\text{potential (volts)}}{\text{resistance (ohms)}}$$

Therefore, different parts of the body exposed to the same voltage will generate a different current because of the differing resistance in different tissues. In general, the least resistance is found in nerves, blood, mucous membranes, and muscles; higher resistance is found in bones, fat, and tendons. Skin has intermediate resistance.

Skin is the primary resistor, and the thicker the skin, the greater the resistance. Wet skin has almost no resistance, and moist mucous membranes have very little resistance, causing significant orofacial injuries in toddlers who put live wires in their mouths.

The pathway of the electrical current through the body determines the type and severity of the injury. Vertical pathways (parallel to the axis of the body) are the most dangerous. A transthoracic (hand-to-hand) pathway may spare the brain but can still be fatal. A saddle transmission through the lower part of the body is rarely fatal but may cause significant morbidity.

In a high voltage injury, the current is carried to the person through an arc before physical contact is made. These can generate very high temperatures (up to 5,000° C), which explains the accompanying severe thermal injuries.

At the cell level, intense electrical impulse causes: electroporation of the cell membrane; cell swelling and rupture; changes in ion channels and pumps; and thermal denaturation of proteins, DNA, and RNA, to name a few. This leads to a coagulative necrosis and a clinical picture similar to crush injury. Research efforts on fluorescent probes and dye-staining techniques to map the area of injury at the cellular/membrane level are ongoing. In the future, these may be beneficial to the surgeon deciding on excision and reconstruction of tissue/organ or amputation. Fractures are common.

Emergency Department Evaluation

Electrical injuries need to be treated as multisystem injuries and approached as such. Prehospital providers need to be cognizant of scene safety and ensure that power sources have been shut off in cases of high voltage wire injuries. When triaging multiple patients, apneic patients should be treated first as they may have central respiratory paralysis with normal cardiac activity. Appropriate c-spine precautions should be observed and other causes of coma—such as hypoglycemia, overdose, CVA, or head trauma—must be considered.

Cardiovascular System

The heart may be involved by direct necrosis of the myocardium and by cardiac dysrhythmias. Tissue necrosis may involve the myocardium, nodal tissue, conduction pathways, and coronary arteries. It is more likely with high voltage and AC injury. Low voltage of 30 to 100 mA with transthoracic or vertical transmission may cause ventricular fibrillation. High voltage of either type may cause asystole. Other dysrhythmias have been reported and may be multifactorial, such as foci of myocardial necrosis, alteration in Na^+/K^+ ATPase concentration, or secondary to anoxic injury where respiratory arrest precedes cardiac injury.

The vascular bed, due to its high water content, is an excellent conductor of electricity. Large vessels may have medial necrosis leading to later aneurysmal formation. Smaller vessels are affected by coagulation necrosis due to thermal injury. Vascular injury in the extremities may lead to compartment syndrome, leading to further compromise of the circulation.

Burns

A variety of burns may be seen as the electrical energy is converted to thermal energy. The severity of the burn depends on the intensity of the current, the surface area involved, and the duration of contact. As a patient may die of ventricular fibrillation at the same exposure that is required to cause second or third degree burns, the victim may die before the burns can develop. The severity of the skin burn cannot be used to determine the degree of internal injury with a low voltage current, as moist skin will offer almost no resistance.

Arcs caused by high voltage current may cause serious burns. Three types of burns may be seen. *Flash* burns due to the heat of the arc, *electrothermal* burns due to the passage of current through the body, and *flame* burns due to ignition of clothing.

Oral burns in children are due to the arcing of the current through the lips as they bite or chew through an electrical wire. This may be full thickness and involve underlying muscle, nerves, and blood vessels. Significant swelling and eschar formation follows and healing with scarring may cause obvious deformity. Involvement of the labial artery may not be obvious until eschar separation occurs days later, causing significant hemorrhage.

Significant burns may lead to significant hemodynamic, cardiovascular, renal, metabolic, and neuroendocrine responses that are seen in burns of more common etiology. They are treated in the same way.

Nervous System

Passage of the electrical current through the brain may lead to injury of the respiratory control center leading to respiratory arrest. Acute cranial nerve injuries and seizures may also occur. Spinal cord transection at C_4-C_8 level may occur with horizontal hand-to-hand transmission. AC current may cause tetany of muscles, giving rise to the *lock-on phenomenon*, which prevents the victim removing his or her hand from the source. Tetany of the respiratory muscles can lead to anoxia and suffocation. Traumatic brain and spinal cord injuries can result from the accompanying fall and secondary brain injury from anoxia may occur. Loss of consciousness, confusion, and retrograde anemia are common. Visual disturbance and deafness may occur.

Transient aphasia, motor paralysis, and peripheral neuropathy are reported and a number of delayed neurological complications, such as cataracts, may develop.

Respiratory

Respiratory arrest is a common cause of death in serious electrical injuries as a result of the ensuing anoxic injury to the brain and heart. Thermal inhalational injuries should be considered and blunt thoracic injuries from blast effect or fall should be investigated.

Kidneys

The kidneys are not usually injured by direct effect of electrical injury but are susceptible to any anoxic/ischemic injury. They are commonly damaged by passage of myoglobin and creatinine phosphokinase (released from damaged muscle) through renal tubules, which may result in acute renal failure.

Skeletal

Fractures may occur from severe muscle contractions or from falls. Upper limb long bones and spinal cord are more commonly involved.

Emergency Department Management

Management requires a combination of acute cardiac life support (ACLS) and acute trauma life support (ATLS) skills. Airway management and cardiac monitoring are addressed immediately in a patient with a significant electrical injury. Physical examination should search for burns, extremity fractures, dislocations, abdominal tenderness/peritoneal signs, level of consciousness, and peritoneal signs. Attention should be paid to looking for spinal cord injury or blunt thoracic/abdominal trauma. Victims exposed to DC current may have visible burns at entry and exit sites. AC current may not cause such burns. Wet skin may offer little resistance to the current, so there may be significant underlying change with little visible change to the skin.

IV fluid resuscitation should be started with Ringers lactate and a Foley catheter inserted for monitoring of hourly urinary output. Significant burns and associated visceral injuries may lead to considerable fluid requirements due to third spacing and ongoing fluid loss. Major myoglobinemia may develop due to muscle destruction and may lead to renal tubular change and renal failure. Aggressive hydration may be required and alkalization of the urine with sodium bicarbonate may be needed.

Burns should be treated in the usual fashion and tetanus prophylaxis considered. Compartment syndrome may develop in an involved extremity leading to the need for emergent fasciotomy. Severely injured limbs may require amputation.

Victims of low voltage injury with normal exam, including normal neurological exam and normal EKG may be discharged home. Those who experienced arrest and/or abnormal neurological or physical exam (including burns or visceral or vascular injuries) require admission with intensive monitoring.

Some controversy exists regarding the need for prolonged EKG monitoring. Currently, EKG monitoring for 24 hours is recommended when there is loss of consciousness, initial abnormal EKG, and a past history of cardiac disease in a victim exposed to high voltage current. Patients exposed to low voltage, with an initial normal EKG and otherwise well, may be safely sent home from the Emergency Department without a prolonged period of cardiac monitoring.

It is also unclear whether workers should be recommended for light duty for a period of time after the exposure.

The actual risk of electrical injury in the pregnant patient is unclear due to the low number of such victims. Fetal mortality varies from 15% to 73%.

Table 130.1 describes the long-term sequelae in electrical injury survivors.

Prevention

The vast majority of electrical injuries are preventable. Education of teenagers (especially males) to avoid climbing electrical poles or accessing transformer stations may lead to a decrease in injuries. Likewise, the public needs to be aware of the significant danger of "live" wires, which may

---

Table 130.1

Long-Term Sequelae in 25% of Survivors

63% Burn sequelae
5% Amputation
18% Neuropsychiatric (such as disorientation, slowing mental processes, PTSD)
12% Sense organs

---

be downed during storms or after accidents. Electrical codes requiring the presence of ground fault circuit interrupters (GFCI) in new dwellings and work places should decrease the number of low voltage injuries. Increased thickness of insulation on wiring and increased public awareness may also be contributory. Occupational exposure remains a problem. In many cases, companies have comprehensive safety procedures, but these may not be fully implemented. Emergency departments are not immune from such hazards and all personnel should be involved in the development and implementation of a safety program, have adequate training in the identification of electrical hazards, and be cognizant of appropriate safety measures.

Lightning

About 100 lightning strikes occur each second in the world and about 100 to 300 lightning fatalities occur in the United States yearly. Most of these occur in the summer months in the South, in the Rockies, along major river valleys, and along the Atlantic coast. However, victims of lightning injuries are rare visitors to most emergency departments. Approximately 90% of victims survive, but up to 74% will experience permanent sequelae and disability. One's lifetime risk of being struck by lightning is 1:3,000.

The current in a lightning bolt may be as high as 30,000 amps with one million or more volts. It is of a very short 1 to 100 millisecond duration, which may limit the injury potential. The severity of injury depends on the secondary heat produced, the voltage of the strike, the duration of contact, the path of the current, the explosive force involved, and the electromagnetic effects of the charge. It is the duration of contact that really determines the type and severity of injury. Due to this usually brief duration of contact, the injuries received by those hit by lightning are usually different than those of victims contacting high voltage electricity.

Three main mechanisms for lightning injury exist. The most severe is a direct strike, either on the victim or through a handheld object, such as a golf club. Much of the current may pass over the skin in a "flashover" pattern. If the body is wet, the current increases and may lead to vaporization of the moisture and the development of an explosive force, which shreds clothing and may blow off the victim's shoes. When a current does enter the body (as may happen at the cranial orifices after a strike to the head), it will pass through the tissue of least resistance. This will include nerves, blood vessels, muscle, and connective tissue.

A *side flash* or *splash* injury may occur when the lightning hits a nearby object and jumps to the victim. This is usually the conclusion involved when multiple fatalities occur among persons grouped together. This may also occur indoors if a victim is using a telephone or electric appliance, or is in a shower as the lightning current hitting the outside of the building may be conducted indoors by these routes.

Ground current injuries occur when lightning enters the ground and then travels outward, hitting a person standing within its radius. The severity of injury in these victims depends on their distance from the point of lightning strike. A *stride potential* develops if a person is standing with their legs apart where the current enters the leg closest to the strike, travels up the trunk, and exits through the opposite leg.

Blunt injury or trauma may occur secondary to the shock wave from the strike or from a resulting fall.

Clinical Effects

Cardiovascular and Respiratory Systems

The primary cause of death is cardiopulmonary arrest. Direct current to the heart may result in asystole but spontaneous recovery may occur. Paralysis of the respiratory center leads to respiratory arrest, which may be prolonged and lead to secondary cardiac arrest because of to the resultant hypoxia. Aggressive resuscitative measures should be initiated as soon as possible in these patients. The victim is not electrically charged and may be approached without fear of electric shock, unlike high voltage electrical injuries. However, lightning can strike the same place twice, resulting in danger to rescuers.

Reverse triage should be initiated in the event of multiple casualties as those who are not in cardiac or respiratory arrest at the scene survive and, therefore, can wait for treatment. Those in arrest may be successfully resuscitated if basic CPR and ALS measures can be commenced. EKG changes such as nonspecific ST changes, QT prolongation, and premature ventricular contractions do occur but generally resolve in a few days.

Vascular spasm may lead to cold, pulseless, mottled extremities, which may resolve over a period of a few hours, without intervention.

Central and Peripheral Nervous System

Central nervous system injuries are common and may be very disabling for survivors. These may include weakness, amnesia and confusion, loss of consciousness, and intracranial injuries such as hematomas or intraventricular hemorrhages. Lightning-induced paraplegia or quadriplegia may occur and resolve in minutes to days. Paresthesias may occur and chronic limb pain is a common sequelae. Neuropsychiatric complications can be particularly disabling such as depression, anxiety, memory deficits, cognitive loss, and post traumatic stress disorder.

Eyes and Ears

Approximately 50% of victims will have eye injuries, usually of the cornea. Cataracts may develop within a few days or may take up to two years to take effect. Transient autonomic disturbance may lead to dilated and/or unreactive, or contracted pupils without an associated head injury.

Tympanic membrane rupture of one or both eardrums is seen in up to 50% of victims. Transient hearing loss and tinnitus are also commonly reported. Chronic ear infections, partial hearing loss, vertigo, and dizziness may occur.

Burns

Extensive skin burns are rare, unlike high voltage electrical injuries. Linear burns may be found along lines of perspiration and deep burns are usually associated with metal objects such as buckles or jewelry. Skin burns may not show distinct entry and exit sites. Severe burns may be seen if clothing is ignited. A rare phenomenon called *ball lightning*, which is a mixture of fire and electricity, may cause extensive burns to the victim.

Skin imprints, pathognomonic for lightning injury, such as Lichtenberg figures, feathering burns, or keraunographic markings may be seen. These results from an electron shower generated by the flashover of current and are not burns per se.

Musculoskeletal System

Injuries may occur from the strike or by the victim being thrown by the blast. Due to the short duration, massive tissue damage as may be seen in high voltage electric injuries is not common. Opisthotonic contraction may occur with the passage of current leading to spinal column and limb fractures, and joint dislocations.

Emergency Department Evaluation

For lone victims who may be amnesic from the event, it may be difficult to ascertain if their injuries are from a lightning strike. The presence of characteristic skin markings, ruptured tympanic membranes, confusion, tattered clothing, and paralysis may offer a clue to the etiology of the injuries.

All patients should be treated with cervical spine precautions with appropriate immobilization. One third of victims will have some form of associated blunt trauma and should be evaluated using ATLS protocols. This may be due to the explosive force of the shock waves or a violent opisthotonic contraction. A thorough physical examination should be conducted looking for vertebral, skull, rib, and extremity fractures and intracranial injuries. Hypotension should be assumed to be due to trauma induced hemorrhage, as hypertension is more common after lightning injuries.

Artificial respiration may need to be supported for many hours after the strike as the respiratory drive may be paralyzed for a prolonged period.

Admission, EKG monitoring, and intravenous lines should be established. Burns, cardiac dysrhythmias, and trauma-induced injuries are treated as usual. Many of the injuries associated with lighting strike resolve spontaneously over time. Psychological sequelae are common and often very disabling. All victims should be referred to the

Lighting Strike and Electric Shock Victims International Support Group, telephone: (910) 346-4708.

Prevention

Lightning is a very dangerous and frequently encountered hazard. A victim's risk of injury is related to their failure to take appropriate precautions. People planning to be outdoors should be cognizant of local weather forecasting and have a plan in place should a storm occur. It is possible to be struck by a storm 10 miles away. Therefore, if you can hear thunder, you should seek shelter. An insulated building with plumbing and wiring is the best choice. If an enclosed metal vehicle such as a car is the only choice, ensure that the windows are up and avoid touching any metal, either inside or outside the vehicle.

Lightning generally strikes the tallest object, so avoid being this object and avoid being close to the tallest object, such as isolated trees or flagpoles. Avoid open fields, open structures, and being in or near water. If you are indoors, turn off and stay away from electrical appliances and fireplaces. Do not use the telephone and avoid metal objects. Stay away from water and wait 30 minutes from the last flash to resume normal activities. If you are in a group outdoors, split up so not all will be affected. If you are caught out in a storm in an open area and are unable to take appropriate shelter, crouch down with your feet together, ideally on the balls of your feet with your hands over your ears. This, however, is a difficult position to maintain for any extended period of time.

Selected Readings

Bailey B, Gaudreault P, Thivierge RL. Experience with guidelines for cardiac monitoring after electrical injury in children. *Am J Emerg Med* 2000;18:671–675.

Bjerke HS, Lintzenich A. *Lightning Injuries.* 2002. Available at: http://www.emedicine.com/med/topic2796.htm. Accessed May 2005.

Blackwell N, Hayllar J. A three-year prospective audit of 212 presentations to the emergency department after electrical injury: with a management protocol. *Postgrad Med J* 2002;78:283–285.

Browne BJ, Gaasch WR. Electrical injuries and lightning. *Emerg Clin North Am* 1992;10:211–226.

Byard RW, Hanson KA, Gilbert JD, et al. Death due to electrocution in childhood and early adolescence. *J Paediatr Child Health* 2003;39:46–48.

Carte AE, Anderson RB, Cooper MA. A large group of children struck by lightning. *Ann Emerg Med* 2002;39:665–670.

Casini V. Overview of electrical hazards. In: *Worker Deaths by Electrocution: A Summary of NIOSH Surveillance and Investigative Findings.* Washington, DC: Department of Health and Human Services (NIOSH), Pub No 98-131, 1998:5–8.

Cherington M. Neurologic manifestations of lightning strikes. *Neurology* 2003;60:182–185.

Chico MS, Capelli-Schellpfeffer M, Kelley KM, et al. Management and coordination of postacute medical care for electrical trauma survivors. *Ann NY Acad Sci* 1999;888:334–342.

Cooper MA, Andrews CJ. Lightning injuries. In: Auerbach PS, ed. *Wilderness Medicine: Management of Wilderness and Environmental Emergencies,* 3rd ed. St. Louis, MO: Mosby, 1995:72-110, 261–289.

Fish RM. Electric injury, part III: cardiac monitoring indications, the pregnant patient, and lightning. *J Emerg Med* 2000;18:181–187.

Garcia CT, Smith GA, Cohen DM. Electrical injuries in a pediatric emergency department. *Ann Emerg Med* 1995;26:604–608.

Hark WT. *The Human Effects of Lightning Strikes and Recommendations for Storm Chasers.* Available at http://www.harkphoto.com/light.html. Accessed May 2005.

Hussman J, Kucan O, Russell C, et al. Electrical injuries: morbidity, outcome and treatment rationale. *Burns* 1995;21:530–535.

Koumbourlis AC. Electrical injuries. *Crit Care Med* 2002;30(Suppl):S424–S430.

Lee RC. Injury by electrical forces: pathophysiology, manifestations, and therapy. *Curr Probl Surg* 1997;34:677–764.

Lewis AM. Understanding the principles of lightning injuries. *J Emerg Nurs* 1997;23:535–541.

Lightning safety. In: *NCAA Committee on Competitive Safeguards and Medical Aspects of Sports. Sports Medicine Guidelines,* 1997–1998 ed. Indianapolis, IN: National College Athletic Association, 1997:12–14.

Price TG. *Electric Shock,* 2002. Available at http://www.emedicine.com/aaem/topic177.htm. Accessed May 2005.

Rabban JT, Blair JA, Rosen CL. Mechanisms of pediatric electrical injury. New implications for product safety and injury prevention. *Arch Pediatr Adolesc Med* 1997;151:696–700.

Rai J, Jeschke MG, Barrow RE, et al. Electrical injuries: a 30-year review. *J Trauma* 1999;46:933–936.

Rosen CL, Adler JN, Rabban JT. Early predictors of myoglobinuria and acute renal failure following electrical injury. *J Emerg Med* 1999;17:783–789.

Shengde G, Yong Y, Gang B. Treatment of severe electrical burns. *Ann NY Acad Sci* 1999;888:60–74.

Van Zomeren AH, ten Duis H-J, Minderhoud JM, et al. Lightning stroke and neuropsychological impairment: cases and questions. *J Neurol Neurosurg Psychiatry* 1998;64:763–769.

Zimmerman C, Cooper MA, Holle RL. Lightning safety guidelines. *Ann Emerg Med* 2002;39:660–664.

Bites and Stings: Insects, Marine, Mammals, and Reptiles

Eunice M. Singletary
Christopher P. Holstege

Almost all classes of the animal kingdom may be responsible for causing disease or injury to humans. This section addresses emergencies resulting from more common encounters by people with arthropods, mammals, marine organisms, and reptiles.

Arthropods

Arthropods are members of the phylum Arthropoda of invertebrate animals. Arthropods have articulated limbs and include several important classes, such as insects and arachnids. The class Insecta includes numerous small segmented invertebrates with a well-defined head, thorax, abdomen, six legs, and typically one or two pairs of wings. Bees, wasps, and ants are all insects. The class Arachnida includes spiders, scorpions, mites, and ticks, have eight legs and no antennae. Patients frequently confuse arthropod bites and stings. Stings are typically caused by the Hymenoptera group of insects via a stinging apparatus, while bites are produced by the jaws of numerous arachnids such as spiders and ticks. Venom production by both insects and arachnids can result in local or systemic toxic reactions or allergic reactions, while nonvenomous bites by arthropods that feed on human blood are frequently responsible for the transmission of infectious diseases.

Insects

Hymenoptera is an order of insects that usually have very thin, transparent wings. The common members of hymenoptera include bees, bumble bees, wasps, hornets, yellow jackets, and ants. Almost all of the hymenoptera have a venom production, storage, and injection apparatus (stinger). Venoms are designed to immobilize and eventually kill their prey. More people die from hymenoptera stings in the United States than from all other animal bite and sting causes combined.[1] Most reactions in humans are due to hypersensitivity, ranging from common minor, local inflammatory effects, to anaphylaxis and cardiovascular collapse. Direct venom toxicity is also responsible for severe anaphylactoid reactions.[2]

Fire ants, or *Solenopsis invicta*, are found throughout the southeastern United States. They live in large colonies and form distinctive mounds. Fire ants attack by biting and fixing its mandibles on the prey. It then rotates its body and inflicts multiple stings in a typical arc-like pattern. Stings are usually localized to the extremities. The sting causes acute localized burning pain, followed by the development of a 1 to 2 mm intensely pruritic sterile pustule within 24 hours. Fire ant venom is 95% piperidine alkaloids and produces histamine release and local tissue necrosis.[3]

Etiology and Pathophysiology

Local or systemic delayed hypersensitivity reactions are usually the result of immunoglobulin (Ig)G and IgM antibody-antigen complex. IgE-mediated reactions result in release of histamine and other mediators thought to be responsible for tissue damage associated with local and systemic reactions. Systemic hypersensitivity findings include: urticaria, vasodilation, increased vascular permeability, bronchospasm, laryngospasm, angioedema, and increased mucous secretions. Individuals with a previous reaction to hymenoptera have a greater likelihood of having another reaction and potentially a worse reaction than before. There are significant antigenic differences between members of Hymenoptera. Thus, an individual may have developed sensitivity to a bee sting and not exhibit the same reaction to a wasp sting.

Emergency Department Assessment

Reactions to hymenoptera stings are classified as local, urticaria without systemic symptoms, and generalized (**Table 131.1**). Local reactions include immediate pain at the sting site, itching, burning, erythema, warmth and varying degrees of soft tissue swelling. Urticaria presents with typical raised scattered wheals or as generalized erythema. Nausea and vomiting may accompany multiple stings. Severe generalized hypersensitivity reactions develop within minutes to a half-hour of the sting. Delayed reactions develop over 2 to 7 days and may resemble serum sickness.

Patient assessment is directed at evaluation of the airway and searching for the described findings of systemic or local hypersensitivity.

Table 131.1

Hymenoptera Allergic Reactions

Local	Urticaria	Systemic
Pain	Wheals	Bronchospasm
Burning	Generalized erythema	Hypotension, tachycardia
Erythema	Nausea, vomiting	
Warmth		Laryngospasm
Edema		Angioedema
Pruritis		Urticaria
		Cardiopulmonary arrest

Emergency Department Management

ED intervention depends on the type of reaction a patient develops. Local reactions are cared for by cleansing the wound and looking for an embedded stinger. Honeybees and occasionally yellow jackets will leave a stinger in the wound. The degree of envenomation increases with time that the stinger remains embedded. Therefore, the stinger should be removed as quickly as possible by whatever means available, such as by scraping with a sterile needle or grasping with tweezers. Use of tweezers to remove a stinger does not increase the envenomation, as previously thought.[4] Treat minor local reactions with oral antihistamines, cool compresses, and analgesics. Large local reactions with significant local edema or multiple stings may benefit from oral or parenteral steroids. Administer

tetanus prophylaxis when indicated, and instruct patients to observe for signs or symptoms of systemic reaction or wound infection following discharge.

Treatment for systemic or severe local reactions is outlined in **Table 131.2**. In general, patients with systemic reactions are admitted for treatment and observation for 24 to 48 hours. For patients with local reactions, antihistamines should be continued for at least 24 hours. Patients receiving steroids in the ED should be discharged on a 4 to 5 day course of oral steroids.

There is no particular treatment available for fire ant stings. Analgesics and antihistamines may alleviate pain and pruritus, as for other hymenoptera stings. Pustules generally last several days. Treat secondarily infected pustules with an antistaphylococcal antibiotic. As for other hymenoptera stings, fire ant allergen-specific immunotherapy may lessen the severity of subsequent systemic reactions.[5]

Arachnids: Spiders

Arachnids of clinical significance for emergency physicians include ticks, spiders, and scorpions. All spiders possess venom, which is neurotoxic and designed to immobilize their prey. A variety of spiders may cause minor local irritation, inflammation, or a local allergic type reaction. In the United States there are only two spiders of importance to the emergency physician: the black widow and the brown recluse. The black widow spider, *Latrodectus mactans*, is more commonly present in the warmer areas of the United States but is found worldwide.[6] The female of the species is small, somewhat round in the ab-

Table 131.2

Management of Hymenoptera Stings

Local	Urticaria	Systemic
• Remove any stinger	• Remove any stinger	• Remove any stinger
• Cool compresses	• Diphenhydramine 50 mg IV or IM	• Cardiac monitor, IV saline
• Diphenhydramine 25–50 mg PO, IM, or IV	• H2 blocker, e.g., cimetidine 300 mg IV	• High-flow oxygen or intubation/ventilatory support
• Tetanus toxoid prn	• Prednisone 60 mg PO or methylprednisolone 1 mg/kg IV	• Trendelenburg position
	• Tetanus toxoid prn	• Epinephrine IM or SQ q15m 0.3–0.5 cc of 1:1,000 (adult), 0.01 mL/kg (children)
		• Epinephrine IV prn 1 mL 1:10,000 slowly (adult), 0.01 mL/kg 1:10,000 (child)
		• Diphenhydramine 1–2 mg/kg (50–75 mg) IV
		• Methylprednisolone 1–2 mg/kg IV
		• Albuterol 0.5 mL (adult), 0.03–0.05 mL/kg (child), 0.5% in 2.5 mL nebulized for bronchospasm
		• H2 blocker, e.g., cimetidine 300 mg IV (adult), 5–10 mg/kg (child)
		• Pressor support, e.g, dobutamine for persistent hypotension
		• Tetanus toxoid prn

domen, and dark, shiny black with a red or yellowish hourglass-shaped marking on the undersurface of the abdomen that becomes more prominent with maturity.

The brown recluse spider, *Loxosceles reclusa,* originally from Central America, is endemic in the United States from southeastern Nebraska through Texas, east to Georgia and southernmost Ohio. In areas where the species is endemic, these spiders can be found and collected in great numbers inside homes. The dorsum of the spider's body has a violin-shaped design that can be very difficult to appreciate. The spider is otherwise small, brownish in color, and nondescript. It moves in short, speedy bursts and does not web.

Emergency Department Evaluation

The venom of a black widow spider is a potent neurotoxin that causes massive release of neurotransmitters from presynaptic nerve terminals. The syndrome that results from envenomation is known as *lactrodectism,* and is characterized by widespread, sustained muscle spasm. Pain from the bite initially varies from none to significant. Local reaction is minimal, with mild induration and erythema at the bite. Symptoms may not progress further. In other cases, dramatic neuromuscular symptoms develop within 30 to 60 minutes following the bite, and include muscle fasciculations and involuntary muscle spasms that usually begin at the bite and propagate proximally. Spasms may involve large muscle groups of the thighs, back, abdomen and/or shoulders. Symptoms may mimic an acute abdomen, or for the case of a bite to the upper extremity, symptoms may mimic angina pectoris. Associated signs and symptoms related to neurotransmitter release include diaphoresis, increased salivation, urinary retention, vomiting, weakness, ptosis, fever and bronchorrhea. Patients appear restless, anxious, clammy, and at times tachypneic. Hypertension is a common finding with envenomation and may be severe.[7–9] Leukocytosis and an elevated creatine phosphokinase (from severe muscle spasm) may be noted on laboratory evaluation. Complete recovery typically occurs within a few days, although pain is reported to persist a week or more.

The venom of the brown recluse spider can produce wound necrosis as well as occasional systemic symptoms. Systemic symptoms are reported in approximately 14% of recluse spider bites.[10] The clinical syndrome that may develop from brown recluse envenomation is known as *loxoscelism.* The venom contains a number of proteins, but sphingomyelinase-D is the most important component producing dermatonecrosis.[11] Recluse spider venom also has a direct effect on endothelial cells, red cells, and platelets.

Most brown recluse spider bites result in a local cutaneous reaction that resolves without intervention. Systemic symptoms are flu-like and may include fever, chills, nausea, vomiting, and arthralgias. Hemolytic anemia with hemoglobinuria has been reported and begins within 24 hours of envenomation.[10,12,13] Thrombocytopenia, renal failure, disseminated intravascular coagulation, and death have also been reported.[14,15] Patients with systemic symptoms should have laboratory evaluation to include a complete blood count, coagulation studies, and urinalysis. Renal and liver function tests should be obtained with severe envenomations.

Spider bites are typically found on areas of the body that correspond with constriction of clothing or an entry point for the spider. The leg is the most frequent site. Pain associated with brown recluse spider bites usually subsides over 6 to 8 hours and is followed by aching, itching and swelling. Ischemia surrounding the bite produces an irregular, violaceous center with a surrounding erythematous "halo." Between the violaceous center and the halo, a white, ischemic ring of vasospasm may be discernible. A vesicle or hemorrhagic bullae may develop in the center of the lesion within 24 to 72 hours. By 1 week the lesion is covered with an eschar. This eschar sloughs after 2 to 5 weeks, creating an ulcer. Lesions vary in size from 1 to 30 cm.

The diagnosis of brown recluse spider bites is most frequently clinical or based on report by the patient of a possible spider bite. Unfortunately, necrotic skin lesions are not infrequently overdiagnosed as brown recluse spider bites.[16] Because a brown recluse spider bite is unlikely in nonendemic regions, emergency physicians should consider the differential diagnoses for patients presenting with ischemic, necrotic, or ulcerative skin lesions (**Table 131.3**). A new ELISA assay for the detection of loxosceles spider venom may be of future benefit in the evaluation of patients presenting with possible brown recluse spider bites.[17]

Emergency Department Management

Treatment of black widow spider bites is aimed primarily at relieving muscle spasm and pain. Narcotic analgesics and intravenous benzodiazepines or methocarbamol are useful and may be required for the first 12 hours. Intravenous calcium gluconate has been advocated in the past but has not proved of benefit and is no longer recommended. Severe hypertension may require parenteral antihypertensives. Rarely, envenomation by the black widow spider can produce shock, coma, or respiratory failure secondary to paralysis. Patients with intractable pain, severe hypertension or other severe systemic symptoms should be admitted to the hospital.

There is a Food and Drug Administration (FDA)-approved black widow spider antivenom: Lyovac or Anti-

Table 131.3
Differential Diagnosis of Ischemic, Necrotic, or Ulcerative Lesions
• Lyme disease
• Lymphomatoid papulosis
• Pyoderma gangrenosum
• Chemical burns
• Cutaneous anthrax
• Necrotizing fasciitis
• Tularemia
• Sporotrichosis
• Brown recluse spider bite

venin (Merck). The antivenom is produced in equine serum, and may produce acute hypersensitivity or delayed serum sickness. Because of the risk of hypersensitivity and limited efficacy, antivenom should only be used in severe envenomations such as those producing seizures, uncontrolled hypertension, respiratory arrest, or in pregnancy.[18]

The approach to treatment of wounds from brown recluse spider bites depends on the severity and stage of presentation. In general, wounds should be cleansed and debrided of necrotic material. Consultation with plastic surgery may be necessary for extensive debridement, excision or full-thickness skin grafting. Topical and systemic corticosteroids have not been found to provide significant benefit.[19] Hyperbaric oxygen (HBO) therapy following venom exposure in animal models has failed to show a benefit.[20,21]

Dapsone, a sulfone antibiotic, is a leukocyte inhibitor that has been shown in experimental animal studies to prevent lesion progression when used within 48 to 72 hours of a bite.[19,22] Other studies have shown no benefit from dapsone, HBO, or cyproheptadine.[21] If dapsone is used, the recommended adult dose is 50 to 100 mg twice daily for 10 days.

Scorpions

Fortunately, there are very few venomous scorpions in the United States. Most are found in Arizona and New Mexico, and are of the *Centruroides* species. The tail of a scorpion is multisegmented, curved, and has a terminal bulbous segment (telson) containing venom sacs and a stinger. Venom from *Centruroides* species is a complex mixture that includes various proteins and neurotoxins. The neurotoxins have sodium channel effects that result in repetitive firing of axons and enhanced release of neurotransmitters. This causes autonomic dysfunction and excessive neuromuscular activity.[23]

Emergency Department Evaluation and Management

Scorpion envenomations vary from minor local irritation to severe systemic syndromes (**Table 131.4**). Symptoms reach maximal severity within 5 hours for adults and 30 minutes for infants, and improve over 9 to 30 hours without antivenom. Most scorpion stings in the southwestern states cause symptoms similar to a local allergic reaction

from a bee sting.[24] Management is directed at general support, including application of cool compresses, use of antihistamines such as diphenhydramine, and analgesics. Unlicensed *Centruroides* antivenom is produced by Arizona State University. Treatment for severe envenomations is primarily via supportive and symptomatic care in an intensive care setting. Consider the use of antivenom for patients with respiratory compromise associated with severe envenomations.

Ticks

Ticks are members of the arachnid family and may be classified as hard ticks (family Ixodidae) or soft ticks (family Argasidae). Hard ticks have a hard plate, or scutum that covers part of the body. Ticks are blood suckers and have three feeding stages: larva, nymph, and adult. Disease is caused in humans through the bite of the tick and transmission of microorganisms. Ixodes scapularis, the deer tick, is the vector for Lyme disease, babesiosis, and human granulocyte ehrlichiosis (HGE). Dermacentor variabilis, the dog tick, is the vector for Rocky Mountain Spotted Fever.

Tick paralysis is an acute, flaccid motor paralysis associated with numerous species of ticks worldwide. The paralysis develops 5 to 6 days after an adult tick attaches, usually to the head or neck, and is seen most frequently in children. Paralysis is ascending, symmetric and flaccid, with loss of deep tendon reflexes.[25] A careful search for the tick, followed by its removal, results in prompt resolution of symptoms within hours to a few days. It is thought that the etiology of the paralysis is a neurotoxin secreted in the saliva of the tick during a blood feeding that blocks release of acetylcholine at the neuromuscular junction, producing symptoms similar to that from botulinum toxin.[26]

Emergency Department Evaluation and Management

Patients present to the emergency department following a tick bite either requesting assistance with removal of a tick, or because of concern for disease transmission associated with a recent asymptomatic tick bite, or due to a local reaction to retained tick mouthparts. A local reaction to a tick bite resembles other insect bites, with formation of a small pruritic nodule, occasionally accompanied by surrounding erythema or induration. Treatment is symp-

Table 131.4

Scorpion Envenomation Signs and Symptoms

Sign	Symptoms
Mild	Pain, burning, itching, mild edema, and erythema
Moderate	Local symptoms plus paresthesias, positive "tap test"
Severe	• Local symptoms plus generalized pain and paresthesias or in contralateral extremities.
	• Difficulty swallowing, blurred vision, slurred speech, involuntary eye movements. Fasciculations, shaking or jerking movements of extremities.
	• Tachycardia, hypertension, hyperthermia.
	• Stridor, pulmonary edema, respiratory failure.
	• Rhabdomyolysis, multiorgan failure, cardiac arrest.

tomatic. Incomplete removal of a tick with retention of mouthparts may cause a foreign body reaction, with formation of a granuloma that can persist for months. Retained mouthparts should be removed if possible, but are not associated with transmission of Lyme disease.[27]

For patients presenting with attached ticks, removal is accomplished by grasping the tick with tweezers as close to the skin as possible, and applying gentle, steady upwards traction.[28] Avoid crushing or squeezing the body, so that infected saliva is not injected into the bite wound. There are dozens of methods for tick removal that have been described in the literature, such as applying nail polish, petroleum jelly, a hot match to the body of the tick, or isopropyl alcohol.[29] None of these methods have a demonstrated advantage over tweezers. A number of commercially available tick removal tools have been shown to be superior to tweezers at removing small, nymphal stage ticks.[30] Successful removal has also been reported after application of 2% viscous lidocaine to attached ticks for 5 minutes, followed by simply wiping off the ticks.[31]

Routine antibiotic prophylaxis against diseases commonly transmitted by ticks is not recommended, as the risk of Lyme disease or Rocky Mountain Spotted Fever is very low. Many physicians, however, have a lower threshold for prophylaxis following deer tick attachment, particularly in pregnant women and in Lyme-endemic regions.[32] The likelihood of infection following tick bites increases with the duration of attachment. Experimentally, few animals become infected with Lyme disease with tick attachment for less than 24 hours, whereas attachment for 72 hours or longer is associated with a higher incidence of disease transmission. Should one decide to use antibiotic prophylaxis in cases where a tick has been attached for 48 to 72 hours, the suggested regimen is a 10 day course of amoxicillin or doxycycline (in the nonpregnant adult).

Mammalian Bites

Etiology and Pathophysiology

One percent of all annual visits to emergency facilities in the United States are the result of animal bites.[33] The most common animal bite in this country is caused by dogs. Cat

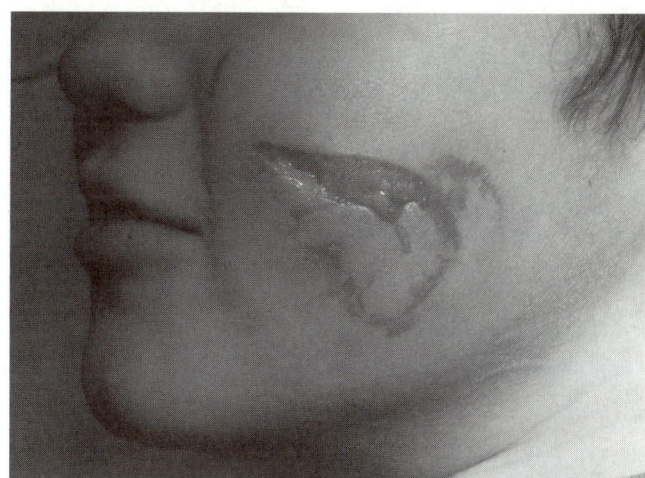

FIGURE 131.1 Dog bite to child's face. (Photo courtesy of E.M. Singletary, MD.)

bites are a close second followed by a multitude of other animal bites.

There are two major pathophysiologic processes associated with animal bites. First, traumatic damage to the tissues results from forces applied by the animals' teeth, jaws, or claws. Most traumatic injuries involve the extremities and include abrasions, lacerations and puncture wounds. In children, injuries involving the head and face are also common (**FIGURE 131.1**). Secondly, infection is a common sequela because of the presence of a multitude of various microorganisms in the mouth and on the paws of the animal. Risk factors for development of infections in common mammal bites are listed in **Table 131.5**.

The rate of infection for nonsutured wounds by dog bites varies in different series from 6.25% to as much as 26%.[34,35] Common pathogens in the mouth of the dog include *Pasteurella canis, Staphylococcus aureus,* species of *Streptococcus,* and various anaerobes.[36] When wound infection from a cat or dog bite occurs less than 8 hours post injury, the most likely infecting organism is *Pasteurella.*[37]

Cats are notorious for producing puncture wounds with their bite rather than lacerations. The fine, sharp teeth of cats can easily penetrate tendon sheaths, joints, or

Table 131.5

Mammalian Bite Wounds at High Risk for Infection

Location	Wound Type	Animal Species	Patient Factors
Hand	Puncture	Cat (esp. hand or lower extremity)	Chronic alcoholism
Wrist	Devitalized or crushed tissue		Immunosuppression
Foot		Human (to hand)	Diabetes mellitus
Over major joint		Pig	Asplenia
Through and through cheek			Peripheral vascular insufficiency
Scalp or face in infant (cranial penetration risk)			Valvular disease/replacement

bones, increasing the risk of infectious tenosynovitis, septic arthritis, or osteomyelitis. The mouth of the cat has similar pathogens to dogs, with *Pastuerella multocida* predominating.[38]

Domestic rodents such as rats and mice as well as wild rodents such as squirrels, chipmunks, and voles can bite. Bites by rodents are usually not significant because their teeth are small and produce minor puncture wounds.

Human bites occur by intention or accident. Most commonly, human bites present as lacerations to the dorsum of the hand. A *fight bite* is a wound that occurs during an altercation with a clenched fist.[39] This position allows the opponent's tooth to pierce the victims' metacarpophalangeal joint or extensor tendon, leading to septic arthritis or tenosynovitis.

The human mouth has a multitude of pathogens, and infections secondary to the human bite are common, particularly when bites are on the extremities.[40] The most common pathogens causing infection from human bites are *Streptococcus viridens, Staphylococcus aureus,* and anaerobes such as *Bacteroides* and *Fusobacterium* species. *Eikenella corrodens* is a gram-negative aerobic bacillus responsible for 10% to 29% of human bite wounds, and is exquisitely sensitive to penicillin, but resistant to penicillinase-resistant penicillins, clindamycin, and some cephalosporins.[41,42]

Emergency Department Evaluation

Patients presenting to triage with animal bites are to be rapidly assessed for signs of life- or limb-threatening injury, particularly small children or when the bite is from a large animal. Care of all animal bites has several common features. First, evaluation of the wound includes historical questions such as the type of offending animal, time of injury, mechanism, tetanus immunization status, and medical conditions that may predispose to subsequent infection.

"Fight bite" wounds typically present over the dorsal surface of a metacarpal-phalangeal joint, and may appear innocuous. When the hand is examined, it is usually examined with the fingers extended. Thus, the potentially injured extensor tendon or intracapsular penetration is not visible at that portion where it was at risk during the impact. Consultation with a hand surgeon should be obtained in cases of suspected joint or tendon penetration by human bites. Obtain soft tissue radiographs to look for retained tooth foreign bodies.

In cases of bites by large dogs of infants and children, the face, skull and long bones are frequently crushed between the jaws of the dog, and appropriate radiographic studies are necessary to determine the presence of fractures as well as to help identify foreign bodies.

Emergency Department Management

The treatment principles for dog, cat, and human bites are all similar (**Table 131.6**) and aimed at decreasing the likelihood of infection, reducing scar formation, and promoting a return to function.

Wounds on the extremities are closed preferably within 6 to 8 hours of injury. Wounds on the face, neck, and

Table 131.6
Treatment Principles for Mammalian Bite Wounds

- Field rinsing/irrigation with tap or drinking water
- Gentle debridement/swabbing of wound for dirt/ foreign objects
- Irrigation with saline, water or 1% povidone iodine under pressure (19 gauge catheter with 35 cc syringe
- Delayed closure of puncture wounds, hand wounds or other high risk wounds
- Tetanus prophylaxis when indicated
- Rabies postexposure prophylaxis when indicated
- Bulky dressing immobilization and elevation for extremity wounds
- Prophylactic antibiotics for high-risk wounds for 5 days
- Follow-up evaluation 24–48 hours post-bite

head, because of the vascularity of those areas, may undergo a more delayed closure. Puncture wounds and small wounds are high-risk for infection, and should be left open in most cases. Gaping and extensive wounds may be loosely approximated. Closure of these wounds is primarily for cosmetic reasons. A number of studies have looked at the rate of infection in mammalian bite wounds closed primarily, with conflicting results. In general, the rate of wound infection for patients with lacerations due to mammalian bites repaired with primary wound closure is only slightly higher than for standard sutured wounds.[43] Antibiotic coverage is indicated in high risk wounds (Table 131.5). Amoxicillin-clavulanate is the first line therapy recommended for cat, dog and human bites, followed by second-generation cephalosporins with anaerobic activity. Due to the relatively low incidence of wound infections in lacerations caused by dog bites, prophylactic antibiotics are not recommended except for high risk wounds.

Human bites must be meticulously cleansed, debrided and irrigated. Avoid primary closure of human bite wounds to the hand due to the high incidence of infection. Broad-spectrum antibiotics are again recommended for all human bites to the hand for up to 5 days.

Marine Organisms

Many marine organisms have developed various systems for attack and defense. Most encounters with marine animals are accidental and can be classified as (1) nonvenomous trauma (e.g., shark bites), or (2) envenomations (e.g., Portuguese man-o-war stings).

Nonvenomous Trauma: Sharks, Barracuda, and Eels

Sharks, barracuda, and moray eels are rarely implicated in bite wounds to humans. It is estimated that only 50 to 100 shark attacks occur annually worldwide. Attacks by sharks on humans are believed the result of misidentification of humans as one of its more traditional preys (e.g., seals). The evaluation and management of wounds from these organisms is the same as for other major trauma. Fractures and hemorrhage are common.

Treatment is as for all major traumas with airway control, resuscitation, and stabilization, followed by evaluation of bite wounds. Typically, wounds are cleansed and packed but not closed primarily. Tetanus toxoid and prophylactic antibiotics are advocated. Suitable choices include penicillin, trimethoprim-sulfamethoxazole, or ciprofloxacin.

Marine Envenomations

With over 12,000 miles of coastline in the United States and its territories, and a steady growth in the popularity of diving, encounters with marine animals are no longer considered unusual. Many marine animals have developed systems for attack and defense that upon accidental exposure to humans result in envenomation. Fortunately, most envenomations are not life-threatening, often presenting only as a minor contact dermatitis. What's unique about encounters with marine organisms is that significant physical trauma commonly accompanies the envenomation. This physical trauma may overshadow symptoms of the envenomation and contribute to associated morbidity and mortality.

Invertebrates

Phylum Cnidaria (Coelenterate) Members of the invertebrates most commonly implicated in envenomations include the coelenterates, which include jellyfish, and the echinoderms, such as sea urchins. Coelenterates (phylum Cnidaria) are divided into three classes:

- Hydrozoa (hydroids, fire corals, Portuguese man-o-war)
- Schyphozoa (true jellyfish)
- Anthozoa (sea anemones)

Although the Portuguese man-o-war is a Hydrozoa, it is commonly discussed with Scyphozoa, or the true jellyfish, because its venom and stinging effects are similar.

Coelenterates envenomate their prey through nematocysts, which are venom-containing organelles located in specialized epithelial cells known as cnidocytes. Nematocysts are located around the mouth and along the tentacles of the animal. The venom of the coelenterates varies among species. They are generally comprised of heat labile polypeptides that may be degraded by proteolytic agents. The venom is believed to destabilize cell membranes through interference with the sodium-potassium pump. Other major actions include hemolysis, muscle paralysis, cardiotoxicity, and dermatonecrosis.

The class Hydrozoa includes hydroids and stinging corals, both of which generally cause various degrees of contact dermatitis, although desquamative eruptions, erythema multiforme, and anaphylaxis have been reported.[44-46] The most dangerous of the hydrozoas is the Portuguese man-o-war (*Physalia physalis*), which is found in the Atlantic Ocean and the Gulf of Mexico during the summer. The portion of the animal that is visible above the surface of the water is the pneumatophore, which is generally 10 to 30 cm in diameter and ranges from blue to purple in color. Dangling from the pneumatophore are the tentacles. Contained within the tentacles are thousands to millions of the venom-filled nematocysts. Three fatal envenomations from *Physalia physalis* have been reported from Florida and North Carolina.[47,48]

Envenomation by the Portuguese man-o-war causes immediate intense pain. The pain is followed by a rash usually described as linear papules or beaded streaks. The rash progresses to erythematous welts within 2 hours and lasts 24 hours. Systemic reactions include nausea, vomiting, headache, myalgias, respiratory distress, cardiovascular collapse, acute renal failure, anaphylaxis, or death.

Treatment consists of initial stabilization and supportive therapy, and prevention of further envenomation. The affected area should be washed at the scene with sea water or normal saline if possible, not fresh water, as the difference in osmolarity may cause further discharge of nematocysts. The area should then be rinsed with 5% acetic acid (vinegar) to neutralize the venom. If acetic acid is not available, appropriate alternatives include isopropyl alcohol and papain (meat tenderizer). The remaining tentacles should then be shaved or scraped off using shaving cream. Local reactions may benefit from topical application of anesthetic ointments, antihistamine creams, or steroid preparations. Administer tetanus prophylaxis if indicated. Oral or parenteral narcotics may be required to control pain. Prophylactic antibiotics are unnecessary. If there is an allergic component, oral antihistamines or steroids may be useful.

Schyphozoa include many species of jellyfish, some of which are extremely dangerous to humans. A number of highly toxic chirodropid (box-shaped jellyfish) such as *Chironex fleckerii* are indigenous to the waters of the Indo-Pacific region. Fortunately, most jellyfish in U.S. waters cause less severe envenomations. Scyphozoa found in the United States include stinging nettles (*Chrysaora quineucirrha*) commonly found in the Chesapeake Bay during mid to late summer, the purple jellyfish (*Pelagia noctiluca*), the more venomous lion's mane jellyfish (*Cyanea capillata*) and more toxic *Chironex* species. *Chiropsalmus quadrumanus* was identified as the culprit in a lethal envenomation of a 4-year-old boy at Galveston Island, Texas, in 1990.[49]

For the majority of jellyfish stings, symptoms are confined to localized pain and rash that resolve over 24 hours. Multisystem reactions are seen more commonly following envenomation by *Chironex, Carybdeid*, and *Physalia* species. Gastrointestinal symptoms include nausea, vomiting, and diarrhea. Headache, malaise, confusion, delirium, coma, seizures, paresthesias and paralysis are potential neurologic symptoms. Cardiopulmonary effects may include dysrhythmias, hypotension, cardiovascular collapse, respiratory distress, bronchospasm, laryngeal edema, and respiratory failure or arrest.[50,51] Musculoskeletal complaints, which are prominent with *Carybdeid* envenomations, include myalgias, muscle spasm, cramping or paralysis.

A symptom complex was recently described in 3 divers who sustained envenomations in South Florida, similar to the Irukandji syndrome, suggesting the presence of small, previously undetected *Carybdeid* species.[52] The Irukandji syndrome is encountered frequently in Australia and includes low back pain, excruciatingly painful muscle cramps in the limbs, abdomen and chest, sweating, anxiety, restlessness, nausea, and headache.[53,54]

Treatment in severe schyphozoa envenomations is directed toward stabilization of vital functions. Aggressive airway control with endotracheal intubation may be necessary. After treatment of life-threatening symptoms, begin decontamination as soon as possible. If decontaminants are not readily available at the scene, first rinse the skin with sea water or saline solution, or with a forceful stream of water to remove nematocysts. Sea water is less likely to result in firing of remaining nematocysts. Decontamination is accomplished by liberal application of either vinegar, baking soda, or dilute (¼ strength) household ammonia. There is some evidence that isopropyl alcohol may induce further discharge of unfired nematocysts, and this is no longer a standard recommended decontaminant. Vinegar and ammonia may be applied continuously by applying a soaked compress. A paste made from unseasoned meat tenderizer or papaya is reported to significantly relieve pain associated with jellyfish stings.[55]

Following decontamination, any remaining tentacles should be removed. This can be accomplished using shaving cream or a baking soda slurry and a razor, or at the scene by using a paste of sand and sea water and a shell or plastic (e.g., credit card).[56]

Hot water immersion of the affected body part at 40° to 41° C provides pain relief for many marine envenomations, including jellyfish.[55] Because jellyfish protein toxins are heat-labile, immersion may allow heat to penetrate the intracutaneous depths to inactivate the venom. Smaller local reactions benefit from application of topical anesthetic ointments or sprays containing benzocaine or 2.5% lidocaine. Hydrocortisone cream or lotion (1%) twice a day is useful for skin reactions. Patients without systemic signs may be discharged with oral analgesics and anti-inflammatories as needed for pain, as well as antihistamines for any allergic component.

Sea anemones are sessile, multicolored animals often found in shallow waters and tidal pools. They have tentacles containing nematocysts that can envenomate humans as well as fish. Envenomation results in a lesion with a pale center and an erythematous or petechial ring. This is followed by increasing edema and ecchymosis. Most lesions resolve in 48 hours. More severe envenomations may result in vesicle formation that can lead to abscess, eschar, or hyperpigmentation. Treatment is the same as recommended for Portuguese man-o-war.

Phylum Echinodermata

Sea Urchins The sea urchin is a free-living echinoderm covered by a hard shell containing multiple irregular spines that may or may not contain venom. Sea urchins that do not possess venom-filled spines have jawed pedicellaria that function to inject the venom. The spines are brittle and break off easily if handled, complicating wound care. Sea urchin venom is poorly characterized but like other marine venoms contains heat-labile high molecular weight toxins, including steroid glycosides, hemolysins, proteases, serotonin and cholinergic substances.[57] Two major types of reactions are seen with sea urchin envenomations. The first is an immediate local reaction that typically presents with burning pain, swelling, and a rash. The spines contain a blue-black dye that may stain the wound but is not of clinical significance. Treatment is with hot water immersion and debridement of any spines. Care should be taken in spine removal as they are very brittle and may crumble in the wound. The wound should be irrigated copiously. Prophylactic antibiotics are generally not needed. A secondary delayed reaction is sometimes seen. This may present with induration, swelling, bony erosion, and granuloma formation. Treatment includes antibiotics and corticosteroids.

Vertebrates

Stingrays

The stingray is considered to be the most common venomous fish involved in human envenomations. It is estimated that approximately 2,000 stings occur annually in North America.[58] Stingrays are generally peaceful bottom dwellers and attacks occur most commonly when a swimmer steps on a stingray buried in the sand. This results in the stingray hurling its barbed tail up in a defensive response.

The barb is serrated and retropointed, and can cause significant lacerations and puncture wounds. Most wounds involve the lower extremities. The barb is covered with heat labile venom composed of a number of toxic compounds including phosphodiesterases, 58-nucleosidase, and serotonin. Symptoms of envenomation include immediate, intense pain that is out of proportion for what may be expected based on the wound alone. The pain usually reaches maximum intensity in about 90 minutes. Potential systemic symptoms include weakness, nausea, muscle cramps, vomiting, peripheral vasoconstriction, cardiac dysrhythmias, respiratory depression, seizures, and coma.

After stabilization of potential life threats, the main goals of treatment are pain control, neutralization of venom, and wound care. Initial irrigation of the wound site should be performed with cold normal saline to wash away existing venom, and the resulting vasoconstriction may slow down further absorption of the venom. The affected area should then be immersed in hot water (up to 113° F) for 30 to 90 minutes, which helps destabilize some of the venom and affords significant pain control. Parenteral narcotics are frequently necessary. If retained portions of the barb or sheath are suspected, the wound should be anesthetized, explored, and debrided. Retained foreign bodies may be visible on plain radiographs. Hot water immersion should be used with caution, if at all, following use of local or regional anesthetics due to the risk of thermal injury. Provide tetanus prophylaxis, if indicated. Due to the risk of infection, the wound should not be closed primarily. Prophylactic antibiotics such as ciprofloxacin, doxycycline or trimethoprim-sulfa are recommended in patients with residual foreign bodies or if the patient is immunosuppressed.[59]

Catfish

Over 1,000 species of fresh and salt water catfish exist worldwide and many are venomous to humans. Catfish possess axillary venom glands and one dorsal and two pectoral fin spines that inflict the envenomation. Some species of catfish produce a proteinaceous toxic epidermal secretion (crinotoxin). The barbs of catfish are retroussé (tip turned up) and thus can produce significant damage and be difficult to remove.[60,61]

The venom contains vasoconstrictive and dermatonecrotic factors. Symptoms frequently include intense pain, paresthesias, and numbness that may last from 30 minutes to 48 hours. Erythema, hemorrhage, edema, cyanosis, and lymphangitis are also common localized findings. Rare systemic effects include fever, weakness, syncope, hypotension, and respiratory distress. Death is rare. Puncture wounds are not infrequently followed by secondary bacterial infections that may take months to heal.[62–64] Treatment of catfish envenomation is as described for stingrays.

Scorpionfish

The family of Scorpaenidae are found worldwide in temperate, tropical, and subtropical climates and include lionfish (Pterois), scorpionfish (Scorpaena), and stonefish (Synanceia). In the United States, reported envenomations are typically the result of encounters by home aquarists who keep lionfish in their tanks.[65] All members of this family have 12 to 13 dorsal spines, 2 pelvic spines, and 3 anal spines. Spines are covered with a loose integumentary sheath that is pushed down the spine when tissue is punctured, compressing the 2 venom glands at the base of the spine and allowing venom to pass up a groove in the spines into the wound. Similar to other marine venoms, venoms from the Scorpaenidae are heat-labile high-molecular weight proteins with antigenic properties. The severity of envenomations appears to be mildest for lionfish, more severe for scorpionfish, and most severe or life-threatening for stonefish.

Lionfish were introduced in the southeast United States in 1994 and have now been spotted by divers from south Florida northward as far as Long Island (**FIGURE 131.2**). As of January 2004, lionfish numbers appear to be increasing between Florida and North Carolina.[66] Following puncture by the spine of a lionfish, there is severe localized pain that frequently is accompanied by swelling. Systemic symptoms include nausea, diaphoresis, difficulty breathing, chest or abdominal pain, weakness, hypotension, and syncope, and were noted in 13% of one series.[67] Treatment of these wounds is similar to other marine envenomations and emphasizes immersion of the puncture wound in hot non-scalding water (45° C, 113° F) for 30 minutes or longer, analgesia, proper wound care, and tetanus prophylaxis.

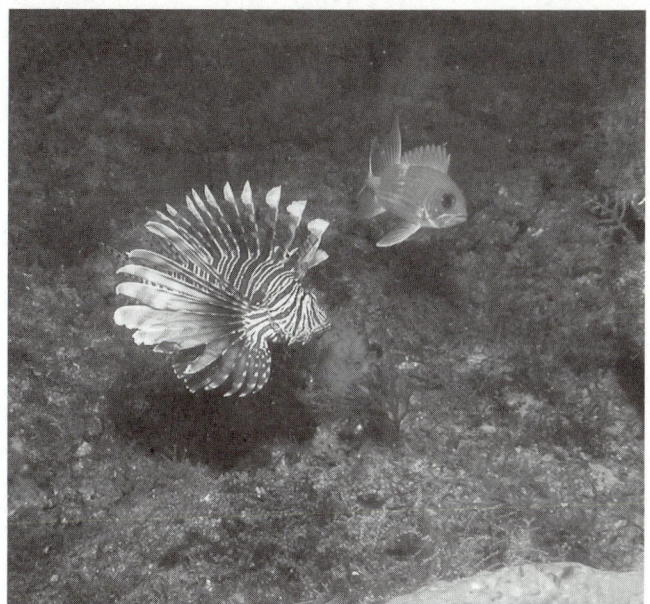

FIGURE 131.2 Lionfish. (Photo courtesy of Douglas E. Kesling, NOAA-NURC/UNCW.)

Crotalid Envenomation

Approximately 3,000 people are reported to suffer poisonous snakebites annually in the United States.[68] Of these envenomations, over 100 were reported to suffer major morbidity from the snakebite. Death occurs in only a few cases a year. Crotalids may be distinguished from other species by their triangular shaped heads, elliptical shaped pupils, and a single row of subcaudal scales. They also possess infrared heat-sensing pits, thus the name "pit viper," which enable them to locate prey and guide the direction of strike.[69]

Pathophysiology

The pathophysiological changes in the crotalid envenomated patient vary because of the species, nutritional status, and age of the snake.[70] The most common problems, accounting for most of the morbidity, involve tissue injury. It is impossible to accurately predict the extent of local tissue damage a patient will develop following a snakebite. Numerous enzymes have been isolated from the venom of snakes.[71–73] The mechanism of each of these enzymes is directed at the breakdown of specific components of the tissue in which the venom has been injected, allowing the venom to penetrate further into the victim's tissues. Coagulopathy is the most frequent cause of death. Snake venoms, because of their complex makeup, have multiple means of disabling the coagulation cascade.

Clinical Presentation

The spectrum of clinical presentation ranges from asymptomatic to cardiovascular collapse and death. Bites from Crotalidae species that do not introduce venom (*dry bites*) have been estimated to occur in up to 20% of exposures.[74] Skin lesions may appear as distinct puncture marks or as faint scratches (**FIGURE 131.3**). Pain is frequently the initial complaint. When envenomation occurs, swelling usually begins within minutes of the bite. Tissue necrosis may follow cyanosis, and bleb formation may occur over the affected areas. In addition to direct tissue damage, rhabdomyolysis, nausea, vomiting, and diaphoresis may be seen.[75] Three distinct snakebite-induced coagulopathies have been reported: venom-induced thrombocytopenia, fibrinolysis, and disseminated intravascular coagulation.[70] Coagulopathy may be manifest as petechia, gastrointestinal bleeding, epistaxis, hemoptysis, and bleeding from wounds or phlebotomy sites.

Treatment

Prehospital

The most important steps to assure a good outcome in the snakebite victim include immobilization and rapid transport of the victim for evaluation by trained medical personnel.[76] It is not necessary to identify the snake and rescuers should not place themselves at risk of a bite in an attempt to capture or kill the snake. Tourniquets, wound incisions, suction, extraction devises, cryotherapy, heat application, electric shock therapy, and wound excision should *not* be performed.[70,77,78]

Emergency Department

The bite area should be gently cleansed. Circumferential measurement at several points along the affected limb

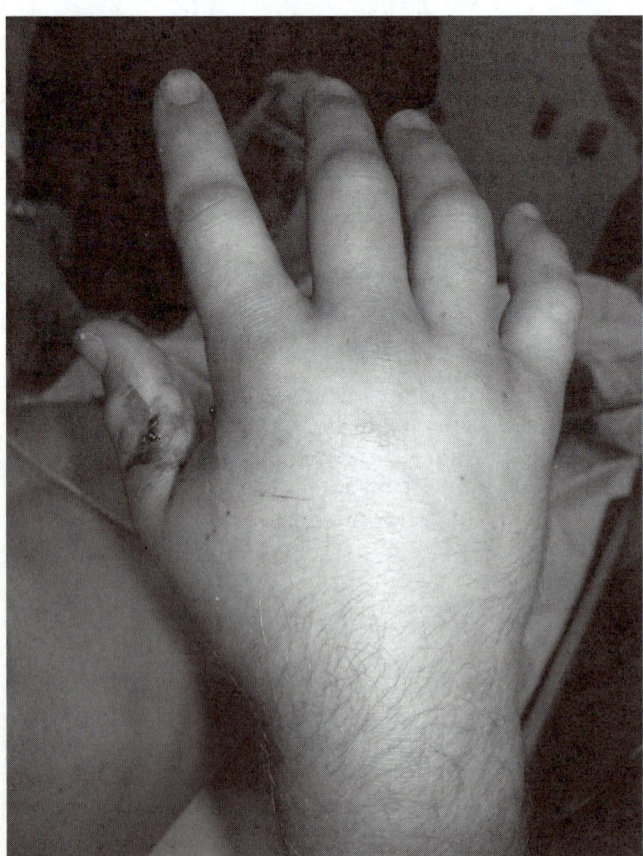

FIGURE 131.3 Rattlesnake bite to thumb. (Photo courtesy of E.M. Singletary, MD.)

should be started shortly after the patient's arrival and repeated with neurovascular checks at hourly intervals until swelling subsides. The bitten extremity should be immobilized with a padded splint and an elastic bandage wrapped gently but firmly from the distal to the proximal aspect of the limb. Elevation to a level above the heart should be achieved.

Hypotension may be caused by fluid loss due to third spacing, vomiting, hemorrhage, or vasovagal effects. Crystalloid administration should begin immediately in these patients and prior to antivenom administration. Pain control usually requires intravenous opioid agents. Prophylactic antibiotics and steroid administration are not recommended.[70] Fasciotomy should not be performed unless elevated muscle compartment pressures are documented and pressures fail to decrease with antivenom.[79,80] Clinically, the snakebite extremity appears nearly identical to an extremity with a compartment syndrome. Victims will have swelling, tense skin, tenderness, paresthesias, and pain with passive motion due to the local inflammatory reaction and not compartment syndrome. Controlled animal studies have shown that fasciotomies are rarely necessary after snakebite and can lead to an potential increased morbidity.[79,81] Administration of antivenom after snake venom injection decreases the rise in compartment pressures and preserves muscle function.

Antivenom

Currently, two snake antivenoms are approved for treating North American crotaline envenomations: equine derived polyvalent IgG (Wyeth-Ayerst Laboratories) and ovine polyvalent Fab immunoglobulin fragments (CroFab from Protherics Inc.). Dosing and mixing of these products can be found on the product insert. Pediatric patients should be treated with the same amount of antivenom as adults, regardless of their weight.

The most critical decision facing the clinician treating snakebite victims is when antivenom therapy is appropriate. Because anaphylaxis and serum sickness have been associated with the use of antivenom (less commonly with ovine polyvalent Fab), potential risk to the patient must be weighed against benefits.[82] The major indications for antivenom therapy are:

1. Rapid progression of swelling
2. Significant coagulation defect
3. Cardiovascular collapse

Attempts have been made to quantitate these signs and symptoms. Generally speaking, swelling that involves the distal 25% of the extremity in the first 1 to 2 hours or a decrease in platelets or fibrinogen of 10% or more below normal may be an indication for antivenom therapy.[70] Patients who are asymptomatic or have minimal symptoms do not require antivenom.

There have been numerous reports of immediate hypersensitivity reactions associated with the use of crotalidae antivenom polyvalent IgG, with incidence rates of 23% to 56% reported.[83] This high reaction rate is due to the large amount of proteins within this partially purified horse antivenom and the presence of the Fc portion of the antibodies. CroFab® is reported to have a lower risk of immediate hypersensitivity reaction with fewer cases of acute allergic reaction reported.[82,84] Serum sickness may occur in patients receiving antivenom. Onset is most common one to two weeks after treatment and manifests as a maculopapular rash, fever, malaise, and arthralgia. Antivenom should *never* be initiated in an area without complete resuscitation capabilities.

Disposition

Patients who remain asymptomatic for four hours and have normal coagulation studies (fibrinogen, fibrin split products, platelets, protime, and partial thromboplastin time) may be released. Symptomatic patients should be considered candidates for hospitalization and the need for antivenom therapy determined.

Elapidae

Elapid snakes are different from the crotalid, with two representatives in the United States: eastern coral snake and the western (Sonoran) coral snake. Snakes that have red and yellow rings in contact with each other are elapid snakes.[85]

Pathophysiology

The bite site typically does not have puncture wounds but rather linear abrasions.[86] The venom of these snakes is primarily a neurotoxin and causes minimal local findings. The venom affects the central nervous system and muscle function. Respiratory failure is usually the cause of death.

Emergency Department Evaluation

Coral snake antivenom is available. Even in absence of the antivenom with appropriate supportive measures such as endotracheal intubation, pressor, and ventilatory support, it is possible to allow time for detoxification of the venom and recovery. The use of antivenom greatly aids the recovery and should be considered in any patient with a bite regardless of symptoms.[87,88] This antivenom is equine serum based and the same precautions as presented for the crotalid bites should be observed.

References

1. Green VA, Siegel CJ. Bites and stings of Hymenoptera, caterpillar and beetle. *J Toxicol Clin Toxicol* 1983;21:491–502.
2. Kontou-Fili K. Patients with negative skin tests. *Curr Opin Allergy Clin Immunol* 2002;2:353–357.
3. Minton SA, Bechtel HB, Erickson TB. North American arthropod envenomation and parasitism. In: Auerbach PS, ed. *Wilderness Medicine*. St. Louis, MO: Mosby, 2001:863–895.
4. Visscher PK, Vetter RS, Camazine S. Removing bee stings. *Lancet* 1996;348:301–302.
5. Stafford CT. Hypersensitivity to fire ant venom. *Ann Allergy Asthma Immunol* 1996;77:87-95; quiz 96–99.
6. Jelinek GA. Widow spider envenomation (latrodectism): a worldwide problem. *Wilderness Environ Med* 1997;8:226–231.
7. Karcioglu O, Gumustekin M, Tuncok Y, Celik A. Acute renal failure following latrodectism. *Vet Hum Toxicol* 2001;43:161–163.
8. Rauber A. Black widow spider bites. *J Toxicol Clin Toxicol* 1983;21:473–485.
9. Woestman R, Perkin R, Van Stralen D. The black widow: is she deadly to children? *Pediatr Emerg Care* 1996;12:360–364.
10. Wright SW, Wrenn KD, Murray L, Seger D. Clinical presentation and outcome of brown recluse spider bite. *Ann Emerg Med* 1997;30:28–32.
11. Boyer L, McNally J, Binford G. Spider bites. In: Auerbach PS, ed. *Wilderness Medicine*. St. Louis, MO: Mosby, 2001:807–838.
12. Eichner ER. Spider bite hemolytic anemia: positive Coombs' test, erythrophagocytosis, and leukoerythroblastic smear. *Am J Clin Pathol* 1984;81:683–687.
13. Hostetler MA, Dribben W, Wilson DB, Grossman WJ. Sudden unexplained hemolysis occurring in an infant due to presumed Loxosceles envenomation. *J Emerg Med* 2003;25:277–282.
14. Bey TA, Walter FG, Lober W, et al. Loxosceles arizonica bite associated with shock. *Ann Emerg Med* 1997;30:701–703.
15. Ginsburg CM, Weinberg AG. Hemolytic anemia and multiorgan failure associated with localized cutaneous lesion. *J Pediatr* 1988;112:496–499.
16. Vetter RS, Bush SP. The diagnosis of brown recluse spider bite is overused for dermonecrotic wounds of uncertain etiology. *Ann Emerg Med* 2002;39:544–546.
17. Gomez HF, Krywko DM, Stoecker WV. A new assay for the detection of Loxosceles species (brown recluse) spider venom. *Ann Emerg Med* 2002;39:469–474.
18. Isbister GK, Graudins A, White J, Warrell D. Antivenom treatment in arachnidism. *J Toxicol Clin Toxicol* 2003;41:291–300.
19. Cole HP 3rd, Wesley RE, King LE Jr. Brown recluse spider envenomation of the eyelid: an animal model. *Ophthal Plast Reconstr Surg* 1995;11:153–164.
20. Beilman GJ, Cerra FB. The future. Monitoring cellular energetics. *Crit Care Clin* 1996;12:1031–1042.
21. Phillips S, Kohn M, Baker D, et al. Therapy of brown spider envenomation: a controlled trial of hyperbaric oxygen, dapsone, and cyproheptadine. *Ann Emerg Med* 1995;25:363–368.
22. Barrett SM, Romine-Jenkins M, Fisher DE. Dapsone or electric shock therapy of brown recluse spider envenomation? *Ann Emerg Med* 1994;24:21–25.
23. Suchard J, Connor D. Scorpion envenomation. In: Auerbach PC, ed. *Wilderness Medicine*. St. Louis, MO: Mosby, 2001:839–862.
24. LoVecchio F, Welch S, Klemens J, et al. Incidence of immediate and delayed hypersensitivity to Centuroides antivenom. *Ann Emerg Med* 1999;34:615–619.
25. Vedanarayanan V, Sorey WH, Subramony SH. Tick paralysis. *Semin Neurol* 2004;24:181–184.
26. Grattan-Smith PJ, Morris JG, Johnston HM, et al. Clinical and neurophysiological features of tick paralysis. *Brain* 1997;120(Pt 11):1975–1987.
27. Rossignol P, Feinsod P. Arthropods directly causing human injury. In: Warren K, Mahmoud A, eds. *Tropical and Geographic Medicine*. New York: McGraw-Hill Information Services Company, 1990:519–532.
28. Edlow JA. Lyme disease and related tick-borne illnesses. *Ann Emerg Med* 1999;33:680–693.
29. Needham GR. Evaluation of five popular methods for tick removal. *Pediatrics* 1985;75:997–1002.
30. Stewart RL, Burgdorfer W, Needham GR. Evaluation of three commercial tick removal tools. *Wilderness Environ Med* 1998;9:137–142.
31. Karras DJ. Tick removal. *Ann Emerg Med* 1998;32:519.
32. des Vignes F, Piesman J, Heffernan R, et al. Effect of tick removal on transmission of Borrelia burgdorferi and Ehrlichia phagocytophila by Ixodes scapularis nymphs. *J Infect Dis* 2001;183:773–778.
33. Medeiros I, Saconato H. Antibiotic prophylaxis for mammalian bites. *Cochrane Database Syst Rev* 2001;CD001738.
34. Callaham M. Prophylactic antibiotics in common dog bite wounds: a controlled study. *Ann Emerg Med* 1980;9:410–414.
35. Callaham ML. Treatment of common dog bites: infection risk factors. *Jacep* 1978;7:83–87.
36. Abrahamian FM. Dog bites: bacteriology, management, and prevention. *Curr Infect Dis Rep* 2000;2:446–453.
37. Keogh S, Callaham ML. Bites and injuries inflicted by domestic animals. In: Aerbach PS, ed. *Wilderness Medicine*. St. Louis: Mosby, 2001:961–978.
38. Talan DA, Citron DM, Abrahamian FM, et al. Bacteriologic analysis of infected dog and cat bites. Emergency Medicine Animal Bite Infection Study Group. *N Engl J Med* 1999;340:85–92.
39. Perron AD, Miller MD, Brady WJ. Orthopedic pitfalls in the ED: fight bite. *Am J Emerg Med* 2002;20:114–117.
40. Lindsey D, Christopher M, Hollenbach J, et al. Natural course of the human bite wound: incidence of infection and complications in 434 bites and 803 lacerations in the same group of patients. *J Trauma* 1987;27:45–48.
41. Goldstein EJ. Bite wounds and infection. *Clin Infect Dis* 1992;14:633–638.
42. Griego RD, Rosen T, Orengo IF, Wolf JE. Dog, cat, and human bites: a review. *J Am Acad Dermatol* 1995;33:1019–1029.
43. Chen E, Hornig S, Shepherd SM, Hollander JE. Primary closure of mammalian bites. *Acad Emerg Med* 2000;7:157–161.
44. Auerbach PS, Hays JT. Erythema nodosum following a jellyfish sting. *J Emerg Med* 1987;5:487–491.
45. Ohtaki N, Oka K, Sugimoto A, et al. Cutaneous reactions caused by experimental exposure to jellyfish, Carybdea rastonii. *J Dermatol* 1990;17:108–114.
46. Veraldi S, Carrera C. Delayed cutaneous reaction to jellyfish. *Int J Dermatol* 2000;39:28–29.
47. Burnett JW, Gable WD. A fatal jellyfish envenomation by the Portuguese man-o'war. *Toxicon* 1989;27:823–824.
48. Stein MR, Marraccini JV, Rothschild NE, Burnett JW. Fatal Portuguese man-o'war (Physalia physalis) envenomation. *Ann Emerg Med* 1989;18:312–315.
49. Bengtson K, Nichols MM, Schnadig V, Ellis MD. Sudden death in a child following jellyfish envenomation by Chiropsalmus quadrumanus. Case report and autopsy findings. *JAMA* 1991;266:1404–1406.
50. Armoni M, Ohali M, Hay E. Severe dyspnea due to jellyfish envenomation. *Pediatr Emerg Care* 2003;19:84–86.
51. Fenner PJ, Williamson JA. Worldwide deaths and severe envenomation from jellyfish stings. *Med J Aust* 1996;165:658–661.
52. Grady JD, Burnett JW. Irukandji-like syndrome in South Florida divers. *Ann Emerg Med* 2003;42:763–766.

53. Fenner P, Carney I. The Irukandji syndrome. A devastating syndrome caused by a north Australian jellyfish. *Aust Fam Physician* 1999;28:1131–1137.

54. Fenner PJ, Williamson J, Callanan VI, Audley I. Further understanding of, and a new treatment for, "Irukandji" (Carukia barnesi) stings. *Med J Aust* 1986;145:569, 572–574.

55. Nomura JT, Sato RL, Ahern RM, et al. A randomized paired comparison trial of cutaneous treatments for acute jellyfish (Carybdea alata) stings. *Am J Emerg Med* 2002;20:624–626.

56. Perkins RA, Morgan SS. Poisoning, envenomation, and trauma from marine creatures. *Am Fam Physician* 2004;69:885–890.

57. Auerbach PS. 2001. Envenomation by aquatic invertebrates. In: Auerbach PS, ed. *Wilderness Medicine*. St. Louis: Mosby, 2001:1450–1487.

58. Auerbach PS. Envenomation by Aquatic Vertebrates. In: Auerbach PS, ed. *Wilderness Medicine*. St. Louis: Mosby, 2001:1488–1506.

59. Isbister GK. Venomous fish stings in tropical northern Australia. *Am J Emerg Med* 2001;19:561–566.

60. Ashford RU, Sargeant PD, Lum GD. Septic arthritis of the knee caused by Edwardsiella tarda after a catfish puncture wound. *Med J Aust* 1998;168:443–444.

61. Taylor DM, Ashby K, Winkel KD. An analysis of marine animal injuries presenting to emergency departments in Victoria, Australia. *Wilderness Environ Med* 2002;13:106–112.

62. Ajmal N, Nanney LB, Wolfort SF. Catfish spine envenomation: a case of delayed presentation. *Wilderness Environ Med* 2003;14:101–105.

63. Baack BR, Kucan JO, Zook EG, Russell RC. Hand infections secondary to catfish spines: case reports and literature review. *J Trauma* 1991;31:1432–1436.

64. Murphey DK, Septimus EJ, Waagner DC. Catfish-related injury and infection: report of two cases and review of the literature. *Clin Infect Dis* 1992;14:689–693.

65. Aldred B, Erickson T, Lipscomb J. Lionfish envenomations in an urban wilderness. *Wilderness Environ Med* 1996;7:291–296.

66. Hare JA, Whitfield PE. An integrated assessment of the introduction of lionfish (Pterois volitans/miles) to the western Atlantic Ocean. In: *NOAA Technical Memorandum NOS NCCOS 2*, NTMNN 2 ed. NOAA National Centers for Coastal Ocean Science, 2003:21. Available at http://shrimp.ccfhrb.noaa.gov/nccos_publications/NCCOS_Tech_Memos.html. Accessed May 2005.

67. Kizer KW, McKinney HE, Auerbach PS. Scorpaenidae envenomation. A five-year poison center experience. *JAMA* 1985;253:807–810.

68. Watson WA, Litovitz TL, Klein-Schwartz W, et al. 2003 annual report of the American Association of Poison Control Centers Toxic Exposure Surveillance System. *Am J Emerg Med* 2004;22:335–404.

69. Gold BS, Barish RA, Dart RC. North American snake envenomation: diagnosis, treatment, and management. *Emerg Med Clin North Am* 2004;22:423–443, ix.

70. Holstege CP, Miller MB, Wermuth M, et al. Crotalid snake envenomation. *Crit Care Clin* 1997;13:889–921.

71. Hong BS. Isolation and identification of a collagenolytic enzyme from the venom of the western diamondback rattlesnake (Crotalus atrox). *Toxicon* 1982;20:535–545.

72. Paine MJ, Moura-da-Silva AM, Theakston RD, Crampton JM. Cloning of metalloprotease genes in the carpet viper (Echis pyramidum leakeyi). Further members of the metalloprotease/disintegrin gene family. *Eur J Biochem* 1994;224:483–488.

73. Moura-da-Silva AM, Laing GD, Paine MJ, et al. Processing of pro-tumor necrosis factor-alpha by venom metalloproteinases: a hypothesis explaining local tissue damage following snake bite. *Eur J Immunol* 1996;26:2000–2005.

74. Russell FE, Carlson RW, Wainschel J, Osborne AH. Snake venom poisoning in the United States. Experiences with 550 cases. *JAMA* 1975;233:341–344.

75. Bush SP, Jansen PW. Severe rattlesnake envenomation with anaphylaxis and rhabdomyolysis. *Ann Emerg Med* 1995;25:845–848.

76. Stewart ME, Greenland S, Hoffman JR. First-aid treatment of poisonous snakebite: are currently recommended procedures justified? *Ann Emerg Med* 1981;10:331–335.

77. Bush SP. Snakebite suction devices don't remove venom: they just suck. *Ann Emerg Med* 2004;43:187–188.

78. Gold BS, Dart RC, Barish RA. Bites of venomous snakes. *N Engl J Med* 2002;347:347–356.

79. Tanen DA, Danish DC, Grice GA, et al. Fasciotomy worsens the amount of myonecrosis in a porcine model of crotaline envenomation. *Ann Emerg Med* 2004;44:99–104.

80. Gold BS, Barish RA, Dart RC, et al. Resolution of compartment syndrome after rattlesnake envenomation utilizing non-invasive measures. *J Emerg Med* 2003;24:285–288.

81. Stewart RM, Page CP, Schwesinger WH, et al. Antivenin and fasciotomy/debridement in the treatment of the severe rattlesnake bite. *Am J Surg* 1989;158:543–547.

82. Holstege CP, Wu J, Baer AB. Immediate hypersensitivity reaction associated with the rapid infusion of Crotalidae polyvalent immune Fab (ovine). *Ann Emerg Med* 2002;39:677–679.

83. Dart RC, McNally J. Efficacy, safety, and use of snake antivenoms in the United States. *Ann Emerg Med* 2001;37:181–188.

84. Dart RC, Seifert SA, Boyer LV, et al. A randomized multicenter trial of crotalinae polyvalent immune Fab (ovine) antivenom for the treatment for crotaline snakebite in the United States. *Arch Intern Med* 2001;161:2030–2036.

85. Gaar GG. Assessment and management of coral and other exotic snake envenomations. *J Fla Med Assoc* 1996;83:178–182.

86. Kitchens CS, Van Mierop LH. Envenomation by the Eastern coral snake (Micrurus fulvius fulvius). A study of 39 victims. *JAMA* 1987;258:1615–1618.

87. de Roodt AR, Paniagua-Solis JF, et al. Effectiveness of two common antivenoms for North, Central, and South American Micrurus envenomations. *J Toxicol Clin Toxicol* 2004;42:171–178.

88. Norris RL, Dart RC. Apparent coral snake envenomation in a patient without visible fang marks. *Am J Emerg Med* 1989;7:402–405.

Toxicologic Disorders

Edward W. Boyer

Introduction

Toxicology is an ever-changing field. New pharmaceuticals are treated by newer antidotes, and adverse reactions to medications are constantly being identified. The mutable nature of the field of toxicology demands that clinicians remain current in their understanding of poisoning and its management. Although the topics described in this section are reflective of the current standard of care, changes in treatment and drug therapy may require that readers check the product information given by the manufacturer for each agent to ensure adequate dosing, the method and duration of administration, and contraindications. Furthermore, clinicians should always consult a Clinical Toxicology Service or Poison Control Center to tap the valuable decision-making ability of these professionals. In this way, the responsibility placed on physicians at the bedside—to rely upon experience and knowledge in treating the patient, as well as selecting the best course of therapy—can be shouldered by experts.

Toxidromes: An Approach to the Poisoned Patient

Darren Menditto
Robert J. Hoffman

A challenging part of caring for poisoned patients is the recognition of signs, symptoms, and a pattern of illness that may allow identification of the responsible class of toxin. Most poisons cause nonspecific constitutional symptoms, such as vomiting or a depressed mental status, which do not suggest a specific offending agent. Several classes of poisons, however, can be identified by a specific constellation of signs and symptoms. These constellations of signs and symptoms are known as *toxidromes,* which is an abbreviation of *toxicologic syndrome.* There are several such well defined and readily diagnosable toxidromes that health care providers should be familiar with. Clinicians should maintain a high index of suspicion in order to recognize poisonings, which may present with nonspecific symptoms, but they should also readily recognize these particular patterns of illness that allow immediate diagnosis of poisoning.

Emergency Department Management

As in other circumstances, addressing airway, breathing, and circulation issues (the *ABCs*) is paramount when caring for poisoned patients. For the poisoned patient, it is necessary to expand the pneumonic to *ABCDE,* with *D* to indicate "dextrose" as a reminder to measure blood glucose in any patient with altered mental status or exposure to a poison capable of causing hypoglycemia, and *E* to indicate "ECG" as a reminder to rapidly assess the electrocardiogram of any patient with abnormal vital signs, symptoms attributable to a cardiovascular poison, or exposure to a poison capable of affecting cardiac function. In circumstances where antidote administration is essential to patient care and may occur prior to the completion of other means of stabilization, such as for cyanide poisoning, the fundamental *ABCDE* care should occur simultaneously and without delay.

In the patient with an altered mental status, after issues of airway, breathing, and circulation have been addressed, other causes of symptoms such as CNS infection, CNS trauma as well as metabolic derangement should be considered and appropriate measures taken until a definitive cause can be determined. Early treatment of a patient with altered mental status includes maintenance of stable vital signs within acceptable limits, adequate oxygenation, and rapid determination of an adequate blood glucose concentration.

History

As rapidly as possible during or after initial stabilization, it is critical to obtain as much information as possible about the exposure. Primary attention should be paid to the identification and quantification of the poison, timing of exposure as well as signs and symptoms subsequent to exposure. Details regarding the nature of exposure, such as an intentional or unintentional ingestion, the location and circumstances in which the patient was found, and the past medical history should also be obtained.

Toxicologic Physical Examination

The secondary survey in a poisoned patient will include focused assessment of the mental status, pupils, skin, bowel, and bladder function (**Table 132.1**). In conjunction with the vital signs, these will most readily assist in the diagnosis of a particular toxidrome. In addition to such a focused exam, a secondary survey will detect trauma, abnormal neurological findings, and unusual breath or body odors.

Toxidromes

Common toxidromes include cholinergic, anticholinergic, sympathomimetics, opioid, and sedative-hypnotic.

Cholinergic

The cholinergic toxidrome is the result of excess stimulation of muscarinic and nicotinic receptors of the central and peripheral nervous system. Cholinesterase facilitates degradation of acetylcholine when released at the synapse in preganglionic junctions of parasympathetic, sympathetic, and myoneural junctions, and the postganglionic junction of the parasympathetic and some sympathetic nervous system. Numerous toxins inhibit cholinesterase. When cholinesterase is inhibited, excess acetylcholine may cause signs and symptoms of cholinergic toxicity.

Table 132.1

Secondary Assessment in a Poisoned Patient

	Anticholinergic	Cholinergic	Sympatho-mimetic	Opioid	Sedative-Hypnotic	Withdrawal from Alcohol or Sedative-Hypnotics
Pupils	Mydriasis	Miosis	Mydriasis	Miosis	Normal	Mydriasis
Skin	Dry, flushed	Diaphoresis	Diaphoresis	Normal	Normal	Diaphoresis, piloerection
Bowel sounds	Decreased	Increased	Normal or increased	Decreased	Normal	Normal
Bladder	Urinary retention	Normal or enuresis	Normal	Normal	Normal	Normal
Mental status	Somnolence, agitation, hallucinosis	Somnolence, agitation, hallucinosis	Agitated	Depressed	Depressed	Agitated, hallucinosis

Features of the clinical presentation can be remembered by the mnemonic DUMBELLS (primarily muscarinic), where the emphasis is placed on the *BBB* symptoms—bradycardia, bronchorrhea, and bronchospasm—because these are the life-threatening problems associated with cholinergic toxicity. Nicotinic effects include fasciculations, muscle cramping, hyporeflexia, and weakness.

The classic features associated with cholinergic poisoning are:

- Diarrhea
- Urination
- Miosis
- Bradycardia, bronchorrhea, bronchospasm
- Emesis
- Lacrimation
- Salivation

Agents that produce the cholinergic toxidrome include:

- Nicotine, carbachol
- Carbamate insecticides
- Cholinergic neuromuscular medicines (edrophonium, neostigmine, physostigmine)
- Nerve agents used in chemical warfare (sarin, soman, tabun)
- Certain mushrooms (*Clitocybe, Inocybe*)
- Organophosphate insecticides
- Pilocarpine

Treatment

Atropine is the mainstay of treatment exerting its effects by blocking acetylcholine at the muscarinic sites. It has no effect on the nicotinic receptors. The goal of atropine therapy is to maintain "atropinization" indicated by drying of secretions, mydriasis, flushing of skin, and tachycardia. Under-dosing of atropine is a common pitfall in therapy. Pralidoxime (2-PAM) is a cholinesterase regenerator that reverses the cholinergic effects at the nicotinic receptors.

Anticholinergic

Anticholinergic symptoms are caused by the antagonism of the central and peripheral cholinergic receptors. Depending on the drug involved, there can be blockade of the muscarinic (most common) nicotinic or both receptors. The classic mnemonic for the anticholinergic toxidrome is "hot as Hades, dry as a bone, red as a beet, blind as a bat, and mad as a hatter."

Physical exam features include:

- Altered mental status that may consist of somnolence, agitation, hallucinosis, or seizure.
- Mydriasis
- Dry mucous membranes
- Tachycardia and hypertension
- Absent bowel sounds
- Urinary retention
- Flushed dry skin and hyperthermia

Agents that cause the anticholinergic toxidrome include many classes of drugs including:

- Antihistamines
- Tricyclic antidepressants
- Antipsychotic drugs (Phenothiazines)
- Antiparkinsonian agents
- Skeletal muscle relaxants (Cyclobenzaprine)
- Scopolamine
- Belladonna alkaloids
- Jimson Weed (*Datura*)

Treatment

Treatment of anticholinergic poisoning is primarily supportive. Benzodiazapines may be used to treat agitation, improve hydration, and as cooling measures for hyperthermia.

Physostigmine is a reversible acetylcholinesterase inhibitor that crosses the blood-brain barrier and can reverse both central and peripheral anticholinergic effects. Physostigmine is contraindicated in TCA overdose as it can potentiate cardiac toxicity and has been reported to cause arrest in patients with TCA toxicity.

Sympathomimetic

Sympathomimetic agents exert their effects through stimulation directly or indirectly on alpha and beta adrenergic receptors in the sympathetic and central nervous systems. The toxidrome seen with sympathomimetic agents is a systemic hyperdynamic state that can also be present in the withdrawal state of ethanol or other sedative-hypnotics.

Clinical features include:
- Agitation
- Mydriasis
- Tachycardia
- Hypertension
- Hyperthermia
- Diaphoresis
- Hyperactive bowel sounds
- Seizures, rhabdomyolysis, and myocardial infarction may occur in severe cases.

Agents that cause the sympathomimetic toxidrome include:
- Amphetamines
- Caffeine
- Cocaine
- Over-the-counter decongestants (phenylephrine, pseudoephedrine, ephedrine, and others)
- Theophylline

The sympathomimetic toxidrome is similar to the anticholinergic toxidrome in many ways. The key in physical differentiation is the skin (diaphoretic vs. dry) and abdominal exam (hyperactive bowel sounds vs. hypoactive bowel sounds).

The primary agents causing sympathomimetic toxicity are amphetamines and similar drugs, such as cocaine and MAO inhibitors. These agents act to increase the release of or potentiate the action of catecholamines or to directly stimulate adrenergic receptors in a manner similar to catecholamines.

Treatment

The treatment of sympathomimetic overdose is primarily supportive. Maintenance of vital signs within acceptable limits may be accomplished with: cooling and adequate hydration for hyperthermia; benzodiazipines, phentolamine, nitrites, or calcium channel antagonists for controlling hypertension; and benzodiazepines for agitation. Cardiac monitoring and cardiac enzymes assessment should occur in the symptomatic patient. Administration of a beta-blocker without concomitant administration of an alpha adrenergic blocker is relatively contraindicated because of the possibility of causing paradoxical increase in blood pressure by creating unopposed alpha adrenergic stimulation. Solitary use of beta-blockers is a well described cause of catastrophic hypertension and even death in patients receiving such treatment.

Opioids

Opioids are classified as natural, semisynthetic, or synthetic. They are commonly encountered in the ED as a result of many legitimate and recreational uses. Opioids have analgesic, euphoric, sedative, and anxiolytic properties. They act by binding to endogenous mu, kappa, delta, sigma, and epsilon receptors in the brain and spinal cord with various clinical effects. In addition to the classic symptoms, opioid toxicity may be associated with hypothermia, bradycardia, hypotension, and noncardiogenic pulmonary edema. Imidazoline medications cause an opioid-like toxidrome that does not reliably respond to naloxone therapy.

The classic opioid toxidrome is a triad of:
- Coma
- Respiratory depression
- Miosis (pinpoint pupils)

Agents associated with the opioid toxidrome include:
- Diphenoxylate
- Fentanyl
- Heroin
- Hydrocodone
- Imidazolines (clonidine, oxymetazoline, tetrahydrolazine), which mimic opioid toxidrome
- Meperidine
- Methadone
- Morphine
- Oxycodone
- Propoxyphene

Treatment

Naloxone is a competitive opiate receptor antagonist that reverses the effects of opioids when administered parenterally, inhalationally, or endotracheally. In the patient with depressed mental status and decreased minute ventilation, control of the airway must be assured. Naloxone administered by the IV route is the most rapid and preferred route of administration. Full immediate reversal should be avoided especially in the habituated user in order to avoid precipitating withdrawal symptoms. A more elegant approach is to titrate small aliquots (0.05 mg to 0.1 mg IV) until adequate spontaneous ventilation occurs. Repeated doses might be required if the ingested opioid has a more prolonged duration of action than the 20 to 60 minute effect of naloxone.

Sedative-Hypnotics

The sedative-hypnotic class of medications works by potentiating the main inhibitory neurotransmitter, gamma-aminobutyric acid (GABA), in the central nervous system. Stimulation of GABA causes sedation, anxiolysis, and striated muscle relaxation. These medications are commonly used for the treatment of anxiety, insomnia, seizures, alcohol withdrawal, conscious sedation, and recreational abuse. The classic toxidrome is one of dose-dependent CNS and respiratory depression. Respiratory depression resulting from benzodiazepine ingestion may be absent or much less prominent than that resulting from other sedative-hypnotic drugs, and often benzodiazepines cause coma with normal vital signs.

Common sedative-hypnotic drugs include:
- Benzodiazepines
- Barbiturates
- GHB (gamma-hydroxybutyrate)

Treatment

Treatment is primarily supportive care and maintenance of vital signs within acceptable limits. Respiratory support may be necessary in circumstances of respiratory depression. Activated charcoal should be given as it binds both benzodiazepines and barbiturates. Flumazenil a competitive benzodiazepine receptor antagonist, does not reliably reverse respiratory depression associated with benzodiazepines, and may precipitate seizures. Flumazenil should not be administered routinely, and should only be considered when there is a specific need and indication. Furthermore, the patient should be known not to be tolerant to benzodiazepines if flumazenil administration is considered.

Selected Readings

Goldfrank LR, Flomenbaum NE, Lewin NA, et al. Vital signs and toxic syndromes. In: Goldfrank LR, Flomenbaum NE, Lewin NA, et al., eds. *Goldfrank's Toxicologic Emergencies,* 7th ed. New York: McGraw-Hill, 2002:255–260.

Hack J, Hoffman RS. General management of poisoned patients. In: Tintinalli JE, Kelen GD, Stapcznski JS, eds. *Emergency Medicine A Comprehensive Study Guide.* New York: McGraw-Hill, 2000:1057–1062.

Kuffner EK. Anticholinergic syndrome. In: Dart RC, Hurlbut KM, Kuffner EK, Yip L, eds. *The 5 Minute Toxicology Consult.* New York: Lippincott Williams & Wilkins, 2000:14–15.

Seifert SA. Cholinergic syndrome. In: Dart RC, Hurlbut KM, Kuffner EK, Yip L, eds. *The 5 Minute Toxicology Consult.* New York: Lippincott Williams & Wilkins, 2000:14–15.

Sharma AN, Benitez JG, Fore C, Allison LG. Toxidromes and vital signs. In: Ling LJ, Clark RF, Erickson TB, Trestrail JH, eds. *Toxicology Secrets,* Philadelphia: Hanley & Belfus, Inc., 2000:10–13.

Gastrointestinal Decontamination

Joshua G. Schier, MD

The principle of gastrointestinal decontamination (GID) is simple: if the toxin cannot be absorbed, then it cannot cause systemic toxicity. There are currently several methods available to the clinician that may enhance elimination from the gastrointestinal tract and/or prevent systemic absorption from the gastrointestinal tract. Whether employment of a particular technique results in a conferred clinical benefit is an entirely different matter. This chapter discusses the most commonly employed GID techniques, their indications/contraindications for usage, and best available evidence for usage.

If the clinician believes some form of GID is necessary, than he or she is faced with other questions such as which form of GID to choose. GID techniques available to the clinician include: orogastric lavage, syrup of ipecac administration, activated charcoal, cathartics, and whole bowel irrigation. The decision to perform GID will depend on several factors: type and amount of drug ingested, time passed since ingestion, and inherent drug properties and pharmacokinetics. In many instances, there may be more than one effective GID technique. In particularly significant poisonings (i.e., those that are commonly life-threatening such as tricyclic antidepressants or sustained release calcium channel blockers), a combination of methodologies may be used. The clinician may be unsure or even unfamiliar with a methodology that seems to be most applicable to the situation. In all cases, the clinician should consult their regional poison control center for individualized guidance.

Gastric Emptying

Gastric emptying (GE) refers to a process or procedure, which is utilized to empty the stomach in order to remove existing drug and thereby prevent its passage into the small intestine where absorption takes place. Gastric emptying is typically done through orogastric lavage or by the induction of vomiting by administration of syrup of ipecac. In considering whether to employ a GE procedure, the clinician should consider several issues in relationship to the ingestion: inherent procedural risk, likelihood of retrieval of a significant amount of drug, benefit gained by removal of that amount, and availability of alternative treatment methodologies (e.g., antidotes or alternate GID technique alone).[1]

Gastric emptying can result in physical removal of drug from the stomach and thereby decrease systemic absorption.[2,3] This does not necessarily correlate with an improved clinical outcome. In fact, there are very few randomized studies evaluating gastric emptying in poisoned patients in which clinical outcome is used as an endpoint.[4-6] These studies have multiple limitations and many of their conclusions are not well-supported by the data presented.[4-6] Based on the current literature, gastric emptying is associated with a clinical benefit in outcome when completed for the sickest patients within one hour from ingestion.[4,6] There is currently insufficient information to determine whether there is a clinical benefit in outcome beyond one hour from ingestion. However, there are selected situations in which GE should be considered.

In the majority of patients, gastric emptying is unlikely to contribute additional benefit when compared to administration of activated charcoal (AC) alone.[7] However, GE should be strongly considered in the following circumstances: (1) ingestion of a potentially life-threatening dose of a severe, difficult to treat poison (such as the tricyclic antidepressants, calcium channel blockers or beta blockers); and (2) severely ill patients who present within one hour of ingestion.[1,4,6,7] It may also be considered in several other selected situations: (1) relatively recent ingestion (<2 h); (2) presence of or ingestion of tablets known to form drug concretions or bezoars (mass of partially digested pill fragments) in the stomach; (3) drugs with anticholinergic properties (since they may delay gastric emptying); (4) if the adsorptive capacity of AC is exceeded by the amount of drug ingested; (5) if the ingested agent is not adsorbed to AC at all; (6) absent or ineffective antidotal therapy; or (7) ingestion of controlled-release drug formulations (theophylline, calcium channel blockers).[1]

Orogastric lavage (OGL) is currently the only accepted gastric emptying procedure (GEP). Ipecac-induced emesis should not be considered as a routine GEP.[8] The reader is referred to selected readings for additional discussion on syrup of ipecac.[1,8] If a GEP is warranted, OGL may be considered if the patient's airway is secure: the patient is awake, alert and in no danger of sudden deterioration *or* the patient is endotracheally intubated. General contraindications include: unsecured airway, ingestion of a caustic substance or hydrocarbon, and patients at risk for gastrointestinal hemorrhage or perforation due to intrinsic disease.[9] The awake, alert adult patient should be placed in the left lateral decubitus position and a 36-40 French tube (in children consider 24-28 French tube) should be used. The length of tube to be inserted should be marked by estimation prior to insertion and coated with a water soluble lubricant.[9] The tube may be then gently inserted into the esophagus through the mouth and placement confirmed by epigastric auscultation of insufflated air.[9] Stomach lavage should be completed with repeated aliquots of warmed normal saline (adults, 250 mL; children, 10 mL/kg), taking care to remove as much as possible from the first aliquot prior to administration of the next.[9] After the lavage fluid is clear of whole or partially-digested drug material, a dose of activated charcoal should be administered, if indicated, and the tube removed.[9]

Activated Charcoal

Activated charcoal can decrease the systemic absorption of many drugs depending on certain factors such as the particular agent, time passed since ingestion, and presence of food in the gastrointestinal tract.[10] It is most effective in preventing absorption if administered within one hour of ingestion.[10] Many of the same methodological concerns discussed earlier in OGL are present in studies that attempt to evaluate the efficacy of AC. However, in most poisonings, the benefits afforded by adsorption of any residual toxin by AC outweigh the risk of administration.[10]

A general guide towards the appropriate initial dose of AC is a 10:1 ratio of AC to drug or 1 g/kg (whichever is larger).[10] Anti-emetic agents and nasogastric tubes may be used to facilitate AC administration.[10] Generally, AC is contraindicated in the following situations: unprotected airway, gastrointestinal disease/dysfunction (perforation, obstruction, or gastrointestinal damage from a caustic ingestion), or when administration increases the risk of aspiration potential (e.g., hydrocarbons).[10] Risks associated with administration are generally minor and gastrointestinal in nature such as nausea and vomiting.[10] The most concerning complication is pulmonary aspiration which can progress to death.

Multiple-dose activated charcoal (MDAC) not only prevents systemic absorption, but also enhances elimination of selected drugs. Drugs that may have elimination enhanced from the GI tract from MDAC tend to have the following properties: (1) they remain in the gastrointestinal tract for extended periods, such as sustained-release formulations or drugs that form bezoars or concretions in the stomach; (2) if a 10:1 ratio of AC to drug cannot be achieved with a single dose (e.g., large dose tablets like 300 mg theophylline tablets); or (3) agents that undergo entero-enteric or enterohepatic recirculation.[1,10,11] Entero-enteric recirculation or "gut dialysis" refers to drugs with long elimination half-lives, small volumes of distribution, and low plasma-protein binding rates. Agents with these properties tend to remain in the intravascular system longer. As they pass

through blood vessels next to the GI tract, they can diffuse across the GI mucosa into the lumen to bind AC down a concentration gradient.[1,10,11] Drugs that undergo entero-hepatic recirculation are absorbed from the GI tract, secreted into bile salts which are then excreted into the GI lumen to facilitate fat absorption.[1,10,11] This recirculation presents an opportunity to bind secreted drug again if AC is present in the GI lumen.[1,10] Published compilations of drugs in which MDAC enhanced elimination/prevented absorption are available.[1,10,11] In fact, MDAC is the only GID technique that is demonstrated to decrease mortality.[12] However, there are very little data in poisoned patients that have examined the correlation of clinical outcome with enhanced elimination and decreased systemic absorption as a result of MDAC therapy for most agents.

Dosing regimens for MDAC are variable and should be individualized to the agent ingested, amount, and patient. As a general guideline, dosing frequency should be approximately every 2 to 4 hours, the repeated dose amount should not exceed 0.5 to 1.0 g/kg, and total number of doses should not exceed 3 to 4.[10,11] Contraindications to MDAC therapy are similar to single dose AC.[10] Intestinal obstruction, although rare, may occur with excessive dosing.[10] The clinician should make sure that if a cathartic is used (many AC preparations contain a sorbitol cathartic also) it is used only once (with the initial dose).

Whole-Bowel Irrigation

The elimination of drugs that remain in the gastrointestinal tract for extended periods of time or are not well adsorbed to AC may be enhanced with whole-bowel irrigation (WBI). These drugs include the controlled-release formulations, especially those with significantly associated morbidity and mortality, such as the calcium-channel and beta-blocker formulations as well as many of the metals (iron, lead, and arsenic).[10,13] WBI should also be considered in bodypackers. Bodypackers are individuals who consume large numbers (typically 50 to 60) of small, well-sealed packages containing illicit drugs with the intention of transporting them across a nation's border undetected. Asymptomatic individuals suspected of or known to be bodypacking should receive WBI to facilitate elimination of packages.[10,13] It may also be considered in selected cases of bodystuffing. Bodystuffers are those individuals who ingest smaller, generally fewer, and much more poorly sealed packets of drugs, usually in hopes of evading criminal prosecution for possession of illegal substances. However, in most minor cases of asymptomatic bodystuffing, a single dose of AC and a short period of observation is adequate.

The only acceptable fluid to perform WBI with is polyethylene glycol electrolyte lavage solution (PEG-ELS) sold commercially under a variety of trade names such as Go-Lytely™. The recommended dosing regimen in adults is 1 to 2 liters per hour (~0.5 L/h in children) until all tablets/packages are eliminated or until the rectal effluent is clear.[10,13] Contraindications to WBI include: unsecured airway, hemodynamic instability, absent bowel sounds, intractable vomiting, and gastrointestinal disease/dysfunction (perforation, ileus, obstruction, etc.).[10,13] Because most people are not able to drink this amount voluntarily, a nasogastric tube should be placed, anti-emetic medications used, and gradual escalation of the oral dose is advised.

Cathartics

A wide variety of cathartic types have been used historically to force drug through the GI tract to prevent systemic absorption. Although cathartic use may influence drug absorption and/or enhance elimination, the effect does not achieve equivalent results when compared to AC alone.[10,14,15] Furthermore, there is no consistent additional benefit from administration of both when compared to AC alone.[10,14]

General contraindications to cathartic administration include: (1) GI disease or dysfunction (obstruction, perforation) or recent surgery; (2) hypotension; (3) absent bowel sounds; (4) electrolyte imbalance; (5) renal insufficiency/failure; (6) caustic ingestion; (7) nontoxic ingestion; and (8) children <1.0 year old.[10,14] There are numerous complications reported from the wide variety of cathartics used throughout history.[10,14]

There are no definite indications for cathartic use in poisonings and routine administration is discouraged. If used, sorbitol-based cathartics are probably the safest and should be given no more than once.

References

1. Smilkstein MJ. Techniques used to prevent gastrointestinal absorption of toxic compounds. In: Goldfrank LR, Flomenbaum NE, Lewin NA, et al., eds. *Goldfrank's Toxicologic Emergencies,* 7th ed. New York: McGraw-Hill, 2002:44–57.
2. Tandberg D, Diven BG, McLeod JW. Ipecac-induced emesis versus gastric lavage: a controlled study in normal adults. *Am J Emerg Med* 1986;4:205–209, 3.
3. Comstock EG, Faulkner TP, Boisaubin EV, et al. Studies on the efficacy of gastric lavage as practiced in a large metropolitan hospital. J Tox Clin Tox 1981;18:581–597.
4. Kulig K, Bar-Or D, Cantrill SV, et al. Management of acutely poisoned patients without gastric emptying. *Ann Emerg Med* 1985;14:562–576.
5. Merigian KS, Woodard M, Hedges JR, et al. Prospective evaluation of gastric emptying in the self-poisoned patient. *Am J Emerg Med* 1990;8:479–483.
6. Pond SM, Lewis-Driver DJ, Williams GM, et al. Gastric emptying in acute overdose: a prospective randomized controlled trial. *Med J Aust* 1995;163:345–349.
7. Bond GR. The role of activated charcoal and gastric emptying in gastrointestinal decontamination: a state of the art review. *Ann Emerg Med* 2002;39:273–286.
8. American Academy of Pediatrics on Injury, Violence, and Poison Prevention. Poison treatment in the home. *Pediatrics* 2003;112:1182–1185.
9. American Academy of Clinical Toxicology. Position statement: gastric lavage. *J Tox Clin Tox* 1997;35:711–719.
10. Howland MA. Antidotes in depth: syrup of ipecac, activated charcoal, cathartics, whole bowel irrigation. In: Goldfrank LR, Flomenbaum NE, Lewin NA, et al., eds. *Goldfrank's Toxicologic Emergencies,* 7th ed. New York: McGraw-Hill, 2002:465–479.
11. American Academy of Clinical Toxicology. Position statement and practice guidelines on the use of multi-dose activated charcoal in the treatment of acute poisoning. *J Toxicol Clin Tox* 1999;37:731–751.
12. De Silva HA, Fonseka MM, Pathmeswaran A, et al. Multiple-dose activated charcoal for treatment of yellow oleander poisoning: a single-blind, randomized, placebo-controlled trial. *Lancet* 2003;361:1935–1938.
13. American Academy of Clinical Toxicology. Position statement: whole bowel irrigation. *J Toxicol Clin Tox* 1997;35:653–662.
14. American Academy of Clinical Toxicology. Position statement: cathartics. 1997;35:743–752.
15. Chin L, Picchioni A, Gillespie T. Saline cathartics and saline cathartics plus activated charcoal as antidotal treatments. *J Tox Clin Toxicol* 1981;18:865–871.

CHAPTER 134

Acetaminophen

Steven D. Salhanick

Acetaminophen (APAP, paracetamol) is the most widely used over-the-counter analgesic and antipyretic in the United States and Europe. Because of its ubiquitous nature, it is also frequently implicated in overdose and is a frequent cause of acute hepatic failure. Every practicing emergency physician will likely be called upon to treat the patient with APAP overdose. Consequently, it is important that emergency physicians have an understanding of the management of APAP overdose and toxicity.

Pharmacology

APAP is rapidly and nearly completely absorbed in the small bowel. Following therapeutic dosing, plasma concentrations peak at approximately one hour, elimination half-life is approximately 1.5 to 2 hours. Virtually all APAP is renally excreted. Roughly 5% is excreted unchanged while 95% is metabolized. There are three main pathways of metabolism. Glucuronidation and sulfonation account for 90% of an absorbed dose; the remaining 5% undergoes reductive metabolism via the hepatic cytochrome P-450 system, primarily CYP 2E1 and 1A2. The resultant metabolite, N-acetyl-para-benzoquinone-imine (NAPQI), is a highly reactive compound that typically conjugates to intracellular glutathione and is eliminated. The volume of distribution is approximately 0.95 L/kg. APAP mechanism of action remains poorly defined. It exhibits only mild inhibition of cyclooxygenase 1 and 2. Recently, cyclooxygenase 3 has been identified, primarily in neural tissue and its action is inhibited by APAP.

Pathophysiology

Overdose of APAP may cause hepatic, renal, and pancreatic injury, but hepatic injury is most common and pronounced. Necrosis of the centrilobular (zone 3) cells progressing to panlobular necrosis in severe cases constitutes the pathology. The exact cause of hepatic injury remains in debate but it is clearly related to the CYP metabolism and/or its metabolites. Toxicity has been described as occurring in two phases: stage 1 is the initial insult and stage 2 is a subsequent inflammatory response that occurs after the drug has been metabolized. The crucial events of stage 1 have undergone intense study over the past 30 years, yet the exact inciting event remains elusive. The most commonly cited theory of APAP toxicity involves excess production of NAPQI due to saturation of the other metabolic pathways coupled with the depletion of glutathione. This allows for the reactive metabolite to bind cellular thiol groups and leads to cell death. NAPQI binding does not always correlate with toxicity, however. Consequently, other theories regarding the cause of APAP toxicity remain under investigation. Notably, these include the production of reactive oxygen species resulting in oxidant stress and lipid peroxidation, peroxynitrate formation, and the resultant oxidative stress and nitrotyrosine-protein binding. Early mitochondrial dysfunction is an important early finding, yet the exact cause is unknown. Stage 2 of toxicity is currently under intense investigation. Many inflammatory mediators including interleukin 10, nitric oxide, and tumor necrosis factor-α have been implicated. It is likely that multiple parallel inflammatory pathways are activated during stage 2 of APAP toxicity.

Presentation

Acute APAP toxicity follows an overdose at a discrete time point and is usually the result of an attempt at self-harm. Acute APAP toxicity has four clinical phases (not to be confused with the aforementioned pathophysiological stages). Phase one occurs immediately after ingestion and typically lasts between 16 and 24 hours. Patients may be asymptomatic or may experience nausea and vomiting. There is no elevation of transaminases at this point. Patients may have a mild elevation in prothrombin time and internal normalized ratio (INR). This has been attributed to a direct effect of APAP and/or the antidote N-acetyl cysteine (NAC) on the vitamin K-dependant clotting factors. This early rise PT/INR has no prognostic significance and should not be treated. Phase two is marked by the rise in transaminases. Phase three occurs at 48 to 72 hours and is marked by signs of hepatic failure including marked rise in prothrombin time, cholestasis, encephalopathy, acidosis, and hyperammonemia. Patients may develop renal failure and pancreatitis. Renal failure occurs due to both hepatorenal syndrome and direct toxicity of APAP on the kidney. Patients who survive phase three will progress to phase four and begin to recover, typically beginning after approximately 96 hours. Complete normalization may take weeks. Complete recovery is the rule.

Patients may present after multiple overdoses due to repeat attempts at self-harm or due to therapeutic misadventure. These are often termed *chronic overdoses*, but acute on chronic is probably more accurate. The course of toxicity is essentially the same as with an acute ingestion, with the exception that the timing of the early phases is less well defined.

Massive ingestions resulting in levels of 800 μg/mL or greater lead to coma and acidosis. The mechanism of toxicity is not known. Data from isolated mitochondria implicate direct inhibitory effect of APAP on mitochondrial energy production.

Clinical Evaluation

Patients may present at any time in the course of toxicity. Given that early signs may be absent or nonspecific, determining ingestion and risk of subsequent toxicity is imperative. Patients who present with a history of intentional overdose of any drug should have a serum APAP level checked due to the ubiquitous nature of APAP. In the case of the single, acute ingestion when time of ingestion can be determined, a serum level obtained between 4 and 24 hours after ingestion can be plotted on the Rumack-Matthews nomogram to determine risk of toxicity (**FIGURE 134.1**). Patients with levels above the higher line (from 200 μg/mL at 4 h to 40 μg/mL at 24 h) have approximately 60% likelihood of hepatic injury as defined by alt or ast > 1,000 IU/L. Most clinicians in the United States use the lower line, as the FDA required a margin of error to prevent errors in history taking prior to approving N-acetyl-cysteine (NAC) as an antidote.

Patients with "chronic" overdose, that is, multiple ingestions, cannot be risk assessed using the nomogram. Those

patients must be assessed by history of ingestion (>150 mg/kg has been suggested to be a toxic threshold) and by assessing for risk factors. Risk factors for hepatotoxicity include chronic exposure to substances that induce CYP 2E1. including ethanol, isoniazid, anticonvulsants, starvation, or recent viral illness. Patients determined to be at risk for APAP hepatotoxicity should have APAP level and baseline hepatic transaminase levels performed. If transaminases are elevated, the patient should be evaluated for evidence of hepatic failure including prothrombin time and clinical evaluation for hepatic encephalopathy. BUN and creatinine should be assayed as well because of the small but significant incidence of renal failure. APAP toxicity should be considered in the differential diagnosis of any patient presenting with acute hepatic failure.

Treatment

Treatment of APAP poisoning consists of decontamination, supportive care, antidote administration, and enhanced elimination. Decontamination consists of the administration of single dose activated charcoal in the usual fashion. No role has been demonstrated for multiple doses of charcoal. Gastric emptying procedures, cathartics, or whole bowel irrigation are not recommended. Charcoal should be administered if there is any possibility that APAP remains in the gut. Some authors have recommended that charcoal administration should not occur concurrently with NAC administration as this will reduce the amount of NAC absorbed. It is reasonable practice to separate the administration of charcoal and NAC by at least one hour if possible; however, no clear clinical benefit has been shown by the practice of delaying antidotal treatment. The clinician should never delay NAC therapy beyond eight hours after ingestion in order to administer charcoal.

Supportive care consists of the standard resuscitative measures, adequate fluid replacement, and any other standard measures dictated by the patient's clinical state. An effort should be made to ensure that the patient is euvolemic in order to ensure that assessment of renal status is accurate. Vitamin K, fresh frozen plasma, and other measures to correct coagulopathy in the absence of hemorrhage should be avoided if at all possible so that assessment of hepatic synthetic function will not be confounded. Sedation should be used judiciously as well to allow the patient's metal status to be monitored.

NAC should be administered to all patients with acute single overdose who have a serum APAP level that puts them at risk for toxicity based on the Rumack-Matthews nomogram. It is important to remember that levels prior to four hours cannot be used to make this determination. Also, patients who present greater that eight hours after their overdose should have NAC administered empirically, as the effectiveness of antidote administration decreases after eight hours. NAC administration may be subsequently discontinued if levels do not warrant treatment. NAC may be given orally or intravenously. Standard dosing requires a loading dose of 140 mg/kg followed by 17 maintenance doses of 70 mg/kg every four hours in the United States. Shorter courses are administered in Europe, Canada, Australia, and in some U.S. centers. It is likely

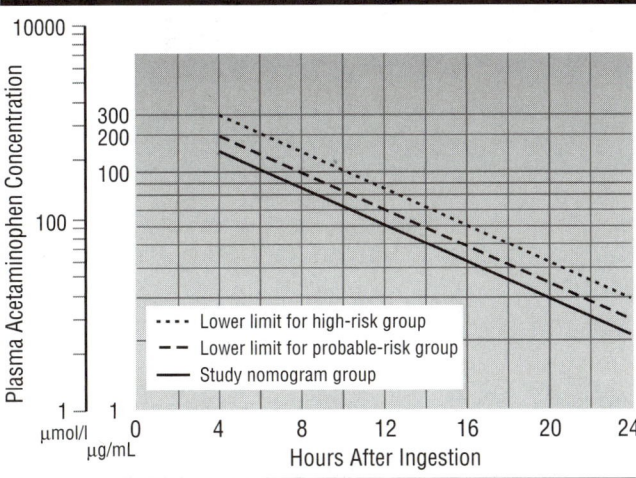

FIGURE 134.1 The Rumack-Matthews nomogram for predicting acetaminophen hepatotoxicity. Levels above the highest line indicate a high likelihood of hepatotoxicity. Levels above the middle line indicate an intermediate likelihood of toxicity. The lowest line is typically used in the United States to determine the need for therapy and allows for error when determining the time of ingestion.

that the trend toward reducing the duration of treatment will continue; however, clinicians not experienced in the management of APAP overdose and toxicity should seek specialty consultation with regard to duration of treatment. Patients who display evidence of hepatotoxicity should continue NAC treatment indefinitely beyond the prescribed course of therapy regardless of APAP level, as there is clear clinical evidence of survival benefit.

Patients with "chronic" overdose for whom the risk of toxicity is difficult to determine should be started on NAC in the standard fashion and observed. If there is no rise in transaminase levels by 24 hours after APAP level has gone to zero, then NAC can be discontinued. Patients with evidence of toxicity should continue treatment until toxicity is resolved.

APAP is amenable to removal by dialysis. Dialysis should be considered for patients who present following massive exposures with levels in the 800 to 1000 μg/mL range, as these patients nearly always succumb to toxicity despite NAC therapy.

Disposition

Patients deemed to require therapy should be admitted to a standard medical bed. In the absence of hepatic failure, intensive care unit admission is generally unnecessary. Patients who display evidence of hepatic failure should be admitted to an intensive care unit. Given the potential for rapid demise, involvement of transplant surgeon should be sought as soon as hepatic synthetic failure becomes evident. Patients who fail to display toxicity after appropriate evaluation and treatment or those who recover from toxicity may be safely discharged. As with any ingestion, the circumstances leading to the overdose should be carefully explored. Patients who have accidentally overdosed should be instructed in the appropriate use of APAP. Patients with intentional overdose should undergo psychiatric evaluation prior to discharge from medical care.

Selected Readings

Harrison PM, Keays R, Bray GP, et al. Improved outcome of paracetamol-induced fulminant hepatic failure by late administration of acetylcysteine. *Lancet* 1990;335:1572–1573.

James LP, Mayeux PR, Hinson JA. Acetaminophen-induced hepatotoxicity. *Drug Metab Dispos* 2003;31:1499–1506.

Keays R, Harrison PM, Wendon JA, et al. Intravenous acetylcysteine in paracetamol induced fulminant hepatic failure: a prospective controlled trial. *BMJ* 1991;303:1026–1029.

Rumack BH. Acetaminophen hepatotoxicity: the first 35 years. *J Toxicol Clin Toxicol* 2002;40:3–20.

Smilkstein MJ, Knapp GL, Kulig KW, et al. Efficacy of oral N-acetylcysteine in the treatment of acetaminophen overdose. Analysis of the national multicenter study (1976 to 1985). *N Engl J Med* 1988;319:1557–1562.

Salicylates

Kavita Babu

Salicylates represent one of the oldest pharmacological therapies known to humans. Even before Hippocrates, the Native Americans and Greeks had discovered the antipyretic and analgesic properties of chewing willow bark (Salix species). Now, salicylate-containing products are essentially ubiquitous in American homes.

The number of cases of salicylate toxicity has steadily decreased in the United States since the 1970s. The association of aspirin therapy with Reye's syndrome in children and the advent of safety packaging have been credited with this decline. The most common salicylate formulations include aspirin (acetylsalicylic acid), antidiarrheal agents (Pepto-Bismol), topical acne medications, muscle liniments, and oil of wintergreen. Herbal preparations containing willow, poplar, or meadowsweet also include varying amounts of salicylates; all of these may be found as ingredients in common body building and weight loss supplements. Notably, the concentration of salicylate in topical preparations and oil of wintergreen makes ingestion of these substances particularly toxic. As little as one teaspoons of oil of wintergreen may cause lethal toxicity in a small child.

Salicylate toxicity occurs at the level of the mitochondria where it uncouples oxidative phosphorylation. The metabolic derangements caused by salicylate toxicity affect every organ system and present with a large variety of symptoms.

Pharmacology

Salicylates produce their antipyretic, anti-inflammatory, and analgesic activities via the irreversible inactivation of cyclooxygenase and subsequent inhibition of prostaglandin synthesis. Aspirin alone has additional antiplatelet activity. It is available in oral, topical, and suppository forms. The recommended dose is 10 to 15 mg/kg every 4 to 6 hours with a maximum recommended daily dose of 80 mg/kg. Aspirin is a weak acid (pKa 3.5) that is absorbed in the stomach and small bowel. Appreciable serum levels occur 30 minutes after a single dose, and peak at 2 to 4 hours postingestion. Therapeutic serum levels of aspirin range from 15 to 30 mg/dL. Once

in the bloodstream, aspirin is rapidly degraded to its active metabolite, salicylic acid, by plasma esterases. Aspirin is highly protein-bound with a small volume of distribution (0.15 kg/L). Metabolism is primarily hepatic with a serum half-life of 2 hours. At low concentrations, the metabolism of aspirin follows first-order kinetics.

Pathophysiology

In toxicity, the pharmacokinetics of aspirin change markedly. Toxicity may be seen in acute overdoses of 150 mg/kg. At high therapeutic and toxic doses, metabolism follows zero-order kinetics as enzyme systems responsible for aspirin metabolism become saturated. Additionally, aspirin toxicity delays gastric emptying, while enteric-coated and sustained release preparations may further prolong absorption. Thus, the half-life of aspirin in overdose may approach 15 to 30 hours. Aspirin may also form intestinal concretions that contribute to prolonged absorption. At high serum levels, protein-binding sites become saturated, leading to increased free aspirin concentrations in the plasma. The metabolic acidosis caused by salicylate toxicity further decreases protein binding. As more aspirin becomes available for tissue distribution, the volume of distribution may increase dramatically.

Once hepatic metabolism is saturated, urinary excretion becomes the primary means of elimination. The amount of aspirin eliminated in the urine varies based on glomerular filtration of the non-ionized drug and active secretion of the ionized form in the proximal tubule. The non-ionized form is then passively reabsorbed from the urine in the distal tubule. In normal renal function, increased urine output improves glomerular filtration and tubular secretion. Alkalinization of the urine favors the ionized form, decreasing the amount of aspirin reabsorbed. Maintenance of euvolemia, adequate urine output and alkaline urine are critical to improving aspirin elimination. Unfortunately, hypovolemia and acidosis are commonly seen in salicylate toxicity, and must be aggressively corrected. Acidemia favors the movement of serum salicylate into the brain and worsens CNS toxicity.

Clinical Presentation

The symptoms of acute salicylate toxicity can be separated into early, middle, and late phases that approximate mild, moderate, and severe intoxication. During the early (mild) phase of toxicity, symptoms of abdominal pain and vomiting predominate. As serum levels increase, salicylates stimulate the medullary respiratory center and cause tachypnea. In adults, respiratory alkalosis is the earliest metabolic derangement. The kidneys respond by increasing urinary output of bicarbonate, and urine pH is typically alkaline at this point. Electrolytes are often normal in the early phase and the degree of hypovolemia may not be fully appreciated. The early neurologic symptoms of salicylate toxicity include tinnitus, headache, vertigo, and lethargy.

The middle (moderate) phase of toxicity begins at 12 to 24 hours after ingestion. In this phase, patients exhibit the classic mixed metabolic derangement associated with salicylate toxicity, respiratory alkalosis, and metabolic acidosis. The patient's initial alkalemia will give way to acidemia without treatment and CNS levels of salicylate rise.

Confusion, agitation, hallucinations, and deafness signal worsening toxicity. Vital sign abnormalities in this phase include hyperthermia, tachycardia, and hypotension secondary to hypovolemia.

The late (severe) phase of toxicity occurs at 24 hours post-ingestion. As the metabolic acidosis progressively worsens, critical CNS dysfunction presents as cerebral edema, seizures, and coma. Patients may develop renal failure and hepatic dysfunction with resultant coagulopathy. Noncardiogenic pulmonary edema results from increased capillary permeability. Cardiac dysrhythmias, congestive heart failure, and hypotension are also seen with this degree of toxicity. Acid-base disturbances and electrolyte abnormalities also contribute to multi-system dysfunction.

Chronic salicylate toxicity and pediatric salicylate overdoses represent two special populations. Chronic salicylate toxicity is much more common in elderly patients and very difficult to diagnose. Noncardiogenic pulmonary edema in an elderly patient should always prompt consideration of salicylate toxicity. The neurological manifestations of chronic salicylate toxicity are protean, including tremor, paranoia, confusion, and papilledema. The mortality of chronic salicylate toxicity has been reported as high as 25%; this is likely due to the occurrence of this toxicity in a susceptible, elderly population as well as increased time to treatment secondary to delayed diagnosis. In children less than four years of age, metabolic acidosis is the most commonly seen metabolic derangement. Chronic salicylate toxicity should be suspected in any child exposed to salicylates who presents with tachypnea, dehydration, or vomiting.

Salicylate levels are helpful in anticipating the course of salicylate toxicity; however, the patient's clinical picture must be the primary determinant of their therapy. A salicylate concentration of 30 mg/dL in a symptomatic patient suggests salicylate toxicity. A level of 100 mg/dL portends severe toxicity. A concentration of 160 mg/dL is associated with high risk of mortality. Salicylate concentrations obtained less than six hours after ingestion may not reflect the true severity of the ingestion. In the symptomatic patient, serial concentrations should be drawn until they begin to fall. If the patient ingested an enteric-coated preparation, inpatient observation may be necessary as levels may peak from six to 30 hours post-ingestion. In chronic toxicity, the utility of salicylate concentration is low except to confirm the presence of salicylates; therapy should be guided by clinical presentation. The general public cannot always reliably distinguish preparations containing acetaminophen and salicylates; in cases of suspected overdose, both levels should be obtained.

Treatment

Management of the salicylate-intoxicated patient must begin with attention to the ABCs. If CNS depression prevents airway protection, or salicylate-induced lung injury causes severe hypoxia, endotracheal intubation is necessary. However, there is real risk for acute deterioration after intubation. An unchecked metabolic acidosis may lead to sudden cardiovascular collapse as the patient loses their ability to compensate with a respiratory alkalosis. *The patient's minute ventilation must be maximized and close attention paid to serial blood pH measurements.*

Monitoring of serum glucose is critical. As metabolic rates increase to compensate for impaired oxidative phosphorylation, glucose and glycogen stores are rapidly utilized. In salicylate toxicity, CNS glucose levels are significantly lower than controls, even in the presence of normal serum glucose. Continuous infusion of a dextrose-containing solution to maintain normoglycemia or even mild hyperglycemia is recommended. Seizures may be a result of hypoglycemia or cerebral edema. After ruling out hypoglycemia, seizures may be treated with benzodiazepines.

The use of charcoal for decontamination in salicylate toxicity has been well studied, but the results are still controversial. Single-dose activated charcoal does reduce the absorption of aspirin at therapeutic doses. Multi-dose activated charcoal may further enhance elimination. Charcoal may be administered at a dose of 1 to 2 g/kg every four to six hours. Early administration of charcoal is necessary as efficacy falls as time from exposure increases. Whole bowel irrigation may be considered in overdose of enteric-coated preparation or in patients whose salicylate levels persistently rise. Patients who present with salicylate toxicity after use of topical preparations should undergo thorough *soap and water* decontamination.

Fluid resuscitation and alkalinization of the urine are the two most essential goals in enhancing salicylate elimination. Patients with salicylate toxicity are typically hypovolemic, from vomiting, tachypnea, hyperthermia, and diaphoresis. The target urine output in patients with normal renal function should be 3 to 5 cc/kg/h. Forced diuresis is not necessary and can worsen cerebral and pulmonary edema. Alkalinization of the urine requires administration of intravenous bicarbonate. In the acidemic patient, a bolus dose of 1 to 2 mEq/kg is indicated. Subsequently, patients must be started on a continuous infusion of bicarbonate (100 to 150 mEq sodium bicarbonate in 1 liter of 5% dextrose in water). The rate of administration in adults is 150 to 200 mL/h (twice the maintenance rate in children), aiming for a target urine pH of 8.0. Serial serum pH measurements must also be obtained; a serum pH greater than 7.55 creates the risk of complications secondary to acidemia. Adequate urinary alkalinization may be difficult or impossible in the face of hypokalemia. However, potassium replacement should not delay the administration of bicarbonate. There is no role for acetazolamide in alkalinizing the urine as it may worsen systemic acidemia and CNS penetration of salicylates.

Extracorporeal means of eliminating salicylates should be considered early in patients who have significant salicylate toxicity. While both hemodialysis and hemoperfusion are effective in eliminating salicylates, hemodialysis can additionally correct electrolyte and acid-base abnormalities. Thus, hemodialysis is preferred. Indications for hemodialysis include any condition that prevents adequate achievement of urinary alkalinization or volume resuscitation, such as renal failure, congestive heart failure, and acute lung injury. Other indications include worsening vital signs or CNS depression, severe-acid base disturbances, persistent electrolyte abnormalities, and salicylate levels greater than 100 mg/dL. If hemodialysis is not available at the treating institution, transfer to a tertiary care center must be arranged.

Patients with suspected salicylate toxicity should be admitted to a highly monitored/ intensive care unit setting. Given the gravity and complexity of severe salicylate toxicity, early consultation with a Poison Center and toxicologist is required.

Selected Readings

English M, Marsh V, Amukoye E, et al. Chronic salicylate poisoning and severe malaria. *Lancet* 1996;347:1736–1737.

Flomenbaum NE. Salicylates. In: Goldfrank LR, Flomenbaum NE, Lewin NA, et al., eds. *Goldfrank's Toxicologic Emergencies*, 7th ed. New York: McGraw-Hill, 2002:507–527.

Kirshenbaum LA. Does multiple-dose charcoal therapy enhance salicylate excretion? *Arch Intern Med* 1990;150:1281–1283.

Temple AR. Acute and chronic effects of aspirin toxicity and their treatment. *Arch Intern Med* 1981;141:364–369.

Yip L, Dart R. Concepts and controversies in salicylate toxicity. *Emerg Med Clin North Am* 1994;12:351–364.

136 | Cocaine

Tamas R. Peredy
Charles McKay

Cocaine (Benzoyl-methyl-ecgonine) is the most potent naturally occurring stimulant and the only naturally occurring local anesthetic. A member of the tropane family (e.g., atropine), this plant alkaloid is present in the mature leaves of the *Erythroxylon coca* shrub native to the Andes region of South America. For centuries it was known by the local natives that the saliva of those who chewed the coca leaves (with co-ingested lime for alkaline extraction) acted as a (1) local anesthetic able to facilitate painful procedures such as skull trephination and (2) a stimulant warding off fatigue and hunger. Following colonization of this region, exportation of the purified hydrochloride salt rose dramatically through the 1800s to meet the increasing demands of Europeans and subsequently North Americans. By beginning of the twentieth century, numerous over-the-counter products at U.S. drug stores contained cocaine as active ingredient. In response, regulatory efforts targeting cocaine included the 1906 Pure Food and Drug Act required ingredient labeling and the 1914 Harrison Tax Act restricting its distribution. Cocaine use remained limited until the late 1970s; after that time, improved distribution systems and the development of new products such as "crack" cocaine led to an increase in abuse of the drug.

Pharmacology

Nasal insufflation ("snorting") remains the most common route of administration. Cocaine powder is water soluble for IV use referred to as *mainlining*. Roughly 10% of regular cocaine users prefer the IV route. Concurrent heroin injection or *speedballing* is common. *Crack* cocaine is a crystalline heat-stable base extracted by local street distributors or addicts using sodium bicarbonate. Of those users who have tried it once, smoking crack is the preferred method of administration in 75%.

Following nasal insufflation, central nervous system (CNS) effects begin within 3 to 5 minutes with a peak plasma level at 60 minutes and persisting for up to 6 hours. Local effects, consisting of nasal mucosal vasoconstriction, limit and prolong cocaine absorption. Cocaine administered by intravenous and inhalational routes produces drug effects within seconds and last 1 to 2 hours. Psychological urges to reproduce the short-lived euphoria may result in a binging pattern of abuse until catecholamine stores are depleted.

Parent compound can be detected in the urine within 30 minutes and for up to 6 to 8 hours following use. Tests for benzoylecgonine typically remain positive for several days but may persist for more than a week following binges.

Physiology

Cocaine blocks the epinephrine and norepinephrine reuptake in the presynaptic neuron resulting in adrenergic excess. Increased levels of sympathomimetic neurotransmitters lead to increased vigilance, agitation, paranoia, and seizures. Repetitive use of cocaine leads to tachyphylaxis, requiring escalating dose to achieve the potent orgasm-like euphoria. Moreover, repetitive cocaine use produces intense psychological cravings.

In the periphery, decreased reuptake leads to increased circulating catecholamines, principally norepinephrine (NE). Stimulation of α and β receptors produces the classic sympathomimetic toxidrome of tachycardia, hypertension, hyperthermia, mydriasis, and diaphoresis. Intense vasoconstriction may result in organ ischemia, particularly the heart, kidney, and gut. Hypertension can lead to vascular catastrophe, including aortic dissection and intracranial hemorrhage.

Clinical Presentations

Irrespective of presenting complaints, initial evaluation of cocaine-abusing patients should include a full set of vital signs including pulse oximetry; patients should also receive continuous cardiac monitoring. Bedside capillary glucose measurements should be performed and hypoglycemia corrected immediately. Visual inspection of the entire patient is necessary to rule out occult trauma. Intravenous fluid resuscitation often will be needed due to increased insensible fluid losses. Any patient with an altered mental status, significant psychiatric history, severe situational stress, or drug ingestion should be evaluated for possible co-ingestants including acetaminophen, alcohol, other street drugs, and prescription medications. Objective studies are dictated by the severity of the intoxication but may include electrolytes, serum osmolality, renal and liver function tests, specific emergently available drug levels including acetaminophen, ethanol level, CPK, type and screen, electrocardiogram, and head CT.

Most patients with cocaine intoxication present with only mild to moderate symptomatology. They may manifest findings of restlessness, tremor, diaphoresis, fasciculations. and other abnormalities consistent with a sympathomimetic toxidrome. Clinicians should remain vigilant, however, for progression of toxicity and sudden cardiopulmonary collapse.

Different routes of administration are associated with specific sequelae. Facial or bilateral palmar thermal burns, carbonaceous sputum, reactive airway disease, and pulmonary barotrauma may arise from smoking cocaine. Pneumomediastinum, pneumothorax, and pneumopericardium are associated with forced inhalation, while perforated nasal septum is seen following insufflation. Intravenous drug abuse may lead to skin foreign body or abscess, phlebitis, cellulitis, venous thrombosis, and acute infectious endocarditis.

Chest Pain

Chest pain—both that suggestive of cardiac origin as well as atypical pain—is the most frequent cocaine-related ED complaint. A number of lines of evidence converge to suggest that *any* patient presenting with cocaine-associated chest pain should be admitted for evaluation and management. First, cocaine use accounts for 25% of myocardial infarctions patients younger than 45 years. Second, the incidence of MI among ED chest pain patients with recent cocaine use is 5% to 10% with another 10% demonstrating reversible myocardial ischemia. Third, crack cocaine use within the previous 24 hours results in a double digit odds ratio increase of an acute cardiac event. Moreover, the absence of risk factors such as family history of heart disease, hypertension, diabetes, or hyperlipidemia does not obviate the need for admission for further evaluation.

The initial EKG is an unreliable assessment tool due to both a high false negative and false positive rate. EKG abnormalities are seen in two thirds of all patients with approximately 40% meeting standard criteria for thrombolytic therapy. Early repolarization and left ventricular hypertrophy are common. Subtle or no EKG changes likely contribute to the inappropriate ED discharge rate 4 times greater than that of the missed MI unrelated to cocaine. Total CK may be misleading due to frequently seen skeletal muscle breakdown, but cardiac specific marker (CK-MB, Troponin I, T) elevations remain useful in identifying myocardial injury.

While under continuous cardiac monitoring, initial treatment modalities include supplemental oxygen, aspirin, benzodiazepines, and nitroglycerin. Calcium channel blockers and phentolamine have been demonstrated to attenuate vasoconstriction and hypertension. The use of β-blockers is contraindicated. Use of sodium nitroprusside and labetolol may be considered to treat hypertension. Heparin is indicated in the setting of unstable angina but should be used with caution if severe hypertension or altered mental status is present. Fibrinolytics therapy has been safely administered but should be used extremely cautiously in light of unreliable EKG findings and excellent patient prognosis without this therapy.

In addition to acute coronary syndromes in the setting of cocaine-induced chest pain, other cardiovascular diagnoses such as aortic or coronary artery dissection, cardiomyopathy, myocarditis, and endocarditis must be considered.

Mental Status Changes

Agitated delirium is a common presentation of acute cocaine intoxication. Unsuccessful verbal de-escalation techniques should prompt consideration for chemical sedation using benzodiazepines. Failure to adequately sedate patients carries the risks of rhabdomyolysis, hyperpyrexia, seizures. and sudden cardiac death. Phenothiazines are relatively contraindicated because this class of drugs inhibits heat dissipation and increases the risk of seizure.

Lethargy and depression following binge cocaine use are common and has been termed the *cocaine washout syndrome*; however. any inability to easily arouse a patient with gentle stimulus should raise suspicion for a possible acute CNS event such as meningoencephalitis, stroke, intracranial (e.g., subarachnoid) hemorrhage, hypertensive encephalopathy, aneurysmal rupture, or dural sinus thrombosis.

Dopamine hyperactivity and subsequent depletion from the basal ganglia (shift in the dopaminergic-cholinergic balance) associated with cocaine use may result in a variety of movement disorders including acute dystonias, tremor, and choreoathetosis (crack dancing). Diphenhydramine is the preferred therapy for acute dystonias, but this agent may exacerbate hyperthermia. Phenothiazines are relatively contraindicated as they further predispose patients to movement disorders, impaired heat dissipation, and increased risk of seizure.

Hyperpyrexia associated with cocaine use is due deranged thermoregulatory capacity and an inability to dissipation heat. Core body temperatures above 104° F (40° C) represent a potential medical emergency requiring the use of cooling techniques such as fans and cool mist.

Cocaine-induced generalized tonic-clonic seizures are seen in up to 10% of addicts presenting to the ED. Seizures can be a harbinger of serious toxicity exacerbating underlying metabolic acidosis, rhabdomyolysis, and hyperthermia. Aggressive treatment with benzodiazepines and fluid resuscitation are needed to avoid renal failure, dysrhythmias, and sudden death. Phenytoin is contraindicated.

Other Clinical Manifestations

Cocaine affects virtually all organ systems. Gastrointestinal effects of cocaine use may include ischemic bowel, hypomotility, ulceration, or frank perforation. Renal failure can occur from acute tubular necrosis, rhabdomyolysis, infarction, or glomerulosclerosis. CT scanning or arteriography may be necessary to ascertain the diagnosis.

Cocaine exerts well-documented effects on fetal development. Obstetric complications of cocaine use include spontaneous abortion, abruptio placentae, premature labor, rupture of membranes, and early delivery. Fetal effects include low birth weight, increased risk of congenital anomalies, seizures, hyperirritability, and long-lasting cognitive impairment. Following birth, neonates may experience significant withdrawal symptoms. Despite the avoidance of intravenous needles, crack cocaine use has led to HIV infectivity rates among regular users equivalent to intravenous drug users, likely due to sexual promiscuity.

Special Considerations

Drug traffickers continue to search for clandestine methods of illegal drug transport. Individuals known as *mules* are paid to ingest large numbers of sealed cocaine balloons for delivery via subsequent defecation after arrival. Many times the lethal dose of cocaine is ingested in carefully sealed latex condom balloons. Expected signs and symptoms of cocaine intoxication from leakage of small amounts of drug may identify the *cocaine body packer.* Drug packets will be visible on plain abdominal radiography in greater than 90% of cases. In the asymptomatic patient, rapid removal of the lethal cargo is best performed by whole bowel irrigation. Initially, 2 liters of a balanced electrolyte solution such as Go-Lytely® is administered via NG and continued at 500 mL/hour until it is believed that all packets have passed. Signs of intestinal obstruction require immediate surgical intervention. Endoscopy, although successful in removing packets, is generally avoided given the potential risk of balloon rupture with manipulation. The body packer should be distinguished from the *cocaine body stuffer,* who hastily swallows the illicit cocaine in order to evade discovery by law authorities. They may present with similar features but are at greater risk of complications within the first few hours, despite smaller amounts of ingested drug, because of the poor packaging. Radiographs are rarely useful in these patients unless the bags were stapled shut. Patients suspected of cocaine ingestion should be considered for ICU admission, particularly in the setting of sympathomimetic symptoms. Resuscitation efforts are similar to those described elsewhere in this chapter.

Conclusions

Cocaine is a drug commonly encountered upon history taking of patients in the emergency department and is often the underlying precipitant of the visit. Clinicians should address vital sign abnormalities during resuscitation including temperature. Special attention should be paid to potential cardiac and neurological toxicity. Severe alterations in acid-base status are common. A broad work-up for delirious patients including a search for co-ingestants is necessary. Medications commonly used in the ED such as β-blockers and phenothiazines may exhibit deleterious effects in cocaine intoxicated patients. Emergency physicians must be aware of their local treatment resources and advocate for abstinence and rehabilitation from illicit drug use. **Table 136.1** is a list of common clinical manifestations of cocaine use.

Table 136.1
Common Clinical Manifestations

System	Clinical Manifestion
Neurologic	Agitated Delirium/Psychosis
	Ischemic or Thrombotic Stroke
	Intracranial Hemorrhage
	Hypertensive Encephalopathy
	Seizure
	Movement Disorder
Cardiovascular	Myocardial Ischemia/Infarction
	Dysrhythmias
	Cardiomyopathy/Myocarditis
	Arterial Dissection or Hemorrhage
Pulmonary	Pulmonary Infarction/Hemorrhage
	Barotrauma
	Reactive Airway Disease
	Pneumonitis
	Pulmonary Edema
Other Organs	Rhabdomyolysis
	Acute Renal Failure
	Bowel Ischemia/Infarction
	Fetal Demise/Spontaneous Abortion

Selected Readings

Aks SE, Vander Hoek TL, Hryhorczuk DO, et al. Cocaine liberation from body packets in an in vitro model. *Ann Emerg Med* 1992;21:1321–1325.

Bauman JL, DiDomenico RJ. Cocaine-induced channelopathies: emerging evidence on the multiple mechanisms of sudden death. *J Cardiovasc Pharmacol Ther* 2002;7:195–202.

Baumann BM, Perrone J, Hornig SE, et al. Randomized, double blind, placebo-controlled trial of diazepam, nitroglycerin or both for the treament of patients with potential cocaine-associated acute coronary syndromes. *Acad Emerg Med* 2000;7:878–885.

Boghdadi MS, Henning RJ. Cocaine: pathophysiology and clinical toxicology. *Heart Lung* 1997;26:466–483.

Brogan WC, Lange RA, Glamann B, et al. Recurrent coronary vasoconstriction caused by intranasal cocaine: possible role for metabolites. *Ann Int Med* 1992;116:556–561.

Catalano G, Catalano MC, Rodriguez R. Dystonia associated with crack cocaine use. *So Med J* 1997. Available at http://www.sma.org/smj1997/octsmj97/17text.htm. Accessed June 2004.

Curry SC, Kolecki PF. Poisoning by sodium channel blocking agents. *Crit Care Clin* 1997;13:829–848.

Erwin MB, Deliargyris EN. Cocaine-associated chest pain. *Am J Med Sci* 2002;324:37–44.

Farre M, De La Torre R, Gonzalez ML, et al. Cocaine and alcohol interactions in humans: neuroendocrine effects and cocaethylene metabolism. *J Pharmacol Exp Ther* 1997;283:164–176.

Fines RE, Brady WJ, DeBehnke DJ. Cocaine-associated dystonic reaction. *J Emerg Med* 1997;15:513–516.

Gawin FH, Ellinwood EH. Cocaine and other simulants, actions, abuse and treatment. *N Engl J Med* 1988;318:1173–1182.

Geyskens P, Coenen L, Brouwers J. The "cocaine body packer" syndrome, case report and review of the literature. *Acta Chir Belg* 1989;89:201–203.

Goodman PE, Rennie WP. Renal infarction secondary to nasal insufflation of cocaine. *Am J Emerg Med* 1995;13:421–423.

Hatsukami DK, Fischman MW. Crack cocaine and cocaine hydrochloride: are the differences myth or reality? *JAMA* 1996;276:1580–1588.

Hoffman RS, Hollander JE. Evaluation of patients with chest pain after cocaine use. *Crit Care Clin* 1997;13:809–828.

Hollander JE. The management of cocaine-associated myocardial ischemia. *N Engl J Med* 1995;333:1267–1272.

Jawahar D, Leo PJ, Anandarao N, et al. Cocaine-associated intestinal gangrene in a pregnant woman. *Am J Emerg Med* 1997;15:510–512.

Lange RA, Cigarroa RG, Flores ED, et al. Potentiation of cocaine-induced coronary vasoconstriction by beta-adrenergic blockade. *Ann Int Med* 1990;112:897–902.

Malbrain ML, Neels H, Vissers K, et al. A massive, near-fatal cocaine intoxication in a body-stuffer. *Acta Clinica Belg* 1994;49:12–18.

McCance EF, Price LH, Kosten TR, et al. Cocaethylene: pharmacology, physiology and behavioral effects in humans. *J Pharmacol Exp Ther* 1995;274:215–223.

Mittleman MA, Mintzer D, Maclure M, et al. Triggering of myocardial infarction by cocaine. *Circulation* 1999;99:2737–2741.

Perron AD, Gibbs M. Thoracic aortic dissection secondary to crack cocaine ingestion. *Am J Emerg Med* 1997;15:507–509.

Riordan M, Rylance G, Berry K. Poisoning in children: rare and dangerous poisons. *Arch Dis Child* 2002;87:407–410.

Roberts JR, Price D, Goldfrank L, et al. The body stuffer syndrome: a clandestine form of drug overdose. *Am J Emerg Med* 1986;4:24–27.

Shanti, CM, Lucas CE. Cocaine and the critical care challenge. *Crit Care Med* 2003;31:1851–1859.

Warner EA. Cocaine abuse. *Ann Intern Med* 1993;119:226–235.

Weber JE, Chudnofsky CR, Boczar M, et al. Cocaine-associated chest pain: how common is myocardial infarction? *Acad Emerg Med* 2000;7:873–877.

Weber JE, Shofer FS, Larkin, et al. Validation of a brief observation period for patients with cocaine-associated chest pain. *N Engl J Med* 2003;348:510–517.

Wilson LD, Shelat C. Electrophysiologic and hemodynamic effects of sodium bicarbonate in a canine model of severe intoxication. *J Toxicol Clin Toxicol* 2003;41:777–788.

137 Opiates and Opioids

Nicole C. Bouchard
Rama B. Rao

Opioids are a class of natural and synthetic agents that are used largely as analgesics, sedatives, cough suppressants, and antidiarrheals. Natural opium derivatives of the poppy plant *Papaver somniferum* are termed *opiates*. Morphine and codeine are both opiates. Semisynthetic agents (e.g., heroin and oxycodone) and synthetic agents (e.g., fentanyl and meperidine) are structurally related to opiates and share binding affinity to opioid receptors. These, along with opiates, comprise the larger classification of opioids. The term *narcotic,* though commonly used in association with illicit drugs of abuse, refers strictly to a drug that induces a somnolent state or *narcosis*.

Opioids produce their clinical effects by binding to specific central nervous system (CNS) receptors that normally bind endogenous opioid peptides such as endorphins, enkephalins, and dynorphins. The mu_1 (opioid) receptor modulates pain, provides analgesia, CNS depression, and euphoria. The mu_2 receptor mediates respiratory depression and decreases in GI motility. Spinal analgesia is mediated by kappa, delta, and mu_2 receptors. Most opioids used in clinical practice are predominantly mu receptor agonists.

Repetitive stimulation of these receptors with chronic opioid use induces tolerance, so higher doses of the drug are required to produce the same clinical effect. Cross-tolerance exists between opioids. Patients who develop tolerance are at risk for both physical and psychological dependence. Abrupt cessation of opioid use or reversal of opioid binding with a competitive antagonist (e.g., naloxone) can result in withdrawal. Clinical manifestations of the opiate abstinence syndrome include rhinorrhea, lacrimation, abdominal cramping, piloerection, yawning, vomiting, and diarrhea. Although opioid withdrawal produces dysphoria and is extremely unpleasant for the patient, it is usually self-limited and is unlikely to cause serious morbidity in alert, adult patients who are able to protect their airway.

Opioid Toxicity

Opioid toxicity or *overdose* is a common presentation in many emergency departments (EDs). Common overdoses involve heroin, methadone, and prescription analgesics. Iatrogenic *oversedation* with opioids also occurs relatively frequently during procedural sedation in the ED. The classic clinical findings in the opioid intoxicated patient include CNS depression, respiratory depression (i.e., hypopnea and bradypnea), miosis, and decreased gastrointestinal (GI) motility. Mid-sized to dilated pupils can be seen with co-ingestants or severe hypoxia. Death is usually from hypoxia or from complications of respiratory depression and sedation.

The primary therapeutic goal in caring for patients with opioid toxicity is reversal of respiratory depression. Apneic patients or those with profound respiratory depression require airway immediate airway management with ventilation with 100% oxygen via bag-valve mask. This serves to both deliver oxygen and decrease PCO_2. Dog models suggest that decreasing hypercarbia through hyperventilation prior to antagonist administration may blunt the catecholamine surge that is associated with abrupt reversal. This may potentially diminish the occurrence of noncardiogenic pulmonary edema (see **Special Considerations** section). When naloxone is used appropriately, intubation can be avoided in most patients.

In patients with presumed oral opioid ingestion, decontamination with activated charcoal (1 g/kg) via nasogastric tube (NGT) should only be administered if the patient is not considered to be an aspiration risk. Aspiration pneumonitis alone or with charcoal is associated with significant morbidity. Serum levels for acetaminophen and salicylate should be sent in all suicidal patients with toxic ingestions as they are common suicidal ingestants as well as common ingredients in many combination analgesic preparations. Drug abusers often co-ingest multiple drugs. A classic example of this is a *speedball* in which heroin and cocaine are used simultaneously. These patients may present sedated with a clinical syndrome ranging from classic opioid toxicity to coma with normal respirations and nonspecific pupil size dependent on the relative amount of each illicit agent. The use of opioid antagonists in these patients may unmask the underlying cocaine intoxication and result in a severely agitated patient. In comatose patients suspected of overdosing on heroin or other illicit substances, titration of naloxone in small increments to an endpoint of adequate respirations can prevent the sudden and uncontrolled agitation that can be associated with antagonist precipitated withdrawal.

Alternatively, patients who do not respond appropriately to adequate doses of opioid antagonist require further investigation of their depressed or altered mental status. Hypoglycemia, sedative-hypnotic agents, CNS infection, or intracranial hemorrhage are etiologies of persistent coma that require consideration and management.

Naloxone Administration

The titration of an appropriate dose of naloxone should be guided by clinical presentation, history of the opioid exposure, and whenever possible, potential for precipitating withdrawal. In the presence of spontaneous respirations, naloxone can be titrated to adequate ventilation in 0.05 to 0.1 mg aliquots. The likelihood of response to naloxone is greatest in patients with a respiratory rate < 12 breaths/min. This dose can be increased if necessary (q1–2 min). The end point of reversal with opioid antagonist should be adequate ventilation and not necessarily complete reversal of sedation. High doses of intravenous or intramuscular naloxone (e.g., 1–2 mg) may be used safely in children and nontolerant individuals. In patients with apnea, artificial ventilation by bag-valve-mask (BVM) can be followed by 1 to 2 mg intravenous naloxone. If BVM is unavailable the empiric dosing with naloxone or intubation should proceed. Naloxone can be given by the intramuscular route when intravenous access is unavailable. Once intubated, naloxone should be avoided. Continuous infusions may be appropriate for patients who overdose with long acting opioids (see below). Patients with the opioid toxidrome and signs of CNS depression with a respiratory rate above 12 breaths/min who have adequate oxygenation do not require immediate reversal. This group can receive either supportive care and close observation, or slow titration of naloxone.

The type and quantity of opioid used, and the route of exposure may affect the naloxone requirements. Most opioids, such as heroin or morphine, require less than a few milligrams of naloxone. Other opioid agents, such as buprenorphine and dextromethorphan may require substantially higher doses. The duration of action of naloxone in the appropriately titrated dose is approximately 30 to 45 minutes. For patients who have recurrent respiratory depression from long acting agents such as methadone, or who are suspected of having large GI stores of opioids, a naloxone infusion can be administered. Two thirds of the dose of naloxone required to achieve the desired clinical response should be administered hourly. Intermittent bolus dosing or infusion dose adjustment may be periodically required. All such patients should be monitored closely and admitted to a critical care environment.

Naloxone is commonly used in both the prehospital and hospital setting to reverse opioid-induced respiratory depression and CNS depression. The typical prehospital use by emergency medical service (EMS) personnel is in the range of 0.4 to 2.0 mg IM or IV. This high dose often precipitates a dramatic and acute withdrawal in the opioid-tolerant individual. Vomiting, aspiration, and severe agitation are common with antagonist-precipitated acute withdrawal. Aspiration is a particular risk following naloxone in opioid-dependent patients with other causes for a depressed level of consciousness.

If acute opioid withdrawal is precipitated by naloxone administration, supportive care is recommended. "Resedation" of an agitated patient in acute withdrawal from naloxone very often leads to an even more profound sedation requiring intubation when naloxone's effects wane.

Longer-acting opioid antagonists such as nalmefene and naltrexone are generally not appropriate for use in the ED secondary to their unpredictable and long duration effect, making withdrawal likely.

Special Considerations

Pulmonary Edema and Medical Complications

Noncardiogenic pulmonary edema is a well described complication of opioid use. Some reported cases of pulmonary edema are attributed to the use of naloxone, via a proposed mechanism that involves a massive catecholamine surge induced by antagonist precipitated withdrawal. It is likely, however, that the etiology is also related to the underlying respiratory status or hypoxic lung injury in these patients. Patients at highest risk for this complication are those with severe respiratory depression or apnea. Pulmonary edema is most likely to occur within the first few hours of opioid intoxication or reversal but delayed onset can occur so these patients should be observed for 24 hours. Signs and symptoms of anoxic encephalopathy may also evolve during this period. All patients with prolonged coma are also at risk for dehydration, rhabdomyolysis, aspiration pneumonia, and compressive neuropathies.

Contaminants and Adulterants

Use of illicit opioids has multiple risks including contaminants or adulterants. Numerous toxic and infectious epidemics have been associated with illicit heroin. In 1995, several cases of anticholinergic toxicity were reported as a result of scopolamine-tainted heroin. Wound botulism, tetanus, and transmission of the human immunodeficiency virus are associated with the use of IV heroin. Clusters, or individual cases of unusual complications from heroin use, should be reported to central agencies such as the local poison control center or health department in order to alert physicians and provide appropriate public health outreach.

Seizures, Dysrhythmias, and Serotonin Syndrome

Seizures and dysrhythmias are uncommon presentations of opioid toxicity. When they occur, they are likely secondary to severe hypoxia. There are, however, certain opioids that can specifically precipitate these events. Propoxyphene, a synthetic opioid with class Ia antidysrhythmic properties, is capable of producing a wide complex tachycardia in overdose. This is most likely to respond to bicarbonate therapy. Acute propoxyphene poisoning can also precipitate seizures, as can both therapeutic dosing and overdose of tramadol. In addition, chronic meperidine use may result in seizures due an accumulation of a neurotoxic metabolite normeperidine. This is especially true in patients with renal failure and in patients receiving high doses of meperidine. Seizure activity can be treated with supportive care and benzodiazepines.

Meperidine and dextromethorphan, because of their unique central serotonergic effects, are associated with serotonin syndrome. Serotonin syndrome, characterized by life-threatening hyperthermia, rigidity, and coarse shaking movements, can develop in patients receiving proserotoninergic agents such as selective serotonin reuptake inhibitors (SSRIs), lithium, clonazepam, or buspirone. Other opioids are not associated with serotonin syndrome. Morphine can be administered to patients taking monoamine oxidase inhibitors (MAOIs) who require pain control without precipitating a serotonergic crisis. Patients taking proserotonergic drugs, especially MAOIs, should not receive meperidine or dextromethorphan.

The many dangerous side effects associated with meperidine have led to a dramatic decrease in its popularity and its removal from many hospital formularies. There is little reason, if any, to use meperidine over other opioids for analgesic purposes.

Buprenorphine

Buprenorphine is a partial opioid agonist with 50 times greater affinity for the mu receptor than morphine. It is relatively resistant to antagonism by naloxone and can readily displace other opioids from mu receptors. Though it is rarely used as an analgesic, it is rapidly replacing methadone as the standard agent for substitution therapy in patients with opioid abuse. These medications are administered sublingually. There may be less ventilatory depression associated with buprenorphine than with full agonist opioids. Some preparations contain naloxone, which has very poor oral/sublingual bioavailability, as a deterrent to diversion of the drug to illicit use. Patients with acute pain who are taking buprenorphine may require very high doses of opioids or regional anesthesia for adequate pain management.

Pediatric Considerations

Unintentional exposure to a single opioid containing tablet can represent a significant risk of apnea in a small child. The onset of respiratory depression can be delayed for many hours, especially in opioid containing antidiarrheal agents. These children can appear deceptively well.

All children with a suspected or confirmed oral exposure to an opioid agent have an airway evaluation and stabilization is necessary, intravenous access established, and admission to a monitored setting for at least 24 hours. Longer acting opioid agents such as methadone require longer observation periods, as clinical effects can last as long as 36 hours after ingestion in children. Gastrointestinal decontamination with 1 g/kg of activated charcoal should only be preformed in awake co-operative children who are not deemed to be at risk for aspiration or intubated children with very large ingestions.

In children presenting with apnea, bag-valve ventilation and either intubation or empiric dosing of naloxone 2 mg can be used. For respiratory depression without apnea, the same 2 mg dose can be used. The 0.1 mg/kg dose that is frequently used in pediatrics is unnecessary, as children are not generally at risk for withdrawal and can tolerate high doses without adverse effect. Children may require a continuous infusion of naloxone, or they may benefit from the use of longer acting opioid antagonists.

Neonates born to opioid-dependent mothers may develop a withdrawal syndrome, which unlike adult withdrawal can be life-threatening. In addition to the clinical manifestations of withdrawal seen in adults, these children can have tremors, seizures, and hypotonia. These children should be managed in a neonatal intensive care unit with anhydrous morphine, diazepam, or phenobarbital at the discretion of the intensivist.

Time to Discharge

Patients presenting with opioid toxicity should be observed until there is certainty that their mental status and respirations remain stable for several hours beyond the duration of the opioid antagonist used. For example, for patients with mild respiratory depression from heroin, who are easily reversed with naloxone and have no other clinical complications or signs or toxicity, a 4 to 6 hour period of observation after naloxone administration is adequate to medically clear the patient for discharge or psychiatric evaluation.

Selected Readings

Goldfrank LR, Weisman RS, Errich JK, et al. A dosing nomogram for continuous infusion intravenous naloxone. *Ann Emerg Med* 1986;15:566–570.

Hoffman JR, Schriger DL, Luo JS. The empiric use of naloxone in patients: a reappraisal. *Ann Emerg Med* 1991;20:246–252.

Hung OL, Hoffman RS. Reversal of opioid intoxication-therapeutic guidelines. *CNS Drugs* 1997;7:176–186.

Nelson LS. Opioids. In: Goldfrank LR, Flomenbaum NE, Lewin NA, et al., eds. *Golfrank's Toxicologic Emergencies,* 7th ed. New York: McGraw-Hill, 2002: 901–917.

Sedative-Hypnotic Agents

Christina Hernon

Background and Epidemiology

Ever since the development of bromide salts in the 1840s, sedative hypnotic agents have been popular drugs for therapeutic or recreational use. Literally thousands of sedative hypnotic drugs have entered clinical practice. It is estimated that approximately 18% to 23% of the United States population has taken a sedative hypnotic agent both with and without a prescription, and members of this drug class are among most commonly prescribed pharmaceuticals in the United States. In the United States in 2003, there were approximately 2.4 million exposures reported to Poison Control Centers; sedative hypnotic agents were the second most frequent class of substances involved in adult exposures with 88,656 cases resulting in 329 deaths.

Pharmacology

In general, sedative hypnotic agents are well absorbed after gastrointestinal administration and possess good bioavailability. The onset of action of these drugs occurs rapidly, often within one hour of oral dosing. Most sedative hypnotic agents are highly protein bound and have relatively large volumes of distribution. The majority undergoes hepatic biotransformation by mixed function oxidases; metabolites are excreted by a variety of mechanisms, including renal elimination. Although barbiturates can induce cytochrome expression, there are few significant pharmacokinetic drug interactions.

Clinical Presentation of Sedative-Hypnotic Overdose

Manifestations of sedative-hypnotic overdose include ataxia, slurred speech, and incoordination, but more severe intoxication is characterized by somnolence or coma. Vital sign abnormalities include hypothermia and hypotension; severe barbiturate poisoning may produce profound hypotension due to depressed myocardial function. Respiratory depression to the point of apnea is uncommon, but may occur in barbiturates poisoning, or in overdose of other sedative-hypnotic agents in the very old or very young. Neurological examination in sedative hypnotic overdose does not demonstrate any lateralizing signs. Severely intoxicated patients who suffer prolonged coma may develop bullae on dependent body surfaces such as the dorsum of the hands. This finding, known as *barb blisters*, arises from prolonged immobilization and has been identified in nearly all overdoses where coma occurs. Depression of mental status may lead to diminished gag reflexes and increase the potential for aspiration of gastric contents.

Management

Supportive care and correction of vital signs remain the mainstay of management for sedative hypnotic overdose. For comatose individuals with absent or poor gag reflex, orotracheal intubation may be indicated to prevent aspiration of gastric contents. Hypotension often responds to intravenous fluids or stimulation, but vasoactive amine pressors such as dopamine may be required to treat severe hypotension. Gastrointestinal decontamination with activated charcoal should be pursued if patients arrive at the emergency department within one hour of ingestion; clinicians should be aware that orotracheal intubation may be needed to prevent aspiration of charcoal. Patients who have elevated serum concentrations of phenobarbital should receive multidose activated charcoal. Protocols such as urine alkalinization to enhance the elimination of phenobarbital are no longer recommended, but phenobarbital is amenable to dialysis in severe intoxication. In general, flumazenil is not recommended for the reversal of sedative-hypnotic associated coma. Seizures are a consequence of flumazenil administration, but because this agent is a GABA antagonist, the recommended therapy—treatment with GABA agonists such as benzodiazepines—may be ineffective.

Diagnosis

The diagnosis of sedative hypnotic overdose must generally be inferred from history and physical examination, because few clinical features are specific sedative hypnotic overdoses. Reliance upon urine drug toxicology testing (*toxic screens*) has severe limitations. While barbiturates often react with the barbiturate portion of the screen, many benzodiazepines produce false negative results. Benzodiazepines that produce positive results on toxic screens possess an oxazepam nucleus such as diazepam and chlordiazepoxide. Electroencephalography should not be utilized to make a determination of brain death in the context of profound barbiturate overdose, as these drugs may demonstrate *reversible* isoelectric waveforms.

Tolerance and Withdrawal

Tolerance to sedative hypnotics is common. In the case of barbiturates, hepatic enzyme induction alone is insufficient to explain the observation that dosing may need to be increased by a factor of up to six to generate the desired therapeutic effect. The tolerance to the effects of sedation and hypnosis is greater than the tolerance to the anticonvulsant effects. As a result, increasing doses lead to more side effects than the commensurate gain in therapeutic effects.

The sedative hypnotic abstinence syndrome produces symptoms are quite variable, but mimic findings of ethanol withdrawal. These clinical signs, which may develop up to two weeks after last use of the drug, are consistent with GABAergic withdrawal. Initial findings include the subtle signs of anxiety or insomnia, followed by: tremor, anorexia, abdominal cramps, nausea, vomiting, orthostatic hypotension, delirium, and progressive seizures. The majority of clinical signs can be effectively treated by restarting the medication, and then tapering its dose to cessation. Seizures should be treated with barbiturate administration, as they are refractory to other anticonvulsant medications such as phenytoin. Notably, the prolonged half life of phenobarbital (up to 12 days) prevents withdrawal from occurring with this drug.

Nonbenzodiazepine Sedatives: Zolpidem, Zaleplon, and Eszopiclone

History

Although benzodiazepines have a remarkable safety profile when compared to earlier sedative-hypnotics such as barbiturates, they are still associated with dependence, next-day sedation, and withdrawal. In 1993, a nonbenzodiazepine agent, zolpidem (Ambien) was introduced in the United States for treating short-term insomnia. It has hypnotic effects but minimal sedation, anxiolytic, or muscle relaxant properties. Since its introduction, additional compounds have appeared on the market; they are structurally dissimilar but maintain a narrow therapeutic profile with minimal disadvantages. Zaleplon (Sonata) and eszopiclone (Lunesta) soon followed. These drugs are structurally unrelated to the benzodiazepines, but mimic the basic chemical structure that allows interaction with the $GABA_A$ receptor. Unlike benzodiazepines, which bind well to virtually all $GABA_A$ receptors, they have distinct specificities for the $GABA_A$ receptor isoforms. Selective binding is thought to mediate the hypnotic effects of the drugs, while minimally affecting other sites on the GABA receptor that are responsible for anxiolytic, anticonvulsant, or muscle-relaxant effects.

Overdose from these drugs produces drowsiness or, in severe poisoning, coma. The general principles that guide treatment of other sedative hypnotic overdoses should be followed for these drugs as well. Interestingly, flumazenil may be used to antagonize zaleplon and zolpidem, but with varying efficacy. Zopiclone has been minimally studied, but appears to fit this categorization, with some reversal after flumazenil.

Selected Readings

Ford M, Delaney KA, Ling L, Erickson T. *Clinical Toxicology*, 1st ed. Philadelphia: WB Saunders Company, 2001.

Goodwin RD, Hasin DS. Sedative use and misuse in the United States. *Addiction* 2002;97:555–562.

Haddad LM, Shannon MW, Winchester JF. *Clinical Management of Poisoning and Drug Overdose*, 3rd ed. Philadelphia: WB Saunders Company, 1998.

Hardman JG, Limbird LE. *Goodman & Gilman's The Pharmacological Basis of Therapeutics*, ed 10. New York: McGraw Hill, 2001.

Olson KR. *Poisoning & Drug Overdose*, 4th ed. New York: Lange Medical Books, 2004.

Club Drugs

Edward W. Boyer

Club drugs include a diverse group of substances that are commonly used by adolescents and young adults desiring to experience alterations of consciousness and perception, enhanced energy, and elevated mood. The most common club drugs are 3,4-methylenedioxymethamphetamine (MDMA; "Ecstasy"), ketamine ("special K"), γ-hydroxybutyric acid ("GHB"), D-lysergic acid diethylamide (LSD), methamphetamine ("crystal meth"), and flunitrazepam (Rohypnol). They are commonly, yet not exclusively, used in the setting of night clubs, raves, and circuit parties. Raves are underground events that are generally held in warehouses or other large venues where law enforcement is unlikely to interfere. Events are advertised via word of mouth or the Internet within the target population, usually heterosexual teens and young adults, a few days prior to the event. Circuit parties by contrast are planned and advertised well in advance. These multi-day events, generally named by colors such as "The White Party," typically recur on an annual basis in a particular major city. They cater mostly to gay and bisexual men in their 20s and often provide a large source of revenue for the host city. Attendees often travel great distances and, therefore, stay in town over an entire weekend, thereby supporting local businesses. Those attending night clubs, raves, and circuit parties frequently use a variety of club drugs to enhance their experience by elevating mood and boosting energy to allow for all night dancing.

The Drug Abuse Warning Network (DAWN) collects data regarding emergency department (ED) visits that mention drug use. The data are collected from 21 representative metropolitan emergency departments in the United States. Although the information collected is illustrative of trends in adverse consequences of drug use that require medical care, a reflection of the incidence and prevalence of club drug use may not appear in this type of surveillance. Therefore, information from the DAWN database must be carefully interpreted. DAWN has identified that visits relating to club drug use are relatively rare when compared with more typical street drugs such as heroin and cocaine. Whereas cocaine accounted for 17% of overall ED drug mentions in 1999, methamphetamine and LSD, the most frequent club drugs reported to DAWN, comprised 0.5% and 1% of overall ED drug mentions in the same year. Although ED visits related to club

drug use are rare, the trend between 1994 and 1999 shows a clear increase in the incidence of certain club drug related cases presenting to health care facilities, particularly GHB and MDMA. Death from club drug use is also quite rare, with the exception of methamphetamine which was associated with 2,601 deaths in the 5 year period from 1994 to 1998. During that same period ketamine and MDMA were associated with 46 and 27 deaths, respectively. The relative rarity of presentation to an ED resulting from club drug use suggests that physicians are likely to be unfamiliar with these substances. Therefore, clinicians are less likely to recognize the specific intoxicant or have the knowledge to treat potential complications. Increasing awareness will enable ED physicians to prepare for such cases when they present.

Drugs

MDMA and Methamphetamine

MDMA ("Ecstasy") is an amphetamine with mild hallucinogenic properties. It was used therapeutically in the 1970s to enhance psychotherapy sessions, but in 1985 the Drug Enforcement Agency (DEA) classified it as a Schedule I substance. The pure drug is a white powder that dealers mold into pills with a unique appearance allowing users to identify the source. Therefore, MDMA tablets appear in a variety of shapes, colors, and symbols. Many dealers cut the drug with other cheaper substances such as caffeine, dextromethorphan, ephedrine, diphenhydramine, etc. Wide variations in MDMA pill content, from 0 mg to 150 mg, may lead to dosing errors and subsequent adverse effects.

The serum concentration peaks 2 hours after ingestion. The half-life averages 8 hours. Metabolism occurs via the hepatic microoxygenase system, specifically CYP2D6. Metabolites as well as a significant portion of unchanged drug (up to 75%) are excreted in the urine. Its central nervous system effects are mediated by its indirect sympathomimetic properties. MDMA causes enhanced release as well as reuptake inhibition of epinephrine, norepinephrine, serotonin, and dopamine. It also appears to have some direct effects on the receptors for these neurotransmitters. Similar actions in the periphery lead to mild tachycardia and hypertension.

After a typical dose of around 100 mg, users experience a calming effect. True hallucinations generally do not occur unless higher doses are used. Altered tactile sensation can lead to the desire for sensual and sexual experiences. Some have referred to it as "the hug drug." Elevation of mood and energy may last for 3 to 5 hours, allowing prolonged uninterrupted dancing and thereby increasing the risk of hyperthermia and dehydration. Most users are aware of this risk and drink copious amounts of water to prevent these complications. However, hyponatremia may develop either as a consequence of water intoxication or the syndrome of inappropriate antidiuretic hormone (SIADH). Those who use repetitive dosing in a short time frame to maintain arousal may be at higher risk of adverse effects. With frequent repetitive dosing or an acute single overdose patients may experience agitation, anxiety, and paranoia. Signs of adrenergic excess such as hypertension, tachycardia, diaphoresis, and tremor are likely to occur. The mode of death may be multifactorial and can include severe hyperthermia, seizures, myocardial infarction, or cerebral hemorrhage.

Methamphetamine has greater sympathomimetic effects than MDMA. It is relatively inexpensive compared to cocaine, and may produce a high which lasts up to 24 hours adding to its popularity. Although production and use of methamphetamine is highest in Western states, particularly California, current trends demonstrate that its use in the Eastern states is rising. Methamphetamine is readily available via oral, rectal, inhalational, and parenteral routes. Toxicity is similar to other amphetamines and includes hypertension, tachydysrhythmias, psychosis, myocardial infarction, and cerebral hemorrhage.

Hallucinogens

Ketamine, also known as "Special K" or "Vitamin K," is a dissociative anesthetic used to produce an "out-of-body" experience that is sometimes referred to by the user as the "K-hole." Ketamine is a glutamate antagonist at N-methyl-D-aspartate (NMDA) receptors in the cerebral cortex and limbic structures. It also causes a mild re-uptake inhibition of catecholamines and dopamine. The drug is typically sold in either powdered or pill form. Nasal insufflation is the most common dosing technique. Users may also ingest the tablets; however, this requires a higher dose. Intravenous administration is a less common mode of administration. The typical insufflation dose of 30 to 75 mg results in sedation and mild hallucinations. Higher doses are associated with dysphoria, inability to process sensory information into a construct of reality (cortical dissociation), agitation, coma, and rarely seizures. Patients presenting to medical care frequently display mild hypertension and tachycardia. Nystagmus and myoclonic motor activity are nearly universal. They may be calm but can become violent depending on their perception of reality. The time course for recovery is dependent on the route of administration. Following intravenous administration users may return to baseline after 15 minutes whereas oral administration may be associated with a high for up to 8

hours. Nasal insufflation produces a high which typically lasts for 45 to 90 minutes.

Lysergic acid diethylamide (LSD) is a synthetic hallucinogen developed in Germany in the 1940s. Although often associated with recreational use in the decade of the 1960s in the United States, a resurgence of use among adolescents has occurred that makes it the second most common ED club drug mention according data from the DAWN report. Users can buy the drug in the form of blotter paper impregnated with LSD, liquid, powder, tablets, or microdots. Although oral administration is most common, sublingual, intranasal, or parenteral routes can be used. The onset of action occurs within 30 to 90 minutes and peaks at 3 to 5 hours. Effects may persist for 8 to 12 hours. The mechanism of action is via stimulation of serotonin and dopamine receptors in the CNS as well as mild enhancement of catecholamine neurotransmission. Shortly after ingestion, users may develop mydriasis, diaphoresis, tachycardia, and hypertension. Subsequently, users develop alterations in perception of various sensory modalities and may experience an "out-of-body" phenomenon. The most common adverse effect is a panic reaction which is accompanied by tremendous anxiety.

Sedative/Hypnotics

Use of γ-hydroxybutyric acid (GHB) and its precursors γ-butyrolactone (GBL) and 1,4-butanediol (1,4-BD) has become epidemic in recent years. This increase in the use of these drugs has been accompanied by multiple adverse events, including several deaths. After the Drug Enforcement Administration classified GHB as a Schedule I substance in 2000, vendors began selling GBL and 1,4-BD in an attempt to avoid legal complications. Currently, GHB occupies a unique Schedule I/III designation; Schedule I applies to nonprescription possession and use, while the Schedule III classification applies when GHB is prescribed for narcolepsy. As GHB for recreational use has become scarce, users often procure precursor compounds from Internet-only companies based outside the United States.

GHB is administered orally in a liquid form. The dose-response curve for GHB is steep, which requires users to carefully measure out doses. Unfortunately, preparations vary in their concentration leading to overdosing. Clinical effects are seen rapidly after the ingestion of as little as 5 cc of GHB or its precursor compounds. Central nervous system effects include lethargy, confusion, and respiratory depression, that are mediated by its enhancement of γ-aminobutyric acid (GABA) neurotransmission and direct stimulation of GHB receptors. Additionally, bradycardia, hypotension, and respiratory arrest may occur. Confusion exists within the literature regarding the existence of epileptiform seizures. Nonepileptic myoclonic jerks are likely the type of abnormal motor activity described in case reports of overdose. Drug effects may last for 5 to 8 hours postingestion. The time-course of intoxication may be altered with co-ingestion of ethanol in patients taking 1,4-BD, which must be converted by alcohol dehydrogenase (ADH) to GHB prior to clinical effect. The user will metabolize the ethanol first and then suddenly become more lethargic once ADH converts 1,4-BD into the active drug GHB.

Flunitrazepam (Rohypnol®) is a short acting benzodiazepine that is no longer available by prescription in the United States. However, the drug can be obtained from Europe or Latin America with relative ease. The tablets come in 1 and 2 mg strengths. Street names for the drug include "Mexican Valium," and "roofies." The drug is characterized by rapid onset of action (within 30 min) and a relatively short duration of action (8 h) owing to its rapid redistribution. As with all benzodiazepines, the toxicity is primarily CNS depression from co-receptor agonism at the GABA chloride ion channel. Flunitrazepam is somewhat unique in its ability to produce amnesia. This can lead to life-threatening respiratory depression, particularly when used in combination with opiates or alcohol.

Testing

Club drugs often fail to elicit a positive response to standard urine immunoassays used by hospital laboratories to detect drugs of abuse. Ecstasy may be identified as a positive amphetamine screen on many commercial assays; however, a significant number of false-negative tests can occur. Methamphetamine is metabolized to amphetamine, which makes a positive result on qualitative urine immunoassays more likely than with MDMA. Clinicians should be aware that a positive amphetamine result on immunoassays may not indicate illicit drug use. Many cough and cold preparations containing structurally similar substances may cross-react with the amphetamine screen. Selegiline, a monoamine oxidase inhibitor (MAOI) used in Parkinson's disease, is metabolized to amphetamine and may lead to confusion. There are no commercially available immunoassays for ketamine or GHB. If confirmation is required, samples must be sent for GC-MS. Similarly, LSD is not detected on routine urine immunoassays and requires GC-MS for confirmation. Given the low doses required for clinical effects with flunitrazepam, urine concentrations of the drug are often below the limit of detection for benzodiazepines. If the diagnosis of flunitrazepam exposure must be documented (alleged rape) clinicians should contact the manufacturer (Roche) for recommendations on assays.

Management

Patients seeking medical care after amphetamine use typically present with a sympathomimetic toxidrome including tachycardia, hypertension, agitation, and possibly hallucinations. Supportive care should include hydration, and sedation with benzodiazepines. Careful attention to vital signs, particularly temperature, is paramount to management. Any attempts at physical restraint must be accompanied by chemical restraint in order to reduce muscle activity and subsequent hyperthermia, acidosis, and death that can occur in the absence of anxiolysis. Patient complaints of chest pain or headache should prompt clinicians to check an electrocardiogram for ischemia and computed tomography (CT) of the brain for hemorrhage, respectively. Laboratory analysis for hyponatremia from MDMA use or rhabdomyolysis from amphetamines is appropriate. Occasionally users may attempt to enhance their "high" by using monoamine oxidase inhibitors in combination with other substances. In this case, severe hypertension may be seen, followed by marked hypotension once endogenous stores of catecholamines are depleted. These rare patients require prolonged Intensive Care Unit monitoring and blood pressure augmentation using pressor agents and antihypertensives alternatively, depending on the hemodynamic status.

Users of ketamine may be brought to medical care as a result of extreme panic relating to hallucinations. A quiet room and benzodiazepine are generally sufficient care. The recovery period following dosing is brief. The same principals apply for LSD except that symptoms may persist for hours and require longer observation.

Coma and respiratory arrest may follow accidental overdose of GHB. Supportive care, particularly mechanical ventilation, is the primary treatment modality. Patients typically awaken from deep sedation quite suddenly within 6 hours of intubation. Self-extubation is common due to the precipitous nature of the recovery. Cardiac monitoring may occasionally reveal bradycardia. However, unless accompanied by hypotension, atropine is generally not required.

Summary

Club drugs including MDMA, methamphetamine, ketamine, LSD, GHB, and Rohypnol are commonly used by attendees of nightclubs, raves, and circuit parties. Users infrequently present to medical care following drug use. Therefore, physicians are less familiar with their clinical presentation, diagnostic testing, and treatment. Although most adverse events related to club drugs are treated with supportive measures, combinations of various agents may lead to unpredictable symptoms, delayed toxicity, and adverse events including death. Clinicians should become familiar with the most commonly used club drugs and their treatment and consider consultation with a toxicologist to assist in the management of these relatively rare poisonings.

Selected Readings

Shannon M. Methylenedioxymethamphetamine (MDMA, "Ecstasy"). *Pediatric Emergency Care* 2000;16:377–380.

Teter CJ, Guthrie SK. A comprehensive review of MDMA and GHB: two common club drugs. *Pharmacotherapy* 2001;21:1486–1513.

Tong T, Boyer EW. Club drugs, smart drugs, raves, and circuit parties: an overview of the club scene. *Pediatr Emerg Care* 2002;18:216–218.

CHAPTER

140   Anticholinergic Agents

Ivan Liang

Anticholinergic agents are competitive antagonists of the neurotransmitter acetylcholine that act specifically at the muscarinic receptor. Acetylcholine is a neurotransmitter used widely in the central and peripheral nervous system, the neuromuscular junction, the autonomic ganglia, and at the effector organs innervated by the parasympathetic nervous system. It has two broad categories of receptors: nicotinic and muscarinic. Nicotinic receptors predominate at the neuromuscular junction and the autonomic ganglia. Muscarinic receptors are used primarily at the effector organs innervated by the parasympathetic nerves, such as the pupils, smooth muscle of the respiratory and gastrointestinal tract, sinoatrial node, and sweat glands. While muscarinic and nicotinic receptors are found throughout the central nervous system, *anticholinergic agents* are more accurately termed *antimuscarinic* for their specific blockade of the muscarinic receptors in both central and peripheral sites. Such inhibition diminishes parasympathetic tone at end organs (including the brain) and results in the well known toxic syndrome.

Anticholinergic agents are found in many formulations of prescription and over-the-counter medications. Atropine is the prototypical anticholinergic agent and can be found in certain antidiarrheal preparations, ophthalmic solutions, and, of course, medications for cardiac resuscitation. Furthermore, antihistamines have anticholinergic properties. They are often the culprit in the patient with altered mental status after an intentional ingestion of an over-the-counter sleeping pill. Almost all such preparations contain diphenhydramine. The American Association of Poison Centers reported over 9,000 intentional diphenhydramine ingestions in 2002, more than the rest of anticholinergics together. Not uncommonly, patients who abuse over-the-counter cold medications will inadvertently become toxic on diphenhydramine or chlorpheniramine when they choose preparations with antihistamines instead of dextromethorphan. In addition, heroin is occasionally cut with scopolamine, resulting in anticholinergic poisoning. Botanical sources, taken accidentally and intentionally, include *Datura strammonium* (jimson weed) and *Atropa belladonna*.

Other medications not commonly thought of as anticholinergic agents will demonstrate such properties in toxic doses. Cyclobenzaprine (muscle relaxant), carbamazepine (anticonvulsant), benztropine (anti-parkinsonian), the phenothiazines (anti-psychotic and anti-emetic), and the newer generation antipsychotics all can produce the anticholinergic symptoms. Tricyclic antidepressants have anticholinergic properties, although often their more serious cardiac toxicity will predominate. Because the types of drugs and formulations that can produce the antimuscarinic findings are so varied, recognition and management of the anticholinergic toxidrome is considered a basic clinical skill to the practice of emergency medicine.

Presentation

Anticholinergic agents are absorbed rapidly from the gastrointestinal tract to produce symptoms within one to two hours of ingestion.

The constellation of physical examination findings are pathogenomic. The classic toxidrome mnemonic associated with anticholinergic poisoning is: blind as a bat (pupillary mydriasis and inability to accommodate), hot as a hare (hyperthermia from inability to sweat), red as a beet (flushed, dry skin), dry as a bone (dry mucous membranes and absent axillary sweat), and mad as a hatter (agitated delirium). Vital signs typically demonstrate sinus tachycardia from vagolytic tone. Blood pressure is normal to slightly elevated. Body temperature may also be elevated as the ability to dissipate heat through perspiration is deranged. Other classic signs include bladder distension from urinary retention, and decreased or absent bowel sounds from diminished gastrointestinal motility. Clinicians should be aware that the anticholinergic toxidrome may be incomplete in its presentation; it is therefore not uncommon for patients to exhibit only one or two of the above findings. The changes in mental status are fairly consistent across all patients, who demonstrate mumbling, incoherent speech, and agitated delirium.

Central anticholinergic signs will usually coincide with the peripheral symptoms. Clinical findings range from mild agitation to combative disorientation with hallucinations and seizures. The classic features include agitated delirium with severe disorientation, myoclonic movements, preoccupation with picking at clothes or hallucinations, and a characteristic response to verbal stimuli. When addressed, the patient may begin with a clear word or two, but then drift into unintelligible mumbling.

Differential Diagnosis

The anticholinergic syndrome is most closely mimicked by sympathomimetic agents (for example, cocaine, amphetamine, phencyclidine) and withdrawal from sedative-hypnotics (alcohol, benzodiazepines, gamma hydroxybutyrate). The absence of diaphoresis and bowel sounds can distinguish the anticholinergic syndrome from the sympathomimetic toxidrome. Coingestions must always be considered, even in unintentional exposures, as anticholinergic agents come in many combination preparations. Nontoxic causes of agitated delirium must also be considered, including encephalitis and meningitis.

Treatment

Patients who are asymptomatic after an exposure to anticholinergic agents should be watched closely. Symptoms should develop within one to two hours. Patients with anticholinergic findings should be placed on cardiac monitoring and intravenous access obtained. Full vital signs and core temperature should be obtained. Provision of emergent supportive measures such as airway protection and cardiovascular resuscitation should be instituted as indicated. Initial serum labs should include electrolytes, blood urea nitrogen, creatinine, glucose, creatine phosphokine, and acetaminophen levels. A 12 lead EKG should be obtained, with close attention paid to the QRS duration.

Seizures should be treated with benzodiazepines such as lorazepam and diazepam; phenobarbitol can be added if seizure activity is refractory. Hyperthermia should be treated with cooling measures. Rhabdomyolysis may complicate the anticholinergic syndrome and should be treated aggressively. Tricyclic antidepressant poisoning may present with anticholinergic findings; they are specifically discussed in another chapter.

Antidotal Therapy

Physostigmine is the antidote for both central and peripheral antimuscarinic toxic syndromes. Physostigmine is a reversible inhibitor of acetylcholinesterase, thus causing higher concentrations of acetylcholine in the synapse by inhibition of its breakdown. Its tertiary amine structure allows it to cross the blood-brain barrier and thus act at central synapses. Other acetylcholinesterase inhibitors, such as neostigmine, pyridostigmine, and edrophonium, have too much polarity to do so.

Physostigmine has been associated with asystole and seizure in several case reports. These patients, however, were seriously poisoned by tricyclic antidepressants.

Overdose of tricyclic antidepressants remains a relative contraindication to use of physostigmine, as does any evidence of cardiotoxicity such as QRS prolongation above 100 milliseconds on EKG or rightward axis deviation (deep R wave in AVR).

As a result of these individual case reports, there is often reluctance to use physostigmine, frequently leading to substitution with benzodiazepines. Several small retrospective studies have investigated the efficacy and safety of physostigmine. Burns et al. retrospectively reviewed 52 patients that presented with an anticholinergic syndrome; 45 were treated with physostigmine, 26 with benzodiazepines, and 19 with both. Physostigmine was effective in controlling agitation (96%) and reversing delirium (87%). Benzodiazepines were only 24% effective at controlling agitation and ineffective at reversing delirium. Rates of side effects were similar in both. Excessive sedation and aspiration events were associated with patients treated with benzodiazepines alone or initially. The only dysrhythmia reported in the series was asymptomatic bradycardia to a rate of 51 in a patient treated with physostigmine. There were no seizures or bronchospasm reported. Similarly, Schneir et al. examined a series of 39 patients who were given physostigmine. Twenty-two patients had full reversal of the syndrome, including all 19 patients who were intoxicated by a known anticholinergic agent. One patient had a seizure after physostigmine administration, although he also had seizures prior to administration. There were no reports of dysrhythmia, bronchospasm, or symptoms of cholinergic excess. Physostigmine was administered to 3 patients with tricyclic antidepressants detected on urine tests without complication; one had a QRS of 138 and a right bundle branch block previously known to exist.

Physostigmine should be administered as a slow intravenous push of 0.5 to 2 mg (pediatric 0.02 mg/kg). Onset of action is within minutes and duration of effect is usually 30 to 60 minutes. Repeat dosing may be necessary. The theoretical risk of creating a syndrome of cholinergic excess can be treated with atropine. Phystostigmine may potentiate depolarizing neuromuscular-blocking drugs (i.e., succinycholine) and may inhibit or reverse action of nondepolarizing agents (such as vecuronium).

Activated charcoal (1 g/kg) can be administered to decontaminate the patient, although its benefits must be weighed against its risks in relation to timing, agitation of the patient, and the possibility of seizure. Administration of activated charcoal can be considered farther into a patient's course because anticholinergic agents slow gastric emptying and, potentially, delay the onset of toxicity. Gastric lavage can be considered for large ingestions presenting early, although it has not been shown to be of benefit. Repeat dose charcoal may increase the risk of charcoal regurgitation and aspiration as decreased gastrointestinal motility is a consequence of anticholinergic poisoning. For varying reasons, hemodialysis and charcoal perfusion are not likely to be of any benefit.

Many patients will present with only mild symptoms that will resolve spontaneously. Patients with more severe symptoms will often require admission for cardiac monitoring, seizure precautions, control of agitation and temperature, and possible repeat antidote dosing. Full assessment is essential, especially for intentional ingestions, including psychiatric evaluation and evaluation for coingestants (especially acetaminophen which is often part of a combination preparation).

Selected Readings

Burns MJ, Linden CH, Graudins A, et al. A comparison of physostigmine and benzodiazepines for the treatment of anticholinergic poisoning. *Ann Emerg Med* 2000;35:374–381.

Dilsaver SC. Antimuscarinic agents as substances of abuse: a review. J Clin Psychopharmacol 1988;8:14–22.

Kirages T, Sule H, Mycyk M. Severe manifestations of Coricidin intoxication. Am J Emerg Med 2003;21:648–651.

Schneir AB, Offerman SR, Ly BT, et al. Complications of diagnostic physostigmine administration to emergency department patients. *Ann Emerg Med* 2003;42:14–19.

Suchard JR. Assessing physostigmine's contraindication in cyclic antidepressant ingestions. *J Emerg Med* 2003;25:185–191.

Beth Cadigan
Edward W. Boyer

Toxic Alcohols

CHAPTER
141

Among the toxic alcohols, methanol and ethylene glycol remain the most poisonous. Ingestion of these materials requires immediate, aggressive intervention to prevent significant end organ damage and death.

Methanol

Methanol, an odorless and colorless liquid, is found in de-icing solutions, windshield washer fluid, solvents, chafing dish heat sources, solvents, and other commercial products. Methanol has no therapeutic uses. Although toxicity has been reported following dermal or inhalational contact, ingestion remains the primary route of exposure. After ingestion, methanol is absorbed rapidly from the gastrointestinal tract. The presence of methanol in blood produces the osmolal gap, the difference between measured and calculated osmolality of the serum. Methanol has a volume of distribution of 0.6 L/kg. Methanol itself is nontoxic; toxicity from methanol ingestion arises from formic acid, a toxic metabolite. Hepatic alcohol dehydrogenase (ADH) oxidizes >95% of methanol to formaldehyde and then formic acid; the remainder is eliminated via the lungs and kidneys. The elimination half-life of methanol is between 14 and 30 hours in untreated patients.

Clinical Manifestations

Initial findings of toxicity include inebriation that is characteristically followed by an asymptomatic period. Within 2 to 30 hours of ingestion (the exact time depends upon the presence of coingested ethanol), patients may exhibit vomiting, severe abdominal pain, back pain, blurred vision, or blindness. Patients may also develop Kussmaul respirations to compensate for an acidosis that is due primarily to the presence of formic acid. Death is likely due to the complication of acidosis or respiratory failure. Among survivors, up to 25% of patients with severe methanol poisoning develop permanent optic nerve damage. Additional sequela of methanol poisoning includes parkinsonism and necrosis of the putamen. Serum methanol concentrations of >20 mg/dL can be expected to generate ocular injury and metabolic acidosis; toxicity has been associated with as little as 10 cc in an adult.

Diagnosis

The diagnosis of methanol poisoning is supported by a history of ingestion as well as the clinical findings of mental status alteration, metabolic acidosis, and visual disturbances. The diagnosis is established, however, by the measurement of serum methanol concentration or by an estimate of the toxin's concentration extrapolated from the osmolar gap. Antidotal therapy is reserved for serum methanol concentrations estimated or measured to be >25 mg/dL, or patients with clinical findings suggestive of methanol poisoning with metabolic acidosis.

Most health care facilities lack the means to directly measure blood methanol concentrations. Clinicians in these facilities must infer the diagnosis from concurrently drawn serum chemistries, serum osmolar gap, and arterial blood gas. The calculated osmolarity consists of twice the serum sodium in mEq, plus the molar sums of the glucose and BUN. Additional molecules—such as toxic alcohols—increase the measured osmolarity to produce an *osmolar gap*, or the difference between the measured and calculated osmolarity. An osmolar gap of 50 mOsm/L is virtually diagnostic of toxic alcohol ingestion. Clinicians should be aware, however, that a normal osmolar gap does not preclude toxic alcohol ingestion, and that it is the change of the osmolar gap from baseline that is most important. A normal osmolar gap may signify a late presentation of poisoning. In these cases obtaining a concurrent arterial blood gas is useful because a pH < 7.10 suggests toxic alcohol poisoning.

Management

If a patient presents soon after a known, large volume ingestion, evacuation of gastric contents using a nasogastric tube should be considered. Intravenous fluids should be administered. Fomepizole (4-MP), which inhibits alcohol dehydrogenase, should be given to all methanol-intoxicated patients with a metabolic acidosis as well as those with elevated methanol concentration (e.g., greater than 25 mg/dL). The use of bicarbonate should be considered to treat acidosis as well. Fomepizole has an interesting pharmacological profile in that it induces its own metabolism, a feature that requires that 15 mg/kg fomepizole be administered intravenously as a loading dose, followed by 10 mg/kg every 12 hours. After 48 hours, however, the dosing interval should be increased to 10 mg/kg every 8 hours.

Patients with a methanol concentration who have received fomepizole must receive hemodialysis; acidotic patients should also be dialyzed after fomepizole administration. Alcohol dehydrogenase is the only effective means of eliminating methanol from the human body; once alcohol dehydrogenase is blocked by fomepizole, methanol must be eliminated by dialysis. Fomepizole itself can be dialyzed, so the antidote must be reloaded following each run of dialysis. Furthermore, the dosing interval for fomepizole must be increased to 10 mg/kg administered every 8 hours. Dialysis should be continued until a methanol concentration of less than 25 mg/dL is achieved.

Ethylene Glycol

Ethylene glycol (EG) intoxication remains one of the most serious poisonings seen in clinical toxicology. Ethylene glycol is found in radiator antifreeze, deicing solutions, and other formulations. Pure ethylene glycol, which has a slightly sweet taste, is odorless and colorless. After ingestion, ethylene glycol is rapidly absorbed from the gastrointestinal tract. The presence of ethylene glycol in blood produces the osmolar gap. Nontoxic itself, ethylene glycol is converted enzymatically to glycolic acid and oxalic acid, which are toxic metabolites. More than 85% of ethylene glycol is oxidized to glycoaldehyde by alcohol dehydrogenase (ADH). Acidosis is attributable to the presence of glycolic, glyoxylic, and oxalic acids. Ethylene glycol is unique among alcohols in that a significant amount is eliminated unchanged in the urine.

Clinical Manifestations

Ethylene glycol poisoning occurs in three phases. The first phase occurs within 3 minutes to 12 hours of ingestion. Patients appear drunk but without the odor of ethanol on the breath. Patients may demonstrate coma, seizure, and tetany due to hypocalcemia. The second phase begins 12 to 14 hours later; patients may demonstrate tachycardia, hypertension, pulmonary edema, and congestive heart failure. Each of these conditions is thought to be due to deposition of calcium oxalate in the pulmonary beds, the myocardium, and vessels. The third phase begins 24 to 72 hours after ingestion and involves flank pain that accompanies acute tubular necrosis. Oliguric renal failure is common.

Diagnosis

The diagnosis of EG poisoning is supported by a history of ingestion as well as the clinical findings of mental status alteration, metabolic acidosis, hypocalcemia, and renal failure. The diagnosis is established, however, by the measurement of serum methanol concentration or by an estimate of the toxin's concentration extrapolated from the osmolar gap. Antidotal therapy is reserved for serum EG concentrations estimated or measured to be >50 mg/dL, or in patients with clinical findings consistent with EG poisoning and metabolic acidosis.

Most health care facilities lack the means to directly measure blood ethylene glycol concentrations. Clinicians in these facilities must infer the diagnosis from a series of concurrently drawn serum chemistries, a serum osmolar gap, and an arterial blood gas. The ingestion of any toxic alcohol can increase the serum osmolarity. The calculated osmolarity consists of twice the serum sodium in mEq, plus the molar sums of the glucose and BUN. Additional molecules—such as toxic alcohols—increase the measured osmolarity to produce an *osmolar gap,* or the difference between the measured and calculated osmolarity. An osmolar gap of 50 mOsm/L is virtually diagnostic of a toxic alcohol ingestion. Clinicians should be aware, however, that a normal osmolar gap does not preclude toxic alcohol ingestion, and that it is the change of the osmolar gap from baseline that is most important. A normal osmolar gap may signify a late presentation of poisoning. In these cases, obtaining a concurrent arterial blood gas is useful because a pH < 7.10 suggests EG poisoning.

Patients who ingest antifreeze may produce—for a brief period—urine that fluoresces under a Wood's lamp. Clinicians must add several drops or urine to filter paper or another absorbent material; glass or plastic may fluoresce if these containers are used. Furthermore, microscopic analysis of the urine may reveal calcium oxalate monohydrate crystals in EG intoxicated patients.

Treatment

Aggressive correction of vital sign and electrolyte abnormalities, hemodialysis, and fomepizole remain the hallmarks of therapy. Patients who present soon after large volume ingestion should receive gastric emptying with a nasogastric tube. Acidosis should be corrected with sodium bicarbonate, and calcium chloride should be used to treat hypocalcemia.

Fomepizole (4-MP), which inhibits alcohol dehydrogenase, should be given to all EG-intoxicated patients with a metabolic acidosis as well as those with elevated EG concentration (e.g., greater than 25 mg/dL). Fomepizole induces its own metabolism, a feature that requires that 15 mg/kg fomepizole be administered intravenously as a loading dose, followed by 10 mg/kg every 12 hours. After 48 hours, the dosing interval should be increased to 10 mg/kg every 8 hours.

Nonacidotic patients with normal renal function and an EG concentration greater than 25 mg/dL who have received fomepizole may not require hemodialysis. This is because

EG undergoes renal elimination; once alcohol dehydrogenase is blocked by fomepizole, the renal beds can eliminate the toxin while fomepizole prevents toxicity. Patients with renal failure or acidosis require hemodialysis and 4-MP. Fomepizole itself can be dialyzed, so the drug must be reloaded following each run of dialysis. Furthermore, the dosing interval for fomepizole must be increased to 10 mg/kg administered every 8 hours. Dialysis should be continued until an EG concentration of less than 25 mg/dL is achieved.

Selected Reading

Toxic alcohols. In *Goldfrank's Toxicologic Emergencies*, 7th ed, page 980–994. New York: McGraw-Hill, 2002:980–994.

142 Abstinence Syndromes: Alcohol

Jeffrey M. Cukor

Over 8 million people are reported to be dependent on alcohol each year in the United States with approximately 500,000 people requiring treatment for withdrawal.[1] The health impacts are tremendous and have led to a greater focus on the detoxification process. Although understating the motivations for drinking and promoting abstinence after cessation of drinking are both essential topics, this chapter focuses on the symptoms of alcohol withdrawal and their management in the acute care setting.

Clinical Presentation

Alcohol is a neurodepressant agent and will generally create a state of neural excitement and autonomic hyperactivity during acute withdrawal. Alcohol withdrawal syndromes can be thought of as along a spectrum ranging from minor withdrawal, to more moderate syndromes including seizures or hallucinations, to the most serious withdrawal syndrome of delirium tremens.

The symptoms of minor alcohol withdrawal center around anxiety and tremulousness and may begin within 6 to 8 hours of stopping or reducing alcohol intake in dependent patients. Alcohol is a short acting agent and symptoms may be triggered by lower than usual alcohol levels, not simply complete cessation.

Other common symptoms include insomnia, nausea and vomiting, mild diaphoresis, headaches, palpitations, and loss of appetite. Examination may reveal an agitated patient with relatively minor increases in heart rate, blood pressure, temperature, and reflexes. Notably, mental status is grossly preserved with an absence of any global confusion. Minor alcohol withdrawal syndromes generally peak within 24 hours and resolve within 1 to 2 days without permanent physical sequelae.

Moderate syndromes of withdrawal include more pronounced autonomic hyperactivity as well as withdrawal seizures and hallucinosis. The seizures tend to occur during the first 48 hours and are usually solitary, generalized and tonic-clonic in nature. These seizures, sometimes referred to as *rum fits*, have been reported to occur as early as 2 hours after alcohol levels begin to fall. They are an uncommon part of withdrawal and are generally treated with benzodiazepines and supportive care. As will be dis-

cussed later, anticonvulsants are not used in this situation. Approximately 3% of individuals having withdrawal seizures will progress to status epilepticus and require more aggressive intervention.[2] Focal or recurrent seizures as well as status should broaden the search for other possible underlying etiologies.

The hallucinations experienced in alcohol withdrawal tend to be visual and begin within the first 12 to 24 hours. It is important to differentiate hallucinations from true *delirium tremens (DTs)* in which there is an accompanying global confusion. A patient experiencing a specific hallucination does not equate with a diagnosis of delirium tremens and does not predict progression to DTs. The hallucinations of alcoholic hallucinosois resolve within 1 to 2 days, and may present as auditory or tactile as well as visual. The relatively early onset and rapid resolution of these hallucinations also helps to distinguish them from DTs in which the symptom onset is generally further delayed (**Table 142.1**).

DTs typically begin 2 to 4 days after alcohol reduction and include roughly 5% of all patients experiencing withdrawal. The hallmark of DTs is global disorientation/confusion along with hallucinations and pronounced agitation. More severe tremors, hypertension, tachycardia, hyperthermia, and diaphoresis are also seen. Progression to DTs is more common in older patients with longer drinking histories who present with an onset of symptoms greater than 2 days after alcohol cessation. Other risk factors include a past history of severe withdrawal or a coexisting acute medical problem.[3] Patients with DTs often suffer from dehydration as well as electrolyte abnormalities, which in the most severe cases can contribute toward cardiac and renal failure.

Treatment

As with all ED patients, the airway should first be assessed and if necessary protected. General supportive therapy would then include administering intravenous fluids (IVF) with repletion of magnesium, potassium, and phosphate as indicated. An oral or IV multivitamin containing folate, and oral or IV thiamine to prevent Wernicke's encephalopathy, should be given. Patients should be assessed for hypoglycemia and treated with dextrose if necessary.

Table 142.1
Timing of Symptoms

Symptoms	Timing of Onset (after drinking reduction)	Resolution
Minor withdrawal	6–36 hours	24–48 hours
Seizures or "rum fits"	6–48 hours	2–48 hours
Specific hallucinations	12–48 hours	24–48 hours
Delirium tremens	48–96 hours	1–5 days after onset

Although serotonin and norepinephrine may also be involved, the symptoms of alcohol withdrawal are most closely related to receptor downregulation of gamma-aminobutyric acid (GABA).[4] As GABA is an inhibitory neurotransmitter, a decrease in GABA receptors results in hyperactivity. Benzodiazepines are therefore the treatment of choice and are the central therapy in all alcohol withdrawal syndromes.

Both diazepam (Valium) and lorazepam (Ativan) are commonly used agents. Ativan is broken down without active metabolites, which is a potential benefit in the advanced cirrhotic patient. Ativan also has a slightly longer anti-epileptic effect. In patients with minor withdrawal, therapy is targeted toward easing symptoms and agitation while maintaining mental status and respiratory drive. Oral Valium (5–20 mg) or Ativan (1–2 mg) may be given every 5 to 10 minutes. The oral doses may be utilized alone, but can also be supplemented with IV boluses. Moderate to severe symptoms necessitate parenteral therapy with 5 to 10 mg of Valium or 1 to 2 mg of Ativan every 5 to 10 minutes until the proper effect is achieved. Massive doses may be required in severe withdrawal, with reports of up to 1 g of Valium needed within the first few hours.[5]

The dosing of benzodiazepines is best determined through a symptom-triggered approach. Study has found that symptom triggered therapy can decrease the amount of medication withdrawing patients need by up to 75% and also decreases the duration of treatment.[6] A commonly used tool is the Clinical Institute Withdrawal Assessment Scale for Alcohol, Revised (CIWA-Ar, see **Table 142.2**). A maximum score of 67 is possible, calculated by looking at degrees of nausea/vomiting, paroxysmal sweats, anxiety, agitation, tremor, headache, auditory, visual and tactile disturbances as well as overall mental status. Scoring is done every 10 minutes (Table 142.2) until a score of less than 10 is achieved, at which point reassessments are done every 1 to 2 hours. CIWA scores between 10 and 15 prompt a 5 mg IV dose of Valium; scores from 16 to 20 yield 10 mg IV Valium, and scores greater than 20 result in a dose of 20 mg of IV Valium.

Adjuvant Therapies

Although data and experience are relatively limited, refractory symptoms warrant the consideration of other medications. Phenobarbital and propofol are excellent choices as they effectively antagonize neuroexcitation, especially if used concurrently with benzodiazepines. The phenobarbital dose is 130 to 260 mg IV every 15 minutes while propofol is administered as a 1 mg/kg bolus. This dose of propofol will require intubation, after which the propofol is further titrated for sedation.

The symptoms of autonomic hyperactivity can be abated with beta-blockers such as atenolol and alpha-2-agonists, such as clonidine. However, unlike the benzodiazepines, neither of these agents has any cross-tolerance with alcohol and, therefore, are unlikely to reduce DTs or seizures. They will, nonetheless, aid in reducing blood pressure and heart rate.

Anticonvulsants, such as dilantin, are not indicated for alcohol withdrawal seizures. In the rare patient who develops status epilepticus, an anticonvulsant can be used acutely with benzodiazepines while a more exhaustive workup is considered to explore the seizures' etiology.

Butyrophenones, like Haldol, should not be used as a solitary agent, as they lower the seizure threshold and are not pharmacologically active at the GABA receptor sites.

Research is currently being conducted on the use of other GABA agonists, such as baclofen; however, a clear indication for use has not yet been established.

Disposition

Patients with minor alcohol withdrawal or an isolated withdrawal seizure may be discharged from the emergency department after an appropriate period of observation. Oral therapy can be considered, with doses of 1 to 2 mg of Ativan three times a day tapered over six days or 30 mg of Valium once a day, also in a six day taper. Risk of overdose must be considered when prescribing outpatient therapy and thus is best coordinated through a physician or clinic.

Patients with moderate or severe alcohol withdrawal syndromes need to be admitted to the hospital and often to the ICU for close monitoring and medication administration. While multiple systems are affected, mortality is often secondary to cardiac dysrhythmia, aspiration pneumonia, or dehydration and renal failure. Cardiac dysrhythmias are associated with withdrawal directly, but may also be caused by associated electrolyte abnormality. Improvements in both monitoring and therapy have reduced the mortality in delirium tremens to approximately 5% to 10%, down from earlier reported rates of 40%.[7,8]

Table 142.2

CIWA-Ar Scale

**Addiction Research Foundation Clinical Institute Withdrawal
Assessment Alcohol (CIWA-Ar)** The scale is not copyrighted and may be used freely.

Patient:	Date: _____ / _____ / _____ y m d	Time: _____ (24 hour clock, midnight + 0:00)
Pulse or heart rate, taken for one minute:		**Blood Pressure:** _____ / _____

NAUSEA AND VOMITING—Ask "Do you feel sick to your stomach? Have you vomited?" Observation.

0 no nausea and no vomiting
1 mild nausea with no vomiting
2
3
4 intermittent nausea with dry heaves
5
6
7 constant nausea, frequent dry heaves and vomiting

TACTILE DISTURBANCES—Ask "Have you any itching, pins and needles sensations, any burning, any numbness, or do you feel bugs crawling on or under your skin?" Observation.

0 none
1 mild itching, pins and needles, burning or numbness
2 mild itching, pins and needles, burning or numbness
3 moderate itching, pins and needles, burning or numbness
4 moderately severe hallucinations
5 severe hallucinations
6 extremely severe hallucinations
7 continuous hallucinations

TREMOR—Arms extended and fingers spread apart. Observation.

0 no tremor
1 not visible, but can be felt fingertip to fingertip
2
3
4 moderate, with patient's arms extended
5
6
7 severe, even with arms not extended

AUDITORY DISTURBANCES—Ask "Are you more aware of sounds around you? Are they harsh? Do they frighten you? Are you hearing anything that is disturbing to you? Are you hearing things you know are not there?" Observation.

0 not present
1 very mild harshness or ability to frighten
2 mild harshness or ability to frighten
3 moderate harshness or ability to frighten
4 moderately severe hallucinations
5 severe hallucinations
6 extremely severe hallucinations
7 continuous hallucinations

PAROXYSMAL SWEATS—Observation.

0 no sweat visible
1 barely perceptible sweating, palms moist
2
3
4 beads of sweat obvious on forehead
5
6
7 drenching sweats

VISUAL DISTURBANCES—Ask "Does the light appear to be too bright? Is the color different? Does it hurt your eyes? Are you seeing anything that is disturbing to you? Are you seeing things you know are not there?" Observation.

0 not present
1 very mild sensitivity
2 mild sensitivity
3 moderate sensitivity
4 moderately severe hallucinations
5 severe hallucinations
6 extremely severe hallucinations
7 continuous hallucinations

Table 142.2 *(continued)*

ANXIETY—Ask "Do you feel nervous?" Observation. 1 mildly anxious 2 3 4 moderately anxious, or guarded, so anxiety is inferred 5 6 7 equivalent to acute panic states as seen in severe delirium or acute schizophrenic reactions	**HEADACHE, FULLNESS IN HEAD**—Ask "Does your head feel different? Does it feel like there is a band around your head?" Do not rate for dizziness or lightheadedness. Otherwise, rate severity. 0 not present 1 very mild 2 mild 3 moderate 4 moderately severe 5 severe 6 very severe 7 extremely severe
AGITATION—Observation. 0 normal activity 1 somewhat more than normal activity 2 3 4 moderately fidgety and restless 5 6 7 paces back and forth during most of the interview, or constantly thrashes about	**ORIENTATION AND CLOUDING OF SENSORIUM**—Ask "What day is this? Where are you? Who am I?" 0 oriented and can do serial additions 1 cannot do serial additions or is uncertain about date 2 disoriented for date by no more than 2 calendar days 3 disoriented for date by more than 2 calendar days 4 disoriented for place and/or person Total CIWA-A Score _____ Rater's Initials _____ Maximum Possible Score 67

References

1. *National Household Survey on Drug Abuse (NHSDA).* Washington DC: Substance Abuse and Mental Health Services Administration (SAMHSA), 1999.
2. Schuckit MA, Tipp JE, Reich T, et al. The histories of withdrawal convulsions and delirium tremens in 1648 alcohol dependent subjects. *Addiction* 1955;90: 1335–1347.
3. Ferguson JA, Suelzer CJ, Eckert GJ, et al. Risk factors for delirium tremens development. *J Gen Intern Med* 1996;11:410–414.
4. Adinoff B. The alcohol withdrawal syndrome: neurobiology of treatment and toxicity. *Am J Addict* 1994;3:227–228.
5. Mayo-Smith MF, Beecher LH, Fisher TL, et al. Management of alcohol withdrawal delirium: an evidence-based practice guideline. *Arch Intern Med* 2004;164:1405–1412.
6. Saitz R, Mayo-Smith MF, Roberts MS, et al. Individualized treatment of alcohol withdrawal. A randomized double blind controlled trial. *JAMA* 1994;272: 519–523.
7. Lohr RH. Treatment of alcohol withdrawal in hospitalized patients. *Mayo Clin Proc* 1995;70:777–782.
8. Yost DA. Alcohol withdrawal syndrome. *Am Fam Physician* 1996;54:657–664, 699. Erratum 1996;54:2377.

Tamas R. Peredy
Charles McKay

Prior to twentieth century drug therapy, patients with psychotic illness suffered from uncontrolled hallucinations and delusions, poor reality awareness, and disorganized thoughts and behaviors. Publicly ostracized, they could look forward to life-long isolation from society in asylums that offered little relief from symptoms. The observation that some intoxicants known to increase dopaminergic neurotransmission (e.g., cocaine, amphetamines) induced "psychotic reactions" led biomedical researchers to hypothesize that excessive dopaminergic neurotransmission was, at least, partially responsible for causing schizophrenia. At the time it was the most common chronic psychotic disorder, affecting more than 1% of the U.S. population. In the early 1950s, the era of modern schizophrenia pharmacotherapy began with the introduction of chlorpromazine (Thorazine®), an antihistamine noted to have significant dopamine (DA) antagonism. This class of *dopamine antagonists* acquired descriptive terms such as major tranquilizers and neuroleptics because of their sedation and psychomotor agitation-relieving properties.

Further investigation into the neurochemical imbalances in schizophrenia led to an understanding that while mesolimbic DA excess accounted for many of the positive symptoms, relative frontal cortex DA hypoactivity was responsible for impaired cognitive processing manifested as social withdrawal, impaired attention, flattened affect, and paucity of speech and activity. Conventional DA antagonists further exacerbated these "negative symptoms."

In 1989, clozapine became the first of six new drugs to date to be approved for the treatment of schizophrenia. Clozapine was welcomed as the first agent to demonstrate efficacy in also relieving negative symptoms. The primary and treatment-refractory efficacy superiority over conventional agents was due to combined modest dopamine type-2 receptor (D_2) and stronger serotonin type-2A receptor ($5-HT_{2A}$) activity. These atypical antipsychotics or *serotonin-dopamine antagonists* are defined by a high $5-HT_{2A}/D_2$ affinity ratio, thus resulting in efficacy against both positive and negative symptoms. Lower relative D_2 affinity at therapeutic doses reduces the incidence of excessive dopamine blockade (extrapyramidal symptoms and neuroleptic malignant syndrome). Functionally selective blockade by newer agents in the mesolimbic versus nigrostriatal tract may further improve the side effect profile. Today, more than 80% of antipsychotic prescriptions written are for one of the newer generation agents. Although mesolimbic DA suppression will likely remain a cornerstone of therapy, further research will better define the influence of excitatory neurotransmitters such as glutamate (NMDA receptor) in the pathophysiology of schizophrenia (**Table 143.1**).

Pharmacology

All antipsychotics are available in traditional oral formulations with rapid absorption within 1 to 2 hours. They undergo significant hepatic first-pass metabolism. Several conventional agents are also available in parenteral form for the control of acutely agitated patients or to control vomiting. Sustained release intramuscular injections of haloperidol and fluphenazine provide outpatient compliance in the more cognitively impaired group. Peak effects from the oral preparations are expected by 4 to 6 hours. The newer agents are highly lipophilic (large V_D) and protein bound. Most antipsychotics undergo extensive P-450 hepatic metabolism; however, multiple metabolic pathways reduce the likelihood of enzyme inhibitor induced toxicity. Long elimination half-lives and active metabolites make qd or bid dosing possible. Only risperidone requires dosage adjustment in renal insufficiency. Drug-drug interactions producing additive side effects such as sedation, hypotension, QT prolongation, and weight gain are clinically important.

Physiology

Dopamine

Dopamine (DA) neurotransmission is distributed throughout the brain with higher concentrations located in the mesocorticolimbic, nigrostriatal, tuberoinfundibular tracts, and area postrema. Ventricular tegmental area neurons in

Table 143.1

Partial List of Typical and Atypical Antipsychotics Marketed in the United States

Potency	Class	Generic Name	Brand Name	Typical Daily Dose Range (mg)	Common Routes of Administration
Conventional					
Low	Phenothiazine, aliphatic	chlorpromazine	Thorazine	100–2,000	PO, IV, IM
	Piperidine	thioridazine	Mellaril	100–600	PO
	Piperazine	mesoridazine	Serentil	100–300	PO
High		fluphenazine	Prolixin	2.5–10	PO, IV, IM (and depot IM)
		perphenazine	Trilafon	8–64	PO
		trifluperazine	Stelazine	5–30	PO, IV
	Diphenylbutyl-piperidine	pimozide	Orap	2–10	
	Thioxanthene	thiothixene	Navane	5–60	PO
	Dihydroindolone	molidone	Moban	50–225	PO
	Dibenzoxazepine	loxapine	Loxapine	20–250	PO, IM
	Butyrophenone	haloperidol	Haldol	5–40	PO, IV, IM (and depot IM)
		droperidol	Inapsine	5–40	PO, IV, IM
Atypical	Dibenzodiazepine	clozapine	Clozaril	300–900	PO
		olanzapine	Zyprexa	10–30	ODT, PO, IM
	Thienobenzodiazepine	quetiapine	Seroquel	300–800	PO
	Benzisoxazole	risperidone	Risperdal	2–6	PO (liq)
	Benzoisothiazoyl-piperazine	ziprasidone	Geodon	40–160	PO, IM
	Quinolinone	aripiprazole	Abilify	10–30	PO

the midbrain, medial to the substantia nigra, synapse with other modulating interneurons that extend to the forebrain prefrontal and frontal cortex, pyramidal neurons and limbic centers. These pathways control (1) cortical executive functions such as planning, problem solving, declarative memory, and sensory gating; and (2) emotional responses of fear (amygdala) and pleasure, for example, kindling or drug craving (nucleus accumbens). Axons from the substantia nigra extend to the corpus striatum, the caudate and putamen (basal ganglia) controlling the initiation and organized control of movement. In the diencephalon, projections to the anterior pituitary gland regulate secretory function. The release of prolactin impacts appetite, libido, and fertility. At the caudal end of the fourth ventricle, the chemoreceptor trigger zone modulated by $5\text{-}HT_3$, D_2 and μ receptors represents the final pathway for nausea and vomiting, receiving a variety of input including vagal stimuli to direct exposure to emetic substances in the blood and CSF.

Serotonin

Serotonin is also widely dispersed throughout the CNS influencing many critical processes. Post-synaptic $5\text{-}HT_{2A}$ antagonism of neurons that run from the raphe nuclei to the substantia nigra and basal ganglia by the atypical antipsychotics partially reverse the D_2 blockade and decrease the incidence of EPS. $5\text{-}HT_{2A}$ antagonism in the frontal cortex is more pronounced with a net effect of enhancing

DA neurotransmission, thus relieving many of the negative cognitive symptoms of schizophrenia. Serotonin also plays an important role in mood regulation (including suicidality). These neurotransmitter effects may explain the oft-seen clinical and therapeutic overlap between psychotic and mood disorders. The atypical antipsychotics are active at a number of other important serotonin receptor subtypes.

Common Side Effects

Movement Disorders

In the nigrostriatal tract, DA-acetylcholine balance can be upset by DA antagonists resulting in (1) *acute dystonia*, which is an uncomfortable or painful twisting spasm of the head and neck musculature potentially effecting swallowing, speech, and respiration; and (2) *akathisia*, an uncomfortable diffuse motor restlessness resulting in agitation or even violence. Anticholinergic medication (e.g., benztropine 1–2 mg PO/IV, diphenhydramine 25–50 mg PO/IV) rapidly and dramatically reestablishes the balance of nigrostriatal dopaminergic and cholinergic activity in acute dystonia. Akathisia responds less completely to benzodiazepines, anticholinergics, opiates and lipophilic beta-blockers (such as propranolol 20–80 mg/day) while drug effects dissipate over several hours. Collectively, the outward manifestations of these movement disorders are known as *extrapyramidal symptoms (EPS)*.

Less acutely, neuroleptics can induce (1) a mostly reversible form of parkinsonism associated with bradykinesia, cogwheel rigidity and tremor; and (2) potentially irreversible tardive dyskinesia (TD), which is characterized by involuntary movements of the tongue, face, trunk, and extremities. The incidence of TD with high potency typical antipsychotic treatment is 5% per year compared with less than 1% per year of treatment with atypical antipsychotics. Other chronic movement disorders include chorea, dykinesias, and tics.

Blockade of the DA tuberoinfundibular tract can lead to elevated prolactin levels (loss of suppression) thought to be responsible for gynecomastia, decreased libido, and infertility. A resulting temperature dysregulation may be responsible for the hyperpyrexia seen as part of malignant hyperthermia (MH) and neuroleptic malignant syndrome (NMS).

QT Prolongation

Heightened postmarketing awareness of the rare arrhythmogenic effects (>1 per 100,000 scripts) due to prolonged ventricular repolarization of some medication combinations has resulted in more than a half dozen manufacturing discontinuations in the last few years. Multiple factors influence the cardiac ventricular repolarization rate normally including: age, sex, time of day, hormonal milieu, electrolyte concentration, genetic polymorphisms and medications (see http://www.qtdrugs.org). Potassium ion channels on the myocyte membrane regulate outward repolarization current (cardiac cycle phase 3). Exacerbated by cardiomegaly and bradycardia, a longer QT interval leads to a greater dispersion of asynchronous repolarization in the ventricular myocardium, increasing the potential for early or delayed depolarizations and extrasystolic beats. EKG markers such as QT duration (best calculated from leads II or V_5), QTc corrected for heart rate, QTc dispersion (time difference between shortest and longest QT) and ΔQT (pre- and post-drug therapy) roughly approximate dysrhythmia risk. Not all causes of significant prolonged QT, however, carry similar increased dysrhythmia risk, for example, hypocalcemia and some very proarrhythmogenic drugs influence QT only slightly (5–10 msec). Psychotropic medication-induced K^+ blockade during the increased sympathetic states such as cardiac ischemia and schizophrenia may potentiate risk. Children are also more susceptible to medication related effects on QT interval.

The upper limit of normal QTc is 450 msec in men and 460 msec in women. QTc > 500 msec and an increase of >60 msec appear predictive of increased risk for torsade de pointes (TdP). Thioridazine, its active metabolite mesoridazine and droperidol have received FDA "black box" warnings due to QT prolongation. Ziprasidone has received a bolded warning. Despite less than 4% of patients on risperidone, olanzapine, and haloperidol having QT prolongation > 60 msec, these drugs have been linked with a slightly increased risk for cardiac arrhythmia and sudden death.

Metabolic Effects

Although the second generation or atypical antipsychotics have an improved profile with regard to movement disorders including potentially irreversible TD, longitudinal studies now are documenting profound long-term metabolic consequences of treatment. These effects may ultimately lead to similar noncompliance seen with earlier agents. These effects include weight gain defined by the FDA as greater than 7% of body mass increase, hyperlipidemia and type 2 diabetes mellitus. Hypertriglyceridemia and insulin resistance may be severe, precipitating acute pancreatitis and diabetic ketoacidosis.

After 12 months of treatment, clozapine and olanzapine were associated with the most weight gain. Quetiapine, risperidone, and haloperidol also exhibited increased obesity. The group most susceptible to weight gain appears to be adolescents. Over half of young patients on clozapine or olanzapine gained more than 7% of their baseline weight. The receptor most linked with weight gain appears to be H_1, which may normally provide gut signals of satiety to prevent overeating. Antagonism of the 5-HT$_3$ receptor also plays a role. Although the precise mechanism is unknown, leptin, a peptide hormone secreted by adipose tissue, may also be affected.

Increases in fasting glucose, increasing insulin resistance and, ultimately, new onset diabetes mellitus are seen particularly with clozapine, olanzapine, and quetiapine. Cases in the literature warn of precipitous diabetic ketoacidosis masquerading as a misperceived exacerbation of underlying psychiatric disease. The mechanism is thought to be that antagonism of the 5-HT$_1$ receptor causes decreased pancreatic β-cell responsiveness. Agonism of the 5-HT$_{2A/C}$ receptors simultaneously causes hyperglycemia. Links between type 2 diabetes and weight gain are clear; however, drug-induced diabetic ketoacidosis (DKA) can occur in the absence of obesity.

Atypical antipsychotics also cause elevations in blood lipids, particularly triglycerides. The most prevalent and pronounced elevations are seen with clozapine and olanzapine, potentially resulting in pancreatitis and the eruption of xanthomas. Patients taking olazapine, risperidone, or quetiapine demonstrated decreased low density lipoproteins (LDLs); however, the beneficial effect was offset by a similar decline in the high density lipoprotein (HDL). The long-term lipid effects combined with weight gain and diabetes increase the risk of acute coronary syndrome and stroke.

Clinical Considerations

Acute Overdose

Suicide remains the leading cause of premature death in schizophrenia. Up to 50% will attempt suicide with a 10% lifetime risk of success 25 times greater than that of the general population. Risk factors include prior attempts, male gender, concurrent depression, substance dependency, and medication noncompliance. As opposed to conventional antipsychotics that do not affect risk, atypical agents reduce suicide attempts by up to 80%. Mechanisms suggested include a direct serotonergic antidepressant effect or indirect effects through improved cognition or substance abuse reduction. Antipsychotic ingestion for self-harm, either alone or with co-ingestant antidepressants, mood stabilizers, anxiolytics, and drugs of abuse, remains a frequent ED encounter. More than three-quarters of antipsychotic ingestions are with atypical agents likely reflecting their market predominance. Poison center data suggest that isolated overdose of these agents are relatively benign, with a mortality rate of less than 1%. Management therefore is mainly supportive and targeted toward co-ingestants. However, accidental ingestion and overdose in nonhabituated adults and children can yield significant toxicity such as coma and respiratory arrest.

The most common effects seen in overdose include CNS depression within 1 to 2 hours manifest as confusion, ataxia, slurred speech, lethargy, and coma. Loss of protective airway reflexes can occur. EPS such as dystonias and akathisia are commonly seen with the initiation of antipsychotic therapy, administration of an anti-emetic phenothiazine such as prochlorperazine or promethazine, use of high potency conventional agents to control acute agitation, and with supratherapeutic doses of some atypical antipsychotics due to therapeutic mishap or intentional overdose. Care must be exercised in administering anticholinergic drugs to relieve dystonia, as this can further exacerbate an anticholinergic delirium seen with low potency agents, clozapine, and olanzapine. Patients with history of recent drug overdose and significantly altered mental status must always be evaluated for the presence of toxic co-ingestants, occult trauma, hypoxia, and hypoglycemia. Hypotension and reflex tachycardia commonly observed usually responds to Trendelenburg positioning and crystalloid infusion of 20 to 40 cc/kg. The use of vasopressors such as epinephrine and dopamine can theoretically worsen hypotension by β stimulation in the face of α blockade. Norepinephrine is therefore recommended. Drugs with additive QT effects such as type I antiarrhythmics should be avoided.

Less common effects encountered include prolonged QT and repolarization abnormalities on EKG. Rarely is intervention necessary even in the face of significant abnormalities. Continuous monitoring and correction of potassium, magnesium, and calcium abnormalities are reasonable steps. The use of sodium bicarbonate in the absence of QRS prolongation may be detrimental as the EKG abnormalities predominantly reflect potassium channel, and not sodium channel blockade. Seizures occur rarely with the antipsychotics and have often been attributed to a lowering of the seizure threshold by phenothiazines. With the exception of clozapine, the atypical antipsychotics likely do not increase the risk of seizures. Treatment of seizures with benzodiazepines is usually sufficient. Transaminase elevations may be present, but are rarely a clinical problem following overdose.

Patients who remain asymptomatic for 4 hours of observation with no other worrisome coingestants can be transferred to the nonmonitored psychiatric area. Those patients, however, who are too somnolent to provide a psychiatric interview or require monitoring for EKG and blood pressure changes should be considered for a short stay admission to the medical ward as symptoms may persist for 12 to 24 hours.

Atypical Antipsychotics

Clozapine (Clozaril®)

The oldest of the atypical antipsychotics, it is now reserved for cases refractory to all other antipsychotics due to its adverse effect profile. Bone marrow suppressive effects mandate frequent CBCs and careful evaluation, particularly in the setting of unexplained fever. Clozapine levels are useful for compliance purposes only. Clozapine may lower seizure thresholds via GABA antagonism. Common side effects include sedation, weight gain, sialorrhea, constipation, tachycardia, and hypotension. Clozapine will cause a false positive on many tricyclic antidepressant (TCA) immunoassays.

Olanzapine (Zyprexa®)

Olanzapine structurally most closely resembles clozapine and is closest in side effect profile. There is significant weight gain, dry mouth, and constipation, but less sedation occurs. An orally dissolving tablet (Zydis ODT) is available for rapid onset in the setting of acute agitation. In overdose, olanzapine may mimic opiate intoxication due to a decreased level of consciousness, hypotension, and miosis (α_2 blockade similar to clonidine) but is unresponsive to nalaxone. Its trade name, Zyprexa®, has been confused by patients with similar-sounding drug names, resulting in medication administration errors.

Risperidone (Risperdal®)

Risperidone is the most widely prescribed antipsychotic in the United States since its introduction in 1994. Doses above 6 mg/d are associated with loss of atypical features and increased EPS. Risperidone is associated with sedation, elevated prolactin, hypotension, and akathisia. Less weight gain occurs. A parenteral form is marketed for acute agitation. Small doses are recommended initially, especially in the elderly due to sedation. Risperidone is the only antipsychotic that requires reduced dosing in renal insufficiency.

Quetiapine (Seroquel®)

This agent is also structurally similar to clozapine but has several orders of magnitude less bone marrow suppression. Quetiapine has the shortest receptor and effective half-life and, thus, twice daily dosing is recommended. It is highly sedating in the overdose setting. Other effects reported include weight gain, prolonged tachycardia, hypotension, hypokalemia, and QT prolongation that may last for hours to several days after ingestion. Aggressive supportive care including IV fluids and airway protection may be necessary. Quetiapine will also produce a false-positive TCA urine immunoassay screen.

Ziprasidone (Geodon®)

This more recent atypical agent on the market has the highest $5\text{-HT}_2/D_2$ ratio exhibiting fewer anticholinergic effects, such as minimal postural hypotension and reflex tachycardia, and metabolic effects. Side effects may include sedation, dyspepsia, hypertension, muscle weakness, and nasal congestion. Rarely, ziprasidone is implicated in the onset of EPS and hyperprolactinemia. Despite demonstrable drug-induced QT prolongation no increased incidence of sudden cardiac death has been reported. Ziprasidone is recommended with food to improve absorption. Its short half-life requires twice daily dosing. A rapid-acting IM formulation every 4 to 6 hours is available for acute agitation. Because of multiple metabolic pathways, fewer drug-drug interactions are seen.

Aripiprazole (Abilify®)

The newest of the atypical drugs, sometimes referred to as a *second generation atypical drug,* provides low level D_2 intrinsic activity (IDA or "dopamine stabilization") allowing for higher D_2 receptor occupancy without the development of EPS at therapeutic doses. The net effect of this constant intrinsic agonist combined with variable affinity for certain dopaminergic neurons called *functional selectivity* has been referred to as agonist trafficking. Few metabolic and cardiac conduction abnormalities are seen chronically. Common side effects include sedation, headache, nausea, constipation, and dizziness. Limited data exists in the overdose setting but EPS may occur. Aripiprazole has a half-life >48 hours. As with many drugs that are metabolized by P-450 CYP3A3/4 and CYP2D6, doses should be reduced when administered with enzyme inhibitors such as some SSRIs, antifungals, and macrolide antibiotics.

Special Considerations

Neuroleptic Malignant Syndrome

Neuroleptic malignant syndrome (NMS) is the rarest and most severe form of EPS. This disorder is usually seen in the few weeks following initial use of the high potency antipsychotics. It is estimated that less than 1% of patients on neuroleptics will experience NMS, which usually occurs within the first month of treatment. Men are affected twice as often as women. Mortality rates of 10% to 20% are reported, probably reflecting a combination of late recognition, inadequate treatment, and underlying illness or fragile health. The syndrome is characterized by temperature elevations, muscle rigidity, lethargy, and rhabdomyolysis. The onset is often subacute, with progressive mental status change and increasing muscular rigidity over hours to days. All features may not be present or occur at the same time; therefore, a high index of suspicion is important. A prior history of NMS to other agents increases its likelihood. Treatment is mainly supportive with cessation of the offending agent(s), efforts to reduce temperature, avoidance of agents such as anticholinergics that prevent heat dissipation, fluid resuscitation, and anxiolysis. A predominance of central effects can be treated with a dopamine agonist such as bromocriptine given via nasogastric tube at 5 mg every 6 to 8 hours. Significant muscular rigidity or rhabdomyolysis, particularly if associated with fever, can be treated with dantrolene (1 mg/kg IV, possibly repeated in 5–10 min, up to 10 mg/kg) in addition to benzodiazepines. Neuromuscular paralysis and intubation are often required.

Selected Readings

Burns MJ. The pharmacology and toxicology of atypical antipsychotic agents. *J Toxicol Clin Toxicol* 2001;39:1–14.

Freedman R. Schizophrenia. *N Engl J Med* 2003;349:1738–1749.

Grunder G, Carlsson A, Wong DF. Mechanism of new antipsychotic medications: occupancy is not just antagonism. *Arch Gen Psych* 2003;60:974–977.

Jibson MD, Tandon R. An overview of antischizophrenic medications. *CNS News* 2001;Nov 15–18.

Labellarte MJ, Crosson JE, Riddle MA. The relevance of prolonged QTc measurement to pediatric psychopharmacology. *J Am Acad Child Adolesc Psychiatry* 2003;42:642–650.

Markowitz JS, Brown CS, Moore TR, et al. Atypical antipsychotics: part II: adverse effects, drug interactions, and costs. *Ann Pharmacother* 1999;33:210–217.

Markowitz JS, Brown CS, Moore TR. Atypical antipsychotics: part I: pharmacology, pharmacokinetics and efficacy. *Ann Pharmacother* 1999;33:73–85.

Meyer JM. Novel antipsychotics and severe hyperlipidemia. *J Clin Psychopharmacol* 2001;21:369–374.

Mullins M, van Zwieten K, Blunt JR. Unexpected cardiovascular deaths are rare with therapeutic doses of droperidol. *Am J Emerg Med* 2004;22:27–28.

Tandon R. Safety and tolerability: how do newer generation "atypical" antipsychotics compare? *Psychiatr Quart* 2002;73:297–311.

Thummel KE, Wilkinson GR. In vitro and in vivo drug interactions involving human CYP3A. *Ann Rev Pharmacol Toxicol* 1998;38:389–430.

van Zwieten K, Mullins ME, Jang T. Droperidol and the black box warning. *Ann Emerg Med* 2004;43:139–140.

Viewed WV. Mechanisms and risks of electrocardiographic QT interval prolongation when using antipsychotic drugs. *J Clin Psychiatry* 2002;63(Suppl 9):18–24.

Wirshing DA. Adverse effects of atypical antipsychotics. *J Clin Psychiatry* 2002;62(Suppl 21):7–10.

Wirshing DA, Boyd JA, Meng LR, et al. The effects of novel antipsychotics on glucose and lipid levels. *J Clin Psychiatry* 2002;63:856–865.

Wirshing DA, Pierre JM, Erhart SM, et al. Understanding the new and evolving profile of adverse drug effects in schizophrenia. *Psychiatr Clin N Am* 2003;26:165–190.

Witchel HJ, Hancox JC, Nutt DJ. Psychotropic drugs, cardiac arrhythmia, and sudden death. *J Clin Psychopharmacol* 2003;23:58–77.

Lithium

Christina Hernon
Edward W. Boyer

Lithium intoxication can arise from long-term therapy or following acute overdose. Small adjustments to a dose or the frequency of administration may produce significant adverse effects. Patients maintained on lithium are at increased risk for toxicity when renal perfusion decreases. Because lithium is renally eliminated, dehydration can lead to increased serum lithium concentrations, particularly when patients remain compliant with medications.

Clinical Manifestations

Although lithium intoxication affects several body systems, neurotoxicity remains the hallmark of severe, acute poisoning.

Central Nervous System

Early signs of lithium intoxication may manifest as serotonergic signs of diarrhea, hyperreflexia, tremor, and myoclonus. Worsening toxicity may present as confusion, agitated delirium, or coma. Mild to moderate lithium intoxication may be distinguished from phenytoin toxicity by the presence of clonus; both conditions may have ataxia and nystagmus, but only patients with lithium poisoning will demonstrate clonus.

Gastrointestinal

Following acute ingestion, patients may develop vomiting and diarrhea.

Cardiovascular

The predominant cardiovascular abnormality in lithium poisoning involves diffuse ST depressions and/or T wave inversions. Complete heart block has been described in massive overdose.

Hematological

Lithium intoxication is associated with leukocytosis with predominant neutrophilia.

Renal

Lithium exerts several effects on the renal beds, the most predominant being nephrogenic diabetes insipidus accompanied by polyuria and polydipsia. Hyponatremia is a common finding in patients with chronic lithium toxicity.

Diagnosis

The diagnosis of lithium intoxication is based upon clinical findings. Lithium possesses a narrow therapeutic index, which means that patients may be intoxicated despite high normal or mildly elevated serum concentrations. A low anion gap may be observed in patients maintained on drug.

Management

Patients with lithium intoxication should receive the following:

1. Discontinuation of lithium.
2. Discontinuation of concomitant diuretics. Thiazide diuretics in particular may alter sodium elimination and should be withheld.
3. Gastrointestinal decontamination. Patients suffering from an acute ingestion should receive polyethylene glycol solutions at a rate of 2 L/h until the rectal effluent is clear. Placement of a nasogastric tube may be required to achieve this rate of administration, and nursing chores may be eased by the application of a rectal tube.
4. Fluid resuscitation. Dehydrated patients should receive half-normal saline (to prevent precipitating hypertonicity that may occur in patients with diabetes insipidus) to restore renal function.
5. Extracorporeal elimination. Patients with severe lithium intoxication should receive hemodialysis. Neurotoxicity from severe lithium poisoning may be persistent, but hemodialysis may mitigate this clinical observation. Patients who therefore meet the clinical criteria for hemodialysis will not improve in several hours to the point that dialysis is not needed. Consequently, obtaining additional lithium concentrations to determine patient condi-

tion are fruitless, particularly since the diagnosis is made primarily on clinical grounds. Consultation with a Clinical Toxicology Service or Poison Control Center can provide specific recommendations to assist in clinical decision-making. Patients who undergo hemodialysis may exhibit a rebound in lithium concentration 2–4 hours following therapy and need additional runs of dialysis.

Selected Reading

Lithium. In: *Clinical Management of Poisoning and Drug Overdose,* 3rd ed. Haddad LM, Shannon MW, Winchester JF, ed. Philadelphia: W.B. Saunders, 1998:467–474.

Tricyclic Antidepressants

Rachel A. Goldstein
Charles McKay

Cyclic antidepressants (CAs) have a variety of clinical indications, including depression, migraine headaches, neuropathic pain, fibromyalgia, and attention deficit hyperactivity disorder. They are prescribed in all age groups and are therefore accessible to household contacts. In 2002, there were 99,860 toxic exposures to antidepressants reported to poison control centers nationwide. Of these, 13,005 were CAs with 118 fatalities. In preschool children, antidepressants are the second most commonly prescribed medication.

Imiprimine, the first CA, was developed in 1950s. During the 1960s to 1980s, CAs were the most commonly prescribed drug for depression. The newer CAs, maprotiline and amoxapine, which have a tetracyclic structure, have less cardiac toxicity than the earlier tricyclic antidepressants. However, neurotoxicity (seizures) is more common.

Pharmacology

The pharmacological mechanisms of action include: inhibition of neurotransmitter uptake (norepinephrine and/or serotonin), sodium channel blocking effects, and inhibition of central sympathetic reflexes. With the exception of desipramine, the CAs have antihistamine properties that contribute to sedation.

Pharmacokinetics

Antidepressants in general are well absorbed from the GI tract, with peak concentrations of most (with a notable exception of maprotiline) occurring within two hours after ingestion of a therapeutic dose. However, CAs taken in overdose may result in delayed absorption secondary to anticholinergic effects, that is, slowed peristalsis.

CAs are lipophilic, widely distributed, and highly protein bound with variable volumes of distribution (15–40 L/kg). Because of this extensive distribution and protein binding, the majority of the absorbed drug is not available for hemodialysis or hemoperfusion. As an example, less than 2% of an ingested dose of imiprimine is present in the blood several hours after overdose.

CAs are primarily metabolized by the liver, with a small fraction being excreted unchanged in the urine. Imiprimine and amitriptyline are metabolized to desipramine and nortriptyline respectively. There are additional metabolites of both tertiary and secondary amines which maintain some pharmacological activity. These metabolites may contribute to toxicity after the first 12–24 hours.

Clinical Manifestations

In general, the CAs have a low toxic threshold, doses of less than 10 times therapeutic daily dose producing severe toxicity. An acute ingestion of 10 to 20 mg/kg or two 50 mg imiprimine tablets in a toddler may be lethal. Therapeutic doses are 2–4 mg/kg/d. In an adult, a dose more than 1 gram can be life-threatening. Initial symptoms tend to be anticholinergic in nature, with increasing drowsiness followed by stupor. The narrow complex tachycardia reflecting the anticholinergic effects may progress in serious overdose with evidence of cardiac conduction abnormalities. Seizures may occur, usually in the setting of significant altered mental status and hypotension. The acidosis precipitated by seizures may be associated with a rapidly worsening clinical situation, with a wide complex tachycardia leading to bradyasystole or ventricular dysrhythmias, and death. As noted earlier, the tetracyclics have little, if any, cardiotoxicity; neurotoxicity therefore occurs in the absence of EKG abnormalities.

Laboratory Assessment

There is little utility in measuring serum CA levels. Most hospital laboratories cannot provide a rapid turnaround for quantitative CA determinations. Although studies have shown that levels of 1000 ng/mL or greater are usually associated with serious poisoning, the rapid onset of clinical and EKG findings preclude these being useful. Commonly available qualitative urine antibody screens, including point of care devices, offer the advantage of a rapid turnaround but suffer greatly from a lack of specificity. In many institutions, a positive tricyclic drug screen is as likely to represent the presence of a cross-reacting substance as it is a CA. Characteristic EKG findings, including a rightward shift in the terminal 40 msec of the QRS (seen as a broad positive R wave in aVR and a deep slurred S wave in Lead I) and QRS widening are the best laboratory indicators of CA toxicity.

Initial Management

Patients with suspected CA overdose should be triaged as high-risk, because of the tendency for these patients to deteriorate quickly. Treatment should be aggressive; rapid intubation is recommended for patients who present with CNS depression and/or significant EKG changes (especially wide-complex tachycardia). Twelve-lead EKG and laboratory tests should be done on all patients. Labs should include electrolytes, glucose, urine toxicology screen (to rule out some other common ingestions or drug abuse history), serum ethanol determination, and an arterial blood gas to determine pH and ventilatory effort.

Generally, patients who will experience life-threatening CA toxicity following overdose will demonstrate abnormal mental status, and conduction and hemodynamic abnormalities within two-three hours of ingestion. A patient who has no evidence of toxicity (including anticholinergic findings) more than six hours after an overdose can be safely assessed as being at low risk for CA toxicity.

Treatment of Cardiac Toxicity

Although CAs may cause changes in the EKG at therapeutic or toxic serum levels, progressive EKG changes are usually seen with increasing clinical illness severity (**FIGURE 145.1**). The most serious of these findings are dysrhythmias, hypotension, and seizures. Hypotension is strongly associated with the development of arrhythmias and pulmonary edema, and is especially found in patients with prolonged QRS intervals and elevated TCA levels. A QRS prolongation of greater than 100 msec and a terminal 40-ms frontal plane axis greater than 120 degrees are the most sensitive predictors of CA overdose. Once cardiotoxicity is evident, the first-line treatment for CA-induced dysrhythmias is serum alkalinization with sodium bicarbonate. By overcoming sodium channel blockade by both sodium loading and altering the channel binding by increased pH, sodium bicarbonate given as a bolus of 1 to 2 mEq/kg IV can reverse the conduction slowing responsible for reentrant dysrhythmias. By extension from this physiological effect and as demonstrated in animal myocardial studies, improved conduction is associated with improved contractility, and hence resolution of this aspect of hemodynamic impairment. To date, available evidence does not support using this therapy prophylactically in the absence of life-threatening cardiovascular toxicity.

Additional pharmacological modalities that have been discussed for CA cardiotoxicity include lidocaine, physostigmine, propanolol, and phenytoin. Lidocaine has membrane-stabilizing properties similar to CAs, which may act to impair conductivity and decrease cardiac conductivity. This is largely a theoretical concern; lidocaine is classified as a Type Ib (rather than Type Ia) agent. Currently, lidocaine is a reasonable choice for ventricular dysrhythmias refractory to sodium bicarbonate. Of note, many patients with a wide complex tachycardia actually demonstrate

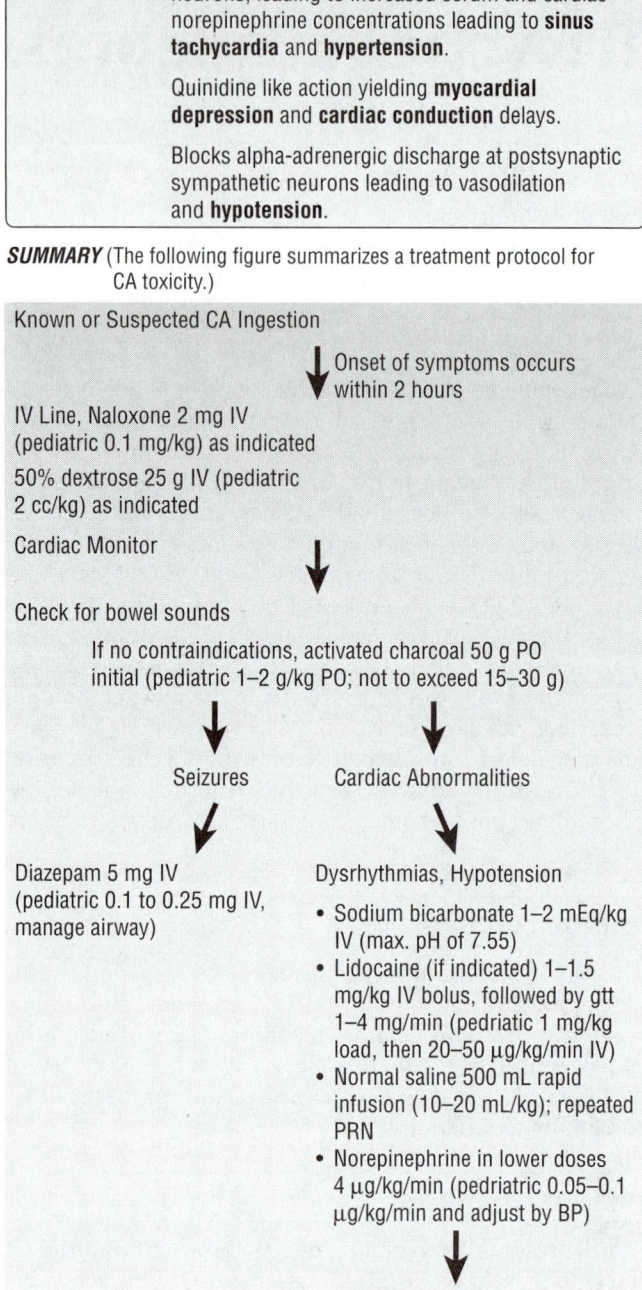

Cardiotoxicity	Atropinelike, anticholinergic effect yielding **sinus tachycardia**.
	Block re-uptake of norepinephrine in adrenergic neurons, leading to increased serum and cardiac norepinephrine concentrations leading to **sinus tachycardia** and **hypertension**.
	Quinidine like action yielding **myocardial depression** and **cardiac conduction** delays.
	Blocks alpha-adrenergic discharge at postsynaptic sympathetic neurons leading to vasodilation and **hypotension**.

SUMMARY (The following figure summarizes a treatment protocol for CA toxicity.)

Known or Suspected CA Ingestion

↓ Onset of symptoms occurs within 2 hours

IV Line, Naloxone 2 mg IV (pediatric 0.1 mg/kg) as indicated

50% dextrose 25 g IV (pediatric 2 cc/kg) as indicated

Cardiac Monitor

↓

Check for bowel sounds

If no contraindications, activated charcoal 50 g PO initial (pediatric 1–2 g/kg PO; not to exceed 15–30 g)

↓ Seizures   ↓ Cardiac Abnormalities

Diazepam 5 mg IV (pediatric 0.1 to 0.25 mg IV, manage airway)

↓ Dysrhythmias, Hypotension

- Sodium bicarbonate 1–2 mEq/kg IV (max. pH of 7.55)
- Lidocaine (if indicated) 1–1.5 mg/kg IV bolus, followed by gtt 1–4 mg/min (pedriatic 1 mg/kg load, then 20–50 µg/kg/min IV)
- Normal saline 500 mL rapid infusion (10–20 mL/kg); repeated PRN
- Norepinephrine in lower doses 4 µg/kg/min (pediatric 0.05–0.1 µg/kg/min and adjust by BP)

↓ Heart Block

Atropine 0.5 mg IV or Temporary Pacer

FIGURE 145.1 Clinical signs and major mechanisms of cyclic antidepressant (CA) toxicity.

aberrant atrioventricular conduction, rather than ventricular dysrhythmia. A clue to this is the narrowing of QRS complexes with the administration of sodium bicarbonate, without a rate change. The proposed utility of physostigmine or propanolol is the longer diastolic recovery time (with reopening of closed, and activation of inactivated sodium channels) imparted by the bradycardia they induce. Propanolol terminated ventricular tachycardia in animal models and humans, but also caused severe hypotension. Physostigmine was more frequently used as a first-line therapy for both neurological and cardiac toxic effects of CA overdose, but its use was discouraged following reports of asystole temporally associated with its administration.

Phenytoin was thought to have antidysrhythmic properties in CA overdose, secondary to it enhancement of atrioventricular and intraventricular conduction as well as decreasing ventricular automaticity. If conduction velocity is increased, CA-initiated reentrant dysrhythmias could be prevented. Studies have not borne this out. Based on available evidence, the use of phenytoin as an antidysrhythmic agent is not recommended with CA-associated widecomplex tachydysrhythmias. The reports of recovery following cardiac arrest due to CA toxicity with prolonged resuscitation emphasize the important role of potentially reversible sodium channel blockade in an otherwise cardiovascularly healthy population.

Treatment of Neurotoxicity

Seizures caused by CA toxicity are usually brief and generalized, occurring soon after ingestion. Because prolonged seizures can result in hypoxia and metabolic acidosis, those that last more than 2 minutes should be treated to prevent potential cardiac disturbances. Benzodiazepines are the first-line treatment; phenytoin should not be used to treat seizure activity. Status epilepticus is not common with CAs with the exception of amoxapine or with other coingestions. In this case, neuromuscular paralysis may be indicated to prevent metabolic acidosis and any cardiac repercussions of cyclic-induced seizures. In the post-ictal

period, broadening of the QRS duration or hypotension can be exacerbated. Recent studies have raised the consideration of prophylactic antiseizure medications (e.g., long-acting benzodiazepines or a slow infusion of phenobarbital) in the subgroup of hypotensive CA-poisoned patients to prevent further cardiovascular deterioration. CA-induced coma will in general display a waxing and waning pattern and will usually resolve within 24 hours, although some cases may persist longer. Other coingestions should be considered in cases of prolonged coma.

Selected Readings

Blackman K, Brown S, Wilkes GJ. Plasma alkalinization for tricyclic antidepressant toxicity: a systemic review. *Emerg Med (Fremantle)* 2001;13:204–210.

Boehnert MT, Lovejoy FH. Value of the QRS duration versus the serum drug level in predicting seizures and ventricular arrhythmias after an acute overdose of tricyclic antidepressants. *N Engl J Med* 1985;22:474–479.

Callahan M, Schumaker H, Pentel P. Phenytoin prophylaxis of cardiotoxicity in experimental amitriptyline poisoning. *J Pharmacol Exp Ther* 1988;245:216–220.

Cusack P, Nelson A, Richelson E. Binding of antidepressants to human brain receptors: focus on a newer generation compounds. *Psychopharmacology* 1994;114:559–565.

Glassman AH. Cardiovascular effects of tricyclic antidepressants. *Ann Rev Med* 1984;35:503–511.

Groleau G, Jotte R, Barish R. The electrocardiographic manifestations of cyclic antidepressant therapy and overdose: a review. *J Emerg Med* 1990;8:597–605.

Hagerman GA, Hanashiro PK. Reversal of tri-cyclic antidepressant induced cardiac conduction abnormalities by phenytoin. *Ann Emerg Med* 1981;10:82–86.

Mayron R, Ruiz E. Phenytoin: does it reverse TCA induced cardiac conduction abnormalities? *Ann Emerg Med* 1986;15:876–878.

Orr DA, Bramble MG. TCA poisoning and prolonged external cardiac massage during asystole. *Br Med J* 1981;283:1107–1108.

Osterhoudt KC. The toxic toddler: drugs that can kill in small doses. *Contemp Pediatr* 2000;17:73–88.

Pentel PR, Bullock M, DeVane CL. Hemoperfusion for imipramine overdose: elimination of active metabolites. *J Toxicol Clin Toxicol* 1982;10:239–248.

Rudorfer MV, Potter WZ. Metabolism of tricyclic antidepressants. *Cell Mol Neurobiol* 1999;19:373–409.

Sasyniuk BI, Jhamandas V. Experimental amitriptyline intoxication. Treatment of cardiac toxicity with sodium bicarbonate. *Ann Emerg Med* 1986;15:1052–1059.

Shannon M, Merola J, Lovejoy F. Hypotension in severe tricyclic antidepressant overdose. *Am J Emerg Med* 1988;6:439–442.

Suchard JR. Assessing physostigmine's contraindication in CA ingestions. *J Emerg Med* 2003;25:185–191.

146 Anticonvulsants

Alberto Perez

Charles McKay

Epidemiology

It is estimated that over 1.5 million Americans suffer from seizure disorders; however, the use of anticonvulsants extends beyond the realm of seizure control. Conditions treated with anticonvulsants (and the most common agents used) include: mood disorders (gabapentin, lamotrigine), withdrawal syndromes (valproic acid, carbamazepine), trigeminal neuralgia (carbamazepine), bipolar disorder (carbamazepine, valorous acid, gabapentin), and migraine prophylaxis (gabapentin).

The AAPCC 2002 annual report implicated anticonvulsants in 35,836 exposures. Of these, approximately 7,200 were classified as moderate or major. The broader clinical use of anticonvulsants such as carbamazepine and valproic acid has been associated with increases in exposure rates.

From a historical view, anticonvulsant therapy began in 1857 with the administration of bromides. Bromides remained the mainstay therapy until phenobarbital was first used in 1912. Phenytoin, the first nonsedating anticonvulsant, was introduced in 1938. The 1960s revolutionized the care of seizing patients with the introduction of benzodiazepines, carbamazepine, and valproic acid. Since 1993, many more anticonvulsants have appeared. These include: gabapentin, felbamate, lamotrigine, levetiracetam, oxcarbazepine, tiagabine, topiramate, and vigabatrin.

Pharmacology and Mechanism of Action

Seizures result from an increase in high-frequency neuronal firing secondary to abnormal sodium channel activity, excessive calcium conduction, increased neuronal excitation, and/or loss of inhibition. Anticonvulsant therapy corrects these abnormalities through blocking voltage-dependent sodium channels, calcium channel blockade, antiglutaminergic/NMDA receptor blockade, and GABA-ergic effects, respectively. **Table 146.1** summarizes the different mechanisms thought to provoke seizures and the putative activity of the anticonvulsants. The emergency department management of the overdosed patient is largely supportive. However, the emergency physician must be cognizant of special considerations pertinent to each of the commonly utilized anticonvulsants.

This chapter focuses mainly on the management of carbamazepine, valproic acid, and phenytoin overdoses. Special considerations for the newer anticonvulsants have been summarized.

Phenytoin

Phenytoin is the first line anticonvulsant for most indications other than absence seizures. It is a preferred anticonvulsant given that it is nonsedating at therapeutic concentrations. It is available in various enteral formulations but may also be given intravenously. The IV formulation is dissolved in propylene glycol. The poor water solubility of this product and the alkaline pH of the parenteral preparation prevent intramuscular use. The soft tissue injury resulting from inadvertent extravasation of this product can necessitate skin grafting. A maximum rate of IV infusion 50 mg/min must be respected to avoid hypotension and local irritation. The development of a phosphate ester derivative of phenytoin, fosphenytoin, has overcome many of these problems.

Phenytoin is a weak base (pKa 8.3) with high protein bonding (90%) that is rapidly absorbed from the gastrointestinal tract. Large overdoses of phenytoin have been associated with prolonged absorption and bezoar formation. Furthermore, clinical conditions that result in significant increases in the free fraction (e.g., hypoalbuminemia, uremia) increase the risk of toxicity from decreased binding of the drug.

Phenytoin undergoes hepatic metabolism. Its major metabolite (parahydroxyphenyl derivative) is inactive but thought to be responsible for hypersensitivity reactions. Phenytoin's hepatic metabolism is characterized by Michaelis-Menton kinetics. At concentrations below 10 mg/L, it follows first-order elimination with a half-life between 6 and 24 hours. At higher doses, enzymatic systems are saturated and elimination becomes dose-dependent (zero-order kinetics) with a half-life of 20 to 60 hours. The kidneys excrete 5% of a therapeutic dose as unchanged drug.

The manifestations of phenytoin toxicity are concentration dependent. Patients will almost uniformly have

Table 146.1
Therapeutic Approach to Seizures

Cause of Seizure	Therapeutic Approach	Drug
Abnormal Sodium Channel	Blockade of Na channel	P,C,VA
		L,F, T,OC,G
Increase Calcium Conduction	Modulation of Ca channels	G
Increase Excitation	Suppression of glutamate-NMDA interaction	
	—competitive glutamate antagonist	F, VA
	—inhibition glutamate release	L, T, P (high doses)
Loss of Inhibition	Increase GABA concentrations	
	—increase release	G
	—inhibit GABA transaminase	V, VA
	—inhibit reuptake	Ti

Abbreviations: C, carbamazepine; G, gabapentin; F, felbamate; L, lamotrigine; Unknown, evetiracetam; OC, oxcarbazeoine; P, phenytoin; Ti, tiagabine; T, topiramate; VA, valproic acid; V, vigabatrin.

neurological dysfunction characterized by cerebellar and vestibular symptomatology. Generally speaking, concentrations of 15 mg/L produce nystagmus; at 30 mg/L patients lead to ataxia; and 50 mg/L often produce lethargy, slurred speech, pyramidal, and extrapyramidal signs. Seizures in the setting of overdose are rare. Atypical manifestations (chorea, opistotonos) have been described in the extremes of ages.

Cardiovascular manifestations such as impairment of myocardial contractility with hypotension, and bradycardia are related to dose and rate of intravenous administration but are due to the diluent, propylene glycol. Cardiovascular manifestations are not observed with enteral administration.

Therapeutic serum phenytoin determinations should be between 10 and 20 mg/L. A free phenytoin fraction should not exceed 2.1 mg/L. Special attention in the interpretation of levels is required in patients with impaired or decreased protein-binding capacity (i.e., neonates, elderly, hypoalbuminemia, hyperbilirubinemia, uremic) and in patients receiving agents that displace phenytoin from proteins (i.e., salicylates, sulfamides, tolbutamide, valorous acid). When indicated a free phenytoin determination should be requested. If a free level is not available, the active phenytoin fraction may be calculated knowing the serum albumin concentration and total phenytoin concentration.

$$\text{Phenytoin} = \frac{\text{measured phenytoin}}{(0.25 \times \text{measured albumin}) + 0.1}$$

The ED management of phenytoin overdose is supportive. A recent ingestion may benefit from activated charcoal. The administration of multiple dose activated charcoal (MDAC) is reported to enhance elimination (gut dialysis); however, the clinical impact of this intervention is unknown and the potential complications of MDAC must be weighed. Given the significant ataxia that may result, close monitoring of the neurological status is warranted. Serial daily serum determinations may be helpful once the patient is admitted. There is no need for cardiac monitoring of patients with phenytoin poisoning. There are no antidotes and no role for enhanced elimination techniques.

Fosphenytoin is a water-soluble ester derivative of phenytoin that lacks the cardiotoxic effects and local tissue damage from the propylene glycol used in parenteral phenytoin formulations. Fosphenytoin is converted to phenytoin within 6 and 16 minutes of injection (1.5 mg of fosphenytoin = 1 mg phenytoin). This agent can also be administered IV at a more rapid rate than phenytoin; however, the time required for conversion of the prodrug may negate any anticonvulsant benefit of more rapid delivery.

Carbamazepine

Carbamazepine is a carbamylated derivative of iminostilbene that was first introduced in 1947. It is related structurally to imipramine, resulting in immunoassay cross-reactivity with tricyclic antidepressant screens. Although carbamazepine ingestions have resulted in death, it is generally regarded as a safe drug with relatively few reported cases of severe toxicity. It is utilized in the treatment of seizures, chronic pain syndromes, migraine prophylaxis, and bipolar disorder, and is considered a first-line anticonvulsant in pregnancy.

Carbamazepine has numerous pharmacologic effects including sedation, anticholinergic, pro-arrhythmic, muscle relaxant, antidiuretic, and antidepressant effects.

Carbamazepine is only available in oral formulation, in solid immediate and sustained release preparations as well as in suspension. The solid formulations are characterized by slow and unpredictable absorption with late peaks in overdose circumstances. The suspension has rapid absorption with resultant peak and therapeutic concentrations within 2 hours; therefore, suspension ingestions may give rise to significant early toxicity, especially in children.

Once absorbed, carbamazepine is rapidly distributed. It is hepatically metabolized by the cytochrome 3A4 system into a primary metabolite, carbamazepine-10, 11-epoxide (CBZE). This active metabolite is not routinely measured and has been thought to contribute significantly to the toxicity since it has a longer half-life than the parent compound. The presence of CBZE may explain the observed lack of correlation between carbamazepine serum concentrations and clinical findings. Carbamazepine auto-induces its metabolism, often forcing adjustments in dosage after the first few weeks of therapy. Carbamazepine also undergoes enterohepatic recirculation. Together, these two features make the half-life of CBZ after an acute ingestion extremely unpredictable.

The manifestations of a CBZ overdose are primarily neurological. These include nystagmus, ataxia, dysarthria, lethargy, and coma, culminating in respiratory depression. Children develop severe manifestations at lower serum levels and develop dystonic reactions, choreoathetosis, and seizures with higher frequency than adults. Coma itself is not associated with a bad outcome. Patients may seize regardless of previous convulsive history. Seizures are usually self-limited and respond to benzodiazepines. Status epilepticus is a rare but ominous complication.

Carbamazepine overdose may produce cardiotoxicity. One third of patients will develop sinus tachycardia secondary to the anticholinergic effects of CBZ. Hypotension, conduction delays (QRS widening >100 msec) and QTc prolongation (>420 msec) have been reported. Limited data suggest ventricular tachycardia that is thought to arise from tricyclic antidepressant-like effects on the myocardium. SIADH has been reported at high carbamazepine levels and occasionally with chronic therapy.

Although there is a rough correlation between high serum concentrations and severity of toxicity, the patient's clinical status emergency clinician must guide management. The diagnosis of CBZ poisoning relies upon clinical findings and is supported by serum determination. Repeated serum determinations are essential given the erratic absorption and possibility of delayed peak. Therapeutic serum concentrations are between 4 and 12 mg/L. Serum CBZ concentrations greater than 40 mg/L in the adult are predictive of coma, seizures, respiratory depression and cardiotoxicity. Children manifest serious toxicity at lower concentrations.

The emergency department management of a carbamazepine overdose is mainly supportive. Activated charcoal is recommended if airway compromise or ileus from the anticholinergic effects is not a limiting factor. MDAC reduces enterohepatic circulation, but should be used judiciously given the concern for ileus and bowel obstruction secondary to inspissated charcoal. Whole bowel irrigation must be considered following recent ingestion of the extended release preparation. The possibility of concretions must be entertained with delayed symptoms or persistently rising levels.

Cardiac monitoring is recommended. No intervention is warranted for the sinus tachycardia but hypotension requires intravenous fluids and possibly vasopressors. Alkalinization of the serum with intravenous boluses of sodium bicarbonate has been described for the rare carbamazepine induced wide complex tachycardia, and is a reasonable intervention given the structural analog to tricyclic antidepressants.

Seizures are usually responsive to benzodiazepines. In the rare event of refractory seizures, phenobarbital is indicated. Phenytoin is not expected to be of any benefit because it shares the same anticonvulsant mechanism as CBZ.

Hemodialysis and charcoal hemoperfusion, although of limited efficacy, may be warranted in situations of severe toxicity (cardiac toxicity, status epilepticus or an ileus that impedes adequate decontamination).

Valproic Acid

Valproic acid (VPA, di-n-propylacetic acid) is a short chain fatty acid–simple branched carboxylic acid. It is prescribed for a variety of conditions including simple, complex absence, complex partial, myotonic seizures, mood stabilizer (bipolar affective disorder), migraine headache prophylaxis, and minor urinary incontinence post-ileoanal anastomosis. The different formulations include capsules, syrup, enteric coated and extended release tablets, and intravenous.

VPA is completely absorbed in the gastrointestinal tract. Peak serum concentrations are reached within hours of ingestion, except with the extended release (ER) formulation where peaks may occur within 24 hours of ingestion. VPA is 90% protein bound at therapeutic levels; however, the protein-bound proportion can decrease dramatically at supratherapeutic levels. The volume distribution is low (0.1–0.5 L/kg). Ninety-five percent of VPA undergoes complex hepatic metabolism. The elimination half-life of valproate at therapeutic doses is 7 to 17 hours; however, this may increase two- or threefold in the setting of an overdose.

The metabolism of VPA can result in carnitine depletion, although the effect of this observation is uncertain in acute overdose. Carnitine depletion impairs long-chain fatty acid transport and interrupts fatty acid β-oxidation. It also has repercussion on efficiency of the urea cycle, citric cycle and gluconeogenesis. The major effect of carnitine depletion is hyperammonia that results from interruption of the urea cycle.

The majority of valproic acid overdoses result in mild self-limiting effects including drowsiness, tachycardia, and vomiting. Large overdoses (greater than 400 mg/kg) may be life-threatening. The manifestations of a large overdose include coma, respiratory depression, cerebral edema, metabolic acidosis, hyperammonemia, bone marrow failure, and circulatory collapse. Cerebral edema has been observed in both acute overdoses and chronic intoxication. The bone marrow suppression observed after an acute overdose usually occurs between 3 and 5 days and resolves spontaneously. The most frequent hematologic manifestation is thrombocytopenia.

Pancreatitis, renal failure, and hepatic failure are rare complications that have been described after an acute overdose. Contrary to carbamazepine and phenytoin, valproic acid is not associated with dysarthia, nystagmus, ataxia, or tremor.

The numerous metabolic abnormalities associated with VPA overdoses include hypernatremia, hypocalcemia, metabolic acidosis, hypocarnitinemia, and hyperammonemia. Thirty-five to 45% of patients on chronic valproic acid therapy will have hyperammonemia (>60 μmol/L).

Valproate-induced hepatotoxicity is a rare but potentially fatal complication that results from altered mito-

Table 146.2
Special Considerations with Newer Antiepileptic Drugs

Drug	Year of Introduction	Special Consideration
Gabapentin	1993	Associated with weight gain
Felbamate	1993	Risk of aplastic anemia and risk of hepatic failure
Lamotrigine	1994	
Levetiracetam	1999	
Oxcarbazepine	1999	Hyponatremia, SIADH
Tiagabine	1997	Almost exclusive hepatic metabolism
Topiramate	1996	Risk of angle closure glaucoma/weight loss/metabolic acidosis
Vigabatrin		
Zonisamide	2000	

chondrial processes secondary to the carnitine deficient state. This entity is usually seen in at risk patients (mental retardation, infants, and polypharmacy drug use) chronically on VPA. Its manifestations are nonspecific and include: lethargy, nausea, vomiting, or worsening seizures.

The ED evaluation following valproate ingestion should include a serum determination (therapeutic levels: 50–100 mg/L). Serial levels should be obtained until a peak is confirmed. An ammonia level should be verified on all patients on VPA presenting with an altered sensorium. Hepatic function tests should also be obtained, especially on patients chronically treated with VPA.

Given that the vast majority of acute valproic acid ingestions are mild and resolve spontaneously, emergent care is largely supportive. In the absence of contraindications, activated charcoal should be given. Although MDAC may decrease half-life from 12 to 48 hours, the clinical significance of this intervention remains unclear. Ingestion of enteric-coated VPA should receive early whole bowel irrigation. Although described, there is no strong clinical evidence supporting naloxone use as an agent able to reverse CNS depression following VPA overdose.

Carnitine supplementation has recently been shown to significantly reduce mortality in valproate-induced hepatoxicity arising from therapeutic dosing but not in overdose. Furthermore, early recognition and treatment were associated with better outcome. Despite the paucity of evidence to support its use in acute overdose, carnitine should be considered in all patients with significant VPA intoxication.

Hemodialysis and charcoal hemoperfusion may be useful in patients with rapid deterioration, hepatic failure, continued absorption refractory to decontamination, or levels >1,000 mg/L.

Newer Antiepileptics

As mentioned earlier, several new antiepileptic drugs have entered service since 1993. There is limited experience with overdoses of these agents. The clinical manifestations following ingestions may be summarized as sedation, slurred speech, ataxia, dizziness, fatigue, and nystagmus. The emergent care of these patients is largely supportive. **Table 146.2** reviews special considerations of these newer anticonvulsants.

Selected Readings

Asconape JJ. Some common issues in the use of antiepileptic drugs. *Semin Neurol* 2002;22:29–38.

AAMT and EAPCCT. Position statement and practice guidelines on the use of multi-dose activated charcoal in the treatment of acute poisoning. *J Toxicol Clin Toxicol* 1999;37:731–751.

Bohan TP, Helton E, McDonald I, et al. Effect of L-carnitine treatment for valproate-induced hepatotoxicity. *Neurology* 2001;56:1405–1409.

Hojer J, Malmlund HO, Berg A. Clinical features in 28 consecutive cases of laboratory confirmed massive poisoning with carbamazepine alone. *J Toxicol Clin Toxicol* 1993;31:449–458.

Isbister GK, Bailit CR, Whyte IM, Dawson A. Valproate overdose: a comparative cohort study of self poisonings. *Br J Clin Pharmacol* 2003;55:398–404.

Mellick LB, Morgan JA, Mellick GA. Presentations of acute phenytoin overdose. *Am J Emerg Med* 1989;7:61–67.

Spiller HA. Management of carbamazepine overdose. *Pediatr Emerg Care* 2001;17:452–456.

Sztajnkrycer MD. Valproic acid toxicity: overview and management. *J Toxicol Clin Toxicol* 2002;40:789–801.

Winnicki RI, Lopancinski B, Szymczak WM., Szymanska B. Carbamazepine poisoning: elimination kinetics and quantitative relationship with carbamazepine 10,11-epoxide. *J Toxicol Clin Toxicol* 2002;40:759–765.

Wyte CD, Berk WA. Severe oral phenytoin overdose does not cause cardiovascular morbidity. *Ann Emerg Med* 1994;5:508–512.

147 Monoamine Oxidase Inhibitors

Eric Adar
Mark Su

History

Monoamine oxidase inhibitors (MAOIs) have been reportedly used as treatment for various medical disorders since the 1950s. Iproniazid, a derivative of isoniazid, was first used for the treatment of tuberculosis. During its initial use, mood elevating properties were noted in many patients. Coincident with this discovery, iproniazid was found to be an inhibitor of the monoamine oxidase enzyme (MAO). In the late 1950s and early 1960s, this medication was administered specifically for the treatment of depression. Despite early enthusiasm in the psychiatric community, the limitations to this class of medications were quickly realized because of a narrow therapeutic window. The decline in the use of MAOIs further sharpened after the discovery of tricyclic antidepressants in the 1960s and again with the advent of the safer selective serotonin reuptake inhibitors (SSRIs) in the 1980s. Today, MAOIs are still used therapeutically for conditions including Parkinson's disease, smoking cessation, and phobias as well as for refractory depression. For this reason, significant toxicity is still likely to occur with these agents. In 2002, the American Association of Poison Control Centers reported 317 exposures to MAOIs, with 50 resulting in adverse reactions and 26 of these were considered major reactions; two deaths were reported. From the toxicology standpoint, MAOIs are fraught with problems that include significant medication and food interactions and may also be life-threatening if taken in overdose. For this reason, suspicion of MAOI toxicity requires a high level of vigilance and prompt recognition of clinical signs and symptoms are crucial.

Pharmacology

Two major subtypes of the monoamine oxidase enzyme exist: monoamine oxidase A (MAO-A) and monoamine oxidase B (MAO-B). These enzymes are concentrated in various regions of the body. Both enzymes can be found in the liver and central nervous system, whereas a higher concentration of MAO-A is found in the gastrointestinal tract, the peripheral nervous system, and placenta. Monoamine oxidase-B,

on the other hand, is more abundant in platelets. The enzyme performs oxidative deamination to deactivate monoamines (i.e., norepinephrine, dopamine, serotonin, etc.).

With most MAO inhibitors, the deactivation process is accomplished via permanent covalent bonding to the enzyme. These irreversible agents maintain their activity until new synthesis of MAO occurs, a process that typically takes eight to ten days. Relatively newer reversible compounds, such as moclobemide (**Table 147.1**), offer some advantages when compared to their older kin including rapid onset, lower incidence of toxicity, or drug interactions, and the lack of necessity for a washout period when terminating the drug and restarting a similar agent.

Several endogenous monoamines are deactivated by MAO including norepinephrine, epinephrine, dopamine, and serotonin. Monamine oxidase inhibitors are believed to exert their antidepressant effect by elevating presynaptic concentration of these catecholamines. Downregulation of serotonin receptors at postsynaptic sites is also believed to be clinically significant. In addition to their MAO inhibiting activity, many of the MAOIs have inherent stimulant activity that contributes to their toxicity in overdose.

Drug Interactions

Many classes of medications have significant interactions with MAOIs. The concomitant use of SSRIs can precipitate the life-threatening serotonin syndrome (see Chapter 143). Deaths have resulted and combined used of these agents should be avoided. Although poorly understood, tricyclic antidepressants have occasionally precipitated toxicity in patients using MAOIs. When taken with MAOIs, TCAs can precipitate a range of symptoms similar to the serotonin syndrome including hyperthermia, restlessness, diaphoresis, seizures, coma, and death. Methylxanthines (e.g., caffeine, theophylline) in combination with MAOIs can cause hyperthermia, agitation, and tremors in animal models and should be avoided as well. Other drugs with serotonergic properties, such as meperidine, have been associated with serotonin syndrome and subsequent intracranial bleeding. Although some concern exists regarding co-administration

Table 147.1

Monoamine Oxidase Inhibitors

	Isoenzyme	MAO Inhibition	Primary Usage
Phenylzine	A and B	Irreversible	Antidepressant
Tranylcypromine	A and B	Irreversible	Antidepressant
Isocarboxazid	A and B	Irreversible	Antidepressant
Procarbazine	A and B	Irreversible (weak)	Chemotherapeutic
Selegiline	B*	Irreversible	Antiparkinsonian
Pargyline[1]	B*	Irreversible	Antihypertensive
Moclobemide[2]	A	Reversible	Antidepressant

*Predominant isoenzyme, selectivity lost in overdose.
[1] Marketing in United States discontinued.
[2]Not FDA approved for use in the United States.
Source: Adapted from Ford, Delaney, Ling, Erickson, eds. *Clinical Toxicology.* St. Louis: Saunders, 2001. Copyright © 2001 W.B. Saunders Company.

of opioids with MAOIs, because the sedative effects of codeine appear to be potentiated by MAOIs, morphine appears to be safe for administration. Monoamine oxidase inhibitors have also been noted to exacerbate the hypoglycemic effects of insulin and sulfonylureas.

A wide variety of over-the-counter medications such as decongestants and appetite suppressants can also have detrimental effects when combined with MAOIs. Pseudoephedrine, dextromethorphan, phenylephrine, and phenylpropanolamine have all been implicated. In addition, decongestant formulas marketed for children and preparations containing phenylpropanolamine may not contain warnings regarding concomitant use of MAOIs. As with prescription medications, nonprescription medications combined with MAOIs may be extremely dangerous.

Food Interactions

Significant interactions with MAOIs can occur with the ingestion of foods rich in tyramine. This exogenous monoamine is normally deaminated in the liver following ingestion. In the presence of a nonselective MAOI, tyramine is able to displace catecholamines from the presynaptic neuron and induces a catecholaminergic surge. Reactions are typically rapid and patients usually become symptomatic within 2 hours. Milder reactions are characterized by elevation of blood pressure, diaphoresis, palpitations, a headache, and at times photophobia. With more severe reactions, a hypertensive crisis, seizures, intracranial bleeding, cardiac ischemia, and rarely death are all possible. Certain foods such as aged cheeses, yeast, and meat extracts, red wine, and Italian broad beans, are rich in tyramine and must be avoided by patients taking MAOIs. Foods with moderate tyramine concentration such as yogurt and avocado also require caution and need to be consumed in moderation.

Overdose

Acute overdose of MAOIs may result in life-threatening toxicity that may be extremely difficult to treat. Patients present with hyperthermia, diaphoresis, tachypnea, tachy-

cardia, and shock. Neurologic signs and symptoms may include headache, confusion, nystagmus, hyperreflexia, tremors, muscular rigidity, and seizures. Furthermore, the signs and symptoms may be delayed up to 12 to 24 hours following ingestion posing an additional clinical challenge. Some patients with hypertensive crisis may have the added complication of intracranial bleeding.

It should be noted that the reversible MAOIs (RIMAs, e.g., moclobemide, brofaromine, cimoxatone, etc.) are generally less toxic and have fewer significant food interactions compared to the irreversible MAOIs. Significant toxicity, however, has been reported from these agents, and although they are currently unavailable in the United States, they may be brought into the country by visitors or travelers.

Diagnostic Evaluation

Monoamine oxidase inhibitor overdose and complications due to food or drug interactions are clinically diagnosed. Adjunctive diagnostic studies are geared toward the diagnosis of concomitant disease processes and to aid in the management of complications. Following the determination of vital signs, pulse oximetry, blood glucose determination and electrocardiography should be rapidly performed. Laboratory tests should be ordered as needed depending on the patient's presentation. Patients presenting in a sympathomimetic state (hyperthermia, diaphoresis, tremors, tachycardia, etc.), require electrolyte determination, blood urea nitrogen, and serum creatinine concentrations to assess kidney function. Serum creatine phosphokinase and urine myoglobin levels can aid in the diagnosis of rhabdomyolysis. Those with suspected risk of cardiac ischemia should have serial cardiac enzyme levels drawn. Patients presenting with altered sensorium or a hypertensive crisis should receive a timely computed tomography scan of the brain to exclude an intracranial bleed; patients with headache, meningismus, or altered mental status should have cerebrospinal fluid determination to exclude infectious etiologies. Serum drug levels of co-ingestants such as acetaminophen and salicylates should also be obtained if suicidal intent is suspected.

Treatment

Patients should be first stabilized with standard resuscitative measures. Following the assessment of airway, breathing, and circulation (the ABCs), supplemental oxygen should be administered and intravenous access secured. Intravenous dextrose should be administered to patients with hypoglycemia.

Activated charcoal should be given for gastrointestinal decontamination to all patients with suspected ingestion who pose a low risk of aspiration. Patients with an altered sensorium or those who pose a high risk of aspiration because of co-ingestants, should have their airway secured before performance of any gastrointestinal decontamination procedure. Orogastric lavage should be strongly considered in patients who are symptomatic from large ingestions and it is believed that pills might still be present in the stomach.

Patients who present with hyperthermia require aggressive external cooling. Antipyretics have little or no efficacy in controlling the body's temperature in this context because the hyperthermia is generally due to psychomotor agitation. Benzodiazepines should be helpful in reducing neuromuscular excitation and may also be effective for the treatment of seizures. Severe hypertension is best treated with a rapidly titratable parenteral agent (e.g., nitroprusside) as hypotension and shock may precipitously occur following initial hypertension in these patients. Hypotension should be initially treated with intravenous fluid boluses with crystalloid, followed by a vasopressor if volume resuscitation fails. When choosing a vasopressor, it is best to avoid indirect acting agents (e.g., dopamine), as these agents rely on endogenous catecholamine stores. Direct acting agents such as norepinephrine and epinephrine are better choices. Cardiac dysrhythmias are best treated with lidocaine or procainamide. Bretylium should be avoided, as it may exacerbate hypotension by further depleting catecholamine stores. Patients who present with a hypertensive crisis in the absence of an overdose may be treated with parenteral phentolamine (or other rapidly acting vasodilator).

Disposition

Given the delay in the presentation of symptoms and the fact that fatal reactions have been reported up to 35 hours following an overdose, all patients with suspected overdose should be admitted to a monitored setting. The recommended observation period is a minimum of 24 hours and the patient should be closely monitored for the signs and symptoms of toxicity as previously discussed. All patients with suspected intentional overdose should be evaluated by a psychiatrist and possibly transferred to an inpatient psychiatric facility at the conclusion of the observation period if no evidence of toxicity occurs.

Patients who present with isolated uncontrolled hypertension in the absence of an overdose, whose blood pressure is successfully controlled in the ED, and have no other significant symptomatology, may be discharged safely after an observation period of four to six hours.

Monoamine oxidase inhibitors are complex agents with significant potential for toxicity from either overdose or interactions with food or drugs. Despite newer and safer alternatives to their use, they are still available and being prescribed. Knowledge of their pharmacologic and toxicologic effects is extremely important to clinicians faced with the task of caring for patients taking these medications.

Selected Readings

Amrein R, Allen SR, Guentert TW, et al. The pharmacology of reversible monoamine oxidase inhibitors. *Br J Psychiatry Suppl* 1989;6:66–71.

Baldessarino RJ. Drugs and the treatment of psychiatric disorders: depression and mania. In: Hardman JG, Limbird LE, Molinoff PB, et al., eds. *Goodman and Gilman's The Pharmacological Basis of Therapeutics,* 9th ed. New York: McGraw-Hill, 1996:431–460.

Feighner JP, Boyer WF, Tyler DL, Neborsky RJ. Adverse consequences of fluoxetine-MAOI combination therapy. *J Clin Psychiatry* 1991;52:87–88.

Harrison WM, McGrath PJ, Stewart JW, Quitkin F. MAOIs and hypertensive crises: the role of OTC drugs. *J Clin Psychiatry* 1989;50:64–65.

Sauter D. Monoamine oxidase inhibitors. In: Goldfrank L, Flomenbaum N, Lewin N, et al., eds. *Goldfrank's Toxicologic Emergencies,* ed 7. New York: McGraw-Hill, 2002:955–965.

Watson WA, Litovitz TL, Klein-Schwartz W, et al. 2003 annual report of the American Association of Poison Control Centers Toxic Exposure Surveillance System. *Am J Emerg Med* 2004;22:335–404.

Beta-Adrenergic Antagonist Toxicity

Boris Khodorkovsky
Mark Su

The β-adrenergic antagonists (β-blockers) are very commonly used for the treatment of various medical conditions including ischemic heart disease, hypertension, hyperthyroidism, glaucoma, migraines, and anxiety. Toxicity is expected because of their widespread use. Epidemiological data from the 2003 American Association of Poison Control Centers Toxic Exposure Surveillance System recorded 15,350 β-blocker exposures, of which 402 cases resulted in major toxicity and 33 deaths were reported.[1]

Pathophysiology

In general, toxicity from β-blockers predominantly results from their effects on the β-adrenergic receptor. When a β agonist binds to the β-adrenergic receptor, there is a G protein (G_s) that activates adenylate cyclase to enhance production of cyclic adenosine monophosphate (cAMP). There is a resultant cascade of events that leads to the opening of calcium channels to increase intracellular calcium influx and subsequent release of calcium from the sarcoplasmic reticulum. Beta receptors are found throughout the body, with a higher concentration of β-1 receptors in the cardiac tissue, β-2 receptors in vascular, pulmonary, and hepatic tissues, and β-3 receptors in adipose tissue. The β-3-adrenergic receptor is involved in the regulation of lipolysis and thermogenesis. The pharmacological effects of β-1, -2, and -3 agonists and antagonists are summarized in **Table 148.1**.

Pharmacokinetics and Toxicokinetics

The β-blockers are a heterogeneous group of agents that produce a wide spectrum of effects on the body. In general, there is rapid absorption from oral preparations in therapeutic doses. In overdose, delays in absorption may be produced secondary to decreased gut motility. Sustained release preparations may also lead to delayed and prolonged absorption. Although therapeutic half-lives of β-blockers range from 30 minutes to 24 hours, in overdose, these times and subsequent toxicity can be significantly lengthened.

Beta-blockers may be cardioselective (effects on the β-1 receptor only) or non-cardioselective (effects on both β-1 and -2 receptors; **Table 148.2**). In general, cardioselective β-blockers are hydrophilic and nonselective agents are lipophilic. Hydrophilic β-blockers (e.g., atenolol) are mainly eliminated by the kidneys, while lipophilic β-blockers (e.g., propanolol, carvedilol) are mainly metabolized in the liver. The importance of these qualities is important in recognizing both the symptomotology and treatment of overdoses. Overdose with lipophilic agents, such as propanolol, can readily produce central nervous system toxicity such as seizures or sedation.

Certain β-blockers have intrinsic sympathomimetic activity (e.g., acebutolol and pindolol). This partial agonism at the β receptor can result in initial increases in blood pressure or heart rate. These agents may be better tolerated in overdose.

Other β-blockers, such as labetalol, pindolol, and propranolol have membrane stabilization properties at high doses similar to the cyclic antidepressants. These effects may result in impaired myocardial contractility and cardiac conduction abnormalities.

Sotalol deserves special mention because it is a class III antidysrhythmic agent. It may be associated with QT interval prolongation even at therapeutic doses. Overdose with this agent can produce premature ventricular contractions as well as potentially lethal ventricular dysrhythmias, including ventricular tachycardia, ventricular fibrillation, and torsade de pointes.

Signs and Symptoms

Signs and symptoms of β-blocker overdose include an extension of their therapeutic effects as well as side effects from other specific pharmacologic properties. The cardiovascular system is commonly affected. Bradycardia is seen early, followed generally by hypotension. In severe cases, patients can develop frank shock with circulatory collapse. Impairment of cardiac contractility and conduction may clinically manifest as congestive heart failure, widening of the QRS complex on electrocardiogram, QT interval prolongation, and asystole. Although depressed cardiac output and hypoglycemia are two of the mechanisms responsible for central nervous system (CNS) depression, lipophilicity of the particular agent also plays a role.[1]

Table 148.1

Beta Receptors (1 and 2), Agonist and Antagonist Effects

	Agonist	Antagonist
β-1 receptor (heart)	• Increase contractility • Increase heart rate • Increase AV node conduction	• Decrease contractility • Decrease heart rate • AV node blockade
β-2 receptor (vasculature, lungs, liver)	• Bronchodilation • Vasodilation • Glycogenolysis • Gluconeogenesis • K^+ cell uptake	• Bronchospasm • Vasoconstriction • Inhibition of glycogenolysis • Inhibition of gluconeogenesis • Hyperkalemia
β-3 receptor (adipose tissue)	• Lipolysis • Thermogenesis	• Inhibition of lipolysis • Hypothermia

Additional metabolic and electrolyte disturbances may occur following overdose of β-adrenergic antagonists. Antagonism of circulating catecholamines results in inhibition of glycogenolysis and gluconeogenesis. Although hypoglycemia occurs more frequently in pediatric overdoses, diabetic adults are also at risk of developing low blood glucose levels. Furthermore, although rarely clinically significant, hyperkalemia is sometimes seen. Blockade of β-2 receptors in the lung can result in respiratory depression, as well as a bronchospasm in patients with reactive airway disease. Several cases of hypothermia have been reported in β-blocker overdose as well.

Evaluation

Routine diagnostic testing is indicated to ascertain severity of overdose as well as to exclude other causes of a patient's presentation. Every patient, especially with altered mental status, should have a bedside blood glucose measurement performed early. An electrocardiogram may show bradycardia, atrioventricular blocks, and QT prolongation. QRS widening may be present in certain β-blocker overdoses, such as pindolol and propranolol, mimicking cyclic antidepressant (CA) overdose. Findings of hyperkalemia will be evidenced by tall T waves and widened QRS on the electrocardiogram (ECG). An arterial blood gas may be helpful in evaluation of shock, respiratory depression, and seizures. Although not necessary for diagnosis of β-blocker overdose, a routine chemistry panel should be sent to obtain the serum potassium level as well as blood urea nitrogen and creatinine concentrations to evaluate renal function. If the cause of bradycardia is unknown and there is an unclear patient history, a serum digoxin level may be added. A chest radiograph is helpful to determine the presence of congestive heart failure and screening for other potentially significant causes of cardiopulmonary disease.

Treatment

Treatment of β-blocker overdose is goal directed. Airway, breathing, and circulation (the ABCs) should be maintained as needed. Every patient with suspected β-blocker overdose should receive supplemental oxygen, have an intravenous access secured, be placed on a cardiac monitor, and have continuous pulse oximetry readings. Gastrointestinal (GID) decontamination should also be considered early in the patient care continuum. Although somewhat controversial, orogastric lavage may be strongly considered if a patient presents within one hour of overdose and the patient is believed to have ingested a significant quantity. This technique of orogastric lavage may also be indicated in a pediatric patient who has ingested a long-acting sustained release β-blocker. Beyond one hour, the indication for orogastric lavage is case dependent. In most cases, single or multiple doses of activated charcoal may be safely administered. Whole bowel irrigation (see Chapter 132 on GI Decontamination) should be performed for sustained release or extended release preparations if gastric lavage is unsuccessful and patient manifests signs of clinical toxicity and/or has ingested large quantities of drug.

Since most β-blocker toxicity manifests as depressed cardiac function, initial treatment is directed to simultaneously counteract bradycardia and hypotension. Bradycardia may initially be treated with intravenous (IV) atropine.[2] The dose of atropine in adults is 0.5 to 1 mg to a maximum total dose of 3 mg. If bradycardia persists, glucagon

Table 148.2

Examples of Various Beta-Blockers and Their Activity at the β-1 or β-2 Receptor

Drug	β-1	β-2
Acebutolol	X	
Atenolol	X	
Betaxolol	X	
Bisoprolol	X	
Labetolol (α-1 antagonist)	X	X
Metoprolol	X	
Nadolol	X	X
Pindolol	X	X
Propranolol	X	X
Sotalol (class III antidysrhythmic)	X	X
Timolol	X	X

is indicated. Glucagon is a β agonist that does not bind to the β receptor. It activates myocardial adenylate cyclase and initiates the same intracellular cascade of events as β agonists do when they bind directly to the β receptor. The physiological end result is an increase in cardiac contractility and chronotropy. Glucagon is administered IV, at a dose of 50 to 150 μg/kg followed by an infusion of 1 and 5 mg/h[3]. Although beneficial effects can be seen immediately, additional doses may be needed to produce the desired effect. Moreover, hypotension is treated initially with IV fluid boluses of crystalloid while closely monitoring for the development of pulmonary edema in susceptible patients. Calcium salts (calcium chloride or calcium gluconate) can be given for persistent hypotension. Direct acting vasopressors (epinephrine, norepinephrine) are indicated in the setting of refractory hypotension and bradycardia. However, because the mechanisms of cardiovascular collapse are multifactorial, involving different effects on the β-1, β-2, and α receptors, one vasopressor alone may not be effective. Several of these agents simultaneously combined may be necessary. In certain cases, phosphodiesterase inhibitors, amrinone and milrinone, have been used to treat β-blocker poisoned patients in whom glucagon therapy was unsuccessful.[4]

New experimental data supports use of high dose insulin in the treatment of severe β-blocker toxicity.[5,6] Insulin administration is thought to alter calcium metabolism in cardiac cells and subsequently improve cardiac contractility. Regular insulin is infused at the rate of 0.5 U/kg/h while glucose is administered at 1 g/kg/h. Concomitant administration of glucose should be undertaken as needed to maintain euglycemia.

In patients who remain hemodynamically unstable despite all of the aforementioned therapies, implementation of an intra-aortic balloon pump is indicated. This therapy has been reported to be used in severe cases of both β-blocker and calcium-channel blocker toxicity.

Hemodialysis and hemoperfusion may be theoretically useful modalities in the extracorporeal elimination of certain β-blockers.[7] However, these techniques are unlikely to be used or considered in the severely poisoned patient because of limited efficacy due to hypotension.

As discussed above, certain β-blockers cause cardiac conduction delays with a prolongation of the QRS complex on the ECG. These phenomena should be treated with IV sodium bicarbonate, at the dose of 1 to 2 mEq/kg intravenous bolus, followed by an IV infusion. Lidocaine is indicated for ventricular tachycardia or ventricular fibrillation and magnesium is indicated in specific ventricular dysrhythmias, such as QT prolongation caused by sotalol and torsade de pointes. While hyperkalemia should be controlled with standard therapies, such as insulin and dextrose infusion, sodium bicarbonate, β-agonists, and calcium salts, hypoglycemia can be easily controlled with dextrose boluses and infusion. Patients with evidence of hypothermia should be warmed with traditional techniques.

Disposition

In most cases of ingestions of immediate release β-blockers, if the patient is asymptomatic, the patient should be observed in the emergency department for 8 to 10 hours. Toxicity usually should be evident within 6 to 8 hours of ingestion. Overdose of sustained release preparations requires prolonged observation and admission for cardiac monitoring. Furthermore, patients with sotalol ingestions may have a delayed presentation of cardiotoxicity and should be admitted. All symptomatic patients, with bradycardia, hypotension, and CNS toxicity, should be admitted to the intensive care unit. Patients with poor cardiac or pulmonary reserve or other significant comorbidities are likely to have a worse outcome in β-blocker overdose. There should be a low threshold to admit these patients for hemodynamic monitoring.

In summary, β-blocker overdose can present with many different signs and symptoms. Early recognition and aggressive treatment can prevent morbidity and mortality in patients with β-blocker toxicity. Appropriate management related to the offending drug should be instituted. The presence of severe signs and symptoms of toxicity should direct admission to intensive care unit or further observation in the emergency department. In the absence of apparent toxicity, there are a multitude of factors to consider, including knowledge of the specific formulation (immediate release vs. delayed release), specific type of β-blocker (e.g., sotalol), age of patient (child or adult), etc., prior to disposition.

References

1. Watson WA, Litovitz TL, Klein-Schwartz W, et al. 2003 annual report of the American Association of Poison Control Centers Toxic Exposure Surveillance System. *Am J Emerg Med* 2004;22:335–404.
2. Mackintosh TF. Propranolol and hypoglycemia. *Lancet* 1967;1:104–105.
3. Albertson TE, Dawson A, deLatorre F, et al. TOX-ACLS: Toxicologic-oriented advanced cardiac life support. *Ann Emerg Med* 2001;37:S78–S90.
4. Howland MA. Antidotes in depth: glucagon. In: Goldfrank LR, et al., eds. *Goldfrank's Toxicologic Emergencies*, ed 7. Norwalk, CT: Appleton & Lange, 1998.
5. Kollef MH. Labetalol overdose successfully treated with amrinone and alpha-adrenergic receptor agonists. *Chest* 1994;105:626–627.
6. Kerns W II, Schroeder D, Williams C, et al. Insulin improves survival in a canine model of acute beta-blocker toxicity. *Ann Emerg Med* 1997;29:748–757.
7. Yuan TH. Insulin-glucose as adjunctive therapy for severe calcium channel antagonist poisoning. *J Toxicol Clin Toxicol* 1999;37:463–474.
8. McVey FK. Extracorporeal circulation in the management of massive propranolol overdose. *Anaesthesia* 1991;46:744–746.

149 Calcium Channel Antagonists

Michael Ganetsky

Calcium channel blockers (CCB) are widely prescribed for hypertension, angina, and supraventricular tachyarrhythmias as well as many other indications. Because of a narrow therapeutic window, the potential exists for significant morbidity and mortality in both large therapeutic dosing as well as overdose. In 2002, 9,585 CCB exposures were reported to poison control centers, 77% of which were unintentional and approximately half were seen at a health care facility. There were 365 major outcomes and 68 deaths.

Physiology

Influx of extracellular calcium into myocardial and smooth muscle cells plays a key role in contraction, automaticity, and conduction. Calcium channel blockers do not affect skeletal muscle, which depends on intracellular calcium stored in sarcoplasmic reticulum and not on influx of extracellular calcium. Depolarization of myocardial and smooth muscle cell membranes activates the L-type calcium channels, which are calcium-specific, voltage-sensitive channels, resulting in a flow of calcium intracellularly down a concentration and electrical gradient. In smooth muscle, calcium binds to calmodulin, activating myosin light-chain kinase, phosphorylating myosin, and allowing it to bind to actin, thus causing shortening of the myofibrils.

Calcium influx performs numerous roles in myocytes. It is critical in excitation-contraction coupling because the magnitude of myocyte contraction is proportional to the rise in intracellular calcium. The plateau (phase 2) of the action potential is due to a slow calcium current that releases larger stores of calcium from the sarcoplasmic reticulum. Calcium then binds troponin C, releasing the inhibition of tropomyosin on actin-myosin interaction, resulting in cell contraction. Conduction across the AV node is dependent on calcium influx because the action potential (phase 0) is largely due to calcium and not sodium as in other myocytes. Calcium currents, presumably through T-type channels, contribute to SA nodal automaticity during spontaneous slow depolarization (phase 4).

Pharmacology

All CCBs in therapeutic use antagonize the L-type calcium channel and thus are considered Vaughn-Williams Type IV antiarrythmic agents. By binding to receptors on the L-type calcium channel found in the myocardium, smooth muscle and pancreas, these drugs decrease the number of open channels and consequently, the amount of calcium influx. This inhibits SA node, AV node, and intracardiac conduction, and decreases contractility in the myocardium. In the vascular smooth muscle, decreases in intracellular calcium concentrations produce vasodilation. Other classes of calcium channels exist, such as the T-type channel. Mibefradil was designed to inhibit both L-type and T-type channels but was withdrawn from the market in 1998 because of serious adverse effects and drug interactions.

Ten CCB are available commercially. They are divided into four classes based on their structure and receptor binding characteristics (**Table 149.1**). All CCB produce vasodilation, but the degree to which they affect myocardial contraction and conduction varies among the individual classes. Verapamil, a phenylalkylamine, has the greatest effect on myocardium, and compared to other CCBs it has the most potential to cause bradycardia and hypotension by inhibiting nodal conduction and decreasing stroke volume as well as systemic vascular resistance. Diltiazem, a benzothiazepine, has moderate conduction effects in myocardium and similar decrease in systemic vascular resistance compared to verapamil; but unlike verapamil, diltiazem tends not to decrease cardiac output except in severe poisoning. The dihydropyridines, such as nifedipine, predominantly affect vascular smooth muscle with minimal effect on the myocardium at therapeutic dosing. Bepridil, a diarylaminepropylamine ether, is a fast sodium channel and potassium channel antagonist (Class I and III antiarrhythmic) as well as a CCB, and can cause prolongation of the QTc and ventricular dysrhythmias.

All oral CCB are well absorbed and have a fairly rapid onset of action (**Table 149.2**). However, the onset of sustained release formulation can be delayed by 6 to 12

Table 149.1

Classes of Calcium Channel Blockers

Class	Drug	Major Effect
Phenylalkylamine	Verapamil	Conduction + contractility
Benzothiazepine	Diltiazem	Conduction > contractility
Dihydropyridine	Amlodipine	Vascular smooth muscle
	Felodipine	
	Isradipine	
	Nicardipine	
	Nifedipine	
	Nimodipine	
	Nisoldipine	
Diarylaminepropylamine ether	Bepridil	Type I and III antiarrhythmic effects

hours. Bioavailability ranges from 5% to 30% due to first-pass metabolism. Calcium channel blockers are hepatically metabolized and excreted in the urine, feces, or bile; hepatic metabolism can be saturated in overdose. Diltiazem is excreted in breast milk in the same concentration as serum. Among the CCBs, metabolites possess clinically insignificant bioactivity except for norverapamil and desacetyldiltiazem. Norverapamil has about 20% of the parent compound's activity, while desacetyldiltiazem has 25% to 50% activity compared to diltiazem. All CCBs are highly protein bound and except for nicardipine, nimodipine, and nifedipine, have a large volume of distribution.

Clinical Presentation

Although the different classes of CCB produce distinct physiological effects in therapeutic dosing, any selectivity between CCB is lost in significant overdose. The hallmarks of severe CCB poisoning are bradycardia, hypotension, hyperglycemia, metabolic acidosis, and acute renal failure; moreover, well-appearing patients may abruptly develop cardiac arrest. Any CCB may produce significant toxicity, although verapamil and diltiazem are most frequently associated with severe poisoning. Fatality from nifedipine and other dihydropyridines is rare.

Bradycardia and hypotension are the most common findings in significant CCB overdose. Suppression of SA and AV nodes, most commonly by verapamil and diltiazem, can result in sinus bradycardia or arrest, atrioventricular block, idioventricular rhythms, junctional escape rhythms, or asystole. Ejection fractions as low as 10% and even complete ventricular standstill occur in severe overdose. Although most CCBs produce bradycardia, patients with nifedipine toxicity initially exhibit a reflex tachycardia; bradycardia, and hypotension develop after worsening poisoning. Hypotension arises from negative ionotropy and systemic vasodilation; these clinical features contribute more to the decrease in cardiac output than does bradycardia.

Electrocardiographic changes seen in CCB overdose include ST elevation, T wave inversion, and nonspecific ST changes. Coronary artery hypoperfusion results in myocardial ischemia. QRS duration is typically not prolonged

Table 149.2

Calcium Channel Blocker Pharmacokinetics

Drug	Onset (min)	Tmax (h)	$T_{1/2}$ (h)
Verapamil	30	1–2.2	3–7
Diltiazem	30–60	2–3	3.5–6
Diltiazem (SR)		6–11	5–7
Amlodipine		6–9	30–50
Felodipine	120–300	2.5–5	11–16
Isradipine	120	1.5	8
Nicardipine	20	0.5–2	2–4
Nifedipine	20	0.5	2–5
Nimodipine		<1	1–2
Nisoldipine		6–12	7–12
Bepridil	60	2–3	24

with CCB toxicity, although bepridil can cause QTc prolongation and ventricular dysrhythmias.

Patients may complain of nausea, dizziness, fatigue, syncope, dyspnea, and chest pain, especially if ischemia is present. Physical exam findings may include mental status changes, seizures, coma, and pulmonary rales. The skin and extremities typically seem well perfused because CCB toxicity causes a warm, vasodilatory shock. Since CCB do not have significant direct CNS activity, mental status change is from cerebral hypoperfusion. Patients tend to preserve cerebral blood flow and maintain some lucidity up until the point of cardiovascular collapse; therefore, any obtunded CCB overdose should be considered either to be severely toxic or to have coingestion. Noncardiogenic pulmonary edema of unclear etiology has also been associated with CCB toxicity.

Hyperglycemia is a common feature of CCB overdose. Pancreatic beta islet cells are stimulated to release insulin by calcium influx, which can be antagonized by large doses of CCB. Functional hypoinsulinemia leads to increased serum glucose concentrations, a laboratory finding that can be used to differentiate CCB from beta-blocker overdose, which can cause hypoglycemia by blunting hepatic catecholamine effects. Hypoinsulinemia may theoretically explain the severe cardiovascular effects found in CCB toxicity. Myocytes utilize free fatty acids for energy in normal metabolism, but switch to glucose oxidation in a stressed state. Therefore, lack of insulin may prevent uptake of glucose in myocytes and smooth muscle cells; once deprived of fuel, these cells are not capable of maintaining contractility and vascular tone.

Severe CCB overdose can cause metabolic acidosis and acute renal failure. The metabolic acidosis is primarily a lactic acidosis secondary to tissue hypoperfusion. The acidosis itself will impair contractility and vascular tone, leading to a cycle of worsening shock. The mechanism of acute renal failure is unclear, but since CCB are not directly nephrotoxic, it is likely from kidney hypoperfusion.

CCBs tend to have a narrow therapeutic window. Poisoning from CCBs has been observed following overdose as well as higher "therapeutic" doses. The risk and severity of toxicity increases with underlying cardiac, kidney or renal disease, extremes of age, and concurrent use of other vasoactive medications, such as beta blockers, digoxin, and nitrates.

Management

The various treatment modalities for CCB overdose are based on case reports, anecdotal evidence, and clinical experience. Even though no prospective controlled trials have been performed, extensive cumulative experience can be used to guide therapy. The goal of management is to increase cardiac output, reverse organ hypoperfusion, and support peripheral vascular tone until the active compound can be metabolized or eliminated.

After assessing the airway, placing intravenous catheters, and beginning continuous cardiac monitoring, management of the poisoned patient begins with an evaluation of hemodynamic status and severity of overdose based on vital signs and quantity of drug ingested. The history should focus on time and amount of ingestion, coingestants, and comorbid illnesses. Physical examination should involve an assessment of mental status, chest auscultation for pulmonary edema and observation of skin and extremity perfusion. Any signs or symptoms of organ hypoperfusion suggest a severe overdose. All patients need a 12-lead electrocardiogram, serum chemistries and other routine toxicologic screens and a Foley catheter to monitor urine output. An anion gap as well as an arterial blood gas can provide a measure of the degree of acidosis.

Serum calcium concentrations are usually normal. Measurement of serum concentrations of the CCBs are generally not helpful because they do not predict toxicity and are not readily available. A chest radiograph provides an additional assessment of pulmonary edema.

Gastric decontamination is important but should not interfere with or delay stabilization of hemodynamic status. Administer a standard dose of activated charcoal without cathartic either orally or by nasogastric tube. Patients should not receive emetics because vomiting may delay gastrointestinal decontamination. Multiple-dose activated charcoal and whole bowel irrigation have been used successfully and are recommended for ingestions of sustained release formulations or when toxicity is present. Their use has theoretical benefits and anecdotal success, but has not been systematically studied. Hemodialysis and hemoperfusion have not been found to improve elimination because most CCB have large volumes of distribution and all are highly protein bound. Orogastric lavage is relatively contraindicated; intoxicated, bradycardic patients who receive a large bore orogastric tube may suffer cardiac standstill if the increase in vagal tone produced by the tube placement further blunts nodal response.

Patients who have asymptomatic bradycardia, are normotensive, and have no signs of organ hypoperfusion can be closely monitored and not treated with vasoactive agents. Initial management of bradycardia with hypoperfusion includes calcium, atropine, and crystalloid boluses if the patient does not have pulmonary edema. Calcium salts improve ionotropy, AV nodal conduction, and blood pressure more so than heart rate. By increasing extracellular calcium concentrations and the transmembrane gradient, intracellular calcium is theoretically increased, although the exact mechanism is unclear. The starting dose is 1 gram of calcium chloride (10 mL of 10% solution) or 3 grams of calcium gluconate (30 mL of 10% solution), which can be repeated every 10 to 15 minutes. Calcium chloride has more than 3 times the elemental calcium of calcium gluconate and produces a more reliable increase in serum calcium, but should not be given through a peripheral vein. Typically, between 3 and 5 amps of a calcium salt may be required for the initial treatment of a moderately intoxicated patient. If the optimal dose of calcium salts is unclear, therapy should be titrated to blood pressure and AV nodal conduction. Large doses, frequent boluses, and continuous infusions are usually needed because the effect of a single bolus is brief and may produce no effect at all in severely poisoned patients. Ionized calcium needs to be measured regularly as hypercalcemia can result in vomiting, confusion, and angina. Approximately one third of patients, especially those with moderate or severe CCB toxicity, will not respond to calcium. Similarly, administration of atropine improves heart rate in less than one third of patients and is typically ineffective in severe toxicity. Atropine may be more effective in mildly toxic patients, patients with SA nodal and not AV nodal suppression, and if he or she was pretreated with calcium. Dosing follows ACLS guidelines and is a safe medication with which to start, but should be abandoned after 2 doses if no effect.

Patients refractory to calcium should be considered for vasopressors, nonpharmacological therapy and hyperinsulinemia/euglycemia therapy (HIE). Dopamine, epinephrine, norepinephrine, isoproteranol, and dobutamine have all been used with inconsistent success. Glucagon, which is considered first line therapy for beta-blocker overdose, has been moderately efficacious for CCB toxicity but also typically fails in severely poisoned patients. The initial dose is 5 to 10mg IV; if an improvement is observed, a glucagon infusion at a rate of 3 to 5 mg/h should be started. Because glucagon and adrenergic agents share a common pharmacological pathway, no clear theoretical advantage exists in the selection of one agent over another. Amrinone and milrinone, both of which are phosphodiesterase inhibitors, can improve ionotropy in CCB overdose, but should be used very cautiously because of the potential for vasodilation and worsening shock.

Transcutaneous or transvenous pacing can be applied to bradycardia resistant to pharmacologic therapy. However, failure to capture and absence of improvement in blood pressure even when capture occurs are frequently reported. Pacing fails to improve hemodynamics because severe CCB toxicity depresses left ventricular contractility as well as impairing automaticity and producing conduction blocks. More invasive treatment options include intra-aortic balloon counterpulsations, cardiopulmonary bypass, and extracorporeal membrane oxygenation (ECMO). Unless resources are readily available and mobilized rapidly, these measures will likely be employed too late to provide hemodynamic support that will result in a meaningful outcome.

One promising therapy for the treatment of severe CCB toxicity is hyperinsulinemia/euglycemia (HIE). The administration of high dose insulin produces striking improvement in blood pressure, ejection fraction, peripheral vascular resistance, and metabolic acidosis. However, HIE may exert minimal effects on bradycardia and conduction blocks. Clinical evidence suggests that the beneficial effects of HIE are maximal when administered early in the clinical course of severe CCB toxicity. Multiple vasopressors can be stopped within hours of starting HIE, even in

severely toxic patients. The exact mechanism is unclear, but theoretically, HIE reverses impaired glucose uptake and permits myocytes and smooth muscle to utilize glucose for fuel, leading to improved contractility and vascular tone. Recommended dosing is Regular Insulin 1 U/kg IV bolus followed by a 0.5 to 1 U/kg/h drip titrated to blood pressure. To prevent hypoglycemia, patients should receive D50 with the initial insulin bolus if euglycemic and maintained on a D10 drip titrated to blood glucose. Remarkably, hypoglycemia is relatively uncommon despite extraordinary doses of insulin. Serum glucose and potassium must be checked often, and potassium repleted if less than 2.5 mEq/dL. HIE appears to be a safe and effective therapy for life-threatening CCB overdose.

Disposition

Disposition of the CCB overdose patient depends on the formulation of the medication and on the presence of signs of toxicity. If the overdose involves a standard release form and the patient is asymptomatic after 6 to 8 hours, they can be safely discharged or referred to psychiatric care. If the patient ingested a sustained release form, they should be monitored on telemetry for 24 hours, even if asymptomatic. A 24 hour hospitalization in asymptomatic pediatric patients is mandatory because a single tablet may be lethal. Special consideration should be given to patients with significant liver and renal disease, who may have delayed metabolism, and for patients concurrently taking beta-blockers, nitrates, or digoxin. Any patient who exhibits signs of toxicity needs to be admitted to an ICU setting because they can rapidly decompensate and need urgent hemodynamic support.

Selected Readings

Boyer EW, Duic PA, Evans A. Hyperinsulinemia/euglycemia therapy for calcium channel blocker poisoning. *Pediatr Emerg Care* 2002;18:36–37.

Boyer EW, Shannon M. Treatment of calcium-channel-blocker intoxication with insulin infusion (correspondence). *N Engl J Med* 2001;344:1721–1722.

Braunwald E, Libby P, Zipes DD, eds. *Heart Disease: A Textbook of Cardiovascular Medicine*, 6th ed. Basel: Elsevier Science, 2001.

Goldfrank LR, Howland MA, Hoffman RS, et al., eds. *Goldfrank's Toxicologic Emergencies*, 7th ed. New York: McGraw-Hill, 2002.

Howarth DM, Dawson AH, Smith AJ, et al. Calcium channel blocking drug overdose: an Australian series. *Hum Exp Toxicol* 1994;13:161–166.

Kerns W, Kline J, Ford MD. Beta-blocker and calcium channel blocker toxicity. *Emerg Med Clin North Am* 1994;12:365–390.

Ramoska EA, Spiller HA, Winter M, Borys D. A one-year evaluation of calcium channel blocker overdose: toxicity and treatment. *Ann Emerg Med* 1993;22:196–200.

Thompson Micromedex™. Available at http://www.micromedex.com. Accessed June 2005.

Watson WA, Lotivitz TL, Rodgers GC Jr, et al. 2002 annual report of the American Association of Poison Control Centers Toxic Exposure Surveillance System. *Am J Emerg Med* 2003;21:353–421.

150 Digitalis

Alberto Perez
Marc Bayer

In 1785, Withering described foxglove (*Digitalis lanata*), as having ". . . *a power over the motion of the heart, to a degree yet unobserved in any other medicine, and that this power may be converted to salutary ends.*" To this day, this description of cardiac glycosides holds true.

Withering recognized the toxicity of foxglove and described the lethal effects of digitalis, the medication distilled from the plant. He warned about the inappropriate use of foxglove and called for the search of a remedy. This life-saving remedy, digoxin specific antibodies (Fab), was first used in a human in 1985. This chapter focuses on aspects of digoxin toxicity that every emergency physician should make their domain.

Digoxin, a cardiac glycoside derived from the leaves of *Digitalis lanata,* is the most commonly prescribed drug for the treatment of heart failure. Digoxin is an inexpensive medication available in oral (solid and elixir) and intravenous formulations.

Between 1995 and 1999, approximately 18,000 exposures with 70 deaths were reported to the American Association of Poison Control Centers. Analysis of the 1999 data revealed that 75% were "therapeutic errors." The 2002 AAPCC report registered almost 3,000 cases of digoxin toxicity, and these numbers are not expected to diminish given the aging population and the unfortunate incidence of preventable heart disease. A common cause of toxicity results from drug-drug interactions in patients on chronic therapy. The introduction of a new medication that interferes with the kinetics (absorption, elimination) may result in increased serum concentrations. Disease states such as hypothyroidism may also predispose to digoxin toxicity.

Exposure to cardiac glycosides may also result from plant and animal exposure. Ingestion of oleander, foxglove, lily of the valley, dogbane, Siberian ginseng, and red squill are well-documented causes of cardiac glycoside toxicity. The ingestion of Bufo toad secretions containing cardioactive bufodienolide-class agents is another reported source of toxicity. The clinical manifestations from plant or animal cardiac glycosides are indistinguishable from those of prescribed formulations. However, in these cases, digoxin levels are either undetectable or low, while their treatment may require large antidote doses.

The clinical indications for digoxin therapy are chronic heart failure and control of ventricular rate in atrial tachyarrhythmias. Recent data indicate that digoxin does not affect mortality in patients with heart failure in normal sinus rhythm although it decreases the number of hospitalizations.

Pharmacology

Digoxin exerts its effects through three mechanisms:
1. Direct antagonism of the Na-K,ATPase pump
2. Neurohumeral
3. Autonomic (sympathoinhibitory)

Digoxin is a potent, highly selective reversible inhibitor of the Na-K,ATPase. The inhibition of the pump results in the intracellular accumulation of sodium with consequent increases in intracellular calcium. The resultant increase in intracellular calcium concentration gives rise to the enhanced inotropism.

The popularity of digoxin in the treatment of heart failure stems from the fact that therapeutic concentrations (1.0–2.0 ng/mL) result in increased inotropy, decreased conductivity between the SA and AV nodes as well as an increase in vagally mediated parasympathetic tone. Digoxin also causes prolongation of the effective refractory period. At therapeutic concentrations, digoxin decreases automaticity and increases the diastolic resting membrane potential.

The neurohumeral effects, which are seen at low doses of digoxin include inhibition of renin release that leads to a natriuretic effect as well as vasodilatation.

At toxic concentrations, excessive increases in intracellular calcium will elevate the resting potential and predispose to dysrhythmias. The resultant slower heart is therefore taxed with increased automaticity. The dysrhythmias associated with digoxin toxicity are numerous and nonspecific. The emergency physician should however recognize that any manifestation of increased automaticity in the face of impaired conduction is highly suggestive of digoxin toxicity.

Digoxin toxicity must be evaluated in conjunction with serum potassium and calcium concentrations. The presence of hypokalemia (usually secondary to concomitant diuretic therapy) increases automaticity whereas hyperkalemia exacerbates the digoxin-induced conduction delays. As the presence of hypercalcemia increases ventricular automaticity and may be synergistic to digitalis, the rapid administration of intravenous calcium in the setting of digoxin toxicity may be detrimental.

Pharmacokinetics and Toxicokinetics

The absorption of digoxin is almost complete resulting in a bioavailability of 70% to 80% for solid preparations and 90% to 100% for elixirs. The distribution of digoxin is biphasic with a principal body reservoir in skeletal musculature (volume of distribution 7–10 L/kg). Therefore, dosing should be based on the estimated lean body mass. Any correlation between serum concentrations and clinical picture should be interpreted at steady state levels, that is, serum determinations 6 hours after ingestion of the last dose. The elimination half-life for digoxin is 36 to 48 hours in patients with normal renal function; therefore digoxin is taken once a day. Digoxin is largely excreted unchanged in the urine. Its excretion is proportional to the glomerular filtration rate; therefore, doses should be adjusted in patients with renal impairment.

Clinical Manifestation

Acute intoxications may have early manifestations or may remain asymptomatic for a period of hours. The patient will usually manifest gastrointestinal symptoms (nausea, vomiting, or abdominal pain) and neurological symptoms (lethargy, confusion, weakness).

The clinical presentation of a chronic intoxication may be deceiving. The early manifestations are nonspecific; nausea, vomiting, anorexia, abdominal pain, and weight loss. Neurological manifestations may include delirium, confusion, dizziness, disorientation, drowsiness, headache, and hallucinations. Classic, but infrequent, visual disturbances include amblyopia, photophobia, scotomas, chromatopsia, and xanthopsia (yellowish visual discoloration).

The most common electrocardiographic manifestations of digoxin toxicity are atrioventricular, junctional or ventricular ectopy, first-degree atrioventricular block, slow ventricular response to atrial fibrillation, or an accelerated atrioventricular junctional rhythm. More severe EKG manifestations include severe bradycardia, high degree heart blocks, and malignant ventricular dysrhythmias. Hypokalemia, hyperkalemia, and hypomagnesium all predispose to dysrhythmias. The emergency physician must be aware that no single ECG abnormality is pathognomonic of digitalis toxicity. However, the presence of both enhanced automaticity and impaired conduction is highly suggestive of digitalis toxicity, even in the presence of therapeutic levels. Thus, accelerated rhythms with conduction delays should make the emergency physician suspicious of digitalis toxicity.

Diagnosis

The diagnosis of digoxin toxicity requires a high index of suspicion, as many patients will display nonspecific manifestations. All patients on digoxin, especially those with altered sensorium or gastrointestinal complaints require determinations of serum digoxin, serum or whole blood potassium, magnesium, and an ECG. The importance of a potassium determination is underlined by the fact that potassium levels have prognostic value. Data prior to the advent of digoxin-specific antibodies clearly demonstrate that serum potassium levels greater than 5 mEq/mL or 5.5 mEq/L in patients with normal renal function were associated with mortality rates of 50 and 90%, respectively.

Management

The initial management of the digoxin toxic patient should be directed at essential ABCs and stabilization of the patient's hemodynamics. Aggressive GI decontamination and measures to effectively enhance elimination should be implemented. Early EKG interpretation and potassium measurements are essential.

Although digoxin is essentially renally excreted through the urine, a significant amount (30%) undergoes enterohepatic recirculation. Therefore, the early administration of activated charcoal not only prevents absorption of recently ingested medication, but also may enhance its excretion through prevention of enterohepatic recirculation. Evaluation of the renal function and efforts to maintain adequate renal perfusion are required. Digoxin is a large molecule with a large volume of distribution and, therefore, hemodialysis and hemoperfusion are of limited utility.

Mild forms of digoxin toxicity such as atrioventricular, junctional or ventricular ectopy, first-degree atrioventricular block, slow ventricular response to atrial fibrillation or an accelerated atrioventricular junctional rhythm will usually respond to atropine.

The standard of care for the treatment of severe digoxin toxicity is the administration of digoxin-specific antibodies (Fab fragments). Fab fragments not only neutralize free digoxin but also cause a rapid and significant decrease in potassium levels as well as an increase in renal excretion of digoxin. The onset of action of Fab fragments can be as rapid as 20 minutes but usually effects are seen within the hour of administration. The emergency physician must have a low threshold to administer Fab fragments in the setting of digoxin toxicity associated with life-threatening dysrhythmias and/or hyperkalemia. Chronic poisoning with associated dysrhythmias, severe GI symptoms, altered mental status, or renal insufficiency requires Fab therapy. Other indications for Fab administration are ingestions of 10 mg or more in an adult and 4 mg or more in a child, as well as poisoning with non-digoxin cardiac glycosides.

Although Fab therapy will effectively treat hyperkalemia, patients should also be treated with insulin and glucose. In the presence of digoxin toxicity and hyperkalemia, the administration of calcium chloride bolus to stabilize the myocardium is disputable. Although many anecdotal and published case reports attest to its safety, the specter of *cardiac tetany* or *stone heart* is omnipresent. Therefore, we do not recommend the rapid administration of calcium chloride for the treatment of hyperkalemia in the presence of digoxin toxicity. Furthermore, we do not recommend the administration of kayexalate if Fab fragments are given since this will result in overcorrection of the serum potassium levels. Since the advent of Fab fragments, pacemaker and cardioversion have almost become obsolete in the treatment of digoxin toxicity.

The number of vials that should be administered can be calculated with the following formula, given a post-distribution digoxin determination:

Number of vials = Digoxin serum concentration
(ng/mL) × patient wt (kg)/100

Conclusion

Cardiac glycosides have a narrow therapeutic window. An aging population and increasing incidence of heart failure may lead to a larger number of patients on digoxin therapy. Emergency physicians must be cognizant that digoxin toxicity may present in very elusive fashion; therefore, a low index of suspicion is required. The early recognition and treatment of digoxin toxicity is life-saving. The emergency physician should not hesitate in treating these patients aggressively.

Selected Readings

Antman EM, Wenger TL, Butler VP, et al. Treatment of 150 cases of life threatening digitalis intoxication with digoxin-specific Fab antibody fragments. *Circulation* 1990;81:1744–1752.

Bismuth C. Hyperkalemia in acute digitalis poisoning: prognostic implications and therapeutic implications. *Clin Toxicol* 1973;3:153–161.

Hauptman PJ, Kelly RA. Digitalis. *Circulation* 1999;99:1265–1270.

Hickey AR, Wenger TL, Carpenter VP, et al. Digoxin immune Fab therapy in the management of digitalis intoxication: safety and efficacy results of an observational surveillance study. *J Am Coll Cardiol* 1991;17:590–598.

Rosen MR. Cellular electrophysiology of digitalis toxicity. *J Am Coll Cardiol* 1985;5: 22A–34A.

Woolf AD, Wenger T, Smith TW, et al. Use of digoxin specific Fab fragments for the severe digitalis intoxication in children. *N Engl J Med* 1992;326:1739–1744.

Centrally Acting Antihypertensive Agents

Adhi N. Sharma
Beth Cadigan

The centrally acting antihypertensives are among the oldest agents used to treat essential hypertension. These agents include clonidine, guanfacine, methyldopa, and guanabenz. Though structurally dissimilar, these agents reduce blood pressure via the same mechanism; stimulation of α_2-adrenoreceptors in the ponto-medullary region, resulting in decreased peripheral sympathetic tone. While popular in the 1960s, these agents were quickly supplanted by newer agents with better side-effect profiles, such as calcium channel antagonists and β adrenergic antagonists. As a result, the centrally acting antihypertensives are infrequently used to manage blood pressure and, with the exception of clonidine, overdose of these agents is a rare phenomenon.

Clonidine is an agonist at both the α_2-adrenoreceptor and the imidazoline receptor. Initially studied as a topical nasal decongestant in the early 1960s, clonidine was found to cause hypotension and was subsequently used in the management of hypertension. Current additional indications for clonidine include: attention deficit/hyperactivity disorder, migraine headache prophylaxis, Tourette syndrome, and management of withdrawal from opioids, nicotine, and ethanol. As a result, clonidine is the centrally acting antihypertensive most commonly used and encountered in overdose. From 2001 to 2002, the American Academy of Poison Control Centers received almost 10,000 reports of clonidine exposures, with 13 deaths ascribed to clonidine. The vast majority of these exposures were in patients less than 19 years of age. Clonidine will be discussed as the prototype for the centrally acting antihypertensives.

Presentation

A number of case reports document an initial sympathetic surge in patients after clonidine overdose. This surge is the result of nonspecific stimulation of peripheral α-adrenoreceptors and resultant vasoconstriction. These patients may present with hypertension, sometimes refractory to treatment. However, the vast majority of patients who overdose on centrally acting antihypertensives present with mental status depression, hypotension, brad-

ycardia, and respiratory depression. Other presenting signs include miotic pupils and hypothermia. Symptoms typically develop within an hour of ingestion, with the exception of methyldopa, a prodrug that requires metabolism to the active forms.

CNS depression is the most common symptom and may vary from lethargy to somnolence, stupor, or coma. Severely depressed mental status is associated with respiratory depression or apnea. Cardiovascular effects are delayed or may not occur at all. Hypotension and bradycardia may be noted several hours after presentation.

Approximately 50% of ingestions result in bradycardia. Other cardiac effects include conduction aberrations ranging from first degree heart block to complete heart block. Cardiac symptoms tend to occur in patients with either underlying conduction abnormalities or in very young patients.

Clinical Assessment

Clonidine overdose is a clinical diagnosis based on the history and physical examination. There are no rapid assays available to aid in the diagnosis. No routine laboratory analysis will yield the diagnosis as there are no hematological or electrolyte disturbances associated with clonidine overdose. When a history of clonidine ingestion is lacking, the clinician may be faced with a patient who appears very much like an opioid overdose: a comatose, apneic patient with pinpoint pupils. Physical clues to opioid abuse such as needle marks or a methadone clinic identification found on the patient are obfuscated by the fact that clonidine is commonly used to treat opioid withdrawal. As such, these patients may have overdosed on opioids, clonidine, or both. In children, a history is usually available to suggest exposure to clonidine.

Initial Management

Initial attention should be placed on the respiratory status of the patient as respiratory depression or apnea may be the presenting symptoms. Often simple tactile stimulation of the patient will be sufficient to improve respirations;

however, endotracheal intubation with mechanical ventilation is occasionally required. Prior to endotracheal intubation, an attempt should be made to reverse respiratory depression with naloxone.

Once the respiratory needs of the patient are met the focus should turn to the patient's cardiovascular status. As cardiac dysrhythmias are common, a 12-lead electrocardiogram (ECG) should be performed and patients should be placed on a cardiac monitor with pulse oximetry measurements. Serial blood pressure determinations should also be made to detect hypotension. Routine laboratory analysis should be performed as well as serum acetaminophen and aspirin concentrations in patients with a history of intentional exposures. Serum glucose determination should be performed in all patients with an altered mental status or hypothermia.

Decontamination is of limited benefit in clonidine overdose unless the patient presents within an hour of ingestion. Gastrointestinal decontamination with charcoal or by other means is of limited benefit due to the typical delay in presentation. Furthermore, these patients are likely to suffer rapid mental status deterioration increasing the risk of charcoal aspiration. Activated charcoal may have some benefit in clonidine patch ingestions, if given early in the patient's course. One method of decontamination that is highly effective is removal of a transdermal clonidine patch. Transfers of clonidine patches from sleeping adults to children have been reported several times. A thorough inspection of the disrobed patient may reveal the offending agent. Other methods of decontamination are unlikely to yield any benefit and may harm the patient and as such are not recommended.

Naloxone administration has yielded variable results in patients with clonidine overdose. As these patients are similar in presentation to patients with an opioid overdose naloxone has been administered to patients with clonidine overdose. The results vary from no response to improved mental status as well as increased respiratory drive, heart rate, and blood pressure. Occasionally, high doses of naloxone (4–10 mg) will be required to reverse clonidine toxicity. Naloxone is essentially devoid of side effects in patients without opioid dependence and therefore, after a small test dose (0.1 mg), escalating doses may be attempted in symptomatic patients with suspected clonidine overdose. The low test dose should preclude the precipitation of acute opioid withdrawal in opioid dependent patients. Naloxone should be reserved for patients with severe mental status and respiratory depression. In this subgroup of patients, a minimal therapeutic benefit may obviate the need for endotracheal intubation. Patients with mild toxicity are unlikely to demonstrate any benefit from naloxone. As naloxone has a brief duration of action relative to clonidine, maintenance of any therapeutic benefit will likely require a continuous infusion.

Atropine has been shown to be effective for severe bradycardia with evidence of hypoperfusion. Again, a continuous infusion may be required to maintain any benefit. For the rare patient who presents with profound hypertension, a direct acting vasodilator such as nitroprusside should be considered when treatment is necessary. Although the hypertension is typically short-lived patients who are symptomatic or with prolonged elevation of blood pressure should be treated. An ultra-short acting vasodilator is ideal as most clonidine toxic patients will develop hypotension, if so the effect of the nitroprusside will terminate rapidly when the drug is discontinued. Therapeutic interventions for patients with hypotension include fluid resuscitation followed by vasopressor therapy (e.g., dopamine) as required. Finally, tolazoline, an obscure α-adrenergic antagonist, has been recommended as antidotal treatment by some authors. Both hemodynamic improvements as well as therapeutic failures with tolazoline therapy have been reported. An adult dose is 5 to 10 mg as an intravenous infusion every 15 minutes as needed to a maximum total dose of 40 mg.

Indications for Consultation

While the management of a patient with a centrally acting antihypertensive overdose is generally supportive, consultation with either a medical toxicologist or a regional poison center may yield several benefits. Consultants can aid in this purely clinical diagnosis when naloxone fails to reverse what seems to be an opioid overdose. They can also aid in naloxone administration as some clinicians may lack experience or feel uncomfortable with escalating doses. As most physicians are unfamiliar with tolazoline, consultants can assist with the appropriate application and dosing of this agent.

Disposition

Clonidine toxicity is variable with regard to the onset and duration of symptoms as well as dose related toxicity. Therefore, any patient with a suspected clonidine overdose should be observed for at least six to eight hours. In the pediatric population this is usually best performed in an inpatient setting. Since low doses of clonidine have resulted in pediatric toxicity, ingestion of even a single pill by a toddler is potentially life-threatening. Any patient who ingests a clonidine patch should be admitted as it is difficult to predict the onset of toxicity in this scenario. Once developed, symptoms typically persist for 24 hours and therefore symptomatic patients should be admitted. All patients admitted for either observation or treatment should be in a closely monitored setting.

Cellular Asphyxiants: Cyanide and Hydrogen Sulfide

CHAPTER

152

Melisa W. Lai
David Osborne

The cellular asphyxiants cyanide (CN) and hydrogen sulfide (HS) are among the oldest known and rapidly acting toxins. Each is a relatively commonly used agent or byproduct of manufacturing and agriculture in the industrialized world; exposures to these toxins can result in significant morbidity and mortality. They act by uncoupling cellular respiration at key points of aerobic energy production. Subsequent induction of anaerobic metabolism and resultant lactic acid production can eventually lead to cardiopulmonary collapse and death unless swift medical intervention and support are instituted.

Cyanide

Cyanide (CN^-) is highly toxic compound with numerous industrial and chemical uses and a notorious history. It was packaged by the Nazis as Zyklon B for use in gas chambers during the Holocaust, was the poison of choice in the 1978 mass suicide of followers of Jim Jones in Jonestown (Guyana Africa), and killed seven people in Chicago in 1983 when it was substituted into common Tylenol® capsules. Cyanide is a necessary component of mining production and plastics manufacturing. It is commonly used for precious metal extraction, metal plating, and photography due to its ability to form soluble bonds with gold and silver. Cyanide is also used for leather tanning and is a key ingredient in the manufacture of organic chemicals such as acrylonitrile and methyl methacrylate used to produce plastics and synthetic fibers. Cyanide is also a product of combustion, and the liberation of hydrogen cyanide gas from burning plastic and synthetics accounts for as many as 5,000 smoke inhalation deaths each year.

Outside of industry, health care providers should be aware that the metabolism of the common venodilator and antihypertensive agent sodium nitroprusside results in cyanide formation in the setting of severe hepatic insufficiency. Xenobiotics also represent another source of CN, with ingested cyanogens being metabolized to cyanide when ingested (**Table 152.1**).

Certain bacteria, fungi, and algae also release cyanide into the environment as metabolic byproducts.

Pathophysiology and Routes of Exposure

Cyanide may be inhaled, ingested, or absorbed topically. As little as 50 ppm of hydrogen cyanide gas can be immediately life-threatening. Ingestion of 2 mg/kg of cyanide salts can be fatal within minutes. Cyanide has a high affinity for the trivalent (Fe^{3+} or ferric) iron, including the ferric core of heme proteins comprising the mitochondrial cytochrome oxidase system. By binding to the cytochrome aa3 complex, cyanide halts oxidative phosphorylation and thus cellular respiration. Once cellular respiration ceases, anaerobic metabolism ensues with concomitant high anion gap lactic acidosis, cardiovascular collapse, coma, and death.

Clinical Presentation and Recognition

Patient history often reveals an occupational source of cyanide exposure. Intentional or malicious ingestions may not be readily apparent. Nonspecific signs and symptoms such as headache, nausea, vomiting, dyspnea, confusion, and seizures may occur in mild to moderate intoxications, while moderate to severely poisoned patients may demonstrate a remarkably abrupt loss of consciousness. The patient may demonstrate an initial hypertension and tachycardia as direct stimulation of the carotid bodies, but this clinical condition often degenerates into hypotension and bradycardia as well as cardiac dysrhythmias. Profound tachypnea may be secondary to lactic acidosis in addition to hypoxia and, to a lesser extent, directly stimulate the respiratory centers by cyanide. Occasionally the health care workers can smell bitter almonds when cyanide toxicity has occurred.

Once in the body 60% of cyanide is protein bound with a volume of distribution of 0.5 L/kg. The main pathways of detoxification and elimination are through enzymatic pathways by rhodanese which sulfonates cyanide to thio-

Table 152.1

Cyanogens of Various Xenobiotics

Amygdalin
  Bitter almonds
  Apricot pits
  Peach pits
  Plum pits
  Pear seeds
  Apple seeds
Linamarin
  Cassava (yucca) plant root

cyanate, a much less toxic compound that is excreted by the kidney. Another pathway of detoxification involves the vitamin B_{12} precursor, hydroxycobalamin (vitamin B_{12a}); when combined with hydrogen cyanide this precursor forms the nontoxic cyanocobalamin (vitamin B_{12}). Cyanide levels are rarely useful in emergency situations as those results are not back in time, however, whole blood levels greater than 0.5–1 mg/L are toxic. This is more useful in those patients on nitroprusside infusions. Blood gas analysis can show a high PaO_2 in the venous blood gas as tissues are unable to extract the oxygen. The patient may demonstrate a significant metabolic acidosis, secondary to lactic acidosis. Therefore, serum lactate level may be useful. As with all suspected poisonings, a toxicology screen should be obtained and for victims of fires or smoke inhalation a carboxyhemoglobin level and methemoglobin level should also be obtained. A baseline hemoglobin level also should be obtained to guide therapy.

Treatment

Decontamination is required as clothes and vomitus or body fluid can emit hydrogen cyanide gas. When cyanide toxicity is suspected, specific cyanide antidote packages are usually available. This antidote package has undergone many name changes (i.e., formerly known as the Lilly kit, it is now referred to as the Taylor kit) but still consists of amyl nitrate, sodium nitrite, and sodium thiosulfate. The amyl nitrate is inhaled or placed under the patient's nose, rapidly produces a mild methemoglobinemia (2%–3%). Once IV access has been obtained, the injection of 300 mg (6 mg/kg in children) of the IV sodium nitrite should be administered. Intravenous nitrite can rapidly produce a severe and even fatal methemoglobinemia of up to 50% and, thus, should only be used in those patients with a very high clinical suspicion of poisoning from cyanide as a single agent. Induction of methemoglobinemia can be fatal in fire victims (i.e., those with a significant carboxyhemoglobin level), those who already have a methemoglobin level from other toxins, and G6PD patients. Cyanide has a greater affinity for methemoglobin than hemoglobin, forming cyanomethemoglobin. It is recommended that the methemoglobin level be maintained below 30% and levels checked an hour after initiation. The sodium thiosulfate is

then infused 12.5 g IV. The thiosulfate is used by rhodanese to catalyze cyanomethemoglobin to thiocyanate and methemoglobin. Thiosulfate is a relatively benign drug that can be given empirically; furthermore, thiosulfate may be used alone as the antidote in fire victims, or those with significant methemoglobinemia. Hyperbaric oxygen therapy is not indicated unless concomitant CO intoxication has occurred. In the case of nitroprusside infusions, it has been recommended to simultaneously infuse sodium thiosulfate at 4 μg/kg/min prophylactically.

Long-term survival and sequelae of CN toxicity depend on the timely administration of the antidote. Obviously, as with CO toxicity, there can be serious neurologic and cardiac sequelae including anoxic brain injury. Other survivors may have peripheral neuropathies as well.

Hydrogen Sulfide

Hydrogen sulfide, commonly known as *swamp gas* or *knock-down gas,* is an extremely toxic, colorless gas with a characteristic rotten egg smell. It is heavier than air and therefore can settle in tanks and reservoirs. It is formed by the anaerobic breakdown of organic materials. It is commonly found in oil fields, natural gas fields, petroleum refineries, waste water treatment plants, pools of sewage or manure, asphalt fumes, carbon disulfide production, mines, hot sulfur springs, paper mills, and commercial fishing holds. The majority of deaths and exposures in the United States are the result of accidental exposures in manure holds and silos.

Hydrogen sulfide inhibits the cytochrome oxidase system to produce cellular asphyxia. It is usually inhaled as a gas. At very low levels of 0.02 to 0.13 ppm, the olfactory nerve can sense the "rotten egg smell," but higher levels of 150 ppm will overwhelm and inactivate the olfactory nerve rendering the victim unaware of the gas. A level above just 15 ppm can cause conjunctival irritation and levels above 70 ppm can cause alkaline eye burns. At levels of 400 ppm, the risk of pulmonary edema and death can occur. Levels of 1,000 ppm are immediately fatal. The gas is an upper airway irritant and skin irritant secondary alkaline formation with water.

The clinical symptoms mimic those of cyanide poisoning with the exception of the upper airway and conjunctival irritation. History again is the key to diagnosis, and the diagnosis of hydrogen sulfide poisoning should be entertained in anyone with abrupt coma shortly after entering a space with limited ventilation. Decontamination and positive pressure ventilatory protection for health care workers should be observed as significant off-gassing may occur. Silver coins on patients with high exposures have been reported to be oxidized and blackened. Patients may have confusion, nausea, vomiting, seizures, coma, respiratory, and cardiac arrest. All patients should receive supplemental oxygen, either by face mask or via endotracheal intubation. Following decontamination, treatment with supportive measures, airway, breathing, intubation, cardiopulmonary resuscitation, intravenous fluids, and pressors may be required.

Detoxification occurs primarily in the liver and the kidneys via sulfide oxidase, and is converted into thiosulfate and sulfate which can be excreted by the kidney. As with cyanide toxicity, methemoglobinemia theoretically may cause the sulfide ions to preferentially bind to methemoglobin. Therefore, use of nitrites may offer some theoretical benefit. However, there is little evidence to support this practice, and the induction of methemoglobinemia has significant risk in an already hypoxic patient. Survivors of hydrogen sulfide toxicity may have neurologic sequelae similar to carbon monoxide and cyanide survivors.

CHAPTER

153 Carbon Monoxide

Gar Ming Chan
Robert S. Hoffman

Carbon monoxide (CO) is an odorless, tasteless, and invisible gas that is the leading cause of unintentional poisoning fatalities in the United States. Unfortunately, CO is also frequently implicated in intentional suicides. These deaths and the neurotoxicity in survivors are largely preventable with simple and inexpensive CO detectors.

Carbon monoxide exposure generally results from one of four sources. Endogenous CO is liberated during the metabolism of heme. Radiolabeled studies demonstrate that the alpha carbon in heme is liberated as a molecule of CO during biotransformation to biliverdin. Although diseases that result in hemolysis may increase carboxyhemoglobin (COHb) levels, these are rarely of clinical significance.

Inhaled CO gas is the most common route of poisoning. CO is liberated from incomplete combustion of carbonaceous fuels including cigarette smoke, wood, charcoal, gasoline, oil, and propane gas. Published reports of poisonings frequently implicate heating enclosed spaces with stoves, charcoal grills, and portable gas heaters. Consequently, seasonal peaks of CO poisoning occur in colder months. Other associated risks include enclosed spaces that involve ice skating rink resurfacers, cabins during recreational boating, makeshift enclosed passenger areas on the back of pickup trucks, and the use of gasoline-powered generators in an enclosed construction space.

Methylene chloride (dichloromethane) is a halogenated hydrocarbon solvent found in household paint strippers, that is metabolized to CO. Exposures have resulted in delayed and prolonged elevations in COHb and significant symptoms, including death. Rarely, desflurane, enfluorane, and isofluorane also result in elevated COHb levels as their difluoromethoxy moiety is degraded to CO in the presence of a carbon dioxide (CO_2) absorbent like Soda lyme and Baralyme. The highest risk for this degradation occurs when the CO_2 absorbent is dry and its water content is low within the anesthetic circuit.

Vertical transmission via the placenta is a consideration in pregnant patients. There are several case reports of stillbirths that were presumed to be from CO poisoning. In a sheep model, fetal hemoglobin binds CO more avidly than maternal hemoglobin and also has a delayed extinction time.

Pathophysiology

The pathologic manifestations of CO poisoning result from several interacting processes. The commonly cited concept of CO producing a functional anemia is only part of the problem. The classic work of Haldane demonstrated that CO binds to hemoglobin with an affinity greater than 200 times that of oxygen. This makes oxygen delivery difficult because oxygen carrying is largely dependent on oxyhemoglobin.

Because of CO's higher affinity to hemoglobin, cooperativity is also disrupted. Thus, if one molecule of CO is bound to a tetramer of hemoglobin, the other three molecules release oxygen poorly. This, and a CO induced reduction in 2,3-diphosphoglycerate, results in a leftward shift of the oxygen dissociation curve. A cleaver investigation refuted the fundamental role of impaired hemoglobin as the central mechanism in CO toxicity. Dogs were given CO until COHb levels rose to greater than 50%, and all died. Animals exchange transfused with the COHb poisoned blood of the dead animals achieved similar COHb values, yet all survived. Thus, other factors are necessary to produce death. In addition to impairing oxygen loading and unloading of hemoglobin, CO prevents oxygen transfer to essential tissues by forming carboxymyoglobin. Finally, by binding to cytochrome oxidase, CO impairs cellular utilization of oxygen that manages to reach the mitochondria. These four factors contribute to CO's lethality.

Carbon monoxide also alters hemodynamics by a dose-dependent increase in heart rate and a decrease in systemic vascular resistance and contractility that cannot be explained by anoxia alone. These effects are thought to contribute to decreased cerebral perfusion and to neurological complications of CO poisoning.

Neurological injury may be related to oxygen delivery and hypotension, but experimental evidence demonstrates that lipid peroxidation resulting from platelet activation, leukocyte adhesion, and the generation of free radicals is required.

Clinical Presentation and Findings

CO poisoning produces clinical signs and symptoms that are similar to common presentations of both benign and life-threatening illnesses. Findings may range from an influenza-like illness and gastroenteritis to myocardial infarction and sudden death. Early papers with controlled CO dosing in human volunteers report that headache is the most common early symptom, followed by nausea and impaired motor skills as dose and time of exposure was increased.

Although specific for CO poisoning, the classic presentation of cherry-red skin is a rare finding that only occurs in near moribund patients. Additionally, the finding of cutaneous bullae suggest CO poisoning, but are not specific to this disorder. Due to the lack of specific signs and symptoms, CO poisoning is an often missed diagnosis.

Because cellular anoxia and impaired metabolic function are the hallmarks of CO poisoning, it often mimics manifestations of ischemic heart disease. Presenting signs and symptoms may include vague chest discomfort which may progress to dyspnea, palpitations, nonspecific electrocardiogram changes, dysrhythmias, and myocardial infarction. Preexisting heart disease is not required to develop cardiac manifestations of CO poisoning although patients with known exercise induced angina require less exertion to exacerbate symptoms in the presence of small elevations of COHb. Seemingly benign symptoms of central nervous system (CNS) manifestations of CO poisoning may include headache and nausea. Alarming CNS signs and symptoms of poisoning include visual disturbances, seizures, ataxia, alterations in mental status, confusion, and coma. Survivors of an initial CO insult may develop persistent neurological symptoms (PNS) or delayed neurologic sequelae (DNS). Reports of PNS and DNS include urinary and fecal incontinence, memory loss, mood disturbances, parkinsonism, irritability, and seizures. The presence of syncope during the exposure is the best predictor of which patients will go on to neurological damage.

Rarer reported findings include retinal hemorrhages, ischemic contractures, oliguric renal failure, and nonspecific findings on the chest radiograph.

Diagnosis and Ancillary Testing

The most accurate way to diagnose CO poisoning is with a high suspicion in the correct clinical setting. Random COHb screening has low sensitivity and only when multiple household members present with similar symptoms suggestive of a CO exposure will the sensitivity of COHb screening increase.

The only readily available confirmatory test of CO poisoning is a blood COHb level. Because little CO is extracted as blood moves across the capillary bed, either venous or arterial blood will suffice. Therefore, arterial blood gas sampling is not routinely needed unless concerns about gas exchange are present. Unfortunately, numerous case reports demonstrate that COHb levels do not accurately reflect the degree of poisoning. It is important to note that in the presence of COHb, the pulse-oximeter overestimates the amount of oxyhemoglobin (O_2Hb). Thus, a normal oxygen saturation measurement by pulse-oximetry does not exclude CO poisoning.

There is a range of normal COHb levels. Generally, healthy nonsmoking patients can have a COHb level up to 5%, while smoking patients may have circulating levels as high as 10%. This range presents a dilemma to the ED physician in that patients may present with "normal" levels but may be poisoned and symptomatic, especially when transport times are long, and patients have been placed on high-flow oxygen. Although the kinetics of COHb have been described, attempts at back-estimating immediate postexposure levels are not useful.

Ancillary tests should include an electrocardiogram and a chest radiograph. Patients with severe neuropsychiatric manifestations of CO poisoning may have characteristic findings on either CT scan or MRI. The most common findings are lesions in the globus pallidus and internal capsule, areas that are highly sensitive to hypoxia. Unfortunately, this late finding is neither sensitive nor specific for CO. Contrast enhancement or other modalities like single photon emission computer tomography (SPECT) may increase sensitivity, but provide their own intrinsic logistic difficulties.

Because survivors of CO poisoning may develop delayed neuropsychiatric illness, a complete neurological evaluation with neuropsychiatric testing (if available) should be performed. While a baseline is essential, it is unclear if these tests need to be performed in the acute setting or whether their findings are predictive of sequelae.

Treatment

The initial emergency department therapy begins with the rapid assessment of the airway and breathing in a potentially seizing or comatose patient. The instant CO poisoning is suspected 100% oxygen therapy should be initiated via a non-rebreather face mask until a blood sample can be obtained to confirm the presence of COHb. Although this will improve oxygen delivery and hasten the elimination of COHb, it probably has no impact on neurological toxicity. When intentional CO poisoning is suspected, the patient should be evaluated and treated for other co-intoxicants.

Patients should be attached to a cardiac monitor to evaluate for dysrhythmias, and have a rapid assessment of their serum glucose. Volume resuscitation may be required as CO has both vasodilatory and negative inotropic effects.

Hyperbaric oxygen (HBO) therapy undisputedly shortens the half-life of COHb from hours to minutes. In addition, it inhibits lipid peroxidation in animals. Futhermore, by raising the PO_2 to nearly 2000 torr, HBO supplies sufficient dissolved oxygen to support metabolism in the absence of hemoglobin. This negates CO's effects both on oxygen's binding to hemoglobin and the leftward shift of the oxyhemoglobin dissociation curve.

Because HBO is a therapy not available in many institutions, it is a precious resource. Although the use of HBO in CO poisoning remains somewhat controversial, the bulk of the theoretical, animal, and human experimental evidence supports the utilization of HBO for patients with serious CO poisoning. However, specific indications have yet to be defined and wide regional variations exist in referral criteria. Some of the generally accepted indications include life-threatening manifestations such as severe neurological impairment and myocardial dysfunction. Syncope, for reasons stated earlier is another common indication. Additionally, arbitrary levels are often used to reflect significant exposure and possible subclinical illness. Other controversial areas include the number of therapies indicated on the time from exposure in which HBO is still likely to be beneficial. It is the opinion of these authors that a single compression of 2.8 to 3.0 atmospheres for the duration of approximately one hour provides the greatest effect when therapy is begun within 6 hours of exposure. Due to regional variations of indications and the importance of early HBO therapy, it is advised to consult a regional poison control center or HBO center.

Special Considerations

Children are an interesting subset of patients because their increased metabolic rate places them at higher risk of CO poisoning. Additionally, some data suggest that children become symptomatic at lower COHb levels than do adults. The pregnant patient presents another challenging scenario for clinicians. Since fetal hemoglobin has a higher affinity for CO than adult hemoglobin, the fetus may scavenge CO from the mother. Furthermore, since the fetus is always relatively hypoxic, catastrophic fetal events can occur at virtually any maternal COHB level. Fortunately, HBO has an excellent safety profile in pregnancy such that more liberal indications may be applied when treating pregnant patients.

Summary

This clinical entity is probably the most preventable environmental toxin. Commercial CO detectors are available for retail purchase and there are products that detect both smoke and CO. Workplace standards exist to protect employee from untoward events from CO, but poisoning continues to be a problem.

The diagnosis of CO poisoning is often overlooked and is associated with significant morbidity if undiagnosed. It continues to be a preventable problem and can be treated effectively only when the diagnosis is considered.

Selected Readings

Cobb N, Etzel RA. Unintentional carbon monoxide-related deaths in the United States, 1979 through 1988. *JAMA* 1991;266:659–663.

Coburn RF. *J Clin Invest* 1966;45:460–468.

Coburn RF. *Acta Med Scand Suppl* 1967;472:269–282.

Douglas C, Haldane J, Haldane J. The laws of combination of haemoglobin with carbon monoxide and oxygen. *J Physiol* 1912;44:275–304.

Goldbaum LR, Ramirez RG, Absalon KB. What is the mechanism of carbon monoxide toxicity? *Aviat Space Environ Med* 1975;46:1289–1291.

Heckerling PS, Leikin JB, Maturen A, Perkins JT. Predictors of occult carbon monoxide poisoning in patients with headache and dizziness. *Ann Intern Med* 1987;107:174–176.

Raphael JC, Elkharrat D, Jars-Guincestre MC, et al. Trial of normobaric and hyperbaric oxygen for acute carbon monoxide intoxication. *Lancet* 1989;2:414–419.

Thom SR, Fisher D, Xu YA, et al. Role of nitric oxide-derived oxidants in vascular injury from carbon monoxide in the rat. *Am J Physiol* 1999;276:H984–H992.

Caustics

Robert J. Hoffman
Brian Rose

There are over 100,000 reported exposures to caustic agents annually in the United States. Caustic toxicity can occur via the following routes of exposure: inhalational, dermal, ocular, oral, and gastrointestinal. Morbidity from caustic exposures ranges from minimally symptomatic to fatal. Appropriate diagnosis and management of caustic exposures may diminish morbidity and mortality and improve long-term function in exposed patients.

Caustic agents include chemical and biological toxins capable of producing histologic damage on contact with tissue as a result of their chemical properties. The most familiar types of caustics are acids and alkali, but there are numerous others including desiccants, vesicants, and protoplasmic poisons. Caustic agents can be found in many commercial forms and common household cleaners. Common types of alkalis include ammonia, calcium hydroxide, sodium hydroxide, and household bleach, which is the most commonly reported agent involved in caustic exposures. Common types of acids include sulfuric acid, hydrochloric acid, chromic acids, and hydrofluoric acid. Hydrofluoric acid is a unique caustic capable of causing severe systemic toxicity and cardiac dysrhythmias due to depletion of calcium and magnesium as well as hyperkalemia.

Pathophysiology

In general, acids and alkalis exert damage as a result of proton donation or acceptance. The determinants of injury after caustic exposure include: pH, particularly when a substance as an extreme pH below 2 or above 12; concentration, with more severe injuries resulting from more concentrated solutions; increased titratable acid or alkali reserve (TAR), which represents the amount of neutralizing agent required to bring the caustic to physiological pH; tissue penetration; duration of contact; volume of caustic involved and, if the caustic is ingested, the amount of food in the stomach and occurrence of vomiting.

Acids and alkalis differ somewhat in the type of injury produced, although there is some overlap in the pattern of injury produced, alkalis typically cause damage by liquefaction necrosis, a process in which saponification and protein disruption allows the caustic to penetrate through layers of tissue.

Acids cause their damage through a process called coagulation necrosis, in which the most superficial layer of damaged tissue forms a tough leathery eschar, preventing deep penetration of the tissue. Acids may cause damage to other organs such as the spleen, liver, biliary tree, and pancreas after being absorbed and distributed systemically.

The classic belief regarding location of injury has been that alkaline substances injure the esophagus and acidic substances injure the stomach. Prospective evaluation has clearly demonstrated that injury in either the esophagus or stomach is possible with both acid and alkali ingestion.

Presentation

Dermal Exposure

These patients have localized pain and typically have apparent burns. Hydrofluoric acid exposure classically may have minimal or even no apparent skin lesions despite complaint of severe pain. Unlike other dermal caustic exposures, hydrofluoric acid may cause severe systemic illness and even death after dermal exposure. Hydrofluoric acid exposures are discussed in detail at the end of this chapter.

Ocular Exposure

Patients with ocular exposures typically have severe pain, although absence of pain is possible and may be the culmination of severe burn. Diminished visual acuity is a poor prognostic sign, as is clouding of the cornea. It is crucial to document the presence of such findings to demonstrate the degree of compromise already present in patients presenting with ocular exposures.

Inhalational Exposure

Patients with inhalational exposures to caustics may present with upper airway irritation, chest pain, stridor, dysphonia, aphonia, dyspnea, bronchospasm, and respiratory distress.

Ingestion

Symptoms resulting from caustic ingestion vary widely, and there may be great disparity between symptomatology, or lack of, and severity of injury. Symptoms occurring in patients after caustic ingestion range from none to severe. Typical findings may include burns to the lips and oropharynx, sometimes with "dribble marks" that are burns to the chin or chest from dribbled or spilled caustic liquid. Pain is a common complaint, and may involve the oropharynx, chest, or abdomen. Ominous signs and symptoms occurring after caustic ingestion include evidence of viscous perforation, constitutional or systemic symptoms including coma, hemodynamic instability, peritoneal signs, and signs of airway compromise.

Symptoms of gastrointestinal injury may include dysphagia, odynophagia, drooling, abdominal pain, chest pain, vomiting, and peritoneal signs if perforation has occurred. Excepting in cases with obvious peritoneal signs, the abdominal examination correlates poorly with the extent of damage after caustic ingestion, and severe injury may be present in patients with little or no abdominal tenderness. Conversely, peritoneal signs are very ominous and suggest serious injury or perforation. Patients may present weeks after ingestion with dysphagia and vomiting from stricture formation.

Predictive Value of Signs and Symptoms

Many attempts have been made to determine the extent of injury in patients that present with minimal symptoms. Fortunately, in children, the group least likely to have the ability to accurately describe subjective symptoms, there are criteria that have excellent negative predictive value with regard to esophageal or gastric injury, and they may be used to determine the need for gastrointestinal endoscopy.

In children with unintentional ingestions of caustic agents, vomiting, drooling, stridor, and the ability to voluntarily take oral liquids can be used as criteria to predict the absence of esophageal or gastric injury. Children with not more than one of these signs and symptoms can be presumed to not have a severe gastrointestinal burn and do not require GI endoscopy. The presence of two or more of these findings does not correlate strongly with presence of injury. However, when such findings are present, endoscopy is warranted to determine the presence or absence of GI burn and to guide management of such burns. These criteria are only applicable to children, and should not be used adults.

Management

Initial management consists of stabilization of the airway and hemodynamic parameters. Patients with exposure by inhalation or ingestion should have vascular access in the event of any rapid decline in stability.

Dermal Exposure

Removing any clothing that might be tainted with the caustic substance and copious irrigation is essential. It is impossible to empirically state what volume of water should be used for irrigation, because this will vary depending on the concentration, volume, viscosity, pH, and titratable reserve of the acid or alkali. A reasonable approach is to have any affected body areas or the entire body washed or showered with water continuously for 15 minutes. At a minimum, the affected area should be irrigated until there appears to be no caustic agent remaining on the patient.

There are certain circumstances for which water is not the diluent of choice for dermal exposure. These include exposure to solid metals, such as sodium, which may react with water in a highly exothermic and potentially explosive manner, and phenol, which may form an adhesive, glue, or gum-like mass that is difficult to remove. Such substances may be removed with the aid of a non-reactive diluent such as polyethylene glycol electrolyte solution (Go-Lytely®).

Ocular Exposure

Decontamination of patients with ocular exposures to caustic agents is crucial to ensuring the best preservation of visual acuity and function. It is critical to immediately irrigate the affected eye with copious quantities of normal saline or water. The recommended manner of doing so is by anesthetizing the eye with a topical anesthetic such as tetracaine, application of an eye lens, such as a Morgan® lens, and irrigating the eye with diluent as quickly as gravity will drain the diluent into the eye. After the initial irrigation, a brief pause to assess gross visual acuity, assessment of ocular integrity, funduscopy, inspection of the cul-de-sacs for caustic material, and pH testing of the eye. Irrigation of the eye should continue with at least 2 liters of fluid per eye or until the pH of the eye returns to normal, approximately pH 7.4. Assessment of the pH should not occur for several minutes after irrigation has ceased, as use of litmus paper before that time will tend to only reflect the pH of the irrigation fluid, rather than the pH of the milieu of the ocular surface.

Penetration of the caustic into the chambers of the eye is possible. It is occasionally necessary to irrigate the anterior chamber of the eye to dilute and flush an alkali that has penetrated the eye. The decision to carry out such a procedure and the actual procedure itself should involve an ophthalmologist.

Inhalational Exposure

Inhalation of caustic agents is unique in that decontamination may safely include administration of neutralizing agents. Combining a neutralizing agent with a caustic is expected to result in an exothermic reaction and copious gas production. Inhalational exposures to caustics involve a relatively minute quantity of caustic agent spread over a very large surface area. For this reason, inhalational exposures to caustic acids may be treated with a nebulized aerosol of neutralizing sodium bicarbonate. Combining 3 mL of an 8.4% sodium bicarbonate solution with 2 mL of normal saline or water makes such a bicarbonate nebulization solution.

Patients with any lower respiratory symptoms should receive supplemental oxygen. Bronchospasm should be managed using bronchodilators. Airway management is discussed below.

Ingestion

Airway compromise is the most urgent problem arising after caustic ingestion or inhalation. Edema or burns of the larynx or vocal cords may rapidly progress to loss of airway patency. Dysphonia, aphonia, and stridor or ominous signs of airway injury, and should trigger immediate action to stabilize and secure the airway. Visualization of the airway and vocal cords is advised in patients with symptoms of airway injury that do not undergo endotracheal intubation or cricothyrotomy. Fiberoptic visualization may be helpful in any of the aforementioned circumstances, as is having present clinicians with expertise in managing difficult airways. Blind nasotracheal intubation is contraindicated due to the risk of inflicting more damage to the already friable tissue.

Decontamination by dilution is often recommended as part of home management, but may be done in hospital as well. It is likely that dilution offers little benefit in the setting of caustic ingestion, because in order to change the pH by 1 point, the solution must be diluted tenfold. For patients with caustic ingestions occurring less than 30 minutes earlier who have not vomited, drinking a small amount of water, approximately 150 mL for an adult and 25 to 150 mL for a child, is reasonable. Any solid or crystalline material in the mouth may be rinsed out, but the patient must spit and not swallow the diluent water. Use of emetic agents is absolutely contraindicated for patients with caustic ingestions.

Neutralization of ingested caustics has classically been discouraged due to concerns over the exothermic reaction and quantity of gas that would result. It is possible that these theoretical concerns are overstated, and recent animal models provide some evidence that neutralization may be safer than previously thought. Until more evidence becomes available, it is recommended that neutralization not be attempted for patients that have ingested caustic agents.

Gastrointestinal decontamination of the stomach contents using a nasogastric tube may be considered for ingestion of large volumes of acids. Evacuation has theoretical benefit because acid injuries occur via coagulation necrosis decreasing the depth of injury and minimizing the risk of iatrogenic perforation. In addition, many deleterious consequences of acid ingestion are due to the systemic effects after absorption, thus it is beneficial to remove any residual acid from the stomach. If performed, a small soft nasogastric tube may cause less damage to the potentially weakened mucosa.

Laboratory Evaluation

Serum chemistry, arterial or venous blood gas analysis, and a 12-lead ECG should be obtained for any symptomatic patient or any patient suspected of ingesting a potentially dangerous caustic. A screening serum acetaminophen assay should be obtained for any patient with intent of self harm.

Imaging

Radiographs of the chest and abdomen may aid in demonstrating pneumothorax, pneumomediastinum, pleural effusion, or intraperitoneal air. Radiographs are not routinely indicated, but should be obtained selectively for patients with symptoms or exposures that may result in viscus perforation. Computerized tomography of the chest and abdomen may aid in detecting organ injuries, but experience with this imaging modality is limited. Endoscopy is the gold standard image for evaluation of caustic ingestion.

Endoscopy

Endoscopy is the gold standard for assessment of the degree of gastrointestinal damage from caustic ingestion and is used to direct the acute therapy. Indications for endoscopy include: (1) any patient considered unreliable to provide an accurate history or accurate information about symptoms, including any patient who has ingested a caustic with intent of self-harm; (2) any patient with second or third degree oral or facial burns; (3) a child with more than one of the following symptoms, including vomiting, drooling, stridor, or failure to take PO liquids as usual.

Frequently, consultant gastroenterologists are reluctant to perform endoscopy on patients in the setting of caustic ingestions. Numerous reasons cited for delaying or refusing endoscopy are offered, typically from clinicians with an inadequate fund of knowledge, or inadequate experience dealing with this type of exposure. It is helpful for the emergency physician to understand the following: Use of an endoscope to evaluate a patient with caustic ingestion will not result in damage or destruction of the endoscope. The notion that an ingested caustic agent can "melt" an endoscope is understandable, but this phenomenon has never been reported. Regarding timing of endoscopy, injury to the gastrointestinal organs occurs very rapidly after exposure. Therefore, there is no need to delay endoscopy for the purpose of ensuring that the injury has fully developed to peak severity. Lastly, although it is possible that a patient with a severe caustic injury may develop viscous perforation while undergoing endoscopy, there is no evidence that this occurs with any greater frequency than in the general population undergoing endoscopy for other reasons. Therefore, endoscopy should be performed expediently on any patient for whom the procedure is indicated.

GI lesions are generally graded by the depth and appearance of the mucosa as put forth by Zarger and colleagues. Grade 0 indicates a normal mucosal appearance; grade I, hyperemia and edema of mucosa; grade IIa, friability, ulcers, hemorrhages, erosions or exudates; grade IIb, similar to IIa with deep discrete or circumferential ulceration; grade IIIa, small scattered necrosis; and grade IIIb, extensive necrosis.

Once the lesions have been graded and mapped by endoscopy, decisions about further treatment may be made. Grade 0 and I injuries can be safely discharged without restrictions providing the ingestion was unintentional and the patient is tolerating food. Patients with grade IIa lesions should be admitted, placed on a soft diet or possibly nasogastric tube feedings, and monitored to ensure that progression is not occurring. Grade IIb lesions and above almost invariably progress to stricture formation, and efforts should be made to help prevent this from occurring. Accordingly, steroid therapy is indicated for such lesions. An appropriate corticosteroid regimen is 2 mg/kg/d of prednisolone in children or methylprednisolone 40 mg every 8 hours in adults. This is continued for 2 to 3 weeks followed by an appropriate taper. Corticosteroid therapy has been demonstrated to aid in preventing stricture formation in patients with grade IIb lesions, and is not beneficial for other types of lesions. In particular, patients with grade III lesions should not receive steroids, as they increase the likelihood of perforation. Any patient receiving corticosteroid therapy should concomitantly receive antibiotics targeted at preventing infection with oral and anaerobic flora. Experimental options for management of grade IIb and higher lesions include endoscopic dilation, esophageal stent placement, N-acetylcysteine, penicillamine, and beta-amino propionitrile therapy.

Patients with evidence of perforation on physical exam, imaging, or endoscopy should have surgical intervention. Operative treatment may allow for repair of perforation, debridement of necrotic tissue, and placement of a gastric or jejunal tube for feeding.

Special Agents

Phenols

Phenols are present in many antiseptic agents and deserve special mention because the mechanism of injury and treatment differs from that of standard caustic exposures. In contrast to other caustics, phenols cause injury by their ability to accept an electron pair to form a covalent bond. This difference alters management of dermal burns in that irrigation should be done with polyethylene glycol solution because water can actually worsen the injury. If water is all that is available for irrigation, it should be mixed with soap. Ingestion of phenol should be managed like other caustic ingestions discussed earlier.

Button Batteries

Button batteries have the potential to cause severe injuries when ingested. As with other ingestions or exposures, airway patency is the primary concern. Urgent bronchoscopy is indicated to remove any battery lodged in the airway. Once airway concerns have been addressed, the physician should obtain neck, chest, and abdominal radiographs in search of the location and size of the ingested battery. If the battery is found in the esophagus, emergent endoscopic removal is necessary because of the high risk of complications. Batteries lodged in the esophagus are very concerning because they can cause pressure necrosis as well as caustic alkaline injury if the battery leaks. If the battery has already passed the pylorus, the patient can be discharged, instructed to strain their stool, and advised to return if they have any abdominal pain, vomiting, or if the battery has not passed in 7 days. Finally, if the battery is in

the stomach, the patient can be discharged with instructions to return within 48 hours for a repeat radiograph to determine if the battery has passed the pylorus. If it remains within the stomach endoscopy should be done to remove the battery. When discharged home, patients may be treated with polyethylene glycol solution in attempt to hasten transit of the battery through the GI tract.

Hydrofluoric Acid and Bifluoride Compounds

Hydrofluoric acid and bifluoride compounds, hereafter referred to only as hydrofluoric acid, can be found in household rust removers and in industrial forms used for glass etching, brick cleaning, petroleum processing, and leather tanning. Damage is caused when free fluoride ions bind with calcium and magnesium causing cell death and necrosis. Hydrofluoric acid does not exert its damage by changes in pH. It is actually a weak acid, which is a property that allows it to remain in an undissociated state, permitting it to penetrate skin.

There is an inverse correlation between the concentration of the hydrofluoric acid and time to onset of pain. Most dilute hydrofluoric acid solutions are concentrations of less than 10%. Pain resulting from such exposures may begin many hours after exposure, typically 12 to 24 hours. Highly concentrated solutions of greater than 50% cause prompt or even immediate pain. Contact with a body surface area as small as 2% to a concentrated solution may be fatal. Moderately concentrated hydrofluoric acid solutions cause pain that begins in an intermediate time frame, usually 2 to 6 hours after exposure.

Dermal burns may be present despite minimal or no changes in skin appearance. Even burns with a benign skin appearance can be extremely painful and life-threatening. Management of dermal burns first consists of copious irrigation with normal saline, water, or lactated Ringer's for at least 15 minutes. Pain in exposed skin is treated by soaking in calcium chloride solution, commercially available calcium gluconate gel, or with a similar gel compounded in the hospital. To compound such a product, combine calcium chloride with a water-soluble lubricant such as Surgilube® or KY® Jelly. The affected skin may be soaked in this gel. Hydrofluoric acid will move from the patient's skin into this gel, and after 30 to 90 minute it may be necessary to replace the gel, as the calcium in the gel progressively becomes chelated by hydrofluoric acid. If topical therapy is adequate for pain relief, this treatment should continue until the patient is pain-free.

If this is inadequate to control the pain 5% calcium gluconate can be injected intradermally into the site. Injections should be done using a 27 gauge needle or smaller, with a concentration of 0.5 cc/cm^2 of skin. Intradermal treatment is often difficult to perform in fingers, which are most frequently involved with topical hydrofluoric acid exposures. If further treatment of an exposed hand or fingers is necessary, an intra-arterial infusion of 10% calcium gluconate diluted in 40 mL normal saline infused over 4 hours can be attempted.

Hydrofluoric acid inhalational injuries are uncommon. Patients may present with a range of complaints from minor upper respiratory tract irritation to stridor and shortness of breath. Suspected inhalational injuries warrant immediate airway evaluation and possible intubation. Nebulized calcium gluconate may be administered for symptomatic relief.

Diligent hemodynamic monitoring is required for any serious hydrofluoric acid exposure or ingestion. Hydrofluoric acid has the ability to cause many electrolyte abnormalities including: hypocalcemia, hypomagnesemia, and hyperkalemia. These abnormalities in turn can cause serious ventricular dysrhythmias and possibly even death. Electrolytes should be monitored frequently and corrected with appropriate measures in order to avoid these dangerous dysrhythmias.

Ingestion of hydrofluoric acid is almost universally fatal, and few patients have ever been reported to survive such exposures. Patients experience severe hypocalcemia, hypomagnesemia, and hyperkalemia, resulting in dysrhythmia and cardiac arrest.

Selected Readings

Appelqvist P, Salmo M. Lye corrosion carcinoma of the esophagus: a review of 63 cases. *Cancer* 1980;45:2655–2658.

Bruno GR, Wallace AC. Caustics. In: Tintinalli JE, ed. *Emergency Medicne. A Comprehensive Study Guide,* 5th ed. New York; McGraw-Hill, 2000:1168–1174.

Nuutinen M, et al. Consequences of caustic ingestion in children. *Acta Pediatr* 1994;83;1200–1205.

Toxicologic Emergencies, 7th ed. New York: McGraw-Hill, 2002:1323–1340.

Schneider SM, Wax PM. Caustics. In: Marx J, Hockberger RS, Ron M, Walls MD, eds. *Rosen's Emergency Medicine: Concepts and Clinical Practice,* 5th ed. Philadelphia: Mosby Inc, 2002:2115–2119.

Sheikh A. Button battery ingestions in children. *Pediatr Emerg Care* 1993;9:224–229.

Zargar SA, Kochhar R, Nagi B, et al. Ingestion of corrosive acids: spectrum of injury to upper gastrointestinal tract and natural history. *Gastroenterology* 1989;97: 702–707.

155 Hydrocarbons

Howard A. Greller
Lewis S. Nelson

Hydrocarbons are an expansive class of organic compounds that are defined by their primary composition of carbon and hydrogen atoms. They are ubiquitous in modern society and can be encountered in industrial, agricultural, automotive, home, and health care environments. Hydrocarbon-containing products include fuels, propellants, oils, solvents, degreasers, lubricants, aerosols, lacquers, refrigerants, paints, polishes, and other cleaning agents. Their omnipresent nature makes them a common source of exposure (both occupationally as well as in the home) and readily abused substances.

Hydrocarbons can be classified toxicologically into four major groups, primarily differentiated by their chemical composition. The first, the aliphatic hydrocarbons, include compounds such as methane, mineral oil, and gasoline. These are straight or branched chain hydrocarbons, often petroleum distillates, which exist either as isolated compounds or as complex mixtures of different length hydrocarbon chains (such as gasoline). These compounds may exist as solids, liquids, or gases and are used, for example, as fuels, degreasers or polishes.

The second group consists of the aromatic hydrocarbons, also typically petroleum distillates. These compounds, such as toluene, contain a benzene ring. They are found in paints, thinners, and other solvents.

The third group, the wood distillates, consists of complex mixtures of aliphatic and aromatic hydrocarbons. This group includes turpentine and pine oil.

The fourth group consists of the substituted hydrocarbons, which in addition to the carbon and hydrogen backbone contain an additional functional group (i.e., a halogen or a hydroxyl group). The diverse nature of this class of compounds is reflected in the variety of products in which they are found. These include ethanol, solvents (methylene chloride), degreasers (carbon tetrachloride), fire extinguishers (trichloroethylene), fumigants (methyl bromide), Freon, and pesticides (DDT), among others.

General Toxicity of the Hydrocarbons

One of the primary toxicities of all volatile or gaseous hydrocarbons is simple asphyxiation caused by the displacement of respirable oxygen. This is most common when hydrocarbons are intentionally inhaled as an agent of abuse.

The ubiquitous nature, ready availability, and low cost of hydrocarbons make them easily accessible to teen and preteens, who abuse them for their euphoric properties. There are three main ways in which volatile hydrocarbons are abused. *Sniffing*, as in the case of typewriter correction fluid, involves the inhalation of the volatile solvent that collects in the headspace of a container. *Huffing* is when a solvent is applied to a cloth that is held over the nose and inhaled. *Bagging* is when a product containing a hydrocarbon propellant (such as spray-paint) is sprayed into a bag. The heavier, particulate matter (the paint) remains attached to the bag, while the atmosphere of the bag contains the gaseous hydrocarbon propellant, which is then inhaled.

As many of these compounds are solvents, they have excellent lipid solubility, and from the blood they readily cross the blood-brain barrier. In the central nervous system (CNS), they act similarly to the inhalational anesthetics (i.e., halothane) and ethanol producing dose-dependent CNS and respiratory depression. Also in a manner similar to ethanol, many of these compounds also cause euphoria, which probably explains their abuse.

The liquid compounds typically have a high potential for aspiration and pneumonitis when ingested, the risk for which is determined by the physicochemical nature of the compound at standard conditions. Hydrocarbons with the combination of a low viscosity and low surface tension carry a higher risk of being aspirated. That is, as the compound becomes less like water, the protective reflexes of the oropharynx are unable to prevent its passage into the respiratory tract. Once in the lungs the hydrocarbons destroy surfactant and lead to atelectasis and chemical pneumonitis.

If ingested, many of the compounds lead to significant gastrointestinal irritation manifesting as nausea and vomiting. This occurs commonly with the wood distillates, the aromatic, and the halogenated hydrocarbons. Combined with the aforementioned CNS depression, this can lead to an increased risk of aspiration and pulmonary toxicity.

Many of the compounds have unique toxicities. Chronic exposure to benzene can lead to aplastic anemia, as well as a thrombocytopenia, multiple myeloma, and acute leukemia. Lindane, a halogenated hydrocarbon pesticide, is a GABA antagonist and can lead to seizures following either dermal exposures or ingestion. Toluene abuse can lead to rhabdomyolysis, leukoencephalopathy, as well as an anion-gap acidosis from its metabolite, hippuric acid. Chronic abuse of toluene leads to a renal tubular acidosis along with associated electrolyte abnormalities such as hypokalemia and hypophosphatemia. Hypokalemia in toluene abusers can be so profound that the patient may present with paralysis. A distinguishing characteristic is that the paralysis of the toluene-abusing patient resolves with correction of the electrolyte abnormality.

The halogenated hydrocarbons also have unique toxicities. Methylene chloride, found in paint remover, is metabolized to carbon monoxide. Patients should be monitored for several hours for the development of signs and symptoms of carbon monoxide poisoning (e.g., headache, tachycardia, metabolic acidosis, and tachypnea). Carbon tetrachloride, a former industrial solvent, may cause fulminant hepatic failure.

Halogenated hydrocarbons possess the ability to "sensitize" the heart to catecholamines. That is, by altering the repolarization of the myocardial tissue via blockade of a potassium channel, the heart is uniquely susceptible to malignant dysrhythmias, such as torsades de pointes.

The myocardial sensitization of halogenated hydrocarbons is best illustrated by *sudden sniffing death,* seen most commonly in young teens. In this scenario, a person abusing a halogenated hydrocarbon is confronted by a stressful experience (i.e., being discovered by parents or police). This leads to a catecholamine surge ("fight or flight") that triggers a malignant dysrhythmia (e.g., torsades, ventricular fibrillation), and sudden death.

Emergency Department Management

The primary management of patients exposed to hydrocarbon products is supportive. In symptomatic patients, close attention should be paid to the respiratory status of the patient, both from a ventilation and oxygenation standpoint. If the patient has a depressed or altered mental status, the cause should not be attributed to hydrocarbon exposure until other causes (e.g., other poisons, central nervous system infection or trauma, etc.) have been eliminated. This is because recovery is generally rapid following inhalational hydrocarbon exposure. Seizure should be managed in standard fashion with airway management and benzodiazepines.

The need for external decontamination depends on the nature of the exposure and the hydrocarbon. In general, patients should be fully undressed as the majority of toxin is removed with the clothing. Strongly consider formal external decontamination of a patient following exposure to a liquid hydrocarbon preparation, since there is often concern for continued dermal absorption. In addition, volatilization of liquid hydrocarbons from the skin may prove problematic for the health care providers. Patients with exposure to solid or gaseous hydrocarbons do not need specific decontamination other than removal of clothing and obvious material.

In situations in which the hydrocarbon is ingested, gastrointestinal decontamination is generally of limited utility and may be potentially harmful. Syrup of ipecac should be avoided as it may raise the risk of aspiration. Many hydrocarbons are rapidly absorbed, and also cause GI irritation and vomiting, rendering typical gastrointestinal decontamination techniques (e.g., activated charcoal, whole bowel irrigation) ineffective. In patients with recent ingestions of large amounts of liquid or systemically toxic hydrocarbons, there may be a role for the placement of a nasogastric tube to remove product that remains in the stomach.

Pulmonary aspiration should be excluded, even in asymptomatic children by performing a chest radiograph at six hours post-arrival. If the radiograph is clear and the child asymptomatic, they can be safely discharged home. Patients with any sign or symptom of respiratory difficulty (e.g., hypoxia, tachypnea, rales, etc.) or radiographic abnormality should be admitted for close monitoring. Acute lung injury is a common result of hydrocarbon aspiration and can be life-threatening. Therapy consists of oxygenation with PEEP, positive pressure ventilation, and may require aggressive support such as extracorporeal oxygenation (ECMO) in severe cases.

Specific testing that should be considered includes serum electrolytes in toluene users, hepatic markers following halogenated hydrocarbon exposure, and a serum acetaminophen level in patients with suicidal intent.

Following halogenated hydrocarbon exposure, patients should have a 12-lead electrocardiogram to evaluate the QTc interval. Although there is no clearly defined role for prophylactic administration of beta-blockers or magnesium in these patients, a prolonged QTc should prompt prolonged observation with telemetry monitoring. A non-perfusing ventricular dysrhythmia should prompt immediate defibrillation, as per standard ACLS protocol. Upon return of spontaneous circulation, therapy includes the use of beta-blockade and magnesium to prevent recurrence of the dysrhythmia.

Conclusion

Hydrocarbon poisoning is common and may occur through a variety of different means. They have a wide-range of toxicity and even the same chemical can produce a variety of effects. Special consideration should be paid to the CNS, myocardial, and pulmonary toxicity of these compounds. Seizures and CNS depression should be managed in a standard fashion. Airway protection, oxygenation, and positive pressure ventilation can address the pulmonary complications of aspiration. Children with unintentional ingestions of a liquid hydrocarbon who remain asymptomatic can be discharged after a normal 6-hour chest radiograph. Defibrillation, magnesium sulfate and beta-blockade should be considered in patients with malignant dysrhythmias as a result of myocardial sensitization from halogenated hydrocarbons. With meticulous supportive care and a focused diagnostic approach, many of these patients can be managed simply.

Selected Readings

Anas N, Namasonthi V, Ginsburg CM. Criteria for hospitalizing children who have ingested products containing hydrocarbons. *JAMA* 1981;246:840–843.

Bass M. Sudden sniffing death. *JAMA* 1970;212:2075–2079.

Nelson LS. Toxic myocardial sensitization. *J Toxicol Clin Toxicol* 2002;40:867–879.

Heavy Metal Poisoning

Ricky Kue

Arsenic

Background

Arsenic is a heavy metal found in that well water and soil contaminated by mining and smelting processes as well as agricultural fertilizers, fungicides, and pesticides. Arsenic is a white powder similar to processed sugar, making it a potential agent for the purpose of intentional poisoning. Despite its history as an agent used for malicious poisoning, arsenic has been used as a treatment for syphilis and is still used today as treatment for trypanosomiasis and amebiasis.

Pharmacology and Pathophysiology

Inorganic arsenic exists as trivalent (arsenite, As^{3+}) and pentavalent (arsenate, As^{5+}) forms. Trivalent arsenic has been reported to be ten to 60 times more toxic than the pentavalent form, likely due to the lipid solubility in the former. Organic arsenic is especially common in seafood and algae but is considered nontoxic. Arsenic has been known to inactivate up to 200 different enzymes, most notably pyruvate dehydrogenase. Arsenic also interferes with cellular glycolysis by binding to sulfhydryl groups in glycolic enzymes. In addition, arsenic can substitute for phosphate in adenosine 5′-triphosphate (ATP) to produce a molecule whose hydrolysis produces no energy for cellular processes. The net result of arsenic poisoning, therefore, is the decoupling of oxidative phosphorylation and decrease in net ATP production. Death has been reported with acute ingestion of doses as low as 100 to 300 mg of trivalent arsenic.

Clinical Features

Acute arsenic overdose is characterized by gastrointestinal symptoms such as nausea, vomiting, and diffuse diarrhea referred to as *choleroid*. The diarrhea from arsenic poisoning, however, has a bloodier appearance than typical cholera-induced diarrhea. Severely poisoned individuals have dramatic fluid losses due to third spacing of fluid and profound GI secretory loss that lead to cardiovascular collapse. Gastrointestinal symptoms often subside within 24 to 48 hours of exposure. In addition, patients may complain of severe abdominal pain that can mimic an acute abdomen. QT prolongation and torsades de pointes have also been described. Common CNS findings include a peripheral neuropathy, ascending paralysis, and encephalopathy with seizures and coma. Notably, the peripheral neuropathy from arsenic intoxication is excruciating, and occurs between 1 to 3 weeks following exposure. Pancytopenia and dermatologic manifestations such as a morbilliform rash have been described.

Diagnosis

Diagnosis is based on a history of exposure with typical clinical symptoms. Arsenic poisoning should be suspected with prolonged or recurrent bloody diarrhea associated with peripheral neuropathy. Blood levels can be varied but are normally less than 5 µg/L. Spot urine levels of >1,000 µg/L or a 24-hour urine collection level of >100 µg/day requires treatment. Seafood, fish, and algae are rich in organic form of arsenic such as arsenobetaine and arsenosugars that can falsely elevate urine levels of arsenic for up to three days. Arsenic is radiopaque and may be seen in radiographs within the GI tract; their absence does not exclude intoxication. Mee's lines, which are 1 to 2 mm transverse white lines on the fingernail, have been described, but this finding occurs several days to weeks following a single, acute exposure; it does not occur in chronic poisoning. Prolonged QT interval can be seen on an electrocardiogram.

Treatment and Disposition

Initial management includes volume resuscitation, and hemodynamic and respiratory support. Clinicians often fail to appreciate the volume of intravenous fluid required for resuscitation; some arsenic-poisoned patients with severe congestive heart failure were underresuscitated despite the administration of 5 L normal saline solution over a 3 hour period. Ventricular dysrhythmias can be treated with lidocaine or phenytoin. Agents that can worsen QT prolongation (including phenothiazines, class IA, IC and III antiarrhythmatics) should be avoided. Whole bowel irrigation should be considered with radiographic evidence of arsenic poisoning. Activated charcoal and hemodialysis has not been shown to be effective unless treating renal failure or a co-ingested agent. Clinicians may consider chelation with dimercaprol (BAL, British anti-Lewisite) given 3 to 5 mg/kg IM every 4 to 6 hours. Dimercaprol is formulated in a peanut oil vehicle, so the absence of peanut allergy must be documented prior to administration. Patients can be transitioned to oral chelation agents (such as dimercaptosuccinic acid) once clinical improvement is realized. Any patient who reports a history of arsenic ingestion, and who has blood vomiting or bloody diarrhea, should be admitted to a monitored setting for further observation. Severely ill patients should be transferred to a tertiary care center.

Mercury

Background

Mercury can be found in fish, thermometers, sphygmomanometers, electrical switches, batteries, electrodes, fluorescent light bulbs, and laboratory chemicals. Several epidemics of mercury poisoning have occurred: the ingestion of methyl-mercury contaminated seed grain in Iraq in 1971 and 1972 as well as two outbreaks in Japan after industrial release of mercury into the Agano River and Minamata Bay. These events have resulted in regulation to mercury disposal regulations and have provided insight into the clinical sequelae of acute mercurial ingestion.

Pharmacology and Pathophysiology

Mercury exists in three distinct species; elemental (metallic) mercury, inorganic mercury salts, and organic mercury. Metallic mercury, also referred to as *quicksilver,* has the potential to be ingested or inhaled since the substance is volatile at room temperature. Over 80% of elemental vapor mercury exposure is absorbed in the lungs and enters the bloodstream where oxidation and binding to sulfhydryl groups occur. The end result is rapid pulmonary dysfunction from direct cellular injury and severe pneumonitis. The half-life of inhaled mercury is about 60 days. Interestingly, only 0.01% of elemental mercury is absorbed through the GI tract, making ingestion an innocuous route of exposure.

Methylmercury is formed from the biotransformation of aquatic sediments that contain inorganic mercury; human exposure usually occurs via the ingestion of fish that have eaten mercury-contaminated aquatic material. Binding to sulfhydryl groups occurs after absorption, leading to an array of irreversible cellular enzyme dysfunction. Although multiple organs are affected by acute methylmercury exposure, the brain is a major target organ resulting in CNS dysfunction.

Inorganic mercury salt exposure occurs from ingestion of salt containing compounds such as soaps, teething powders, and creams. The acute lethal dose is about one to 4 grams. Inorganic mercury toxicity, unlike organic or elemental mercury is corrosive to the gastrointestinal tract. Cell membrane permeability has been experimentally shown with inorganic mercury exposure and is also nephrotoxic.

Clinical Features

Most clinical features of mercury toxicity depend on the mercury species. Acute ingestion of inorganic mercury salts produces corrosive gastritis, abdominal pain. Gastrointestinal fluid loss and hemorrhage can be substantial and lead to cardiovascular collapse, shock, and intestinal necrosis. Renal failure arises from a combination of fluid loss and acute tubular necrosis. Subacute exposure to mercury salts in children produces acrodynia, a constellation of findings that includes painful, red, swollen digits accompanied by photophobia, irritability, asthenia, and hypertension.

Organic and elemental mercury ingestion commonly results in CNS symptoms such as irritability, tremor, paresthesias, ataxia, memory dysfunction, and erethism (bizarre behavior such as excessive shyness or aggression). Vapor exposure from elemental mercury results in rapid onset of shortness of breath, fevers, and chills that progress into a chemical pneumonitis with subsequent edema formation and ARDS.

Diagnosis

History of exposure or ingestion with appropriate clinical symptoms leads the diagnosis. Serum mercury concentrations are useful in establishing exposure, but urine mercury levels are preferred for the assessment of inorganic mercury exposure. In the case of organic mercury exposure, methylmercury undergoes biliary excretion and enterohepatic recirculation with over 90% being excreted in the feces. Measuring urine concentration to assess organic mercury exposure is futile. In persons without occupational exposure, normal urine and serum levels of metallic and inorganic mercury are usually less than 10 µg/L. In acute ingestions, levels are usually greater than 500 µg/L. With organic mercury, symptoms occur with serum levels greater than 200 µg/L. Serum mercury concentrations here do not correlate with toxicity.

Treatment and Disposition

Treatment of metallic, inorganic, or organic mercury exposure requires immediate decontamination with removal from the source environment and reducing any further exposure from contaminated clothes, gut exposure, and avoidance of worsening vaporization of metallic mercury (i.e., vacuuming spills). Aggressive support of respiratory and circulatory function, including intubation, volume resuscitation, and hemodynamic support, is necessary in acute inhalation of mercury vapors. In the case of inorganic mercury ingestion, rapid fluid resuscitation and GI decontamination should be instituted. This includes whole bowel irrigation, and orogastric lavage. Ingestion of metallic mercury is innocuous as elemental mercury undergoes minimal GI absorption, a clinical feature that obviates the need for gut decontamination. Activated charcoal may be given, but its benefit is not established.

Chelation with oral dimethylsuccinic acid (DMSA) or intravenous DMPS may enhance elimination of organic mercury or absorbed metallic mercury. DMPS may minimize renal injury, thus treatment should be rapidly instituted if inorganic mercury ingestion is suspected. Chelation with dimercaprol (British anti-Lewisite, BAL) should be avoided because this chelating agent may paradoxically increase the brain burden of mercury following organic mercury exposure and exacerbate toxicity.

Acute intoxications are most severe with inorganic ingestions or inhalation of metallic mercury. These patients require admission and supportive care. Asymptomatic patients can be followed closely in an outpatient setting with serial urinary levels.

Iron

Background

Iron is a common substance found in many nutritional supplement formulations and has found use in the treatment of anemia, iron deficiency, prenatal, and daily vitamins. It remains one of the most common causes of pediatric poisonings and almost all reported cases are due to accidental ingestion. Toxicity is dependent of the amount of elemental iron ingested. The amount of iron, in turn, depends whether the ingested formulation is ferrous sulfate, ferrous gluconate, and ferrous fumarate. These compounds contain about 20%, 33%, and 12% elemental iron, respectively. Pediatric formulations including children's multivitamins with usual range of elemental iron around 10 to 18 mg per tablet. Most adult preparations including prenatal vitamins contain anything from 36 to 60 mg of elemental iron per tablet. Given the frequency of accidental iron ingestions, the FDA required the packaging of iron supplements containing more than 30 mg per tablet as individual doses to reduce the likelihood of toxicity.

Pharmacology and Pathophysiology

Iron is an essential co-factor in numerous cellular activities and has the ability to accept and donate electrons readily. It plays a vital role in the function of hemoglobin, myoglobin and any cellular function requiring the activity of cytochromes and oxygen-binding molecules. Similarly, it is dangerous for its role in generating free-radicals that produce cellular damage.

After oral administration and gastrointestinal absorption, ferrous iron in serum gets bound to transferrin. Humans have no physiological mechanism for elimination of iron. After significant overdose, transferrin is 100% saturated and excess iron accumulates as free iron in the serum. As ferrous iron is absorbed, it is converted to ferric iron at the expense of releasing hydrogen ions into the bloodstream. Hepatocyte absorption of iron results in the generation of free radicals that leads to the uncoupling of oxidative phosphorylation, anaerobic metabolism and lactic acidosis. Iron induces arterial vasodilation as well as venous pooling resulting in decreased oxygen delivery, further shock and acidosis. Free iron has also been reported as a direct myocardial toxin that inhibits myocardial activity and contributes to shock. Symptoms are unlikely when less than 20 mg/kg of elemental iron has been ingested. Ingestion of 20 to 60 mg/kg has resulted in mild to moderate symptoms and greater than 60 mg/kg is potentially lethal.

Clinical Features

Classically, iron overdose has been described in five stages. In the first stage, direct gastrointestinal corrosion produces abdominal pain, nausea, bloody vomitus, and bloody diarrhea. Vomiting occurs within 80 minutes of ingestion in 90% of all symptomatic patients. The absence of these symptoms after six hours of observation with ingestion of <20 mg/kg essentially excludes iron toxicity.

The second stage is characterized by a relatively asymptomatic period that can last from 12 to 24 hours. Abnormal vital signs and acidosis may nonetheless persist. Most patients recover, but some progress to stage three, a clinical state characterized by shock, acidosis, lethargy, coma, seizures, and/or cardiovascular collapse. Multiorgan involvement with hepatic failure, coagulopathy, and heart and renal failure can occur.

The fourth stage occurs 2 to 5 days after ingestion and manifests as fulminant hepatic failure with elevation in transaminases and ammonia levels as well as hypoglycemia and coagulopathy. Stage five occurs up to one month after ingestion and involves recovery from iron's corrosive effects. Typically, pyloric or bowel stenosis obstruction occurs.

Diagnosis

Correlation of clinical symptoms with a history of ingestion is helpful in establishing a diagnosis. Clinicians should suspect iron intoxication in patients who have bloody vomitus, bloody diarrhea, and an elevated anion gap metabolic acidosis. A serum iron level drawn four hours postingestion is most useful in evaluating the potential severity of exposure. Levels greater than 500 μg/dL are associated with severe toxicity while levels up to 300 μg/dL are generally associated with mild toxicity. A level between 300 and 500 μg/dL is associated with moderate toxicity. A second level drawn six to eight hours later should be considered in patients who have ingested enteric-coated or sustained-release formulations. Levels drawn after the institution of deferoxamine can be falsely low and thus unhelpful. Total-iron binding capacity (TIBC), serum glucose measurement, or white blood cell counts do not correlate with toxicity. Most iron formulations except children's multivitamins are considered radiopaque and visible on radiographs. The absence of radiographic evidence of iron ingestion, however, does not exclude the diagnosis.

Treatment and Disposition

Most patients with an ingestion history of <20 mg/kg who remain asymptomatic after six hours of observation can be discharged safely. Symptomatic or hemodynamically unstable patients should receive aggressive fluid resuscitation and hemodynamic support. Activated charcoal does not bind to iron and is not recommended unless another substance has been co-ingested. Whole bowel irrigation should be considered to assist in gastrointestinal decontamination. Large ingestions of iron tablets may produce a mass that adheres to the stomach wall; occasionally these concretions must be removed by gastrotomy.

Deferoxamine should be immediately instituted in these patients and considered in patients ingesting greater than 90 mg/kg or who have a serum level greater than 500 μg/dL. Hypotension can occur and usually responds to a decrease in administration rate. Deferoxamine binds with iron to form a water-soluble compound ferrioxamine, which is renally excreted and dialyzable. Endpoints of deferoxamine chelation include clearing of the typical "vin rosé" color, resolution of symptoms, and return of iron levels to normal range. ARDS and *Yersinia* sepsis has been associated with prolonged chelation therapy with deferoxamine. All patients receiving deferoxamine should be admitted to an ICU setting.

Selected Readings

Banner W, Tong TG. Iron poisoning. *Pediatr Clin North Am* 1986;33:393–409.

Beckman KJ, Bauman JL, Pimental PA, et al. Arsenic-induced torsades de pointes. *Crit Care Med* 1991;19:290–292.

Black J, Zenel JA. Child abuse by intentional iron poisoning presenting as shock and persistent acidosis. *Pediatrics* 2003;111:197–199.

Clarkson TW, Laszlo M, Myers GJ. The toxicology of mercury-current exposures and clinical manifestations. *N Engl J Med* 2003;349:1731–1737.

Counter SA, Buchanan LH. Mercury exposure in children: a review. *Toxicol Appl Pharmacol* 2004;198:209–230.

Eto K. Pathology of Minamata disease. *Toxicol Pathol* 1997;25:614–623. Erratum 1998;26:741.

Fine JS. Iron poisoning. Review. *Curr Probl Pediatr* 2000;3:71–390.

Gurzau ES, Corneliu N, Gurzau AE. Essential metals—case study on iron. *Ecotoxicol Environ Safety* 2003;56:190–200.

Hilfer RJ, Mandel A. Acute arsenic intoxication diagnosed by roentgenograms. Report of a case with survival. *N Engl J Med* 1962;266:663–664.

Morris CC. Pediatric iron poisoning in the United States. *South Med J* 2000;93:352–358.

Ratnaike RN. Acute and chronic arsenic toxicity. *Postgrad Med J* 2003;79:391–396.

Riordan M, Rylance G, Berry K. Poisoning in children 3: common medicines. *Arch Dis Child* 2002;87:400–402.

Schoolmaster WL, White DR. Arsenic poisoning. *South Med J* 1980;73:198–208.

Siff JE, Meldon SW, Tomassoni AJ, et al. Usefulness of the total iron binding capacity in the evaluation and treatment of acute iron overdose. *Ann Emerg Med* 1999;33:73–76.

Tenenbein M, Kopelow ML, deSa DJ. Myocardial failure and shock in iron poisoning. *Hum Toxicol* 1988;7:281–284.

Warkany J, Hubbard DM. Acrodynia and mercury. *J Pediatr* 1953;42:365–386.

Hypoglycemic Agents

Jessica Fulton
Lewis S. Nelson

Diabetes mellitus (DM) is a metabolic disorder resulting in hyperglycemia and occurs as a consequence of insulin deficiency, insulin resistance, or both. Treatment options include insulin and oral antidiabetic drugs, which may be classified as either hypoglycemic agents (i.e., sulfonylureas and benzoic acid derivatives) or antihyperglycemic agents (i.e., biguanides, α-glucosidase inhibitors, and thiazolidinediones). This chemically heterogeneous group of antidiabetic agents has the ability to cause toxicities unique to each drug in addition to hypoglycemia.

Pharmacology and Pathophysiology

Oral Hypoglycemic Agents

Sulfonylureas

Chlorpropamide (Diabinese), glipizide (Glucotrol and Glucotrol XL), glyburide (Micronase, Diabeta, and Glynase), and glimepiride (Amaryl) are several members of the class of oral hypoglycemic agents called the *sulfonylureas*. Following ingestion, sulfonylureas undergo rapid absorption from the gastrointestinal (GI) tract. The parent compound then undergoes hepatic metabolism with the formation of active metabolites that are responsible for the long duration of action of these agents. Metabolite elimination is generally renal. Therefore, diminished hepatic and renal function may lead to hypoglycemia.

Sulfonylureas stimulate a specific receptor on adenosine 5′-triphosphate (ATP)-sensitive potassium (K^+) channel in pancreatic β cells. This results in closure of this K^+ channel and enhanced insulin release in response to the glucose-related rise in intracellular ATP. Note that in the absence of glucose, excessive insulin release should not occur. Hepatic effects of sulfonylureas include a decreased clearance of insulin by the liver and decreased glycogenolysis, adding to the hypoglycemic effect.

The adverse event most commonly associated with sulfonylureas is clinical hypoglycemia. Other adverse effects include the syndrome of inappropriate antidiuretic hormone (SIADH), cholestatic jaundice, agranulocytosis, thrombocytopenia and anemia, and disulfiram type reactions.

As a class, the sulfonylureas in overdose may cause delayed hypoglycemia, with reports of onset at 48 hours following chlorpropamide ingestion and 24 hours following exposure to the newer agents.

Drug interactions with sulfonylureas occur as either pharmacokinetic interactions (i.e., alterations in drug absorption, distribution, metabolism, and elimination), or pharmacodynamic interactions (i.e., alteration of blood glucose levels by changing insulin release or action). Aspirin and cimetidine are examples of drugs that pharmacokinetically interact with sulfonylureas. Aspirin displaces the sulfonylurea from plasma proteins and cimetidine inhibits hepatic enzymes that metabolize sulfonylureas. Thus, both interactions potentiate hypoglycemia. Phenytoin, rifampin, and barbiturates can decrease the serum levels, and thus the hypoglycemic effects, of sulfonylureas through hepatic enzyme induction. Furosemide, thiazides, and glucocorticoid steroids are examples of agents that have pharmacodynamic interactions with sulfonylureas. These drugs inhibit insulin release from the pancreas and thereby increase blood glucose levels.

Prandial Glucose Regulators

Repaglinide (Prandin) and nateglinide (Starlix) are non-sulfonylurea oral hypoglycemic agents with a similar mechanism of action to the sulfonylureas. Their major clinical distinction from the sulfonylurea agents is that they are taken just prior to a meal, are quickly effective, and have a short duration of effect. Accordingly, there are no reports of severe hypoglycemia to date, although their similarity to the sulfonylureas clearly presents this possibility. Repaglinide excretion is mostly biliary while nateglinide's is largely renal, suggesting caution in appropriate situations.

Oral Antihyperglycemic Agents

Biguanides

Metformin (Glucophage, Glucophage XR) is the only biguanide available in the United States. It is prescribed for the treatment of diabetes both alone and in combination with other oral antidiabetic agents such as glyburide (Glucovance).

Noninsulin-dependent diabetics have an increase in the activity of glycoprotein PC-1, which is ultimately responsible for decreased insulin sensitivity and therefore decreased glucose uptake in skeletal muscle and adipocytes. Metformin improves insulin sensitivity in these tissues through inhibition of PC-1. It also decreases hepatic glucose output by interfering with gluconeogenesis. Control of serum glucose is similar to that of the sulfonylureas without causing hypoglycemia.

The most life-threatening toxicity associated with metformin as well as with its predecessor phenformin, is metabolic acidosis with an elevated lactate. This complication most commonly occurs with therapeutic dosing in the setting of impaired renal function, although it may rarely be seen with normal renal function or following overdose. Although the pathogenesis has yet to be completely elucidated, it is suggested that the increased metformin tissue burden in the presence of renal dysfunction causes an elevated lactate through inhibition of aerobic metabolism and suppression of gluconeogenesis. Patients with metformin-associated metabolic acidosis usually require treatment with large amounts of sodium bicarbonate and hemodialysis. Because of its almost exclusive renal elimination, the drug is contraindicated in patients with renal dysfunction and should be stopped for at least 48 hours following administration of IV radiologic contrast pending confirmation of renal function. Because a dose-response relationship is not well characterized, all patients with metformin overdose should be observed for 6 hours.

Thiazolidinediones

Following the FDA withdrawal of troglitazone (Rezulin) from the market in 2000 because of its association with severe liver toxicity, only two currently available thiazolidinediones remain: pioglitazone (Actos) and rosiglitazone (Avandia). Like metformin, these drugs increase insulin sensitivity in skeletal muscle and adipose tissue while also reducing hepatic glucose production. As such, hypoglycemia should not be expected with drugs of this class. Although not yet noted, hepatotoxicity from the two available thiazolidinediones remains a possibility.

α-Glucosidase Inhibitors

Acarbose (Precose), miglitol (Glyset), and voglibose (Takeda) make up a class of oral antihyperglycemic agents that inhibit α-glucosidase enzymes present in the brush border of the small intestine. Due to the subsequent poor absorption of undigested sugars, bloating, diarrhea, and abdominal pain are common. As expected based on their mechanism, there are no reports of hypoglycemia or severe toxicity following overdose of α-glucosidase inhibitors.

Insulin

Endogenous insulin is released from the β cells of the pancreas in response to an elevation in blood glucose and binds to specific receptors on cell surfaces of skeletal muscle, cardiac muscle, and adipose tissue. This leads to stimulation of carbohydrate metabolism as well as protein synthesis and lipogenesis. Both the lack of insulin synthesis in insulin-dependent DM (IDDM) and the insulin re-

Table 157.1

Duration of Action of Commonly Used Types of Insulin

Insulin	Duration of Action (h)
Insulin Lispro (Humalog)	<5
Regular	5–8
Semilente	12–16
Lente	18–24
Mixtard (Novolin 70/30, Humulin 70/30) 70% isophane 30% regular	24
NPH	18–24 h
Insulin Glargine (Lantus)	>24 h (basal levels only)
Protamine Zinc Insulin	24–46 h
Ultralente	20–36 h

sistance seen in noninsulin-dependent DM (NIDDM) provide a basis for exogenous insulin use.

Following injection, time of onset, peak, and duration of action differ depending on the insulin preparation (**Table 157.1**). In overdose, the kinetics of insulin are less predictable and present the possibility for delayed-onset hypoglycemia independent of the dose or type injected. This is in part due to altered absorption of insulin from its depot in the subcutaneous tissue. Insulin is metabolized by the liver with a small percent excreted unchanged by the kidneys.

Clinical Assessment and ED Management in Overdose

Initial Presentation

History and Physical Exam Findings

The most common clinical presentation of patients with hypoglycemia is altered mental status. However, because hypoglycemia may occur concomitantly with other medical conditions, the differential diagnosis and evaluation must be kept broad and include, but not be limited to, structural, infectious, metabolic, and toxicologic causes.

Most emergency department (ED) patients with hypoglycemia are insulin-using diabetics who have inadequate food intake. Also common are diabetic patients who use sulfonylureas and develop comorbid illness. It should be noted that hypoglycemia in oral hypoglycemic users is rarely due simply to missed meals. In the nondiabetic adult or child, intentional or unintentional exposure to an oral hypoglycemic or insulin may also result in consequential hypoglycemia. As discussed earlier, hypoglycemia should not be attributed to the biguanides, α-glucosidase inhibitors, or thiazolidinediones.

The brain is acutely sensitive to low blood glucose and in an effort to combat hypoglycemia will activate the sympatho-adrenal axis, causing release of the counterregulatory hormones: epinephrine, norepinephrine, glucagons, and growth hormone. As a result, the typical clinical findings of hypoglycemia are tachycardia, diaphoresis, confusion, agitation, tremor, altered mental status, coma, seizure, and occasionally focal neurological deficits.

Initial Interventions/Definitive Treatment

In general, for the stable patient with mild signs and symptoms suggestive of hypoglycemia, a bedside test for blood glucose concentration should be done. Normal plasma glucose levels are between 70 and 150 mg/dL, although poorly controlled diabetics may develop symptomatic hypoglycemia with numerically normal blood glucose concentrations. If measurement cannot be accomplished rapidly or if the patient presents with serious findings of presumed hypoglycemia, an intravenous bolus dose of 0.5 to 1.0 g/kg of dextrose should be administered empirically. In an adult, start with 100 mL of 50% dextrose (50 g of dextrose); in a child start with 2 to 4 mL/kg of 25% dextrose; and in an infant start with 2 to 4 mL/kg of 10% dextrose and repeat until resolution of hypoglycemia. As dextrose provides only a very small amount of calories (i.e., 100 calories in 50 mL of 50% dextrose), it is imperative that the patient eats as soon as possible following the initial resuscitation phase. For similar reasons, continuous infusions of low concentration glucose solutions, while often used, are not likely to prevent recurrent hypoglycemia.

Blood glucose concentrations should be determined every 1 to 2 hours after initial control for several hours, every 4 to 6 hours thereafter, and as needed based on clinical findings. In the absence of numerical or clinical hypoglycemia, the duration of serum glucose monitoring should be for at least as long as the duration of action of the drug. Bolus glucose therapy often results in rebound hypoglycemia because of robust pancreatic insulin release in response to the transiently elevated blood glucose concentration. Therefore, it is common to administer octreotide to patients with sulfonylurea-induced hypoglycemia following the restoration of euglycemia with bolused dextrose, particularly those with recurrent hypoglycemia.

Octreotide is a well-tolerated long-acting analog of somatostatin that suppresses insulin secretion from the β cells of the pancreas. It reduces dextrose requirements and prevents the hyperinsulinism associated with dextrose therapy. In adults, 50 μg and in children 1 to 1.5 μg/kg of octreotide is administered subcutaneously following an initial episode of sulfonylurea-induced hypoglycemia and every 6 hours thereafter for at least 24 hours. It should be noted that patients receiving octreotide may still require dextrose or food to maintain euglycemia. Following discontinuation of octreotide, blood glucose should be monitored for 24 hours prior to discharge.

Diazoxide is less effective, more complicated to use (e.g., infusion), and associated with more side effects than octreotide, so it should only be used if octreotide is not available.

Activation of glycogenolysis and gluconeogenesis through administration of glucagon should not be considered unless intravenous access cannot be obtained. Glucagon's efficacy requires adequate hepatic stores of glycogen, which will likely be low. Glucagon is given subcutaneously or intramuscularly 1 mg in adults, 0.5 mg in children, and 50 μg/kg in infants. Glucagon commonly causes vomiting, which may be problematic if the patient does not rapidly arouse.

In the case of chlorpropamide toxicity, where 20% of the drug is excreted unchanged in the urine, alkalinization of the urine to a pH of 7 to 8 enhances drug elimination and reduces the drug's half-life.

Finally, in the setting of any oral antidiabetic medication exposure, GI decontamination with 1 g/kg activated charcoal may be beneficial in the awake and alert patient who presents within several hours of ingestion.

Disposition

All patients who present to the ED with intentional or unintentional sulfonylurea overdose or sulfonylurea-induced hypoglycemia should be admitted to the hospital for 24 hours regardless of symptoms. In a child, ingestion (or even suspicion) of even a single pill mandates admission for observation. Hospitalization is recommended after unintentional overdose of long-acting insulin preparations as well as those with persistent hypoglycemia after short or intermediate-acting preparations. Because the kinetics of insulin absorption after large overdoses of any preparation are unpredictable, admission is suggested. Continued neuropsychiatric symptoms despite correction of hypoglycemia require further evaluation. Psychiatric evaluation should be considered for all cases of intentional overdose.

Selected Readings

Boyle PJ, Justice K, Krentz AJ, et al. Octreotide reverses hyperinsulinemia and prevents hypoglycemia induced by sulfonylurea overdoses. *J Clin Endocrin Metab* 1993;76:752–756.

Harrigan RA, Nathan MS, Beattie P. Oral agents for the treatment of type 2 diabetes mellitus: pharmacology, toxicity, and treatment. *Ann Emerg Med* 2001;38:68–78.

Howland MA. Antidotes in Depth. In: Goldfrank LR, Flomenbaum NE, Lewin NA, et al., eds. *Goldfrank's Toxicologic Emergencies*, 7th ed. Stamford, CT: Appleton & Lange, 2002:611–613.

Malouf R, Brust JC. Hypoglycemia: causes, neurological manifestations, and outcome. *Ann Neurol* 1985;17:421–430.

McLaughlin SA, Crandall CS, McKinney PE. Octreotide: an antidote for sulfonylurea-induced hypoglycemia. *Ann Emerg Med* 2000;36:133–138.

Shorr RI, Ray WA, Daugherty JR, et al. Incidence and risk factors for serious hypoglycemia in older persons using insulin or sulfonylureas. *Arch Intern Med* 1997;157:1681–1686.

Methemoglobinemia

Melisa W. Lai

Methemoglobinemia is an uncommon but distinct cause of central cyanosis in the absence of hypoxemia or cardiovascular compromise. It occurs when a significant concentration of hemoglobin (Hb) is oxidized to methemoglobin (MetHb).

When the iron atoms of a hemoglobin molecule encounter a powerful oxidizing agent, iron loses an electron and switches from the ferrous (2+) to ferric (3+) state, turning Hb to MetHb (**FIGURE 158.1**). MetHb cannot bind oxygen, so as the MetHb concentration of blood rises in relation to Hb concentration, the oxygen-carrying capacity of blood diminishes and results in tissue hypoxia.

Pathophysiology

Iron in deoxyhemoglobin constantly undergoes a cycle of oxidation and reduction. This cycle affects only 1% to 3% of Hb at any given time and produces a steady-state level of 1% to 2% MetHb. Oxidative stresses are countered by NADH/NADPH-dependent reductase enzymes which return iron from a ferric (3+) to ferrous (2+) state (**FIGURE 158.2**). Methemoglobin production is directly related to the body's NADH-dependent reductase capacity. Methemoglobinemia occurs when enzymatic reductase activity is exceeded by heme iron oxidation.

The four main pathways to MetHb production are detailed in **Table 158.1**, and **Table 158.2** lists examples of compounds that can produce methemoglobinemia.

Recognition and Diagnosis

Methemoglobinemia most commonly presents as cyanosis unresponsive to supplemental oxygen. However, depending on a patient's actual MetHb concentration, inciting agent and timing of presentation, secondary effects of tissue hypoxia or of the inciting agent may predominate (e.g., vasodilation from nitrite administration).

Clinical manifestations of tissue hypoxia are dependent on the ratio of MetHb to Hb and thus the oxygen-carrying capacity of all hemoglobin in the blood. Cyanosis is apparent in the nonanemic patient when MetHb concentration

reaches 1.5 g/dL, in contrast to the 5 g/dL of deoxyhemoglobin needed to produce the appearance of cyanosis from deoxyhemoglobin. Most patients, even if cyanotic, will not become symptomatic until the proportion of MetHb rises above 20% total hemoglobin (**Table 158.3**).

History often suggests exposure to an oxidative/reducing agent (Table 158.2). All cyanotic infants should have methemoglobinemia included on their differential diagnosis as all infants have a relative NADH-reductase deficiency (~50% of adult levels). Similarly, patients with a known history of hemoglobin M or inherited enzyme reductase deficiency should raise suspicion for methemoglobinemia.

The most notable physical exam finding is generalized cyanosis, which can manifest as muddy brown/dark mucous membranes before proceeding to global skin discoloration. Some observers have described the skin discoloration seen in methemoglobinemia as "slate-gray" in contrast to the bluish skin seen in cyanosis.

Arterial blood gas co-oximetry confirms the diagnosis of methemoglobinemia. Bedside testing in the ED may nonetheless prove more efficient and practical: a drop of patient's blood left to dry on white filter paper should be compared to a "control" drop of normal blood. MetHb produces a characteristic chocolate-brown color. Pulse oximetry will be depressed and unlikely to change with the administration of supplemental oxygen. At MetHb levels >30% total Hb, pulse oximetry may read a constant 85%, but this finding may depend upon the age of pulse oximeters used for readings.

Other bedside testing protocols have been proposed that are for various reasons impractical and unlikely to be of use in the ED. Bubbling oxygen through venous blood and watching for a color change to bright red indicates a normal Hb-MetHb ratio but raises issues of body fluid exposure and blood-borne pathogens. Potassium cyanide (KCN) added to venous blood diluted to 1:100 in deionized water will produce a pink color change in methemoglobinemia, but the difficulty in obtaining approval for the use of KCN in the ED as the impracticality of proper dilution of blood makes this method impractical.

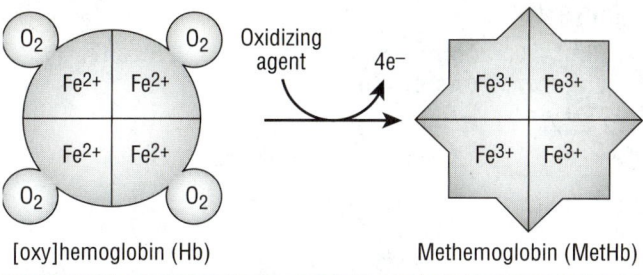

FIGURE 158.1 Hemoglobin with heme iron in a 2+ valence (ferrous) state is able to bind oxygen. If the heme irons are oxidized to their ferric state, hemoglobin becomes methemoglobin and is unable to bind oxygen.

Emergency Department Management

Emergency Department management of methemoglobinemia is focused on maximizing oxygen saturation of deoxyhemoglobin and decreasing the half-life of MetHb. Patients with cyanosis or difficulty breathing should receive supplemental oxygen. A persistent pulse oximetry reading of 85% or no improvement in oxygen saturation or cyanotic appearance with supplemental oxygen should raise suspicion for methemoglobinemia.

Methylene blue may be administered to patients without glucose-6-phosphate-dehydrogenase (G6-PD) deficiency as an antidote to methemoglobinemia. The half-life of MetHb is only one hour when undergoing reduction via NADH-dependent cytochrome b5 reductase alone. Methylene blue uses an alternative *NADPH*-dependent reductase path to accelerate heme iron reduction (**FIGURE 158.3**). Administration of methylene blue may increase the rate of heme iron reduction up to sixfold. Administer 1 to 2 mg/kg methylene blue IV over 5 minutes, q1hr × 2 to a maximum of 7 mg/kg. Improvement is usually noted within the first 30 minutes of administration. Clinicians should note, however, that administration of methylene

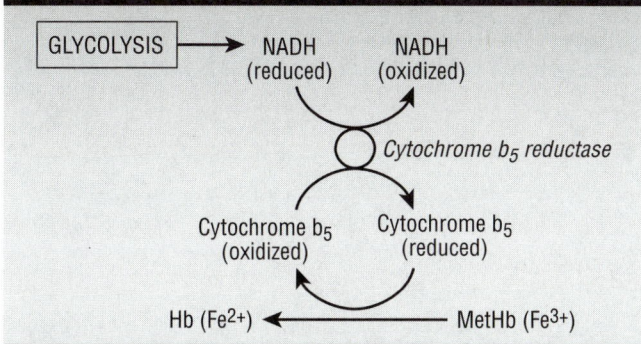

FIGURE 158.2 Reduction of methemoglobin with its ferric (3+) heme iron to hemoglobin and its ferrous (2+) heme iron is accomplished by the donation of an electron from cytochrome b5. Cytochrome b5 is oxidized in the process and regenerates its reducing properties by accepting an electron donated by NADH. NADH cannot reduce cytochrome b5 without the NADH-dependent cytochrome b5 reductase.

Table 158.1
The Four Main Pathways to MetHb Production

1. Congenitally abnormal hemoglobin: Hemoglobin M
   - Hemoglobin M is passed as an autosomal dominant trait affecting either the alpha or beta chain of hemoglobin; homozygous Hb M affecting both alpha and beta chains is incompatible with life.
   - Amino acid substitution (often a tyrosine for histidine) near the heme iron facilitates iron oxidation
2. Inherited enzyme deficiencies: *NADH-dependent cytochrome b5-reductase* and *cytochrome b5* deficiency
   - Deficiency of either cytochrome b5 or its reducing enzyme, cytochrome b5-reductase, decreases reduction of MetHb back to Hb (Figure 158.2)
3. Nitrite (NO_2), other oxidants and oxygen-reducing compounds
   - Nitrites are a common oxidizing source of MetHb production
     - Common sources: *poppers* of amyl and butyl nitrite used to enhance sexual stimulation (slang: locker room bang, bolt, thrust, flash, highball); arc welding combustion; explosives; anaerobic fermentation of crops in silos; well water in Midwest from irrigation run-off
   - Reducing agents paradoxically produce methemoglobinemia by reducing oxygen to a free radical or water to H_2O_2 which then oxidizes hemoglobin.
4. "Sensitive" hemoglobin: *Blue baby syndrome*
   - Bacteria in the immature gastrointestinal tracts of infants convert nitrate (NO_3) to the powerful oxidant nitrite (NO_2)
   - Infants have a relative NADH-dependent reductase deficiency (only 50% of adult levels) and are more susceptible to oxidative injury

---

blue produces a dramatic but transient depression in pulse oximetry.

Caution should be exercised during methylene blue administration, as doses greater than 7 mg/kg can paradoxically produce free radical formation leading to further methemoglobin production. Infants receiving methylene blue require especially careful monitoring because they have a relative NADH-reductase deficiency. Also, methylene blue should not be administered to patients with G6-PD deficiency for two reasons:

1. Patients with G6-PD deficiency are "resistant" to methylene blue. G6-PD is the initial enzyme of the hexose monophosphate (HMP) shunt that generates NADPH needed for glutathione production; with a relatively insufficient amount of G6-PD, the HMP shunt does not provide the NADPH needed for *NADPH-dependent MetHb reductase* to reduce methylene blue.

Table 158.2

Chemicals and Medications That Can Produce Methemoglobinemia

Phenols	Arsine gas
Menthol	Rifampin
Nitrite	Primaquine
Naphthalene	Hydrogen peroxide
Dapsone	Nitroglycerin
Aniline dyes	Pyridium
Cobalt	Methylene blue*

*Methylene blue is also the antidotal therapy for treatment for methemoglobinemia.

Table 158.3

Signs/Symptoms Corresponding to Percent Concentrations of MetHb Compared to Total Body Hb

Percent	Signs and Symptoms
5%–10%	Asymptomatic, normal color
15%	Cyanotic
30%	Headache, dizziness
60%	Lethargy, respiratory distress, seizures
>70%	Cardiopulmonary arrest, death

2. G6-PD deficient patients are more susceptible to RBC lysis from oxidative stress than those without the enzyme deficiency. These patients lack the G6-PD for efficient glutathione production to protect red blood cell (RBC) membranes from oxidation by oxygen free radicals. Methylene blue's reducing capability creates oxygen free radicals which damage RBC membranes and lead to hemolysis.

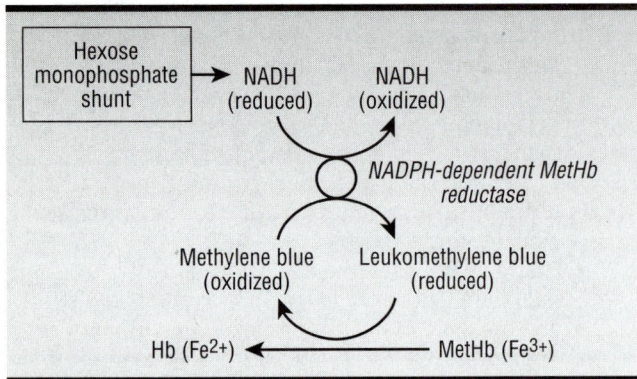

FIGURE 158.3 NADPH-dependent reduction of methylene blue converts it to its active electron donator form, leukomethylene blue. Reduced methylene blue donates an iron to the ferric (3+) methemoglobin heme iron to convert it to the ferrous (2+) state. Only hemoglobin with ferrous heme iron has the capacity to bind and carry oxygen.

Adjunctive Therapies

Severe cases of methemoglobinemia may benefit from exchange transfusion by removing and replacing MetHb with Hb. Exchange transfusion also offers the advantage of removal or dilution of toxin causing oxidative stress as well as hemolyzed erythrocytes and their contents.

Hyperbaric oxygen therapy has also been used, primarily in conjunction with exchange transfusion, to increase oxygen availability to hypoxic tissue. Multidose activated charcoal has been used in methemoglobinemia seen in patients with adverse reactions to dapsone, where a metabolite that undergoes enterohepatic circulation can produce persistent methemoglobinemia.

Indications for Consultation

All suspected cases of methemoglobinemia should be referred to a medical toxicologist and the regional poison control center.

Selected Readings

Bradberry SM. Occupational methaemoglobinemia. Mechanisms of production, features, diagnosis and management including the use of methylene blue. *Toxicol Rev* 2003;22:13–27.

Keys C, Keller HW. Methemoglobinemia. In: Aghababian R, ed. *Emergency Medicine: the Core Curriculum.* New York: Lippincott-Raven, 1998.

Price D. Methemoglobinemia. In Goldfrank LR, ed. *Goldfrank's Toxicologic Emergencies,* 7th ed. New York: McGraw-Hill, 1996.

Schofstall J. Methemoglobinemia. Emedicine. Available at http://www.emedicine.com/med/topic1466.htm. Accessed June 2005.

Organophosphate Poisoning

Steven B. Bird

Since the terrorist attack on the Tokyo subway system in 1995 and the ongoing threat of chemical weapons, the medical and military communities have an increased interest in the prevention, recognition, and treatment of casualties due to organophosphorous agents. Despite these concerns, the overwhelming majority of poisonings occur with commercially available products. According to the 2002 AAPCC Toxic Exposure Surveillance System database, there were more than 13,000 reported organophosphate/carbamate exposures in the United States, but few deaths. By far, the greatest burden of these agents is borne by the developing world. It is estimated that worldwide more than 3,000,000 people are exposed each year to organophosphate and carbamate compounds, with up to 300,000 fatalities. Cases of organophosphate toxicity have been described following the ingestion of rat poison, exposure to agricultural pesticides, ingestion of contaminated fruit, flour, and cooking oil, and wearing of organophosphate-contaminated clothing.

Although organophosphates and carbamates are structurally unique, they have similar commercial uses and mechanisms of action, and produce similar toxicities. The use of the term *organophosphate* herein also refers to carbamates, unless specifically indicated.

History of Organophosphate Development

Organophosphate compounds were first synthesized in the early twentieth century. In the 1940s, Germany military scientists began experimentation with several organophosphorous nerve agents (e.g., tabun [GA], sarin [GB], soman [GD]), but they were never used to wage chemical warfare. Commercial interest in organophosphates as insecticides began with the development of tetraethyl pyrophosphate (TEPP) in 1943 and parathion in 1944. The medical applications of organophosphates and carbamates include the reversal of neuromuscular blockade (neostigmine, pyridostigmine, edrophonium), and the treatment of glaucoma, myasthania gravis, and Alzheimer's disease (echothiophate, pyridostigmine, tacrine, and donepezil). The use of organophosphates as insecticides has steadily declined since the late 1950s largely due to the development of less toxic carbamates (**Table 159.1**).

Mechanism of Action

Organophosphate compounds contain carbon and phosphorous acid derivatives. These agents are absorbed through the respiratory and GI tracts, and, because of their significant lipophilicity, dermal absorption can be significant. The clinical and toxicologic effects of organophosphates are due to their actions at cholinergic synapses, where organophosphates inhibit and bind irreversibly to cholinesterase, the enzyme responsible for the degradation of acetylcholine. Over a period of time that depends upon the specific organophate, cholinesterase undergoes a conformational change known as "aging" that renders it impervious to reactivation by antidote. Other enzymes such as neuropathy target esterase (NTE) are also inhibited by certain organophosphates.

Carbamate compounds are derived from carbamic acid. Like organophosphates, carbamates are absorbed by all routes of exposure. Unlike organophosphates, these agents are *reversible* cholinesterase inhibitors; carbamates spontaneously hydrolyze from the cholinesterase enzymatic site within 48 hours. Carbamates also poorly penetrate the blood-brain barrier. Therefore, carbamate toxicity in equivalent doses to organophosphates tends to be more benign and shorter in duration than organophosphate toxicity (**Table 159.2**).

Clinical Effects

Acute Toxicity (Cholinergic Crisis)

Acute toxicity from organophosphates presents with manifestations of cholinergic excess. Primary toxic effects involve the autonomic nervous system, neuromuscular junction, and the CNS. The most noticeable clinical features of acute organophosphate toxicity involve the autonomic nervous system, which is mediated by both muscarinic and nicotinic acetylcholine receptors. The parasympathetic nervous system is particularly dependent on acetylcholine regulation because both the autonomic ganglia and end organs of the parasympathetic nervous system are regulated by nicotinic and muscarinic cholinergic receptor subtypes, respectively. As a result, the clinical features of acute toxicity primarily re-

Table 159.1
Potency of Common Organophosphates

Hazard	Common Name (Proprietary Name)
Extremely hazardous Class Ia (oral LD_{50} < 5 mg/kg in rats)	Disulfoton (Disyston) Fonofos (Dyfonate) Hexachlorobenzene (HCB) Mevinphos (Phosdrin) Parathion, ethyl and methyl (Parathion-E and Metcide) Sulfotep (Bladaflun, Di-thione)
Highly hazardous Class Ib (oral LD_{50} 5–50 mg/kg in rats)	Dichlorvos (DDVP, Vapona) Monocrotophos (Bilobran, Monocron)
Moderately hazardous Class II (oral LD_{50} 50–500 mg/kg in rats)	Chlorpyrifos (Dursban) Diazinon (Spectracide, Dia-zide, Gardentox) Dichlofenthion (Mobilawn, Bromex, Nemacide) Dimethoate (De-Fend, Dicap, Dimet) Fenthion (Baytex, Entex, Ti-gurvon, Spotton, Lyaoff) Trichlorfon (Dylox, Dipterex, Neguvon)
Slightly hazardous Class III (LD_{50} > 500 mg/kg in rats)	Acephate (Orthene) Malathion (Cythion, Lar-bofoa, Malamar) Propanil (Arrosol, Wham EZ)

Common names are given first. An incomplete list of proprietary pesticide names are given in parentheses. For a complete list see *The WHO Recommended Classification of Pesticides by Hazard and Guidelines to Classification 2000-2002.* Available at http://www.who.int/pcs/docs/Classif_Pestic_2000_2002.pdf. Accessed June 2005.

Table 159.2
Potency of Carbamates

Hazard	Common Name (Proprietary Pesticide)
Extremely hazardous Highly hazardous	Aldicarb (Temik) Carbofuran (Furadan) Methiocarb (Mesurol, Draza) Methomyl (Lannate, Nudrin)
Moderately hazardous	Carbaryl (Adios, Dicarbam, Sevin) Pirimicarb (Pirimor, Aphox, Rapid) Propoxur (Baygon)

Common names are given first. An incomplete list of proprietary pesticide names are given in parentheses. For a complete list see *The WHO Recommended Classification of Pesticides by Hazard and Guidelines to Classification 2000–2002.* Available at http://www.who.int/pcs/docs/Classif_Pestic_2000_2002.pdf. Accessed June 2005.

semble parasympathetic stimulation and include brady-cardia, miosis, lacrimation, salivation, bronchorrhea, bronchospasm, urination, emesis, and diarrhea. Diaphoresis occurs because sweat glands are regulated through sympathetic activation of postganglionic muscarinic receptors. At times, however, mydriais and tachycardia (due to direct sympathetic stimulation or hypoxia) may be observed because sympathetic ganglia also contain nicotinic receptors.

Fasciculations, muscle weakness, and paralysis may be observed in acute organophosphate poisoning via acetylcholine stimulation of nicotinic receptors at the neuromuscular junction. This mechanism is analogous to the depolarizing effects of succinylcholine in producing neuromuscular blockade. Finally, nicotinic and muscarinic receptors have been identified in the brain and may contribute to the CNS respiratory depression and clinical findings of lethargy, excitability, seizures, and coma.

Cardiac arrhythmias, including heart block and QTc prolongation, have been observed in organophosphate poisoning. Acute pancreatitis is an occasional presentation following poisoning and is thought to result from cholinergic stimulation of acinar pancreatic gland secretion.

Onset and duration of toxicity varies depending on the agent of poisoning, the route of absorption, enzymatic conversion to active metabolites, and the lipophilicity of the organophosphate. After oral or respiratory exposure to organosphosphates, most patients develop signs or symptoms within 3 hours. However, dermal absorption has been reported to delay the onset of symptoms up to 12 hours from exposure. Lipophilic agents such as dichlofenthion, dimethoate, fenthion, and malathion are also associated with delayed onset of symptoms (up to 5 days) and prolonged illness (greater than 30 days), which may be related to rapid adipose fat uptake and delayed redistribution from the fat stores. Many organophosphate insecticides have a characteristic petroleum or garlic-like odor, which may be helpful in establishing the diagnosis in an unknown exposure.

Fatalities from organophosphate poisoning generally result from respiratory failure due to a combination of depression of the CNS respiratory center, neuromuscular weakness, excessive respiratory secretions, and bronchoconstriction. Survivors of acute organophosphate poisoning may have permanent neurobehavioral deficits that persist after recovery. These include deficits in memory and abstract thought, as well as symptoms consistent with Parkinsonism.

Intermediate Syndrome

A subset of organophosphate poisoned patients develops a distinct neurologic disorder 24 to 96 hours post-exposure. This disorder, termed the "intermediate syndrome," consists of neck flexion weakness, decreased deep tendon reflexes, cranial nerve abnormalities, proximal muscle weakness, and respiratory insufficiency. With adequate ventilatory care, most patients appear to have complete resolution of their neurologic dysfunction within 2 to 3 weeks. Clinical deterioration and improvement appear to correlate with plasma and red blood cell acetylcholinesterase levels. Nerve conduction studies on patients with intermediate syndrome reveal unique postsynaptic abnormalities that differentiate this disorder from delayed neurotoxicity. Risk factors for the development of intermediate syndrome include exposure to a highly fat-soluble organophosphate and may be related to inadequate doses of oximes. The intermediate syndrome has not been described following carbamate poisoning.

Delayed Neurotoxicity

Delayed neurotoxicity typically occurs 1 to 3 weeks following an organophosphate exposure. Affected patients present with transient, painful "stocking-glove" paresthesias followed by a symmetrical motor polyneuropathy characterized by flaccid weakness of the lower extremities that ascends to involve the upper extremities. Sensory disturbances are usually mild. Delayed neurotoxicity primarily affects distal muscle groups; but in severe neurotoxicity, proximal muscle groups may also be affected. Electromyograms and nerve conduction studies of affected patients reveal decreased firing of motor conduction. Histopathologic sections of peripheral nerves reveal Wallerian (or "dying-back") degeneration of distal, large axons.

The risk of developing delayed neurotoxicity is independent of the severity of acute cholinergic toxicity. Some organophosphates, such as parathion, are potent cholinergic agents but are not associated with delayed neurotoxicity. Other organophosphates, such as triorthocresyl phosphate (TOCP), produce few clinical signs of cholinergic excess but are frequently implicated in causing delayed neurotoxicity. Carbamates are not associated with the development of delayed neurotoxicity.

The mechanism of delayed neurotoxicity may involve organophosphate-induced inhibition of neuropathy target esterase (NTE). This enzyme, which is found in the brain, peripheral nerves, and lymphocytes, is responsible for the metabolism of various esters within the cell.

Most cases of mild delayed neurotoxicity improve with time, but permanent disability—an upper motor neuron syndrome with spasticity of the lower extremities—usually follows in severe cases.

Treatment

Initial approach to the organophosphate or carbamate poisoned patient should focus on maintaining the patient's airway and prompt anticholinergic therapy (see below). Early endotracheal intubation and mechanical ventilation should be considered. Organophosphate-induced seizures should be treated with a benzodiazepine. There is no evidence that phenytoin has any effect on organophosphate-induced seizures. In fact, prophylactic diazepam has been shown to decrease neurocognitive dysfunction after organophosphate poisoning. This finding, in part, led to the US military development of a 10 mg autoinjector for diazepam.

In cases of topical exposure with potential dermal absorption, aggressive decontamination with complete removal of the patient's clothes and vigorous irrigation of the affected areas should be performed. Irrigation with a dilute 0.5% sodium hypochlorite solution may be more effective than saline or water because organophosphates and carbamates are hydrolyzed at alkaline pH. The patient's clothes and belongings should be discarded as they absorb organophosphates and reexposure may occur even after washing. In cases of early presentation after an organophosphate ingestion, nasogastric lavage may be considered. Activated charcoal should also be considered in cases of organophosphate and carbamate ingestions. Forced emesis is contraindicated because of the risk of aspiration and seizures.

Further evaluation of the organophosphate poisoned patient should include an assessment for signs of respiratory dysfunction including bronchorrhea, bronchoconstriction, and neuromuscular dysfunction including fasciculations and weakness. For moderate to severe cholinergic toxicity, atropine should be administered beginning at a dose of 2 to 5 mg IV for adults and 0.05 mg/kg IV for children. Atropine competes with acetylcholine at muscarinic receptors, preventing cholinergic activation. If no effect is noted, the dose should be doubled every 3 to 5 minutes until muscarinic signs and symptoms are alleviated; atropine dosing should be titrated to the therapeutic endpoint of the clearing of respiratory secretions and the cessation of bronchoconstriction. Tachycardia and mydriasis are inappropriate markers for therapeutic improvement as they may instead indicate continued hypoxia or sympathetic stimulation. In patients with severe poisoning, hundreds of milligrams of atropine by bolus and continuous infusion may be required for several days.

Since atropine does not bind to nicotinic receptors, it is ineffective in treating neuromuscular dysfunction. Pralidoxime (2-PAM), a cholinesterase reactivating agent, is effective in treating both muscarinic and nicotinic symptoms and should be given to all patients with cholinergic toxicity, patients with neuromuscular dysfunction, or patients with exposures to organophosphates known to cause delayed neurotoxicity. No controlled studies of optimal pralidoxime dosing for poisoned humans exist, but current recommendation for initial IV bolus therapy with pralidoxime is 1 to 2 g for adults and 25 to 50 mg/kg (based on severity of symptoms) for children. Pralidoxime should be administered slowly over 30 minutes since too-rapid administration has rarely been associated with cardiac arrest and slow administration prevents the muscle weakness (including respiratory muscles) that results from rapid inhibition of acetylcholinesterase by pralidoxime. After the initial bolus dose, the pralidoxime dose should be repeated every 6 hours for 24 to 48 hours or may be given as a continuous infusion of at least 3.2 mg/kg/h for adults and 10 to 20 mg/kg/h for children. More severe poisonings are associated with larger volumes of distribution of pralidoxime. Therefore, continuous IV dosing should be adjusted to patient severity and symptoms. If rapidly available, serial red blood cell acetylcholinesterase concentrations may be valuable in determining the efficacy of oxime-induced acetylcholinesterase regeneration. Pralidoxime should not be administered without concurrent atropine administration. Although no specific treatment has been shown to prevent intermediate syndrome or delayed neurotoxicity, early treatment with pralidoxime theoretically may be of benefit for these conditions.

The clinician should avoid the use of pharmacological agents that may induce or exacerbate seizures or worsen neuromuscular weakness. In particular, succinylcholine should be avoided as a neuromuscular blocking agent for endotracheal intubation. Succinylcholine, like acetylcholine, is metabolized by cholinesterase. In the setting of organophosphate or carbamate poisoning, the duration of paralysis after succinylcholine may be greatly prolonged.

In general, the diagnosis and treatment of organophosphate and carbamate poisoning rests on clinical evaluation and response to treatment. Serial laboratory assay of red blood cell cholinesterase and plasma cholinesterase may be helpful in confirming response to treatment and occasionally to confirm the diagnosis. With clinical improvement, cholinesterase levels should increase appropriately.

Admission Criteria

The decision to admit a patient to the hospital following an organophosphate or carbamate exposure should be based on the type of exposure and severity of the poisoning. Asymptomatic, nonsuicidal patients with exposures to short-acting organophosphates or exposures to carbamates can be released after a minimum of 4 to 6 hours of observation with appropriate follow-up and discharge instructions. In contrast, asymptomatic patients with exposures to organophosphates with delayed onset of symptoms such as the lipophilic organophosphates, fenthion or malathion, may require hospitalization for 24-hour observation. Any patient who requires treatment with atropine or pralidoxime should also be admitted to the hospital for at least 24-hour observation. Physicians are reminded that the intermediate syndrome may be delayed for several days.

Selected Readings

Aboud-Donia MB, Lapadula DM. Mechanisms of organophosphorus ester-induced delayed neurotoxicity: type I and type II. *Annu Rev Pharmacol Toxicol* 1990;30: 405–440.

DeBleeker JL, DeReuck JL, Wilems JL. Neurological aspects of organophosphate poisoning. *Clin Neurol Neurosurg* 1992;94:93–103.

Dunn MA, Sidell FR. Progress in medical defense against nerve agents. *JAMA* 1989;262:649–652.

Eddleston M. Patterns and problems of deliberate self-poisoning in the developing world. *QJM* 2000;93:715–731.

Rosenstock L, Keifer M, Daniell WE, et al. Chronic central nervous system effects of acute organophosphate pesticide intoxication. *Lancet* 1991;338:223–227.

Senanayak N, Karalliedde L. Neurotoxic effects of organophosphorous insecticides: an intermediate syndrome. *N Engl J Med* 1987;316:761–763.

Tafuri J, Roberts J. Organophosphate poisoning. *Ann Emerg Med* 1987;16:193–202.

Mushroom Poisoning

Sage W. Wiener
Robert J. Hoffman

There are old mushroom hunters and there are bold mushroom hunters, but there are no old, bold mushroom hunters.

—ANONYMOUS

Background

Only about 2% of the 5,000 mushroom species found in the United States are considered poisonous. Of these, only about 20 species are considered lethal, with over 90% of reported fatalities due to a single species: *Amanita phalloides*. Although reporting biases make it difficult to assess the true incidence of mushroom exposures and poisonings, 8,722 cases were reported to Poison Centers in 2002. Within this limited data set, there were no deaths attributed to mushrooms in 2001, and only five in 2002. However, of cases that are reported, unintentional pediatric exposures predominate. Because most of these children never actually ingest a significant amount of toxin, these statistics may mislead clinicians into underestimating the danger to a patient who truly ingests a toxic mushroom. Even though ingestion of a single mushroom from the cyclopeptide group is potentially fatal, pediatric exposures due to exploration and hand-to-mouth behavior are generally benign. In fact, the only children reported to suffer significant illness or death from mushroom poisoning have been exposed by eating food cooked with toxic mushrooms. Most clinically significant cases of mushroom poisoning result from foraging. Typically, immigrants may mistake toxic American mushrooms for similar-appearing edible mushrooms from their own countries. Once again, because adults actually intend to consume the mushrooms, they account for most fatalities, despite the fact that 80% of reported exposures involve children.

Mushroom Identification

There are numerous techniques available to identify an unknown mushroom, although most are arcane to anyone but a professional mycologist. The geographic location, type of terrain, time of the year, and structural appearance of the mushroom may all help in identification. If patients were foraging, it also helps to know what type of mushrooms they were looking for. If a sample is available, after structural features are noted, the stem may be cut off, and the cap placed on a piece of paper with alternating black and white bands. A bowl is placed over the mushroom so that spores may settle without disturbance by air currents. After several hours, the pattern is "fixed" with hair spray or fixative for cervical cytology. This *spore print* can be used by mycologists to identify a mushroom. Spores may also be tested with several drops of 10–12 N hydrochloric acid. A blue color ("the Meixner reaction") indicates the presence of amatoxin, although this is not definitive, as other tests are preferred by mycologists. The absence of a blue color does not exclude another type of poisonous mushroom.

It is potentially dangerous to base clinical decisions on amateur identification of a mushroom. In fact, an attempt to validate the use of an electronic database (Poisindex®) to identify mushrooms resulted in numerous misidentifications. When patients present after an unknown mushroom ingestion, the regional Poison Control Center should be contacted, as it may assist with mushroom identification and/or in locating a mycologist. Although an attempt should always be made to contact an expert mycologist (consider a university botany or plant pathology department or local botanical gardens), they may not be routinely available when actual patients present after ingesting a potentially toxic mushroom. Furthermore, identification may be difficult and time-consuming even when a mycologist is involved. Fortunately, most mushroom ingestions result in recognizable clinical patterns of toxicity, such that identification of the mushroom itself is often not necessary.

Recognizable Patterns of Toxicity by Specific Mushroom Groups

There is no universally agreed-upon system of classifying mushroom toxins. Groupings can be based either on clinical toxicological features or taxonomy. Many equally valid schemas are available, but we have adapted the system used by most clinicians. This system groups mushrooms by their toxic components: cyclopeptides, gyromitrin, muscarine, coprine, muscimol/ibotenic acid, psilocybin, gastrointestinal irritants, orellanine, allenic norleucine, and an as-yet unidentified myotoxin.

Cyclopeptide-Containing Mushrooms

This group contains many mushrooms of the *Amanita* genus, such as *Amanita phalloides, A. virosa,* and *A. verna,* as well as species of the *Lepiota* and *Gallerina* genera. These mushrooms contain about sixteen different amatoxins and phallotoxins, complex molecules known as cyclopeptides. **α-Amanitin**, the most important in human toxicity, interferes with mRNA synthesis by inhibiting RNA polymerase II.

Amanita mushrooms are notable in that they are highly developed mushrooms, with a cup at the base, a ring around the stem, and scales on the cap, all of which are remnants of veils that play a protective role during the development of the mushroom fruiting body. These features may not be obvious at some stages of mushroom development, leading to ingestion of equally toxic immature forms of these mushrooms by unlucky foragers. An excellent gallery of *A. phalloides* photographs illustrating these features is available online at: http://www.bioimages.org.uk/HTML/T2111.htm (Accessed June 2005).

The clinical presentation after cyclopeptide ingestion is divided into three phases. The first phase begins 5 to 24 hours after ingestion and is characterized by nausea, vomiting, and severe watery diarrhea. In phase II, between 12 and 36 hours after ingestion, patients improve if given good supportive care. Two to six days after ingestion, patients enter phase III of toxicity, characterized most significantly by hepatic necrosis, with liver enzyme elevation, hyperbilirubinemia, and jaundice. Liver failure may lead to hypoglycemia, encephalopathy, coma, and ultimately death (even with current advances in therapy, the mortality rate is reported to be 20%–30%). Associated renal and pancreatic injury may also be present.

Treatment for cyclopeptide poisoning consists both of good supportive care, decontamination, and possibly specific "antidotal" therapy, although the latter is controversial. Supportive care should consist of aggressive volume repletion and provision of adequate glucose to maintain euglycemia. Because α-amanitin has significant enterohepatic circulation and good binding to activated charcoal (AC), multiple dose AC should be administered. It may be given either by bolus dosing 1 g/kg orally every 2 to 4 hours or as a continuous infusion by nasogastric tube. Several therapies improve outcome in animal models, but there are as yet few data to support their clinical use. These include intravenous penicillin G (1 million units/kg/d) and silibinin (milk thistle), 5 mg/kg/d orally. It should be noted that seizures may result at these doses of penicillin. Other therapies that have as yet failed to show promise in humans include cimetidine, N-acetylcysteine, forced diuresis, hemodialysis, plasmapheresis, exchange transfusion, hemofiltration, and hemoperfusion, although many of these modalities continue to have their advocates.

It is difficult to implement treatment strategies based on the available data. Two clinical scenarios will help illustrate this point. For the patient who presents early (less than 2 h) after a known *A. phalloides* ingestion, aggressive gastrointestinal decontamination should be performed with orogastric lavage followed by multiple dose AC. If available, plasmapheresis, hemoperfusion or hemodialysis should be considered. Silibinin should be given (if not available in the hospital pharmacy, it can usually be obtained from a health food, nutrition, or vitamin store). If silibinin is not available, penicillin G should be given. For the patient who presents 12 hours after a known *A. phalloides* ingestion or with late gastrointestinal symptoms and a history suggestive of such an ingestion, the patient should get multiple dose AC (with antiemetics if necessary). Silibinin should be given, with penicillin as an alternative as in the first scenario.

Liver transplantation offers the last hope for patients with fulminant hepatic failure from cyclopeptide intoxication. Criteria for transplant are not well-established, but referral to a transplant center should be considered for patients who present with evidence of severe hepatotoxicity (encephalopathy, coagulopathy, azotemia) before they become too unstable for transfer.

Gyromitrin (Monomethyl-Hydrazine)-Containing Mushrooms

Poisoning from this group of mushrooms is extremely uncommon in the United States, but it is more common elsewhere, particularly Central Europe, although the mushroom is found commonly near the Great Lakes. Foragers seeking the highly desirable morel may ingest mushrooms of the species *Gyromitra esculenta* (the false morel), which, like the morel, is often described as "brain-like." The mushroom (like others of the genus *Gyromitra*) contains **gyromitrin**, a toxin that is metabolized to monomethyl-hydrazine. This metabolite shares its mechanism of toxicity with isoniazid, interfering with pyridoxine-mediated conversion of glutamate to gamma-amino-butyric acid (GABA). Perhaps because the toxin must first be metabolized, presentation tends to be delayed, often 6 to 12 hours after ingestion. Symptoms initially include such non-specific findings as nausea, vomiting, diarrhea, headache, cramps, and dizziness. Ultimately, the lack of inhibitory GABA tone may lead to seizures, and late findings may also include delirium or coma. Treatment is the same as for isoniazid toxicity. Benzodiazepines such as lorazepam are initial therapy for seizures, followed by pyridoxine (vitamin B_6) 5 g IV (70 mg/kg up to 5 g in a child).

Muscarine-Containing Mushrooms

Mushrooms of the genera *Clitocybe* and *Inocybe* contain **muscarine**, an acetylcholine analog with a long history (muscarinic acetylcholine receptors were first defined by their affinity for this compound). Muscarinic effects can be recalled with the mnemonic "**SLUDGE**," for salivation, lacrimation, urination, defecation, GI distress, and emesis. Bronchorrhea, bronchospasm, and bradycardia are the potentially serious muscarinic manifestations, and miosis may also occur. These effects typically present within 30 minutes to 2 hours after ingestion and last for several more hours. Symptoms are generally mild and self-limited, and rarely require more than supportive care. Atropine may be considered for severe symptoms, with doses of 0.5 to 1 mg in adults or 0.02 mg/kg in children, infused slowly IV, titrating to the drying of secretions as an endpoint.

Muscarine does **not** cause any nicotinic symptoms (weakness, fasciculations, paralysis), and the presence of any such symptoms strongly suggests contamination with an organophosphate or carbamate pesticide agent, rather than toxicity from the mushroom itself.

Coprine-Containing Mushrooms

Coprinus atramentarius, and other mushrooms of this genus, are often consumed because of their similar appearance to the edible "Inky Cap" (*Coprinus comatus*). *C. atramentarius* contains a toxin **coprine** that is metabolized in several steps to **cyclopropanone hydrate**, a competitive inhibitor of aldehyde dehydrogenase. Those who consume the mushroom without ethanol suffer no ill effects. Those who consume ethanol as much as 72 hours after these mushrooms suffer a disulfiram-like effect, with flushing, nausea, and vomiting. Supportive care with fluids and antiemetics, and ethanol abstinence for three days is the only treatment necessary.

Muscimol/Ibotenic Acid-Containing Mushrooms

The fly agaric, *Amanita muscaria,* has a long history of use by indigenous peoples from Central Europe to Central America. It has a distinctive appearance, inspiring many children's book illustrators, with a red/orange cap covered with white specks. Despite its name, this psychoactive mushroom is neither muscarinic nor antimuscarinic, although it does contain trace amounts of muscarine. The toxin **ibotenic acid** and its metabolite **muscimol** are thought to be the active components, although some have suggested that bufotenin may also be present. Interestingly, ibotenic acid is a glutamate (an excitatory neurotransmitter) agonist whereas muscimol is a GABA (an inhibitory neurotransmitter) agonist. The onset of symptoms is within 30 minutes to 2 hours after ingestion and the duration ranges from 4 to 14 hours. Principal effects include mental status depression, ataxia, and questionable hallucinations, progressing to obtundation. Hysteria, hyperkinetic behavior, and seizures or myoclonic twitching are more common findings in children, presumably from glutamatergic effects of ibotenic acid. Supportive care is generally all that is required, although seizures and other glutamatergic manifestations should be treated with benzodiazepines.

Psilocybin and Psilocin-Containing Mushrooms

Enthusiasts of hallucinogenic drugs may intentionally consume "magic mushrooms" or "shrooms" for their psychoactive effects. These mushrooms contain the toxins **psilocybin** and **psilocin**. *Psilocybe cubensis, P. caerulescens, Conocybe cyanopus, Panaeoulus foenisecii, Gymnopilus spectabilis,* and *Psathyrella foenisecii* may be found growing wild in many parts of the United States, but they are now more often cultivated. This is because the spores contain no toxin, so their possession and sale are legal. Psilocybin and psilocin are indoles resembling serotonin, and ingestion of these toxins produce 5-HT$_2$ agonist effects similar to LSD. Hallucinations, anxiety, and dysphoria are common symptoms, and tachycardia, mydriasis, and tremor may be noted on physical examination. These patients rarely come to the hospital, but reassurance and benzodiazepines are generally the only therapy required for those patients who do. More severe effects such as seizures, renal failure, and myocardial infarction have rarely been reported, although it is doubtful that these resulted from direct action of hallucinogenic mushrooms alone. One death was attributed to hallucinogenic mushrooms in 2002, although no details were provided in the report.

Gastrointestinal Irritants

A large number of mushroom species, typically "green gills" or "little brown mushrooms," contain varied and poorly understood toxins that result in gastrointestinal symptoms, such as nausea, vomiting, diarrhea, and abdominal discomfort. These symptoms appear early, typically within 30 minutes to three hours of ingestion, and last 6 to 24 hours. Although this is uncomfortable for the patient, there are rarely long-term sequelae, and treatment is symptomatic and supportive, including antiemetics and volume resuscitation.

Orelline/Orellanine-Containing Mushrooms

Mushrooms of the genus *Cortinarius* including *C. rainierensis, C. speciosissimus,* and *C. orellanus* contain the bipyridyl toxins **orelline** and **orellanine**. Ingestion of these mushrooms is common in Europe, with toxicity first described in Poland. No cases have yet been documented in the United States (although *C. rainierensis,* a North American species, contains the toxins). Nephrotoxicity typically presents in a delayed fashion. The first symptoms, occurring 24 to 36 hours after ingestion, are nonspecific, including headache, nausea, vomiting, chills, and myalgias. Marked polydipsia develops between 3 and 17 days after exposure, and is associated with tubular toxicity to the kidneys, with rapid progression to fibrosis and interstitial nephritis. There is no specific therapy for this toxicity, but hemodialysis is used for the resultant renal failure. Most patients will ultimately recover renal function. For the rare patients who do not recover, renal transplant is a potential consideration.

Allenic Norleucine-Containing Mushrooms

Until recently, all mushroom exposures resulting in early GI symptoms were considered benign. In recent years, however, reports of 13 cases of acute renal failure from *Aminita smithiana* after early GI symptoms (20 min to 12 h) has led to a change in outlook. All cases were from the Pacific Northwest, where foragers seeking the appetizing matsutake mushroom ingested the similar-appearing *A. smithiana.* This mushroom contains **allenic norleucine**, an amino acid toxin that results in nausea, vomiting, diarrhea, and abdominal cramping acutely, followed by delayed onset of renal failure 2 to 6 days later. There is no specific therapy, so supportive care and hemodialysis for those with renal failure are the only treatments. Some have suggested hemodialysis or hemoperfusion acutely for those with early symptoms and evidence (either by history or mushroom identification) of *A. smithiana* ingestion, but there is currently no evidence to support this approach. There is no reported mortality from this poisoning, and all reported patients had return of renal function within 4 to 6 weeks.

Myotoxic Mushrooms

Twelve patients were reported to develop delayed non-traumatic rhabdomyolysis after ingesting large quantities of *Tricholoma equestre* for three consecutive days. Although this fungus is also found in the United States, where it is known as the yellow-knight fungus, all reported cases so far have occurred in France. Although the toxin has not yet been identified, extracts of the mushroom has induced creatine phosphokinase (CPK) elevation experimentally in a mouse model. Patients presented with fatigue, myalgias, and proximal muscle weakness 1 to 3 days after ingestion. Over the next few days, patients developed worsening rhabdomyolysis, with dark urine and leg stiffness as well as facial erythema, nausea, and profuse sweating. CPKs higher than 600,000 IU/L were reported. Three of the 12 patients ultimately died of what appeared to be cardiac rhabdomyolysis. There is not yet any specific therapy for this exposure.

Approach to the Patient with Ingestion of an Unknown Mushroom

Patients who present to the hospital after ingesting a potentially toxic mushroom should be approached systematically. An algorithm summarizing this approach is shown in **FIGURE 160.1**. First, asymptomatic children with exposures from hand-to-mouth behavior do not need hospital evaluation. Adults who present will generally have symptoms. A thorough history should be obtained, including the timing of mushroom ingestion, the specific symptoms, whether others are ill, and most importantly, if more than one type of mushroom was consumed. In parallel with this process, attempts should be made to identify the mushroom, either through history, or more ideally through obtaining a sample. The regional poison control center and any available mycologist should be consulted to assist with identification and management. Most adult patients should receive GI decontamination with AC, and gastric emptying should only be considered for patients without significant vomiting and a history suggesting a life-threatening ingestion. As discussed above, extracorporeal removal should also be considered for such patients, and silybinin should be given. Any patient with symptoms after ingesting multiple types of mushrooms should be managed with AC and admission for observation. The following sections describe procedures that can be applied to patients who are symptomatic after ingestion of a single type of mushroom.

Patients Who Present with Early Symptoms (<3 Hours After Ingestion)

Patients with early symptoms can be assessed based upon the type of symptoms they present in the ED. Patients with neuropsychiatric symptoms such as hallucinations or alteration in mental status can be presumed to have ingested a psilocybin/psilocin-containing or muscimol/ibotenic acid-containing mushroom, and can be managed supportively with benzodiazepines if indicated. Patients with early gastrointestinal symptoms are addressed differently depending upon where they were exposed. Patients outside the Pacific Northwest are likely to have ingested a gastrointestinal irritant or coprine or muscarine-containing mushroom, and can be managed supportively unless they manifest significant muscarinic signs and symptoms, in which case atropine may be considered. If symptoms persist, these patients should be treated as if they had delayed symptoms and admitted for observation. In patients with early GI symptoms in the Pacific Northwest, *A. smithiana* must be considered. These patients should get GI decontamination with AC. They should be admitted and followed closely for renal toxicity over the following week. Some sources advocate early hemodialysis or hemoperfusion if there is a strong suspicion of this ingestion.

Patients Who Present with Symptoms 5 to 24 Hours After Ingestion

Patients who present with GI symptoms that begin more than 5 hours after ingestion are highly likely to have ingested a significant toxin such as α-amanitin, gyromitrin, or allenic norleucine. Antiemetics should be given to permit the administration of AC. Patients with history suggesting *G. esculenta* ingestion or those with seizures should be treated with pyridoxine. These patients should all be admitted for observation and serial liver enzyme and creatinine determination.

Patients Who Present With Late Symptoms (>24 Hours After Ingestion)

Patients who first develop symptoms more than 24 hours after ingestion are likely to have ingested an α-amanitin, gyromitrin, orelline/orellanine, allenic norleucine, or myotoxin-containing mushroom. All of these patients require admission and should be followed for renal and hepatic injury. Those with symptoms or exposure suggestive of gyromitrin ingestion should be treated with pyridoxine. CPK should be checked in those with muscle symptoms.

Conclusion

Although mushroom poisoning is rare in the United States, significant morbidity and mortality may result. Most fatalities are due to amanitin-containing species such as *A. phalloides*. Although identification may be difficult, every effort should be made to obtain material and seek expertise for analysis. The regional poison center

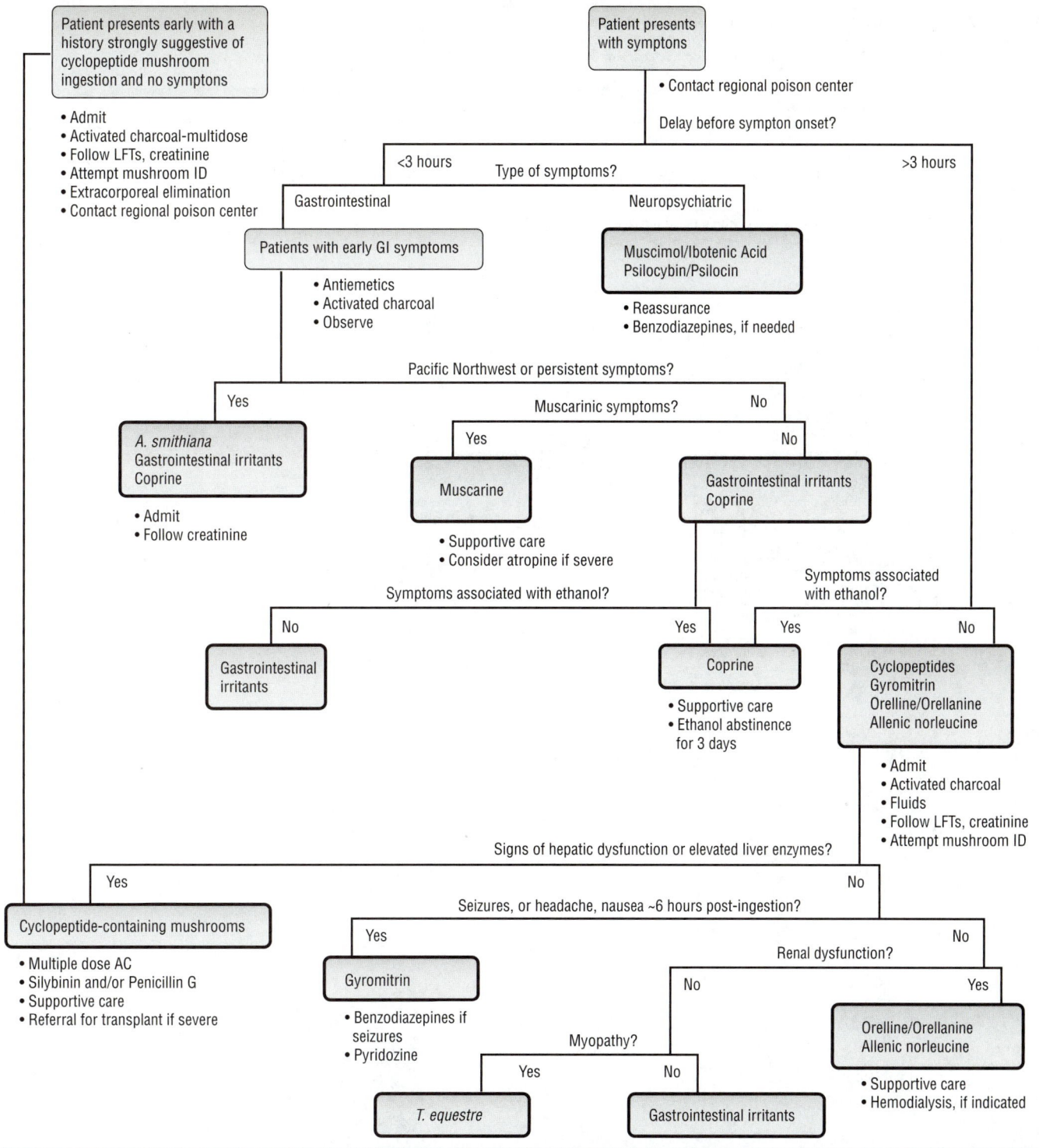

FIGURE 160.1 An algorithmic approach to the patient with a mushroom ingestion. Note that this is a guide only. Coingestants may complicate the process, and symptoms may be due to ingestions other than mushrooms. Management decisions should involve the regional poison center.

should be contacted and a mycologist consulted, if available. If identification is not possible, management decisions can be made based on clinical grounds. Patients with symptoms less than three hours after ingestion of a single type of mushroom are likely to have a relatively benign course unless they are from the Pacific Northwest or if their symptoms persist. All patients who present with late symptoms should be admitted, decontaminated, and observed for consequential toxicity.

Selected Readings

Bedry R, Baudrimont I, Deffieux G, et al. Wild-mushroom intoxication as a cause of rhabdomyolysis. *N Engl J Med* 2001;345:798–802.

Benjamin DR. Mushroom poisoning in infants and children: the *Amanita pantherina/muscaria* group. *J Toxicol Clin Toxicol* 1992;30:13–22.

BioImages: The Virtual Field-Guide (UK). Available at http://bioimages.org.uk/html/T22111.html. Accessed on June 2005.

Fischbein CB, Lipscomb JW, Mueller GM, Leikin JB. Field test of the new fungal identification system in Poisindex®. *Vet Hum Toxicol* 1993;35:204–206.

Fiume L, Stirpe F. Decreased RNA content in mouse liver nuclei after intoxication with α-amanitin. *Biochim Biophys Acta* 1966;123:643–645.

Floersheim GL. Treatment of human amatoxin mushroom poisoning: myths and advances in therapy. *Med Toxicol* 1987;2:1–9.

Goldfrank LR. Mushrooms. In: Goldfrank LR, Flomenbaum NE, Lewin NA, et al., eds. *Goldfrank's Toxicologic Emergencies,* 7th ed. New York: McGraw-Hill, 2002: 1115–1128.

Karlson-Stiber C, Persson H. Cytotoxic fungi—an overview. *Toxicon* 2003;42: 339–349.

Lampe KF. Toxic fungi. *Ann Rev Pharmacol Toxicol* 1979;19:85–104.

Lindell TJ, Weinberg F, Morris PW, et al. Specific inhibition of nuclear RNA polymerase II by α-amanitin. *Science* 1970;170:447–449.

Spoerke DG, Rumack BH, eds. *Handbook of Mushroom Poisoning: Diagnosis and Treatment,* 2nd ed. Boca Raton, FL: CRC Press, 1994.

Warden CR, Benjamin DR. Acute renal failure associated with suspected *Amanita smithiana* mushroom ingestions: a case series. *Acad Emerg Med* 1998;5: 808–812.

Watson WA, Litovitz TL, Rodgers GC, et al. 2002 annual report of the American Association of Poison Control Centers Toxic Exposure Surveillance System. *Am J Emerg Med* 2003;21:353–421.

Weisman JS, Abeles RH. Mechanism of inhibition of aldehyde dehydrogenase by cyclopropanone hydrate and the mushroom toxin coprine. *Biochemistry* 1979;18:427–435.

Wieland T. Poisonous principles of mushrooms of the genus *Amanita. Science* 1968;159:946–952.

882   SECTION XX: TOXICOLOGIC DISORDERS

Traumatic Disorders

Richard V. Aghababian
Peter Angood
Harry L. Anderson III

Introduction

In 2001, injuries accounted for the fifth highest number of deaths in the United States behind diseases of the heart, malignancies, cerebrovascular diseases, and chronic obstructive pulmonary diseases. Approximately 157,078 persons died from an unintentional injury in the United States, with 44,332 of these deaths being caused by motor vehicle accidents. It should be noted that injuries accounted for the majority of deaths in individuals of ages 1 to 34. These data indicate that injuries are the principal cause of death for the younger segment of the U.S. population. During this same period, a total of 27,551,362 persons who sustained nonfatal unintentional injury were seen in emergency rooms. Efforts to prevent the accidents and assaults that cause injury to this segment of the population, along with efforts to provide effective medical intervention when injury has occurred, increase the number of young adults who will go on to live long and productive lives.

Team Response

The goal of emergency personnel is to keep the victims of trauma alive and stable from the time the patient first receives medical care until definitive intervention in the emergency department (ED), operating room, and/or intensive care unit can be provided. To optimally achieve this goal in a consistent manner, emergency medical personnel must be organized into teams in which each individual role and specific tasks are well defined. The caregivers on the team must act according to prospectively designed multidisciplinary patient care protocols that are constantly subjected to evaluation in order to assure that quality of care is being provided.

Trauma team members include:
- Emergency Medical Services (EMS) personnel
- Emergency nurses
- Emergency physicians
- Trauma surgeons
- Specialty surgeons
- Anesthesiologists
- Critical care personnel
- Rehabilitation teams

Usually the first members of the team to encounter the patient are emergency medical technicians (EMTs). Whether the EMT has been trained to the basic or paramedic level, the initial assessment should involve a systematic survey of the patient's medical condition and the circumstances surrounding the accident. The primary survey in the prehospital setting must focus on the status of the victim's airway, breathing effort, circulatory integrity and neurologic status. Because the absence of an intact airway or adequate breathing effort can lead to death in a matter of minutes, repositioning of the airway (with proper attention to immobilization of the cervical spine), intubation, and/or assisted ventilation may be immediately life-saving. Assessment of the victim's level of neurological function may provide clues to the presence of intracranial or spinal cord injury. Progressive deterioration of neurologic function during the stabilization and transport phases provides strong evidence for progression of accident-related hemorrhage or swelling of the central nervous system. Assessment of the accident scene can provide valuable information about the forces applied to the body at the time of injury.

At the scene of an accident it is often difficult to perform a thorough patient assessment. When the victim is found in a badly damaged motor vehicle on a busy highway, it may be best to perform a primary survey, implement necessary stabilization procedures, and move the victim to the ambulance for rapid transport to an ED or trauma center. In such cases, further patient survey or stabilization can be done en route. When immediate transport is not feasible or in mass casualty situations where some victims must wait in line for the transport, the EMT can perform a secondary survey in the field. The intention of the secondary survey is to carefully re-inspect the victim for more subtle findings that were missed during the primary survey. To find possible concealed injuries, the head, torso, and extremities must be visibly inspected, or at least palpated, for abnormalities.

When transport time exceeds 5 minutes, the EMT should resurvey the patient at regular intervals to note any changes in airway, breathing, circulatory, and neurological status from the line of the initial survey. Resuscitation of victims at the scene is also necessary when the victim requires prolonged extrication or when the EMT must care for mass casualty victims awaiting transport. The physician providing medical control should be familiar with the limitations inherent to field care, the level of training of the prehospital personnel and system treatment protocols.

Assessment of the accident scene can provide valuable information about the forces applied to the body at the time of injury. Upon arrival in the ED, the emergency department team receiving the patient should also perform an initial survey. If the patient is intubated, the status of the endotracheal tube should be first ascertained. Pulse oximetry, capnometry, and possibly blood gas analysis can aid in evaluating the effectiveness of oxygenation and ventilation. A comprehensive survey in the ED of victims of blunt trauma should be performed immediately after the airway is secure, breathing has been assessed, excessive bleeding has been controlled, and fractures have been stabilized. Careful inspection of the scalp, back, pelvic area, and rectum may reveal injuries that were not apparent at the scene of injury.

Periodic reassessment of the victims of trauma in the ED is essential. In busy trauma centers occult injuries may not become apparent for hours, despite efforts to properly prioritize patients for imaging studies or diagnostic procedures.

Triage of the Trauma Victim

At the scene of injury with multiple victims, following the primary survey and initial stabilization, victim triage determines the order in which patients will be moved from the scene by transport vehicles. Triage decisions often determine the equipment and personnel that will be used to accomplish the patient transfer (helicopter vs. ground ambulance, for example). In the hospital, a similar triage process is used to determine the order in which victims in the ED will be sent to the operating room or given access to diagnostic imaging equipment.

The complexity of the triage process is determined by the conditions at the scene of injury, the degrees of injury of the victims, and the number of victims that require medical care. In any civilian situation requiring the triage process, the triage officer should be the most experienced medical person at the scene. This individual must have some familiarity with the epidemiology of injuries so as to provide accurate prediction of which patients need the quickest possible access to emergency care. In a mass casualty setting, some victims may seem to have injuries of greater severity than is the case when they are assessed in the hospital. This is referred to as *overtriage*. Some patients may be triaged to a hospital that does not have the personnel (e.g., a neurosurgeon) or facilities (e.g., a burn unit) to handle the patient's immediate and long-term needs. Such situations may result in the patient requiring a second transport before receiving appropriate management. It is therefore best that the triage officer be familiar with the personnel and equipment of the medical facilities in the region.

Shock in the Trauma Victim

CHAPTER

161

Richard V. Aghababian
Peter Angood
Harry L. Anderson, III

Shock is a term used to indicate the presence of clinical evidence of inadequate perfusion of end organs. The presence of shock following an injury is an indication to the trauma team that serious injury is likely, and the patient is in need of careful assessment and resuscitation measures. In most circumstances, the body is able to adjust to diminished blood flow to organs via nervous system-directed vasoconstriction in nonessential vascular beds. In addition, blood sequestered in capacitance vascular beds, such as the splanchnic and lower extremity venous beds, and protein-rich fluid in extracellular space is drawn back into the circulation. Clotting cascades are activated at bleeding sites. Over time, clotting along with vasoconstriction to the skin and subcutaneous tissue decreases blood loss from external wounds. Clot formation may also slow bleeding from sharp penetrating wounds to vascular organs. The mechanisms described serve to maintain blood flow to essential organs such as the brain and heart for a period after injury. Resuscitation that is begun while protective reflexes are aiding the victim may lead to victim stabilization and survival. When circulatory volume is lost rapidly, as occurs when major vessels are torn or severed, those compensatory mechanisms are inadequate. Death results in a matter of minutes unless bleeding is controlled and resuscitation efforts are started immediately Resuscitation efforts are futile following trauma if the resultant injuries cannot be repaired surgically or otherwise.

When shock is not reversed by resuscitative efforts, the decreased tissue perfusion results in organ ischemia and the accumulation of the byproducts of an anaerobic metabolism. Metabolic byproducts along with the electrolytes exiting dying cells are released in the circulation, which leads to the development of metabolic acidosis and derangement in serum electrolyte levels. Immediate resuscitative efforts for victims of trauma are directed at minimizing further loss of blood, restoring circulatory volume, maintaining proper levels of glucose and oxygen available to tissue for aerobic metabolism, and monitoring the victim for complications of accumulated metabolic abnormalities.

Shock has been divided into four categories based on the alteration in normal physiology that has occurred. Three of these four forms of shock—hypovolemic, cardiogenic, and neurogenic—can be observed immediately following serious injury. The fourth form, septic shock, may appear as a late complication of injury.

Hypovolemic Shock

Hypovolemic shock is usually the result of internal or external blood loss from injuries to blood vessels or vascular organs. This form of shock may also occur as a result of the loss of large amounts of protein-containing fluids following extensive burns. As well, hypovolemic shock may occur in patients experiencing massive loss of fluids from the gastrointestinal tract. In the face of hypovolemic shock, the uninjured heart attempts to compensate for decreased circulatory volume by beating faster to maintain cardiac output. The blood pressure falls while the pulse rises. Decreased cutaneous blood flow produces pallor and coolness of the skin, particularly at the extremities. The Advanced Trauma Life Support (ATLS) classification of hemorrhagic shock appears in **Table 161.1**.

Cardiogenic Shock

Cardiogenic shock follows injury to the heart, pericardium, and great vessels. Blunt cardiac injury is usually the result of severe blunt trauma transmitted through the chest wall. Since the injured heart muscle is unable to contract normally, the volume of blood ejected from the left ventricle decreases and blood pressure falls even though circulatory volume has not changed. Pressure in the venous system rises, eventually resulting in pulmonary congestion and distension of venous system. Jugular vein distension resulting from cardiogenic shock in the trauma victim may on occasion be confused with venous distension secondary to tension pneumothorax. Venous distension in the face of tension pneumothorax is a result of impeded venous return to

Table 161.1

ATLS Classification of Hemorrhagic Shock

Degree of Hemorrhage	Class I Very Mild	Class II Mild	Class III Moderate	Class IV Severe
Blood volume loss	<15%	15%–25%	26%–39%	≥40%
Cardiovascular	HR normal or mildly ↑, normal pulses, normal BP	Tachycardia, peripheral pulses may be ↓, normal BP	significant tachycardia thready peripheral pulses, ↓ BP	severe tachycardia thready CENTRAL pulses, significantly ↓ BP
pH	normal	normal	metabolic acidosis	significant acidosis
Respiratory	RR normal	tachypnea	moderate tachypnea	severe tachypnea
CNS	slightly anxious	irritable, confused, or combative	irritable, lethargic, or diminished pain response	lethargic, coma
Skin	warm, pink, capillary refill brisk	cool extremities, mottled, delayed cap. refill	cool extremities, mottled or pallor, prolonged cap. refill	cold extremities, pallor or cyanosis
Kidneys	normal urine output	oliguria, increased specific gravity	oliguria, increased BUN	anuria

the right side of the heart caused by elevated intrathoracic pressure.

Neurogenic Shock

Neurogenic shock may be observed when severe injury to the central nervous system has occurred. As a result of the injury the nervous system control of vascular tone is lost or impaired. Peripheral arterial resistance decreases, and inability to regulate vessel wall tone in the venous systems results in the pooling of blood in capacitance spaces such as the splanchnic bed. Although the circulatory volume is unchanged, blood pressure falls. Peripheral vasoconstriction does not occur; therefore, the skin is warm and pink. Since circulatory volume is unaffected, the pulse is generally not elevated and may, in fact, be paradoxically slow due to unmatched parasympathetic tone.

Septic Shock

Septic shock is a result of the increased circulatory demand produced by fever and toxic metabolites that accompany certain systemic infections. Although metabolism may be increased, circulatory volume is unchanged. Patients generally have warm, dry skin, and a bounding pulse, which may be elevated or normal.

Shock should be anticipated by EMTs and by the medical staff managing trauma victims in the field when blood loss, chest injury, or CNS injury is observed or suspected, even though the initial blood pressure is within the normal range. Decreasing blood pressure, deteriorating mental status, cutaneous vasoconstriction, and increasing pulse observed after the initial assessment should prompt immediate reevaluation for occult injuries.

Selected Readings

Advanced Trauma Life Support (ATLS) for Doctors, 6th ed. Chicago: The American College of Surgeons, 2004.

Moore EE, Feliciano DV, Mattox KL, eds. *Trauma,* 5th ed. New York: McGraw-Hill Professional, 2004.

Initial Assessment and Management of the Trauma Victim

Richard V. Aghababian
Peter Angood
Harry L. Anderson III

The major causes of death in the prehospital period are severe CNS injury, massive hemorrhage, or respiratory failure caused by airway obstruction or mechanical impairment of ventilation. Patients who die from severe head injury in the field for the most part are either nonsalvageable or die as a result of loss of control of their airway and the resultant respiratory compromise. Maintaining oxygenation and preventing hypercarbia are critical in the management of all trauma victims, particularly those who have sustained head injury. Evaluation of the airway is the first concern. If the patient has lost the ability to protect the airway or the airway is endangered by swelling, fluids, or collapse, it should be secured with endotracheal intubation. After securing the airway, ventilation should be assisted with a bag-valve mask device, and high-flow supplemental oxygen should be administered. Ventilation should be confirmed by auscultation of bilateral breath sounds, capnometry, and monitoring oxygen saturation via pulse oximetry if available.

Axial spine injury should be suspected in any patient who has sustained trauma. The cervical spine is particularly vulnerable. Any patient who has sustained an injury above the clavicle, a head injury resulting in loss of consciousness, or an injury resulting from a high-speed accident should be presumed to have a spinal column injury. Immobilization of the entire patient should be maintained until screening roentgenograms are obtained, and fractures or dislocations have been excluded. Injudicious movement or manipulation may result in more injury. Vascular access should be obtained in all trauma victims with obvious injury as well as those whose mechanism of injury suggests the potential for internal injury. Ideally, access should be obtained with two large-bore (14–16 gauge) intravenous catheters. In patients requiring resuscitation, an initial fluid bolus of 1000 to 2000 mL (20 mL/kg in the pediatric population) of an isotonic electrolyte solution should be rapidly administered. Lactated Ringer's solution is usually the fluid of choice; however, normal saline is acceptable. Normal saline in very large volumes, as may be required in trauma resuscitation, may result in a hyperchloremic acidosis. The amount of fluid administered varies depending on the patient's response to resuscitation, evidence of end-organ perfusion and oxygenation, and transport time to the hospital. As stated before, there continues to be controversy regarding the administration of fluid resuscitation to victims of penetrating trauma. Currently, however, the standard of care is to administer fluids to all hypotensive trauma patients in the field regardless of the mechanism of injury.

Patients who have been involved in accidents that require prolonged extrication, such as severe motor vehicle accidents, building collapse at construction sites, or entrapment in industrial or farm machinery, present a special problem for the EMT. Initial assessment and treatment cannot wait until the patient has been fully extricated. This often requires the EMT to climb into the vehicle or equipment to gain access to the patient. Caution must be taken not to endanger the lives of the rescuers. Once the patient is reached, initial assessment of the ABCs (airway, breathing, and circulation) should begin. The cervical spine should be immobilized immediately, even if simply with inline traction. The airway should be secured, intravenous access obtained, and fluid administration initiated. It should be recognized that there are situations where hemorrhage or airway problems may result in death if the patient is not immediately extricated. In such cases, treatment must focus on the problem that is the greatest immediate threat to the patient's life, and further assessment and treatment must wait.

Trauma patients may be subject to several environmental stresses after their injury. Patients are often exposed to the weather and rapidly lose heat to the environment, particularly if they are wet. Infusion of fluids cooler than body temperature, in addition to shock, can contribute to hypothermia. All patients should be kept covered and warm as much as possible. Conversely, patients who have had prolonged heat exposure may have hyperthermia. Active cooling should not be instituted in the field unless the patient's temperature is greater than 105° F. Depending on the environment in which the accident took place, consideration may also have to be given to the presence of toxic gases or other substances that may have contaminated the victim. Besides removing the patient from the area as soon as possible, the patient may have to undergo decontamination procedures or hyperbaric therapy.

Initial Management of the Trauma Victim

The emergency physician should be immediately called to assess victims of serious trauma. In trauma centers with in-house trauma teams, the decision to call the trauma team should be based on the description of the patient provided by the EMTs or by the emergency physician following the performance of an initial survey. The trauma team should be assembled before the patient arrives if the patient is described to be in shock, in need of immediate resuscitative intervention, or if predetermined criteria for trauma team activation are met (**FIGURE 162.1**).

Whether the victim is transported by EMS personnel or appears unannounced, the emergency physician is responsible for the care of the patient. The direction of the ED staff and other trauma team members is the responsibility of the on-duty emergency physician during the initial assessment and stabilization phase. As the patient's injuries are diagnosed and definitive treatment has begun, the emergency physician may turn over care of the patient to the trauma team attending surgeon or on-call surgeon, who agrees to accept responsibility for the patient in the hospital. Because an emergency physician is available 24 hours a day, 7 days a week, it is essential that the emergency physician be assigned the initial responsibility for trauma victims delivered to the ED. The exact point at which responsibility should be shifted from the emergency physician to the surgeon is determined by the severity of the injury, the need for immediate surgical intervention, and the availability of the surgeon and the operating room facilities. When circumstances do not permit the adequate management of trauma victims at the receiving facility, it is the responsibility of the emergency physician to stabilize the victim to the degree that is possible and arrange transfer to a medical facility capable of managing the victim's injuries. Transfer arrangements should follow predetermined protocols. Copies of medical records and the results of ancillary tests should accompany the patient. The receiving facility must agree to accept the patient in transfer.

The initial ED survey performed by the emergency physician for victims of severe trauma repeats some of steps taken in the field during the primary survey. During the initial phase of assessment, the cervical spine could be stabilized if injury is a possibility. The emergency physician should once again check the status of the airway and assure the adequacy of ventilation. When evidence of blunt chest trauma is present, pneumothorax and flail chest must be ruled out by physical examination. Pulse oximetry provides further information about the adequacy of ventilation. Oropharyngeal foreign bodies should be sought when facial trauma is evident.

The presence of hypotension due to blood loss suggests a loss of at least 20% of the victim's blood volume (see Chapter 161, Table 161.1), and blood samples should be sent for type and cross-match immediately. Traditional teaching has been that type O negative or type-specific blood along with isotonic solution should be administered if the blood pressure continues to drop because of uncontrolled hemorrhage. When massive transfusion is required, calcium, clotting factors, and platelets will be depleted. Calcium replacement, fresh frozen plasma, and platelet transfusion are usually necessary.

While performing the ED assessment, the emergency physician should attempt to obtain information about the circumstances producing the injuries and the patient's relevant medical history. Information about medications, allergies, and preexisting medical conditions may provide clues to the cause of a motor vehicle accident or a fall from a height.

Preexisting medical conditions/medications may have an impact on victims of trauma. It is important for the emergency physician to elicit a history of preexisting conditions and to be prepared to handle subsequent complications that may arise as a result. When the patient is unable to provide information, medical alert bracelets or family members may be helpful. Jehovah's witnesses' religious convictions forbid them to accept blood or blood products. Albumin, immune globulins, and clotting factors are a matter of individual conscience, but there is no objection to using non-blood alternatives such as low molecular weight dextrans or Haemaccel (cross-linked gelatin polypeptides). All patients who are mentally competent have the right to refuse transfusion therapy even if it means death. In the unconscious patient, where informed consent cannot be obtained, the presence of a Jehovah's witness card stating the patient's convictions and signed by the patient is felt to be adequate documentation of assent to withhold transfusion therapy.

With the continuing growth in organ transplant programs, there is an increasing need for organ donors. Trauma patients who have sustained irreversible injury may have healthy organs that potentially could benefit patients who are awaiting transplant. It is the responsibility of the organ procurement agency who is dealing with the surviving family to discuss the option of organ donation. If the family is receptive, the appropriate personnel (in most local it is only the regional organ procurement agency who may approach a family) can be summoned to meet with the family to discuss this option in more detail.

Indications for Consultation

After the emergency physician evaluates and stabilizes a trauma patient, arrangements must be made for definitive care. A general surgeon experienced in the care of multiple trauma is usually the most appropriate individual to assume responsibility of care from the emergency physician. Consultation should be made to the general surgeon immediately after initial resuscitation and stabilization. When a patient is known to have sustained injuries that will require immediate surgical intervention, such as penetrating abdominal injury or an evisceration, it is appropriate to consult the general surgeon as soon as this information is confirmed. The emergency physician, however, must still remain responsible for the initial resuscitation and stabilization, after which the care may be transferred to the general surgeon. Other situations that may require immediate consultation to a specialist other

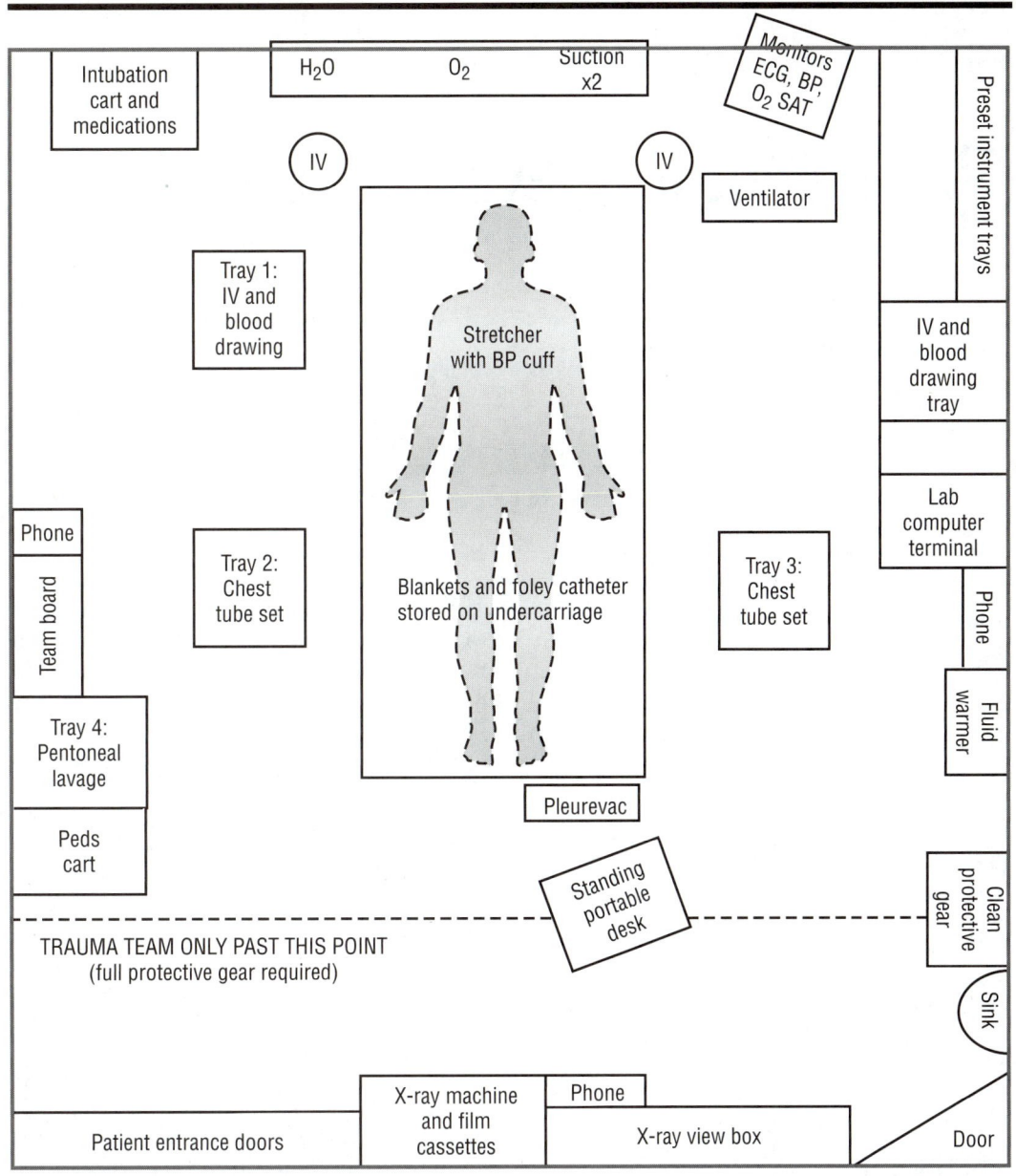

FIGURE 162.1 Diagram of a typical trauma resuscitation area. *Source:* From Committee on Trauma, American College of Surgeons. *Resources for the Optimal Care of the Injured Patient.* Chicago: American College of Surgeons, 1999.

than a general surgeon during the initial resuscitation phase include severe head injury (neurosurgery) and penetrating trauma to the chest (cardiothoracic surgery). Other services such as orthopedics, plastic surgery, ENT, and ophthalmology, while important to the overall care of the patient, generally are not needed during the initial phase of resuscitation, but rather should be consulted after specific needs have been identified. Many multiple-trauma patients will require admission to a critical care setting where consultation with intensivists can be obtained. In patients with complex medical problems, consultation with an internist may be necessary to assist in the management of these problems, and to stabilize the patient for urgent or elective surgery.

Selected Readings

Advanced Trauma Life Support (ATLS) for Doctors, 6th ed. Chicago: The American College of Surgeons, 2004.

Committee on Trauma, American College of Surgeons. *Resources for the Optimal Care of the Injured Patient.* Chicago: American College of Surgeons, 1999.

Moore EE, Feliciano DV, Mattox KL, eds. *Trauma,* 5th edition. New York: McGraw-Hill Professional, 2004.

Radiologic Evaluation

Richard V. Aghababian

Peter Angood

Harry L. Anderson III

Standard Plane Radiography

Patients with serious injuries, those with a major mechanism of injury, and those with potential multisystem trauma should undergo plane film evaluation of their cervical spine, chest, and pelvis. The proper timing of these studies varies with the clinical scenario and is ultimately decided by the trauma team leader. Additional plane films are obtained as deemed necessary. In the less seriously injured patient, plane films are ordered based on the history and physical examination and the emergency physician's index of suspicion for particular injuries.

Cervical Spine

Bony injury to the cervical spine (C-spine) and the potential for spinal cord injury represent two of the greatest concerns to the trauma patient. A good-quality lateral C-spine film reveals approximately 85% of significant C-spine injuries and can be performed early in the management of a trauma patient. Alignment, bones, cartilage, and soft tissues must be carefully evaluated. Most commonly a single lateral C-spine film is obtained during the initial evaluation, resuscitation, and stabilization phases of patient care, with remaining views (odontoid, anteroposterior [AP], and optionally the oblique views) completed when the patient's condition is stabilized. The lateral C-spine film also provides useful information to assist in decision making if active airway control is required and the clinical situation allows time to perform the study. CT scanning of the C-spine may be necessary to radiographically evaluate the bony detail (obese patients, significant degenerative disease, inability to visualize C7-T1 levels, etc.).

Strict immobilization must be maintained at all times until the cervical spine is cleared of significant injuries both radiographically and clinically. Stable injuries require urgent spine team (orthopedic or neurosurgical) consultation, while unstable injuries or those associated with neurologic findings mandate emergent orthopedic and/or neurosurgical consultation.

Chest

The chest radiograph often provides vital information that can dramatically alter the management of the trauma patient. In the multiply injured patient, an AP chest x-ray performed in the supine position is usually the first thoracic study obtained.

The lung fields must be assessed for any signs of pneumothorax, hemothorax, or pulmonary contusion. In the setting of penetrating trauma, a globular cardiac silhouette should be presumed to represent hemopericardium until proven otherwise. The course of the trachea and main stem bronchi can give clues to the presence of injuries to these structures. Careful evaluation of the mediastinum is critical if there is any potential for injury to the great vessels. In particular, one should assess for mediastinal widening, blurring of the borders of the aortic knob, rightward displacement of the trachea or nasogastric tube (if present), downward displacement of the left main stem bronchus, narrowing of the carinal angle, and apical capping. These findings may represent aortic injury and when present, usually warrant further evaluation (**FIGURE 163.1**). Clinical suspicion alone *without* chest radiograph abnormality is sufficient reason to further evaluate the aorta and great vessels.

Additionally, any radioopaque foreign bodies should be identified and localized. All visible bony structures must be inspected for signs of injury. The presence of gas in the soft tissues or mediastinum is another significant finding, usually representing injury to the tracheobronchial tree or penetrating injury through the thoracic wall.

If the clinical situation permits, the initial supine film is often followed by an upright chest film that can more reliably reveal some abnormalities, particularly hemo- or pneumothoraces, and mediastinal abnormalities.

Pelvis

Pelvic fractures can result in considerable morbidity and mortality, testifying to the degree of force involved in the injury-causing incident. A single AP view of the pelvis is

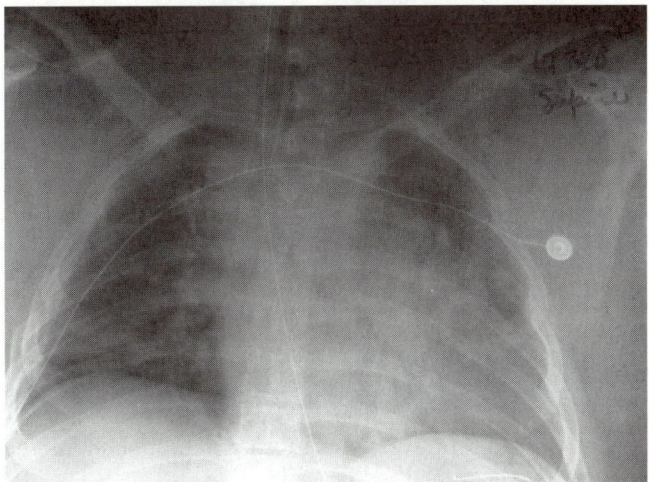

FIGURE 163.1 Anteroposterior view of chest radiograph with a widened mediastinum in a motor vehicle crash victim. Subsequent arch aortography confirmed thoracic aortic rupture just beyond the left subclavian artery.

obtained, and in the hands of a skilled interpreter is usually sufficient to diagnose any significant injury to the bony pelvis. In addition to examining for any disruption of the normally smooth bony cortices, one should also look closely for any asymmetry or widening of the sacroiliac joints as well as signs of bony injury to the sacrum (which may manifest only as subtle irregularities in the normal smooth curve of the sacral ala). Widening of the symphysis pubis is a very important finding as it represents disruption of the pelvic ring. Stable fractures represent fractures that do not disrupt the pelvic ring or do so in only one location. Unstable pelvic fractures involve disruption of the pelvic ring in two or more places, giving rise to at least two separate fragments that may be independently mobile. Unstable fractures are associated with increased rates of associated injuries and significantly higher morbidity and mortality.

The most significant injury associated with pelvic fractures is bleeding from the arterial and venous vascular beds that lie within the pelvis. This bleeding is often retroperitoneal and brisk, and can easily lead to death. Adjacent organ systems, particularly the genitourinary and lower gastrointestinal tracts, are subject to injury and require careful evaluation.

Stable pelvic fractures require urgent orthopedic consultation. Unstable pelvic fractures require emergent orthopedic consultation for reduction. If bleeding is present and continues despite reduction, arteriography with selective arterial embolization may be of benefit. Some advocate the use of military antishock trousers (MAST) for temporary splinting of suspected unstable pelvic fractures. More recently, external fixation or the use of a corset-like device at the pelvis (T-POD) are typically selected for major pelvic disruption.

Skull

Plane film evaluation of the skull and face of the trauma patient has been largely replaced by CT. There may still be

some role for plane films in the evaluation of isolated facial injuries, particularly those of the zygoma and mandible.

Spine

Thoracic, lumbar, and sacral spine films are ordered frequently on the injured patient. Some indications for these include: significant direct trauma to the spine, spinal pain, or tenderness, a step-off or other detectable deformity, other spinal fractures (especially in the setting of axial-load injuries), neurologic deficit at the thoracic/lumbar/sacral level, and calcaneus fractures secondary to falling in a standing position. The evaluation of spinal films is similar to that noted for cervical spine films above. Spinal fractures warrant emergent spine team consultation, and if a neurological deficit is present, a neurosurgeon should be emergently consulted. Strict spinal immobilization must be maintained at all times.

Extremities

A wide variety of extremity fractures may be present in an injured patient, and some of these are associated with significant morbidity and mortality (e.g., midshaft femur fractures). Bony injuries to the extremities can occur with relatively little force. Radiographic examination should be undertaken when the patient has a history of an injury mechanism capable of producing a bony injury and signs and symptoms of fracture or dislocation. These include deformity, pain, swelling, ecchymosis, decreased motion of a joint, bony tenderness, and inability to tolerate axial loading. In addition to abnormalities of the bones themselves, the emergency physician must be alert to the presence of other more subtle radiographic signs of injury, such as soft tissue swelling or joint effusion, which may indicate an occult fracture or ligamentous injury.

Abdomen

There is little utility for plane films of the abdomen in the management of the trauma patient, except for localization of foreign bodies such as bullets.

Urethrogram

Retrograde contrast urethrogram is indicated in the evaluation of patients with suspected urethral injuries, including patients with clear evidence of direct trauma to the penis, blood at the urethral meatus, inability to void, and patients with anterior pelvic injuries. The procedure can be performed in the ED. Urgent consultation with a urologist is required.

Esophagogram

Contrast esophagography may be used in the evaluation of the patient with a penetrating neck injury. There is still some debate about which patients warrant mandatory exploration and which can be evaluated by other means. Esophagoscopy is another method used to evaluate the esophagus after penetrating trauma. If the decision is made to perform an esophagogram, most trauma surgeons recommend the use of Gastrografin rather than barium as the contrast agent because it causes fewer complications if it enters the mediastinum.

Intravenous Pyelography

Intravenous pyelography (IVP) has been used in the past to assess the kidneys and urinary tract in patients with gross hematuria or suspected renal injury. The current trend is toward using contrast-enhanced CT for these purposes.

Computed Tomography Scanning

The continued development of the technology of CT scanning has led to great advances in the speed of the procedure and in the quality of the images produced. CT scan plays a proven valuable role in the evaluation of the injured patient.

Head

Computed tomography has radically altered the management of patients with acute head injuries. It has replaced the technique of observation with a quick and reliable test that accurately identifies the vast majority of significant intracranial injuries.

There is ongoing study as to delineating which patients require CT scan of the head after head injury. In patients with open or depressed injuries of the skull or patients with altered level of consciousness, the decision is easily made. It is in the setting of mild-to-moderate closed head injury with brief or no associated loss of consciousness in a patient, who is now neurologically intact, that the issue is more difficult to settle.

CT scans of the head are very sensitive in detecting traumatic injury to the skull and brain. An experienced physician should interpret the scan, looking for any evidence of fractures, epidural or subdural hematoma, subarachnoid hemorrhage, intraparenchymal hemorrhage, edema, mass effect, or herniation. Most of these are well visualized without the aid of intravenous contrast. All require emergent neurosurgical consultation.

Face

CT scanning has largely replaced plane film studies in the evaluation of orbital and facial trauma. It is very effective at revealing retroorbital and orbital processes as well as providing detailed information on even the most complex facial fractures. Common indications include deformity, midface instability, massive facial trauma, and orbital entrapment.

Abdomen/Pelvis

The advent of CT scanning has led to a marked reduction in exploratory laparotomy rates and is proven to have decreased morbidity and mortality in the trauma setting. Contrast-enhanced abdominal CT scanning plays its greatest role in the setting of blunt abdominal trauma. It provides detailed information on both the solid and hollow viscera as well as the peritoneal and retroperitoneal space. Pelvic studies allow visualization of the lower genitourinary tract and gastrointestinal tract.

Many sets of criteria have been proposed as indications for abdominal CT scanning in the injured patient. It is helpful to remember general considerations when deciding whether to pursue this diagnostic option. First and foremost, the patient must be hemodynamically stable. If so, abdominal CT scanning should be considered in any patient whose history and physical examination is suspicious for intraabdominal injury or who has the potential for intraabdominal injury but is difficult to evaluate (e.g., secondary to altered mental status from alcohol or drugs, spinal cord injury, or paralysis/sedation). All such scans should be performed with both oral and intravenous contrast and, given the subtleties in interpretation, should be read by a well-trained radiologist.

CT scans of the abdomen are excellent at revealing solid-organ injuries. The liver, spleen, pancreas, and kidneys are all well visualized. Hollow-organ injuries can be more subtle in appearance, but extravasation of contrast from these organs is diagnostic of rupture or perforation. Free fluid (usually blood from acute hemorrhage) is readily seen in the peritoneum and retroperitoneum. This information, taken together with the patient's clinical status, can help guide decisions about laparotomy. Some advocate that an ultrafast helical (late generation) abdominal CT scanner located adjacent to the trauma room might safely replace peritoneal lavage as a diagnostic test, even in the setting of hemodynamic metastability.

Chest

CT scanning of the chest in the trauma setting plays its greatest role in the evaluation of great vessel injuries, and ongoing research suggests helical chest CT scan may replace angiography as the gold standard in diagnosing aortic injuries. All chest CT scans must be performed with well-timed intravenous contrast and with as little motion artifact as possible.

Current indications for chest CT scan in the acutely injured patient include patients with potential great vessel injury and abnormal mediastinal findings on chest x-ray (see above) who are otherwise stable, and patients with thoracic injuries that are unclear or poorly defined by plane films where better understanding of the injury would potentially alter patient management. In addition to providing useful information about the mediastinum, chest CT scan can also visualize the chest wall (e.g., rib fractures), lungs (e.g., pulmonary contusion), pleural space (e.g., hemo- or pneumothoraces), tracheobronchial tree (e.g., disruption), and diaphragm (e.g., traumatic rupture).

Bone

CT scan provides accurate and detailed three-dimensional views of bony structures. It is frequently employed as an adjunct to plane films in the evaluation of bony injuries, either when such an injury is strongly suspected but not seen on plane films or when more detailed information is needed on identified fractures. This is frequently the case with fractures of the spine, pelvis, hip, scapula, calcaneus, distal tibia (pilon fractures), or tibial plateau.

Angiography

Contrast Angiography

Contrast angiography still plays an established role in the evaluation of vascular injuries in the trauma patient. However, recent studies suggest that as the technologies of CT scan, magnetic resonance angiography, and vascular ultrasound improve, these modalities may replace contrast angiography under most conditions. Alternatives to angiography are being actively pursued because it is an invasive procedure and involves intravenous contrast administration, both of which increase complication rates. It is also personnel intensive and requires highly specialized equipment and specially trained radiologists for accurate interpretation.

Contrast angiography is now considered the gold standard for investigation of potential thoracic aorta injuries, although helical CT scan may replace it (see above). It is also employed in the setting of penetrating zone I and zone III neck injuries to assess the carotid arteries. Arteriography of the extremities is performed when there are penetrating injuries near major vascular structures, fractures that alter perfusion despite reduction, and posterior knee dislocations. Selected pelvic fractures require arteriography, particularly those that are associated with continued hemorrhage despite reduction.

Magnetic Resonance Imaging (MRI)

MRI provides very detailed anatomical information, particularly on the soft tissues that are imaged by CT scan. Its utility in the setting of acute trauma is restricted, however, by limited ready availability and the fact that only specialized equipment can accompany the patient into the testing room because of the very powerful magnetic fields generated.

Currently, in the setting of acute trauma, MRI is employed only for the evaluation of spinal cord injuries, especially when a level of spinal injury cannot be established by plane radiography or CT scan. It also has utility as a follow-up test for diffuse axonal injury of the brain, where it outperforms CT scanning.

Magnetic resonance angiography (MRA) uses the same technology to evaluate vascular structures. Research is under way to determine its proper application in the trauma setting, but currently there are no clear indications for its use.

Ultrasonography

Ultrasound is appealing to practitioners of emergency medicine because of its favorable technical aspects, and this holds true for the assessment of the acutely injured patient. It is virtually without risk to the patient, can be quickly performed at the bedside, and meaningful diagnostic information can be gathered with relatively little training. Its role in the practice of emergency medicine is expected to increase.

Attention has recently been focused on the use of ultrasonography in detecting intraabdominal injury in the victim of blunt trauma, so called *focused abdominal sonography for trauma (FAST)*. It is clear that it is imperfect in assessing the visceral organs themselves, but FAST has been demonstrated to be quick and accurate in detecting free fluid (blood) in the peritoneum. In many hospitals FAST has replaced diagnostic peritoneal lavage as the test of choice in identifying abdominal hemorrhage in the hemodynamically unstable patient. FAST will be covered in more detail in a later section.

Ultrasound can also be used to evaluate the heart and great vessels of victims of thoracic trauma. *Transthoracic echocardiography (TTE)* can quickly establish a diagnosis of hemopericardium, and can identify cardiac wall motion abnormalities seen in both blunt (e.g., blunt cardiac injury) and penetrating injuries. *Transesophageal echocardiography (TEE)* can accurately identify aortic injuries.

Selected Readings

Advanced Trauma Life Support (ATLS) for Doctors, 6th ed. Chicago: The American College of Surgeons, 2004.

Mirvis SE, Shanmuganathan K, eds. Imaging in Trauma and Critical Care, ed 2. Philadelphia: Elsevier Science, 2003.

Moore EE, Feliciano DV, Mattox KL, eds. *Trauma,* 5th ed. New York: McGraw-Hill Professional, 2004.

CHAPTER

164 Head Injuries

Richard V. Aghababian
Peter Angood
Harry L. Anderson III

Head trauma is a common problem often initially evaluated in the ED. In cases of minor head trauma, the emergency medicine physician must provide the appropriate evaluation and observation to ensure that the patient does not develop complications from undiagnosed intracranial bleeding (**FIGURE 164.1**). When a patient presents significant head trauma, the physician must act expediently to stabilize the patient and perform the necessary diagnostic procedures to determine the appropriate medical and surgical interventions. The importance of rapid recognition and evaluation cannot be overemphasized. Delaying necessary intervention by minutes may result in a significant defect in intellect, affect, or a disability in coordination that may affect the patient detrimentally for the rest of his or her life. Of all traumatic injuries, head trauma results in the most morbidity and mortality.

The brain is contained within a bony encasement that provides a solid barrier to the external environment and therefore significant protection. However, the benefit of the skull is offset in instances of internal bleeding as there is no means of outward expansion. Injury to the brain results from rapid deceleration, acceleration, rotation, or a combination of these events. Traumatic brain injury is a multifactorial event resulting from both mechanical (primary injury) and ischemic (secondary injury) insults. Primary injury is the direct neuronal destruction and/or axonal disruption from the initial traumatic force. Secondary injury results from directive bleeding and compression, cerebral edema, hypotension, or hypoxia.

Axonal injury is caused by the sudden acceleration and deceleration of the brain mass containing neuronal axons. It occurs at the time of the direct brain insult and can be most easily viewed as stretching and breaking of the axons. Diffuse white matter injury is associated with anatomic disruption of axons throughout both cerebral hemispheres. This primary shearing injury is associated with high mortality and substantial neurologic disability. Despite severe shearing injury, the brain most often appears grossly normal on CT scan. However, 1 to 2 weeks after injury widespread axonal transection may be seen on microscopic examination of the white matter. The distor-

tional forces causing primary injury may also be great enough to tear intraparenchymal capillaries, superficial subdural bridging veins, or epidural arteries in the brain. Axonal injury that occurs at the time of impact may result in irreversible damage. Many of these patients present in coma to the ED; the prognosis of those who remain in prolonged coma is poor.

Epidural Hematoma

Hemorrhage between the inner table of the skull and the dura mater most commonly arises from a tear in the middle meningeal artery or one of its branches. Arterial bleeding strips the dura from the undersurface of the bone and produces a hematoma that may progressively increase in size and compress the underlying brain. Although epidural hematoma is a result of arterial bleeding, on occasion an epidural hematoma may occur from a lacerated major dural venous sinus. Since venous sinus pressure is low, a venous epidural hematoma only forms in the presence of a depressed skull fracture that creates a space in which the blood can collect. Patients may present to the ED in a number of clinical states: (1) in a coma; (2) awake but with a decreased Glasgow Coma Score (GCS; **Table 164.1**); or (3) awake and alert following a loss of consciousness at the time of trauma. As epidural hematoma may progress rapidly and compress brain tissue, rapid recognition of this entity is one of the foremost priorities in the ED.

Subdural Hematoma

Subdural hematoma develops primarily when bridging veins from the cortex to the dura mater or to venous sinuses are torn. Intracerebral bleeding extends into the subdural space and may also cause a subdural hematoma. A subdural hematoma may be quite large despite bleeding of venous origin. The collection of blood is located beneath the dura mater and overlies the arachnoid and the brain. The mechanism of injury resulting in a tear of bridging veins is usually due to acceleration and decelera-

Table 164.1		
The Glasgow Coma Score (GCS)		
Type of Response	**Points**	**Presentation**
Best Eye Response (maximum 4 points)	1	No eye opening
	2	Eye opening to pain
	3	Eye opening to verbal command
	4	Eyes open spontaneously
Best Verbal Response (maximum 5 points)	1	No verbal response
	2	Incomprehensible sounds
	3	Inappropriate words
	4	Confused
	5	Oriented
Best Motor Response (maximum 6 points)	1	No motor response
	2	Extension to pain
	3	Flexion to pain
	4	Withdrawal from pain
	5	Localizes painful stimulus
	6	Obeys commands

The individual scores of the three exam components are added together to arrive at the GCS (range 3–15 points).

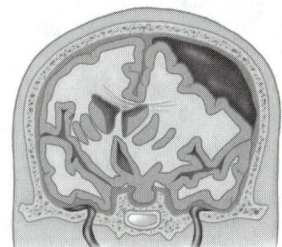
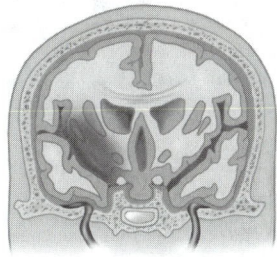
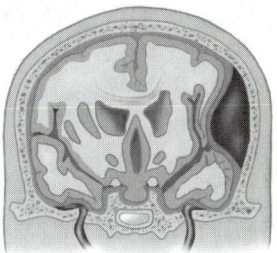

Subdural

Intracerebral   Epidural

FIGURE 164.1 Subdural, intracerebral, and epidural hematoma. The anatomic location of these lesions have present as distinguishable appearance on CT scanning. *Source:* Used with permission from AAOS. *Emergency Care and Transportation of the Sick and Injured,* 8th ed. Sudbury, MA: Jones and Bartlett, 2002:697, Figure 30-15.

tion. Patients with brain atrophy as a result of chronic diseases or age are particularly susceptible to the development of subdural hematoma. These patients' bridging veins span a greater distance and are more readily torn. A common occurrence in the ED is the alcoholic who presents with relatively minor head trauma and has sustained a subdural hematoma. If not recognized early, this may result in catastrophic consequences. The typical hematoma usually becomes symptomatic within the first 24 hours of injury. However, a small number may not become symptomatic until 24 hours to 2 weeks after the initial injury. Rare reports of a subdural hematoma remaining asymptomatic for up to 6 weeks have been reported. In the case of a chronic subdural, the hematoma is initially small and then later it becomes encased with a fibrous membrane, liquefies, and may gradually enlarge.

Intracerebral Hemorrhage

Blood vessels may be torn within the brain parenchyma resulting in hematoma formation. The most common location is in the temporal or frontal lobes. Combined contusion and internal hemorrhage can produce an expanding mass that leads to brain stem herniation. Most cases of intracerebral hemorrhage with a decreased GCS are monitored simply with a neurosurgical pressure monitor, commonly referred to as a bolt. Other patients with significant symptoms need neurosurgical debulking of the injured brain tissue.

Subarachnoid Hemorrhage

Subarachnoid hemorrhage is the most common abnormality found on CT scan following head injury and results from contusion to the brain surface. Small subarachnoid hemorrhages result in little clinical significance. However, a large subarachnoid hemorrhage may cause cerebral vasospasm or acute hydrocephalus.

Penetrating Injury

Penetrating injury, currently less common than blunt head trauma, evokes a much more significant response from ED personnel. Injuries from knives and ice picks into the brain generally cause damage by lacerating arteries with resultant internal hemorrhage. On occasion, these objects may transect significant neuronal tracks, resulting in focal signs. High-speed penetrating wounds from bullets directly destroy neuronal tissue within their path with adjacent tissue damaged by a shock effect (**FIGURE 164.2**). Finally, internal bleeding with resultant shift may cause damage. It is difficult to predict the prognosis of most patients with penetrating injuries until after a CT scan is obtained.

Skull Fractures

The significance of a skull fracture results in its indicating the severe force that the head sustained and the high risk for serious intracranial pathology. Basilar skull fractures

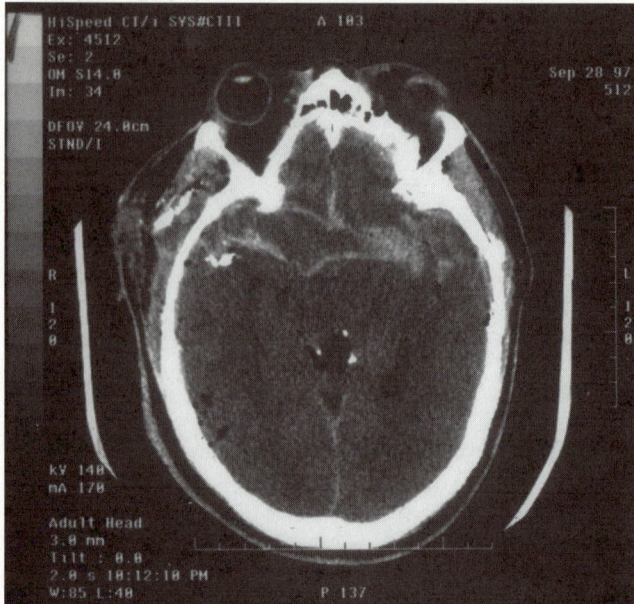

FIGURE 164.2 Transcranial gunshot wound. Fracture fragments, pneumocephalus, and parenchymal hemorrhage are seen within the path of the bullet. This injury was not survivable.

are common and are diagnosed clinically as the CT scan often is unable to identify the fracture. Clinical findings include hemotympanum, otorrhea, Battle's sign, cerebrospinal fluid (CSF) rhinorrhea, or raccoon's sign. Any single sign or combination of signs is indicative of the diagnosis. However, many of these signs take several hours to develop and may not be present at the time of the immediate ED evaluation. Depressed skull fractures are classified as either open or closed depending on whether the overlying skin is lacerated or intact. Although all skull fractures require neurosurgical consultation, open skull fractures are most significant, as they often require antibiotics and aggressive irrigation. Depression of more than 5 mm usually results in a clinical injury requiring operative repair (**FIGURE 164.3**).

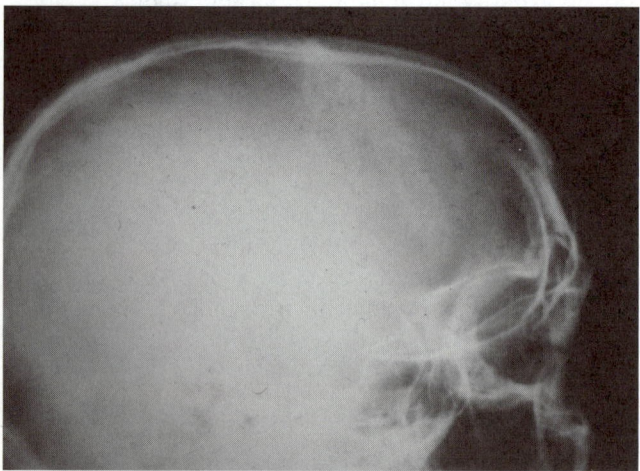

FIGURE 164.3 Lateral plane film of the skull revealing a depressed frontal fracture.

Minor Head Trauma

The vast majority of patients who present to the ED with head injuries present with minor head trauma. These patients have sustained blunt injury to the head with a resultant jarring of the brain. Some of these patients have experienced a transient loss of consciousness immediately following the blunt head impact. This type of injury has been characterized as a concussion. Although the exact pathophysiology of a concussion is unclear, it has been hypothesized that in severe cases there is a degree of axonal stretching. The stretching and associated edema (in part) contributes to the so-called *postconcussive syndrome,* described below. A small set of patients who present with minor head trauma may actually develop more severe pathology (subdural or epidural hematoma), making this type of patient one of the more difficult to evaluate.

Emergency Department Evaluation

The speed of the ED assessment is dependent on the patient's presenting condition. The patient's GCS (Table 164.1) should be recorded immediately upon presentation to the ED. Patients who are alert and awake and have a GCS of 15 usually provide a window of time for assessment. However, any patient with a decreased level of consciousness, localizing signs, or coma must be evaluated rapidly. In addition, these patients must be treated as they are evaluated. Care should be taken to avoid a delay in diagnosis of intracranial injury, as a delay in diagnosis of both epidural and subdural hematoma has been shown to increase the patient's morbidity. The history of the injury may provide important clues that assist in appropriate management of the patient and may be obtained from the paramedics, family members, or any bystander who witnessed the injury. In addition to the mechanism of injury, the time of injury, the presence of a lucid interval, and the history of any drug or alcohol use should be noted. Serial examinations throughout the patient's stay in the ED are of critical importance, as any deterioration in neurological state should be rapidly addressed and treated. A key piece of history is whether the patient was actually witnessed to have lost consciousness. Many patients have brief amnesia and confuse this with loss of consciousness when asked directly.

Neurological Examination

The neurological examination is essential in establishing the severity of head injury. The importance of a detailed and thorough neurological examination of the patient cannot be overemphasized. Repeated examinations are necessary to determine if the patient is stable or potentially deteriorating. The examination should begin with an evaluation of all the cranial nerves. In patients who are alert and awake, asymmetric pupils are common and are not indicative of intracranial pathology. However, a mass lesion is suggested by the patient who presents with equal, reactive pupils and subsequently develops asymmetrical pupils. Brain stem function can be tested by checking corneal reflexes. This reflex originates in the pons with the afferent limb conducted by the ophthalmic branch of the fifth cranial nerve and the efferent limb by the facial nerve.

In addition, oculocephalic (doll's eyes maneuver) or ocular vestibular responses (ice water calorics) are important in testing the integrity of the brain stem. Oculocephalic reflexes should not be tested until bony or ligamentous injury to the cervical spine has been excluded. Careful testing of sensation and motor strength of the extremities is extremely important. This examination should include the movements of all four extremities with sensation of light touch. Partial spinal cord lesions such as anterior cord syndrome may preserve light touch and temperature while eliminating pain. Therefore, a more detailed evaluation that includes all the neurological parameters such as pain, temperature, light touch, and vibration should be completed. In addition, coordination and detailed movements of each extremity should be elicited as well as determining reflexes of the knees, ankles, elbows, and wrists.

Emergency Department Intervention for Specific Injuries

Herniation

Herniation occurs as intracranial pressure (ICP) elevates, displacing portions of the brain. Multiple locations of herniation may occur, with uncal herniation being the most readily identified. Uncal herniation results as some type of mass forces the temporal lobe through the tentorial falx, compressing the ipsilateral oculomotor nerve and the contralateral cerebral peduncle. Clinically, the patient presents with a fixed, dilated pupil and contralateral hemiparesis. Therapy is aimed at temporarily decreasing ICP while the patient immediately undergoes head CT scanning. Hyperventilation decreases ICP through cerebral vasoconstriction and is the fastest method to initially decrease ICP. However, it should only be viewed as a temporizing measure as it may be detrimental to many patients by causing cerebral ischemia if excessive. A reasonable goal is a $PaCO_2$ of 30 mm Hg. Intravenous mannitol may also be used to decrease ICP and should be given to all patients with a dilated pupil and asymmetrical motor examinations. Definitive therapy involves resolution of the source of intracranial pressure by surgical means following the CT scan. In those patients who are rapidly deteriorating and unable to enter the CT suite, ED burr holes may be performed by qualified personnel on the side of the dilated pupil.

GCS of 8 or Less

Patients with severe head injury are often suffering from multiple system trauma and, thus, a dedicated pathway must be followed. The initial survey is followed by the secondary survey and a rapid, focused neurological examination. Rapid stabilization of the patient is imperative as both hypoxia and hypotension have been shown to increase morbidity and mortality in patients with head injury. Endotracheal intubation with administration of 100% oxygen and hyperventilation has been the mainstay of initial management. Patients should be loaded with an anticonvulsant (phenytoin) to prevent complications from posttraumatic seizures, while the administration of steroids offers no benefit to patients with intracranial injury and should be avoided. Immediate head CT scanning and early neurosurgical consultation are mandatory.

Rapid-sequence intubation of the head-injured trauma patient should be conducted to minimize any adverse effects to the patient. The patient should be preoxygenated with 100% oxygen to establish an oxygen reserve. Elevation of ICP may occur with intubation, and specific therapy is aimed at preventing this response. Pretreatment with a defasiculating dose of vecuronium (0.01 mg/kg IV) may blunt the rise of ICP in response to succinylcholine. Lidocaine (1.5 mg/kg IV) and fentanyl (3–5 mg/kg IV) is given 2 to 3 minutes prior to intubation, which aids in blunting the rise in ICP associated with laryngoscopy. Sedation is accomplished with thiopental (3 mg/kg IV) as this agent decreases both ICP and cerebral oxygen consumption. Paralysis is accomplished with succinylcholine (1.5 mg/kg IV). Intubation should be performed with inline cervical immobilization to avoid worsening a cervical spine fracture. In patients suffering from multisystem trauma who may potentially become hypotensive, etomidate (0.3 mg/kg IV) should be substituted for thiopental as it offers less cardiovascular depression.

GCS of 9 to 13

Patients with a GCS ranging from 9 to 13 are considered to have moderate head injury. Up to 20% of patients in this group deteriorate while in the emergency room and, thus, aggressive management is warranted. All patients require emergent CT scanning, with neurosurgical consultation, and hospital admission is required for those patients with abnormal CT scan results. Although intubation is not routinely performed in this group, careful observation of the patient's airway is required to prevent episodes of hypoxia, hypoventilation, or aspiration.

GCS 14 to 15

There continues to be debate in the medical literature about which patients with minor head trauma require head CT scan in the ED. The debate is driven by the need to immediately identify all patients with potentially serious injury versus increasing demands to cut escalating medical costs. Most clinical experience in patients with a history of loss of consciousness (LOC)/amnesia and a GCS of 14 or 15 has been anecdotal, and practices have varied regionally. A consistent approach in recent scientific literature provides for better overall patient care.

Patients presenting with a GCS of 14 and a history of LOC in general should have a head CT scan. A second management option is to observe the patient. If the patient improves and their sensorium clears, no CT scan is obtained. This option is often taken in head trauma patients who are intoxicated. However, in the authors' opinion, observation may delay the diagnosis of intracranial bleeding.

GCS 15

Several recent studies have helped provide guidance on which patients with a GCS of 15 and history of LOC need a head CT scan. In this group approximately 0.2% of patients have intracranial bleeding that requires neurosurgical intervention. Patients at risk may be identified by one or more of the following risk factors: (1) nausea or vomiting, (2) severe headache, (3) signs of depressed skull fracture, or (4) significant external scalp injury. By following these guidelines, all at-risk patients can be identified and the use of head CT scans may be reduced by 60%.

Penetrating Trauma

The evaluation of patients with penetrating injury to the head proceeds as with all trauma patients. Resuscitation with stabilization of both the patient's blood pressure and airway take first priority. Early endotracheal intubation is required in all patients with a GCS of 8 or less to avoid secondary insult to the brain. Care must be taken during the examination to identify all entry/exit wounds including any distal to the head injury. Skull films may be obtained during the initial resuscitation, although an immediate head CT scan provides the most information. Both intravenous antibiotic and anticonvulsant administration are recommended in patients with injuries penetrating the skull. Penetrating foreign bodies should be removed from the skull in the operating room and not in the ED. Poor prognostic indicators include posterior fossa wounds, transcranial wounds that injure both cerebral hemispheres, and a GCS of 3 to 5. Regardless of the patient's prognosis, aggressive treatment is warranted as the patient may become an organ donor.

Postconcussive Syndrome

Following head injury, a subset of patients continues to have chronic, ongoing neurological problems collectively referred to as the *postconcussive syndrome*. This is a difficult area of research as it is often difficult to determine a precise pathophysiological or psychiatric cause of these problems. However, enough data exist to show that many patients have no psychiatric dysfunction and yet have significant problems.

Following head injury, patients may develop chronic recurrent headaches that are difficult to control and result in repeated evaluations by physicians. Additional subsets of patients develop problems with memory and concentration, which may persist for months. One study showed a decrease in cognitive ability in a large percentage of patients who had sustained head trauma. A number of patients have increased emotional distress following head injury, which may last for years. These will need to be treated symptomatically and other underlying causes must be evaluated.

Selected Readings

Advanced Trauma Life Support (ATLS) for Doctors, 6th ed. The American College of Surgeons. Chicago, 2004.

Harris JH Jr, Harris WH. *The Radiology of Emergency Medicine,* 4th ed. Philadelphia: Lippincott Williams and Wilkins, 2000.

Mirvis SE, Shanmuganathan K, eds. Imaging in Trauma and Critical Care, ed 2. Philadelphia: Elsevier Science, 2003.

Moore EE, Feliciano DF, Mattox KL, eds. *Trauma,* 5th ed. New York: McGraw-Hill Professional, 2004.

Spine Injuries

Peter Angood
Harry L. Anderson III

In the United States, there are approximately 10,000 new cases (40 to 50 per 1 million population) of spinal injuries each year. They most commonly result, in descending order of frequency, from motor vehicle collisions, falls, sporting injuries, and penetrating trauma. The initial mortality is estimated at 50%. Most deaths are to high cervical cord damage or associated injuries.

Overall, spinal fractures lead to spinal cord injury in an estimated 10% to 20% of patients. In cervical vertebral injury, the incidence of associated spinal cord damage reaches almost 50%. In approximately 10% of patients, spinal cord injury is seen in the absence of detectable fractures. Once a spinal cord lesion is suspected, it must be determined whether the neurological deficit is complete or incomplete. A complete lesion implies total loss of motor and sensory function. Any preservation of function may indicate that the lesion is incomplete with a better prognosis and perhaps amenable to neurosurgical intervention. The spinal column is a series of 33 vertebrae: 7 cervical, 12 thoracic, 5 lumbar, 5 sacral (fused), and 4 coccygeal (fused) vertebrae connected by fibrous ligaments. Intervertebral disks, consisting of a central nucleus pulposus surrounded by an outer annulus fibrosus, provide cushioning and flexibility to the vertebral column. The spinal cord travels within the spinal canal, a ring formed by the pedicles and laminae. Sensory, motor, and autonomic impulses travel through nerves that course through the vertebral foramina. The cord begins at the foramen magnum and ends at the second lumbar vertebra where it becomes the *conus medullaris*. The *cauda equina* is a structure consisting of nerve roots emerging from the *conus medularis* and *filum terminale*.

Stability of any segment of the spine is affected by both osseous and ligamentous structures and their ability to maintain mechanical relationships and, hence, neurological function in the presence of physiologic stresses on the spine. The anterior column includes the anterior two thirds of the vertebral body, the anterior part of the annulus fibrosis, and the anterior longitudinal ligament. The middle column encompasses the posterior third of the vertebral body, the posterior part of the annulus fibrosus, and the posterior longitudinal ligament. The posterior column is composed of facet joints, the neural arch, the spinal canal, and posterior ligaments. The intact middle and posterior columns are most instrumental in maintaining stability. Injuries that destabilize these columns carry a high likelihood of associated spinal cord damage. The craniocervical junction is supported by a series of specialized ligaments. The atlantooccipital joint is served by the tectorial membrane and posterior atlantooccipital membrane. The odontoid is attached via the apical (dentate) ligament to the foramen magnum and by the alar ligaments to the occipital condyles. The transverse ligament travels through the ring of the atlas behind the odontoid, securing its position. Disruption of this ligament presents a very unstable condition. The ring of the atlas is approximately 3 cm in anteroposterior (AP) diameter. Steel's rule of thirds reminds us that 1 cm is occupied by the odontoid, 1 cm by the spinal cord, and the remaining 1 cm is potential space that allows for some displacement of the odontoid without spinal cord damage. The vascular supply to the spinal cord is through various tributaries of the vertebral arteries and thoracolumbar aorta. The great radicular artery of Adamkiewicz is an anastomotic vessel that provides flow to the watershed areas ofC1, T4, and L1. Injury to this and other vessels can cause neurologic deficits not explained by the recognized level of spinal fracture. Hematoma formation can cause additional damage through compression.

Mechanism of Injury

Forces acting on the spine during trauma include flexion, lateral flexion, extension, distraction, and axial loading. Most often, forces act in combination to produce undue stress and injury to the spine. Hyperflexion injuries lead to fatalities at a much more frequent rate than hyperextension injuries. Certain events predictably lead to well-described mechanisms of injury. For example, diving accidents result in injury from a flexion and axial loading. Rear-end collisions cause hyperextension injuries, and head-on collisions typically lead to hyperflexion. It is important to obtain as much detailed information as is available from the patient, witnesses, or paramedics regarding the circumstances that led to injury. Certain congenital and acquired conditions, such as rheumatoid arthritis, congenital spinal stenosis, ankylosing spondylitis, and Down's syndrome, make the spine less able to withstand forces applied to it even during minor trauma.

Radiological Examination

Several modalities are available to evaluate the patient with a potential or recognized spinal injury. These include plane radiographs, CT scanning, conventional tomography, MRI, and myelography.

Plane radiographs are generally the first and often only study required. A standard cervical series includes the lateral, AP, and open-mouth odontoid views. The lateral view can detect approximately 80% of all cervical injuries. The AP and odontoid views raise the sensitivity to 92% and negative predictive value to 99% in the detection of fractures in this portion of the spine. Coned-down and swimmer's views should be added to the standard series to visualize the complete cervical spine and cervicothoracic junction as needed. Additional views available include flexion/extension and oblique views and they help serve to rule out ligamentous injury and injury to the posterior elements, respectively.

CT scan can be used to augment information obtained through standard radiography. When combined with plane films, sensitivity and negative predictive value for the detection of spinal injuries approaches 100%, which is helpful in the evaluation of suspicious areas and areas not well visualized on plane films alone. Routine scanning of the C1 to C3 area in patients with significant head trauma is controversial. This is advocated by some authors because of the difficulty in evaluating this area with plane films in the uncooperative patient. However, it can be argued that this is a low-yield procedure given the low incidence of unstable fractures and the inherent limitations of CT scan in detecting small fractures. CT scan is helpful in the assessment of established fractures and to determine the integrity of the spinal canal and posterior elements. The scout view may be helpful in demonstrating alignment abnormalities. It is better than plane films at detecting most fractures including burst fractures, soft tissue swelling, disk herniation, and bony fragments. The radiation exposure and patient movement are less than with other modalities, though it significantly more expensive. It is limited in the identification of horizontally oriented fractures, although the thin slice (1.5 mm) technique is more sensitive than the standard slice (3 to 4 mm). Additionally, three-dimensional (3D) CT scan reconstruction of structures promises to overcome certain disadvantages of standard CT scan. Conventional tomography is used on occasion when CT scan is not available or insufficient. It is superior to CT at demonstrating horizontally oriented fractures, subluxation, dislocation, and fractures of the lateral masses, articular processes, and vertebral bodies.

MRI is the preferred procedure in patients with findings suggestive of spinal cord injury. Its use has demonstrated a higher prevalence of spinal canal intrusion than previously suspected, and is also helpful in defining ligamentous disruption and locked facets. Its use is restricted to patients who are not on metallic life support and monitoring systems or who have metallic implants such as pacemakers, cerebral aneurysm clips, and other foreign bodies, particularly ophthalmic.

Myelography is also used concurrently with CT for the evaluation of incomplete spinal cord injuries due to suspected compression of the cord. It requires the injection of metrizamide, a nonionic contrast material, into the thecal space through a high cervical approach. This technique serves to delineate the spinal cord and demonstrate any lesions caused by disk herniation or other space-occupying lesions.

Radiological Features

Lateral View

A helpful mnemonic has been developed that can be used to inspect the various structures seen on the lateral C-spine view. The ABCSs are used to remind us to examine alignment, bones, cartilage, and soft tissues. The following review is organized to fall within this scheme as much as possible (**FIGURE 165.1**).

Alignment   Alignment is assessed using the normally smooth curves of the anterior vertebral contour, posterior vertebral contour, and spinolaminal lines as well as the posterior cervical line, which connects the spinous processes of C1, C2, and C3. Loss or slight reversal of cervical lordosis is most often due to paravertebral spasm, degenerative arthritis, or immobilization itself. However, it may also be a subtle clue to a potentially unstable injury. Anterior subluxation of one vertebral body over its subjacent should not exceed 3.5 mm. Greater displacement is

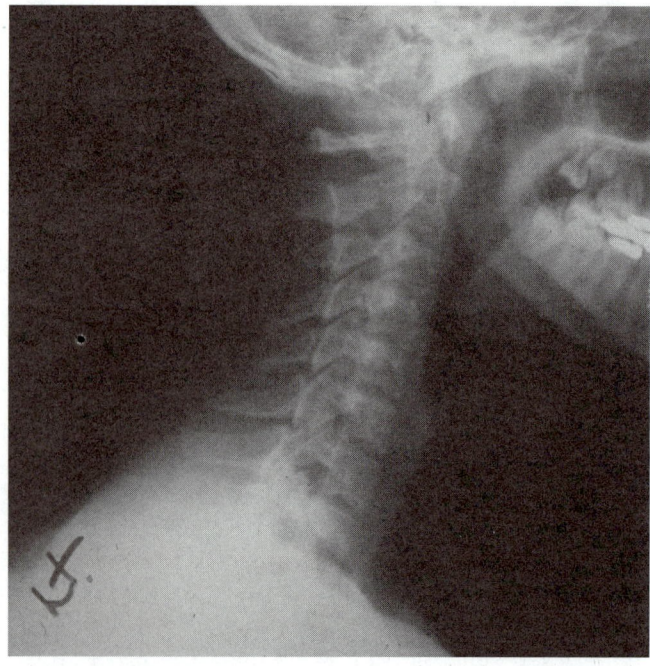

FIGURE 165.1 Normal lateral view of the cervical spine.

considered abnormal and potentially unstable. At C2 there may normally be up to 2 mm posterior displacement of the spinolaminal line. A Hangman's fracture, bilateral fracture of the *pars interarticularis* of C2, should be suspected if the base of any of the spinous processes of Cl to C3 falls >2 mm anterior or posterior to the posterior cervical line, particularly in a child. The lines drawn posteriorly from the spinous processes tend to converge to a point behind the neck, and divergence, known as fanning, should be regarded as a sign of potential instability.

The adequacy of the spinal canal is determined in part by its dimensions. A preliminary evaluation can be performed on the lateral plane film. The anterior margin is defined by the posterior vertebral contour line and the posterior margin by the spinolaminal line. Its radiographically augmented diameter should be at least 13 mm wide in adults to accommodate the spinal cord.

Attention should then turn to the craniocervical junction for signs of possible dislocation or subluxation. Several guidelines have been advanced to assist in this determination. Most involve the anterior margin of the foramen magnum, the basion, a landmark discernible in at least 90% of lateral C-spine films. In the absence of dislocation or subluxation, it lies within 5 mm directly above the tip of the odontoid.

Bones   The height and configuration of each of the vertebral bodies require careful consideration. Look for loss of height of the anterior and posterior margins as clues to wedge or compression fractures. The caudal-anterior margin should be examined for teardrop fractures, and the relationship between the facets or fractures of the laminae and spinous process. Some dens fractures may be detected on the lateral view.

Cartilage   Three sets of potential spaces require particular attention: the predental space, intervertebral spaces, and interspinous spaces. The *predental* space is the area seen directly anterior to the dens, behind the anterior arch the atlas. Measurements <3 mm in adults and <4 mm in children are considered normal. An interval of >3 mm is consistent with transverse ligament deficiency and >5 mm indicates rupture, a very unstable situation. All ligaments are presumed tom if the interval measures >10 mm. The intervertebral spaces should be equal in their anterior and posterior height. Examine closely for the presence of any small bony fragments of teardrop fractures. The interspinous spaces should be roughly equal, except at C4 to C6 where they tend to be slightly narrower.

Soft Tissues   Prevertebral soft tissues are then assessed for the presence of swelling, indicating possible hematoma. These are more common in injuries of the anterior columns. Several measurements are considered helpful in the determination of abnormal soft tissue swelling. More than 7 mm is considered abnormal at C2, but small hematomas are characteristic of odontoid and compression fractures. At C3 to C4, 5 mm or one half of the width of the vertebral body is within the range of normal. The C6 prevertebral soft tissues after the age of 15 should mea-

sure less than 22 mm, and in children, less than 14 mm. At this level, the width of the vertebral body can also be used as a guideline for the upper limit of normal. False-positive distention is seen with flexion/extension, swallowing, crying, pooled secretions, nasogastric tubes, and endotracheal tubes. At the thoracolumbar level, soft tissue swelling that accompanies fractures may obscure the psoas shadow.

Anteroposterior View   The AP view is considered adequate if there is visualization of the C3 to C7 spinous processes. It yields information through alignment of the spinous processes, height and configuration of the vertebral bodies, and intervertebral spaces as well as the transverse processes (**FIGURE 165.2**).

Odontoid View   The odontoid view is a required portion of the standard series as it is the only view that effectively demonstrates the atlantoaxial joint. One must look for symmetry of the lateral masses and spaces surrounding the odontoid projection. The odontoid itself is to be examined for any signs of fracture. The Mach band is an artifact created by the base of the occiput and often mistaken for a dens fracture. The *os odontoideum* is an entity of controversial origin that may be seen in this view and may represent malunion of a fracture or failure of the ossification center of the dens. Suspicion of a Jefferson fracture through the ring of the atlas, with or without rupture of the transverse ligament, is raised by the presence and dimension of overhang of the lateral masses of C1 over the body of C2 (**FIGURE 165.3**).

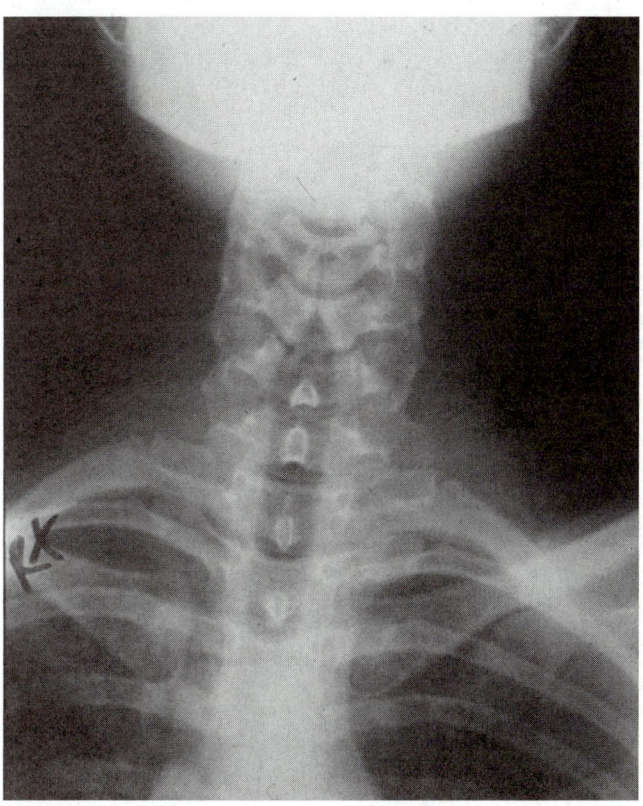

FIGURE 165.2 Normal anteroposterior (AP) view of the cervical spine.

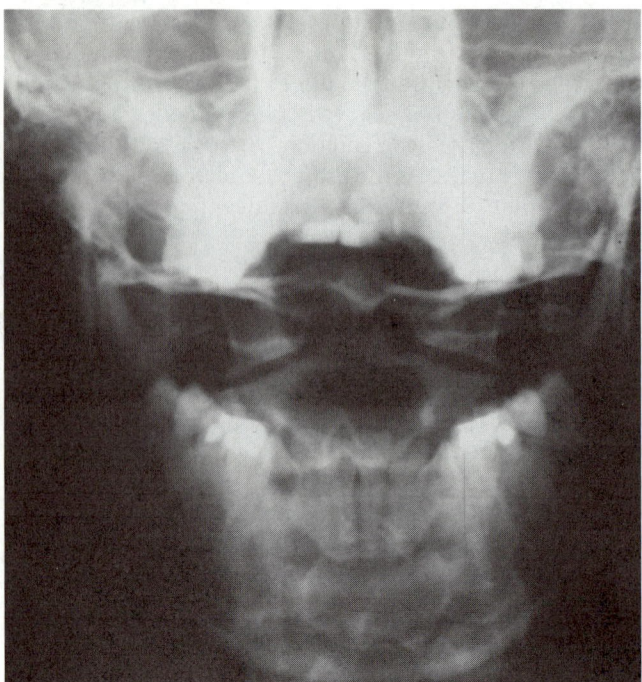

FIGURE 165.3 Normal odontoid view of the cervical spine.

Evaluation of the posterior cervical line may be used to rule out pathology. Likewise, the vertebral bodies at an early age appear somewhat compressed anteriorly and are often mistaken for simple wedge fractures. It is useful to compare the appearance of several different levels and inspect for soft tissue swelling if this is in question.

A Jefferson fracture can be mistakenly diagnosed in the child with pseudo spread of the lateral masses of C1 due to growth discrepancies. The predental space is slightly wider than in the adult, but should be less than 4 mm. It has a V-shaped appearance in flexion due to ligamentous laxity. In addition, ossification centers are often confused with fractures. The emergency physician should be aware of their location and expected age of fusion.

Severe spinal cord injury may occur in the pediatric population even in the absence of associated fracture. These injuries are referred to as spinal cord injury without radiological abnormality (SCIWRA). This is due to the natural elasticity of the pediatric vertebral column, which is vulnerable to deformation without fracture. Children younger than 8 years of age are most at risk. In one published study, over 50% of the injuries that caused paralysis had a delayed onset of symptoms, potentially as late as 4 days after trauma.

Cervical Spine Injury Patterns

The rare survivors of injuries at the occipitoatlantoaxial complex are infrequently afflicted with neurological deficit due to the relatively larger dimensions of the spinal canal at this level. Those patients who do succumb to these injuries do so early and primarily because of the associated injury to the spinomedullary junction. Dislocation follows rupture of the tectorial membrane and is manifested by widening of the atlantooccipital gap (tip of the odontoid to the basion) to more than 5 mm. Fractures of the occipital condyles are rare and often missed, as they are difficult to visualize on plane films of the adult spine.

Fractures of the Cl ring may occur individually or in combination. An isolated fracture of the posterior neural arch of the atlas occurs by an extension mechanism and is generally considered stable. A Jefferson fracture is the eponym used for the four ring fractures of C1 (two posterior, two anterior) that result from axial loading. This is usually a stable fracture unless the transverse ligament is ruptured, which is suggested on the lateral view by widening of the predental space and on the odontoid view by overhang of the lateral masses by greater than 7 mm. Deficits attributable to neural loss from this injury are rare.

Dislocations involving the C1 to C2 joint are rare but somewhat more common in patients with Down syndrome and rheumatoid arthritis. Complete separation of the transverse ligament may present as anterior dislocation of C1 on C2, but is rarely seen without an associated fracture of C2. In the rare instances of isolated apical and alar ligament disruption, a posteriorly dislocated atlas is seen. Rotatory subluxation of this joint is seen in both traumatic and nontraumatic conditions. Torticollis (or wry-neck) constitutes rotatory displacement and occurs fairly commonly in children. It may follow viral infec-

Additional Views Lateral flexion and extension views of the cervical spine should be considered in the neurologically intact patient who presents subtle alignment abnormalities without obvious signs of instability on the lateral view or in patients with persistent significant neck pain on examination. It must be stressed that the patient, without any assistance from the examiner or technician, is allowed to flex and extend the neck.

Flexion is more effective if the patient is asked to extend the chin outward prior to flexing. Any neurological symptoms or increase in pain should lead to prompt termination of the procedure and replacement of the cervical immobilization collar. These patients are best studied by CT scan or other modalities.

Oblique views, while standard at some institutions, need to be considered primarily for the evaluation of posterior elements in suspected fracture or misalignment. The vertebral foramina are best visualized on this projection and this may be helpful in a patient with radicular symptoms.

The Pediatric Cervical Spine

The pediatric cervical spine, due to a proportionately larger head, increased ligamentous laxity, and differently shaped facets, is more prone to high cervical injury than the adult spine. Lateral films should be obtained with slight padding of the upper back and shoulders to prevent inadvertent flexion due to the large occiput. Some radiological findings are characteristic of the pediatric spine and at times disconcerting to the clinician. Pseudo subluxation of C2 on C3 is seen in 25% and is due to more relaxed ligaments and flattened facet joints in normal children under 8. It may also be seen at the C3 to C4 level.

tions, which perhaps serve to temporarily weaken the ligaments that support these structures. Patients present with their head laterally flexed and rotated at least 45 degrees. This position is quite painful and distressing to the patient. Occasionally, rotatory atlantoaxial subluxation and dislocations are caused by trauma. Complete dislocation is associated with severe, and often fatal, spinal cord damage. The radiographic findings for both the spontaneous and traumatic conditions are similar, but trauma is more likely to have associated neurological compromise. On the lateral view, one mass may have the appearance of lying anterior to the dens appendage. On the odontoid view, severe rotation is seen, with significant asymmetry and magnification of one of the lateral masses.

Traumatic spondylolisthesis of the axis, the Hangman's fracture, results from rapid deceleration with resulting cervical hyperextension (**FIGURE 165.4**). In the modem era, most are caused by high-speed, head-on automobile collisions. This injury is considered mechanically unstable, but cord damage tends to be minimal. It consists of fractures of the pars interarticularis pedicles bilaterally with anterior subluxation of the C2 body and, occasionally, retrolisthesis of the posterior elements on C3. Most are clearly visible on plane films. Minimally displaced fractures may require CT for detection. Soft tissue swelling may cause respiratory compromise.

Odontoid fractures are fairly common and result from complex mechanisms. Approximately 80% may be attributable to flexion; 20% are due to extension. These are usually classified into three types: Type I fractures affect the tip of the dens, are uncommon, and heal well. Type II fractures involve slight distraction of the odontoid process from the body of the axis. It is the most common and also the most problematic, with a high incidence of nonunion due primarily to interruption of the blood supply to the tip of the dens. Type III fractures are through the body of the axis, below the junction of the dens itself. This leads to some controversy regarding the classification of this injury as a dens fracture. Neurological abnormalities are seen in approximately 25% of patients, but are usually minor.

Axial loading with slight flexion leads to the simple wedge fracture, which is a stable condition without associated deficits unless compression is greater than 40%. There is damage only to the superior end plate with loss of anterior height. The ligaments and the integrity of all columns remain intact. A compression burst fracture is a more extensive injury caused primarily by axial loading while the spine is straightened. The anterior and posterior end plates suffer from some degree of impaction with resultant loss of height throughout the vertebral body. There is involvement of the anterior and middle columns. On the lateral view, there is characteristic loss of height and misalignment of the posterior vertebral contour line. On AP radiographs, a vertically oriented fracture through the vertebral body may be seen, as well as widening of the span between pedicles. The spinal cord is at risk from impingement by bony fragments and thus a CT scan is mandatory in the evaluation of these injuries.

Hyperextension injuries may entail primarily soft tissue damage or extension teardrop fractures. In young adults, the C5 to C6 region is most commonly affected; in individuals suffering from osteoporosis, involvement of C2 is seen. The anterior ligamentous structures are most at risk and at times completely disrupted, as best demonstrated by MRI. There may be posterior disk herniation as well, with associated neurologic findings. Typically these take the form of the central cord syndrome. There is usually normal alignment of the vertebrae with slight widening of the intervertebral space anteriorly. The extension teardrop fracture results from avulsion of the anteroinferior aspect of the vertebral body by the anterior longitudinal ligament. Although it involves the upper cervical spine in most instances, in diving accidents it tends to affect the C5 to C7 disk spaces primarily.

Hyperflexion injuries include pure soft tissue injury (whiplash) and flexion teardrop fractures. Whiplash injuries usually affect the C5 to C6 region of the cervical spine. There may be a spontaneously reduced subluxation that is not apparent on radiological studies. The posterior ligamentous complex is most vulnerable and damage may be severe. Instability may be suggested by fanning of the posterior processes and 1 to 3 mm of anterior subluxation. Some authors report delayed healing with chronic pain. Flexion teardrop fractures are among the most unstable of all cervical injuries and most occur in the lower cervical vertebrae, primarily at the C5 to C6 interspace. They are caused by extreme flexion with complete disruption of all soft tissues at the affected joint. Frequently they are accompanied by neurological findings consistent with the anterior cord syndrome because of backward displace-

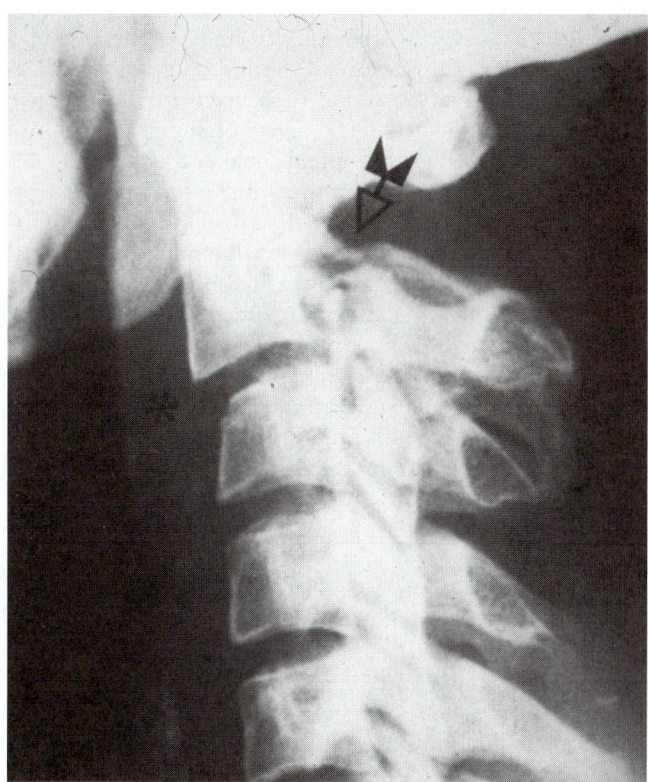

FIGURE 165.4 Hangman's fracture.

ment of the posterior fragments. A small, triangular compression fragment can be seen on the caudal-anterior aspect of the body with significant soft tissue swelling.

Unilateral facet disorders, including subluxation, dislocation, or fractures, occur most commonly at C4 to C7 and are due to flexion and rotation. They are considered a stable injury although occasionally there may be neurological deficits related to nerve root compression. These usually resolve after reduction is accomplished. On lateral plane films, the articular processes assume a "bowtie" configuration because of superimposition and rotation of the facets at the level of injury. Associated laminae or facet fractures are often overlooked due to their subtle appearance. A subluxation of approximately 25% of the width of the body is characteristic (**FIGURE 165.5**). On the oblique views, there is disruption of the normal relationship of the laminae, which is often described as shingles on a roof. The anteroposterior view may demonstrate a marked misalignment of the spinous processes above the disruption from those below it. These injuries are easily demonstrated by CT scan, which also visualizes the vertebral foramina.

Bilateral facet dislocation is a severe soft tissue injury and very unstable. It results from extreme hyperflexion with displacement of both facets of one vertebra over and anterior to those of the subjacent. There is complete disruption of the ligamentous structures supporting all three columns, often with an associated herniated intervertebral disk. This results in anterior subluxation of at least 50% of the vertebral body. Abnormal fanning of the spinous processes is seen on lateral view.

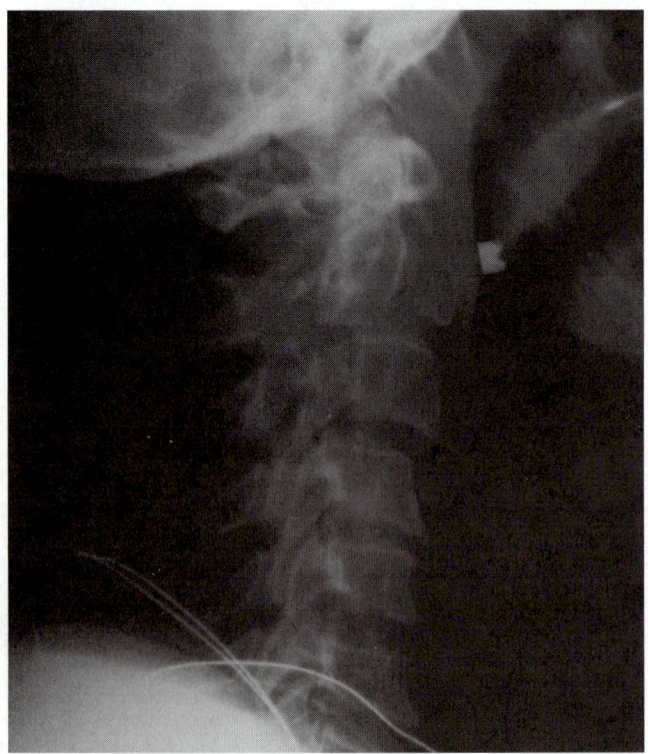

FIGURE 165.5 Fracture dislocation of C2 and C3.

Pillar fractures are caused by extension and rotation leading to compression of the articular mass of one vertebra by the one directly above it. They are usually unilateral and are stable neurologically and mechanically. They are best visualized on pillar views that are taken at a 30- to 45-degree angle from the AP beam direction. Lamina fractures are best demonstrated on oblique views where their normally intact ellipse is seen to be disrupted. Although mechanically stable, these injuries may result in vertebral artery disruption.

Transverse process fractures, although innocuous in appearance, may have accompanying brachial plexus and vascular injuries. These complications are seen primarily with fractures that extend into the foramen, where they may damage the vertebral arteries. They are best seen on the AP view, but CT scan may be necessary. Angiography is recommended when vascular compromise is suspected.

Spinous process avulsion fractures of the lower cervical and high thoracic vertebrae may result generally from rapid hyperflexion, extension, or direct trauma. They are called *clay shoveler's fractures* and are considered mechanically and neurologically stable. The resulting fractures occur at C7, T1, or C6, in that order of frequency.

Thoracic Spine Injury Patterns

There are significant structural characteristics of the thoracic spine that make it relatively resistant to injury. Consequently, when enough force is exerted on the thoracic spine to cause osseous or ligamentous damage, one must expect severe accompanying injuries of surrounding organs. Due to its inherent curvature, the thoracic spine is not very susceptible to compression. Additionally, the angle of the facet joints limits rotation, making these injuries quite unusual as well. Any axial loading is translated into a flexion force with resultant wedge compression fractures. Disk herniation tends to be rare in the thoracic spine, but there is a high incidence of spinal cord injury due to the relatively small spinal canal at this level.

It is important that the entire spine be palpated for areas of tenderness or step-offs before declaring it free of injury. Immobilization of the entire spine must be observed until this point. Radiographic valuation of the thoracic spine begins with AP and lateral plane films. The AP view must be inspected for alignment of the spinous processes and pedicles. Soft tissue changes consistent with a paraspinal hematoma include mediastinal widening and apical capping. These findings are the same as those seen with aortic disruption and may lead to diagnostic errors. On the lateral view, integrity of the bony structures including vertebral bodies, spinous processes, and pedicles must be ascertained. The intervertebral spaces and interspinous process distance should be well maintained.

The most common thoracic fracture is the wedge compression fracture. The incidence is higher in patients with osteoporosis, and T12 is the most commonly affected of the thoracic vertebrae. The mechanism of injury is a combination of flexion and axial loading. If the compression of the anterior segment is less than 50%, the injury is considered mechanically stable. Neurological deficits are rare unless associated with extensive posterior disk herniation. Fracture-dislocations of the thoracic spine are the product of considerable force transmitted to the spine through hyperflexion. There is tremendous ligamentous damage with often complete disruption of all columns. As a consequence, there generally is at least partial spinal cord injury.

Thoracolumbar Injuries

The lower thoracic and lumbar spines are functionally and structurally alike and hence are subject to similar forces. The high pliability of this junction allows it to act as leverage for much of the movement of the lower body. The primary forces to which it is subject are flexion, extension, and rotation. As with the thoracic spine, true axial loading is not possible. The spinal canal is wider once again and the spinal cord has ended at this level. Nonetheless, the nerve roots remain susceptible to damage. A reported 15% of patients with calcaneus fractures have concurrent thoracolumbar lesions.

Simple wedge compression fractures are common and considered stable if the compression is less than 40% and there are no neurological deficits, as with all other vertebral levels. Burst fractures, with involvement of the middle and anterior columns, jeopardize the spinal cord and nerve roots particularly if there is some disruption of the posterior column. They result from pure flexion or extension forces. Diagnosis is often readily apparent, and is first suggested by loss of height of the vertebral body with disruption of the posterior vertebral line on lateral radiograph. CT scan evaluation is mandatory to determine the presence and degree of spinal canal narrowing. The most common thoracolumbar wedge fracture in the elderly is at T12.

The Chance fracture, in reality, is a fracture-dislocation injury that results from flexion and distraction. It is most commonly seen in victims of motor vehicle collisions who are restrained only by a lap belt. The flexion thus occurs over the lap belt, and the forward propulsion results in distraction of the spine. The posterior and middle columns are disrupted primarily as a consequence of the distraction and the anterior column is compressed. These fractures have a very high incidence of associated intraabdominal injuries. On AP imaging, the outlines of the laminae at the affected level appear discontinuous. On lateral view, there may be a transverse fracture noted through the laminae; the spinous process may also be involved. CT imaging is necessary to fully delineate the extent of the injury. These fractures are mechanically unstable and appear restricted to the T12 to L2 region.

Occasionally, all three columns of the spine are disrupted by a shearing mechanism. These injuries are uncommon but are associated with complete spinal cord injury. Injuries due to simple extension are very rare and result in disruption of the anterior and middle columns; at times the posterior elements are also compressed.

Transverse process fractures are more frequent than commonly suspected and are easily missed on cursory examination of the plane films. They are not inherently unstable or damaging, but are often associated with pelvic fractures or injury to the kidneys, ureters, and major intraabdominal vessels. Spinous process fractures may also be subtle and missed. They can be seen on both lateral and AP views with close review. They have no associated neurological deficits. Most often they result from direct trauma.

Spondylolysis refers to the congenital faulty union of the *pars interarticularis* of the lumbar spine. It may also result from sports-related trauma in young athletes. It can be detected on oblique views of this region of the spine, using the outline of the *pars interarticularis* and articular processes, which resemble a Scottish terrier dog. The neck of the dog corresponds to the pars interarticularis; it has a severed appearance in spondylolysis. This defect is more prominent in spondylolisthesis, where the superior segment of the vertebral body slides forward on the inferior segment. It is seen in approximately half of those patients diagnosed with spondylolysis and can lead to chronic pain.

Sacral and Coccygeal Injuries

Sacral injuries are rare and result from direct trauma or shear forces and are often seen in conjunction with pelvic fractures. They are of concern because of associated neurological problems that may result from injury to the lower sacral nerves. Patients may present with symptoms of sciatica or perianal anesthesia with impairment of bladder control. Coccygeal injuries also may result from direct trauma, usually as a result of a fall. Aside from the subsequent pain and discomfort, these injuries are often of limited clinical consequence unless there are associated rectal tears. The diagnosis is clinical, and radiological studies are not indicated; treatment is primarily symptomatic.

Management of Patients with Suspected or Known Spinal Injuries

One of the fundamental goals in the care of the patient with potential or recognized spinal injury is the avoidance of spinal cord damage extension. Immobilization is essential and must begin in the prehospital setting, continuing throughout the evaluation. The semirigid collar alone is not adequate to immobilize the spine. The head and neck position must be secured through the use of a spine board, adhesive tape or Velcro straps, and sandbags. Other commercially manufactured products are available that will provide immobilization comparable to that offered by halo-vest outfits.

Airway management is challenging in trauma patients with suspected cervical spinal injuries who are immobilized and whose own ability to maintain the airway is compromised by positioning and potentially severe neurological deficits. Clinicians must be cognizant of the high risk of aspiration in these patients. The spinal board should be used to turn the patient to either side should emesis occur. The controversy regarding the safety of orotracheal intubation in this setting persists, but most authors agree that executed with care and in-line stabilization, this procedure represents perhaps the safest maneuver for airway control. Alternatively, blind nasotracheal intubation performed by an experienced practitioner remains an option in the spontaneously breathing patient. The treating physician must be prepared for emergent surgical airway procedures, including cricothyrotomy and tracheostomy. Whichever technique is deemed best, taking control of the airway early and assuring adequate pulmonary ventilatory volumes is crucial in the patient with spinal injury.

Hemodynamic instability in the trauma victim may result from thoracic, abdominal, and pelvic injuries. It may also represent spinal shock due to interruption of sympathetic outflow pathways after spinal injury. The loss of visceral and peripheral autonomic control and uninhibited parasympathetic impulses leads to hypotension and paradoxical bradycardia with loss of cutaneous vasoconstriction and bladder control. It is partially responsive to cautious fluid and vasopressor administration. Low-dose atropine may be necessary should bradycardia be profound and refractory.

Several pharmacological modalities under investigation are aimed at limiting the extent of neurological deficits in patients with spinal cord injuries. A full description of these is beyond the scope of this discussion but include methylprednisolone, naloxone, nimodipine, and thyrotropin. Of those agents, methylprednisolone is currently widely used, and although benefits have not been conclusively proven, results of various studies have been promising if started within the first 8 hours after injury. The present regimen consists of methylprednisolone given at 30 mg/kg IV in the first hour with a continuous dose of 5.4 mg/kg/hour IV for 23 hours.

Patients with spinal column injuries with or without cord damage must be carefully evaluated for the presence of other life- or limb-threatening conditions. Assessment of these conditions may be hindered by the patient's altered mentation, distracting pain, and anxiety. Additionally, altered sensory and motor pathways may interfere with the evaluation of the abdomen or extremities. Careful examination and additional studies, including CT scan, ultrasound, and diagnostic peritoneal lavage, can assist in the elucidation of further injury. Supportive measures for all patients should include placement of a nasogastric tube and a Foley catheter, unless there are specific contraindications. Measures to prevent early skin damage from pressure points must be initiated in the ED.

Selected Readings

Advanced Trauma Life Support (ATLS) for Doctors, 6th ed. Chicago: The American College of Surgeons, 2004.

Harris JH Jr, Harris WH. *The Radiology of Emergency Medicine,* 4th ed. Philadelphia: Lippincott Williams and Wilkins, 2000.

Mirvis SE, Shanmuganathan K, eds. Imaging in Trauma and Critical Care, ed 2. Basel: Elsevier Science, 2003.

Moore EE, Feliciano DV, Mattox KL, eds. *Trauma,* 5th ed. New York: McGraw-Hill Professional, 2004.

Facial Injuries

Harry L. Anderson III

Facial injuries are a source of great concern to patients and family and must be carefully approached by the emergency physician. Both blunt and penetrating trauma may be seen, often in conjunction with other injuries. It is important to perform a complete examination without allowing a highly visible facial injury to distract one's attention. Furthermore, midface fractures alone will not lead to respiratory compromise and embarrassment. Facial injuries are rarely life-threatening and, once diagnosed, may await patient resuscitation and stabilization of injuries that have higher morbidity and mortality associated with them. Airway management, ensuring breathing and circulation, and intraabdominal or intrathoracic catastrophes remain top priorities (**FIGURE 166.1**). The emergency physician's identification of specific facial injuries is crucial to ensure appropriate management. Many surgical sub specialties overlap in management of injuries to this area, including trauma surgery, interventional radiology, neurosurgery, oral and maxillofacial surgery, plastic surgery, and otolaryngology. The available services and consultants will determine which of these specialists manages these patients at any given hospital.

The facial bones serve several purposes. They surround and protect the eyes, provide sinus air spaces to lighten the skull, warm inspired air, give resonance to the voice, protect sensory nerves, and provide a framework to the muscles of the face. Much like a modern automobile, the eloquence of the skeletal structure of the face allows magnitudes of energy to be dissipated upon impact in order to protect the contents of the skull (**FIGURE 166.2**).

The supraorbital, infraorbital, and mental nerves emerge from their foramina in nearly a straight line drawn from the pupil to the corner of the mouth. Fractures along this line are therefore likely to produce a sensory deficit over their distribution. This can be a subtle clue to the presence of fracture when suspicion is high but no step-off or motor deficit is found on examination. Fractures may affect any of the functions of the facial bones, and knowledge of the injury pattern seen with each type of fracture facilitates identification of fractures when present. Facial trauma is usually caused by blunt trauma, either from a direct blow or as part of diffuse trauma, frequently a motor vehicle crash (MVC). The nasal bones, mandible, and zygoma are most suscepti-

ble to fracture, while the supraorbital ridges are least susceptible of the facial bones. Over half of MVC victims have associated facial trauma. Many patients with facial trauma have an altered level of consciousness, whether from intoxication or from brain injury, making a thorough and careful examination paramount (Figure 166.1).

Frontal Sinus

The force required to fracture the frontal bone frequently results in associated injuries in the area, including orbital and nasal injuries, and injuries to the ethmoid sinus and cribriform plate. Fracture of the frontal wall may be palpable as a step-off or facial crepitus, or may be obscured by edema and missed on initial examination only to heal with an unsightly depression. Posterior wall fracture may tear the dura with CSF rhinorrhea and frontal lobe injury as a result. CT scan reveals both anterior and posterior wall fractures. Cribriform plate injury should also be suspected in the patient with CSF rhinorrhea. Both sinus and cribriform plate injuries should be treated with prophylactic antibiotics (penicillin or clindamycin) and consultation to the appropriate surgical specialist. When cribriform plate injury is suspected, avoid nasal instrumentation to prevent inadvertent intracranial placement of nasogastric catheters or endotracheal tubes.

Mandibular Fractures

The mandible is second only to nasal bones in frequency of fracture. The arc shape of the mandible makes it susceptible to multiple fractures since forces are transmitted along the ramus. Mechanism of injury may help to predict the site of a fracture; direct blows are more likely to result in fractures of the body and angles while higher velocity trauma is more likely to produce fractures of the body and condyles. The importance of identifying these fractures early lies in the ability to protect the airway. Bilateral and even some unilateral fractures of the mandible can occlude the airway of the supine patient. This often occurs in the trauma patient who is lying supine for spine precautions. Those patients who do not warrant spine precautions should be transported sitting upright protecting

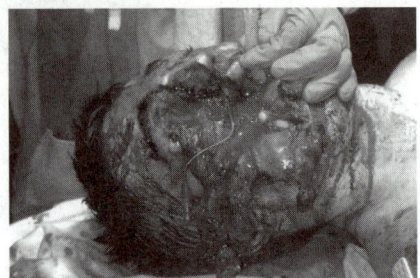

FIGURE 166.1 Shotgun wound to face. Despite the horrific appearance of some facial injuries, the first priorities include cervical spine immobilization and securing an effective airway.

their airway. The ability to identify a 1 to 2 mm malocclusion is an important clinical sign of mandibular fracture. In the patient unable to cooperate fully with the examiner, palpation internally and externally looking for step-off and discontinuity, focal pain, laceration, ecchymosis, and bleeding from intraoral laceration or avulsed teeth may help to pinpoint a fracture. Inability to open and close the mouth fully, loss of bite strength, malocclusion, or an asymmetric opening may be another important clue to a mandible fracture.

After ensuring that the airway is patent and the patient has been stabilized, complete radiographic studies will delineate the fracture. These may include posteroanterior (PA), oblique, and reverse Townes views or Panorex, if available. CT scan may be helpful in showing condylar fractures. The crucial factor in repair of mandibular fractures is restoration of proper occlusion. In rare patients this may require no more than a full liquid diet and careful following of bite position; more commonly, interdental fixation alone or in conjunction with open reduction and internal fixation may be required as decided by the consultant. Antibiotics are prescribed for open fractures as indicated by intraoral bleeding, avulsed teeth, ear canal lacerations, or in areas with tightly adherent mucosa. Penicillin and/or clindamycin in the nonallergic patient remain the drugs of choice for coverage of intraoral flora.

Mandibular dislocation may be seen in trauma or after forceful opening of the mouth as in yawning. Bilateral dislocations are more common and present with inability to close the mouth. Unilateral dislocations may present with asymmetric mouth excursion. In both cases, masseter muscle spasm tends to hold the mandible in its dislocated position. After excluding associated fracture and establishing adequate analgesia and relaxation, the mandible may be reduced by the emergency physician. This is best accomplished by placing the thumbs, wrapped in gauze for protection, on the lower molars and exerting gentle steady downward force. Sometimes an upward rotation of the mandible is helpful in allowing the condyles to return to their correct position.

Maxillary Fractures

Maxillary fractures are less common than mandibular fractures, but are commonly seen in multisystem trauma. One may see massive hemorrhage in conjunction with midface fractures, usually in association with sinus fractures. This hemorrhage may be controlled by fracture reduction; anterior and posterior packing and anterior traction on the posterior packing may also be necessary. Examining for injury to the maxillae includes observation of asymmetry of the face, malocclusion of the teeth noted by the patient, and testing for midface stability by stabilizing the forehead with one hand and grasping the upper alveolar ridge with the other hand and attempting to rock the maxilla.

The LeFort fractures (named after the French surgeon, Leon Clement LeFort [1829–1893]) classify the amount of instability: the LeFort I is a separation of the upper alveolar ridge from the face; the LeFort II begins at the bridge of the nose and extends across the maxillary arch medial to the zygoma; the LeFort III is total craniofacial separation, extending from the bridge of the nose across the orbits and the zygomatic arches. The pattern may be asymmetric, with LeFort II aspects on one side and LeFort III characteristics on the other. The airway must be carefully evaluated in LeFort II and III fractures. Facial films are helpful assessing these fractures, but CT scan with coronal and sagittal reconstructions is becoming the study of choice to delineate precisely the injuries and plan the repair. This being said, coronal films are impossible in the acute trauma patient as the position of the patient with the neck extended is prohibited until the spine has been cleared.

Associated injuries with these types of fractures include cerebrovascular injuries. Therefore, the literature clearly supports 4-vessel angiography for the increased risk of blunt carotid and vertebral artery injury in those with multiple facial fractures. Carotid duplex and CT angiography is unreliable in diagnosing grade I and some grade II injuries. The two studies that recently compared CT angiography versus 4 vessel angiography could only demonstrate a 50% and 68% sensitivity demonstrating the lack of accuracy of CT angiography. Still, a multi-institutional, randomized, prospective trial, is currently being put together to closely re-examine this issue as well as the safety of conventional angiography.

Also associated is carotid cavernous sinus injury. These are dealt with by interventional radiology and emergent embolization. Consultation with a highly skilled interventional radiologist is mandatory, and not all centers will have such radiologists on staff. For maxillary fractures, surgical consultation to the appropriate specialist while the patient is in the ED is mandatory. Antibiotics are indicated when sinus spaces have been entered.

Nasal Fractures

The nasal bones, the most fragile and vulnerable of the facial bones, are also the most commonly fractured, usually by direct blow. Swelling, discoloration, tenderness, epistaxis, nasal deviation, and widening may all be seen in the patient with suspected nasal fracture. Internal examination may reveal septal deviation or hematoma. More serious nasal fractures may present with widened intercanthal distance, foreshortening of the nose, periorbital emphy-

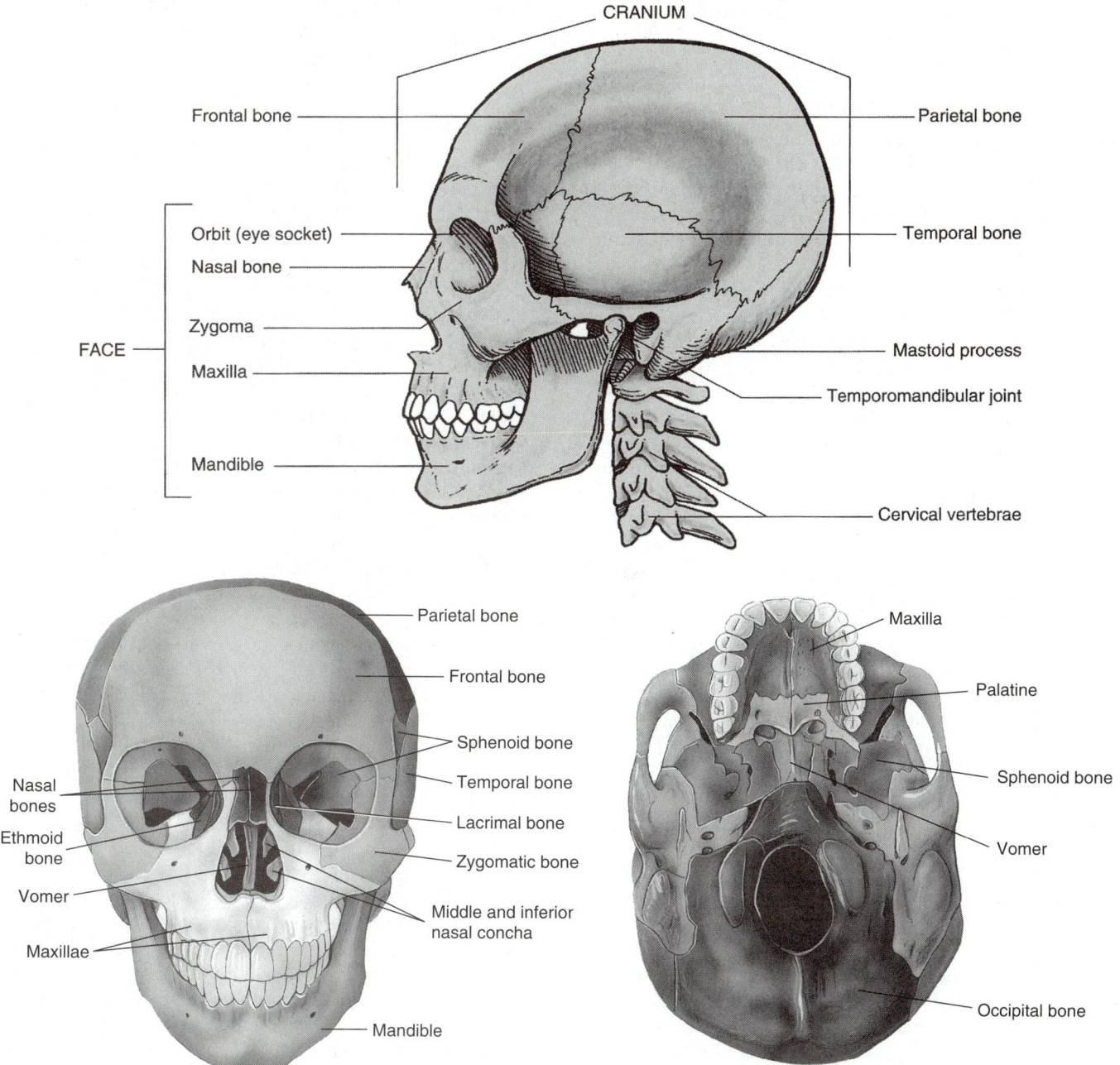

FIGURE 166.2 Bones of the (A) face and (B) skull. *Source:* Used with permission from Jones and Bartlett Publishers. *Emergency Care and Transportation of the Sick and Injured,* 8th ed. Sudbury, MA: Jones and Bartlett Publishers, 2002:603 (Figure 26-1), 84 (Figure 4-5).

sema, or CSF rhinorrhea. Plane films of the nose may show the fracture. Clinical management is guided by the examination. Obvious deviation of the septum may be manually reduced. Septal hematoma must be drained and a compressive packing applied to prevent pressure necrosis of the cartilaginous septum with resultant saddle nose deformity.

Most cases of traumatic epistaxis stop spontaneously and require no intervention. Posterior nasal hemorrhage, however, can carry significant blood loss. Posterior nasal packing should be performed by a surgeon and if warranted, intranasal balloon tamponade is another adjunct. In any case, where the mucosa is violated, prophylactic

antibiotics may be a consideration to prevent toxic shock. The literature concerning this practice is mixed, although it leans against prophylaxis and more toward dressing changes. Most patients can be discharged after arranging follow-up with an otolaryngologist or a plastic surgeon. The decision of whether to reduce the fracture immediately or several days later, after the swelling has subsided but before union begins, varies with each consultant.

Orbital Fracture

The recessed position of the orbits below the protection of the frontal ridge somewhat compensates for the fragility of the bones, but a direct blow below the frontal ridge from an object such as a fist or baseball may impact directly against the globe and the orbital walls. The loose connective tissue in this area permits such a degree of swelling that timely and thorough evaluation is essential before swelling precludes visualization of the eye. The most commonly fractured of the orbital walls is the inferior wall. With a significant fracture, the inferior rectus muscle may herniate through the floor of the orbit, limiting extraocular movement and resulting in diplopia and enophthalmos. In one third to one half of cases, the floor fracture extends into the medial wall. The medial orbital wall is the thinnest of the walls, and may present with similar symptoms to a floor fracture, except that the diplopia is horizontal rather than vertical. In both cases, CT scans with coronal cuts are the preferred study to delineate the extent of entrapment.

The patients may be observed for 1 to 2 weeks with surgical intervention indicated for persistent diplopia and marked enophthalmos. Orbital roof fractures are uncommon and frequently extend into the frontal or zygomatic complexes. The anterior cranial fossa may be involved also, so careful ophthalmic and neurologic examinations in conjunction with CT scan of both coronal and axial cuts to define extent and type of fracture are essential; if the inner table is involved, a combined neurosurgical and ophthalmic procedure is necessary. The orbits may also be involved in zygomatic and midface fractures, which are discussed below. In a case in which the sinuses are entered, prophylactic antibiotics are indicated.

Dental Fractures and Avulsions

Dental injuries may extend from total tooth loss to subtotal avulsion, tooth fracture, alveolar fracture, and related soft tissue injuries. The examination must therefore include soft and hard tissues to look for lacerations, ecchymosis, and mobility. Avulsed teeth must be accounted for to ensure they are not in the patient's soft tissues or airway. This may require soft tissue films of the cheeks, neck, chest, or abdomen in addition to careful examination and exploration of any intraoral lacerations. When the teeth are found, they should be gently rinsed to remove debris and transported in moistened gauze or the cooperative patient's buccal cavity. Avulsed teeth should be replaced as soon as possible; the odds of successful reimplantation diminish every minute the tooth is out of the socket. The exception is deciduous teeth, which should not be replaced or they may interfere with later eruption of permanent teeth. Mobile teeth may be left in place unless there is a risk of aspiration; soft diet and time will generally permit healing. Highly mobile teeth may be splinted with wire or tooth-bonding products. Tooth fractures are classified I to V from enamel (Class I) and dentin (Class II) injuries not involving the nerve and requiring no treatment to Class III, exposed pulp, and Classes IV and V, exposed nerve, which require palliative treatment in the ED, with further studies to determine whether extraction is needed.

Antibiotics are indicated with fractures associated with mucosal injury. Alveolar fractures vary from minimally mobile to totally nonviable. Treatment likewise varies, from an-

tibiotics and soft diet for minimally mobile fractures, to fixation by splinting or maxillomandibular fixation for severely mobile fractures, and debridement of nonviable tissue.

Zygomatic Fractures

The zygoma is one of the most commonly fractured facial bones, involved in approximately one fourth of all facial injuries. It may fracture at any point of attachment to the frontal, temporal, or maxillary bones; through the arch; or body fracture at all points of attachment produces the tripod fracture. Clinical findings may include facial asymmetry, depression and tenderness of the orbital rim, diplopia (either horizontal or vertical), hyperesthesia over the distribution of the infraorbital nerve, and trismus from impingement on the coronoid process of the mandible. Ocular injury may be seen in 10% to 20% of these fractures. Nondisplaced fractures need no surgical treatment. Antibiotics are indicated when the sinuses are involved. Displaced fractures must be reduced by either closed or open methods.

Soft Tissue Facial Injuries

Careful management of soft tissue injuries is essential to permit optimal recovery. In addition to consideration produced by every type of injury, including determination of tetanus prophylaxis in all patients with a break in skin integrity and rabies status in cases of animal bites, facial injuries have unique requirements. Important structures lie so close to the surface that a seemingly minor injury may have long-term sequelae if not approached properly. Careful reapposition of structures such as the vermilion border of the lip, the eyebrow, eyelid margins, nostril margins, parotid duct, lacrimal apparatus, and facial nerve is critical. The vascularity of the face is such that even seemingly nonviable tissue may survive if handled gently, so aggressive debridement is contraindicated. Standard soft tissue injury management techniques may be employed with a few special exceptions. Because of the improved vascularity, older and more contaminated lacerations may be closed on the face; such lacerations elsewhere on the body would not be treated this way. The patient should have tetanus prophylaxis updated if necessary and the wound should be thoroughly cleaned. Superficial lacerations may be closed with fine nonabsorbable interrupted sutures.

Complex Facial Lacerations

Large or stellate lacerations require more careful closure. Thorough exploration and examination to assess sensorimotor function and exclude retained foreign body is essential. Lacerations that penetrate galea or interrupt muscle must be closed in layers to promote tamponade and to prevent cephalohematoma formation. These injuries may require a brief course of prophylactic antibiotics. If the wound edges gape widely, subcutaneous absorbable sutures will take tension off the skin edges. This may require undermining the edges to permit apposition. The abundant vascularity encourages healing of what might elsewhere be marginally viable tissue, so debridement should be minimal and cautious, although obviously devitalized tissue and ragged edges may be removed to permit a clean repair. The decision when to seek surgical consultation depends on facts such as the type of injury, availability of consultants, the ED physician's experience, the current ED volume, and patient preference.

Severe Abrasions

Careful cleansing of abrasions is especially important on the face, where traumatic tattooing will be distressing to the patient. This may require topical anesthesia to permit thorough cleansing. Gentle scrubbing may not suffice to remove particulate matter; a fine needle or scalpel tip may be required to remove as much as possible. Antibiotic ointment may facilitate removal of oil-based material. Care must be taken to avoid converting the partial thickness abrasion into a full-thickness injury either by too vigorous scrubbing or by later infection; thus, meticulous wound care is important. Sterile technique should be observed during the cleansing and debridement to prevent introduction of contaminants.

Parotid Gland/Duct Injuries

The parotid gland may be injured in deep laceration posterior to the anterior border of the masseter muscle. The gland itself does not need to be sutured, but the facial nerve runs inside the gland, and injury to the nerve should be carefully sought by a specialist if the gland is injured. The parotid duct runs from the body of the gland and empties into the mouth at Stenson's duct opposite the first maxillary molar. Injury to the parotid duct is often seen in association with damage to the buccal branch of the facial nerve. Parotid duct injury may be suspected with the presence of clear liquid in the wound or by gently exploring the duct opening with a fine flexible probe. If the duct is injured, it should be repaired over a stent. Salivary fistulae that may form with injury to gland or duct usually resolve spontaneously.

Facial Nerve Injuries

Facial nerve injury may be suspected by anatomic landmarks and examination. Indicators of trauma to the nerve include muscle paralysis and sensory deficit. Once identified, the injury to the temporal branch may result in eyelid paralysis and corneal exposure. Proximal injury should merit early surgical consultation and subsequent attempt at operative repair under magnification; injury medial to the midpupillary line is not usually repaired because nerve regeneration may occur at this level, and significant muscle innervation will be lost.

Selected Readings

Fonseca RJ, Walker RV, Betts NJ, et al., eds. *Oral and Maxillofacial Trauma,* 3rd ed. Basel: Elsevier, 2005.

Mirvis SE, Shanmuganathan K, eds. *Imaging in Trauma and Critical Care,* 2d ed. Basel: Elsevier Science, 2003.

Ophthalmologic Injuries

Mark L. Shapiro

Trauma to the orbital contents requires careful management to avoid permanent disability averting the possible loss of vision requires meticulous examination for identification of injuries and aggressive management of time-dependent therapies. Damage to the eye may be sustained by direct or penetrating injury or by injury to the surface of the eye through directly toxic exposures. In nearly all cases, an ophthalmologist should be involved in the follow-up care, if not consulted while the patient is in the ED.

The ophthalmological system can be approached in many ways, but a systematic approach must be adopted for consistent and complete evaluation of the eye. Visual acuity evaluation is the first test of eye function. Next, the lids and lashes must be examined for signs of infection or inflammation, including lid eversion. Extraocular muscle function is tested and visual fields are examined; confrontational direct assessment is most readily available in the ED. The sclera and conjunctiva are then observed for injection, foreign bodies, or discharge. The cornea and anterior chamber must be examined directly and with the slit lamp to assess anterior chamber depth, presence of cells, clarity of the cornea, and presence of foreign bodies. The pupil and iris may be inspected for regularity and reactivity, including the presence of afferent pupillary function (consensual reactivity of one pupil when the other is exposed to light). The fundoscopic examination looks at the vitreous for presence of hemorrhage, at the retinal vessels for venous pulsations, for hypertensive changes such as silver wire changes, and the retinal background for exudates or hemorrhage. The disk is observed for clear margins or lack thereof, which may indicate papilledema, a marker for elevated intracranial pressure. Finally, if there is no suspicion of penetrating globe injury, intraocular pressure is tested.

Corneal Abrasion or Laceration

Corneal injury is the most common ophthalmic condition seen in the ED. Most patients present with complaints of foreign body sensation. In many cases, the foreign body has left the eye but a retained foreign body must be carefully sought. Frequently, clear light and slit lamp examination may not reveal the injury until fluorescein stain is applied and illuminated with cobalt blue light under a slit lamp, when the stain will collect in the irregularities including the cornices and corneal injuries. Corneal laceration should be patched and immediately referred to ophthalmology for repair without further manipulation of the globe. If no other injury is present and the anterior chamber is intact, corneal abrasions may be treated symptomatically. Topical anesthetics such as tetracaine and proparacaine facilitate examination but should not be given to the patient to use at home, since anesthetized corneas may sustain further injury without alerting the patient. A mydriatic agent may be applied to dilate the pupil if the patient does not need to drive. However, if neurological injuries or deficits are noted, it is of the utmost importance to alert the neurosurgical team that mydriatic agents have been used, as this will obscure or obviate the exam. A topical antibiotic ointment, which provides some lubrication under the lid, is usually given. Whether to patch the eye depends on whether the patient must drive home and on the preference of the treating physician and ophthalmologic consultant. Oral pain medication may be required for 1 to 2 days. The patient may be discharged with ophthalmology follow-up in 24 hours. Most corneal abrasions heal within 24 to 48 hours.

Foreign Bodies Involving the Eye

Foreign bodies may come from a variety of sources, including metal, wood, and dirt, and can be broadly grouped into corneal and intraocular. Corneal foreign bodies can usually be seen either with direct examination or after fluorescein stain. Vertical linear abrasions are seen with a foreign body trapped under the lid. These foreign bodies may be removed after topical anesthesia in a number of ways. A damp sterile cotton swab may be gently swept across the object or under both lids if no foreign body is clearly visualized. If this is unsuccessful, an eye spud or hypodermic needle may be used to lift the foreign body off the eye. Irrigation may help to remove the foreign body. More firmly embedded foreign bodies may require immediate ophthalmologic evaluation to extricate them. Bodies that penetrate beyond the epithelium have an increased chance of producing scarring.

Metal objects must be removed promptly to avert formation of a rust ring around the metal, which will remain after the object is removed. To facilitate the removal of some metallic object without further injury to the eye, a magnet is extraordinarily useful. The rust ring may need to be debrided with a burr or scraped off with a needle by the emergency physician or the ophthalmologic consultant; removal is often easier after 24 hours because of corneal softening. The risk of creating further damage and producing scarring in the visual axis must be evaluated when deciding how aggressively to attempt removal of the foreign body and the rust ring; if the visual axis is affected, the decision should be discussed with an ophthalmologist. After the foreign body is removed, the residual corneal abrasion may be treated as outlined above. If the foreign body was vegetable or organic, the increased risk of infection outweighs the benefit of patching.

Iritis

Blunt trauma can cause irritation to the iris, leading to an inflammatory reaction in the anterior chamber. This can be a cause of unilateral red eye and may manifest as pain, photophobia, and blurred vision. Pupillary constrictor spasm may leave the pupil smaller than the contralateral one. Cells and flare may be seen in the anterior chamber on slit lamp examination. Treatment consists of long-acting mydriatic and cycloplegic drops and ophthalmologic referral.

Hyphema

Traumatic hyphema describes blood in the anterior chamber from tearing of ciliary or iris vessels. Hyphema is classified according to the quantity of blood present, which may vary from microscopic specks to filling the anterior chamber. The symptoms are similar to iritis but may include somnolence and lethargy. The blood layers out if the patient is upright, facilitating diagnosis. Traumatic mydriasis may coexist and must be differentiated from an afferent papillary defect, suggesting optic nerve injury, by the swinging flashlight test. The most common complication is rebleeding, usually within 2 to 5 days, but corneal staining, synechiae formation, and elevated intraocular pressure from outflow obstruction may occur. Treatment includes immediate ophthalmologic consultation, bed rest with the head of the bed elevated above 45 degrees, avoidance of eye activity, eye shield, avoidance of Valsalva maneuvers, and antiemetics and analgesics. Mydriatics prevent synechiae formation; beta-blocker drops control elevated intraocular pressure. Small hyphemas may be treated on an outpatient basis, but most require admission for therapy and close following of the intraocular pressure and slit lamp examinations.

Lens Dislocation

The zonule fibers that tether the lens in place behind the iris may be disrupted by blunt trauma, resulting in subluxation or complete dislocation. Loss of visual acuity results. The edge of the lens may be seen after pupillary dilation. A trembling of the lens, *iridodonesis,* may be seen after rapid eye movements. A posteriorly dislocated lens may be seen on fundoscopic examination. The anteriorly dislocated lens in the anterior chamber may cause acute angle closure glaucoma, necessitating emergent repair; otherwise, these may be patched and referred to the ophthalmologist for repair.

Retinal Detachment

Blunt trauma can also cause retinal tears and detachment immediately or delayed by months or years. Symptoms include flashing lights and visual field cuts. A dilated funduscopic examination is necessary. Treatment includes head positioning to prevent progression and emergent consultation for possible surgical correction.

Penetrating Globe Injuries

Intraocular foreign bodies should be suspected with a history of high-speed projectiles and loss of vision. Penetration of the cornea or globe represents a surgical emergency. Associated findings may include loss or cornea contour, shallow anterior chamber, positive Seidel's test in which a rivulet of clear liquid emerges through heavy fluorescein staining from the site of injury, an irregular pupil, prolapsed iris through the corneal laceration, hyphema, or lens opacification. Intraocular pressure is diminished but should not be measured because of the risk of increased loss of globe contents. Imaging studies should be obtained; CT scan is the study of choice but plane films may also be helpful. The composition of the object will affect treatment decisions; inert materials such as glass may be left in place. Metal causes a local reaction and usually needs to be removed. Organic matter has a high associated incidence of infection and must be removed; prophylactic antibiotics must be given. If soil contamination is present, Bacillus coverage must be included in the antibiotic considerations.

Eyelid Lacerations

The skin, orbicularis muscle, and tarsal plate are the three layers of the eyelid. Palpebral conjunctiva lies below the tarsal plates, necessitating a four-layered closure in lacerations that transect the tarsal plate. In the upper eyelid, the *levator palpebrae superioris* lies behind the orbicularis and inserts near the upper margin of the tarsus forming the upper lid fold; absence of this fold may be a clue to injury of the levator. The presence of orbital fat in a laceration indicates violation of the orbital septum and mandates ophthalmologic consultation. Coexisting injuries and foreign bodies must be sought and ruled out; radiography of the orbits may be helpful. The lids must be gently cleansed. Local anesthetic may be used for small lacerations but it blurs the margins. Regional supraorbital or infraorbital anesthesia provides analgesia without exacerbating existing edema and obscuring landmarks. The wound must be explored and layers identified; if the levator and septum are intact, the skin and orbicularis can be closed as a single layer. Lacerations that involve the tarsal plate, lid margin, *levator palpebrae,* orbital septum, or canthal angles should be referred to a specialist for surgical repair.

Lacrimal Duct Injuries

The nasolacrimal duct drains tears from the medial aspect of both upper and lower lids. Penetrating trauma to the medial aspect of the eyelid, especially between the medial canthus and the lacrimal punctum, can damage the canalicular apparatus. The lacrimal duct must be probed to establish patency; it must be repaired over a stent if it has been violated. Immediate referral to ophthalmology is indicated to avoid permanent tearing over the cheek.

Corneal Burns

Topical corneal damage from toxic exposure requires aggressive prompt therapy to minimize damage. Severity of injury depends on concentration of chemical and duration of exposure. Immediate copious exposure is indicated in chemical exposure until pH testing returns to normal. Acid injury leads to a coagulation necrosis, limiting depth of penetration of injury. Copious irrigation is immediately instituted. Sequelae include corneal and conjunctival scarring, uveitis, and glaucoma. Follow-up with ophthalmology is indicated within 24 hours.

Alkali injury is a devastating injury, because the liquefaction necrosis produced permits deep penetration of ongoing damage. Copious irrigation can diminish injury and should be started immediately. Irrigation should continue until the measured pH remains 7.4 for 30 minutes after irrigation has ceased; this may require liters of irrigant. Topical antibiotics, cycloplegics, and steroids may also be indicated and should be instituted in consultation with ophthalmology. Acute injury occurs in the first 3 days after exposure and is graded according to the degree of limbal and corneal ischemia. Early sequelae include corneal edema and elevated intraocular pressure. Late injury results from corneal breakdown with ulceration and perforation possible. Lid damage may result in sagging and adhering of the lower lid or ectropion.

Ultraviolet (UV) corneal injury may be seen in people who are exposed to increased ultraviolet radiation such as welders and skiers who fail to wear UV protective eye protection. The patient may complain of diffuse pain or foreign body sensation. The eyes appear injected, and increased tearing may be noted. Fluorescein staining reveals multiple punctate areas of uptake most concentrated between the palpebral fissure. Treatment is supportive as for corneal ulceration; antibiotic ointment, optional patching of the more affected eye, pain medication, and ophthalmological follow-up in 24 hours are usually offered to the patient.

Selected Readings

Gossman MD, Roberts DM, Barr CC. Ophthalmic aspects of orbital injury: a comprehensive diagnostic and management approach. *Clin Plast Surg* 1992;19:71–85.

Kuhn F, Morris R, Witherspoon CD. *Ocular Trauma: Principals and Practices.* Kuhn F, Pieramici D, eds. Stuttgart: Thieme Publishers, 2002.

Michel FK, Sulewski ME. Focused assessment of the patient with eye trauma: The Essentials. *Top Emerg Med* 2000;22:1–8.

Otologic Injuries

Mark L. Shapiro

Otologic trauma is common in all age groups. Injury may affect any of the three parts of the ear. The cochlea and vestibular apparatus of the inner ear may be injured with temporal bone fracture or barotrauma. The middle ear and tympanic membrane show injury with barotrauma, foreign body, thermal, and blunt trauma. External canal and auricle injury are seen with thermal, blunt, and penetrating trauma.

Lacerations

Careful wound care and meticulous tissue handling may permit satisfactory healing of even significant lacerations as long as no tissue is lost. Anesthesia may best be obtained by a ring block around the base of the auricle, leaving tissue undistorted by anesthetic. Margins must be carefully reapproximated to prevent notching of the rim. Lacerated cartilage can be pulled gently together with a few stitches of absorbable suture; overlapping the edges may minimize notching. The skin may be closed with finer suture, and a compressive dressing, padding the auricle apart from the head, can be applied over antibiotic ointment. Significant tissue loss can be repaired with primary flap or wedge resection, or staged reconstruction may be attempted later with denuded cartilage, which may be stored in a subcutaneous pocket. All of these repairs should be referred to a specialist. Delayed complications include infection and tissue necrosis, leading to defects and deformities.

Subperichondrial Hematoma

A direct blow to the auricle may result in auricular hematoma, often seen in contact sports, most notably in wrestling. The hematoma must be completely evacuated either by aspiration or incision and drainage. A compressive dressing is then applied to prevent reaccumulation. The most feared complication of this condition is cartilage necrosis and loss with subsequent scarring and deformity, the so-called cauliflower ear.

Tympanic Membrane Perforation

Many mechanisms can lead to tympanic membrane rupture, including barotrauma, foreign body, and aggressive canal exploration. The defect is usually centrally located and irregular. Symptoms include pain, transient vertigo, tinnitus, and hearing loss. Otomicroscopy is indicated within 1 to 2 days. Irrigations and local medications are contraindicated. Healing is usually uneventful and without scarring, and wounds heal within 2 months.

Selected Readings

Ishman SL, Friedland DR. Temporal bone fractures: traditional classification and clinical relevance. *Laryngoscope* 2004;114:1734–1741.
Nolle C, Todt I, Seidl RO, Ernst A. Pathophysiological changes of the central auditory pathway after blunt trauma of the head. *J Neurotrauma* 2004;21:251–258.
Pelkonen O, Tikkakoski T, Luotonen J, Sotaniemi K. Pulsatile tinnitus as a symptom of cervicocephalic arterial dissection. *J Laryngol Otol* 2004;118:193–198.

CHAPTER

169 Neck and Upper Airway Injuries

Mark L. Shapiro

Few emergency situations have more potential for rapid deterioration than penetrating neck trauma, because esophageal, pulmonary, vascular and/or neurological injuries may be present. Patients may appear deceptively stable, but can rapidly decompensate, requiring urgent airway intervention or control of bleeding. Most patients who die with isolated neck wounds die of massive blood loss (50%) or airway compromise, or from resultant neurological deficit. In a patient with penetrating neck trauma, the emergency physician must be prepared for active airway intervention, including surgical airway intervention. Early intubation before deterioration should be undertaken in the presence of any indication of potential airway compromise. Control of bleeding and volume resuscitation should be addressed rapidly; emergent operative intervention may be required and immediate surgical consultation is imperative.

Penetrating neck wounds can produce significant morbidity and mortality because of the exposure of many vital structures in a region that provides little protection from injury. There are multiple fascial compartments that can limit bleeding, but can also contribute to airway compromise. The cervical visceral fascia surrounding the esophagus and thyroid also serves as a conduit for contaminants to pass into the mediastinum. The neck can be divided into two compartments: the superficial compartment is external to the platysma and does not contain any major vessels or nerves; the deep compartment beneath the platysma contains the vital structures of the neck.

Traditionally, the neck topography has been divided into two triangles: the anterior triangle is bordered by the posterior border of the sternocleidomastoid muscle (SCM), inferior mandible, and the midline to the manubrium; the posterior triangle is bordered by the SCM, the trapezius, and the clavicle. Most serious injuries are in the anterior triangle. Alternatively, the neck can be divided into three zones to help guide evaluation of vascular injuries.

Zone I is defined as the area between the clavicle and the cricoid cartilage (**FIGURE 169.1**). Injuries in this area have the highest mortality. In life-threatening injuries, the structures most frequently involved are the great vessels of the superior mediastinum. Angiography is helpful in identifying injured vessels in this zone. Injuries to this zone may also involve the esophagus, spinal cord, and lung. A high suspicion for pneumothorax or hemothorax should be maintained. *Zone II* is the area between the cricoid cartilage and the angle of the jaw. Up to 80% of penetrating neck injuries occur in Zone II, but mortality is low with these injuries because of the ease of surgical exposure and ability to control vascular injuries, which are the most common injuries in this zone. Structures at risk for injury in this zone include the carotid artery, jugular vein, pharynx, larynx, and trachea (**FIGURES 169.2** and **169.3**). *Zone III* consists of the area between the angle of the base of the skull. This is the least common injury, but has high morbidity, since obtaining exposure of the involved structures here frequently penetrates the pharynx and angiography is usually required to evaluate to the distal internal carotid artery. Other important structures in this region include the jugular vein, parotid gland, cranial nerves, spinal cord, and intracranial vessels.

Approximately 30% of penetrating neck wounds involve more than one zone, and injury may extend beyond the zone involved in the entrance wound, especially when the injury is caused by a missile wound. Up to the time of World War II (WWII), most experience with penetrating neck wounds came from the military and primarily involved gunshot wounds and shrapnel injuries. Since WWII, there has been an increase in civilian injuries, with approximately 43% involving guns and 52% stab wounds. Among children, 16% are from animal bites, usually dogs. Gunshot wounds, especially from high-velocity weapons, have a higher likelihood of causing indirect injury secondary to kinetic energy ($k = \frac{1}{2} mv^2$) imparted to the surrounding area.

High-velocity missiles include shrapnel and bullets from civilian rifles of military weapons. These missiles are subject to tumble and fragmentation, and cause extensive damage with high rates of infection. These wounds should all be explored and debrided. Low-velocity wounds inflicted by handgun, birdshot, or buckshot are more prone to have erratic pathways, and missiles may ricochet off bones, causing injury distant to the entrance wound. Handgun wounds to the neck have 2% to 6% mortality.

Stab wounds have lower mortality than gunshot wounds but may result in significant vascular injuries. These wounds often present with shock, active hemor-

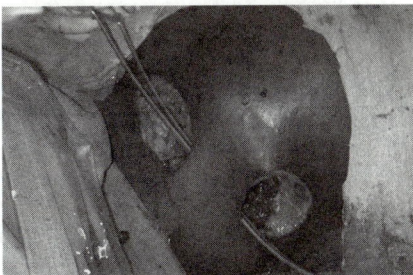
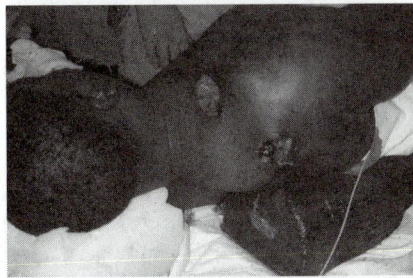
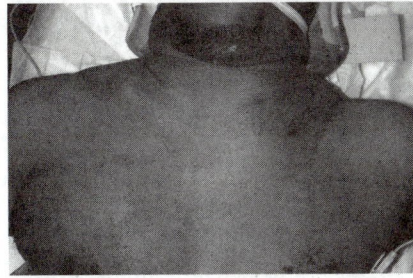

FIGURE 169.1 Injuries in Zone I. (A) Gunshot wound in the neck. (B) Lateral view of panel (A). (C) Note swelling in the neck.

rhage, or a history of significant blood loss on the scene. Complete and partial cord transection can occur, and cranial nerve lacerations occur in 5% of stab wounds to the neck, most commonly of the facial nerve. In some cases, blunt trauma is associated with laceration, impalement, or deep penetrating trauma to the neck.

Airway Injuries

Airway compromise in patients with penetrating neck trauma can occur for several reasons. Expanding hematoma can compress or displace the trachea or hypopharynx. Direct injury of the pharynx, larynx, or trachea may cause local edema, and active hemorrhage into the airway can occur. Injuries to Zone I of the neck can result in violation of

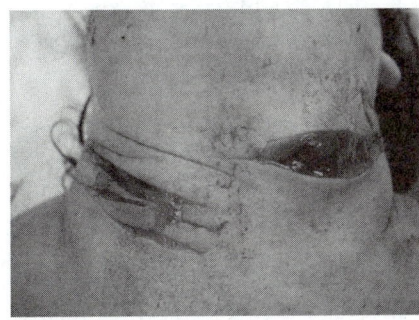

FIGURE 169.2 Lacerations of the neck caused by a knife.

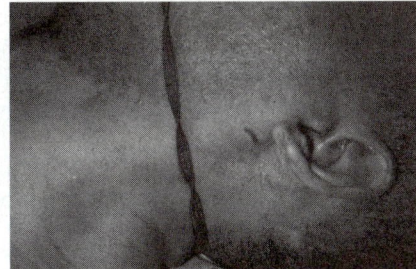

FIGURE 169.3 Trauma to the ear.

the pleural cavity with subsequent pneumothorax or hemothorax. Rarely, injury to the phrenic or recurrent laryngeal nerve can disrupt air flow. Aspiration and vomiting are additional risks to be considered.

Vascular Injuries

Vascular injuries may involve direct or indirect trauma. Direct injuries include partial or complete transection, intimal flaps, arteriovenous fistula, or pseudoaneurysm. Indirect injuries include spasm, external compression, contusion, or thrombosis. The most commonly injured vessel is the internal jugular vein, and the most commonly injured artery is the carotid artery, particularly the common and internal divisions. Signs of arterial injury include absence of pulses or asymmetric pulses, large or expanding hematoma, bruits, or thrills. Air embolus secondary to venous injury is rare but may be lethal. If high suspicion for significant vascular injury exists, immediate surgical consultation is indicated. Alternatively, if low suspicion for arterial injuries exists, angiography can be performed. In some studies, color flow Doppler imaging is being evaluated as an alternative to angiography. With Zone 1 neck injuries, subclavian artery injury with subsequent hemothorax should be suspected.

Neurological Injuries

Although neurological structures are injured relatively infrequently, neurological injuries are a cause of significant morbidity and mortality, and can be from direct injury to the spinal cord, or indirectly from cerebrovascular accidents secondary to vascular injuries such as carotid artery dissection. Spinal cord injury is noted to be a poor prognostic factor. Some 3% of penetrating neck injuries involves damage to the spinal cord, and other neurological structures at risk for injury include the brachial plexus, spinal accessory, hypoglossal, vagus, phrenic, and facial nerves. The sympathetic chain ganglia are also at risk, but lie posterior to the carotid sheath and are somewhat protected by it. Therefore, a thorough neurological evaluation should be performed in any patient with penetrating neck trauma to look for evidence of spinal cord, cranial nerve, or CNS injury.

Esophageal Injuries

Esophageal injuries are infrequent because the esophagus is somewhat protected by its location between the pharynx and spine. However, delayed diagnosis in esophageal injuries may result in adverse outcome, particularly in the event of an esophageal injury with communication to the mediastinum. Therefore, adequate exploration or a diagnostic workup is essential. Contrast studies can be used to elucidate injuries to the esophagus. The barium esophagogram is more sensitive than the Gastrografin esophagogram; however, barium can be introduced into the mediastinum causing a severe mediastinitis. Therefore, a Gastrografin swallow should be performed initially, followed by a dilute barium solution. This is helpful only if positive, however, as esophagoscopy has a high false-negative rate (up to 25%). Examination of the esophagus directly with a rigid endoscope has been shown to have 89% sensitivity and 95% specificity.

Signs of impending airway compromise include hoarseness, stridor, hemoptysis, significant subcutaneous emphysema, hypoxia, or an expanding neck hematoma. Extreme agitation should always be interpreted as evidence of impending airway compromise. Objective evidence of an expanding hematoma may be subtle, but comparison with the anatomy of the opposite side of the neck can be helpful, and loss of definition of the sternocleidomastoid is often seen. Patients leaving the ED for further studies such as angiography should be closely monitored, and prophylactic intubation should be considered.

Endotracheal intubation of patients with penetrating neck injuries can be challenging. Blood or vomitus in the pharynx can obscure the view; suction should be immediately available. Rapid-sequence intubation may be contraindicated in patients with associated injuries to the face or jaw that can interfere with mask ventilation. If these patients are cooperative, nasotracheal intubation may be the preferred approach, but patients with shock, head injury, or intoxication may be agitated and unable to cooperate with attempts at nasotracheal intubation. Disturbance of clots can produce ongoing hemorrhage, and the possibility of creating false passages are additional risks with blind intubation attempts. Distorted anatomy, either from direct injury to the airway or compression from an adjacent hematoma, can compound the difficulty. If initial attempts at orotracheal or nasotracheal intubation are unsuccessful, a surgical airway should be attempted. Cricothyrotomy is one possible approach, but if the injury is below the cricoid cartilage (e.g., laryngeal fracture), a tracheostomy may be necessary. Preparation of equipment for a surgical airway should be done before attempts at rapid sequence intubation are begun.

Breathing

After establishment of an airway, the adequacy of ventilation should be assessed. A chest radiograph should be part of the evaluation of all patients with significant penetrating neck injury. Difficulty with ventilation or oxygenation may imply pneumothorax or hemothorax, but correct placement of the adjunctive airway must be confirmed. A chest tube should be immediately placed in any patient with ventilatory compromise secondary to hemothorax or pneumothorax.

Circulation

Acute management of significant blood loss from penetrating neck trauma includes direct pressure to control ongoing bleeding and aggressive fluid and blood resuscitation. At least one intravenous line should be placed in the lower extremity if subclavian injury is suspected. Circumferential pressure dressings must be avoided, as should blind clamping of blood vessels in open wounds. Significant pharyngeal bleeding may be temporarily managed by packing the pharynx with gauze, or inflation of a Foley or Fogarty catheter balloon after an airway has been established. Neck wounds that extend through the platysma should not be probed, as clots may be dislodged, resulting in significant bleeding. Pumping blood loss from an arterial wound may be controlled with a sterile gloved finger placed into the wound; however, the person holding pressure on the wound should be prepared to accompany the patient to the operating room to maintain direct pressure. If air embolism is suspected, the patient should be placed in left lateral decubitus in Trendelenburg's position.

Mandatory Versus Selective Exploration

Currently, controversy exists regarding definitive management of penetrating neck wounds. Prior to WWI, patients without symptoms were observed, but this resulted in a high mortality rate of 11% to 15%. Between WWI and WWII, mandatory exploration was performed if the platysma was violated, resulting in a 4% to 7% mortality rate, but at a substantially increased cost. Today, mortality rates approach 1% because of improvements in anesthesia, antibiotics, and resuscitation, regardless of whether mandatory or selective exploration is used. Although some physicians continue to explore all neck wounds, many now use selective exploration based on clinical estimates of injury and the zone of the neck within which the injury lies.

Wounds that do not cross the platysma can be treated in the same fashion as any superficial laceration, but any wound that penetrates the platysma has the potential to damage the vital structures of the neck. Initial wound evaluation should be limited to establishing whether the platysma is violated. Blind probing of the wound may dislodge clots, leading to uncontrollable hemorrhage. It is generally agreed that surgical exploration is called for if the patient is unstable or exhibits any signs or symptoms of significant injury. In the stable patient with a Zone I or Zone III injury and indication for exploration, angiography should be performed preoperatively to assist in planning surgical strategy. In Zone II injuries, adequate exposure can be obtained to obviate the need for angiographic evaluation.

Controversy revolves around the stable asymptomatic patient with a wound that penetrates the platysma. Angiography is generally recommended by most authors in a stable patient with a Zone I or Zone III injury, but some authors suggest that Zone II injuries require exploration. Proponents of mandatory exploration of Zone II injuries argue that there is a high incidence of reported positive findings (40% to 50%), morbidity of exploration in this region is low, undetected injuries have devastating consequences, and a significant time delay usually occurs before angiographic studies are completed. Most authors advocating selective exploration of Zone II injuries also advocate angiography in lieu of exploration in this group, but a recent study suggests that Zone II injuries may be managed by physical examination alone without arteriography or ultrasonography.

Laryngotracheal Injuries Associated with Neck Trauma

Blunt trauma to the neck, most commonly resulting from motor vehicle injuries, may result in injury to the larynx. Airway obstruction is the most serious complication of these injuries. The examination in the awake and cooperative patient begins with assessing the voice, particularly hoarseness, odynophagia, cough, and hemoptysis, and looking for swelling and loss of landmarks. Indirect laryngoscopy is difficult in the trauma patient. Fiberoptic laryngoscopy is the examination of choice in the acute evaluation of the trauma patient. It is commonly accepted that the most complete examination of the larynx is done with a rigid laryngoscope in the operating room; however, recent studies state that flexible bronchoscopy is equivocal. CT scan is sensitive for laryngotracheal injury, showing fractures, hematoma, dislocations, and disruptions of the larynx. Airway management is paramount in these patients; the precise method of securing the airway varies with the patient's clinical picture, the physician's experience, and the materials available. Endotracheal intubation, fiberoptic guidance, and cricothyrotomy are among the airway options for immediate control of the airway, but tracheotomy will often be required eventually. Mucosal lacerations of the larynx and trachea may be suspected with hemoptysis and cough. Direct visualization will be necessary to assess these injuries. Open repair is usually required for large lacerations. Small lacerations without vocal cord involvement may be managed expectantly by the surgical team.

Laryngeal and Tracheal Injury

Vocal cord injury may manifest with voice changes hoarseness, or increased work of breathing. Direct laryngoscopy is necessary to determine whether injury is apparent. Vocal cord injuries require open repair after tracheostomy.

If the injuries to the larynx are unstable or multiple fractures exist, operative repair may need to include stenting to permit adequate healing. Silastic molds or Teflon stents may be used to support the laryngeal framework. Stents may need to be affixed to the larynx for up to 3 months in severe fractures.

Complete transection of the trachea is a surgical emergency that can manifest itself with massive subcutaneous emphysema and progressive airway compromise. In this situation, emergent tracheostomy is warranted to control the airway and relieve the compressive effect. If the tracheal transection is low, the distal ends may retract into the chest, further complicating an already stressful situation. Tracheal hooks to secure the distal end, once placed, should not be released until the airway is secure.

Selected Readings

Advanced Trauma Life Support (ATLS) for Doctors, 6th ed. Chicago: The American College of Surgeons, 2004.

Biffl WL, Ray CE Jr, Moore EE, et al. Noninvasive diagnosis of blunt cerebrovascular injuries: a preliminary report. *J Trauma* 2002;53:850.

Cothren CC, Moore EE, Biffl WL, et al. Anticoagulation is the gold standard therapy for blunt carotid injuries to reduce stroke rate. *Arch Surg* 2004;139: 540–546.

Demetriades D, Theodorou D, Cornwell E. Transcervical gunshot injuries: mandatory operation is not necessary. *J Trauma* 1996;40:758–760.

Mattox K, Feliciano DV, Moore EE. Penetrating and blunt neck trauma. In: *Trauma*, ed 4. Norwalk, CT: Appleton and Lange, 1999:437–450.

Miller PR, Fabian TC, Croce MA, et al. Prospective screening for blunt cerebrovascular injuries: analysis of diagnostic modalities and outcomes. *Ann Surg* 2002;236:386.

Moore EE, Feliciano DV, Mattox KL, eds. *Trauma*, 5th ed. New York: McGraw-Hill Professional, 2004.

Srinivasan R, Haywood T, Horwitz B, et al. Role of flexible endoscopy in the evaluation of possible esophageal trauma after penetrating injuries. *Am J Gastroenterol* 2000;95:1725–1729.

170 Chest Injuries

Harry L. Anderson III

Of the 157,078 unintentional deaths each year, thoracic injury is the primary cause of death in 25%, and a contributing factor in an additional 25% to 50% of these deaths. Thoracic injury is second only to head injury as a leading cause of traumatic deaths. Blunt chest trauma victims are primarily males in the third decade of life. Motor vehicle accident is by far the leading cause or disabling injury and death. A slight decline in these statistics has been noted with the implementation of reduced highway speed limit, seat belt and air bag use, and improved vehicular safety. Falls also contribute significantly to blunt thoracic injuries. Severe blunt chest trauma without appreciable chest wall injury can also occur in the context of nonpenetrating ballistic injuries or blast and shock wave loading from bombings. Unfortunately, these injuries might become more prevalent as terrorist activities continue to increase. Blunt chest trauma has higher morbidity and mortality than penetrating trauma, as patients are likely to have sustained injuries to multiple organs.

Penetrating chest trauma may be from either gunshot or stab wounds. Victims are likely 17- to 30-year-old males from inner city environments. In 2001, there were 11,671 deaths in the United States due to gunshot wounds. Active crime prevention and education targeted at the at-risk population have led to a decline of these types injuries in some U.S. cities.

The thorax is encased by the chest wall. Intrathoracic structures/organs include the heart, lungs, respiratory trees, esophagus, and major vessels. The caudal extent of the thorax is defined by the diaphragm, which separates it from the abdominal cavity. Trauma to the chest can cause injury to any of these thoracic structures.

Injuries to the Chest Wall

Fifty percent of patients with significant thoracic trauma have injuries to chest wall structures. These injuries can range from an isolated rib fracture to life-threatening flail chest. They are often missed initially due to more emergent conditions, but because of their proximity to underlying cardiopulmonary structures, even seemingly minor injuries can lead to life-threatening complications.

Penetrating Chest Injuries

The management of penetrating chest wounds has evolved to a large extent from the experience gained through military casualties. The mortality from penetrating chest wounds has decreased from 56% during World War I to 3% during the Vietnam War partly because of improved transportation, which allowed a higher percentage of critically injured patients to reach the hospital alive. In the civilian setting, handguns and knives are the most common causes of penetrating injuries, although other objects such as ice picks, staples, and nail guns, and other sharp objects have been implicated. It is estimated that 40% of those suffering from penetrating trauma have thoracic injuries. Improved prehospital care in the form of airway and resuscitation management as well as prompt field recognition and management of the complications of penetrating chest injuries, such as sucking chest wound and tension pneumothorax, have resulted in the presentation of more severely injured but alive patients to the ED (**FIGURE 170.1**).

The extent of injuries sustained by the patient depends on the mechanism of injury and the locations of the wounds. Gunshot wounds are more likely to cause extensive tissue damage, with often unclear trajectories, and possible gross contamination with foreign bodies. A functional anatomic classification dividing wound locations as either central or peripheral and upper or lower (thoracoabdominal) is useful and can guide management. Central wounds are defined within the following boundaries: the midclavicular lines laterally, the clavicles and sternal notch superiorly, and the costal margins and xiphoid inferiorly. The upper and lower regions are separated by the nipple line. Generally, central wounds may involve the heart and great vessels, the trachea and main stem bronchi, the esophagus, and the spinal cord. Lower wounds should alert the ED to potential injuries to the liver, spleen, pancreas, vascular structures, and the diaphragm. However, entry and exit wound sites may not predict the actual trajectory of the injury, and all transmediastinal wounds (i.e., when the trajectory of the wound traverses the mediastinum) should be treated as central

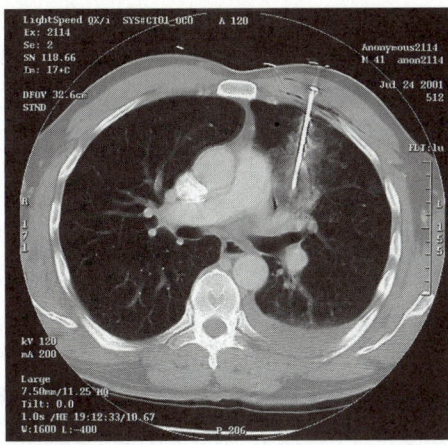

FIGURE 170.1 Computed tomography scan of the chest in a patient who sustained a nail gun injury to the left chest. Pulmonary contusion and hemorrhage are evident on the CT scan.

wounds. Peripheral wounds are defined as lateral to the midclavicular line, with the upper and lower boundaries defined by the tip of the scapula posteriorly and the sixth intercostal space laterally.

The patient's presentation may vary from minimal signs and symptoms requiring observation only to cardiac arrest requiring airway control, massive resuscitation, and ED thoracotomy. With upper peripheral wounds, patients may present with signs and symptoms of a pneumothorax or hemothorax. Instability is likely secondary to hemorrhage or tension pneumothorax. Tube thoracostomy is often the definitive treatment except in 5% to 10% of cases where operative thoracotomy is required. Urgent thoracotomy is indicated for massive and ongoing hemorrhage, a persistent air leak, or an esophageal injury. Hemodynamically stable patients with initially normal chest radiograph are observed for delayed hemothorax and/or pneumothorax. Patients with stab wounds should have a repeat hematocrit and chest radiograph 3 hours after arrival. Approximately 90% of these studies are expected to be normal, and these patients can be discharged from the ED. Patients with peripheral gunshot wounds are usually admitted and observed for longer periods of time. Close range gunshot wounds are often grossly contaminated and have extensive tissue damage; thus, operative intervention is generally required.

Patients with centrally located wounds tend to have serious injuries to vital organs requiring surgical intervention. The majority of unstable patients have either cardiac tamponade or exsanguinating hemorrhage from cardiac or great vessel injuries. Pericardial tamponade is most often associated with stab wounds to the chest. The classic findings of Beck's triad, *pulsus paradoxus,* and Kussmaul's sign are seldom present and not helpful in ED diagnosis of acute pericardial tamponade from penetrating trauma. Ultrasonography has been proven useful in the rapid diagnosis of significant pericardial effusion, and, if positive, pericardiocentesis followed by definitive pericardiotomy in the operating room is needed. ED pericardiocentesis should be performed only on patients in extremis or if time

to operating room management is prolonged. It should be performed as a temporizing therapeutic procedure, and not as a diagnostic procedure, because pericardiocentesis has an accuracy of about 50%. ED thoracotomy has been shown to improve survival in the presence of penetrating chest injuries under specific circumstances. Patients who sustained low-velocity injuries (e.g., stab wounds) with rapidly deteriorating vital signs in the ED have the highest survival rates. Patients with injuries from blunt trauma and those with penetrating injuries without signs of life or vital signs in the field have no meaningful recovery; hence, ED thoracotomy should not be performed. Patients with penetrating trauma who arrest at the scene or en route requiring prolonged cardiopulmonary resuscitation also have near 100% mortality following ED thoracotomy.

Stable patients with penetrating injuries to the central thoracic areas require extensive workup. Various combinations of angiography, esophagoscopy, and bronchoscopy may be warranted depending on clinical presentation. These patients should be carefully monitored for any sudden deterioration, and immediate intervention should be readily available. Given the potential for life-threatening injuries to vital organs, these patients should be admitted for observation pending the results of these diagnostic studies.

Patients with penetrating wounds in the thoracoabdominal region, either central or peripheral, need to be evaluated for intraabdominal and diaphragmatic injuries. Gunshot wounds involving the abdomen should be explored in the operating room. Hemodynamically unstable patients also need surgical intervention. Depending on the patient's presentation and clinical status, workup on the subset of stable patients may include diagnostic peritoneal lavage and/or CT of the abdomen, intravenous pyelography, or contrast-enhanced CT enema. Simple observation has also been advocated for patients with asymptomatic stab wounds to the thoracoabdominal regions.

Impalement injuries to the chest involve either attachment of the patient to the impaling object or retained foreign body (e.g., a knife) at the site of the wound. If at all possible, patients should be transported with the foreign body in place so as not to disturb the tamponade effect and risk uncontrolled bleeding in the field. These objects should be removed in the operating room under a controlled environment.

Fractures

Rib Fractures

Studies have reported a 4% to 10% incidence of rib fractures in all trauma patients admitted to level 2 and nontrauma centers. Since rib fractures are often missed on radiograph, the actual incidence is probably higher. Most rib fractures are caused by motor vehicle accidents, followed by falls and athletics injuries. Studies by automotive safety engineers have defined the point of maximal weakness of the thoracic cage at 60-degree rotation from the sternum. This has important implications, as 32% of passenger car fatalities occur in lateral impact crashes. There are two unique types of rib injuries associated with sports. First rib fracture at the shallow groove where the subclavian artery passes over the bone has been associated with throwing injuries, postulated secondary to powerful contraction of the scalene muscles. Floating rib (ribs 11-12) fractures are avulsion fractures of the attachments of the external oblique muscles. Minimal or no trauma can also lead to rib fractures in patients with severe osteopenia or bony metastases.

In some instances, rib fractures may be a marker for severe injuries. The presence of three or more rib fractures on radiograph has been identified by some as an indication for tertiary care. One study showed mortality doubled from those without rib fracture to those with three or more. Mortality is also significantly increased in the elderly and the young. Associated increased incidences in pulmonary contusion, cardiac injury, splenic and hepatic injuries, pneumothorax, hemothorax, and flail chest have been noted. Of note, increased incidence of aortic injury has not been associated with either first or second rib fractures or multiple rib fractures.

Point tenderness over fracture site, bony crepitus, splinting, and pain with movement, respiration, and cough are all hallmarks of rib fractures. Compression in the anteroposterior or lateral directions away from the injured site can cause severe pain. Pulse oximetry should be obtained and arterial blood gas may be necessary depending on the degree of respiratory distress and underlying pulmonary disease. Cardiac monitoring or ECG may be obtained if cardiac injury is suspected. Chest radiograph may miss 30% to 50% of rib fractures. The upright posteroanterior projection provides the highest yield. Rib radiographs are rarely indicated. The chest radiograph should be evaluated for pneumothorax, hemothorax, pulmonary contusion, mediastinal hematoma, subcutaneous emphysema, and rib fractures. Fractures of the rib cartilage and costochondral dislocation are not seen by chest radiograph.

If two or more adjacent rib fractures are present, a flail segment may be present and should be evaluated accordingly. Fracture of four or more ribs should trigger a search for potential severe intrathoracic injuries. If ribs 7 to 12 are involved, intraabdominal injuries need to be ruled out. Fracture of ribs 1 or 2 does not automatically require arteriography. Recent studies have not shown an association between isolated fracture of rib 1 or 2 and thoracic aortic injury. However, there may be some increased incidence of subclavian artery injury with first and second rib fractures. Further studies should be guided by evidence of neurovascular deficits and significant fracture displacements.

Atelectasis and pneumonia are potential complications of rib fractures. Aggressive pain management ranging from oral analgesics to intercostal blocks to thoracic epidural may be used depending on the patient's needs. Pulmonary toilet consisting of deep breathing, postural drainage, incentive spirometry, and chest physiotherapy are mandatory in order to lower the risk of postinjury pneumonia. Bronchodilator has also been advocated. A return to modified usual daily activity is preferred over strict bed rest. Binders, tapes, and other restrictive devices are not recommended. Hospital admission should be considered for the young and the elderly, those with other debilitating comorbid diseases, and those with multiple rib fractures. A stay at an observation unit may be warranted in order to optimize pain management, pulmonary toilet, and monitor for potential development of pulmonary contusion.

Sternal Fractures

The incidence of sternal fractures ranges from 3% to 15% of blunt chest trauma; 58% to 80% occur in the upper or midportion of the sternum. The mechanism involves either a direct blow to the anterior chest or hyperflexion. An association with steering wheel impact has been established. A great amount of force is required to fracture the sternum and hence an isolated sternal fracture is rare. It has been reported that a 75% incidence of head trauma is associated with sternal fracture. Two thirds of sternal fractures have associated injuries including myocardial contusion, pulmonary contusion, head injury, ruptured diaphragm, flail chest, and sternal clavicular dislocation. Controversy exists regarding the association of blunt cardiac injury with sternal fracture. Reported association ranges from 18% to 62%. This may be due to the variability in diagnostic criteria as well as the extent to which these injuries are suspected. Interestingly, recent studies have not shown any established relationship between sternal injury and thoracic aortic injury. Sternal fracture is often missed in the presence of more severe associated injuries. Mortality is 25% to 45% and is secondary to the associated injuries.

The diagnosis of sternal fracture is clinical. The patient complains of severe chest pain. Inspection of the anterior chest wall may show bruising and deformity. Palpation of the injured site may define a step off or crepitus. A lateral supine radiographic view of the chest establishes the diagnosis and can be easily obtained on a recumbent trauma patient. Chest CT scan may be needed to assess for sternal clavicular dislocation, which is associated with more severe injuries. Given the potential high association with blunt trauma to the heart, an ECG should be obtained and, if abnormal, cardiac echocardiography may be warranted.

Patients with an isolated nondisplaced sternal fracture and a normal ECG can be treated with aggressive pain management and cardiac monitoring for 6 to 12 hours postinjury to rule out significant arrhythmia prior to discharge. Twenty-four–hour admission to an observation unit should be strongly considered. In patients with displaced or overriding sternal fractures, surgical consultation should be obtained, as early operative fixation may be indicated. These patients are at higher risks for other associated injuries and evaluation should be guided by clinical presentation. They should be admitted to an inpatient monitored bed for continued observation, evaluation, and treatment of associated injuries.

Flail Chest

Flail chest is defined as fracture of two or more adjacent ribs at two or more locations each. Functionally it is defined by a loss of chest wall stability with paradoxical inward chest movement of the flail segment with inspiration and outward movement with expiration. This pathologic motion results in ineffective respiration and an increased work of breathing. More importantly, association of this injury with parenchymal injury of the lungs and pulmonary contusion is reportedly greater than 50%. One study shows that the mortality of pulmonary contusion or flail chest alone is 16% whereas the mortality increases to 42% when both are present. Patients with moderate-to-severe pulmonary contusions associated with flail chest have an increased risk of pneumonia as compared to those with lesser parenchymal damage. Elderly patients, with their less compliant chest and increased likelihood of underlying disease, have an increased risk of complication and fatality.

Flail chest is diagnosed by inspection and palpation. However, this is one of the most commonly missed chest injuries with up to 30% missed in the initial 6 hours. A high index of suspicion is needed with the examiner looking actively for signs and symptoms of this potentially life-threatening injury. The patient should be completely disrobed and the chest inspected for paradoxical chest movements. A light directed tangentially across the chest wall may assist in the evaluation. The chest should then be palpated for tenderness and crepitus. Paradoxical movement may not be apparent in patients with hypotension and splinting or in intubated patients. The examiner may also be distracted by other more obvious injuries. Chest radiograph should be evaluated for multiple rib fractures, pulmonary contusion, hemothorax, pneumothorax, subcutaneous emphysema, and mediastinum hematoma. Pulse oximetry and arterial blood gas should be obtained. ECG and cardiac monitoring may be needed if cardiac injuries are suspected.

There has been significant controversy regarding the treatment of flail chest over the past 40 years. It has evolved from mandatory mechanical stabilization to internal stabilization by intubation to the currently advocated trend of selective intubation with aggressive pulmonary toilet and pain management. Pain control can be achieved by patient-controlled analgesia, intercostal nerve blocks, intrapleural catheters, and epidural catheters. Depending on the patient's condition, pulmonary toilet ranges from frequent suctioning, postural drainage, chest therapy, and incentive spirometry, to bronchoscopy. Some have advocated mechanical ventilation when PaO_2 is less than 60 mm Hg in room air or less than 80 mm Hg with supplemental oxygen. However, effective pain control, correction of underlying hemothorax and/or pneumothorax, and a trial of continuous positive airway pressure (CPAP) may eliminate the need for intubation. Intubation is recommended in patients with shock or closed head injury, patients requiring immediate operation, patients with severe initial pulmonary dysfunction, and patients with deteriorating pulmonary status. Placement of chest tube on the side of multiple fractures is recommended in intubated patients. Judicious resuscitation aimed at euvolemia is important. There are currently no data to support the use of steroid or prophylactic antibiotic coverage. Given the significant morbidity and mortality of this injury, all these patients should be admitted initially to an ICU setting.

Clavicular Fracture and Dislocation

Clavicular fracture is usually secondary to a fall or direct blow to the clavicle. These fractures most commonly occur in the middle third of the clavicle. In the context of major chest trauma, clavicular fracture is associated with pneumothorax, hemothorax, and ipsilateral humeral and scapula fractures. Patients need to be evaluated for injury to the subclavian vessels and the brachial plexus. Callus formation at the fracture site may compress these structures. A pseudoaneurysm of the subclavian artery has been reported after clavicular fracture. Traumatic dislocation of the sternoclavicular joint is unusual because of the density of the ligamentous attachments and it represents fewer than 1% of all dislocations. It is most commonly secondary to massive direct trauma to the anterior chest wall driving the medial end of the clavicle posteriorly or posterolaterally. Posterior dislocation is clinically relevant due to its association with manubrium fracture and the proximity to the innominate vessels and the trachea.

Diagnosis of clavicular fracture is clinical. The patient is inspected for the presence of hematoma, ecchymosis, and deformity. Severe point tenderness, crepitus, and asymmetry of the clavicles are noted on palpation. Displaced fractures are easily recognized on chest radiographs. Nondisplaced fractures require special angled frontal views. Dislocation is difficult to diagnose by chest radiograph and is best evaluated with one or two axial CT scan images through the level of the sternoclavicular joints.

Most clavicular fractures can be managed nonoperatively by either a sling or a figure-eight brace. Nonunion is rare. Immobilization and pain control is the mainstay of therapy. In dislocation of the sternoclavicular joint, reduction under conscious sedation or anesthesia is usually indicated. In posterior dislocation, tracheal injury with near-complete airway obstruction may be present. Emergent manual reduction with a sandbag or rolled towel under the upper thoracic spine may be needed.

Thoracic Aortic Disruption

Approximately 15% to 23% of victims of motor vehicle accidents in the United States each year have rupture of the thoracic aorta at autopsy. The mechanism of injury is classically attributed to severe horizontal deceleration (i.e., high-speed, head-on collision, and ejection from a vehicle), which creates shear forces at the aortic isthmus, the junction between the relatively mobile aortic arch and the fixed descending aorta. Recently, a higher incidence of thoracic aortic injury (*T-bone collision*) has been noted in victims involved in severe broadside collisions than has been previously suspected. These injuries have also been associated with vertical deceleration from falls from great heights. Other causes include external cardiac massage, fracture dislocation of the thoracic spine, direct kick by animals, and displaced fractures of the sternum, ribs, and clavicles causing direct laceration of the aorta. Of note, recent reviews of the data have not demonstrated an increased risk of thoracic aortic disruption with isolated first or second rib fracture or with sternal fractures. However, four- and ninefold increases in aortic rupture have been noted with pelvic fracture and anteroposterior compression-type pelvic fracture, respectively.

Rupture of the thoracic aorta through the intima, media, and adventitia results in exsanguination and immediate death in 75% to 90% of cases. Those who survive have maintained integrity of the adventitia or have fragile perivascular hematoma around the injured site and are at risk for complete rupture. Autopsy data from 1958 have shown that without repair, 12.5% to 20% of initial survivors will die within 6 hours, 30% will die within 24 hours, and more than 50% will die within 1 week of initial rupture; 70% to 86% of injuries occur at the aortic isthmus, just distal to the left subclavian artery, 13% to 20% have injuries in multiple aortic sites, and 8% to 23% have injuries to the ascending aorta and the aortic arch.

The clinical presentation of aortic disruption is varied. Complete open rupture presents in traumatic arrest. Rupture of the ascending arch into the pericardium may present as cardiac tamponade. The patient with aortic disruption may also present without any external evidence of chest trauma (up to 50%) and with normal vital signs. Chest pain, midscapular back pain, and shortness of breath are the most common symptoms. Stridor or hoarseness and dysphagia are uncommon but may result from compression of the laryngeal nerve and esophagus, respectively. Extremity pain due to ischemia and lower extremity paralysis may occur as dissection progresses. On physical examination, generalized hypertension may be seen secondary to stretching of aortic sympathetic fibers. Pseudocoarctation or decreased blood pressure in the left arm occurs in only 5% of patients with disruption of the aortic isthmus. Upper extremity hypertension with diminished femoral pulses has been described but is absent in most cases. A harsh systolic murmur may be heard over the precordium or posterior interscapular area. Precordial ecchymosis may be evident in 12% to 43% of patients.

The chest radiograph is the best initial screening test for aortic disruption, and if the patient is hemodynamically stable and there is no vertebral injury, a posteroanterior upright chest film should be obtained. Significant discrepancy exists regarding the value of chest radiographic signs in detecting aortic injury. An increased width in the mediastinum is found in 50% to 92% of aortic rupture, with a specificity ranging from 10% to 59% (see Chapter 163, Figure 163.1). A subjective interpretation of mediastinal widening is more reliable than direct measurement. Various authors have advocated using various groupings of radiographic signs to improve on reliability. One source found loss of the aortic knob outline, loss of the descending aortic outline, and widening of the mediastinum to be most predictive, whereas another group believes that shift of nasogastric tube to the right, shift of the trachea to the right, and downward shift of the left main stem bronchus to be statistically significant findings. A normal chest radiograph does not exclude an aortic injury, as one study showed that 7% of patients with

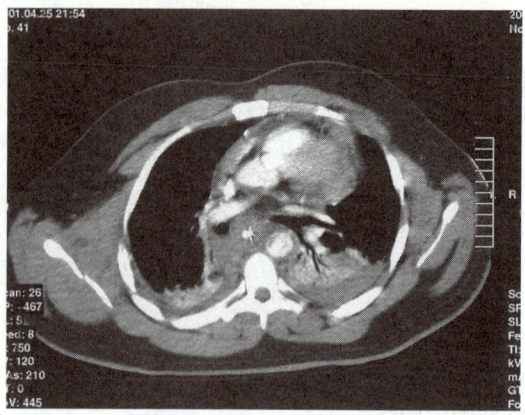

FIGURE 170.2 Computed tomography scan of the chest in blunt thoracic trauma revealing intimal disruption in the lumen of the aorta.

aortic injury had a normal mediastinum on chest radiograph. Other diagnostic options include: routine CT scan, helical or spiral CT scan (**FIGURE 170.2**), transesophageal echocardiography (TEE), digital subtraction angiography (DSA), and biplane aortography.

The arch aortogram remains the gold standard, but the procedure entails a significant time delay (**FIGURE 170.3**). It is the most accurate in detecting and localizing tears in the thoracic aorta. DSA has been the diagnostic study of choice in many institutions as it requires less time and less contrast material. Nevertheless, there is concern about its sensitivity in visualizing small intimal flaps. TEE can be performed quickly and in the resuscitation areas. However, one recent study showed a sensitivity of 63% and a specificity of 84% in TEE performed by staff cardiologists to evaluate for aortic injury in blunt trauma patient. Given the time sensitivity and significant morbidity and mortality of these injuries, additional studies are needed before this modality can be used to rule out aortic injury. Its role in patients with facial trauma and cervical spine injuries

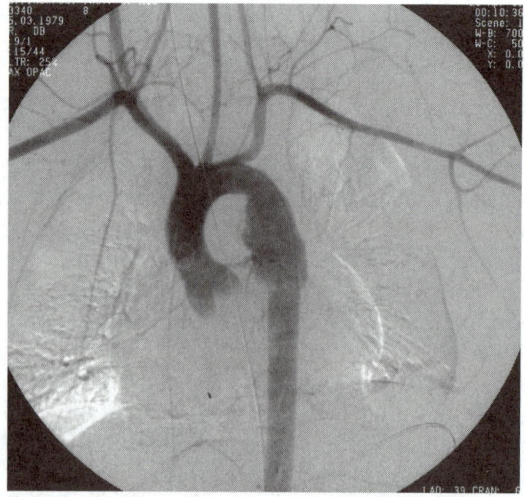

FIGURE 170.3 Arch aortography in blunt thoracic trauma with aortic injury. There is pseudoaneurysmal disruption of the aorta at the descending portion of the aortic arch (beyond the left subclavian artery).

also needs to be addressed. The use of conventional CT to evaluate aortic injury is controversial. Technical limitations due to slice thickness, motion artifacts, and artifacts from nasogastric and endotracheal tubes can make intimal defects difficult to see. Its use should be limited to stable patients with an equivocal chest radiograph when the mechanism and clinical suspicion is low for traumatic thoracic aortic injury. Helical CT can more precisely delineate arterial lesions, and in one prospective study where 1,518 helical CT scans were performed and follow-up aortography was done in those with an abnormal mediastinum or aorta, helical CT scan reportedly had 100% sensitivity and 81.7% specificity as compared to 94.4% and 96.3%, respectively, for aortogram. However, the negative predictive value of this modality for aortic injury has not been defined.

After initial resuscitation and stabilization, medical treatment aimed at controlling or reducing stress on the aortic wall should be instituted in patients with suspected aortic injury. Such treatments include treatment of hypertension, adequate sedation and pain control, and spine immobilization. Aortography should be performed emergently. Surgery is indicated for definitive repair of most arterial lesions. Nonoperative management has been reported with increasing frequency since 1981, and is recommended only for patients with severe neurological deficit or multiorgan system failure, or in those with benign lesions (e.g., small intimal defect alone or without significant false aneurysm).

Blunt Cardiac Injury (Myocardial Contusion)

Blunt cardiac injury is characterized by patchy areas of muscle necrosis and hemorrhagic infiltrate that is recognizable at surgery or autopsy. It covers a spectrum of cellular damage ranging from microscopic changes to massive tissue necrosis. The lack of standard diagnostic criteria other than pathological has led to large variability in its reported incidence and in the sensitivity and specificity of diagnostic studies for blunt cardiac injury. The reported incidence varies from 3% to 76% in studies of blunt chest trauma. The clinical significance of blunt cardiac injury is also unclear. A wide variety of atrial and ventricular dysrhythmias has been associated with blunt cardiac injury. Most related events are nonfatal arrhythmias, and aggressive pursuit of this diagnosis with costly and time-consuming tests in hemodynamically stable and asymptomatic patients is not warranted. Transient reduction in cardiac output may be seen in 50% to 75% of patients with significant myocardial contusion. However, cardiac failure is rare. The mortality and morbidity of blunt cardiac injury is closely correlated with the severity of other associated injuries. Complications include thromboembolism from mural thrombus, myocardial rupture, cardiac tamponade, ventricular aneurysm, and constrictive pericarditis. Mechanisms of injury include a direct blow to the heart, crush injury between the thoracic spine and the sternum, and increased intrathoracic pressure transmitted against a closed glottis.

Symptoms are variable and may be masked by the presence of other injuries. Most patients complain of nonpleuritic chest pain. Reportedly, 73% of patients have external evidence of chest trauma. Tachycardia is the most common sign of blunt cardiac injury and is seen in about 70% of these patients. Palpation of the chest wall may reveal crepitus and tenderness. Auscultation may reveal a new murmur or a friction rub.

Electrocardiography is neither sensitive nor specific for blunt cardiac injury. It is relatively insensitive to right ventricular damage and can remain normal despite pathologic evidence of injury. In addition, up to 50% of patients with abnormal ECG have other etiologies for the abnormalities. The relative risk of dysrhythmia as a function of ECG changes is not currently known. Hence, the ECG is recommended as a screening examination in patients in whom blunt cardiac injury is suspected. Its findings should be correlated with the clinical condition of the patient.

The routine use of cardiac enzyme in patients suspected of blunt cardiac injury is not recommended. This laboratory test is neither sensitive nor specific, and its result difficult to interpret. Elevation of isoenzymes of creatine kinase with muscle and brain subunits (CK-MB) is not predictive of cardiac complications. A recent study has evaluated the use of cardiac troponin I as a marker of traumatic cardiac injury on the basis that this regulatory protein is found in cardiac tissue only and its plasma level is not affected by skeletal muscle injury. Results suggest that this test is highly sensitive; however, the clinical relevance of troponin I elevation in this clinical context is not clear. Other modalities such as radionuclide angiography and echocardiography allow for evaluation of wall motion abnormalities and, in the case of radionuclide angiography, ejection fractions of both ventricles. Both techniques are rapid, noninvasive, and can be done at the bedside, although they are usually not readily available. Again, the clinical implication of a positive study is not known, although these studies may provide a measure of cardiac output in the multiply injured patient who requires surgery.

The management of patients with suspected blunt cardiac injury has evolved in the past few years. Recent studies have shown that in young healthy patients with suspected myocardial contusion from chest trauma, clinically significant events are rare. Additionally, no life-threatening dysrhythmias have been reported beyond 12 hours. Patients may be stratified on the basis of age, underlying comorbid diseases, other associated injuries, and symptoms, and managed accordingly. Older and unstable patients, patients with prior cardiac diseases, and patients with significant ECG changes suggestive of ischemia and new conduction defects should be admitted to an ICU setting and monitored. Supplemental oxygen and analgesic should be administered. Fluid resuscitation, antiarrhythmics, and pressors are used as clinically needed. Further evaluation with echocardiography may be needed on selected patients. Stable patients younger than 45 years of age who have no prior cardiac disease, nonspecific ECG findings, and no other associated injuries may be admitted for 24 hours to an observation unit and monitored. Asymptomatic patients with a normal ECG do not need to be admitted and require no further workup.

Pulmonary Contusion

Pulmonary contusion is seen in 30% to 75% of blunt thoracic traumas, usually in motor vehicle accidents when the chest strikes the steering wheel or car door. Other mechanisms include falls from great heights, blast injuries, and nonpenetrating high-velocity missile wounds. Isolated pulmonary contusions occur less frequently than in association with other thoracic or extrathoracic injuries. Isolated pulmonary contusions have mortality estimated at 5% to 16%, whereas this can increase fivefold with even one associated extrathoracic injury. Most common complications are pneumonia and sepsis, and these significantly worsen the prognosis.

Pathologically, pulmonary contusion is defined by injuries to the alveolar-capillary walls. The extent of intraalveolar and interstitial hemorrhage depends on the degree of injury. Atelectasis and consolidation in the adjacent normal lung can occur secondary to reflex increased in mucus secretions, to blood and edema fluid in the bronchial trees, and to increase capillary permeability. Clinically, this is manifested as a decrease in lung compliance, increase in pulmonary vascular resistance, and increased alveolar-arterial oxygen difference.

Clinical presentation is variable and may range from asymptomatic, to dyspnea and tachypnea, and to hypoxic and hypercapneic, and in respiratory failure. A high index of suspicion is needed as this entity can present insidiously and evolve over a period of time. Patients may complain of shortness of breath, chest pain, or hemoptysis. Physical examination may reveal rales or decreased breath sounds. Oxygenation should be monitored with pulse oximetry. Arterial blood gas is helpful in the diagnosis of pulmonary contusion. Chest radiograph findings lag behind clinical signs and symptoms. Pulmonary contusion may present initially as a patchy irregular streaky infiltrate. This picture evolves over the next 4 to 6 hours and the rapidity of change predicts the severity of the contusion. The diagnosis can be made by chest radiograph together with clinical presentation. CT of the chest is not needed, although it may be useful in assessing other associated thoracic injuries.

Treatment of pulmonary contusion is similar to that for flail chest. Management of both disease entities has changed drastically over the last 40 years. Stabilization of the chest is no longer the goal of therapy. Respiratory support, aggressive pulmonary toilet, and pain management are the mainstay of therapy. Respiratory support varies depending on the patient's condition and may include supplemental oxygen by face mask, CPAP, or mechanical ventilation. The use of intravenous fluid resuscitation has been a matter of debate, although agreement exists that adequate resuscitation in a trauma patient is essential but that overhydration should be avoided. Clinical improve-

ment with the use of steroid has yet to be proven and its use is not recommended. Similarly, there is no role for prophylactic antibiotics.

Rupture

Esophageal Rupture

Esophageal rupture following blunt trauma is rare. Rupture of the cervical esophagus has been reported with cervical spine fracture. Most thoracic esophageal injuries occur from anteroposterior compression of the chest with simultaneous closure of the cricopharyngeal and gastroesophageal sphincters. The pathophysiology is similar to that observed for Boerhaave's syndrome. The esophagus has no serosal lining and, hence, perforation leads to direct contamination of the mediastinum. Rupture most commonly occurs in the left lateral wall of the distal thoracic esophagus where it is weakest. Spillage of contents into the mediastinum or pleural space can cause severe inflammatory responses with exudation of fluid, sepsis, and potential shock, respiratory failure, and death.

A high index of suspicion is required to diagnose esophageal injury in a traumatic patient with multiple injuries. Substernal pleuritic pain with radiation to the neck and shoulders is the most common symptom. Dysphagia, odynophagia, tachypnea, and tachycardia may also be present. As mediastinal air dissects over the heart, it may be heard as a rhythmic Hamman's crunch. As the dissection of air progresses, it may become evident as subcutaneous emphysema most commonly found in the cervical region and in the supraclavicular fossa. Palpation of these areas for crepitus is important. Late findings include fever and hypotension.

Chest radiograph should be evaluated for pneumothorax, pneumomediastinum, pleural effusion, or subcutaneous emphysema. Lateral soft tissue radiograph of the neck may show air or esophageal contents around the esophagus and the trachea. Confirmation of perforation is obtained by contrast esophagogram. In most cases, a water-soluble contrast such as Gastrografin is administered first. A barium contrast study is carried out if the initial study is negative, as it allows for better mucosal definition. Endoscopy can also be used to assess these injuries. Accuracy depends on the size and location of the perforation and the skill of the endoscopist. Early diagnosis is key to the outcome of esophageal injuries as delay results in a significant increase in mortality. Treatment consists of fluid resuscitation, broad spectrum antibiotic coverage, nasogastric decompression, and definitive surgical repair.

Diaphragm Rupture

The reported incidence of diaphragmatic rupture is reportedly 1% to 3% of patients suffering from blunt chest trauma. Between 70% and 90% of patients with blunt diaphragmatic injuries have multiple associated injuries; hence, a significant number of diaphragmatic ruptures are missed initially. Of patients undergoing laparotomy or thoracotomy for traumatic injuries, 4% to 6% have diaphragmatic injuries. Mechanism of injury is primarily from motor vehicle accidents with minor contributions from falls and crushing injuries. An increased intraabdominal or intrathoracic pressure is transmitted to the diaphragm, leading to rupture. A predominance of the rupture occurs on the left side secondary to hepatic protection on the right and the inherent weakness of the left hemidiaphragm at points of embryonic fusion. However, a more even distribution may be seen with more severe trauma.

The clinical presentation of diaphragmatic rupture may be classified by three phases depending on the time of diagnosis. The *acute phase* is defined as up to 14 days after injury and patients may complain of chest pain radiating to the left shoulder, shortness of breath, or abdominal pain. However, these signs and symptoms are often overshadowed by other findings, and the diaphragmatic defect is often discovered during laparotomy or thoracotomy undertaken for associated injuries. If the diagnosis is not made during the initial hospitalization, the disease progresses to the latent phase. Patients may be either asymptomatic or have chronic or intermittent vague abdominal pain. These symptoms are often worse after meals and are exacerbated in the supine position. This phase may last from months to years until complications develop and the disease progresses to the obstructive phase. In the *obstructive phase,* herniated viscera become strangulated and may progress to ischemia, necrosis, and perforation with ensuing sepsis and death. A mortality rate of 30% has been noted in patients who present in the late obstructive phase.

Radiograph of the chest is helpful in the diagnosis of 40% to 50% of patients with diaphragmatic hernia. However, initial radiograph may be normal in 25% of these patients. Chest film should be reviewed for bowel gas, loops of bowels, and the tip of the nasogastric tube above the diaphragm. Pleural effusion, pneumothorax, elevated hemidiaphragm, or small mediastinal shift may be evident. CT scan and ultrasound have not proven useful. MRI allows for better visualization but is difficult to access. The recommended study is barium upper GI series or barium enema to demonstrate bowel above the diaphragm or points of obstruction. Diagnostic peritoneal lavage is often performed in these patients, but reportedly 15% to 25% of diaphragmatic ruptures are missed even if 5,000 red blood cells are considered a positive result for rupture. Liver and spleen scans can be obtained when herniation of these organs is suspected.

Once the diagnosis is established, surgical treatment should be promptly instituted but should not precede more urgent diagnostic or therapeutic measures for other associated injuries. A nasogastric tube should be passed for decompression. In patients presenting in the obstructive phase, airway management, fluid resuscitation, and broad-spectrum antibiotics may be needed as operative management is being arranged.

Tracheobronchial Tree Injuries

Tracheobronchial injury is seen in 1% to 2% of patients sustaining blunt trauma, and in less than 1% of blunt thoracic trauma. It has been reported that 75% to 100% of these patients have associated injuries, particularly concomitant esophageal and spinal column injuries. Combined tracheobronchial and great vessel injuries are rare. Postulated mechanisms of injury include rapid deceleration causing shear forces at sites of fixation, increased compressive intrathoracic pressures leading to lateral traction on the carina, and compression of the airway between the sternum and the vertebral column against a closed glottis leading to increased intrabronchial pressures. About 80% of these injuries occur near the carina (approximately 1 inch or 2.5 cm from the carina), at the distal trachea, or near the origin of a main stem bronchus. Mortality depends on the extent of the injury and the severity of other associated injuries, but overall mortality has been reported as 30% and mortality in the first hour as 50%.

Clinical presentation varies depending on the location of the injury. Rupture of the proximal trachea may cause airway obstruction and hemoptysis. Disruption of the distal trachea and proximal main stem bronchi, which are extrapleural, can present with mediastinal, subcutaneous, and cervical emphysema. The respiratory trees distal to the proximal main stem bronchi are intrapleural, and rupture of these may cause a pneumothorax that persists despite correctly placed tube thoracostomy. Patients may present with dyspnea, dysphonia, hoarseness, subcutaneous emphysema, and hemoptysis. Most patients do not present with respiratory distress; hence, a high index of suspicion is needed, and the ED physician or trauma surgeon should actively search for the above signs and symptoms. Chest and soft tissue of the neck radiographs should be reviewed for pneumothorax, pneumomediastinum, deep cervical emphysema, subcutaneous emphysema, and abnormal placement of the orotracheal tube. The constellation of persistent pneumothorax, massive air leak, and atelectatic lung in the presence of a well-placed, functioning tube thoracostomy is highly specific for intrathoracic airway rupture. Although small lesions may be missed, fiberoptic bronchoscopy is the diagnostic tool of choice for tracheobronchial injuries.

Treatment of these injuries, as in all traumas, should follow ATLS protocol with immediate attention to ABCs (airway, breathing, circulation). Patients with respiratory distress and hemoptysis should be intubated with a fiberoptic bronchoscope if conditions permit. If this is unsuccessful, a surgical airway is required. Tension pneumothorax (a clinical diagnosis that should not delay treatment by obtaining a CXR), should be immediately treated with needle thoracocentesis followed by tube thoracostomy. Stable pneumothorax can be treated with tube thoracostomy. Persistent air leak may require selective intubation of the uninvolved bronchus followed by operative repair of the lesion.

Pneumothorax

The lung is held fully expanded against the chest wall with negative pressure within the potential space between the visceral and parietal pleura. Air entering this space results in a pneumothorax, which collapses lung tissues and results in a ventilatory and perfusion defect, because blood circulated to the area of collapsed lung is not oxygenated.

Simple Pneumothorax

A pneumothorax is defined as *simple* or *closed* when there is no communication between the atmosphere and the pleural space. A leak from the lung results in air entry into the potential pleural space. This is most often seen in association with rib fractures after blunt chest trauma or from compressive impact to the chest against a closed glottis, resulting in a sudden increase in intraalveolar pressure.

The clinical presentation is variable. Most common complaints are shortness of breath and sharp chest pain, with the degree of dyspnea dependent on the patient's underlying health and pulmonary reserve. Physical examination may reveal decreased breath sounds on auscultation and hyperresonance on percussion over the involved side. Subcutaneous emphysema may also be evident. The chest radiograph confirms the diagnosis. If the patient's condition permits, an initial upright inspiratory film should be obtained and, if negative, should be followed by an expiratory film. A pneumothorax is defined as small if it occupies less than 15% of the pleural cavity, a moderate one is between 15% and 60%, and a large one is greater than 60%.

In the absence of other complications, patients with a small pneumothorax who are asymptomatic, otherwise healthy, and not requiring general anesthesia or positive pressure ventilation can safely be observed in the hospital without tube thoracostomy. Any respiratory compromise or increase in the size of the pneumothorax would mandate immediate placement of a chest tube. Other indications for tube thoracostomy are moderate to large pneumothorax, symptomatic patients, recurrence of pneumothorax after chest tube removal, associated hemothorax, bilateral pneumothoraces, and tension pneumothorax.

Open Pneumothorax

A pneumothorax is defined as open when there is direct communication between the atmosphere and the pleural space. In some instances, air can be heard rushing in and out of the defect, thus the name *sucking chest wound*. These defects of the chest wall are often associated with penetrating trauma and when they are larger than approximately two-thirds the diameter of the trachea, air passes preferentially through the defect, causing severe ventilatory disturbances.

Initial treatment requires occlusion of the chest wall defect with an occlusive dressing taped on three sides, providing a flutter-type valve effect, thus converting an open pneumothorax to a closed one. The dressing should be applied at end expiration to evacuate as much air as possible from the pleural cavity. Care should be taken to avoid completely sealing the dressing as this can convert the injury into a tension pneumothorax. A chest tube should then be placed away from the wound site to re-expand the lung. Definitive surgical repair of the chest wall defect is usually required.

Tension Pneumothorax

A tension pneumothorax occurs when a one-way-valve air leak results from injury to the lung or from a chest wall de-

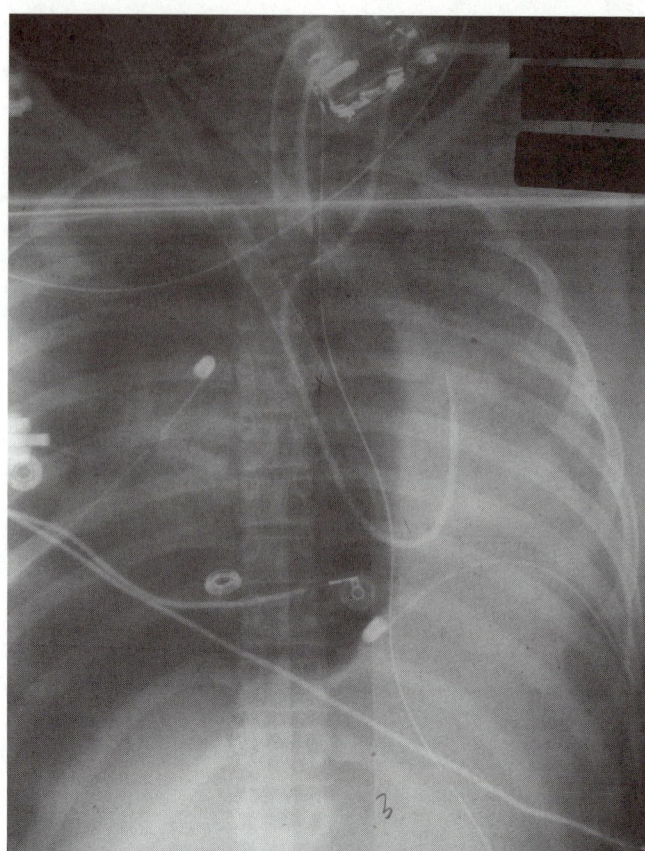

FIGURE 170.4 Tension pneumothorax in an ICU patient. A large pneumothorax on the right side has shifted the mediastinum to the left, compressed the left lung, and in doing so, has resulted in hypotension and a life-threatening emergency.

fect. Progressive accumulation of air in the pleural cavity produces collapse of the ipsilateral lung, contralateral shift of the mediastinum, and increase in intrapleural pressure, leading to a decrease in venous return. Mechanism of injury is similar to those causing simple and open pneumothoraces. Clinically, the patient often experiences progressive dyspnea, tachycardia, cyanosis, and ultimately, vascular and respiratory collapse (**FIGURE 170.4**).

The physical signs of patients with tension pneumothorax are usually striking. Patients are tachycardic, tachypneic, with tracheal shift away from the affected side, and absent breath sounds with hyperresonance on the ipsilateral side. Hypoxemia is noted early on and hypotension and pulseless electrical activity (PEA) are likely preterminal events. If the diagnosis is suspected clinically, needle decompression of the affected side should be carried out immediately, followed by tube thoracostomy. A chest radiograph is not needed for the diagnosis of tension pneumothorax.

Hemothorax

Hemothorax results from the accumulation of blood in the potential pleural space. It can present as a complication of either blunt or penetrating chest trauma and is often associated with other injuries. The extent of blood loss depends on the source of bleeding, which may be from the chest wall, the parenchyma of the lung, the great vessels, or the heart. Bleeding from the chest wall and the lung parenchyma is likely self-limited, whereas those from the arteries and the heart are likely to require operative management.

Physical presentation is variable depending on the size of the hemothorax. The patient may be asymptomatic or in hypovolemic shock. Tachypnea and dyspnea may be present secondary to other associated injuries such as a pneumothorax or fractured ribs or mediastinal shift from a massive hemothorax. Patients may have diminished or absent breath sounds on auscultation and dullness on percussion. If the patient's clinical condition permits, an upright chest radiograph is preferred. Blunting of the costophrenic angles requires at least 250 to 500 mL of fluid in the upright position. Chest radiograph in the supine position, which is the study most often obtained in the acute situation, is less accurate in the diagnosis of hemothorax, but should be suspected if the hemithoraces are grayish in appearance with a mechanism consistent with the clinical picture.

Treatment of significant hemothorax requires simultaneous resuscitation and drainage of the accumulated blood. A large bore chest tube (sizes 36 to 40 French) should be placed and autotransfusion devices used, if available. The initial amount drained and the rate of continued bleeding dictate either conservative management or thoracotomy. If 1,000 to 1,500 mL is immediately evacuated, an immediate thoracotomy should be carried out to locate and treat the source of hemorrhage. If bleeding continues at greater than 200 mL/h for more than 4 hours, or if bleeding increases with time, or if the patient remains hypotensive or deteriorates despite adequate resuscitation and in the absence of any other source of hemorrhage, a thoracotomy should also be performed immediately. It is also important to optimize a patient's coagulopathy during the resuscitation as acidemia and hypothermia profoundly contribute to ongoing blood loss.

Selected Readings

Advanced Trauma Life Support (ATLS) for Doctors, 6th ed . Chicago: The American College of Surgeons, 2004.

Mirvis SE, Shanmuganthan K, eds. *Imaging in Trauma and Critical Care,* 2d ed. Basel: Elsevier Science, 2003.

Moore EE, Feliciano DV, Mattox KL, eds. *Trauma,* 5th ed. New York: McGraw-Hill Professional, 2004.

Mark L. Shapiro

The patient with abdominal trauma may present a diagnostic and management challenge to even the most experienced physician. Both history and physical examination, usually the cornerstone of the diagnostic process, may be equivocal or even misleading. The physician must use, or at least consider, all of the tools available including history, physical examination, labs, radiographs, CT scan, angiography, ultrasonography, contrast studies, diagnostic peritoneal lavage (DPL), diagnostic laparoscopy, exploratory laparotomy, and—most importantly—vigilant observation. The goal of evaluation and management is focused solely on resuscitation and recognition of the need for surgical intervention as opposed to specific diagnosis of injuries. These patients have the potential for significant morbidity and mortality, and missing any injury, not being quick enough, or not being aggressive enough with treatment could have serious implications for the patient. An organized, efficient, and effective approach to these clinical situations can substantially alter morbidity and mortality risks as well as increase hospital resource utilization and reduce health care costs.

Blunt trauma may involve a variety of possible mechanisms including motorcycle accidents, motorcycle accidents, pedestrian accidents, bicycle accidents, falls, assaults, or sports injuries. There are multiple biomechanical mechanisms involved in injuries, including direct impact, deceleration injury (traction beyond the capacity of a fixed point in the body), and crush injury. Penetrating injuries may be from gunshot wounds (handguns, rifles, shotguns) or stabbing with a knife or other pointed, sharp object capable of impaling the body. Glass fragments, scissors, ice picks, screwdrivers, and other objects may result in serious injury. Penetrating injuries may also occur secondary to explosive or blast injuries that may be occupation or home related, such as firecracker accidents, homemade bombs, and explosives. Multiple forces are involved in these injuries including direct missile penetration, missile fragment disbursement, after the initial penetration, and subsequent cavitation that secondarily damage surrounding tissues of organs with high water content (i.e., liver, spleen, and kidney).

The most frequently injured organ following blunt trauma is the spleen (46%), with liver injuries being the second most frequent (33%). Certain situations are considered risk factors for significant intra-abdominal injury with hypotension, acidosis, respiratory insufficiency, and depressed mental status being obvious clues to pending instability. In addition, certain injury patterns are significantly associated with intra-abdominal injury including pelvic ring disruption, abdominal wall injury, femoral fracture, hip dislocation, head injury, or any intrathoracic injury.

Anatomical Considerations

Assessment of the abdomen is influenced by its anatomical features and may be conceptualized as four distinct regions: the intrathoracic abdomen, the true abdomen, the pelvic region, and the retroperitoneal abdomen. The *intrathoracic abdomen* lies beneath the rib cage and, encompasses the diaphragm, liver, spleen, and stomach. Injury to the lower ribs necessitates ruling out injury to these organs. The accessibility of this area to palpation is severely limited and complicates its evaluation. The *pelvic abdomen* contains the urinary bladder, urethra, rectum, small intestine, and gynecological organs. Although the bony pelvis protects this area to a certain extent, it also predisposes these structures to injury when pelvic fracture exists. The physical examination is often unreliable in this area, and minimal findings are likely even in situations of serious injury. The *retroperitoneal area* includes the kidneys, ureters, pancreas, aorta, vena cava, and two thirds of the duodenum. In all of these anatomical areas, other ancillary tests which may aid in diagnosis include IVP, upper gastrointestinal contrast studies, cystography, angiography, and CT scanning; however, the FAST exam and DPL will not assess the retroperitoneum. Finally, the *true abdomen* (the middle free portion of the abdomen), is more accessible to the examiner and injury in this anatomic area more reliably manifests with pain and abnormalities on examination.

Initial Stabilization

The fluid used to resuscitate a patient with abdominal trauma should initially be crystalloid, reserving blood products for hypotensive patients not responding adequately to crystalloid. Although multiple fluid types have been studied, lactated Ringer's is considered the ideal solution as demonstrated by Velanovich in 1989 and later by Choi in 1999 in prospective investigation.

With a pH of physiologic proportions and isotonic, this fluid is most compatible with resuscitation of the head injured as well. Issues such as hyperchloremic metabolic acidosis are obviated with large fluid resuscitations with 0.9% NS. However, many centers are looking at the measurable benefits of hypertonic saline for resuscitation. In fact, this fluid has improved benefit over lactated Ringer's in recent studies looking at mortality. It remains to be seen as more institutions become comfortable with this particular fluid how it will compare over time to other traditional methods as well as which formulation will become standard (3% or 7.5% saline). One thing has been proven by many investigations: albumin has no role in initial resuscitative efforts.

Patient Symptoms and Mechanism of Injury

If symptoms are obtainable, they may include light-headedness from volume loss or pain if peritoneal irritation has occurred. Pain may be referred from the diaphragm area to the shoulder on the corresponding side (Kehr's sign) or may be referred from the retroperitoneal area to the testicle in cases of duodenal or pancreatic injury. Other symptoms may include nausea secondary to peritoneal irritation or hypovolemia and dyspnea secondary to diaphragmatic irritation, gastric distention, or herniation of intraperitoneal organs into the chest cavity. Hypotension and/or bradycardia may be due to gastric distention—a vagal reflex—from aggressive bag-valve masked ventilation.

History can also be derived from other sources including paramedics, bystanders, and family. The mechanism is the most important historical information. Motor vehicle crashes make up 75% of blunt mechanisms. Key information to seek for MVCs includes the position of the patient in the vehicle, seat belt use, interior and exterior car damage, steering wheel deformity, air bag inflation, ejection, and prehospital course (loss of consciousness, hypotension, abnormal vital signs). Interior and exterior damage, however, is not very reliable. The vehicles of today are constructed much more safely in that deceleration injuries occur over a longer period of time. This is to say that at impact, the energy is dissipated over time as well as through multiple fragments of the vehicle. This is a sharp contrast to the motor vehicles of the 1970s and earlier, when they were not made to fall apart, and actually remained intact and the high energy forces were transmitted directly to the occupants. Past medical history may be important to consider, particularly if the patient has cardiovascular disease, a coagulopathy, or is pregnant. An allergy to medication or contrast media is also important to know.

Physical Examination

The physical findings in abdominal trauma range from seemingly insignificant to profoundly unstable and require a careful, thorough, and vigilant evaluation. The ab-

dominal assessment should not be ignored in the presence of other obvious traumatic injury. Similarly, in situations of obvious abdominal trauma, it is just as critical to completely evaluate the patient for coexisting injury. Vital signs should be continuously monitored in the seriously injured patient. An early drop in blood pressure is most often due to solid visceral injury or severe pelvic fracture. Any patient with hypotension following a blunt trauma mechanism should definitely be assumed to have intraperitoneal hemorrhage until confidently excluded.

Any patient in shock, with disruption of the abdominal wall or free air below the diaphragm on the chest radiograph, should be moved to the operating room for surgical evaluation and laparotomy. Further, any patient with physical signs and symptoms compatible with peritoneal irritation, including involuntary guard, rebound tenderness, or significant abdominal tenderness, should be considered for emergent laparotomy. But even these physical signs lack 100% specificity and may be due to lower rib fracture or even thoracoabdominal wall contusions.

The physical examination is notoriously unreliable for diagnosis of intra-abdominal injury in the trauma patient. Approximately 50% of patients with significant intra-abdominal injuries do not show peritoneal signs on physical examination. The examination may be complicated by distracting injuries and psychological distress, and the nature of the abdominal pain. Although rarely there will be identifiable localized pain, the pain may be diffuse or even referred, as in the case of diaphragmatic irritation being referred to the shoulder or trapezius ridge, or pancreatic irritation being referred to the back. In alert patients with visceral injury, abdominal tenderness is present in roughly 90%. Tenderness elicited by palpation may be absent or minimal during the early stages injury; therefore, the importance of serial abdominal examinations cannot be overemphasized. A palpable mass suggests the presence of a rectus hematoma.

The physician should not forget the simple examination of the appearance of the abdomen, regardless of the mechanism. Any discoloration of the skin and subcutaneous tissues may be signs of occult intra-abdominal injury and should be noted. Although classically delayed signs, ecchymosis of the flank (Turner's sign) or periumbilical ecchymosis (Cullen's sign) strongly suggest retroperitoneal injury (**FIGURES 171.1** and **171.2**). Any other contusions are suspect as well, including seat belt marks. Abdominal injury is caused by lap seat belts themselves in

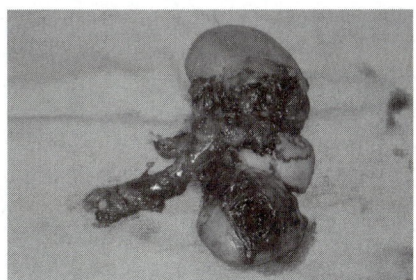

FIGURE 171.1 Dissection of kidneys and bladder following second degree blunt trauma.

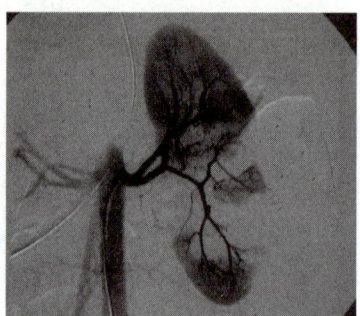

FIGURE 171.2 Angiogram showing traumatic renal fracture.

roughly one third of the cases, and most commonly results in hollow viscus injury. Abdominal distention should also be noted and considered suspicious for pneumoperitoneum or peritoneal irritation. Again, this physical observation is not specific and may be present secondary to gastric dilation or ileus, or urinary bladder distention. The physician should not overlook examination of the perineal area and back, even for patients going to the operating room emergently, because the diagnosis may affect operative management.

There may be secondary effects that present more impressively such as intestinal obstruction secondary to duodenal hematoma or, even more commonly, respiratory compromise secondary to gastric distention, diaphragm irritation, or herniation of abdominal contents into the chest cavity. For those who invest in auscultation of bowel sounds among the cacophony in the trauma bay, bowel sounds may be considered a clinical parameter of intra-abdominal injury with markedly decreased or absent bowel sounds reported in 65% to 93% of patients with visceral injury diagnosed at laparotomy. There are also other etiologies for lack of bowel sounds including ileus, as occurs with vertebral fractures, or listener error. If bowel sounds are auscultated in the thoracic cavity, diaphragmatic injury with subsequent herniation of abdominal contents into the thoracic cavity should be suspected.

A urinary catheter should be placed if urinary output needs to be quantified or if the patient is unable to void on his or her own. It must be noted if blood is present at the urethral meatus or if hematuria is present. The urinary catheter should not be placed in these patients until a urethrogram has been performed and urethral injury has been ruled out. However, if the catheter is already in place when the blood is noted, it should not be removed.

A rectal examination should also be performed prior to Foley catheter placement to rule out the presence of gross or occult blood, subcutaneous emphysema, or a high riding prostate suggesting urethral injury. If the position of the prostate is abnormal, a urethrogram should be done emergently. If blood or emphysema is found, this finding has a high correlation with intra-abdominal injury.

Unless severe maxillofacial trauma is present, a nasogastric tube is placed to decompress the stomach, evaluate for the presence of blood, and decrease the chance of aspiration. None of these physical clues is completely sensitive or specific, and, in many situations, the physician must rely more heavily on diagnostic testing. In the alert patient, active bowel sounds and a soft abdomen without distention or tenderness is reassuring for conservative management without further diagnostic endeavors. Regardless, a patient who has endured a significant injury mechanism should be followed clinically with serial abdominal examinations or CT scan for nearly definitive rule out of intra-abdominal injury. Additional conservative management must involve keeping the patient NPO, serial hemoglobin assays as well as white blood cell (WBC) counts, use of minimal pain medication. Additional laboratory data to assist with resuscitative efforts include the arterial blood gas (ABG) and a lactic acid level. Chiefly, the base deficit should be followed as one of many possible endpoint of resuscitation. Bishop, Abou Khalil, Scalea, and subsequently Porter highlighted this measurement in previous investigations.

Diagnostic Testing

Laboratory Data

Hematological values and a baseline electrolyte panel with liver and renal function tests are useful for comparison to subsequent values, which may indicate occult injury. Most importantly, a change in hemoglobin may reflect acute hemorrhage. Serial measurements may also be helpful for assessment of continued hemorrhage. Leukocytosis up to 12,000 to 20,000 cells/mm^3 may occur within several hours of a major traumatic injury due to tissue damage, hemorrhage, peritonitis, or epinephrine-induced demargination. Serum amylase is nonspecific and lacks sensitivity; however, an increase should lead to suspicion of pancreatic, proximal small bowel or genitourinary tract injury. Coagulation studies are important for assessment of preexisting abnormalities and assessment in patients requiring massive transfusions. Arterial blood gases, urinalysis, and urine drug screen should be considered when appropriate.

Plane Radiographs

The use of routine chest, lateral cervical spine, and anteroposterior pelvic x-ray films has been recommended by some textbooks, as well as the American College of Surgeons ATLS program. Pelvic radiographs are included due to the consideration that there are few external manifestations of pelvic fractures, and these patients do generally have a higher incidence of abdominal injuries. However, recent studies have found a sensitivity, specificity, and diagnostic accuracy of above 95% for the physical examination in diagnosis of pelvic fractures in the patient alert enough for a reliable physical examination. Pelvic injury should be investigated if there is altered mental status or an equivalent physical examination. Although pelvic fractures are indeed associated with an increased incidence of intra-abdominal visceral injury, an isolated pelvic fracture can cause similar large amounts of blood loss.

The chest radiograph is helpful initially for identifying pneumothorax or hemothorax or free air. Wide mediastinum (>8 cm) is an indication for chest CT scan and/or aortography. Other features on the chest radiograph can demonstrate foreign bodies (including endotracheal tubes, central lines, nasogastric tubes), pulmonary contusions, fractured calcifications around the aortic arch, fractured ribs. Once the chest x-ray is seen and no correctable abnormality is identified (pneumothorax, hemothorax), the patient can be transported to the CT scanner or floor.

Computed Tomography (CT Scan)

Clinical circumstances determine the preferred method of evaluation; however, all trauma patients must be carefully evaluated with a low threshold for CT scan if there is any suspicion of abdominal injury. The CT scan is highly accurate (99%) and specific (94.7%), and it has the potential to not only diagnose and localize injuries, but also grade organ injury and hemoperitoneum. The CT scan is most sensitive for diagnosis of injury of the liver, spleen, kidneys, bony structures, and the retroperitoneal area. It is less sensitive for bowel (chiefly duodenal) and pancreas injuries.

The use of oral and intravenous contrast provides information about any hollow viscus, kidney, ureter, or bladder injury. The CT scan is most suitable in hemodynamically stable cases. Making a decision as to how the abdomen will be evaluated must be done quickly and with consideration of the entire clinical picture. In general, the physician must use sound clinical judgment to assess each individual case regarding the most appropriate method. DPL is mandatory in cases involving hemodynamic instability, and clearly, if surgery is already indicated, time should not even be wasted performing a DPL. If the patient is both hemodynamically stable and the GCS is 14 to 15, the most logical option to evaluate injury is a CT of the abdomen. The specificity and sensitivity are marginally greater than those of DPL. In comparison to the rate of nontherapeutic diagnostic laparotomy following CT versus DPL, less are reported following CT (19%) compared to DPL (25%).

Potential complications of evaluating the patient by CT scan include deterioration of the patient in the scan room and allergic reaction to the contrast dye. Although allergic reaction is uncommon, clinical deterioration while out of the ED is a real risk and potentially disastrous.

Diagnostic Peritoneal Lavage

Diagnostic peritoneal lavage (DPL) is the preferred evaluation method for unstable patients. Compared to the CT scan, the DPL may be performed either by open (direct visualization), semiclosed, or closed technique. Preparation to perform the DPL involves not only gathering of the appropriate surgical materials, but also placement of a urinary catheter and nasogastric tube for decompression of the bladder and the stomach prior to initiating the DPL. An upright or lateral decubitus radiograph should be obtained to check for free air because the procedure itself introduces free air into the abdominal cavity.

After proper sterile preparation and local anesthesia with lidocaine, with epinephrine to control local bleeding, one of several techniques can be performed. For the closed technique, a small skin incision is made and a trocar placed. The Seldinger technique is employed to place the DPL

catheter into the peritoneal cavity. Alternatively, for the semiclosed or Hasson technique, the skin incision is carried down to the rectus fascia that is visualized by the physician prior to puncture into the peritoneal cavity. For the open technique, the incision is carried all the way down to the peritoneum itself, approaching by careful dissection though the layers of tissue. For this technique, the physician directly views the peritoneum as the DPL catheter is placed. Of these, the preferred method is the semiopen technique, which can be completed not only expediently, but also with fewer complications. The standard incision should be in the midline, approximately 1 cm inferior to the umbilicus in nongravid females and those without a suspicion for a pelvic fracture in which decompression of a retroperitoneal hematoma may lead to the patient hemorrhaging for the rest of their life. However, a paramedian or supraumbilical incision site is also acceptable. For all of these techniques, attention to meticulous hemostasis is imperative to avoid false-positive lavage results.

If no blood is found on aspiration, 1,000 mL of crystalloid solution is instilled into the peritoneum through the DPL catheter (15–20 mL/kg), agitated externally, then drained, by placing the fluid collecting bag below the level of the patient's abdomen. If the return of fluid is inadequate, the position of the patient may be changed to reverse Trendelenburg's position, or the position of the catheter may be redirected. This is easier than it sounds, however. Once the seal is broken and air is introduced into the line, siphoning the fluid out is most difficult. An aliquot of this fluid may be sent for laboratory analysis including cell count and differential, Gram stain, amylase, alkaline phosphatase, vegetable matter, and bile.

Disadvantages of the DPL include its invasive nature and suboptimal diagnosis of diaphragmatic rupture, retroperitoneal injury, and pelvic injury. It gives no information about the type or grade of organ injury. False results may occur and are mainly due to traumatic catheter insertion, pelvic fractures, and retroperitoneal hematoma. Studies have demonstrated a negative exploratory laparotomy incidence up to 5% in patients with false-positive results. False-negative results may also occur, but are primarily in cases of either retroperitoneal injury or hollow visceral injury, in which less hemorrhage is produced and inflammatory response delayed.

Relative, but not absolute, complications to performing a DPL include previous abdominal surgery, pregnancy, morbid obesity, advanced hepatic dysfunction with portal hypertension, coagulopathy, or pelvic fracture. Generally, the procedure may still be performed safely and when anatomic contraindications exist, the technique is modified. For example, for patients with pelvic fractures, the DPL should be performed by supraumbilical incision as the DPL fluid may be falsely positive if the catheter goes through a pelvic hematoma. This complication could lead to catastrophic consequences as the contained hematoma would be decompressed and the patient runs the risk of exsanguination. For patients with a past surgical history of only one uncomplicated laparotomy, the DPL is usually safe if performed at a site away from the previous incision, avoiding the right lower quadrant area to eliminate future confusion with appendectomy. However, multiple prior laparotomies are a contraindication to DPL and render the results less sensitive secondary to possible loculation of intra-abdominal fluid due to adhesions. In these cases, the patient must be evaluated either by CT scan, exploratory laparotomy, or conservative management, if appropriate.

Although rare (0–1.6%), complications of the DPL procedure include bleeding, infection, hematoma, bowel perforation, vascular injury, bladder injury, dehiscence, or hernia. Perforations of the bowel are most common and may especially be a risk when gaseous distention of the gastrointestinal tract occurs with bag ventilations. Standard precautions and proper technique minimize all of these risks (**Table 171.1**).

If the DPL is indeterminate and the physical examination is ambiguous, the patient likely warrants a celiotomy, or possibly a diagnostic laparoscopy. Initially, however, a CT scan with intravenous contrast for optimal resolution is considered the single most helpful test for evaluation of abdominal trauma if the patient is stable enough.

Ultrasonography

Although the exact role of ultrasonography has not been perfected, academic centers have begun to use ultrasonography in the ED to evaluate the abdomen and pericardial space in the trauma patient. Ultrasound is a noninvasive but high-yield procedure when performed by an experienced and trained physician for the evaluation of the trauma patient. Ultrasonography by a competent operator has been demonstrated to be equivalent to the DPL in some studies and is already the standard in many European trauma centers. Compared to CT scan and similar to DPL, ultrasound is a quick method of evaluation. It takes only 1 to 5 minutes to perform and requires little or no interruption in the resuscitation efforts. Immediate ultrasonography may be performed concomitantly with the remainder of the resuscitation procedures in the trauma bay, requiring little space at the patient's bedside.

Limitations to ultrasonography include morbid obesity, subcutaneous emphysema, confinement of intraperitoneal blood secondary to adhesions, differentiation of blood from

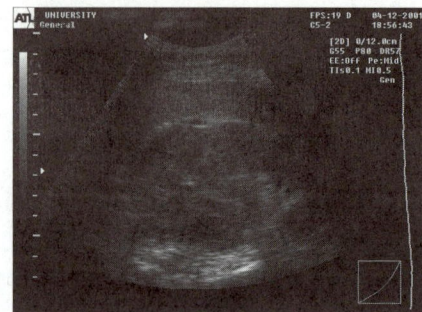

FIGURE 171.3 Sonogram showing the irregularity of a diaphragm with a finger exposed through the defect.

ascites, and inadequate assessment of the pancreas or early bowel injury. Most authors suggest three major acoustic windows using a 3.5-MHz transducer: the Morrison's pouch view, a left upper quadrant view, and a pelvic view. A subcostal view is an additional view recommended by some. Basically, the sonographer looks for free intraabdominal free fluid. Fluid will appear anechoic or black, on the ultrasound screen.

Morrison's pouch is the potential anatomical space between the liver and the right kidney where fluid may collect between Gerota's fascia and Glisson's capsule of the liver. It is viewed with the 3.5-MHz probe placed in a vertical position immediately inferior to the right subcostal margin (**FIGURE 171.3**).

The left upper quadrant view is obtained by placing the probe in a vertical position inferior to the left subcostal margin for visualization of the paracolic gutter around the left kidney and spleen. This view requires a more posterior position compared to the right view.

The pelvic cul-de-sac view or Douglas's pouch should theoretically be the most dependent area and the most sensitive view for detection of intraperitoneal fluid. However, this view is optimal only with bladder distention, which would provide a perfect acoustic window for ultrasound wave transmission and displace any bowel loops potentially interfering with the examination (**FIGURE 171.4**).

Ultrasonography detects a threshold amount of intraperitoneal fluid as low as 100 to 200 mL. An anechoic strip measuring 0.5 cm corresponds to approximately 500 mL of fluid. More experienced and talented ultrasonographers may be able to detect specific organ injury; however,

---

Table 171.1

Interpretation of Diagnostic Peritoneal Lavage (DPL) Fluid

Positive
10 mL gross blood upon initial aspiration
>100,000 RBCs in blunt trauma
>10,000 RBCs in penetrating trauma*
Presence of bile, stool, vegetable fiber in effluence
>500,000 WBCs/mm³
Cannot read print on the opposite side of the infusate bag**

---

*Some institutions will accept >1000 so that the likelihood of a missed injury is greatly attenuated.
**This is a general rule of thumb and is not an evidenced based mechanism. It is commonly accepted in the face of hemodynamic lability.

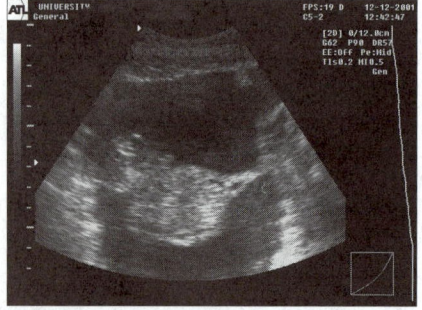

FIGURE 171.4 Sonogram showing diaphragm repair.

the goal of ultrasound in the trauma bay is to detect the presence of free fluid in a hypotensive patient. Ongoing research continues to define the ultimate role of ultrasound in the evaluation of the trauma patient, but preliminary studies have been favorable with relation to accuracy of diagnosis, expediency of patient care, and outcome.

Other Studies

Other diagnostic studies may be considered. Water-soluble contrast studies may be useful for the diagnosis of gastrointestinal and rectal injuries. Endoscopic retrograde cholangiopancreaticography (ERCP) is useful for evaluation of the pancreas and its ductal system in a non-urgent fashion. Angiography for evaluation of blunt abdominal trauma is useful to evaluate renal vascular pedicle injury, splenic and hepatic injuries with blush, and for embolization of bleeding vessels secondary to pelvic fracture.

Diagnostic laparoscopy is an additional option for evaluation of the abdomen, but not proven to be superior to CT scan, DPL, or ultrasound. Most surgeons have a great deal of experience with this technique and it may even be performed in the ED or intensive care unit. Indications are essentially the same as for the DPL. The procedure is limited and may be technically complicated if there are adhesions secondary to prior abdominal surgery. In addition, on rare occasion, carbon dioxide gas introduced into the peritoneal cavity may potentially cause gas emboli or pneumothorax. Advantages of diagnostic laparoscopy include direct visualization of intraabdominal organs and opportunity for the immediate repair of any injuries visualized. At present, research has not confirmed or defined the usefulness of the procedure.

Specific Abdominal Injuries

Penetrating Abdominal Trauma

Multiple objects may be responsible for penetrating trauma to the abdomen. The intra-abdominal area is at risk when violated between the boundaries of the pelvis inferiorly, the fourth intercostal space anteriorly, the sixth intercostal space laterally, and the scapular tip posteriorly. Concomitant thoracic violation is present in 15% to 46% of abdominal injuries. Stab wounds of the abdomen are most commonly located in the upper quadrants, left more often than right, with multiple wounds present 20% of the time. The most commonly injured intra-abdominal organ resulting from penetrating trauma is the liver.

If the penetration is in the back or the flank, diagnosis of retroperitoneal injury may be a challenge. Due to the proximity of the retroperitoneal organs and their relatively fixed position, penetration of the peritoneal cavity from the retroperitoneum constitutes a severe injury. A triple-contrast CT scan with intravenous, oral, and rectal contrast may be useful, but this is controversial.

The initial resuscitation is the same as in blunt abdominal trauma. A careful search should be undertaken for any evidence of penetrating trauma as these wounds may be exceptionally small or inconspicuous. Nevertheless, failure to note a penetrating wound, which may be present even in the absence of conforming history, may be calamitous. If any wound is found, a search for a corresponding exit wound should be undertaken. The back should always be examined carefully at the very end of the primary survey, even if the patient is being transferred to a trauma center. Plane radiographs may aid in localization of foreign bodies and missiles. Indications for immediate laparotomy are hemodynamic instability, signs of peritoneal irritation, evisceration, diaphragmatic injury, and gastrointestinal bleeding.

Between 70% and 90% of patients with visceral injury have RBC counts of 100,000 cells/mm^3 or greater in the lavage fluid. Patients with lower counts can be observed over 12 to 24 hours, with attention to ruling out hollow viscera injury. If clinical observation is not feasible, laparotomy may be necessary. Interpretation of the DPL in cases of penetrating trauma involving the lower chest or diaphragm is significantly different and even 1,000 red blood cells (RBCs)/mm^3 is considered positive by some. If the physician suspects diaphragmatic involvement, 5,000 RBCs/mm^3 should be the lower level threshold. Penetrating trauma to the lower chest with peritoneal penetration, by virtue of its mechanism, penetrates the diaphragm and requires surgical repair.

In general, nonballistic penetrating abdominal trauma can be selectively managed, and operative intervention may not be necessary. A rough estimate of the incidence of severity of injury is the *rule of thirds:* one third has no peritoneal violation, one third penetrate the peritoneum but do not really require intraabdominal surgical treatment, and one third require surgical repair. Stab wounds generally produce direct injury and laceration of tissue. Immediate laparotomy is indicated if there is evisceration of abdominal contents, peritoneal signs on physical examination, or persistent hypotension. Otherwise, these patients may be managed on an individual basis, without routine surgical exploration. However, local exploration is absolutely mandatory, and should be done utilizing local anesthesia to ensure complete and thorough examination to rule out the presence of foreign body, penetration of the anterior fascial layer, or vascular damage. Blind manipulation of the wound is not recommended. Injection of contrast medium into the wound is also not recommended, as it is not adequate to rule out peritoneal injury, and it increases the risk of infection.

Most experts recommend laparotomy if a stab wound causes blood loss, peritoneal signs are present, or if there is evisceration of abdominal contents. In cases of evisceration, the abdominal contents should be covered with moist sterile dressings and replacement should be attempted only in situations of moderate-to-severe compromise tissue viability and delay in surgical exploration.

The stable and alert patient with an isolated stab wound with no peritoneal penetration may be observed clinically. It is also acceptable to perform a CT scan for flank wounds as well as to help delineate the tract and possible peritoneal violation. The trend in management of penetrating superficial injuries has been toward decreasing unnecessary laparotomy but still maintaining a low incidence of delayed injury manifestation.

Ballistic Injuries

Although most commonly caused by firearm-related injuries, ballistic injuries can include multiple types of propelled missiles, including flying objects or fragments, explosive bombs, shotguns, or handguns. The severity of the injury depends on the kinetic energy ($k = \frac{1}{2} mv^2$), or the mass of the projectile and the square of its velocity. Projectile velocities are separated into three categories: low, medium, and high. Low-velocity missiles travel slower than 1,000 feet per second, medium-velocity between 1,000 and 2,000 feet per second, and high-velocity greater than 2,000 feet per second. The actual velocity at the time of impact is most important and is directly related to the distance from which it was fired, the muzzle velocity, and the trajectory and mass of the bullet itself. For shotgun injuries, the key variable is distance.

The mechanics of the damage caused in the body varies with the type of weapon and involves both direct and indirect tissue damage. At higher velocities, the bullet creates a cavitary passage as it passes through tissues with high water content such as the central nervous system or liver or spleen; however, this tract tends to cavitate transiently in those tissues with less water content such as muscle or skin. The diameter of cavitation can be as large as three times the diameter of the missile.

Gunshot wounds may result in the forcing of external contaminants into the wound and increase the risk of subsequent infection if not adequately irrigated and debrided. Routine antibiotic prophylaxis is arguably indicated in addition to tetanus toxoid. Appropriate antibiotic choices include cefoxitin or ampicillin/sulbactam, covering a polymicrobial range of organisms.

In contrast to stab wounds, ballistic injuries result in significant intra-abdominal injury in approximately 75% to 80% of cases. Most patients die due to either complications of hemorrhage and shock, or multiple organ injury. Fluid resuscitation is highly important. Indications for laparotomy include hemodynamic instability, suspected peritoneal violation, back or flank wounds which are not superficial, significant gastrointestinal bleeding, evidence of diaphragmatic penetration, or positive lavage fluid.

Abdominal Wall Injury

The most common abdominal wall injuries following blunt trauma are simple hematoma and abrasion. A rectus muscle hematoma may be palpable as a mass in the abdominal wall and is best evaluated by CT scan. Abdominal wall disruption is a rare injury, with flank and anteroinferior defects being the most common anatomical locations. The defect may be full-thickness, with or without evisceration, or may be a defect of the musculoaponeurotic layers only, resulting in an acute traumatic abdominal wall hernia. In addition to anterior evisceration, a second site of potential evisceration is from the anus.

The management and repair of abdominal wall disruptions presents a challenge to the surgeon as the primary repair is often unsuccessful due to the related tissue destruction. The incidence of associated intra-abdominal injuries is high and should be addressed in the usual manner, depending on the stability of the patient.

Solid Organ Injury

Liver

Liver injury is commonly seen following blunt and penetrating trauma of the abdomen as well as lower thoracic injury. It is the most commonly injured organ following penetrating abdominal trauma and the second most commonly injured organ resulting from blunt abdominal trauma. Patients with a history of hepatomegaly or chronic obstructive pulmonary disease may have an increased risk secondary to an increased amount of liver mass below the right costal margin of the rib cage.

The seriousness of the liver injury itself depends largely on the mechanism of injury and may cause critical hemodynamic instability. In cases of blunt abdominal trauma, there may be a massive amount of blood loss requiring large volumes of crystalloid and blood transfusion for resuscitation. Types of liver injury include laceration, intraparenchymal hematoma, subcapsular hematoma, contusion, vascular damage, or biliary duct transection. Blood and bile may spill into the peritoneal cavity following severe liver injury and cause significant peritoneal irritation. The major hepatic vessels may be involved, and blood loss can be massive. The physical examination is unreliable in many patients, and even the alert patient with less severe liver injury may complain only of abdominal pain and referred pain to the right shoulder. The clinician must be alert and watchful for existing or pending hypotension. The maxim is the more severe the liver injury, the more likely that additional organs have been injured as well. Morbidity and mortality are directly related to multiple organ injuries and reports range widely from 4% to 70%. Liver injury severity may be quantified on a five-grade classification scale by CT scan, and conservative management may be an option for less severe liver lacerations.

Delayed presentations following liver injury include chemical peritonitis and traumatic hematobilia, and hyperpyrexia. Chemical peritonitis develops secondary to persistent bile leakage into the peritoneal cavity over a period from days to approximately 1 month after the injury. The patient presents with often vague abdominal discomfort, distention, peritoneal signs, and jaundice. Traumatic hematobilia develops from persistent hemorrhage leading to increased intrahepatic pressure, parenchymal tissue damage, and backup of blood into the biliary tract. The patient typically presents 3 days to 2 years after the traumatic event with upper or lower gastrointestinal bleeding, abdominal discomfort, and jaundice. Initial diagnosis is often accomplished with ultrasound by the erudite practitioner, or CT scan. Subsequently, the patient is referred to angiography for angioembolization and ERCP or transhepatic cholangiographic drainage.

Spleen

The spleen is the most frequently injured intra-abdominal organ in blunt trauma. Twenty percent of patients with lower left rib fractures have an associated splenic injury. The patient presents with symptoms and signs of hemorrhage including tachycardia, hypotension, dizziness, syncope, nausea, abdominal pain, left upper quadrant tenderness, and perhaps external ecchymoses. Kehr's sign, or referred pain to the left shoulder, may be present. Although peritoneal signs are helpful when present, up to 50% of patients with splenic injury have a normal abdominal examination.

The plane chest radiograph obtained early in the resuscitation may provide clues regarding the existence of a splenic injury. Lower rib fractures, increased splenic shadow, elevated left hemidiaphragm, or medial and inferior displacement of the gastric bubble are soft signs that may be present with splenic injury.

Mechanisms resulting in splenic injury vary widely from apparently minor trauma to significant direct blows resulting from sports injuries, road accidents, or assaults. The spleen may be compressed and may rupture in any of these cases; however, an enlarged spleen is particularly susceptible to disruption following even minor trauma. Pathologically, the splenic parenchyma may be lacerated, contused, or fractured. The pedicular vessels may also be disrupted.

Recently, more conservative management of splenic injuries has been pursued for adults as well as children, primarily because of the acknowledgment of the risks of post-splenectomy infection and sepsis. The estimated risk for overwhelming post-splenectomy sepsis (OPSS) in adult patients is small (0.025%), but real. In children, the risk is much higher. Conservative management of splenic injuries has been the standard of care for children and has been successful due to the relatively thicker splenic capsule in children. Depending on the hemodynamic status of the patient and the severity of the splenic injury, the surgeon may choose nonoperative management, splenorrhaphy, or splenectomy. Splenic injuries are graded by CT scan as described by a four-grade classification. In more severe injury, splenorraphy with hematoma stabilization may be an option, allowing preservation of the spleen. These patients are then monitored very carefully to ensure that the postoperative course is not complicated by secondary bleeding or abscess formation. If a splenectomy is performed, the patient is at a slightly increased risk of an encapsulated bacterial infection that is theoretically preventable with immunization against organisms such as *Streptococcus* sp., *Meningococcus* sp., and *Haemophilus influenzae*.

Interestingly enough, Pneumovax efficacy is only about 77% (Butler 1993). Functional antibody response to the vaccine is improved in those individuals when administered 14 days after traumatic splenectomy, than for those vaccinated 1–7 days after splenectomy (Shatz 1998). OPSS rarely occurs in those patients who underwent splenectomy for trauma. The incidence of delayed splenic rupture is unknown, but thought to be 10% to 20%. These cases are most likely due to contained, self-controlled hemorrhage and result from progressive accumulation of blood. They will be diagnosed by serial abdominal examinations and serial hematocrit determinations.

Pancreas

Pancreatic injury can be difficult to diagnose. Injuries are more common following penetrating injuries; however, blunt traumatic mechanisms may cause crush injuries in which the pancreas may be compressed over the vertebral bodies and even divided. When a CT scan of the abdomen is obtained and/or plane film reveal a Chance fracture (shearing injury of a low thoracic or upper lumbar vertebrae), it is of the utmost importance for the physician to review the CT scan once more to convince her or himself that a pancreatic injury does not exist. Pathologically, the injuries range from isolated contusions or lacerations to involvement and damage to the ductal system, complete transection of the pancreas, or associated duodenal rupture. The release of irritating pancreatic enzymes or hemorrhage may cause peritoneal signs, or more commonly mild tenderness to palpation. Classically, the physical examination may initially improve followed by return or worsening of discomfort within the first 6 hours. If the diagnosis is not made early, the enzymes continue to leak into the abdominal cavity providing an excellent bacterial medium for abscess formation. In addition, pseudocysts may form secondary to the autodigestive properties of the pancreatic enzymes.

Although significantly lacking in sensitivity and specificity, the serum amylase is elevated in approximately 75% of pancreatic injury due to blunt mechanism and 27% due to penetrating trauma. Leukocytosis is proportional to the severity of peritonitis. Other helpful diagnostic studies include Gastrografin contrast study and CT scan. Morbidity and mortality vary with diagnostic delays and associated injuries.

Hollow Viscus Injury

The hollow viscus organ where injury most commonly occurs following abdominal trauma is the colon. Stomach and duodenal injuries, although less common, may also occur and are associated with pneumoperitoneum, hemoperitoneum, or blood in the nasogastric tube drainage. Overall, most hollow viscus injuries occur secondary to penetrating trauma mechanisms. There is approximately 17% incidence of colonic injury following penetrating abdominal trauma and 4% incidence following blunt abdominal trauma.

Hollow viscus injuries following blunt trauma occur due to compression, shearing at fixed points, or acute increases in intraluminal pressure such as that following seat belt constriction during accident impact. An increase in intraluminal pressure classically occurs when the patient was wearing the lap belt improperly. As in when it does not lie across the anterior superior iliac spines. Subsequently, the C-loop of the duodenum suffers from increased intraluminal pressure as the proximal and distal portions are literally crushed against the spinal vertebrae. This leaves only one spot for the closed loop to decompress, that area generally is along the antimesenteric border. This can be a catastrophic injury. Pathologically, the duodenum may be perforated or an intramural hematoma may develop. Mucosal or submucosal tears also occur. The colon may develop contusions, lacerations, or transection. The vulnerability of a hollow viscus segment to compression injury correlates with its relative immobility.

The patient classically presents with a history of being a restrained back-seat passenger and a physical examination demonstrating early signs of peritoneal irritation. Tenderness may be mild and diffuse. Peritoneal signs occur due to spillage of intestinal contents into the peritoneal cavity, but may be absent if the injury is isolated to the retroperitoneal portion of the duodenum. Patients with a significant crush or laceration injury of the retroperitoneal duodenum may demonstrate retroperitoneal air on the plane radiograph or CT scan, an elevated amylase level, or extravasation of dye on a contrast study. In recent reviews of CT scanning of the abdomen however, oral contrast was not found to be beneficial in identifying duodenal injuries. In fact, those patients identified with duodenal injuries were noted to have free air and no extraluminal contrast. Furthermore, those patients who did receive contrast had a delay in obtaining the CT scan and had more complications with aspiration of gastric contents that included the oral contrast. More often, evidence of injury in the retroperitoneal duodenum is slow to develop in cases of less severe injury, such as duodenal hematoma, and diagnosis may be delayed for up to several days. The delayed presentation consists of intestinal obstruction and obstructive jaundice if the ampulla of Vater is involved. Often, the duodenal hematoma is incidentally diagnosed during laparotomy and, if not significant enough to cause obstruction, can be managed conservatively without drainage. Surgical correction may be emergently needed if obstruction develops.

A gastrointestinal injury may be diagnosed by DPL, CT scan, or water-soluble gastrointestinal contrast studies. DPL lavage fluid demonstrates elevated amylase levels in most cases. Water-soluble (Gastrografin) contrast must be used for contrast studies any time disruption of a hollow viscus is suspected. Again, if the patient is unstable, operative exploration should be expedited in lieu of definitive diagnosis preoperatively.

One important injury site to recognize prior to operative exploration is the rectum, because it is extraperitoneal and injury may not be as readily apparent. The rectum must be evaluated by both palpation and hemoccult testing. Sigmoidoscopy or rectal contrast administered just prior to the abdominal CT scan could also be considered. Bony penetration secondary to a pelvic or coccygeal fracture is an open fracture and could lead to serious contamination, potentially escalating into life-threatening sepsis. If rectal penetration is detected, the patient must receive broad spectrum antibiotics in the ED, as prophylactic antibiotic coverage of anaerobes and coliforms has been demonstrated to significantly decrease the incidence of critical infection and sepsis after traumatic injury. If the injury is not diagnosed preoperatively, the chance of detection intraoperatively is nearly nonexistent.

Vascular Injury

Patients with intra-abdominal vascular injuries following trauma present with hypotension, and there is the poten-

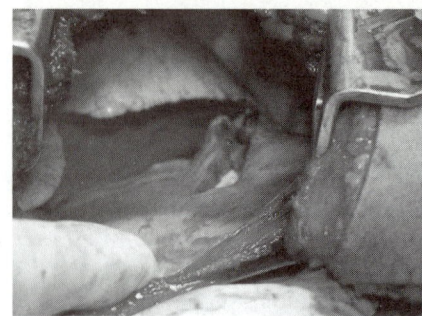

FIGURE 171.5 Photograph of an irregularity of a diaphragm with finger exposed through the defect.

tial for significant amounts of blood loss. Retroperitoneal location may afford the benefit of anatomical tamponade, increasing the chance of survival. The only preoperative way to control the hypotension is with control of the hemorrhage, perhaps with military antishock trousers (MAST) in the most desperate of times. These are often the patients whom have improved outcomes from the "scoop and run" measures executed by the EMTs and paramedics that Mattox described. Infusing fluids rapidly may increase the patient's blood pressure and possibly dislodge a clot on a major vessel. In this instance, hypotension is a life-saving maneuver the body utilizes in times of severe extremes. Because the key to operative management is both proximal and distal vessel control, the patient is emergently taken to the operating room and prepped from chin to just below the knees. When massive amounts of blood loss is expected, the perfusion team should be called for preparation of cell saving and autotransfusion equipment. At least 10 units of blood and blood product to control dilutional coagulopathy should be made available.

Penetrating trauma causes most cases of intra-abdominal vascular injury resulting in contusions, intimal tears, lacerations, perforations, or transection of major blood vessels. Contusions and intimal tears may not lead to significant blood loss; however, potential complications include thrombosis and pseudoaneurysm formation.

Diaphragmatic Rupture

Probably one of the most difficult diagnosis to make early in the hospital course is diaphragmatic rupture. The typical mechanism is the crush injury to the lateral chest wall. The abdominal contents may herniate into the chest cav-

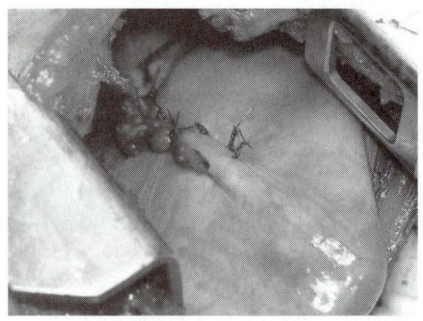

FIGURE 171.6 Photograph of diaphragm repair showing sutures.

ity or even strangulate. If a liver or spleen laceration is present, the defect allows blood to accumulate in the thoracic cavity, compromising respiratory function and leading to massive hemothorax. The chest radiograph may demonstrate subtle blurring of the diaphragm or small pleural effusion, or a nasogastric tube in the hemithorax; however, the injury may also be diagnosed by CT with reconstructed images or with contrast studies identifying a dumbbell shaped pattern of a hollow viscus. The injury more commonly occurs on the left side (65%–90%) with gastric herniation found greater than 50% of the time, followed by herniation of the colon, omentum, spleen, and small intestine. The treatment is surgical repair, either open or laparoscopic (**FIGURES 171.5** and **171.6**).

Selected Readings

Abou-Khalil B, Scalea TM, Trooskin SZ, et al. Hemodynamic responses to shock in young trauma patients: need for invasive monitoring. *Crit Care Med* 1994; 22:633–639.

Bishop MH, Shoemaker WC, Appel PL, et al. Prospective randomized trial of survivor values of cardiac index, oxygen delivery, and oxygen consumption as resuscitation endpoints in severe trauma. *J Trauma Inj Infect Crit Care* 1995;38: 780–787.

Butler JC, Breiman RF, Campbell JF, et al. Pneumococcal polysaccharide vaccine efficacy. *JAMA* 1993;270:1826–1831.

Gonzalez RP, Turk B, Falimirski ME, Holevar MR. Abdominal stab wounds: diagnostic peritoneal lavage criteria for emergency room discharge. *J Trauma* 2001; 51:939–943.

McKenney MG, McKenney KL, Hong JJ, et al. Evaluating blunt abdominal trauma with sonography: a cost analysis. *Am Surg* 2001;67:930–934.

Nagy KK, Roberts RR, Joseph KT, et al. Experience with over 2500 diagnostic peritoneal lavages. *Injury* 2000;31:479–482.

Porter JM, Ivatury PR. In search of the optimal end points of resuscitation in trauma patients: A review. *J Trauma Inj Infect Crit Care* 1998;44:908–914.

Rozycki GS, Ochsner MG, Schmidt JA, et al. A prospective study of surgeon-performed ultrasound as the primary adjuvant modality for injured patient assessment. *J Trauma* 1995;39:492–498.

Scalea TM, Maltz S, Yelon J, et al. Resuscitation of multiple trauma and head injury: role of crystalloid fluids and inotropes. *Crit Care Med* 1994;22:1610–1615.

172 Upper and Lower Extremity Injuries

Harry L. Anderson III

Proper diagnosis, treatment, and disposition of extremity injuries is an essential aspect of emergency medicine. Traumatic injury can be divided into fractures, dislocations, and soft tissue injuries. The role of the emergency physician is to treat these disorders in a timely fashion so that future function is not compromised. In addition, the proper consultation can only be made after a rapid, accurate diagnosis.

General Principles and Definitions

Fractures

A fracture is defined as a break in the bony cortex of bone, and is named according to its appearance on a radiograph.

- *Transverse:* fracture line bisects the long axis of the bone.
- *Oblique:* fracture line travels obliquely down from one cortex to the other.
- *Spiral:* fracture line travels in a spiral fashion down the long axis of the bone.
- *Comminuted:* fracture line includes one or more pieces broken off from the bone.

Further definitions of a fracture should include *degree of displacement. Nondisplaced* indicates no deviation of the cortex from the long axis of the bone. If the fracture is displaced, the degree of displacement as well as angulation and direction may be of importance in diagnosing possible neurovascular compromise.

The alignment and apposition of the fracture should be properly described. *Alignment* refers to the long axis of each fragment in relation to the other, while *apposition* refers to the degree of contact between each fragment. Valgus and varus refers to the angulation of one fracture segment. When the bony segment angles away from the midline, it is termed *valgus* and when toward the midline it is termed *varus. Impaction* refers to axial loading of force causing a fracture to impact on itself.

Open versus closed fractures must be correctly diagnosed so that proper irrigation and antibiotic prophylaxis can be done. An open area near to a fracture site should be probed to ensure there is no tracking down to the fracture.

In addition, all open fractures must have a deep wound culture done prior to irrigation and antibiotic use.

Fractures in Children

Pediatric fractures represent unique challenges to diagnosis. Unlike adult bones, pediatric bones have more elasticity and, depending on age, may have growing end plates that are not yet fused, called *epiphyses.* Because of their elasticity, a child's bones can take a greater amount of force before breaking than an adult's. A *greenstick fracture* is one that results from this eased elasticity and is unique to children. This fracture induces a bending and angulation of the bone without breaks in the cortex. These can be subtle and require special attention to bony angulation or deformity that should not be there.

Salter and Harris described a classification system used to define fracture involving the epiphysis in children. A *Salter I fracture* does not involve fractures of bone but a widening of the epiphysis. A *Salter II fracture* is most common and involves a small, usually triangular, fracture of the metaphysis accompanied by a widening of the epiphysis. *Salter III* involves a break through the articular surface and a separation of the epiphysis. *Salter IV* includes fractures of both the metaphysis and articular surface with widening of the epiphysis. A *Salter V* fracture involves the articular surface impacting on the metaphysis.

Dislocations

Dislocations occur when two normally articulating bones do not maintain their proper alignment. A dislocation involves a complete disruption of the articulation, whereas a subluxation involves a partial disruption with part of the articulating surface of each bone not in proper alignment. Whenever a dislocation is suspected, radiographs are required to ensure there is not a concurrent fracture.

Soft Tissue Injury

In the absence of bone fracture, soft tissue injury must be considered. This injury pattern carries with it its own pitfalls for the emergency physician. One must be able to ensure there is not a more serious injury than appears to be present. One potential hazard is compartment syndrome, but this entity rarely occurs in the emergency department. However, as a result of resuscitation (especially a massive resuscitation), it is likely to develop earlier in crush injuries and ischemic injuries.

The ideas of alkalinization of the urine and the addition of furosemide or mannitol are inappropriate and not supported by contemporary literature. This especially holds true for the initial management and resuscitative phase, as these maneuvers would obviously be counterproductive. The goal, should rhabdomyolysis or myoglobinuria be suspected, is to maintain a urinary output of 100 mL/h. Nonetheless, the clinician must look for the four Ps—pain, pulselessness, pallor, and paresthesia—although not all of these may be present in every case.

Another soft tissue injury that the clinician needs to be aware of is the Morel-Lavalle type injury. This typically occurs with pelvic fractures. The etiology is due to an infected hematoma that develops along the lateral thigh. The orthopedic surgeons must be aware of this as they follow the patient and be prepared to intervene early on in the patient care continuum. It is not uncommon that the emergency medicine physician finds this patient in the ER after the patient has been discharged and arrives with complaints of a cellulitic and painful thigh. This constitutes a surgical emergency.

Examination of Extremity Injuries

The goal of ED evaluation of extremity trauma is to preserve function of the limb. Most extremity injuries are diagnosed during the secondary survey. When an injury is identified, the emergency physician should go through a methodical investigation of the area. First, the injury should be observed for any obvious deformity or lacerations. If a break in the skin is present near a deformity, an open fracture should be assumed. The physician should take a culture of the wound prior to further treatment.

Following the observation, the extremity should be palpated from above to below the injured part to examine for point tenderness over bone and tenderness or firmness over muscle bodies. All involved joints should be interrogated for pain or deformity with movement. The next step is to assess all extremity injuries for neurovascular integrity. Distal pulses should be evaluated and a complete neurologic examination documented.

Radiological Examination

The affected area should be radiographed as well as one joint above and below. Usual views include AP, lateral, and oblique, though different views should be used depending on the injury (**FIGURE 172.1**). Following routine radiographs, some fractures may warrant CT evaluation. Orthopedic consultation should be done prior to CT scans.

Upper Extremity Injuries
Hand
Fractures of the phalanges and metacarpals should be properly splinted and referred to a hand specialist within 1

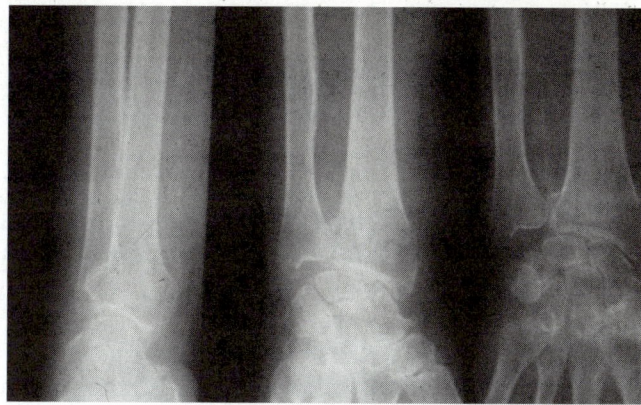

FIGURE 172.1 Radiograph of a Colles fracture of the wrist.

to 2 days. Fractures that are intraarticular and involve 30% or more of the joint surface may require internal fixation for correction. Phone consultation, anatomical splinting, and follow-up are required. Any injury involving multiple metacarpal fractures, severe soft tissue damage, or deformity should have immediate hand surgery consultation.

A *mallet finger* may occur when a flexion injury of the distal interphalangeal joint ruptures the extensor tendon at its insertion on the distal phalanx. This can occur on any of the digits. The finger should be splinted with the distal and proximal interphalangeal joints in extension. Hand surgery consultation should occur immediately. Usually splinting in extension for 6 weeks is adequate treatment unless a bony avulsion of the distal phalanx has occurred, in which case splinting in hyperextension is the treatment of choice.

A *boutonniere deformity* is caused by a flexion injury to the proximal interphalangeal joint or a crush injury to that joint. This injury causes a disruption of the anchoring system of the extensor tendon, allowing the tendons to migrate toward the volar aspect of the hand. This results in flexion of the proximal interphalangeal and extension or hyperextension at the distal interphalangeal joint when the finger extensor muscles are contracted. Treatment for this deformity includes splinting the proximal interphalangeal joint in extension for 6 to 8 weeks and follow-up with a hand surgeon.

DeQuervain's tenosynovitis is a condition affecting the compartment for the first dorsal extensor tendons, the *tensor pollicis brevis,* and the *abductor pollicis longus* on the radial aspect of the wrist. This injury is most often seen in overuse syndromes. A diagnostic test is Finkelstein's test, performed by placing the thumb in a flexed position in the palm and deviating the wrist in the ulnar direction. This will elicit pain as the extensor tendons are pulled through the affected compartment. This condition is treated with splinting and local corticosteroid injections.

Wrist
The carpal bones may be fractured or dislocated and may accompany hand injuries. Lunate and perilunate dislocations are commonly seen in wrist injury. In addition, all

hand injuries should be assessed for snuffbox tenderness. By exerting pressure in the anatomical snuffbox and eliciting pain, the clinician can diagnose scaphoid injury despite a normal radiograph. All patients with snuffbox tenderness should be placed in a thumb spica splint and followed up with an orthopedist for suspected occult fracture. This is essential to prevent the very serious complication of avascular necrosis of the scaphoid sometimes seen in scaphoid fractures.

Kienbock's disease is avascular necrosis of the lunate bone. This is seen in fractures of the bone, which often has sole blood supply from the volar aspect. This is most often seen in patients with congenital shortening of the lunate. Any fracture or suspected injury of the lunate requires splinting and orthopedic follow-up.

Elbow

Fractures of the proximal radius may be difficult to diagnose. The patient complains of diffuse elbow pain after trauma. Radiography may fail to demonstrate a fracture; however, the telltale "sail" sign of fat pad disruption is often present. Fractures of the proximal ulna usually result from direct trauma to the elbow, unlike other fractures of the elbow that may result from indirect trauma. The proximal ulna makes up the largest bone of the distal elbow and therefore when a fracture occurs, a large amount of force has been applied to the arm. Because of this, the emergency physician should look for accompanying fractures or dislocation of the elbow. If there is dislocation of the joint or displacement of more than 2 mm closed, and if that fails, open reduction should be performed with orthopedic consultation.

Monteggia's fracture is a proximal midshaft fracture of the ulna with accompanying dislocation of the radial head, most commonly anteriorly. The radial head dislocation is often missed on radiograph. This fracture may cause injury to the deep branch of the radial nerve. Treatment usually involves internal fixation after closed reduction of the radial head.

Nursemaid's elbow is a radial head subluxation and is often seen in children between the ages of 1 and 4 years. The injury is most commonly caused by someone abruptly pulling on the child's arm; hence, the commonly used name. The injury is often diagnosed by a history of such an injury resulting in the child's crying and unwillingness to use the arm. Radiographs should only be done if the mechanism of injury is not known. Treatment is simple and dramatic. The clinician should grasp the child's elbow with one hand, placing the thumb over the radial head and exerting gentle pressure. The other hand grasps the child's wrist and supinates the forearm while flexing the elbow and providing gentle traction on the wrist. The child will cry during this quick procedure, but if it is done successfully, the child will begin using the arm within 2 or 3 minutes.

Upper Arm and Shoulder

Humerus fractures are often seen in falls in the elderly or accompanying multiple traumas. The supracondylar fracture, a serious injury often accompanied by neurovascular compromise, occurs just proximal to the olecranon fossa but does not violate the joint. The supracondylar fracture, especially if caused by an extension mechanism, may have concurrent neurovascular injury, including occlusion or disruption of the brachial artery. The neurovascular integrity of the arm must be assessed and the fracture treated expeditiously to avoid further compromise. If the radial pulse is absent or diminished, such injury must be assumed. Closed or open reduction to restore anatomical alignment should be followed by arteriography to assess vascular damage. If vascular compromise is not diagnosed, then prolonged ischemia can cause Volkmann's contracture.

Proximal humerus fractures should be assessed for neurovascular compromise, as with all fractures; however, in the absence of gross deformity most can be treated conservatively with sling and swathe and orthopedic follow-up. Fracture of the surgical neck is uncommon but may result in avascular necrosis of the head of the humerus and should have orthopedic consultation after neurovascular assessment.

Acromioclavicular separation commonly occurs in trauma when an abrupt force has been exerted on the lateral shoulder. This injury pattern is often seen in sports such as hockey and football, as well as in motor vehicle accidents. The clavicle is displaced forward or backward and the shoulder joint slumps downward. This injury is diagnosed by tenderness over the acromioclavicular joint and radiography. A Type I injury has normal anatomical position on the radiograph when done with and without the patient holding weights. Types II and III may involve displacement of this joint. Types I and II are often treated with a sling and swathe, while Type III may be treated with the same or with open surgical reduction. This decision should be made by the orthopedic consultant.

Shoulder dislocations are the most common dislocations to present to the ED. Although rare, shoulder dislocations can be associated with or mimicked by humerus fractures, and therefore all suspected dislocations should have pre- and postreduction x-rays. Greater than 95% of dislocations are anterior and can be reduced within the ED. Patients with posterior dislocations and those anterior dislocations that cannot be reduced with conscious sedation in the ED should be sent to the operating room for either reduction under general anesthesia or open reduction.

Clinical Highlights

Lower Extremity

Foot

Isolated phalangeal and metatarsal fractures of the foot are most often treated conservatively with splinting or in some cases a hard-sole shoe, and orthopedic follow-up in 2 to 3 days. If the articular surface is involved, the joint may require fixation, and orthopedic consultation and follow-up are required. Interphalangeal dislocations may occur and are often easily reduced with traction of the distal toe. After such a procedure the toe should be "buddy taped" to the adjacent toe for a period of 2 to 3 days.

A fall from a height onto the feet should prompt the emergency physician to suspect a calcaneus fracture, which is the most common cause of such an injury. If fracture is suspected clinically, radiography should be done. If a fracture is seen, often a CT scan is needed to evaluate the full extent of the fracture. In addition, one should pay particular attention to the other foot as well as to the knees and spine, as there may be an occult fracture from the axial force from the fall.

A commonly missed injury is the Lisfranc fracture-dislocation usually from a fall onto a plantar-flexed foot. There is fracture of the middle cuneiform with dislocation of the lateral four metatarsals. The patient presents with a diffusely swollen, tender foot. On radiograph, the fracture may be easily seen, but the dislocations missed. The most reliable finding on radiograph aiding in the diagnosis is separation for the first and second metatarsals at their base. Most of these injuries require open reduction and internal fixation (ORIF).

Ankle

Ankle fractures are most often treated conservatively with splinting and orthopedic follow-up. The emergency physician should be aware of some pitfalls in treating ankle injuries. Most commonly missed fractures of the ankle occur on the dome, the superior aspect of the talus, and the anterior process of the talus, so particular attention should be paid to those areas on the x-ray. Whenever an ankle sprain or fracture is diagnosed, the proximal fibula should be palpated, and if tender, radiographs obtained.

In addition, rupture of the gastrocnemius tendon, or Achilles tendon, should always be suspected in patients exhibiting posterior ankle pain after a short fall or jump onto a slightly plantar-flexed foot. This injury is commonly seen in a patient who has been sedentary and, recently began participating in sports, such as basketball or running. The tendon is not stretched sufficiently prior to activity and is not flexible, making it prone to injury. The Thompson test is used to assess the integrity of this tendon. With the patient lying prone, the foot is allowed to hang off the end of the stretcher and relaxed. The body of the gastrocnemius muscle is grasped and squeezed. If the tendon is intact, the foot will plantar flex with this maneuver. In addition, the insertion of the tendon should be palpated for tenderness and for the presence of a defect. Ankle dislocations can be seen in severe, direct traumatic injury, such as a motorcycle accident where the foot and ankle are impacted onto the road, and are almost always associated with fractures and are often open. The most common of these is a posterior dislocation of the talus on the tibia (**FIGURE 172.2**). Although these fracture/dislocations almost always require ORIF, rapid reduction in the trauma room may be required to restore neurovascular integrity.

Knee

A large direct force to the knee may cause fractures of the distal femur, tibia, or fibula. The distal femur may be intercondylar, between the condyles, or supracondylar, above the condyles (**FIGURE 172.3**). These fractures may

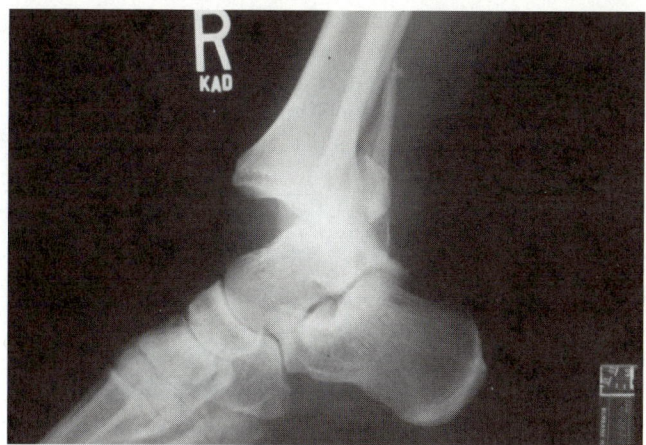

FIGURE 172.2 Radiograph showing dislocation of the ankle.

cause disruption of the peroneal nerve. Immediate orthopedic consultation should be obtained.

Fractures of the proximal tibia, or tibial plateau, are the most common fractures of the knee. They result most often from a medial or lateral force causing the femur to impact the tibia. There may also be associated ligamentous or meniscus injury. If the injury is nondisplaced, immobilization alone is sufficient treatment. Displaced fractures of the tibial plateau require ORIF. The tibial tuberosity is where the quadriceps tendon inserts and may be fractured with a sudden extension of the knee against force. In addition, this may cause a quadriceps tendon rupture, which is diagnosed by pain and a palpable defect just proximal to the anterior aspect of the knee, and weakness and pain with extension of the knee. A quadriceps rupture requires surgical intervention.

A patella fracture most often occurs with a direct blow on the knee, such as against the dashboard of the car during an accident. These fractures may require surgical correction, depending on the extent of the fracture and its alignment. If the patient is unable to extend the leg at the knee, the retinaculum may have been disrupted, mandating surgical correction. If the extensor mechanism of the knee is intact, immobilization is curative treatment. Patellar subluxation most often occurs laterally and results in the lock-knee syndrome. A true locked knee may occur from a meniscus tear, resulting in trapped cartilage limiting movement of the knee. Patients with a chroni-

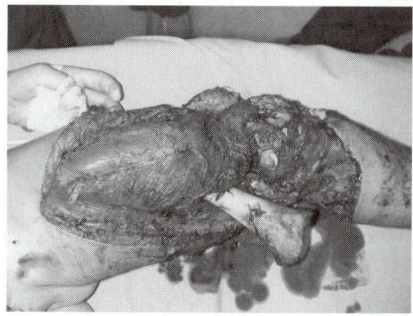

FIGURE 172.3 Photograph of an open femur fracture from a second degree motorcycle crash.

cally subluxing patella may report that their knee will suddenly and unexpectedly freeze, causing them pain and putting them at risk for further trauma from a fall. Often the patella will spontaneously reduce prior to arrival in the ED, and the diagnosis is made based on the history as well as on the presence of a loose patella. A chronically subluxing patella should be followed up with an orthopedics specialist, as they may require surgical repair. Knee dislocations are rare, but are serious results of a large amount of force in the form of a direct blow. The ligaments around the knee are very strong and must be disrupted in order for this dislocation to occur. These dislocations are most often accompanied by significant concurrent traumatic injuries. Anterior dislocations result from a hyperextension injury. Posterior dislocations are often seen in motor vehicle accidents when the patient's knee strikes the dashboard. There is a high rate of vascular injuries with this dislocation, mandating emergent reduction, even in the field if prolonged transport time to a trauma center is suspected. Though the presence of pulses is a good diagnostic sign, it does not rule out vascular in-

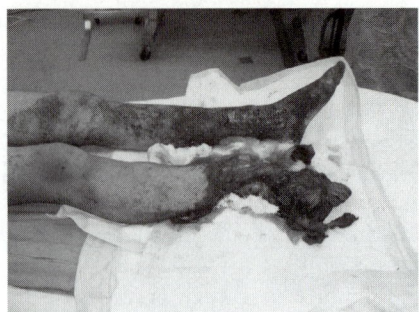

FIGURE 172.4 Photograph showing an antipersonnel mine injury.

jury. All knee dislocations should undergo angiography to rule out injury (**FIGURE 172.4**).

Selected Readings

Harris JH Jr, Harris WH. *The Radiology of Emergency Medicine.* 4th ed. Philadelphia: Lippincott Williams and Wilkins, 2000.
Mirvis SE, Shanmuganathan K, eds. *Imaging in Trauma and Critical Care,* 2d ed. Basel: Elsevier Science, 2003.
Moore EE, Feliciano DV, Mattox KL, eds. *Trauma,* 5th ed. New York: McGraw-Hill Professional, 2004.

Hip and Pelvic Fractures

Harry L. Anderson III

Hip Fractures

Fractures of the proximal femur are defined by their anatomical location. Femoral head fractures are the least common; they involve fracture through the most proximal part of the femur, and may involve the articulating surface. Most of these are seen in younger patients involved in motor vehicle collisions (MVCs). Type I femoral head fracture has only one fracture line and fragment, while Type II fracture is comminuted and has one or more resulting fragments. These fractures may be accompanied by dislocations and must be reduced urgently.

Femoral neck fractures are subdivided into four types, using the Garden classification. *Type I* is an impacted fracture where only trabeculae may be disrupted; *Type II* is nondisplaced, but completely through the neck; *Type III* is similar to Type II with some displacement; and *Type IV* is comminuted or with complete displacement. Avascular necrosis of the femoral head is a relatively common occurrence after a displaced femoral neck fracture.

Intertrochanteric fractures occur between the greater and lesser trochanters. These fractures are outside of the joint capsule, and therefore have less morbidity associated with them. Subtrochanteric fractures are less common fractures of the hip and occur distal to the lesser trochanter. Fractures of the shaft of the femur do not involve the hip; however, they are often comminuted and displaced, and may be associated with large amounts of blood loss into the thigh.

Treatment of displaced hip fractures includes immobilization, pain control, and orthopedic consultation. The consultant may request in-line traction to be started in the ED, which often provides relief of pain. Femoral shaft fractures are also treated with traction. A grossly deformed femur should be reduced in the ED so that the reservoir for blood loss created by the distorted anatomy is reduced.

Hip dislocations are most commonly (~90%) posterior dislocations and result from a direct blow along the long axis of the femur. They are sometimes associated with acetabular fractures. Anterior fractures result from a forced abduction. Hip dislocations can often be diagnosed by the position of the leg. With an anterior dislocation of the hip, the leg is usually flexed and externally rotated, while with a posterior dislocation, the leg is often flexed and adducted. Treatment includes assessment of neurovascular integrity and orthopedic consultation.

Dislocations must be reduced quickly. Anterior dislocations are sometimes associated with avascular necrosis of the femoral head, while posterior dislocations can cause injury to the sciatic nerve. Closed reduction of hip dislocations can often be accomplished. The patient is placed on the floor or on the stretcher while the physician stands above him and puts traction on the leg while the pelvis is being held by an assistant. In an obturator dislocation (a form of anterior dislocation), the knee is kept flexed to relax the hamstrings, while the thigh is flexed, abducted, and internally rotated. In the pubic form of anterior dislocation, the hip is internally rotated and hyperextended.

Pelvic Fractures

Pelvic fractures can represent a significant source of morbidity and mortality in the victim of blunt trauma. A major injury to the normally stable pelvic ring testifies to a degree of force that is capable of producing life-threatening injuries both within and distant from the pelvis.

Anatomy

The pelvic ring is composed of two symmetrical innominate bones (formed at maturity by the union of the ilium, ischium, and pubis) and the sacrum. The innominate bones connect to one another anteriorly at the symphysis pubis. In the posterior midline lies the sacrum, joined to each innominate bone by the sacroiliac joints. In addition to protecting the lower abdominal and pelvic organs, the pelvis is an important load-bearing structure, transmitting weight from the axial skeleton to the lower extremities (when standing) or the ischial tuberosities (when sitting). It also serves as a point of attachment for numerous muscles of the abdomen, back, pelvis, and lower extremities. Within the pelvic ring lie parts of the gastrointestinal and genitourinary tracts as well as important neurovascular structures. Significant pelvic trauma can be associated with injuries to these structures, and anatomical relationships must be kept in mind when evaluating the patient with pelvic injuries.

Mechanism of Injury

Nearly all injuries to the bony pelvis are caused by blunt trauma, and pelvic fractures can be broadly divided into low-energy and high-energy fractures depending on the mechanism of injury.

Low-energy fractures generally occur in one of two settings. The first is that of a fall from a standing or seated position onto a bony prominence, resulting in an isolated fracture to the pelvis. This type of injury often occurs in elderly, osteopenic patients. The second is that of excessive strain on a muscle that inserts into the pelvis, resulting in an avulsion fracture at the point of tendon insertion. These fractures are typically seen in athletes, particularly those whose skeletons have not yet fully matured.

High-energy fractures generally result from motor vehicle accidents, falls from heights, and crush injuries. These fractures are usually more complex than low-energy fractures, often result in instability of the pelvic ring, and are exclusively responsible for the associated injuries that can cause significant morbidity and mortality in this setting.

Classification

A number of classification systems have been proposed for pelvic fractures. The system currently accepted by the American Academy of Orthopedic Surgeons is a modification of one first published in 1988 by Tile. It is based on the roles that direction of force, anatomy, and stability play in the evaluation and management of pelvic fractures. It is important to remember that unstable fractures pose the greatest threat to the patient. Like all such classification systems, this system is helpful in understanding the causation of pelvic fractures and guiding their treatment, but does not replace the judgment of a skilled clinician when managing individual patients.

Presentation

Patients with low-energy injuries usually present with a history of a mechanism of injury as described above as well as focal pain. Swelling, ecchymosis, erythema, and focal tenderness may also be present. With avulsion injuries there is often pain associated with contraction of the involved muscle.

As stated above, patients with high-energy injuries present after motor vehicle accidents, falls, and crush injuries. If conscious, these patients complain of significant pain in the pelvis, lower back, buttocks, or hips. They are usually unable to stand. Concomitant distracting injuries or intoxication may limit the reliability of the history. In patients with altered mental status or spinal neurologic deficits, the presence of a pelvic fracture should be assumed until definitively excluded. Physical findings include pelvic deformity or instability, abnormal position of the lower extremities, swelling, and ecchymosis. The abdomen, perineum, genitals, rectum, and lower back must be carefully examined. Signs of associated injuries include evidence of hypovolemia, abdominal distention, signs of retroperitoneal hemorrhage, evidence of injury to the lower gastrointestinal or genitourinary tracts, and neurovascular deficits of the lower extremities.

Evaluation

A single anteroposterior plane film of the pelvis reveals approximately 85% of bony pelvic injuries. All bony cortices must be examined for disruption. The width of the symphysis pubis should be measured (normally <6 mm). Injuries to the sacrum may be poorly seen on this view. The sacroiliac joints must be specifically inspected for asymmetry or widening (normal width <5 mm). Fractures of the sacral body are often evidenced only by subtle disruption of the arcuate lines. Inlet and outlet views of the pelvis are more sensitive in revealing sacral fractures and may be obtained if initial evaluation suggests such an injury.

Computed tomography plays a valuable adjunctive role in the evaluation of pelvic fractures. It provides highly detailed images of the complex bony structure of the pelvis and reliably visualizes even very small, nondisplaced fractures. It is especially useful in the evaluation of known or suspected sacral fractures which it readily identifies, and acetabular fractures. CT scan also provides important information regarding associated injuries, particularly hemorrhage.

Associated Injuries

Bleeding is the only immediately life-threatening complication of pelvic fractures and is responsible for the vast majority of deaths related to these injuries. Unstable fractures can disrupt the arterial and venous beds that lie within the pelvis, resulting in hemorrhage that is often retroperitoneal and therefore difficult to identify. Such bleeding should be presumed in any patient with evidence of a fractured pelvis and signs of hypovolemia.

As described above, the pelvic contents are prone to injury when the bony pelvis is disrupted, and associated injuries to these structures must be sought. The gastrointestinal, genitourinary, and nervous systems are particularly vulnerable. The specific injuries and their treatment are discussed elsewhere in this book.

Treatment

Low-energy injuries (isolated fractures and avulsions) are usually adequately managed with conservative care including bed rest, pain control, and physical therapy. Consultation and early follow-up with an orthopedic surgeon are recommended.

The management of high-energy or unstable pelvic fractures is a more pressing concern to the emergency physician. These patients are best treated as severely injured trauma patients, and involvement of a designated trauma team is warranted. If such services are unavailable, transfer to a trauma center should take place as soon as the patient's clinical status permits. Treatment of the patient's pelvic injuries must be appropriately prioritized and coordinated with the management of other injuries. An orthopedic surgeon should in all cases be emergently consulted. The variety of associated internal injuries that may be present is great, and their management is discussed in relevant sections of this book.

If associated hemorrhage has been excluded, then definitive care of the fracture is provided by the consulting orthopedist. The emergency physician must in the meantime maintain pelvic immobilization while addressing any other issues. Associated hemorrhage, if present, represents a potential threat to the patient's life and must be aggressively managed.

There may remain some role for the use of the pneumatic antishock garment (PASG), also known as military antishock trousers (MAST), in the initial management of patients with known or suspected unstable pelvic fractures, especially if associated with evidence of hypovolemia. They help to reduce and stabilize the fractures, which in turn can help control hemorrhage. Their use may be most justified in the prehospital setting, particularly when long transport times are involved. There are drawbacks to their application, however, and no clear consensus exists as to the particular instances in which they should be employed.

For the emergency physician, the mainstay of treatment of hemorrhage associated with pelvic fractures, as with any patient suffering significant blood loss, is aggressive intravascular volume resuscitation. Other more definitive methods of controlling associated bleeding include placement of an external fixation device, open reduction and external fixation, and angiography-guided selective arterial embolization. These techniques require the involvement of specialist consultants. Which technique is chosen depends on the clinical situation, the opinion of the consultant, and the capabilities of the institution.

Types of Pelvic Fractures

Pubic Rami

Fractures to the pubic rami can be isolated low-energy fractures or may be one component of a more significant high-energy fracture pattern. An isolated superior or inferior pubic ramus fracture is the most common pelvic fracture, and typically results from a fall onto the buttocks. Treatment is conservative. Fractures through both the superior and ipsilateral inferior pubic rami represent disruption of the pelvic ring at that point but constitute a stable fracture pattern unless accompanied by another fracture in the pelvic ring (**FIGURE 173.1**).

Straddle

Bilateral double pubic ramus fractures are dubbed straddle fractures, as they are often the result of falling onto a hard object (e.g., fence, rim of bathtub) that is between the legs. They are unstable fractures and result in associated injuries, particularly of the lower urinary tract or bowel, in up to one third of cases. Perineal findings are common.

Iliac Crest

Low-energy stable fractures of the iliac crest include avulsion fractures at sites of tendinous insertion. The Duverney fracture (also called the stove-in or pelvic wing fracture) is a high-energy but stable injury and involves an isolated fracture through the pelvic wing. It results from a

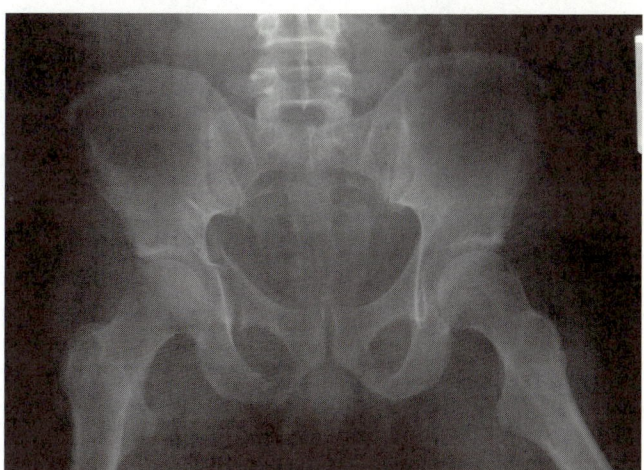

FIGURE 173.1 Radiograph showing a fracture of the right inferior pubic ramus.

lateral compressive force and can be associated with injury to adjacent viscera. The fracture fragment off of the iliac crest may be unstable, mimicking pelvic ring instability on physical examination.

Fractures through the ilium typically involve the iliac crest. These are high-energy injuries that represent pelvic ring disruption and are often associated with disruption of the pelvic ring at another point. Concomitant visceral injuries are frequently present.

Malgaigne

The definition of a Malgaigne fracture varies somewhat among physicians. Here the term refers to an injury pattern involving a disruption through both the anterior and posterior pelvis with resultant instability of the intervening fragment. The anterior disruption typically involves the symphysis pubis or pubic rami, while the posterior

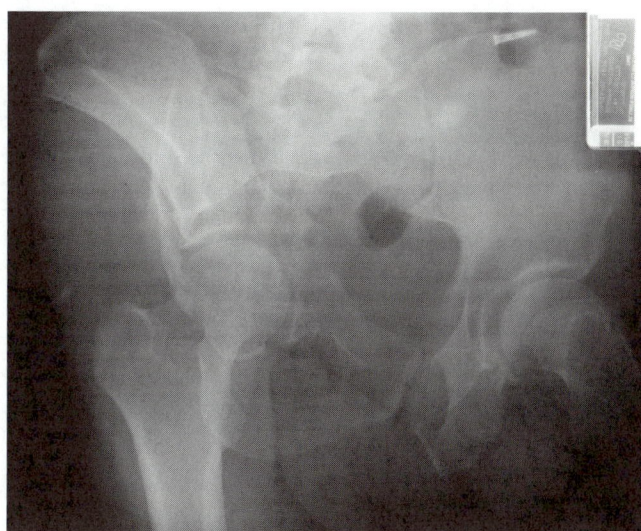

FIGURE 173.2 Oblique view of the pelvis demonstrating disruption of the anterior pelvis, the right acetabulum, and the right sacroiliac joint.

component involves the sacrum, sacroiliac joint, or ilium. These fractures result from vertical shear forces, usually from a fall from a height onto the lower extremities (i.e., in a standing or kneeling position). They are the least common of the major pelvic fractures. These high-energy, unstable fractures are associated with significant concomitant injuries. Morbidity and mortality rates are high (**FIGURE 173.2**).

Selected Readings

Harris JH Jr, Harris WH. *The Radiology of Emergency Medicine,* 4th ed. Philadelphia: Lippincott Williams and Wilkins, 2000.

Mirvis SE, Shanmuganathan K, eds. *Imaging in Trauma and Critical Care,* 2d ed. Basel: Elsevier Science, 2003.

Moore EE, Feliciano DV, Mattox KL, eds. *Trauma,* 5th ed. New York: McGraw-Hill Professional, 2004.

Genitourinary Injuries

Peter Angood

Trauma to the genitourinary (GU) system and the potential hemodynamic consequences resultant from these injuries may be easily underestimated due to the concealed, retroperitoneal location of many of its structures. The magnitude and complexity of multisystem involvement of the significantly traumatized patient create a diagnostic diversion, resulting in missed or delayed diagnoses. Since genitourinary injuries usually occur along with other truncal injuries, the clinical picture at presentation is often obscure. GU trauma may present as generalized abdomen tenderness, flank or back pain, hematuria, hypovolemic shock, or even no symptoms. To illustrate, it's not difficult to imagine overlooking a renal contusion or a posterior urethral transection in a patient with a Glasgow Coma Scale equal to 7, a flail segment, and an open, comminuted femur fracture. Although many of these injuries do not represent an immediate threat to life, they are associated with long-term morbidity and delayed hemodynamic compromise. These injuries are present in 3% to 10% of patients with blunt or penetrating trauma. GU pathology is relatively common in the trauma victims.

The spectrum of GU injuries is fairly limited. Most frequently, errors in management arise from failure to diagnose, as opposed to treatment errors following their detection. These injuries are often subtle and must be found. The key to prompt diagnosis and appropriate management is awareness. The primary components of the GU system requiring urgent evaluation in any trauma patient are the kidneys, ureters, bladder, and urethra.

Renal Injuries

The kidneys are highly vascular organs, subsequently carrying the highest risk of hemorrhage and hemodynamic sequelae of all the organs included in this system. Their location is retroperitoneal, with the lower ribs and the muscles of the back providing protection from blunt forces. Trauma to the kidneys results from direct force to the back, flank, or abdomen, with penetrating trauma accounting for approximately 5% of injuries. Renal injuries can include contusions, lacerations, fragmentation, and pedicle injuries. Most common are the parenchymal contusions accounting for approximately 85% of all injuries. Renal vascular injuries are the most life threatening. The kidney is relatively fixed in position in the retroperitoneum. Unfortunately, the renal vasculature is not. Shearing forces in blunt abdominal trauma may disrupt renal blood flow and result in significant retroperitoneal and intra-abdominal hemorrhage.

Diagnostic Testing

After years of debate, the recent literature has provided valuable data defining the standard of care in many of these issues. Often, the patient's urological diagnostic needs are delayed to achieve acute hemostasis and treat other acute traumatic pathology. These cases pose little complexity in the acute diagnostic evaluation of the GU system. If the patient requires emergent exploratory laparotomy mandated by signs of peritoneal irritation or persistent hemodynamic compromise, three options remain: direct exploration without radiographic evaluation; rapid injection or one-shot intravenous urogram en route to the operating room; or postsurgical observation with subsequent radiographic evaluation. Patients requiring postsurgical evaluation include those with signs of persistent urologic injury such as elevations in blood urea nitrogen and creatinine, gross hematuria, inability to void, and abdominal findings such as masses, peritoneal irritation, suprapubic, and/or flank tenderness or contusions consistent with urine extravasation or abscess/hematoma formation. Following surgical stabilization, the patient's clinical course will guide the clinician's need for further diagnostics.

A common diagnostic dilemma encountered by the emergency physician is which radiographic modality to employ when evaluating the stable trauma victim with the potential for injury to the kidney, ureters, or bladder. Diagnostic studies to evaluate the kidneys after trauma can include plane films, intravenous pyelogram (IVP), computed tomography (CT), and ultrasound. Plane films offer limited information but can give subtle signs such as loss of renal or psoas shadows, or fracture of lower ribs. Traditionally, IVP has been the study of choice to evaluate renal trauma since it can be done on an unstable patient in the ED. IVP gives a comparison study of one kidney with the other and can indicate renal injury through delay of excretion of contrast. Intravenous contrast-enhanced CT scan has now become the study of choice. In trauma, CT scanning can be used to evaluate all abdominal injuries, and not just renal injuries. Odds are that a patient with GU injuries will have other abdominal injuries requiring CT for evaluation. CT provides more information per study than IVP; CT scans provide functional and anatomical information about the kidneys as well as other valuable information about other structures. Proper screening to determine the necessity for urological evaluation is essential. Many patients will undergo CT scan of the abdomen for evaluation of abdominal pain without peritoneal signs or with significant mechanism of injury to raise the index of suspicion for intra-abdominal pathology. Following CT of the abdomen, no further evaluation of the kidneys, ureters, or bladder is needed as this modality has proven to be very effective in the detection of retroperitoneal and intraperitoneal pathology.

Urologic Injuries

In evaluating those patients with suspected isolated urologic injuries, without suspicion of concomitant abdominal trauma, the most important question to ask is, "Which patients require radiological evaluation?" Hematuria is the cardinal marker of renal injury, and the severity of hematuria usually parallels the magnitude of renal injury. Previous data supported emergent/urgent urologic evaluation for microscopic hematuria of 50 red blood cells (RBCs) per high power field (hpf). Subsequent data suggested a more discriminating approach using 100 RBCs/hpf. As this debate has evolved, the current literature recommends that adult patients with microscopic hematuria do not require emergent/urgent GU evaluation unless it is accompanied by hypotension. This hypotension may also include transient hypotension reported by emergency medical services (EMS) personnel. Furthermore, these cases of uncomplicated microscopic hematuria usually resolve spontaneously. However, all of these patients should be referred for urological follow-up to confirm resolution of their hematuria. The pediatric population should be treated with a lower threshold for investigation.

Special Consideration: Children

Because of their anatomical disadvantages, children are very susceptible to intra-abdominal injuries. Blunt renal injuries are responsible for 90% of renal injuries in children. Some investigators have reported the kidney as the most common organ injured in blunt abdominal trauma in childhood, and that children should receive formal investigation regardless of the degree of hematuria present following significant blunt renal trauma. To date, no strong data support the screening of the pediatric population as we do adults with suspected renal injuries. Although IVP is likely to be as effective as CT scan in elucidating injuries of the kidneys, ureters, and bladder, CT scan should always be considered because of the vulnerability of the pediatric abdomen and the propensity for multiple organ injuries.

Radiographs

IVP and CT scanning have shared well-documented success for the evaluation of the kidneys, ureters, and bladder. Although IVP and CT are well respected, ultrasonography is rapidly finding a permanent place in the radiological evaluation of the trauma victim. Currently, that role appears to be one of bedside screening for hemoperitoneum, kidney, and bladder injuries. If readily available at the bedside, and perhaps incorporated into the secondary survey, ultrasound may help screen for injuries requiring emergency/urgent surgical explorations or more definitive radiologic examination. Although it is the least expensive modality, the diagnostic accuracy of ultrasound in the face of blunt renal trauma has been reported to be as low as 41%, compared to IVP with 80.8% accuracy.

Ureteral Injury

Ureteral injuries are rare but may occur from blunt or penetrating trauma. Ureteropelvic disruption is the most common ureteral injury and should be suspected with lumbar vertebrae fractures. Urinalysis may or may not reveal hematuria. Urinalysis may be normal in up to 50% of patients. IVP should be performed to rule out extravasation of contrast dye. Urgent surgical repair is required if ureteral injuries are revealed since the risk of nephrectomy increases with time.

Blunt trauma to the lower urinary tract is usually associated with pelvic fractures. Obvious signs are blood at the urethral meatus, a high-riding prostate, difficulty in voiding, or a perineal hematoma. At times, these signs may not be present because bladder rupture can occur in a full bladder without a pelvic fracture. Urethral injuries are divided into anterior urethral injuries (the penis and urethra below the urogenital diaphragm) and posterior urethral injuries (the urethra above the urogenital diaphragm). Injuries to the posterior urethra may result in incontinence and impotence. If Buck's fascia is injured in anterior urethral injuries, urine may extend into the penis and scrotum.

Evaluation of suspected posterior urethral injury is addressed with very little controversy. Patients with pelvic fractures, nonpalpable or high riding prostates, gross hematuria, scrotal or labial hematoma, inability to void, or obvious urethral injury should be studied via retrograde cystourethrogram. Retrograde urethrography can be performed by inflating the balloon of a Foley catheter 2 to 3 cm into the urethra with the instillation of 30 cc of water-soluble contrast. Extravasation of the contrast or no contrast evident in the bladder is evidence of urethral disruption. This may be followed with a voiding cystourethrogram. Positive findings suggestive of urethral disruption include contrast media extravasation into surrounding tissues and lack of contiguous contrast flow. One should not blindly insert a Foley catheter into a patient with suspected urethral or bladder injury; a urethrogram or cystourethrogram should be performed first.

Genital Injury

Scrotal and testicular injuries occur from direct trauma, most commonly sporting injuries or straddle injuries. Injuries range from minor testicular contusions and hematoma to testicular rupture. The testes are protected by the cremasteric reflex and the tunica albuginea. Testicular injury usually results from compression of the testes against the symphysis pubis. The injury results in a hematocele and the patient presents with a tender, enlarged scrotum, taking on a bluish hue. Physical examination may be limited in evaluation of testicular injuries due to local swelling and tenderness. If physical examination cannot provide accurate information, diagnostic studies such as ultrasonography and radionuclide scanning should be pursued. Radionuclide scanning offers the benefit of providing information on function of the testes. Treatment for minor hematoma or contusion can be treated conservatively with ice packs and scrotal support. Recent information recommends exploration and evacuation of blood clots for large hematoma and testicular rupture. Penetrating injuries to the testes universally require surgical exploration. The sooner surgical repair can be performed, the more likely testicular function can be preserved.

Penile trauma is rare, presenting as simple lacerations or penile fractures. In either case, a urethrogram should be obtained to rule out urethral injury if suspected. Penile fracture presents as a painful, discolored, and swollen penis. Surgical evacuation of the blood clot that has formed is necessary. Zipper injuries of the penis are best treated with cutting of the median bar of the zipper, which will cause the zipper to fall apart. Manipulation of the zipper in attempts to unzip it will only result in increased pain and infrequent success.

Vaginal injuries must be suspected in trauma patients presenting with vulvar/perineal hematoma, or swelling. Careful pelvic examination must be performed to rule out urethral, vulvar, vaginal, and/or rectal injuries. Vulvar and vaginal trauma may result in significant bleeding and hypotension. Initial therapy should be addressed to hemodynamic stability with intravenous fluids. Again, careful physical examination will lead to the source of bleeding. Appropriate screening by the emergency physician is the key to successfully diagnosing injuries of the genitourinary system. Clinicians must be mindful of the presence of urologic injuries while treating the multiply injured patient. Detection and treatment of more life-threatening injuries must be a patient management priority, not an excuse for overlooking the subtleties of urinary system injury.

Selected Readings

Bandi G, Santucci RA. Controversies in the management of male external genitourinary trauma. *J Trauma* 2004;56:1362–1370.

Nance ML, Lutz N, Carr MC, et al. Blunt renal injuries in children can be managed nonoperatively: outcome in a consecutive series of patients. *J Trauma* 2004;57:474–478.

Villas PA, Cohen G, Putnam SG III, et al. Wallstent placement in a renal artery after blunt abdominal trauma. *J Trauma* 1999;46:1137–1139.

Wessells H, Suh D, Porter JR, et al. Renal injury and operative management in the United States: results of a population-based study. *J Trauma* 2003;54:423–430.

175 Cutaneous Injuries Including Crush Injuries

Harry L. Anderson III
Peter Angood
Marc Gautreau

Approximately 10 million wounds are seen each year in the nation's EDs with many requiring meticulous wound care and closure. The general goals of wound care are to minimize the risk of infection, optimize cosmetic appearance, and restore strength and function to the affected part. However, there are still more than 500,000 wound infections and complications per year, leading to considerable costs and patient morbidity. The quality of the initial wound care directly influences the outcome. Thus, it is imperative that the emergency physician be knowledgeable in the aspects of wound physiology and healing as well as have the technical expertise for basic wound care and closure techniques.

Physiology

Typical wound healing is an orderly but complex process that begins almost immediately after the initial insult. The stages of coagulation, inflammation, epithelialization, fibroplasia, and scar maturation characterize all wounds that extend below the epithelium. Once the skin is disrupted, platelets initiate the coagulation cascade in addition to releasing chemotactic factors to initiate and enhance the inflammatory steps. Capillaries surrounding the area become more permeable and allow the migration of white blood cells (WBCs) to the site of injury. Epithelial cells begin to migrate early in the repair process and may cover the wound as early as the first 24 to 48 hours.

Phagocytosis of dead tissue, debris, and bacteria occurs by neutrophils and monocytes. Between the second and fourth days, neovascularization begins and chemotactic factors stimulate the fibroblasts to begin synthesizing collagen. This starts the process of scar formation or *fibroplasia*. After initial retraction, the wound edges will begin to contract during the third to fourth day. By about day 7 the collagen production has peaked and the tensile strength of the wound will increase dramatically. In this early stage, the wound has only 5% of its ultimate tensile strength. Because of the disorganized way collagen is initially laid down, it will take another 1 to 2 years before the collagen is remodeled and the scar reaches its maximum strength.

It is important to note that the final appearance of the scar cannot be predicted until at least 4 to 6 months into its remodeling stage. Patients should be made aware of the time needed for complete recovery during the initial evaluation and before any scar revision is contemplated.

Initial Evaluation

History

A complete history should include a detailed review of the circumstances surrounding the wound including the mechanism of injury, the timing of the event, associated injuries, and prehospital care, if any. Certain mechanisms such as blunt or crush injuries, high pressure injection injuries, and bite wounds may radically change the management.

Several factors affect initial wound care and may inhibit proper wound healing, including the mechanism and the timing of the wound, wound contamination, the initial wound care and closure technique, and associated conditions of the patient. A thorough past medical history should be obtained, focusing on those aspects that could affect wound healing and treatment such as comorbidities, current medications, allergies, and immune status.

Mechanism of Injury

Most cutaneous wounds are caused by three mechanisms: shearing, compression, and tension forces. The mechanism of injury effects both the initial wound management and the potential for infection.

Shearing forces are those caused by sharp objects and typically lead to lacerations. This imparts little energy, thus minimizing damage to the surrounding tissues. Simple lacerations of this nature are generally repaired by primary intention, have a lower risk of infection, and have cosmetically acceptable scars.

Tension forces are caused by blunt injuries exerted at less than 90 degrees to the skin surface. These injuries typically result in avulsions. They impart a greater amount of destructive energy to the surrounding tissues. Avulsion injuries are also at greater risk for ischemia unless the base of the avulsion is relatively large and well preserved. Thus tension forces increase the risk for wound infection and scar formation.

Compression injuries are the result of forces applied at 90 degrees to the skin surface. This typically imparts substantial energy to the surrounding tissue and leads to ragged and stellate wounds if the force is sufficient to tear skin. These injuries have a greater amount of devitalized tissue, which increases the likelihood of infection and often unacceptable scarring. These wounds frequently require extensive debridement and irrigation.

Age of the Wound

In general, the risk of wound infection increases as delays in wound cleansing and decontamination increase. Any wound that has been open for more than 12 hours poses a significant risk of infection if closed in a primary fashion. However, all wounds requiring closure need to be evaluated in their own context regardless of the timing of the event. For example, the physician may choose to close most wounds of the face even after 24 hours have elapsed to achieve the best cosmetic result. Scalp wound closure may also be safely extended more than 12 hours. On the other hand, some wounds may be unsuitable for closure regardless of the timing, such as puncture wounds and heavily contaminated wounds of the extremities.

Patient Factors Affecting Wound Care

Several patient factors, including comorbid illnesses, may affect the way a wound is managed. It is generally felt that conditions such as diabetes, peripheral vascular disease, malnutrition, cirrhosis, and uremia may adversely affect or delay the healing process.

Several drugs have been implicated in delayed wound healing because of their effect on the inflammatory process or their propensity to cause hematoma formation. These include corticosteroids, nonsteroidal anti-inflammatory drugs (NSAIDs), penicillamine, colchicine, and antineoplastic agents.

Keloid formation is an excessive accumulation of scar tissue that extends beyond the borders of the original wound. This condition is more common in blacks and dark-skinned people. The most common sites are the ears, lower abdomen, sternum, and upper extremities.

Examining the Wound

The wound should be examined with sterile technique and preferably under local or regional anesthesia. Every wound should be examined for associated structural injuries. This includes neurological and vascular examinations of the injured area. Capillary refill, peripheral pulse quality, and skin color should be noted. Strength testing, range of motion, and sensory testing (including two-point discrimination of the digits) should be documented. A thorough visual and tactile examination of the wound needs to be done to appreciate subtle tendon lacerations or palpable bony irregularities that might otherwise be missed. This sometimes requires surgical extension of the wound incision for proper inspection.

Most new wounds need some degree of active hemostasis. This can usually be done by direct pressure over the wound site with sterile gauze. Epinephrine is a good vasoconstrictor and, when combined with a local anesthetic, prolongs anesthesia as well as provides some degree of hemostasis.

Electrocautery is available in many EDs and is an excellent choice for hemostasis of bleeding vessels less than 2 mm in diameter. This form of hemostasis requires a relatively dry field, and active suctioning by an assistant is often needed. Bipolar cautery causes 30% less tissue necrosis in the surrounding area and is usually preferred over monopolar cautery. Self-contained battery-powered cautery is available and is very easy to use. It is very convenient but can cause excessive tissue damage if used extensively, and it should not be used on finger or toe injuries. Bleeding vessels greater than 2 mm in size, and refractory to direct pressure should be ligated with absorbable suture. Because of the proximity of the nerves to the vessels and the potential for neuropraxia or permanent nerve damage, ligature and cautery techniques are best avoided in the hands and feet.

Hemostasis can also be achieved by a tourniquet mechanism. For example, when exploring digits, a Penrose drain tightened around the digit can often achieve a bloodless field. A blood pressure cuff inflated to 70 mm Hg above the systolic blood pressure and then clamped can give adequate hemostasis for extremity wounds. The time of tourniquet placement must be documented and is generally safe for up to 30 minutes to an hour on an extremity or digit.

Gelatin foam, fibrin foam, and other hemostatic materials are very useful in small wounds with continuous oozing. These work well with small, complete skin avulsions of the fingers, which have a tendency for prolonged capillary bleeding. For excessive bleeding from scalp wounds, Raney scalp clips are excellent hemostatic devices that are easy to use and very fast to apply. They are applied along the scalp edge by a special applicator to tamponade the bleeding. Once the bleeding is controlled, the wound can be closed by sequentially removing the clips from the part of the wound edge being repaired.

Detecting Foreign Bodies

Nearly every wound needs to be explored for foreign bodies (FBs). The physician should assess the potential for FB presence and determine the best method of locating it. Low-risk wounds such as those caused by a sharp, intact metallic edge or knife often require only basic irrigation and cleansing. However, deep splinters of wood, teeth, dirt, clay, and other organic materials will most certainly cause infection, and the exploration should be carried out diligently. This often requires extension of the wound with an incision, extensive probing, and cleansing.

The most common and cost-effective adjunctive technique is plane radiographs. This generally requires multiple projections to localize the FBs. It is also helpful to place two needles in the area of the FB. The needles should be at 90 degrees to each other. These can serve as directional landmarks when trying to determine the position of the FB in relation to the x-ray. It is also better to use an underpenetrated technique. If the history suggests a radioopaque FB, this is the test of choice. Metallic objects are demonstrated quite well. The exception to this is aluminum, which can be difficult to detect on plane films especially if it has dimensions less than 0.5 mm. Glass can sometimes be detected on plane films. Gravel, teeth, and a few plastics can also be detected on plane films. Organic material such as wood splinters and thorns are poorly visualized on plane films. Xeroradiography has been investigated but shown to be no better than plane films and is not typically available to the emergency physician.

Although CT scan and MRI are available, they have limited usefulness in detecting FBs. CT scan may define subtle soft tissue changes and it generally detects the same substances as plane films. MRI may be more sensitive for wood and plastic FBs. MRI should not be used if metallic FBs are suspected.

Ultrasound (US) is becoming more readily available to the ED physician and is rapidly becoming the modality of choice for the hard-to-find FB. This is especially true with FBs composed of plastic or wood. US has about a 90% sensitivity and specificity for these types of FBs. In areas with many echogenic structures such as the hands and feet, US becomes less useful. US should be done before manual wound exploration since the presence of gas in tissue obscures the US images. Fluoroscopy has also been utilized, although it is rarely readily available.

Wound Preparation

Once a history and physical examination has addressed the life- and limb-threatening injuries, a complete functional and neurovascular examination should be performed. The wound should be anesthetized by local or regional methods prior to wound cleansing, irrigation, or exploration. Patients should be supine for the examination because fainting is a common occurrence. The physician should work in a comfortable position, and universal precautions should always be used, including sterile gloves, face and eye shielding, and a protective gown or garment. Shaving the body hair around the wound leads to an increase in the rate of infection. Hair around the wound may be clipped if it is interfering with the wound closure. Surgical gel can be applied to hair around the wound to mat down any troublesome strands. Sterile drapes or a single fenestrated drape are used to border the wound site after the surrounding skin has been cleansed.

Wound Cleansing

The two accepted methods of wound cleaning are mechanical scrubbing and irrigation. Soaking a wound in an antiseptic solution is inadequate and may increase the risk of wound infection. The area surrounding the wound should be scrubbed and any particulate matter and tissue debris should be removed. Scrubbing the area around the wound should be done with an antiseptic solution, the most common being 10% povidone-iodine solution (not the surgical scrub). This particular solution has been implicated in supporting fungal growth and has since been proven inferior to chlorhexidine with isopropyl alcohol.

Commercially available antiseptics should be applied only to intact skin. They should not be used as irrigant solutions. Most of the antiseptic solutions are toxic to exposed tissue and may inhibit wound healing.

Scrubbing the inside of the wound may lead to tissue damage and increased inflammation. This should be reserved for those wounds that are heavily contaminated or have embedded particulate matter that cannot be removed by irrigation alone. If the internal surface of the wound requires scrubbing, then a fine-pore sponge should be used to minimize tissue damage. Patients with road rash abrasions may have extensive areas of embedded particulate matter. This often requires extensive scrubbing of the wound, which can be extremely painful. Viscous lidocaine over the abraded area is often helpful, and conscious sedation is frequently needed.

"Dilution is the solution for pollution." Irrigation has been well proven as the most effective modality of open wound cleansing. Normal saline is the irrigant of choice. Antiseptic dilutions of 1% povidone have shown promise but should not be used near mucous membranes. Full-strength antiseptics should not be used as wound irrigants. The recommended amount of irrigant for an average-size wound is estimated to be—but not limited to—between 100 and 300 mL. This number is only a guideline and a heavily contaminated wound should be irrigated with much more than this amount of fluid.

Wound irrigation is not effective unless there is sufficient hydraulic force applied when delivering the irrigant solution. IV irrigation under gravity will deliver less than 10 psi. A handheld syringe with an 18-gauge catheter attached can deliver up to 25 to 40 psi and is a quite effective, low-tech irrigating system. Some manufactures have developed a convenient ring-handled irrigation syringe attached to an IV via a one-way valve. There are pulsatile jet irrigation systems also available that are capable of 50 to 70 psi and of delivering an extraordinary amount of irrigant in a very short amount of time. These systems are relatively cumbersome and should be reserved for those wounds that are extensive and heavily contaminated.

Debridement

Debridement of devitalized and severely contaminated tissue is done to improve wound healing and cosmesis. Sharp dissection of wound edges is usually performed with a scalpel and forceps or skin hooks. Debridement is also done to transform a ragged laceration into a linear wound to hasten the repair and lessen the scar. Wounds with clean sharp edges usually need no debridement. Most wounds are closed readily after debridement, but if excessive skin tension becomes an issue after tissue removal, then undermining the edges may help. If excessive skin tension is the result of the debridement, then even a transformed, linear wound may heal with a worse scar than its ragged counterpart.

If possible, it may be best to forgo debridement in areas such as the eyebrows, lips, and eyelids. Maintaining the symmetry of these structures is cosmetically and functionally important. These areas also tend to heal remarkably well. In some areas of the body circumferential excision of the entire wound may be useful. For example, a heavily contaminated wound of the trunk could be completely excised, making primary closure feasible.

Wound Closure

Most uncomplicated wounds can be managed with primary closure in the ED. Some wounds are at great risk for infection and should be managed by secondary intention. Several factors such as age of the wound, contamination, and the presence of severe crush injuries and bite injuries need to be weighed when assessing the risk of infection. Healing by secondary intention implies the wound will be cleansed in the standard fashion but left open and allowed to heal without approximation of the wound edges. Secondary healing involves much more inflammation, scarring, and contracture.

Another alternative is to close the wound in a delayed fashion. Once a contaminated wound is thoroughly cleansed, irrigated, and debrided, it may be packed with sterile, wet-saline gauze pads and dressed. The dressing and packing are changed daily. Antibiotics are often prescribed but have not proven useful during this period. The wound should be rechecked in 3 to 5 days. Healing wounds gain resistance to infection during this period. If the wound is not infected after this time, then the edges can be approximated with standard closure techniques (delayed primary closure). The edges can also be excised before closure (secondary closure). Cosmetic results are usually the same as if the wound were closed by primary intention.

Suturing

Suturing is the primary method of wound closure in most situations. Suturing technique is covered extensively in other textbooks; however, some basic principles need mentioning.

Suturing Materials

There are several ways to categorize suture material, but the two most commonly used are *nonabsorbable,* which is typically used to close the outer layer of skin, and *absorbable,* which is generally used for closure of deep layers of the wound. The absorbable types can be natural or synthetic. They are made from cow or sheep serosa and submucosa (plain gut and chromic gut), polyglycolic acid (Dexon), or polyglactin (Vicryl and coated Vicryl). The nonabsorbable types include silk and a variety of synthetic materials such as nylon, Dacron, polyester, polyethylene, and polypropylene. Sutures can also be classified as monofilament or multifilament and braided.

Absorption and reactivity are important characteristics of any suture material. Suture that maintains its strength in tissue for at least 60 days is considered nonabsorbable. Suture that is degraded before 60 days is considered to be absorbable. Of the absorbable types, plain gut lasts 10 to 40 days, except in the oral cavity, where it lasts only 3 to 5 days. Gut suture treated with chromium trioxide lasts 15 to 60 days. Vicryl maintains its strength for 60 to 90 days and Dexon 120 to 200 days.

All sutures create a host inflammatory reaction that can increase the risk of wound infection. The least reactive of the absorbable sutures are the polyglycolic types and the polyglactin type, while gut sutures have the greatest reactivity. Of the nonabsorbable sutures, polypropylene is the least reactive and silk the most reactive.

Practically speaking, most wounds can be closed using only a few types of sutures. Fascial closure is typically done with absorbable 3-0 or 4-0 suture materials, although it is acceptable to use low-reactivity, nonabsorbable types. Subcutaneous closure is typically done with absorbable 3-0 to 4-0 sutures, while skin closure is done with 3-0 to 5-0 nonabsorbable types.

There is much leeway in the selection of suture materials. For example, most clinicians prefer a smaller-caliber suture on facial closure, such as 5-0 to 6-0 sutures. Eyelids require a very fine suture, such as 6-0 to 7-0, while wounds that may be subject to considerable tension may require 2-0 to 4-0 sutures.

Closures

Most wounds can be closed with a single cutaneous layer. Scar formation is related to wound tension; thus, most wounds that are deep or gaping should be closed in several layers. This technique reduces tissue tension, closes the deep spaces, and may lower the risk of infection. One begins with the deep muscle layers, closing the fascia only. One should not attempt suture through the friable belly of the muscle. The next layer is the subcutaneous layer; suturing this layer reduces the tension on the outermost layer of closure. Sometimes it may be necessary to undermine the wound edges with sharp or blunt dissection to reduce tension on the skin edges. The final layer is the cutaneous closure.

The depth and width of each suture should be the same on either side of the wound edge. This will keep the surface even and minimize scarring. The wound edges should be slightly everted and the wound edges should be approximated with no more than the tension necessary to appose the two sides.

Facial Wounds

Special mention should be made of facial wound repair. Wounds of the face bring added anxiety to the patient for obvious cosmetic reasons. Wound closure of the face also requires some important details that need to be considered to obtain the best cosmetic result.

Facial lacerations require attention to certain closure principles to produce an acceptable cosmetic result. First, debridement should be very conservative. In fact, most facial wounds have excellent vascular supply, and even tenuous wound edges may survive without infection or necrosis. When wounds are perpendicular or oblique to the natural skin lines, the increased tension will result in a less acceptable cosmetic effect. There is less scarring in wounds that are parallel to natural skin lines.

Another very important principle is wound tension. Most deep facial wounds should be closed in a multilayer fashion in order to reduce the tension on the epithelial stitch. The subcutaneous layer should be repaired with thin absorbable suture so as to approximate the outer wound edges within 2 to 3 mm of each other before final closure. It is also important that the subcutaneous repair leaves the wound edges exactly parallel in depth before final closure. This can be accomplished by adjusting the depth of each bite. By taking a deeper bite on the shallow wound edge, one can elevate this edge to meet the opposing wound edge. The opposite is also true—a more shallow bite may be able to depress a wound edge that was originally too high to line up with its opposing wound edge.

Once the wound has been adequately approximated, the epithelial closure can be accomplished with 6-0 nonabsorbable suture. Either a running or interrupted technique is acceptable. Outer sutures should be no more than 2 to 3 mm apart and 2 to 3 mm from the wound edge. Excessive tension on the suture will increase scarring. A subcuticular approach may be used, but there is some controversy as to whether this has a superior cosmetic effect. The closing suture can also be reinforced with wound tape.

Sutures should be removed in 4 to 5 days and reinforced with wound tape strips if necessary. During healing, the debris and scab that forms on the wound should be gently cleansed with dilute hydrogen peroxide or sterile water to reduce scarring. The patient should be instructed to refrain from sunbathing, and exposing the healed skin to sun for at least 6 months, since this can enhance the scarring. Sunblock may be helpful. Consultation with a plastic surgeon may be necessary for complex wounds.

Surgical Staples

Surgical staples are an excellent technique for wound closure if the wound is properly selected. Appropriate wounds are linear lacerations with sharp edges on the, chest, back, abdomen, or extremity. High cost is the primary disadvantage to stapling, and staples are not used for deep-layer closure. The deep layers need basic suturing before staples are applied. Staples should never be used on the face, neck, hands, or feet. Staples should also be avoided in closing scalp lacerations, since they provide little hemostasis to the very thick and vascular skin of the scalp. A running, interlocked closure of heavy (2-0), nonabsorbable suture is best used here. Staples should also be avoided if the patient is a candidate for CT scan, since they will cause artifact in areas undergoing radiological survey.

The primary advantage to stapling is the speed at which relatively large wounds can be closed. Stapling carries the same risk of infection as suturing and equal wound healing properties. Staples are left in for the same duration as sutures. Staple removal can be done in the office setting, but the patient should receive a staple remover prior to discharge since many offices may not stock them.

Wound Tape

The use of wound tape strips has increased over the past several years. This method of wound closure has advantages over staples and sutures, including a reduced need for anesthesia, greater resistance to wound infection, evenly distributed tissue tension, no suture marks, ease of application, and no need for suture removal.

Primarily this technique is used on superficial, straight lacerations in areas with very little tissue tension. Gaping tissue must be approximated with deep suturing before taping. Taping can also be used as an adjunct to sutured skin closure and to support the wound after early suture removal. It should not be used on ragged, nonlinear wounds under excessive tissue tension. Moist intertriginous areas, palms, soles, scalp, or bearded areas are better areas for suturing than for surgical tape strips. Never place tape strips circumferentially around a digit.

The basic procedure is quite simple, but a few key points need mentioning. As with any wound, proper selection and thorough cleansing is required. Meticulous drying of the wound edges is needed for the tape to function. Before application, benzoin or mastisol may be applied to the intact skin only, and allowed to dry briefly. These act as adhesives, and purportedly increase the performance of the tape. However, the manufacturer does not recommend the use of additional adhesives over and above that on the tape strip itself. The tape is then cut to lengths that will overlap the wound edges by 2 to 3 cm. Enough strips are placed to appose the edges but not completely cover the wound. Cross strips may be applied to strengthen the closure.

The strips should be kept clean and dry and may be left in place for up to 2 weeks. No dressing should be applied over the tape unless the patient is a small child and at risk of prematurely removing the tape.

Surgical Adhesive (Skin Glue or "Super Glue")

N-2-butylcyanoacrylate is a tissue adhesive that polymerizes upon contact with water. This is a method of wound closure that is quite fast and convenient. Pain is typically less and cosmetic results are similar to traditional methods of closure. Although this technique has been used in other countries, it is still under study in the United States. Tissue adhesive is only for superficial wounds in areas of very little skin tension. It should not be used near the eyes or over joints.

The wound is prepared and cleansed in the usual manner. The wound edges are manually approximated and the adhesive is dripped onto the wound edge lengthwise or across the long axis. The adhesive is not applied to the internal walls of the wound. The wound is supported for I minute and then can be reinforced with tape.

Hair Tying

Although rarely used, hair tying is mentioned here as a novel technique to close a scalp wound. After proper wound cleansing, hair at the wound edges is rolled into small bundles on either side of the wound. Using standard knot tying technique, the hair is tied across the wound with corresponding bundles so that the wound edges are approximated. This technique should not be used on grossly contaminated or contused wounds. Wound separation may be slightly more common.

Drains

Drains are sometimes used prophylactically in wounds in accumulating pus or blood. In practice, the drain is a foreign body; increasing inflammation at the drain site also increases the likelihood of retrograde contamination. If the physician is concerned about infection, intense cleansing, adequate debridement, and closure are a better alternative. Splinting a wound is often useful to avoid undue stress wound that is over a joint or involves a tendon. The splint should generally be applied for the first 5 to 7 days across the wound. However, delicate repairs or soft tissue wounds that involve tendons may need to be splinted for longer amounts of time. Splinting can also reduce any postprocedure pain.

Incision and Drainage

Cutaneous abscess drainage is a very common procedure in the emergency room, accounting for approximately 1% to 2% of the visits. Incision and drainage procedures are primarily used for the treatment of abscesses, but the same techniques apply to drainage of mature hematomas and subcutaneous fluid collections.

A cutaneous abscess is a discrete collection of pus surrounded by inflammation and granulation tissue. Although the skin is highly resistant to infection, abscesses have been noted in virtually every part of the body. Most abscesses are polymicrobial, with the predominant organism being staphylococcal species. Certain areas of the body form abscesses with a higher incidence of anaerobic organisms, such as the perianal area. With recurring abscesses one should consider uncommon etiologies and conditions such as underlying osteomyelitis, retained foreign bodies, and the presence of *Mycobacterium* or *Actinomyces* infection. Regardless of the bacteriology of the abscess, the treatment is generally the same. With the exception of a few situations, antibiotics have not proven to be useful before or after drainage.

The presentation of an abscess is usually pain, redness, and swelling at the site. A tender, fluctuant mass can often be felt. The abscess may be spontaneously draining. Sometimes, in early abscess formation, the collection of pus has not formed and the area may only be indurated and painful. It is often prudent to allow the abscess to mature for 24 hours before an incision and drainage is performed. This allows better localization of the abscess and may help confirm the diagnosis. An abscess may lead to bacteremia. The patient should be assessed for systemic toxicity and treated accordingly. Unless the patient appears septic or is immunocompromised, it is unnecessary to perform routine Gram's stain and cultures of abscesses. These tests usually show a polymicrobial infection and rarely change the management. Gram's stains are occasionally helpful in a recurring abscess that has been refractory to treatment.

The basic incision and drainage procedure begins by prepping the wound in standard fashion. Although it is impossible to maintain sterility during the procedure, this is still recommended. Proper anesthesia is often difficult to attain. Infiltrating the dome with a thin needle will provide adequate anesthesia for the incision, but due to hyperemia, local infiltration will often not be effective enough to completely anesthetize the walls of the abscess. Nerve blocks and field blocks usually provide a better result. It is often necessary to provide some parenteral analgesia or even conscious sedation for extensive or time-consuming procedures. Nitrous oxide is also an excellent adjunct to analgesia. Occasionally the patient will not tolerate the procedure, or the abscess may be too involved to drain in the ED. It is often best that these selected patients be treated in the operating room under heavy sedation or general anesthesia.

Once the wound has been properly anesthetized, an incision is made that spans the diameter of the abscess dome. Drainage is usually spontaneous but it is very important to probe the wound and break up the smaller loculated pockets of pus that are found deep in the abscess. This is best performed with a curved hemostat protected by gauze. Bleeding is generally minimal and oozing generally halts with light packing. Most clinicians irrigate the abscess cavity with saline, but this has not been proven to affect the outcome.

The wound is then loosely packed with gauze stripping. The wound should not be packed too tightly and should be loose enough to allow liberal drainage. There is no proven efficacy in using gauze impregnated with an antiseptic solution. The incision is then covered lightly with sterile gauze to absorb excess drainage.

The packing is left in for 24 to 48 hours. With very small abscesses and reliable patients, the packing can be removed at home without further follow-up. However, the packing should be rechecked and removed by a clinician. It is often necessary to repack larger wounds or ones that are still actively draining pus. These patients should be rechecked every 24 to 48 hours until the packing is removed. Once the packing is removed, the wound can heal by secondary intention.

Antibiotics are unnecessary in the uncomplicated abscess. Any abscess complicated by cellulitis and lymphangitic streaking should be treated with appropriate antibiotics to cover *Staphylococcus* and *Streptococcus* species. Although it has not been proven to be useful, most physicians empirically cover immunocompromised patients with antibiotics. The risk for endocarditis after incision and drainage is unknown, but it has been shown that a significant number of patients have a transient bacteremia after the procedure. The American Heart Association has recommended antibiotic prophylaxis for any patient with a cardiac lesion that puts them at high risk for endocarditis.

Crush Injuries

Crush injury occurs when muscle tissue is compressed by great force for a long period of time, generally more than four hours. This scenario is most frequently seen in building collapse, when the rescue of entrapped victims is prolonged. While rare in common emergency department practice, crush injury syndrome, a systemic illness, can be a major concern during disasters in which there is widespread structural collapse, such as in earthquakes. Aggressive treatment must begin before the extrication is complete if the patient is to be afforded the best chance of recovery. In fact, crush injuries are among the very few circumstances in which the presence of an emergency physician or trauma surgeon at the scene may be appropriate, especially if advanced life support EMS capable of establishing large bore vascular access is not available.

Several physiological mechanisms contribute to the development of crush injury. Muscle tissue dies if it is ischemic for more than about four hours due to the interruption of its vascular supply. Some cells are disrupted immediately by the force of the compression injury, and release their intracellular components. Those cells that are not immediately lysed but experience the direct force of the compression will become ischemic within the first hour, generating lactic acid as they switch to anaerobic metabolism. Ultimately, these cells will also begin to release toxic products of lysis. It is this release of toxins that is responsible for the systemic effects of crush injury, primarily acidosis and hyperkalemia that may lead to dysrhythmias and myoglobinemia and eventually to acute renal failure. Myoglobin is an intracellular pigment protein that precipitates in the distal nephron, obstructing nephron flow and is also apparently directly toxic to tubular epithelium. Other toxins such as prostaglandins and leukotrienes may contribute to pulmonary injury and possible ARDS. Early treatment is aimed at ameliorating the effects of these toxins.

Signs and Symptoms

Crush injury should be suspected in any patient who sustains sufficient compressive force to compromise vascular supply to a complete extremity or large portion of an extremity for at least one hour, but more typically after about four hours. The affected limb may not appear severely injured upon first examination. Paralysis of the extremity, often mistaken for a spinal cord injury; severe pain, especially after extrication; and some pallor and swelling are all hallmarks of crush injury. These physical findings are virtually indistinguishable from those of compartment syndrome, a frequent complication of crush injury. Distal pulses may or may not be present, but their presence should not be taken for evidence of sufficient muscle cell perfusion. Urine may appear dark red or brown, indicating the presence of myoglobinuria.

Evaluation

Laboratory analysis will reveal hyperkalemia released from the intracellular stores into the blood as cells are lysed. Serum CPK will also be elevated and can be used as a marker of severity. Levels above 75,000 correlate with increased incidence of renal failure and mortality. Urinary levels of myoglobin will likewise be elevated. Urine output must be monitored carefully, with a urine output of 150 cc/h maintained. A decrease in the serum calcium, caused by an influx of calcium into damaged cells, will aggravate the cardiac toxicity of hyperkalemia. A twelve lead EKG will give an approximation of the extent of elevation of potassium, and it is changes in the EKG that govern treatment of hyperkalemia rather than the level itself.

As anaerobic metabolism occurs in ischemic muscles, lactic acidosis results. As cells lyse, other organic acids are released, furthering the progression of metabolic acidosis.

The release of thromboplastin may lead to disseminated intravascular coagulation, a grave finding which greatly worsens the prognosis. Plain film x-rays to evaluate for fractures in the affected limbs are required, and angiography may also be needed to assess the damage to the vascular system.

Treatment

As noted above, it is crucial to begin aggressive resuscitation before extrication has been achieved. Sudden decompression of the limb will result in massive reperfusion, causing a sudden increase in acidosis. Many victims have succumbed to lethal dysrhythmias immediately after removal from their entrapment. Normal saline should be infused at a rate of 1,500 cc/h through a large bore catheter. Lactated Ringer's solution, which contains potassium, should theoretically be avoided given the risk of elevated potassium levels. If EMS personnel cannot gain access to the peripheral circulation, a central line should be placed, even if this involves a physician responding to the scene. Extrication may need to be delayed until vascular access and fluid resuscitation has been accomplished. Patients with significant crush injury are critically ill, and should be transported to a trauma center for definitive care.

Compartment syndrome is a frequent, but not universal complication of crush injury. Compartment syndrome may occur in the forearms, legs, thighs or buttocks, and is the result of excess pressure in the relatively rigid osseofacial spaces compressing the arterial supply to the limb. All the symptoms and complications of ischemic muscle necrosis may result. Diagnosis is made by passive stretching of the muscles in the involved compartment, producing severe pain. Diminished two-point discrimination is also a consistent finding in those patients who can cooperate with this test. The diagnosis is confirmed by direct measurement of intra-compartmental pressures with a needle manometer; pressures of 30–45 mm Hg are strongly suggestive.

Treatment of compartment syndrome has traditionally been fasciotomy. Incisions made along the long axis of the affected compartment(s) release the pressure, allowing return of vascular flow. The decision to proceed with fasciotomy should be made by an experienced surgeon, because the procedure carries a high complication rate, including severe hemorrhage and sepsis. Many surgeons now defer fasciotomy unless compartment pressure is so elevated that arterial supply is occluded. Attention should also be given to the risk of reperfusion complications as noted above.

Once fluid resuscitation has taken place, attention turns to preventing the renal failure secondary to myoglobinuria and the dysrhythmias due to hyperkalemia. Alkaline diuresis with the osmotic diuretic mannitol or the use of loop diuretics have both been advocated, but each has drawbacks. Mannitol may result in volume overload, while loop diuretics acidify the urine. Dialysis may be necessary; for this reason the patient should be admitted to a facility where emergency dialysis is available.

The cardiotoxic effects of hyperkalemia are treated with IV calcium to stabilize the conducting system of the heart. Excess potassium is removed by dialysis or an exchange resin such as Kaexalate. Insulin and glucose are frequently used to transfer potassium back into cells, but it should be remembered that the source of the potassium in these patients is cells that have been destroyed, and cannot take the potassium back.

Some authors believe there is a role for hyperbaric oxygen in the treatment of crush injury. This application remains poorly tested; its main facility may be in the long-term care of poorly healing wounds in patients whose cardiac and renal function has been stabilized. As such, the decision to transfer a patient to a facility with hyperbaric capabilities is not one that need involve the ED physician.

Occasionally, where rescue personnel have decided that the situation is so unstable that there is little hope of extricating the entrapped extremity without extraordinary risk to the patient and rescuers, or if the limb is so mangled that salvage is extremely unlikely, a field amputation may be required. True informed consent is not possible given the circumstances, but the decision should ideally be agreed upon by at least two experienced physicians, such as trauma surgeons, emergency physicians, or orthopedic surgeons. The most experienced available operator available should perform the procedure, but it should not be unduly delayed for the arrival of additional personnel. A regional nerve block or intramuscular ketamine may be used for anesthesia. If possible, the limb is elevated for two minutes, a tourniquet is applied, and a guillotine amputation is performed. Revision may take place in the operating room.

Selected Readings

Rowe K. Hyperbaric oxygen therapy: what is the case for its use? *J Wound Care* 2001;10:117–121.

Smith J, Greaves I. Crush injury and crush syndrome: a review. *J Trauma* 2003; 54(Suppl 5):S226–S230.

Marc Gautreau

Incidence

The incidence of burns has declined sharply in the past 40 years to slightly more than 1 million injuries per year. About 4,500 result in death, a 60% decline in the fatality rate from 1971 to 1998, according to the American Burn Association. About 700,000 annual emergency department visits result in about 45,000 admissions, half to specialized burn centers. The average extent of surface area burned admitted to a burn center is 14%; more than half of all admissions to burn centers involve less than 10% total body surface area (TBSA). About 6% of burn center admissions die; most fatalities have inhalation injury.

Burn Classification

There are typically three characteristics of burns by which they are classified; thickness, surface area burned and mechanism, that is, thermal versus chemical or radiation. Body surface area is most critical in triaging the severity of burns worse than first degree. All patients with burns must first be assessed for airway problems and associated injuries such as toxic exposures, smoke inhalation, and trauma as well as comorbidities that might complicate care of the burn patient.

While burns have been traditionally classified as first, second, or third degree, current emphasis on requirements for healing have simplified the classification into partial thickness (first and second degree), which heal spontaneously, and full thickness (third and fourth degree), which requires skin grafting. The older classification remains widely used, and is presented below.

First-degree burns are limited to the epidermis. The skin is red, warm, and very tender and may be slightly edemetous. The patient will complain of pain or pruritus. While blistering may sometimes occur, they generally heal without scarring. The classic sunburn is the most frequent manifestation of first-degree burns. Pain lasts two or three days, and the damaged epithelium sloughs away in 5 to 10 days.

Second-degree burns are of two types. The first type is the superficial partial-thickness burn, which involves both the epidermis and the papillary portion of the dermis.

These burns often present with thin-walled blisters that are quite painful. They rarely scar and typically heal within 2 to 3 weeks. The second type is the deep partial thickness burn. These burns involve the epidermis, papillary dermis, and the deeper reticular dermis. The burned area is often red or even blanched and has thick blisters with decreased sensation. They tend to heal with hypertrophic scarring and are at risk for contractures across joints. They often progress to third degree burns, sometimes as a result of infection. Skin grafting often improves the outcome of these deep partial thickness burns. Patients with deep partial thickness burns are now grafted earlier than in the past, taking advantage of recent advances in skin graft technology.

Third-degree or full-thickness burns involve the complete epidermal and dermal layer. The capillary layer is destroyed and the burn takes on a leathery, white appearance. The area over the burn is insensate, although areas surrounding the full thickness burn may be partial thickness and therefore be quite painful. These burns require skin grafting.

Fourth-degree burns involve all layers of the skin including the underlying fascia, muscle, or bone. These require extensive debridement and inevitably lead to dysfunction of the involved part.

Burns may deepen in the first 24 to 48 hours after presentation. Residual heat from the initial insult may continue the burning process, and edema developing in the first days following a burn may cause further ischemic injury to areas with tenuous vascular supply. While it is appropriate to cool minor burns with tepid water or saline immediately after onset, severe burns should be covered with dry sterile dressings to prevent heat loss.

Total body surface area (TBSA) burned is most often estimated using the rule of nines. Each body part is assigned a certain percentage of the total surface area based on multiples of nine. The head represents 9% TBSA, the chest 18% TBSA, the back 18% TBSA, the arms 9% TBSA each, and the legs are 18% each. The perineum is the exception, representing 1% TB SA. The same system is used for infants and children with some modifications as shown. It is best to separately estimate the percentage of both partial- and full-thickness burns. For children, the Lund-Browder chart is more appropriate, as it provides an age specific estimation of the relative contribution of each anatomical area to surface area.

The American Burn Association has established guidelines for the classification of burned patients based on the TBSA involved and the depth of the burn. The minor burn category includes partial-thickness burns of <10% TBSA in children or the elderly, <15% in healthy adults, or any full-thickness burn of <2% TBSA. This category does not include burns that present a cosmetic or functional risk to the patient; thus, these burns can usually be managed on an outpatient basis. The moderate-burn category includes partial-thickness burns with 15% to 20% TBSA in adults and 10% to 15% TBSA in children and the elderly. This category excludes any burn that poses a cosmetic risk or involves the eyes, ears, face, feet, hands, or perineum. It also excludes patients with other trauma, inhalation injury, or electrical burns. These patients require hospitalization and possible transfer to a specialized burn unit.

The major-burn category is characterized by full-thickness burns >10% TBSA, and partial-thickness burns of >25% TBSA in adults or >20% TBSA in children and adults over 50 years of age. This category also includes burns to a compromised host (e.g., immunosuppression, diabetes). This category also includes high-voltage electrical burns, burns associated with major trauma or inhalation injury, burns caused by caustic chemical materials, burns to an immunocompromised host, and burns that will result in cosmetic or functional disfigurement of the face, feet, hands, or perineum.

Approach to the Burn Patient

The history in any burn should include mechanism of injury and length of time the patient was exposed to smoke. Firefighters can often assist in determining the type of fuel and whether the patient was trapped in a building for any length of time. A careful assessment of comorbidities should be done, including immunocompromise, diabetes, cardiac disease and pulmonary disease. Any patient with suspected pulmonary involvement or smoke inhalation should have oxygen saturation monitored and carboxyhemoglobin concentration measured.

Assessment of the airway is the absolute priority in all burn patients. Any patient burned to the face or who has been exposed to super-heated gases in a burning building must be presumed to have airway compromise until proven otherwise. Continual reassessment is mandatory, as patients may develop increasing airway edema well after presentation. Some clues to impending airway compromise are soot around the nares or in the pharynx, singed nasal hair or the development of wheezing, throat tightness or dysphagia. The physician should maintain a low threshold for airway intubation and mechanical ventilation because progressive airway edema may make late oral intubation impossible.

Pulmonary compliance may be reduced by lung or airway damage, or by chest wall burns that impede expansion. High pulmonary end expiratory pressures and/or escharotomy may be required. Escharotomy is a procedure

easily performed by the emergency physician, and should not be delayed for surgical consult or deferred for transfer to a burn or trauma center. Longitudinal incisions are performed along the anterior axillary line from the clavicle to the costal margin. The incision is made to the depth of subcutaneous fat. No analgesia is required through full thickness burns, and minimal local bleeding can be controlled with direct pressure or electrocautery. Vascular compromise of a limb, indicated by loss of peripheral pulses and Doppler signals, is another indication for escharotomy. If deeper fasciotomy is required, the procedure should be performed by an experienced surgeon.

Burns result in significant third spacing of intravascular fluids, causing a relative hypovolemia. The mechanism is thought to be increased capillary permeability due to the release of vasoactive substances from injured tissue. Volume resuscitation is central to the management of any patient with burns exceeding 20% TBSA. Large bore (14–18 gauge) IV access should be established and lactated Ringer's solution infused according to the Parkland Formula: 4 cm^3/kg body weight/% TBSA. The first half is given in the first eight hours after the occurrence of the injury; the second half in the following 16 hours. Crystalloid resuscitation continues until capillary permeability has returned to normal states, usually 24 hours post burn. Adequacy of resuscitation is based upon monitoring of vital signs, urine output and mentation; the use of pulmonary artery catheterization probably contributes little. There is no evidence supporting the use of hypertonic saline in the resuscitation of burn patients.

Heat loss is a critical problem in the burn patient, and steps to prevent hypothermia should begin in the prehospital setting. The ambulance should be well heated, to a level uncomfortable to the crew, and the transport cot should be lined with warm blankets both under and on top of the patient. Upon notification of the impending arrival of a burn patient, the resuscitation room should be made similarly warm.

Pain medication should not be withheld from any patient, and those with severe burns may require high doses of narcotics.

Burn Wound Care

Minor burns should initially be cleaned gently with normal saline. While some authors advocate leaving blisters intact, those that interfere with function should be aspirated. Blisters that have broken should be debrided of necrotic skin and dressed.

Most minor burn wounds can be treated in open or closed fashion. The open fashion involves simple wound cleansing and then application of a topical antibiotic or aloe vera. A good combination for minor facial burns is to apply a mixture of one-half aloe vera and one-half bacitracin ointment. Most burns of the face, neck, and hands can be managed this way. If there is a risk of frequent contamination or if the patient wants the wound dressed for cosmetic reasons, then the closed method may be better.

The closed method refers to the utilization of various dressings to cover the burn. Synthetic dressings, biologic dressings, or simple gauze dressings are available; however, no one dressing seems to be superior to the others. The basic technique is to cover the wound with fine mesh gauze or a commercially available dressing. The key is to have the dressing remain moist but prevent pooling of fluids at the wound site. Typically, an initial layer is applied to the wound, which becomes adherent to the surface. An outer layer of fluffed gauze is placed over this layer. Fluid passes out onto the surface of the first layer and it is absorbed by the fluffed gauze to prevent fluid buildup at the wound site. The dressing is lightly wrapped and checked in 24 to 48 hours. The fluffed gauze is then taken down while the initial layer remains adherent to the wound. If there is no sign of infection or exudate buildup, then the initial dressing may be left in place and the outer layers changed. The wound can be rechecked every other day. After 7 to 10 days the initial dressing should be less adherent and can be removed if the wound has epithelialized. If there is any fluid buildup or the wound begins to look infected, then the dressing should be removed completely and the wound should be gently washed. After this, the dressing should be changed once a day and the wound should be washed during each change.

Some authors recommend 12-hour dressing change with an antibiotic such as Silvadene or bacitracin. Gauze is impregnated with the antibiotic and applied to the burn. The burn is rechecked in the usual fashion. Some opponents to this method feel that antibiotic residue loses its efficacy at the burn site and can increase the incidence of infection. The patient should be instructed to remove all residual antibiotic ointment before reapplying a fresh dressing.

Special mention should be made of coal tar burns. Coal tars are used in road asphalt and roof pitching; they are heated into liquid form for ease of use. When coal tar contacts skin, it rapidly cools and becomes adherent to the underlying skin and hair. It rarely causes full-thickness burns. One should immediately cool the tar with water, but if this is done, removing the tar may be quite difficult due to the adherence to the skin. The tar can be emulsified by polyoxyethylene sorbitan. This is a water-soluble emulsifying agent found in Neosporin and bacitracin preparations. This can be applied to the wound and eases the removal of tar. Most of the tar can be removed during the initial visit; however, if some tar remains, then Neosporin can be applied liberally and the tar removal can be completed at a subsequent visit.

Patients should have their tetanus status updated if necessary, and most patients will need oral analgesics if outpatient care is considered.

Selected Readings

Brown MD. Hypertonic versus isotonic crystalloid for fluid resuscitation in critically ill patients. Review. *Ann Emerg Med* 2002;40:113–114.

Burn Incidence. In: Roberts JR, Hedges JR. *Clinical Procedures in Emergency Medicine,* 3rd ed. Philadelphia: American Burn Association, W.B. Saunders Company, 1998. Available at http://www.Ameriburn.org. Accessed June 2005.

Sheridan RL. Burns. Review. *Crit Care Med* 2002;30(Suppl 11):S500–S514.

Sheridan RL, Tompkins RG. What's new in burns and metabolism. Review. *J Am Coll Surg* 2004;198:243–263.

Trauma in Pregnancy

Richard V. Aghababian
Peter Angood

Harry L. Anderson III
Mark L. Shapiro

Trauma complicates 7% to 10% of all pregnancies and has become the leading cause of maternal death during pregnancy in many urban areas. Although pregnancy does not affect the maternal outcome following trauma, trauma does alter the fetal outcome as both the rate of placental abruption and fetal loss increase. Initial management of the pregnant trauma patient follows the same protocols as the nonpregnant patient, because treating the mother treats the fetus and potentially prevents fetal death. However, anatomical and physiological changes occur with pregnancy, and knowledge of these alterations is imperative for appropriate diagnosis and management. Difficulty may arise in identifying maternal injuries during pregnancy as the usual physical examination findings of injury are often absent. The pregnant trauma patient is also subject to a unique set of injuries including uterine rupture, placental abruption, amniotic fluid embolism, and occult Rh sensitization. Thus, the presentation of the pregnant trauma patient requires a team approach involving not only the emergency medicine physician but often the trauma surgeon and the obstetrician for appropriate management.

An important concept always to remember when evaluating female trauma patients in the ED is that all women of childbearing age should be assumed to be pregnant until proven otherwise. This practice will not only guide the physician in management decisions but will also avoid unnecessary complications for the patient and the physician.

Anatomical, Physiological, and Laboratory Changes with Pregnancy

Multiple cardiovascular changes occur during pregnancy, resulting in a hyperdynamic, low-resistance state. Heart rate increases by 15 to 20 beats/min. Cardiac output begins to increase at 10 weeks' gestation and may approach 6 to 7 L/min during the third trimester. The 40% increase in cardiac output results in a systolic flow murmur in 90% of women during their third trimester. At the same time peripheral vascular resistance decreases. These hemodynamic changes result in a 10 to 15 mm Hg decrease in both systolic and diastolic blood pressures in the first and second trimester, but by the third trimester blood pressure

levels may return to prepregnancy values. Circulating blood volume increases by 50%, allowing the mother to tolerate a significant hemorrhage (35% of total blood volume) without alterations in vital signs. Alterations in the electrocardiogram are primarily due to an elevated diaphragm and result in a shift of the QRS axis 15 degrees to the left. Nonpathologic Q waves may occur in leads III and a VF and T waves may be flattened or inverted in lead III.

Pulmonary changes occurring with pregnancy result in a decreased maternal pulmonary reserve with the patient less able to tolerate insult. Functional residual capacity decreases. An increase in tidal volume produces an increased minute ventilation and an average decrease in $PaCO_2$ by 10 mm Hg. The kidneys compensate for this respiratory alkalosis by excreting bicarbonate, and maternal buffering capacity is subsequently decreased. The increased tidal volume also elevates the maternal PaO_2 by an average of 10 mm Hg. However, an increase in maternal oxygen consumption by 25% during pregnancy results in decreased maternal oxygen reserve. Diaphragmatic elevation during the third trimester may increase lung markings on chest radiograph.

Multiple hematological changes occur during pregnancy. The 50% increase in maternal blood volume is compensated only by a 25% increase in red blood cell mass. The result is the "anemia of pregnancy" as the average hematocrit during the third trimester is 34%. A leukocytosis occurs resulting in an average white blood cell count of 12,000 to 18,000/mm^3, primarily composed of neutrophils. International normalized ratio (INR) and activated partial thromboplastin time (aPTT) remain unchanged despite an increase in coagulation factors. However, the pregnant patient is hypercoagulable and at an increased risk for deep venous thrombosis.

Gastrointestinal changes that occur must be recognized when managing pregnant trauma patients. Decreased motility of the gastrointestinal tract is secondary to the increased circulating progesterone and its relaxant effects on smooth muscle. All pregnant patients therefore should be considered to have a full stomach and at high risk for aspiration. Lower esophageal sphincter tone decreases, which increases the risk of reflux. The enlarging uterus stretches the peritoneum, decreasing its sensitivity to pain. Conditions normally resulting in peritoneal irritation such as bowel perforation and hemoperitoneum may present with normal physical findings in the pregnant patient. The gravid uterus elevates and compresses the bowel against the diaphragm, protecting it against injury from blunt trauma. However, multiple loops of bowel may be injured from penetrating trauma. As mentioned previously, the diaphragm is elevated 4 cm from its normal position, which is important when performing tube thoracostomy. Placing the chest tube at the fourth intercostal space rather than the normal 5th intercostal space may avoid placement in the abdomen.

Changes in the urinary system include a decrease in BUN and creatinine secondary to an increased glomerular filtration rate. The ureters dilate and displace laterally. The bladder elevates out of the pelvis and becomes an intra-abdominal organ by the twelfth gestational week, increasing its risk of injury from trauma.

The nonpregnant uterus is 7 cm in length, weighs 75 g, and ultimately becomes a 40 cm, 1,000 g organ at term. Blood flow to the uterus increases from 60 mL/min in the nonpregnant state to 600 mL/min during the third trimester. At the twelfth week of gestation, the uterine fundus rises to the level of the pubis and by the twentieth week to the level of the umbilicus. From 20 to 31 weeks, the gestational age roughly equates the fundal height, allowing a rapid estimation of fetal maturity. By the thirty-sixth gestational week, the uterus reaches its maximum size as it approaches the costal margin.

Fetal lie is variable during the first and second trimester with the fetus protected by the amniotic fluid, which absorbs energy from the trauma. By the third trimester, the amount of protection afforded by the amni-otic fluid decreases as the fetus occupies a larger percentage of the uterine cavity. The fetal head presents caudally during the third trimester as it prepares to engage the cervical canal prior to delivery and is at higher risk of crush injury against the pelvis (**FIGURE 177.1**).

Pelvic veins progressively engorge with blood as the pregnancy progresses. A life-threatening amount of retroperitoneal hemorrhage may occur with trauma to this area. The symphysis pubis begins to widen by the seventh month of pregnancy leading to a potential incorrect diagnosis of pelvic diastasis as the distance between the pubic rami may increase to 20 mm during the third trimester.

Abdominal Trauma

Blunt Abdominal Trauma

Blunt abdominal trauma occurring during pregnancy most often results from motor vehicle accidents, falls, or assaults. The incidence of occurrence for these mechanisms of injury is distributed equally throughout the 40 weeks of gestation except for falls, which most commonly occur after 32 weeks' gestation as pregnancy alters the patient's stability. Assaults are more likely to result in pregnancy complications than other mechanisms of blunt injury, as the uterus is often the object of the assault.

As with the nonpregnant trauma patient, the most frequently injured abdominal organs are the spleen and liver. Despite the ability of an enlarged uterus to absorb traumatic energy and protect intra-abdominal contents, massive hemoperitoneum may occur. An increased difficulty in diagnosing these injuries may occur secondary to the peritoneum's decreased sensitivity and the lack of change in maternal vital signs despite major blood loss. Indications for exploratory laparotomy when intra-abdominal injuries are suspected to be present are unchanged from the nonpregnant patient, as the operation does not alter fetal outcome.

Pelvic fractures and retroperitoneal bleeding cause particular concern in the pregnant patient, and exsanguination from these injuries is a common cause of maternal death. A combination of increased pelvic blood flow during pregnancy and the pressure the gravid uterus exerts on the inferior vena cava result in venous hypertension of the pelvic veins, and the patient with pelvic fractures may rapidly lose 4 to 5 L of blood from lacerated pelvic veins.

Preterm contractions are the most common sequelae following blunt trauma. Prostaglandins and arachidonic acid released from traumatized uterine cells stimulate the uterus to contract. Administration of tocolytics is controversial, as the majority of contractions related to trauma resolve spontaneously and without therapy. The 10% of traumatic contractions that continue usually relate to placental abruption, fetal injury, or major uterine injury, and tocolytics are contraindicated in these conditions.

Uterine rupture may occur following a major traumatic force. A higher incidence of rupture occurs in the presence of pelvic fractures or a prior cesarean section. Resultant maternal mortality is approximately 10%, whereas fetal

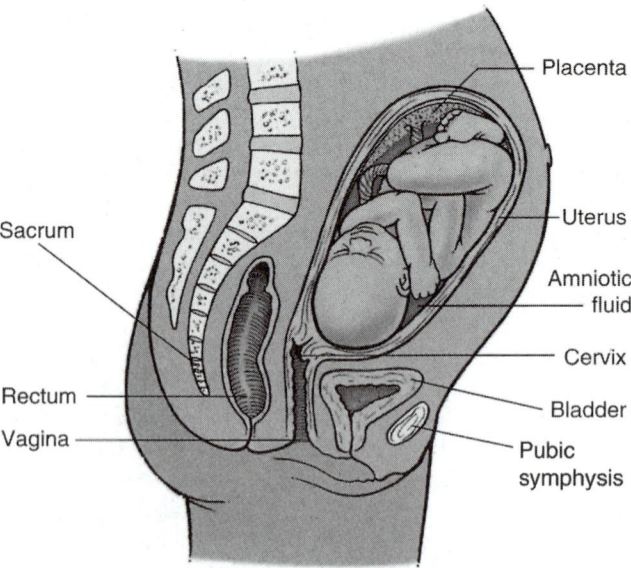

FIGURE 177.1 Anatomic relationships of the near term fetus within the mother. *Source:* Used with permission from the American Academy Orthopedic Surgeons. *Emergency Care and Transportation of the Sick and Injured,* 8th ed. Sudbury, MA: Jones and Bartlett Publishers, 2000:492, Figure 20-1.

mortality is almost universal. Palpation of fetal parts outside the uterus is diagnostic. Radiographic evaluation may include abdominal radiographs, which may identify fetal bones outside of the uterus, or ultrasound, which is the gold standard for diagnosing this condition.

Placental abruption occurs as a portion of the placenta separates from the uterine wall prior to the onset of normal labor. It may complicate up to 38% of pregnancies with major injuries and 4% with minor injuries. The mechanism of abruption results from the highly elastic properties of the uterus contrasted with the inelastic properties of the placenta. As the uterus is compressed and folded the unyielding placenta is sheared away from the uterine wall. The resulting decreased uterine blood flow impairs fetal nutrient and waste exchange, and if significant the fetus becomes hypoxic and acidotic. Unfortunately, abruption may occur without evidence of trauma to the abdomen. Fetal mortality increases as the degree of separation increases, approaching 100% if the abruption is greater than 50%. The classic triad of placental abruption includes vaginal bleeding, abdominal pain, and uterine irritability, but this triad only presents in half of the cases. Other indications of placental abruption include tetanic uterine contractions and fetal distress. Maternal complications include disseminated intravascular coagulation from the release of thromboplastin and severe hemorrhage, as 2 L of blood may be sequestered between the uterus and placenta without vaginal bleeding. Maternal death is rare, occurring in less than 1% of cases.

Amniotic fluid embolism occurs as amniotic fluid enters maternal venous circulation. The exact pathophysiology is unknown but is thought to be a response to activation of the maternal immune response. Diagnosis is based on the clinical presentation of dyspnea, hypoxia, and hypotension. Chest radiography may reveal diffuse pulmonary infiltrates. Supportive treatment is required as no specific therapy is available.

The most common cause of fetal death from blunt trauma is often quoted secondary to maternal death, but series show placental abruption to be the most common cause. Injuries to the fetus, rare during the first and second trimester, occur primarily during the third trimester as the protective abilities of the amniotic fluid diminish. The head is the most commonly injured fetal organ because it is often compressed against the maternal pelvis. Skull fractures with cortical contusions and subdural hematoma are the common head injuries identified at autopsy. Abdominal injuries most commonly involve contusions of the fetal solid viscera, whereas fetal hollow viscus injury is rare.

The use of seat belts during pregnancy has raised much controversy in recent years, because of concern about possible increased injury to the uterus and fetus from the lap belt. Presently it is recommended for mothers to wear seat belts during their pregnancy, as seat belts prevent maternal death. Proper usage of the seat belt must be stressed. The lap portion of the belt should ride across the anterior iliac spine, thus positioning itself at the lower uterine edge. If the belt is over the uterus, fetal head trauma may occur due to compression of the head between the lap belt and the sacral promontory. Use of the shoulder harness is recommended and may help decrease the severity of lap-belt–related injuries.

Penetrating Abdominal Trauma

Penetrating injury to the abdomen is most often secondary to gunshot wounds but may also occur following knife injuries. The incidence of self-inflicted gunshot wounds aimed at the uterus in an attempt to abort the pregnancy has unfortunately increased in recent years. The nongravid uterus is rarely injured by penetrating abdominal trauma because of the protection afforded by the pelvis, but in the pregnant patient, the likelihood of uterine injury increases as the pregnancy progresses and the uterus protrudes beyond the pelvic brim. Reports show the incidence of fetal injuries from gunshot wounds to be between 59% and 89% with a fetal mortality rate of 47% to 71%. Once initial stabilization of the patient with penetrating abdominal injury occurs, further diagnostics and management rests with the surgical consultant.

Management of gunshot wounds to the abdomen traditionally involves immediate exploratory laparotomy. Recently, several authors have suggested conservative management for stable patients when the bullet is lodged in the uterus. Criteria for nonoperative management include injuries where the entrance site is below the fundus, the bullet is visualized via radiographs in the uterus, the abdominal and rectal examinations are normal, the mother and fetus are stable, and there is no hematuria.

Stab wounds to the abdomen are likewise categorized by the entrance location. As with gunshot wounds, operative management is mandatory for entrance wounds above the fundus, which penetrate the anterior fascia as both multiple bowel injuries and visceral injuries may occur. Management of wounds below the fundus may be with DPL, ultrasound, and/or serial abdominal examinations. When compared to gunshot wounds, stab wounds involving the uterus result in better fetal outcomes.

Burns

Pregnancy does not alter maternal outcome after burn injury. However, fetal outcome is dependent on the extent of maternal burn injury as well as the complications resulting from the burn. Burns less than 20% result in little fetal or maternal morbidity. However, as the percentage of burn increases, the incidence of preterm labor and fetal mortality also increases, with fetal mortality becoming universal if the maternal burn exceeds 50% of total body surface.

Initial management of the pregnant burn patient is the same as that of the nonpregnant patient. However, aggressive fluid resuscitation is particularly important or uterine blood flow may decrease with concomitant fetal distress. Fluid resuscitation with lactated Ringer's follows the formula 4 cc/kg/percent of total body area (%TBSA), with half the resuscitative fluid given over the first 8 hours and the remaining half over the next 16 hours. Recommendations for admission to a burn center are similar but more liberal than those for the nonpregnant patient. Silver sulfadiazine may cause kernicterus, and its use should be avoided in the late third trimester.

All patients with evidence of smoke inhalation require evaluation for carbon monoxide poisoning. Fetal hemoglobin binds carbon monoxide more aggressively than maternal hemoglobin, resulting in fetal carboxyhemoglobin levels 10% to 15% higher than maternal levels. Initial treatment involves administration of the highest concentration of oxygen possible. Indications for hyperbaric oxygen treatment include maternal levels >20%, fetal distress, or the presence of neurologic symptoms.

Electrical Injury

There are few documented cases of electrical injuries involving pregnant patients. Electrical injuries may involve either direct current, as from a lightning strike, or more commonly alternating current, as from a household appliance. Regardless of the mechanism, the fetus is much less tolerant of electrical insult than the mother.

Household appliance injuries involve the passage of an electrical current from the hands to the feet, and subsequently current travels directly through the uterus and fetus. Fetal death may be as high as 73% from an electrical shock. Fetal complications including intrauterine growth retardation and oligohydramnios have been documented in surviving infants.

Lightning injuries are rare. A review of 12 cases documented immediate fetal death in five cases, with the remainder progressing to normal deliveries. At autopsy no fetal or placental injuries were documented, suggesting potential cardiac rhythm disturbance as the cause of fetal death. All pregnant women should be advised to seek medical care following an electrical injury regardless how trivial. Management of electrical injuries involves initial stabilization and treatment of the mother. Fetal evaluation should include fetal monitoring and ultrasound with obstetrical consultation.

Maternal Abuse

Physical abuse during pregnancy is unfortunately a common occurrence. Up to 20% of teenage girls and 14% of women experience some form of physical abuse during their pregnancy. These patients often present to the ED for evaluation following trauma but may not volunteer the exact mechanism of injury unless directly questioned about abuse. Complications to the pregnancy beyond the immediate trauma include low birth weight infants and late entry into prenatal care. It is imperative that any pregnant patient presenting with evidence of trauma be questioned about potential abuse. Direct questioning, without the patient's partner present, has been shown to increase the number of positive responses by threefold. Patients who have been abused require information on counseling, and many states have statutes requiring police notification of domestic violence.

Evaluation and Treatment

As with all trauma patients, a thorough history should be obtained from both the patient and those giving prehospital care. The patient's prenatal history and problems with prior pregnancies should also be ascertained. The date of the last menstrual period and expected date of confinement allow estimation of fetal maturity. The patient should be questioned about the sensation of fetal movement and any abdominal pain or contractions. The loss of fetal movement following trauma is highly suggestive of fetal injury. The patient should be asked about the passage of any fluid or blood from the vagina.

History should include the mechanism of the injury, including any direct trauma to the abdomen. A history of seizure while driving may not only elicit the cause of the motor vehicle accident but suggests a diagnosis of eclampsia that may require urgent delivery. If a seat belt was worn, the patient should be questioned about the position of the belt on the abdomen. The time of the last meal should be noted, but all pregnant women should be considered to have a full stomach.

As with all trauma patients, the primary survey focuses on the ABCs of resuscitation with fetal examination delayed to the secondary exam. Oxygen delivery is paramount in the pregnant patient, and all patients should be placed on supplemental oxygen. Although increasing inspired oxygen concentration does little for the normal mother, it can significantly increase fetal oxygen concentration, as the fetus normally operates at the low end of the oxyhemoglobin dissociation curve. Maternal heart rate normally increases during pregnancy, so tachycardia is not unexpected, but a heart rate greater than 115 beats/min raises concerns about other causes. Maternal hypotension and shock requires early identification and aggressive treatment, because fetal mortality approaches 80% as the mother shunts blood away from the uterus in a self-protective manner.

After 20 weeks' gestation, the enlarged uterus may compress the inferior vena cava resulting in the supine hypotension syndrome. Blood return to the heart is compromised and hypotension results. Cardiac output may drop by 28% with a decrease in systolic blood pressure of 30 mm Hg. Initial treatment includes manual displacement of the uterus off the inferior vena cava. If this maneuver is unsuccessful, the left lateral tilt position may be attempted. Care must be taken not to compromise spinal precautions if there is concern of spinal injury. In such cases, it may be preferable to leave the patient on a backboard, slanted to the left at a 30° angle.

Hypotension not responsive to the above maneuvers warrants aggressive fluid resuscitation. The pregnant patient is relatively hypervolemic prior to trauma so hypotension from hemorrhage implies major blood loss. Lactated Ringer's solution has been shown to be most effective in improving fetal oxygenation when compared to other crystalloids and should be the initial fluid of choice for resuscitation. The clinician should have a low threshold for blood transfusion to restore vascular stability in the pregnant patient. Vasopressors should be avoided if possible, because of vasoconstriction of the uterine vessels. If vasopressors are required for stabilization of the patient's pressure once volume replacement is obtained, ephedrine is most often used, as it has been shown to improve fetal acidosis secondary to hypotension in animal models. Low-dose dopamine ($5 \mu g/kg/min$) may increase arterial pressure with very little effect on the uterine circulation, but as dosages are increased uterine circulation diminishes.

Rapid sequence intubation with the Sellick maneuver is recommended when airway management is necessary. Thiopental (class C), ketamine, and etomidate (class C) are induction agents that may be used in pregnancy. Succinylcholine and vecuronium are class C drugs that may be given for paralysis. Benzodiazepines are to be avoided, if possible, as they are class D. Preoxygenation with 100% FiO_2 is essential prior to intubation as maternal functional residual capacity is reduced and rapid desaturation occurs without adequate preoxygenation.

Pregnant patients presenting in cardiac arrest are managed as per advanced cardiac life support (ACLS) guidelines. Closed-chest CPR is routinely performed on patients in the supine position; however, adequate blood flow may be difficult to produce in pregnant patients for several reasons. The inferior vena cava may compress the uterus, inhibiting venous return to the heart, and the uterus may steal blood from vital organs during CPR. For these reasons, a thoracotomy is often indicated if there is no initial response to therapy. Thoracotomy with direct cardiac massage not only improves coronary and cerebral perfusion but also improves perfusion to the uterus.

The secondary survey proceeds along the same algorithm as for any trauma patient; however, special attention must be placed on the obstetrical examination. The fundal height is measured from the symphysis pubis to the fundus and should be documented on serial exams. Expanding fundal heights are suggestive of placental abruption. The uterus should be palpated for the presence of contractions and tenderness and for evidence of fetal movement. Between 10 and 14 weeks' gestation, fetal heart tones may be auscultated with a Doppler and by 18 weeks with a standard stethoscope. The rate should be documented on serial examinations. Normal fetal heart rate is between 120 and 160 beats per minute. The presence of fetal bradycardia suggests fetal distress that may be due to fetal or placental injury as well as to maternal blood loss.

A pelvic examination is mandatory. If the patient is stable and there is evidence of ruptured membranes, a sterile speculum examination is recommended. Leakage of amniotic fluid may be identified by pooling of fluid in the vaginal vault, a positive nitrazine test, or by ferning of the dried vaginal fluid. If vaginal bleeding is present, the source may be secondary to vaginal mucosal tears, but is most likely from the uterus. In the trauma patient, third trimester uterine bleeding is likely placental abruption; however, placenta previa should be ruled out with ultra-sound prior to a pelvic examination. Cervical dilation, effacement, and fetal presentation should all be documented once a bimanual examination can be performed.

Laboratory analysis in the pregnant trauma patient suffering major injury includes a complete blood count, chemistries, blood typing, coagulation panel, and urinalysis. Anemia of pregnancy is not unexpected, but profound anemia is abnormal and a source of blood loss should be sought. Abnormal coagulation factors may suggest disseminated intravascular coagulation (DIC) from placental abruption. There is evidence that both low bicarbonate and elevated lactate levels correlate with poor fetal outcome. Tetanus immunoglobin and toxoid is both safe and appropriate in pregnancy when indicated.

Radiation exposure from radiographs is often a concern. Complications from fetal exposure to radiation *in utero* are dependent on the amount of radiation and the gestational age at the time of exposure. From 0 to 2 weeks' gestation, the fetus is relatively resistant to the teratogenic and growth retardive effects of radiation, but is highly susceptible to the lethal effects of radiation. From 2 to 8 weeks' gestation, the embryo is subject to teratogenic, growth retardation, and neoplastic effects of the radiation. From 8 to 40 weeks' gestation, risks of teratogenic effects are minimal, but fetal risks of growth retardation, CNS dysfunction, and neoplastic effects continue. Regardless of the risks, pregnant patients should have all appropriate x-ray studies.

Several important concepts apply to the pregnant patient when radiographic studies are being considered. If possible, informed consent should be obtained before radiographic studies, but it is not essential. The risk of fetal injury is virtually unchanged if the total fetal dosage is less than 10 rad (10,000 millirads). Shielding of the maternal abdomen is mandatory as fetal exposure may be decreased by 75%. In general, x-rays focused more than 10 cm away from the uterus are not harmful due to scatter of the beam.

Radiation dosages for x-ray studies vary depending on the type of radiograph obtained and should be remembered when ordering particular films. Cervical spine, chest, and extremities x-rays are all safe as they result in a <5 mrad exposure to the fetus. However, pelvic and lumbar spine films expose the fetus to 1,000 mrad and 300 mrad, respectively. Head CT scanning is relatively safe as fetal exposure is <50 mrad. However, abdominal CT scanning should be avoided if at all possible as a CT scan limited to the upper abdominal exposes the fetus to 3,000 mrad, and if the pelvis is included the fetus may be exposed up to 10,000 mrad.

Real-time ultrasound allows assessment of both the fetus and the uterus. Gestational age, fetal heart rate, and fetal movement may be documented. Placental location and amniotic fluid volume may also be assessed. Use of ultrasound for detecting placental abruption has only a 50% sensitivity and should not be solely relied up to detect this entity. Acute hemorrhage sequestered between the placenta and uterus may have the same echogenicity as the placenta resulting in the high false-negative rate of ultrasound for placental abruption.

Ultrasound is used more frequently in many trauma centers for the detection of intra-abdominal injury and has replaced DPL at many locations. Ultrasound is beneficial in that it is rapid and detects hemoperitoneum in over 90% of cases. The presence of free fluid in Morrison's pouch or the pelvis mandates further diagnostic measures such as abdominal CT, DPL, or exploratory laparotomy. However, evidence of ultrasound's efficacy for detecting intra-abdominal injury during pregnancy has not been definitive.

Diagnostic peritoneal lavage may be safely used to identify intra-abdominal injuries in the pregnant patient, but the technique requires alteration. A supraumbilical approach using an open technique is recommended to avoid the enlarged uterus. Laboratory analysis of the dialysate is unchanged from the nonpregnant patient.

Fetal evaluation requires cardiotocodynamometry. Continuous, noninvasive monitoring of both fetal heart rate and uterine contractions allows for the early detection of fetal and placental injuries and is the gold standard for detecting placental abruption. Monitoring the fetus may not only detect fetal/placental injuries, but fetal bradycardia may be the first sign of maternal blood loss. Regardless of how trivial the mechanism, all pregnant trauma patients beyond 24 weeks' gestation require 4 to 6 hours of continuous monitoring. From 20 to 24 weeks' gestation, monitoring is controversial as emergency cesarean delivery is not indicated for fetal distress. Proponents for monitoring from 20 to 24 weeks' gestation argue that the presence of fetal distress may be the first indicator of occult maternal blood loss.

Initiation of monitoring should begin immediately after the mother is stabilized. Greater than eight contractions per hour places the patient at risk for abruption and monitoring for an additional 24 hours is required. Loss fetal beat-to-beat variability and late fetal decelerations indicate potential fetal distress.

Medications routinely used in trauma patients must be evaluated for their risk and benefits during pregnancy. Pain control following injuries and sedation for procedures are often required. Narcotics are safe as they are class B. However, if delivery is imminent, maternal narcotics cause fetal respiratory depression, and may require treatment of the newborn with Narcan. Patients requiring conscious sedation may be treated with fentanyl and low dose etomidate. Dilantin may be used without fetal harm for short-term seizure prophylaxis (1 week) in head injury patients.

Patients with minimal trauma who are discharged from the ED require explicit instructions and close follow-up. The patient should be instructed to record fetal movements (normal 4/h), and an appointment with an obstetrician should be scheduled. Immediate return to the hospital is required for signs of labor, decreased fetal movement, vaginal bleeding, or possible membrane rupture.

Fetomaternal Hemorrhage

Fetomaternal hemorrhage (FMH) occurs in 8% to 30% of trauma patients as placental integrity is disrupted and fetal blood cells enter maternal circulation. Potential complications include maternal Rh sensitization, neonatal anemia, fetal death from exsanguination, and fetal cardiac arrhythmias. Risk of maternal Rh sensitization may occur if an Rh-negative mother is exposed to as little as 1 cc of Rh-positive fetal blood cells.

The Kleihauer-Betke (KB) test determines the quantity of fetal red blood cells in maternal circulation. By eluting the hemoglobin from maternal red blood cells with citric acid and staining the hemoglobin in fetal red blood cells, the KB test determines a ratio of fetal blood cells to maternal blood cells in a sample of maternal blood. This ratio can then be extrapolated to the amount of fetal blood that entered the maternal circulation by using the following formula: FMH (mL) = maternal blood volume (5 L) $\times$ stained cells (fetal RBC)/unstained cells (maternal RBC). The KB test is limited by its low sensitivity, as hemorrhages less than 5 mL do not routinely test positive. Therefore, to avoid occult maternal Rh sensitization, all pregnant patients who are Rh negative require RhoGAM even if the KB test is negative. Unfortunately, the KB test has not been shown to be predictive of fetal outcome following trauma.

RhoGAM is an immunoglobin that protects the Rh negative mother from Rh sensitization. A standard dose of RhoGAM (300 μg) protects the mother from 30 mL of fetal blood and should be given within 72 hours of fetomaternal hemorrhage. Prior to 16 weeks of gestation, fetal circulation is less than 30 mL, and thus the total hemorrhage is of less concern when determining the dosage of RhoGAM.

Emergency Department Perimortem Cesarean Section

Emergent cesarean section may be required on the patient following traumatic arrest (hysterotomy). This procedure has the potential benefits of salvaging a viable fetus, and improving both maternal circulation and response to resuscitation. Infant survival and prognosis is inversely proportional to the amount of time from maternal arrest to delivery, and neurological complications are the most common sequelae. The best prognosis is offered if the infant is delivered within 5 minutes of maternal arrest, but infant survival has been documented with delivery as long as 23 minutes after maternal arrest. The selection criteria for ED cesarean section are maternal arrest and gestational age greater than 24 weeks. Gestational age may be quickly estimated by measuring fundal height. Although accurate, ultrasound should not be used to determine gestational age in this setting as it can result in unnecessary delay. If possible, consent should be obtained from the family, but this also should not delay delivery.

The ED trauma cesarean section is a rapid, simple procedure. A vertical midline incision is taken from the xiphoid process to the pubis. The uterus is identified and a generous vertical midline incision is made through the upper uterine segment and extended distally with scissors. The infant is withdrawn from the uterus and resuscitation is performed on the infant as necessary. Maternal cardiopulmonary resuscitation should be continued throughout the cesarean section, and upon successful delivery of the infant the mother's status should be reassessed. Improvement in maternal circulation often occurs once the fetus is removed from the uterus, thus increasing the possibility of successful resuscitation of the mother after delivery of the fetus.

Selected Readings

Mirvis S, Shanmuganathan K, eds. Imaging in Trauma and Critical Care, 2d ed. Basel: Elsevier Science, 2003.

Moore EE, Feliciano DV, Mattox DV, eds. *Trauma,* 5th ed. New York: McGraw-Hill Professional, 2004.

178 | Pediatric Injuries

Ruben Peralta

Michael Hirsh

Trauma is the leading cause of death and disability in the 1- to 14-year-old age groups. The 22 million injuries suffered by children each year translate into an economic impact of more than 15 billion dollars annually. More productive work years of life are lost because of pediatric trauma than all other pediatric diseases combined. With the large number of deaths and permanent disabilities attributed to pediatric trauma, it must be addressed and included as an inextricable component of trauma care.

Special Considerations

Mechanism of Injury

Blunt trauma accounts for 90% of pediatric injuries. Although falls overall are the most common form of pediatric injury, motor vehicular crashes (MVC) are the most common cause of death in children. Other leading causes of death are drowning, burn, and penetrating trauma.

Infants, toddlers and preteen children have small enough body masses such that they become ready projectiles when tossed around the inside cab of a crashing motor vehicle or when struck by one as pedestrians. The disproportionate distribution of weight in the cranial region makes the head the prime area of impact. Adolescents frequently demonstrate "adult physiology" in their responses to injury, but their emotional and psychosocial makeup demands a pediatric-friendly resuscitation approach.

Management

Although the priorities and assessment of an injured child are the same as in the adult patient, children differ anatomically and physiologically from adults, and the treatment, equipment, and management of their cases must take these differences into account. There are a number of excellent systems (i.e. Broselow system) available that help organize the approach to the pediatric trauma patient by their weight estimate. This can be an excellent time saver in the trauma bay. It cannot be assumed that the same procedures routinely used on adults can be used on pediatric patients.

Emergency and Trauma Resuscitation

A team approach is essential in the initial management and resuscitation of the injured child.

Primary Survey

The primary survey must involve evaluation of the child's airway and breathing and circulation (A-B-C-D-E) as described by the ATLS protocol (Table 178.1).

There are some critical differences in the ABC's of the child that are worth emphasizing.

A is for Airway In preadolescent children, >75% of the unsuccessful resuscitations revolve around inability to secure the airway properly. The airway in this age group is a much more difficult entity to master without experience and practice. The airway in children is short, anterior and encroached upon by the natural craniofacial disproportionality that all leads to more difficult access. Inexperience with pediatric intubation should lead prehospital caregivers to try bag-valve mask as a method to temporarily oxygenate and ventilate without causing great delays in the field with unsuccessful intubation techniques. Esophageal intubation in children is ineffective as by insufflating the stomach one reduces the effectiveness of the abdominal wall breathing that most children in this age group perform preferentially.

One feature in the child that can help improve ventilation is the fact that children up to the age of ten are obligate nasal breathers. The nasopharynx can therefore be a critical pathway for ventilation. It should be cleared with suctioning and nasal airways as well as oral airways can be used with bagging the patients to augment oxygen delivery. Face masks should cover the nares as well as the mouth. Another corollary of this anatomic feature is that the child with extensive nasofacial trauma may be an early candidate for surgical airway.

The surgical airway in a child is not one done routinely, but every year pediatric patients are saved by accessing the slit-like cricothyroid membrane just inferior to the "Adam's Apple" in the neck. A temporizing measure in the field that can be done if conditions do not favor an open cricothyroidotomy is the needle puncture of the mem-

Table 178.1

The ABCDE Protocol for First Survey of Children with Trauma

Airway and cervical spine stabilization
1. Anatomical considerations
   a. Shorter neck
   b. Larynx is smaller and more anterior
   c. Shorter trachea
   d. Epiglottis is floppy
   e. Larger tongue
2. Intubation (oro-tracheal) with in-line cervical spine immobilization.
   The cervical spine must be immobilized until cervical spine injury can be excluded.
   a. Nasotracheal intubation is *NOT* recommended
   b. Recommended airway size = (16 + age in yrs)/4 = internal tube diameter in mm. Approximate estimate is size of fifth phalanx at base
   c. Use of uncuffed tubes in children under eight (8) years of age to minimize tracheal trauma is recommended.
   d. Taped tube at 3 times (size of tube) at the lips.
   e. Surgical cricothyroidotomy via needle or open technique is recommended, if unable to obtain airway.

Breathing
Assessment for adequacy of lower chest and abdominal rise, as infants and children are diaphragmatic breathers.
  Gastric distension, abdominal, and diaphragmatic trauma can compromise ventilation.

Circulation
1. Children have significant cardiovascular reserve. Therefore, signs of shock may not present until there is a blood loss of greater than 30%.
2. Evaluate for shock, not just BP alone:
   a. Heart rate
   b. Cap refill
   c. Mental status
   d. Extremities: pulses, cap refill, temperature, and turgor.
   e. Urine output
3. A palpable pulse roughly correlates with a systolic blood pressure over 80 mm Hg.
4. Vascular access could be a difficult task in an injured child.
   a. Percutaneous peripheral intravenous access
   1. Bilateral 20-gauge IV catheter should be placed in bilateral extremities.
   2. Intraosseous infusion if unavailable to obtain peripheral access. Allows rapid fluid administration in children younger than 6 years. Medial tibia plateau is the preferred location.
   3. Fluid resuscitation: For shock, crystalloid fluid boluses of 20 mL/kg are given rapidly. If after 3 boluses signs of shock have not been corrected, start pack red blood cells. It should be given using 10 mL/kg boluses, Type 0 for boys and type $0^{(-)}$ for girls.

Disability
1. Rapid neurologic examination to evaluate patient disability using AVPU system or Glasgow Coma Scale (GCS). (modified for nonverbal children).
2. AVPU system: A—alert; V—responds to verbal stimuli; P—responds to painful stimuli; and U—unresponsive.

Exposure
1. Fully undress the patient to assess for hidden injuries. Hypothermia should be avoided because of the increase in the metabolic requirement of a child.
2. Use of warm ambulance, helicopter, and trauma bay. Keep the patient covered. Use warm fluids.

This protocol was developed by the ATLS. Used with permission.

brane with a 12 or 14 gauge IV catheter. This will oxygenate about 90% effectively and ventilate 65% effectively until definitive care is available.

B is for Breathing The baseline rate of breathing in children is higher than in their adult trauma patient counterparts. Establish a rate of 20–30 with even higher rates a consideration in infants. Overventilation is ill advised, as the flimsy mediastinal structures in the child are very vulnerable to shift from the barotrauma that causes pneumothoraces. The person assigned to bag the child should look at the child's sternum and opt for excursions of no more that 1 cm to prevent this phenomenon.

Another important difference in the breathing apparatus of the child is the dependence on abdominal wall musculature rather than the chest intercostals to stoke the diaphragm to ventilate. This means that a child who has had an abdominal injury may present as respiratory failure. Another pitfall in management are the problems that ensue from vigorous bagging or crying in the pediatric trauma patient leading to massive gastric dilatation. This too will cause ineffectual abdominal wall breathing. Intubation may become necessary in these children, and this should include Nasogastric tube insertion to decompress the stomach. The formula used to calculate the endotracheal tube size is $16 +$ (age in years)/4. A good check on the ET tube sizing that results from this formula is holding the chosen tube size up against the child's fifth digit nail. This is a very accurate estimate of pediatric airway size. The tube should be taped at the lips at approximately $3 \times$ the ET tube size.

C is for Circulation

It seems odd to say but one of the most commonly made mistakes made in the resuscitation of pediatric trauma patients is failure to recognize the presence of shock. This is in part due to compensatory mechanisms in a child that make the systolic blood pressure maintain a steady state for quite some time before deterioration in this vital sign is noted. When intravascular volume is depleted from hemorrhage in the pediatric trauma patient, the child's baroreceptors, working with their pristine, atherosclerosis-free arterial beds, can effectively maintain central perfusion by raising systemic vascular resistance and shutting down useless beds of circulation (i.e., the extremities). Meanwhile the central perfusion to the brain, heart and kidneys are preserved. The heart rate can also be raised as high as 220 beats/min in order to maintain the cardiac output and central intravascular perfusion. Fully 40% of the child's intravascular volume can be depleted before this compensatory mechanism breaks down and the systolic blood pressure, estimated in the child to be $70 + 2 \times$ (age in years), begins to fall. There are two important corollaries from this physiologic process:

1. The pediatric trauma patient who is "normotensive" may still be in shock and one must learn the hemodynamic assessment of a child to determine this.
2. The pediatric trauma patient is truly hypotensive is decompensating rapidly and needs to be in a pediatric trauma center, in an OR, or in a pediatric ICU for maximal resuscitation and hemorrhage cessation.

The overall hemodynamic assessment of a child is performed taking the following parameters into account:

1. Vital Signs
   a. Heart Rate—can be as high as 220 and still be considered sinus tachycardia
   b. Systolic Blood Pressure—do not overact to sub-100 numbers—this is a norm until the children reach the ages of 10-12.
2. Skin
   a. Texture/Turgor—clammy
   b. Temperature—cold
   c. Color—mottled, pale, cyanotic
   d. External Hemorrhage—Aggressively identify and treat with digital pressure applied directly for 5-10 minutes continuously. Particularly in the scalp, large volumes of blood loss can occur if this is not done promptly and properly.
3. Capillary Refill—should be <2 sec
4. Central vs Peripheral Pulse Pattern—compare carotids to the radials and femorals to the pedal pulses. If

the peripheral pulses are comparatively weak, this indicates compensation for hemorrhagic shock
5. End Organ Perfusion
   a. Central Nervous System—altered mental status with or without head injury may indicate poor perfusion
   b. Renal—urine outputs are critical to monitor—may require Foley catheter insertion into the bladder. Recommended urine outputs are 2 cc/kg/hr for children <2, 1 cc/kg/hr for ages 2–13, and $\frac{1}{2}$ cc/kg/hr for ages >13. This reflects the fact that the immature kidney requires more perfusion to clear the nitrogenous wastes of the infant than the older kidney does.

If after the above assessment the determination is made that the child is indeed in shock, then fluid resuscitation must be begun. It does not usually need to be begun immediately upon arrival at the injury scene however. Much precious time can be wasted attempting futilely to start an IV on a child in a cold, dark, roadside injury scene when these lines can be problematic even in the best in-hospital situations. The prioritization in the field should be to secure the airway, scoop up the child, and run to the trauma center for IV access there.

Where to turn for IV access is a tough part of pediatric trauma resuscitation. IVs can be hard to come by in a vasoconstricted, crying child in which there is great anxiety for both child, parents, and caretakers. The current recommendations are to attempt a peripheral IV anywhere one becomes available—the "Any Port in a Storm" theory. This is not the time to let the most inexperienced person try their hand. The vein they blow may be the last good one. In infants, the scalp can be an important source for veins as well. After 90 seconds of attempts, the patient should undergo placement of a central venous line in the groin if a skilled practitioner is available. Sometimes this practitioner will prefer a cutdown in the saphenous in the ankle or groin. If this skilled person is not available, an intraosseus line can be placed. This device is usually placed in the tibial plateau just medial and inferior to the tibial tuberosity of the leg (do not use a leg that is fractured), or the anterior superior iliac crest in the abdomen. The sternum can also be used in older children. Although current recommendations is to use this access in the age group <7 years, success with this technique has been demonstrated even in adults.

The fluid resuscitation given to the children is once again done by weight. Threee crystalloid fluid boluses of either Ringer's lactate or normal saline are given in aliquots of 20 cc/kg. After administration of each, the hemodynamic profile should be assessed to determine if a repeat bolus is needed. After 1 or 2 the pediatric patient usually settles down well. If a third is still not adequate, then the patient should begin boluses of 10 cc/kg of type-specific packed red blood cells for up to 4 times, or essentially $\frac{1}{2}$ the child's blood volume (80 cc/kg).

In infants under 1 year, stored glycogen is depleted form the stress of a trauma quite rapidly. It is therefore quite possible that failure to respond to resuscitation can be secondary to hypoglycemia. In this age group, one of the boluses of crystalloid should contain D5 as well, or at least care must be taken to check a stat glucose shortly after beginning resuscitation to ensure that these levels are adequate.

D is for Disability There are a number of Pediatric Trauma Scoring Systems, as well as a modified Glasgow Coma Scale for non-verbal children to optimize evaluation. The most important determinant is the Secondary Survey, outlined below.

E is for Exposure Children have much more exposed body surface area and much less insulating fat than their adult counterparts do, leaving them very prone to hypothermia. Keeping ambulance bays, helicopters, trauma resuscitation areas, radiology, and OR suites warmed can help reduce this. Administered fluids should be warmed and blankets should be applied liberally during resuscitations. Only expose the part of the body that is in need of assessment or treatment to minimize heat loss. This can help eliminate one important source of poor response to resuscitation.

Secondary Survey

Identification of all other injuries begins after the completion of primary survey, establishment of resuscitation priorities, and after life-threatening injuries have already been managed. This represents a head to toe evaluation of the entire patient.

Family member presence often is helpful in reducing the stress of the frightened and injured child.

Diagnostic Studies

Children who are injured should undergo the following examinations:

- Initial trauma radiologic series as with adults (lateral C-spine, chest, pelvis)
- CT scan if hemodynamically stable—CT without IV contrast for head, and with IV contrast for thoracoabdominopelvic studies
- Other modalities (DPL and FAST) have a limited role (only in hemodynamically unstable patients)
- Angiography maybe also therapeutic in the control of bleeding from pelvicfractures and for blunt splenic/hepatic trauma with blush on CT.

Specific Pediatric Injuries

Head Trauma

The leading cause of death and disability among children is head trauma, with falls being the most frequent etiology. Children may have significant trauma without skull fracture. Scalp lacerations in children can be significant sources of hemorrhage and should be controlled concurrent with the neurologic evaluation.

Child abuse should be ruled out in children aged two and younger with head injury. Shaken baby syndrome usually shows little evidence of external injury, but can include subdural, subarachnoid hemorrhage, retinal hemorrhage, occipital skull fractures, and posterior rib fractures.

Early CT scan imaging may show little evidence of injury. Frequent neurological examination is a key component in the detection of head injury.

The Glasgow Coma Score (and its modified version for non-verbal children) is used to clinically assess the degree of traumatic brain injury. GCS scores of 13–15 indicate mild injury, 9–12 indicate moderate injury, and 3–8 indicate severe injury.

The initial insult to the brain is called the primary injury. Only injury prevention can curtail this problem. Treatment of head injury therefore revolves around efforts to minimize the secondary injury to the brain, i.e., the potential expansion or deterioration of the originally injured brain area. Secondary injury can result form hypoperfusion form shock or from hypoxia from inadequate ventilation.

Treatment should avoid hypoxia, hypoventilation, hypotension, and fluid overload in order to avoid secondary injury. Intracranial pressure (ICP) monitors should be used early in severe (all) and some moderate injuries (usually with a CT documented lesion). A neurosurgical consult is mandatory for patients with GCS < 8 or patients with CT findings. Availability of neurosurgical expertise has become a major criteria for transfer of pediatric trauma patients to Pediatric Trauma Centers.

Spinal Cord Injury

Spinal chord injury is relatively uncommon in young children, but the most frequent involvement is in the C1–C2 portion of the spine. The thoracic and lumbar spine may be associated with lap-belt syndrome. Because of the increased flexibility of the spine and spinal column in younger children, and the disproportionately weighty skull sitting atop this flexible spine, spinal cord injury without radiological abnormalities (SCIWORA) accounts for the majority of cervical spinal injuries in children under the age of 8. This involves contusion to the spinal column with or without hemorrhage that doesn't appear on routine radiographic testing. It is almost always accompanied by neck pain and tenderness +/− neurologic deficit.

In performing cervical spine clearance in the pediatric trauma patient, the child should be awake and responsive without distracting injuries or sedation.

Children with suspected spinal cord injuries undergo administration of IV steroids, although the data for amelioration of spinal injuries in children is less compelling than in adults.

Thoracic Trauma

The majority of thoracic injury (90%) is due to blunt trauma and this type of injury is the second leading cause of traumatic death in children. Serious intrathoracic injuries may present without rib fractures because of the greater compliance of the chest wall and increased mobility of mediastinal structures. As with this injury in adults, emergency department thoracotomy should be performed selectively. The presence of rib fractures indicates the presence of a high impact injury to the focal area of chest. If the mechanism of injury described doesn't support this impact, the possibility of intentional injury (child abuse) should be suspected.

Abdominal Trauma

Ninety percent of abdominal trauma is blunt. The spleen is the most commonly injured abdominal organ and the liver is the second most common. With hematuria, although a nonspecific finding, the physician should suspect genitourinary trauma and evaluate for this possibility. If hematuria occurs after a "minor" trauma, then rule out renal malignancy.

The most common pitfall of abdominal assessment in the pediatric trauma patient is the crying child who develops a massive gastric dilitation. This condition can cause four major sequellae:

1. The patient's abdomen may appear rigid and tense, fooling the practitioner into suspicion of a more serious intra-abdominal injury
2. Respiratory embarrassment may occur
3. Vagal stimulation may lead to reflex bradycardia. If the patient has concomitant head injury, this may lead to false impression of impending increased intracranial pressure crisis as seen with the Cushing reflex (bradycardia with hypertension)
4. The massively over distended stomach can cause vomiting and then aspiration in the immobilized, supine trauma patient.

All four of these scenarios can be avoided by early nasogastric tube insertion.

Ninety percent of pediatric abdominal trauma can be managed non-operatively. Injuries to the spleen, liver, kidney, pancreas, and duodenum fit this category. An exception to this non-operative management schema is caused by the success injury prevention advocates have had in encouraging parents to keep their children in motor vehicles strapped into seat belts. Unfortunately, up to 75% of the time, the mode of restraint used is used incorrectly. The seat belt triad, an injury complex in which there is an umbilical level seat belt-induced abdominal wall contusion along with back pain (with or without neurologic deficit) and abdominal pain, is a common pattern that needs to be recognized early. Up to 80% of children with this triad have an intra-abdominal injury most often to a hollow viscus that will not show up on Abdominal CT immediately if at all. These patients most often require laparoscopy or laparotomy for complete evaluation and treatment.

The frequency of non-operative management in these pediatric trauma patients should lull any caregivers into the acceptability of management of these patients without pediatric surgical/trauma expertise. The non-operative treatment modality works only at a center where operative treatment can rapidly be activated in the event of hemodynamic instability.

Pediatric Orthopedic Injuries

Orthopedic injuries are actually the most common injuries seen in Pediatric Trauma. They are infrequently life threatening. Pediatric bones are more flexible and can bend a great deal before breaking. They can break incompletely (greenstick fractures) and in odd orientations (spiral fractures). They can also break along growth plates. These types of injuries may not cause a great deal of outward extremity deformity, so that a careful centimeter by centimeter exam of the extremities is necessary, taking care to note any areas of tenderness (particularly at the growth plates). Open fractures need to be treated operatively within six hours of injury to reduce risk of osteomyelitis or septic arthritis. The supracondylar elbow fracture is also in need of emergent attention, as failure to reduce and evaluate for possible vascular compromise from brachial artery injury can lead to limb loss.

Disposition

The decision of whether to admit the pediatric trauma patient or transfer the patient to a Pediatric Trauma Center should be made early and with collaboration of the trauma surgeon. The overall condition of the patient, the complexity of the injury complex, the presence of suspicion of maltreatment, the need for pediatric critical care are all reasons for transfer to the Pediatric Trauma Center. The mode of transport chosen will also depend on the patients condition, the distance between facilities, and the weather conditions. All suspected cases of child abuse must be reported at the treating facility (see Chapter 87).

Injury Prevention Programs

Because 90% of all pediatric injury is preventable, emergency department and trauma centers play an important role in reducing the impact of injury by participating in prevention programs. Hospital-based injury surveillance is insufficient due to the fact that they only identify those patients that survive to reach a trauma center. At the University of Massachusetts Medical Center, many programs are already in place. *Injury Free Coalition for Kids of Worcester, Car Seat Safety Program,* and *Guns for Goods Program,* are a few examples of the effective programs in place for Worcester and the surrounding communities.

Selected Readings

Cantor RM, Callahan JM, eds. Pediatric emergency medicine: current concepts and controversies. *Emerg Med Clin North Am* 2002;20:1–27.

Committee on Trauma, American College of Surgeons. *Advance Trauma Life Support Student Manual.* Chicago: American College of Surgeons, 1997.

Hauda WE II. Pediatric trauma. In: Tintinalli JE, Keenen GD, Stapczynski S, et al., eds. *Emergency Medicine, A Comprehensive Study Guide,* 6th ed. New York, McGraw Hill, 2004:1542–1549.

Injury Free Coalition for Kids of Worcester, MA. Available at http://www.injuryfree. org. Accessed June 2005.

Klein MD, Long JA. Trauma in infants and children. In: Wilson RF, Walt A, eds. *Management of Trauma, Pitfalls and Practice,* 2d ed. Baltimore: Williams & Wilkins, 1996:128–145.

National Pediatric Trauma Registry-Fact Sheets. Available at http://www.nptr.org/.

Rutkauskas JJ, et al., eds. Special considerations for the pediatric emergency patient. *Emerg Med Clin North Am* 2000;18:539–548.

Tepas JJ III, ed. Caring for the injured child: modern concepts and emergency challenges. *Surg Clin North Am* 2002;82:263–447.

Administration

John C. Moorhead

Introduction

Emergency physicians practice in a complex health care system. Approximately 30% of all resources are devoted to the administrative aspects of the system. Creating an environment to support optimal clinical outcomes as well as patient and staff satisfaction and safety requires the participation of all members of the team, in collaboration with pre-hospital and hospital staff. Physicians should provide leadership for physician-specific issues as well as overall system improvement processes. Although specific administrative roles are often assigned to individual members of the group, a general understanding of the administrative aspects of care may prevent system errors and contribute to physician wellness and career satisfaction.

Hospital Medical Staff

Michael T. Rapp

In the United States, the organized medical staff plays an integral and well-established role within the hospital structure. This derives from the early collaborative relationship between hospitals and physicians. Hospitals were established by members of the community and were governed by an elected or appointed board of lay persons. The board selected interested physicians to attend patients in the hospital.

As medical care developed, hospitals became more and more necessary for the care of patients. Physicians increasingly brought patients to the hospital rather than to seek to provide care elsewhere. Although the hospital governing body had legal control over the hospital, it lacked the expertise to supervise the medical care rendered within the institution. Hospitals, therefore, were encouraged to have an organized medical staff who would be responsible for the medical care rendered.

Through the medical staff structure, physicians could practice independently at facilities where they had no financial or employment relationship. Yet the medical staff structure also provided accountability to the governing body for the medical care rendered in the hospital. Over time, the requirement for an organized medical staff was incorporated into hospital accreditation and other standards. Today, the Joint Commission on Accreditation of Healthcare Organization (JCAHO) standards, hospital licensing laws, and Medicare regulations all require hospitals to have an organized medical staff. Because of the fact that nearly all hospitals seek JCAHO accreditation, JCAHO medical staff standards play a major role in determining the organization and functions of hospital medical staffs.

Purposes and Function

Generally, the medical staff's purpose is to promote quality care in the hospital. It does this by providing a structure through which physicians and other practitioners may organize, interact, relate to the governing body, and fulfill various specific functions.

A primary responsibility delegated to the medical staff is the delineation of privileges. Through this process the medical staff is directly involved in deciding who may

practice at the hospital and what they may do. Although the governing body retains the final responsibility for authorizing practice in the hospital, medical staff recommendations on privileging are normally accepted in a well functioning hospital.

Another major role of the medical staff is to provide oversight of physicians and other independent practitioners. Through a variety of means, the medical staff works to assure that the work of the practitioners meets the standards sought in the hospital.

The JCAHO specifies a number of other medical staff functions. These include providing leadership in performance improvement and patient safety activities; participating in measurement, assessment, and improvement of other specific processes; and providing oversight in analyzing and improving patient satisfaction. Examples of processes that medical staff involvement must review are the use of medications, the use of blood and blood components, and the use of operative and other procedures.

Duties of the medical staff are to:
- Delineate the scope of privileges for physicians and other licensed independent practitioners
- Provide oversight of quality of care, treatment, and services for those it credentials and privileges
- Provide leadership in performance improvement and patient safety activities
- Participate in process measurement, assessment, and improvement within the organization

Structure

The medical staff structure is that of an organized self-governing body. Self-governance, however, does not signify that the medical staff is completely independent. Rather, the medical staff is accountable to the ultimate authority of the governing body.

Medical staff bylaws specify both the medical staff structural organization and its relationship to the governing body. The bylaws are designed to provide a framework within which medical staff members can act with a reasonable degree of freedom and confidence. As such, they define a system of mutual rights and responsibilities to which both the medical staff members and governing body must adhere. Several courts have decided that medical staff bylaws create a contractual relationship between the medical staff members and the governing body.

The JCAHO has a major role in determining the structure and function of the medical staff by specifying particular provisions that must be included in the medical staff bylaws. Among the most significant JCAHO requirements is the stipulation that neither the medical staff nor the governing body will unilaterally amend the medical staff bylaws. This provision has a major role in preserving autonomy for the medical staff. The JCAHO also requires, in the bylaws, a fair hearing and appeal mechanism, a provision for selecting and removing medical staff officers, and the structure and function of the medical staff executive committee.

According to the JCAHO, a mechanism for how certain other items are determined must be in the bylaws. These include the mechanism for establishing and enforcing criteria and standards for medical staff membership; the mechanism for establishing and enforcing criteria for delegating oversight responsibilities to practitioners with independent privileges; the mechanism for establishing and maintaining patient care standards; and the mechanism for credentialing and delineation of clinical privileges. Many medical staffs will believe, however, that the bylaws should contain the specifics rather than just the mechanism for determining important items.

The complexity of a medical staff's structure depends on the hospital's complexity and the preferences of the medical staff and governing body. Although JCAHO standards require that all hospitals have an executive committee, the organizational structure is left to the particular hospital to decide, subject to state law. Hospital medical staff bylaws typically do provide for various medical staff committees because fulfilling medical staff functions is often difficult without a committee structure.

The medical staff is normally headed by a chief of staff or president of the medical staff who is elected by the medical staff for a fixed term. The chief of staff represents the interests of medical staff members to the governing body and to the hospital administration. The chief of staff will normally appoint members of medical staff committees, chair the executive committee, and serve as the representative of the medical staff to the governing body, particularly on major matters.

Most medical staffs are organized according to departments, although this is not a JCAHO requirement. At times, hospitals have a separate clinical department for each specialty. In other cases specialties may be grouped. For example, most surgical specialties may be included as sections within a single department of surgery. Where the size of the medical staff is small, seemingly unrelated specialties may be placed in a single department.

A department chair typically has an automatic seat on the executive committee of the medical staff. This direct representation provides a specific spokesperson for the members of the specialty or group of specialties comprising the department. Some consultants currently recommend small numbers of clinical departments, each composed of multiple specialties. The stated goal is to streamline the medical executive committee and to make it smaller and more efficient. Departmental status can be of great importance for a specialty, however. Thus, the implications of accepting such a recommendation should be carefully considered.

Within the medical staff structure, medical staff members are usually categorized by activity level. Active staff members usually provide most of the care and provide the leadership of committees and medical staff offices. Physicians on the active medical staff are accorded all rights and responsibilities of the medical staff, including the right to vote and hold office. The associate medical staff is for more junior members and a midpoint between courtesy and active. Physicians on the courtesy staff typically only use the hospital occasionally, and are not desirous of the opportunity to vote and serve in leadership positions on the medical staff. Other special categories of medical staff membership can include consulting or honorary members.

The executive committee, as the only required committee, has a primary role related to medical staff activities. All medical staff departments and other medical staff committees report to the medical executive committee. The executive committee makes recommendations directly to the governing body on such matters as appointments and reappointment to medical staff membership, adoption of medical staff policies, and corrective action. Finally, the executive committee may act for the medical staff in the intervals between medical staff meetings.

Traditionally medical staff membership was limited to physicians and dentists. In recent years, however, the number and types of licensed practitioners who desire to have privileges at the hospital has significantly increased. This has resulted in further consideration as to which practitioners should be allowed to be members of the medical staff, what privileges they should have, and what role the medical staff should have in credentialing and privileging such individuals.

The JCAHO's resolution of the matter in its standards has several components. First, the JCAHO leaves to the governing body and the medical staff the decision as to criteria for medical staff membership. In other words, the medical staff bylaws may reserve membership to physicians and dentists or it may expand membership. Second, the JCAHO states that privileges and medical staff membership are not necessarily synonymous. Thus, a particular practitioner may have privileges without medical staff membership or may have medical staff membership without privileges.

Due to the variety of practitioners in a hospital and their roles, the JCAHO has sought to distinguish those who function independently from those who function under supervision or direction. To do this, the JCAHO has adopted the term *licensed independent practitioner,* which is defined as "any individual permitted by law and by the organization to provide care, treatment, and services, without direction or supervision."

For medical staff purposes, the medical staff must credential and privilege all licensed independent practitioners. In addition, licensed independent practitioners must be included in medical staff membership (although not necessary all categories of licensed independent practitioners). With regard to practitioners who are not independent of supervision and direction, the medical staff may or may not be directly involved in their credentialing and privileges, and may or may not include them as members of the medical staff.

Structure of the medical staff:

- Self-governing
- Reports to and is accountable to the governing body.
- Organized and operates as defined in a set of bylaws defining its role in hospital setting
- Neither the medical staff nor governing body may unilaterally amend medical staff bylaws
- Medical Executive Committee required by JCAHO standards
- Departmental structure optional
- Membership criteria determined by governing body and medical staff
- Membership may or may not be limited to physicians and other licensed independent practitioners

Credentialing

The JCAHO requires that the medical staff must credential and privilege all independent licensed practitioners. This process derives from the hospital's obligation to assure patients that physicians and others practicing at the hospital are reasonably qualified and competent, given the scope of practice permitted.

As defined by the JCAHO, credentialing consists of a series of activities designed to collect relevant data that serve as the basis for decisions regarding hospital privileges and medical staff membership. The specific information gathered as part of the credentialing activity can vary among hospitals provided that the credentialing criteria are explicit. JCAHO required criteria include primary source verification and documentation of current licensure, relevant training or experience, current competence, and ability to perform the privileges requested. In addition, the information gathered must include any pending or prior challenges to any of the credentials.

The credentialing process for initial appointment is generally exhaustive and can be very time consuming given the necessity for primary source information. It is, therefore, advisable for physicians to maintain specific information throughout their career as to their professional activities so that it will be available to them when needed for credentialing. In addition, it is advisable to allow a large amount of time for the credentialing process for any initial appointment.

Physicians must be reviewed for renewal of privileges and medical staff reappointment at least every 2 years according to JCAHO standards. The credentialing process for reappointment can differ from the original appointment, and usually does because at reappointment the hospital will have more information on the physician from internal sources.

The Health Care Quality Improvement Act of 1986 requires that the National Practitioner Data Bank be queried at the time of initial medical staff appointment and initial granting of clinical privileges, and at least every 2 years thereafter for any physician or other practitioner granted clinical privileges. The data bank maintains information reported to it as required regarding medical malpractice payments, licensure disciplinary actions, adverse clinical privilege actions taken by a health care entity including hospitals, and adverse actions affecting professional society membership.

The application of the Americans with Disability Act to medical staff credentialing is somewhat unclear. The act strictly speaking only relates to employees. However, it has been interpreted as applying to medical staff members as well. The act would prevent the medical staff from making certain inquires that relate to disabilities prior to offering the physician membership on the hospital medical staff. Once the initial offer is made, inquiry can be made, but then there would need to be reasonable accommodation for the physician related to a disability.

Although the Act may prohibit inquiry as to specific health matters or disability at the application stage, it appears to allow inquiry as to the ability of the applicant to perform the specific privileges requested without specific reference to health status. In the credentialing process, hospitals typically do require some statement to the effect that the applicant has the physical and mental ability to discharge the patient care responsibilities requested.

Credentialing

- Consists of a series of activities designed to collect relevant data that serve as the basis for decisions regarding hospital privileges and medical staff membership.
- Medical staff is responsible for credentialing and privileging of all independent licensed practitioners.
- JCAHO standards require recredentialing every two years.

Privileging

Privileging is the process of granting setting specific authority to engage in patient care activities. Thus, the granting of privileges is based not only on the individual's qualifications to exercise the specific privileges, but also on the type of procedures, care, and treatment to be performed or provided within the proposed setting. In other words, the granting of privileges depends in part on an institutional decision to allow and support a particular type of patient care activity in the institution.

The privileging process starts with the medical staff's development of the criteria for privileges. This may include such benchmarks as board qualification or certification for general privileges in a specialty. Privileging criteria are necessary to provide objectivity to the privileging of applicants, which are used to evaluate the specific credentialing information from the applicant.

Several recent developments have led to challenging issues involving physician privileging in hospitals. One is the perceived need by some hospitals to introduce economic criteria into the privileging process due to hospital financial challenges. Physicians generally oppose any such criteria not directly related to professional competence and performance. The JCAHO has dealt with this issue by requiring that privileging decisions consider criteria that are directly related to the quality of care. Where criteria are used that may be unrelated to quality of care, treatment, and services or professional competence, the JCAHO requires evidence that the impact of the resulting decisions on quality be evaluated. As such, decisions based purely on economic factors (economic credentialing) would appear to be contrary to JCAHO standards.

Another important recent development is the delivery of health care services through telemedicine. By this means, practitioners may provide services related to patients at distant hospital sites. To deal with telemedicine in a flexible manner, the JCAHO provides that the primary credentialing and privileging process is the responsibility of the originating site rather than each recipient hospital. However, medical staffs at both originating and recipient sites are expected to recommend those clinical services that may be provided through a telemedical link.

Finally, the threat of disruption of health care services through terrorism has led the JCAHO to develop a category of privileges called *disaster privileges*. In this case, the credentialing and privileging criteria are greatly relaxed compared to what is normally required. In this way, hospitals are allowed to dispense with unrealistic requirements in such unusual circumstances.

Privileging:
- The process of granting setting specific authority to engage in patient care activities.
- Privileges are delineated for each independent licensed practitioner.

Physician Discipline

If the quality of care rendered by a person with clinical privileges is not at the level expected by the medical staff, there are numerous steps that may be taken in response: education, developing rules and policies to standardize the clinical care, putting systems in place to improve quality, or a focused review of the practitioner's work. In addition, the biannual reappointment process allows privileges to be modified, based on the required periodic assessments.

Occasionally, however, more specific corrective action is needed. In these circumstances, disciplinary action can take various forms. These may include a letter of reprimand, restriction of privileges, required supervision short of suspension, or removal from the medical staff. Often a factor considered is whether the matter will need to be reported to the National Practitioner Data Bank. Final disciplinary action (after hearings and appeals), which extends for more than 30 days, must be reported. State laws also govern the circumstances where disciplinary action must be reported to the state licensing board. At times these standards are more strict than the reporting requirements of the National Practitioner Data bank.

The grounds and procedures for disciplinary action are normally found in the bylaws of the medical staff. Typically, the grounds are limited to professional conduct,

competence, and quality of care. Ideally, disciplinary action is based on objective, standardized review of clinical care derived from the formalized processes established by the medical staff and the hospital to review quality of care in the hospital. Discipline based on a bad case rather than a pattern of clinical care that objectively is different from established patterns of practice often is difficult to support and may lead to arbitrary or unreasonably harsh disciplinary action.

The procedures for disciplinary action can vary from hospital to hospital. However, the general procedure will involve a complaint process, investigation, involvement of the departmental chair, and a recommendation by the medical executive committee to the governing body. Prior to an adverse recommendation by the medical executive committee there is typically an opportunity for a fair hearing, and some appeal process prior to a final decision by the governing body.

The JCAHO standards require that the medical staff bylaws contain a fair hearing and appeal process for any adverse decisions regarding reappointment, denial, reduction, suspension, or revocation of privileges that may relate to quality of care, treatment, and service issues. As stated by the JCAHO, the mechanisms for fair hearing and appeals processes are designed to allow the affected individual a fair opportunity to defend her- or himself regarding the adverse decision to an unbiased hearing body of the medical staff, and an opportunity to appeal the decision of the hearing body to the governing body. On the other hand, JCHAO standards do not require any specific fair hearing or appeal procedures. Despite this, frequently hospitals do comply with the specific procedures stated in the Healthcare Quality Improvement Act of 1986. This Act provides hospitals with antitrust exemption for adverse peer review action, if the hospital complies with the specified hearing procedures.

While the JCAHO provision regarding fair hearing may appear to be broad, it is noteworthy that the JCHAO standards do not require a fair hearing with respect to initial privileges or initial medical staff appointment. Moreover, the provisions of exclusive contracts generally override the JCAHO requirement for fair hearings and appeals. Thus, physicians subject to certain contractual provisions in exclusive contracts frequently find their opportunity to practice at a hospital may be terminated through the action of a hospital official without any access by the physician to a fair hearing or appeal procedure.

Physician Discipline:
- JCAHO standards require medical staff bylaws to contain a fair hearing and appeal mechanism
- Health Care Quality Improvement Act delineates procedures for fair hearing and appeal
- Hospital disciplinary action lasting more than 30 days must be reported to National Practitioner Data Bank

Policy and Procedures

In addition to its bylaws, rules, and regulations, the medical staff frequently adopts policies and procedures that govern the work of its members. The formality of the process for adopting policies and procedures is less than for bylaws and, therefore, easier to adopt and modify. By developing such rules, the members of the staff can standardize certain processes and thereby promote quality care and assure compliance with external laws, regulations, and accreditation requirements.

Although a policy is somewhat different than a procedure, the two are frequently merged into one document. The policy portion sets forth the general approach of the organization as to a particular subject. For example, the policy portion may state that the medical staff will comply with the requirements of 1986 Emergency Medical Treatment and Active Labor Act (EMTALA). The procedural portion of the document may then state the procedures for such compliance. Relative to EMTALA, this may include how triage will be conducted, who will be responsible for the medical screening exam, the procedure for transferring patients, and other such details.

Policies and procedures can pertain to the entire medical staff or only a segment, such as a clinical department. The procedure for adopting such policies would typically be stated in the bylaws of the medical staff. If such documents are to affect the entire medical staff or more than one component, the policy and procedure would need to be adopted by either the medical executive committee, which represents the entire staff, or by the medical staff itself. If the policy is only to affect a certain department, the bylaws might provide that the department has the authority to adopt the policy itself. However, because even policies of a single department may impact members of other medical staff departments, medical staff bylaws frequently require that departmental policies be approved by the medical executive committee.

In addition to medical staff policies and procedures, hospitals normally have many other such policies. These can include administrative policies, adopted by the hospital administration, nursing policies, adopted by the nursing division, and policies affecting certain patient care areas such as the intensive care unit or the emergency department. Policies affecting particular patient care areas are often adopted jointly by the medical and administrative director of the area.

In view of the number of policies within a hospital and its various administrative and clinical departments, there can be overlap, confusion, and even conflict among policies. From the perspective of the medical staff, it is important to be aware of the various policies and work to avoid such problems.

Policies and procedures may have importance in legal proceedings. Failure to adhere to one's own policies can be the most direct evidence of negligence in professional liability cases. Therefore, it is important to be cautious in drafting policies and procedures. They must be reasonable and must actually be followed. Otherwise, if there is an untoward event, the policy may provide a sole basis for legal liability. It is also important that policies be accessible to staff members and be reviewed on a regular basis for modification or rescission.

Care is especially necessary in drafting medical staff policies that affect the entire medical staff. It is essential that the

policy contain appropriate exceptions or modifications for particular areas or departments, particularly the emergency department. As an example, a medical staff policy on moderate sedation that requires four to eight hours of fasting prior to administration of the sedation may be appropriate for the operating suite for elective cases, but not be appropriate for the emergency department.

Although policies and procedures have risks associated with their adoption, they can also provide protection to the individual practitioners and care givers. For instance, when the medical staff or hospital adopts policies on matters that are controversial in hospital or medical practice, the individual practitioner may be protected from liability by following an institutional policy.

Policies and Procedures:
- Allow standardization of processes
- Promote quality care and compliance with external laws, regulations, and accreditation requirements
- Can define standard of care for a particular institution

Departmental/Interdepartmental Interaction

Departments within a hospital include both administrative and medical staff departments. Administrative departments provide for the hospital facility, supplies, and nursing as well as other support personnel. Administrative department heads are responsible for budgeting, employment decisions, and supervision. Medical staff departments, on the other hand, are responsible for the clinical performance of department members and others with clinical privileges. Department chairs and their members also provide input on decisions within the scope of responsibility of the administrative departments.

The interaction among administrative and clinical departments can be complex. A given medical staff department may need to interact with several administrative and clinical departments. The emergency service is a good example because its personnel must interact with virtually all hospital administrative and clinical departments.

The chair of a medical staff department has primary responsibility for interaction of members within the department, interaction with other departments, and the integration of the clinical service into the operations of the hospital. As a result, the chair of the clinical department must be very skilled in dealing with the numerous individuals with whom the chair may be involved.

With regard to the internal department matters, the principal responsibility of the chair is to recommend to the medical staff the criteria for clinical privileges that are relevant to the care provided in the department, and recommending clinical privileges for each member of the department. Among the more common intradepartmental issues are conflicts deriving from competition among its members. It is essential that the departmental chair be evenhanded in dealing with all members, regardless of their practice affiliation. Should differences arise within a department that cannot be resolved by the chair, they would become the responsibility of the medical staff executive committee.

As for interaction among medical staff departments, a common problem is a difference of opinion between specialties as to the appropriate clinical scope of practice of another. A key advantage of departmental status for any specialty is that its chair is responsible for recommending the criteria for privileges for its members. This limits the impact of the opinion of the chair of another specialty in another department as to the scope of practice of a particular specialty.

Departmental/Interdepartmental Interaction:
- Hospitals have both administrative and clinical departments
- Chair of clinical department has primary role in departmental/interdepartmental interaction

Selected Readings

American Medical Association. *Physician Guide to Organization Medical Staff Bylaws*, ed 2. Chicago: AMA, September 2002. The latest document is available at http://www.ama-assn.org. Accessed June 2005.

California Medical Association. Model Medical Staff Bylaws. June 2003. The latest bylaws are available at http://www.cmanet.org. Accessed June 2005.

Joint Commission on Accreditation of Healthcare Organizations. *2004 Hospital Accreditation Standards Manual*. Oak Brook, IL: Joint Commission Resources, 2004. The latest HAS are available at http://www.jcrinc.com/publications.asp?durki=8141&site=4&return=77. Accessed June 2005.

Fundamentals of Emergency Medicine Practice Groups

James M. Brown
Manisha Gupta

Emergency medicine is a relatively new and rapidly evolving specialty. Although emergency physicians began the business by independently contracting with hospitals, staffing groups emerged that controlled a large number of hospital contracts. These staffing groups evolved into today's large contract groups. Large groups offer economies of scale, reliable staffing, stable administrative support systems, and an easy entry into practice for physicians unable or unwilling to make the entrepreneurial sacrifices required to start an independent group practice or to become a partner in an existing practice. The convenience that large groups offer to physicians comes at a price, however. Positions offered by these groups often require some surrender of autonomy in practice, lack of control over reimbursement for physician services, lack of job security and stability, and sometimes even restriction of medical staff privileges. Understanding issues regarding emergency medicine group practices requires a basic understanding of the history of emergency medicine, the elements unique to emergency medicine practice, the emergence and influence of contract management groups, the relationship of emergency medicine practice groups to hospitals, the relationship of individual emergency physicians to practice groups, the business fundamentals of emergency medicine, and the rudiments of contracts.

A Brief History of Emergency Medicine

The clinical and business aspects of emergency medicine developed simultaneously during a period of rapidly increasing demand for emergency care. In early post-World War II America, most hospital admissions were elective. Availability and quality of emergency care varied widely. "Emergency Rooms" (ERs) were often that in the literal sense, and were staffed by a nurse with the doctor on-call from home. Multiple factors led to a steadily increasing demand in emergency care, however. The rapidly growing population became more mobile. As the "house call" became obsolete, the demand for care in emergency rooms grew, and ER visits quadrupled between 1955 and 1971. During this time, emergency rooms were often staffed by rotating rosters of physicians with active staff privileges,

regardless of specialty or training. Some of these physicians began to limit their practice strictly to emergency medicine.

In 1961, four physicians in Alexandria, Virginia left their practice of general medicine to staff the Alexandria Virginia Hospital continuously, thereby becoming the first group of physicians to staff an emergency department exclusively. This model of exclusively practicing in the emergency room became known as the Alexandria Plan. In the same year, groups in Pontiac and Flint, Michigan also formed to continuously staff emergency departments, but maintained their office practices as well. This model of practice became known as the Pontiac Plan. No formal training or educational programs in emergency medicine existed until the first national meeting of emergency physicians took place in Arlington in 1968. Emergency medicine became the twenty-third specialty to be recognized by the American Board of Medical Specialties in 1979. Demand for emergency care far outpaced the number of residency-trained emergency medicine specialists available to staff emergency departments. Corporations holding multiple hospital contracts rapidly emerged, paying physicians a fixed hourly rate, billing and collecting their professional fees, while keeping the balance as profit. Physician credentials, quality of care, and quality of the physicians' workplace in this environment were erratic.

Demand for emergency care continues to grow. The annual number of ED patient visits increased to 108 million in 2000. As of 1999, only 62% of physicians practicing emergency medicine were residency trained or board-certified. It is likely that the shortage of residency-trained physicians to staff emergency departments will persist for years to come. So far, the void between demand for emergency care and availability of residency-trained and board-certified emergency physicians continues in part to be filled by national and regional groups of various sizes, some of which hold hundreds of contracts. Such groups provide many readily available opportunities for employment. Many of these positions, however, lack democratic group structure, long-term stability, and opportunity to become a partner in the group. Many of these positions do not require residency training or board certification in emergency medicine. Change in group structure may occur gradually as the number of residency-trained and board-certified physicians increases.

Elements Unique to Emergency Medicine Practice

Hospital-based specialties include emergency medicine, anesthesiology, pathology, and radiology. No specialty is more restricted to the hospital environment than emergency medicine, however. The *emergency department* is essentially the only location where emergency medicine is practiced. There are a relatively fixed number of emergency departments. Unlike clinics, emergency departments are open 24 hours a day, seven days a week. Compared to emergency physicians, physicians practicing in clinic environments may have greater control over their physical environment, the patient base, and their administrative and clinical staff. Except as specified in the contract, emergency physician groups may have little control over the environment and staff provided by the hospital. In clinical practices, the patient-physician relationship is one of mutual choice. In emergency medicine, physicians must treat all patients who come to the emergency department. The demographics of the patient base are primarily dependent upon the location and reputation of the hospital, not the credentials or preferences of the emergency physicians.

Relationship of Practice Groups to Hospitals

In the ideal world, every hospital would provide an excellent facility and staff, and the physician group would continuously provide an adequate number of the best-qualified emergency medicine specialists to practice in the department. Economic realities may dictate otherwise. Like most contracts, agreements between hospitals and groups include numerous compromises. The hospital provides a physical facility, nursing and ancillary staff, medication, equipment, supplies, registration, and may provide documentation services. Physician groups provide physician staffing, a director, clinical policies and procedures, documentation policies, performance improvement activities, and malpractice coverage. Contracts between hospitals and physician groups must at a minimum cover these basic provisions. Many groups perform their own coding, billing, and collecting, although under some circumstances the hospital may perform these services. Hospital administrators with their fiscal eye on the bottom line may opt to contract with the lowest bidder rather than a group of emergency medicine specialists committed to providing high quality care.

Relationship of Physicians to Practice Groups

The majority of physicians in other specialties are owners in whole or in part of their practices. Physicians who are not partners work as either independent contractors or employees. From the legal perspective, an employee is any person who is subject to the will of the employer regarding the type and manner of work done. Physician employees of hospitals or practice groups may enjoy benefits packages and freedom from self-employment taxes, but may surrender the right to control their professional fees. To be considered truly independent contractors, physicians must meet numerous IRS guidelines. A trend toward employer-employee relationship between physicians and contract groups is growing.

Physicians working as independent contractors or employees enter a practice in which many fundamental decisions have already been made. Group structure and governance varies widely and must be evaluated on an individual basis. One striking characteristic of emergency medicine is the widespread willingness of its practitioners to work for others instead of becoming partners in a practice. As of 1997, emergency medicine was the specialty with the lowest number of self-employed physicians (21.6%), the highest number of independent contractors (25.5%), and one of the highest number of physician employees (52.9%). Radiology and anesthesiology, also dependent on the hospital for their practice environment, both show a much stronger practice ownership. Many emergency physicians choose simple contracts promising little more than an hourly wage, paid malpractice insurance, and a promise for a minimum number of monthly clinical hours. Larger, more detailed contracts may promise better reimbursement or benefits packages but may also contain undesirable clauses such as surrender of due process rights and restrictive covenants. *Due process* refers to formal procedures by which adverse actions against a physician regarding employment or hospital staff privileges are addressed. *Restrictive covenants* refers to an agreement that limits the right to practice employment, either in a given facility or geographic area, for a period of time after termination of employment or contract termination. A more specific term is *non-compete clause*.

The hospital contract holder, whether a contract management group or simply a local individual, has the advantage of controlling access to an emergency department. Contracts offered to physicians may be structured in a way to maximize the power and profit of the hospital contract holder. Vigilance prior to signing any contract is required, but a physician applying for a position as an independent contractor or group employee often has limited leverage to alter the contract.

Democratic Practice Groups

Democratic principles can exist in a broad range of group organization structures. No exact definition of *democratic group* exists, however. The model democratic group envisioned by many emergency physicians is a group equally owned by physicians who work in a partnership structure. It may be true that clinical, administrative, and financial autonomy can only be obtained through practice ownership, but the sacrifices and personal risk required to start a practice are formidable. **Table 180.1** provides a sample of

Table 180.1

Sample of Activities Required to Form a Democratic Group

Form a partnership or corporation.

Develop bylaws.

Elect a board of directors.

Develop a business strategy.

- Assess start-up costs.
- Obtain start-up funding (requires personal financial risk by physicians).
- Establish procedures for coding, billing, and collecting.
- Form a plan for physician reimbursement.
- Estimate other practice costs such as malpractice insurance.

Select a hospital and negotiate a contract including:

Contract period and termination provisions

Group responsibilities to the hospital

- Physician hours of coverage
- Minimum physician credentials
- Directorship issues
- Participation in hospital committees and medical staff activities
- Performance improvement
- Documentation
- Compliance
- Physician duties outside the ED.

Hospital responsibilities to the group

- Physical facility
- Nurse and ancillary staffing
- Medication, equipment, supplies
- Work areas and call rooms
- Miscellaneous provisions such as meals and parking.

Develop administrative and clinical policies and procedures.

Develop a model contract between the group and individual physicians including:

- Rights and responsibilities
- Entry and exit plans
- Initial employment status
- Physician scheduling policy
- Reimbursement for clinical and administrative duties
- Benefits (insurance, CME, retirement plan, vacation, etc.)
- Pathway to partnership
- Distribution of shares
- Process for termination of physician with cause
- Process for termination by physician, without restrictive covenants.

Develop and negotiate contracts between the group and party payers.

---

the basic tasks required to start a practice group. Each of these tasks translates into a significant investment of time or expense. Emergency physicians wishing to enjoy the privileges of democratic process in their relationship with a group should be aware of all the elements required to form and maintain a true democratic practice group, and be prepared to offer the same personal risk and sacrifice as their peers.

The Business of Emergency Medicine

The elements necessary to form a practice group hint at the business of emergency medicine. From a health care perspective, emergency departments exist because real emergencies occur and a platform is needed to respond to them. From a business point of view, emergency departments exist because hospitals need a portal for unscheduled admissions and can profit from fees for emergency services they provide. Hospital emergency departments and emergency physician groups depend on each other, but each has its own interests. Each will try to structure the relationship to their own advantage. Hospitals cannot necessarily be expected to subsidize unprofitable physician groups. In general, the physicians must be able to generate sufficient revenue to pay for their own operations. Every physician should become familiar with the coding, billing, and collecting process.

Rudiments of Contracts

A contract is "a legally enforceable agreement, express or implied" (From *Business Law*, Barron's Educational Series, Inc., 2004). This broad definition implies that a contract may include virtually any legal conditions to which both parties agree. When evaluating a contract, both what is included and what is omitted are important. Refer to "development of contract between group and individual physicians" in Table 180.1. At a minimum, a democratic group contract will address each of these issues in detail. When approaching contracts, physicians must understand the structure and function of a democratic practice group, the rudiments of reimbursement and compliance, and the nature of the business of emergency medicine. Physicians should estimate the potential value of their own financial contribution to the group and negotiate accordingly. In most cases, physicians should review the contract with an attorney or senior physician with extensive experience in evaluating emergency physician employment contracts. Perhaps most importantly, physicians must understand their own needs and wants, to assess whether or not they will be comfortable in the clinical and business culture of a particular group.

Conclusion

The literature regarding emergency medicine practice groups is characterized by a dearth of current and objective information. Currently, an increasing number of practices are staffed by residency-trained specialists, but the supply of specialists is unlikely to supply the entire demand for emergency care in the near future. As emergency medicine continues to mature, a trend toward emergency physicians taking control of their practice may emerge. Meanwhile, graduating residents should recognize themselves as true specialists, be aware of current workplace realities, and make informed decisions when entering practice.

Selected Readings

American Academy of Emergency Medicine, multiple authors. *Democratic Groups.* Available at www.aaem.org

American College of Emergency Physicians. Emergency Medicine Practice Committee. *Starting a Democratic Emergency Department Group.* April 2001. Available at www.acep.org

ACEP Reimbursement Committee. *The Fundamentals of Reimbursement: What Every Graduating Resident Should Know Before Starting Practice.* Available at: www.acep.org

Augustine J, Kellerman A. The emergency medicine workforce study: more questions than answers. *Ann Emerg Med* 2002;40:16–18.

Fisher BA, Wittlake WA. Future of the emergency physician: subject or citizen? *Am J Emerg Med* 2000;18:102–107.

Moorhead J, Gallery ME, Hirshkorn C, et al. A study of the workforce in emergency medicine: 1999. *Ann Emerg Med* 2002;40:3–15.

Fundamentals of Physician Contracts

Michael A. Peterson

What Is a Contract?

The primary purpose of a contract is to maintain a good relationship between two parties. A contract accomplishes this by defining the specifics of the relationship so that conflict is minimized. A contract is only an adjunct to a relationship; it cannot create a good relationship from a bad one, nor in and of itself destroy a good relationship. A good business relationship is a key component to a satisfying working environment, and a good contract is helpful in maintaining that good relationship. Unfortunately, half of all emergency physicians report being victims of unfair business practices at some time in their careers. A carefully constructed contract can help avoid this frustrating situation.

The second purpose of a contract is to enforce promises made between parties. When disagreements cannot otherwise be resolved, legal action may result. When this occurs, the relationship has invariably been harmed. A contract that allows a relationship to end in major conflict or in court should be viewed as a failure.

In emergency medicine, a single individual or group of individuals contracts with a hospital to supply emergency physicians to staff the emergency department. This contract is referred to as the *hospital contract* and the individual or group of individuals is known as the *contract holder*. The contract holder in turn may contract with individual emergency physicians; these contracts are known as *emergency physician contracts*. This section discusses general issues in emergency physician contracts. There are other specific contractual issues related to democratic group structure, including partnership requirements and *buy in* periods, which are beyond the scope of this chapter.

What If a Contract Holder Wants Me to Work Without a Contract?

If you enter into any relationship where there are complex issues, a potential for misunderstanding, or the possibility of a significant loss to either party in the relationship, then a contract is essential. An emergency medicine (EM) position certainly fits this description. Working without a contract is known as *employment-at-will*. In an employment-at-will relationship, the contract holder can fire you on the spot for any

reason if he or she so chooses. Without a contract, you may lose your job unexpectedly, have your income reduced or interrupted, or have little recourse if you are treated unfairly. If you choose to work with no contract, at a minimum you should draft a letter outlining what you understand will be expected of you and review it with the contract holder. Such a document may not be binding in court but it will help uncover any misunderstandings before you start working.

Evaluating a Contract

When you are considering a new position and it comes time to sign a contract, seek the advice of an experienced attorney. Although this chapter will help you understand some of the language in a typical contract, it cannot replace a thorough review by an attorney. Read over your contract beforehand, make notes about anything you don't understand, and take these notes with you to the attorney's office. It's important that the language in the contract is clear and understandable to you. Vague, nonspecific, or inconsistent language in a contract may lead to misunderstandings and tension with the contract holder.

Hire the attorney on an hourly basis and anticipate spending 1 to 2 hours overall. Remember, a good attorney is not inexpensive. Consider it an investment in your working relationship. When choosing an attorney, pick carefully: you want someone who knows about emergency medicine contracts in general and preferably someone who is familiar with typical contract language in your area. Emergency physician contracts often include controversial and potentially harmful language that may have significant consequences. Choose someone who has sufficient expertise to be of value to you. You can find such an attorney by soliciting a recommendation from your local or national emergency medicine society or from other emergency medicine physicians whom you trust.

Will I Be Able to Make Changes to My Contract?

It is true that "everything is negotiable." The other side in a negotiation will often try to make you think that things are not negotiable, employing such phrases as "this is a standard contract" or "this is the same contract that everyone else signs." When it comes to contracts, however, nothing is "written in stone." The corollary to "everything is negotiable" is that many things are not worth negotiating; the time and energy spent to change them is not worth what you'll get in return. You, in consultation with your attorney, have to decide what is important enough to change and what you are likely to get changed.

Typical negotiations in emergency medicine do not involve a lot of back and forth over the contract. You review your contract and decide what you want to change, and then submit your changes. One simple technique is to return a signed contract with language corrected as you and your attorney see fit. The contract holder has a contract immediately if he agrees to the changes. It doesn't hurt to ask: the worst that can happen is that the contract holder says "no." You then have the choice of accepting or negotiating the terms.

Do You Really Know What Your Whole Job Is?

There is more work to be done in an emergency department than just patient care. The contract should be specific about *all* the duties of your position. Look for the following in your contract:

1. What are your expected administrative duties? How much time are they expected to consume? What are the minimum attendance requirements for ED group meetings, hospital staff meetings, and your assigned committee meetings? You'll want to know how often you'll be expected to come in on your "days off" from clinical duties.

2. Do you have required teaching duties? How much preparation time will they require? Preparation time for teaching usually far exceeds the actual time spent teaching.

3. Are you required to cover other areas of the hospital while you are working in the ED (such as "codes" on the floor, ICU procedures, or obstetrics)? Will you be adequately protected from a medicolegal standpoint when you provide these additional services?

4. Are you required to be "on-call" to the ED when you are not in the ED? Will you be required to wear a beeper, or be located within a certain distance of the hospital? On-call responsibilities can make quite a dent in your personal life and restrict your ability to travel.

5. What is the minimum number of clinical hours you will be assigned per month? If this is not specified in your contract, you may find your clinical hours being cut back. This is one way you can essentially be fired without receiving notice.

Compensation

When you work in an ED under a contract with a contract holder, you usually agree to give up the rights to all fees from patients whom you see, in return for agreed upon pay from the contract holder. This is known as *reassignment* and is a common practice in emergency medicine. You agree to this reassignment in contracts you sign from various insurance companies and other *third party payers* such as Medicare. In many instances, you are not given access to the amount of these fees or "charges" billed in your name. This is known as working with *closed books*. Notably, both the American College of Emergency Physicians and the American Academy of Emergency Medicine have policy statements supporting an emergency physician's right to know what is billed and collected on his or her behalf. A closed book arrangement may be agreeable to you if your pay package is satisfactory and is determined independent of collections. If, however, part of your pay or bonus is determined by *collections* (the amount of money that the group actually receives from patients for your services), you should have the right to review and preferably audit these collections to determine if you are being paid as promised. Make sure that, if bonuses are based on certain events (e.g., number of patients seen, group profits, etc.), you have the ability to independently audit those events. Have your lawyer help you construct appropriate language in your contract. Whatever the method of compensation for your position is, it should be clearly and concretely laid out in the contract. Disagreements over pay can be very ugly.

Benefits

Benefits are the equivalent of money, so make sure they are listed in your contract. Many benefits are essential and if they aren't provided to you, then you will be purchasing them with your own money. Benefits are only given to employees, whether you are employed by the contract holder or directly by the hospital. Independent contractors aren't provided benefits, but are usually paid more so they can purchase benefits on their own. Benefits packages vary significantly from position to position. **Table 181.1** shows typical benefits and the frequency with which they are included as part of an emergency medicine pay package.

Table 181.1
List of Benefits Provided by Emergency Medicine Employers

Commonly Provided
- Retirement plan with or without matching contributions
- Continuing medical education (CME) allowance
- Relocation allowance

Less Commonly Provided
- Medical Insurance
- Dental Insurance
- Life Insurance
- Disability Insurance

Occasionally Provided
- Paid vacation
- Paid sick time
- Business expense reimbursement
- Severance package

Malpractice Insurance

Most contract holders cover their members with malpractice insurance. How insurance is paid for varies; one common way is for the contract holder to deduct a few dollars from your pay for each clinical hour worked. Your contract should state who pays for malpractice insurance and exactly the limits of coverage. Check that the coverage limits are typical for the practice of emergency medicine in your area. Verify that you are specifically named as an insured, and that you will receive a copy of the certificate of insurance as a record. Malpractice suits are often filed months or years after the fact, so having proof of insurance is important should you change positions in the interim.

The contract should also state who pays for the malpractice insurance *tail* (i.e., the purchase of additional coverage should you leave the position) if one is required by your policy. The contract holder often pays this fee, and it can be quite expensive. If the contract holder is paying for the tail, ensure that the minimum length of the tail is stipulated in the contract. A tail that is only one or two years long may be too short and force you to pay out of pocket for additional coverage.

Termination

All relationships, even the best, must eventually end. Contracts also must end. This is called *termination*, and how and when this occurs should be defined in the contract. Most contracts specify the length that a contract is valid, usually for one or more years. At the end of this period the contract *expires* unless certain conditions are met. The best contract for an EM physician is an *automatically renewing* contract. Automatically renewing means that unless certain specific actions are taken, the contract automatically renews at expiration. If you have an automatically renewing contract you may want to insert the proviso that compensation or other issues may be renegotiated prior to automatic renewal.

A contract may be terminated before it expires through action of either one of the parties. Termination prior to expiration can be *without cause*, meaning you can quit or the contract holder can fire you for no specific reason, or *with cause*, meaning a certain event has to occur before the contract is terminated. Terminations prior to expiration usually occur *with notice*, meaning there is a period of time between the notification of one of the parties that they wish to terminate the contract and the time it is terminated. This allows time to look for a new job or a new employee before termination. Termination can also be *automatic*, meaning that if a certain event occurs termination is immediate. This is usually reserved for severe events like losing your medical license, assaulting a patient, etc. All reasons for automatic termination and termination for cause should be clearly stated, objective, and reasonable. Vague terms such as termination for *unprofessional behavior* should be avoided. You may want to include in the contract some conditions in which you, the emergency physician, could terminate the contract immediately (without notice). An example of grounds for automatic termination on your side might be failure of the contact holder to pay you.

It is also important to be aware of how termination affects your benefits. Do you lose all retirement contributions made by the contract holder if termination comes before a certain time has passed (i.e., those contributions are not *vested*)? Will your malpractice tail still be paid? Will you have to return part of your relocation allowance or contract signing bonus if you leave early? These issues should be addressed in the contract.

Due Process

Lack of due process clauses is an area of controversy in emergency medicine contracts. *Due process* refers to the right to appeal the loss of medical staff membership. For any doctor to provide patient care services at a hospital, she or he must become a member of the medical staff. The medical staff has its own rules and regulations, and helps to run the medical operation of the hospital. Termination of membership from the medical staff is considered to be a significant event. It is so significant that members of the medical staff usually have the right to due process, usually a hearing, before their membership is terminated.

Many emergency physicians sign contracts giving up their right to due process. In fact, 15% of EM physicians report being terminated without due process at some time in their career. Contracts often stipulate that if your contract is terminated, you automatically lose medical staff membership. Depending on your location, such action may prompt a negative report to the National Practitioner Databank. Another concern is that if the contract holder loses his contract with the hospital, you may lose your medical staff membership even if your contract with the contract holder has not been terminated. Continuing to work at that hospital will require you to reapply for membership. Clauses limiting your right to due process should be removed from your contract.

The Non-Compete Clause

The non-compete clause is another controversial EM contract issue. A *non-compete* clause states that if your contract is terminated, you are prohibited for a defined period of time (usually a couple of years) from working for any other contract holder at your hospital or at any other hospital within a certain geographic radius. The idea behind this clause is that it prevents anyone from "stealing" the contract from the current contract holder. If a new contract holder were to take over the hospital contract, the non-compete clause would prevent them from hiring you or anyone else who is working for the current contract holder.

A non-compete clause can affect you negatively even if you or someone else in the group is not trying to take over the contract. If your contract is terminated for any reason, you may be unable to work in the local area for several years, including another hospital within the same town. This is true even if through no fault of yours the contract holder loses his contract with the hospital. In this case, you, the hospital, or the new contract holder often must pay the old contract holder to *buy out* the non-compete clause. "Buy outs" can cost tens of thousands of dollars per physician. A new contract holder may find it more cost effective to hire someone else rather than to buy out your non-compete clause, leaving you without a job.

If the contract holder doesn't want to remove the non-compete clause, try to negotiate for a *non-interference* clause instead, which basically states that you won't compete for the contract. If this doesn't work, at least try to figure out how termination will affect your ability to keep working in the area. Look at the geographic area you would be excluded from. Will it mean you have to move if you are terminated? Also, does the clause prevent you from working at other facilities that are part of the same hospital system? If so, then you may be prevented from working at hospitals outside the restricted radius, even in other cities. If someone tells you not to worry about a non-compete clause because it isn't enforceable, you need to know that this is not necessarily true. One out of every ten emergency physicians has lost a job, been forced to move, or had to pay compensation as a result of a non-compete clause.

In Summary

A contract is a tool to help maintain a good working relationship. Don't look at the contract as a hammer to take to court, but rather as an instrument to avoid misunderstandings and therefore avoid court. When you end up in court, everybody loses (except the attorneys). Read and make sure you understand what is in your contract and invest in good legal help to forge the best contract you can. Your goal is to maximize the chance of a long, smooth, and productive business relationship.

Selected Readings

American Academy of Emergency Medicine. 1997. Position statement on open books. Available at www.aaem.org.

American College of Emergency Physicians. 1999. Policy # 400151: Emergency physician contractual relationships. Available at www.acep.org.

American College of Emergency Physicians. 2001. Policy # 400284: Emergency physician rights and responsibilities. Available at www.acep.org.

American Academy of Emergency Medicine. 2004. AAEM contract guidelines for emergency physicians. Available at http://www.aaem.org/contractissues/guideline.shtml. Accessed June 2005.

Cohen H. *You Can Negotiate Anything.* New York: Bantam Books, 1980.

Plantz SH, Kreplick LW, Panacek EA, et al. A national survey of board-certified emergency physicians: quality of care and practice structure issues. *Am J Emerg Med* 1998;16:1–4.

West R. 2001. *Contracts 101: Employment at Will/Good Faith and Fair Dealing.* http://www.aaem.org/contractissues/contracts101.shtml. Accessed February 1, 2005.

Wood J, ed. *Contract Issues for Emergency Physicians.* Irving, TX: Emergency Medicine Residents' Association, 2000.

Performance Monitoring and Improvement

Timothy J. Reeder
Nicholas H. Benson

The dire need for quality in emergency medical care was a driving force for the establishment of our specialty. During our evolution, there have been great strides in developing a body of knowledge, operational processes, and physical plants to respond to emergent medical needs. In recent years, the health care system and our specialty have been challenged by patients, policy makers, and the business community to ensure quality of care.

Defining quality is difficult as it is subjective and can be defined in different ways based on the perception of the respondent; patient, physician, hospital, heath care organization, or regulatory agency. This section will describe the evolution of *performance improvement (PI)*, the system infrastructure for PI, tools for performing PI, peer review, and examples of improvement efforts.

Background

PI can be described as an organized, ongoing, planned process for identifying, monitoring and improving systems in order to obtain a quality outcome. It is best performed in a multidisciplinary manner. The outcome is defined by the organization and can be related to indicators such as patient satisfaction, accuracy of diagnosis, resource utilization, or patient throughput. While PI is the term used more recently, several terms have been used in the past.

Quality assurance (QA), an early term used to describe the process of establishing standards, monitoring adherence to these standards, and developing programs or policies to address deviations from these standards, was focused almost exclusively on the performance of individuals and very little on the system and environment for providing care. Based on the work of Demming, Juran, and others, there was recognition of the importance of a *systems* based approach to quality. QA moved away from placing blame on an individual to looking for systemic situations and environments that lead to poor quality. With this evolution, the terms continuous quality improvement (CQI) and total quality management (TQM) began to appear. TQM describes a management or operational *style,* while CQI refers to *processes and activities* designed to address quality issues. Both approaches focus on the system,

environment and process in place, rather than an individual's actions. A goal of CQI is to improve the outcome of the entire process rather than only those cases that exceed an established threshold. A central tenet of CQI is to reduce the variability in the outcomes that result from variability in organizational systems.

More recently, the term *performance improvement (PI)* has been used. This development moves beyond simply a structure and process for improvement, and focuses on improved clinical outcomes. The purpose of PI programs is to enhance the performance of the system and individuals and to align improvement activities to the core mission of the organization. A PI program helps develop the optimal path for achieving the desired outcomes.

Description of PI

A PI program requires both philosophical and structural elements to ensure success. The most important philosophical element is a firm and demonstrable commitment by organizational leadership to the PI process. Leaders must develop a culture that supports innovative thinking, interactive problem solving, and an appreciation of institutional systems that work to deliver care. There must be adequate resources to fund the PI process and to implement the necessary changes identified by participants. The organizational environment must foster a culture of quality and ensure each individual's commitment to overall success. Finally, all participants must know and accept the definition of quality of the process or product involved.

Several structural elements are required. Multidisciplinary teams must be responsible and accountable for continuous identification, planning, implementation, and monitoring improvement activities. They must meet on a regular basis and have knowledge of and access to the variety of tools available for the PI process. In health care organizations, the full integration of these groups across the organization is required for accreditation by the Joint Commission on Accreditation of Healthcare Organizations.

Data Needs

Accurate data collection and analysis are critical for PI. Objective data must be used to drive decision-making.

One difficulty in health systems is the lack of easily retrievable, electronic data that links clinical, financial, and outcome information. A successful PI program must have support from information systems personnel. It is difficult to make significant process improvement changes relying solely on data from hand-reviewed medical records. One advance in ED data collection has been the use of electronic tracking and documentation systems. Although these systems may provide limited clinical data, they can report many demographic and time related throughput data elements.

With the improvement of data collection and reporting, new tools and analytical methods are required to understand and improve processes. Organizations must understand the key concept of process *variation*. In any system, especially health care, any given process will produce a range of outcomes. The process may be patient length of stay, timing of medication administration, or blood culture contamination rate. Variation is the degree that a process deviates from the norm. This variation can be *random*, a result of the process itself, or *non-random*, resulting from identifiable special circumstances. For example, a hospital might have both pills and spray nitroglycerin that can be given for angina. Random variations would be the time interval for the physician to write the order and the nurse to see the order. A non-random variation is that the spray must be sent from pharmacy while the pills are in the ED. Therefore, the spray has a longer elapsed time from order to patient delivery. One of the primary goals of PI is to reduce both random and non-random variation in the system; this is called bringing a process into *control*. Gaining control of a system implies a level of efficiency, reliability and reproducibility of outcome from the system and its processes.

PI Tools

In some cases, an out of control, dysfunctional process is readily evident and requires little study before a solution is designed and implemented. More often, a system is very complicated and a failure to completely understand the process and issues involved will result in wasted or even inappropriate improvement efforts. Many techniques and tools have been developed to study systems, describe processes, identify sources of variation, gather and analyze data, and plan and monitor improvements. These tools and techniques are described in more complete detail in other sources, but here are a few of the more common tools and techniques.

Many techniques are available to identify and organize improvement efforts, but one commonly used is the FOCUS-PDCA cycle. The steps involved in this process include:

- Find a process to improve
- Organize a team
- Clarify the process
- Understand the causes of variation
- Select the improvement
- Plan the improvement
- Do the data collection

- Check the data for improvement
- Act to hold the improvements

Other tools can be used to assist with the improvement process, within the framework of a FOCUS-PDCA.

Flow charts are graphical representations used to describe a process and identify sources of variation. These diagrams use various symbols to illustrate the process and depict the various steps needed for completion. Flow charts help teams break down the process into its components, understand the current process, visually display the process, and comprehend how decisions and branch points affect downstream actions. Flow charts are a vital first step in helping teams understand a complex process and can be helpful to challenge established practices and brainstorm potential solutions (**FIGURE 182.1**).

Cause-and-effect (fishbone or Ishikawa) *diagrams* are a graphic display to help elucidate and organize various sources of variation in a process. Using this technique, the process under review is identified and main causes of variation are identified. Elements that contribute to variation

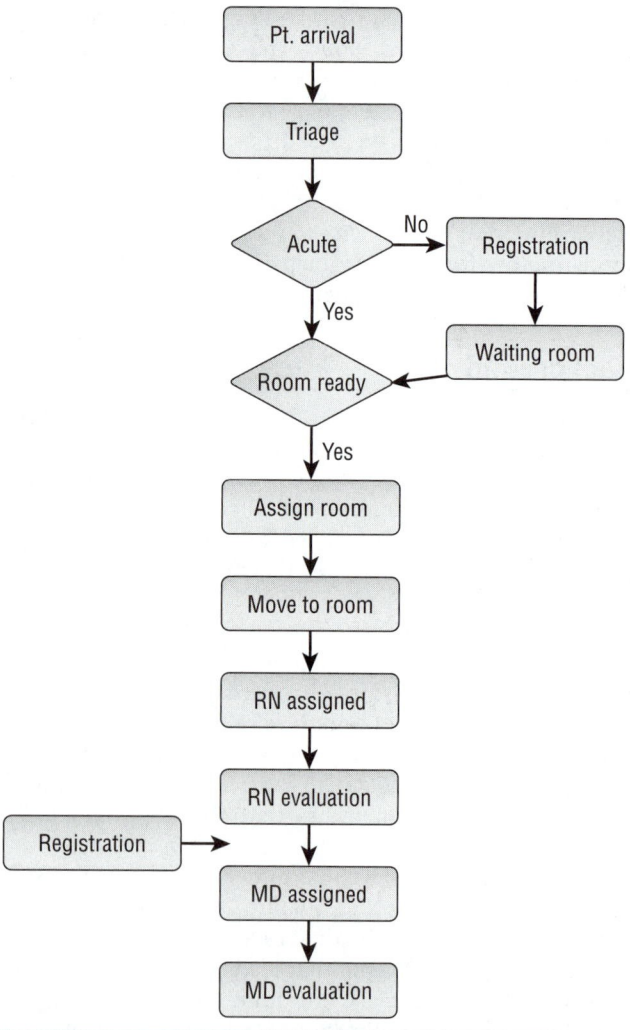

FIGURE 182.1 Flow chart showing steps from patient arrival to physician evaluation.

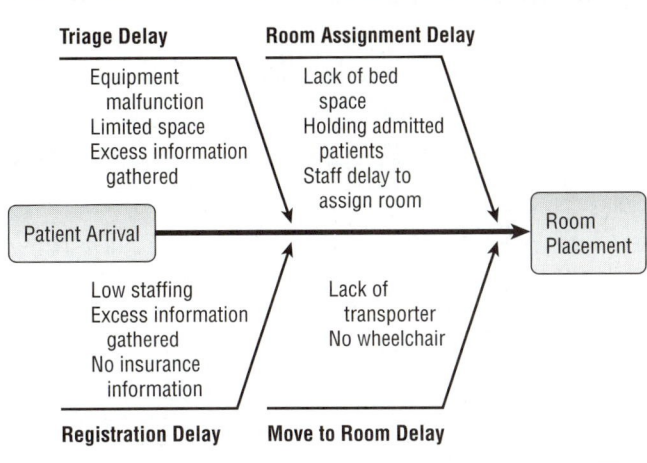

FIGURE 182.2 Cause and effect diagram showing causes of delay from patient arrival to placement in a room.

are identified. An important element of this tool is to ensure that there is a true cause and effect relationship between the elements and the variation (**FIGURE 182.2**).

Histograms (frequency plots) are bar charts that display the frequency distribution of the outcome of a process. To create histograms, the outcome is plotted in equal units on the x-axis and the number of observations in each outcome is plotted on the y-axis. The charts readily show the distribution, range, center, and outline of the results of the process. Repeated histograms over time will demonstrate reductions in variation resulting from successful PI efforts (**FIGURE 182.3**).

Pareto charts are a special type of histogram that assigns percentiles to the specific causes identified from cause-and-effect diagrams. The causes are listed sequentially with the largest percentile on the left and decreasing order to the right. Charts often use an individual frequency on the left axis and a cumulative frequency on the right.

Pareto charts are helpful to gain consensus on sources of variation and to prioritize improvement efforts.

Time plots (run charts) are graphic displays of the outcome of a process over time. Plotting the average of the data over a time period creates these graphs. The plots are helpful to watch for trends in data and identify changes in outcome. They also identify variation in the process outcome.

Control charts are a special type of time plot with upper and lower control limits. These additional lines help identify both random and non-random variation. Derivation of these control limits is beyond the scope of this book. Random variation is depicted by the intrinsic movement of the trend line. Non-random variation is evident when the process moves outside the upper and lower control limits (**FIGURE 182.4**).

Computer simulations are more recent innovations that allow programmers to develop a computer model of ED processes and operations. The modeling is based on probability theory and allows predictions to be made about flow, throughput, staffing and many other variables. This information allows the study of process changes and their impact prior to undergoing a major effort to change the physical plant or operations. The major disadvantages to simulations are the cost and time to develop, build and test the computer model.

Computerized simulator manikins allow clinicians to practice clinical scenarios in the setting of the simulation lab. Learners are encouraged to try new approaches and can make mistakes without endangering patients. Both the simulator manikins and the modeling routines allow PI teams to test out action plans in a safe environment prior to real-time implementation.

Peer Review

Peer review is a critical element for all PI programs. Physician actions and behaviors have a large impact on ED operations and outcomes. Peer review involves systematic review of specific cases for all physicians. Data on utilization, effectiveness, and outcomes must be collected, summarized, and reported in a physician specific manner. Sharing comparison data is a successful method to change physician behavior and improve outcomes. Through an

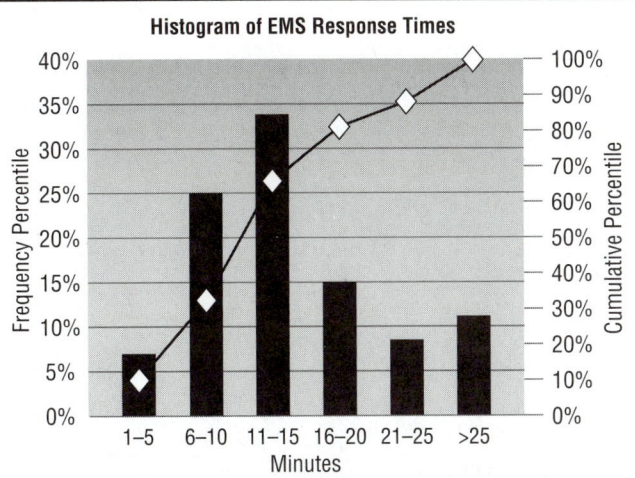

FIGURE 182.3 Histogram showing EMS response times.

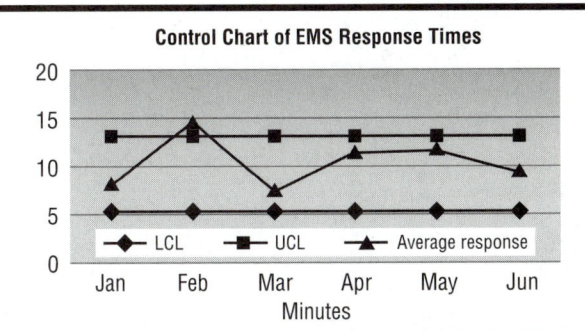

FIGURE 182.4 Control chart of EMS response times. LCL, lower control limit; UCL, upper control limit.

educational approach, peer review can be successful at minimizing practice variation, in the development of treatment algorithms, and improving the outcome of all patients. It is important that peer review activities be viewed, not in a punitive nature as the case in the days of quality assurance, but in the spirit of education, consensus building, and system improvement.

Conclusion

The quest for quality in Emergency Medicine is critical to ensure excellent clinical care, patient safety, and successful emergency departments. A comprehensive PI program requires both a cultural and structural institutional commitment to quality. Using a systems approach, many tools are available to support multidisciplinary teams describe processes, gather, and analyze data and implement quality improvement initiatives. Quality emergency care was a founding tenet of our specialty and with consistent effort it will remain a guiding principle.

Selected Readings

Barnard C, Eisenberg J. *Performance Improvement: Winning Strategies for Quality and JCAHO Compliance,* 2nd ed. Marblehead, MA: Opus Communication, 2000.

Carey RG, Lloyd RC. *Measuring Quality Improvement in Healthcare: A Guide to Statistical Process Control Applications.* Milwaukee, WI: ASQ Press, 2001.

Institute of Medicine, eds. *Crossing the Quality Chasm: A New Health System for the 21st Century.* Washington, DC: National Academy Press, 2001.

Kohn LT, Corrigan J, Donaldson MS, eds. *To Err is Human: Building a Safer Health System.* Washington, DC: National Academy Press, 1999.

Lighter DE, Fair DC, eds. *Principles and Methods of Quality Management in Health Care.* Gaithersburg, MD: Aspen Publishers, 2000.

McLaughlin CP, Kaluzny AD, eds. *Continuous Quality Improvement in Health Care: Theory, Implementation, and Applications.* Gaithersburg, MD: Aspen Publishers, 1994.

Polsky SS, ed. *Continuous Quality Improvement in EMS.* Dallas, TX: American College of Emergency Physicians, 1992.

Scholtes PR, Joiner BL, Streibel BJ. *The Team Handbook,* 2nd ed. Madison, WI: Oriel Inc.: 1996.

Siegel DM, Crocker PJ, eds. *Continuous Quality Improvements in Emergency Departments.* Dallas, TX: American College of Emergency Physicians, 1994.

Wheeler DJ. *Understanding Variation: The Key to Managing Chaos.* Knoxville, TN: SPC Press, 1993.

Patient Safety and Quality Assurance in Emergency Medicine

Cherri Hobgood
Carrie Vice

Error in Medicine

The publication of the Institute of Medicine (IOM) report *To Err is Human* placed error in medicine at the forefront of the U.S. public health and health policy debate.[1] This report summarized previously published data demonstrating that errors in medicine are numerous and expensive. Considered in terms of human life and health care dollars, the figures were staggering; costing the U.S. health care system more than 9 billion dollars and more than 100,000 lives annually.[1]

Errors in the classification of cause of death has been the subject of debate,[2] and no one will deny the importance of the issue. This chapter discusses patient safety in the emergency department (ED), and identifies the principles and practices of quality assurance that can assist in making the ED a safer place for all our patients.

Magnitude of the Problem

The IOM estimates that error, defined as "failure of a planned action to be completed as intended or the use of a wrong plan to achieve an aim," costs the American health care system from 9 to 19 billion dollars and more than 100,000 human lives per year.[1] There are few data that define ED error rates; however, three large inpatient studies provide some insight. Their usefulness to understanding errors in the ED is limited because all of these studies included only hospital-admitted patients. In each study, the ED was responsible for a small percentage of all adverse events (range 1.5%–3%), and the clinical setting had the highest rate of preventable errors with serious consequences.[3-5] One more recent estimate extrapolated from one U.S. tertiary care teaching hospital suggested that 18 million errors and 360,000 adverse events occur in our emergency departments annually.[6] In 1999, more than 102.8 million patients were treated in U.S. emergency departments, a 14% increase from 1992.[7] Because the number of patients treated in our emergency departments continues to grow, efforts that focus on improving patient safety in the ED will play an increasingly key role in improving the quality of all U.S. health care.

Types of Errors

Health care has been identified as a "high-hazard" industry[8] and the ED has been described as a practice prone to error.[9] Terms and definitions used to describe error can be confusing; the knowledgeable practitioner is encouraged to review and use the nomenclature and the definitions provided by the IOM to describe events within their clinical contexts. This nomenclature is presented in **Table 183.1**. In studies of inpatients, the most common nonoperative error types were diagnostic error, medication error, and therapeutic misadventures.[3,5] Analysis of errors from a national sample in Australia suggests that cognitive errors were more likely to result in permanent disability and to have been preventable.[5] Bates' classification of 247 adverse drug events (ADE) and 194 potential adverse drug events in two Boston teaching hospitals demonstrated that 28% of all ADEs were deemed preventable, but among the most serious ADEs, 42% were preventable.[10] In one study of ED error, the top three error domains were diagnostic studies, administrative procedures, and pharmacotherapy.[6] Among the most significant of all ED errors are those of delayed or missed diagnoses. This is the error type most likely to lead to disability and death, and accounts for about half of all litigation brought against emergency physicians. The three primary types of diagnostic error— no-fault errors, system errors, and cognitive errors—are described in **Table 183.2**.[11]

Cognitive Performance and Error

The types of errors that occur in medicine are also identifiable in other fields and have been well described by cognitive scientists. Two pioneers, Rasmussen and Jensen, defined a model of cognitive performance in 1974[12] that was later expanded and detailed by Reason.[13] They describe three types of cognitive error: skill-based, rule-based, and knowledge-based.

Skill-Based Cognition

Skill-based performance describes actions that are performed with little conscious thought on the part of the clinician. The action is based on predefined plans or

Table 183.1

Institute of Medicine's Patient Safety and Adverse Event Nomenclature

Term	Definition
Safety	Freedom from accidental injury.
Patient Safety	Freedom from accidental injury; involves the establishment of operational systems and processes that minimize the possibility of error and maximizes the probability of intercepting errors when they occur.
Accident	An event that damages a system and disrupts the ongoing or future output of the system.
Error	The failure of a planned action to be completed as intended or the use of a wrong plan to achieve an aim.
Adverse Event	An injury caused by medical management rather than by the underlying disease or condition of the patient.
Preventable Adverse Events	An injury that is attributable to error.
Negligent Adverse Events	A subset of adverse events that meet the legal criteria for negligence.
Adverse Medication Event	An adverse event due to or caused by a medication or pharmacotherapy.
Active Error	Errors that occur at the front line and whose effects are felt immediately.
Latent Error	Errors in design, organization, training, or maintenance. Often these are due to management or senior level decisions. When expressed, these errors result in operator errors but may have been hidden, dormant in the system, for lengthy periods of time prior to their appearance.

Source: Used with permission from Kohn LT, Corrigan JM, Donaldson MS, eds. *To Err is Human: Building a Safer Health System.* Washington, DC: National Academy Press. 2000:xxi, 287.

Table 183.2

Categories of Diagnostic Failures

No Fault
Lack of complete information transfer from patient
Insufficient medical information available about a new disease
Patient noncompliance
Illness is silent or masked
Atypical presentation of illness
Inconsistent confusion or lack of clarity of symptoms by patient
System Fault *(occurs at any level in the system of care delivery)*
Technical
Insensitive, inaccurate, or inappropriately performed test
Equipment failure
Lack of correct equipment
Organizational
Absence of policies or inadequate policies
Lack of backup expertise
Inefficiencies in care delivery
Lack of training or supervision
Failure to coordinate care
Defective communication
Excessively stressful work environment
Cognitive Fault *(occurs at the level of the diagnostician)*
Inadequate knowledge
Incomplete data gathering or information processing
Faulty clinical reasoning
Biased heuristics

Source: Used with permission from Graber M, Gordon R, Franklin N. Reducing diagnostic errors in medicine: what's the goal? *Acad Med* 2002;77:981–992.

instructions. Examples of skills-based activities in our daily lives are brushing one's teeth or driving a car, actions that require little conscious input in order for the events to be accomplished. In the same way, auscultation of a chest, prepping a procedure site, or suturing a wound may be performed by an experienced clinician with very little conscious thought for the steps in the process.

Rules-Based Cognition

Rules-based cognitive actions require linking the clinical data with a known rule. These rules are unique to each clinician and are based on education, anecdotal experience, assimilation of clinical data, or clinical guidelines. Other rules are empirically derived and have broader application. Examples of empirically derived clinical decision rules are the Ottawa ankle rule and the Canadian C-spine rule[14,15] for patients with suspected ankle or neck injuries, respectively. Application of these clinical rules guides the clinician in the decision about the need for radiographs.

Knowledge-Based Cognition

In situations where rules are not useful, clinicians use knowledge-based cognitive performance. Like rule-based cognition, knowledge-based performance is a conscious course of action. It differs from rule-based cognition by its requirement for interpretation of new data in the context of a previously defined domain of knowledge. This type of cognition is most often used in the process of diagnostic reasoning and clinical decision making and is often identified as analytic thought.

With the acquisition of additional training and experience, a provider's clinical skills advance and their cognitive functioning undergoes a transformation. As clinical experience increases the practitioner's exposure to the myriad of clinical scenarios, there is a resultant decrease in the need for knowledge-based cognitive function. Experienced clinical providers are more likely to use rules or skill-based functions to resolve a clinical problem as compared to novice providers, who are more likely to use knowledge-based cognitive function.[13]

Error Classification

A classification system of errors can be derived from the model of cognitive performance presented above. These error types are skill-based errors, known as *slips and lapses,* or rule and knowledge-based errors, called *mistakes.*[13] Slips are a breakdown in the planned execution of an observable action sequence often as a result of a interruption or disturbance. Lapses are memory failures resulting in the failed implementation of a plan. Rule-based mistakes occur during problem solving when the wrong rule is applied or selected, or is applied incorrectly. Knowledge-based mistakes result from similar processes: incomplete or incorrect knowledge, flawed analytical processes, or incorrect application of the knowledge.

Croskerry uses the following three themes to classify error in the ED setting: procedural, cognitive, and affective.[16] Procedural error occurs during the performance of procedures in the ED (e.g., suturing, chest tube, or central line placement). Cognitive errors are those that arise anywhere within the decision-making domain of ED clinical management. Affective error results when the emotions (or the affective state) of the provider disproportionately influence the clinical decision-making process.

Why Is the ED Error-Rich?

Numerous studies have identified contributing factors for the high rates of ED error, but application of knowledge from the disciplines of cognitive science, organizational psychology, and human factors engineering are particularly applicable. *Error producing conditions (EPCs)* and *violation producing behaviors (VPBs)* have been identified in medicine.[13,17] EPCs in the ED result from the unique properties of the clinical science, such as high levels of diagnostic uncertainty, high decision density, and high clinician cognitive load. EPCs also result from the organization of the system of care delivery in the ED. Examples include frequent interruptions, distractions, shift-changes with transitions of care, staff fatigue, overcrowded conditions, poor equipment, and ergonomic design of the ED. These are common problems across all emergency departments.

Another key source of error in the ED relates to characteristics of the individual clinician. These violation-producing behaviors (VPBs) occur because clinical and interpersonal behavior is influenced by characteristics of the individual, such as gender and age, and also by personality traits such as confidence levels, risk-taking behaviors, and the responsiveness to authority. Performance impairment may result from these and other personality variables and maladaptive decision-making choices.[13] Errors arising as a result of EPCs and VPBs are common in most EDs.

Reason[13] also classified errors or systems failures as either active or latent. Active failures are those that cannot be easily predicted and are committed by people with direct patient contact. They may be any type of cognitive error, affective error, or VPB. Latent failures are systems errors that are not expressed directly and may lie "latent" within the system for years. Latent failures are the results of decisions made by management, designers, and procedure writers, among others. These strategic and management decisions need not be mistakes, but they can create opportunities for active failures or weaknesses in the system.[18] Examples of active and latent failures are presented in **Table 183.3**. Recent studies suggest that in the ED, many documented errors are inconsequential.[6] Error reduction techniques in other systems, such as aviation and nuclear power, imply that careful scrutiny of these errors along with data from near misses will provide significant amounts of information useful for systems improvement.[19]

Solutions From Other Fields

The recognition that error is inevitable with a subsequent focus on error reduction has led to remarkable transformations in fields such as nuclear power and aviation.[20] These industries are similar to medicine in terms of operating characteristics and high hazard potential yet suffer

Table 183.3	
Active and Latent Failure Types	
Active Failures[a]	**Latent Failures**[b]
Cognitive Errors	Excessive workloads/ inadequate staff
Slips	Inadequate knowledge/ experience/training
Lapses	Lack of supervision
Mistakes	High stress environment
Rule based	Poor communication systems
Knowledge based	Poor maintenance of work environment
Violations	Rapid organizational change
Low morale	Conflict between institutional mission and values
Poor examples from senior staff	Production pressure
Maladaptive decision styles	Overcrowding
Authority gradient	Poor feedback
Over- or under-confidence	Poor design characteristics
Risk taking behaviors	

[a]Committed by those whose actions have immediate adverse consequences (e.g., direct patient care providers; sharp end).
[b]Because of the actions or decisions of those not directly involved in the workplace (e.g., management and/or senior clinicians; blunt end).
Source: Used with permission from Reason J. Human error: models and management. *BMJ* 2000;320:768–770; Vincent C, Taylor-Adams S, Stanhope N. Framework for analyzing risk and safety in clinical medicine. *BMJ* 1998;316:1154–1157.

far fewer mishaps.[19] These types of organizations have been identified as high-reliability organizations,[21] where safety is maintained by an system-wide organizational culture that fosters and maintains resilience of operations despite the occurrence of human error.[21] High reliability organizations promote this culture of safety and systems improvement by first acknowledging that error is inevitable and will always occur.[18] In aviation, for example, error management is based on a sequential understanding of the nature and extent of error, evaluating the conditions and behaviors that prevent or mitigate error followed by training personnel to identify conditions and use behaviors which result in reduced error rates. Health care has been slower to recognize the inevitability of error and the result is a culture which still endorses individual responsibility over systems responses.[1] This cultural milieu limits the development of specific training in error identification and reduction.[20] If we are to be successful in transforming medicine into a high reliability organization, it will require a cultural paradigm shift.[18,20]

Systems of Safety

A specific safety analysis framework has been proposed by Vincent et al. to evaluate adverse incidents in clinical medicine.[22] This framework consists of seven aspects of clinical care: institutional context, organizational and management, work environment, teams and teamwork, individuals, tasks, and patients (**Table 183.4**). Interventions designed to improve safety can be organized and focused at specific levels within this framework.[22,23]

Prevention, recognition, and mitigation are three universal strategies for reducing incidents and adverse events. Prevention may take the form of identifying latent errors in the system and eradicating these errors prior to expression. An example might be reorganizing medications in the Pyxis® (Cardinal Health, Dublin, OH) to prevent selection of a similar but fundamentally different agent, and eradicating look-alike medication vials. The second strategic defense—recognition—is designed to make unintended events easily recognized and therefore offer the opportunity for cure prior to an adverse event affecting a patient. Repeating back verbal orders (or a *check-back*), which was recently mandated by the Joint Commission on Accreditation of Healthcare Organizations 2003 safety standards, is an example of a recognition strategy.[24] The third strategy—mitigation—focuses on the ability to recover from errors by lessening their damage. For example, anticipating the need for rescue airway equipment when respiratory depressant medications are given and having the equipment handy would allow mitigation of an adverse medication event.

Other approaches such as process simplification or forcing functions can be used to support any of the three strategies. Process simplification has been shown to significantly increase the reliability of procedures, for example, decreasing the number of steps in a drug delivery process such as fibrinolytic dosing regimens.[25,26] Another general method is the application of constraints (or *forcing functions*). These design changes make it harder to perform the

Table 183.4

Vincent's Hierarchy of Factors Influencing Clinical Practice

Factor	Component Factors
Institutional Context	Economic context—national, regional, and institutional
	Regulatory agenda (JCAHO, CMS, etc.)
	Legal constraints (malpractice)
Organizational and Management Factors	Organizational mission and values
	Organizational culture and administrative hierarchy
	Financial constraints and solvency
Work Environment Factors	Workload and staffing allocation
	Provider skills mix
	Administrative/managerial/leadership support
	Shift work and circadian pattern
Team Factors	Communication, both verbal and written
	Leadership
	Teamwork training and team structure
Individual (Staff) Factors	Skill level
	Training
	Individual health of providers
Task Factors	Task design and clarity
	Protocol availability
	Accuracy of results
Patient Factors	Complexity of presenting complaint
	Acuity of illness
	Language and communication skills
	Social and cultural traits

Source: Used with permission from Vincent C, Taylor-Adams S, Chapman EJ. Framework for analyzing risk and safety in clinical medicine. *BMJ* 1998;320:777–781.

wrong action. For example, mechanical pieces are engineered so that they are unable to connect to improper equipment or a computerized forcing function such as decision support systems integrated into medication ordering systems. These decision support systems inform, educate, and restrict the improper dosing of medications.[27] Other approaches and strategic improvements to emergency care delivery can be identified using the processes of continuous quality improvement.

Continuous Quality Improvement

Continuous quality improvement (CQI), also known as *total quality management (TQM)*, has been used for decades in business to define customers' needs and make companies more productive and profitable. Only recently has the health care system started to incorporate these practices and it has not yet attained full acceptance.[28] CQI has been defined in many ways. Some define CQI as "a model for reducing defects in a system that affects an outcome of quality." Others believe that it is a means of "meeting or exceeding the customer's expectations." In the health care arena, Berwick has stated that the ultimate goal of CQI is to obtain an unprecedented level of performance.[29]

The key feature of any CQI process is the application of a scientific system of continuous evaluation designed to improve the daily work of the organization. This section of the chapter will examine the history of CQI, introduce the basics of the CQI process, and provide examples of integrating CQI and research in emergency medicine.

History

W. Edwards Deming, a statistician who worked in Japan after World War II (WWII), is considered by many to be the father of CQI. Deming worked there during a time in which Japanese products were considered to be low in quality, and he helped Japanese businesses to improve their quality by applying statistical methods. In a brief span of three decades, his methods transformed the international reputation of quality for Japanese products. Simply stated, Deming's philosophy was that improving process was the only way to improve quality.[30] Deming's 14 essential points for CQI are elucidated in **Table 183.5**; They emphasize a focus on leadership, training, pride, and removing barriers between staff members.[31]

Another pioneer in the field of CQI, Joseph Juran, developed the *quality trilogy*. The first stage of the trilogy is to identify the customers and their needs. The second

stage establishes guidelines to meet those needs. Thirdly, quality improvement is to be ongoing to ensure the highest level of performance.[32] This seminal work of Deming and Juran, along with the work of others such as Armand Feigenbaum,[33] laid the groundwork for the CQI process.

CQI Processes

CQI was born out of the basic fundamentals of *quality assurance (QA)*. QA focuses on the application of established standards, monitoring organizations for the adherence to these standards, and the development of programs to reduce deviations from these standards.[34] QA specifically examines structure, process, and outcome in an attempt to "assure" quality. Although the QA process allowed a more centralized approach to quality management, many believed that assuring quality, especially in the medical field, was impossible, and that any attempt to do so meant holding employees to standards that could not possibly be met. Furthermore, the QA process invited external organizations to evaluate the care delivery system for possible breeches in quality, which led to an "us versus them" mentality that hindered open communication and change. Although this QA system was a marked improvement from monitoring methods of the past, many believed that QA needed to evolve so that it could also measure improvements over time. From this evolution, continuous quality improvement (CQI) was developed. This transition to the CQI process signaled two important changes: (1) health care had moved away from the blame and shame mentality that had hampered previous QA efforts; (2) the transition to CQI signaled an understanding that quality is a dynamic process that requires the continuous efforts of the entire system to insure improvement.

CQI in Action

The CQI ideal has evolved since its creation and several rules for a properly functioning CQI system are in place. First, the system must be internally driven; change must come from the individuals within the system. When people are given responsibility for their own work and actions, they are more likely to take great pride in their work and strive for a more efficient system. Secondly, one must recognize that care can only be improved and not guaranteed. This tenet allows individuals to be held up to a standard that is reasonable to achieve, and recognizes there is much that can be learned from individual and system errors. Next, the primary focus must be placed on systems first and individuals second. Because changes in systems have the biggest possibility of imparting the greatest overall effect, implementation of a new system or a change in the existing system will affect many customers. This is not to say that individuals that are performing outside the norm should not be addressed, only that the majority of the time should be spent on systems analysis. Another important facet of a successful CQI implementation is that organization-wide involvement is imperative. The system, in this case the emergency department, cannot run independently. Instead, it relies on other departments such as radiology, laboratories, consult teams, housekeeping, and many others when caring for patients. Any discussion of

---

Table 183.5

Deming's 14 Essential Points for CQI

1. Create constancy of purpose for improvement of product and service
2. Adopt the new philosophy
3. Cease dependence on mass inspection
4. End the practice of awarding business on price tag alone
5. Improve constantly and forever the system of production and service
6. Institute training
7. Institute leadership
8. Drive out fear
9. Break down barriers between staff areas
10. Eliminate slogans, exhortations, and targets for the work force
11. Eliminate numerical quotas
12. Remove barriers to pride in workmanship
13. Institute a vigorous program of education and retraining
14. Take action to accomplish the transformation

Source: Used with permission from Deming E. *Out of the Crisis*. Cambridge, MA: Massachusetts Institute for Technology Center for Advanced Engineering Study, 1993.

system changes should include all parties responsible. Along with the importance of CQI being organization-wide, it should also be centered on patient care. Prior to the implementation of CQI, departments were often responsible for their own quality assurance, and interdepartmental discussions of cases were not commonplace; therefore, departments could pass the blame to other departments when there was a systems breakdown. In contradistinction to this approach, CQI advocates a multidisciplinary focus to patient care where all responsible parties are involved in discussions centered on improving outcomes.

Four Steps of CQI

When implementing the CQI system to improve patient care, at least four steps must be completed. First, a problem must be identified and defined; it may occur from specific patient encounters, chart reviews, etc. A group or committee must be formed that comprises representatives from all involved patient care areas to evaluate this potential problem and discuss changes that can be made for improvement. Next, possible alternative solutions to the identified problem are discussed and implemented. Finally, the new system is checked for effectiveness, stressing the continuous basis of change, which is paramount to the CQI process. Continuous monitoring of the success of the implementation phase should be carried out in an on-going manner, with particular attention paid to the detection of unintended consequences or outcomes.

CQI and Research

Not only is continuous quality improvement being used in hospital systems to implement change, its effects are also being proven in the research sector.[35,36] These approaches have benefited from the delineation of the 6 domains of quality identified by the IOM: effective, timely, efficient, safe, patient-centered, and equitable care (**Table 183.6**).[37] Through the CQI process, hospitals have taken their cue from the business sector in an attempt to improve management, efficiency, communication, and thus patient care. Hospitals that have been proactive in developing organization-wide CQI programs have proven their effectiveness and set the stage for a revolution in quality management. In the future, the benefits of CQI will continue to be documented in both the business and research realms.

Summary

Emergency care, like safety, is a dynamic process that requires constant attention to promote the safest and the highest quality care. Improving emergency care requires the integration of CQI process with application of the knowledge and solutions gained from other fields such as organizational psychology and human factors engineering. Initiatives designed to improve patient safety in the ED should focus on minimizing error-producing conditions and violation-producing behaviors, and improving the resilience of the system to manage the unexpected. Insurance of sustained successful efforts to improve requires an ongoing analysis of the way work in the ED is actually performed, effective utilization of the tools of CQI, and the application of high quality research techniques.

Table 183.6

The Institute of Medicine's Six Aims for Quality Improvement

Aim Health Care Should Be	Definition
Safe	Avoiding injuries to patients from care that is intended to help.
Effective	Providing services based on scientific knowledge. (Avoiding underuse and overuse)
Patient-centered	Providing care that is respectful of and responsive to individual patient preferences, needs, and values and ensuring that patient values guide all clinical decisions.
Timely	Reducing waits and sometimes harmful delays for both those who receive and those who give care.
Efficient	Avoiding waste, in particular waste of equipment, supplies, ideas, and energy.
Equitable	Providing care that does not vary in quality because of personal characteristics such as gender, ethnicity, geographic location, and socioeconomic status

Source: Used with permission from Committee on Quality Health Care In America. *Crossing the Quality Chasm: A New Health System for the 21st Century.* Washington, DC: National Academy Press, 2001.

References

1. Kohn LT, Corrigan JM, Donaldson MS, eds. *To Err is Human: Building a Safer Health System.* Washington, D.C.: National Academy Press, 2000;xxi, 287.
2. McDonald CJ, Weiner M, Hui SL. Deaths due to medical errors are exaggerated in Institute of Medicine report. *JAMA* 2000;284:93–95.
3. Brennan TA, Leape LL, Laird NM. Incidence of adverse events and negligence in hospitalized patients. Results of the Harvard Medical Practice Study I. *N Engl J Med* 1991;324:370–376.
4. Thomas EJ, Studdert DM, Burstin HR, et al. Incidence and types of adverse events and negligent care in Utah and Colorado. *Medical Care* 2000;38:261–271.
5. Wilson RM, Harrison BT, Gibberd RW, Hamilton JD. An analysis of the causes of adverse events from the Quality in Australian Health Care Study. *Med J Aust* 1999;170:411–415.
6. Fordyce J, Blank FS, Pekow P, et al. Errors in a busy emergency department. *Ann Emerg Med* 2003;42:324–333.
7. Burt CW. 1992-1999. Trends in Hospital Emergency Department Utilization: United States. *Vital Health Stat* 2001;13:1–34.
8. Gaba D. Structural and organizational issues in patient safety: a comparison of health care to other high-hazard industries. *Calif Manage Rev* 2000;43:83–102.
9. Croskerry P, Sinclair D. Emergency medicine: a practice prone to error. *Can J Emerg Med* 2001;3:271–276.
10. Bates DW, Cullen DJ, Laird N, et al. Incidence of adverse drug events and potential adverse drug events. Implications for prevention. ADE Prevention Study Group. *JAMA* 1995;274:29–34.
11. Graber M, Gordon R, Franklin N. Reducing diagnostic errors in medicine: what's the goal? *Acad Med* 2002;77:981–992.
12. Rasmussen J. Mental procedures in real-life tasks: a case study of electronic troubleshooting. *Ergonomics* 1974;17:293–307.
13. Reason J. *Human Error.* Cambridge, UK: Cambridge University Press, 1990.
14. Stiell IG, Greenberg GH, Wells GA, et al. Prospective validation of a decision rule for the use of radiography in acute knee injuries. *JAMA* 1996;275:611–615.
15. Stiell IG, Wells GA, Vandemheek KL, et al. The Canadian C-spine rule for radiography in alert and stable trauma patients. *JAMA* 2001;286:1841–1848.

16. Croskerry P. Cognitive forcing strategies in clinical decision-making. *Ann Emerg Med* 2003;41:110–120.
17. Reason J. 1997. Managing the Risks of Organizational Accidents. Aldershot, UK: Ashgate Publishing Co.
18. Reason J. Human error: models and management. *BMJ* 2000;320:768–770.
19. Barach P, Small SD. Reporting and preventing medical mishaps: lessons from non-medical near miss reporting systems. *BMJ* 2000;320:759–763.
20. Leape LL. Error in medicine. *JAMA* 1994;272:1851–1857.
21. Roberts K. Some characteristics of high-reliability organizations. *Organization Science* 1990;1:160–177.
22. Vincent C, Taylor-Adams S, Stanhope N. Framework for analyzing risk and safety in clinical medicine. *BMJ.* 1998;316:1154–1157.
23. Vincent C, Taylor-Adams S, Chapman EJ, et al. How to investigate and analyse clinical incidents: clinical risk unit and association of litigation and risk management protocol. *BMJ* 2000;320:777–781.
24. Joint Commission on Accreditation of Healthcare Organizations. *2003 National Patient Safety Goals.* Oakbrook Terrace, IL: Joint Council on Accreditation of Healthcare Organization, 2002.
25. Richards CF, Cannon CP. Reducing medication errors: potential benefits of bolus thrombolytic agents. *Acad Emerg Med* 2000;7:1285–1289.
26. Cannon CP. Thrombolysis medication errors: benefits of bolus thrombolytic agents. *Am J Cardiol* 2000;85:17C–22C.
27. Bates DW, Cohem M, Leape LL, et al. Reducing the frequency of errors in medicine using information technology. *JAMA* 2001;8:299–308.
28. Hsia DC. Medicare quality improvement: bad apples or bad systems? *JAMA* 2003;289:354–356.
29. Berwick DM. Continuous improvement as an ideal in health care. *N Engl J Med* 1989;320:53–56.
30. Deming E. *Out of the Crisis.* Cambridge, MA: Massachusetts Institute for Technology Center for Advanced Engineering Study, 1993.
31. Walton M. *Deming Management at Work.* New York: Perigee, 1990.
32. Juran J. The quality function. In: Juran J, Gryna F, eds. *Juran's Quality Control Handbook.* New York: McGraw-Hill, 1988.
33. Feigenbaum A. *Total Quality Control,* ed 3. New York: McGraw-Hill, 1991.
34. Blumenthal D, Kilo CM. A report card on continuous quality improvement. *Milbank Quart* 1998;76:625–48, 511.
35. Magid DJ, Rhodes KV, Asplin BR, et al. Designing a research agenda to improve the quality of emergency care. *Acad Emerg Med* 2002;9:1124–1130.
36. Bizovi KE, Wears R, Lowe RA. Researching quality in emergency medicine. *Acad Emerg Med* 2002;9:1116–1123.
37. Committee on Quality Health Care in America. *Crossing the Quality Chasm: A New Health System for the 21st Century.* Washington, DC: National Academy Press, 2001.

Fundamentals of Physician Billing, Coding, and Compliance

Jonathan E. Siff

Medical reimbursement is a complex process involving multiple providers and payors with complex, sometimes conflicting rules. Historically, medical training has given little attention to this aspect of medicine. Physicians who are in practice quickly learn that these issues are extremely important on a day-to-day basis. This chapter briefly reviews the basics of coding and compliance.

Inside the Numbers

Anyone who has looked at a professional medical bill has noted a variety of number or codes on the bill. These generally fall into two groups: physician services and diagnosis codes. The codes allow standardization among providers, payors, and patients for reporting the services provided and the diagnosis associated with those services.

Current Procedural Terminology (CPT) reports physician services, including procedures, using a five-digit code.[1] About 80% of emergency physician (EP) reimbursement is based on five codes, the 9928x series: 99281-99285.[1,2] These codes are usually referred to by their last digit; for example, a level 3 visit refers to 99283. The group of CPT codes referring to physician visits, including the 9928x series is generally called *Evaluation and Management codes* ("E/M," spoken as "E and M codes"). The *Resource Based Relative Value Scale (RBRVS)* is a system that assigns relative values (RVUs) to services based on the resources used, and the physician effort and risk involved with that service. Once the total RVU value has been assigned for a given procedure, this is multiplied by the annual conversion factor (CF) for services. This CF is determined annually by the Centers for Medicare and Medicaid Services (CMS).[2] Many private payors use the RVU system as a starting point for their payment arrangements.

Each procedure or visit is assigned a related diagnosis code or codes. These codes are based on the *International Classification of Diseases (ICD)* and currently the *ICD-9* is being widely used. This assigns a 3 to 5 digit code to every diagnosis, allowing for standardized diagnoses and simplification of epidemiological research.[3]

Charting and Coding

The ED physician chart is divided into several sections: History, Exam, Course, and Disposition. The chart should convey all aspects of the patient visit.

The history section should detail the patient's presenting complaints and convey an accurate picture to subsequent providers of why the patient was seen. The history begins with the *chief complaint,* which is why the patient came to the ED in his or her own words. The details of the chief complaint are called the *history of present illness (HPI)*. The HPI should cover a number of components including the location of the problem, severity, timing, modifying factors, quality, duration, context, and the signs and symptoms associated with the problem. The second segment of the history section is the *review of systems (ROS)*. Items from some or all of the 14 standard body systems are reviewed with the patient and documented. The extent of the ROS should be based on the presenting problem. When the EP performs a complete review of systems (all 14 systems), they may report the pertinent positive and negative findings and then state that, "The remainder of the review of systems is negative," which gives them credit for a "complete" review of systems. The third part of the history is the past medical/surgical, family, and social histories *(PFSH)*. For the PFSH, the patient's ongoing or past medical conditions, surgical history, relevant medical histories of family members, and the patient's social history are reviewed. The social history is age-dependent and may include: use of tobacco, alcohol, or drugs; grade in school; marital status; employment; birth history; and/or other items pertinent to the chief complaint. Patients presenting to the emergency department may be unable to give a complete history and in some cases they are unable to give any history. The documentation rules recognize this problem in emergency medicine and provide a solution that gives the EP credit for a complete history. The provider should document what is known from all sources including the patient, EMS staff, family, etc., and then chart that, "A complete history and review of systems could not be obtained due to . . ." (fill in the reason the patient was unable to provide the history such as unconscious, confused, intubated, etc.). This is called the *Level 5 Caveat*.[4]

The *physical exam (PE)* section of the chart is documentation of the provider's examination of the patient. The exam is based on the presenting complaint and history and should document pertinent positive and negative findings. The extent of the PE is based on the number of body areas or organ systems examined. Most commonly, the organ systems are documented, including: General, Eyes, Ears/Nose/Mouth/Throat, Cardiovascular, Respiratory, Gastrointestinal, Genitourinary, Musculoskeletal, Skin, Neurologic, Psychiatric, and Hematologic/Lymphatic/Immunologic systems.[1]

The next section of the chart is the *Medical Decision Making (MDM)*. This outlines the thought process and decision-making process used by the physician during the encounter. It is MDM that truly defines the level of service. MDM is the process of combining knowledge and experience that physicians learn during residency and throughout their careers. The complexity of selecting management and establishing the diagnosis are quantified by the evaluation of three areas: (1) number of diagnosis or management options; (2) amount and/or complexity of data to be reviewed; and (3) risk of complications and/or morbidity or mortality. Documentation of the patient's ED course, the provider's thought process during the encounter, the patient's response to treatment, consults with other providers, and results of ancillary testing are all extremely important to include in the documentation. Patients who are sent home should have detailed instructions for when to return to the ED or when to follow up with their regular physician. All charts must also support the medical necessity of any services provided.

Once the physician chart is complete, the chart is ready to be coded and billed. Patient encounters are billed based on the amount of work and resources provided and documented by the physician. Complex or admitted patients generally will be a Level 5 visit. To bill this level, an "extended" HPI with four of the components noted above, a "complete" ROS, which is generally considered ten or more systems, at least two components of PFSH, eight organ systems on PE, and a high level of MDM are generally required. Patients who are more complex in their differential, require diagnostic testing, radiography, consults, and/or discussions with other providers or family, are considered higher level for MDM.

Many EPs hire certified coders or use the services of a large company that specializes in professional billing, while some providers do their own coding. The use of professional coders and billing personnel provides specially trained people to free physicians for clinical work. The generation of appropriate codes is time consuming and requires significant training to keep current with the frequent rule changes and optimized reimbursement strategies. Regardless of who does the billing, the physician is always responsible for what ends up billed in their name.

Compliance

A compliance program is designed to assure quality within an organization's framework. It establishes rules for internal controls and monitors the organization's conduct to prevent or subsequently address inappropriate activity. The purpose of the compliance plan is to insure that the entity will not inadvertently, negligently, or illegally engage in illegal activity. Each group of providers—whether of one physician, multiple physicians, or a hospital-based group—should have a compliance program in place. The compliance plan should address seven key elements that are outlined by the office of the inspector general's model for compliance programs. These are: (1) compliance standards and procedures; (2) oversight responsibilities; (3) education and training; (4) developing effective lines of communication; (5) monitoring and auditing; (6) enforcement and discipline; and (7) response and prevention. If through a compliance program an entity discovers credible evidence of its own misconduct, that entity must report such conduct to the appropriate agencies. Generally, self-reporting will result in greatly reduced penalties because the entity is making efforts to fix the problem. One of the biggest risks the provider can undertake is not to follow their own plan.[5]

References

1. *Current Procedural Terminology 2004 Standard Edition*. American Medical Association Press, 2005. Available at http://www.ama-assn.org/ama/pub/category/3884.html. Accessed June 2005.
2. American College of Emergency Medicine. *Fundamentals of Reimbursement: What Every Graduating Resident Should Know*. Available at http://www.acep.org/webportal/PracticeResources/IssuesByCategory/Reimbursement/default.htm. Accessed June 2005.
3. *ICD-9-CM Expert for Physicians*, vol 1, 2. Salt Lake City, UT: Igenix/St. Anthony Publishing/Medicode, 2002.
4. *Principles of CPT Coding*, ed 2. AMA Press, 2001. Available at http://www.ama-assn.org/ama/upload/mm/372/6/doc. Accessed June 2005.
5. OIG Compliance Program for Individual and Small Group Physician Practices, *Federal Register* 2000;65:59434–59452. Available at http://oig.hhs.gov/authorities/docs/physician.pdf. Accessed June 2005.

185 Regulatory Issues

James M. Brown
Manisha Gupta

No man's life, liberty or property are safe while the legislature is in session.

JUDGE GIDEON J. TUCKER (1866)

Physicians labor for many years to master the art of patient care, which is rightfully the focus of their everyday work. But in the background lurks a complex web of regulatory issues, which can directly impact decisions physicians make at the bedside and impose specific burdens on the hospitals in which they practice. Physicians must have a basic knowledge of fundamental regulatory issues and understand the responsibilities these regulations impose on their practice. This chapter introduces federal regulatory issues that have a direct impact on the day-to-day practice of emergency medicine.

Federal Regulatory Issues

History

The federal government asserts its authority over medical practice primarily by requiring recipients of federal funds to follow certain regulations. An early example was the Hill-Burton Act of 1946. The goal of this act was to increase access to quality health care by subsidizing construction of hospitals. However, the Hill-Burton act also mandated that any hospital receiving funds must provide (with certain limits) medical care to all persons, regardless of their ability to pay. This principle was echoed in the Emergency Medicine Transfer and Active Labor Act (EMTALA), whose mandates extend to all hospitals that participate in the Medicare program. The Health Insurance Portability and Accountability Act of 1996 (HIPAA) is the first broad federal law that applies to all health care providers, whether or not they receive federal funds.

Titles XVIII and XIX of the Social Security Act, better known as the Medicare and Medicaid Bill, were signed in 1965 by then President Lyndon Johnson. This act made the federal government the largest single payer of health care costs in the United States, resulting in a substantial expansion of federal regulatory authority. The Medicare and Medicaid programs were administered by separate agencies in the federal Department of Health, Education, and Welfare. In 1977, the Health Care Finance Administration (HCFA) was created to administer both the Medicare and Medicaid programs. HCFA changed its name to Centers for Medicare & Medicaid Services (CMS) in 2001.

The federal government garnered more direct authority with the passage of the Health Insurance Portability and Accountability Act (HIPAA) in 1996. The Administrative Simplification portion of this act imposes national standards on the electronic transmission, security, and privacy of health information. HIPAA standards apply to all health care providers, not just those receiving funds from CMS.

This chapter covers the three main federal regulatory issues facing today's physicians: CMS documentation guidelines, EMTALA, and HIPAA. Each issue will be covered separately, with an emphasis on how these regulations directly impact the practicing emergency physician.

CMS: Medicare and Medicaid Documentation Guidelines

The Centers for Medicare and Medicaid Services (CMS) is a federal agency within the U.S. Department of Health and Human Services. CMS is responsible for Medicare, Medicaid, State Children's Health Insurance Program (SCHIP), HIPAA, and the Clinical Laboratory Improvement Amendments (CLIA). The primary impact CMS regulations have on the practice of emergency medicine is through documentation guidelines. The first set of formal guidelines became effective in 1995. These regulations do not directly impact bedside care, but they do require that the elements of care be documented to a level of detail sufficient to justify the subsequent claim to CMS. Physicians supervising medical students and residents must also follow specific documentation guidelines. Failure to adhere to these guidelines can result in denial of claims or an investigation by the Office of the Inspector General for potentially fraudulent claims.

Compliance with CMS documentation guidelines requires at least a rudimentary understanding of the coding and claims process. Current Procedural Terminology (CPT) is a uniform coding system for health care providers developed by the American Medical Association. The first version was introduced in 1966. It was quickly adopted by third party payers, including CMS. Revised annually, it is published in both paper and software editions. CPT consists of a set of 5-digit codes, which describe two categories of work done by physicians. Evaluation and Management (E&M) codes describe work done by physicians in the process of performing a history and physical examination, formulating a differential diagnosis, ordering and interpreting tests, ordering therapeutic interventions, and making a diagnosis and disposition. Procedure codes describe work physicians do with their hands. Seven E&M codes pertain to emergency medicine: 99281–99285 (often referred to as "level" 1-5) and 99291–99292 (critical care). Virtually every procedure performed by emergency physicians is described by a procedure code, from simple laceration repair (12001) to endotracheal intubation (31500).

International Classification of Diseases is a coding system developed by the World Health Organization to record morbidity and mortality data. The first edition was published in 1948 and the ninth revision (ICD-9) was published in 1977. ICD-9-CM ("clinical modification") became the single accepted classification for hospital diagnosis indexing in 1979. This system was designated by HCFA in 1988 as the coding system physicians must use in describing diagnoses made on claims.

Coding is the process of taking physician documentation of the patient encounter, converting it into CPT and ICD-9-CM codes, and entering these onto claims forms. Most emergency medicine practices employ coders or contract this service to a separate coding and billing company. The process by which their documentation is turned into claims is therefore transparent to most emergency physicians. CMS firmly asserts that individual physicians are responsible for the veracity of claims made under their provider numbers, regardless of who codes the charts and submits the claims. Emergency physicians must understand both CMS documentation guidelines and the processes by which their charts are coded and billed. These processes vary between practices and facilities.

The 1995 documentation guidelines were developed jointly by HCFA and the AMA based on CPT codes. These guidelines specify the fundamental elements of documentation and utilize a system by which these elements are tallied to justify a claim for a given CPT evaluation and management code. Elements of the history, physical examination, and medical decision-making are defined along with a system for counting these elements. Critical care codes are based exclusively on time and acuity.

Because of widespread resistance, the use of revised documentation guidelines introduced in 1997 is optional. Work on a set of guidelines based on clinical vignettes rather than a counting system has been in progress since 1997. It is likely that new guidelines will be released in the near future. Physicians must be familiar with current documentation guidelines and be prepared to deal with changes as they arise. Of note, many third party payers adopt CMS guidelines or follow them closely. Current guidelines and information on work in progress are available at the CMS Web site (http://www.cms.gov).

Key Points

1. Each physician is responsible for all billing done under his/her provider number. Each physician is individually responsible for understanding CMS regulations and remaining compliant with them.
2. Care provided must be supported by documentation.
3. Billed services must be provided as documented to avoid charges of fraud and abuse.
4. Emergency physicians should be familiar with the coding, billing, and claims process used by their practice group, including the group's compliance plan.

Emergency Medical Transfer and Active Labor Act (EMTALA)

Every physician must be familiar with the mandates of EMTALA, but emergency physicians deal directly with these mandates daily. Emergency physicians should be knowledgeable of EMTALA requirements and maintain strict adherence to its rules. Failure to do so places the physician and the hospital at risk for civil penalties and loss of Medicare reimbursement.

EMTALA was enacted in 1985 as a part of the Common Omnibus Budget Reconciliation Act (COBRA). Concern over the "dumping" (transferring or refusing to treat patients because of their financial status) led to its inception. COBRA pertains both to emergency medical care and the continuation of group health insurance of individuals losing or transferring employment. EMTALA imposes regulations regarding the emergency medical care and transfer of patients presenting to emergency departments. These regulations apply to hospitals, emergency physicians, and physicians on-call to the hospital. An inherent problem with this regulation, however, is that no funds are appropriated to compensate hospitals or physicians for providing the required care. Thus, the fiscal responsibility for care under EMTALA is shifted onto providers under the threat of fines, civil liability, and loss of participation in the Medicare program. The statute is composed of five basic components: medical screening examination; necessary stabilizing treatment; restriction of transfers until stabilization is complete; enforcement; and nondiscrimination.

Medical Screening Examination

A hospital with an emergency department must provide an appropriate medical screening examination within the capability of the hospital's emergency department to anyone who comes to the facility and requests medical care. The medical screening examination must be conducted by hospital-appointed staff deemed suitable for these tasks. In the event of a conflict, CMS has the authority to decide whether this appointed staff member is appropriate. As a matter of practice, the person performing the medical screening examination is usually the emergency physician on duty.

An emergency medical condition is defined as "a medical condition manifesting itself by acute symptoms of sufficient severity (including severe pain) such that the absence of immediate medical attention could reasonably be expected to result in" one of the following:

- Placing the health of a person (or her unborn child) in serious jeopardy;
- Serious impairment to bodily functions;
- Serious dysfunction of any bodily organ or part.

A more detailed expansion of these definitions is not given; it is left to hospitals and practitioners to determine if these conditions are met.

Necessary Stabilizing Treatment for Emergency Medical Conditions and Labor

When an emergency medical condition is determined to exist, the hospital must provide "such further medical examination and such treatment as may be required to stabilize the medical condition" within the capabilities of the hospital or transfer the patient to a facility having the capacity to provide the necessary care. Stabilization is defined as providing "such medical treatment of the condition to assure, within reasonable medical probability, that no material deterioration of the condition is likely to result from or occur during the transfer of the individual from a facility."

Individuals may refuse treatment or transfer. Hospitals are deemed to have met the requirements of EMTALA if the patient or legally responsible person refuses treatment or transfer after being informed of the risks and benefits of the proposed treatment or transfer plan. The hospital must take all reasonable steps to procure signed documentation when the patient refuses treatment or transfer.

Restriction of Transfers Until Stabilizing Care Is Provided

Transferring a patient with an emergency medical condition that has not yet been stabilized may be done under EMTALA only when specific conditions are met:

1. The patient or responsible party may request a transfer in writing after having been informed of the hospital's EMTALA obligations.
2. A physician must certify in writing that the potential benefits of the transfer outweigh the risks to the patient or unborn child.
3. The receiving facility must have available space and qualified personnel for the treatment of the patient.
4. Acceptance by the receiving facility must be obtained.
5. A detailed copy of the medical record including observations, diagnostic tests, and preliminary diagnoses must accompany the transferred patient.
6. The transfer must be affected through qualified personnel and transportation equipment.
7. A woman in labor is not deemed to be stabilized until the fetus and placenta have been delivered.

EMTALA requires hospitals to "maintain a list of physicians who are on call for duty after the initial examination to provide treatment necessary to stabilize and individual with an emergency medical condition." If the emergency physician determines that the services of an on-call physician are required, he may transfer the patient if the on-call physician fails or refuses to appear. The on-call physician is then subject to penalties under EMTALA.

Enforcement

EMTALA's enforcement provisions are aimed at both hospitals and physicians who violate the statute. An individual or another hospital may sue the hospital (not the physician) for recovery of monetary losses arising from a violation. EMTALA imposes no federal criminal penalties, but several states have statutes imposing criminal penalties for inappropriate transfers.

The Department of Health and Human Services (DHHS) is responsible for enforcing EMTALA. Within DHHS, CMS can terminate a violating hospital's Medicare agreement, effectively imposing a financial death sentence on the hospital. CMS notifies the Office of the Inspector General (OIG) of all individuals and hospitals found guilty of a violation. The OIG may impose monetary penalties of up to $50,000 on physicians or hospitals and terminate physicians' participation in Medicare or Medicaid. Only CMS can terminate a hospital's Medicare agreements.

Ten regional CMS offices receive EMTALA complaints, which may be filed by any individual or hospital. Hospitals are required to report any transfer that may be a violation of EMTALA. The report may be made to CMS or an appropriate state agency. State agencies are required to report all potential violations to CMS. EMTALA enforcement is entirely complaint-driven; no investigative or enforcement actions are taken unless a complaint is received. CMS protects the identities of complainants. Complaints are investigated through state health departments or other state agencies responsible for hospital licensure. Enforcement therefore varies by state and region. CMS proceedings contain no due process or appeal mechanisms.

Nondiscrimination

Participating hospitals may not refuse an appropriate transfer. A hospital having specialized capabilities or serving as a regional referral center in rural areas must accept any individual in transfer if the hospital has the capacity to treat that individual.

Over the years, the original EMTALA statute was criticized for being vague on many key points. Significant revisions were introduced in September 2003 in an attempt to clarify some of the issues in question. The new regulation elaborates on the role of the hospital and physician with regard to hospital-owned facilities off-campus, hospital-owned ambulance regulations, outpatient visits to the ED, on-call coverage, and inpatient admissions. The following paragraph summarizes the important points of CMS's new "final rule" regarding interpretation of EMTALA.

EMTALA does not apply to hospital-operated off-campus facilities not meeting the definition of a dedicated emergency department. Prior interpretations burdened these facilities with providing a medical screening examination and meeting EMTALA requirements for transfer. In a similar manner, hospital-owned ambulances operating according to community-wide EMS protocols may transport patients to other facilities. Hospitals are not required to conduct comprehensive medical screening examinations for patients presenting with clearly nonemergent complaints such as a request for suture removal. Physicians are permitted to be on-call simultaneously at more than one hospital provided appropriate back-up plans have been established. EMTALA obligations end when an individual has been admitted to the hospital, with the expectation that the hospital's clinical policies provide adequate protection to inpatients. Sanctions for inappropriate transfers do not apply to hospitals located within an area experiencing a national emergency.

"Administrative simplification" is an oxymoron.

(ANONYMOUS)

Health Information Privacy and Portability Act (HIPAA)

Two decades of effort to standardize claims and transactions of information within the health care data management industry culminated in the passage of the Health Insurance Portability and Accountability Act (HIPAA). The industry first initiated efforts in 1975 to develop a standard claim form, resulting in the UB-82 seven years later. The success of this standard form, and later the HCFA 1500 claim form, lent credence to the idea that standardized forms could be implemented on a national basis. The Workgroup for Electronic Data Interchange, formed under the direction of HHS Secretary Louis Sullivan in 1991, issued a report in 1992 estimating potential health care administrative savings of $40 billion over six years if standard electronic formats were adopted for claims and other health data transmission. This finding prompted industry leaders to seek congressional sponsorship to implement the proposed standards. Representatives David Hobson and Thomas Sawyer authored administrative simplification provisions and attached them to a health insurance portability bill authored by Senators Edward Kennedy and Nancy Kassebaum. HIPAA is a massive bill consisting of five titles. The relatively small portion of this act under Title II, "Subtitle F: Administrative Simplification" contains the provisions regarding electronic transmission, privacy, and security of health information with which health care providers are now required to comply. It is these provisions to which health care providers refer when using the term "HIPAA." All further mention of HIPAA in this chapter refers only to Title II, Subtitle F, and the regulations developed under the direction of these provisions.

HIPAA is best understood by keeping in mind its history, purpose, and process by which its mandates are implemented, rather than by focusing on complex details. HIPAA's stated purpose is to improve Medicare, Medicaid, and the efficiency and effectiveness of the health care system "by encouraging the development of a health information system through the establishment of standards and requirements for the electronic transmission of certain health information."

To accomplish this goal, HIPAA calls for the development of "standards for information transactions and data elements," and "standards with respect to the privacy of individually identifiable health information." *All HIPAA regulations are a direct consequence of standards developed under these two broad categories.* The development of these standards is a complex and lengthy process. HIPAA charges the Secretary of the Department of Health and Human Services with the responsibility of implementing its standards. Following extensive review, a Notice of Proposed Rule Making is published in the *Federal Register.* Public comments are accepted for 60 days following publication. Modifications to the proposed rule are made based on these comments. The Final Rule, along with a summary of the comments, responses, and changes made based on the comments is published in the *Federal Register.* Once published, final rules carry the weight of federal law. Following publication of a final rule, the compliance deadline is 24 months for most organizations. Small health organizations have a 36-month compliance deadline. The provisions known as "administrative simplification" are therefore a multilayered, extensive, complex, and ongoing effort.

Table 185.1

Key Administrative Requirements of HIPAA

Minimum necessary standard	Covered entities must make reasonable efforts to limit protected health information (PHI) to the minimum necessary to accomplish the intended purpose of the disclosure. *"Minimum necessary" standard does not apply when PHI is used by a provider for treatment.*
Notice of Privacy Practices for Protected Health Information	Individuals have a right to adequate notice of the uses and disclosures of PHI. A detailed list of elements required in this notice is included in HIPAA.
Uses and Disclosures of PHI	PHI may be used for treatment, payment, and health care operations purposes without specific consent for each use, once the Notice of Privacy Practice has been provided and initial consent to use PHI has been signed. Specific exceptions are provided for treatment of emergencies.
Personnel Designations	Privacy official, security official, and person to receive complaints must be designated.
Training	Train all members of workforce with access to individually identifiable health information.
Safeguards	Administrative, technical, and physical safeguards to protect the PHI from unauthorized access, alteration, deletion, and transmission.
Policies and Procedures	Must implement and maintain polices and procedures with respect to PHI.

HIPAA applies to health plans, health care clearinghouses, and providers who transmit any health information in electronic form. An emergency physician with minimal administrative responsibilities may be unaware of the extensive requirements HIPAA places on health care practices. Compliance with HIPAA standards requires adherence to specific administrative requirements and specific security procedures. Key administrative requirements are summarized in **Table 185.1**. HIPAA's security rule requires each covered entity to develop administrative, technical, and physical safeguards to protect health information. Despite its vast size and scope, HIPAA's regulations are mainly the responsibility of practice groups, billing companies, and hospitals. HIPAA has little effect on the manner in which the practicing emergency physician uses health information at bedside. The primary focus of Administrative Simplification is standardization of data transactions, not modification of clinical practice. The privacy section of HIPAA was included because Congress recognized the challenges to the confidentiality of health information presented by the increasing complexity of the health care industry, and by advances in health care information systems and communication. The first privacy rule encountered significant protests by health care providers due to perceptions that, if literally enforced, the consent requirements for use of protected health information would impede timely patient treatment. The modified privacy rule issued in August 2002 deleted the requirement that patient consent must be obtained prior to using their private health information for routine health care purposes.

HIPAA preempts existing state privacy laws, but only when HIPAA imposes a higher standard of privacy. Physicians who have not encountered problems complying with existing privacy laws are unlikely to encounter problems solely due to HIPAA. After the required Notice of Privacy Practices is provided to the patient, the modified privacy rule allows exchange of protected health information for purposes of treatment, payment, or operations in essentially the same manner as existed prior to HIPAA.

The development of the policies, training of the privacy officer, and training of other personnel required by HIPAA demands a significant commitment of time and effort. Emergency department policies must be tailored to each individual facility and integrated with hospital HIPAA compliance policies. Group partners and directors responsible for this task will probably require the help of a consultant. Groups performing their own billing must also ensure that their software is compliant with electronic transaction and code set standards.

Table 185.2 summarizes HIPAA's requirements regarding common privacy issues emergency physicians might encounter during patient care.

Table 185.2	
Emergency Medicine Scenarios Involving Protected Health Information	
Notice of Privacy Practices	Providers must make a reasonable effort to inform each patient of their rights regarding the use of PHI. This requirement is satisfied by providing a written Notice of Privacy Practices, which must also be posted in the waiting area. *Once this notice is provided, no further consent from the patient is required to use PHI for treatment, payment, or health care operations purposes.*
Triage	Use of sign-in sheets is allowed. OCR asserts that only the name is necessary; the chief complaint should be omitted because it is not necessary for the purpose of signing in.
Waiting room	Calling out patients' names is allowed as an "incidental disclosure," provided the facility has implemented reasonable safeguards and applied the minimum necessary rule. Each patient must be provided a written notice of the facility's privacy policy. The entire privacy policy must be posted in a readily visible location.
Status boards	"Minimum necessary" rule allows a status board to contain information necessary to maintain a functioning board, whether electronic or white board. There is no specific guidance regarding what information may be on the board to meet minimum necessary standard. Reasonable safeguard and security standards apply. HIPAA allows providers to develop policies and procedures regarding access to PHI appropriate for their individual facilities.
Access to charts	HIPAA imposes no significant changes in chart handling. As specified in prior privacy laws, charts must be handled in such a way as to protect private health information. Incidental disclosures resulting from the chart being next to doors are allowed if reasonable safeguard standard has been applied.
Room partitions	Retrofitting of curtained or non-soundproofed rooms is not required. HIPAA affirms that reasonable safeguards in work areas should be exercised to prevent disclosure of private health information. Each facility must determine what precautions are reasonable.
Discussions with family and friends	Common sense prevails. HIPAA does not prohibit discussions with family or friends the patient has brought with them. Physicians may exercise professional judgment in determining the level of disclosure necessary for treatment of each individual patient.

Note: "OCR" refers to the United States Department of Health and Human Services Office for Civil Rights. Most of this table is derived from their answers to frequently asked questions on privacy rights under HIPAA.

Table 185.2

Emergency Medicine Scenarios Involving Protected Health Information—continued

Discussions with other providers	The Privacy Rule recognizes these conversations are necessary and may incidentally be overheard by others in the treatment area. No burden other than existing privacy laws and current privacy standards is imposed. Specific authorization from the patient is not required once the Notice of Privacy Practices has been provided.
Obtaining old records	A case-by-case justification for obtaining the entire old record is not required for treatment purposes, including obtaining a copy of the record from another facility.
Transfers	EMTALA requires that the entire record of treatment along with diagnostic studies must accompany the transferred patient. As in conversations with other providers, the HIPAA "minimum necessary" disclosure requirement does not pertain to emergency treatment. No rules on handling the medical record during transport are specified.
Disposal of documents	Covered entities must have formal policies and procedures for disposal of hardware and electronic materials containing PHI. No specific requirement exists for disposal of paper documents, other than the rule requiring reasonable safeguards to prevent disclosure of PHI. Each facility must develop its own policy regarding destruction of paper documents. HIPAA does not recommend a specific method.
Medical photography	Specific authorization is required for photography if individually identifiable information will be included in the photograph (such as the patient's face). If PHI is not included HIPAA has no rule regarding photography; existing state laws may apply.
Fax transmittals	Protected health information may be disclosed to other health care providers for treatment purposes by fax and other means. Reasonable and appropriate means to safeguard the faxed information should be used.
E-mail	Similar to fax transmittals. For treatment purposes, e-mail discussions with other involved providers are allowed. Encryption is an "addressable" security issue, meaning each facility may develop its own policy on encryption requirements. Consider placing PHI in a password-protected ZIP file attached to the e-mail.
Development of policies and procedures	Each covered entity must develop its own policies and procedures regarding disclosure of personally identifiable information. No single standard is imposed on all providers.
Communicable disease reporting	Reporting of communicable diseases required under existing laws is not limited by HIPAA.
Keeping a personal log of interesting cases	Keeping such a log is not specifically prohibited, but the physician must guard its privacy to the same standard as the formal patient record. If a lapse in protective safeguards allows unauthorized access to PHI, the individual physician may be liable to the civil and criminal penalties of HIPAA. HIPAA's Security Rule applies if the log is kept on any electronic device. HIPAA differentiates between violations due to "reasonable cause" and "willful neglect," but defending a complaint could be costly in terms of time, effort, and expense to the physician. State laws may also govern keeping of private logs. HIPAA makes specific provisions for "de-identifying" PHI, which if properly implemented would allow keeping a record of interesting cases but make it impossible to trace the case back to an individual.
Law enforcement	PHI may be released to report crime on the premises, report crime in emergencies, or to identify suspects or victims of crime. Disclosure must be limited to the identity, location, and description of perpetrators or victims.
Domestic violence and abuse	PHI regarding victims may be released to agencies authorized to receive reports of domestic abuse. Release of PHI regarding suspected abusers is limited to information for identification only.
Child abuse	As above, but HHS makes a specific exemption deferring to existing state laws requiring the reporting of suspected child abuse without respect to the wishes of the child, parents, or guardians.
Decedents	PHI may be released to professionals who might handle the body of the deceased (121), including funeral directors, coroners, or medical examiners.

HIPAA Key Points

1. HIPAA is a very large law. The "Administrative Simplification" portion of Title II is the portion of HIPAA that directly affects health care providers.
2. HIPAA consists of an act of Congress and a set of regulations published by the Secretary of the Department of Health and Human Services. The regulations are a perpetual work in progress; significant modifications and additions are a certainty.
3. HIPAA's main burden is the administrative development of policies and implementation of standards and procedures. Each covered entity is responsible

for the development of policies and procedures covering a very broad and expanding list of topics. Use of clinical information for treatment purposes is not significantly impacted by HIPAA. Methods of access to that information may be impacted by HIPAA security rules.

Conclusion

Federal regulations affecting the practice of emergency medicine are currently expanding and will continue to do so in the foreseeable future. Physicians may find federal regulations intrusive and even threatening. The best approach to compliance is to acquire a fundamental understanding of the reasons for the development of each regulation, and to keep up with the ever changing requirements they impose. Acquiring an understanding of the ways by which policies evolve may motivate physicians to participate in the complex process of developing future legislation.

Selected Readings

Bitterman RA. *Providing Emergency Care Under Federal Law: EMTALA*. Dallas: American College of Emergency Physicians, 2000:1.

Consolidated Omnibus Budget Reconciliation Act of 1985 (COBRA). Pub. L. No. 99-272, Title IX, Section 9121, 100 Stat 167 (1986). The Emergency Medical Treatment and Active Labor Act is found in 4 pages under "miscellaneous provisions" of COBRA. See 42 U.S.C. Sec. 1395dd. Title 42—The Public Health and Welfare, Chapter 7—Social Security, Subchapter XVIII—Health Insurance for the Aged and Disabled, Part C—Miscellaneous Provisions.

Draft OIG Compliance Program for Individual and Small Group Physician Practices. *Federal Register* 2000;65:36820.

Education materials: Your frequently asked questions on privacy. *Federal Register* 2003;68:8380. HHS Office for Civil Rights Available at http://www.hhs.gov/ocr/hipaa/. Accessed June 2005.

Goedert J. *HIPAA's Long and Winding Road*. Health Data Management, March 2003. Available at http://www.healthdatamanagement.com/html/current/PastIssueStory.cfm?PostID=14319&PastMonth=March&PastYear=2003. Accessed June 2005.

Health Insurance Portability and Accountability Act of 1996, Pub. L. No. 101-191.

Health Insurance Portability and Accountability Act of 1996, Pub. L. 104–191.

Medicare Program; Clarifying Policies Related to the Responsibilities of Medicare-Participating Hospitals in Treating Individuals With Emergency Medical Conditions; Final Rule. Thomas E. Hamilton, Director, State Survey and Certification Group, CMS/Center for Medicaid and State Operations. Memorandum to State Survey Agency Directors regarding EMTALA interim guidance. November 7, 2003. Available at http://www.acep.org/library/pdf/sc0410.pdf. Accessed June 2005.

OCR Guidance Explaining Significant Aspects of the Privacy Rule. Available at http://www.hhs.gov/ocr/hipaa/privacy.htmlhttp://www.hhs.gov/ocr/hipaa/. Accessed June 2005.

Standards for Privacy of Individually Identifiable Health Information; Final Rule. C.F.R. Parts 160 and 164. *Federal Register* 2002;67.

Ethics and Professionalism

Andrew R. Barnosky
Bradley J. Uren

The foundation of the practice of medicine is the physician–patient relationship. It is a distinctly special and unique relationship in which the health and future well being of one human being is placed into the hands of another, as a result of existential human needs that have arisen in the former, and the uniquely specialized body of knowledge and skills possessed by the later. It represents that circumstance in which the "patient" is the individual in need, and where a therapeutic relationship with a physician is entered into which is founded on trust, a trust that the physician will suspend self-interest and act in the best interest of the patient. It is a trust based on the assumption that the primacy of patient welfare will motivate and guide the physician, in all of the decisions and actions, which may be undertaken in caring for the patient.

It is within the context of this professional relationship that the ethical duties and virtues guiding the appropriate motives and actions of the physician may be circumscribed and defined. It is this relationship that forms the undeniable basis of professionalism in medicine: a relationship which is intimately tied to the universal human experience of vulnerability, and our common respect for the inestimable value of human life and health.[1,2] The doctor–patient relationship is the foundational base of the healing professions, and the elements of professionalism form the bedrock of the social contract of physicians to all members of society.

Professionalism and Professions Defined

Professionalism has been defined in a variety of contexts and by several different organizations. The American Board of Internal Medicine defines professionalism as "those attitudes and behaviors that serve to maintain patient interest above physician self-interest." It has likewise been referred to as "a set of values, attitudes, and behaviors that results in serving the interests of patients and society before one's own."[5] Although a variety of professional organizations have crafted definitions of this concept, regardless of authorship, the *primacy of patient welfare* serves as a guiding theme through all definitions of professionalism.

Professionalism is a concept which articulates that in order for medicine to be an honorable profession, its practitioner's attitudes and behaviors must consistently elevate the patient's interest above the self-interest of the profession or its members. It is considered as representing the highest ideals, virtues, attitudes, and ethical actions of the members of the medical profession. It reaffirms the fiduciary obligation of the physician to act in an unwavering advocacy role for the benefit of the patient under circumstances that require total trust, good faith, and honesty. It dignifies the philosophy that physicians have pursued careers in medicine with high-minded caring and advocacy motives, and a desire to preserve altruism, and that financial gain has tradiationally been held as a secondary consideration. It recognizes that the relationship between doctors and patients are optimal when patients trust physicians and believe that physicians will consistently work in their best interest. Professionalism acknowledges that the stability of the medical profession is derived from the public trust, which is necessary in maintaining the integrity of medicine's relationship to the public, and hence its future. It promotes the concept that aggregate doctor–patient relationships represent the basic infrastructure of society's trust in medicine.

"Professionalism" and "membership within a profession" have some similarities, yet significant differences between the two exist, and they are worthy of explanation. A profession has been defined as "an occupation that regulates itself through systemic, required training and collegial discipline, that has a base in technical, specialized knowledge, and that which has a service rather than a profit orientation enshrined in its code of ethics."[6] The professions have long been recognized to consist of three essential characteristics: expert knowledge (as distinguished from a practical skill), self-regulation, and a fiduciary responsibility to place the needs of the client ahead of the self interests of the practitioner.[7] Although the number of professions has varied somewhat with changing social, economic, intellectual, and political circumstances over the past several centuries, the professions have traditionally consisted of medicine, law, and theology (ministry). Notwithstanding the passage of time, it is apparent that the time-honored distinguishing *ideal* characteristics of professions today remain essentially the same: the acquisition of a specialized body of knowledge by the group's members, self-regulation, accountability, and—most importantly—*service above self*.

While all physicians are unquestionably members of the profession of medicine, it is understandable that simply being a member of a profession does not guarantee that one incorporates "a set of values, attitudes, and behaviors that result in serving the interests of patients and society before one's own."[4] In this light, professionalism and professional membership have significant potential differences. Membership in a profession, in and of itself, does not mean that all of its members value individual and public health more than other social good, and remain motivated to work hard even when the financial rewards for such efforts may not be great.[1] Likewise, "membership" does not necessarily assure that such individuals adhere to high ethical and moral standards, evince core humanistic values, demonstrate a lifelong commitment to excellence, and exercise accountability for themselves and their colleagues. Rather, it is *professionalism* (as opposed to simply membership within a profession) that represents these esteemed virtues, ideals, and actions. In a normative sense, it is unquestionably desired that all members of any profession would themselves exhibit high levels of professionalism, yet it is known that this is not universally true. Internal and external forces can and do pose challenges to professionalism for medicine in general, and certainly emergency medicine in particular.

Challenges to Professionalism in Emergency Medicine

The virtues and attitudes of professionalism, and the core ethics of caring, appear to be a significant portion of the belief system held by physicians during some or all of their careers. Given the historical status of medicine as an honorable profession, when we become physicians, we undertake a series of specific moral obligations, a number which are unquestionably demanding, particularly in the specialty of emergency medicine. The nature of the doctor–patient relationship is such that it is born from the intuitional knowledge of our inherent vulnerability as persons, with pervasive uncertainties regarding a future of health or illness, and on our commonly held respect for the value of human life and health.[1] Certainly, in no area of medicine is the concept of vulnerability more prevalent than in emergency medicine and, likewise, in no other specialty field of medicine is the social contract between physicians and the public as strong. In this regard, the virtues and ethics of professionalism in emergency medicine have served as a structurally stabilizing and morally protective force in society.

But while the ideals of professionalism are part of the core belief system of physicians in general, voices representing many interests within and outside of medicine are calling for a renewed sense of professionalism.[2] Although a variety of factors have precipitated this call for renewal, the great majority of issues are in some circumstance reflective of the social, economic, political, and cultural trans-formation of modern medicine and health care delivery systems in virtually all industrialized countries.

In the discipline of emergency medicine, growing awareness of evolving challenges to professionalism in the United State had prompted the Society for Academic Emergency Medicine to initiate a project entitled, "Professionalism in Emergency Medicine."[8] With the support of the American Board of Emergency Medicine, the American College of Emergency Physicians, the Emergency Medicine Resident Association, the American Academy of Emergency Medicine, and the Association of Academic Chairs of Emergency Medicine, this document was intended to describe proper behavior and attitudes of the ideal practitioner of emergency medicine. As such, it identified those attitudes and behaviors that enhance trust by placing the patient's interest above all other interests, inherently stipulating that the primacy of patient welfare should be the prevailing interest in decision-making in the context of the physician-patient relationship in emergency medicine.[8]

In a like manner, meetings among the European Federation of Internal Medicine, the American College of Physicians—American Society of Internal Medicine, and the American Board of Internal Medicine resulted in the voicing of their shared view that medicine's commitment to the patient continues to recognize increasing challenges by external forces of change within representative societies.[9] In this light, meetings among these internal medicine organizations resulted in the development of the Medical Professionalism Project, which eventually resulted in a Charter on Medical Professionalism.[9] This charter has been an attempt to enlist all physicians worldwide (regardless of specialty) to live by a set of precepts of professionalism, and to resist competing external interests that threaten each physician's commitment to patient welfare.[9] It is a document that had been developed through the consensus of a broad plurality of physicians, in the hopes that its principles and commitments could be expanded to all specialization fields in medicine, thereby covering *all* physicians. The efforts on behalf of those involved on the work on professionalism through Medical Professionalism Project of the American Board of Internal Medicine, and the Project on Professionalism of the Ethics Committee of the Society of Academic Emergency Medicine, have provided much direction in the renewal and rejuvenation of professionalism to physicians specializing in emergency medicine.

The doctor–patient relationship is truly unique in emergency medicine, and the changing face of medicine in both the United States and the industrialized world has posed increasing challenges in holding the primacy of patient welfare as the exclusive overriding interest in decision-making for emergency physicians. Increasingly, other interests appear at the bedside of patients in the ED, and the intrusion that these competing interests bring to bear on the fiduciary obligation of the physician as well as their increasing number continue to pose enlarging challenges in this regard. On the financial side, emergency physicians find that the resolve of their professional integrity is increasingly stressed by issues of institutional cost containment efforts, managed care directives, restrictive transfer policies, hospital admission avoidance policies, prescribing restrictions, and other issues that manifest themselves as a desire to constrain the upward spiral of health care costs. Although many of these issues are unavoidable as the result of a desire to achieve a just allocation of finite resources in a culture with increasing demands for health care services, some of the competing interests to professionalism are recognized as the direct result of the profit motive for medical services, often delivered unequally in a market-based health care economy. Avoidance of liability and the consequences of medical malpractice litigation promote risk-aversion strategies among physicians in general that, although in some circumstances may be beneficial in promoting error reduction, can bring maladaptive incursions into the physician–patient relationship. An ever-increasing population of inadequately insured individuals who are incapable of receiving primary care in the traditional fashion can unfavorably impact the advocacy role that all physicians play on these individuals' behalf. Emergency department overcrowding impacts the timeliness in the development of physician–patient relationship, limits the duration of physician–patient interaction, and can impact physician advocacy efforts in a number of ways. Admittedly, there are additional factors in a growing list of challenges to professionalism in emergency medicine whose enumeration is not the purpose of this chapter. Yet it stands to reason that as health care systems in the industrialized world grow in scientific, technical, and administrative complexity (amid aggressive escalating resource constraint efforts), it is probable that a variety of new competing interests will continue to manifest themselves at the bedside between the patient and the emergency physician.

Need for Professionalism in Emergency Medicine

The demand for professionalism is unquestionably high in the specialty of emergency medicine. In no other branch of medicine is the physician–patient relationship more time limited and challenging. Physicians and patients are often thrust together in the context of an acute medical emergency, without prior opportunities for either party to consider the multiple facets of the professional relationship prior to entering into it. Catastrophic illness and injury occur with unpredictability to all persons, with little ability on the patient's part to choose a physician. Patients who are without insurance or inadequately insured, and individuals without financial resources who have had difficulty receiving preventive care or disease management in the early stages of symptom onset, often have no other choice for care, and present when the situation is urgent to the emergency department. Physicians are often faced with little time to develop rapport, with a patient population that varies widely in numbers, demands, acuity, severity, communication abilities, and levels of consciousness. Individuals who are marginalized due to physical or intellectual infirmity, socioeconomic compromise, and those at the ends of the life continuum represent members of vulnerable populations, and the challenges and demands for rapport and integrity within these physician–patient relationships are great.

The demands for technical competency in emergency medicine are very great. An emergency physician must be able to possess a comprehensive fund of knowledge and to utilize it effectively and efficiently in the clinical environment. Prioritization of illness, effective triage strategies, and the need for multi-tasking are great. The demand for high technical competency in the performance of a wide variety of critical procedures is high. The expectations that society has on its emergency physician and, hence, the expectations that emergency physicians have for themselves, are quite high.

The obligations to act in the best interest of patients is inextricably tied to the optimization and integrity of the physician–patient relationship, and the competency of practitioners of emergency medicine. The preservation of the trust of patients and society can only occur through the maintenance of a deep commitment to professionalism. When a profession has the trust of society, it is granted the authority to control who enters the profession, who is granted the authority to regulate and discipline members of the profession, and who bears accountability and responsibility of practice decisions.[4]

As the transformation stresses inherent in health care evolution continue, the commitment to professionalism in emergency medicine is necessary to both manage change and to retain the core values of our profession. Our purpose as emergency physicians will continue to be driven by our core values. The profession must recall that, "purpose serves as a point of reference. As long as we keep purpose in focus in both our organizational and private lives we are able to wander through the realms of chaos, make decisions about what actions will be consistent with our purpose, and emerge with a discernible pattern or shape to our lives."[10]

Principles and Commitments of Medical Professionalism

As specified in the Charter on Medical Professionalism, the ongoing renewal and preservation of professionalism in medicine is based on the delineation of a set of principles to which all members of the medical profession should aspire.[9] In addition to a set of core principles, a series of specific commitments can be derived, and the adherence to them can promote professionalism and the overall integrity of the profession. The three main principles of professionalism include the principle of the primacy of patient welfare, the principle of patient autonomy, and the principle of social justice. The set of professional responsibilities that highlight further the core attitudes and behaviors necessary for professionalism, include:

1. The commitment to professional competence
2. The commitment to honesty with patients
3. The commitment to patient confidentiality
4. The commitment to maintaining appropriate relationships with patients
5. The commitment to improving quality of care
6. The commitment to improving access to care

7. The commitment to a just distribution of finite resources
8. The commitment to scientific knowledge
9. The commitment to maintaining trust by managing conflicts of interest
10. The commitment to professional responsibilities

The application of these core principles and commitments to professionalism in the practice of emergency medicine are as follows.

The Principles of Professionalism

The Principle of the Primacy of Patient Welfare

The primacy of patient welfare is the core principle of professionalism. It defines the overarching fiduciary obligation of the emergency physician in the doctor–patient relationship in its most elementary sense. This principle states that the physician shall suspend self interest and allow the interest of the patient and his or her welfare to be the guiding principle in medical decision-making and advocacy on behalf of the patients. Although it is recognized that a multitude of competing interests may present themselves within the context of this relationship, adhering to the primacy of patient welfare means that the emergency physician will channel his/her attitudes and behaviors to relegate all non-advocacy interests in a subjugated position relative to advocating for the needs of the patient. This obviously does not mean that the interests of third-party payors, institutional policies and directives, and other driving administrative and economic forces within the medical-administrative context need be completely ignored, as this is most often impossible and unrealistic. It simply states that the primacy of patient welfare is the most superior interest in this balance, and the emergency physician need to forever hold this as the lens through which patient care is viewed, allowing it to set the priorities regarding ethical medical decision-making and physician advocacy to serve the goals of medicine in this relationship. Conflicts which arise in this circumstance include inappropriate requests for the transfer of patients, ineffective on-call schedules, and unwilling participation of specialty back-up physicians, risk aversion practices by emergency and on-call physicians which fail to promote the patient's best-interest, directives of managed care organizations and other third payers which may be poorly aligned with ethically appropriate management decisions involving treatment and disposition of patients, staffing ratios of emergency physician and nurses that may be financially advantageous yet inappropriate to manage patient volumes, restrictive institutional admission policies, and others. In retrospect, it is quite understandable that the development of federal regulations such as the Emergency Medical Treatment and Active Labor Act were developed specifically to address the lowering of the professional standards of some health care institutions and physicians regarding the ethical disposition and transfer of some of our most vulnerable patients.[11]

Holding the primacy of patient welfare as paramount in the physician–patient relationship promotes a degree of altruism that contributes to trust. This is a principle that cannot be compromised by social or societal pressures, market forces, administrative requirements, or political expediency.

The Principle of Patient Autonomy

Respect for patient autonomy is one of the cornerstones of ethical practice in medicine. This principle holds that emergency physicians will respect the decisions and liberty interests of the patients they care for, and promote honest dialogue with patients to allow them to make truly informed consent-based decisions. Autonomy engages patients in medical decision-making, and fosters the practice of informing patients of their health-related situation in a manner in which they understand their diagnosis, and subsequently informing them of the variety of options for treatment (including no treatment), while enhancing their understanding of the benefits and burdens of these various courses of therapy. It is through respecting autonomy that, when patients are unable to participate in medical decision making and give informed consent due to impaired decisional-capacity, that appropriate surrogate decision makers are sought to act in the best interests of patients. Patient autonomy has driven the push for advanced directives, and the right of patients to assign, through durable power or attorney designation, an individual of their choosing to decide for them. It is through autonomy that "Emergency Doctrine" legislation has been drafted in allowing the justification of physician paternalism when life-threatening emergencies exist, and where the physician must act in the best interest of individuals so compromised.[12] Respect for autonomy allows the patient's decision to be paramount in health care decisionmaking, providing that those decisions are in accord with customary ethical practice and not demanding of inappropriate or futile care.

The Principle of Social Justice

Of all of the specialty fields in medicine, emergency medicine unquestionably has been at the forefront in the promotion of social justice. Emergency departments throughout the industrialized world are open at all times, their external signage representing an implicit contractual relationship between emergency physicians and the public of a willingness to evaluate and care for all individuals, regardless of race, color, ethnicity, citizenship, health-insurance status, or the personal resources of those in need. Market forces, societal pressures, and administrative exigencies should not compromise emergency medicine's quest for social justice, and the profession must continue to promote adequate and equitable emergency services and continue to work toward the elimination of systematic barriers to access. Patients must continue to be treated without bias or judgment, and without regard for socioeconomic status or position. Members of the specialty of emergency medicine should continue to work to promote processes of care, which foster the well being for all members of society. Distributive justice demands fairness and equity in the process of allocating health care resources under urgent and emergent conditions. In this regard, emergency physicians have a responsibility to promote efficiency in delivering care, eliminate unnecessary and inappropriate diagnostic testing and therapies, minimize that which is marginally beneficial, and work toward waste reduction. The virtuous emergency physician will become involved in advocacy activities, both within and without the context of the physician–patient relationship, which promote fairness in health care, and attempt to diminish health care disparities in individuals or groups.

The Set of Professional Responsibilities

Commitment to Professional Competence Emergency medicine is a specialty that has high standards for professional competence. The body of information in the clinical specialty continues to expand, and the fund of knowledge requirements on its practitioners is demanding. The quality of care which emergency physicians are able to deliver is dependent on the maintenance of clinical skills and a comprehensive knowledge base. Embracing a commitment to continuation of learning throughout one's professional life is necessary for the maintenance of professional competence. Loss of conscientiousness, and the reluctance or failure of an otherwise competent physician to fulfill professional obligations, signifies the loss of a commitment to professional competence. Not only individual physicians, but the entire profession must adopt this pattern of lifelong learning, and members from the ranks of the specialty must continue to adopt leadership roles in this regard; the desire to develop and promote continuous board certification methodologies is considered by many a step in this regard.

Emergency physicians with impaired or declining competence need to be identified and appropriately cared for, for the benefit of themselves and the potential patients they might treat inappropriately. Whether physician impairment is due to declining cognitive abilities from organic illness, substance abuse, or other etiologies, emergency physicians so identified need compassionate management which may include temporary or permanent removal from the work force. Self-regulation is a privilege awarded the professions by society, and curtailment of the activities of some emergency physicians is sometimes required. Trust is the bedrock not only of the doctor–patient relationship, but also the relationship of emergency medicine to society. Erosion of trust through a decline in the commitment to individual emergency physicians or their collective body erodes the public trust, which undermines to integrity of the specialty and the profession.

Commitment to Honesty with Patients Honesty is as integral as professional competence in retaining the trust that society places in emergency physicians. Honesty with patients entails the principles of informed consent, in that it is incumbent on the emergency physician to provide each patient with a reasonable enough base of knowledge to make an appropriate informed decision about a proposed course of therapy. Not allowing patients to voice their wishes as participants in their own care is an abuse of power. Honesty is dependent on effective communication, as com-

munication is an essential factor in initiating and maintaining rapport in the professional relationship. Effective communication requires a willingness to understand cultural differences, and entails both effective listening as well as effective verbal and non-verbal communication. Humility is a virtue that enhances communication and rapport, in that it enhances the respect of patients that is a necessary requirement to honest relationships. Arrogance is an offensive and inappropriate display of superiority that must be avoided at all costs because it makes empathy and honesty difficult and diminishes objective self-doubt.

Errors are a common part of medical practice and when they occur, patients need to be informed and involved in an honest and comprehensive dialogue. An honest and well-intentioned analysis of past medical mistakes is a forthright and sincere attempt to diminish future occurrences, and promotes public confidence in medicine.

Honesty and integrity are necessary in dealing not only with patients, but also with insurers, members of regulatory and governmental agencies, hospital administrators, and others. Professional areas in which the requirement for honesty is high additionally includes medical record accuracy, expert witness testimony, the privileging and credentialing of emergency medicine colleagues, responsible authorship, curriculum vitae preparation, and letters of recommendation.

Commitment to Patient Confidentiality Confidence and trust in the physician–patient relationship is enhanced through the patient's belief that information relayed to the physician will be held in confidence. Breach of patient confidentiality in any form is an abuse of power, and in addition to a high degree of discretion in communicating patient information held in confidence, emergency physicians need to continually work toward developing procedures and safeguards that uphold confidentiality. The electronic medical record and computerized information systems pose ongoing challenges in this regard, yet with the exception of the need to yield to public health concerns when appropriate, physicians must continue to strive for achieving high degrees of confidentiality. In the event that patients lack decisional capacity, ethical issues surrounding the preservation of confidentiality need to be extended to designated surrogates.

Commitment to Maintaining Appropriate Relationships with Patients As a result of illness, injury, disability, psychosocial difficulties, or socioeconomic issues, many emergency patients are vulnerable. Patient vulnerability in the context of the doctor–patient relationship creates an imbalance of power where the physician may be deemed to be a powerful and authoritarian figure. Exploitation in this situation needs to be avoided at all costs. Sexual interactions between physicians and patients subvert the goals of the physician–patient relationship, may exploit the vulnerability of the patient, may interfere significantly with the physician's objective judgment regarding medical decision-making, and has the potential of being detrimental to the patient's well-being.[13] In addition to sexual exploitation, patients should never be exploited for personal financial gain or any other private personal interest of the physician.

Commitment to Improving Quality of Care In addition to maintaining technical and knowledge competence through ongoing training and lifelong education, emergency physicians need to actively engage in continuous quality improvement efforts as an ongoing process to enhance care in the emergency department. Such activities are often linked to the reduction of error, with concomitant improvement in the goals of medicine and the outcomes of care delivered. Ongoing efforts directed at the utilization of evidence-based medicine by individual physicians and the specialty incorporate the prevailing scientific wisdom into the care provided to patients. Self-regulation of those who enter and exit from the specialty, based on fair and objective assessment of competency, signifies the commitment to improving the quality of health care delivered to the public. Emergency physicians should actively participate in the development of measures to assess the professional quality of care performed by themselves, as well as within the institutions and systems in which they practice.

Commitment to Improving Access to Care Departments of emergency medicine have a long and proud history of providing an enlarging safety net to an ever-growing segment of the population in need. It is the only health care service whose doors never close. Yet despite a desire to promote a consistent pattern of fair and universal access, challenges continue to present themselves. The Emergency Medical Treatment and Active Labor Act alluded to earlier was a legislated remedy to one such challenge to emergency department access.

Departmental overcrowding presents an increasing barrier to care for many persons in needs of care, and emergency physicians need to continue in advocacy roles via driving institutional and governmental leadership to facilitate solutions. The changing health care environment resulting from health maintenance and managed care organization directives has challenged care access to some, and emergency physicians may need to continue to invest advocacy efforts in this regard. Justice demands the fair and equitable triage of patients according to severity of illness, and denotes the rapidity with which care need proceed. Issues regarding citizenship, immigration status, race, culture, ethnicity, religion, socioeconomic level, or payor status should never promote differential decision-making on the part of the emergency physician. Although the challenges that exist in securing appropriate out-patient follow-up for many ED patients remain a broad societal issue, to the extent that emergency physicians might facilitate optimal out-patient referral outcomes in this realm, they should make the attempt. The information transfer challenges which language barriers pose represents an access issue and physicians should request the use of interpreters when available.

Commitment to a Just Distribution of Finite Resources Just health care should be adequate and equitable to all persons, and physicians should be conservatively judicious in the ordering of health care resources in both diagnostic and treatment realms. While distributive justice requires equal treatment without regard to bias or discrimination, emergency physicians should work towards improved efficiency and the reduction of unnecessary tests and treatments. In this regard, evidence-based medicine in EM has been pivotal the development of optimal care guidelines. Given the growing population marginalized and underserved persons, the extremely virtuous emergency physician might join other colleagues in primary care through medical service volunteerism and social engagement.

Commitment to Scientific Knowledge Medicine's contract with society is based in part on our ability to acquire and utilize scientific knowledge in an appropriate manner. Emergency physicians need to join colleagues in other disciplines in promoting scientific inquiry, and utilizing the information obtained to promote standards that foster higher quality care for the populations we serve.

Commitment to Maintaining Trust by Managing Conflicts of Interest Conflicts of interests occur between the emergency physician and those of their patients or the public. Suspension of self-interest reduces the conflict, whereby the welfare of patients and the public takes precedence over the interests of the emergency physician; these include the interests of status, financial gain, power, and personal pleasure. A major area of conflicts of interests involves the pharmaceutical industry, both in breaching the boundaries between academic medicine and the for-profit industry, and gifts to physicians.

The relationships between industry and opinion leaders should always be disclosed, especially when the latter determine the criteria for conducting and reporting clinical trials, writing editorials or therapeutic guidelines, or serving as editors of scientific journals.[13] Regarding gifts from the pharmaceutical industry, it is important to bear in mind the interactions between the marketing of pharmaceuticals and the influence that such companies have on undergraduate medical education and training as well as the practicing physician. In this manner, the Council on Ethical and Judicial Affairs of the American Medical Association has recommended that gifts accepted by physicians (1) should primarily entail a benefit to patients and should not be of substantial value; (2) should be related to the physician's work; and (3) that subsidies should not be accepted to pay for costs for travel, lodging personal expenses, or compensation for lost earnings while the physician is engaged in continuing medical education.[13]

Authority granted to members of the profession entails the responsibility to use that power wisely. Emergency physicians should never enter into relationships where income is tied to resource utilization. In like fashion, deliberate falsification (lying) or misrepresentation (fraud) to achieve an inappropriate gain is the antithesis of professionalism (and, needless to say, illegal).

Commitment to Professional Responsibilities Emergency physicians must bear accountability in their relationship with the patients as well as in their relationship to the specialty. As a group, they should work collaboratively to promote the maximal quality of patient care, to maintain respect for each other, and to participate in the process of self-regulation (including the discipline and re-mediation of members who have failed to meet professional standards).[9] The process of determining the standards of practice needs to be defined from within the specialty, recognizing that failure to do so will erode the public trust, diminish the integrity of the specialty, and force an external regulatory body to replace the profession's self-regulatory privilege. Exercising accountability for all emergency medicine colleagues through internal assessment (and the acceptance of external scrutiny) is the core foundation of organizational professional responsibilities.

Professionalism in Teaching

All specialty fields of medicine have a responsibility to make provisions for the health care needs of future generations through the education of new members of the specialty. Our implicit social contract with the public health community entails a responsibility to promote intergenerational solidarity, that is, to act in a manner where high quality emergency medical care may be provided to generations that follow, through the comprehensive education of the medical students and residents of today. It thus becomes the obligation of present emergency physicians to foster the education and growth of younger colleagues who will, near the completion of their training, evince core humanistic values including honesty and integrity, caring and compassion, altruism and empathy, respect for others, and trustworthiness.

Role modeling is considered as one of the most significant aspects in the socialization process in medical education. The "hidden curriculum" is very real and each and every interaction that occurs within a training program can modify and form the behaviors of future emergency physicians, where the underlying culture promotes only those values which are considered important.[14] Academic emergency physicians must promote an internal culture in the academic health center which better enforces the values that medical educators wish to impart. Teachers who engage in the intimidation and humiliation of their students create a hostile environment, which not only discourages participation, but also fosters the likelihood of these individuals engaging in such behavior at a later point in their professional career. The prevailing culture evolves not by what is verbally expressed, but by the accepted behavior and attitudes of its members. Teaching physicians who role-model adherence to high ethical and moral standards have the greatest influence on promoting a subsequent generation of physicians who adhere to high degrees of professionalism.

Professionalism in Research

A portion of emergency medicine's commitment to present and future societal needs mandates continued efforts in scholarship and research aimed at acquiring new knowledge. Such efforts, while intended to improve the health of groups of individual and the public at-large, nonetheless need to be balanced with regard of ethical standards of clinical research. In this regard, research needs to be evaluated within a coherent ethical framework in which customary requirements are met.[15] Such requirements include "(1) value—enhancements of health or knowledge must be derived form the research; (2) scientific validity—the research must be methodologically rigorous; (3) fair subject selection—scientific objectives, not vulnerability or privilege, and the potential for and distribution of risks and benefits should determine communities selected as study sites and the inclusion criteria for individual subjects; (4) favorable risk-benefit ratio—within the context of standard clinical practice and the research protocol, risks must be minimized, potential benefits enhanced, and the potential benefits to individuals and knowledge gained for society must outweigh the risks; (5) independent review—unaffiliated individuals must review the research and approve, amend, or terminate it; (6) informed consent—individuals should be informed about the research and provide their voluntary consent; and (7) respect for enrolled subjects—subjects should have their privacy protected, the opportunity to withdraw, and their well-being monitored."[15]

Professionalism in Administration

When an emergency physician assumes a leadership role in either institutional or business administration, additional professional ethical obligations and responsibilities are undertaken. In this circumstance, it is the relationship between the physician leader and his/her physician colleagues that is central, and although requiring a different moral focus than the traditional doctor–patient relationship, it is a relationship that remains aligned in the vision of promoting the integrity of emergency medicine as a professional specialty.

A health care system that exists in a market-based capitalistic economy creates a variety of employment arrangements for emergency physicians. This fosters an opportunity for medical ethics and the ethics of business to at-times run into conflict, and where the pursuit of self-interest becomes a moral hazard to be avoided by all ethical physician leaders and professional corporate entities. Regardless of the employment vehicle in which emergency physicians find themselves, they are entitled to practice in a fair business environment that guarantees substantive and procedural due process, honesty and justice in reimbursement practices, administrative fairness, accountability, non-exploitation of colleagues, respect for others, and trustworthiness. In order to maintain professionalism, loyalty to the primacy of patient welfare must be the penumbral and final guiding vision. To the extent that the realization of this vision is dependent on a fair and reasonable administrative/practice environment for emergency physicians, a "business enterprise that sustains itself through practices that are harmful to patients, colleagues, or society must be opposed by individual emergency physicians and their professional organizations."[15]

Conclusion

Professionalism in emergency medicine consists of maintaining those attitudes, and demonstrating those behaviors where the interests of the patient are held above all other competing interests. The integrity of the medical profession as a whole, and emergency medicine in particular, is based upon the solid retention of the public trust during periods of health care transformation, in which the dynamics of the doctor–patient relationship undergo varying stresses. The foundation of the public trust is based on the degree of professionalism exhibited by members of the medical profession. The leading principles of professionalism in medicine include the primacy of patient welfare, patient autonomy, and justice.

Emergency departments remain the "front door" for access to heath care for many persons in the industrialized world, and having become an ever-expanding "safety net" for a variety of marginalized and vulnerable populations, the demands for professionalism will always remain high. As the continued transformation of health care poses innumerable stresses on professionalism in medicine, emergency physicians must remain vigilant in maintaining the primacy of patient welfare as our guiding vision.

References

1. Wynia MK, Latham SR, Kao AC, Emanuel LL. Medical professionalism in society. *N Engl J Med* 1999;341:1612–1616.
2. Pelligrino ED, Thomasma DC. *A Philosophical Basis of Medical Practice.* Oxford, UK: Oxford University Press, 1981.
3. American Board of Internal Medicine. *Project Professionalism.* Chicago: ABIM, 1995:2.
4. Adams J, Schmidt T, Sanders A, et al. Professionalism in emergency medicine. *Acad Emerg Med* 1998;5:1193–1199.
5. Renolds PP. Professionalism in residency. *Ann Internal Med* 1991;91:91–92.
6. Starr P. *The Social Transformation of American Medicine.* New York: Basic Books, 1984.
7. Ludmerer KM. Instilling professionalism in medical education. *JAMA* 1999;282:881–882.
8. Schneider SM, Hamilton GC, Moyer P, Stapczynski JS. Definition of emergency medicine. *Acad Emerg Med* 1998;5:348–351.
9. ABIM Foundation, ACP-ASIM Foundation, European Federation of Internal Medicine. Medical professionalism in the new millennium: a physician charter. *Ann Intern Med* 2002;136:243–246.
10. Wheatley MJ. *Leadership and the New Science.* San Francisco: Berrett-Koehler, 1992:36.
11. *Emergency Medical Treatment and Active Labor Act* (42 U.S.C.S. 1395dd), the "Patient Dumping" Act. Available at http://njatty.net/focus-on-patient-dumping-act.htm. Accessed June 2005.
12. Iserson KV, Sanders AB, Mathieu D, eds. *Ethics in Emergency Medicine,* ed 2. Tuscon AZ: Galen Press, 1995.
13. American Medical Association Council on Ethical and Judicial Affairs. *Code of Medical Ethics 150th Anniversary Edition.* 1996-97;Section 8.14:130. Available at www.ama-assn.org/meetings/ public/annual01/call_to_order.pdf. Accessed June 2005.
14. Ludmerer KM. *Time to Heal: American Medical Education from the Turn of the Century to the Era of Managed Care.* New York: Oxford University Press; 1999.
15. Emanuel EJ, Dwindle D, Grady C. What makes clinical research ethical? *JAMA* 2000;238:2701–2711

Physician Wellness

Kristin E. Harkin

The real moment of success is not the moment apparent to the crowd.

GEORGE BERNARD SHAW (1856–1950)

Physicians, by definition, are promoters of wellness. However, it requires a conscious, concerted effort for physicians to maintain their own health and well-being. It is a necessity that seldom is taught in training. In short, wellness is the quality or state of being in good health, and all that good health incorporates (body, mind, and spirit).

Well-being is influenced by personal happiness and professional satisfaction. You know you are professionally satisfied when most of the time you look forward to going to work during your commute into the workplace.

Scheduling

Be grateful for each new day. A new day that you have never lived before. We can squander, neglect, or use it. Life will be richer or poorer by the way we use today.

RALPH WALDO EMERSON (1803–1882)

Your schedule is your life. It is key to your personal and professional happiness. Your time is the most valuable commodity you have and time management is the ultimate skill.

Shift work is the reality that the emergency physician faces. Many studies have confirmed the adverse effects of shift work on physical and mental health. Working swing shifts shortens life expectancy and increases the likelihood of peptic ulcer disease, hypertension, cardiovascular mortality, infertility in women, rate of work-related accidents and errors (e.g., car accidents), depression, drug and alcohol abuse, and higher divorce rates.

Shift work has a definitive effect on sleep patterns. There are four distinct stages of sleep: Stage 1 is a brief transition period; Stage 2 is a deeper sleep period; Stages 3 and 4 are comprised of slow wave sleep (SWS) and rapid eye movement sleep (REM). SWS is essential for physical recuperation; it decreases throughout adulthood and may be absent in the elderly. Growth hormone is secreted during SWS. Those deprived of it complain of fatigue and muscle aches. REM sleep is crucial for psy-

chological well-being. Those deprived of it complain of irritability and moodiness. Cerebral blood flow is increased more during REM sleep than during wakefulness. Dreams occur during REM sleep. Shift workers who have fragmented sleep or shorter sleep are often deprived of REM sleep.

Alertness is an absolute at work and is related to temperature variations. Humans function best when their normal temperature is highest, which is typically during the middle of the wakeful period. Total sleep time, adequate SWS time, and regularity of schedule influence alertness as well. A siesta is better than napping at other times of the day as it is rich in REM.

Circadian rhythms reflect the body's natural rhythms due to hormonal changes that result in fluctuations in body temperature. For the best overall productivity, minimizing circadian rhythm conversion is key. Clockwise shift rotation is preferred (days, evenings, nights). Productivity decreases for an average of two days after working night shifts as the circadian rhythm cycle reconverts from night peaking to day peaking. Circadian rhythms do not fully reset from the normal day peaking to night peaking until the third night shift in a row, which is why it is better to do no more than two night shifts in a row at the most. Doing single night shifts are still better and easier to readjust one's circadian rhythm. Having 48 hours off between night and day shifts is a necessity. If one is forced to do many night shifts in a row, however, it is better to do them all in one month rotations to allow circadian stabilization.

Twelve-hour shifts are preferred by most younger physicians to allow more complete days off. However, it is harder to reset the biological clock over a 12-hour adjustment than an 8-hour adjustment. Often, swaps are necessary, yet too many shifts in a row are exhausting (physically and mentally). Moreover, returning from a much needed vacation an entire full day before one's return to work, as opposed to late the night before, prevents you from returning to work drained, which is probably how you felt before you even left!

Go to sleep as soon as possible after working a single night shift and force yourself to get up after four hours. This will enable you to sleep the next entire night because you will be sleepy at your usual bedtime. Sleeping longer than four hours will impede the next night's sleep, often causing REM deprivation. Moreover, if you do not fall asleep within 30 minutes, then get out of bed and do an activity conducive to sleep (i.e., read). By sleeping several hours before your night shift and then no more than four hours after it, you will not reset your circadian rhythm and you will avoid the physiological drain of recuperation from the time change.

Pharmaceuticals that assist in falling asleep decrease the proportion of REM sleep, and many promote drug dependence. Unfortunately, there is no perfect solution. Alcohol decreases the proportion of REM sleep as well, thus ensuing poor quality sleep. Central nervous system stimulants, such as nicotine and caffeine, impede the onset of sleep and normal sleep stage progression, resulting in fragmented sleep. You should thus avoid caffeinated beverages four hours prior to sleeping.

Finally, do not forget the value of room darkening shades, white noise fans, and the silence button on your telephone!

Time Management

In life, we have either reasons or results …

PETER MCWILLIAMS (1950–2000)

Time management is the best gift you can give yourself. Emergency physicians are masters of multitasking. However, to truly succeed in maintaining wellness, one has to make a personal mission statement and honor it. It describes who you are, what your values are, and what you want to do in your life. This one step will enable everything else to fall into place. This necessitates much soul searching and honest introspection.

Once you have made your personal mission statement, you can set realistic goals that honor your priorities. Your life goals should be just that: about all aspects of life, including personal relationships and work. Make a "to do" list for every day, but schedule in downtime to ensure it is reasonable. Schedule enough time to get the daily chores of living done (such as exercising, grocery shopping, getting your car inspected, and paying bills on time), and keep long-term projects on task by scheduling appropriate deadlines for objectives along the way. Most importantly, it is essential to regularly assess and modify goals as needed to ensure they remain in line with one's priorities.

One of the hardest phrases everyone needs to learn is how to say "no." Do not fall into the trap of being a people-pleaser and over-committing yourself in every aspect of your life. Each opportunity is just that—an opportunity to succeed or fail. If the task or project is not in accord with your mission statement then tactfully decline. Granted, some obligations must be honored and some sacrifices must be made. However, it is wiser to not go overboard and pay the price of disappointing them and yourself in failing to do a good job or failing to balance your other, more important projects in life. When appropriate, delegate tasks and finally, avoid procrastination.

Lifestyle

You have to have emptiness before it can be filled. You have to exhale before you can inhale.

TOM YEOMANS

Physicians are experts in delayed gratification. Many long years have been sacrificed to train for the job you practice today. Nevertheless, delayed gratification should not last perpetually and become a way of life itself. It is easy to let a career in medicine consume you. Consider hiring assistants to perform tasks that you normally would have before you had a demanding full-time occupation, such as a cleaning person, a landscaper, and a contractor for home projects and renovations. It may not be worth the few dollars you save by doing it yourself, unless you truly enjoy doing these tasks and find them relaxing. Household production research has recently expanded and weighing time versus cost will help you determine what price to put on your personal time. You are your own best article of trade.

At the same time, it is tempting to overindulge. Be careful to not lock yourself into maintaining a lifestyle that you simply cannot afford. There is no worse feeling than being bound to a lifestyle above your means where you are forced to work extra hours to maintain it, yet not have enough time to live and enjoy it. It is easy to develop a never-ending sense of emptiness that is always looking to be filled, often by material goods, which simply results in working more and living less. You should not sweat the small stuff. However, when the small stuff (expensive clothes, costly dinners, and extravagant travel) starts adding up to large sums, you might want to rethink them when they are equivalent to a half-day's pay or more. Take an inventory of all the unused items in your closet, garage, or attic, and remember them when the purchasing impulse strikes. Think twice before you buy a home or new car and question whether you really need the one you have chosen. Living above your means is a definite prescription for unhappiness.

Emergency physicians have remarkable flexibility in lifestyle options. There are very few absolute limitations, most of which are self-imposed. By setting up impossible standards, one will always fail.

Health

Be kind to your knees, you'll miss them when they're gone. Enjoy your body … don't be afraid of it, or what other people think of it, it's the greatest instrument you'll ever own.

BAZ LUHRMANN (1962–)

Simply put, your health is an absolute priority. There is no leeway or latitude here. You only have one you, and you are the only who can take care of it. You cannot function effectively over a lifetime, under the extraordinary levels of physical and mental stress that the emergency department requires, without first taking care of yourself. Often, physicians care less for themselves than they do for their own patients. Time constraints may restrict and frank denial may cloud physicians into not taking care of themselves.

It is a conscious decision to choose life-enhancing options. It requires emotional commitment to follow through with them, as they are tested daily. The rewards of these conscious choices are a sense of energy, well-being, and freedom. Endorphins are rewarding. Nothing compares to feeling well.

To this end, the obvious tenets hold true. Avoid smoking, excessive drinking, and drug use. Do not use unhealthy surrogates, such as food, as a stress-reducer or alternate for taking the time to care for yourself. Eat a balanced diet, low in salt. Work is often busy with no downtime, lending itself to diets high in sugar, fat, and caffeine. Quick meals of fast foods are readily available, easily consumed while standing, rapidly deliver an immediate sense of satiety, and exponentially raise one's cholesterol unnecessarily. Anticipation of imminent interruption looms in the back of one's mind while eating, preventing one from fully relaxing and digesting. Take vitamins to offset an imperfect diet.

Exercise is essential for both one's physical and mental well-being. It enhances the immune system. Find what works for you and stick with it. Whatever activity you enjoy that gives you weight resistance is the one you need to do on a consistent basis. Resistance training is important for bone density, muscle toning, and joint function. Aerobic exercise will help prevent the fatigue from standing on your feet an entire shift.

Exercising in the morning before a shift is a great way to start your day and prepare yourself for the day's activities. Others prefer exercising after a shift to release the day's tensions. Hire a personal trainer to get yourself started on a fitness program or to keep yourself motivated in following one. Invest in home equipment or join a gym. Do whatever it takes, but this is one area where you absolutely must succeed. A few dollars now will help reduce your cardiovascular risk later, which is a bigger expense. Stretch before, during, and after your shifts. It will make you feel better and may even make them feel as if they are going by faster.

Wear comfortable clothes and especially comfortable shoes during your shifts. If you are not at ease, you will not get that intubation as easily. Make sure you are warm enough for your night shifts when your circadian rhythm drops your body temperature at 3 AM. Take the time to practice universal precautions. You are your only true overseer of this effort.

Schedule regular check ups. Make sure you get your timely mammograms, colonoscopies, and cholesterol profiles. Request help when you need it, either from family or friends, colleagues, or professional counselors.

Finally, massages, facials, manicures/pedicures, saunas, and acupuncture can help relieve those tired muscles after the most harrowing of shifts. Meditation may also help. But, throughout it all, do not forget to breathe. Oxygen is the best nutrient you can give your cells.

Aging

People grow old only by deserting their ideals. Years may wrinkle the skin, but to give up interest wrinkles the soul.

DOUGLAS MACARTHUR (1880–1964)

Aging is inevitable. You can embrace it or fear it. The latter makes it more difficult to accept the changes that come with time. Continual growth is essential. Grow in every way. Stretch yourself—physically and intellectually. Keep your mind sharp. Read for work and also enjoyment. Cultivate your interests both inside and outside of medicine. Learn how to speak Italian, take a cooking class, grow a garden, decorate your home, volunteer in a shelter, or become active in your place of worship. Sing. Pursue another degree. Remain active. Be present. Process your experiences. Learn from them. Respect them.

Alterations in hearing, vision, reflexes, and stamina make it more difficult to work in the emergency department and to cycle the clock in rotating shifts. If you are on prescription medications, make sure you take them and adjust them as appropriate for your shifts. Get enough sleep. Eat well. Continue to exercise.

Be good to yourself and understand that what you did when you were 20 is not what you can safely do at 60. Accept the aging process. Enjoy the true wisdom, inner peace, and quiet that only comes with age. Embrace tranquility. Welcome the satisfaction that is found in a life well lived. Smile at the wrinkles. Overlook the failures.

Be open to career transitions and alternative work opportunities in emergency medicine. Be willing to make changes. Opportunity knocks every day—it is just a matter of recognizing it. You may discover a new role for yourself in administration, education, community relations, or even public office.

One of the difficulties in accepting age is that others age with you, notably those you care about. It is very stressful to endure a family illness, to assume the care of an aging parent, or to become the caregiver or provider for significant others who previously used to care for themselves.

There is no perfect formula or recipe for living a life of meaning, success, and longevity. By continuously evaluating and modifying your goals, you will not find yourself in a mid-life crisis, looking for the answers to life's questions. You will come to realize that success does not require arrival.

Financial Management

The way I see it, if you want the rainbow, you gotta put up with the rain.

DOLLY PARTON (1946–)

It is easy to postpone financial planning, but you should start as early as possible, even during training. Money does not define who you are, and it is important to not lose sight of that concept.

Plan ahead because life is full of surprises. Dividing financial planning into three different phases of life will help you plan accordingly. The first phase—the transition period—is the time from the last year of residency to the fifth year of practice. Much happens during this phase professionally, with growth as an attending and the completion of the boards. This is paralleled by dramatic growth financially. It is essential to create a budget and spend suitably. Many will buy a new car, buy a home, pay off credit card debts, and pay off school loans. This requires strategy. Moreover, during this period you should purchase maximum disability insurance, adequate life insurance to cover your dependents, and an umbrella policy as an adjunct to your homeowners or automobile insurance. You should take advantage of insurance benefits offered by your employer. If you need to purchase professional liability insurance, research all options. Utilize pretax savings by contributing the maximum to your retirement plans. The earlier you invest in retirement contributions, the faster you will realize financial independence. Begin estate planning by compiling a will and trust.

Phase two is a period of greatest income. This is the time to accumulate significant wealth. During this phase, you should supplement retirement objectives, save money for your children's educations, and accelerate debt payments (such as paying off the mortgage you secured in phase one). Invest in stocks and mutual funds. Professional advice is strongly suggested for this area, unless you are truly adept in following the market. Choose your advisor wisely.

Phase three is the pre-retirement/retirement period. It commences five years before retirement. During this time, you must decide how to allocate your investment portfolio that you have worked so hard to accumulate. Retirement is a significant period of your life where you will live in a manner different than you have been used to. Living on a fixed income will be an adjustment. Think about how you are going to spend your free time. Your portfolio needs to balance the increase of inflation and taxation. Retirement distribution should stress flexibility. Estate planning is now a priority, and an attorney can help greatly. Options to reduce estate tax need to be explored, such as irrevocable life insurance trusts, gifts to individuals, and charitable gifts to those in need.

Burnout

Sometimes you're ahead, sometimes you're behind … the race is long, and in the end, it's only with yourself.

BAZ LUHRMANN

Medicine is a vocation. It is not your identity. Plan your career; do not let it plan you. You should sincerely love the job you choose and feel good about the work you do, otherwise, it is not fun and you will not last in the profession. Do not get trapped into thinking that your paycheck defines your self-worth or the perceived status of your position determines your real value. Your personal happiness and self-fulfillment are what matter most. You are whole and complete outside of medicine. Live with intention.

Burnout is a state of exhaustion that results from intense work in emotionally draining situations over time. It is a depletion of one's spirit that is felt physically and emotionally. Burnout is a gradual process that does not happen overnight. It is found in individuals under constant pressure.

Chronic fatigue, emotional exhaustion, cynicism, feelings of helplessness and hopelessness, depersonalization, and perceived lack of control over one's working conditions are common symptoms of burnout. Fatigue and emotional exhaustion were expected in training. This concept of martyrdom is then reinforced in the workplace when one places the needs of their patients before their own. Work overload and the difficulty in continuously meeting this volume contribute to the development of this phenomenon. Burnout is often seen in doctors who are very successful in their careers and who over-achieve. Such altruism in the extreme can thus lead to feelings of resentment or anger. These thoughts are frequently repressed, only to later manifest in feelings of frustration and irritability.

Once in this downward spiral, it is difficult but not impossible to recover. Fear of incompetence is a common feeling in physicians and learning to say "I don't know" is crucial. No one is perfect. Accept that. There will always be someone that knows more about a specific area of the body, because the emergency physician is not limited to one body region, and the breadth and depth of this knowledge is exhausting.

Know when to schedule a vacation, and take a real one. Continuing medical education conferences are not vacations. Furthermore, leisure is not relaxation. Take the time to rest the mind and the body. In a quiet setting, reflect and renew by processing your feelings. Feel your fears; cry your tears. Don't repress them. Ask for help when you need it.

Longevity

To leave the world a bit better whether by a healthy child, a garden patch, or a redeemed social condition;
To know even one life has breathed easier because you have lived.
This is to have succeeded.

RALPH WALDO EMERSON

We are fortunate enough to truthfully do this every day and feel the incredible, unrivaled rewards of relieving someone's pain. It really does not get any better than that. It is a gift that we all have been given, worked to develop, and continue to practice every day.

The best way to predict your future is to make it. You have to fall a few times before you learn to walk. Never forget that *you* are the one in control of your life! You have got what it takes—it has been in you all along, just waiting for you to find it. Decide upon the values that are most important to you, and live by them always. Never compromise them or give them up, even when it seems as though that is the only way to get what you want. You may win in the short term, but never in the long run. Learn to prize what truly is of value and live your life for yourself.

Selected Readings

Flanagan PJ. Manage your finances one phase at a time. *Resid Staff Physician* 2003;1(suppl):12.

Guzzardi LJ. Financial planning. In: Andrew LB, Pollack ML, eds. *Wellness for Emergency Physicians*. Chicago: American College of Emergency Physicians 1995:17–20.

Harkin KE. *Taking Care of Yourself*. Empire State EPIC. New York State Chapter. Chicago: American College of Emergency Physicians 2004;21.

Harkin KE, Moorhead JC. Choosing a career in emergency medicine. In: Harkin KE, Cushman JT, Wei HG, eds. *Emergency Medicine: The Medical Student Survival Guide*. Irving, TX: Emergency Medicine Residents' Association, 2001:7–8.

Koltonow SH. Physician Well-being. In: Tintinalli JE, Kelen GD, Stapczynski JS, eds. *Emergency Medicine: A Comprehensive Study Guide*, ed 5. New York: McGraw-Hill, 2000:1943–1948.

Margulies JL, Pollack ML. Developing a healthy lifestyle. In: Andrew LB, Pollack ML, eds. *Wellness for Emergency Physicians*. Chicago: American College of Emergency Physicians, 1995:24–26.

Menapace C. Can you put a price on personal time? *Resid Staff Physician* 2003:13(Suppl).

Perina DG, Chisholm CD. Physician wellness in an academic career. In: Hobgood C, Zink B, eds. *Emergency Medicine: An Academic Career Guide*, ed 2. Irving, TX: Society for Academic Emergency Medicine and Emergency Medicine Residents' Association, 1999:53–58.

Pollack ML, Pollack FS. Health, diet, and exercise. In: Andrew LB, Pollack ML, eds. *Wellness for Emergency Physicians*. Chicago: American College of Emergency Physicians, 1995:21–23.

Slapper DD, Mazur N. Career planning and longevity. In: Andrew LB, Pollack ML, eds. *Wellness for Emergency Physicians*. American College of Emergency Physicians, 1995:3–7.

Whitehead DC. Using circadian principles in emergency medicine scheduling. In: Andrew LB, Pollack ML, eds. *Wellness for Emergency Physicians*. American College of Emergency Physicians, 1995:8–13.

188 Faculty Development

Nicholas J. Jouriles

Faculty development is important for the evolution of all emergency physicians' careers. While traditionally thought of as only applying to academicians, successful faculty—or personal—development is the hallmark of growth and success in each emergency physician's career. In academics, the emergency physician's institution provides the ground rules for success. In non-academic careers, the skills needed by individual emergency physicians to grow and succeed in their careers are defined by the individual and the situation.

Academic Emergency Medicine

In academics, the institution (usually a medical school or university) defines the criteria for success usually as academic promotion and tenure. Universities have formal structures for these achievements, including bylaws and committee review. The traditional "up or out," publish or perish system is still common at many universities. The award of tenure is seen as a protection of academic freedom. Department chairs must ensure that good junior faculty members appointed at the assistant professor level eventually receive promotion and tenure.

Tenure is based on the candidate's record of performance in the areas of teaching, research, and service. The most important aspect by far is research. Publication quality is more important than quantity. While one theoretically could be tenured after publishing only a single landmark publication, most institutions count and judge the number of publications of which the candidate is the first author. In addition, publications can be judged by the number of times they are cited as a reference in subsequent publications.

The specific number of publications needed for promotion varies from institution to institution; 10 to 15 first-author publications of original scientific work is a good benchmark for most universities. Books, book chapters, case reports, and monographs may count, but usually not with the same weight as original scientific research. Unfunded research and presentations at scientific meetings are also considered.

Extramural funding of research from sources that evaluate proposals on a peer-reviewed competitive basis, such as the National Institutes of Health (NIH) or Centers for Disease Control (CDC), usually provide very convincing evidence of the quality and importance of the scholarly activity.

Teaching is also important, and most universities value medical student teaching over resident teaching. Faculty members seeking promotion must list all courses and the number of students taught, including an estimate of total student contact hours. The quality of teaching must be documented through student feedback and peer evaluation.

Many universities now offer an alternative to the traditional tenure tract, often termed *the clinician educator tract*. In this tract, there is usually less pressure to perform and publish research. Faculty members in this tract are promoted based on service and excellence in either teaching or research. Evidence of teaching awards or publications related to educational efforts constitutes excellent evidence of activity worthy of academic promotion.

Because teaching and service are the basis of promotion, it is imperative that faculty in this tract meticulously document their activities. A well-constructed portfolio that documents teaching and service is a great way to accomplish this task. The portfolio should be started early in one's career and updated weekly. Ideally, it should be organized based on the university's criteria for promotion. In that way, all relevant information can be quickly collated when presented to the promotions committee. An informal meeting with the promotions committee chair early in one's career can provide invaluable insight about how to succeed at the task of promotion.

Skills vital to an academic emergency physician's development include teaching, curriculum development, research, and the ability to compete for grants. In addition, computer skills, time management, and rudimentary business acumen are important.

Teaching and curriculum are fundamental to academics, but most physicians learn by emulating role models. Simple educational techniques increase the chances of success. Curriculum and teaching based on learning objectives and meaningful evaluation of the learner have the best chance for success.

Research skills are dependent on an inquisitive mind and a grasp of the scientific method. While background information such as statistical analysis is taught in formal courses, mentoring is probably the best way to ensure a successful research career.

Computer skills such as word processing, communication skills, information gathering/analyzing, and presentation graphics are mandatory for all academic emergency physicians. Time management is important, because there is never enough time to do all that is needed. Emergency physicians should be very good at this skill, for effective time management is a series of prioritizations.

Academic emergency physicians should take advantage of the common resources provided by the institution such as libraries, secretarial support, multidepartmental research opportunities, and workshops on teaching skills, curriculum development, and grant writing.

The junior faculty member and the chair must work out an effective strategy for balancing research, teaching, and service. It is very helpful to place objectives and long-term strategy in writing. The chair should provide mentors, ensure financial support for research, and protect research time for the junior faculty member.

Providing start-up resources for research should be part of the department's budget. This may mean that a portion of the department's clinical revenue needs to be allocated for new faculty members. This prudent investment in junior faculty improves recruitment and retention, which ultimately strengthens the whole department. In some institutions, seed grants are also available.

New faculty members should receive few, if any, committee assignments or administrative responsibilities. Committee work can be a "time robber" for junior faculty, as that time could be spent more productively working on grant preparation, research, teaching, or publications.

Individual Career Development

Career development is also important for non-academic emergency physicians. Most physicians receive little or no formal training for the administrative aspects of their careers. To be successful, emergency physicians must continuously acquire new skills. Any course of personal professional development must be planned. There should be both short- and long-term goals. Once the emergency physician determines his/her long-term goals, it becomes easier to decide what steps need to be taken to get there. Short-term goals are those steps.

In deciding goals, a careful assessment of what resources are needed helps to avoid failure. Issues such as over-commitment and personal or family conflict should be considered. Time, money, and effort are all resources that physicians must spend with extreme caution. Young emergency physicians often have commitments to spouse and children that must be factored into the equation.

Knowledge and skills can be acquired by self-instruction, short courses, attending seminars given by professional organizations, enrolling in formal courses of instruction sponsored by universities or business schools, or by accepting tasks from professional organizations.

Mentoring is an important concept for junior emergency physicians. A mentor should have documented accomplishments. An academic mentor can help interpret the literature, suggest projects that need to be done, identify funding sources, and provide critical reviews of grant applications and manuscripts before they are submitted. In some cases, a laboratory will also be available. A mentor for the non-academic emergency physician can help with clinical practice, business and management skills.

An often-overlooked aspect of career development is orientation to a new job. Each emergency physician should be provided an orientation for each new job that focuses on the culture and mission of the institution or group. A successful orientation will ease the transition of the new emergency physician into the group. It will also clarify expectations and requirements. The more one knows about one's job the more effective—and successful—one can be.

Summary

To succeed, emergency physicians must evolve with their careers. Since institutional and group values and rewards change over time, the individual must develop skills that will survive an entire career. Matching self-development with the objectives and rewards of one's employer will lead to long-term success and satisfaction.

Selected Readings

Farrell SE, Digioia NM, Broderick KB, Coates WC. Mentoring for clinician-educators. *Acad Emerg Med* 2004;11:1346–1350.

Jouriles NJ, Kuhn GJ, Moorhead JC, et al. Faculty development in emergency medicine. *Acad Emerg Med* 1997;4:1078–1086.

Kuhn GJ. Faculty development: the educator's portfolio: its preparation, uses, and value in academic medicine. *Acad Emerg Med* 2004;11:307–311.

Propp DA, Glockman S, Ueharra DT. ED leadership competency matrix: an administrative management tool. *Am J Emerg Med* 2002;21:483–488.

Rust G, Taylor V, Morrow R, et al. The Morehouse faculty development program: methods and 3-year outcomes. *Fam Med* 1998;30:162–167.

SUBJECT INDEX

A

ABC (airway/breathing/circulation)
ABCDE Protocol for First Survey of Children
    with Trauma, The, Table 178.1, 971
Abdominal
    /GI disorders, 43-45
    imaging, trauma patients, 46-57, 70-74,
        855-859, 890-893
    injuries, 930-939
    malignancies, 75-83
    radiology for FB localization, 890-893
    trauma, pediatric, 608-613, 970-974
    x-rays/CT imaging for hydrocarbon toxic-
        ity-related perforations, 855-859
Abnormal Uterine Bleeding, Table 123.1, 715
Abnormality(ies)
    blood cell production, 267-271
    bone, 375-381
    electrolyte
      in AML, 280-285
        pediatric, 585-593
    muscle, 393-395
    radiographic, after liquid hydrocarbon
        aspiration, 701-704
    uterine bleeding, 713-722
Abortion, 461-475
Abrasion(s)
    corneal, 240-251, 912-914
    facial, 907-911
Abruptio placenta, 461-475
Abscess(es)
    Bartholin gland, 713-722
    brain, 444-449, 450-458
    felon, 396-399
    large bowel, 84-88
    lateral, nail skin fold, 396-399
    liver, 58-65
    ovarian, 483-488
    pancreatic, 70-74
    parameningeal, 444-449
    peridontal, 235-239
    perirectal, 89-94
    peritonsillar, 235-239
    retropharyngeal, pediatric, 496-506
    S. aureus infections, 161-162
    TOA, 713-722
    visceral, 660-663
Abstinence syndromes, 816-819
Abuse, child, 543-549, 608-613, 970-974
Academic emergency medicine,
    1024-1025
Acalculous cholecystitis, AIDS-related,
    341-364
Accelerated hypertension, 148-155
Access to medical records, 1011-1018
Accident scene assessment of traumatic
    injuries, 885-886
Acetaminophen (APAP) poisoning,
    792-794
Achalasia treatment, 46-57
Acid
    -base disturbances, diagnosis, 179-184
    ingestion, 46-57

Acidosis
    hemodialysis, 813-815
    lactic, 179-184
    metabolic, 179-184
    pediatric metabolic, 507-528, 585-593
    respiratory, 179-184
Acinar tissue loss in pancreatitis, 70-74
Acne, 159-160
Acquired immunodeficiency syndrome
    (AIDS), *See also* AIDS
    diseases (rheumatic fever, collagen vascular
        diseases, dermatomyositis,
        polymyositis, Reiter's syndrome,
        rheumatoid arthritis), 291-297
    Hodgkin's disease inpatients, 264-266
    nephritis, 58-65
    prevention/post exposure prophylaxis,
        341-364
Acromioclavicular separation, 940-944
ACS-Associated Symptoms, Table 17.3, 100
ACS Signs and Symptoms: Clinical
    Conditions to Consider in the
    Differential Diagnosis, Table 17.2,
    100
Activated charcoal decontamination
    anticholinergic agent toxicity, 810-812
    drug overdose therapy, 830-833
    multiple-dose, properties, 789-791
    oral opioid ingestion, 802-804
    sedative-hypnotic medication overdose,
        785-788
ACTH (adrenocorticotropic hormones),
    185-186, 585-593
Active and Latent Failure Types, Table 183.3,
    997
Acute
    angle closure glaucoma, 444-449
    appendicitis (AA), 75-83
    bacterial
      conjunctivitis therapy, 240-251
      prostatitis, 723-727
    bronchitis, 685-687
    cardiac life support (ACLS), 766-770
    chest syndrome, sickle cell anemia,
      pediatric, 570-573
    closed angle glaucoma (ACG), 240-251
    cocaine intoxication-induced mental state
      changes, 798-801
    coronary syndrome (ACS) complications
      of hypertension, 148-155
    decompensated heart failure (ADHF),
      117-124
    gastritis, 46-57
    glomerulonephritis (GN), 651-654
    gout, 382-385
    hematogeneous osteomyelitis, 375-381
    hyperglycemia, 365-371
    intermittent porphyria, 426-430
    interstitial nephritis (AIN), 664-665
    life-threatening event (ALTE), 496-506
    lumbosacral strain, 386-390
    lung injury, transfusion-related, 272-279
    lymphocytic leukemia (ALL), 280-285

    malaria, 329-335
    mesenteric ischemia (AMI), 75-83
    motor
      axonal neuropathy (AMAN), 422-425
      sensory axonal neuropathy
        (AMSAN), 422-425
    mountain sickness (AMS) management,
      759-765
    myeloid leukemia (AML), 280-285
    myocardial infarction (AMI)
      adult, 97-116, 134-147
      pediatric, 9-13
    necrotizing ulcerative gingivitis (ANUG),
      235-239
    otitis media (ACM), pediatric, 550-569
    pancreatitis, 70-74, 187-196
    pulmonary edema, 117-124
    renal failure (ARF), 179-184, 574-584,
      651-654, 660-663, 666-672
    respiratory distress syndrome (ARDS),
      705-706, 707-709
    retroviral infection, 291-297
    rheumatic fever, 291-297
    rhinosinusitis, 226-234
    spinal cord compression, 431-433
    stroke, 444-449
    trauma life support (ATLS), 766-770
    tubular necrosis (ATN), 651-654, 666-672
    urethritis, gonoccocal infection-induced,
      309-328
    viral hepatitis, 58-65
Acyanotic congenital heart defects, pediatric,
    529-542
Adenocarcinomas (AC), esophageal, 46-57
Adenomyosis, 713-722
Adenovirus-causing conjunctivitis, 240-251
Adhesives, surgical, 952-959
Adjuvant therapy
    alcohol withdrawal, 816-819
    methemoglobinemia, 870-872
Administration
    leadership in the emergency department,
      975-1025
    professonalism, 1011-1018
Admission and Discharge Criteria, Table
    110.3, 658
Adnexal torsion, 713-722
Adolescent(s)
    blood pressure measurement, 148-155
    STDs among, 574-584
Adrenal
    diseases, 177-216
    hyperplasia, pediatric congenital, 585-593
    insufficiency
      diagnosis, 185-186
      symptom of Sheehan's syndrome, 211-212
Adult(s)
    blood pressure measurement, 148-155
    cardiopulmonary resuscitation, 3-8
    epiglottitis, 235-239
    intestinally-absorbed botulism, 309-328
    pulmonary arrest patient resuscitation, 1-13
Advanced Cardiac Life Support (ACLS), 3-8

Hypopyon, abnormal fluid collection, external eye, 240-251
Hypospadias, 723-727
Hypotension
  acute infection process-related, 365-371
  dialysis patients, 673-676
  drug-related, 440-443
Hypothermia, 739-752
Hypothermia: Predisposing Factors, Table 127.4, 744
Hypothyroidism, symptom of Sheehan's syndrome, 211-212
Hypovolemic shock, 885-886
Hypoxia
  stress at high altitudes, 759-765
  tissue, 179-184

I

Iatrogenic botulism, 309-328
Ileus
  adynamic, 75-83
  gallstone, 66-69, 75-83
Iliac crest, 945-948
Imaging
  acute pyelonephritis, 655-659
  angiographic, intracranial lesions, 403-414
  CT
    abdominal, 46-57
    cerebral atrophy, 341-364
    cerebrovascular disorders, 403-414
    CNS
      lymphoma, 341-364
      tumors, 450-458
    emphysema, subcutaneous, 219-220
    fascia, deep, 396-399
    gallbladder, 66-69
    headache, 444-449
    hydrocarbon toxicity-related perforations, 855-859
    neuroimaging, 291-297, 440-443
    osteomyelitis, 375-381
    PE, 697-700
    PID, 713-722
    pituitary apoplexy, 211-212
    /plane radiography, for trauma patients, 890-893
    SAH early detection, 444-449
    SBO, 75-83
    spinal
      cord, 431-433
      injuries, 431-433, 899-906
      stenosis, 386-390
    trauma patients, 890-893
    /US, septic shock patients, 365-371
  Doppler, for PE, 697-700
  genitourinary injuries, 949-951
  hepatocellular carcinoma, 58-65
  MRI
    angiography, 403-414
    central
      nervous system tumors, 450-458
      seventh nerve lesions, 415-418
    cerebral atrophy, 341-364
    hepatocellular carcinoma, 58-65
    infratentorial tumors, 450-458
    MS, 419-421
    myelography, spinal injuries, 899-906
    myocardial perfusion, 97-116
    nervous system disorders, 401
    neuroimaging, 291-297
    osteomyelitis, 375-381

pituitary apoplexy, 211-212
soft tissue, 890-893
spinal
  injuries, 899-906
  stenosis, 386-390
stroke syndrome exclusion with, 148-155
nuclear lung scans, 697-700
pediatric fractures, 594-602
plane radiography/CT, trauma patients, 890-893
pyelogram (IVP)
  genitourinary injuries, 890-893, 949-951
  intravenous, 890-893, 949-951
radiographic, for chronic rhinosinusitis, 226-234
US
  during pregnancy, 461-475
  pediatric
    testicular flow assessment, 574-584
    upper GI series, 507-528
X-ray
  abdominal, 70-74
  chest, 117-124, 127-128, 129-130, 131-133, 651-654, 685-687, 697-700, 707-709, 855-859, 890-893, 916-919, 930-939
  gastric tumors, 46-57
Immediate on-scene care, catastropic disaster, 26-28
Immune
  system disorders, 289-306
  thrombocytopenic purpura, 257-263
Immunization
  DPT, 309-328
  influenza, 341-364
  mumps, 341-364
Immunosuppressive medication complications, 298-300
Imperforate hymen, 713-722
Impetigo, 161-162
Impetigo-like infection, 166-167
Inborn metabolism errors, pediatric, 585-593
Incident Command System (ICS), 17-22
Incision(s)
  drainage, 952-959
  epidermoid inclusion cysts, 171
Indicated Antibiotics for Suspected Acute Bacterial Rhinosinusitis, Table 51.6, 233
Indication for Pacemaker Placement, Table 17.7, 113
Indications for Skeletal Survey, Table 98.5, 612
Individual career development for emergency medicine physicians, 1024-1025
Infant(s)
  GI bleeding, 507-528
  intestinally-absorbed botulism, 309-328
Infection(s)
  acute retroviral, 291-297
  anal canal, 89-94
  bacterial, 161-162, 309-328, 685-687
  bite wound, 771-782
  blood transfusion-related, 272-279
  C. albicans, 163-164
  C. pneumoniae, 309-328
  C. psittaci, 309-328
  CAP, 691-695
  cardiac transplantation, 298-300
  chlamydial, 309-328
  conjunctivitis, 240-251
  CSF shunt, 434-439

DISC, 386-390
EAC, 221-222
erysipelas, 396-399
extragenital, 483-488
eye, 240-251
fungal, 163-164, 221-222, 341-364
genital chlamydial, 309-328
gonococcal, 309-328
Gram positive/negative sepsis, 365-371
H. pylori, 46-57
head/neck, 219-220
HPV, HIV patients, 341-364
impetigo-like, 166-167
intertriginous, 341-364
M. catarrhalis, 685-685, 691-695
malarial, 329-335
muscle tissue, 396-399
mycoplasma, erythromycin treatment, 172
oral candidiasis, 235-239
parasitic, 165, 329-335
pediatric
  CNS, 543-549
  lower respiratory tract, 496-506
  sweat gland, 240-251
  systemic, 543-549
  upper airway, 496-506
  urinary tract, 550-569
pseudomonal, 434-439
puerperal, 483-488
retroviral, 291-297
soft tissue, 396-399
streptococcal pharyngitis, 651-654
systemic, pediatric, 543-549
toxoplasmosis, 329-335
urinary tract
  general, 43-45
  male, 723-727
vascular access site, dialysis patients, 673-676
viral, 166-167, 240-251, 341-364
Infectious
  arthritis, 382-385
  clotting complications, 272-279
  diseases, 307-371, 550-569
  esophagitis, 46-57
  mononucleosis (IM), 341-364
  pneumonia, 705-706
  proctitis, 89-94
  vasculitis, 169
Infection Criteria Guidelines for the Use of Drotregcogin (XIGRIS®), Table 67.2, 370
Inflammation, lacrimal/melbomian glands, 240-251
Inflammatory
  bowel disease (IBD), 75-83, 172
  esophageal disorders, 46-57
  liver disease, 58-65
  muscle disease, 291-297
Influenza
  -induced meningitis, 434-439
  viruses, 341-364
Informed consent, 647-648
Infratentorial tumors, 450-458
Ingestion, caustic agents, 855-859
Inhalation of caustic agents, 855-859
Initial Approach to a Patient with Presumed ACS, Table 17.6, 109
Injury(ies)
  abdominal, 930-939
  acute lung, transfusion-related, 272-279

Urologic injuries, 949-951
Urticaria, 170, 301-306
Uterine
atony/rupture, 483-488
bleeding, dysfunctional, 713-722
function, 713-722
inversion, 476-482
prolapse, 713-722
ruptures, 476-48, 963-969
tumors, 713-722

V

Vaccination(s)
AIDSVAX HIV trials, 291-297
pediatric
H. influenza, 570-573
S. pneumoniae, 570-573
postexposure, for hepatitis B, 728-731
rabies, 341-364
rubella, 341-364
Vaginal
discharge, 713-722
foreign bodies, 713-722
tears during intercourse, 732-735
Valves, mitral, stenosis, 131-133
Valvular disease, 131-133
Varicella (chicken pox), pediatric, 550-569
Varicella
chickenpox, 166-167, 550-569
-zoster virus (VZV), 221-222, 341-364
Varices
esophageal, 46-57
gastric, 46-57
Varicoceles, 723-727
Variola, DNA virus causing smallpox, 35-40
Vascular
access site infections, dialysis patients,
673-676
bleeding, head/neck, 219-220
disease
collagen, 291-297
ischemic, 461-475
peripheral, 156-158
injuries, 890-893, 930-939
Vaso-occlusion in sickle cell disease pediatric
patients, 570-573
Vein(s)
central retinal, occlusion, 240-251
deep, thrombosis, 156-158
Venereal disease, 732-735
Venous
catheters, 450-458
Doppler examination of PE, 697-700
thromboembolisms (VTE), 156-158,
697-700
thrombosis
deep, 461-475, 660-663
mesenteric, 75-83
Ventricular
ectopy, 134-137
fibrillation, 3-8, 97-116, 134-147
septal defect, pediatric, 529-542

tachycardia, 3-8, 134-147
Ventriculoatrial shunt (AV), 434-439
Ventriculomegaly, 434-439
Ventriculoperitoneal (VP) shunts, 434-439
Vertebrate envenomation, 771-782
Vertigo, alternobaric, 753-758
Vesicular/bullous lesions, 173
Vestibular neuronitis (labyrinthitis), 223-225
Vincent's Hierarchy of Factors Influencing
Clinical Practice, Table 183.4, 998
Viral
exanthems, 550-569
hepatitis, acute, 58-65
infections, 166-167, 240-251, 341-364
Viral Exanthems, Table 92.14, 568
Virus(es)
adeno-, conjunctivitis-causing, 240-251
coxsackie-, varicella-mimicking, 166-167
cytomegalo-
esophagitis, 46-57
liver, 58-65
DNA, smallpox-causing, 35-40
echo-, varicella-mimicking, 166-167
Epstein-Barr, 58-65, 291-297, 341-364
herpes simplex, 46-57, 166-167
human
immunodeficiency, 291-297
papilloma, 166-167
influenza, 341-364
Jakob-Kreutzfeldt, 341-364
papilloma in HIV patients, 291-297
paramyxo-, 341-364
pox-, 166-167
RNA, 58-65
varicella
-mimicking, 166-167
-zoster, reactivation, 221-222
variola, DNA, causing smallpox, 35-40
west Nile, 272-279
Visceral
abscesses, 660-663
intraabdominal injuries, 930-939
Visual disturbances, cranial nerve disorder-
induced, 415-418
Vital Sign Normal Values in Pediatric
Patients, Table 2.1, 11
Vitamin
B1 deficiency, 204-205
B12 deficiency, 204-205
D deficiency/excess, 204-205
K insufficiency impairing coagulation,
257-263
Vitreous hemorrhage, 240-251
Volvulus
gastric, 46-57
midgut, pediatric, 507-528
Vomiting
bilious, pediatric, 507-528
CNS tumor-induced, 450-458
von Willibrand's disease (vWD), 257-263,
272-279
Vulvar hematomas, 483-488
Vulvovaginitis, 713-722

W

Warts, plantar, 166-167
Water
homeostasis, 187-196
replacement, hypernatremia therapy,
187-196
shortages, clean, death-causing in Dafur,
Sudan, 23-25
Webs, esophgeal, 46-57
Wellness, physician, 1019-1023
Well's Clinical Parameters for VTE, Table
119.2, 698
Wernicke's
encephalopathy prevention, 816-819
-Korsakoff syndrome, 204-205
syndrome, 415-418
West Nile virus (WNV), 272-279
White blood cell count (WBC), 280-285
WHO/REAL Classification of the Non-
Hodgkin's Lymphomas, According
to Clinical Aggressiveness, Table
55.3, 266
Whole-bowel irrigation, 789-791
Withdrawal
from intoxication substances, 628-630,
816-819
symptoms, neonatal, 802-804
Wolff-Parkinson-White (WPW) syndrome,
134-147
World Health Organization (WHO) classification, non-Hodgkin's lymphoma,
264-266
Wound(s)
bite infections, 771-782
botulinum, 309-328
burn dressings, 960-963
care, 952-959
closure, 952-959
FBs, 952-959
infectious, post C section, 483-488
penetrating
thoracoabdominal, 920-929
neck, 219-220, 916-919
stab, laparotomy for resultant blood loss,
930-939
thoracoabdominal penetrating, 920-929
Wrist injuries, 940-944

X

X-ray imaging, *See also* Radiography
abdominal, 46-57, 70-74
chest, 117-124, 127-128, 129-130, 131-133
Xenobiotic cyanogens, 849-851

Y

Yersinia pestis, 309-328, 507-528

Z

Zeis gland infection, 240-251
Zygomatic fractures, 907-911

DRUG INDEX

A

Abciximab, 97-116
Abilify®, 619-624
Acebutolol, 837-839
Acetaminophen, 58-65, 70-74, 226-234, 301-306, 386-390, 391-392, 444-449, 759-765, 792-794
Acetic acid, 166-167, 221-222, 771-782
Acetylcholine, 688-690, 810-812
Acetylcholine inhibitor, 89-94
Acetylcholinesterase, 810-812
Actos, 867-869
Acyclovir, 46-57, 58-65, 89-94, 166-167, 172, 240-251, 341-364, 574-584
Adenosine, 97-116, 134-147, 298-300
Adrenergic inhibitors, 148-155
Agenerase, 291-297
Albendazole, 89-94, 426-430
Albuterol, 301-306, 496-506, 666-672, 679-684, 685-687
Alcohol, 625-627
α-blockers, 209-210, 816-819
Altepase (Rt-PA), 403-414
Amaril, 867-869
Amikacin, 341-364
Aminoglycosides, 240-251, 309-328, 329-335, 422-425, 434-439
Aminophylline, 685-687
Amiodarone, 3-8, 9-14, 58-65, 97-116, 134-147, 529-542
Amitriptyline, 58-65, 391-392
Amlodipine, 840-843
Amoxapine, 827-829
Amoxicillin, 31-34, 89-94, 226-234, 309-328, 341-364, 382-385
Amoxicillin-clavulanate, 161-162, 235-239, 496-506, 550-569, 691-695, 771-782
Amphetamines, 543-549
Amphotericin, 291-297, 341-364
Amphotericin B, 280-285
Ampicillin, 58-65, 309-328, 341-364, 444-449, 496-506, 507-528, 550-569, 655-659, 723-727
Ampicillin-Sulbactam, 550-569
Amrinone, 840-843
Amygdalin, 849-851
Analgesics, 43-45, 226-234, 235-239, 257-263, 386-390, 391-392, 444-449, 574-584, 603-607, 771-782
Anesthetics, 491-495, 625-627
Angiotensin-converting enzyme (ACE) inhibitor, 3-8, 70-74, 97-116, 298-300, 301-306, 529-542
Antacids, 46-57
Anthralin, 159-160
Antiarrhythmics, 3-8, 625-627
Antiasthmatics, 625-627

Antibiotics, 9-14, 35-40, 43-45, 46-57, 58-65, 66-69, 75-83, 127-128, 129-130, 131-133, 159-160, 161-162, 171, 172, 173, 221-222, 223-225, 226-234, 235-239, 280-285, 309-328, 336-340, 341-364, 375-381, 396-399, 444-449, 496-506, 507-528, 550-569, 594-602, 625-627, 679-684, 691-695, 713-722, 728-731, 739-752, 759-765, 771-782, 894-898, 907-911, 912-914, 952-959
Anticholinergics, 46-57, 159, 625-627, 679-684, 685-687, 688-690, 810-812
Anticonvulsants, 450-458, 543-549, 585-593, 625-627, 810-812, 816-819, 830-833, 894-898
Antidepressants, 46-57, 543-549, 625-627, 633-637, 785-788, 789-791, 810-812, 827-829
Antidysrhythmias, 837-839
Antiemetics, 43-45, 46-57, 444-449
Antiepileptics, 830-833
Antifungals, 163-164, 280-285, 341-364
Antihistamines, 166-167, 168, 226-234, 272-279, 301-306, 625-627, 771-782, 785-788, 810-812, 820-824
Antihypertensives, 625-627, 847-848
Anti-inflammatories, 46-57, 58-65, 66-69, 257-263, 291-297, 301-306, 341-364, 375-381, 382-385, 386-390, 391-392, 507-528, 550-569, 570-573, 574-584, 625-627, 660-663, 666-672, 679-684
Antimicrobials, 226-234, 444-449, 550-569, 723-727
Antiparkinsonian agents, 625-627, 785-788, 810-812
Antipruritics, 550-569
Antipsychotics, 46-57, 450-458, 619-624, 628-630, 638-639, 785-788, 810-812, 820-824
Antipyretics, 166-167, 739-752
Antitoxin, equine botulinum, 309-328
Antiviral agents, 625-627, 707-709
Anxiolytics, 628-630, 638-639, 642-646
Argatroban, 97-116, 286-287
Aripiprazole (Abilify®), 619-624, 820-824
Arsenic poisoning, 863-866
Artemisinin, 329-335
Aspirin, 3-8, 97-116, 257-263, 529-542, 550-569, 795-797, 867-869
Atenolol, 134-147, 816-819, 837-839
Ativan, 134-147, 440-443, 543-549, 638-639, 816-819

Atovaquone-proguanil, 329-335
Atropine, 3-8, 31-34, 134-147, 298-300, 529-542, 847-848
Avandia, 867-869
Azathioprine, 58-65, 70-74, 419-421
Azithromycin, 89-94, 226-234, 309-328, 329-335, 496-506, 550-569, 574-584, 688-690, 691-695, 713-722, 723-727
Aztreonam, 483-488, 655-659

B

Bacitracin, 159-160
Baclofen, 444-449
Barbiturates, 257-263, 666-672, 785-788, 805-806
Belladonna alkaloids, 543-549, 785-788, 810-812
Benzathine, 89-94
Benzimidazoles, 426-430
Benzisoxazole, 820-824
Benzodiazepines, 134-147, 309-328, 440-443, 450-458, 543-549, 628-630, 638-639, 666-672, 739-752, 785-788, 807-809, 816-819, 827-829
Benzoisothiazoyl-piperazine, 820-824
Benzoyl peroxide, 159-160, 161-162
Benztropine, 810-812
Bepridil, 840-843
β-blockers, 3-8, 97-116, 117-124, 131-133, 134-147, 159-160, 298-300, 301-306, 422-425, 625-627, 679-684, 688-690, 816-819, 837-839
β-lactam, 434-439, 688-690, 691-695
Betaxolol, 837-839
Bicarbonate, 187-196, 813-815, 666-672
Bismuth, 46-57
Bisoprolol, 837-839
Bitolterol, 679-684
Botulinum toxin, 89-94
Breutal, 603-607
Buproprion (Zyban, Wellbutrin), 633-637
Buspirone, 802-804
Butyrophenone, 820-824

C

Caffeine, 543-549, 834-836
Calcium
  channel blockers (CCBs), 46-57, 89-94, 97-116, 131-133, 298-300, 529-542, 785-788, 789-791, 840-843
  chloride, 187-196, 666-672, 813-815
  gluconate, 476-482, 666-672
Cannabis, 625-627

V

Valacyclovir, 46-57, 89-94, 166-167, 341-364, 574-584
Valium, 134-137, 440-443, 476-482, 543-549, 638-639, 816-819, 827-829
Valproic acid (Depakote), 58-65, 70-74, 633-637, 830-833
Vancomycin, 75-83, 280-285, 444-449, 507-528, 550-569, 570-573, 691-695
Vasodilators, 129-130
Vasopressin, 3-8, 9-14, 46-57, 365-371
Vasopressors, 403-414
Venlafaxine (Effexor), 633-637

Verapamil, 134-147, 298-300, 444-449, 529-542, 840-843
Versed, 603-607
Vigabatrin, 830-833
Viracept, 291-297
Voriconazole, 291-297

W

Warfarin, 156-158, 257-263, 286-287, 697-700
Wellbutrin, 633-637

X

Xenobiotics, 849-851

Z

Zaleplon, 805-806
Zidovudine, 58-65
Ziprasidone, 619-624, 820-824
Zoloft, 633-637
Zolpidem, 805-806
Zonisamide, 830-833
Zyban, 633-637
Zyprexa®, 619-624, 633-637, 820-824

INDEX of TABLES

WIDENER UNIVERSITY WOLFGRAM LIBRARY CHESTER, PA

LOOKING FOR WAYS TO HELP SAVE YOUR INSTITUTION TIME AND MONEY?

eACLS™: ACLS Renewal Training Made Easy

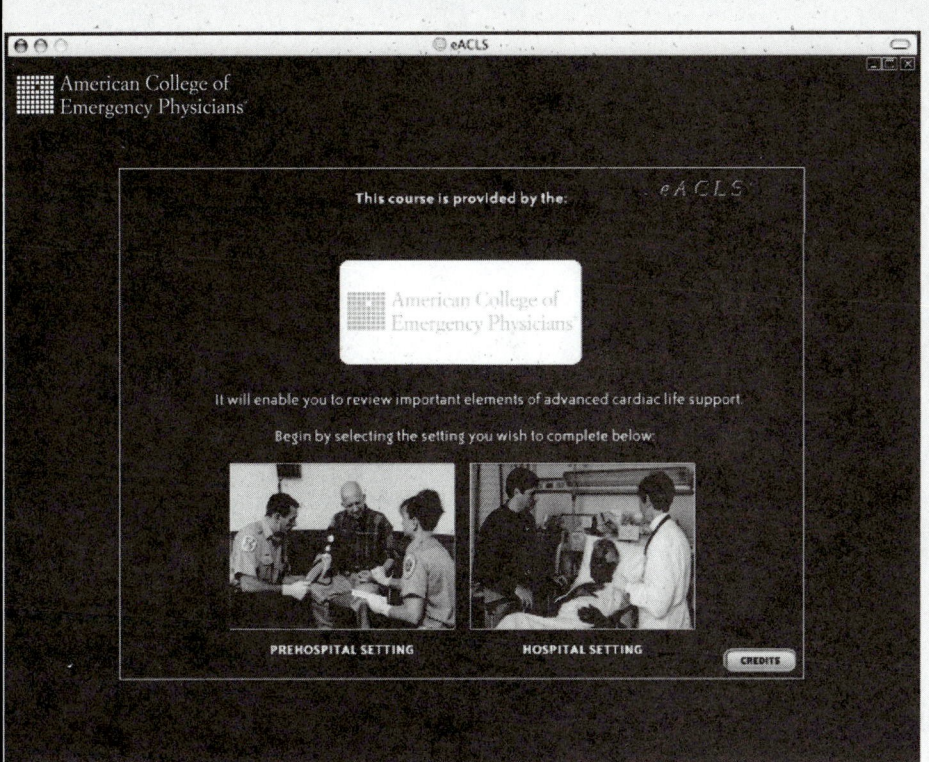

Save *time*, *money*, and get *superior training* with eACLS™

Experience the new standard in advanced cardiac life support (ACLS) training, brought to you by the American College of Emergency Physicians and Jones and Bartlett Publishers.

eACLS™ provides an electronic case-based approach to ACLS training. eACLS™ is a highly interactive, innovative program that includes more than 200 live-action video clips and 500 photos and animations.

Learn more about the advantages of eACLS™ Visit www.eACLS.com today!

Earn An ACLS Course Completion Card, Simply:

1. Complete the didactic portion of the eACLS™ course at www.eACLS.com.

2. Upon successful completion of the didactic portion, Course Completion acknowledgement and Continuing Education credits are immediately provided.

3. Users can print out and/or email the Course Completion acknowledgement and Continuing Education credits to the Institution Course Coordinator.

4. Skills verification can be completed easily and conveniently at the institution's location.

5. Upon successful completion of both didactic and skills portions, users can receive an ACEP eACLS™ wallet-sized Course Completion Card from the institution.

JONES AND BARTLETT PUBLISHERS
BOSTON   TORONTO   LONDON   SINGAPORE
40 Tall Pine Drive, Sudbury, MA 01776 • Phone: 800-832-0034 • Fax: 978-443-8000 • Email: info@jbpub.com

LEARN MORE ABOUT THE PATIENTS

According to recent statistics, about 34% of calls for emergency medical services involve patients over the age of 60. Conversely, pediatric calls account for less than 10% of emergency calls.

Whether you are treating an infant or an older adult, Jones & Bartlett has the resources you need.

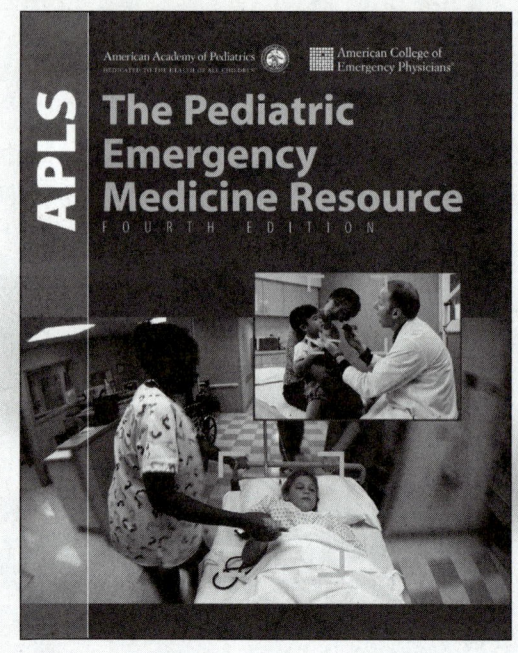

ISBN: 0-7637-3316-4
The definitive pediatric emergency medical resource!

NATIONAL CONTINUING EDUCATION PROGRAMS

PLACE YOUR ORDER TODAY!

Your order is risk-free. If you are not satisfied with your order, return it within 30 days for a full refund.

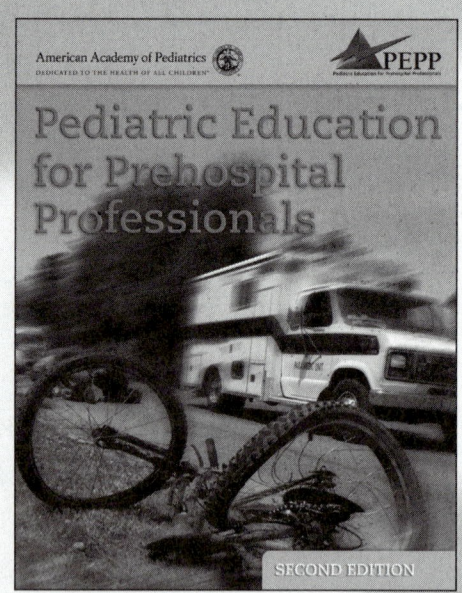

ISBN: 0-7637-2684-0

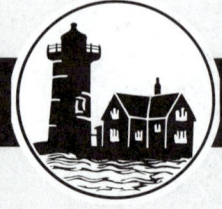

Jones ar

Phone: 800-832-00

OU SEE THE MOST... AND THE LEAST!

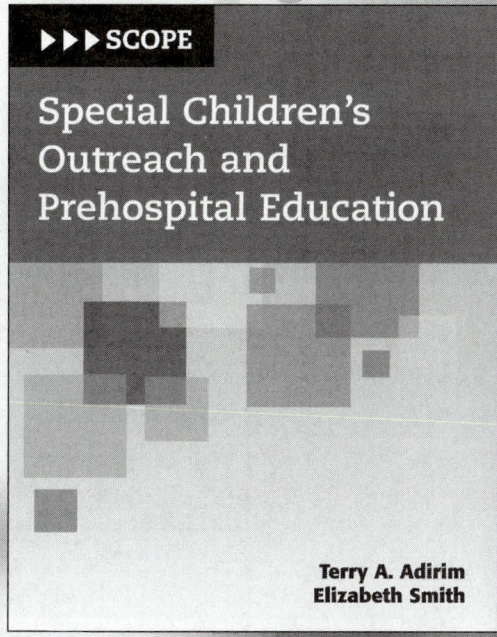

▶▶▶ SCOPE

Special Children's Outreach and Prehospital Education

Terry A. Adirim
Elizabeth Smith

ISBN: 0-7637-2468-8
Prepare for treating children with special health care needs!

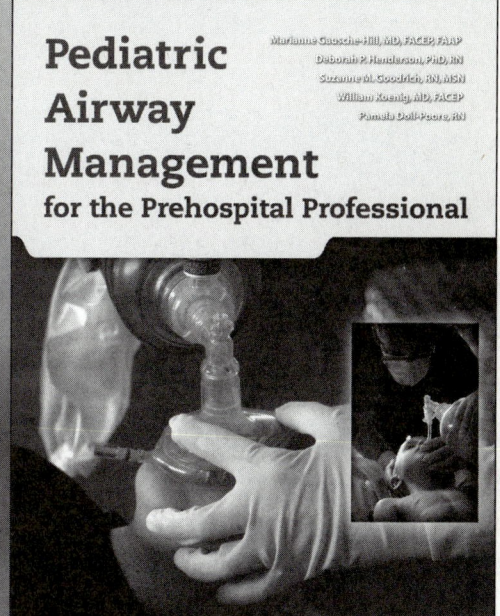

Pediatric Airway Management for the Prehospital Professional

Marianne Gausche-Hill, MD, FACEP, FAAP
Deborah P. Henderson, PhD, RN
Suzanne M. Goodrich, RN, MSN
William Koenig, MD, FACEP
Pamela Doll-Poore, RN

ISBN: 0-7637-2066-6
Master the challenges of a pediatric airway!

DESIGNED TO MEET YOUR TRAINING NEEDS!

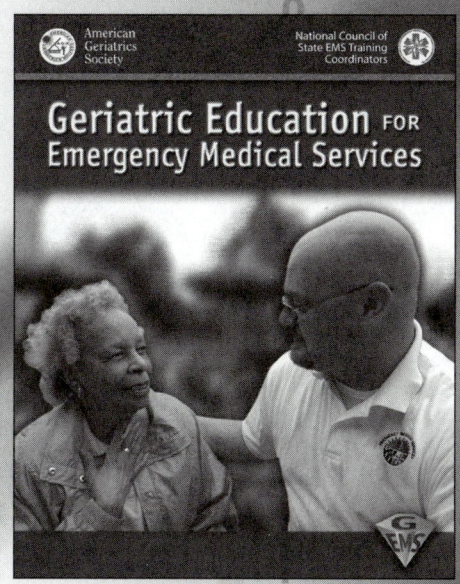

Geriatric Education FOR Emergency Medical Services

ISBN: 0-7637-2086-0

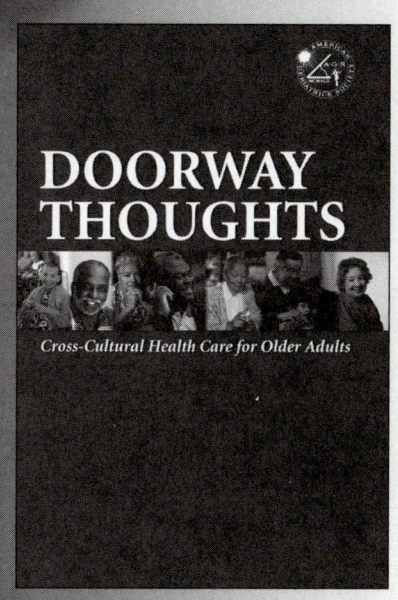

DOORWAY THOUGHTS

Cross-Cultural Health Care for Older Adults

ISBN: 0-7637-3338-5

artlett Publishers

Web: www.jbpub.com

THE DEFINITIVE RESOURCE ON EMERGENCY MEDICAL SERVICES SYSTEMS!

Principles of EMS Systems is the only resource to provide the latest information on timely topics such as EMS for Children, Rural EMS, Trauma Systems, and Response to Terrorist Incidents. This resource provides a complete education on what the components of an EMS system are and how they interrelate.

American College of Emergency Physicians
Paperback • 362 pages
© 2006
ISBN: 0-7637-3382-2

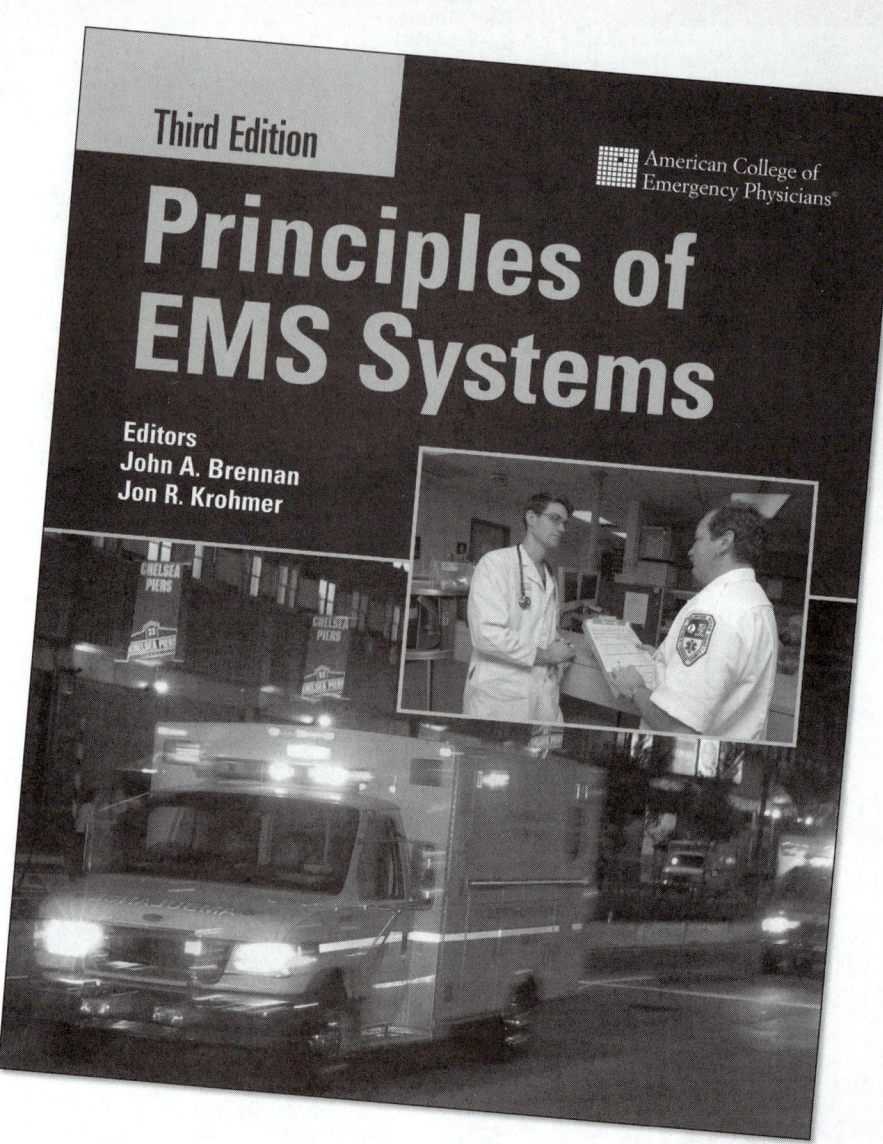

A must-have for EMS providers, police, fire departments, emergency physicians, emergency departments, and hospitals!

ORDER TODAY!

Call 1-800-832-0034 or visit www.jbpub.com

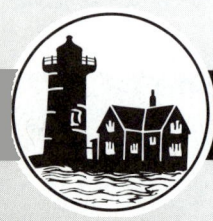

Jones and Bartlett Publishers

PHONE: 800-832-0034 • WEB: WWW.JBPUB.COM

NEW EDITION
OF IDEAL RESOURCE OFFERS TIMELY, EVIDENCE-BASED INFORMATION

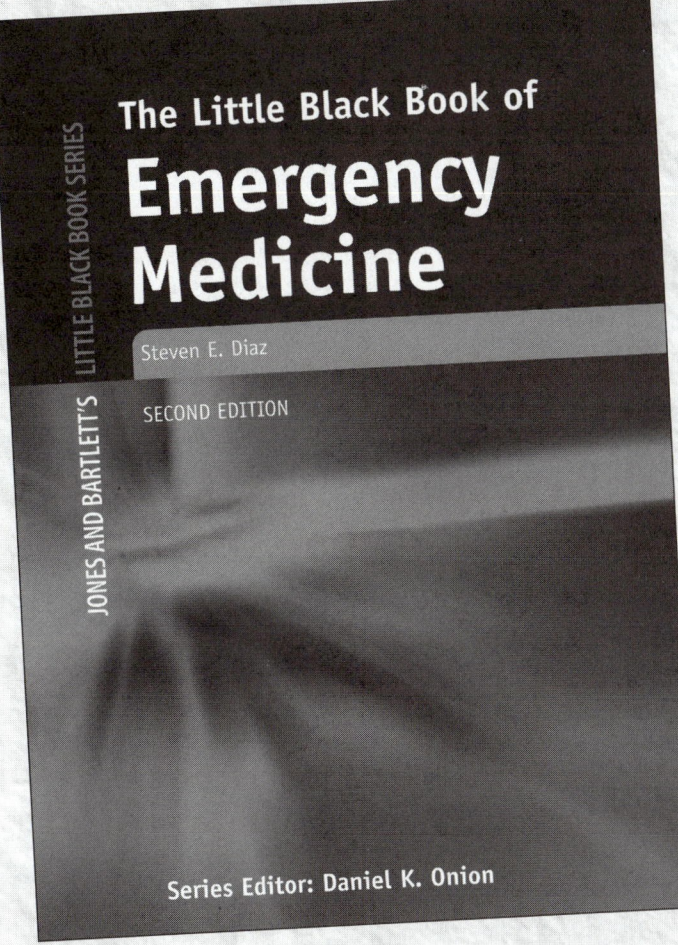

The Little Black Book of Emergency Medicine

Steven E. Diaz, MD, MaineGeneral Medical Center
ISBN: 0-7637-3456-X • Price: $39.95*
Paperback • 525 Pages • © 2006

Thoroughly revised and updated, the second edition of this pocket-sized handbook provides comprehensive, concise, evidence-based information on diagnosing and treating illness and injury in the emergency setting. *The Little Black Book of Emergency Medicine* is a convenient resource offering quick access to vital information and makes a great reference for solving pressing problems on the ward or in the clinic.

Also Available in PDA Format!

To learn more about this and other titles in *The Little Black Book* series, please visit www.jbpub.com.

ORDER YOUR COPY TODAY RISK-FREE!*

Jones and Bartlett Publishers

PHONE: 800-832-0034 • WEB: WWW.JBPUB.COM

*Price subject to change. Shipping and sales tax will be applied to your order.
If you are not completely satisfied with your order, return it within 30 days for a full refund.

Become a master of ECGs!

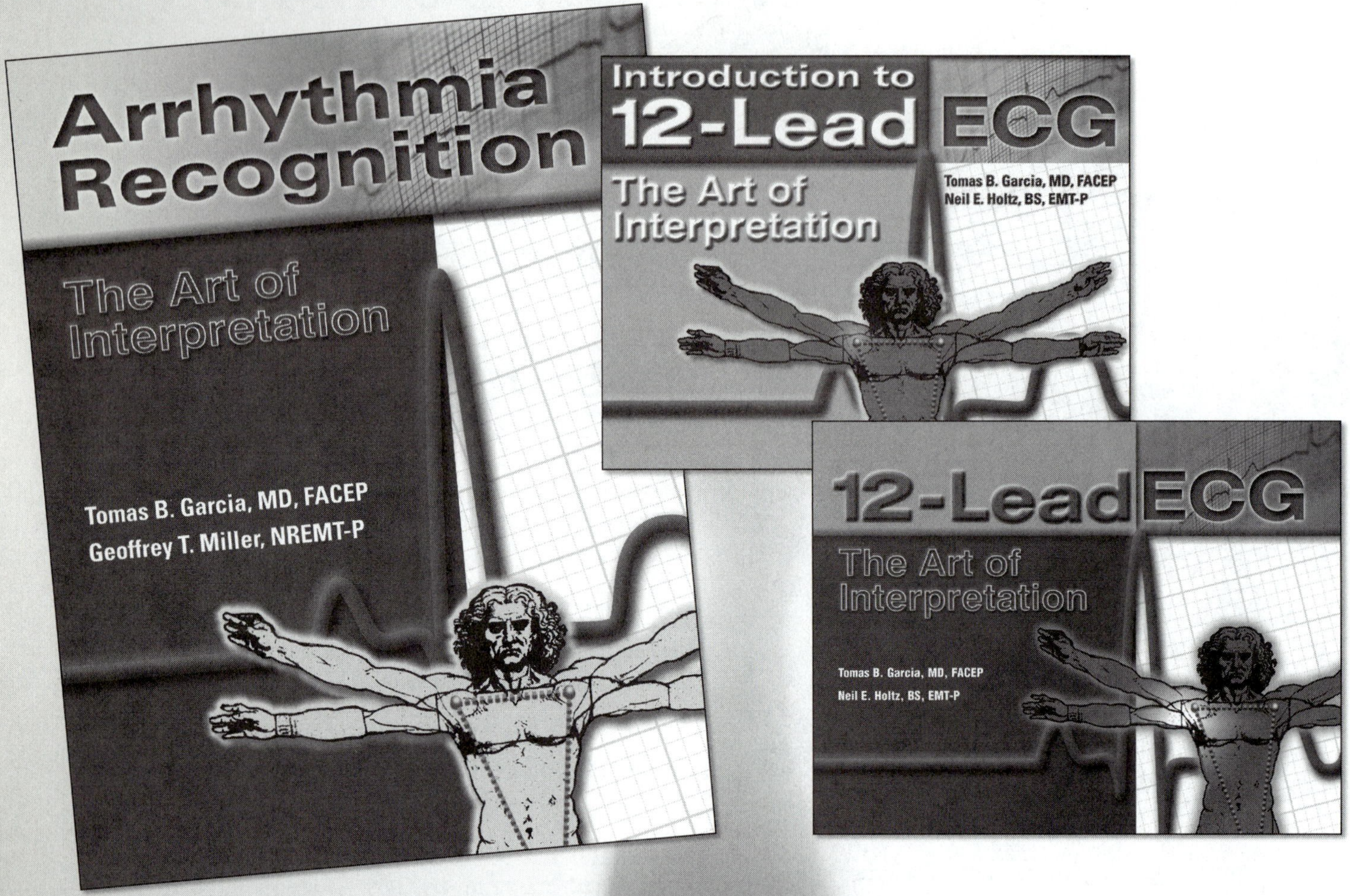

Interpreting electrocardiograms (ECGs) can be a difficult task. This series will bring you from beginner to expert by taking this complex subject and making it simple!

Arrhythmia Recognition, IBSN: 0-7637-2246-4
Introduction to 12-Lead ECG, IBSN: 0-7637-1961-7
12-Lead ECG, IBSN: 0-7637-1284-1

Order online today at www.12LeadECG.com or call 1-800-832-0034.

 **Jones and Bartlett Publishers**

PHONE: 800-832-0034 • WEB: WWW.JBPUB.COM

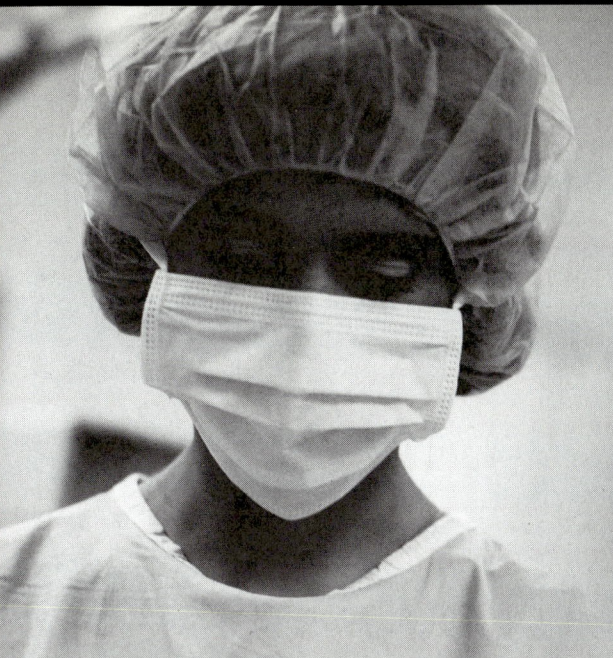

AMERICAN ASSOCIATION *of* CRITICAL-CARE NURSES

and

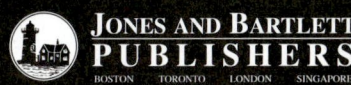

JONES AND BARTLETT PUBLISHERS
BOSTON   TORONTO   LONDON   SINGAPORE

Announce the Newly Revised Protocols Series!

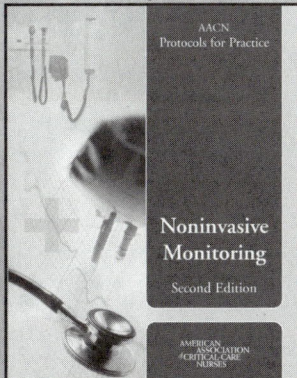

AACN PROTOCOLS FOR PRACTICE:
Noninvasive Monitoring, Second Edition

Edited by: **Suzanne M. Burns**, RN, MSN, RRT, ACNP, CCRN, FAAN, FCCM

ISBN: 0-7637-3825-5
$99.95* (Sugg. US List)
Paperback • © 2006

AACN Protocols for Practice: Noninvasive Monitoring delineates the evidence for using devices for noninvasive patient monitoring of blood pressure, heart rhythms, pulse oximetry, end-tidal carbon dioxide, and respiratory waveforms. These protocols guide clinicians in the appropriate selection of patients for use of the device, application of the device, initial and ongoing monitoring, device removal, and selected aspects of quality control.

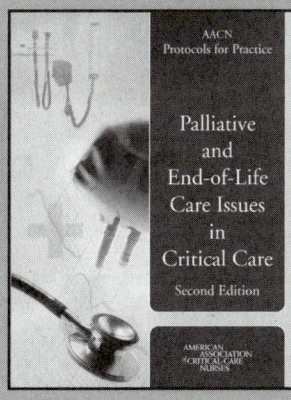

AACN PROTOCOLS FOR PRACTICE:
Palliative and End-of-Life Care Issues in Critical Care, Second Edition

Edited by: **Justine Medina**, RN, MS **Kathleen Puntillo**, RN, DNS, FAAN

ISBN: 0-7637-4027-6 • $99.95* (Sugg. US List) • Paperback • © 2006

Palliative and End-of-Life Care Issues in Critical Care sets forth the evidence-based guidelines for providing appropriate end-of-life and palliative care. The *Protocols* equip critical care nurses to effectively manage the following:

- symptom management
- family issues and intervention
- withholding and withdrawing life support
- communication and conflict resolution
- caring for the caregiver

Coming Soon in the *AACN Protocols for Practice* series:

- Care of the Mechanically Ventilated Patient
- Creating a Healing Environment
- Medication Administration
- Hemodynamic Monitoring
- Care of the Cardiovascular Patient
- Symptom Management

For more information visit: http://nursing.jbpub.com or http://www.aacn.org today!

Mail to: Jones and Bartlett Publishers • 40 Tall Pine Drive • Sudbury, MA 01776

Phone: 1-800-832-0034 • Fax: 978-443-8000 • Email: info@jbpub.com • Visit: www.jbpub.com

*Prices subject to change and do not include shipping or sales tax. If you are not completely satisfied with your order, please return within 30 days for a full refund or replacement copy.

2003 AJN Book of the Year Award Winner!

Contains more pathoph~~ysiology, gr~~owth and development, and embryological considerations than any other pediatric emergency nursing book currently on the market!

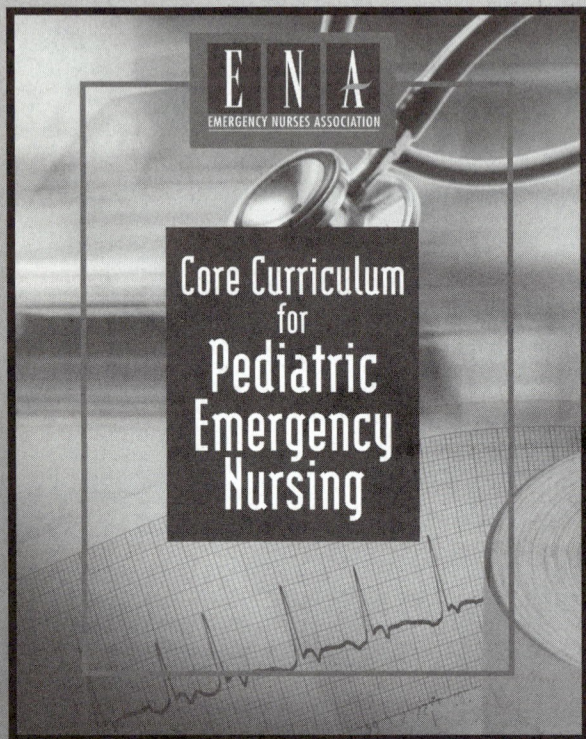

Core Curriculum for Pediatric Emergency Nursing

Emergency Nurses Association (ENA)

ISBN: 0-7637-0176-9 • $66.95* (Sugg. US List)
Paperback • 619 Pages • © 2003

This unique text serves as the foundation for pediatric emergency nursing practice and pediatric trauma care. ***Core Curriculum for Pediatric Emergency Nursing*** contains comprehensive coverage for topics related to psychosocial issues, health promotion, discharge instructions, and the nursing process in caring for children in the emergency department setting.

Core Curriculum for Pediatric Emergency Nursing:

- Integrates the nursing process with pediatric physiology and psychosocial theories.
- Follows an organized format for consistency of content that includes normal physiology, pathophysiology, the nursing process, and psychosocial considerations.
- Stresses the differences in treating children versus adults and other considerations such as growth and development and respecting parental involvement in care.
- Includes chapters on management, the future of pediatric emergency nursing, and common complaints.

About the Author:

Emergency Nurses Association (ENA) is the specialty nursing association serving the emergency nursing profession through research, publications, professional development, and injury prevention. In the 30 years since Judith Kelleher and Anita Dorr founded the Association, ENA has grown larger, stronger and more influential each year. ENA's mission is to provide visionary leadership for emergency nursing and emergency care.

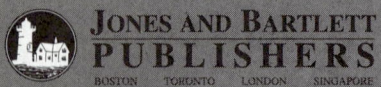

JONES AND BARTLETT PUBLISHERS
BOSTON TORONTO LONDON SINGAPORE

For more information visit: http://nursing.jbpub.com

Mail to: Jones and Bartlett Publishers • 40 Tall Pine Drive • Sudbury, MA 01776

Phone: 1-800-832-0034 • Fax: 978-443-8000 • Email: info@jbpub.com • Visit: www.jbpub.com

*Prices subject to change and do not include shipping or sales tax. If you are not completely satisfied with your order, please return within 30 days for a full refund or replacement copy.